Pediatric Endocrinology

Clinical Pediatrics

Series Editor

Fima Lifshitz

Miami Children's Hospital
University of Miami School of Medicine
State University of New York
Health Science Center at Brooklyn
Pediatric Sunshine Academics
and Sansum Medical Research Institute

Additional Volumes in Preparation

Pediatric Endocrinology

FOURTH EDITION
REVISED AND EXPANDED

EDITED BY

Fima Lifshitz

Miami Children's Hospital, University of Miami School of Medicine
State University of New York Health Science Center at Brooklyn
Pediatric Sunshine Academics
and Sansum Medical Research Institute

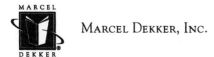

MARCEL DEKKER, INC.

NEW YORK • BASEL

Library of Congress Cataloging-in-Publication Data

A catalog record for this book is available from the Library of Congress.

ISBN: 0-8247-0816-4

This book is printed on acid-free paper.

Headquarters

Marcel Dekker, Inc.
270 Madison Avenue, New York, NY 10016
tel: 212-696-9000; fax: 212-685-4540

Eastern Hemisphere Distribution

Marcel Dekker AG
Hutgasse 4, Postfach 812, CH-4001 Basel, Switzerland
tel: 41-61-260-6300; fax: 41-61-260-6333

World Wide Web

http://www.dekker.com

The publisher offers discounts on this book when ordered in bulk quantities. For more information, write to Special Sales/Professional Marketing at the headquarters address above.

Current printing (last digit):
10   9   8   7   6   5   4   3   2   1

PRINTED IN THE UNITED STATES OF AMERICA

To the cycle of life,
the new generation

To my grandchildren,
Jonah and Rebecca

About the Series

"Clinical Pediatrics" is a series of books designed to continually update the knowledge of the practicing pediatrician in diverse areas of the specialty. Each volume in the series addresses rapidly developing topics that are changing the attitudes and treatment approaches of the clinician. The chapters comprising the volumes represent the state of the art on the various subjects from the vantage point of recognized experts in the field.

The books already published in this series are *Common Pediatric Disorders, Congenital Metabolic Diseases, Antimicrobial Therapy in Infants and Children, Food Allergy, Metabolic Bone Disease*, and *Pediatric Endocrinology*. The first edition of the last book was published in 1985, the second edition in 1990, and the third edition in 1996. This book has become the most sought-after reference book in the field, making necessary an updated fourth edition. This fourth edition of *Pediatric Endocrinology* is the ninth book in the Clinical Pediatrics series. It is an updated, improved, and greatly expanded version, which covers the field in a comprehensive manner to update clinicians on the numerous recent advances in pediatric endocrinology. The most frequent encounters by pediatricians are covered and reviewed in a practical, patient-oriented, yet scientific style, making it an invaluable resource for pediatricians and specialists alike.

These books serve as the foundation for the volumes that will follow, each complementing the others. Together, they will constitute a comprehensive review of the most recent developments in pediatrics.

Fima Lifshitz

Foreword

The fourth edition of *Pediatric Endocrinology* is designed according to the same concept as that of the first three, but it far exceeds the very significant accomplishments of the previous editions. The first three editions, each of which was more complete and broadly informative than the last, were written for a diversified audience of general pediatricians, pediatric endocrinologists, geneticists, and others. Each of these texts became the most used and sought-after in the field in the United States and throughout the world. *Pediatric Endocrinology* became established as the most respected book on the subject, dating back to the publication of the first edition in 1985. A review of the content of this, the fourth edition, reveals an even more improved text. Each chapter is written by highly respected clinicians who are also investigators in the topics covered. The book has a very practical clinical approach, yet it provides comprehensive coverage of all the major endocrine glands and diseases. The content of each of the various chapters is fully inclusive, which augments the value of the presentation of each subject. The balance between the clinical material and the physiology, physio-pathophysiology, and treatment information is ideal. The review of each topic is as updated as is feasible in constructing a book of this magnitude.

Readers and users of this text will be pleased and appreciative of the effort and successful accomplishment of Dr. Lifshitz and his colleagues who edited and authored this fourth edition. Dr. Lifshitz has again demonstrated his insight and capability as an accomplished educator for students at all levels. Congratulations on this contribution, a legacy to pediatric endocrinology!

Robert M. Blizzard, M.D.
Professor and Chairman Emeritus
The University of Virginia School of Medicine
Charlottesville, Virginia, U.S.A.

As the number of pediatric endocrinologists continues to grow worldwide, so does the scope of the field. The spectrum of pediatric endocrinology has expanded to encompass genetics, nutrition, immunology, biochemistry, and psychology. In addition, the explosive increase in numbers of patients seen in today's pediatric endocrine clinics reflects the heightened awareness of the role of hormones in health and disease in children. Molecular genetic studies completed since the last edition of the book have further elucidated the etiology of many endocrine and metabolic disorders. These new studies have been incorporated into the chapters of the fourth edition, edited by our friend and colleague, Dr. Fima Lifshitz. New chapters have been added to this edition, while existing chapters have been updated, creating a thorough yet succinct book.

I would like to congratulate Dr. Lifshitz who, again, has assembled the foremost specialists in all areas of pediatric endocrinology to create this book, which has become indispensable to pediatric clinicians and researchers alike.

Maria I. New, M.D.
Weill Medical College of Cornell University
New York Presbyterian Hospital
New York, New York, U.S.A.

Preface

The more you practice what you know, the more you know what to practice.

W. Jenkins

The fourth edition of *Pediatric Endocrinology* is a comprehensive book in the field designed to meet the needs of the practicing physician, yet it is written at a level suitable for the subspecialist. The 43 chapters of this book are completely updated and the information contained provides state-of-the-art knowledge in all areas of the specialty. There have been multiple changes in the field since 1985 when the first edition was published. The most important advances were incorporated into the previous editions and were brought to the clinicians in didactic, practical chapters. Each contained comprehensive discussions addressing all clinical situations encountered in the practice of this subspecialty. The fourth edition of *Pediatric Endocrinology* constitutes the culmination of the experience and accomplishments reflected in previous editions. It is a mature, seasoned book that reflects the continuous growth and accumulated wisdom of the 63 contributors. Their knowledge is eloquently transmitted in each chapter.

As in previous editions, the book is divided into seven parts, each dealing with a major area of childhood endocrinology: "Growth and Growth Disorders," "Adrenal Disorders and Sexual Development Abnormalities," "Thyroid Disorders," "Disorders of Calcium and Phosphorus Metabolism," "Hypoglycemia and Diabetes Mellitus" and "Miscellaneous Disorders." The final part includes an updated chapter on dynamic tests used by pediatric endocrinologists, as well as one with a more complete collection of newer and updated reference charts and tables utilized to assess patients with growth disorders and endocrine alterations. Additionally, there are two new chapters of current interest; one on reimbursement issues with a coding supplement, and another on using the Web to obtain information on genetic and hormone disorders. These should make it easier for the busy practitioner to care for children with pediatric endocrine disorders. Also included are new conceptual chapters on major topics in the field not covered in previous editions, i.e., worrisome growth, multiple endocrine neoplasia syndromes, hyperlipoproteinemias, hypertension, and supplements to enhance athletic performance.

Each of the 43 chapters of this book contains sufficient material to cover the topic in its entirety and impart new information to enhance the knowledge of the practitioner and the subspecialist. It provides the reader with the most updated and pertinent information to address questions asked in the care of patients with endocrine and endocrine-related disorders. From pathophysiology to treatment, there is a succinct and clear description of the subject in each chapter. The book fully encompasses the daily problems seen in pediatric endocrine practices.

The field of pediatric endocrinology has rapidly advanced and changed very significantly in many aspects, not only in medical knowledge and the scientific basis of endocrinology. The practice of the specialty has also evolved and changed radically, together with changes brought about by "managed health care." It has changed the way we care for our patients and the way we practice our specialty, as well as many other aspects of our practice. Not all of these changes have been positive. One of the most significant casualties has been the transmission of the knowledge accumulated by prominent academic pediatric endocrinologists. As the editor of this book I experienced first-hand this sad state of affairs. Since the last edition was published in 1996, the support for teaching endeavors in many institutions has virtually vanished, and the academic pediatric endocrinologist is now an endangered species. Many of our colleagues have moved to other areas and away from clinical academic practices, and those who stayed work on a battlefront and have no time to invest in teaching endeavors. Those who contributed to this book did so on their own time, often against the implicit wishes and mandates of administration. The current constraints of the health care system have also taken a toll in academic programs. It praises productivity in other areas, not in teaching, nor in writing and transmitting knowledge through a chapter in a book. Even secretarial support was often not available to some contributors for this activity.

Thus, I am particularly and evermore grateful to my colleagues who revised and updated their chapters, and to those who provided new sections for this book. They all made very significant contributions, which continue to make this book a most valuable and necessary tool for pediatricians and pediatric endocrinologists alike. I believe this edition was brought forth with much more effort and commitment than previous ones, and I profusely thank all the contributors; without their dedication and talent there would not be a fourth edition. Hopefully the cycle of healthcare will continue to evolve and to move forward positively. I wish that in the future the academic pediatric endocrinologist will be given the recognition and support that are deserved. This will allow us to devote energy to enhancing our knowledge and passing it on to practicing physicians for the health of our children.

Fima Lifshitz, M.D.

Contents

Contents

Contents   xvii

Contents

VII. ADDITIONAL INFORMATION AND RESOURCES

Contributors

Jose E. Abdenur, M.D. Associate Scientific Director, Foundation for the Study of Neurometabolic Diseases, and Associate Professor of Biochemistry, University of Buenos Aires School of Dentistry, Buenos Aires, Argentina

Ramin Alemzadeh, M.D., FAAP Associate Professor, Section of Pediatric Endocrinology & Diabetes, and Director, Children's Diabetes Program, Department of Pediatrics, Medical College of Wisconsin, Milwaukee, Wisconsin, U.S.A.

David B. Allen, M.D. Professor and Director of Endocrinology and Residency Training, Department of Pediatrics, University of Wisconsin Medical School, Madison, Wisconsin, U.S.A.

Albert Altchek, M.D. Clinical Professor with Tenure of Obstetrics, Gynecology, and Reproductive Science, and Chief of Pediatric and Adolescent Gynecology, Mount Sinai School of Medicine and Hospital, New York, New York, U.S.A.

Dorothy J. Becker, M.D. Professor of Pediatrics and Director, Division of Endocrinology, Diabetes & Metabolism, University of Pittsburgh School of Medicine and Children's Hospital of Pittsburgh, Pittsburgh, Pennsylvania, U.S.A.

Gary D. Berkovitz, M.D. Professor of Pediatrics and Chief, Pediatric Endocrinology, Mailman Center for Child Development, University of Miami School of Medicine, Miami, Florida, U.S.A.

Diego Botero, M.D. Attending in Endocrinology, Children's Hospital, and Instructor in Pediatrics, Harvard Medical School, Boston, Massachusetts, U.S.A.

Frederieke M. Brouwers, M.D. Research Fellow, Unit on Clinical Neuroendocrinology, Pediatric and Reproductive Endocrinology Branch, National Institute of Child Health and Human Development, National Institutes of Health, Bethesda, Maryland, U.S.A.

Thomas O. Carpenter, M.D. Professor, Department of Pediatrics, Yale University School of Medicine, and Attending Physician, Yale–New Haven Hospital, New Haven, Connecticut, U.S.A.

Adriana A. Carrillo, M.D. Fellow in Pediatric Endocrinology, Jackson Memorial Hospital, University of Miami School of Medicine, Miami, Florida, U.S.A.

Maribel Cedillo, B.S. Research Nutritionist, EMTAC, Inc., Miami, Florida, U.S.A.

Fred Chasalow, Ph.D. Former Chief of Pediatric Endocrine Research and Former Director of Pediatric Endocrine Laboratory, Maimonides Medical Center, Brooklyn, New York, U.S.A.

Ellen Lancon Connor, M.D. Assistant Professor, Division of Pediatric Endocrinology and Diabetes, Department of Pediatrics, University of Wisconsin, Madison, Wisconsin, U.S.A.

Giulia Costi, M.D. Endocrine Fellow, Juvenile Diabetes Program, Department of Pediatrics, Weill Medical College of Cornell University, New York Presbyterian Hospital, New York, New York, U.S.A.

Richard M. Cowett, M.D. Former Chief, Division of Neonatology, Children's Hospital, Youngstown, and Professor, Department of Pediatrics, Northeastern Ohio Universities College of Medicine, Rootstown, Ohio, U.S.A.

John S. Dallas, M.D. Associate Professor and Director, Division of Pediatric Endocrinology, Department of Pediatrics, University of Texas Medical Branch–Galveston, Galveston, Texas, U.S.A.

Marco Danon, M.D. Staff Attending, Department of Medical Education, Miami Children's Hospital, Miami, Florida, and Associate Professor, Department of Pediatrics, State University of New York, Brooklyn, New York, U.S.A.

Allan L. Drash, M.D. Professor Emeritus of Pediatrics, University of Pittsburgh School of Medicine and Children's Hospital of Pittsburgh, Pittsburgh, Pennsylvania, U.S.A.

Graeme Eisenhofer, Ph.D. Staff Scientist, Clinical Neurocardiology Section, National Institute of Neurological Disorders and Stroke, National Institutes of Health, Bethesda, Maryland, U.S.A.

Oscar Escobar, M.D. Assistant Professor, Division of Endocrinology, Department of Pediatrics, University of Pittsburgh School of Medicine and Children's Hospital of Pittsburgh, Pittsburgh, Pennsylvania, U.S.A.

Hussien M. Farrag, M.D. Assistant Professor of Pediatrics, Tufts University School of Medicine, and Division of Newborn Medicine, Department of Pediatrics, Baystate Medical Center, Springfield, Massachusetts, U.S.A.

Thomas P. Foley, Jr., M.D. Professor, Department of Pediatrics, School of Medicine, and Professor of Epidemiology, Graduate School of Public Health, University of Pittsburgh and Children's Hospital of Pittsburgh, Pittsburgh, Pennsylvania, U.S.A.

S. Douglas Frasier, M.D. Emeritus Professor, Division of Endocrinology, Department of Pediatrics, UCLA School of Medicine, Los Angeles, California, U.S.A.

Joseph M. Gertner, M.B., M.R.C.P. Vice President, Clinical Research, Serono Inc., Rockland, and Division of Endocrinology, Department of Medicine, Children's Hospital, Boston, Massachusetts, U.S.A.

Lucia Ghizzoni, M.D., Ph.D. Assistant Professor, Department of Pediatrics, University of Parma, Parma, Italy

Judith G. Hall, O.C., M.D., F.R.C.P.(C.), F.A.A.P., F.C.C.M.G., F.A.B.M.G. Professor of Pediatrics and Medical Genetics, Department of Pediatrics, University of British Columbia, and British Columbia Children's Hospital, Vancouver, British Columbia, Canada

Julie R. Ingelfinger, M.D. Professor of Pediatrics, Harvard Medical School; Senior Consultant in Nephrology, Massachusetts General Hospital for Children, Massachusetts General Hospital; and Deputy Editor, *New England Journal of Medicine*, Boston, Massachusetts, U.S.A.

Muhammad A. Jabbar, M.D. Associate Professor, Department of Pediatrics, Hurley Medical Center, Michigan State University School of Medicine, Flint, Michigan, U.S.A.

Christian A. Koch, M.D., F.A.C.E. Investigator and Attending Physician, Pediatric and Reproductive Endocrinology Branch, National Institute of Child Health and Human Development, National Institutes of Health, Bethesda, Maryland, U.S.A.

Winston W. K. Koo, M.B., F.R.A.C.P. Professor of Pediatrics, Obstetrics and Gynecology, Department of Pediatrics, Hutzel Hospital and Children's Hospital of Michigan, Wayne State University, Detroit, Michigan, U.S.A.

Roberto L. Lanes, M.D. Coordinator, Pediatric Endocrine Unit, Hospital de Clinicas Caracas, and Professor, Post Graduate Courses in Pediatrics and Endocrinology, Hospital Central "Dr. Carlos Arvelo," Universidad Central de Venezuela, Caracas, Venezuela

Peter A. Lee, M.D., Ph.D. Professor of Pediatrics, Pennsylania State College of Medicine, The Milton S. Hershey Medical Center, Hershey, Pennsylvania, U.S.A.

Fima Lifshitz, M.D. Former Chief-of-Staff and Chair of Nutrition Sciences, Miami Children's Hospital, Professor of Pediatrics, University of Miami School of Medicine, Miami, Florida; State University of New York Health Science Center at Brooklyn, Brooklyn,

New York; President, Pediatric Sunshine Academics; and Senior Nutrition Scientist and Director of Pediatrics, Sansum Medical Research Institute, Santa Barbara, California, U.S.A.

Noel K. Maclaren, M.D.   Professor, Department of Pediatrics, and Director, Juvenile Diabetes Center, Weill Medical College of Cornell University, New York Presbyterian Hospital, New York, New York, U.S.A.

Joseph A. Majzoub, M.D.   Chief, Division of Endocrinology, Children's Hospital, and Professor of Pediatrics, Harvard Medical School, Boston, Massachusetts, U.S.A.

Claude J. Migeon, M.D.   Professor of Pediatrics, Division of Pediatric Endocrinology, Johns Hopkins University School of Medicine, and Children's Medical and Surgical Center, Johns Hopkins Hospital, Baltimore, Maryland, U.S.A.

Louis J. Muglia, M.D., Ph.D.   Division of Pediatric Endocrinology and Metabolism, St. Louis Children's Hospital, and Associate Professor of Pediatrics, Molecular Biology and Pharmacology, and Obstetrics and Gynecology, Washington University School of Medicine, St. Louis, Missouri, U.S.A.

E. Kirk Neely, M.D.   Clinical Associate Professor, Division of Pediatric Endocrinology, Stanford University Medical Center, Stanford Medical School, Stanford, California, U.S.A.

Maria I. New, M.D.   Professor and Chairman, Department of Pediatrics, and Chief, Pediatric Endocrinology, Weill Medical College of Cornell University, New York Presbyterian Hospital, New York, New York, U.S.A.

Karel Pacak, M.D., Ph.D., D.Sc.   Chief, Unit on Clinical Neuroendocrinology, Pediatric and Reproductive Endocrinology Branch, National Institute of Child Health and Human Development, National Institutes of Health, Bethesda, Maryland, U.S.A.

Songya Pang, M.D.   Professor of Pediatrics and Chief of Pediatric Endocrinology, Department of Pediatrics, University of Illinois at Chicago College of Medicine, Chicago, Illinois, U.S.A.

Jaakko Perheentupa, M.D., Ph.D.   Professor (Emeritus) of Pediatrics and Former Director, Hospital for Children and Adolescents, University of Helsinki, Helsinki, Finland

John A. Phillips III, M.D.   Director, Division of Medical Genetics, David T. Karzon Professor of Pediatrics, and Professor of Medicine and Biochemistry, Vanderbilt University School of Medicine, and Adjunct Professor of Microbiology, Meharry Medical College, Nashville, Tennessee, U.S.A.

Robert Rapaport, M.D.   Emma Elizabeth Sullivan Professor and Director, Division of Pediatric Endocrinology and Diabetes, Mount Sinai School of Medicine, New York, New York, U.S.A.

Raphaël Rappaport, M.D.   Professor Emeritus, Departments of Pediatrics and Developmental Biology, Hôpital Necker–Enfants Malades, Paris, France

Bridget F. Recker, R.N., Ed.M., C.C.R.C.   Research Coordinator, University Physicians Group–Endocrine Division, Staten Island University Hospital, Staten Island, New York, U.S.A.

David L. Rimoin, M.D., Ph.D.   Steven Spielberg Chair of Pediatrics and Director, Medical Genetics–Birth Defects Center, Cedars–Sinai Medical Center, and Professor of Pediatrics and Medicine, UCLA School of Medicine, Los Angeles, California, U.S.A.

Russell Rising, M.S., Ph.D.   Senior Research Scientist, EMTAC, Inc., Miami, Florida, U.S.A.

Scott A. Rivkees, M.D.   Associate Professor of Pediatric Endocrinology, Department of Pediatrics, Yale University School of Medicine, New Haven, Connecticut, U.S.A.

Alan D. Rogol, M.D., Ph.D.   Professor of Clinical Pediatrics, University of Virginia, Charlottesville, and Clinical Professor of Internal Medicine, Medical College of Virginia, Richmond, Virginia, U.S.A.

Arlan L. Rosenbloom, M.D.   Distinguished Professor Emeritus, Department of Pediatrics, University of Florida College of Medicine, Gainesville, Florida, U.S.A.

Ron G. Rosenfeld, M.D.   Oregon Credit Union Endowment Professor and Chair, Department of Pediatrics, and Professor, Department of Cell and Developmental Biology, Oregon Health and Science University, and Physician-in-Chief, Doernbecher Children's Hospital, Portland, Oregon, U.S.A.

Daphne Sack-Rivers   Research Assistant, Division of Pediatric Endocrinology and Diabetes, Mount Sinai Hospital, New York, New York, U.S.A.

Mordechai Shohat, M.D.   Professor of Pediatrics and Genetics, and Director, Department of Medical Genetics, Rabin Medical Center —Beilinson Campus, Petah Tikva, Israel

Janet H. Silverstein, M.D.   Professor and Chief, Division of Pediatric Endocrinology, Department of Pediatrics, University of Florida College of Medicine, Gainesville, Florida, U.S.A.

Elisabeth Thibaud, M.D.   Gynecologist, Pediatric Endocrinology and Gynecology Unit, Department of Pediatrics, Hôpital Necker– Enfants Malades, Paris, France

Guy Van Vliet, M.D.   Professor, Department of Pediatrics, University of Montreal, and Chief, Endocrinology Service, Sainte-Justine Hospital, Montreal, Quebec, Canada

David A. Weinstein, M.D., M.M.Sc.   Assistant in Endocrinology, Children's Hospital, and Instructor in Pediatrics, Division of Endocrinology, Harvard Medical School, Boston, Massachusetts, U.S.A.

Martina Weise, M.D.   Head, Endocrinology and Diabetes Section, Institute for Drugs and Medical Devices, Bonn, Germany

Kurt Widhalm, M.D.   Professor of Pediatrics and Clinical Chemistry, Division of Neonatology, Intensive Care and Congenital Disorders, Department of Pediatrics, University of Vienna, Vienna, Austria

William E. Winter, M.D.   Professor, Department of Pathology, Immunology and Laboratory Medicine; Medical Director, Department of Pediatrics and Department of Molecular Genetics and Microbiology; Section Chief, Clinical Chemistry; and Director, Pathology Residency Training Program, University of Florida College of Medicine, Gainesville, Florida, U.S.A.

Joseph I. Wolfsdorf, M.B., B.Ch.   Senior Associate in Medicine, Attending Physician in Endocrinology, and Director, Diabetes Program, Children's Hospital; and Associate Professor of Pediatrics, Harvard Medical School, Boston, Massachusetts, U.S.A.

Donald Zimmerman, M.D.   Professor of Pediatrics, Mayo Medical School, and Consultant in Pediatric Endocrinology and Metabolism, Mayo Medical Clinic, Rochester, Minnesota, U.S.A.

Online References Cited in Text

Pediatric
Endocrinology

1

Worrisome Growth

Fima Lifshitz

Miami Children's Hospital and University of Miami School of Medicine, Miami, Florida; State University of New York Health Science Center at Brooklyn, Brooklyn, New York; Pediatric Sunshine Academics; and Sansum Medical Research Institute, Santa Barbara, California, U.S.A.

Diego Botero

Children's Hospital and Harvard Medical School, Boston, Massachusetts, U.S.A.

I. THE GENERAL PROBLEM

One of the primary concerns of pediatricians is the appropriate growth of their patients. Parents and children also worry about "growth" as evidence of good health. Several conditions, as discussed later, may alter the height, weight, and growth progression of a patient; these must be diagnosed and treated. However, there are other problems in being short, even when the body size is only mildly affected. Indeed, any person who is below average height (in the United States 5 feet 9 inches for men and 5 feet 5 inches for women) may also experience a number of psychosocial difficulties. Dwarfs have these problems to a greater degree, with various amounts of tolerance and rejection according to the different customs and beliefs of the locality in which they live. Recent medical research on the subject questioned whether short stature is a handicap (1) or whether this is a problem that requires growth hormone therapy (2). Also there are issues concerning the quality of life and the potential benefits that may be attained by increasing adult height (3). There are additional questions about the reasons for internalizing behavior problems and/or poor social skills of short stature individuals. All these concerns challenge the justification for extraordinary means of treating a short-stature child. It has been postulated that growth hormone treatment in short children is an issue beyond medicine, involving many aspects best resolved at present by a research approach (4, 5).

However, there is ample evidence of prejudice in our society towards the short person. The psychosocial prejudice toward the short person transcends age, gender, race, creed, and financial status: all short people may be victims of discrimination. This seldom mentioned form of prejudice, like sexism or racism, is well established in this country and may be prevalent throughout the world. It has been called heightism. (The reader is referred to the book *The Height of Your Life*, by Ralph Keyes, for a very comprehensive and interesting review of this problem.) This book approaches heightism in a wry and humorous fashion. It highlights facts regarding height so basic to our relationships with others that we have ceased to think about them. It is from this book that the following comments have been extracted.

So pervasive is the bias against short people that no one notices it—no one, that is, except the short person. The English language illustrates this bias clearly. Feisty is the classic example, a word normally used in tandem with "little." Distinguished, by contrast, may not be synonymous with "tall" but rarely is used to refer to short persons. Other very important phrases remind us regularly of the importance of height: compare "looks up to" and "looks down upon." The question is always; how tall are you, instead of the neutral, what is your height? The song "Short People" by Randy Newman describes those below-average in height who have "grubby little fingers" and "dirty little minds" with "no reason to live." This song is a spoof of bigotry with a catchy tune, yet it made the hit parade. The composer meant it as a joke; of course, he is 5 feet 11 inches!

Height is one of the most important traits both parties try to match when it comes to selecting a personal relationship. In romantic matters, little men are "cut down to size." An ideal lover is never short, and at present both genders seem to feel that in relationships the male should be taller than the female. Even Sandy Allen, who at 7 feet 71/2 inches is certified by *The Guinness Book of World Records* as the tallest woman in the world, was quoted as saying, "I've got this old-fashioned idea, I will never marry anyone smaller than I am." She never married. Thus, the tall man seems to have all of womankind to choose from, whereas the short man appears to be limited to short women. Indeed, there may be more interreligious and interracial marriages than there are couples in which the man is shorter than the woman. The former Secretary of State Henry Kissinger was acknowledged as a truly unusual phenomenon because he married a taller woman. Rewards for being tall in our society include money. Business, it seems, is interested in short men mostly as customers for elevator shoes. The president of the Mutual Life Insurance Company surveyed its policyholders and found a nearly perfect correlation between body height and policy value. Several studies have pointed out that taller persons earn higher salaries. Corporate recruiters also tend to choose the taller of two equally qualified applicants. Even when he succeeds, despite the odds against him, the short person is often accused of being a "Little Napoleon."

Height is more than a mere statistic: for men it is a measure of manhood. Height brings acknowledgment, deference, and power. Big and strong are, from childhood, considered nearly the same word. The dominant figures in advertisements and legendary figures in the movies are usually represented by tall people. Height is equated with power to such a degree that it plays a very important role in politics. Most US presidents have not been short; the shortest was James Madison at 5 feet 4 inches. Only six other presidents were slightly below the present average height. Americans have usually favored the taller political candidate. As a matter of fact, the taller of the two major presidential candidates is usually sent to the White House. There have been only four exceptions. In 1924, Calvin Coolidge (5 feet 10 inches) defeated John Davis (5 feet 11 inches); in 1972, Richard Nixon (6 feet) defeated George McGovern (6 feet 1 inch), in 1976 Jimmy Carter (5 feet 6 inches) defeated Gerald Ford (6 feet 1 inch). In the 2000 election, both candidates were over 6 feet tall, but George W. Bush, who is slightly shorter than Al Gore, won the election only by a Supreme Court decision, while the popular vote went to the taller Mr. Gore by a substantial margin. In this, as in most presidential elections, the American public voted by the inch. However, this form of prejudice may also transcend the United States. For the first time in the history of Mexico, the very tall opposition candidate Mr. Vicente Fox defeated the official shorter presidential candidate of the PRI Party in the 2000 election. This was a very unusual accomplishment since the PRI party had held power consecutively for over 75 years.

Although human esthetics and social tastes clearly favor tallness, nature shows no such preference. Anthropologists estimate that, for most of history, natural selection kept adult male heights within a range below our current averages. Supporting the natural selection process, infants' skeletons, which are abundant in old graveyards, are rather tall; in fact their length is comparable to our present norms. Some experts think that these two phenomena are related. It seems that environmental problems were more detrimental to youngsters destined to be large, and only those destined to be small survived the rigors of malnutrition and disease. Ashley Montagu, in *Human Evolution*, wrote: "At least in part the recent increase in overall size visible in the modern adult population is due to the fact that improved standards of food and medical care have allowed genetic combinations to survive which would have been selected against in ages past."

II. THE MEDICAL PROBLEM

Pediatricians are often consulted by parents worried about short stature in their children. This term needs definition. "Short stature" has been defined as height below the third percentile; therefore, 3% of normal children would be classified as being short. "Dwarfism," the severe form of short stature, is defined as height below 3 standard deviations (SD) from the mean. The population selected for reference is important when judgments are made about the shortness of an individual. A number of different reference charts have been used in this country in recent decades, each varying somewhat from others because of the representative population from whom the data were derived (e.g., predominantly rural children from Iowa vs. Boston city children). A revision of the 1977 National Child Health Survey growth percentile was recently completed and was published in May 2000 by the Center for Disease Control and Prevention (CDC) (*www.cdc.gov/ growthcharts*). These growth charts are included in the chapter of Reference Charts in this book (Chapter 43). These new charts are recommended for use as an enhanced instrument to evaluate the size and growth of children (6).

These charts are based on more up-to-date improved data gathered from the National Health Examination Surveys (NHANES I, II, and III) with five supplementary data sources. They feature several noteworthy items including the inclusion of 3rd and 97th percentiles. In addition, these charts contain data extending to 20 years of age, and they better represent the current growth patterns of the population. One other important contribution is that there is better continuity between 2–3 years and the >2 years growth in the charts. The new 2000 CDC percentiles have been adjusted slightly to account for the fact that recumbent length should be greater than the stated differences of 0.8 cm in the national surveys. Another significant consequence of updating the data is that the new percentiles of the CDC tend to be a bit higher for weight from 0 to 2 years. The 2000 growth charts also include body mass index (BMI) values of years 2 and older.

Although these growth charts constitute an important advancement over the previous charts used (1977 NCHS percentiles), they are not ideal for use in all infants and children. In particular they may misdiagnose the normalcy of growth in some young children as discussed below, including constitutional short stature or breastfed babies. These growth charts show average growth patterns of height and weight gain during specific periods in life (i.e., adolescent growth spurt). These percentile charts were based on cross-sectional data that effectively average growth across different periods. In individual patients the developmental stage of puberty will therefore make the pattern of growth vary in accordance with it, and that is not shown in the charts. In theory, useful supplementary growth charts for the pubertal periods are available, but these data were derived from nonrepresentative samples recorded a long time ago. Another concern with the CDC 2000 graphs is that it is hard to visualize the metric numbers in the axis, and the grids are not easy to follow. Therefore in this book we have published an improved version of those graphs. (See Chapter 43 for Reference Charts).

A program for monitoring the growth of children has been prepared by the Eurogrowth Study Group (*www.eurogrowth.org*). This is excellent for individually tracking the physical growth of children from birth to 36 months of age (7). It allows the monitoring and the plotting of individual growth data, calculates growth velocity, provides body mass index centiles, measures influences of breastfeeding on growth, modifies growth by midparental height, corrects growth for gestational age of premature infants, calculates Z scores, and offers multilingual access (8–11). It is a highly recommended tool to assess growth in children up to 36 months of age.

Pediatricians know that most children with mild short stature eventually become average-sized adults; however, some children have serious growth disturbances that may prevent them from reaching normal adult size. The Newcastle study in England (12) supported the need for an explanation of the cause of short stature in all children whose height falls below the third percentile. Almost half of the 5000 infants born in Newcastle in 1960 were measured for height at age 10. The height of 111 children fell below the third percentile: 16 were found to have a previously unsuspected organic disease as a cause of short stature. These findings demonstrate that it is unusual for a "normal" child to have a height below the third percentile, although most of these children may be healthy. However, it may also be inferred that in 10–15% of children who are short, a pathological condition may be found to account for the short stature. Therefore, the cause of short stature should always be investigated in all children whose height is below the 3rd percentile and more importantly in those who fail to grow at appropriate growth rates.

Growth-related disorders are also the most frequent problems encountered by pediatric endocrinologists. Pediatricians often seek consultation to help in the diagnosis and management of children with growth disturbances and these children are referred to pediatric endocrinologists. Even in a pediatric endocrine referral center, a large proportion of patients with short stature are usually healthy children. At times children are referred for short stature although they are of normal height. This may be because of either poor, inaccurate measurements, or because of the need of a pediatric endocrinologist to reassure a patient or family when a child is growing in the lower end of the normal range. A pathological condition accounted for poor growth and/or short stature in about one-third of the short-stature patients seen in a tertiary referral center (13).

III. DIAGNOSIS OF SHORT STATURE

In most instances of short stature a diagnosis is usually made, although in some patients the cause of short stature may defy the differential diagnosis of numerous experts. The different causes of short stature in children are listed in Table 1. This classification differentiates most forms of short stature into two main categories: short patients who are normal and short patients who have an abnormality that produces the short stature and poor growth. These basic concepts should be considered in the diagnosis of all short patients. That is, one must differentiate between the short child who is healthy and growing normally from those who are sick and not growing well. This is most important, since a clinician must determine if a short child is subject to a pathological cause, which must be diagnosed to provide adequate treatment, from one who may only need reassurance without a major work-up. Each of these two possible categories of short stature denotes not only the cause but also the pathophysiological process involved and the prognosis for final adult height. The specific applicable situation should be recognized by the physician before subjecting the patient to expensive and complicated investigations.

Other classifications to determine the different categories of short patients have been used by pediatric endocrinologists. For example, familial or genetic short stature was referred to as "intrinsic shortness." Constitutional growth delay was called "delayed growth," and all other disorders resulting in poor growth were called "attenuated growth" and/or "normal variance short stature" (14). Other authors have used the term "idiopathic short stature" to describe short individuals who are growing poorly, who have no demonstrable functional abnormality in growth hormone secretion, and whose parents are normal in height (15). Idiopathic short stature often implies a continuum of growth hormone insufficiency, not clearly demonstrable by the classic biochemical criteria (Chapters 2, 3 and 41). However, these terms to classify short patients are unnecessary because the two categories proposed above are inclusive and sufficient to understand and clarify growth problems.

A specific diagnosis can usually be made to define the patient's condition by appropriate observations. These include accurate measurements over time and specific comprehensive testing when the usual laboratory data do not define the diagnosis.

Table 1 Causes of Short Stature

Normal
    Constitutional growth delay
    Genetic-familial short stature
    Constitutional growth delay and familial short stature
Pathological
    Nutritional
        Hypocaloric
        Chronic inflammatory bowel disease
        Malabsorption
        Celiac disease
        Zinc deficiency
    Endocrine
        Hypothyroidism
        Isolated growth hormone deficiency
        Hypopituitarism
        Excess cortisol
        Precocious puberty
    Chromosome defects
        Turner syndrome
        Down syndrome
    Low birth weight short stature (intrauterine growth
            retardation)
        Sporadic
        Characteristic appearance
            Russell-Silver syndrome
            De Lange syndrome
            Seckel bird-headed dwarfism
            Dubowitz syndrome
            Bloom syndrome
            Johanson-Blizzard syndrome
    Bone development disorders
        Achondroplasia
        Chondrodystrophies
        Other skeletal disorders
    Metabolic
        Mucopolysaccharidosis
        Other storage disorders
    Chronic disease
        Chronic renal disease
        Chronic liver disease
        Congenital heart disease
        Pulmonary (cystic fibrosis, bronchial asthma)
        Poorly controlled diabetes mellitus
        Chronic infections (including human
                immunodeficiency virus infection)
    Associated with birth defects or mental retardation
        Specific syndromes
        Nonspecific defects
    Psychosocial
    Chronic drug intake
        Glucocorticoids
        High-dosage estrogens
        High-dosage androgens
        Methyphenidate
        Dextroamphetamine

Pediatric endocrinologists believe that short stature by itself may not be of concern for the individual, if he or she is healthy. However, there is ample evidence that height may play a role in the risk for adult-onset disease. For example, in large population studies it was found that short stature raises the risk for coronary heart disease. The Physician Health Study (16), the Framingham Study (17), and the Royal Canadian Health Force Study (18) showed that the size of the individual was important as a risk factor for myocardial infarction in adults. Although the mechanisms for the increased risk were not elucidated, they may be related to the size of the coronary arteries, which would be expected to be smaller in shorter individuals. Thus, they would be more prone to be blocked by atherosclerotic plaque than in taller adults who would have larger arteries.

IV. GROWTH PATTERNS

A. Growth Progression

The most important tool to assess growth problems in a short child is to evaluate the pattern of growth. Growth is a continuous process that starts at conception and ends with fusion of the epiphysis after pubertal development is completed. At any time during this process there may be variations or alterations in growth progression. These can only be identified with accurate measurements over time. Unfortunately, the most frequent method of measuring height, using a flip-up horizontal bar on a weighing scale, is subject to great errors caused by the child's slumping posture and considerable variation in the angle of the horizontal bar. Children should be measured standing upright and fully extended against a wall or firm vertical structure to which a properly mounted, accurate measuring device is attached. A steel tape measure, properly affixed to the wall, serves this purpose well and economically. The child stands shoeless, heels down, as erect as possible, and with the head directly forward. The back of the head, chest, gluteal area, and heels should touch the vertical surface. A firm object (e.g., a carpenter's angle) is then placed at a right angle over the top of the head and against the wall above the head. A Harpenden stadiometer (Holtain Limited, Crymych, Dyfed, UK), which determines height accurately (within 0.25 cm) is the most sophisticated instrument (19). However other devices are less expensive and/ or are comparable in accuracy to the more expensive Harpenden stadiometer (20).

Thus previous height and weight data are useful and very important in the assessment, if these measurements are accurate. The data must be plotted on standard growth charts to evaluate the pattern of growth. A normal pattern of growth may be defined as a pattern of progression of height and weight compatible with established standards for age, and that is appropriate for the genetic potential of the individual. It should also be appropriate for the various growth patterns of specific patients, stages of development, racial groups and population types (19–28) (Chapter 43).

On the other hand, pathological growth should always be considered in children who do not grow well regardless of height (Fig. 1). Any child who falls behind in growth across major percentiles in the chart should be evaluated, even when the height is not below the 3rd percentile (29). It must be kept in mind that growth is not continuously linear, but instead occurs in steps between saltation and stasis (30). Therefore, growth progression over a long period of time is more informative than extrapolations based on shorter periods of time. The growth rate varies according to the seasons, generally being fastest in the spring and summer. The growth rate in the fastest 3-month period is two to three times higher, but could be up to seven times the height increment during the slowest growth period in the other months (31, 32). Therefore, growth progression should be evaluated over a period of at least 6 months to 1 year (15). In addition, there is a great variation in the growth at different stages of life. In the first year of life, linear growth is very fast: a total of approximately 25 cm is gained. However, the rate of growth declines rapidly over the first year, from 38 cm/year in

the first 2 months to 28 cm/year at 4 months of age and 12 cm/year at 1 year of age (33). In the second year of life it is 10 cm/year, in the third through fourth years 7 cm/year, and in the fifth through sixth years 6 cm/year. From then on to puberty it is 5 cm/year (31, 32). Guidelines for abnormal growth rates adjusted for chronological age are as follows: fewer than 7 cm/year under age 4 years, fewer than 6 cm before age 6, and fewer than 4.5 cm from 6 years until puberty. At this stage growth acceleration ensues. Pubertal growth spurt occurs during early puberty and before menarche in girls (Tanner stages II–III), during which time they grow at a mean velocity of 10.3 cm per year. The pubertal growth period is longer in boys than in girls. The growth data of each patient must be plotted on the appropriate chart for that particular child. As mentioned above, new standards for the general population have been established and the recent CDC growth charts are recommended for use (5). In addition, growth velocity charts may be helpful because these take into account different stages of growth such as pubertal growth spurt. As mentioned above, the Eurogrowth Program is an excellent tool for use in infants up to 36 months of age, as it considers most variables that may influence growth progression at this stage in life (7–11).

However, monitoring weight gain in short-stature patients is as important as following the height progression. Changes in weight progression may precede alterations in height increments in certain conditions such as nutritional dwarfing and obesity (34–37). Therefore, monitoring height alone does not provide sufficient information to assess a growth pattern, as discussed in the section of nutritional growth retardation. Accurate weight measurements should be made on a regular hospital weighing scale. An infant should be stripped of clothes and diapers, and older children should wear a hospital gown or light clothing. These measures minimize inaccuracies resulting from variability in clothing weight, which varies with season. Adherence to these rules is important if we are to take note of changes in weight over time.

B. Genetic Potential

The genetic potential of the child should be considered in the evaluation of the present growth pattern. Any deviation from the expected height for the family should be worrisome (38). For this purpose, formulas and standards for target height for the family and predicted adult height have been developed. The following formulas provide an easy way of estimating the target height:

For males: (mother's height + 13 cm
+ father's height) divided by 2
For females: (father's height − 13 cm
+ mother's height) divided by 2

This formula provides the midparental height ±2 SD (1 SD would be equivalent of about 5 cm). However, It

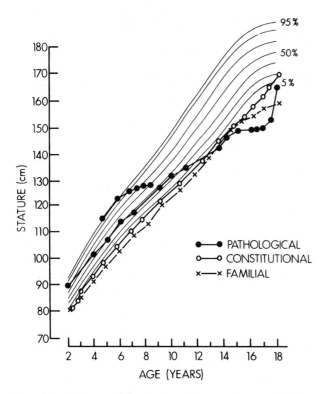

Figure 1 The growth patterns of three patients with short stature and one patient with pathological growth disorder who nevertheless was of normal height. The patient with pathological short stature received treatment at age 17 and attained catch-up growth. (From Ref. 13.)

is important to remember that the parents' heights should be measured and not guessed.

The target height obtained by this method is then applied to the 20-year line of the gender-appropriate growth chart. The projected height is determined by extrapolating the child's growth along his or her own channel. If the projected final height is within 5 cm of target or midparental height, the child's height is appropriate for the family. On the other hand, if the difference between the target and the projected height is more than 5 cm, a pathological cause should be considered.

A simple way of evaluating whether a child is within the normal limits of height for the family is to compare the stature of the patient with the midparental height in charts developed specially to assess the correlation coefficient of these variables (38) (Fig. 2). This correlation coefficient changes little between ages 2 and 9 years. For this norm, a simple chart plotting the age in relation to parents' heights can be constructed with the usual percentile for the family stature. Figure 2 depicts charts of three patients with different diagnoses. Patient A's height falls on the third percentile, and his parents' heights midpar-

ental have an average of 157 cm. The position of this patient's stature in the chart is between the 10th and 25th percentiles. Thus, for the population at large, this patient would be small, but he would be appropriate for his immediate family. Therefore, this patient may have familial short stature. In contrast, patient B, who has the same height as patient A, has parents of average height (midparental height 167 cm). This means that patient B is actually very short for the family and requires further work-up. Patient C is a more extreme case: his parents are actually tall. Although this patient's height is equal to that of the other two patients, his stature falls more than 3 SD from the family norm.

In addition to the projected target height, the predicted adult height should also be considered in the evaluation of the short child. There are three popular methods of calculating a child's predicted adult height. These are based on the fact that in a normal individual, there is a direct correlation between the degree of skeletal maturation and the time of epiphyseal closure, which is the event that ends skeletal growth. Predictions of ultimate height consider the fact that the more delayed the bone age is for the chronological age, the longer the time before epiphyseal fusion ends further growth. However, predictions of ultimate adult height are not totally accurate and are of limited value in children with growth disorders, since the predictions vary if children do not grow at normal rates. The data also may not be accurate for short patients from very short parents' (39). It has been shown that children from very short parents may end up taller in adult stature, and their target height and their predicted height may be underestimated.

The Bayley-Pinneau method is the most commonly used method to assess the predicted height (40). This method is based on the postulate that skeletal age at the time of the radiograph study correlates well with the proportion of adult height that the child will achieve. This correlation is more accurate after 9 years of age. The Tanner-Whitehouse (TW) method utilizes TW standards for the assessment of the bone age (41). In addition to bone age, this method takes into consideration actual height, chronological age, parental heights, and, in girls, the occurrence of menarche. The third method used in predicting adult height is the Roche-Wainer-Thissen (RWT) method. This method gives attention to the weight or nutritional status of the child (42). Additionally, recumbent length is used instead of standing height. The five predictor variables in this method are recumbent length, weight, bone age, chronological age, and parental heights.

One of the main sources of inaccuracy of adult height prediction is the inaccuracy of the bone age estimation. A small difference in bone age determination can lead to a great difference in height prediction, especially during the pubertal growth spurt (43). Comparability studies of the various methods of adult height prediction suggest that the RWT method is the most accurate, but it involves the

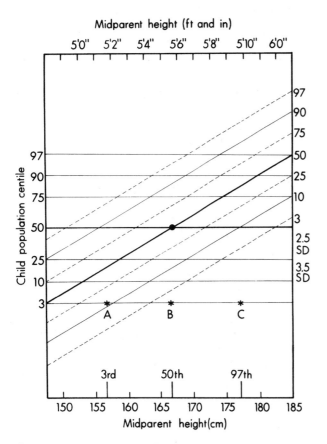

Figure 2 The Tanner standards for height of girls and boys from 2 to 9 years in relation to parents' height. (From Ref. 48.)

greatest amount of calculation. Its inaccuracy increases with age, and it therefore should not be used when more than half of the bones are adult (42, 43). In general, height prediction methods differ with respect to their accuracy and their tendency to overestimate or underestimate adult height (43). However, height prediction, as such, is useful only in children with normal growth rates and has limited usefulness in children who are not growing at normal rates. The calculation of target height for the family and the predicted adult height (by all three methods) can be done by computer programs developed for this purpose (ARC Software). Currently several manufacturers of growth hormone provide software at no cost to the clinician with which to follow patients with growth problems and the means to assess the information needed for a precise diagnosis.

C. Bone Maturation

In order to assess properly the predicted adult height, accurate bone maturation patterns are necessary. The two most commonly used methods of assessing the maturation or skeletal age are the Greutich and Pyle (G–P) (44) and the Tanner-Whitehouse (TW2) methods (41). The former method utilizes standards derived from US children living in Cleveland; the latter was derived from British children (45). The G–P method of assessing bone age is usually done by comparing an x-ray film of the frontal view of the left hand and wrist with given standards of the G–P atlas. The TW2 method is always done by assigning scores to each of the 20 hand bones, including the radius, ulna, carpals, metacarpals, and phalanges, depending on their stage of maturation. The total score determines the bone age. The advantage of the TW2 method over the G–P method is that it appears to be more objective. Moreover, it can differentiate bone age up to one-tenth of a year, whereas the G–P method gives only a rough approximation, with intervals of 6–12 months between the standards. Thus, the TW2 method is more sensitive in following small changes in bone age, but it is more time-consuming and few clinicians used it.

Studies comparing the two methods of bone age determination in the same ethnic population among children aged 2–24 years suggest that the median G–P skeletal ages were markedly greater than the corresponding chronological ages, particularly from 6 to 9 years in boys, and from 4 to 8 years in girls (45). The differences between these scales could be a result of real differences in the rates of skeletal maturation in the different populations. Studies were also done to determine whether there are significant differences among methods of evaluating skeletal age in relation to the group of bones studied. The results showed that when bone age is assessed by examining all the bones, but excluding the carpals, there is a high correlation with the bone age detected by measuring the maturation of all bones, including the carpals (45).

The bone maturation pattern is also helpful in differentiating the type of short stature. The bone growth in children with constitutionally delayed growth is slightly retarded (2, or at the most, 3 years), and it is usually proportional to height. When adolescence begins and the growth spurt occurs, the bone age increases proportionally to height. The bone age in patients with familial or genetic short stature is seldom retarded more than 1 year compared with chronological age, and it usually follows a normal maturation pattern. In contrast, there may be a marked bone age delay in children with pathological short stature, such as hypothyroidism, growth hormone deficiency, or chronic disease. The bone age may be even further behind than that expected for height. A short adolescent with sexual infantilism and a bone age maturation delay greater than 3 years is more likely to have pathological short stature, such as that caused by hypopituitarism or hypothyroidism. The degree of the delay may also reflect the length of time the patient has had the disease.

D. Body Proportions

Aside from body weight, height, and bone progression, attention must be given to the changes in body proportions during growth (46). The skeleton does not grow in a completely proportional manner. At birth, the upper to lower body ratio is 1.7. As the legs grow, the ratio becomes 1.0 by 10 years of age. If growth plates close early, as in precocious puberty, the proportions are those of a child, with short limbs compared with the trunk. On the other hand, if growth is prolonged as in hypogonadism, the limbs are longer compared with the trunk (47). Various types of tubular bone alterations are often found among short patients (48). These categorize patients into specific diagnostic groups and potential treatments. Thus, aside from accurate measurement of height, weight, and target and predicted height, every child who presents with a growth problem should be evaluated for disproportionate limb or trunk shortening. This information helps to narrow the differential diagnosis, including ruling out skeletal dysplasia. A detailed anthropometric evaluation of a child's body segments is indispensable.

The arm span should be measured with the patient standing against a flat wall, the arms stretched out as far as possible to create a 90 degree angle with the torso. The distance between the distal ends of both middle phalanges is measured to determine the arm span. Normally, the arm span is shorter than the height in boys under the age of 10–11 years and in girls under 11–14 years, after which the arm span becomes longer than the height. The average adult male has an arm span about 5.3 cm greater than his height, and the adult female has an arm span 1.2 cm greater than her height (Chapter 43). Conditions that adversely affect the vertebrae may result in growth retardation and disproportionately long arms. Children with arm spans that are disproportionately longer than their heights should also be evaluated for scoliosis.

Determination of the upper and lower body segment is also essential because skeletal dysplasias that result in growth problems are usually characterized by disproportionate shortening of the lower limbs or spine (Chapter 4). This can be done by measuring the distance between the upper border of the symphysis pubis and the floor in a patient who is standing against a flat wall in the proper position for height measurement. This measurement is difficult to obtain accurately, because the superior border of the symphysis pubis is not easy to locate and palpate, particularly in some obese patients. Preferably, the sitting height can be measured to represent the upper segment, using a Harpenden sitting table (Holtain Ltd.). The patient is asked to sit on the table with the back of the knees touching the table edge. The vertical unit is then moved close to the patient's back and the patient positioned so that the entire back, including the back of the head, touches the vertical surface. The sitting height is indicated by a counter, and the sitting height to standing height ratio, or relative sitting height, is calculated and multiplied by 100. The normal absolute and relative sitting heights of the different ages and sexes are listed in chapter on Reference Charts (Chaper 43). Conditions that cause disproportionate limb shortening include achondroplasia, hypochondroplasia, and Turner syndrome. On the other hand, the trunk height may be disproportionally shorter than the limbs in scoliosis or in spondyloepiphyseal dysplasia (Chapter 4).

The determination of rhizomelia should be made by accurate measurements of the proximal and distal segments of the limbs. This is important to assess for skeletal dysplasias, some of which may present clinically as short stature, without any other associated feature, such as mild hypochondroplasia or short-limbed short stature of genetic or familial nature (48). Disproportion between the upper arm and forearm length may be determined by measuring the shoulder-to-elbow (SE) length and the elbow-to-metacarpal length (EMC; Fig. 3) using an anthropometer. For SE length, the blades of the anthropometer are positioned from the midshoulder to the distal end of the humerus, with the elbow at a 90 degree angle and the upper arm next to the lateral side of the chest. To obtain the EMC length, the blades are positioned from the tip of the elbow to the distal end of the third metacarpal of the closed hand. Normally, the SE/EMC ratio is about unity. Rhizomelia is present if this ratio is lower than 0.98 (48). The presence of shortening of specific bones may likewise lead to the diagnosis of certain syndromes, such as type E brachydactyly (49), Turner syndrome (50), or pseudopseudohypoparathyroidism (51). These patients may be seen by the physician because of short stature and must be differentiated from those with familial genetic and short stature in whom metacarpal bone shortening and other tubular bone shortenings are very prevalent (48, 52).

To detect metacarpal shortening, a ruler is placed in front of the patient's fist. In most of the normal population the three knuckles of the third, fourth, and fifth fingers touch the ruler simultaneously. In brachymetacarpia V, however, there is a gap of 2 mm or more between the fifth knuckle and the edge of the ruler, as shown in Figure 4. This clinical observation has been confirmed radiologically (52). In patients with Turner syndrome and pseudopseudohypoparathyroidism, fourth metacarpal shortening is frequent. This can be detected radiologically and clinically in a manner similar to that used to detect fifth metacarpal bone shortening (50, 51). There is a gap be-

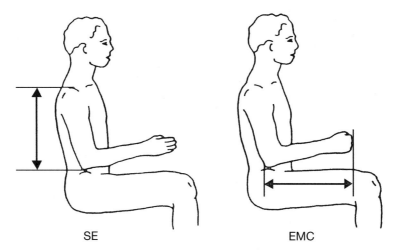

Figure 3   Measurement of shoulder-to-elbow length (SE) and elbow-to-end-of-third metacarpal length (EMC) is shown using an anthropometer. SE is the distance between the shoulder and the tip of the elbow, whereas EMC is the distance between the tip of the elbow and the distal end of the third metacarpal on a closed fist. (From Ref. 48.)

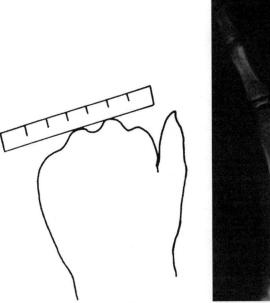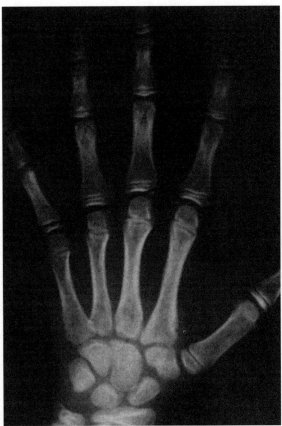

Figure 4 A straight ruler is applied against the distal ends of the third, fourth, and fifth metacarpals of a tightly closed fist. The clinical observation of brachymetacarpia V was confirmed radiologically when the fifth metacarpal bone failed to intercept a straight line connecting the distal ends of the third and fourth metacarpal bones by more than 2 mm. (From Ref. 52.)

tween the fourth knuckle and the edge of the ruler, which touches the third and fifth knuckles simultaneously. Standards at various ages for all body parts have been established (46), and the handbook of auxological measurements should be a part of every physician's reference library to help in the evaluation of growth problems and other syndromes.

Recently the so-called SHOX gene was located in the short arm of the sex chromosome. This acronym stands for short stature homebox and defines a deficiency of one copy of the SHOX gene (53). It is believed to be the cause of some forms of short stature, including Turner syndrome (54) and Leri Weill syndrome (55). It is believed to play a significant role in growth problems with disproportionate short limbs and tubular bones alterations, particularly in patients with Madelung deformity (i.e., shortening and bowing of the radius with dosral subluxation of the distal ulna, and partial foreleg anomalies) (53). It remains to be established whether SHOX plays a role in other more common forms of short stature, such as children with brachymetacarpia or milder forms of rhi-

zomelia. This test is now available for clinicians (*www. esoterix.com*).

E. Physical and Dental Examinations

Aside from obtaining accurate anthropometric measurements, a detailed physical examination may help to elucidate the cause of short stature or growth failure. Specific stigmata are present in common dysmorphology syndromes, such as Russell–Silver syndrome, Williams syndrome, Turner syndrome, and Prader-Willi syndrome (49). Signs of chronic illness should be looked for, such as pallor, dry skin, abnormal hair texture, splenomegaly, enamel hypoplasia, or dental caries. An important part of the physical examination that may provide insight into a child's maturational development is evaluation of dental age. Tables 2 and 3 list the ages at which primary and secondary teeth are expected to erupt (56). Remember that there are wide variations in the time of eruption, which may be affected by local and environmental factors, such as the size of the jaw, position of the unerupted teeth, and premature loss of deciduous teeth (57).

Table 2 Average Age at
Eruption of Primary Teeth

Tooth	Age (months)
Central incisor	6–9
Lateral incisor	7–10
Canine	16–20
First molar	12–16
Second molar	20–30

Children with growth hormone deficiency or un-treated hypothyroidism usually have a significantly delayed dentition or abnormal teeth (i.e., hypodontia, usually of the upper incisors), potentially associated with the epidermal growth factor gene on chromosome 4 (58–59). Mild delays in dental progress may occur in constitutional delay of growth and development.

V. CONSTITUTIONAL GROWTH DELAY

The most common cause of short stature and sexual infantilism in the adolescent is constitutionally delayed growth and sexual development. This diagnosis constitutes a large proportion of the growth disorders seen by pediatric endocrinologists. The total incidence in the population may even be higher, because pediatricians usually do not refer these patients to an endocrinologist. This entity is characterized by short stature as a variant of normal growth. These patients are the typical "slow growers" and

Table 3 Average Age at Eruption of Secondary Teeth

Tooth	Age (years)
Maxilla	
Central incisor	7–8
Lateral incisor	8–9
Canine	11–12
First premolar	10–11
Second premolar	10–12
First molar	6–7
Second molar	12–13
Third molar	17–25
Mandible	
Central incisor	6–7
Lateral incisor	7–8
Canine	9–11
First premolar	10–12
Second premolar	11–12
First molar	6–7
Second molar	11–13
Third molar	17–25

"late bloomers," with a familial prevalence. Often it is recognized long before adolescence, when sexual development is not yet a concern. The child with constitutional delay of growth and development typically is characterized by a deceleration of growth occurring during the first 2 years of life, followed by normal growth progression paralleling a lower percentile curve throughout the rest of the prepubertal years, until a late catch-up growth or growth spurt occurs in adolescence (Fig. 5). Fathers usually report a similar pattern of growth and delayed puberty. Patients with constitutional growth delay usually follow a familial pattern of growth; growth delay is itself inherited from multiple genes from both sides of the family. There may be no short stature in the family, but there may be similar growth patterns. Usually it occurs in boys, only occasionally in girls. The diagnosis of constitutional growth delay in girls should be made only after eliminating other possibilities of pathological growth patterns (60).

In a longitudinal study it was clearly shown that growth progression in patients with constitutional growth delay slows within the first 3–6 months of life (61). Both height and weight gain decelerate, and infants destined to have constitutional growth delay downcross percentiles until age 2–3 years (62). Thereafter, they grow at a normal rate until adolescence. This type of recanalization of growth is also seen in infants with familial short stature (see below). However, body weight progression differs between the two types of infants. In patients with constitutional growth delay, body weight gain slows, whereas in those with familial short stature it does not. Thus, patients with constitutional growth delay appear to fail to thrive with body weight deficits for length, whereas infants with familial short stature maintain a normal, or even an excess, body weight for length. These growth patterns are maintained throughout childhood, but before puberty patients with constitutional growth delay patients exhibit body weight gain and recover the body weight deficits for height before exhibiting sexual development (62). These data suggest that in constitutional growth delay there may be an association with suboptimal nutrition at the time that weight progression decreases in infancy.

Of interest is that in developing countries suboptimal nutrition was shown to produce a growth pattern similar to that of constitutional growth delay (63). In children with growth failure due to primary malnutrition, when the nutritional intake improved, growth resumed at a lower percentile, as in patients with constitutional growth delay. Once there was downregulation of the growth, the patients canalized their growth at a lower level than that before the nutritional insult. A similar pattern of growth retardation may be induced in experiments with rats subjected to suboptimal nutrition. When given a low-protein diet they ceased growing. When a normal dietary intake was provided they resumed growth at an appropriate rate, but in a lower percentile (64). In these rats there were long-

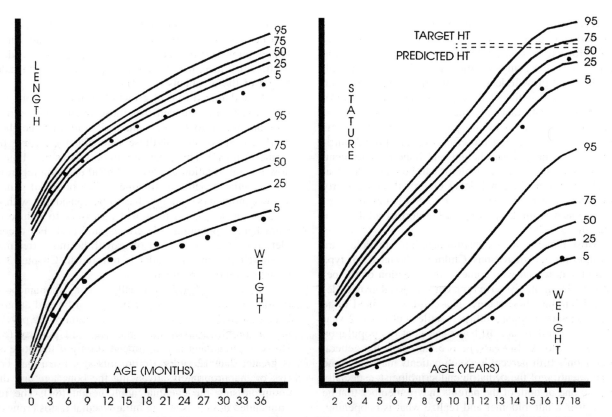

Figure 5 Constitutional growth retardation. Left: Note the readjustment of the growth channel and weight percentile in early infancy. Right: Note the progression of height and weight below, but parallel to, the lower percentile. Body weight deficits for height are evident. There is delayed pubertal growth spurt eventually leading to normal predicted adult stature, which is in range for the target height. (From Lifshitz F, Tarim O, Worrisome growth patterns in children. Int Pediatr 1994; 9:181–188.)

term alternations in growth hormone and insulin secretion after the temporary dietary protein restriction in early life. These alterations in the neurosecretory axis, together with subnormal insulin secretion, likely correlated to the lack of catch-up growth. These data suggest that the down-regulation of growth in the early life of patients with constitutional growth delay may also be nutritionally related, although it is not clear why these infants would ingest insufficient nutrients for growth at this stage of life. These patients appear to have failure to thrive, and the differential diagnosis may be difficult while the recanalization of growth is taking place.

Patients with constitutional growth delay may also show an apparent deviation from the normal curve sometime between 10 and 14 years. However, this may represent merely the difference between the prepubertal child with constitutional delay of growth and development and the average child already having a pubertal growth spurt. There is also a 2–4 year delay in skeletal maturation, retarded sexual development, and a 60–90% incidence of a familial history of delayed growth and pubertal development (65). The mechanism of this phenomenon is still unclear. Some investigators consider it the result of a tran-

sient or partial growth hormone deficiency (66–68). Other groups believe that it is the result of permanently diminished growth hormone secretion during sleep (69) or modifications in the region of the IGF-I gene (70). Some investigators think that the growth hormone alterations in these patients are caused by a deficiency of testosterone or estrogen, which are known to stimulate the production and secretion of growth hormone (71). In most patients with constitutional growth delay, however, there are no abnormalities in growth hormone secretion, nor are there any other detectable endocrine alterations (72). However, some authors believe that there may be a partial growth hormone insensitivity (73).

Although children with constitutional delay attain a normal height during adulthood, they generally end up along the lower end of the normal height for their family (74, 75). Studies have shown that in boys with untreated constitutional delay in growth and puberty, there was no significant difference between final and predicted adult height, but there was a significant difference between final height and measured midparental height. Thus, although these boys reach their predicted height, they were short for their families (74, 76). This is probably the result of the lower peak height velocity attained by later maturers than normal or early maturers (77). Other factors may play a role: for example, the selection for presentation to the clinic probably accounts for the finding that children with constitutional growth delay do not, on the average, attain the average percentile of their parents as expected (74). This may indicate that only the smallest of the sibships come to the attention of the physician (65). Also, this could be due to the possible effects of suboptimal nutrition (62) on the ultimate height and bone development. Based on various data available, it can be concluded that a child with constitutional delay of growth and puberty with a target or predicted height of 3 SD below the population mean is unlikely to reach the normal adult range of height (75, 78).

Most patients with constitutional growth delay are also short for genetic reasons. Children who have this type of short stature and who come to the attention of the pediatric endocrinologist have both constitutional growth delay and familial short stature. If a child is destined to be an average-sized adult (50th percentile) but has a 2 year delay as a child, at age 10 he or she is at the population fifth percentile. At 14 years, he is 5 cm below the general population's fifth percentile. Such patients may not come to the attention of the pediatric endocrinologist, especially because one or both of the parents may remember that he or she was a late bloomer and realize what is happening. On the other hand, if a patient is destined to reach only the 10th percentile as an adult and is 2 years late as a child, then at age 14 he would be about 2–3 cm below the third percentile, that is, more than 2 SD below the mean, and therefore likely to be referred for an endocrinological work-up. The typical boy with this syndrome is otherwise healthy, 10 years of age, and with the height and bone age of an average 8 year old. At the age of 12 (2 years later), height age and bone age are appropriate for age 10 years. Linear and skeletal growth remain consistent, but delayed, until his adolescent growth spurt takes place and secondary sexual characteristics appear. This condition is often difficult to diagnose when the patient is first seen unless measurements at various earlier ages are available, and follow-up height increments are assessed. The main concern with these patients is the psychological aspect of both the short stature and the lack of secondary sexual characteristics. In severe cases there may be a defective self-image and social withdrawal.

Treatment of patients with constitutional growth delay with or without familial short stature is controversial. The practicing physician is now under mounting pressure to prescribe human growth hormone (hGH) for short children who are not deficient in this hormone. The medical literature contains reports of improved growth with this treatment in "normal short children" who are experiencing a variety of combinations of constitutional delay and familial short stature (14, 79). To date, there is no definite evidence that even when such children transiently respond with improved growth rates with growth hormone treat-

ment, or any growth-promoting agent for that matter, there will be a permanent beneficial effect on ultimate stature. Papers published in recent literature on this subject demonstrate that there may be a mild improvement of the adult height of these patients (80, 81).

A randomized trial of growth hormone in short–normal girls clearly showed that those treated with growth hormone for up to 10 years attained an ultimate height of 5–10 cm above that of those who did not receive this medication (82). These data are important as the clinician now has information to base a clinical decision regarding the potential benefits of treatment. The potential gain of a few centimeters in height has to be considered with regard to the long-term treatment necessary to induce the extra height, potential side effects, and cost. For a complete review of the subject of growth hormone treatment of short children, the reader is referred to Chapter 3 on growth hormone treatment.

Although puberty eventually occurs spontaneously, treatment with testosterone in boys for a limited duration is recommended primarily for amelioration of the psychological problems associated with delayed puberty (83). However, treatment is recommended only if the bone age is greater than 12 years. Before this age, there may be a risk of inappropriately advancing the bone age and thus compromising the eventual adult height (84). The recommended dosage is 50 mg intramuscular testosterone enanthate or 170 mg of the cypionate form every month for 4–6 months. The 6 month course can be repeated if puberty does not progress spontaneously. Methyltestosterone may be used, but it may have potential toxicity to the liver. The use of anabolic steroids has been utilized to stimulate growth as well as to promote sexual development (85–89). Ideally, this should promote both these objectives with minimal side effects and without danger of damage to the gonads or a decrease in the patient's final adult height. In addition, there seems to be a psychological advantage to inducing puberty in patients who might otherwise have very delayed maturation.

Treatment with these medications should be reserved for patients who have attained the psychological development appropriate for puberty. Therapy may not be indicated in any patient with a chronological age of under 12 years or a bone age under 10 years. One should always keep in mind that anabolic steroids given for short periods may accelerate growth and bone maturation, but will not increase ultimate height. In fact, they may even prevent attainment of maximum height potential. Fluoroxymesterone is an anabolic compound that seems to be the best growth-promoting agent available. Long-term studies have shown that this drug causes accelerated growth without adversely causing rapid bone maturation or compromising adult height. For a comprehensive review of the effects of oxandrolone on growth, the reader is referred to an excellent article published elsewhere (89).

Aside from androgens and anabolic steroids, other pharmacological agents that have been used in the treatment of these children who are not growth hormone deficient include propranolol, clonidine, and dopaminergic drugs, such as L-dopa (levo-dopa) and bromocriptine (90–93). Clonidine treatment of constitutional short stature improved the growth of some, but not all patients treated, nor in placebo-controlled studies (91–93). Other drugs used include luteinizing hormone-releasing hormone administration at physiological intervals to stimulate testosterone production by means of pituitary gonadotropin secretion (68). However, these regimens are expensive and cumbersome. Although these drugs have been shown to increase growth hormone secretion, the growth-promoting effects are debatable. Also, long-term studies on their effect on the final height of children treated by such drugs are not promising (89, 93).

The decision to use pharmacological intervention must necessarily be based on the patient's emotional outlook and the severity of delay. Most children with constitutional delay of growth and development are able to cope with this condition, if they are properly reassured about their ultimate height and development. This diagnosis, by definition, presages eventual normal maturity and height without medical intervention. A good deal of

caution is warranted when treating such a benign alteration, although the induction of more rapid maturation with medications is an immediate reward. A careful assessment of the nutritional intake is recommended, with particular attention to deficits in micronutrients, iron, and calcium, since these patients may have decreased bone density as adults (94). If deficits are uncovered, nutritional therapy is recommended.

VI. FAMILIAL SHORT STATURE

Familial short stature has also been defined as genetic short stature. These patients are short throughout life and are short as adults, but characteristically they grow at normal rates in their own percentile (see Fig. 1); however, their height is within normal limits when allowance is made for parental heights (95). The growth of these patients in infancy reveals that growth channels were reduced some time between 6 and 18 months of age (62) (Fig. 6). After 2–3 years of age growth assumes a steady channel below the fifth percentile. This is because a child's size at birth is mostly determined by maternal fac-

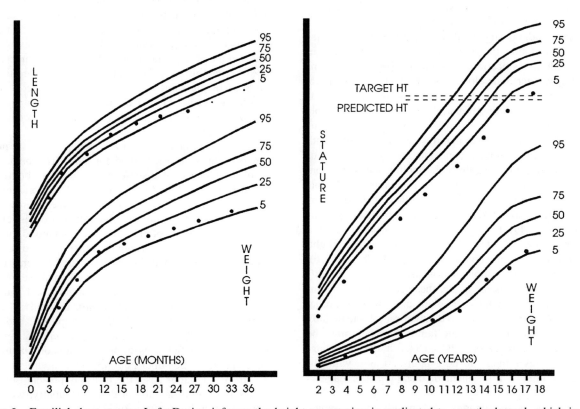

Figure 6 Familial short stature. Left: During infancy, the height progression is readjusted to growth channel, which is more appropriate for the genetic potential. Right: The new height percentile is maintained without further fall-off from the lower percentile, and the weight is appropriate for height. Note that short stature is life-long and there is no catch-up growth in puberty. The predicted height of the patient is in range for the target. (From Lifshitz F, Tarim O, Worrisome growth patterns in children. Int Pediatr 1994; 9:181–188.)

tors. After 6 months, the genetic influence predominates, and therefore a child who was born of average size may now shift to lower channels because his or her parents are of short stature. In contrast to patients with constitutional growth delay, these infants gain weight at a steady rate, do not exhibit weight deficits for height, and have no bone age delay (62).

The bone age of patients with familial short stature is consistent with their chronological age, although usually there is a component of constitutional delay in growth and development. The diagnosis of familial short stature is made when the child's height is normal, when allowance is made for parental heights, or the predicted adult height falls within the target range for the family. Tubular bone alterations were described as significantly more prevalent in children with familial short stature children and adults than in the normal height population (48). These tubular bone alterations include fifth metacarpal bone shortening (brachymetacarpia V, Figs. 3 and 4), rhizomelia, and disproportionate shortening of the arms and lower limbs. Most children and adults with familial short stature had two to four types of tubular bone alterations, whereas most individuals with normal stature had either none or only one type of tubular bone defect. A direct linear relationship was observed between the degree of shortening of the fifth and first metacarpal bones, but not of the other metacarpal bones (48).

These findings suggest that in some patients with familial short stature there may be an inherited defect in endochondrial ossification, which is the major process involved in tubular bone elongation and increase in stature. This defect may result not only in overall decrease in stature but also in disproportionate limb shortening. Patients with familial short stature may show a heterogeneous group of conditions, which manifest as short stature, with or without minor tubular bone alterations, and with or without disproportionate limb shortening, and/or present short stature with no other stigmata. For example, patients with type E brachydactyly have no other skeletal abnormalities except short stature and metacarpal and metatarsal shortening (49). Hypochondroplasia, particularly when mild, may only manifest as short stature with a slight, disproportionate limb shortening and brachydactyly (96). Unless careful observations and measurements of the different body segments are made, these patients can be underdiagnosed as having only plain and simple familial short stature. In these cases, a detailed radiological study and segregation analysis of the family members must be done. The availability of SHOX-DNA studies for diagnostic purposes remains to be established as a valid indicator for clinical assessment of these types of patients (53–55).

Although it is important to consider the parents' heights in evaluating a child's short stature, it should be remembered that a parent's stature is not necessarily familial or genetic (39). Stature also depends on a multitude of environmental factors that may have affected a parent's growth, including nutrition, drugs, and illness (97). Thus, considering the heights of the parents' siblings and parents, as well as obtaining a medical history of the parents, are also important before making a diagnosis of simple familial short stature (95). In these patients as in children with constitutional growth delay, there is pressure to consider treatment to increase growth and attain an increased ultimate height. As mentioned above, evidence is now available demonstrating a small potential gain in height with prolonged growth hormone therapy (80–82). In normal girls with genetic short stature given this medication for up to 10 years, there was a mean gain of 5–10 cm in ultimate adult height compared with the group not treated (82). However, the cost of such prolonged therapy to gain a very modest height increment should always be kept in mind, as well as other potential side effects.

VII. PATHOLOGICAL SHORT STATURE

Pathological short stature is the least frequently occurring but most serious cause of short stature. Pathological short stature should be suspected in children who do not grow normally, those with a growth velocity of less than 4.5 cm/year after 6 years of age, and in those with marked short stature. Bone maturation is usually quite delayed, often behind that expected for height. These patients usually fail to develop sexually, and the prognosis for ultimate height is dependent on the specific diagnosis (see Table 1). Pathological short stature has accounted for over one-third of the short patients referred to a pediatric endocrinology center (13). This incidence is high compared with the general population (12), but appropriate for a referral center.

It is essential to recognize these patients. A precise diagnosis must be established for early treatment. Often the only evidence of disease is the growth abnormality. The disturbances found to account for the short stature in these children may vary depending on the interest of the pediatric endocrine center to which the patient is referred. The causes are most often endocrine, metabolic, or nutritional disturbances. Undoubtedly, other alterations known to interfere with growth in children, such as renal or cardiac, predominate in patients referred to these types of subspecialty centers. The specific pathological causes of short stature due to hypopituitarism, as well as Turner syndrome are reviewed in detail in Chapters 2 and 9. Individuals with Turner syndrome have sex chromosome abnormalities and often present because of short stature. The karyotype could be either pure 45,XO or a variety of mosaicism. In the latter case, the girl may present only with short stature with or without delayed puberty, with none of the dysmorphic features of Turner syndrome (Chapter 10). The pathogenesis of the short stature is unclear, but recent studies suggest a functional abnormality of the hypothalamic–pituitary axis. During an overnight study of their nocturnal growth hormone secretion patterns, children with Turner syndrome had a significantly decreased number and frequency of peaks compared with normal children. Moreover, their responses to acute growth-hormone-releasing hormone (GHRH) stimulation are lower. This abnormal growth hormone neuroregulation is thought to be caused by the absence of gonadal steroids (98). Human growth hormone, anabolic steroids, and low-dose estrogen therapy, alone or in combination, have been recommended for increasing these patients' heights (Chapters 3 and 10) (99–101).

Other chromosomal defects can lead to short stature, the most common autosomat abnormality being Down syndrome. This anomaly is also the most common malformation in humans; it occurs with an incidence of 1:600. These children follow a typical growth pattern (see Chapter 43: Growth Charts) and have obvious dysmorphic features. The average adult female height is about 57 inches, and the average adult male is about 61 inches. Patients have a tendency to be overweight beginning in late infancy and throughout the remainder of the growing years (25). Growth and weight gain may also be affected by a concomitant congenital heart defect. The underlying cause of short stature remains unexplained; however, low circulating levels of insulin-like growth factor I (IGF-I) and diminished provoked and spontaneous growth hormone secretion have been reported in some patients (102, 103). However, most of the studies performed on Down syndrome patients in regard to hGH secretion were done without consideration of body composition, excess fat being a known cause of decreased growth hormone secretion (104). Thus, caution is encouraged in interpreting the results of growth hormone testing in these patients or using them in justifying treatment with growth hormone. Growth hormone treatment of a small number of patients with Down syndrome has resulted in an accelerated short-term linear growth and an increase in head circumference. However, careful and cautious evaluation of the safety, efficacy, and ethical ramifications of growth hormone treatment of children with Down syndrome is recommended before embarking on this form of intervention (105).

Short stature associated with congenital anomalies is also seen with bone diseases classified as skeletal development disorders, which result in disproportionate short stature are discussed in Chapter 4. The primary error leading to the disease may affect either the cartilaginous or the bone-forming stage of bone development. More than 250 different types of bone dysplasia are known, but the cause of most of these is unknown. The classification is therefore based largely on morphological criteria rather than metabolic or molecular ones (106, 107). This disproportion seen in many skeletal dysplasias may have therapeutic implications because some bones grow better than others. Therefore, growth-promoting agents may accentuate the disparity among the various bones.

One group of conditions characterized by severe short stature and typical dysmorphic features is occasionally referred to as primordial dwarfism because no specific cause for the short stature is defined, and no skeletal dysplasia is identifiable. Short stature is prenatal in onset, these children are born small for gestational age, and skeletal age is retarded (58). The most notable among the causes of primordial dwarfism is Russell–Silver syndrome, described independently by Silver in 1953 and Russell in 1954. Skeletal asymmetry is a distinct feature of this disorder, as is clinodactyly of the fifth finger and small triangular face with downturning of the corners of the mouth. Café-au-lait spots are usually present. De Lange syndrome typically is characterized by mental retardation, microbrachycephaly, bushy eyebrows and synophrys, and long, curly eyelashes. Patients have a small nose, anteverted nostrils, high arched palate, micrognathia, hirsutism, delayed dentition, micromelia, phocomelia and/or oligodactyly, hypospadias, undescended testes, and hypoplastic external genitals. There may or may not be associated endocrinopathies (108).

Bloom syndrome is characterized by mild microcephaly with dolichocephaly, malar hypoplasia, and facial telangiectaticerythema. There may be a mild mental deficiency and immunoglobulin deficiency. Death is usually caused by a lymphoreticular malignancy (58). Johanson-Blizzard syndrome is characterized by varying degrees of intellectual impairment. Clinical characteristics include hypoplastic or aplastic alae nasi, hypoplastic deciduous teeth, and absent permanent teeth. They may have cryptochoridism, micropenis, imperforate anus, hydronephrosis, septate or double vagina, primary hypothyroidism, and/or pancreatic insufficiency (58). Seckel syndrome is characterized by microcephaly, mental deficiency, premature synostosis, receding forehead, prominent nose, micrognathia, low-set and malformed ears, relatively large eyes with downslanting palpebrat fissures, clinodactyly of the fifth finger, and dislocation of the radial head and/or hips. These patients are referred to as bird-headed dwarfs because of the disproportionately large nose size in comparison with the mandible and face (58). Finally, Williams syndrome is characterized by varying degrees of mental retardation, medial eyebrow flare, short palpebral fissures, depressed nasal bridge, epicanthal folds, periorbital fullness of subcutaneous tissues, blue eyes, anteverted nares, long philtrum, and prominent lips with open mouth. Nails are hypoplastic, and there may be cardiovascular anomalies, including supra-alveolar aortic stenosis, pulmonary artery stenosis, ventricular or atrial septal defects. There may also be renal artery stenosis, hypertension, and hypoplasia of the aorta (58).

VIII. INTRAUTERINE GROWTH RETARDATION

Intrauterine growth retardation (IUGR) refers to a pathological condition found in infants who have low birth weight (LBW) for their gestational age as a result of different genetic and/or environmental influences during gestation. The Third National Health and Nutrition Examination Survey showed an overall 8.6% prevalence of U.S. newborns who are small for gestational age (SGA) of all live births (109). Elsewhere the prevalence of this condition is approximately 3% (110).

IUGR is especially important because of the higher incidence of morbidity and mortality in such children and the potential long-term complications of IUGR in adults. Infants with LBW are 5–10 times more likely to die in the first year of life than are normal birth weight infants (111, 112). Those who survive may present neurological and developmental disabilities, and have an increased risk of reduced rate of postnatal growth with ultimate short stature. Although some IUGR babies may grow and develop normally and attain normal stature as adults, about 10–15% do not exhibit catch-up growth and remain short throughout life (109). The association of IUGR with several adult-onset disorders has also been described and is currently the aim of broad research. An increased incidence of hypertension, cardiovascular and cerebrovascular disease, noninsulin-dependent diabetes mellitus (NIDDM), and lipid disorders have been reported in adults with clinical antecedent of LBW (113–120).

IUGR has been defined most commonly as a birth weight of under the 10th percentile for the gestational age (121–123). This weight cutoff has been criticized for allowing an overestimation of the real incidence of this disorder, since this implies that 10% of normal infants will have a birth weight below the 10th percentile. However, there is a significant increased risk for fetal death in those with birth weights between the 10th and the 15th percentiles (124), but up to 70% of all SGA infants may be constitutionally small fetuses expressing their genetic potential, and may not be at risk for perinatal mobidity or mortality. The remaining 30% are growth-restricted infants because of various pathological conditions, and are at risk for an adverse outcome (125–128). The standards for fetal growth developed by Brenner et al. (129), which included 30,772 deliveries made at 21–44 weeks gestation, are very useful to evaluate the presence or absence of IUGR.

A. Etiology

Normal uterine growth depends on the genetic potential of the fetus modulated by environmental, hormonal, and other biological factors, including maternal health and nutrition (130). Infants of small parents tend to be small, with maternal size having the greatest influence (131). Several factors play an important role in the etiopathogenesis of IUGR. Fetal growth failure may be due to extrinsic factors, mainly maternal, or to intrinsic fetal growth retardation. The extrinsic factors occur later in pregnancy as a result of placental disorders or maternal disease, which compromise the delivery of oxygen and nutrients

to the fetus. Of special importance is the nutritional status of the mother, as this has major implications on fetal growth. Chronic undernutrition, more prevalent in developing countries, is responsible for a large population of infants with IUGR worldwide. Different outcomes are observed according to the stage of fetal development at which maternal malnutrition takes place (132, 133). Early fetal malnutrition may affect growth permanently by reducing cell proliferation and size. A decrease of the cell size with preservation of cell population is the pathological consequence of later malnutrition, which might also result in growth deficit. Infants exposed to early fetal malnutrition have LBW and are symmetrically small (proportionate IUGR). Undernutrition in late pregnancy results in an asymmetrically growth-retarded infant whose head circumference is preserved as a result of a physiological adaptation (brain-sparing phenomenon), by which a major selective blood flow is directed to the brain (130).

There is undoubtedly an association between maternal weight status and infant birth weight (134). Adequate prenatal care and improved maternal nutrition, through balanced calorie or protein supplementation, leads to an overall increase in infant birth weight and to a decreased rate of LBW deliveries in at-risk populations (135). These guidelines have been endorsed by the American College of Obstetricians and Gynecologists (136) and used by the supplement food programs for Women, Infants, and Children (137). Previous nutritional guidelines recommended a gain of 22–27 pounds for women of all weight categories. Currently, the Institute of Medicine recommends for underweight women (body mass index < 19.8 kg/m^2) a weight gain of 29–40 pounds; for average women (body mass index between 19.8 and 26 kg/m^2) 25–35 pounds; and for overweight women (body mass index between 26 and 29 kg/m^2) 15–25 pounds (134). These recommendations for weight gain during pregnancy have been associated with a decreased incidence of LBW (133–137).

Other maternal risk factors associated with IUGR include maternal short stature, early menarche, short interpregnancy interval, and high maternal parity. Maternal constraints of fetal growth that result in IUGR may be multigestational, an effect that may take several generations to correct (131). Often several other conditions overlap, such as chronic malnutrition and substance abuse, tobacco smoking, and alcohol ingestion (139). Mothers who live at high altitudes (>3000 m) may have systemic hypoxemia that could account for the LBW. Other maternal illnesses can impair the fetal growth because of systemic hypoxemia, including cardiac disease (mainly cyanotic type), sickle cell disease, or severe asthma. Proteinuric hypertension during pregnancy also is often complicated by growth retardation.

Intrinisic fetal factors that tend to reduce the size of the baby for gestational age include various infectious agents. These are usually responsible for early onset of IUGR, and have more severe consequences, such as agents associated with the TORCH syndrome (toxoplasmosis, other infections, rubella, cytomegalovires, herpes simplex). Of these, rubella and cytomegaloviruses are the most important identifiable agents associated with marked fetal growth retardation. These viral agents reduce cell number and subsequent birth weight by simultaneously inhibiting cell division and producing cell death (140).

Chromosomal abnormalities, including Down syndrome, trisomy 13, trisomy 18, Turner syndrome, and other major congenital malformations are other intrinsic factors that compromise the growth and development of the fetus (141). Chromosomal aberrations and single-gene defects often result in fetal growth failure by interfering with cell division. Several syndromes cause multiple congenital malformations and are associated with IUGR (141). As mentioned above, this group of conditions is characterized by IUGR and typical dysmorphic features, which at times are identified at birth (58). Included are patients with Russell–Silver, De Lange, Bloom, Johnson-Blizzard, and Williams syndromes.

The role of imprinting genes on fetal growth is another area of interest in the causation of IUGR. Kohler et al. (142), reported the first imprinting gene (*grf1*) to be implicated only in postnatal growth control. It codes for a protein (Grf-1) found exclusively in the hypothalamus and acts as an important regulator of synthesis and release of growth hormone (GH). The Grf-1 protein is not detected in the fetus and is only slightly detectable at birth, but is clearly present on the second postnatal day. Analysis of heterozygous mutant mice for this gene confirmed that *grf1* is an important imprinted gene whose deletion leads to a significant postnatal growth deficiency that persisted in adult mice. In contrast to other imprinting genes implicated in fetal growth, *grf1* is the first to be related exclusively to postnatal growth control.

B. Hormonal Influences

Neither growth hormone nor thyroid hormones are important regulators of fetal growth. Insulin has a major effect on growth and size at birth, mostly during the third trimester when it stimulates fetal lipogenic activity, including a rapid accumulation of adipose tissue. Insulin induces protein synthesis and hepatic glycogen deposition, increases nutrient uptake and utilization, and has a direct anabolic effect. In general, growth-restricted infants are characterized by fetal hypoglycemia, which limits insulin secretion and fetal glucose production with increased protein breakdown. This reduces protein accretion, which results in slow growth. In addition, insulin plays a permissive role in the release of different growth factors from placental tissues (143). The placental lactogen, a structural related placental peptide that has many GH-like actions, also seems to play an important role in fetal growth. Maternal serum concentrations of placental lactogen rise significantly in the third trimerster, parallel with a rise in serum IGF-I (144, 145).

IGF-I and IGF-II, which in the fetus function independently of pituitary GH, also have important effects on the growth and differentiation of various tissues. There is a positive correlation between the serum levels of IGF-1 and birth weight (146, 147). Insulin-like growth factor levels are regulated in a reciprocal direction by maternal nutritional status. Alterations in the GH–IGF axis have been reported in infants with IUGR (147, 148). Evidence exists that GH, IGF-I, and insulin-like growth factor-binding protein 3 (IGFBP-3) are regulated in a different way in SGA infants than in infants whose birth weight is appropriate for gestational age (147). There is an inverse relation between the levels of IGF-I, its major transporter, IGFPB-3, and birth weight. The cord levels of IGF-I and IGF-II are lower in SGA infants than in neonates whose weight is appropriate for gestational age (145). Also, higher basal levels of serum GH and a higher GH response to the growth-hormone-releasing hormone have been reported in SGA infants, which might be indicative of GH resistance or insensitivity (148). In IUGR infants who achieve catch-up growth, levels of IGF-I and IGFBP-3 normalize. By midchildhood, higher serum concentrations of IGF-I have been found in this group of children than in normal control subjects. This may reflect a stage of GH resistance that could be the result of a different reprogramming of the IGF-I axis than that occuring in utero (149).

Other potential factors may play a role in fetal growth. Weber et al. (150) found clear evidence of a relationship between birth month and body size at 18 years of age, with maximal height obtained in children born in spring and minimal height obtained in children born in autumn. The underlying physiological mechanism for this effect might involve the light-dependent activity of the pineal gland. Melatonin is active during the prenatal period via transplacental passage, and its cyclic production in the newborn is already established by 9–15 weeks after birth.

Recent studies (151, 152) have shown that leptin, the product of the *ob* gene, a hormone produced in adipose tissue, may play a role in the nutritional homeostasis of the fetus and in fetal growth. The hormone has been detected in fetal blood as early as the 18th week of gestation. No relationship has been found between maternal and fetal serum leptin levels. The birth weight and the body mass index correlate strongly with the serum concentration of leptin in infants (152). Infants who are SGA have a serum leptin concentration equivalent to half of the values found in infants whose weight is appropriate for gestational age. In infants who are large for gestational age, the concentration of leptin is likewise three times higher than in infants who are SGA. Although not universally reported, there seems to be a gender correlation for leptin levels, with higher serum concentrations in female infants (151). Leptin levels are influenced significantly by fatty mass and are highly related to nutritional status during the fetal and neonatal periods. The role of this hormone in the postnatal growth of infants with IUGR remains to be elucidated.

C. Assessment of Growth in Fetuses and Infants

The detection in utero of fetuses with IUGR may maximize the chance of survival and reduce their chance of morbidity and mortality. Ultrasound can detect up to 80% of fetuses with IUGR with great precision. However, there may be an incidence of 20% false-positive results (153). Several measurements have been implemented via ultrasound to make a diagnosis of IUGR: fetal abdominal circumference, biparietal diameter, head circumference, and skeletal length. In order to detect abnormalities in fetal growth, at least two serial ultrasound measurements should ideally be taken before the 26th week of gestation. Doppler ultrasound measurement of fetal cardiac output, systemic blood flow, and organ supply (particularly with respect to placental circulation) is a powerful tool in identifying IUGR fetuses at risk of acidemia. Cordocentesis to measure lactate concentration in fetal blood is one of the earliest markers of fetal distress. A significant correlation exists between elevated and midtrimester β-core fragment levels of human chorionic gonadotropin and IUGR, comparable to third-trimester ultrasound and superior to maternal serum analytes (154). This could be a promising new tool for the early prediction of IUGR in at-risk populations.

At birth, the ponderal index (PI) (birth weight (g) $\times$ 100/length (cm)$^{-3}$) is a measurement of proportionality that is simple and easily available. It has been used to determine the symmetry of infants with IUGR. Infants with low PIs have been exposed to short periods of malnutrition that compromises mostly the weight but not the length or the head circumference (disproportionate IUGR). On the other hand, infants with "normal" PIs are proportionate at birth and may have been exposed to a more chronic injury in utero. The ratio of midarm to head circumference, which reflects somatic muscle and fat stores, has been proposed as a better predictor of mobidity than PI (155).

D. Postnatal Growth and Outcome

It is important to recognize that infants with IUGR even without any major disability may fail to catch up, and their IUGR may be a cause of short stature (156). It has been shown that 15–20% of infants with IUGR will have short stature by the age of 4 years and 7.9% will have short stature at 18 years of age. Infants with IUGR usually experience catch-up growth during the first 2 years of life, with most infants achieving this growth in the first 6 months of life (109). Of those children who do not show

catch-up growth, 50% will remain short as adults (125). However the most important determinants of the final height of infants with IUGR are unknown. Leger et al. (157) reported in a longitudinal study involving 213 SGA infants that the most important factors determining final height were parental height (especially the mother's stature) and birth length, rather than variables such as gender, birth weight, or PI.

Strauss et al. (158) evaluated a cohort of infants born with IUGR and found no differences in terms of risk factors (birth weight, birth length, head circumference, PI, maternal weight gain, maternal size, placental size, smoking, toxemia, or hypertension) between the infants who showed catch-up growth and those who did not, suggesting that genetic factors rather than environmental events account for the persistent effects of IUGR on growth. The importance of a genetic contribution is supported by the increased prevalence of IUGR within some families and the discovery of single-gene mutations in IGF-1 in some infants with IUGR (159). The Third National Health and Nutrition Examination Survey (109) showed a tendency of infants who were SGA at birth to be shorter and to have smaller head circumferences despite catch-up growth. In general, after an initial period of rapid growth, infants who were SGA at birth can be expected to attain growth around the 25th percentile in early childhood. Unlike term infants who are SGA, LBW infants who are born preterm usually show poorer progress. Infants with IUGR attain 80% of catch-up growth in the first 6–8 months of life (111). In those in whom catch-up growth does not take place, final stature may be compromised.

However, the postnatal growth of IUGR infants often is compromised by failure to thrive (FTT). The incidence of FTT in IUGR infants appears to be high, and it is often difficult to determine if such infants are growing normally after birth without experiencing catch-up growth or if they have FTT. Kelleher et al. (160) reported an incidence of 19.7% of FTT in a cohort of 914 preterm infants with LBW who were evaluated for 3 years. Infants who experienced FTT remained smaller on all growth parameters (weight, length, and head circumference) at 36 months of age compared to their matched controls. On the other hand, IUGR infants who are labeled as experiencing FTT may be growing appropriately and may be subjected to unnecessary diagnostic and therapeutic studies (13). One example of normal growth in IUGR misdiagnosed as FTT is shown in Figure 7. The weight and length of this patient were plotted on a growth chart for normal children, not on the specific IUGR growth charts available for these infants. However, a simple examination of the anthropometric measurements of this patient ruled out the diagnosis of FTT. The patient tripled his weight by 1 year of age and quadrupled it by 2 years. His length likewise progressed well and remained proportional to weight throughout. A careful evaluation of the growth pattern and weight gain elucidated the differential diagnosis.

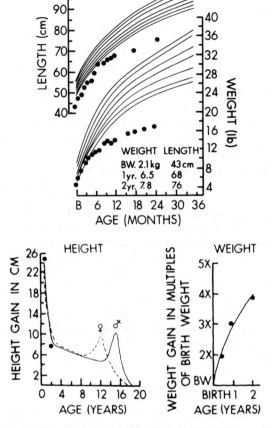

Figure 7 Top. Growth patterns of a patient with intrauterine growth retardation. Bottom. The growth velocity is plotted against normal standards. Note that this patient did not have failure to thrive nor was it suspected because he was growing at a normal velocity. (From Ref. 13.)

The diagnosis of FTT cannot be sustained when the birth weight is tripled within the first year of life. This rate of growth is the one that occurs in normal children. However, this infant did not exhibit catch-up growth. Infants with IUGR who start with a tremendous size deficit and who do not exhibit catch-up growth may be expected to remain proportionally small thereafter. Aside from the absence of catch-up growth, these children with IUGR may undergo early puberty and be unusually short as adults (161). Often these children may be forced to increase calorie intake in order to grow more in length to no avail.

However if weight gain progression does not occur at a normal rate, FTT must be considered. Because infants with IUGR often have other associated abnormalities such as neurological, cardiac, or pulmonary disorders, these may contribute and compromise growth and/or lead to

FTT. Frequently these patients also present oral motor dysfunction (162) resulting in "poor feeding." Nutrient intake in LBW infants is difficult at best, and most often does not meet the recommended dietary intakes (163). There is an accumulated nutrient deficit during the first few weeks of life of energy, protein, and other nutrient alterations that has an impact on infants' growth. The long-term consequences of this accumulated nutrient deficit may be important: as much as 45% of the growth variation was related to this. Thus, IUGR infants must be carefully monitored to ensure an adequate intake, which should allow for their maximum growth after birth. This is particularly important because growth hormone was recently approved for treatment of such infants, and this should not be undertaken without appropriate nutrient intake.

Growth failure in IUGR children is a new Food and Drug Administration (FDA)-approved indication for HGH therapy (Chapter 3). With the availability of unlimited amounts of biosynthesized HGH, the possibility of improving the final adult stature of children with IUGR by giving daily injections of HGH has been assessed in several studies (164–173). Although long-term results of HGH therapy in children with IUGR are not yet available, some studies have shown a short-term growth benefit after 2–4 years of HGH therapy (164–173). A clear dose–response effect to HGH was also shown (169–171). Dosages from 0.4–1.2 U/kg have been implemented, with a better growth response occurring with the highest dosages of HGH. However, some studies have shown that by using high dosages of HGH (>1.2 U/kg) accelerated skeletal maturation occurs. This could minimize the long-term benefits of the initial growth response (161) and the final height of IUGR subjects may not differ with and without growth hormone treatment (174).

High dosages of HGH have been used in infants with IUGR based on the hypothesis of a state of HGH insensitivities in this group of patients, which might be overcome by administering elevated dosages of the hormone. The use of high dosages of HGH in infants with IUGR is only recent and although HGH seems to be well-tolerated, long-term side effects have not been ruled out. Taking into consideration some data showing a potential risk for hyperinsulinism in infants and children with IUGR (115, 117–119), and since one of the potential side effects of GH therapy is the induction of insulin resistance, the use of high dosages of HGH in these patients must be viewed with caution.

Although some of these studies have shown promising results with HGH therapy, this form of treatment has only been implemented for a relatively short period of time, and no long-term data on the beneficial effects on final adult height are yet available (169). In most of these studies administration of HGH was started in patients over 2 years of age (171). To date, it is not known if there may be a better chance to induce a higher level of recanlization of growth with an earlier onset of HGH therapy.

E. Long-Term Effects

IUGR may have important long-term consequences, resulting in increased morbidity and mortality in adulthood. Experiments using animals (175, 176) indicate that transient events in fetal and early life might lead to permanent and significant changes in physiology and metabolism later in life. These studies have shown that undernutrition during critical period of rapid growth in fetal and early life may permanently modify the structure and physiology of different organs, including that of the endocrine pancreas, liver, and blood vessels, changing their structure and physiology permanently. In this way, hormonal physiology and tissue sensitivity could be definitely compromised, leading to disease in adult life, a phenomenon called "programming" (177). Hales and Barker (178), in their "thrifty phenotype" hypothesis, have pointed out how prenatal nutrition has an effect on fetal development that becomes evident in adulthood. This hypothesis has been supported by animal experiments. Pregnant rats fed with isocaloric, protein-restricted diet have offspring with lower birth weights, decreased β-cell mass, decreased islet vascularization, and impaired insulin response (176). This damage might be irreversible if a normal diet after birth does not restore a proper insulin response by adulthood. Thus, permanent endocrine dysfunction is one consequence of initial in utero nutritional insult.

Epidemiological and long-term follow-up studies have shown an inverse relation between birth weight and several adult-onset diseases (178, 179). A higher percentage of essential hypertension, impaired glucose tolerance, NIDDM, ischemic heart disease, high serum triglycerides, and low serum high-density lipoprotein concentration (syndrome X) has been reported in adults with a clinical history of LBW (180). These studies have shown a reduction in insulin response in prepubertal children and adults with a history of IUGR. The lower sensitivity to insulin seen in infants with IUGR might indicate that insulin resistance is present during childhood even without clinical manifestations. Low birth weight secondary to malnutrition during fetal development might be associated with abnormalities in muscle structure and function, which could interfere with glucose uptake, normally induced by insulin. Thus the β-cells must produce larger amounts of insulin to keep serum glucose levels within the physiological range, which in the course of time could lead to their exhaustion. Previous studies (177–180) have shown an association of several cardiovascular risk factors with insulin resistance. Thus, the presence of insulin resistance in children with IUGR could be a risk factor for the development not only of adult-onset NIDDM (117–119) but also of cardiovascular disease. A higher prevalence of arterial hypertension, high serum triglyceride concentrations, and low concentrations of high-density

lipoprotein cholesterol is found in adults with antecedent of LBW (177).

A threefold increased risk of NIDDM in men over 60 years of age with the clinical antecedent of IUGR was reported in a Swedish study (118). A recent study of a cohort of 70,000 women from the Nurses' Health Study (117) likewise found a strong inverse correlation between birth weight and NIDDM among more than 2000 confirmed cases of NIDDM. Women who weighed less than 5 pounds at birth had a relative risk for NIDDM of 1.83, compared with a risk of 0.83 in women who weighed more than 10 pounds at birth.

It is evident that growth restricted newborns are not all created equally (181). In recent years HGH trials have demonstrated an apparent beneficial effect on patients with noncomplicated IUGR treated after 2 years of age for 2–4 years. Most of these studies (171) have shown recanalization and improvement of height, although long-term data demonstrating gain in adult height are lacking. Whether an improved height attained with HGH treatment could ameliorate some of the long-term sequelae of IUGR in adult life is not known at present. However, in very stunted IUGR patients, it can be expected that psychological adjustment could improve with treatment that results in increased height.

IX. FAILURE TO THRIVE

The term, "failure to thrive" (FTT) is used to describe infants and young children whose body weight and weight gain are substantially less than those of their peers. It is defined as growth deceleration to a point below the third percentile in weight; a child who has fallen across two or more percentiles; or a child whose weight is less than 80% of the ideal weight for age.

FTT accounts for 1–5% of tertiary hospital admissions for patients less than 1 year of age (182). Many more children, perhaps 10%, are managed as outpatients by physicians throughout the United States (183). Despite its established status in medical terminology, the concept of FTT lacks a clear definition and should be considered a sign or symptom, not a diagnosis or a disease (184).

Children with FTT are typically diagnosed in the first few months of life and their illness may persist for years. All FTT infants have physiological alterations due to malnutrition, but the causes can be categorized as organic or nonorganic (185). Organic FTT (OFTT) involves infants who have specific diagnosable disorders. It is only identified in 20% to 40% of children hospitalized with FTT and even less frequently in outpatient clinics.

Non-organic failure to thrive (NOFTT) is a subtype of FTT that accounts for the majority of infants with FTT, although the percentage varies from institution to institution. NOFTT does not imply a specific cause, but merely suggests that the cause is primarily external to the infant (186). In addition, there may be an overlap between OFTT and NOFTT owing to the presence of minor infections, vomiting, and diarrhea together with behavioral problems and altered eating behavior. Therefore, several authors have questioned the adequacy of this dichotomous view, suggesting the need for a third category: so-called mixed cause (187, 188). NOFTT is more than a growth problem. Children with NOFTT present a low rate of weight or length gain, delayed development, abnormal behavior, and distorted caretaker–infant interaction.

Failure to thrive can be due to a variety of disorders that may have little in common except for poor body weight. Each one of them must be recognized and treated accordingly (189–191). However, the goals of nutritional rehabilitation are similar regardless of the cause. On the other hand, pediatricians should always be aware of different patterns of growth in the first years of life that can present as factitious failure to thrive (192). These patterns include patients with constitutional growth delay and/or familial short stature. Because the size of an infant at birth is more related to maternal size and intrauterine influences than to genetic factors, in some children an adjustment in growth velocity greater than 25% (across two percentile lines) takes place as a recanalization of normal growth. A significant decrease in growth rate in these conditions may represent a physiological event in the first years of life and does not necessarily indicate FTT. Also, patients with IUGR may mimic the symptoms of FTT as described above.

A. The Breastfed Baby

Caution must also be taken in labeling an infant who is exclusively breastfed as having FTT. Because growth charts for breastfed infants are not usually used, a normal growth pattern of a breastfed baby may seem to be lower on the growth channel of the most frequently used growth charts, which are based on studies of infants who were mostly formulafed (193, 194). To date, no clear data would warrant discouraging breastfeeding of an infant whose growth seems to deviate across channels in such growth charts. Human milk is the ideal and most readily available nutrient, and should therefore be continued and encouraged as much as possible. However, breastfeeding alone may not be adequate for a particular child who indeed may be failing to gain weight appropriately (195–197). Breast feeding must be closely monitored to ensure that adequate lactation is present and that the infant thrives at an appropriate rate as plotted on growth charts specific for breastfed babies (11).

The effect of prolonged breastfeeding on growth is controversial. One study (194) demonstrated that exclusively breastfed infants had slower length velocity after 3 months of age than infants who were weaned early and given formula plus solids. This trend was more obvious at 9 months of age. In this study, relative weight for length had no deficit. The growth of breastfed and formulafed infants from 0 to 18 months of age was investigated in the so-called DARLING study (198). The mean weight of breastfed infants was shown to drop below the median of the formulafed group between 6 and 18 months of age. In contrast, length and circumference values were similar between the two groups. The results of the study showed that breastfed infants gain weight more slowly than formulafed infants from similar socioeconomic and ethnic backgrounds during the first 9 months of life.

A comprehensive assessment of the effects of prolonged breastfeeding on children's growth was performed by Grummer-Strawn (199). In this retrospective analysis of 13 studies, eight reported negative relationships between breastfeeding and growth, two found a positive effect, and three showed mixed results. Even if prolonged breastfeeding is found to impair weight gain, the protection that breast milk offers against infection and other health benefits would argue in favor of preserving the policy of encouraging human milk feedings as the main food, (sole feeding for the first 4–6 months of life), particularly where sanitary conditions are poor. Prolonged breastfeedings also provide beneficial impact on birth spacing, mother–child interactions, infections, allergies, other morbidities, and infant mortality.

B. Clinical Findings

In the NOFTT syndrome, both inadequate nutrition (i.e., nature) and distorted social stimulation (i.e., nurture) contribute to poor weight gain, delayed development, and abnormal behavior. The clinical characteristics of infants with this type of FTT include small for age, thin for length, wide-eyed expression or gaze aversion, thin chests, wasted buttocks, prominent abdomen, hanging folds under the arms, expressionless face, decreased vocalization, gross motor activity, and response to social stimuli; lack of cuddling, and clenched fists.

There is evidence that NOFTT infants may present a combination of biological vulnerability, environmental difficulties, and be the products of parents with poor marital relationships (200, 201). Infants with this type of FTT are more passive, more likely to sleep through meals or take longer to finish their meals, and more likely to be diagnosed as hypotonic. There is also evidence that NOFTT infants receive less appropriate developmental stimulation at home and have developmental delays.

Developmental delays have also been linked to oral–motor dysfunction (OMD), which is frequently found in FTT children. When children with FTT were compared with children of the same developmental age with cerebral palsy, the oral–motor profiles were remarkably similar. It has been hypothesized that children with OMD might have subtle neurodevelopmental disorders (202). At 20 months of age, FTT infants were twice as likely to show mental developmental quotients less than 80 (200). The infants also showed less sociability. The clinician evaluating a child with FTT must also consider that prenatal factors may play a role in causing the problem. The possibility of prenatal exposure to psychoactive substances needs to be ascertained, including exposure to alcohol, tobacco, and other drugs (203). There may also be signs of neglect, abuse, or illness in infants with FTT. It should be kept in mind that confirmation of the diagnosis of NOFTT is always based on a positive growth and behavioral response to treatment.

C. Nourishing and Nurturing

Every child who fails to thrive has either not taken, has not been offered, or has not retained adequate energy to meet his or her nutritional needs. However, FTT infants prove that nourishment involves much more than ingestion of food. In most instances NOFTT results from a disruption in nurturing practices that ultimately affects the child's ability to obtain proper nourishment. These nurturing factors include parental beliefs and their concept of nutrition. Also the infant's behavior or adverse social or psychological environments may contribute to an inadequate nurturing environment, leading to NOFTT. Therefore, direct observation of mother–infant feeding and their social interaction is a necessary part of the evaluation. A careful nutritional evaluation must also be performed, which should include collecting dietary intake from a 24 h dietary recall or, more accurately, a food diary for 3–7 days. It should also address meal frequency, feeding patterns, and an assessment of all fluids given. It is also valuable to determine whether any particular food was restricted or promoted i.e., "no junk food," increased fruit juice consumption (204–208), or if there are vegetarian practices (209–211).

Often the diet record suggests that the child is receiving adequate calories for weight and length, but not for age. This level of intake allows the infant to maintain current weight but does not provide sufficient nutrients for growth. Sometimes the dietary intake is adequate in calories and protein, but is deficient in specific nutrients, such as iron, zinc, and/or other micronutrients, resulting in growth faltering (212–215). Supplementation studies have demonstrated that improvements in nutrient intake result in improved growth, including bone mineralization and maturation (216–218).

Particular attention should be paid to the presence of nonspecific symptoms, such as intermittent vomiting, spitting up, diarrhea, and frequent upper respiratory tract infections. These may be present in infants with NOFTT and in other organic conditions (i.e., gastroesophageal reflux) (219). So-called feeding difficulties may also lead to decreased nutrient intake in NOFTT infants (220). These infants exhibit unusual behaviors, such as wide-eyed staring, gaze avoidance, fist clenching, and apathy toward their caregivers. Although apathy and decreased motor activity are recognized behaviors in malnourished infants (221, 222), many of the abnormal behaviors of patients with NOFTT are not attributable to malnutrition alone.

Some nutritional alterations may influence the infant's behavior. Iron deficiency during infancy has been associated with anorexia, irritability, and lack of interest in their surroundings (223, 224). Zinc deficiency may likewise compound the course of FTT and excess lead ingestion may complicate the clinical picture even before the lead blood levels reach a toxic concentration. NOFTT infants were shown to have lead blood levels in a range formerly thought to be safe (i.e., 15–20 mg/dl) (225). These elements should be monitored in all FTT patients and treatment should be given when alterations are demonstrated.

If decreased nutrient intake is found to be the cause of inappropriate weight gain, the question becomes: Why are insufficient amounts of food consumed by infants with NOFTT? Are these infants simply not offered enough? Do the infants fail to signal hunger or satiety? Do they have a poor appetite or refuse food?

D. Neglect and Deprivation

In frequent cases, parental stress affects the way infants interact with their mothers (190–192). The quantity and quality of social and emotional stimulation between mother and child may be decreased even before clinical evidence of FTT is apparent. Many mothers of NOFTT infants are depressed, come from lower socioeconomic groups, lack a support group, and/or are themselves under multiple stresses. Mothers from higher socioeconomic groups may also lack the emotional strength or motivation to interpret or respond to the needs of their infant. As more mothers become engaged in work outside of the home or involved in activities that are independent of their family responsibilities, their children may not be getting the appropriate attention to meet their needs for nurturing (226).

Psychosocial deprivation may also lead to FTT in infants (227–229). It has long been known that neglect and deprivation may lead to FTT. King Frederick in Sicily was interested in learning the innate language of humans. Consequently he isolated infants to learn what language they would speak spontaneously. These children did not thrive and thereafter died due to lack of communication and attention (230, 231). Also, it has long been known that infants often died and did not thrive in foundling homes (232–236) or hospitals (237, 238). A classic example of the role of nurturing influencing somatic growth was described by Waddissom (236). She described the experience of two German orphanages run by women of different personalities. The children under the care of the unpleasant, aggressive woman who did not render nurturing care did not thrive, whereas those under the care of the woman with opposite personality traits grew well. Both groups had similar dietary intakes. These patients usually have no hormonal disturbances such as growth hormone deficiency to account for poor growth, and they usually recover when sufficient nourishment and nurturing is given.

E. Infantile Anorexia

An infant behavior that typically leads to FTT is infantile anorexia nervosa, which is characterized by food refusal, extreme food selectivity, and undereating despite parental efforts to increase the infant's food intake. The onset of this disorder usually is between 6 months and 3 years of age, with peak prevalence around 9 months of age (239). The feeding difficulties stem from the infant's thrust for autonomy; a striking observation in these infants is their willfullness. Mother and infant become embroiled in conflicts over autonomy and control, which manifest primarily during feeding time. This conflict leads to a battle of wills over the infant's food intake. Characteristically, parents mention that they have tried "everything" to get the infant to eat. Chatoor and colleagues (240) hypothesized that this separation-related conflict interferes with the infant development of somatopsychological differentiation. The process of differentiating somatic sensations, such as hunger or satiety, from emotional feelings, such as affection, anger, or frustration, is clouded by noncontingent responses by the parents to cues coming from the infant. As a result of this confusion, the infant's eating becomes controlled by emotional experiences instead of by physiological needs. The focus of the treatment is on improving communication between the parents and the infant to facilitate the process of separation and individuality. In a cognitive–behavioral approach, the therapist explains to the parents the infant's behavior and suggests ways to positively modify and structure mealtimes to facilitate growth.

F. Laboratory Findings

Poor nutrition and psychosocial factors are by far the most frequent factors leading to NOFTT. Therefore, laboratory tests offer limited value in determining the causes of growth deficiency and should only be used when the findings from the history and physical examination indicate something organic or possible nutritional alterations. In some cases, the child's bone age should be determined to facilitate the process of ruling out systemic chronic diseases or a hormonal abnormality. This measurement may also be of help as a baseline for future growth and bone development progression.

Unless organic disease is suspected, detailed testing should be reserved for patients in whom management of nutritional and psychosocial problems does not result in the expected improvement in the rate of growth. It has long been known that fewer than 1% of laboratory tests showed an abnormality that helped identify the cause (241). However, laboratory evaluation of the nutritional status should be comprehensive to assess for deficiencies that are not clinically apparent (242). Such an evaluation should include iron deficiency, which may be responsible for anemia and some of the long-term complications of FTT even when there is no anemia (212–221).

If weight gain does not occur soon after advice is given to the parent(s) about feedings, the child needs to be evaluated more intensely. Usually these patients are admitted to the hospital to have possible organic alterations ruled out, and most importantly simultaneously to receive appropriate nutritional intake to induce weight gain and thus to verify that the patient has the capacity to grow well (243).

G. Management

In the past, hospital care was routinely recommended as part of the initial management of FTT patients. The goals were to ensure an adequate dietary intake, to observe the child's behavior, and watch the family–child interactions. Despite today's economic constraints, hospital care is justified when the patient has not responded to appropriate outpatient management; the severity of the malnutrition warrants it; or abuse, neglect, or both are suspected. A meta-analysis of NOFTT found that hospitalization significantly improved growth recovery and sustained catch-up growth (244). However, an aggressive outpatient management program may also be appropriate (245). The use of a multidisciplinary team usually offers special advantages in the rapid correction of undernutrition and developmental progress in children with NOFTT (246).

Nutritional therapy of FTT children has several goals: (a) achieving ideal weight for height; (b) correcting nutrient deficits; (c) allowing catch-up growth; (d) restoring optimal body composition; and (e) educating parents in the nutritional requirements and feeding or the child. Regardless of why a child fails to thrive, effective nutritional management consists primarily of providing enough calories to achieve a positive energy balance and growth. The World Health Organization Expert Consultation on Energy and Protein Requirements recommended that "whenever possible, energy requirements should be based on measurement of expenditure rather than intake" (247). The standard energy expenditure prediction equations were all derived from data accumulated from healthy children. Thus they may underestimate about one-quarter of the true energy requirement for infants with FTT (248).

Because nutritional intervention is usually the focus in treating children with FTT, high-calorie, adequate protein feeding has been advocated for many years. With this treatment the child recovers more rapidly, the stay in the hospital is shorter, and more children can be treated in a given period of time at less cost. Nurses or trained therapists should feed the infant initially to allow identification of a feeding problem and to ensure that intake will be adequate. Proper feeding of the FTT child can be achieved most often with infant formula that is given in sufficient quantities to meet the child's specific nutrient needs. Protein and other types of supplementation are usually not needed, but some products can be used when indicated.

Tube feedings are indicated only in cases of severe malnutrition or failure to induce weight gain in the hospital. They may be necessary if the child is severely debilitated, metabolically unstable, or requires immediate restoration of fluid and electrolyte balance. Tube feedings may be useful for children with NOFTT as a temporary behavior modification modality, or in patients who fail to respond to other methods of nutritional rehabilitation (249).

Many clinical trials have indicated that supplementation with micronutrients improves weight gain in growth-faltering patients. Single-nutrient deficiencies are cumbersome to document and micronutrient deficiencies commonly coexist. For example, iron deficiency may be present without iron deficiency anemia, and zinc deficiency may be difficult to document by the lack of a good indicator. Yet clinical trials of iron supplementation have positive effects on weight gain, linear growth, and psychosocial behavior (212, 221, 250). Similar studies have revealed positive effects with zinc supplementation on growth as well as on morbidity and severity of infections in children. (251–256). Vitamin and mineral deficiencies sometimes become evident only after the infant starts growing and gaining weight. Therefore a multivitamin–mineral preparation that includes iron and zinc is recommended for all undernourished children.

Nutritional rehabilitation for these children must accomplish catch-up growth, which is defined as the acceleration in growth that occurs when a period of growth retardation ends and favorable conditions are restored. Catch-up growth in FTT depends on the provision of calories, protein, and other nutrients in excess of normal requirements. Children need 25–30% more energy and nearly double the amount of protein for catch-up growth (257). The extent to which nutritional rehabilitation can restore normal body size and composition is a critical subject. Returning to one's previous growth curve does not indicate achievement of a normal body composition (258).

H. Recovery

During the recovery period, parental nutrition education programs are extremely important. When families with psychosocial maladaptations are revealed to be major contributors to FTT, the physician must discuss these behaviors in a nonjudgmental way, so that guilt is not increased or compliance endangered. Parents should be reassured, and support should be provided for correction of the problems as much as possible.

To improve their infant's eating habits, parents should be introduced to inpatient treatment programs for food-refusing infants (259). Parents and infant may have to be separated at meal times. The nurse must feed the child with structured, time-limited meals. Parents are to be given individual therapy and afterwards be reintroduced to the feeding situation. Parents must be educated regarding the catch-up growth process and long-term growth goals for their child. The baseline appearance of a cachectic child may bias the family's perception of recovery.

The misperception that the recovering child is too plump may result in an abrupt diet change and abandonment of high-calorie feedings.

In all instances and at all stages of the evaluation and treatment of FTT, a "working alliance" between key family members and professionals must be established (260). Developing such relationships can be a challenge and it requires the availability and commitment of multidisciplinary teams to assist the family in the treatment of NOFTT.

Continued treatment after discharge from the hospital is necessary and the infant should be evaluated at regular intervals for a long time. Growth, development, and social behavior must be carefully and continually monitored. Temporary placement in a more favorable setting within the family or in a foster care environment may be necessary if the immediate family is judged as incapable of following through on the recommended management.

I. Long-Term Outcome

A few systematic long-term studies of growth and development in NOFTT infants have been carried out. The longest follow-up study on growth found a difference between former FTT children and control children when the relationship between the height and weight ages of the children were compared with their chronological ages (261). Of the children with FTT, 6 of 14 were 1 or more years below their chronological age for height and weight. In the comparison group it was 1 child out of 14. Studies of catch-up growth show that NOFTT children continue to do poorly developmentally despite increased weight. A study by Singer showed that even after extended hospitalization, NOFTT infants manifested persistent intellectual delays at a 3 year follow-up examination, despite maintenance of weight gains achieved during early hospitalization (262).

These children remained significantly behind their control group in language development, reading age, and verbal intelligence. They also scored lower than the control group on a social maturity rating.

J. Special Considerations

The physician faces specific additional problems when dealing with a NOFTT patient in the managed health care environment. The diagnostic coding of such children is fraught with so-called Catch-22 dilemmas (263). Medical, nutritional, developmental, and/or psychiatric diagnosis may be utilized, but no optimal classification and coding scheme exists for use in these patients. The rapid growth of managed care also has significant implications for access to care, quality of services, reimbursement, and payment for health care. The special needs of these patients amplify the issues and challenges in ensuring that managed care is an effective component of community resources that foster healthy growth and development (264). These patients are at risk for concurrent illness and adverse development outcomes. A healthier child ultimately requires fewer services and indirect benefits may also occur with fewer health care expenditures and lifelong productivity.

X. NUTRITIONAL GROWTH RETARDATION

The single most important cause of growth retardation worldwide is poverty-related malnutrition (265). When suboptimal nutrition is continued for prolonged periods of time, stunting of growth occurs as the main clinical picture (266, 267). However, nutritional growth retardation (NGR), as found in pediatric endocrine practices in the United States, is usually not the result of poverty-related malnutrition. NGR and delayed sexual development among suburban upper middle class adolescents is most often a result of self-restrictive nutrient inake (35, 268). Also, poor growth and inadequate nutrition have been found in such systemic problems as chronic inflammatory bowel disease (CIBD) and celiac disease (CD) (269, 270). Children with NGR are generally referred to the pediatric

endocrinologist because of short stature or delayed puberty. Therefore, pediatricians and pediatric endocrinologists need to recognize NGR and become familiar with its causes and treatment.

A. Diagnosis

Pediatric endocrinologists usually evaluate linear growth accurately in the assessment of patients with short stature, but often little consideration is given to body weight progression. Although the importance of evaluating the pattern of stature increments throughout life in the differential diagnosis of short stature cannot be overemphasized, the assessment of the progression of body weight is equally relevant to be able to recognize NGR. Figure 8 illustrates this point.

This 15-year-old boy was referred to the endocrine clinic with short stature of unknown cause. He was healthy in all other respects, and the only presenting symptom was deteriorating linear growth. On examination, both his height of 146.9 cm and weight of 37.6 kg were below the fifth percentile. No body weight deficit for height was evident, and sexual development was de-

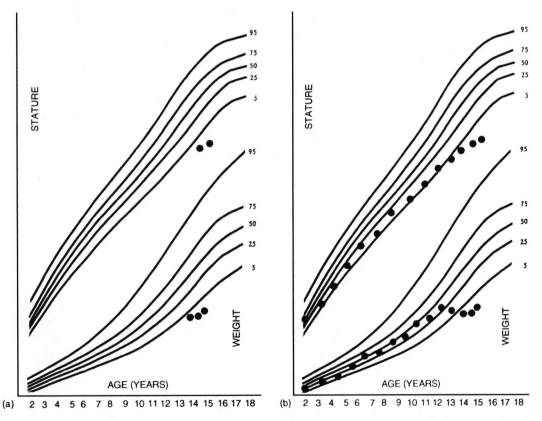

Figure 8 a. The patient was referred because of short stature. Initially, the heights and weights depicted were the only available data. Signs of sexual development were absent. b. Complete growth data for the patient, who began dieting at 12 years of age. (From Ref. 272.)

layed (Tanner stage 1). The initial measurements provided by the referring pediatrician indicated a decreasing growth rate with appropriate weight gain that was progressing just below the fifth percentile (Fig. 8a). However, after additional growth data were obtained and all height and weight records were compiled, a typical picture of nutritionally related growth retardation emerged (Fig. 8b). At 12 years of age, his weight gain ceased, which subsequently resulted in deceleration of linear growth and pubertal delay. Review of his nutritional intake showed that he was consuming only approximately 60% of his estimated energy needs based on age and gender. He was an athletic boy who described a desire to remain slim and avoid obesity, a syndrome that was discovered in 1983 (34).

The Wellcome Trust classification differentiates NGR from other types of malnutrition characterized by wasting and stunting (271). The anthropometric criteria for ND stipulate low weight for age with minimal deficit in weight for height. By these criteria, it may be difficult to differentiate NGR children from those who have familial short stature or constitutional growth delay. Cross-sectional data in these normal children may also demonstrate weights below the mean for age. Only the longitudinal progression of body weight and height can more clearly reveal NGR (272), which may occur even when there is weight-for-height excess (273). In NGR there is a deteriorating linear growth and/or delayed sexual development associated with inadequate weight gain (Fig. 9a,b) (34, 268, 272). This pattern of growth is seen in organic forms of NGR, as in chronic inflammatory bowel disease (274), as well as in nonorganic forms, that is, ingestion of restrictive diets (207). Furthermore, although concern is heightened when weight or height measurements fall below the fifth percentile, deterioration across percentiles of weight and height may also indicate NGR, even when height and weight are above the fifth percentile. With nutritional rehabilitation, catch-up growth is usually achieved.

The analysis of body weight progression may be the most important clue to diagnosis of NGR in patients with short stature (Fig. 9a,b). The calculation of theoretical weights and heights based on previous growth percentiles may be used to compare current anthropometric indices quantitatively with previously established patterns of weight and height progression (Fig. 9a). Theoretical weight is defined as the weight the patient should have had at the time of the examination, if the patient had continued to gain weight along the previously established percentile during the premorbid growth period (272). Body weight for height deficits are not common in NGR, but there is often a body weight deficit for theoretical weight (Fig. 9a,b). In contrast, short patients without NGR, such as those with constitutional growth delay, continue to gain weight along established percentiles and the body weight at the time of assessment is equal to the theoretical body weight (Fig. 9c).

The growth patterns of NGR must also be differentiated from normal variations in growth that may occur as a result of variations in frame size, feeding practices, or constitutional factors that may resemble NGR. Most normal children exhibit minimal deficits or excesses in body weight in proportion to height and grow along established percentiles (275). These constitutional variations in body weight are usually within one or two major percentiles of the height; they represent variations in frame size and do not necessarily reflect over- or undernutrition. The body weight and height increments of a child with constitutional thinness are depicted in Figure 10. Although his body weight was two major percentile lines below the height percentile, representing more than 20% body weight deficit for height, the adolescent grew and developed normally. A body weight deficit for height that remains constant and permits normal growth to proceed along a set percentile cannot be construed as abnormal. In contrast, a fall in growth associated with a poor rate of weight gain may indicate NGR, even without an appreciable body weight deficit for height (Figs. 8b,9a).

The pattern of growth and weight gain in NGR differs from that of children with constitutional growth delay or familial short stature. The latter type of patients grow at constant rates, and their weight progression is also maintained in their respective percentiles after 3 years of age, as described above. In infancy, the pattern of growth and weight gain among constitutional growth delay and NGR may be indistinguishable. However, the children with constitutional growth delay usually recanalize their growth and gain weight and height over time at appropriate levels, and do not exhibit any nutritional intake alterations. There may likewise be confusion at this stage in life between NGR and the breastfed infants. The latter gain at appropriate rates when their length and weight are plotted in specific growth charts for this type of infant as described above.

Patients with nutritional growth retardation do not appear to be wasted, and the biochemical parameters of nutritional status, including serum levels of retinol-binding protein, prealbumin, albumin, transferrin, and triiodothyronine (T3) levels, do not differentiate NGR patients from those with familial or constitutional short stature (276). Other indices of malnutrition, such as the urinary creatine–height index or urinary nitrogen/creatinine ratio, do not usually reflect abnormalities. The reason is that NGR patients have adapted to their suboptimal nutritional intake and they maintain homeostasis by decreasing growth, thereby reaching an equilibrium with preservation of all nutritional markers. We also showed that IGF-1 levels could not differentiate NGR patients from those with familial constitutional short-stature (276). This is in contrast to other studies, which measured IGF levels and their binding proteins (IGFBP) in fasting and in varying levels of nutritional intake, both in rodents and in humans (277–286).

These studies showed that IGF-I is reduced in children with protein–calorie malnutrition and in rats chronically deprived of nutrients. Reductions in IGF-I concentrations were observed in fasted volunteers (281). However, the degree of nutritional insufficiency in NGR is not as severe as that observed in protein–calorie malnutrition or fasting. The amount of nutrient restriction in NGR may impair growth by altering other cellular mechanisms without affecting the serum IGF-I levels. Because the energy restriction is mild, and NGR children consume sufficient dietary protein, IGF-I concentrations may be preserved within a range appropriate for bone age development. Likewise, studies in rats showed IGF-I concentrations to be maintained within normal ranges or to improve rapidly when diets containing 15% protein and 90% of the total energy requirements were consumed (287, 288). Serum IGF BP-3 concentrations are likewise de-

creased in prolonged fasting and/or protein deficiency states (284). However, alterations in IGFPB-3 levels in more subtle forms of suboptimal nutrition like that observed in NGR have not yet been studied.

On the other hand, we reported that NGR patients show decreased activity of erythrocyte Na$^+$, K$^+$-ATPase compared with familial short-stature children (276). This enzyme is involved with the active transport of sugars and amino acids and with cellular thermogenesis. It normally accounts for approximately one-third of the basal energy requirements (289). A diminished energy intake lowers the basal metabolic rate (290) and decreases Na, K-ATPase activity (291). Thus, it may be a good marker of NGR. Because anthropometric parameters may be lacking or inaccurate and biochemical markers may not be sufficient to detect NGR, a more sensitive test is required for diagnosis. Erythrocyte Na$^+$, K$^+$-ATPase activity may offer

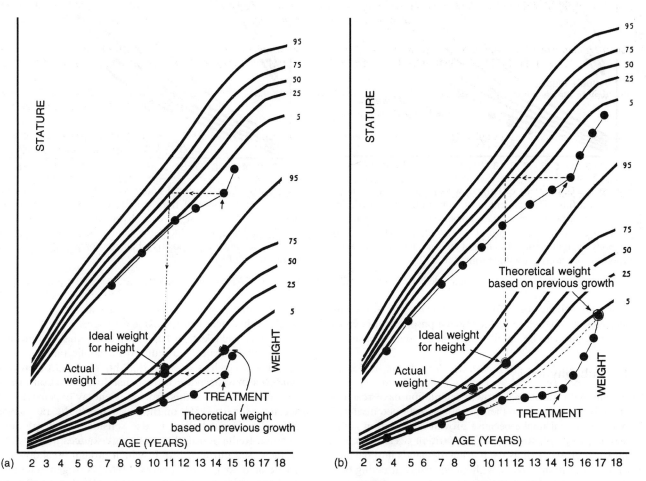

Figure 9 Growth pattern of nutritional dwarfing (a,b) compared with constitutional growth delay (c). a. Body weight gain and height progression decreased after 10 years of age. Extrapolated weight after age 14 years revealed a body weight deficit based on previous growth percentile. However, there was no body weight deficit for height; with nutritional rehabilitation, there was recovery in weight gain and catch-up growth. b. In another patient there is a body weight deficit for height, but the deficit for theoretical weight is more marked. (From Ref. 272.)

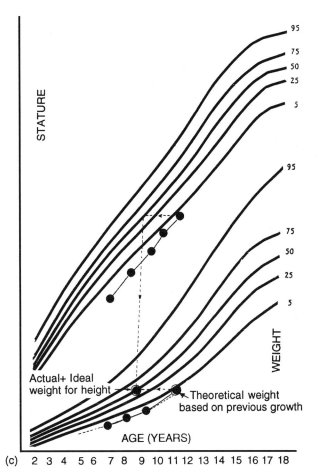

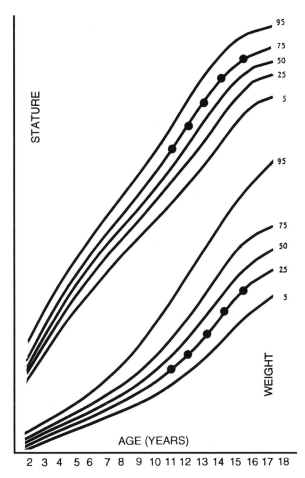

Figure 9 Continued. c. Patient who does not have nutritional dwarfing. This patient, with constitutional growth delay, shows a body weight gain consistently along the lower percentile, with no deviation in growth. Note that there was no body weight deficit for height or for theoretical weight based on previous growth. (From Ref. 272.)

Figure 10 Constitutional underweight for height. Note the constant progression of both height and weight in the same percentiles for at least 4 years. Even though there is body weight deficit for height, there cannot be malnutrition because there must be a positive balance for growth to occur. (From Ref. 272.)

such a diagnostic tool. To date, however, this assay has not been widely available for clinical purposes, it is cumbersome, and can be applied only on a research basis.

B. Pathophysiology

Patients with nutritional growth retardation have reached an equilibrium between their genetic growth potential and their nutritional intake because growth deceleration is the adaptive response to suboptimal nutrition (292, 293). Diminished growth brings the nutrient demands into balance with the nutritional intake without adversely affecting biochemical or functional homeostatic measures. Of course, there are limits to these adaptive possibilities. If nutritional deprivation becomes more severe, acute malnutrition may be superimposed on the chronic state, leading to NGR. In such patients, malnutrition would be reflected by

altered anthropometric measurements, such as weight and skinfold thickness or biochemical indices.

It has been known for many years that diminished energy intake leads to a reduced metabolic rate even before there is a loss of body weight. The rate of protein synthesis may decrease in response to a reduction in energy intake, because this process is energy expensive and accounts for 10–15% of the basal metabolic rate (294, 295). Protein catabolism is also sensitive to energy deprivation. Reduction in dietary energy sources may lead to an increased nitrogen flux in which protein breakdown is accelerated to provide energy (296). Nitrogen retention markedly increases during nutritional rehabilitation of malnourished children (295, 297). In addition, nutritional recovery normalizes the excretion of amino acids (296) and increases the rate of protein synthesis (298). In NGR, the result of the altered rates of protein turnover and nitrogen retention may be the cessation of normal growth as an adaptive response to the decreased intake. In addition to suboptimal energy intake, various mineral and vitamin deficiencies have been implicated in the causes of NGR, as discussed below.

However, it remains controversial whether decreased body size is an advantageous adaptation to a limited food supply or whether adverse health and functional impairments result (292, 293). It has been demonstrated that physical activity is decreased with a 20% decrease in energy consumption (299), but other functional impairments are more difficult to assess. The decreased growth velocity nevertheless constitutes a functional compromise per se, which should be detected and treated as early as possible.

C. Endocrine Adaptation

The changes in the endocrine system in response to undernutrition are adaptive in nature and largely revert to the "normal" state after nutritional status is improved (300). Undernutrition may involve single or multiple micronutrient deficiencies, and thus any one or a combination of deficits could be the primary problem leading to the endocrine alterations. A detailed description of the hormonal alterations in malnutrition has been published elsewhere (272, 300). However, it must be remembered that most studies have been conducted in severely malnourished patients, which may not accurately reflect more subtle forms of suboptimal nutrition leading to NGR. For example, although circulating growth hormone (GH) levels are increased in severe malnutrition, we have shown that pubertal NGR children show decreased overnight growth hormone secretion and prepubertal subjects have an increased growth hormone response to growth-hormone-releasing hormone (GHRH) stimulation (72). An interesting finding is that body composition is a significant determinant of spontaneous growth hormone secretion. In normal children with short stature, the degree of adiposity modifies spontaneous growth hormone secretion and alters the amplitude of growth hormone pulses in puberty and the number of pulses in prepubertal children (72). Indeed, NGR may be easily confused with growth hormone deficiency or neurosecretory dysfunction if the deterioration in weight progression is overlooked (Fig. 11). These patients respond to nutritional rehabilitation and do not require HGH treatment.

D. Causes

1. Organic Causes

Various pathological conditions that lead to decreased nutritional intake or malabsorption may cause NGR (301). Crohn's disease, celiac disease, and cystic fibrosis are some of the relatively more common pathological conditions. However, any alteration that reduces energy intake or excess energy expenditures may lead to decreased growth. Also included are cardiac or renal diseases. When

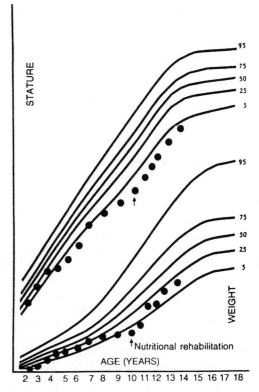

Figure 11 Nutritional dwarfing or growth hormone deficiency? The patient was diagnosed to have GH deficiency at age 10 years because of poor growth. However, because of inadequate weight gain associated with decreased growth increments, therapeutic trial with an adequate diet was tried in lieu of growth hormone. Note the catch-up growth after the initiation of nutritional rehabilitation. (From Ref. 272.)

the dietary intake is disturbed, as in patients with cleft palate or other developmental disabilities, there may also be NGR. The acquired immunodeficiency syndrome and human immunodeficiency virus (HIV) infection were also shown to be associated with short stature and poor growth, that preceded any other manifestation of disease (Chapter 37) (302). However, the growth data in HIV-infected patients clearly indicate NGR because body weight progression failed to proceed at appropriate rates even before any other symptom of the disease was apparent (303). It is very likely that anorexia and decreased intake of nutrients lead to suboptimal nutrition in HIV-infected patients and cause NGR, even before other signs and symptoms of the disease become apparent.

Chronic inflammatory bowel disease (CIBD) is usually associated with impaired linear growth, retarded skeletal maturation, and delayed sexual development. This problem is estimated to occur in 5–10% of pediatric patients with ulcerative colitis and 25% of patients with Crohn's disease (304, 305). Growth failure may be the first indication of CIBD and may precede disease-related symptoms (306). Therefore, the diagnosis of CIBD should always be considered in children who cease to grow adequately, even in the absence of gastrointestinal complaints. Although the pathogenesis is influenced by age at onset, duration of disease, disease activity, and medication intake, suboptimal nutrition is now recognized as the primary factor in growth failure in Crohn's disease (274). Multifactorial nutritional alterations include a decreased nutrient intake, impaired absorption of nutrients, specific nutrient deficiencies, and enhanced protein losses through the gastrointestinal tract. Decreased energy intake in children with CIBD has been associated with anorexia and the early satiety and discomfort that accompany eating.

The total daily calorie intake of CIBD patients usually is not above the recommended dietary allowance (RDA) for height age (306). Multiple studies have documented catch-up growth when adequate energy is provided (304, 305). Various forms of nutritional support (parenteral, elemental, or complex diet) have been employed, often resulting in decreased disease activity and improved growth (307–309). In addition to energy and protein deficits, other nutritional alterations may affect growth in patients with CIBD. Iron deficiency, particularly when there is blood loss through the stools, may compound anorexia and poor growth (310). These patients also may have magnesium deficiency (311) and zinc deficiency (312). It has been shown that large enteric losses of zinc occur in CIBD patients who have diarrhea and small bowel disease. In addition, zinc absorption may be reduced. Therefore, nutritional rehabilitation is essential for the treatment of CIBD patients. This may reverse the growth retardation and even improve the disease itself (313–314).

Growth failure in association with gastrointestinal symptoms is common in children with active CD. It has been shown that up to 55% of patients with CD were below the third percentile for height and up to 60% were below the same percentile for weight. Failure to thrive was present in 25% of children with celiac disease at the time of diagnosis (315, 316). However, several investigators have reported short stature as the sole manifestation of CD (270, 315–317). These asymptomatic patients were considered to have so-called occult celiac disease. The prevalence of asymptomatic CD is highly variable. It was reported to be present in up to 8% in some studies (270, 316), whereas in others it was higher: 24 and 48% (315, 317). This may be the result of geographic differences in the prevalence of the disease and/or the level of suspicion in recognizing these patients. The incidence of CD in the western New York area, estimated by serum IgA–endomysial antibody, has been reported to be 1:3752 (318).

The recognition of occult CD is dependent on the alertness of the clinician to consider this entity as a cause of short stature. Many asymptomatic CD patients have a history of diarrhea at an early age or have iron deficiency. They may also have other alterations when studied (e.g.,

increased stool fat, antigliadin, and antiendomysial antibodies, low serum folate and ferritin levels) that point to the possibility of CD (319–321) as the cause of short stature. Although various methods may be used for screening purposes, these are not diagnostic of CD (315, 317, 318). Therefore, a small bowel biopsy is the "gold standard" for the diagnosis of this disease, and should be performed in every short child showing NGR from unidentified causes. A history of diarrhea during the first year of life and/or the presence of iron deficiency in a short patient should also warrant consideration of CD and therefore of a small bowel biopsy. The diagnosis of CD should be confirmed by documentation of catch-up growth with weight and height gain after institution of a gluten-free diet, which is the only treatment available for the disease. Long-term studies of children with CD suggest that those who do not comply with the diet have significantly lower mean heights and weights and a greater abnormality of the intestinal mucosa than those who are compliant.

2. Nonorganic Causes

The prevalence of nonorganic NGR leading to malnutrition and poor growth in affluent communities is unknown. Only those patients whose height is markedly impaired have been recognized thus far. However, suboptimal nutritional intake may result in a fall in height within the normal percentiles that may elude medical attention. In a survey of 1017 high school students from a middle-class parochial school, a high incidence of low-weight students was reported. More than 25% of these students weighed less than 90% of their ideal body weight for height, but only 1.8% of them had growth patterns suggestive of NGR (275). In a pediatric endocrine clinic in a referral center in the same geographic area, we detected more than 300 patients with NGR.

The most common causes (73%) of nutritional alterations that resulted in NGR and delayed sexual development among adolescents referred to us were nonorganic. There were patients in whom a specific fear or health belief was identified as the cause of the poor nutritional intake leading to short stature (207, 226, 268, 272). A fear of obesity or a fear of hypercholesterolemia was specifically verbalized by some. However, most patients with nonorganic NGR expressed preoccupations that involved similar issues of body weight and cholesterol and concern with a so-called healthy dietary intake. They avoided excess dietary fat and cholesterol and what they termed junk food (272). Regardless of the reason for the inadequate nutritional intake, the result in these children was NGR.

These patients with inadequate dietary intake appeared to be free of severe psychopathology. They did not meet the inclusion criteria for severe eating disorders, such as anorexia nervosa or bulimia nervosa. Moreover, in a controlled, double-blind, prospective study, it was demonstrated that these children did not have behavioral or psychosocial deviations and did not differ from a group of normal or short-stature children (322). Thus, we concluded that the dietary habits that led to NGR were a result of the prevalence of current health beliefs and preoccupation with slimness, weight control, and the search for longevity through the intake of idealized diets (35, 205, 207).

A recent national survey found that 31% of fifth grade girls have dieted (323). Abramovitz and Birch explored 5-year-old girls' ideas, concepts, and beliefs about dieting (324). They found that 34–64% of the girls had ideas about dieting and weight loss and understood the link with body shape. Girls' knowledge about how people diet is inappropriate. These included descriptions of modified eating behaviors, such as drinking diet shakes, sodas, eating more fruits and vegetables, special foods, and restrictive eating behaviors. Mothers seem to be modeling both health-promoting and health-compromising eating behaviors to their daughters. Girls whose mothers reported current or recent food restrictions were more than twice as likely to have ideas about dieting (324). Another factor found to influence girls' ideas, concepts, and beliefs about dieting is family history of overweight. The media was also mentioned by 55% if the children as a source of dieting ideas (325).

Neumark recently published results from a national survey examining weight-related behaviors among 6728 American adolescents in grades 5–12 (323). Almost half of the female population (45%) and 20% of male adolescents reported dieting. Older female adolescents were significantly more likely to diet than younger ones. Dieting was reported by 31% of 5th graders and increased consistently to 62% among 12th graders. The largest increase was among female adolescents between the 8th (40%) and 9th (53%) grades. Thirteen percent of the girls and 7% of the boys reported disordered eating behaviors. In another study, Neumark found that in 3832 adults and 459 adolescents from four regions of the United States, a high percentage of them reported weight control behaviors. Based on gender, weight control behaviors were found in 56.7% of adult women, 50.3% of adult men, 44.0% of adolescent girls, and 36.8% of adolescent boys (326).

Moses et al. showed that high school adolescents in an affluent suburban location were dieting at a very high rate (327). Forty-one percent of the adolescents were dieting on the day of the survey. Sixty-seven percent of all the adolescents had made on their own important dietary efforts during the past 4–8 weeks. Dieting occurred in normal-weight and underweight students. About 30% of dieters were among the underweight and normal weight for height. However, the proportion of the overweight students who were dieting was relatively low: 50–60%.

Children not only diet but also worry about their body appearance and distorted proportions about weight. More and more children are concerned and dissatisfied with their body image. Studies have shown that 55% of girls and 35% of boys in grades 3–6 want to be thinner (328).

The Children's Version of the Eating Attitude Test showed a negative correlation with children's BMI. It was found that 4.8% of them had scores suggestive of anorexia nervosa. Stice et al. found that eating disturbances that emerged during childhood led to inhibited and secretive eating, overeating, and vomiting. Maternal body dissatisfaction, internalization of the thin ideal, dieting, bulimic symptoms, and maternal and paternal body mass prospectively predicted the emergence of childhood eating disturbances. Infant feeding behavior and body mass during the first month of life also predicted the emergence of eating disturbances (329).

Parents who worry about their children becoming overweight may set the stage for a vicious cycle. Johnson and Birch found those parents who control what and how much their children eat may impede energy self-regulation and put these children at a higher risk for being overweight (330). Furthermore, the Framingham Children's Study showed that children whose parents had high degrees of dietary control had greater increases in body fatness than did children whose parents had the lowest levels of dietary restraint and noninhibition (331).

A distorted perception of ideal body weight, manifested as below appropriate body weight for height, is very prevalent among high school students. Adolescents often know what their ideal weight should be, but some prefer to be 10% less than their ideal weight for their height (327). Health-compromising behaviors and the fear of obesity may have detrimental consequences in children. Inappropriate nutrient intake may lead to NGR, failure to thrive, and various other nutritional problems (326).

There is also a high prevalence of extreme measures taken by high school students to avoid obesity throughout the country (327, 332, 333). In addition to dieting, they may have inappropriate eating habits and purging behaviors. These data indicate just how powerful and important it is for adolescents to achieve an ideal slim and trim figure. Young persons, even when they are not overweight, diet to avoid obesity at a time when they are still growing and developing (35, 327, 332, 333). Regardless of their physical needs, they strive to reach a thin ideal, consequently developing nutritional short stature (35, 327). In addition to growth retardation, other potential medical complications may be associated with excessive dieting, binging, and purging: electrolyte disturbances, dental enamel erosion, acute gastric dilation, esophagitis, enlargement of the parotid gland, aspiration pneumonitis, and pancreatitis.

However, it must be kept in mind that the population at large is also quite concerned about cholesterol and preoccupied with diets to lower cholesterol levels (334). These concerns are also prevalent among children (335). The medical profession and the American Academy of Pediatrics have also recommended a low-fat–low-cholesterol diet for the population at large in an effort to prevent adult-onset diseases. However, there are potential harmful consequences of feeding children with adult diets (334). A low-fat–low-cholesterol intake may lead to nutritional short stature (35, 335) and nutrient deficits (272). A recent study confirmed our observations demonstrating that children on low-fat, low-cholesterol diets can easily ingest inadequate nutrient intake (336).

Careful assessment of weight and height progression will clearly identify children who are not gaining weight and growing appropriately (204, 268, 301, 327). An awareness by health care providers and pediatric endocrinologists of the prevailing eating attitudes and behaviors among adolescents in the population of their practice's area may help detect the adolescent at risk for more serious problems. Simple tests and questionnaires may help to identify the patient with eating disorders (337). The 24 h dietary recall may identify short-stature patients who have inappropriate dietary intake. Patients with obesity constitute another group of children who often diet. Although these children usually do not present to the pediatric endocrinologist because of poor growth, when obesity occurs in association with short stature there may be concerns about their health. A variety of endocrine disorders may affect obese children who do not grow well (Chapter 28). Diet-related growth failure may be uncovered by a careful history, thereby eliminating other concerns. Weight loss is associated with a negative balance that does not allow growth in height even if the child is obese (338). Therefore, during the treatment of obesity in children, allowances must always be made to maintain a balance between the need of a patient to lose weight and the nutritional requirements that allow growth in height.

Nutritional rehabilitation for NGR of nonorganic origin requires providing the patient with adequate caloric and nutrient intake for the restoration of previous growth patterns. Initially, estimation of energy requirements should be based on the age- and gender-specific RDA using the patient's theoretical weight. Adequate intake of protein usually accompanies sufficient caloric intake, but care should be taken that micronutrient intakes meet the RDA. If results of biochemical tests reveal specific deficiencies, such as iron or zinc, these nutrients should be supplemented. Some patients may not be willing or able to consume a completely balanced diet and may require a multivitamin and mineral supplement. A careful diet history can elucidate food preferences and eating patterns that can be used to devise an appropriate dietary plan. Our experience has been to offer general dietary suggestions rather than to prescribe a specific diet. Frequent follow-up visits provide an opportunity to revise and update dietary recommendations and to obtain weight and height measurements.

Although the appropriate diet can be easily determined, successful intervention requires a change in dietary patterns and possibly health beliefs as well. Increasing the caloric density of the child's diet often involves raising the dietary fat content to at least 30–35% of calories. The increase in fat consumption may concern both the child and the parent, especially in patients who fail to grow because of dieting. The assurance that an appropriate nutritional intake will result in normal growth, without producing obesity, is necessary supportive therapy. This is of particular concern in the initial stages of the treatment, when weight increases rapidly, whereas no noticeable effect on height is observed.

3. Vitamin and Mineral Deficiencies

Regardless of NGR's cause, patients may present with multiple vitamin and mineral deficiencies that contribute to growth failure (272, 335). There may be generalized malnutrition with multiple macro- and micronutrient deficits, or there may be more specific nutritional alterations, as discussed below.

Vitamin A is an important nutrient for gene expression of growth hormone. Studies have shown an improvement in linear growth in some subsets of supplemented children (339). A study in Java found that children who consumed small frequent amounts of vitamin A in fortified monosodium glutamate experienced greater height gain but similar weight gain to control children (340). In the Sudan, dietary vitamin A intake, but not vitamin A supplements given once every 6 months, was positively associated with greater weight gain and with linear growth of children (341, 342). This suggests that small daily supplements of vitamin A may be beneficial over and above the benefits imparted by periodic doses of vitamin A. However, in other intervention studies, vitamin A supplements had no effect on either linear growth or weight gain even when other vitamins and nutrients in addition to vitamin A were supplemented. In a large placebo-controlled study in Tamil Nadu, India, children were visited every week and given a small dose of vitamin A or a placebo. In spite of a large protective effect against mortality, the supplements had no effect on growth (343).

Multiple postulated mechanisms link other vitamin deficiencies with poor growth. These include iron, folate, and/or B_{12} deficiency, which lead to poor oxygen delivery to tissues, and to multiple metabolic pathways that alter protein synthesis leading to impaired growth. Furthermore, there may be anorexia and inappropriate intake in iron deficiency. Iron supplementation in school children demonstrated beneficial effects on appetite, growth, and anemia (344, 345). Vitamin-D-deficiency rickets can, of course, present with growth failure and osteomalacia.

In several prospective cohort studies in developing countries, the onset of stunting coincided with dietary deficiencies of several micronutrients, including iron, zinc and iodine (346). Height deficits were associated with chronic deficits in energy and protein, as well as suboptimal zinc levels. Multiple micronutrient deficiencies may explain why supplementary feeding programs that aimed at only increasing energy and protein intake resulted in limited physical growth (347).

Growth retardation caused by zinc deficiency in humans was first reported by Prasaad et al. in 1963. The patients had remarkably short stature and hypogonadism. They were shown to have zinc deficiency documented by decreased zinc concentrations in plasma, erythrocytes, and hair. Studies with ^{65}Zn revealed that plasma zinc turnover was greater, the 24 h exchangeable pool was smaller, and the excretion of ^{65}Zn in stool and urine was less in the growth-retarded subjects than in the controls (348). Further studies showed that the rate of growth was greater in patients who received supplemental zinc than in those receiving only an adequate animal protein diet (349). Since then, many cases of marginal or moderate growth impairment in children with zinc deficiency as a consequence of inadequate zinc intake have been reported from various parts of the world (350, 351). It appears that zinc deficiency is prevalent throughout the world in both developed and developing countries. Favier indicated that, depending on the country, 5–30% of children had moderate zinc deficiency, responsible for small-for-age height (352). Those reports showed positive effects of oral zinc supplementation on growth velocity in children with zinc deficiency (349–352).

It is also well known that zinc deficiency in pregnant women causes fetal growth retardation. Kirksey et al. revealed a significant correlation between maternal plasma zinc concentrations measured at midpregnancy and birth weight (353). Neggers et al. reported that the prevalence of low birth weight (LBW) infants was significantly higher (eight times) among women with serum zinc concentrations in the lowest quartile in early pregnancy, independent of other risk factors (354). However, the effects of zinc supplementation in pregnancy are not clear. It is now speculated that zinc supplementation during pregnancy might be beneficial only in populations that are zinc deficient and at high risk of poor fetal growth (355).

Marginal zinc deficiency seems to be prevalent in infancy. Michaelsen et al. examined zinc intake and status in healthy term infants from birth to 12 months of age in Denmark, and found suboptimal zinc status in many subjects during late infancy. They also reported that serum zinc level at 9 months was positively associated with growth velocity during the period from 6 to 9 months (356).

The zinc status in short-stature patients with normal GH secretion was tested by body zinc clearance studies to detect the marginal zinc nutriture, and to evaluate the effects of oral zinc supplementation (357). This Japanese study indicated that about 60% of short children had marginal zinc deficiency. Oral zinc supplementation was effective on height gain in short boys with marginal zinc deficiency, but not in girls. There was also a significant correlation between the body zinc clearance values and percentage increases in the growth velocity after oral zinc supplementation, indicating that oral zinc supplementation was most effective on height gain (357). The reason for

such a high incidence of marginal zinc deficiency in Japanese short children may be mainly the recent prevalence of precooked food, snacks, and convenience foods in their diets. In 1993 Nakamura et al. conducted an age-matched control study showing that oral zinc supplementation was effective in improving the growth rate in short children with marginal zinc deficiency. They reported that oral zinc supplementation induced increases of serum IGF-1, osetocalcin, and alkaline phosphatase activity (358).

There have been a few reports on the relationship between zinc deficiency and GH secretory insufficiency. Nishi et al. described a 13-year-old Japanese boy with growth disturbance who had partial GH deficiency due to chronic mild zinc deficiency. His diet was low in animal protein and consisted primarily of rice and vegetables, because he disliked meats, fish, eggs, and dairy products that were rich sources of zinc. His plasma zinc level and GH responses to the pharmacological stimulation tests were low. After 3 months of oral zinc supplementation, however, his growth velocity improved without GH replacement therapy, and his plasma zinc levels and GH responses to those tests increased to the normal range (359).

The mechanism by which zinc deficiency causes growth disturbance has been controversial. Zinc is required for activities of more than 300 enzymes (zinc metalloenzymes), in which zinc is located at the active site, including DNA polymerase, RNA polymerase, and thymidine kinase. Because these enzymes are important for nucleic acid and protein synthesis and cell division, zinc may be essential for growth. Furthermore, several hundred zinc-containing nucleoproteins are probably involved in gene expression of various proteins (349, 360).

Zinc deficiency may adversely affect GH production and/or secretion (359). Since zinc has an important role in protein synthesis, IGF-1 synthesis can be impaired by zinc deficiency. Ninh et al. reported that low IGF-1 levels in zinc-deprived rats were closely associated with decreased hepatic IGF-1 gene expression and with a diminuation of liver GH receptors and circulating GH-binding protein (GHBP). They also suggested that decreased hepatic GH receptors and/or GHBP concentrations might be responsible for the decline of circulating IGF-1 in zinc-deficient animals (361).

The presence of a large amount of zinc in bone tissue suggests that zinc plays an important role in the development of skeletal systems (362). Retardation of bone growth is a common finding in various conditions associated with zinc deficiency. Zinc has a stimulatory effect on bone formation and mineralization (363). Zinc is required for alkaline phosphatase activity and the enzyme is mainly produced by osteoblasts whose major function is to provide calcium deposition in bone diaphysis. The administration of vitamin D3 or zinc produced a significant increase in bone alkaline phosphatase activity and DNA content was synergistically enhanced by the simultaneous treatment with zinc (363). The receptors for 1,25-dihydroxyvitamin D3 were shown to have two zinc fingers at the site of interaction with DNA (364). One possible function of zinc is to potentiate the interaction of the 1,25-dihydroxyvitamin D_3 receptor complex with DNA at that site. Zinc also directly activates aminoacyl-tRNA synthetase in osteoblasts, and it stimulates cellular protein synthesis. Moreover, zinc has an inhibitory effect on osteoclastic bone resorption by suppressing osteoclast-like cell formation from marrow cells (362).

Zinc deficiency should be considered as a causative factor in some children with unexplained short stature. Oral zinc supplementation should be considered as the growth-promoting therapy for children with short stature once the status of their zinc nutrition is established. Not all zinc intervention studies have found improved growth patterns in subjects receiving supplements. Rosado et al. performed a randomized clinical trial among young Mexican children, comparing daily doses of iron, zinc, both, or placebo (365). Others have also reported no effect of zinc supplementation on growth rates (366, 367), and some have hypothesized that the presence of multiple micronutrient deficiencies may be at least in part to blame (368, 369). Prentice reported that zinc supplementation failed to show beneficial effects on height gain in Guatemalan children, although the relatively short supplementation period of 25 weeks might have been insufficient to detect subtle changes in growth velocity (370). A systematic review of 25 clinical trials that evaluated the impact of zinc supplementation on growth found a significant pooled effect of an increment of 0.22 standard deviations (SD) on height and 0.26 SD on weight (371). The greatest impact of zinc supplementation was found in stunted children (in whom an increase of 0.49 SD was found in height), and in those with low initial zinc concentrations.

XI. LABORATORY AIDS IN DIFFERENTIATING SHORT STATURE

Any patient who falls below the third percentile in height and/or has decreased growth rates (falling across the major percentiles) should receive a complete diagnostic evaluation. Because there are multiple causes of short stature and growth retardation, laboratory investigation should be geared toward confirming or ruling out the differential diagnoses based on information obtained from history and physical examination. It is important to assess, in addition to the growth rates: history of chronic illness and medications, midparental and target height, birth size, growth pattern, nutritional state, pubertal stage, body segment proportions, bone age, and predicted adult height. The following simple laboratory screening tests may be performed: urinalysis, urine metabolic screening, hemoglobin, hematocrit and ferritin levels, measurement of sedimentation rate and creatine phosphokinase (CPK), ve-

nous blood gases with simultaneous urine pH, liver and kidney function tests, and antigliadin and antiendomyacil antibodies.

A karyotype is imperative in every girl with short stature, even in the absence of the stigmata of Turner syndrome. Children who demonstrate skeletal abnormalities on physical examination deserve evaluation for metabolic bone disease, such as mucopolysaccharidosis, mucolipidosis, and gangliosidosis (Chapter 4). In addition, skeletal abnormalities should be looked for in accordance with body proportion alterations detected on physical examination (i.e., hypochrondroplasia) (46, 58, 95).

Endocrine causes of short stature and/or poor growth may be determined by evaluating thyroid function and assessing the hypothalamic–pituitary axis (Chapters 2, 3, and 38). Examination of the eye grounds and visual fields should be done, but a magnetic resonance imaging (MRI) scan may be necessary if hypopituitarism is considered. A thorough nutritional assessment should be made if there is a growth pattern of NGR. If zinc deficiency is suspected, serum zinc levels may be obtained, but they are usually not sufficient to establish the diagnosis. Other tests may be necessary before treatment is instituted as described above.

A number of tests to assess growth hormone status have been devised using various provocative tests: insulin, L-dopa, arginine, clonidine, and other agents (372). Growth hormone is secreted at intervals and random growth hormone measurements are useless. Estrogen and/or androgen priming before provocative testing is also useful in Tanner I or Tanner II children to differentiate between GH deficiency and constitutional growth delay (373, 374). A frequent test is to measure GH after exercise (375). Pituitary function may also be evaluated comprehensively using a combined hormonal stimulation test (376). This utilizes sequentially administered insulin or arginine or L-dopa, thyrotropin-releasing hormone, and gonadotropin-releasing hormone. In addition, deficiency of GHRH may be ruled out by giving human pituitary GHRH and evaluating the patient's growth hormone response. So-called neurosecretory growth hormone dysfunction can be determined by performing an overnight growth hormone study and assessing growth hormone pulsatile secretions under physiological conditions, such as sleep.

The indications for this test are for those patients who may demonstrate a normal growth hormone response to pharmacological stimuli, but may not be able to secrete growth hormone under physiological conditions (377–379). However, there is no completely reliable test for diagnosing or excluding growth hormone deficiency in short children (Chapters 2, 3). IGF-I and IGFBP levels are decreased in growth hormone deficiency and may help in differentiating short children with growth hormone deficiency (380–383). However, these tests are not useful in NGR or younger patients. Measuring levels of GHBP or

IGFBP may also help differentiate the different conditions, as well as IGF levels and their response to exogenous growth hormone administration. Details of the foregoing tests and procedures are described in Chapter 41. However, it should be kept in mind that growth measurements over time are better guidelines than many of the tests mentioned above. Indeed without the clinical growth data, the results of the tests are hard to interpret.

XII. FINAL CONSIDERATIONS

Short children and their parents face a number of specific psychosocial problems. These problems are frequently associated with the developmental stage of (384) the child's life. The parents frequently have difficulty in accepting the child's height and in treating the child according to age level. By 7 or 8 years of age the child usually has become acutely aware of his or her short stature. The teenage years are much more difficult for the short-stature child than for the child of normal or mildly abnormal height. The problems of short stature are often compounded by lack of sexual development and withdrawal from heterosexual social activities or by other transition periods, such as moving to a new school or community. Despite these developmental problems, the short individual frequently makes an adequate adjustment to life as an adult (384).

Other issues transcend the purely developmental aspects of short stature, such as the general personality mechanisms of the small child and his or her parents. Of importance are the school achievements of such children and the specific techniques they develop in coping more effectively with their environment. One of the most important problems of short people is being treated in an infantile manner, appropriate for their size, but not for their age. Some short people respond to being treated as a younger child by behaving immaturely (Peter Pan reaction). Others rebel against being pampered and sometimes develop various neurotic and psychosomatic symptoms, including denial, withdrawal, phobias, and compensatory fantasies. Still others find a more satisfactory solution in the reaction of "mascotism."

Frankness (diplomatic rather than brutal) is desirable in counseling short and dwarfed people about their situation in life. They are then able to plan the future realistically, to discuss the taboos that beset them, and to perfect techniques in dealing with silly comments about their size and age. Emotional deprivation and neglect may cause a certain type of dwarfism (385). This may be the primary problem and, when resolved, growth occurs. Short stature is not typically associated with intellectual defect (386). Dwarfed people may expect to be employed and, under some circumstances, graduate from college. Short people can meet one another by joining such organizations as Little People of America, P.O. Box 622, San Bruno, CA 94006; the Human Growth Foundation, Inc., 4607 David-son Drive, Cherry Lane, MD 20815; or Magic, 1327 North Harlem Drive, Oak Park, IL 60302. They may legitimately hope for romance, marriage, and a successful sex life and should consider help regarding their height through the use of footwear that may increase their size without other major procedures or therapies (Elevators, Richlee Shoe Co., P.O. Box 3566, Frederick, MD 21705, Tel 1-800-290TALL).

ACKNOWLEDGMENT

This work was supported in part by Pediatric Sunshine Academics.

REFERENCES

1. Kranzler JH, Rosenbloom AL, Proctor B, Diamond F, Watson M. Is short stature a handicap? A comparison of the psychosocial functioning of referred and non-referred children with normal stature and children with short stature. J Pediatr 2000; 136:96–102.
2. Sandberg DE, Brook AE, Campos SP. Short stature: a psychosocial burden requiring growth hormone therapy? Pediatrics 1994; 94:832–840.
3. Sanberg DE. The quality-of-life benefits of growth hormone-increased final height: what do we know? Endocrinologist 2001; 11:8S–14S.
4. Bort LLE, Mul D. Growth hormone in short children: beyond medicine? Acta Paediatr 2001; 90:69–73.
5. Macklin R. Growth hormone in short children: medically appropriate treatment. Acta Paediatr 2001, 90:5–6.
6. Roberts SB, Dallal GE. The new childhood growth charts. Nutr Rev 2001; 59:31–36.
7. Haschke F, van't Hof MA, the Euro-Growth Study Group. Euro-Growth references for length, weight and body circumferences. J Pediatr Gastroenterol Nutr 2000; 31 (suppl 1) S14–38.
8. Van't Hof MA, Haschke F, the Euro-Growth Study Group. Euro-Growth References for body mass index (BMI) and weight for length (WfL). J Pediatr Gastroenterol Nutr 2000; 31 (suppl 1) S48–59.
9. Van't Hof MA, Haschke F, Darvay S, the Euro-Growth Study Group. Euro-Growth references on increments in length, weight, head- and arm circumference during the first three years of life. J Pediatr Gastroenterol Nutr 2000; 31 (suppl 1) S39–47.
10. Freeman V, van't Hof MA, Haschke F, the Euro-Growth-Study Group. Patterns of milk and food intake during the first three years of life. The Euro-Growth Study. J Pediatr Gastroenterol Nutr 2000; 31 (suppl 1) S76–85.
11. Haschke F, van't Hof MA, the Euro-Growth-Study Group. Euro-Growth references for breastfed boys and girls: the influence of breastfeeding and solids on growth until 36 months of age. J Pediatr Gastroenterol Nutr 2000; 31 (suppl 1) S60–71.
12. Lacey KA, Parkin JM. Causes of short stature. A community study of children in Newcastle-upon-Tyne. Lancet 1974; 1:42–45.
13. Lifshitz F, Cervantes C. Short stature. In: Lifshitz F, ed. Pediatric Endocrinology, 3rd ed. New York: Marcel Dekker, 1996:1–18.

14. Rudman D, Kutner MH, Blackstone RD, Cushman RA, Bain RP, Patterson JH. Children with normal variance short stature: treatment with human growth hormone for six months. N Engl J Med 1981; 305:123–131.

15. Rekers-Mombarg LT, Karel GH, Massa GG, Wit JM. Influence of growth hormone treatment on pubertal timing and pubertal growth in children with idiopathic short stature. J Pediatr Endocrinol Metab 1999; 12:611–616.

16. Hebert PR, Rich-Edwards JW, Manson JE, Ridker PM, Cook NR, O'Connor GT, Buring JE, Hennekens CH. Height and incidence of cardiovascular disease in male physicians. Circulation 1993; 88:1437–1443.

17. Kannam JP, Levy D, Larson M, Wilson PW. Short stature and risk for mortality and cardiovascular disease events. The Framingham Heart Study. Circulation 1994; 90: 2241–2247.

18. Krahn AD, Manfreda J, Tate RB, Mathewson FA, Cuddy TE. Evidence that height is an independent risk factor for coronary artery disease (the Manitoba Follow-Up Study). Am J Cardiology 1994; 74:398–399.

19. Tanner JM, Whitehouse RH, Marubini E, Resele L. The adolescent growth spurt of the boys and girls of the Harpenden Growth Study. Ann Hum Biol 1976; 3:109–126.

20. Roche AF, Guo S, Baumgartner RM, Falls RA. The measurement of stature. Am J Clin Nutr 1988; 47:922.

21. Taranger J, Bruning B, Claesson I, et al. Skeletal development from birth to 7 years. In: Taranger J, ed. The Somatic Development of Children in a Swedish Urban Community. Acta Paediatr Scand (Suppl) 1967; 258:98–108.

22. Tuddenham RD, Snyder MM. Physical growth of California boys and girls from birth to eighteen years. Univ Calif Pubi Child Dev 1954; 1:183–364.

23. Horton WA, Rotter JI, Rimoin DL. Standard growth curve for achondroplasia. J Pediatr 1978; 93:435–438.

24. Babson SO, Benda GI. Growth graphs for the clinical assessment of infants of varying gestational age. J Pediatr 1976; 89:814–820.

25. Cronk C, Crocker AC, Pueschel SM, Shea AM, Zackai E, Pickens G, Reed RB. Growth charts for children with Down syndrome: 1 month to 18 years of age. Pediatrics 1988; 81:102–110.

26. Lyon AJ, Preece MA, Grant DB. Growth curve for girls with Turner syndrome. Arch Dis Child 1985; 60:932–935.

27. Horton WA, Hall JG, Scott CI. Growth curves for diastrophic dysplasia, spondyloepiphyseal dysplasia and pseudoachondroplasia. Am J Dis Child 1982; 136:316–319.

28. Witt DR, Keena BA, Hall JG, Allanson JE. Growth curves for height in Noonan syndrome. Clin Genet 1986; 30:150–153.

29. Brook GGD, Hindmarsh PC, Healy MJR. A better way to detect growth failure. Br Med J 1986; 293:1186.

30. Lampl M, Veldhuis JD, Johnson ML. Saltation and stasis: a model of human growth. Science 1992; 258:801–803.

31. Tanner JM, Whitehouse RH, Takaishi M. Standards from birth to maturity for height, weight, height velocity and weight velocity in British children. Arch Dis Child 1966; 41:613–616.

32. Tanner JM, Whitehouse RH. Clinical longitudinal standard for height, weight, height velocity, weight velocity and stages of puberty. Arch Dis Child 1976; 51:170–171.

33. Guo S, Roche AF, Fomon SJ, Nelson SE, Chumlea WC, Rogers RR, Baumgartner RN, Ziegler EE, Siervogel RM.

Reference data on gains in weight and length during the first two years of life. J Pediatr 1991; 119:355–362.

34. Pugliese MT, Lifshitz F, Grad G, Fort P, Marks-Katz M. Fear of obesity: a cause of short stature and delayed puberty. N Engl J Med 1983; 309:513–518.

35. Lifshitz F, Moses N, Cervantes C, Ginsberg L. Nutritional dwarfing in adolescence. Semin Adolesc Med 1987; 3: 255–266.

36. Desai ID, Garcia-Tavares ML, Dutra de Oliveira BS, Desai MI, Romero LS, Vichi FL, Duarte FA, Dutra de Oliveira JE. Anthropometric and cycloergometric assessment of the nutritional status of the children of agricultural migrant workers in Southern Brazil. Am J Clin Nutr 1981; 34:1925–1934.

37. Trowbridge FL, Marks JS, Lopez de Romana G, Madrid S, Boutton TW, Klein PD. Body composition of Peruvian children with short stature and high weight-for-height. Implications for the interpretation of weight-for-height as an indicator of nutritional status. Am J Clin Nutr 1987; 46:411–418.

38. Tanner JM, Whitchouse RH, Marshall WA, Carter BS. Prediction of adult height from height, bone age, and occurrence of menarche, at ages 4 to 16, with allowance for midparent height. Arch Dis Child 1975; 50:14–26.

39. Luo ZC, Albertsson-Wikland K, Karlberg J. Target height as predicted by parental heights in a population-based study. Pediatr Res 1998; 44:563–571.

40. Bayley N, Pinneau SR. Tables for predicting adult height from skeletal age: revised for use with the Greulich-Pyle hand standard. J Pediatr 1952; 40:423–441.

41. Tanner JM, Whitehouse RH, Cameron N, Marshall WA, Healy MJR, Goldstein H. Assessment of Skeletal Maturity and Prediction of Adult Height (TW$_2$ Method). London: Academic Press, 1983.

42. Roche AF, Wainer H, Thissen D. The RWT method for the prediction of adult stature. Pediatrics 1975; 56:1026–1033.

43. Lenko HL. Prediction of adult height with various methods in Finnish children. Acta Pediatr Scand 1979; 68:85–92.

44. Greulich WW, Pyle SI. Radiographic Atlas of Skeletal Development of the Hand and Wrist. Stanford, CA: Stanford University Press, 1950.

45. Roche AF, Davila GH, Leyman SL. A comparison between Greulich-Pyle and Tanner-Whitehouse assessment of skeletal maturity. Radiology 1971; 98:273–280.

46. Hall JG, Froster-Iskenius U, Allanson J. Handbook of Normal Physical Measurements. Oxford, UK: Oxford University Press, 1989.

47. Albanses A, Stanhope R. Does constitutional delayed puberty cause segmental disproportion and short stature? Eur J Pediatr 1993; 152:293–296.

48. Cervantes C, Lifshitz F. Tubular bone alterations in familial short stature. Hum Biol 1988; 60:151–165.

49. Beresma D. Birth Defects Compendium, 2nd ed. The National Foundation March of Dimes. New York: Alan R. Liss, 1982:151–152.

50. Archibald RM, Findy N, DeVito F. Endocrine significance of short metacarpals. J Clin Endocrinol Metab 1959; 19:1312–1322.

51. Van der Werf Ten Rosch JJ. The syndrome of brachymetacarpal dwarfism ("pseudopseudohypoparathyroidism") with and without gonadal dysgenesis. Lancet 1959; 1:69–71.

52. Cervantes CD, Lifshitz F, Levenbrown J. Radiologic an-

thropometry of the hand in patients with familial short stature. Pediatr Radiol 1988; 18:210–214.

53. Musebeck J, Mohnike K, Beye P, Tonnies H, Neitzel H, Schnabel D, Gruters A, Wieacker PF, Stumm M. Short stature homebox-containing gene deletion screening by fluorescence in situ hybridisation in patients with short stature. J Pediatr 2001; 160:561–565.

54. Ballabio A, Bardoni B, Carrozzo R, Andria G, Bick D, Campbell L, Hamel B, Ferguson-Smith MA, Gimelli G, Fraccaro M, Maraschio P, Zuffardi O, Guioli S, Camerino G. Contiguous gene syndromes due to deletions in the distal short arm of the human X chromosome. Proc Natl Acad Sci USA 1989; 86:10001–10005.

55. Belin V, Cusin V, Viot G, Girlich D, Toutain A, Moncla A, Vekemans M, Le Merrer M, Munnich A, Cormier-Daire V. SHOX mutations in dyschondrosteosis (Leri-Weill syndrome). Nat Genet 1998; 19:67–69.

56. Stewart RE, Horton WA, Eteson DJ. General concepts of growth and development. In: Stewart RE, Barber TK, Troutman KC, Wei SHY, eds. Pediatric Dentistry: Scientific Foundations and Clinical Practice. St. Louis: CV Mosby, 1982:3–34.

57. Duterloo HS. An Atlas of Dentition in Childhood. London: Wolfe Publishing, 1991:93–96.

58. Jones KL: Smith's Recognizable Patterns of Human Malformation, 5th ed. Philadelphia: WB Saunders, 1997:592.

59. Murray JC, Bennett SR, Kwitek AE, Small KW, Schinzel A, Alward WL, Weber JL, Bell GI, Buetow KH. Linkage of Rieger syndrome to the region of the epidermal growth factor gene on chromosome 4. Nat Genet 1992; 2:46–49.

60. Veitia R, Ion A, Babaux S, Jobling MA, Souleyreaux N, Ennis K, Ostrer H, Tosi M, Meo T, Chibani J, Fellous M, McElreary K. Mutation and sequence variants in the testes-determining region of the 4 chormosome in individuals with a 46XY female phenotype. Hum Genet 1997; 99:648–652.

61. Horner JM, Thorsson AV, Hinz RI. Growth deceleration patterns in children with constitutional short stature: an aid to diagnosis. Pediatrics 1978; 62:529–534.

62. Vaquero-Solans C, Lifshitz F. Body weight progression and nutritional status of patients with familial short stature with and without constitutional delay in growth. Am J Dis Child 1991; 146:296–302.

63. Galler JR, Ramsey F, Solimano G. A follow-up study of the effects of early malnutrition in subsequent development in physical growth and sexual maturation during adolescence. Pediatr Res 1985; 19:518–523.

64. Harel Z, Tannenbaum GS. Long-term alterations in growth hormone and insulin secretion after temporary dietary protein restriction in early life in the rat. Pediatr Res 1995; 38:747–753.

65. Bierich JR. Constitutional delay of growth and development. Growth Genet Horm 1987; 3:9–12.

66. Gourmelen M, Pham-Huu-Trung MT, Girard F. Transient partial hGH deficiency in prepubertal children with delay of growth. Pediatr Res 1979; 13:221–224.

67. Kastrup KW, Andersen H, Eskildsen PC, Jacobsen BB, Krabbe S, Petersen KE. Combined test of hypothalmic–pituitary function in growth-retarded children treated with growth hormone. Acta Paediatr Scand (Suppl) 1979; 227: 9–13.

68. Clayton PE, Shalet SM, Price DA. Endocrine manipulation of constitutional delay in growth and puberty. J Endocrinol 1988; 116:321–323.

69. Bierich JR, Brogmann G, Schippert R. Assessment of

70. Schneid H, Le Bouc Y, Seurin D, Gourmelen M, Cabrol S, Raux-Demay MC, Girard F, Binoux M. Insulin-like growth factor-I gene analysis in subjects with constitutionally variant stature. Pediatr Res 1990; 27:488–491.

71. Link K, Blizzard RM, Evans WS, Kaiser DL, Parker MW, Rogol AD. The effect of androgens on the pulsatile release and the twenty-four-hour mean concentration of growth hormone in pre-pubertal males. J Clin Endocrinol Metab 1986; 62:159–164.

72. Abdenur JE, Publiese MT, Cervantes C, Fort P, Lifshitz F. Alterations in spontaneous growth hormone secretion and the response to GH-releasing hormone in children with non-organic nutritional dwarfing. J Clin Encocrinol Metab 1992; 75:930–934.

73. Attie KM, Carlsson LM, Rundle AC, Sherman BM. Evidence for partial growth hormone insensitivity among patients with idiopathic short stature. J Pediatr 1995; 127: 244–250.

74. Preece MA, Greco L, Savage MD, Cameron N, Tanner JM. The auxology of growth delay. Pediatrics 1981; 15–76.

75. LaFranchi S, Hanna CE, Mandel SH. Constitutional delay of growth: expected versus final adult height. Pediatrics 1991; 87:82–87.

76. Crowne EC, Shalet SM, Wallace WHB, Eminson DM, Price DA. Final height in boys with untreated constitutional growth delay in growth and puberty. Arch Dis Child 1990; 65:1109–1112.

77. Hagg U, Taranger J. Pubertal growth and maturity pattern in early and late maturers. A prospective longitudinal study of Swedish urban children. Swed Dent J 1992; 16: 199–209.

78. Ranke MB, Aronson AS. Adult height in children with constitutional short stature. Acta Paediatr Scand (Suppl) 1989; 362:27–31.

79. Von Vliet G, Styne PN, Kaplan SL, Grumbach MM. Growth hormone treatment for short stature in children. N Engl J Med 1983; 309:1016–1023.

80. Hintz RL, Attie KM, Baptista J, Roche A, for the Genentech Collaborative Group. Effect of growth hormone treatment on adult height of children with idiopathic short stature. N Engl J Med 1999; 340:502–507.

81. Buchlis JG, Irizarry L, Crotzer BC, Shine BJ, Allen L, MacGillivray MH. Comparison of final heights of growth-hormone-treated vs. untreated children with idiopathic short stature. J Clin Endocrinol Metab 1998; 83: 1075–1079.

82. McCaughey ES, Mulligan J, Voss LD, Betts PR. Randomised trial of growth hormone in short normal girls. Lancet 1998; 351:940–944.

83. Rosenfeld RG, Northcraft GB, Hintz RL. A prospective, randomized study of testosterone treatment of constitutional delay of growth and development in male adolescents. Pediatrics 1982; 69:681–687.

84. Lee PA, O'Dea L. Primary and secondary testicular insufficiency. Pediatr Clin North Am 1990: 37:1359–1387.

85. Strickland AI. Long-term results of treatment with low-dose fluoxymesterone in constitutional delay of growth and puberty and in genetic short stature. Pediatrics 1993; 91:716–720.

86. Bettmann HK, Goldman HS, Abramowics MN, Sobel EH. Oxandrolone treatment of short stature, effect on predicted matrix adult height. J Pediatr 1971; 79:1018–1023.

87. Buyukgebiz A, Hindmarsh PC, Stanhope R, Preece MA, Brook CGD. Long term outcome of oxandrolone treatment in boys with constitutional delay of growth and puberty. J Pediatr 1990; 117:588–591.

88. Blethen SL, Gaines S, Welden V. Comparison of predicted and adult heights in short boys: effects of androgen therapy. Pediatr Res 1984; 18:467–469.

89. Blizzard RM, Hindmarsh PC, Stanhope R. Oxandrolone therapy: 25 years experience. Growth Genet Horm 1991; 4:1–6.

90. Chihara K, Kodama H, Kaji H, Kita T, Kashio Y, Okimura Y, Abe H, Fujita T. Augmentation by propanolol of growth hormone-releasing hormone-(1-44)-NH$_2$-induced growth hormone release in normal short and normal children. J Clin Endocrinol Metab 1985; 61:229–233.

91. Pintor C, Cella SC, Loche S, Puggioni R, Corda R. Locatelli V, Muller EE. Clonidine treatment for short stature. Lancet 1987; 1:1226–1230.

92. Allen DB. Effects of nightly clonidine administration on growth velocity in short children without growth hormone deficiency: a double-blind, placebo-controlled study. J Pediatr 1993; 122:32–36.

93. Pescovitz OH, Tan E. Lack of benefit of clonidine treatment for short stature: a clonidine therapy of non-growth hormone deficient patients: double-blind, placebo trial. Lancet 1988; 2:874–877.

94. Finkelstein JS, Klibanski A, Neer R. A longitudinal evaluation of bone mineral density in adult men with histories of delayed puberty. J Clin Endocrinol Metab 1996; 81:1152–1155.

95. Tanner JM, Goldstein H, Whitehouse RH. Standards of children's height at ages 2 to 9 years allowing for height of parents. Arch Dis Child 1970; 45:755–762.

96. Hall B, Spranger J. Hypochondroplasia: clinical and radiological aspects in 39 cases. Radiology 1979; 133:95–100.

97. Gebhardt-Henrich SG. Heritability of growth curve parameters and heritability of final size: a simulation study. Growth Dev Aging 1992; 56:23–34.

98. Bermasconi S, Ghizzoni L, Volta C, Morano M, Giovanelli G. Spontaneous growth hormone secretion in Turner's syndrome. J Pediatr Endocrinol 1992; 5:101–105.

99. Raiti S, Moore WV, Van Vliet G, Kaplan SL. Growth-stimulating effects of human growth hormone therapy in patients with Turner syndrome. J Pediatr 1986; 109:944–949.

100. Ross JL, Long lM, Skerda M, Cassorla F, Kurtz D, Loriaux DL, Cutler GB Jr. Effect of low doses of estradiol on 6-month growth rates and predicted height in patients with Turner's syndrome. J Pediatr 1986; 109:950–953.

101. Rosenfeld RG, Frane J, Attie KM, Brasel JA, Burstein S, Cara JF, Chernausek S, Gotlin RW, Kuntze J, Lippe BM, et al. Six-year results of a randomized, prospective trial of human growth hormone and oxandrolone in Turner syndrome. J Pediatr 1992; 121:49–55.

102. Anneren G, Gustavson KH, Sara VR, Tunemo T. Growth retardation in Down syndrome in relation to insulin-like growth factors and growth hormone. Am J Med Genet (Suppl) 1990; 7:59–62.

103. Torrado C, Bastian W, Wisniewski KE, Castells S. Treatment of children with Down syndrome and growth retardation with recombinant human growth hormone. J Pediatr 1991; 119:478–483.

104. Lifshitz F. Commentary. Growth Genet Horm 1993; 9:1011.

105. Allen DB, Frasier SD, Foley TP Jr, Pescovitz OH. Growth hormone for children with Down syndrome. J Pediatr 1993; 123:742–743.

106. Spranger J. Classification of skeletal dysplasias. Acta Paediatr Scand (Suppl) 1991; 377:138–142.

107. Rimoin DL. International nomenclature and classification of the osteochondrodysplasias. International Working Group on Constitutional Diseases of Bone. Am J Med Genet 1998; 79:376–382.

108. Schwartz ID, Schwarts KJ, Kouseff BG, Becru BB, Root AW. Endocrinopathies in Cornelia de Lange syndrome. J Pediatr 1990; 117:920–922.

109. Hediger, MI, Overpeck MD, Maurer KR, Kuczmanski, RJ, McGlynn A, Davis WW. Growth of infants and young children born small or large for gestational age: findings from the third national health and nutrition examination survey. Arch Pediatr Adolesc Med 1998; 152:1225–1231.

110. Albertsson-Wikland K, Karlberg J. Natural growth in children born small for gestational age with and without catch-up growth. Acta Paediatr Suppl 1994; 399:64–70.

111. McCormick M. The contribution of low birth weight to infant mortality and childhood morbidity. N Engl J Med 1985; 312:82–90.

112. McIntire DD, Bloom SL, Casey BM, Leveno KJ. Birth weight in relation to morbidity and mortality among newborn infants. N Engl J Med 1999; 340:1234–1238.

113. Barker DJP, Gluckman PD, Godfrey KM, Harding JE, Owens JA, Robinson JS. Fetal nutrition and cardiovascular diseases in adult life. Lancet 1993; 341:938–941.

114. Williams S, St. George IM, Silva PA. Intrauterine growth retardation and blood pressure at age seven and eighteen. J Clin Epidemiology 1992; 45:1257–1263.

115. Leger J, Levy-Marchal C, Bloch J, Pinet A, Chevenne D, Porquet D, Collin D, Czernichow P. Reduced final height and indications for insulin resistance in 20 year olds born small for gestational age: regional cohort study. Br Med J 1997; 315:341–347.

116. Laor A, Stevenson DK, Shemer JG, Rena S, Daniel S. Size at birth: maternal nutritional status in pregnancy, and blood pressure at age 17. Br Med J 1997; 315:449–453.

117. Rich-Edwards JW, Colditz GA, Stampfer MJ, Willett WC, Gillman MW, Hennekens CH. Birthweight and the risk for type 2 diabetes mellitus in adult women. Ann Intern Med 1999; 130:278–284.

118. Litheil HO, McKeigue PM, Berglund L, Mohsen R, Lithell UB, Leon DA. Relation of size at birth to non-insulin dependent diabetes and insulin concentrations in men aged 50–60 years. Br Med J 1996; 312:406–410.

119. Hofman PL, Cutfield WS, Robinson EM, Bergman RN, Menon RK, Sperling MA, Gluckman PD. Insulin resistance in short children with intrauterine growth retardation. J Clin Endocrinol Metab 1997; 82:402–406.

120. Barker DJP, Gluckman PD, Robinson JS. Fetal origins of adult disease: report of the first study group. Sydney, 29–30 October, 1994. Placenta 1995; 16:317–320.

121. Lubchenko LO, Hanaman C, Dressler BE. Intrauterine growth as estimated from live born birth weight data at 24–42 weeks of gestation. Pediatrics 1963; 32:793–800.

122. Usher R, McLean F. Intrauterine growth of live born Caucasian infants at sea level: standards obtained from measurements in 7 dimensions of infants born between 25 and 44 weeks of gestation. Pediatrics 1969; 74:901–910.

123. Goldberg RL, Cutter GR, Hoffman HJ, Foster JM, Nelson KG, Hauth JC. Intrauterine growth retardation: standards for diagnosis. Am J Obstet Gynecol 1989; 161:271–277.

124. Seeds JW, Peng T. Impaired growth and risk of fetal death: is the tenth percentile the appropriate standard? Am J Obstet Gynecol 1998; 178:658–667.

125. Karlberg J, Albertsson-Wikland K. Growth in full-term small-for-gestational-age infants: from birth to final height. Pediatr Res 1995; 38:733–739.

126. Wright K, Dawson JP, Fallis D, Vogt E, Lorch V. New postnatal growth grids for very low birth weight infants. Pediatrics 1993; 91:922–926.

127. Cooke RJ, Ford A, Werkman S, Conner C, Watson D. Postnatal growth in infants born between 700 and 1,500 g. J Pediatr Gastroenterol Nutr 1993; 16:130–135.

128. Casey PH, Kraemer HC, Bernbaum J, Tyson JE, Sells JC, Yogman MW, Bauer CR. Growth patterns of low birth weight preterm infants: a longitudinal analysis of a large, varied sample. J Pediatr 1990; 117:298–307.

129. Brenner WE, Edelman DA, Hendricks CH. A standard for fetal growth for the United States of America. Am J Obstet Gynecol 1976, 126:555–564.

130. Singer DB, Sung CJ, Wigglesworth JS. Fetal growth and maturation: with standards for body and organ development. In: Wigglesworth JS, Singer DB, eds. Textbook of Fetal and Perinatal Pathology. Boston: Blackwell Scientific Publications, 1996:11–47.

131. Klebanoff MA, Mairik O, Berendes HW. Second generation consequences of small-for-dates birth. Pediatrics 1989; 84:343–347.

132. Godfrey K, Robinson S, Barker, DJP, Osmond C, Cox V. Maternal nutrition in early and late pregnancy in relation to placental and fetal growth. Br Med J 1996; 312:410–414.

133. Luke S, Gillespie B, Min S-J, Avni M, Witter FR, O'Sullivan MJ. Critical periods of maternal weight gain: effect on twin birth weight. Am J Obstet Gynecol 1997; 177:1055–1062.

134. Abrams B, Selvin S. Maternal weight gain pattern and birth weight. Obstet Gynecol 1995; 86:163–169.

135. Food and Nutrition Board, Institute of Medicine (United States). Nutrition During Pregnancy and Lactation. Washington: National Academy Press, 1990:1–233.

136. American College of Obstetricians and Gynecologists. Nutrition During Pregnancy. Washington: American College of Obstetricians and Gynecologists, 1993 (Technical bulletin no. 179).

137. Brown HL, Watkings K, Hiett KA. Fetus–placenta–newborn; the impact of the women, infants and children food supplement program on birth outcome. Am J Obstet Gynecol 1996; 174:279–283.

138. Cogswell ME, Serdula MK, Hungerford DW, Yip R. Gestational weight gain among average-weight and overweight women—what is excessive? Am J Obstet Gynecol 1994; 172:705–712.

139. Tudehope DI. Neonatal aspects of intrauterine growth retardation. Fetal Med Rev 1991; 3:73–85.

140. Berge P, Stagno S, Federer W, Cloud G, Foster J, Utermohlen V, Armstrong D. Impact of asymptomatic congenital cytomegalovirus infection on size at birth and gestational duration. Pediatr Infect Dis J 1990; 9:170–175.

141. Khoury MJ, Erickson JD, Cordero JF, McCarthy BJ. Congenital malformations and intrauterine growth retardation: a population study. Pediatrics 1988; 82:83–90.

142. Kohler M, Moya-Sola S, Autusti J. Imprinted gene in postnatal growth role. Nature 1998; 393:125–126.

143. Krook A, Brueton L, O'Rahilly S. Homozygous nonsense mutation in the insulin receptor gene in infant with leprechaunism. Lancet 1993, 342:227–228.

144. Furlanetto RW, Underwood LE, Van Wyk JJ, Hanweger S. Serum immunoreactive somatomedine-C is elevated in late pregnancy. J Clin Endocrinol Metab 1979; 47:695–698.

145. Freemark M, Comer M, Mularoni T, D'Ercole AJ, Granois A, Kodack L. Nutritional regulation of the placental lactogen receptor in fetal liver: implications for fetal metabolism and growth. Endocrinology 1989; 125:1504–1512.

146. Leger J, Noel M, Limal JM, Czernichow P, for the Study group of IUGR. Growth factors and intrauterine growth retardation: II: serum growth hormone, insulin-like growth factor (IGF)-1 and IGF binding protein 3 levels in children with intrauterine growth retardation compared with normal control subjects: prospective study from birth to two years of age. Pediatr Res 1996; 40:101–107.

147. Cance-Rouzaud A, Laborie S, Bieth E, Tricoire J, Rolland M, Grandjean H, Rochiccioli P, Tauber M. Growth hormone, insulin like growth factor-1 and insulin-like growth factor binding protein-3 are regulated differently in small-for-gestational-age and appropriate-for-gestational-age neonates. Biol Neonate 1998; 73:347–355.

148. Lassarre C, Hardouing S, Daffos F, Forestier F, Frankenne F, Binoux M. Serum insulin-like growth factors and insulin-like growth factor binding proteins in normal subjects and in subjects with intrauterine growth retardation. Pediatr Res 1991; 29:219–225.

149. Job JC, Chatelain P, Rochiccioli P, Ponte C, Oliver M, Sagard L. Growth hormone response to a bolus injection of 1-44 growth-hormone-releasing hormone in very short children with intrauterine onset growth failure. Horm Res 1990; 33:161–165.

150. Weber GW, Prossinger H, Horst S. Height depends on month of birth. Nature 1998; 39:754–755.

151. Jaquet D, Leger J, Levy-Marchal C, Oury JF, Czernichow P. Ontogeny of leptin in human fetuses and newborns effect of intrauterine growth retardation on serum leptin concentrations. J Clin Endocrinol Metab 1998; 83:243–246.

152. Marchini G, Fried G, Ostlund E, Gagenas L. Plasma leptin in infants: relations to birth weight and weight loss. Pediatrics 1998; 101:429–432.

153. Chang TC, Robson SC, Boys RJ, Spencer JAD. Prediction of the small for gestational age infant: which ultrasonic measurement is best? Obstet Gynecol 1992; 80:1030–1038.

154. Bahado-Singh R, Oz U, Kovanchi E, Lernik E, Flores D, Singh-Basra D, et al. Mid-trimester maternal uterine marker for the prediction of subsequent IUGR. Am J Obstet Gynecol 1999; 180 (suppl II):174–175.

155. Georgieff MK, Sasanow SR, Chockalingam UM, Pereira GR. A comparison of the mid-arm circumference/head circumference ratio and the ponderal index for the evaluation of newborn infants after abnormal intrauterine growth. Acta Paediatr Scand 1988; 77:214–219.

156. Peralta-Carcelen M, Jackson DS, Goran MI, Royal SA, Mayo MS, Nelson KG. Growth of adolescents who were born at extremely low birth weight without major disability. J Pediatr 2000; 136:633–640.

157. Leger J, Limoni C, Collin D, Czernichow P. Prediction factors in the determination of final height in subjects born small for gestational age. Pediatr Res 1998; 43:808–812.

158. Strauss RS, Dietz WH. Growth and development of term children born with low birth weight: effects of genetic and environmental factors. J Pediatr 1998; 133:67–72.

159. Woods KA, Camacho-Hubner C, Savage MO, Clark AJL. Intrauterine growth retardation and postnatal growth failure associated with deletion of the insulin-like growth factor I gene. N Engl J Med 1996; 335:1363–1367.

160. Kelleher KJ, Casey PH, Bradley RH, Pope SK, Whiteside L, Barret KW, et al. Risk factors and outcomes for failure to thrive in low birth weight preterm infants. Pediatrics 1993; 91:941–948.

161. Arisaka G, Arisaka M, Kiyokawa N, Shimizu T, Nakayama Y, Yabuta K. Intrauterine growth retardation and early adolescent growth spurt in 2 sisters. Clin Pediatr 1986; 25:559–561.

162. Reilley SM, Skuse DH, Wolke D, Stevenson J. Oral-motor dysfunction in children who fail to thrive: organic or non-organic. Dev Med Child Neurol 1999; 41:115–122.

163. Embleton NE, Pang N, Cook RJ. Postnatal malnutrition and growth retardation: an inevitable consequence of current recommendations in preterm infants? Pediatrics 2001; 107:270–273.

164. Fjellestad-Paulsen A, Czernichow P, Brauner R, Bost M, Colle M, Lebouc JY, Lecronu M, Leheup B, Limal JM, Raux MC, Toublanc JE, Rappaport R. Three-year data from a comparative study with recombinant human growth hormone in the treatment of short stature in young children with intrauterine growth retardation. Acta Paediatr 1998; 87:511–517.

165. Chaussain JL, Colle M, Landier F. Effects of growth hormone therapy in prepubertal children with short stature secondary to intrauterine growth retardation. Acta Paediatr Suppl 1994; 399:74–75.

166. Coutant R, Carel JC, Letrait M, Bouvattier C, Chatelain P, Coste J, Chaussain JL. Short stature associated with intrauterine growth retardation: final height of untreated and growth-hormone-treated children. J Clin Endocrinol Metab 1998; 83:1070–1074.

167. Boguszewski M, Albertsson-Wikland K, Aronsson S, Gustafsson J, Hagenas L, Westgren U, Westphal O, Lipsanen-Nyman M, Sipila I, Gellert P, Muller J, Madsen B. Growth hormone treatment of short children born small-for-gestational-age: the Nordic Multicentre Trial. Acta Paediatr 1998; 87:257–263.

168. Chernausek SD, Breen TJ, Frank GR. Linear growth in response to growth hormone treatment in children with short stature associated with intrauterine growth retardation: The National Cooperative Growth Study experience. J Pediatr 1996; 128(suppl):22–27.

169. de Zegher F, Albertsson-Wikland K, Wilton P, Chatelain P, Jonsson B, Lofstrom A, Butenandt O, Chaussain JL. Growth hormone treatment of short children born small for gestational age: metanalysis of four independent, randomized, controlled, multicentre studies. Acta Paediatr Suppl 1996; 417:27–31.

170. Job JC, Chaussain JL, Job B, Ducret JP, Maes M, Oliver M, Ponte C, Rochiccioli P, Vanderschueren-Lodeweyckx M, Chatelain P. Follow-up of three years of treatment with growth hormone and one of post-treatment year, in children with severe growth retardation of intrauterine onset. Pediatr Res 1996; 39:354–359.

171. Botero D, Lifshitz F. Intrauterine growth retardation and long-term effects on growth. Curr Opin Pediatr 1999; 11: 340–347.

172. Butenandt O, Lang G. Recombinant human growth hormone in short children born small for gestational age. J Pediatr Endocrinol Metab 1997; 10:275–282.

173. de Zegher F, Maes M, Gargosky SE, Heinrichs C, Caju M, Thiry G, De Schepper J, Craen M, Breysem L, Lof-

strom A, Jonsson P, Bourguignon JP, Malvaux P, Rosenfeld RG. High-dose growth hormone treatment of short children born small for gestational age. J Clin Endocrinol Metab 1996; 81:1887–1892.

174. Zucchini S, Cacciari E, Balsamo A, Cicognani A, Tassinari D, Barbieri E, Gualandi S. Final height of short subjects of low birth weight with and without growth hormone treatment. Arch Dis Child 2001; 84:340–343.

175. Persson E, Jansson T. Low birthweight is associated with elevated adult blood pressure in the chronically catheterized guinea pig. Acta Physiol Scand 1992; 145:195–196.

176. Dahri S, Snoeck A, Reusens-Billen B, Hoet JJ. Effect of a low protein diet during pregnancy on the fetal rat endocrine pancreas. Biol Neonate 1991; 40(suppl 2):115–120.

177. Lucas A. Programming by early nutrition in man. In: Barker DJP, ed. The Childhood Environment and Adult Disease: CIBA Symposium 156. Chichester, UK: John Wiley, 1991:38–55.

178. Hales CN, Barker DJ. Type 2 (non-insulin dependent) diabetes mellitus: the thrifty phenotype hypothesis. Diabetologia 1992; 35:444–446.

179. Barker DJP, Hales CN, Fall CHD, Osmond C, Phipps K, Clark PMS. Type 2 (non-insulin-dependent) diabetes mellitus, hypertension and hyperlipidemia (syndrome X): relation to reduced fetal growth. Diabetologia 1993; 36:62–67.

180. Bao W, Srinivasan SR, Wattigney WA, Berenson GS. Persistence of multiple cardiovascular risk clustering related to syndrome X from childhood to going adulthood: the Bogalusa Heart Study. Arch Intern Med 1994; 154:1842–1847.

181. Kramer MS, Platt R, Yang H, McNamara H, Usher RH. Are all growth-restricted newborns created equal(ly)? Pediatrics 1999; 103:599–602.

182. Porter B, Skuse D. When does slow weight gain become 'failure to thrive'? Arch Dis Child 1991; 66:905–906.

183. Mitchell WG, Gorrell RW, Greenberg RA. Failure-to-thrive: a study in a primary care setting. Epidemiology and follow-up. Pediatrics 1980; 65:971–977.

184. Wilcox WD, Nieburg P, Miller DS. Failure to thrive: a continuing problem of definition. Clin Pediatr 1989; 28: 391–394.

185. Rosenn DW, Loeb LS, Jura MB. Differentiation of organic from non-organic failure to thrive syndrome in infancy. Pediatrics 1980; 66:698–704.

186. Frank DA, Zeisel SH. Failure to thrive: mystery, myth and method. Contemp Pediatr 1993; 2:114.

187. Edwards AGK, Halse PC, Parkin JM, Waterson AJ. Recognizing failure to thrive in early childhood. Arch Dis Child 1990; 65:1263–1265.

188. Skuse DH. Non-organic failure to thrive: a reappraisal. Arch Dis Child 1985; 60:173–178.

189. Kirkland RT. Failure to Thrive. In: Oski FA, De Angelis CD, McMillan JA, Feigin RD, Warshaw JB, eds. Principles and Practice of Pediatrics, 2nd ed. Philadelphia: JB Lippincott, 1994:1048–1050.

190. Leung AK, Robson WL, Fagan JE. Assessment of the child with failure to thrive. Am Fam Phys 1993; 48: 1432–1438.

191. Powell GF. Failure to thrive. In: Lifshitz F, ed. Pediatric Endocrinology, 3rd ed. New York: Marcel Dekker, 1996: 121–130.

192. Lifshitz JZ, Lifshitz F. Failure to thrive. In: Lifschitz CL, ed. Pediatric Gastroenterology and Nutrition. New York: Marcel Dekker, 2001:301–326.

193. Sheard NF. Growth pattens in the first year of life: what is the norm? Nutr Rev 1993; 51:52–54.

194. Salmenpera L, Peerheentupa J, Slimes MA, Exclusively breast-fed healthy infants grow slower than reference infants. Pediatr Res 1985; 19:307–312.

195. Hill PD. Insufficient milk supply syndrome. Clin Issues Perinat Womens Health Nurs 1992; 3:605–612.

196. Motil KJ, Sheng HP, Montandon CM. Case report: failure to thrive in a breast-fed infant is associated with maternal dietary protein and energy restriction. J Am Col Nutr 1994; 13:203–208.

197. Weston JA, Stage AF, Hathaway P, Andrews DL, Stonington JA, McCabe EB. Prolonged breast-feeding and nonorganic failure to thrive. Am J Dis Child 1987; 141: 242–243.

198. Dewey KG, Heining MJ, Nommsen LA, Peerson JM, Lonnerdal B. Growth of breast-fed infants from 0 to 19 months: the DARLING Study. Pediatrics 1992; 89:1035–1041.

199. Grummer-Strawn LM. Does prolonged breast-feeding impair child growth? A critical review. Pediatrics 1993; 91: 766–771.

200. Wilensky DS, Ginsberg G, Altman M, Tullchinsky TH, Ben Yishay F, Auerbach JA. A community-based study of failure to thrive in Israel. Arch Dis Child 1996; 75: 145–148.

201. Altemeier WA, O'Connor SM, Sherrod KB, Vietze PM. Prospective study of antecedents of nonorganic failure to thrive. J Pediatr 1985; 106:360–365.

202. Reilly SM, Skuse DH, Wolke D, Stevenson J. Oral–motor dysfunction in children who fail to thrive: organic or nonorganic? Dev Med Child Neurol 1999; 41:115–122.

203. Frank DA, Wong F. Effects of prenatal exposures to alcohol, tobacco and other drugs. In: Kessler DB, Dawson P, eds. Failure to Thrive and Pediatric Undernutrition— A Transdisciplinary Approach. Baltimore: Brookes Publishing Co., 1999:275–280.

204. Pugliese MT, Weyman-Daum M, Moses N, Lifshitz F. Parental health benefits as a cause of non-organic failure to thrive. Pediatrics 1987; 80:175–182.

205. Lifshitz F. Children on adult diets. Is it harmful? Is it healthful? J Am Coll Nutr 1992; 11:845–905.

206. McCann JB, Stein A, Fairburn CG, Dunger DB. Eating habits and attitudes of mothers of children with non-organic failure to thrive. Arch Dis Child 1994; 70:234–236.

207. Lifshitz F, Tarim O. Nutritional dwarfing. Curr Probl Pediatr 1993; 23:322–326.

208. Smith MM, Lifshitz F. Excessive fruit juice consumption as a contributing factor in non-organic failure to thrive. Pediatrics 1993; 93:438–443.

209. Campbell M, Lofters WS, Gibbs W. Rastafarianism and the vegan syndrome. Br Med J 1982; 285:1617–1618.

210. Roberts IF, West RJ, Ogilvie D, Dillon MJ. Malnutrition in infants receiving cult diets: a form of child abuse. Br Med J 1979; 1:296–298.

211. Sanders TA, Reddy S. Vegetarian diets and children. Am J Clin Nutr 1994; 59 (suppl): 1176S–1181S.

212. Latham MC, Stephenson LS, Kinoti SN, Zaman MS, Kurz KM. Improvements in growth following iron supplementation in young Kenyan school children. Nutrition 1990; 6:159–165.

213. Cavan KR, Gibson RS, Grazioso CR, Isalgue AM, Ruz M, Solomons NW. Growth and body composition of periurban Guatemalan children in relation to zinc status: a cross-sectional study. Am J Clin Nutr 1993; 57:334–352.

214. Hadi H, Stoltzfus R, Dibley MJ, Moulton LH, West KP Jr, Kjolhede CL, Sadjimin T. Vitamin A supplementation selectively improves the linear growth of Indonesian preschool children: results from a randomized controlled trial. Am J Clin Nutr 2000; 71:507–513.

215. Allen LH. Nutritional influences on linear growth: a general review. Euro J Clin Nutr 1994; 48 (Suppl 1):S75–S89.

216. Martorell R. Results and implications of the INCAP follow-up study. J Nutr 1995; 125:1127S–1138S.

217. Caulfield LE, Himes JH, Rivera JA. Nutritional supplementation during early childhood and bone mineralization during adolescence. J Nutr 1995; 125:1104S–1110S.

218. Pickett KE, Haas JD, Murdoch S, Rivera JA, Martorell R. Early nutritional supplementation and skeletal maturation in Guatemalan adolescents. Nutrition 1995; 125: 1097S–1103S.

219. Vandenplas Y, Lifshitz JZ, Orenstein S, Lifschitz CL, Shepherd RW, Casaubon PR, Muinos RI, Fagundes-Neto U, Garcia Aranda JA, Gentles M, Santiago JD, Vanderhoof J, Yeung CY, Moran JR, Lifshitz F. Nutritional management of regurgitation in infants. J Am Coll Nutr 1998; 17:308–316.

220. Ramsay M, Gisel EG, Boutry M. Non-organic failure to thrive: Growth failure secondary to feeding-skills disorder. Dev Med Child Neurol 1993; 35:285–297.

221. Dobbing J. Vulnerable periods in developing brain. In: Dobbing J, ed. Brain, Behavior and Iron in the Infant Diet. New York: Springer-Verlag, 1990.

222. Wachs TD. Relation of mild-to-moderate malnutrition to human development: Correlational studies. J Nutr 1995; 125 (8 Suppl.):2245S–2254S.

223. Idjradinata P, Pollitt E. Reversal of developmental delays in iron-deficient anemic infants treated with iron. Lancet 1993; 341:1–4.

224. Pollitt E, Oh S. Early supplementary feeding, child development and health policy. Food Nutr Bull 1994; 15: 208–214.

225. Bithoney WG. Elevated lead levels in children with non-organic failure to thrive. Pediatrics 1986; 78:891–895.

226. Lifshitz F, Moses-Finch N, Lifshitz JZ. Failure to Thrive in Children's Nutrition. Boston: Jones & Bartlett, 1991: 253–270.

227. Krieger I. Food restriction as a form of child abuse in 10 cases of psychosocial deprivation dwarfism. Clin Pediatr (Phila) 1974; 13:127–133.

228. Krieger I, Mellinger RC. Pituitary function in the deprivation syndrome. J Pediatr 1971; 79:216–225.

229. Whitten C, Fischoff J. Evidence that growth failure from maternal deprivation is secondary to undereating. JAMA 1969; 209:1675–1682.

230. Krieger I. Endocrines and nutrition in psychosocial deprivation in the USA: comparison with growth failure due to malnutrition on an organic basis. In: Gardner LI, Amacher P, eds. Endocrine Aspects of Malnutrition: Marasmus, Kwashiorkor and Psychosocial Deprivation. Santa Ynez, CA: Kroc Foundation, 1973:129–162.

231. Krieger I, Whitten CF. Energy metabolism in infants with growth failure due to maternal deprivation under-nutrition, or causes unknown. J Pediatr 1969; 75:374–379.

232. Gardner LI. Deprivation dwarfism. Sci Am 1972; 227: 76–82.

233. Green WH. Psychosocial dwarfism: psychological and etiological considerations. Adv Clin Child Psychol 1986; 9:245–278.

234. Bakwin H. Loneliness in infants. Am J Dis Child 1942; 62:30–40.

235. Talbot NB, Sobel EH, Burke BS, Lindemann E, Kaufman SB. Dwarfism in healthy children, its possible relation to emotional, nutritional and endocrine disturbances. N Engl J Med 1947; 236:783–793.

236. Widdowson EM. Mental contentment and physical growth. Lancet 1951; 1:1316–1318.

237. Spitz R. Hospitalism, an inquiry into the genesis of psychiatric conditions in early childhood. Psychoanal Study Child 1945; 1:53–74.

238. Spitz R. Hospitalism, a follow-up report. Psychoanal Study Child 1946; 2:113–117.

239. Chatoor I, Egan J. Non-organic failure to thrive and dwarfism due to food refusal: a separation disorder. J Am Acad Child Psychiatry 1983; 22:294–301.

240. Chatoor I, Egan J, Getson P, Menvielle E, O'Donnell R. Mother–infant interactions in anorexia nervosa. J Am Acad Child Adolesc Psychiatry 1988; 27:535–540.

241. Benjamin DR. Laboratory tests and nutritional assessment. Protein–energy status. Pediatr Clin North Am 1989; 36:139–161.

242. Figueroa-Colon R. Clinical and laboratory assessment of the malnourished child. In: Suskind RM, Lewinter-Susking L, eds. Textbook of Pediatric Nutrition, ed. 2. New York: Raven Press, 1993:191–205.

243. Berwick DM, Levy JC, Kleinerman R. Failure to thrive. Diagnostic yield to hospitalization. Arch Dis Child 1982; 57:347–351.

244. Fryer GE Jr. The efficacy of hospitalization of non-organic failure to thrive children: a meta-analysis. Child Abuse Neglect 1988; 12:375–381.

245. Casey PH, Wortham B, Nelson JY. Management of children with failure to thrive in a rural ambulatory setting: epidemiology and growth outcomes. Clin Pediatr 1984; 23:325–330.

246. Bithoney WG, McJunkin J, Michalek J, Snyder J, Egan H, Epstein D. The effect of a multidisciplinary team approach on weight gain in non-organic failure-to-thrive children. J Dev Behav Pediatr 1991; 12:254–258.

247. World Health Organization. Energy and Protein Requirements. Report of a Joint FAO/WHO/UNU Expert Consultation. WHO Technical Report Series No. 724. Geneva: World Health Organization, 1985.

248. Sentongo TA, Tershakovec AM, Mascarenhas MR, Watson MH, Stallings VA. Resting energy expenditure and prediction equations in young children with failure to thrive. J Pediatr 2000; 136:345–350.

249. Ramsay M, Zelaso PR. Food refusal in failure to thrive infants: nasogastric feeding combined with interactive-behavioral treatment. J Pediatr Psychol 1988; 13:329–347.

250. Angeles IT, Schultnick WJ, Matulessi P, Gross R, Sastroamidjojo S. Decreased rate of stunting among anemic Indonesian preschool children through iron supplementation. Am J Clin Nutr 1993; 58:339–342.

251. Black RE. Therapeutic and preventive effects of zinc on serious childhood infectious diseases in developing countries. Am J Clin Nutr 1998; 68:476S–479S.

252. Sazawal S, Black RE, Jalla S, Mazumdar S, Sinha A, Bhan MK. Zinc supplementation reduces the incidence of acute lower respiratory infections in infants and preschool children: a double-blind controlled trial. Pediatrics 1998; 102:1–5.

253. Muhe L, Lulseged S, Mason KE, Simoes EA. Case–control study of the role of nutritional rickets in the risk of developing pneumonia in Ethiopian children. Lancet 1997; 349:1801–1804.

254. Umeta M, West CE, Haidar J, Deurenberg P, Hautvast JG. Zinc supplementation and stunted infants in Ethiopia: a randomised controlled trial. Lancet 2000; 355:2021–2026.

255. Bhutta ZA, Black RE, Brown KH, Gardner JM, Gore S, Hidayat A, Khatun F, Martorell R, Ninh NX, Penny ME, Rosado JL, Roy SK, Ruel M, Sazawal S, Shankar A. Prevention of diarrhea and pneumonia by zinc supplementation in children in developing countries: pooled analysis of randomized controlled trials. Zinc Investigators' Collaborative Group. J Pediatr 1999; 35:689–697.

256. Rosado JL, Lopez P, Munoz E, Martinez H, Allen LH. Zinc supplementation reduced morbidity, but neither zinc nor iron supplementation affected growth or body composition of Mexian preschoolers. Am J Clin Nutr 1997; 65:13–19.

257. Whitehead RG, Biol FL. Protein and energy requirement of young children living in the developing countries allow for catch-up growth after infections. Am J Clin Nutr 1977; 30:1545–1547.

258. Reeds PJ, Jackson AA, Picou D, Poulter N. Muscle mass and composition in malnourished infants and children and changes seen after recovery. Pediatr Res 1978; 12:613–618.

259. Chatoor I. Infantile anorexia nervosa: a developmental disorder of separation and individuation. J Am Acad Psychoanal 1989; 17:43–46.

260. Sturm L, Dawson P. Working with families—an overview for providers. In: Kessler DB, Dawson P, eds. Failure to Thrive and Pediatric Undernutrition—A Transdisciplinary Approach. Baltimore: Brookes Publishing Co., 1999:65–76.

261. Oates RK, Peacock A, Forrest D. Long-term effects of non-organic failure to thrive. Pediatrics 1985; 75:36–40.

262. Singer L. Long-term hospitalization of non-organic failure-to-thrive infants: patient characteristics and hospital course. J Dev Behav Pediatr 1987; 8:25–31.

263. Casey PH. Diagnostic coding of children with failure to thrive. In: Kessler DB, Dawson P, eds. Failure to Thrive and Pediatric Undernutrition—A Transdisciplinary Approach. Baltimore: Brookes Publishing, 1999:281–286.

264. Hess CA. Managed care as part of family-centered service systems. In: Kessler DB, Dawson P, eds. Failure to Thrive and Pediatric Undernutrition—A Transdisciplinary Approach. Baltimore: Brookes Publishing, 1999:287–302.

265. Torun B, Viteri FE. Protein energy malnutrition. In: Shils ME, Young VR, eds. Modern Nutrition in Health and Disease, 7th ed. Philadelphia: Lea & Febiger, 1988:746–773.

266. Nikens PR. Stature reduction as an adaptive response to food production in Mesoamerica. J Archaeol Sci 1976; 3:21–41.

267. Stin WA. Evolutionary implications of changing nutritional patterns in human populations. Am Anthropol 1971; 73:1019–1030.

268. Lifshitz F. Nutrition and growth. In: Paige DM, ed. Clinical Nutrition. Nutrition and Growth Supplement 4. St Louis: CV Mosby, 1985:40–47.

269. Kelts DO, Grand RJ, Shen G, Watkins JB, Werlin SL, Boehme C. Nutritional basis of growth failure in children and adolescents with Crohn's disease. Gastroenterology 1979; 76:720–727.

270. Stenhammar L, Fallstrom SP, Jansson G, Jansson U, Lindberg T. Cocliac disease in children of short stature

without gastrointestinal symptoms. Eur J Pediatr 1986; 145:185–186.

271. Keller W, Fillynore CM. Prevalence of protein–energy malnutrition. World Health Stat Q 1983; 36:129–167.

272. Lifshitz F, Tarim O, Smith MM. Nutrtional growth retardation. In: Lifshitz F, ed. Pediatric Endocrinology, 3rd ed. New York: Marcel Dekker, 1996:103–120.

273. Trowbridge FL, Marks JS, Lopez de Romana G, Madrid S, Boutton TW, Klein PD. Body composition of Peruvian children with short stature and high weight-for-height: implication for the interpretation for weight-for-height as an indicator of nutritional status. Am J Clin Nutr 1987; 46:411–418.

274. Kirschner BS. Nutritional consequences of inflammatory bowel disease on growth. J Am Coll Nutr 1988; 7:301–308.

275. Pugliese MT, Lifshitz F, Grad G, Fort P, Marks-Katz M. Fear of obesity: a cause of short stature and delayed puberty. N Engl J Med 1983; 309:513–518.

276. Lifshitz F, Friedman S, Smith MM, Cervantes C, Recker B, O'Connor M. Nutritional dwarfing: a growth abnormality associated with reduced erythrocyte Na+, K+ ATPase activity. Am J Clin Nutr 1991; 54:1–7.

277. Clemmons DR, Underwood LE. Nutritional regulation of IGF-I and IGF binding proteins. Annu Rev Nutr 1991; 11:393–412.

278. Thissen JP, Underwood IE, Maiter D, Maes M, Clemmons DR, Ketelslegers JM. Failure of insulin-like growth factor-1 (IGF-I) infusion to promote growth in protein-restricted rats despite normalization of serum IGF-I concentrations. Endocrinology 1991; 128:885–890.

279. Clemmons DR, Thissen JP, Maes M, Ketelslegers JM, Underwood LE. Insulin-like growth factor-I (IGF-1) infusion into hypophysectomized or protein-deprived rats induces specific IGF binding proteins in serum. Endocrinology 1989; 125:2967–2972.

280. Clemmons DR, Underwood LE, Dickerson RN, Brown RO, Hak LJ, MacPhee RD, Heizer WD. Use of somatomedin-C/insulin-like growth factor I measurements to monitor the response to nutritional repletion in malnourished patients. Am J Clin Nutr 1985; 41:192–198.

281. Merimee TJ, Zapf J, Froesch ER. Insulin-like growth factors in the fed and fasted states. J Clin Endocrinol Metab 1982; 55:999–1002.

282. Underwood LE, Thissen JP, Moats-Staats BM, et al. Nutritional regulation of IGF-I and postnatal growth. In: Spencer EM, ed. Modern Concepts of Insulin-like Growth Factors. New York: Elsevier, 1991:37–47.

283. Donhue SP, Phillips LS. Response of IGF-I to nutritional support in malnourished hospital patients: a possible marker of short-term changes in nutritional status. Am J Clin Nutr 1989; 50:962–969.

284. Ranke MB, Blum WF, Frisch H. The acid-stable subunit of insulin-like growth factor binding protein (IGFBP-3) in disorders of growth. In: Drop SLS, Hintz RL, eds. Insulin-like Growth Factor Binding Proteins. Amsterdam: Excerpta Medica, 1989:103–113.

285. Guler HP, Zapf J, Schmid C, Froesch ER. Insulin-like growth factors I & 11 in healthy man. Estimations of half-lives and production rates. Acta Endocrinol (Copenh) 1989; 121:753–758.

286. Phillips LS, Unterman TG. Somatomedin activity in disorders of nutrition and metabolism. Clin Endocrinol Metab 1984; 13:145–189.

287. Phillips LS, Young HS. Nutrition and somatomedin. 1. Effect of fasting and re-feeding on serum somatomedin

288. activity and cartilage growth activity in rats. Endocrinology 1976; 99:304–314.

288. Phillips LS, Orawski AT, Belosky DC. Somatomedin and nutrition. IV. Regulation of somatomedin activity and growth cartilage activity by quantity and composition of diet in rats. Endocrinology 1978; 103:121–124.

289. Golden M, Jackson AA. Chronic severe under-nutrition. In: Olson RE, Broquist HP, Chichester CO, Darby WJ, Kolbye AC Jr, Stalvey RM, eds. Present Knowledge in Nutrition. Washington, DC: Nutrition Foundation, 1984: 57–67.

290. Byung PY. Update on food restriction and aging. Rev Biol Res Aging 1985; 2:435–443.

291. Patrick J, Golden M. Leukocyte electrolytes and sodium transport in protein energy malnutrition. Am J Clin Nutr 1977; 30:1478–1481.

292. Montage A, Brace C. Human Evolution, 2nd ed. New York: Macmillan, 1977.

293. Beaton GH. The significance of adaptation in the definition of nutrient requirements and for nutrition policy. In: Blaxter KL, Waterlow JC, eds. Nutritional Adaptation in Man. London: Libbey, 1985:219–232.

294. Poehlman F, Melby CL, Badylak SF. Resting metabolic rate and post-prandial thermogenesis in highly trained and untrained males. Am J Clin Nutr 1988; 47:793–798.

295. Waterlow JC, Golder M, Picou D. Protein turnover in man. Am J Clin Nutr 1977; 30:1333–1339.

296. Read WW, McLaren DS, Tchalian M, Nassar S. Studies with 15 N-labelled ammonia and urea in the malnourished child. J Clin Invest 1969; 48:1143–1149.

297. Waterlow JC, Golden MH, Garlick PJ. Protein turnover in man measured with 15N-Comparison of end products and dose regimens. Am J Physiol 1978; 235(2):EI65–EI74.

298. Golden M, Waterlow JC, Pilou D. The relationship between dietary intake, weight change, nitrogen balance, and protein turnover in man. Am J Clin Nutr 1977; 30: 1345–1348.

299. Viteri FE, Torun B. Nutrition, physical activity and growth. In: Ritzer M, Apsia A, Hall K, eds. The Biology of Normal Human Growth. New York: Raven Press, 1981:269–273.

300. Lifshitz F, Brasel JA. Nutrition and Endocrine Disease. In: Kappy MS, Blizzard RM, Migeon C, eds. Wilkins Diagnosis and Treatment of Endocrine Disorders in Childhood and Adolescence. Springfield, IL: Charles C Thomas, 1994:535–573.

301. Alemzadeh R, Pugliese M, Lifshitz F. Disorders of puberty. In: Friedman SB, Fisher M, Shonberg SK, eds. Comprehensive Adolescent Health Care. St. Louis: Quality Medical Publishing, 1992:187–205.

302. Brettler DB, Forsberg A, Bolivar E, Brewster F, Sullivan J. Growth failure as a prognostic indicator for progression to acquired immunodeficiency syndrome in children with hemophilia. J Pediatr 1990; 117:584–588.

303. Gertner JM, Kaufman FR, Donfield SM, Sleeper LA, Shapiro AD, Howard C, Gomperts ED, Hilgartner MW. Delayed somatic growth and pubertal development in human immunodeficiency virus-infected hemophiliac boys: hemophilia growth and development study. J Pediatr 1994; 124:896–902.

304. Kirschner BS, Sutton MM. Somatomedin C levels in growth impaired children and adolescents with chronic inflammatory bowel disease. Gastroenterology 1986; 91: 830–836.

305. Belli DC, Seidman E, Bouthillier L, Weber AM, Roy CC, Pletinex M, Beaulieu M, Morin CL. Chronic intermittent elemental diet improves growth failure in children with Crohn's disease. Gastroenterology 1988; 94:603–610.

306. Kanoff ME, Lake AM, Bayless TM. Decreased height velocity in children and adolescents before the diagnosis of Crohn's disease. Gastroenterology 1988; 94:1523–1527.

307. Seidman E, LeLeiko N, Ament M, Berman W, Caplan D, Evans J, Kocoshis S, Lake A, Motil K, Sutphen J, et al. Nutritional issues in pediatric inflammatory bowel disease. J Pediatr Gastroenterol Nutr 1991; 12:424–438.

308. Lindor KD, Fleming CR, Burnes JU, Neslon JK, Listrup DM. A randomized prospective trial comparing a defined formula diet, corticosteroids, and a defined formula diet, corticosteroids, and a defined formula diet plus corticosteroids in active Crohn's disease. Mayo Clin Proc 1992; 67:328–333.

309. Logan RF, Gillon J, Ferrington C, Ferguson A. Reduction of gastrointestinal protein loss by elemental diet in Crohn's disease of the small bowel. Gut 1981; 22:383–387.

310. Daum F, Aiges KW. Inflammatory bowel disease in children. In: Lifshitz F, ed. Clinical Disorders in Pediatric Gastroenterology and Nutrition. New York: Marcel Dekker, 1980:145–168.

311. LaSala MA, Lifshitz F, Silverberg M, Wapnir RA, Carrera E. Magnesium metabolism studies in children with chronic inflammatory disease of the bowel. J Pediatr Gastroenterol Nutr 1985; 4:75–81.

312. Nishi Y, Lifshitz F, Bayne MA, Daum F, Silverberg M, Aiges H. Zinc status and its relation to growth retardation in children with chronic inflammatory bowel disease. Am J Clin Nutr 1980; 33:2613–2621.

313. Morin CL, Roulet M, Roy CC, Weber A. Continuous elemental enteral alimentation in children with Crohn's disease and growth failure. Gastroenterology 1980; 79:1205–1210.

314. Motil KJ, Grand RJ, Maletskos CJ, Young VR. The effect of disease, drug and diet on whole body protein metabolism in adolescents with Crohn's disease and growth failure. J Pediatr 1982; 101:345–351.

315. Groll A, Candy DCA, Preece MA, Tanner JM, Harries JT. Short stature as the primary manifestation of coeliac disease. Lancet 1980: 22:1097–1099.

316. Cacciari E, Salardi S, Volta U, Biasco G, Lazzari R, Corazza GR, Feliciani M, Cicognani A, Partesotti S, Azzaroni D, et al. Can antigliadin antibody detect symptomless coeliac disease in children with short stature? Lancet 1985; 1:1469–1471.

317. Rosenbach Y, Dinari G, Zahavi I, Nitzan M. Short stature as the major manifestation of celiac disease in older children. Clin Pediatr (Phila) 1986; 25:13–16.

318. Rossi TM, Albini CH, Kumar V. Incidence of celiac disease identified by the presence of serum endomysial antibodies in children with chronic diarrhea, short stature, or insulin-dependent diabetes mellitus. J Pediatr 1993; 123:262–264.

319. Ashkenazi A, Branski D. Pathogenesis of celiac disease. Part 1. Immunol Allergy Pract 1988; 10:227–234.

320. Ashkenazi A, Branski D. Pathogenesis of celiac disease. Part 2. Immunol Allergy Pract 1988; 10:268–277.

321. Ashkenazi A, Branski D. Pathogenesis of celiac disease. Part 3. Immunol Allergy Pract 1988; 10:315–323.

322. Sandberg DE, Smith MM, Fornari V, Goldstein M, Lifshitz F. Nutritional dwarfing: is it a consequence of disturbed psychosocial functioning? Pediatrics 1991; 88:926–933.

323. Neumark-Sztainer D, Hannan P. Weight-related behaviors among adolescent girls and boys: results from a national survey. Arch Pediatr Adolesc Med 2000; 154:569–577.

324. Abramovitz B, Birch L. Five-year-old girls' ideas about dieting are predicted by their mothers' dieting. J Am Diet Assoc 2000; 100:1157–1163.

325. Schur E, Sanders M, Steiner H. Body dissatisfaction and dieting in young children. Int J Eat Disord 2000; 27:74–82.

326. Neumark-Sztainer D, Rock CL, Thornquist MD, Cheskin LJ, Neuhoser ML, Barnett MJ. Weight-control behaviors among adults and adolescents: associations with dietary intake. Prev Med 2000; 5:381–391.

327. Moses N, Banilvy M, Lifshitz F. Fear of obesity among adolescent girls. Pediatrics 1989; 83:33–398.

328. Vanderwall JG, Thelen MH. Eating and body image concerning obese and average weight children. Addiction Behav 2000; 25:775–778.

329. Stice E, Agras W, Hammer L. Risk factors for the emergence of childhood eating disturbances: a five-year prospective study. Int J Eat Disord 1999; 25:375–387.

330. Johnson S, Birch L. Parents' and children's adiposity and eating style. Pediatrics 1994; 93:653–661.

331. Hood MY, Moore LL, Sundarajan-Ramamurti A, Singer M, Cupples LA, Ellison RC. Parental eating attitudes and the development of obesity in children. The Framingham Children's Study. Int J Obes 2000; 24:1319–1325.

332. Storz NS, Greene WI. Body weight, body image and perception of fad diets in adolescent girls. J Nutr Ed 1983; 15:15–18.

333. Killen JD, Taylor CB, Telch MJ, Saylor KE, Maron DJ, Robinson TN. Self-induced vomiting and laxative and diuretic use among teenagers: precursors of the binge–purge syndrome. JAMA 1986; 255:1447–1449.

334. Tarim O, Newman TB, Lifshitz F. Cholesterol screening and dietary intervention for prevention of adult-onset cardiovascular disease. In: Lifshitz F, ed. Childhood Nutrition. Boca Raton, FL: CRC Press, 1995:13–20.

335. Lifshitz F, Moses N. Nutritional dwarfing: growth, dieting and fear of obesity. J Am Coll Nutr 1988; 7:368–376.

336. Kaistha A, Deckelbaum RJ, Starc TJ, Couch SC. Overrestriction of dietary fat intake before formal nutritional counseling in children with hyperlipidemia. Arch Pediatr Adolesc Med 2001; 155:1225–1230.

337. Garner DM, Garfinkel PE. The eating attitudes test: an index of the symptoms of anorexia nervosa. Psychol Med 1979; 9:273–279.

338. Dietz WH, Hartung R. Changes in height velocity of obese pre-adolescents during weight reduction. Am J Dis Child 1985; 139:704–708.

339. Hadi H, Stoltzfus RJ, Dibley MJ, Moulton LH, West KP Jr, Kjolhede CL, Sadjimin T. Vitamin A supplementation selectively improves the linear growth of Indonesian preschool children: results from a randomized, controlled trial. Am J Clin Nutr 2000; 71:507–513.

340. Muhilal-Permeisih HD, Idjradinata YR, Muherdiyantiningsih D. Vitamin A-fortified monosodium glutamate and health, growth and survival of children: a controlled field trial. Am J Clin Nutr 1988; 48:1271–1276.

341. Fawzi WW, Herrera MG, Willett WC, Nestel P, el Amin A, Mohamed KA. Dietary vitamin A intake in relation to child growth. Epidemiology 1997; 8:402–407.

342. Fawzi WW, Herrera MG, Wilett WC, Nestel P, el Amin A, Mohamed KA. The effect of vitamin A supplementa-

tion on the growth of preschool children in the Sudan. Am J Public Health 1997; 87:1359–1362.

343. Rahmathullah L, Underwood BA, Thulasiraj RD, Milton RC. Diarrhea, respiratory infections, and growth are not affected by a weekly low-dose vitamin A supplement: a masked, controlled field trial in children in southern India. Am J Clin Nutr 1991: 54:568–577.

344. Latham MC, Stephenson LS, Kinoti SN, Zaman MS, Kurz KM. Improvements in growth following iron supplementation in young Kenyan school children. Nutrition 1990; 6:159–165.

345. Lawless JW, Latham MC, Stephenson LS, Kinoti SN, Pertet AM. Iron supplementation improves appetite and growth in anemic Kenyan primary school children. J Nutr 1994; 124:645–654.

346. Allen LH. Malnutrition and human function: a comparison of conclusions from the INCAP and nutrition CRSP studies. J Nutr 1995; 125:1119S–1126S.

347. Beaton G, Ghassemi H. Supplementary feeding programs for young children in developing countries. Am J Clin Nutr 1982; 35:864–916.

348. Prasad AS, Miale A, Farid Z, Sandstead HH, Schulert AR. Zinc metabolism in patients with the syndrome or iron deficiency anemia, hepatosplenomegaly, dwarfism and hypogonadism. J Lab Clin Med 1963; 61:537–549.

349. Prasad AS. Zinc deficiency in women, infants and children. J Am Coll Nutr 1996; 15:113–120.

350. Hambidge KM, Hambidge C, Jacobs M, Baum JD. Low levels of zinc in hair, anorexia, poor growth, and hypogeusia in children. Pediatr Res 1972; 6:868–874.

351. Slonim AE, Sadick N, Pugliese M, Meyers-Seifer CH. Clinical response of alopecia, trichorrhexis nodosa, and dry, scaly skin to zinc supplementation. J Pediatr 1992; 121:890–895.

352. Favier AE. Hormonal effects of zinc on growth in children. Biol Trace Elem Res 1992; 32:383–398.

353. Kirksey A, Wachs TD, Yunis F, Srinath U, Rahmanifar A, McCabe GP, Galal OM, Harrison GG, Jerome NW. Relation of maternal zinc nutriture to pregnancy outcome and infant development in an Egyptian village. Am J Clin Nutr 1994: 60:782–792.

354. Neggers YH, Cutter GR, Acton RT, Alvarez JO, Bonner JL, Goldenberg RL, Go RC, Roseman JM. A positive association between maternal serum zinc concentration and birth weight. Am J Clin Nutr 1990; 51:678–684.

355. Osendarp SJM, van Raaij JMA, Arifeen SE, Wahed MA, Baqui AH, Fuchs GJ. A randomized, placebo-controlled trial of the effect of zinc supplementation during pregnancy on pregnancy outcome in Bangladeshi urban poor. Am J Clin Nutr 2000: 71:114–119.

356. Michaelsen KF, Samuelson G, Graham TW, Lonnerdal B. Zinc intake, zinc status and growth in a longitudinal study of healthy Danish infants. Acta Paediatr 1994; 83:1115–1121.

357. Kaji M, Gotoh M, Takagi Y, Masuda H, Kimura Y, Uenoyama Y. Studies to determine the usefulness of the zinc clearance test to diagnose marginal zinc deficiency and the effects of oral zinc supplementation for short children. J Am Coll Nutr 1998; 17:388–391.

358. Nakamura T, Nishiyama S, Futagoishi-Suginohara Y, Matsuda I, Higashi A. Mild to moderate zinc deficiency in short children: effect of zinc supplementation on linear growth velocity. J Pediatr 1993; 123:65–69.

359. Nishi Y, Hatano S, Aihara K, Fujie A, Kihara M. Transient partial growth hormone deficiency due to zinc deficiency. J Am Coll Nutr 1989; 8:93–97.

360. Nishi Y. Zinc and growth. J Am Coll Nutr 1996; 15:340–344.

361. Ninh NX, Thissen JP, Maiter D, Adam E, Mulumba N, Ketelslegers JM. Reduced liver insulin-like growth factor-I gene expression in young zinc-deprived rats is associated with a decrease in liver growth hormone (GH) receptors and serum GH-binding protein. J Endocrinol 1995; 144:449–456.

362. Yamaguchi M. Role of zinc in bone formation and bone resorption. J Trace Elem Exp Med 1998; 11:119–135.

363. Yamaguchi M, Inamoto K. Differential effects of calcium-regulating sulfate hormones on bone metabolism on weanling rats orally administered zinc sulfate. Metabolism 1986; 35:1044–1047.

364. McDonell DP, Mongelsdorf DJ, Pike JW, Haussler MR, O'Malley BW. Molecular cloning of complementary DNA encoding the avian receptor for vitamin D. Science 1987; 235:1214–1217.

365. Rosado JL, Lopez P, Munoz E, Martinez H, Allen LH. Zinc supplementation reduced morbidity, but neither zinc nor iron supplementation affected growth or body composition of Mexican preschoolers. Am J Clin Nutr 1997; 65:13–19.

366. Bates CJ, Evans PH, Dardenne M, Prentice A, Lunn PG, Northrop-Clewes CA, Hoare S, Cole TJ, Horan SJ, Longman SC. A trial of zinc supplementation in young rural Gambian children. Br J Nutr 1993; 69:243–255.

367. Meeks Gardner J, Witter MM, Ramdath DD. Zinc supplementation: effects on the growth and morbidity of undernourished Jamaican children. Eur J Clin Nutr 1998; 52:34–39.

368. Rosado JL. Separate and joint effects of micronutrient deificiencies on linear growth. J Nutr 1999; 129:531S–533S.

369. Hambidge MK. Zinc deficiency in young children. Am J Clin Nutr 1997; 65:160–161.

370. Prentice A. Does mild zinc deficiency contribute to poor growth performance? Nutr Rev 1993; 51:268–270.

371. Brown KH, Peerson JM, Allen LH. Effect of zinc supplementation on children's growth: a meta-analysis of intervention trials. Bibl Nutr Dieta 1998; 54:76–83.

372. Shalet SM, Toogood A, Rahim A, Brennan BM. The diagnosis of growth hormone deficiency in children and adults. Endocr Rev 1998; 19(2):203–223.

373. Deller JJ, Boulis MW, Harriss WE, Hutsell TC, Garcia JF, Linfoot JA. Growth hormone response patterns to sex hormone administration in growth retardation. Am J Med Sci 1979; 259:292–296.

374. Martin LG, Clark JW, Connor TB. Growth hormone secretion enhanced by androgens. J Clin Endocrinol Meta 1968; 28:425–428.

375. Greene SA, Torresani T, Prader A. Growth hormone response to a standardized exercise test in relation to puberty and stature. Arch Dis Child 1987; 62:53–56.

376. Pugliese M, Lifshitz F, Fort P, Cervantes C, Recker B, Ginsberg L. Pituitary assessment in short stature by a combined hormone stimulation test. Am J Dis Child 1587; 141:556–561.

377. Bercu BB, Shulman DJ, Root AW, Spiliotis BE. Growth hormone provocative testing frequently does not reflect endogenous GH secretion. J Clin Enocrinol Metab 1986; 63:709–716.

378. Rose SR, Ross JL, Uriarte M, Barnes KM, Cassorla FG, Cutler JB Jr. The advantage of measuring stimulated as

compared with spontaneous growth hormone levels in the diagnosis of growth hormone deficiency. N Engl J Med 1988; 319:201–207.

379. Lanes R. Diagnostic limitations of spontaneous growth hormone measurements in normally growing prepubertal children. Am J Dis Child 1989; 143:1284–1286.

380. Blum WF, Ranke MB, Kietzmann K, Gauggel E, Zeisel HJ, Bierich JR. A specific radioimmunoassay for the growth hormone-dependent somatomedin-binding protein: its use for diagnosis of GH deficiency. J Clin Endocrinol Metab 1990; 70:1292–1298.

381. Hasegawa Y, Hasegawa T, Aso T, Kotoh S, Tsuchiya Y, Nose O, Ohyama Y, Araki K, Taranka T, Saisyo S, et al. Usefulness and limitation of measurement of insulin-like growth factor binding protein-3 (IGFBP-3) for diagnosis of growth hormone deficieiency. Endocrinol Jpn 1992; 39:585–591.

382. Sklar C, Sarafoglou K, Whittam E. Efficacy of insulin-like growth factor-I and IGF-binding protein-3 in predicting the growth hormone response to provocative testing in children treated with cranial irradiation. Acta Endocrinol (Copenh) 1993; 129:511–515.

383. Smith WJ, Nam TJ, Underwood LE, Busby WH, Celnicker A, Clemmons DR. Use of insulin-like growth factor binding protein-2 (IGFBP-2), IGFBP-3 and IGF-1 for assessing growth hormone status in short children. J Clin Endocrinol Metab 1993; 77:1294–1299.

384. Sandberg DE. Short stature: intellectual and behavioral aspects. In: Lifshitz F, ed. Pediatric Endocrinology, 3rd ed. New York: Marcel Dekker, 1996:149–162.

385. Blizzard RM, Bulatovic A. Syndromes of psychosocial short stature. In: Lifshitz F, ed. Pediatric Endocrinology, 3rd ed. New York: Marcel Dekker, 1996:83–94.

386. Meyer-Bahlburg HFL. Short stature: psychological issues. In: Lifshitz F, ed. Pediatric Endocrinology, 2nd ed. New York: Marcel Dekker, 1990:173–196.

2

Hypopituitarism and Other Disorders of the Growth Hormone and Insulin-Like Growth Factor Axis

Arlan L. Rosenbloom
University of Florida College of Medicine, Gainesville, Florida, U.S.A.

Ellen Lancon Connor
University of Wisconsin, Madison, Wisconsin, U.S.A.

I. INTRODUCTION

Disorders involving the growth hormone (GH) pathway result in insulin like growth factor-I (IGF-I) deficiency or ineffectiveness and may be congenital or acquired. Congenital GH deficiency is associated with structural malformations of the central nervous system, hypothalamus, or pituitary. IGF-I deficiency/resistance may result from genetic defects involving critical factors in the embryological development of the pituitary or in the cascade from hypothalamic stimulation of GH release to completion of IGF effects on growth. Acquired abnormalities affecting the GH/IGF axis range from damage to the hypothalamic–pituitary region from tumors, infection, autoimmune disease, or radiation to a broad spectrum of chronic conditions characterized by catabolism.

The frequency of GH deficiency (GHD) has been estimated in various studies to range from 1:4000 to 1:10,000 (1). Estimates based on clinic referral populations are inherently biased. An excellent population-based study of 80,000 schoolchildren in Salt Lake City documented growth rates over 1 year; of the 555 children who were below the third percentile in height and had growth rates <5 cm/year, 16 had previously undiagnosed GHD. Combined with known instances in the population (i.e., children being treated for GHD), this gave a prevalence estimate of 1:3500 in the school-age population (2). An estimate of relative contributions of organic and idiopathic or genetic causes can be gleaned from the large post marketing databases of manufacturers of recombinant human (rh) GH. Among >20,000 children being treated with rhGH registered in the National Cooperative Growth Study, ~25% of those with proven GHD had an organic

cause. Nearly half of these (47%) were central nervous system (CNS) tumors, including craniopharyngioma, 15% were CNS malformations, 14% septo-optic dysplasia, 9% leukemia, 9% CNS radiation, 3% trauma, 2% histiocytosis, and 1% CNS infection (3). Comparable findings were obtained in the European postmarketing surveillance study (Kabi International Growth Study; KIGS). Some 22% of approximately 15,500 children with GHD had an organic cause, congenital in 24% of this subgroup. The most common central malformation was empty sella, accounting for 37%, followed by septo-optic dysplasia in 24% of those with congenital organic GHD. Among the 76% of patients with organic GHD considered acquired, craniopharyngioma accounted for 24% and other CNS tumors for 30%, leukemia 16%, histiocytosis 3.5%, trauma 3%, and CNS infection 1% (4).

II. PITUITARY GLAND, GROWTH HORMONE, AND IGF-I

A. Embryology of the Pituitary Gland

The pituitary, traditionally considered the "master gland," appears early in embryonic life. At 3 weeks' gestation, the ectodermal stomodeum of the embryo develops an outpouching anterior to the buccopharyngeal membrane. This outpocketing is Rathke's pouch, which usually separates from the oral cavity and will give rise to the adenohypophysis of the pituitary gland. An evagination of the diencephalon then gives rise to the neurohypophysis of the pituitary gland. In rare cases, the primitive oral cavity origin of the pituitary results in a functional pharyngeal adenohypophysis (5). The fetal pituitary gland consists of the pars distalis (anterior lobe), pars nervosa (posterior lobe), and the pars intermedia (6). Secretion of pituitary hormones can be detected as early as week 12 in the fetus, and some of these hormones are found within the pituitary by 8 weeks' gestation (7). Average newborn pituitary weight is 100 mg.

Differentiation of the primordial pituitary gland requires a cascade of factors to be expressed in critical temporal and spatial relationships. These include extracellular signaling factors from the adjacent diencephalon that initiate anterior pituitary gland development from the oral ectoderm, and transcription factors that control pituitary cell differentiation and specification. Several homeodomain transcription factors directing embryological development of the anterior pituitary have been found to have mutations that result in congenital defects affecting the synthesis of GH and one or more additional pituitary hormones (9, 10).

The homeobox gene expressed in embryonic stem cells (HESX1) is important in development of the optic nerve, as well as of the anterior pituitary. HESX1 has also been referred to as the Rathke's pouch homeobox gene (Rpx). The three mutations that have been described account for a small minority of instances of septo-optic dysplasia with variable GH and other pituitary deficiencies (11).

LIM-type homeodomain proteins (named for the 3 homeodomain proteins lin-11, Islet-1, and mec-3), known as LHX3 accumulate in the Rathke pouch and the primordium of the pituitary and are thought to be involved in the establishment and maintenance of the differentiated cell types (12). Only four patients in two families have been described with mutations of this transcription factor, which results in deficiencies of all pituitary hormones except adrenocorticotropin, and cervical spine rigidity indicating extrapituitary function for this factor (13).

Prophet of Pit1 (PROP1) represses HESX1 expression at the appropriate time and is required for initial determination of pituitary cell lineages, including gonadotropes and those of Pit1 (GH, thyroid-stimulating hormone [TSH], prolactin [PRL]). Nine recessive mutations have been described in PROP1 that result in GH, PRL, TSH, gonadotropin, and variable adrenocorticotropin (ACTH) deficiency. Eleven recessive and four dominant mutations have been reported affecting the Pit1 gene, with resultant GH, PRL, and TSH deficiency (10, 14).

Somatotroph development is also dependent on hypothalamic GH-releasing hormone (GHRH). Mutation in the gene encoding the GHRH receptor results in severe GH deficiency (15, 16).

B. Functional Anatomy of the Pituitary Gland

The adult pituitary weighs 0.5 g and has average dimensions of 10 × 13 × 6 mm (Fig. 1). The pars intermedia is vestigial in the adult, except in pregnancy. The adenohypophysis receives hormonal modulating signals from the hypothalamus, transmitted from ventromedial and infundibular nuclei axons that terminate in the hypophyseal portal system. These signals result in production of specialized cells of the pars distalis of ACTH by 8 weeks gestation, TSH by 15 weeks gestation, somatotropin (GH) by 10–11 weeks gestation, prolactin by 12 weeks, and the gonadotropes, luteinizing hormone (LH) and follicle-stimulating hormone (FSH) by 11 weeks,. The pars distalis has at least three distinct hormone-producing cell populations classified by staining characteristics (8). Fifty percent of the cells are chromophobes, 40% are characterized as acidophils, and the remainder as basophils. Acidophils secrete GH or prolactin. Basophils secrete TSH, LH, FSH, or ACTH. Some basophils have a positive periodic acid–Schiff (PAS) base reaction: these are the cells that secrete the glycoproteins LH, FSH, or TSH. Although chromophobe cells arc known to produce ACTH in the rat pituitary, the role of these cells in the human pituitary remains unclear.

Anterior pituitary hormones enter the portal venous system to drain into the cavernous sinus, enter the general circulation, and ultimately exert long-distance influence over their respective target organs. PRL has an effect on lactation through direct effects on breast ductal tissue. ACTH stimulates the adrenal cortical production of cortisol and affects renal reabsorption of water. TSH promotes growth of the thyroid and production of thyroxine. LH and FSH stimulate gonadal maturation and hormonal cycling. GH exerts indirect growth effects through the elaboration of IGF-I in the liver, direct growth effects on bone, and direct metabolic effects, primarily in adipose tissue. Although the pars intermedia had been identified as a site of possible melanocyte-stimulating hormone (MSH) production, more recent studies suggest that MSH is actually being produced in the pars distalis and enters the portal venous system to exert a distant effect on skin pigmentation (17).

The pars nervosa, or infundibular process, and the infundibulum, or neural stalk, comprise the neurohypophysis. The infundibulum consists of the pituitary stalk and median eminence and is the direct connection to the hypothalamus. The neurohypophysis receives, stores, and releases two important hormones produced in the hypothalamus. These hormones, oxytocin and arginine vasopressin, originate in the supraoptic and paraventricular nuclei of the hypothalamus. The 100,000 axons of these nuclei are unmyelinated and form the supraopticohypophyseal tract that transports oxytocin and vasopressin to be stored in the posterior lobe of the pituitary (7, 18).

The rich blood supply of the pituitary gland is subject to interruption during periods of severe hypotensive stress and hypoxia, resulting in the Sheehan syndrome of hypopituitarism. This is classically described after intrapartum hypotension, but is possible in any hypovolemic crisis or increased intracranial pressure episode, as in hypopi-

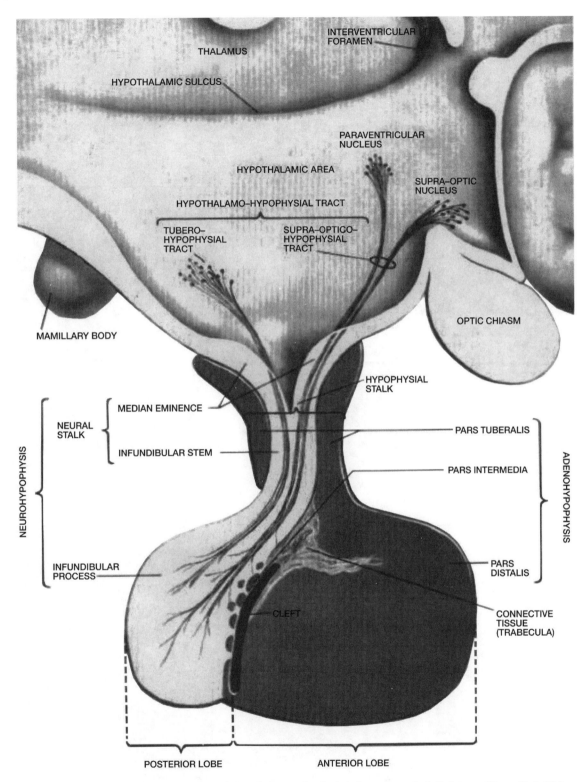

Figure 1 Diagrammatic illustration of the pituitary gland, showing anatomical divisions. (From Ref. 20.)

tuitarism following recovery from cerebral edema (19). The internal carotid arteries supply the vascular branches that bathe the pituitary. The right and left superior hypophyseal arteries, which branch into anterior and posterior divisions, supply the median eminence and infundib-

ulum. The neurohypophysis and stalk are supplied by the right and left inferior hypophyseal arteries. The hypophyseal portal vessels, which originate from capillary beds in the median eminence and infundibular stem, supply the pars distalis (Fig. 2) (18, 20).

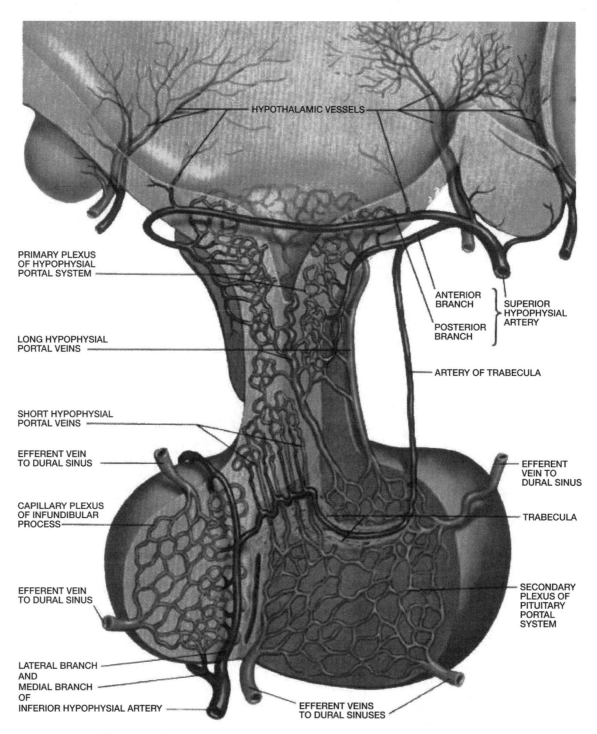

Figure 2   Diagrammatic illustration of pituitary blood supply. (From Ref. 20.)

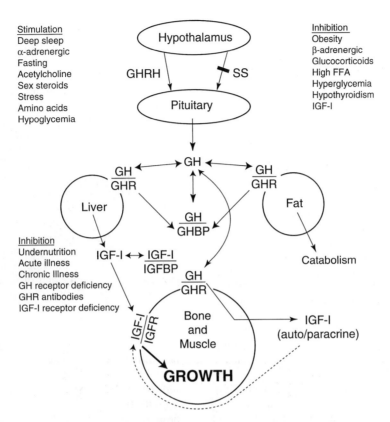

Figure 3 Simplified diagram of the GH-IGF-I axis involving hypophysiotropic hormones controlling pituitary GH release, circulating GH binding protein and its GH receptor source, IGF-I and its largely GH-dependent binding proteins, and cellular responsiveness to GH and IGF-I interacting with their specific receptors. (Reprinted from Trends in Endocrinology and Metabolism, vol. 5, Rosenbloom AL, Guevara-Aguirre J, Rosenfeld RG, Pollock BH, Growth in growth hormone insensitivity, pages 296–303. © 1994, with permission from Elsevier Science.)

C. Biochemistry and Physiology of the GH/IGF-I/IGF-Binding Protein Axis

1. GH

Human GH is a single-chain, 191 amino acid, 22 kD protein, containing two intramolecular disulfide bonds (21). Release of GH from the anterior pituitary somatotrophs is controlled by the balance between stimulatory GHRH and inhibitory somatostatin (SS) from the hypothalamus (Fig. 3). This balance is regulated by a variety of neurological, metabolic, and hormonal influences; numerous neurotransmitters and neuropeptides are involved. These include vasopressin, corticotropin-releasing hormone, thyrotropin-releasing hormone, neuropeptide Y, dopamine, serotonin, histamine, norepinephrine, and acetylcholine, which respond to various circumstances that affect GH secretion such as sleep, fed–fasting state, stress, and exercise. Other hormones including glucocorticoids, sex steroids, and thyroid hormone also influence secretion of GH. These various influences are important in the evaluation of GH secretion, which may give abnormal results despite normal somatotroph function.

Stimulation of GH release by GHRH is via specific GHRH receptors. A number of synthetic hexapeptides, referred to as GH-releasing peptides (GHRPs), have been developed that act on other receptors to stimulate GH release (22, 23). The naturally occurring ligand for the GHRP receptor, ghrelin, has been isolated and cloned (24). Ghrelin is unique among mammalian peptides in its requirement of a posttranslational modification for activation. This involves addition of a straight chain octanyl group conferring a hydrophobic property on the N terminus that may permit entry of the molecule into the brain. Similarly to synthetic GHRPs, ghrelin binds with high affinity and specificity to a distinct G protein-coupled receptor (25). Unlike GHRH, ghrelin is synthesized primarily in the fundus of the stomach (24), as well as in the hypothalamus (26) and its receptor is more widely distributed than that of GHRH. Ghrelin may have widespread metabolic effects in addition to being synergistic with GHRH in the stimulation of GH release.

Some 75% of circulating GH is in the 22 kD form. Alternative splicing of codon 2 results in a deletion of 11 amino acids and formation of a 20 kD fragment accounting for 5–10% of secreted GH. Other circulating forms include deamidated, N-acetylated, and oligomeric GH. About 50% of GH circulates in the free state, the rest bound principally to GH binding protein (GHBP). Because the binding sites for the radioimmunoassay of GH are not affected by the GHBP, both bound and unbound GH are measured (27).

2. GHBP

A high-affinity GHBP was identified in rabbit and human serum in the mid-1980s (28), and separate reports in 1987 found this binding protein to be absent in the sera of patients with GH resistance (29, 30), who were identified by high circulating GH concentration with a clinical picture of severe GH deficiency. The recognition that circulating GHBP in rabbit serum corresponded to liver cytosolic GHBP was followed by the purification, cloning, and sequencing of human GHBP (31). The human GHBP was found to be structurally identical to the extracellular hormone-binding domain of the membrane bound GH receptor (GHR). The entire human GHR gene, localized to the proximal short arm of chromosome 5, was subsequently characterized (32). The GHR was the first to be cloned of a family of receptors that includes the receptor for prolactin and numerous cytokine receptors. Members of this family share ligand and receptor structure similarities, in particular the requirement that the ligand bind to two or more receptors or receptor subunits and interact with signal transducer proteins to activate tyrosine kinases (33).

In humans, GHBP is the proteolytic product of the extracellular domain of the GHR. This characteristic permits the assaying of circulating GHBP as a measure of cellular-bound GHR, which usually correlates with GHR function. The GH molecule binds to cell surface GHR, which dimerizes with another GHR so that a single GH molecule is enveloped by two GHR molecules (34). The intact receptor lacks tyrosine kinase activity, but is closely associated with JAK2, a member of the Janus kinase family. JAK2 is activated by binding of GH with the GHR dimer, which results in self-phosphorylation of the JAK2 and a cascade of phosphorylation of cellular proteins. Included in this cascade are signal transducers and activators of transcription (STATs), which couple ligand binding to the activation of gene expression, and mitogen-activated protein kinases (MAPK). Other effector proteins have also been examined in various systems. This is a mechanism typical of the growth hormone/prolactin/cytokine receptor family (27, 35).

The GH receptor in humans is also synthesized in a truncated form (GHRtr) lacking most of the intracellular domain. Although the quantity of this GHRtr is small relative to the full-length GHR, release of GHBP from this isoform is increased (36). Some of the changes in body composition that occur with GH treatment in GH deficiency may be related to changes in the relative expression of GHR and GHRtr (37).

3. IGF-I

Most of the growth effect that gives GH its name is indirect, via stimulation of IGF-I production, primarily in the liver (38). IGF-I is a 70 residue single-chain basic peptide, and IGF-II a slightly acidic 67 residue peptide. Their structure is similar to that of proinsulin: A and B chains connected by disulfide bonds and a connecting C-peptide, but unlike the posttranslational processing of insulin, there is no cleavage of the C-peptide. The two IGFs share approximately two-thirds of their possible amino acid positions and are 50% homologous to insulin (39, 40). The connecting C-peptide is 12 amino acids long in the IGF-I molecule and 8 amino acids long in IGF-II, and has no homology with the comparable region in the proinsulin molecule. The IGFs also differ from proinsulin in having carboxy terminal extensions. These similarities and differences from insulin explain the ability of IGFs to bind to the insulin receptor and insulin's ability to bind to the type 1 IGF receptor, as well as the specificity of IGF binding to the IGFBPs.

4. IGFBPs

Hepatic IGF-I circulates almost entirely bound to IGF-binding proteins (IGFBPs), with <1% being free. The IGFBPs are a family of 6 structurally related proteins with a high affinity for binding IGF. At least 4 other related proteins with lower affinity for IGF peptides have been identified and are referred to as IGFBP-related proteins (41). The principal BP, IGFBP-3, binds 75–90% of circulating IGF-I in a large (150–200 kD) complex consisting of IGFBP-3, an acid-labile subunit (ALS), and the IGF molecule. ALS and IGFBP-3 are produced in the liver as a direct effect of GH. The remainder of bound IGF is in a 50 kD complex with mostly IGFBP-1 and IGFBP-2. IGFBP-1 concentrations are controlled by nutritional status as reflected in insulin levels, with the highest IGFBP-1 concentrations found in the fasting, hypoinsulinemic state. The circulating concentration of IGFBP-2 is less fluctuant and partly under the control of IGF-I; levels are increased in IGF-I deficiency due to GH insensitivity, but increase further with IGF-I therapy (42).

The actions of IGFBPs are under intense investigation (38, 43, 44). The IGFBPs modulate IGF action by controlling storage and release of IGF-I in the circulation and influencing its binding to its receptor, facilitate storage of IGFs in extracellular matrices, and exert independent actions. IGFBPs 1, 2, 4, and 6 inhibit IGF action by preventing binding of IGF-I with its specific receptor. The binding of IGFBP-3 to cell surfaces is thought to decrease its affinity, effectively delivering the IGF-I to the type 1 IGF receptor. IGFBP-5 potentiates the effects of IGF-I in a variety of cells. Its binding to extracellular matrix proteins allows fixation of IGFs and enhances binding to hydroxyapatite. IGFs stored in such a manner in soft tissue may enhance wound healing. IGF-independent mechanisms for IGFBP-1 and IGFBP-3 proliferative effects have been demonstrated in vitro and nuclear localization of IGFBP-3 has been reported. In addition to IGFBP phosphorylation and cell surface association determining the influence of IGFBPs, specific protease activity, particularly affecting IGFBP-3, is also important in the modulation of IGF action in target tissues. The proteolytic activity may alter the affinity of the binding protein for IGF-I, resulting in release of free IGF-I for binding to the IGF-I receptor (38, 43, 44).

5. IGF Receptors

IGF binding involves three types of receptors: the structurally homologous insulin receptor and type 1 IGF receptor and the distinctive type 2 IGF-II/mannose-6-phosphate receptor (Fig. 4). Splice variants and atypical forms occur but have not been found to have physiological significance, Insulin/IGF-I hybrid receptors, however, are ubiquitous and may be the most important receptors for IGF-I in some tissues (44).

The type 1 IGF-I receptor and insulin receptor are heterotetramers consisting of two alpha subunits that contain the binding sites and two beta subunits containing a transmembrane domain, an ATP-binding site, and a tyro-

sine kinase domain comprising the signal transduction system (44). The IGF-I receptor is able to bind IGF-I and IGF-II with high affinity but the affinity for insulin is approximately 100-fold less. Although the insulin receptor has a low affinity for IGF-I, IGF-I is present in the circulation at molar concentrations 1000 times those of insulin. Thus, even a small insulin-like effect of IGF-I could be more important than that of insulin itself, were it not for the IGFBPs that control the availability and activity of IGF-I. In fact, intravenous infusion of rhIGF-I can induce hypoglycemia, especially in the IGFBP-3-deficient state (45). It is not known why IGF-II and M6P share a receptor. This receptor differs from the type 1 receptor in binding only IGF-II with high affinity, IGF-I with low affinity, and insulin not all (44).

D. Role of IGF-I in Growth

The importance of IGF-I in normal intrauterine growth in humans has been demonstrated in a single patient with a homozygous partial deletion of the IGF-I gene (46), and in a second patient with inactivating mutations of the IGF-I receptor (47), both having severe intrauterine growth

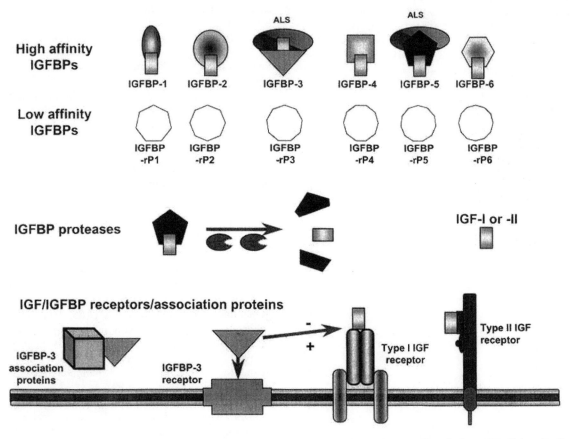

Figure 4 Components of the IGF-IGFBP-IGF/IGFBP receptor axis. (Reprinted from Collett-Solberg PF, Cohen P. Genetics, chemistry, and function of the IGF/IGFBP system. Endocrine 2000; 12:121–136, with permission from Humana Press.)

retardation. Cord serum IGF-I and IGF-II concentrations correlate with birth weight and are significantly increased in large for gestational age infants compared with appropriate for gestational age newborns (48). Intrauterine IGF-I synthesis, however, does not appear to be GH dependent, because most patients with genetically determined severe IGF-I deficiency, due to GHRH defects, GH receptor deficiency (GHRD), or GH gene mutations, have normal or only minimally reduced intrauterine growth. Standard deviation score (SDS) for length declines rapidly after birth, however, in these conditions, demonstrating the immediate need for GH-stimulated IGF-I synthesis for postnatal growth (49). Growth velocity in the absence of GH is approximately half normal (49).

The metabolic and growth effects of GH and IGF-I are compared in Table 1. In addition to direct protein-sparing effects and synthesis and release of IGF-I from the liver, GH stimulates autocrine and paracrine production of IGF-I in other tissues, primarily bone and muscle (Fig. 3). GH has a direct effect on differentiation of prechondrocytes into early chondrocytes, which in turn secrete IGF-I. This local IGF-I stimulates clonal expansion and maturation of the chondrocytes, resulting in growth (50). It is estimated that 20% of GH-influenced growth is the result of the direct effect of GH on maturing bone and the autocrine/paracrine production of IGF-I in this tissue (51). Treatment studies of children with GHRD given IGF-I compared to GH-deficient patients treated with GH support this hypothesis (52, 53). IGF-II is considered an important growth factor in utero, but its role in extrauterine life is unclear; concentrations of IGF-II in serum parallel those of IGF-I.

III. CLASSIFICATION OF DISORDERS INVOLVING THE GH/IGF-I AXIS

The classification in Table 2 is based on the fundamental role of IGF-I, with *primary IGF-I deficiency* referring to

genetic and acquired defects in IGF-I synthesis, *secondary IGF-I deficiency* including congenital and acquired GH insensitivity, *tertiary IGF-I deficiency* including congenital and acquired forms of GH deficiency, and *IGF-I insensitivity*.

IV. CONGENITAL GH DEFICIENCY

A. Hypothalamic–Pituitary Malformations

Anterior and posterior pituitary deficiencies associated with various congenital syndromes affecting the hypothalamus, the pituitary, or both may be discovered through magnetic resonance imaging (MRI) of the hypothalamus and pituitary gland. These abnormalities may result in apparent deficiencies in infancy or not until later in childhood.

Anencephaly has long been recognized as a cause of an ectopic, hypoplastic, or malformed pituitary gland (54, 55). Slightly less severe in the clinical spectrum of major cranial malformations, holoprosencephaly is commonly associated with hypothalamic defects resulting in pituitary hormone deficiency. Associated defects can range from cyclopia to hypertelorism, with varying coexistent defects, including palatal or lip clefts, nasal septal aplasia, or, in surviving older children, a single central incisor (56, 57). Schizencephaly, sometimes identified by MRI during evaluation of gait disturbance, can also be associated with hypothalamic–pituitary malformation. Lastly, even isolated cleft lip or palate may be associated with hypothalamic or pituitary defects (58, 59).

Septo-optic dysplasia (SOD) is another malformation syndrome closely associated with hypopituitarism (60). At least 50% of children with SOD have hypopituitarism (54, 61). A child identified as having SOD should be referred to a pediatric endocrinologist for monitoring or testing. In its most severe form, SOD is associated with hypoplasia or absence of the optic nerves or chiasm, agenesis or hypoplasia of the septum pellucidum, and hypothalamic defects, and is known as deMorsier syndrome (59, 62–64). Typically, growth failure due to GH deficiency becomes apparent between 6 and 18 months of age.

Other specific, rare genetic syndromes can be associated with hypopituitarism. Rieger's syndrome, the result of a transcription factor gene mutation, results in hypopituitarism associated with coloboma of the iris, glaucoma, and dental hypoplasia (65, 66). Pallister Hall syndrome is associated with hypothalamic hamartoma-blastoma, micropenis, cryptorchidism, and postaxial polydactyly (67). Because MRI is used increasingly in the evaluation of children with unexplained neurological findings, additional genetic syndromes affecting the structural integrity of the hypothalamic–pituitary axis may be recognized. The use of MRI has led to the recognition that many children thought to have idiopathic GH deficiency actually have abnormal posterior pituitary or stalk regions (68).

Table 1 Metabolic Effects of GH and IGF-I

	GH	IGF-I
GH secretion	—	Decreased
IGF-I production	Increased	—
IGFBP-1	Decreased	Decreased
IGFBP-2	Decreased	Increased
IGFBP-3	Increased	No effect
Insulin: secretion	Increased	Decreased
sensitivity	Decreased	Increased
Hepatic glucose output	Increased	Decreased
Muscle glucose uptake	Decreased	Increased
Lipolysis	Increased	No effect[a]
Nitrogen balance	Increased	Increased
Protein synthesis	Increased	Increased

[a]Decreased with very high dosages.

Table 2 Classification of IGF-I Deficiency and IGF-I Resistance with Clinical and Biochemical Features

Condition	GHD[a]	Ht SDS	Biochemistry			
			GH	GHBP	IGF-I	IGFBP-3
Primary IGF-I Deficiency						
Congenital						
Defect in IGF-I synthesis	No	−6.9 (IUGR)	High	Normal	Very low	Normal
Acquired						
Alagille syndrome (12)	No	Varies	High	High	Low	Normal
Secondary IGF-I Deficiency						
Congenital						
GH receptor deficiency	Yes	−4 to −12	High	Low/nml/high	Very low	Low
GH–GHR signal transduction defect	Yes (Arab) No (Pakistani)	−3.4 to −6	High	Normal	Very low	nml/low
Acquired						
Catabolic states/chronic illness	No	Normal–low	High	Low/nml	Low	nml/low
Tertiary IGF-I Deficiency						
Congenital						
GHRH receptor deficiency	No	−4.3 to −8.9	Low	Normal	Low	Low
GHD	Yes	≤3	Low	Normal	Low	Low
Acquired						
GH inhibiting antibodies	Yes	−3 to −8.5	Low	Normal	Low	Low
GHD	Yes	Varies	Low	Normal	Low	Low
IGF-I Insensitivity						
Congenital						
IGF receptor deficiency	No	Severe/IUGR	High	Normal	High	High
IGF–IGFR signal transduction defects	No	−2 to −4.6	Normal	?	High	?

[a]Phenotype.

Ht SDS, standard deviation score for height.

Some children found to have hypopituitarism have MRI findings of an interrupted pituitary stalk. The lesion may be congenital and accompanied by varying degrees of diabetes insipidus or anterior pituitary deficiencies. Other instances are probably acquired during trauma and may show some recovery of function later.

Hypothalamic dysfunction may explain the not infrequent finding of the short child with abnormal growth velocity and delayed bone age who, to the surprise of the endocrinologist, has a normal response to provocative GH testing. Some investigators have surmised that these children, while able to produce GH in response to pharmocological stimuli, fail to have adequate daily secretion of GHRH and thus, GH (69). This may be particularly true for a subset of children: those who have had prophylactic intracranial irradiation for leukemia (70). Children with GH deficiency following cranial radiation were found to respond to GHRH administration with augmented levels of GH (71).

Spontaneous GH secretion testing for this neurosecretory disorder can be cumbersome, requiring an indwelling catheter and the obtaining of frequent spontaneous growth hormone samples over a 24 h period or a nocturnal 12 h period. For this reason and because GHRH is not a commercially available therapeutic option, common practice is to pursue a trial of GH therapy, usually for 6 months, in the short child with poor growth velocity and normal provocative GH testing results.

Another example in which the phenotype of GH deficiency may be hypothalamic in origin is the child with Prader–Labhart–Willi syndrome (PLWS), resulting from partial deletion of chromosome 15 or maternal uniparental disomy (i.e., the loss of paternally derived genetic material on chromosome 15). PLWS results in a phenotype of variable short stature, hypothalamic obesity, hypotonia, and hypogonadism (72). GH therapy results in an increase in lean body mass and growth velocity sustained over the 2 years of reported trials of therapy (73).

The empty sella syndrome is frequently found by MRI during the evaluation of children with isolated growth hormone deficiency or panhypopituitarism, but is only a finding in 2% of healthy children (74). Mild elevation of serum prolactin may be observed. The empty sella is the enlarged pituitary fossa, the size of which has been altered by herniated arachnoid contents. An empty sella may be a primary or secondary finding (75). Secondary causes include surgery, irradiation, and tumor. The actual pituitary tissue is flattened against the fossa wall, leading to varying degrees of hypopituitarism.

Prenatal and postnatal injuries are known to result in the birth of some infants with hypopituitarism (76). Breech delivery is also associated with hypopituitarism, but may be the result rather than the cause of hypopituitarism (77). Support for this hypothesis includes the finding of microphallus in some newborn boys with perinatal asphyxia (78, 79), suggesting inadequate prenatal gonadotropin, GH, or both. In some instances, however, perinatal asphyxia may compromise pituitary blood flow with subsequent ischemic pituitary damage.

B. Hereditary Forms of GH Deficiency

Although studies of GH response with GHRH and GH-releasing peptides indicate a hypothalamic basis for many instances of GHD, no defects have been described that affect GHRH synthesis (80). Numerous mutations have been described, however, affecting homeodomain transcription factors for pituitary development, the GHRH receptor, and GH genes.

1. Pituitary Differentiation Factors

As noted in the section on pituitary differentiation, *HESX1* and *LHX3* are factors involved in differentiation of the Rathke pouch into distinctive pituitary cell types. A missense mutation of *HESX1* has been described in a single family with septo-optic dysplasia, agenesis of the corpus callosum, and anterior hypopituitarism. Heterozygous members of the family were unaffected. Three siblings having deficiency of all pituitary hormones but adrenocorticotropin were found to be homozygous for a missense mutation in the *LHX3* gene. A single patient with the same hormonal status in another family had an intragenic deletion that predicted a severely truncated protein lacking the entire homeodomain (13). One of these patients had an enlarged anterior pituitary, whereas the others had pituitary hypoplasia. All four had rigidity of the cervical spine resulting in limited rotational ability of the head.

Some instances of multiple pituitary hormone deficiency (MPHD) have been attributed to dominant and recessive mutations of the gene for pituitary transcription factor, POU1F1 (formerly referred to as Pit-1), which is critical for the differentiation of somatotrophs, thyrotrophs, and lactotrophs. Recessive mutations, of which seven have been reported, result in varying degrees of loss of DNA binding or transcriptional activation functions (10). Mechanisms for the effects of the four dominant mutations are less readily explained, one involving enhanced binding of the mutant to GH and PRL promoter sites, another impairing distal enhancer activation; mechanisms for the other two mutations remain unexplained. Affected patients have intact ACTH, LH, and FSH function (81). Such occurrences have also been characterized by a small or normal sella turcica (82, 83). Since the original description of a Pit1 mutation in 1992 (84), only a few cases have been reported.

A similar phenotype to that found in POU1F1 mutation is caused by mutation of the PROP1 gene in the Ames dwarf mouse. This gene encodes a paired-like homeodomain protein expressed briefly in embryonic pituitary and necessary for POU1F1 expression (85). Thus, it was anticipated that mutation of the PROP1 gene in humans would result in a clinical picture similar to that with POU1F1 mutations. It was demonstrated in several families, as well as in sporadic cases, however, that mutation of the PROP1 gene can cause gonadotropin deficiency in addition to somatotropin, thyrotropin, and prolactin deficiency (86–88). In the families described by Nader et al. (89) in 1975, and by Parks et al. (90) in 1978, now recognized to be families with PROP1 deficiency, MPHD was associated with sellar enlargement. In a few instances in which this mass has led to surgical intervention, histological examination indicates proliferation of undifferentiated connective tissue (91). This phenomenon does not appear to be genotype specific and varies within the families of the same genotype (Fig. 5); the clinical importance is the need to differentiate this pituitary enlargement from adenoma, craniopharyngioma, or other tumor. Adrenocorticotropin deficiency may result from progressive deterioration of the pituitary or be specific to certain mutations, suggesting a role for PROP1 in the differentiation or maintenance of corticotroph cells (92).

Homozygosity for a GA or an AG deletion in the sequence 296GAGAGAG in exon 2 of PROP1, originally noted in one of the first four families with PROP1 deficiency reported by Wu et al. (86), is the most common of the eight recessive mutations that have been described, reported in patients from Russia (87, 93), Turkey (93), Jamaica (91), the United States (93), Brazil (91, 93), and Dominican Republic (94). The series of three dinucleotide repeats appears to be a mutational hot spot, with susceptibility to misalignment of DNA, generating slippage and deletion independently in different populations. Another mutational hot spot also results in a 2 bp deletion in exon 2 (149delGA) that leads to the same serine to stop codon change at codon 109. It is present as a compound heterozygote with the 296delGA mutation in children with MPHD from four Russian families (10). The 296GAdel mutation represents a severe loss of function mutation. The altered sequence predicts a protein of 108 amino acids with a frameshift and truncation in the second α-helix of the DNA-binding domain. When expressed in a mouse PROP1 context, the recombinant protein lacks detectable DNA-binding and transcriptional activation activities (86). The severity of the hormone deficiency phenotype is compatible with the complete loss of PROP1 activity.

PROP1 mutations are an important cause of MPHD, in contrast to the situation with POU1F1 mutations. Of 52 Polish patients with MPHD, 33 had mutations in

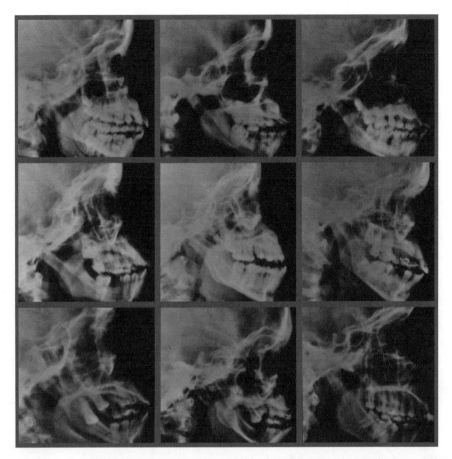

Figure 5 Lateral skull films for sellar area in patients with familial anterior hypopituitarism due to PROP1 deficiency, from left to right and top to bottom: ages 17, 21, 23, 27, 29, 33, 38, 40 years, and normal sister age 22 years (third row, right). The first, fourth, and fifth subjects have sellar enlargement for height and bone age. (Reprinted from Rosenbloom AL, Selman-Almonte A, Brown MR, Fisher DA, Baumbach L, Parks JS: Clinical and biochemical phenotype of familial anterior hypopituitarism from mutation of PROP-1 gene. J Clin Endocrinol Metab 1999; 84:50–57; © The Endocrine Society.)

PROP1, and none in POU1F1; all 11 multiplex families had mutations, while 17 of 27 isolated cases did (10). Of 73 subjects with MPHD in Switzerland, 35 had PROP1 mutations, including all who were affected in 17 multiplex families (95).

2. GHRH Receptor Defects

Reports of mutations of the GHRH receptor gene come from inbred populations in India, Pakistan, and Brazil (15, 96–99). The first two families reported consisted of two children each from Indian Muslim families not known to be related, one of which was consanguinous (96, 97). These patients were homozygous for a G to T transversion at position 265 of the GHRH-R gene, which introduces a premature stop codon at residue 72, a mutation that was also found in 18 Pakistani patients who were part of a multiply consanguinous pedigree (15). The largest group of patients described thus far, 105 white patients of Por-

tuguese descent from an inbred population in northeastern Brazil, exhibit homozygosity for a different splice site mutation (98, 99).

As expected, individuals with GHRH receptor mutations have severe short stature and high-pitched voices. There is mild delay in sexual maturation but fertility has been demonstrated for both males and females (who require delivery by cesarean-section). One affected couple had an obligatorily affected but otherwise normal child. A number of clinical features differentiate subjects with GHRH receptor mutation from individuals with related conditions of severe isolated GH deficiency or GH insensitivity. GHRH-receptor-deficient patients have a normal penis size before puberty, whereas microphallus is typical of patients with GH deficiency and insensitivity. Unlike congenital GHD and GHRD, history of hypoglycemia has not been elicited in any of the populations with GHRH receptor deficiency and there is minimal or no facial hypoplasia or prominence of the forehead (Figs. 6, 7). The Pakistani patients had asymptomatic low blood pressure and relatively small head sizes, but this has not been noted in the other reports. In further contrast to GHD and GHRD, central adiposity is uncommon and body proportions are normal in those with GHRH receptor mutation. A further interesting difference from GHRD is that there is no difference in the markedly low levels of IGF-I, IGF-II, and IGFBP-3, or the elevated levels of IGFBP-2 between prepubertal and adult individuals (15). In GHRD, IGF-I, IGF-II, and IGFBP-3 levels are significantly greater and IGFBP-2 concentrations significantly lower in adults than in children (100, 101).

3.   Isolated (I) GHD

Four autosomal recessive disorders, an autosomal dominant mutation, and an X-linked form of IGHD have been identified (102).

1.   IGHD IA is a recessive condition caused by heterogeneous defects of the gene for GH (GH-1), and is the most severe form of GHD. Defects of the GH-1 have included gene deletions, and frameshift and nonsense mutations (1, 103–107). Because these individuals have complete GHD with no exposure to endogenous GH, the administration of rhGH results in formation of anti-GH antibodies and cessation of growth response after a few months in most, but not all patients (1, 108–110). In an Italian family with three affected children, two showed high-titer antibodies and ceased responding to exogenous GH, while the third sibling continued to respond and had low-titer antibodies (111).

2.   IGHD IB is also an autosomal recessive condition differing from IGHD IA by the presence of detectable levels of endogenous GH and, consequently, continued response to rhGH administration without the development of anti-GH antibodies. This form of IGHD results from mutations affecting splicing of the GH-1 gene. These rare mutations have been described in Middle Eastern consanguineous families. The result of some of these mutations can be complete absence of measurable circulating GH, thought to be due to loss of anti-GH antibody-binding sites necessary for the radioimmunoassay reaction. The presence of some GH-related protein has been supported by the absence of development of anti-GH antibodies when these patients are treated with rhGH (97). In an Arab Bedouin family from Israel with IGHD IB, carriers of the mutant GH-1 allele were significantly shorter than those who were homozygous normal; one-third of 33 heterozygotes, but only 1 of 17 normal homozygotes had stature >2 standard deviations (SD) below the mean (112).

3.   IGHD II is differentiated from IGHD I because it is inherited in an autosomal dominant mode, the result of dominant negative mutations of the GH1 gene. Affected individuals typically have an affected parent and respond well to rhGH administration. Most of the mutations that have been described associated with this form

of IGHD are in intron 3 of the GH gene and alter splicing of GH mRNA with skipping or deletion of exon 3. It is not clear why these mutations prevent expression of normal GH from the unaffected allele (the dominant negative phenomenon) (113–115). With one of the splice mutations, resulting in del32-71-GH, transfection studies in neuroendocrine cell lines demonstrated suppression of wild-type GH by the mutant as a posttranslational effect caused by decreased stability rather than decreased synthesis of the wild-type GH (116).

4.   IGHD III is inherited in an X-linked manner. It is associated with agammaglobulinemia in some but not all families, suggesting contiguous gene defects on the long arm of the X chromosome as a cause of some instances of IGHD III (117).

5.   Bioinactive GH. The presence of immunologically detectable but biologically ineffective GH has been proposed for a number of reported patients with the appearance of GHD, normal levels of radioimmunoassayable GH in the circulation, and low concentrations of IGF-I (118). Radioreceptor assay for GH in these cases has indicated lower concentrations than in the radioimmunoassay, and therapeutic response to rhGH is comparable to that in IGHD (118, 119). A mutation resulting in a heterozygous single amino acid substitution in the GH1 gene has been described in a patient thought to have bioinactive GH. Although there was an abnormal GH peak on isoelectric focusing, there was also a normal one and the patient shared this mutation with his normal father, suggesting that it was not pathological (120). In quest of a molecular defect in such patients, 200 children with short stature found to have GH sufficiency were reviewed. Three were identified who had short stature and growth velocities consistent with GHD, but elevated basal and stimulated levels of immunoassayable GH, and low concentrations of IGF-I and IGFBP-3 in the serum. A rat lymphoma cell proliferation assay and an immunofunctional assay for GH gave abnormally low responses compared to results on the radioimmunoassay (RIA). High-resolution sequencing of both strands of the coating region and display sites of genomic DNA and sequencing of the CD did not reveal GH-1 gene mutation in any of the patients. It was postulated that the reduced biological activity of abnormal translation product could be due to posttranslational processing in these patients (121).

V.   ACQUIRED GH DEFICIENCY

A.   Tumors

By far the most common cause of acquired GH deficiency in children is tumor. Craniopharyngiomas account for the greatest number of tumors causing GH deficiency, but several other benign or malignant tumors can also be responsible for the deficient state (122–124). Benign lesions that damage the hypothalamic–pituitary axis include pi-

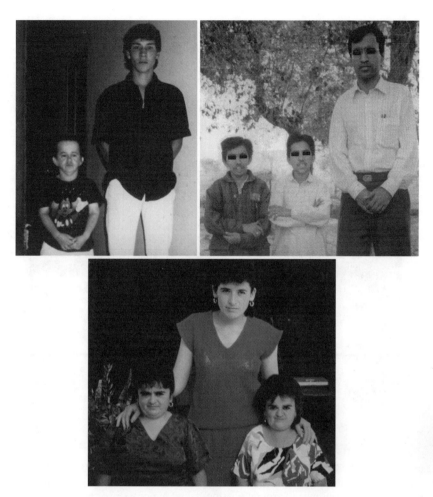

Figure 6 Comparison of patients with GHRD and GHRH receptor deficiency. Upper left: 30-year-old man with GHRD (Laron syndrome), height 106 cm (−10.8 SDS), with 17-year-old brother, height 162 cm (−2.1 SDS). Upper right: 21-year-old twins with GHRH receptor deficiency, heights 119 and 118 cm (−8.8, 8.9 SDS) and normal adult from region (height 168 cm). Lower: 27-year-old woman with GHRD, height 106 cm (−9.4 SDS), 24-year-old unaffected sister, height 155 cm (−1.4 SDS), and 25-year-old affected sister, height 112 cm (−8.4 SDS). Note in patients with GHRD family resemblance but with marked foreshortening of the face, prominence of the forehead, obesity, in men, frontotemporal baldness, and relatively short upper extremities. In contrast, the men with GHRH receptor deficiency have normal facies and body proportions, without obesity. (Upper right photo reprinted from Maheshwari HG, Silverman BL, Dupuis J, Baumann G. Phenotypic and genetic analysis of a syndrome caused by an inactivating mutation in the GH-releasing hormone receptor: dwarfism of Sindh. J Clin Endocrinol Metab 1998; 1983:4065–4074; © The Endocrine Society.)

tuitary adenoma, Rathke's cleft cyst, and arachnoid cyst (125). Primary malignant tumors that can affect this region include dysgerminomas, germinomas, meningiomas, and gliomas (126). Although metastatic tumor is a more common cause of GH deficiency in adults than in children, childhood Hodgkin's disease or nasopharyngeal carcinoma can metastasize to the pituitary or hypothalamus (126). Signs and symptoms of primary or metastatic malignancies and benign intracranial lesions can be visual loss (particularly bitemporal hemianopsia, for optic chiasm lesions), papilledema, headache with sleep or on awakening, emesis, and behavioral changes (126). Lesions

in the hypothalamus may additionally cause hypersomnolence, appetite changes, or diabetes insipidus (127). Weight loss may result from appetite loss or excess fluid losses from diabetes insipidus. Symptoms of prolactin excess, including amenorrhea or galactorrhea, may occur, because of the loss of dopamine inhibition from the hypothalamus.

1. Craniopharyngioma

Two-thirds of craniopharyngiomas are found in a suprasellar location. The tumor most likely arises from rem-

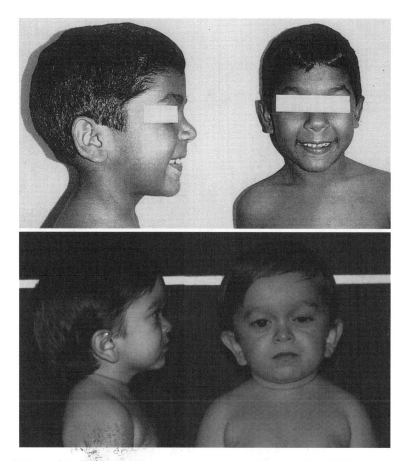

Figure 7 Top: 7-year-old boy with GHRH receptor deficiency, height 95 cm (−5.2 SDS) and weight 12 kg (5th percentile for height) with bone age 3 years, spontaneous and stimulated GH concentrations <1.5 μg/L, and serum IGF-I concentration below the level of measurability. Note absence of frontal bossing, facial hypoplasia, or truncal obesity. Bottom: 8-year-old boy with GHRD, height 78.9 cm (−9.1 SDS) and weight 9.2 kg (5th to 10th percentile for height) with a bone age of 3.3 years, spontaneous serum GH concentration 31 μg/L (immunoradiometric assay), IGF-I 8 ng/ml (2 SD range for age 52–222, for bone age 20–79), IGFBP-3 141 ng/ml (2 SD range for age 2400–5800, for bone age 1180–3280), and IGFBP-2 500% of normal. Note small facies, frontal bossing, depressed nasal bridge and truncal obesity, despite low weight percentile. Ptosis (left) has been seen in ∼15% of Ecuadorian patients with GHRD.

nants of the invagination of the embryonic stomodeum that gives rise to the adenohypophysis in the fetus. However, some neuropathologists believe the tumor could instead arise from metaplastic squamous epithelial cells in the adenohypophysis (125). The tumor accounts for 6–10% of all pediatric brain tumors and is most common from ages 5 to 15 years, but a second peak in incidence is seen in adults ages 50–70 years (123). MRI imaging often shows a calcified lesion, and histopathological examination reveals an encapsulated, oil-containing cystic tumor of squamous epithelial cells that show keratinization. The high cholesterol content of the tumor aids in identification on MRI. In one series, 95% of patients with craniopharyngioma had at least one anterior pituitary hormone deficiency at diagnosis, and 38% had hyperprolactinemia (122). Diabetes insipidus does not usually occur preoperatively (128). In the Jenkins series, nearly two-

thirds of patients had tumor recurrence, which correlated with cyst size. The best long-term prognosis is seen in patients with purely cystic lesions, and patients with tumor symptoms before the age of 5 years may have a worse prognosis than older patients (124). After initial surgical resection, virtually all patients with craniopharyngioma have hypopituitarism. Sleep and appetite centers in the hypothalamus may be damaged by the tumor or by the attempted resection. Hyperphagia and resultant obesity tend to correlate with damage to the ventromedial and/or paraventricular nuclei (125), and this excess nutrition may result in normal or supranormal growth velocity despite profound GH deficiency.

In a series of 20 patients with craniopharyngioma reported by Jenkins, 19 of 20 had GH and gonadotropin deficiencies at diagnosis (122). Thirteen patients had secondary or tertiary hypothyroidism, and 10 had ACTH deficiency. None of the patients had diabetes insipidus before surgical resection.

With surgical resection, nearly all patients with craniopharyngioma will have at least temporary vasopressin deficiency. The development of further pituitary deficiency depends upon degree of tumor resection (129), which will also influence long-term survival. With attempted complete removal of the tumor (without subsequent radiation), 42% of patients have tumor recurrence (124). Gross total resection of the tumor gave a 90% cure rate in another series, but about one-third of patients experienced behavioral problems, appetite or sleep dysfunction, and memory deficits postoperatively (126). Near-total excision followed by fractionated radiotherapy may provide the best prognosis (130, 131).

2. Rathke Cleft Cyst

A Rathke cleft cyst (RCC) is a benign lesion believed to arise from Rathke's pouch remnants, neuroepithelium, or metaplastic anterior pituitary cells (132). The lesion is generally intrasellar and may result in hypopituitarism, neurological findings, or visual deficits (125). The lesion is often mucoid and may contain cuboidal, columnar, or ciliated epithelium. It may be difficult to differentiate from a craniopharyngioma or arachnoid cyst . In one series, 81% of patients with RCC had preoperative hypopituitarism, 60% had neurological dysfunction, and 38% had visual losses (132). As in craniopharyngioma, hyperprolactinemia may result from loss of dopamine inhibition of prolactin secretion.

3. Arachnoid Cleft Cyst

The arachnoid cleft cyst (ACC) usually occurs in an intrasellar location and may be difficult to identify preoperatively. ACC occurs typically in older patients than does craniopharyngioma or RCC. The cyst is lined by arachnoid cells and contains cerebrospinal fluid. It is either a congenital lesion or an acquired lesion that occurs when the diaphragma sella permits herniation of the arachnoid membrane. The endocrine prognosis is worse for ACC than RCC or craniopharyngioma, most likely due to more chronic, high-pressure damage to the adenohypophysis by the cyst (132).

4. Pituitary Adenoma

Although more common in adults than in children, the pituitary adenoma may cause hypopituitarism in children by pressure damage to surrounding normal pituitary tissue. Five to 6% of childhood pituitary tumors are adenomas and may occur in isolation or as part of multiple endocrine neooplasia type I (133). More than half of these adenomas are prolactinomas; the remainder may secrete ACTH or GH, or may be nonfunctioning (134). Histopathological evaluation often reveals areas of hemorrhage within the adenoma; hemorrhage may cause pituitary ap-

oplexy, and, if longstanding, the hemorrhagic areas may become cystic. (133).

B. Other Causes of Acquired GH Deficiency

A variety of other causes of acquired GH deficiency have been identified. Among the mechanical causes of GH deficiency are trauma with or without skull fracture, irradiation for therapy of malignancy, and surgery. Hemorrhage into the pituitary or hypothalamus may cause hypopituitarism and has been reported in patients receiving chronic anticoagulant therapy as well as in those with pituitary apoplexy. Inflammatory processes resulting in hypopituitarism include autoimmune hypophysitis, infectious diseases resulting in meningitis or encephalitis, and infiltrative processes such as sarcoidosis, histiocytosis X, and hemochromatosis. Cerebral edema occurring with diabetic ketoacidosis has also been reported to result in hypopituitarism (19, 135).

1. Head Trauma

Following significant head trauma, 40% of patients may have transient or permanent vasopressin deficiency (127). On occasion, apparently permanent anterior hypopituitarism has spontaneously resolved months after the head injury (136). Varying degrees of other pituitary hormonal deficiencies may be seen. Hypopituitarism may result from direct structural damage to the hypothalamus or pituitary or because of hypovolemia with severe blood loss or increased intracranial pressure. Hypopituitarism may occur after seemingly minor head trauma (137) and should always be a diagnostic consideration in the evaluation of the child abuse victim with head trauma.

2. Radiation Therapy

Current CNS oncological radiation includes conventional radiation, as well as proton-beam, gamma knife, and yttrium-90 or gold-198 radiotherapy. All of these therapies may cause pituitary insufficiency (127, 138). With conventional radiation of 50 Gy for 4 weeks for pituitary adenoma, 11 of 22 patients developed hypopituitarism within 4.2 years (139). Head and neck irradiation, or "mantle" radiation for lymphoma, may lead to pituitary deficiencies as well (140). It is prudent to evaluate growth velocity, weight gain, and, in pubertal age patients, pubertal progression, at frequent intervals in the first 5 years following radiation to the head.

3. Pituitary Apoplexy

Pituitary apoplexy has been described in patients with pituitary adenomas and in women in the immediate postpartum period (141). It may also occur in severely dehydrated patients with diabetes mellitus, trauma, or intracranial pressure changes, or in patients undergoing chronic anticoagulation or radiation therapy (127, 142). Postpartum apoplexy is known as Sheehan's syndrome.

Apoplexy is due to hemorrhage or infarct into an adenoma or into normal pituitary tissue, with subsequent hypopituitarism. Failure to recognize the signs of ACTH deficiency resulting from apoplexy can have fatal consequences. Patients may have severe headache ("the worst of my life"); diplopia or visual loss; deficits of cranial nerves III, IV, or VI; sensorium changes; or hypotension. Diagnosis is confirmed by findings on computed tomographic (CT) scan or MRI.

4. Inflammatory Disease

Autoimmune or lymphocytic hypophysitis has been described in patients with autoimmune polyglandular syndrome, in postpartum women, and as an isolated finding (143, 144) . Diagnosis can be difficult to confirm but may be based on the finding of pituitary antibodies (not commercially available) or of lymphocytic infiltration on pituitary biopsy (145). Patients with meningitis or encephalitis may also develop hypopituitarism with bacterial, viral, or fungal infections (146). Infiltrative diseases uncommonly cause hypopituitarism in children, but may result from histiocytosis X, sarcoidosis, or hemochromatosis due to chronic blood transfusions for thalassemia (147). A thickened pituitary stalk may suggest the diagnosis on MRI. Children with histiocytosis X initially have diabetes insipidus (DI) without other hormonal deficiencies and with a thickened pituitary stalk (148). The child with histiocytosis and DI often has unusual, desperate, water-seeking behaviors, such as drinking from flower vases or pets' water dishes. Subsequently, GH deficiency, alone, or with other pituitary deficiencies, may occur.

5. Deprivation Syndrome

Failure to thrive thought to result from lack of nurturing in infants raised in institutions was described as anaclitic depression (149). Talbot et al. (150) initially suggested that growth failure can occur beyond infancy associated with emotional deprivation and characterized by subtle nutritional inadequacy. The spectrum of pathology associated with growth failure in dysfunctional settings has been referred to as deprivation, maternal deprivation, emotional deprivation, or environmental deprivation dwarfism, psychosocial dwarfism, and hyperphagic short stature. Fifteen years after the report of Talbot et al., Patton and Gardner (151, 152) stressed the importance of historical information in defining some instances of growth failure as a truly psychosomatic disorder. They speculated that the problem could be attributed to hypothalamic influences on the pituitary secretion of GH, undernutrition as a result of neglect, diminished appetite resulting from depression and lethargy, or decreased intestinal motility and absorption due to nutritional and emotional factors.

Deprivation dwarfism was later described as a triad of extreme short stature, voracious appetite, and markedly delayed sexual maturation in nine patients who had had feeding difficulties in infancy, persistent sleep problems, and whose parents had serious psychological disturbances; growth improved markedly with foster placement (153). The clinical syndrome was further described in 13 children initially thought to have idiopathic hypopituitarism to include, in addition to high degrees of social disruption and pathology in the family and severe growth failure, bizarre eating and drinking behavior by history, sleep disturbances, malabsorption with foul-smelling stools, delayed speech, and abdominal protuberance. The children ate out of garbage cans, "stole" food, gorged, and ate from the pets' dishes. They drank from toilet bowls, glasses filled with dishwater, rain pools, and old beer cans holding stagnant water. Removal from the home was associated with growth acceleration and behavioral improvement. Emotional factors, malabsorption, inadequate nutrition, and hypopituitarism were all considered as possible contributors (154). Endocrinological evaluation indicated frequent deficiency in adrenocorticotropin and GH with return of GH responses to normal; occasional patients had normal GH values, but it was not recognized at that time that recovery of GH secretion might occur very early after removal from the home (155). Others confirmed deficient GH and ACTH responses to hypoglycemia in children, but not infants, with the deprivation syndrome and noted that some children had normal or elevated serum GH concentrations at the time of admission, reminiscent of the range of possibilities with malnutrition (156).

Two important investigations published in 1969 addressed the question of whether environmental or maternal deprivation, in the presence of adequate nutrition, could result in growth failure. Rhesus monkeys, shown to be extremely dependent on maternal attention and physical play for normal behavioral development, were provided an ad libitum diet, but deprived of all social contact and environmental stimulation from birth, including direct human contact except that required for maintenance and experimental measures. Despite developing persistent behavioral abnormalities including autistic posturing, fear, inability to engage in social play and, after maturity, to engage in social and sexual activity, their growth was completely normal (157).

A remarkable prospective study was carried out by Whitten et al. of 16 human infants aged 3–24 months referred for growth failure, who were of normal weight at birth (158). During a 2-week period of initial hospitalization with minimal mothering and plentiful calories, and a period of high-intensity mothering, comparable weight recovery occurred. In the home setting, provision of adequate calories supervised by a home visitor, described to the family as a study protocol rather than supervision, also resulted in adequate gain. Some of the mothers admitted that the amount of food consumed was considerably greater than they had been providing. Other mothers have likewise admitted to intentional starvation as a form of

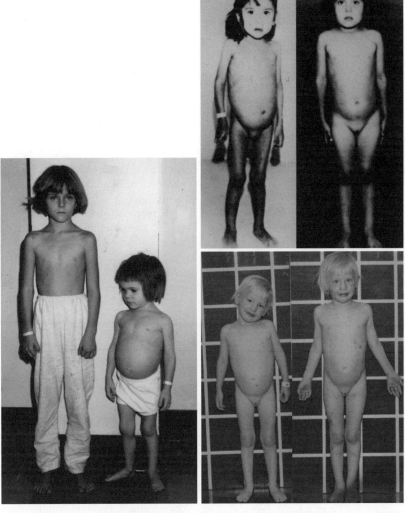

Figure 8 Three children with deprivation syndrome. Left: 7-year old daughter (on right) of psychotic parents, with hepato-megaly and lack of normal social behavior, standing with a normal-sized age mate. Right upper: daughter of alcoholic single mother, this 5-year-old was thought to have gluten-induced enteropathy to explain her short stature (height SDS −4.1, height age 2 years 4 months). In the care of her grandmother, she gained 20 lbs in 10 months, nearly doubling her weight, and grew 7-1/4 inches (height SDS −1.2, height age, 4 years 8 months). Right lower: 5-year-old thought to have GHD to explain severe short stature (height SDS −5); when she returned 6 months later to start pituitary GH injections, she had grown 4 inches and it was learned that her social situation had changed dramatically after the initial hospitalization.

abuse, or to avoid having the child get sick, bloated, throw up, or have loose stools (159). Extensive studies of mothers of affected infants and children have demonstrated a range of pathology affecting mothering skills and character (160, 161).

In a review of 185 patients hospitalized for evaluation of failure to thrive, 50% could be attributed to environmental deprivation, corresponding precisely to the percentage noted 20 years earlier by Talbot et al. (150). Or-

ganic causes were suggested by history and physical examination; only 1.4% of laboratory studies performed were of diagnostic value and only if there was a specific indication for the test from the clinical evaluation (162).

The frequent observation of disturbed sleep patterns in these children suggests that their growth failure might be related in part to a failure of nocturnal GH secretion, dependent on the attainment of deep sleep (163). Polygraphic sleep recordings soon after hospital admission in children with psychosocial dwarfism demonstrated a gross deficit of stage IV sleep and a decrease in the overall slow-wave sleep episodes, both stage III and IV. After 3–15 weeks in the new environment and with growth recovery, stage IV sleep returned (164). More recent studies have demonstrated progressive improvement in GH pulse amplitude, with maintenance of the individual's characteristic pulsatility (165, 166).

The deprivation syndrome can now be recognized as a social pathology resulting in chronic undernutrition and secondary endocrine deficiencies, primarily GH and ACTH, which are readily reversible with provision of adequate food intake (Fig. 8). Removal from the home temporarily or permanently is usually necessary, particularly for older children. Infants with failure to thrive often have mothers who mean well, but are immature, dependent, and insensitive to their infants' needs; counseling and support may make it possible for the child to thrive in the home (161). In the few recognized instances in which exogenous GH has been administered to children with deprivation syndrome, responses been been nil to much less than typical of GH deficiency, as one might expect in the context of noncompliance and undernutrition (167, 168).

VI. CONGENITAL GH INSENSITIVITY

A. GH Receptor Deficiency (GHRD)

Following the initial report (169) of three Yemeni Jewish siblings "with hypoglycemia and other clinical and laboratory signs of GH deficiency, but with abnormally high concentrations of immunoreactive serum growth hormone," 22 patients were reported from Israel, all Oriental Jews, with an apparent autosomal recessive mode of transmission in consanguineous families (170). These reports preceded the recognition of the critical role of cell surface receptors in hormone action and it was postulated that the defect was in the GH molecule these patients were producing. This impression was substantiated by the observation of free fatty acid mobilization, nitrogen retention, and growth in patients being administered exogenous GH (170). These effects may have been due to other pituitary hormones in the crude extracts administered or to nutritional changes in the investigative setting. In the first patient reported outside of Israel, in 1968, there was no response to exogenous GH, leading to the hypothesis that the defect was in the GH receptor (171). This hypothesis was substantiated by the failure to demonstrate sulfation factor activation with exogenous GH administration, reported in 1969 (172) and reports in 1973 and 1976 that the patients' GH was normal on fractionation, in its binding to antibodies, and in its binding to hepatic cell membranes from normal individuals (173–176). In vitro demonstration of cellular unresponsiveness to GH was demonstrated by the failure of erythroid progenitor cells from the peripheral blood of two patients to respond to

exogenous GH (177). The failure of radioiodine-labeled GH to bind to liver cell microsomes obtained from biopsy of two patients with Laron syndrome confirmed that the defect was in the GHR (178). The two reports of absent GHBP in sera of patients with Laron syndrome (29, 30) appeared just before the publication of the finding that GHBP was the extracellular domain of the cell surface GHR (31).

Mutations of the GHR have provided insight into its physiology. Thirty-six distinct mutations in the extracellular and transmembrane domains produce a clinical picture of severe GH/IGF-I deficiency in the homozygous state or as compound heterozygotes, whereas two dominant negative mutations of the intracellular domain result in a milder clinical syndrome. Some individuals described with features of GH resistance appear to have defective signal transduction by the GH–GHR complex. Knowledge of the biology and signaling of the GHR has attracted extensive research interest because GH is a powerful regulator of somatic growth, mitogenesis, and metabolism, with a wide variety of effects on target cells, all mediated by the GHR, which is expressed in 40 different tissues.

The structure of the human GHR gene is depicted in Figure 9. There are eight variants (V1–V8) contributing to the 5′ untranslated region (UTR), followed by nine coding exons (exons 2–10). Exon 2 encodes the last 11 base pairs of the 5′-UTR sequence, an 18 amino acid signal sequence, and the initial five amino acids of the extracellular hormone binding domain. Exons 3–7 encode the extracellular hormone-binding domain, except for the terminal 3 amino acids of his domain, which are encoded by exon 8. Exon 8 further encodes the 24 amino acid hydrophobic transmembrane domain and the initial four amino acids of the intracellular domain. Exons 9 and 10 encode the large intracellular domain. Exon 10 also encodes the 2 kb 3′-UTR. Four of the alternative 5′-UTRs of the human gene have been cloned from genomic DNA, indicating that each was encoded by a separate exon. It has been suggested that this variability serves to regulate translational efficiency of the mRNAs (179). The human GHR is unique in existing in an alternative splice isoform that excludes exon 3; this deletion has no demonstrable effect on GHR function (180).

The report of the characterization of the GHR gene included the first description of a genetic defect of the GHR, a deletion of exons 3, 5, and 6 (32); recognition that the exon 3 deletion represented an alternatively spliced variant without functional significance resolved the dilemma of explaining deletion of nonconsecutive exons. No other exon deletions have been described in patients with GHI, but the additional defects of the GHR gene that have been described in association with GH insensitivity (GHI) include eight nonsense mutations, 14 missense mutations, five frame shift mutations, 10 splice mutations, and a unique intronic mutation resulting in insertion of a pseudoexon (181). The functional insignificance of exon 3 is emphasized by the fact that no mutations affecting this exon have been associated with GHI. Neither have functional mutations been described in exon 2. A number of other mutations have been described that are either polymorphisms or have not occurred in the homozygous or compound heterozygous state.

The point mutations that result in severe GHI when present in the homozygous state or as a compound heterozygote are all associated with the typical phenotype of severe GHD. All but three of the defects result in absent or extremely low levels of GHBP. Noteworthy is the D152H missense mutation that affects the dimerization site, thus permitting production of the extracellular domain in normal quantities but failure of dimerization at the cell surface, which is necessary for signal transduction and IGF-I production (182). Two defects that are close to (G223G) or within (R274T) the transmembrane domain result in extremely high levels of GHBP (183–185). These defects interfere with the normal splicing of exon 8, which encodes the transmembrane domain, with the mature GHR transcript being translated into a truncated protein that retains GH-binding activity but cannot be anchored to the cell surface.

As noted, all these homozygous defects and the four compound hetorozygotes, whether involving the extracellular domain or the transmembrane domain and whether associated with very low or unmeasurable GHBP, result in a typical phenotype of severe GHD. In contrast, the intronic mutation present in the heterozygous state in a mother and daughter with relatively mild growth failure (both SDS for height −3.6), and resulting in a dominant negative effect on GHR formation, is not associated with

other phenotypic features of GHD. This splice mutation preceding exon 9 results in an extensively attenuated, virtually absent intracellular domain (184). Japanese siblings and their mother have a similar heterozygous point mutation of the donor splice site in intron 9, also resulting in mild growth failure compared to GHRD, but with definite, although mild, phenotypic features of GHD (185). GHBP levels in the white patients were at the upper limit of normal with a radiolabeled GH-binding assay (184) and in the Japanese patients twice the upper limit of normal, using a ligand immunofunction assay (185).

These heterozygote GHR mutants transfected into permanent cell lines have demonstrated increased affinity for GH compared to the wild type full-length GHR, with markedly increased production of GHBP. When cotransfected with full-length GHR, a dominant negative effect results from overexpression of the mutant GHR and inhibition of GH-induced tyrosine phosphorylation and transcription activation (184, 186). Naturally occurring truncated isoforms have also shown this dominant negative effect in vitro (36, 187, 188).

A novel intronic point mutation was discovered in a highly consanguineous family with two pairs of affected cousins with GHBP-positive GHI and severe short stature, but without the facial features of severe GHD or GHRD. This mutation resulted in a 108 bp insertion of a pseudoexon between exons 6 and 7, predicting an in-frame, 36 residue amino acid sequence. This is a region critically involved in receptor dimerization (189).

Of just over 250 reported cases of typical GHRD, ethnic origin is known for 232 (181). Of these, nearly 50% are Oriental Jews as described in the original report, or known descendants of Iberian Jews who converted to

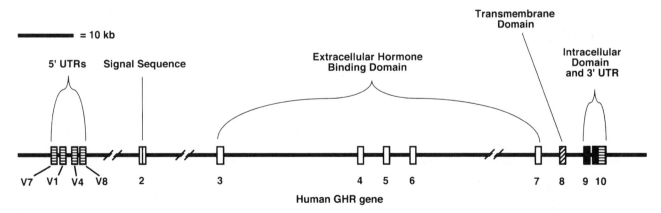

Figure 9 Diagram of the growth hormone receptor gene. The black horizontal line represents intron sequence, diagonal breaks in the lines indicate uncloned portions of the intron, and the boxes represent exons, which are enlarged for clarity. Exons with horizontal stripes, untranslated regions of the transcripts; vertical striped exon, signal sequence; open exons, hormone-binding domain; diagonal striped exon transmembrane domain; solid exons, intracellular domain. (Reprinted from Edens A, Talamantes F. Alternative processing of growth hormone receptor transcripts. Endocrine Reviews 1998; 19:559–582; © The Endocrine Society.)

Catholicism during the Spanish Inquisition. The latter make up the largest cohort (n = 70) and the only genetically homogeneous group. All but one subject have the E180 splice site mutation that is shared with at least one Israeli patient of Moroccan heritage. Most of the other defects appear to be highly family-specific, with the R43X mutation that is seen in a single Ecuadorian patient, two other nonsense mutations (C38X, R217X), and the intron 4 splice mutation being the only ones thus far described that appear in disparate populations, on different genetic backgrounds, indicating mutational hotspots (190). Because the molecular defect in the GHR has been identified in about one-third of the patients with GHRD outside of Ecuador, it is likely that the list of mutations will continue to grow and provide further insight into the function of the GHR.

B.   Partial GHI

GH resistance might be expected to occur in an incomplete form, analogous to insulin resistance, androgen insensitivity, or thyroid hormone resistance. Affected children might have growth failure with normal or slightly increased GH secretion, variable but usually decreased GHBP levels, decreased IGF-I concentrations, but not as severely reduced as in GHD or GHRD, and might respond to supraphysiological dosages of GH. It might also be expected, given the need for dimerization of the GHR for signal transduction, that certain mutations could have a dominant negative effect in the heterozygous state.

Credibility for a heterozygous defect as a cause of short stature requires the demonstration of functional significance, not only by transfection of the mutant allele but also by cotransfection with wild-type GHR gene, to approximate the circumstance in vivo. Goddard et al. (191) have identified six mutations in eight children with short stature (SDS for height −5.1-−2.0) and normal or increased stimulated GH levels. One patient had compound heterozygosity involving a novel mutation in exon 4 (E44K) and a mutation in exon 6 previously associated with GHRD in the homozygous state (R161C). Two other patients were heterozygous for this mutation. The other five patients included two who were heterozygous for the same novel mutation in exon 7 (R211H), and one each with novel mutations of exon 5 (C122X), exons 7 (E224D), and exon 10 (A478T). Expression in vitro of these four novel mutations involving the extracellular domain has shown functional effects, although cotransfection studies have not yet been reported. The defect involving exon 10 has not been expressed in vitro. Other defects without demonstrable significance have been described involving exon 10 (192–194). None of these putative partial GHI patients had the clinical phenotype of GHD. Five of the eight patients were treated with GH and had variable improvement in growth velocity, from slight to dramatic, in the first year (191). This variable response

could be due to GH resistance or to the fact that the patients were not GH/IGF-I deficient.

The subjects studied by Goddard et al. were selected from the large Genentech National Cooperative Growth Study database in pursuit of the question raised by the observation that GHBP concentrations are low in children with idiopathic short stature (ISS; i.e., short children without a recognizable syndrome or GHD). Using a ligand-mediated immunofunction assay Carlsson et al. (196) studied a large number of short children with known causes of growth failure such as GHD and Turner's syndrome, or ISS, and compared their GHBP concentrations in serum to those of normal controls. Ninety percent of the children with ISS had GHBP concentrations below the control mean and nearly 20% had concentrations that were 2 standard deviations or more below the normal mean for age and gender. Whether the distribution of GHBP concentrations in children with unexplained short stature indicates that partial GH resistance is a common cause of short stature remains to be demonstrated.

If heterozygous mutations of the GHR ultimately prove to be one cause of partial GH resistance, this would explain only a very small proportion of cases of idiopathic short stature. This impression is supported by a review of 37 patients who had relatively high GH responses to insulin and failure to increase IGF-I concentrations in the serum after several days of GH administration. GHBP concentrations were normal. Only one patient in this group failed to demonstrate a growth response to exogenous GH. The authors concluded that partial GH insensitivity was likely to be a rare cause of unexplained short stature (196).

The possibility of an effect of heterozygosity for a mutation known to cause GHRD in the homozygous state was explored in the unique Ecuadorian cohort with GHRD, which comprises a large population with a single mutation, permitting genotyping of numerous first-degree relatives. There were no significant differences in stature between carrier and homozygous normal relatives, indicating a lack of influence of heterozygosity for the E180 splice mutation of the GHR (197). A more general indication of the lack of influence of heterozygosity for GHR mutations involving the extracellular domain on growth comes from studies of the large multicenter European-based GHI study. In both the European and Ecudorian populations the stature of parents and of unaffected siblings does not correlate with statural deviation of affected individuals (197, 198), while an expected high correlation exists between parents and unaffected offspring (197). If the mutations that cause growth failure in the homozygous state also affected growth in heterozygotes, heterozygous parents and predominantly heterozygous siblings would have height SDS values that correlated with those of affected family members. In the Ecuadorian families, there was no difference in height correlations with parents between carriers and homozygous normal offspring (197).

C. Growth Hormone–GH Receptor Signal Transduction Failure

Evidence of a post-GHR defect in three siblings of Palestinian Arab origin has been presented by Laron et al. (199). The children had typical features of severe GHD, but normal GHBP and IGFBP-3 levels with severe IGF-I deficiency. The molecular defect has yet to be identified. In contrast to these patients, four GHBP-positive children from two unrelated Pakistani families, who had high GH, low IGF-I, and low IGFBP-3 serum concentrations, had no phenotypic features of Laron syndrome except for short stature, which was less severe than in typical GHRD (200). Fibroblasts from the children in one of the families demonstrated failure to activate part of the GH-signaling pathway (201).

VII. ACQUIRED GH INSENSITIVITY

Acquired resistance to GH is a ubiquitous adaptation in a number of protein catabolic states such as malnutrition, poorly controlled diabetes mellitus, and chronic renal disease. Growth failure is a variable result. GHBP is diminished for reasons that remain unexplained in these conditions, with elevated GH concentrations, decreased IGF-I, and normal to decreased IGFBP-3 concentrations. IGFBP-1 concentrations are elevated and reflect the catabolic state, and in those with diabetes, relative insulin deficiency (202). Children with end-stage renal disease, in addition to having decreased GHBP, normal or elevated GH, and low normal IGF-I concentrations, have high concentrations of IGFBP-3 , IGFBP-1, and IGFBP-2, thereby decreasing IGF-I bioavailability (203). These catabolic or chronic disease conditions may affect the GH–IGF-I axis in a manner comparable to the sick euthyroid syndrome. In the case of renal disease, the excess binding of IGF-I is not sufficient reason for invoking a GH-resistant explanation.

VIII. PRIMARY IGF-I DEFICIENCY AND IGF-I RESISTANCE

A. Congenital IGF-I Synthetic Defect

A single case of defective IGF-I synthesis due to a gene deletion has been described in a patient with a homozygous partial deletion of the IGF-I gene. His profound intrauterine growth retardation (IUGR) persisted into adolescence and he had sensorineural deafness with mental retardation (46). The absence of the craniofacial phenotype of severe GHD and the presence of normal IGFBP-3 in this patient, despite unmeasurable levels of IGF-I, indicates that the craniofacial features and low IGFBP-3 of GHD and GHR deficiency are related to an absence of the direct effects of GH that do not act through the medium of IGF-I synthesis. It is also noteworthy that profound IUGR and mental retardation are not characteristic of GHD or GHRD (204, 205), but IGF-I knockout mice have defective neurological development as well as growth failure (206). Thus, IGF-I production in utero does not appear to be GH-GHR dependent. Elevated GH levels would be expected in this circumstance as a result of the absence of IGF-I suppression of somatostatin; diurnal levels of GH were high, with an overnight GH peak of 171 ng/ml (46).

B. Acquired IGF-I Synthetic Defect

Alagille syndrome (chronic intrahepatic cholestasis) is associated with moderate growth failure in 50% of instances along with elevated GH and GHBP levels, and normal IGFBP-3 levels. Thus, this does not appear to be a GH-resistant state but one involving failure of IGF-I generation due to hepatic dysfunction (207).

C. Congenital IGF-I Receptor Defect

Defects in the IGF type I receptor or in the IGF receptor signal transduction pathway have been hypothesized in several patients. IGF-I resistance has been invoked as a cause of short stature in the Pygmy people, demonstrated by failure of response of T cells from such patients to IGF-I in vitro; the absence of IGF-I elevation that should accompany such resistance, however, requires explanation (208).

Loss of a single allele for the IGF receptor caused by distal long arm deletion of chromosome 15 fails to abolish in vitro effects of IGF-I and, therefore, would not appear to explain short stature in affected patients (209). Homozygous IGF-I receptor deletion is probably lethal (210).

Three patients have been reported with normal or high GH levels and elevated IGF-I levels. In two of these patients, normal bioactivity was demonstrated for the circulating IGF-I and fibroblasts from skin biopsies of these patients responded normally to recombinant IGF-I (211–213). It was hypothesized that these patients might have a tissue-specific (i.e., skeletal) IGF-I unresponsiveness. Such an explanation could also be invoked to explain the findings of normal IGF-I levels, lack of response to exogenous GH, and normal fibroblast response to IGF-I in those patients with heterozygous deletion of the IGF-I receptor gene (209).

A systematic examination for mutations in the IGF-I receptor was pursued in 38 children with IUGR who remained <2 SD for length after 18 months of age. This group was selected for study because IGF-I receptor knockout mice have more severe IUGR than do IGF-I knockout mice. A single patient was identified with compound heterozygosity for mutations resulting in amino acid substitutions. He had severe IUGR (birthweight 1420 g at 38 weeks), poor postnatal growth, and elevated concentrations of IGF-I and integrated GH concentration when prepubertal, consistent with IGF-I resistance. The location of the mutations was within a putative ligand-binding domain (47).

IX. DIAGNOSTIC EVALUATION

A. Clinical Assessment

Children should be evaluated for growth problems based on the following criteria:

> Height velocity <25th percentile for >6 months
> Downward crossing of percentiles on growth chart after age 18 months
> Height below −2 SD for age
> Height below genetic potential (−2 SD below midparental height)
> Bone age delay comparable to height age

Evaluation should begin with a complete history, including consideration of the mother's pregnancy (illness, toxins, alcohol/drugs used, gestation), perinatal events, birth weight and length, signs of chronic disease or abnormality in psychosocial status, and growth history. Family history of growth and pubertal timing are important, and parental heights should be measured, if possible. Calculation of midparental and target heights provides a context for determining the child's growth potential, based on current bone age and height, and whether, in fact, there is an abnormality.

Midparental height is calculated as:

$$\text{Girls:} \quad \frac{(\text{father's height} -13 \text{ cm}) + \text{mother's height}}{2}$$

$$\text{Boys:} \quad \frac{(\text{mother's height} +13 \text{ cm}) + \text{father's height}}{2}$$

Target height = midparental height ±2 SD (1 SD = 5 cm)

Height needs to be measured against the wall, using a fixed scale and a right-angle device against the head, with the back of the head, spine, and heels against the wall or device without flexion of the legs. Head circumference should also be measured and compared to standard curves for age and size. Body proportions can be determined by measuring span from middle fingertip to middle fingertip of the outstretched arms, and upper to lower segment calculated by measuring the distance from the top of the symphysis pubis to the floor with the legs slightly apart and straight. This distance is subtracted from total height to obtain the upper segment. Major and minor anomalies should also be looked for as clues to syndromes associated with small stature; the presence of a dysmorphic syndrome, however, does not obviate the possibility of concomitant GHD.

Accurate weight is important because the endocrine causes of growth failure result in height deviation that is greater than that of weight, so that such individuals often have greater than normal weight for height. The physical examination should also assess pubertal status and look for any signs of chronic illness, typically associated with low weight for height.

The typical somatic features of severe secondary and tertiary IGF-I deficiency, listed in Table 3, are not cause specific (Fig. 10). Many, if not most, such patients, including those with GHRH receptor deficiency, GH gene deletion, and GHRD, have normal intrauterine growth. SDS for length declines rapidly after birth in severe GHD or GHRD (Fig. 11) indicating the GH dependency of extrauterine growth. It was formerly thought that the first 6 months of infantile growth was not GH dependent, but this was based on inadequate data in severe GHD. Growth velocity with severe GHD or GHRD is approximately half normal (Fig. 12). Occasional periods of normal growth velocity, as noted in Figure 12, may be related to improved nutrition (214).

Despite normal sexual maturation in isolated secondary or tertiary IGF-I deficiency, the pubertal growth spurt is minimal or absent, as documented in some of the most extensive available data, in subjects with GHRD from Israel and Ecuador (49, 215). The adolescent growth spurt is GH-dependent, reflected in significantly elevated circulating levels of GH and IGF-I compared to preadolescence and adulthood (216). Among 24 Israeli patients with GHRD followed from infancy to adulthood, persistent growth beyond the normal time of adolescence was seen only in boys. In the Ecuadorian population girls also showed this phenomenon (Fig. 11). Adult stature in GHRD varies from −12 to −5.3 SD in Ecuadorian patients and −9 to −3.8 SDS in others in the literature, using the US standards (49). This is a height range of 95–124 cm for women and 106–141 cm for men in the Ecuadorian population. This wide variation in the effect of GHRD on stature was seen not only within the affected population but also between affected siblings. This intrafamilial variability has also been described with severe GHD due to GH gene deletion (108) and between those having the same mutations in the GHRH receptor (15). With multiple pituitary hormone deficiency, resulting in failure of adolescence, growth may continue into the 30s and 40s (Fig. 13).

Children with familial causes of IGF-I deficiency may be recognized by knowledgeable family members at birth because of craniofacial characteristics of frontal prominence, depressed nasal bridge, and sparse hair, as well as small hands or feet, and hypoplastic fingernails. Decreased vertical dimension of the face is typical of severe GHD or GHI and has been demonstrated in GHRD by computer analysis of the relationships between facial landmarks in all patients, including those with normal appearing facies. This foreshortening is particularly apparent

Table 3 Clinical Features of Severe IGF-I Deficiency Due to GH Deficiency or GH Receptor Deficiency

Growth
    Birth weight: normal; birth length; usually normal
    Growth failure, from birth, with velocity 1/2 normal
    Height deviation correlates with (low) serum levels of IGF-I, -II, and IGFBP-3
    Delayed bone age, but advanced for height age
    Small hands or feet
Craniofacial characteristics
    Sparse hair before age 7; frontotemporal hairline recession all ages
    Prominent forehead (bossing)
    Head size more normal than stature, with impression of large head
    "Setting sun sign" (sclera visible above iris at rest) in 25% <10 years of age
    Hypoplastic nasal bridge, shallow orbits
    Decreased vertical dimension of face
    Blue scleras
    Prolonged retention of primary dentition with decay; normal permanent teeth, may be crowded; absent third molars
    Sculpted chin
    Unilateral ptosis, facial asymmetry (15%); only reported in GHRD
Musculoskeletal/body composition
    Hypomuscularity with delay in walking
    Avascular necrosis of femoral head (25% of GHRD)
    High-pitched voices in all children, most adults
    Thin, prematurely aged skin
    Limited elbow extensibility after 5 years of age
    Children underweight to normal for height, most adults overweight for height; marked decrease of ratio of lean mass to fat
        mass, compared to normal, at all ages
    Osteopenia indicated by dual energy x-ray absorptiometry
Metabolic
    Hypoglycemia (fasting)
    Increased cholesterol and LDL-C
    Decreased sweating
Sexual development
    Small penis in childhood; normal growth with adolescence
    Delayed puberty
    Normal fertility

when patients are compared with their unaffected relatives (Figs. 6, 7) (217). Blue scleras, the result of decreased thickness of the scleral connective tissue, permitting visualization of the underlying choroid, were originally described in Ecuadorian patients with GHRD, and subsequently recognized in other populations with GHRD, as well as in GHD (94, 204, 218, 219).

Hypomuscularity is apparent in radiographs of infants with GHRD, and is thought to be responsible for delayed walking, despite normal intelligence and timing of speech onset (100). Radiographs of children who are GH-deficient or insensitive also suggest osteopenia; dual-photon absorptiometry and dual energy x-ray absorptiometry in children and adults confirm this. Limited elbow extensibility is an unexplained phenomenon seen in most patients over 5 years of age with GHRD or severe GHD. It is an acquired characteristic, absent in younger children and increasing in severity with age (94, 100). Although children may appear overweight, those with GHRD, and some with

GHD, are underweight to normal weight for height, while most adults, especially females, are overweight with markedly decreased lean to fat ratios (Figs. 6, 7, 10) (100).

Symptoms of hypoglycemia, including convulsions, particularly in infancy, are common in children with isolated GHD, MPHD, and GHI, indicating the critical importance of direct metabolic effects of GH in the fasting state: increasing hepatic glucose output, decreasing glucose uptake, and increasing lipolysis (Table 1, Fig. 3). Persistent physiological jaundice of infancy has also been noted with GHD. Decreased sweating has been described in GHD and documented by pilocarpine electrophoresis in patients with GHRD. The subjects had significantly reduced sweat secretion rates and elevated sweat electrolyte concentrations, indicating that sweat gland function is under the influence of the GH–IGF-I axis (220).

Severe GHD is associated with small penis size with normal penile growth at adolescence or with testosterone treatment in childhood. This is also true of GHRD but,

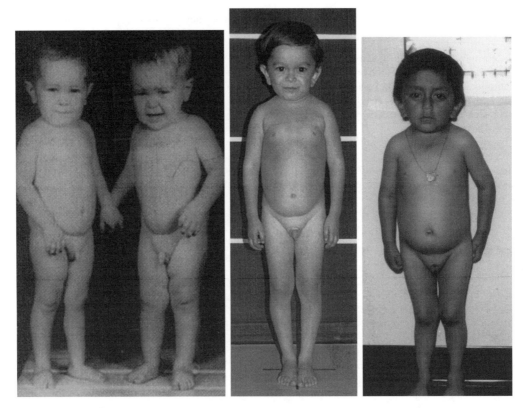

Figure 10 Similar phenotype for GH gene deletion, left; GH receptor deficiency, center; and idiopathic combined pituitary hormone deficiency (GH, thyroid), right. Left: Argentinian brothers with type I-A familial GHD, aged 2 yrs 11 months (left) and 5 years (right), demonstrating marked heterogeneity of the growth effect despite common genetic cause; the height SDS for the younger boy was −7.1 and for the older boy −8.6. (Reprinted from Rivarola MA, Phillips JA III, Migeon CJ, Heinrich JJ, Hjelle BJ: Phenotypic heterogeneity in familial isolated growth hormone deficiency type I-A. J Clin Endocrinol Metab 1984; 59:34–40; © The Endocrine Society.) Center: Subject at 9.4 years of age, with a bone age of 3.5 years, has a height SDS −9.1; despite the appearance of obesity, his weight for height is just under the third percentile. Right: Boy at 8-1/2 years, with a bone age of 2 years, has a height SDS −8.5 and weight for height well below the third percentile, approximately 4 SD below the mean. These patients are clinically indistinguishable despite their distinctive diagnoses; all show prominent foreheads, immature facies with foreshorting, the appearance of obesity, particularly truncal, despite reduced weight for height, and small phallus.

for as yet unexplained reasons, not in severe GH–IGF-I deficiency resulting from functional mutations of the GHRH-R (15). Although puberty may be delayed 3–7 years in some 50% of individuals with isolated GHD or GHRD, there is normal adult sexual function with documented reproduction by males and females (100).

There is no evidence that GHD per se results in intellectual impairment. Studies that do not account for the ascertainment bias related to the cause of the GHD, or the effects of other deficiencies in multiple pituitary hormone deficiency, can be misleading. Intellectual impairment was originally considered a feature of the Laron syndrome (221). Among 18 affected children and adolescents with Laron syndrome administered the Wechsler Intelligence Scale for Children, only 3 had IQs within the average range (90–110); of the remaining 15 subjects, three were in the low–average range (80–89), three in the borderline range (70–79), and nine in the intellectually disabled range (<70). These studies were done without family controls, so that the possibility of other factors related to consanguinity that might affect intellectual development could not be addressed. In a follow-up study 25 years later, the investigators re-examined eight of the original 18 patients and four new patients with GHRD, excluding five patients with mental disabilities who were in the original study (222). This group had mean verbal and performance IQs of 86 and 92 on the Wechsler scale without evidence of visual motor integration difficulties noted in the earlier group, but there was a suggestion of deficient short-term memory and attention. The investigators hypothesized that early and prolonged IGF deficiency might impair normal development of the central nervous system, or that hypoglycemia common in younger patients may have had a deleterious effect.

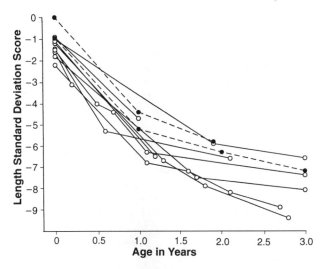

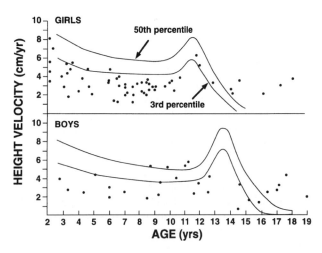

Figure 11 Length SD scores of nine girls from Ecuador (open circles, solid lines) and two brothers from southern Russia (solid circles, dashed lines) with known birth lengths, evaluated over the first 2–3 years of life. (Reprinted from Trends in Endocrinology and Metabolism, vol. 5, Rosenbloom AL, Guevara-Aguirre J, Rosenfeld RG, Pollock BH, Growth in growth hormone insensitivity, pages 296–303, © 1994, with permission from Elsevier Science.)

Figure 12 Growth velocities of 30 Ecuadorian patients (10 males) with GH receptor deficiency; repeated measures were at least 6 months apart. (Reprinted from Trends in Endocrinology and Metabolism, vol. 5, Rosenbloom AL, Guevara-Aguirre J, Rosenfeld RG, Pollock BH, Growth in growth hormone insensitivity, pages 296–303, © 1994, with permission from Elsevier Science.)

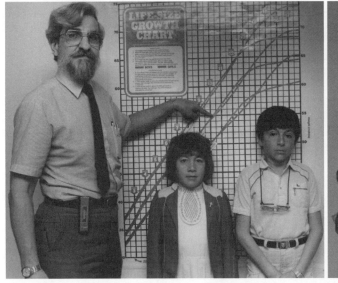

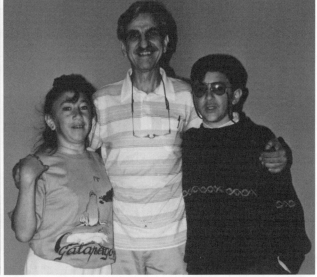

Figure 13 Adult Ecuadorian siblings with multiple pituitary hormone deficiency demonstrate persistence of responsiveness to growth promotion effects of exogenous GH. Left: 33.4-year-old woman with SDS for height −5.9 and bone age 11 years, and 31.7-year-old man with height SDS −5.6 and bone age 13.5 years, with investigator at time of diagnosis. Right: The woman at 37.1 years of age with a bone age of 13.5 years: she has received thyroid and cortisol replacement for 3.7 years, rhGH for 2.6 years (until 14 months previously), and low dosages of estradiol for the past 2.6 years; her height SDS is now −2.5, an increase of 3.4 SDs. The man at age 35.4 years with SDS for height SDS −3.0, an increase of 2.6 SDs, and bone age 15.8 years; he has also received thyroid and cortisol replacement since diagnosis, rhGH until 6 months previously and incremental testosterone since 1 year after diagnosis.

The recent description of intellectual impairment with severe IGF-I deficiency due to partial deletion of the IGF-I gene added concern about potential effects of severe IGF-I deficiency in utero (46). Nonetheless, patients with severe IGF-I deficiency due to GH gene deletion or GHRH receptor deficiency have not been intellectually impaired (15, 108). Sporadic anecdotal reports of patients with GHRD suggested a normal range of intelligence. The collective data from the European IGF-I treatment study group, which includes a wider range of clinical abnormality than either the Ecuadorian or Israeli populations, note a mental retardation rate of 13.5% among 82 patients, but formal testing was not carried out (198). Here again, the high rate of consanguinity was proposed as an explanation; hypoglycemia could not be correlated with these findings.

In the Ecuadorian GHRD cohort, exceptional school performance was reported among 51 affected individuals of school age or older who had attended school, with 44 typically in the top three places in their classes and most thought to be as bright or brighter than the smartest of their unaffected siblings (223). The first controlled documentation of intellectual function in a population with GHRD was in the Ecuadorian patients, a study of school-age individuals compared to their close relatives and to community controls. No significant differences in intellectual ability could be detected among these groups, using nonverbal tests with minimal cultural limitations. It was hypothesized that the exceptional school performance in this population might have been related to the lack of social opportunities due to extreme short stature, permitting greater devotion to studies and superior achievement in school for IQ level (205).

The clinical findings of intellectual impairment with IGF-I gene deletion (46) and intellectual normality with GHRD is consistent with gene disruption studies in mice. The IGF-I-deleted mouse is neurologically impaired, while the GHRD mouse is behaviorally normal (224). Thus, while GH-independent IGF-I synthesis appears necessary for normal brain development in utero, GH-dependent IGF-I production is not necessary for normal brain development and function.

B. Laboratory Evaluation

The methods for GH testing include provocative stimulation with arginine, insulin, clonidine, l-DOPA, and glucagon, frequently with propranolol priming, and physiological testing with exercise or serial sampling. Priming with sex steroids is often done, especially in late prepub-

Table 4 Reference Values (ng/ml) for IGF-I and IGFBP-3 According to Age and Sex (after age 7 years—F/M)

Age (years)	Mean IGF-I	−2 SD IGF-I	Mean IGFBP-3	−2 SD IGFBP-3
0	27	5	1874	1040
1	35	8	2058	1107
2	56	20	2153	1248
3	59	20	2203	1180
4	69	25	2321	1578
5	97	37	2628	1789
6	119	45	2862	1862
7	172/170	44/54	3913/3329	2190/1699
8	236/170	50/52	3840/3478	2497/2371
9	227/192	44/64	3413/3604	575/2265
10	270/131	94/37	3982/3244	2371/3244
11	308/137	93/30	4540/3396	2494/2041
12	387/219	126/63	4413/3666	2074/2167
13	459/329	216/83	4134/4334	2260/2616
14	481/519	271/183	4246/4354	2592/1946
15	473/518	254/335	4332/4028	2710/1495
16	431/519	192/401	4570/4842	3225/3435
17	412/372	253/210	4001/4152	2183/2065
18	408/499	223/206	4078/4810	1846/3235
19	335/397	182/168	4218/4752	2049/2495
20	255/434	86/267	4398/4554	2446/3214

Source: Adapted from the Meet-the-Professor session handouts for the Endocrine Society 81st Annual Meeting, June 12–15, 1999, Clinical Utility of IGF and IGFBP Measurements by Ron G. Rosenfeld, M.D.

ertal children. GH secretion is pulsatile throughout the day, with the usual concentration being low, typically below the limits of sensitivity of most assays. Thus, random GH samples are not helpful unless they are elevated, which might occur as a result of the stress of venipuncture. These various stimuli provoke GHRH release, suppress somatostatin, or work in combination. Serial sampling studies have not been helpful in diagnosis (225). Exercise must be standardized in terms of VO_2 max, which is difficult to accomplish.

The problems with GH testing are:

Response only correlates with successful GH treatment when there is unequivocal deficiency (226).

Deficient GH response to stimulation is seen without endocrine disease, for example, in malnutrition, and during the slow growth phase of preadolescence.

There is great variability in the assay from laboratory to laboratory. The monoclonal immunoradiometric assay results in values that are approximately two-thirds those of the polyclonal assay (227).

There is great intraindividual variability in response from day to day, including nocturnal profiles (228).

Responses vary with age and body mass (229).

The definition of a normal response is arbitrary.

In view of these difficulties with GH testing, the measurement of GH-dependent IGF-I and IGFBP-3 for the diagnosis of GHD has been proposed as a functional bioassay. These substances have low or no circadian variation. They are present in sufficient concentration to minimize difficulties with assay sensitivity. They vary with nutritional status and in disease states, however, and there is wide age variation (Table 4). They may also be normal in children with GHD resulting from brain tumors.

Two studies have looked at the usefulness of IGF-I and IGFBP-3 measurements. Based on results of peak stimulated GH and mean nocturnal GH concentrations, Nunez et al. (230) organized 104 short-statured patients into three groups: GHD (<7 μg/L) , borderline (7–10 μg/L, or nocturnal GH below -2 SD of mean for age and pubertal stage), and idiopathic short stature (ISS, >10 μg/L). Confirmed was the earlier finding that nocturnal GH monitoring had little diagnostic value (225). IGF-I and IGFBP-3 concentrations, expressed as SD scores, correlated with peak stimulated GH but with wide scatter and primarily as a result of the strong correlations in the GHD group. Although means differed, there was not a significant difference between IGFBP-3 concentrations among patients in the three diagnostic groups, and only the GHD group differed in IGF-I mean concentration from the other two. The practical application of these findings was to use IGF-I for initial testing, with a criterion of -1.0 SD to identify a subgroup that would include 88% of those

with GH deficiency, 71% of borderline GHD, and 46% of ISS. With IGF-I and IGFBP-3 above -1.0 SD, 68% of ISS would be identified as not requiring GH testing. Evaluation of growth velocity over the next 3–6 months will identify those children requiring further testing.

In a study that classified 203 children into one of two groups, GHD and normal on the basis of response to provocative testing, IGF-I and IGFBP-3 concentrations were found to correlate with peak GH response. In children <10 years of age with GHD, however, IGF-I concentrations were below the cutoff of -2 SD in only half, for a sensitivity of 53.3%. IGFBP-3 gave a comparable sensitivity of 60% and the combination was even less sensitive (46.6%). Specificity, however, was nearly 100% for both IGF-I and IGFBP-3. In 10–20-year-olds specificity and predictive value of these measures were generally lower (231).

C. GHD

GHD may be considered with the following findings or circumstances:

Other systemic causes of growth failure ruled out
Subnormal growth rate
Progressive decline in height percentile
Delayed bone age
Low IGF-I, IGFBP-3
Poor GH response to stimulation
Predisposing condition (e.g., brain irradiation, optic atrophy)
Other evidence of pituitary dysfunction (e.g., neonatal hypoglycemia, microphallus, midfacial hypoplasia, central adiposity, single central incisor)

Consensus guidelines for the diagnosis and treatment of GHD in childhood and adolescence were developed by the GH Research Society in October 1999 (232). The process of evaluation of the GH-IGF axis was summarized as follows:

In a child with slow growth, whose history and auxology suggest GHD, testing for GH/IGF-I deficiency requires IGF-I/IGFBP-3 levels and GH provocation tests after hypothyroidism has been excluded. In suspected isolated GHD, two GH provocation tests (sequential or on separate days) are required. In those with defined CNS pathology, history of irradiation, MPHD or a genetic defect, one GH test will suffice. In addition, an evaluation of other pituitary function is required. In patients who have had cranial irradiation or malformations of the hypothalamic–pituitary unit, GHD may evolve over years and its diagnosis may require repeat testing of the GH–IGF axis.

It is recognized, however, that some patients with auxology suggestive of GHD may have IGF-I and/

or IGFBP-3 levels below the normal range on repeated tests, but GH responses in provocation tests above the cut-off level. These children are not classically GH deficient but may have an abnormality of the GH–IGF axis and, after the exclusion of systemic disorders affecting the synthesis or action of IGF-I, could be considered for GH treatment.

An MRI (or CT scan) of the brain with particular attention to the hypothalamic–pituitary region should be carried out in any child diagnosed as having GHD.

Conclusion

The diagnosis of severe GHD is usually straightforward, as there are well-defined clinical, auxological, biochemical, and radiological abnormalities. However, the diagnosis of moderate GHD can be associated with normal values within the IGF axis and a normal MRI. It is very important that the response to GH treatment be carefully reviewed, particularly in those patients with moderate GHD.

D. GHRD

GHRD is readily diagnosed in its typical and complete form because of severe growth failure; the somatic phenotype of severe GHD; elevated serum GH levels; and marked reduction in IGF-I, IGF-II, and IGFBP-3 concentrations, with increased concentrations of IGFBP-1 and IGFBP-2. Most such individuals will also have absent to very low concentrations of GHBP, although the less common GHBP-positive forms make absence of GHBP an important but not essential criterion. As noted in Table 2, some of the biochemical features of GHRD may be shared by conditions associated with acquired GH insensitivity, such as malnutrition and liver disease. In a large multinational study designed to identify patients for replacement therapy with recombinant human IGF-I (rhIGF-I), a scoring system was developed that assigned one point for each of the following:

Height >3 SD below mean height for age
Basal GH >2.5 μg/L
Basal IGF-I <50 μg/L
Basal IGFBP-3 <-2 SD
IGF-I rise with GH (0.05 mg/kg/day $\times$ 4 days) <15 μg/L
IGFBP-3 rise with GH stimulation <0.4 mg/L
GH binding <10% (based on binding of ^{125}I-hGH)

A score of 5 out of the possible 7 was considered diagnostic for GHRD. This standard resulted in identification of 82 patients from 22 countries who reflect a wide variability for each criterion. Particularly noteworthy was that height SDS range was up to -2.2 (233). These criteria recognize the age and gender (after age 7 years) variation of IGFBP 3 by using a standard of $\leq$2 SD but,

oddly, designate a fixed standard for IGF-I that falls within the range of normal for children under age 7 (Table 4).

As noted above, the presence of a homozygous mutation or a compound heterozygous mutation affecting the GHR usually provides definitive diagnosis. Thirty-one of the 82 patients reported by Woods et al. (198) underwent a genetic study of the GHR, of whom 27 had abnormalities affecting both alleles of the GHR gene, in association with clinically and biochemically unequivocal GHRD. Identification of heterozygous mutations, however, is not necessarily helpful because, as noted earlier, polymorphisms have been described that appear to have no phenotypic consequences.

X. TREATMENT

A. GHD

1. History

The history of GH therapy for the treatment of GHD now spans more than 40 years. In 1958, Raben reported the first use of human pituitary-derived GH for replacement therapy in a child with hypopituitarism (234). Until the advent of recombinant GH products for general use in 1985, GH therapy was in very limited supply and subject to many interruptions, because of the limited supply of human pituitary gland and the absence of effects of GH extracted from the pituitary glands of other mammalian species. As a result, only a very select group of patients could be treated. These children had unmistakable GHD, having failed to respond to at least two GH stimulation tests using extremely stringent criteria. Treatment with as little as 2.5 units once weekly was effective in improving growth velocity (235, 236); however, overall, children were suboptimally treated because of relatively low dosage and intermittent therapy due to limited supplies. At best, they achieved an adult height -2 to -2.5 standard deviations below the normal means (237, 238).

Use of pituitary-derived GH came to a rapid halt in 1985 with the recognition of Creutzfeldt–Jakob disease (CJD) in recipients of pituitary-derived GH (239, 240). CJD is a rare prion disease with a long latency period, transmitted by the pituitary-derived product to at least 70 former patients. Affected individuals develop neurological degeneration and dementia. Diagnosis is difficult, requiring brain biopsy. There is no therapy (241, 242).

Fortunately for patients with GDH, rhGH (a 192 amino acid product) entered formal testing in 1981 and was approved for use by the Food and Drug Administration in 1985. With the advent of recombinant product, a continuous, unlimited supply of GH became available for the more optimal treatment of children with GHD. Such a large and reliable supply has allowed physicians to seek the best dosages and treatment intervals and to verify the safety of therapy.

2. Guidelines of GH Therapy

In patients with GHD, GH therapy provides the best growth velocity response in the first 12 months of therapy (three to five times pretreatment velocity), and improved velocity (above pretreatment levels) is maintained throughout the duration of therapy. Continuous therapy in a dosage range of 0.15–0.30 mg/kg/week, divided into six or seven daily doses per week, optimizes response, and the long-term result is further improved by early initiation of therapy (before the age of 6 years) (243–248). Some investigators recommend that therapy be given at bedtime, because GH secretion in normal children is maximal during sleep (232). Standard of care dictates that children being treated currently are evaluated every 3–6 months by endocrinologists familiar with monitoring for efficacy and safety. The ultimate objective of therapy, of course, is to normalize adult height, but considerable debate remains surrounding the definition of "normal."

3. Adult GH Therapy

Although his or her epiphyses are fused, the adult with GHD nevertheless may benefit from continuation of GH replacement therapy, at a much smaller dose than that used to stimulate growth. Long-term monitoring of adults with GHD has revealed a striking physical profile in the absence of continued therapy, an increased risk for obesity, for lipid disorders, and for significant cardiovascular morbidity and mortality (249, 250). Recognition of the role of GH in lipolysis, muscle strength, and generalized well-being in adults has led to acceptance of the use of rhGH in management of adults with hypopituitarism (251). The observation that the recently appreciated cardiovascular risk factor of elevated serum homocysteine is improved in men with GHD treated with GH suggests a mechanism for the increased risk with GHD (252, 253). Current guidelines include cessation of growth-promoting GH therapy in the patient who has reached adult height. Because spontaneous resolution of GH deficiency has been documented in 50–80% of patients, particularly those with isolated GHD, any adult being considered for adult GH replacement therapy should undergo provocative GH stimulus testing within 6 months of cessation of GH therapy (251). An adult patient diagnosed with any pituitary deficiency should likewise undergo GH stimulation testing, because of the recognized benefits of identification and treatment of adult-onset GHD.

4. Safety Issues

Long-term, worldwide use of rhGH has allowed endocrinologists to monitor and document the relative safety and rarity of side effects associated with the recombinant product. Unlike pituitary-derived GH, recombinant GH does not carry a risk of human infectious contamination. Large-scale collaborative efforts, such as the National Cooperative Growth Study (NCGS) sponsored by Genentech and the KIGS (Kabi International Growth Study) sponsored by Pharmacia and Upjohn are permitting endocrinologists to share and analyze data regarding safety and efficacy of rhGH, in therapy of hypopituitarism and other growth-deficient states.

In 1998, Root et al. (244) summarized the North American NCGS experience in the use of recombinant human GH in more than 20,000 children, of whom 44% had idiopathic GH deficiency and 13.8% had organic GH deficiency. This evaluation, like the others that preceeded and followed it, confirmed the general safety of GH in patients who do not have other underlying risk factors (particularly malignancy or genetic syndromes in which malignancy is a frequent feature).

Side effects that have been reported in patients receiving recombinant human GH are listed in Table 5. Salt retention with peripheral edema is sometimes noted with initiation of GH therapy. Pseudotumor cerebri has been noted to occur in some patients in the first 5 years of therapy (254). It is more common in patients with renal insufficiency or Chiari malformation. Typically, symptoms resolve with temporary cessation of therapy and generally do not recur when therapy is reintroduced a week or more later. Some investigators advocate resumption of GH therapy at lower doses with gradual increases to the presymptomatic level.

Prepubertal gynecomastia has been reported in some children treated with GH (255). Twenty-five percent of patients with GHD may have falling T4 levels after starting GH replacement therapy, necessitating regular assessment of serum thyroxine levels during GH therapy (256). GH antibodies develop in some patients, but diminution of growth response beyond that normally expected with continued therapy does not occur, except in the rare patient with type IA GHD. Scoliosis is sometimes seen, particularly during the period of peak growth velocity, and can compromise final height in some patients. Slipped capital femoral epiphysis (SCFE) may occur with therapy, possibly reflecting a growth effect rather than an adverse effect of GH (257); children with long-standing IGF-I deficiency may be at greater risk of this complication.

Table 5 Reported Side Effects of Growth Hormone Treatment

Growth of nevi
Peripheral edema
Pseudotumor cerebri
Gynecomastia
Pancreatitis
Slipped capital femoral epiphysis
Scoliosis
GH antibody formation
Hypothyroidism
Hyperinsulinism
Glucose intolerance/type 2 diabetes

Among GHRD patients from Ecuador, 25% had radiological evidence of Legg-Perthes disease (100). Therefore, careful monitoring for knee pain, hip pain, or limp should be a part of each clinic visit, and patients' families should be instructed to report any joint symptoms or gait changes. Pancreatitis is a rare side effect of GH therapy, but should be suspected in the patient with recurrent abdominal pain and emesis (258).

Although hyperinsulinemia may occur in response to GH therapy, glucose intolerance or diabetes has been considered rare. A retrospective analysis of the KIGS database found 85 of 23,333 children reported as having abnormal glucose metabolism, 43 of which were confirmed using American Diabetes Association (ADA) criteria. Eleven of the 43 had type 1 diabetes, consistent with expected frequency for the population, whereas 18 had type 2 diabetes and 14 impaired glucose tolerance, giving an incidence of type 2 diabetes of 34.4:100,000 years of GH treatment. The type 2 diabetes was not associated with obesity and did not clear up with discontinuation of GH (259). The authors' rejection of half of the patients diagnosed by their physicians as having glucose intolerance or diabetes reflects the more stringent criteria of the ADA than those of the WHO that these European investigators were more likely to be using. Even without this consideration, this is an approximately 20-fold greater incidence than expected in a largely white population (260). Similar observations have not been reported from the NCGS database.

The mitogenic potential of GH has led to careful monitoring and considerable concern about whether GH therapy might increase a patient's risk of malignancy or of tumor recurrence if a patient has had a primary malignancy. Studies to date have not revealed an increase in cancer risk for patients receiving GH replacement therapy. Although an increase in size of nevi can be seen, there has been no increase in melanoma formation. Careful analysis of a cluster of cases of leukemia in Japanese patients receiving GH therapy and similar extensive evaluation of nine cases in the United States and Canada revealed that the number of cases was not different from that expected for the general population (261–263). In the US/Canadian cohort, six of the patients had risk factors for leukemia (262). Specific examination of risk for patients with treated malignancies has not demonstrated that GH increases tumor recurrence risk (264). Patients with malignancy should not receive GH therapy during the acute phase of the malignancy and should be disease-free for at least 1 year after successful surgery, radiotherapy, or chemotherapy before starting GH therapy (265). Patients who have had malignancies or who have syndromes in which malignancy is a known component should have close monitoring by an endocrinologist, oncologist, neurosurgeon, or geneticist at frequent intervals.

The development of a purified, relatively safe rhGH product has allowed many patients with hypopituitarism to attain normal height and health. The availability of rhGH has also permitted many non-GH-deficient short children, including those with a variety of genetic syndromes, to receive GH therapy in hopes of improving their final height. For those children, therapy has had varying degrees of success.

B. GHI/GHRD

Soon after the cloning of the human IGF-I cDNA, human IGF-I was synthesized by recombinant DNA techniques (rhIGF-I) (266, 267). Subcutaneous preparations of rhIGF-I became available in 1990. Results have been reported for 67 patients with GHI treated with rhIGF-I for 12 months or longer. Five of these patients had GH gene deletion with acquired GHI due to GH inhibiting antibodies (53). The rest had primary GHI, including Pakistani and Arab patients thought to have postreceptor defects.

1. Dose–Response

In the European multicenter study (268), responses to twice-daily doses varied, but average dosage was similar to that used in the North Carolina (53, 269, 270) and Ecuadorian (52, 271) study populations. As predicted from short-term studies, IGFBP-3 levels did not increase during long-term treatment with rhIGF-I. In the only direct comparison of dosages, there was no difference in growth response between 80 μg/kg body weight and 120 μg/kg twice daily, apparently defining a plateau effect (52). Improvement in mean height SDS over 2 years was 1.2 in the European study, 1.5 for the higher dosage and 1.3 for the lower dosage in Ecuador, and 1.3 in the North Carolina study. The European multicenter study and Ecuadorian study patients achieved two-thirds of their improvement in the initial year (Table 6). In the Israeli patients treated with single daily injections of rhIGF-I (120 μg/kg), there was an improvement of only 0.4 SDS during the first year of treatment, with no further improvement for the 6 patients completing 2 years of therapy (272). This supports the rationale for twice-daily administration, which was based on kinetic studies in normal controls.

Comparison of growth response of 22 rhIGF-I treated GHRD patients and 11 GH-treated GHD patients in the same setting demonstrated mean growth velocity increment in those with GHRD to be 63% of that achieved with GH treatment of GHD in the first year and less than 50% in the second and third years (52). The North Carolina group has reported IGF-I treatment responses after 6.5–7.5 years in five children with GHRD and three with GHI from antibody formation (53). The inadequate growth response compared to GH treatment of GHD persisted over this longer term treatment period, with a mean improvement in height SDS of only 1.4 (from −5.6 to −4.2), thus only sustaining the improvement of the first 2 years of treatment, as noted in Table 6. The most recent report from the European study described 17 patients treated for 48 months or longer. Overall increase in height SDS was 1.67 ± 1.16, suggesting modest continued im-

Table 6 IGF-I Treatment of Children with GH Insensitivity for 1 Year or Longer

Number (males)	Age (yrs)	IGF-I dose (μg/k)	Ht SDS[g]				Source (reference)
			Start	1 year	2 year	4–7.5 yrs	
26 (14)	3.7–19.6	40–120 bid	−6.8 (1.6)	−6.1 (1.5)	X	X	Europe (268, 273)
18 (10)[a]	3.7–16.7	40–120 bid	−6.4 (1.7)	−5.6 (1.6)	−5.2 (1.9)	X	
17 (9)[a]	3.7–13.4	40–120 bid	−6.5 (1.3)	−5.8 (1.5)	−5.4 (1.8)	−4.9 (1.8)	
2 (1)[b]	18/17.5	120 bid	−8.0/−9.1	−7.1/−7.9	X	X	Ecuador (52, 271, 274, 275)
16 (5)	4.7–17.1	120 bid	−8.5 (1.3)	−7.5 (1.1)	−7.0 (1.2)	X	
7 (2)	3.1–15.2	80 bid	−8.0 (1.8)	−7.2 (1.8)	−6.7 (1.8)	X	
21 (6)[c]	3.1–17.1	80–120 bid	−8.1 (1.2)	−7.3 (1.2)	−6.7 (1.4)	−6.3 (1.3)	
9 (6)[d]	0.5–14.6	150–200/d	−5.6 (1.5)	−5.2 (1.7)	X	X	Israel (272)
6 (4)[e]	0.5–14.6	150–200/d	−6.2 (1.5)	−6.0 (1.6)	−5.8 (1.2)	X	
8 (6)[f]	2.3–11	80–120 bid	−5.6 (1.1)	NA	−4.5 (1.3)	−4.2 (1.9)	North Carolina (53, 269)

[a]Same cohort as all 26.
[b]Also treated with GnRH analog.
[c]Same cohort as above.
[d]Patient age 0.5 excluded because rapid growth first 6 months of life before treatment (18 cm/yr).
[e]Same cohort as all 9.
[f]5 with GHRD, 3 with GHD IA and antibody-induced GHI.
[g]SD in parentheses.
NA, not available.

provement over time in this group, but still markedly less than expected with GH replacement therapy (273). Studies in Ecuador noted correlation of growth acceleration with trough levels of serum IGF-I, obtained before the 12 hourly injection (52). Also noted was an increase in body weight for height; in the European study, the gain in BMI correlated with improvement in SDS for height. In the North Carolina patients, fat mass increased with treatment and was thought to reflect high-dosage IGF-I insulin-like effects during peak times following IGF-I injection (53).

The lesser rate of response to IGF-I in GHI/GHRD than to GH in GHD could be attributable to failure to increase IGFBP-3 and ALS levels, a direct GH effect. However, three children who had defective IGF-I synthe-

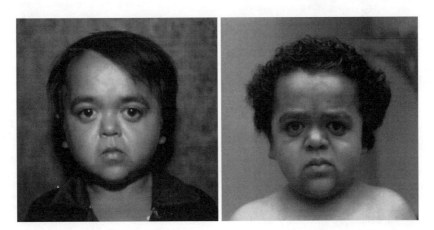

Figure 14 Face and hair changes in 17.7 year old patient (bone age, 13 years) with GHRD during 6 months treatment with IGF-I, 120 μg/k twice daily and depot GnRH agonist begun at age 16.5 years. (Reprinted from Rosenbloom AL. IGF-I treatment of growth hormone insensitivity. In: Rosenfeld RG, Roberts CT (eds.). The IGF System: Molecular Biology, Physiology, and Clinical Applications. Copyright 1999, with permission from Humana Press, Totowa, NJ; pp. 739–769.)

sis attributed to a postreceptor defect did not grow better while receiving IGF-I than did subjects with GHRD, despite their normal IGFBP-3 levels (199, 272). Furthermore, acromegaloid facial changes in some patients (Fig. 14) indicate that the amount of IGF-I reaching tissues is supraphysiological (53, 271, 273). The more likely explanation for the relatively modest growth response is the absence of the direct GH effects at the growth plate. These effects include epiphyseal prechondrocyte differentiation, increased responsiveness to IGF-I, and enhancement of local production of IGF-I that stimulates clonal expansion of the differentiating chondrocytes (50, 51). Of great interest would be studies of the administration of recombinant IGFBP-3 with rhIGF-I. The pursuit of further treatment studies with rhIGF-I, however, is limited by the decision of manufacturers to no longer produce IGF-I.

2. Adverse Events

Hypoglycemia is frequent in children with GHRD, and was a concern with rhIGF-I treatment because of the very low IGFBP-3 levels resulting in greater amounts of free IGF-I. Severe hypoglycemic episodes have been reported in the European treatment study (268). During a 6-month placebo controlled trial of rhIGF-I treatment in children with GHRD, however, there was no difference in the frequency of hypoglycemia between placebo and treatment groups (274). Headache is a frequent complaint among treated patients, but also did not vary in frequency between placebo-treated and rhIGF-I-treated patients (268). Pain at the injection site is common and injection into lumps may result in cessation of response. Tachycardia, reflecting the inotropic effect of IGF-I (276), is uniformly present early in treatment, but clears after several months (277). Less frequent side effects include parotid swelling, facial nerve palsy, lymphoid hyperplasia that may require tonsillectomy or adenoidectomy, papilledema, and pseudotumor cerebri. Coarsening of the facial features with mandibular hyperplasia and excessive weight gain are also seen in some patients (278, 279). Hyperandrogenism, with oligomenorrhea or amenorrhea, acne, and elevated serum androgens, has been described in prepubertal and young adult patients given single daily injections of rhIGF-I (280).

REFERENCES

1. Rimoin DL, Philips JA III. Genetic disorders of the pituitary gland. In: Rimoin DL, Connor JM, Pyeritz RE, eds. Principles and Practice of Medical Genetics. 3d ed. New York: Churchill Livingstone, 1997:1331–1364.
2. Lindsay R, Feldkamp M, Harris D, Robertson J, Rallison M. Utah growth study: growth standards and the prevalence of growth hormone deficiency. J Pediatr 1994; 125:29–35.
3. Kemp S. Growth hormone deficiency. Emed Pediatr 2000; http://www.emedicine.com/ped/topic1810.htm.
4. Chatelain P. Trends in the diagnosis and treatment of short stature as revealed by KIGS. In: Ranke MB, Wilton P, eds. Growth Hormone Therapy in KIGS-10 Years' Experience. Heidelberg: Johann Ambrosius Barth Verlag, 1999:11–20.
5. Weber FT, Donnelley WH, Behar RL. Hypopituitarism following extirpation of a pharyngeal pituitary. Am J Dis Child 1977; 131:525–528.
6. Sadler TW. Langman's Medical Embryology. 5th ed. Philadelphia: Williams & Wilkins, 1985:353–355.
7. Heimer L. Hypothalamus and the hypothalamohypophyseal system. In: The Human Brain and Spinal Cord. New York: Springer-Verlag, 1983:295.
8. Junqueira LC, Carneiro J. Basic Histology. 3rd ed. Los Altos, CA: Lange Medical Publications, 1980:410–420.
9. Cohen LE. Genetic regulation of the embryology of the pituitary gland and somatotrophs. Endocrine 2000; 12:99–106.
10. Parks JS, Brown MR, Hurley DL, Phelps CJ, Wajnrajch MP. Commentary: Heritable diseases of pituitary development. J Clin Endocrinol Metab 1999; 84:4362–4370.
11. Dattani M, Martinez-Barbera J-P, Thomas PQ. Mutations in the homeobox gene HESX1/HESX1 associated with septo optic dysplasia in human and in mouse. Nat Genet 1998; 19:125–133.
12. Zhadanov AB, Bertuzzi S, Taira M, Dawid IB, Westphal H. Expression pattern of the murine LIM class homeobox gene *Lhx3* in subsets of neural and neuroendocrine tissues. Dev Dyn 1995; 202:354–364.
13. Netchine I, Sobrier M-L, Krude H, Schnabel D, Maghnie M, Marcos E, Duriez B, Cacheux V, Moers A, Goossens M, Grüters A, Amselem S. Mutations in *LHX3* result in a new syndrome revealed by combined pituitary hormone deficiency. Nat Genet 2000; 25:182–186.
14. Hendriks-Stegeman BI, Augustijn KD, Bakker B, Holthuizen P, van der Vliet PC, Jansen M. Combined pituitary hormone deficiency caused by compound heterozygosity for two novel mutations in the domain of the Pit 1/POU1F1 gene. J Clin Endocrinol Metab 2001; 86:1545–1550.
15. Maheshwari HG, Silverman BL, Dupuis J, Baumann G. Phenotypic and genetic analysis of a syndrome caused by an inactivating mutation in the GH releasing hormone receptor: dwarfism of Sindh. J Clin Endocrinol Metab 1998; 83:4065–4074.
16. Murray RA, Maheshwari HG, Russell EJ, Baumann G. Pituitary hypoplasia in patients with a mutation in the growth hormone-releasing hormone receptor gene. Am J Neuroradiol 2000; 21:685–689.
17. Evans VR, Manning AB, Bernard LH, Chronwall BM, Millington WR. Alpha-M-S-hormone and N-acetyl-β-endorphin immunoreactivities are localized in the human pituitary but are not restricted to the zona intermedia. Endocrinology 1994; 134:97–106.
18. Pickering BT. The neurosecretory neurone: a model system for the study of secretion. Essays Biochem 2978; 14:45–81.
19. Keller RJ, Wolfsdorf JI. Isolated growth hormone deficiency after cerebral edema complicating diabetic ketoacidosis. N Engl J Med 1987; 316:857–859.
20. Netter FH. Endocrine system and selected metabolic diseases. In: The CIBA Collection of Medical Illustrations. Vol. 4. Chicago: RR Donnelley and Sons, 1981:4–5.
21. Lewis UJ, Singh RNP, Tutwiler GH, Sigel MB, VanderLaan EF, VanderLaan WP. Human growth hormone: a complex of proteins. Recent Prog Horm Res 1980; 36:477–508.
22. Bowers CY, Momany F, Reynolds GA, Hong A. On the in vitro and in vivo activity of a new synthetic hexapeptide that acts on the pituitary to specifically release growth hormone. Endocrinology 1984; 114:1531–1536.

23. Goth MI, Lyons CE, Canny BJ, Thorner MO. Pituitary adenylate cyclase activating polypeptides, growth hormone (GH) releasing peptide and GH releasing hormone stimulate GH release through distinct pituitary receptors. Endocrinology 1992; 130:939–944.

24. Kojima M, Hosada H, Date Y, Nakazato M, Matsui H, Kangawa K. Ghrelin is a growth hormone releasing acetylated peptide from stomach. Nature 1999; 402:656–660.

25. Bowers CY. Unnatural growth hormone-releasing peptide begets natural ghrelin. J Clin Endocrinol Metab 2001; 86: 1464–1469.

26. Korbonits M, Bustin SA, Kojima M, Jordan S, Adams EF, Lowe DG, Kangawa K, Grossman AB. The expression of the growth hormone secretagogue receptor ligand ghrelin in normal and abnormal human pituitary and other neuroendocrine tumors. J Clin Endocrinol Metab 2001; 86:881–887.

27. Postel-Vinay M-C, Kelly PA. GH receptor signalling. Bailliere's Clin Endocrinol Metab 1996; 10:323–326.

28. Ymer SI, Herrington AC. Evidence for the specific binding of growth hormone to a receptor like protein in rabbit serum. Mol Cell Endocrinol 1985; 41:153–161.

29. Daughaday WH, Trivedi B. Absence of serum growth hormone binding protein in patients with growth hormone receptor deficiency (Laron dwarfism). Proc Natl Acad Sci USA 1987; 84:4636–4640.

30. Baumann G, Shaw MA, Winter RJ. Absence of plasma growth hormone-binding protein in Laron-type dwarfism. J Clin Endocrinol Metab 1987; 65:814–816.

31. Leung DW, Spencer SA, Cachianes G, Hammonds RG, Collins C, Henzel WJ, Barnard R, Waters MJ, Wood Wl. Growth hormone receptor and serum binding protein: purification, cloning and expression. Nature 1987; 330:537–543.

32. Godowski PJ, Leung DW, Meacham LR, Galgani JP, Hellmiss R, Keret R, Rotwein PS, Parks JS, Laron Z, Wood WI. Characterization of the human growth hormone receptor gene and demonstration of a partial gene deletion in two patients with Laron-type dwarfism. Proc Natl Acad Sci USA 1989; 86:8083–8087.

33. Kelly PA, Nagano M, Sotiropoulos A, Lebrun J-J, Touraine P, Goujon L, Dinerstein H, Ferrag F, Buteau H, Pezet A, Esposito N, Finidori J, Postel-Vinay M-C, Edery M. Growth hormone-prolactin receptor gene family. In: Shiverick KT, Rosenbloom AL, eds. Human Growth Hormone Pharmacology: Basic and Clinical Aspects. Boca Raton, FL: CRC Press, 1995:13–28.

34. de Vos AM, Ultsch M, Kossiakoff AA. Human growth hormone and extracellular domain of its receptor: crystal structure of the complex. Science 1992; 255:306–312.

35. Campbell GS. Growth-hormone signal transduction. J Pediatr 1997; 131:S42–S44.

36. Dastot F, Sobrier ML, Duquesnoy P, Duriez B, Goosens M, Amselem S. Alternative spliced forms in the cytoplasmic domain of the human growth hormone (GH) receptor regulate its ability to generate a soluble GH binding protein. Proc Natl Acad Sci USA 1996; 93:10723–10728.

37. Fisker S, Kristensen K, Rosenfalck AM, Pedersen SB, Ebdrup L, Richelsen B, Hilsted J, Christiansen JS, Jørgensen OL. Gene expression of a truncated and the full-length growth hormone (GH) receptor in subcutaneous fat and skeletal muscle in GH-deficient adults: impact of GH treatment. J Clin Endocrinol Metab 2001; 86:792–796.

38. Rajaram S, Baylink DJ, Mohan S. Insulin-like growth factor-binding proteins in serum and other biological fluids: regulation and functions (Review). Endocr Rev 1997; 18:801–831.

39. Rinderknech E, Humbel RE. The amino acid sequence of human insulin like growth factor I and its structural homology with proinsulin. J Biol Chem 1978; 253:2769–2772.

40. Rinderknech E, Humbel RE. Primary structure of human insulin like growth factor II. FEBS Lett 1978; 89:283–287.

41. Baxter RG, Binoux MA, Clemmons DR, Conover CA, Drop SLA, Holly JMP, Mohan S, Oh Y, Rosenfeld RG. Recommendations for nomenclature of the insulin-like growth factor binding proteins superfamily. J Clin Endocrinol Metab 1998; 83:3213.

42. Vaccarello MA, Diamond FB Jr, Guevara-Aguirre J, Rosenbloom AL, Fielder PJ, Gargosky S, Cohen P, Wilson K, Rosenfeld RG. Hormonal and metabolic effects and pharmacokinetics of recombinant human insulin-like growth factor-I in GH receptor deficiency/Laron syndrome. J Clin Endocrinol Metab 1993; 77:273–280.

43. Siddle K, Soos MA. Alternative IGF related receptors. In: Rosenfeld RG, Roberts CT Jr, eds. The IGF System: Molecular Biology, Physiology, and Clinical Applications. Totowa, NJ: Humana Press, 1999:199–226.

44. Collett-Solberg PF, Cohen P. Genetics, chemistry, and function of the IGF/IGFBP system. Endocrine 2000; 12: 121–136.

45. Rosenbloom AL. IGF-I treatment of growth hormone insensitivity. In: Rosenfeld RG, Roberts CT, eds. The IGF System: Molecular Biology, Physiology, and Clinical Applications. Totowa, NJ: Humana Press, 1999: 739–769.

46. Woods KA, Camacho-Hübner C, Savage MO, Clark AJL. Intrauterine growth retardation and postnatal growth failure associated with deletion of the insulin-like growth factor I gene. N Eng J Med 1996; 335:1363–1367.

47. Abuzzahab MJ, Goddard A, Grigorescu F, Lautier C, Smith RJ, Chernausek SD. Human IGF-I receptor mutations associated with intrauterine and postnatal growth retardation. 82nd Annual Meeting of the Endocrine Society, Toronto, June 21–24, 2000.

48. Giudice LC, de Zegher F, Gargosky SE, Dsupin BA, de las Fuentes L, Crystal RA, Hintz RL, Rosenfeld RG. Insulin like growth factors and their binding proteins in the term and preterm human fetus and neonate with normal and extremes of intrauterine growth. J Clin Endocrinol Metab 1995; 80:1548–1555.

49. Rosenbloom AL, Guevara-Aguirre J, Rosenfeld RG, Pollock BH. Growth in GH insensitivity. Trends Endocrinol Metab 1994; 5:296–303.

50. Isaksson OGP, Lindahl A, Nilsson A, Isgaard J. Mechanism of the stimulatory effect of growth hormone on longitudinal bone growth (review). Endocr Rev 1987; 6: 426–438.

51. Daughaday WH, Rotwein P. Insulin-like growth factors I and II: peptide, messenger ribonucleic acid and gene structures, serum and tissue concentrations. Endocr Rev 1989; 10:68–91.

52. Guevara-Aguirre J, Rosenbloom AL, Vasconez O, Martinez V, Gargosky SE, Rosenfeld RG. Two year treatment of GH receptor deficiency (GHRD) with recombinant insulin-like growth factor-I in 22 children: comparison of two dosage levels and to GH treated GH deficiency. J Clin Endocrinol Metab 1997; 82:629–633.

53. Backeljauw PF, Underwood LE, GHIS Collaborative Group. Therapy for 6.5–7.5 years with recombinant insulin like growth factor I in children with growth hormone insensitivity syndrome: a clinical research center study. J Clin Endocrinol Metab 2001; 86:1504–1510.

54. Grumbach MM, Gluckman PD. The human fetal hypothalamic and pituitary: the maturation of neuroendocrine mechanisms controlling secretion of fetal pituitary growth

hormone, prolactin, gonadotropins, adrenocorticotropin-related peptides and thyrotropin. In: Tulchinsky D, Little AB, eds. Maternal and Fetal Endocrinology. Philadelphia: WB Saunders, 1994:193–261.

55. Lemire RJ, Beckwith JB, Warkeny J. Anencephaly. New York: Raven, 1978.

56. Hintz RL, Menking M, Sotos JF. Familial holoprosencephaly with endocrine dysgenesis. J Pediatr 1968; 72: 81–87.

57. Lieblich JM, Rosen SE, Guyda H, Reardan J, Schaaf M. The syndrome of basal encephalocele and hypothalamic–pituitary dysfunction. Ann Intern Med 1978; 89:910–916.

58. Rudman D, Davis T, Priest JH, Patterson JH, Kutner MH, Heymsfield SB, Bethel RA. Prevalence of growth hormone deficiency in children with cleft lip or palate. J Pediatr 1978; 93:378–382.

59. Izenberg N, Rosenblum M, Parks JS. The endocrine spectrum of septo-optic dysplasia. Clin Pediatr 1984; 23:632–636.

60. Hoyt WF, Kaplan SL, Grumbach MM, Glaser JS. Septo-optic dysplasia and pituitary dwarfism. Lancet 1970; 1: 893–894.

61. Kaplan SL, Grumbach MM. Pathophysiology of GH deficiency and other disorders of GH metabolism. In: LacCauza C, Root AW, eds. Problems in Pediatric Endocrinology, Serono Symposia. Vol. 32. London: Academic Press, 1980:45.

62. Jacquemin C, Mullaney PB, Bosley TM. Ophthalmological and intracranial anomalies in patients with clinical anophthalmos. Eye 2000; 14:82–87.

63. Wilson DM, Enzmann DR, Hintz RL, Rosenfeld G. Cranial computed tomography in septo-optic dysplasia: discordance of clinical and radiological features. Neuroradiology 1984; 26:279–283.

64. Willnow S, Kiess W, Butenandt O, Dorr HG, Enders A, Strasser-Vogel B, Egger J, Schwarz HP. Endocrine disorders in septo-optic dysplasia (deMorsier syndrome)—evaluation and followup of 18 patients. Eur J Pediatr 1996; 155:179–184.

65. Semina EV, Reiter R, Leysen NJ, Alward WL, Small KW, Datson NA, Siegel-Bartelt J, Bierke-Nelson D, Bitoun P, Zabel BU, Carey JC, Murray JC. Cloning and characterization of a novel bicoid-related homeobox transcription factor gene, RIEG, involved in Rieger syndrome. Nat Genet 1996; 14:392–399.

66. Kleinmann RE, Kazarian EL, Raptopoulos V, Braverman LE. Primary empty sella and Rieger's anomaly of the anterior chamber of the eye: a familial syndrome. N Engl J Med 1981; 304:90–93.

67. Biesecker LG, Abbott M, Allen J, Clericuzio C, Feuillan P, Graham JM Jr, Hall J, Kang S, Olney AH, Lefton D, Neri G, Peters K, Verloes A. Report from the workshop on Pallister-Hall syndrome and related phenotypes. Am J Med Genet 1996; 65:76–81.

68. Argyropoulo M, Perignon F, Brauner R, Brunelle F. Magnetic resonance imaging in diagnosis of growth hormone deficiency. J Peds 1992; 120:886–891.

69. Spiliotis B, August G, Hung W, Sonis W, Mendelson W, Bercu BB. Growth hormone neurosecretory dysfunction: a treatable cause of short stature. JAMA 1984; 251:2223–2230.

70. Oliff A, Bode U, Bercu BB, DiChiro G, Graves V, Poplack DG. Hypothalamic–pituitary dysfunction following CNS prophylaxis in acute lymphoblastic leukemia: correlation with CT scan abnormalities. Med Pediatr Oncol 1979; 7:141–151.

71. Lustig RH, Schriock EA, Kaplan SL, Grumbach MM. Effect of growth hormone release in children with radi-

ation-induced growth hormone deficiency. Pediatrics 1985; 76:274–279.

72. Angelo M, Castro-Magana M, Uy J. Pituitary evaluation and growth hormone therapy in Prader-Willi syndrome. J Pediatr Endocrinol 1991; 4:167–172.

73. Myers SE, Carrel AL, Whitman BY, Allen DB. Sustained benefit after two years of growth hormone on body composition, fat utilization, physical strength and agility, and growth in Prader-Willi syndrome. J Pediatr 2000; 137: 42–49.

74. Shulman DI, Martinez CR, Bercu BB, Root AW. Hypothalamic–pituitary dysfunction in primary empty sella syndrome in childhood. J Pediatr 1986; 108:540–544.

75. Rapaport R, Logrono R. Primary empty sella syndrome in childhood: association with precocious puberty. Clin Pediatr 1991; 30:466–471.

76. Craft WH, Underwood LE, Van Wyk JJ. High incidence of perinatal insult in children with idiopathic hypopituitarism. J Pediatr 1980; 96:397–402.

77. Maghnie M, Larizza D, Triulzi F, Sampaolo P, Scotti G, Severi F. Hypopituitarism and stalk agenesis: a congenital syndrome worsened by breech delivery? Horm Res 1991; 35:104–108.

78. Lovinger RD, Kaplan SL, Grumbach MM. Congenital hypopituitarism associated with neonatal hypoglycemia and microphallus: four cases secondary to hypothalamic hormone deficiencies. J Pediatr 1975; 87:1171–1181.

79. Brown RS, Bhatia V, Hayes E. An apparent cluster of congenital hypopituitarism in central Massachusetts: magnetic resonance imaging and hormonal studies. J Clin Endocrinol Metab 1991; 72:12–18.

80. Perez Jurado LA, Phillips III JA, Francke U. Exclusion of growth hormone-releasing hormone gene mutations in familial isolated growth hormone deficiency by linkage and single strand conformation analysis. J Clin Endocrinol Metab 1994; 78:622–628.

81. Parks JS, Brown MR, Abdul-Latif H, Kinoshita E. Abnormalities of the pituitary-specific transcription factor-1 gene and protein. Clin Pediatr Endocrinol 1995; 4:33–39.

82. Phelan PD, Connelly J, Martin FIR, Wettenhall HN. X-linked recessive hypopituitarism. Birth Defects 1971; 7: 24–27.

83. Adler-Bier M, Pertzelan A, Laron Z, Lieberman E, Moses S. Multiple pituitary hormone deficiencies in eight siblings of one Jewish Moroccan family. Acta Paediatr Scand 1979; 68:401–404.

84. Tatsumi K, Miyai K, Notomi T, Kaibe K, Amino N, Mizuno Y, Kohno H. Cretinism with combined hormone deficiency caused by a mutation in the PIT1 gene. Nat Genet 1992; 1:56–58.

85. Sornson MW, Wu W, Dasen JS, Flynn SE, Norman DJ, O'Connell SM, Gukovsky I, Carriere C, Ryan AK, Miller AP, Zuo L, Gleiberman AS, Andersen B, Beamer WG, Rosenfeld MG. Pituitary lineage determination by the Prophet of Pit-1 homeodomain factor defective in Ames dwarfism. Nature 1996; 384:327–333.

86. Wu W, Cogan JD, Pfaffle RW, Dasen JS, Frisch H, O'Connell SM, Flynn SE, Brown MR, Mullis PE, Parks JS, Phillips JA 3rd, Rosenfeld MG. Mutations in PROP1 cause familial combined pituitary hormone deficiency. Nat Genet 1998; 18:147–149.

87. Fofanova OV, Takamura N, Kinoshita E, Parks JS, Brown MR, Peterkova VA, Evgrafov OV, Goncharov NP, Bulatov AA, Dedov II, Yamashita S. A mutational hot spot in the Prop-1 gene in Russian children with combined pituitary hormone deficiency. Pituitary 1998; 1:45–49.

88. Fofanova O, Takamura N, Kinoshita E, Parks JS, Brown MR, Peterkova VA, Evgrafov OV, Goncharov NP, Bulatov AA, Dedov II, Yamashita S. Compound heterozygous

deletion of the PROP1 gene in children with combined pituitary hormone deficiency. J Clin Endocrinol Metab 1998; 83:2601–2604.

89. Nader S, Fisher JA, Doyle FH, Mashiter K, Joplin GF. Familial dwarfism: case report. Postgrad Med J 1975; 51: 676–681.

90. Parks JS, Tenore A, Bongiovanni AM, Kirkland RT. Familial hypopituitarism with large sella turcica. N Engl J Med 1978; 298:698–702.

91. Parks JS, Brown MR, Baumbach L, Sanchez JC, Stanley CA, Gianella-Neto D, Wu W, Oyesika N. Natural history and molecular mechanisms of hypopituitarism with large sella turcica. Proceedings, Endocrinological Society 80th Annual Meeting, New Orleans, LA, 1998:471.

92. Agarwal G, Bhatia V, Cook S, Thomas PQ. Adrenocorticotropin deficiency in combined pituitary hormone deficiency patients homozygous for a novel PROP1 deletion. J Clin Endocrinol Metab 2000; 85:4556–4561.

93. Cogan JD, Wu W, Phillips JA 3rd, Arnhold IJ, Agapito A, Fofanova OV, Osorio MG, Bircan I, Moreno A, Mendonca BB. The PROP-1 2bp deletion is a common cause of combined pituitary hormone deficiency. J Clin Endocrinol Metab 1998; 83:3346–3349.

94. Rosenbloom AL, Selman-Almonte A, Brown MR, Fisher DA, Baumbach L, Parks JS. Clinical and biochemical phenotype of familial anterior hypopituitarism from mutation of PROP-1 gene. J Clin Endocrinol Metab 1999; 84:50–57.

95. Deladoey J, Fluck C, Buyukgebiz A, Kuhlmann BV, Eble A, Hindmarsh PC, Wu W, Mullis PE. "Hot spot" in the PROP1 gene responsible for combined pituitary hormone deficiency. J Clin Endocrinol Metab 1999; 84:1645–1650.

96. Wajnrajch MP, Gertner JM, Harbison MD, Chua SCJ, Leibel RL. Nonsense mutation in human growth hormone-releasing hormone receptor causes growth failure analogous to the little (lit) mouse. Nat Genet 1996; 12: 88–90.

97. Netchine I, Talon P, Dastot F, Vitaux F, Goossens M, Amselem S. Extensive phenotypic analysis of a family with growth hormone (GH) deficiency caused by a mutation in the GH-releasing hormone receptor gene. J Clin Endocrinol Metab 1998; 83:432–436.

98. Salvatori R, Hayashida CY, Aguiar-Oliveira MH, Phillips III JA, Souza HO, Gondo RG, Toledo SPA, Conceicao MM, Prince M, Maheshwari HG, Baumann G, Levine MA. Familial dwarfism due to a novel mutation of the growth hormone-releasing hormone receptor gene. J Clin Endocrinol Metab 1999; 84:917–923.

99. Hayashida CY, Gondo RG, Ferrari C, Toledo SPA, Salvatori R, Levine MA, Ezabella MCL, Abelin N, Gianella-Neto D, Wajchenberg BL. Familial growth hormone deficiency with mutated GHRH receptor gene: clinical and hormonal findings in homozygous and heterozygous individuals from Itabaianinha. Eur J Endocrinol 2000; 142: 557–563.

100. Rosenbloom AL, Guevara-Aguirre J, Fielder PJ, Gargosky S, Rosenfeld RG, Diamond FB Jr, Vaccarello MA. Growth hormone receptor deficiency/Laron syndrome in Ecuador: clinical and biochemical characteristics. In: Laron Z, Parks JS, eds. Lessons from Laron Syndrome (LS) 1966–1992. Pediatr Adolesc Endocrinol 1993; 24:34–52.

101. Rosenbloom AL, Guevara-Aguirre J, Fielder PJ, Gargosky S, Cohen P, Rosenfeld RG. Insulin-like growth factor binding proteins-2 and -3 in Ecuadorian patients with growth hormone receptor deficiency and their parents. In: Laron Z, Parks JS, eds. Lessons from Laron Syndrome (LS) 1966–1992. Pediatr Adolesc Endocrinol 1993; 24: 185–191.

102. Moseley CT, Phillips JA III. Pituitary gene mutations and the growth hormone pathway. Semin Reprod Med 2000; 18:21–29.

103. Vnencak-Jones CL, Phillips JA III, Chen EY, Seeburg PH. Molecular basis of human growth hormone gene deletions. Proc Natl Acad Sci USA 1988; 85:5615–5619.

104. Vnencak-Jones CL, Phillips JA III, De-fen W. Use of polymerase chain reaction in detection of growth hormone gene deletions. J Clin Endocrinol Metab 1990; 70: 1550–1553.

105. Mullis PE, Akinci A, Kanaka C, Eble A, Brook CGD. Prevalence of human growth hormone-I gene deletions among patients with isolated growth hormone deficiency from different populations. Pediatr Res 1992; 31:532–553.

106. Duquesnoy P, Amselein S, Gounnelen M, LeBouc Y, Goossens M. A frameshift mutation causing isolated growth hormone deficiency type IA. Am J Hum Genet 1990; 47:A 110.

107. Cogan JD, Phillips JA III, Sakati N, Frisch H, Schober E, Milner RDG. Heterogeneous growth hormone (GH) gene mutations in familial GH deficiency. J Clin Endocrinol Metab 1993; 76:1224–1228.

108. Rivarola MA, Phillips III JA, Migeon CJ, Heinrich JJ, Hjelle BJ. Phenotypic heterogeneity in familial isolated growth hormone deficiency type 1A. J Clin Endocrinol Metab 1984; 59:34–40.

109. Laron Z, Kelijman M, Pertzelan A, Keret R, Shoffner JM, Parks JS. Human growth hormone gene deletion without antibody formation or arrest during treatment: a new disease entity? Isr J Med Sci 1985; 21:999–1006.

110. Matsuda I, Hata A, Jinno Y, Endo F, Akaboshi I, Nishi Y, Takeuchi S, Takeda M, Okada Y. Heterogeneous phenotypes of Japanese cases with a growth hormone gene deletion. Jpn J Hum Genet (Jinrui Idengaku Zasshi) 1987; 32:227–235.

111. Ghizzoni L, Duquesnoy P, Torresani T, Vottero A, Goossens M, Bernasconi S. Isolated growth hormone deficiency type 1A associated with a 45-kilobase gene deletion within the human growth hormone gene cluster in an Italian family. Pediatr Res 1994; 36:654–659.

112. Lieberman E, Pesler D, Parvari R, Elbedour K, Abdul-Latif H, Brown MR, Parks JS, Carmi R. Short stature in carriers of recessive mutation causing familial isolated growth hormone deficiency. Am J Med Genet 2000; 90: 188–192.

113. Cogan JD, Phillips JA III, Schenkman SS, Milner RDG, Sakati N. Familial growth hormone deficiency: a model of dominant and recessive mutations affecting a monomeric protein. J Clin Endocrinol Metab 1994; 79:1261–1265.

114. Cogan JD, Ramel B, Lehto M, Phillips III J, Prince M, Blizzard RM, de Ravel, TJL, Brammert M, Groop L. A recurring dominant-negative mutation causes autosomal dominant growth hormone deficiency. J Clin Endocrinol Metab 1995; 80:3591–3595.

115. Binder G, Ranke MB. Screening for growth hormone (GH) gene splice-site mutations in sporadic cases with severe isolated GH deficiency using ectopic transcript analysis. J Clin Endocrinol Metab 1995; 80:1247–1252.

116. Lee MS, Wajnrajch MP, Kim SS, Plotnick LP, Wang J, Gertner JM, Leibel RL, Dannies PS. Autosomal dominant growth hormone (GH) deficiency type II: the del32-71-GH deletion mutant suppressor secretion of wild-type GH. Endocrinology 2000; 141:883–890.

117. Moseley CT, Philips III JA, Wajnrajch MP, Gertner JM, Moshang T, Saenger P, Leibel RL. Isolated growth hormone (GH) deficiency, type 11 (IGHD 11) caused by substitution of arginine by histidine in C-terminal portion of

the GH molecule. Proceedings, Endocrinological Society 80th Annual Meeting, San Francisco CA, 1996:2–313.

118. Kowarski AA, Schneider JJ, Ben-Galim E, Weldon W, Daughaday WH. Growth failure with normal serum RIAGH and low somatomedin activity: somatomedin restoration and growth acceleration after exogenous GH. J Clin Endocrinol 1978; 47:461–464.

119. Valenta LJ, Sigel MB, Lesniak MA, Elias AN, Lewis UJ, Friesen HG, Kershnar AK. Pituitary dwarfism in a patient with circulating abnormal growth hormone polymers. N Engl J Med 1985; 312:214–217.

120. Takahashi Y, Kaji H, Okimura Y, Goji K, Abe H, Chihara K. Brief report: short stature caused by a mutant growth hormone. N Engl J Med 1996; 334:432–436.

121. Binder G, Benz MR, Elmlinger M, Pflaum C-D, Strasburger CJ, Ranke MB. Reduced hGH (hGH) bioactivity without a defect of the GH-1 gene in three patients with rhGH responsive growth failure. Clin Endocrinol 1999; 51:89–95.

122. Jenkins JS, Gilbert GJ, Ang V. Hypothalamic–pituitary function in patients with craniopharyngioma. J Clin Endocrinol Metab 1976; 43:394–399.

123. Bunin GR, Witman PA, Preston-Martin S, Davis F, Bruner JM. The descriptive epidemiology of craniopharyngioma. J Neurosurg 1998; 89:547–551.

124. Curtis J, Daneman D, Hoffman HJ, Ehrlich RM. The endocrine outcome after removal of craniopharyngioma. Pediatr Neurosurg 1994; 21(Suppl 1):24.

125. Shin JL, Asa SL, Woodhouse LJ Smyth HS, Ezzat S. Cystic lesions of the pituitary: clinicopathological features distinguishing craniopharyngioma, Rathke's cleft cyst, and arachnoid cyst. J Clin Endocrinol Metab 1999; 84:3972–3982.

126. Robertson PL. Pediatric brain tumors. Primary Care 1998; 25:323–339.

127. Vance ML. Hypopituitarism. N Engl J Med 1994; 330: 1651–1662.

128. Lafferty AR, Chrousos GP. Pituitary tumors in children and adolescents. J Clin Endocrinol Metab 1999; 84: 4317–4323.

129. Sklar CA. Craniopharyngioma: endocrine sequelae of therapy. Pediatr Neurosurg 1994; 21(Suppl 1):120–123.

130. Scott RM, Hetelkidis S, Barnes PD, Goumnereroval L, Tarbell NJ. Surgery, radiation, and combination therapy in the treatment of childhood craniopharyngioma—a 20-year experience. Pediatr Neurosurg 1994; 21(Suppl 1): 75–81.

131. Fahlbusch R, Honegger J, Paulus W, Huk W, Buchfelder M. Surgical treatment of craniopharyngiomas: experience with 168 patients. J Neurosurg 1999; 90:237–250.

132. Rout D, Rao VRK, Radhakrishnan VV. Symptomatic Rathke's cleft cyst. Surg Neurol 1983; 19:42–45.

133. Kunwar S, Wilson CB. Pediatric pituitary adenomas. J Clin Endocrin Metab 1999; 84:4385–4396.

134. Thapar K, Kovacs K, Laws ER, Muller PJ. Pituitary adenomas: current concepts in classification, histopathology, and molecular biology. Endocrinologist 1993; 3:41–57.

135. Rosenbloom AL. Intracerebral crises during treatment of diabetic ketoacidosis. Diabetes Care 1990; 13:22–33.

136. Eiholzer V, Zachmann M, Gnehm HE, Prader A. Recovery from posttraumatic anterior pituitary insufficiency. Eur J Pediatr 1986; 145:128–130.

137. Bevenga S, Campenni A, Ruggeri RM, Trimarchi F. Clinical review 113: hypopituitarism secondary to head trauma. J Clin Endocrin Metab 2000; 85:1353–1361.

138. Constine LS, Woolf PD, Cann D, Mick G, McCormick K, Raubertas RF, Rubin P. Hypothalamic-pituitary dysfunction after radiation for brain tumors. N Engl J Med 1993; 328:87–94 (erratum 328:1208).

139. Snyder FJ, Fowable BF, Schatz NJ, Savino PJ, Gennarelli TA. Hypopituitarism following radiation therapy of pituitary adenomas. Am J Med 1986; 81:457–462.

140. Samaan NA, Vieto R, Schultz PN, Maor M, Meoz RT, Sampiere VA, Cangir A, Ried HL, Jesse RH Jr. Hypothalamic, pituitary, and thyroid dysfunction after radiotherapy to the head and neck. Int J Radiat Oncol Biol Phys 1982; 8:1857–1867.

141. Barkan AL. Pituitary atrophy in patients with Sheehan's syndrome. Am J Med Sci 1989; 298:38–40.

142. Cardosa ER, Peterson EW. Pituitary apoplexy: a review. Neurosurgery 1984; 14:363–373.

143. Cheung CC, Ezzat S, Smith HS, Asa SL. The spectrum and significance of primary hypophysitis. J Clin Endocrinol Metab 2001; 86:1048–1053.

144. Crock PA. Cytosolic autoantigens in lymphocytic hypophysitis. J Clin Endocrinol Metab 1998; 83:609–618.

145. Unluhizarci K, Bayram F, Colak R, Ozturk F, Selcuklu A, Durak AC, Kelestimur F. Distinct radiological and clinical appearance of lymphocytic hypophysitis. J Clin Endocrinol Metab 2001; 86:1861–1864.

146. Sano T, Kovacs K, Scheithauer BW, Rosenblum MK, Petito CK, Greco CM. Pituitary pathology in acquired immunodeficiency syndrome. Arch Pathol Lab Med 1989; 113:1066–1070.

147. Vannasaeng S, Fucharoen S, Pootrakul P, Ploybutr S, Yansukon P. Pituitary function in thalassemic patients and the effect of chelation therapy. Acta Endocrinol (Copenh) 1991; 124:23–30.

148. Schmitt S, Wichmann W, Martin E, Zachmann M, Schoenle EJ. Pituitary stalk thickening with diabetes insipidus preceding typical manifestations of Langerhans cell histiocytosis in children. Eur J Pediatr 1993; 152: 399–401.

149. Spitz RA, Wolff K. Anaclitic depression. Psychoanalyt Stud Child 1946; 2:313–337.

150. Talbot NB, Sobel EH, Burke BS, Lindemann E, Kaufman SB. Dwarfism in healthy children: its possible relation to emotional nutritional and endocrine disturbances. N Engl J Med 1947; 236:783–793.

151. Patton RG, Gardner LI. Influence of family environment on growth: the syndrome of "maternal deprivation." Pediatrics 1962; 30:957–962.

152. Patton RG, Gardner LI. Growth Failure in Maternal Deprivation. Springfield, IL: Charles C Thomas, 1963.

153. Silver HK, Finkelstein M. Deprivation dwarfism. J Pediatr 1967; 70:317–324.

154. Powell GF, Brasel JA, Blizzard RM. Emotional deprivation and growth retardation simulating idiopathic hypopituitarism. I. Clinical evaluation of the syndrome. N Engl J Med 1967; 276:1271–1278.

155. Powell GF, Brasel JA, Blizzard RM. Emotional deprivation and growth retardation simulating idiopathic hypopituitarism. II. Endocrinologic evaluation of the syndrome. N Engl J Med 1967; 276:1279–1283.

156. Krieger I, Mellinger RC. Pituitary function in the deprivation syndrome. J Pediatr 1971; 79:216–225.

157. Kerr GR, Chamove AS, Harlow HF. Environmental deprivation: its effect on the growth of infant monkeys. J Pediatr 1979; 75:833–837.

158. Whitten CF, Pettit MG, Fischoff J. Evidence that growth failure from maternal deprivation is secondary to undereating. JAMA 1969; 209:1675–1682.

159. Krieger I. Food restriction as a form of child abuse in ten cases of psychosocial deprivation dwarfism. Clin Pediatr 1974; 13:127–133.

160. Fischoff J, Whitten CF, Pettit MG. A psychiatric study of mothers of infants with growth failure secondary to maternal deprivation. J Pediatr 1971; 79:209–215.

161. Evans SL, Reinhart JB, Succop RA. Failure to thrive. A study of 45 children and their families. J Am Acad Child Psychiatry 1972; 11:440–457.
162. Sills RH. Failure to thrive. The role of clinical and laboratory evaluation. Am J Dis Child 1978; 132:967–969.
163. Karacan I, Rosenbloom AL, Williams RL, Finley WW, Hursch CJ. Slow wave sleep deprivation in relation to plasma growth hormone concentration. Behav Neuropsychiatry 1971; 2:11–14.
164. Guilhaume A, Benoit O, Gourmelen M, Richardet JM. Relationship between sleep stage IV deficit and reversible HGH deficiency in psychosocial dwarfism. Pediatr Res 1982; 16:299–303.
165. Stanhope R, Adlard P, Hamill G, Jones J, Skuse D, Preece MA. Physiological growth hormone (GH) secretion during the recovery from psychosocial dwarfism: a case report. Clin Endocrinol 1988; 28:335–339.
166. Albanese A, Hamill G, Jones J, Skuse D, Matthews DR, Stanhope R. Reversibility of physiological growth hormone secretion in children with psychosocial dwarfism. Clin Endocrinol 1994; 40:687–692.
167. Tanner JM, Whitehouse RH, Hughes PCR, Vince FP. The effect of human growth hormone treatment for 1 to 7 years on growth of 100 children, with growth hormone deficiency, low birth weight, inherited smallness, Turner's syndrome, and other complaints. Arch Dis Child 1971; 46:745–782.
168. Frasier SD, Rallison ML. Growth retardation and emotional deprivation: relative resistance to treatment with human growth hormone. J Pediatr 1972; 80:603–609.
169. Laron Z, Pertzelan A, Mannheimer S. Genetic pituitary dwarfism with high serum concentration of growth hormone—a new inborn error of metabolism? Isr J Med Sci 1966; 2:152–155.
170. Laron Z, Pertzelan A, Karp M. Pituitary dwarfism with high serum levels of growth hormone. Isr J Med Sci 1968; 4:83–94.
171. Merimee TJ, Hall J, Rabinovitz D, McKusick VA, Rimoin DL. An unusual variety of endocrine dwarfism: subresponsiveness to growth hormone in a sexually mature dwarf. Lancet 1998; 2:191–193.
172. Daughaday WH, Laron Z, Pertzelan A, Heins JN. Defective sulfation factor generation: a possible etiological link in dwarfism. Trans Assoc Am Physicians 1969; 82:129–138.
173. Bala RM, Beck JC. Fractionation studies on plasma of normals and patients with Laron dwarfism and hypopituitary gigantism. Can J Physiol Pharmacol 1973; 91:845–852.
174. Eshet R, Laron Z, Brown M, Arnon R. Immunoreactive properties of the plasma hGH from patients with the syndrome of familial dwarfism and high plasma IR-hGH. J Clin Endocrinol Metab 1973; 37:819–821.
175. Tsushima T, Shiu RPC, Kelly PA, Friesen HG. Radioreceptor assay for human growth hormone and lactogens: structure-function studies and clinical applications. In: Raiti S. Advances in Human Growth Hormone Research. Bethesda, MD: USPHS, USPHS-DHEW publication 74-612, 1973:372–387.
176. Jacobs LS, Sneid DS, Garland JT, Laron Z, Daughaday WH. Receptor-active growth hormone in Laron dwarfism. J Clin Endocrinol Metab 1976; 42:403–406.
177. Golde DW, Bersch N, Kaplan SA, Rimoin DL, Li CH. Peripheral unresponsiveness to human growth hormone in Laron dwarfism. N Engl J Med 1980; 303:1156–1159.
178. Eshet R, Laron Z, Pertzelan A, Arnon R, Dintzman M. Defect of human growth hormone receptors in the liver of two patients with Laron-type dwarfism. Isr J Med Sci 1984; 20:8–11.

179. Edens A, Talamantes F. Alternative processing of growth hormone receptor transcripts. Endocr Rev 1998; 19:559–582.
180. Pantel J, Machinis K, Sobrier ML, Duquesnoy P, Goossens M, Amselem S. Species-specific alternative splice mimicry at the growth hormone receptor locus revealed by the lineage of retroelements during primate evolution. A novel mechanism accounting for protein diversity between and within species. J Biol Chem 2000; 275:18664–18669.
181. Rosenbloom AL. Physiology and disorders of the growth hormone receptor (GHR) and GH-GHR signal transduction. Endocrine 2000; 12:107–119.
182. Duquesnoy P, Sobrier M-L, Duriez B, et al. A single amino acid substitution in the exoplasmic domain of the human growth hormone (GH) receptor confers familial GH resistance (Laron syndrome) with positive GH-binding activity by abolishing receptor homodimerization. EMBO J 1994; 13:1386–1395.
183. Sobrier M-L, Dastot F, Duquesnoy P, Kandemir N, Yordam N, Goossens M, Amselem S. Nine novel growth hormone receptor gene mutations in patients with Laron syndrome. J Clin Endocrinol Metab 1997; 82:3705–3709.
184. Ayling RM, Ross R, Towner P, Von Laue S, Finidori J, Moutoussamy S, Cuchanan CR, Clayton PE, Norman MR. A dominant-negative mutation of the growth hormone receptor causes familial short stature. Nature Genet 1997; 16:13–14.
185. Iida K, Takahashi Y, Kaji H, Nose O, Okimura Y, Abe H, Chihara K. Growth hormone (GH) insensitivity syndrome with high serum GH binding protein levels caused by a heterozygous splice site mutation of the GH receptor gene producing a lack of intracellular domain. J Clin Endocrinol Metab 1998; 83:531–537.
186. Iida K, Takahashi Y, Kaji H, Takahashi MO, Okimura Y, Nose O, Abe H, Chihara K. Functional characterization of truncated growth hormone (GH) receptor (1-277) causing partial GH insensitivity syndrome with high GH-binding protein. J Clin Endocrinol Metab 1999; 84:1011–1016.
187. Ross RJ, Esposito N, Shen XY, Von Laue S, Chew SL, Dobson PR, Postel-Vinay MC, Finidori J. A short isoform of the human growth hormone receptor functions as a dominant negative inhibitor of the full-length receptor and generates large amounts of binding protein. Mol Endocrinol 1997; 11:265–273.
188. Amit T, Bergman T, Dastot F, Youdim MBH, Amselem S, Hochberg Z. A membrane-fixed, truncated isoform of the human growth hormone receptor. J Clin Endocrinol Metab 1997; 82:3813–3817.
189. Metherell LA, Munroe PB, Bjarnason R, Johnston LB, Rose SJ, Caulfield MJ, Savage MO, Clark AJ. Growth hormone (GH) insensitivity, without the phenotype of Laron syndrome and with normal GH binding protein (GHBP), caused by a novel intronic point mutation in the human GH receptor (GHR) gene. 82nd Annual Meeting of the Endocrine Society, Toronto, June 21–24, 2000.
190. Rosenbloom AL, Guevara-Aguirre J. Lessons from the genetics of Laron syndrome. Trends Endocrinol Metab 1998; 9:276–283.
191. Goddard AD, Covello R, Luoh S-M, Clackson T, Attie KM, Gesundheit N, Rundle AC, Wells JA, Carlsson LMS. Mutations of the growth hormone receptor in children with idiopathic short stature. N Engl J Med 1995; 333:1093–1098.
192. Kou K, Lajara R, Rotwein P. Amino acid substitutions in the intracellular part of the growth hormone receptor in a patient with the Laron syndrome. J Clin Endocrinol Metab 1993; 76:54–59.

193. Iida K, Takahashi Y, Kaji H, Onadera N, Takahashi MO, Okimura Y, Abe H, Chihara K. The C422F mutation of the growth hormone receptor gene is not responsible for short stature. J Clin Endocrinol Metab 1999; 84:4214–4219.
194. Chujo S, Kaji H, Takahashi Y, Okimura Y, Abe H, Chihara K. No correlation of growth hormone receptor gene mutation P561T with body height. Eur J Endocrinol 1996; 134:560–562.
195. Carlsson LMS, Attie KM, Compton PG, Vingcol RV, Merimee TJ, The National Cooperative Growth Study. Reduced concentration of serum growth hormone-binding protein in children with idiopathic short stature. J Clin Endocrinol Metab 1994; 78:1325–1330.
196. Cotterill AM, Camacho-Hubner C, Duquesnoy P, Savage MO. Changes in serum IGF-I and IGFBP-3 concentrations during the IGF-I generation test performed prospectively in children with short stature. Clin Endocrinol 1998; 48:719–724.
197. Rosenbloom AL, Guevara-Aguirre J, Berg MA, Francke U. Stature in Ecuadorians heterozygous for the growth hormone receptor (GHR) gene E180 splice mutation does not differ from that of homozygous normal relatives. J Clin Endocrinol Metab 1998; 83:2373–2375.
198. Woods KA, Dastot F, Preece MA, Clark AJL, Postel-Vinay M-C, Chatelain PG, Ranke MB, Rosenfeld RG, Amselem S, Savage MO. Extensive personal experience. Phenotype:genotype relationships in growth hormone insensitivity syndrome. J Clin Endocrinol Metab 1997; 82:3529–3535.
199. Laron Z, Klinger B, Eshet R, Kaneti H, Karasik A, Silbergeld A. Laron syndrome due to a post-receptor defect: response to IGF-I treatment. Isr J Med Sci 1993; 29:757–763.
200. Freeth JS, Ayling RM, Whatmore AJ, Towner P, Price DA, Norman MR, Clayton PE. Human skin fibroblasts as a model of growth hormone (GH) action in GH receptor-positive Laron's syndrome. Endocrinology 1997; 138:55–61.
201. Freeth JS, Silva CM, Whatmore AJ, Clayton PE. Activation of the signal transducers and activators of transcription signaling pathway by growth hormone (GH) in skin fibroblasts from normal and GH binding protein-positive Laron syndrome children. Endocrinology 1998; 139:20–28.
202. Rosenbloom AL. Hot topic. The GH-IGF-I axis and diabetes complications. Pediatr Diabetes 2001; 2:66–70.
203. Powell DR. Effects of renal failure on the growth hormone insulin like growth factor axis. J Pediatr 1997; 131:S13–S16.
204. Rosenbloom AL, Savage MO, Blum WF, Guevara-Aguirre J, Rosenfeld RG. Clinical and biochemical phenotype of GH receptor deficiency/Laron syndrome. Acta Paediatr [suppl] 1992; 380:58–61.
205. Kranzler JH, Rosenbloom AL, Martinez V, Guevara-Aguirre J. Normal intelligence with severe IGF-I deficiency due to growth hormone receptor deficiency: a controlled study in genetically homogeneous population. J Clin Endocrinol Metab 1998; 83:1953–1958.
206. Beck KD, Powell-Braxton L, Widmer H-R, Valverde J, Hofti F. IGF-I gene disruption results in reduced brain size, CNS hypomyelination, and loss of hippocampal granule and striatal parvalbumin-containing neurons. Neuron 1995; 14:717–730.
207. Bucuvalas JC, Horn JA, Carlsson L, Balistreri WF, Chernausek SD. Growth hormone insensitivity associated with circulating growth hormone-binding protein in children with Alagille syndrome and short stature. J Clin Endocrinol Metab 1993; 76:1477–1482.
208. Geffner ME, Bersch N, Bailey RC, Golde DW. Insulin-like growth factor I resistance in immortalized T cell lines from African Efe pygmies. J Clin Endocrinol Metab 1995; 80:3732–3738.
209. Siebler T, Lopaczynski W, Terry CL, Casella SJ, Munson P, DeLeon DD, Phang L, Blakemore KJ, McEvoy RC, Kelley RI, Nissley P. Insulin-like growth factor I receptor expression and function in fibroblasts from two patients with deletion of the distal long arm of chromosome 15. J Clin Endocrinol Metab 1995; 80:3447–3457.
210. Jain S, Golde DW, Bailey R, Geffner ME. Insulin-like growth factor-I resistance. Endocr Rev 1998; 19:625–646.
211. Lanes R, Plotnick LP, Spencer EM, Daughaday WH, Kowarski AA. Dwarfism associated with normal serum growth hormone and increased bioassayable, receptor-assayable and immunassayable somatomedin. J Clin Endocrinol Metab 1980; 50:485–488.
212. Heath-Monnig E, Wohltmann HJ, Mills-Dunlap B, Daughaday WH. Measurement of insulin-like growth factor I (IGF-I) responsiveness of fibroblasts of children with short stature: identification of a patient with IGF-I resistance. J Clin Endocrinol Metab 1987; 64:501–507.
213. Momoi T, Yamanaka C, Kobayashi M, Haruta T, Sasaki H, Yorifuji T, Kaji M, Mikawa H. Short stature with normal growth hormone and elevated IGF-I. Eur J Pediatr 1992; 151:321–325.
214. Crosnier H, Gourmelen M, Prëvot C, Rappaport R. Effects of nutrient intake on growth, insulin-like growth factors, and their binding proteins in a Laron-type dwarf. J Clin Endocrinol Metab 1993; 76:248–250.
215. Laron Z, Lilos P, Klinger B. Growth curves for Laron syndrome. Arch Dis Child 1993; 68:768–770.
216. Rose SR, Municchi G, Barnes KM, Kamp GA, Uriarte MM, Ross JL, Cassorla F, Cutler GB Jr. Spontaneous growth hormone secretion increases during puberty in normal girls and boys. J Clin Endocrinol Metab 1991; 73:428–435.
217. Schaefer GB, Rosenbloom AL, Guevara-Aguirre J, Campbell EA, Ullrich F, Patil K, Frias JL. Facial morphometry of Ecuadorian patients with growth hormone receptor deficiency/Laron syndrome. J Med Genet 1994; 31:635–639.
218. Rosenbloom AL, Guevara-Aguirre J, Rosenfeld RG, Fielder PJ. The little women of Loja: growth hormone receptor-deficiency in an inbred population of southern Ecuador. N Engl J Med 1990; 323:1367–1374.
219. Rosenbloom AL, Berg MA, Kasatkina EP, Volkova TN, Skorobogatova VF, Sokolovskaya VN, Francke U. Severe growth hormone insensitivity (Laron syndrome) due to nonsense mutation of the GH receptor in brothers from Russia. J Pediatr Endocrinol Metab 1995; 8:159–165.
220. Main KM, Price DA, Savage MO, Skakkebae NE. Decreased sweating in seven patients with Laron syndrome. J Clin Endocrinol Metab 1993; 77:821–823.
221. Frankel JJ, Laron Z. Psychological aspects of pituitary insufficiency in children and adolescents with special reference to growth hormone. Isr J Med Sci 1968; 4:953–961.
222. Galatzer A, Aran O, Nagelberg N, Rubitzek J, Laron Z. Cognitive and psychosocial functioning of young adults with Laron syndrome. Pediatr Adolesc Endocrinol 1993; 24:53–60.
223. Guevara-Aguirre J, Rosenbloom AL. Psychosocial adaptation of Ecuadorian patients with growth hormone receptor deficiency/Laron syndrome. In: Laron Z, Parks JS, eds. Lessons from Laron Syndrome (LS) 1966–1992. Pediatr Adolesc Endocrinol 1993; 24:61–64.

224. Zhou Y, Xu BC, Maheshwari HG, He H, Reed M, Loz-kowski M, Okada S, Cataldo L, Coschigamo K, Wagner TE, Baumann G, Kopchick JJ. A mammalian model for the Laron syndrome produced by targeted disruption of the mouse growth hormone receptor/binding protein gene (the Laron mouse). Proc Natl Acad Sci USA. 1997; 94: 13215–13220.

225. Rose SR, Ross JL, Uriarte M, Barnes KM, Cassorla FG, Cutler GB Jr. The advantage of measuring stimulated as compared with spontaneous growth hormone levels in the diagnosis of growth hormone deficiency. N Engl J Med 1988; 319:201–207.

226. Lin T-H, Kirkland RT, Sherman BM, Kirkland JL. Growth hormone testing in short children and their re-sponse to growth hormone therapy. J Pediatr 1989; 115: 57–63.

227. Reiter EO, Morris AH, Macgillivray MH, Weber D. Var-iable estimates of serum growth hormone concentrations in different radio assay systems. J Clin Endocrinol Metab 1988; 66:68–71.

228. Donaldson DL, Hollowell JG, Pan F, Gifford RA, Moore WV. Growth hormone secretory profiles: variation on consecutive nights. J Pediatr 1989; 115:51–56.

229. Kamp GA, Manasco PK, Barnes KM, Jones J, Rose SR, Hill SC, Cutler GB Jr. Low growth hormone levels are related to increased body mass index and do not reflect impaired growth in luteinizing hormone-releasing hor-mone agonist-treated children with precocious puberty. J Clin Endocrinol Metab 1991; 72:301–307.

230. Nunez SB, Municchi G, Barnes KM, Rose SR. Insulin-like growth factor I (IGF-I) and IGF-binding protein-three concentrations compared to stimulated and night growth hormone in the evaluation of short children—a clinical research center study. J Clin Endocrinol Metab 1996; 81: 1927–1932.

231. Juul A, Skakkebaek NE. Prediction of the outcome of growth hormone provocative testing in short children by measurement of serum levels of insulin-like growth factor I and move insulin-like growth factor binding protein 3. J Pediatr 1997; 130:197–204.

232. Growth Hormone Research Society. Consensus guidelines for the diagnosis and treatment of growth hormone (GH) deficiency in childhood and adolescents: summary state-ment of the GH Research Society. J Clin Endocrinol Me-tab 2000; 85:3990–3993.

233. Woods KA, Savage MO. The Laron syndrome: typical and atypical forms. Bailliere's Clin Endocrinol Metab 1996; 10:371–387.

234. Raben MS. Treatment of pituitary dwarfism with human growth hormone. J Clin Endocrinol Metab 1958; 18:901–903.

235. Rosenbloom AL. Growth hormone replacement therapy. JAMA 1966; 198:364–368.

236. Rosenbloom AL, Riley WJ, Silverstein JH, Garnica AD, Netzloff ML, Weber FT. Low dose single weekly injec-tions of growth hormone: response during the first year of therapy of hypopituitarism. Pediatrics 1980; 66:272–276.

237. Burns EC, Tanner JM, Preece MA, Cameron N. Final height and pubertal development in short stature children with idiopathic growth hormone deficiency, treated for between 2 and 15 years with human growth hormone. Eur J Pediatr 1981; 137:155–164.

238. Tanner JM, Whitehouse RH. Growth response of 26 chil-dren with short stature given growth hormone. Br Med J 1967; 2:69–275.

239. Underwood LE, Fisher DA, Frasier SD, et al. Degenera-tive neurologic disease in patients formerly treated with human growth hormone—report of the Committee on Growth Hormone Use of the Lawson Wilkins Pediatric Endocrine Society, May 1985. J Pediatr 1985; 107:10.

240. Brown P. Human growth hormone therapy and Creutz-feldt-Jakob disease: a drama in 3 acts. Pediatrics 1988; 81:85–92.

241. Fradkin JE. Creutzfeldt-Jakob disease in pituitary growth hormone recipients. Endocrinologist 1993; 3:108–114.

242. Gibbs CJ, Joy A, Heffner R, et al. Clinical and patholog-ical features and laboratory confirmation of Creutzfeldt-Jakob disease in a recipient of pituitary-derived human growth hormone. N Engl J Med 1985; 81:85–92.

243. Kastrup KW, Sandahl-Christiansen J, Koch Anderson J, Orskov H. Increased growth rate following transfer to daily s.c. administration from 3 weekly IM injections of human growth hormone in growth hormone deficient chil-dren. Acta Endocrinol 1983; 104:148–152.

244. Root AW, Kemp SF, Rundle AC, Dana K, Attie KM. Ef-fect of long term recombinant growth hormone therapy in children—the National Cooperative Growth Study, 1984–1994. J Pediatr Endocrinol Metab 1998; 11:403–412.

245. Rosenbloom AL, Knuth C, Shulman D. Growth hormone by daily injection in patients previously treated for growth hormone deficiency. South Med J 1990; 83:653–655.

246. Smith PJ, Hindmarsh PC, Brook CGD. Contribution of dose and frequency of administration to the therapeutic effect of growth hormone. Arch Dis Child 1988; 63:491–494.

247. Furlanetto RW, Drug and Therapeutics Committee of the Lawson Wilkins Pediatric Endocrine Society. Guidelines for the use of growth hormone in children with short stat-ure. J Pediatr 1995; 127:857–867.

248. MacGillivray MH, Baptista J, Johanson A. Outcome of a four-year randomized study of daily vs. three times weekly somatotropin treatment in prepubertal naive growth hormone-deficient children. Genentech Study Group. J Clin Endocrinol Metab 1996; 81:1806–1809.

249. Salomon F, Cuneo RC, Hesp R, Sonksen PH. The effects of treatment with recombinant human growth hormone on body composition and metabolism in adults with growth hormone deficiency. N Engl J Med 1989; 321:1797–1803.

250. Bates AS, Van't Hoff W, Jones PJ, Clayton RN. The effect of hypopituitarism on life expectancy. J Clin Endocrinol Metab 1996; 81:1169–1172.

251. Growth Hormone Research Society. Consensus guidelines for the diagnosis and treatment of adults with growth hor-mone deficiency: summary statement of the Growth Hor-mone Research Society Workshop on Adult Growth Hor-mone Deficiency. J Clin Endocrinol Metab 998; 83:379–381.

252. Rosen T, Bengtsson BA. Premature mortality due to car-diovascular disease in hypopituitarism. Lancet 1990; 336: 285–288.

253. Sesmilo G, Biller BMK, Llevadot J, Hayden D, Hanson G, Rifal N, Klibanski A. Effects of growth hormone (GH) administration on homocysteine levels in men with GH deficiency: a randomized control trial. J Clin Endocrinol Metab 2001; 86:1518–1524.

254. Malozowski S, Tanner LA, Wysowski D, Fleming GA. Growth hormone, insulin-like growth factor I and benign intracranial hypertension. N Engl J Med 1993; 329:665–666.

255. Malozowski S, Stadel BV. Prepubertal gynecomastia dur-ing growth hormone therapy. J Pediatr 1995; 126:659–661.

256. Rosenbloom AL, Netzloff ML, Garnica AD, Weber FT. Replacement therapy with human growth hormone

(hGH): efficacy of low dosage and need for routine thyroid replacement. Acta Paediatr Belg 1979; 32:173–179.

257. Blethen S, Rundle AC. Slipped capital femoral epiphysis in children treated with growth hormone: a summary of the National Cooperative Growth Study experience. Horm Res 1996; 46:113–116.

258. Malozowski S, Hung W, Scott DC. Acute pancreatitis associated with growth hormone therapy for short stature. N Engl J Med 1995; 332:401–402.

259. Cutfield WS, Wilton P, Bennmarker H, Albertsson-Wikland K, Chatelain P, Ranke MB, Price DA. Incidence of diabetes mellitus and impaired glucose tolerance in children and adolescents receiving growth hormone treatment. Lancet 2000; 355:610–613.

260. Rosenbloom AL. Hot topic. Fetal growth, adrenocortical function, and the risk for type 2 diabetes. Pediatr Diabetes 2000; 1:150–154.

261. Watanabe S, Tsunematsu Y, Fuminoto J, Komiyama A. Leukemia in patients treated with growth hormone (Letter). Lancet 1988; 1:1159–1160.

262. Lawson Wilkins Pediatric Endocrine Society. Addendum to minutes of the Drug and Therapeutics Committee, Washington, D.C., July 1991.

263. Fradkin JE, Mills JL, Schonberger LB, Wysowski DK, Thomson R, Durako SJ, Robison LL. Risk of leukemia after treatment with pituitary growth hormone. JAMA 1993; 270:2829–2832.

264. Ogilvy-Stuart AL, Ryder WD, Gattamneni HR, Clayton PE, Shalet SM. Growth hormone and tumour recurrence. Br Med J 1992; 304:1601–1605.

265. American Academy of Pediatrics. Considerations related to the use of recombinant human growth hormone in children. Pediatrics 1997; 99:122–129.

266. Jansen M, van Schaik FMA, Ricker AT, Bullock B, Woods DE, Gabbay KH, Nussbaum AL, Sussenbach JS, Van den Brande JL. Sequence of cDNA encoding human insulin-like growth factor I precursor. Nature 1983; 255:306–312.

267. Niwa M, Sato Y, Uchiyamo F, Ono H, Yamashita M, Kitaguchi T. Chemical synthesis, cloning and expression of genes for human somatomedin-C (insulin-like growth factor I) and [5a]val somatomedin-C. Ann NY Acad Sci 1986; 469:31–52.

268. Ranke MB, Savage MO, Chatelain PG, Preece MA, Rosenfeld RG, Blum WF, Wilton P. Insulin-like growth factor I improves height in growth hormone insensitivity: two years' results. Horm Res 1995; 44:253–264.

269. Backeljauw PF, Underwood LE. Prolonged treatment with recombinant insulin-like growth factor-I in children with growth hormone insensitivity syndrome—a clinical research center study. J Clin Endocrinol Metab 1996; 81:3312–3317.

270. Backeljauw PF, Underwood LE. Prolonged treatment with recombinant insulin-like growth factor-I (rhIGF-I) in

children with growth hormone insensitivity syndrome (GHIS): 4 year update. Horm Res 1997; 48(suppl 2):15 (abstract 58).

271. Martinez V, Vasconez O, Martinez A, Moreno Z, Davila N, Rosenbloom AL, Diamond FB, Backrach L, Rosenfeld RG, Guevara-Aguirre J. Body changes in adolescent patients with growth hormone receptor deficiency receiving recombinant human insulin-like growth factor I and luteinizing hormone-releasing hormone analog: preliminary results. Acta Paediatr 1994; Suppl 399:133–136.

272. Klinger B, Laron Z. Three year IGF-I treatment of children with Laron syndrome. J Pediatr Endocrinol Metab 1995; 8:149–158.

273. Ranke MB, Savage MO, Chatelain PG, Preece MA, Rosenfeld RG, Wilton P. Long-term treatment of growth hormone insensitivity syndrome with IGF-I. Results of the European Multicentre Study. The Working Group on Growth Hormone Insensitivity Syndromes. Horm Res 1999; 51:128–134.

274. Guevara-Aguirre J, Vasconez O, Martinez V, Martinez AL, Rosenbloom AL, Diamond FB Jr, Gargosky SE, Nonoshita L, Rosenfeld RG. A randomized double-blind, placebo-controlled trial of safety and efficacy of recombinant insulin-like growth factor-I in children with growth hormone receptor deficiency. J Clin Endocrinol Metab 1995; 80:1393–1398.

275. Rosenbloom AL, Guevara-Aguirre J. Four year treatment results with rhIGF-I in 21 Ecuadorian children with growth hormone receptor deficiency (GHRD). NCGS 15th Annual Meeting, Scottsdale, AZ, October 4–7, 2001.

276. Donath MY, Sutsch G, Yan X-W, Piva B, Brunner HP, Glatz Y, Zapf J, Follath F, Froesch ER, Kiowski W. Acute cardiovascular effects of insulin-like growth factor I in patients with chronic heart failure. J Clin Endocrinol Metab 1998; 83:3177–3183.

277. Vasconez O, Martinez V, Martinez AL, Hidalgo F, Diamond FB, Rosenbloom AL, Rosenfeld RG, Guevara-Aguirre J. Heart rate increase in patients with growth hormone receptor deficiency treated with insulin-like growth factor I. Acta Paediatr Suppl 1994; 399:137–139.

278. Backeljauw PF, Kissoondial A, Underwood LE, Simmons KE. Effects of 4 years treatment with recombinant human insulin-like growth factor-I (rhIGF-I) on craniofacial growth in children with growth hormone insensitivity syndrome (GHIS). Horm Res 1997; 48(suppl 2):40 (abstract 243).

279. Leonard J, Samuels M, Cotterill AM, Savage MO. Effects of recombinant insulin-like growth factor-I on craniofacial morphology in growth hormone insensitivity. Acta Paediatr 1994; Suppl 399:140–141.

280. Klinger B, Anin S, Silbergeld A, Eshet R, Laron Z. Development of hyperandrogenism during treatment with insulin-like growth factor-I (IGF-I) in female patients with Laron syndrome. Clin Endocrinol 1998; 48:81–87.

3

Growth Hormone Treatment

David B. Allen

University of Wisconsin Medical School, Madison, Wisconsin, U.S.A.

I. INTRODUCTION

Human growth hormone (GH) was first used more than 30 years ago to stimulate growth in a child with hypopituitarism (1). Subsequently, a limited supply of pituitary glands from which GH could be extracted and purified required that GH therapy be restricted to children with the most severe and unequivocal GH deficiency. Strict, arbitrary laboratory criteria were established to identify patients likely to derive the greatest benefit from scarce GH. Delays in diagnosis and treatment, interruptions in therapy, and dosage restrictions were common during this time. Consequently, while GH accelerated growth of these individuals, adult statures were usually less than average (2–4).

In 1985, the first case of Creutzfeld-Jakob disease (CJD) in patients who had received GH was recognized; investigation disclosed that pituitary glands from which the GH was derived were contaminated with subviral particles. Distribution of pituitary-derived GH was stopped. Subsequently, in the United States, CJD was diagnosed in seven recipients of GH distributed by the National Hormone and Pituitary Program (5, 6). It was fortunate that 192 amino-acid biosynthetic GH, first tested in the United States in 1981, was approved by the Food and Drug Administration (FDA) in 1985 (7) and a second 191 amino-acid biosynthetic GH was approved in 1987. The production of GH by biological systems (*Escherichia coli* and, more recently, mammalian cells [8]) transplanted with the GH gene yields a virtually unlimited supply of GH.

Biosynthetic GH therapy eliminated the risk of CJD and offered children with severe GH deficiency an opportunity for optimal treatment. Children with milder forms of inadequate GH secretion, previously excluded from receiving GH, could be treated. Increased availability of recombinant DNA-derived GH has also allowed investigation of its growth-promoting effects in poorly growing children who do not fit traditional definitions of growth hormone deficiency (GHD), many of whom were previously believed to be unresponsive to GH treatment. In addition, metabolic effects of GH apart from linear growth promotion are now being studied extensively, leading to new indications for GH therapy.

Abundance of GH has added complexity to decisions about treatment of stature disorders. Human growth hormone *augmentation* therapy has now been added to GH *replacement* therapy, thus expanding the traditional boundaries of endocrinology endeavors, in which missing hormones are replaced and excessive hormones production suppressed. Advantages conferred by increased height in social, economic, professional, and political realms of Western society are well documented. Concern about social and psychological harm of short stature, and hope for effective therapy, have resulted in increased referrals for growth-promoting therapy. However, data confirming that stature per se is a primary determinant of psychological health are limited, although some have reported a higher frequency of underachievement, behavior problems, and reduced social competency in short-statured children (9). Neuroendocrine dysfunction (e.g., classic growth hormone deficiency), rather than stature itself, may correlate most closely with psychological and scholastic impairment (10). Although the physiological benefits of GH supplementation to children with severe GH deficiency *appear* obvious, data confirming the efficacy of GH therapy in improving the quality of life of non-GH-deficient recipients are scarce (11).

For many children, GH treatment will be appropriate therapy after the cause, concerns of patients and parents, and likelihood of success have been assessed. For most short children, however, efforts to build self-esteem through parental support, judicious selection of activities, and counseling will be more effective than injected GH therapy. The decision to institute long-term GH therapy should include both careful physical and psychological evaluation, to determine whether the degree of disability and likelihood of therapeutic benefit justify investment of the required emotional and monetary resources. Although experience has shown that side effects appear minimal, other possible effects remain unknown. Unexpected benefits may also be found.

The spectrum of disorders for which GH has been prescribed and the number of children receiving treatment (Table 1) continue to increase. In this chapter, we review aspects of GH treatment for severe, "classic" GH deficiency, including recent information on nongrowth metabolic effects of GH for adult GH-deficient individuals. Treatment of various short-stature conditions and catabolic disorders with GH is also considered, reflecting the recent proliferation of investigations of the metabolic and growth-promoting effects of GH in non-GH-deficient individuals. Possible risks and ethical issues related to GH therapy are also addressed.

II. GROWTH HORMONE PHYSIOLOGY

Human growth hormone is secreted by the anterior pituitary gland throughout life under the primary influence of stimulatory growth hormone-releasing hormone (GHRH) and inhibitory somatostatin (SRIH). Both of these regulatory peptides are synthesized in and released from the hypothalamus. The cyclical pulsatile secretion of GH is a response to a coincident decline in SRIH release and abrupt increase in GHRH secretion, modified by the input of neurotransmitters and the metabolic status upon the hypothalamus and somatotroph (12). Both GH and insulin-like growth factor-1 (IGF-1) exert positive feedback on SRIH secretion, and GH exerts negative feedback on GHRH secretion. Growth hormone is released in response to sleep, exercise, and relative hypoglycemia. Sleep-associated pulses of GH release usually occur in the first 30–60 min of sleep, and can occur at any time of day when individuals reach stages 3 and 4 of slow-wave sleep. Vigorous exercise for 15–20 min provokes a significant GH surge in 90% of normal children. Since surges in GH are more prolonged in physically unfit than in fit individuals performing comparable work, exercise-induced GH release appears more related to physical stress than to exercise *per se*. Psychological stress, such as venipuncture or general alarm, also produces GH elevations. Rises in GH occur with the postprandial decline of blood glucose concentration, and GH secretory surges occur more often in the hours preceding meals than those following meals (13).

Human growth hormone is synthesized and stored in acidophils of the pituitary gland and accounts for as much as 8% of pituitary weight. About 80% of secreted GH has a 191-amino acid sequence and molecular weight of 22 kD; the other 20% is approximately 20 kD and is produced by alternate gene splicing, which deletes amino acids 32–46 from the RNA. Human growth hormone is found in pituitary gland and plasma as monomers, dimers, and oligomers. Many other variants of GH, including proteolytically cleaved, N-acetylated, and deamidated forms, may also be found either as physiological variants or products of the extraction process. Because GH is species-specific, animal GH other than that from primates is ineffective in humans. Circulating GH-binding protein (GHBP) complexes about 50% of GH and probably acts as a modulator of release and distribution to tissues (14).

Table 1 Growth Disorders, Illnesses, and Metabolic Conditions for which hGH Treatment has been Investigated.

Familial short stature	Catabolic states
Constitutional delayed growth	Postoperative wound healing
[a]Intrauterine growth retardation:	Burns
Russell-Silver syndrome	Regenerative or reparative states
[a]Turner syndrome	Fractures
Skeletal dysplasia	Peripheral nerve damage
Hypochondroplasia	Neural tube defects
Achondroplasia	Spina bifida
Spondyloepiphyseal dysplasia	Myelomeningocele
Multiple epiphyseal dysplasia	Chronic illness
Hypophosphatemic	Glucocorticoid-dependent disorders (renal transplantation,
Miscellaneous syndromes	juvenile rheumatoid arthritis, asthma)
Noonan syndrome	Chronic renal failure
[a]Prader-Willi syndrome	Cystic fibrosis
Down syndrome	AIDS wasting
[a]Growth hormone deficiency in	Inflammatory bowel disease
adults	Aging

[a]FDA-approved indication for GH therapy.

GHBP shows immunological identity with the extracellular domain of the GH receptor, and concentrations of GHBP are low in patients with GH receptor deficiency (15). The regulation of GHBP remains uncertain; gonadal steroids such as estrogen increase GHBP activity, while GH secretory status appears to play a minor role (16).

Serum GH concentrations are high in full-term and premature infants during the first 24 h of life, averaging 50–60 ng/ml and resulting from both enhanced frequency and amplitude of pulses (17). In full-term, but not in premature infants, GH levels fall after 48 h. Thereafter, growth hormone concentrations reflect pulsatile secretion, which occurs more often and with higher peaks during infancy, diminishes during childhood, and is lowest in late prepubertal childhood and in adults. Spontaneous puberty in boys or androgen treatment of prepubertal boys results in significant increases in GH release (18). This sex-hormone-induced augmentation of growth hormone secretion is primarily an amplitude-modulated phenomenon, although more frequent GH peaks do occur (19). It is interesting, however, that testosterone's effect on pubertal growth may be largely independent of changes in circulating GH (20). Stimulation of the somatotropic axis by testosterone is partly dependent upon its aromatization to estradiol; GH levels in adult women are higher than in men and rise in men when they are given estrogens (21).

The very short half-life (less than 20 min) of circulating GH requires that blood sampling be carried out at frequent intervals to identify peaks. Studies of children indicate that normal and short stature are both associated with a broad range of GH secretion patterns (22). Whereas it was previously thought that a bimodal distribution of GH secretion discretely separated normal from abnormal, it is now clear that (with the rare exception of *complete* GH deficiency secondary to GH gene deletion or abnormalities of expression) a continuum of "inadequate" GH secretion likely spans classic and partially GH-deficient children, children with delayed growth and puberty, and other poorly growing children who pass provocative tests but still secrete less GH than their peers. An asymptotic relationship between growth velocity and spontaneous GH secretion has been postulated for short children (23). This spectrum of GH insufficiency, in which there are varying degrees of abnormal GH secretion, creates enormous difficulty in interpreting tests of GH secretion.

III. GROWTH HORMONE EFFECTS

The objective of GH therapy traditionally has been to increase the growth rate and adult height of short-statured GH-deficient children. The effectiveness of this therapy has been assessed through achievement of normal growth velocity and height. Although linear growth promotion remains the focus of GH therapy, additional metabolic effects of GH are being actively investigated for their po-

tential clinical application. The major indirect actions of GH are anabolic and growth-promoting, mediated by insulinlike growth factors (principally IGF-1), and include cell proliferation and protein synthesis in both skeletal and nonskeletal tissues. The IGFs are a family of peptides with molecular weight similar to insulin that have insulinlike activity. Circulating IGFs are produced primarily by the liver in response to GH stimulation, and circulate bound to larger carrier proteins (IGFBPs) with molecular weight of 28–150 kDa. Since most organs synthesize IGFs, their action may occur within their cells of synthesis (autocrine), on cells in the immediate area (paracrine), and at distant sites (endocrine). A complex interplay of IGF production rates, clearance, and degree of binding to various IGFBPs modulates the levels and systemic activity of free IGFs (24).

The most apparent metabolic effect of GH is stimulation of linear growth in children prior to epiphyseal fusion. The relative roles of GH and IGF-1 in stimulating bone growth may be most accurately described by a so-called dual effect model of GH action, in which GH stimulates cartilage precursor cells first to differentiate and subsequently to produce, and become responsive to, autocrine and paracrine mitogenic effects of IGF-1 (25). The wide distribution of receptors for IGF-1, and the fact that blood levels of IGFs are higher than in any tissue, suggest that the endocrine function may also be important. However, administration of IGF-1 to hypophysectomized rats does not promote growth equivalent to that of GH (26). IGF-1 also participates in negative feedback regulation of GH secretion by stimulating hypothalamic somatostatin secretion (27) and by inhibiting the action of GHRH (28).

IGF-1 levels correlate with the clinical state of GH deficiency, sufficiency, or excess. Serum IGF-1 levels are low in utero and in infancy, increase with age in both boys and girls, reach maximum values during puberty (earlier and higher in girls than boys), and decline to adult values as adolescence is completed. Although often used as part of the assessment of hypopituitarism, IGF-1 levels do not exclusively reflect GH production and are age-dependent. Concentrations of IGF-1 correlate more closely with bone age and puberty (29) than with chronological age. Hypothyroidism, malnutrition, poorly controlled diabetes, and chronic disease diminish secretion of IGF-1. Thus, a low serum IGF-1 level is consistent with, but not diagnostic of, GH deficiency. The normally low levels of IGF-1 in infants and young children preclude its diagnostic utility for classic GH deficiency in this age group. Given these limitations, the use of IGF-1 alone as a screening test for GH status is of little diagnostic value. However, the Growth Hormone Research Society recently recommended measurement of IGF-1 and IGFBP3 in addition to provocative GH testing as a means of identifying children with abnormalities in the GH/IGF axis not detected by standard tests.

Other metabolic effects of GH can be described as anabolic, lipolytic, and diabetogenic (Fig. 1). Growth-hormone-induced growth acceleration is facilitated by concomitant enhancement of protein synthesis in bone, cartilage, skeletal muscles, the erythropoietic system, and other major organs. Administration of GH produces positive nitrogen balance, increased amino acid transport into cells, increased intracellular RNA, and decreased urea production and blood urea nitrogen (BUN) levels. The metabolic efficacy of total parenteral nutrition is also enhanced by GH (30). A high-normal or mildly elevated BUN level and low serum phosphorus and alkaline phosphatase level are usually observed in GH deficiency and reverse with GH treatment. Effects on mineral metabolism include increased intestinal calcium absorption and urinary calcium excretion and reduced urinary phosphate excretion (31). Bone density and levels of osteocalcin, procollagen type 1, and 1,25-dihydroxyvitamin D are reduced in GH-deficient children and increase with long-term GH therapy (32).

Growth hormone receptors and expression of GH receptor mRNA have been demonstrated in both preadipocyte cultures and mature adipocytes. Some actions of GH in adipose tissue are mediated directly through interaction with the GH receptor, while others are mediated indirectly through IGF1. These actions include inhibition of differentiation of immature adipocytes to mature adipocytes; enhancement of lipolysis and site-specific free fatty acid release from adipose tissue; and inhibition of lipoprotein lipase and stimulation of hormone sensitive lipase (33). Consequently, GH-deficient children tend to demonstrate increased, predominantly abdominal, subcutaneous fat that lessens and becomes more peripheral during therapy with exogenous GH. Non-GH-deficient children also display reduction in overall body fat during GH therapy. The mechanism by which GH reduces adipocyte size in vivo remains unclear, but in vitro studies suggests that GH increases the basal rate of lipolysis and depresses reesterification of free fatty acids (34).

The effects of GH on carbohydrate metabolism are complex. Intravenous administration of GH causes an acute fall in blood glucose, most likely reflecting enhanced transport of glucose into adipose and skeletal muscle cells. GH is pivotal for the maintenance of normal glucose homeostasis in infants, but this critical role is markedly diminished in older children and adults. In a child with GH deficiency, insulin secretion is diminished, related in part to pancreatic islet cell hypoplasia. Glucose tolerance tests may reveal impaired ability to dispose of a carbohydrate load. However, fasting hypoglycemia can also occur in such patients because of heightened sensitivity to insulin. Administration of GH reduces sensitivity to insulin, thereby correcting hypoglycemia, and increases insulin secretion. Chronic administration of GH results in compensatory hyperinsulinemia and is associated with the development of insulin resistance. In summary, the combined effects of GH on both the release of and response to insulin create states of altered carbohydrate intolerance in situations of either GH deficiency or excess.

IV. GROWTH HORMONE DEFICIENCY

The classic presentation of severe growth hormone deficiency is characterized by marked growth retardation, diminished growth velocity, delayed skeletal maturation, absence of other explanations for growth retardation, and subnormal secretion of GH, both physiological and in response to provocative stimuli. Genetic (e.g., altered GH or GHRH gene), anatomical or congenital (e.g., midline cranial defects, septo-optic dysplasia, vascular malformations), and acquired abnormalities of the hypothalamus and pituitary (e.g., craniopharyngioma, glioma, histiocytosis) are identifiable in many affected children. Evaluation of pituitary gland anatomy using magnetic resonance imaging has revealed a spectrum of more subtle morphological abnormalities associated with the diagnosis of GH deficiency (35). Irradiation or chemotherapy for malignancies and traumatic brain injury also cause organic hypopituitarism, and accounts for an increasing incidence of GH deficiency as survival of these patients improves. In spite of this growing list of causes, most children with GH deficiency still are designated as *idiopathic*, often due to apparently defective hypothalamic regulation of GH release, rather than inability to synthesize GH. It is likely that further improvement in imaging techniques will reveal additional organic lesions contributing to this dysfunction.

Idiopathic GH deficiency usually occurs sporadically but may be familial (36). Its frequency has been reported to be from 1:4000 children to 1:60,000 (37, 38). Although the latter figure is similar to the treated population in the United States before 1985, the true incidence of classic GH deficiency is probably in the range of 1:10,000. These estimates are complicated by the fact that, with the exceptions of GH gene deletion and severe pituitary or hypothalamic dysfunction, GH deficiency is partial, rather than complete. The incidence of GH deficiency is likely to continue to rise due to improved prolonged survival of children who have received radiation therapy for malignancies.

Arbitrary laboratory criteria currently provide a technical distinction between GH deficiency and GH sufficiency, even though it is generally accepted that there is no meaningful physiological distinction between children whose provoked GH levels fall slightly above or below laboratory threshold values. Evidence is accumulating to support the notion that GH deficiency is not a distinct entity, but rather a spectrum of disorders of GH pulsatility. A continuum of GH secretion may span essential absence of GH, partial GH deficiency, and a spectrum of so-called normal GH secretion. Some investigators have found significant correlations between spontaneous GH secretion

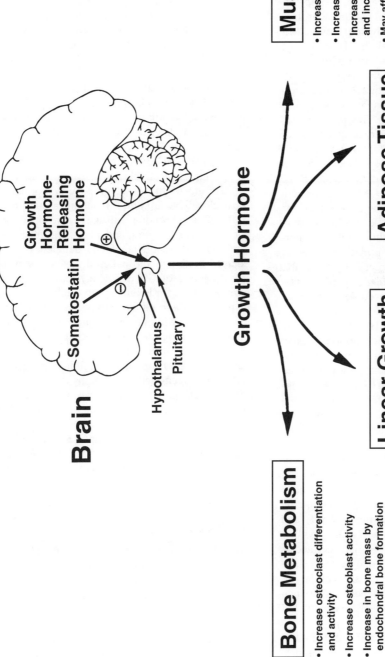

Figure 1 Multiple sites of growth hormone action.

and statural growth rates (39) while others have not (40). The blurring of what was once thought to be a clear distinction between GH deficiency and sufficiency has combined with the luxury of available, expensive GH to create new opportunities, uncertainties, and controversies in GH therapy.

Profoundly GH-deficient infants and young children may present initially with hypoglycemia. This is more commonly associated with adrenocorticotropin (ACTH) deficiency and hypocortisolism, but hypoglycemia may persist in spite of glucocorticoid replacement. Prompt administration of GH is necessary to prevent the neurological sequelae of persistent or recurrent hypoglycemia. Microphallus occurring in the newborn with GH deficiency most often, but not invariably, is associated with gonadotropin deficiency. Since GH is largely responsible for phallic growth after the first few months of life, (untreated) isolated GH deficient males may display poor phallic growth during early childhood. This problem can be effectively treated with GH and very small doses of androgen. Growth velocity may be mildly or severely impaired, depending on the degree of GH deficiency and/or presence of accompanying hormonal deficiencies. Bone age is usually delayed in patients with GH deficiency, but is often less delayed than height age (age for which the child's height is average). Bone age is less delayed in isolated GH deficiency than with multiple pituitary hormone deficiencies. So-called catch-up growth, a period of supranormal growth velocity often observed particularly during early GH treatment, is accompanied by skeletal maturation proportion to growth achieved, leading to the *appearance* of accelerated bone age advancement.

At least half the children with GH deficiency were described in 1968 as having an isolated hormonal defect (41). This proportion has steadily risen as more children with partial or neurosecretory GH deficiency have been recognized and diagnosed. A rise in GH secretion and increase in growth velocity observed following pulsatile GHRH administration in many of these patients indicates that deficient hypothalamic regulation of pituitary GH secretion is the cause of GH deficiency in many patients with isolated GH deficiency (42). However, GH deficiency is often accompanied by deficiencies of other anterior pituitary hormones: adrenocorticotrophic hormone (ACTH), thyroid stimulating hormone (TSH), luteinizing hormone (LH), follicle-stimulating hormone (FSH) and posterior pituitary antidiuretic hormone (ADH, synthesized in hypothalamic nuclei). Hypopituitarism, defined as the deficient production or release of one or more hormones from the pituitary, may be primary or secondary to hypothalamic dysfunction. When deficiencies other than GH occur, they are, in decreasing order of frequency, LH and FSH, TSH, and ACTH (43).

Deficiency in ADH, manifested as diabetes insipidus, usually occurs in acquired GH deficiency (e.g. craniopharyngioma, surgical trauma) or congenitally as part of

the septo-optic dysplasia (SOD) syndrome. In contrast to anterior pituitary hormones, ADH is synthesized in the hypothalamus and transported to and stored for release in the posterior pituitary, which is embryologically distinct from the anterior pituitary. Consequently, with the exception of SOD, deficiency of ADH is rarely seen with idiopathic hypopituitarism. On the other hand, extensive surgery for pituitary tumors will usually result in ADH deficiency (if it was not present before) and variable but usually progressive loss of other pituitary hormonal secretion (44). A combination of less extensive surgery and irradiation, or irradiation alone, has been recommended as a more moderate approach to treatment of such patients. However, the gradual development of impaired GH secretion is also observed in many children who undergo cranial irradiation for neoplasms of the central nervous system (45). With radiation of the hypothalamic–pituitary axis, GH is the first hormone to be affected and the degree of hormonal deficit is related to the radiation dosage (46). In one study, 5 years following 3.75–42.5 Gy radiation therapy, all patients were GH deficient; gonadotropin, ACTH, and TSH were deficient in 91%, 77%, and 42% of patients, respectively (47).

Timing of the onset of puberty normally is related most closely to a child's reaching a state of maturation (rather than chronological age) corresponding to a bone age of 10–11 for girls, and 11.5–12.5 for boys. Late recognition and treatment of GH deficiency often result in delayed bone age and pubertal development. In addition, late diagnosis of GH deficiency may not allow sufficient treatment time for height age to catch up to bone age prior to puberty; these children may experience rapid pubertal development without an adequate pubertal increment in height, resulting in reduced adult stature. LH-releasing hormone agonist therapy, which can slow or stop pubertal advancement, or aromatase inhibitor therapy, which may reduce estrogen-mediated epiphyseal plate closure, may offer effective means of "reclaiming" the time required for sufficient growth, but further controlled studies are needed to evaluate the efficacy of these treatments. A preferable option includes prompt recognition of GH deficiency and optimization of GH dosage and schedule, which facilitate both the achievement of normal prepubertal height and entrance into puberty at a more appropriate chronological age.

A. Treatment

For over 30 years, the diagnosis of GH deficiency was based on the analysis of serum GH levels following at least two provocative stimuli. The limited amount of available pituitary-extracted GH dictated that few short children could be treated. Criteria were established by national committees of the National Pituitary Agency (which later became the National Hormone and Pituitary Program [NHPP]) to ensure that the most severely affected GH-deficient children would receive GH treatment. Thus, only very short, very slowly growing children who had very low GH levels on stimulation tests qualified for GH therapy, and these children were treated only until a height within −2 to −2.5 standard deviations (SD) of normal adult height was reached. This meticulous rationing of scarce GH to the most severely affected children maximized the overall benefit that could be derived from this therapy.

Improved pituitary collection and extraction strategies increased availability of GH during the 1970s and, as a result, criteria for treatment were relaxed. Whereas stimulated levels of GH less than 3–5 ng/dl were originally considered to be sufficiently subnormal to indicate GH deficiency, the threshold GH level required for this diagnosis gradually rose to 7 ng/dl, then 10 ng/dl, and, in some clinics, to 12 ng/dl. Currently, children with levels in the higher subnormal range and children with normal stimulated GH levels but low spontaneous GH secretion are now designated as having "partial" GH deficiency.

Interpretation of tests for GH is also complicated by laboratory variation. Whereas the NHPP originally provided uniform material, standards, and methodology for GH testing, later commercialization of GH assays methods created significant variation in laboratory values for GH in a single blood sample. Today, expanding definitions of so-called partial GH deficiency variations in GH assays, and unlimited GH availability have transformed the historically clearly defined and tightly regulated practice of diagnosing and treating GH deficiency into a rapidly evolving and controversial endeavor.

Growth failure caused by severe GH deficiency is a universally accepted therapeutic indication for GH treatment. Treatment of growth failure due to partial GH deficiency, defined by subnormal stimulated GH levels, has also become accepted practice. However, it is now widely recognized that children with partial or subtle defects in the secretion of GH are difficult to identify, and no individual assessment of GH secretion or GH-associated biochemical finding unerringly detects such subjects (48). A single provocative test for GH (a necessary but not sufficient criterion for these diagnoses) appears to lack both specificity and sensitivity in identifying GH insufficiency. In children of normal stature, stimulated GH levels may be <7 ng/ml in as many as 20% (49). Specificity may be increased by performance of a second provocative test. On the other hand, a normal GH response to provocative stimuli does not guarantee sufficient spontaneous GH to maintain normal growth.

Attempts to define milder forms of GH through frequent blood sampling and analysis of spontaneous GH secretion pattern have led to the development of elaborate mathematical techniques for their interpretation. Children with subnormal GH secretion following cranial irradiation, who may pass provocative GH testing, may be identified solely by this frequent sampling method. (Over time, classic GH deficiency occurs in many of these patients

[50].) However, determination of spontaneous GH secretion requires considerable time, expense, and technical help, and is complicated by technical difficulties, disturbed daily and nighttime routines of the patients, and lack of reproducibility (51). Current methods have been criticized for their inability to differentiate normal children from short, GH-responsive children, and even from classic GH-deficient children. In summary, measurement and analysis of spontaneous GH secretion are sometimes helpful in identifying GH-sufficient subjects, but adds little in most instances to provocative tests in the identification of the GH-deficient child. With either test, the notion of a discrete cutoff level of GH secretion that reliably differentiates GH deficiency from normal is historical, and has limited relevance to current practice of pediatric endocrinology. The diagnosis of mild forms of GH insufficiency depends primarily upon clinical perception; laboratory tests of GH secretion provide ancillary information that help to confirm or disprove that clinical diagnosis.

Whom to treat for isolated idiopathic GHD and for how long is further complicated by the fact that most children who are treated with GH do not have permanent or complete GHD, but have insufficient secretion of GH to support normal childhood growth. When children with isolated GHD are retested after GH replacement therapy has been interrupted, 30–70% will have a normal GH response. Children with a previous diagnosis of partial GHD (i.e., peak stimulated GH levels of 5–10 μg/L or low 24-h integrated GH secretion) are particularly likely to have normal results on posttreatment testing (52).

Various studies of time of initiation, dosage, and frequencies of GH administration have advanced progress toward optimal treatment of GH deficiency during childhood. Subcutaneous daily GH administration is currently preferred, with the average GHD child in the United States receiving initial treatment with 0.3 mg/kg/week divided into six or seven doses. GH preparations are essentially equivalent, but vary in preparation and delivery. They include lyophilized GH that is mixed with a sterile diluent, pre-mixed GH solutions in a multiple dose vial, GH pen/needle delivery system, a nonneedle delivery system, and a depot preparation given every 2–4 weeks. Intranasal preparations are being developed (53). Since growth before puberty is a major determinant of final adult height, early initiation of GH treatment allows more complete normalization of height prior to puberty and an improved final height prognosis (54). There can be a temptation to defer injection therapy in young children in order to minimize discomfort and inconvenience, but the available evidence strongly supports early recognition, referral, diagnosis, and treatment of severely GH-deficient patients as an important step to optimizing their growth potential.

Increasing the dosage of GH improves growth rate; a dose–response equation derived from treatment of children of all ages with various degrees of GH deficiency reveals a logarithmic relationship between GH dosage and growth rate for thrice weekly dosages ranging from 0.015 to 0.1 mg/kg (55). The variation around the mean of each of these growth rate points is great, attesting to the poorly understood contribution of factors other than GH levels to the normal linear growth process. Other studies of daily GH injections confirmed the relationship between growth rate and so-called conventional doses of GH (56). A recent study using 0.025, 0.05, and 0.1 mg/kg *daily* in prepubertal severely GHD children showed significantly greater growth velocities and gains in cumulative height SDS in the 0.05 and 0.1 mg/kg/day groups compared with the 0.025 mg/kg/day group after 2 years of treatment. There were no significant differences between the 0.05 and 0.1 mg/kg/day groups (57). The serum IGF1 response to GH is also dose-dependent, continuing to rise as GH is administered in doses above currently prescribed levels (58). Results of epidemiological studies that suggest an association between high serum IGF1 levels and the incidence of malignancy have prompted a recommendation that IGF1 and IGFBP3 levels be monitored on a regular basis. A younger age, greater delay in height age and bone age, and greater severity of GH deficiency based upon provocative testing each correlate with improved *initial response* to GH therapy. Using multiple regression analysis, variables that have positive effects on *adult height* of GH-treated patients include taller parents, more frequent GH injections, longer duration of GH treatment, taller height at start of GH treatment, and greater severity of GH deficiency.

Increased frequency of GH administration improves growth rate, suggesting the so-called pulsing message of GH to its target cells, in addition to adequacy of GH levels, enhances linear growth. When the same weekly dosage is given in daily injections, rather than three times per week, an improvement in first-year growth rate of about 1.5 cm/year is observed (59). On the other hand, subcutaneous administration of depot preparations of GH at every-other-week intervals, has also been shown to increase growth rates effectively nearly to the same degree (60). Nocturnal administration, which more closely mimics physiological GH secretion, may also add to efficacy (61), although this is not consistently observed. Regardless of the regimen chosen, the effect of GH wanes with time, and the first year of treatment usually produces the greatest growth increment. Following this early phase of rapid growth, short-term increased replacement doses of GH renews catch-up growth without adverse metabolic effects (62). Seasonal variation in growth rate during GH therapy, with peaks in the summer and nadirs in the winter (North American population), has also been described (63).

Children who have undergone removal of craniopharyngioma frequently experience growth acceleration in the absence of measurable GH. This phenomenon may be attributable to postoperative nutritional excess and hyperinsulinemia (64), although other mechanisms (e.g., GH variants, IGFs) are also postulated (65). Polyphagia and significant weight gain are usually also observed. Although supplementation with GH is not required to sustain linear growth, body composition analysis reveals increased fat mass and decreased lean mass typical for the GHD state. Avoidance of excessive cortisol replacement therapy is extremely important in these individuals. This growth pattern may persist, allowing attainment of normal adult stature without GH therapy, but GH may nevertheless be indicated to improve body composition and other metabolic consequences of GHD.

The distinct augmentation of GH pulsations and increased production rates that occur during normal puberty raise the question of whether GH replacement dosages also should be increased during puberty. Insufficient dosage and frequency of GH administration has been shown to permit epiphyseal closure in GH-deficient adolescents prior to adequate catch-up growth, thereby reducing expected adult height (66). In one study, doubling the dosage of GH during puberty did not significantly change growth rate, but did tend to advance pubertal maturation (67). On the other hand, a larger and more recent randomized trial showed that an increase in dosage to 0.7 mg/kg/week (in contrast to conventional dosage recommendations of 0.18–0.35 mg/kg/week) improved growth rates, near-adult height, and height SDS in GHD adolescents without evident adverse effects (68). Since the cost of such treatment must be balanced with the possible added benefit achieved, the most effective frequency and dosage of GH therapy during puberty is yet to be determined.

Children treated with GH may experience transient or persistent declines in serum thyroxine (T4) levels; in approximately 25%, T4 levels become abnormally low and may impair response to GH. Thyroid function tests should be monitored periodically (especially early) during GH therapy to ensure detection of secondary T4 deficiency and prevent this treatable cause of a poor response to GH. Cortisol supplementation may also impair the growth response to GH; as little as 7.5–10 mg/day of hydrocortisone may be growth-suppressive in a school-aged child. Thus, when ACTH deficiency has been documented, the dosage of daily cortisol replacement therapy should be reduced to a level sufficient to prevent symptoms of fatigue and lack of energy. In prepubertal children, these replacement levels are quite low, and some children with idiopathic hypopituitarism, even with evidence for ACTH deficiency, will not need cortisone replacement in the absence of illness or stress.

Testosterone or other anabolic agents will enhance the growth velocity of a prepubertal GH-deficient child taking GH, but (except for boys with microphallus) should not be given if the bone age is less than 9 years, and then in very low dosages initially. Treatment for the purpose of virilization in a boy who is gonadotropin-deficient should be initiated after bone age approximates 11–12 years with low-dosage (e.g., 50 mg) testosterone enanthate intramuscularly per month to prevent accelerated epiphyseal maturation. Dosages can be gradually increased to adult replacement levels (e.g., 200–300 mg testosterone enanthate every 3–4 weeks) over the next several years. It has recently become clear that estrogens have a potent effect on bone age acceleration in patients with Turner syndrome, and may have an accelerating effect on the growth resulting from GH therapy. The androgen oxandrolone, which cannot be aromatized to estrogen, in low dosages has also been useful in accelerating growth rate in both boys and girls. Future management of short stature during puberty may include other measures (e.g., aromatase inhibitors) designed to reduce epiphyseal-maturing estrogen effects while preserving growth-accelerating effects of GH and androgens.

B. Effects of Treatment

With early diagnosis, careful attention to accompanying hormonal deficiencies, and progressive dosage adjustments, children with GH deficiency reach normal adult height (Fig. 2) (69). Bone age will advance with GH treatment, but usually not more than height age. Linear growth often accelerates faster than bone age following initiation of GH therapy, leading to increases in predicted final height. Even with successful long-term GH therapy, however, correction of disabling short stature does not consistently normalize the psychosocial outcome for adults with GH deficiency (70). Psychosocial counseling, which increases both therapeutic compliance during childhood and social outcome during adulthood (71), should be a consistent adjunct to parenteral GH administration.

The consequences of severe GH deficiency (GHD) in adult life and the beneficial effect of replacement therapy are increasingly well established. Accurate selection of appropriate candidates for adult GH treatment, and the transition of their care from pediatrics to adult medicine, require careful consideration of several issues. Since the

majority of children who are diagnosed as GHD and treated with GH do not have permanent GHD, anticipatory counseling regarding possible lifelong treatment should be focused on children with panhypopituitarism and those with severe isolated GHD associated with central nervous system abnormalities. Appropriate timing for termination of so-called growth-promoting GH therapy should be guided by efforts to balance the high cost of late-adolescent treatment with the attainment of reasonable statural goals. Confirmation of GHD following provocation with appropriate stimuli (i.e., not clonidine) is appropriate for all candidates for adult GH therapy. Testing of the GH axis can be performed within weeks of GH cessation, but confirmation of an emerging adult GHD state with body composition, blood lipid, and quality of life assessments may require 1 or more years of pretreatment observation. Although it remains unclear whether such a period of observation is needed or even advisable for late adolescents with unequivocal panhypopituitarism, it is likely that a transition from growth-promoting to adult replacement dosages of GH therapy without interruption will be recommended. Selection of patients for lifelong adult GH replacement therapy will present diagnostic, therapeutic, and ethical dilemmas similar to those arising from treatment of childhood GHD. The experience and expertise of pediatric endocrinologists in diagnosing and treating GHD should be offered and utilized in the identification and transitioning of appropriate patients to adult GH therapy (72).

V. IDIOPATHIC SHORT STATURE AND CONSTITUTIONAL GROWTH DELAY

For every short child who has impaired GH secretion, many more are short for other reasons. Parental concerns about the disadvantages of their child's short stature are legitimized by a "heightist" premise in modern America:

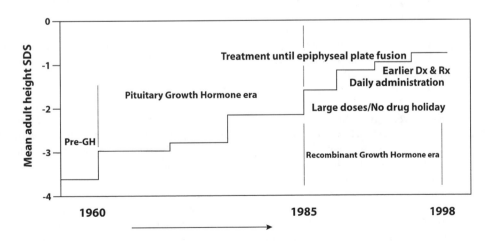

Figure 2 Progress in efficacy of childhood GH treatment. (Adapted from Ref. 69.)

to be tall is good and to be short is to be stigmatized (73). The preponderance of white males in the GH-treated population suggests that these social pressures give rise to ascertainment of short-statured patients biased by gender, race, and socioeconomic status (74). Stigmatization based upon height begins in childhood. Feelings of incompetence and low self-esteem may arise from the short child's struggle with stature, although these problems may depend as much on the projection of parental perceptions of their child's vulnerability and immaturity as on short stature per se (75). Future studies investigating improvement in *quality of life*, as well as improved stature growth, of non-GH-deficient children treated with GH will be of paramount importance.

Since the previous edition of this text, the medical literature has been replete with reports of non-GH-deficient children treated with GH, and numerous studies continue to investigate new indications for GH (Table 1). Many extraordinarily short children have overlapping diagnostic conditions (e.g., familial short stature and constitutional growth delay), which complicate interpreting the response of a specific condition to GH therapy. Specific disorders that have undergone investigational trials to date, some of which are currently approved indications for GH therapy, are discussed in the following sections.

The prospect that GH therapy may accelerate growth and increase adult height of markedly short but otherwise healthy children has generated great interest and debate. Serum GH concentrations are usually normal in these children; however, children with severe constitutional growth delay (CGD) may demonstrate temporary failure to secrete GH in response to stimuli, which normalizes with pubertal progression or induction (76). The finding that 30–70% of adults diagnosed as GH deficient during childhood have normal GH levels later suggests that this phenomenon is more common than generally recognized. Thus, repeat provocative testing for GH following short-term sex hormone treatment is advisable before considering a commitment to GH therapy for most near-pubertal patients who fit clinical criteria for CGD.

Administration of GH at dosages used to treat GH deficiency increases growth velocity in the majority of these children throughout at least 3 years of treatment. A controlled study reported that mean growth velocity increased during the first year from 5.3 to 7.4 cm/year and height SD score increased by 0.63 in GH-treated children compared with no change in velocity or SD score for untreated children (77). Growth rates declined during each successive year of therapy and, in one study, approximated pretreatment growth velocity by the fourth year (78). In a more recent study, however, daily GH therapy during years 2 and 3 sustained growth rates of 7.6 and 7.2 cm/year respectively, compared with baseline growth rate of 4.6 cm/year (79). Short, non-GH-deficient children who demonstrate sustained acceleration of growth rate when given GH therapy tend to attain prepubertal heights

that are closer to, but do not exceed, their genetic height potential (80).

Information regarding the efficacy of GH in improving the final height of children with idiopathic short stature (ISS) or CGD is now accumulating. Since height at onset of puberty is a more important determinant of adult height than pubertal growth (because prepubertal growth normally contributes 85% of final height), the most effective GH therapy will require substantial growth acceleration prior to puberty. Increases in standardized Bayley–Pinneau predictions of adult height have been consistently reported during prepubertal GH therapy, but these gains do not improve substantially during treatment of pubertal subjects. Puberty generally appears to occur at expected time in GH-treated children with ISS or CGD, but an accelerated tempo of puberty has been noted in boys (81) and an earlier age of onset in girls (82). This possible decrement in height acquired during puberty probably accounts for reports of *actual* final heights of GH-treated children that fall short of earlier more optimistic height predictions (83). Alternative strategies include administration of a higher dosage of GH for 2 years prior to puberty to achieve normalization of adolescent height, precluding the need for GH therapy during puberty (84). Long-term GH therapy in non-GHD adolescents may increase insulin resistance, but not impaired glucose tolerance or hyperlipidemia (85).

How effective is GH therapy at increasing adult height of non-GHD individuals? Of several studies published in the mid-1990s, only two reported final heights greater than pretreatment predicted heights and only one reported an improved proportion of subjects with final height greater than the midparental target height (86). On the other hand, a more recent study of 80 non-GHD children treated with GH (highly variable duration of treatment) showed a mean increase in SD score for height from −2.7 to −1.4. The mean (±SD) difference between predicted adult height (using Bayley–Pinneau method) before treatment and achieved adult height among boys was 5.0 ± 5.1 cm and 5.9 ± 5.2 cm for girls; still, only a few subjects achieved their midparental target height (87). Thus, it appears that long-term GH treatment of non-GHD short children at currently recommended dosages can lead to statistically significant increases in final height in *some* children. Unfortunately, in this and other studies, no clinical (e.g., pretreatment growth rate) or biochemical (e.g., overnight endogenous GH secretion) determinants reliably predicted the individual response to GH therapy. Consequently, whether improvements in final height due to GH therapy alone are *sufficiently likely or clinically significant* to justify cost and commitment to several years of therapy is still debatable.

Novel approaches to the treatment of idiopathic short stature include concomitant suppression of pubertal hormones using GnRH agonist therapy and reduction of estrogen production using aromatase inhibitors. A recent study reported that combined gonadotropin releasing hormone agonist/growth hormone (GnRH/GH) therapy for 3 years resulted in gains in predicted height of 8–10 cm without demonstrable side effects (88). Final height data on these patients are not yet available, and current expense of such treatment is formidable. Anecdotal evidence regarding effectiveness of aromatase inhibitor therapy exists (89), but long-term studies in pubertal boys are just beginning.

VI. TURNER SYNDROME AND NOONAN SYNDROME

Between 95 and 100% of girls with Turner syndrome (TS) experience growth failure, and the untreated mean final height of these patients is 143 cm (90), approximately 20 cm below the female average of the corresponding ethnic group. Growth curves for TS have been developed by European investigators, and results in North American patients closely match these data (91). Individual's height percentiles on this TS curve do not change from childhood to adulthood if patients remain untreated. During childhood, average growth velocity is 4.44 cm for each year of bone age advancement. The lower final height results from the combined effects of mild intrauterine growth retardation, a lack of a pubertal growth spurt (due to ovarian failure to produce estrogens), and growth failure during childhood due to abnormalities in growth plate cartilage (92) and a possible resistance to the

action of GH. Studies clearly show that TS patients do not have classic GH deficiency, although endogenous GH levels (93, 94) and urinary GH levels (95) are below normal after the age of 8 years.

With the exception of GH-deficient children, girls with TS have received the longest trials of GH therapy (up to 10 years). Numerous studies have demonstrated that GH, with or without anabolic steroids, can accelerate growth in girls with TS (96–98). During subsequent years of treatment, growth rates declined but remained higher than those of untreated girls. In one cohort, 14 of 17 girls receiving GH alone equaled or exceeded their original projected adult heights, while 41 of 45 girls receiving combined oxandrolone–GH therapy did so. The mean height of girls who completed a mean of 7.6 years of GH therapy (n = 17) was 150.4 cm, a gain of 8.4 cm over the expected average height, while those treated with GH plus oxandrolone (n = 43) achieved a mean final height of 152.1 cm, representing an average gain of 10.3 cm over predicted height without treatment (Fig. 3) (99). These results suggest that an adult height above the lower limit of normal for American women (150 cm) is now an attainable goal for many girls with this syndrome. Somewhat more modest effects on total height gain (e.g., mean 0.7 SD increase) are also reported, particularly when estrogen treatment was initiated prior to 14 years of age (100). These data have led to regulatory approval for the use of GH to treat the short stature of TS in many countries worldwide (including the United States). Critical fac-

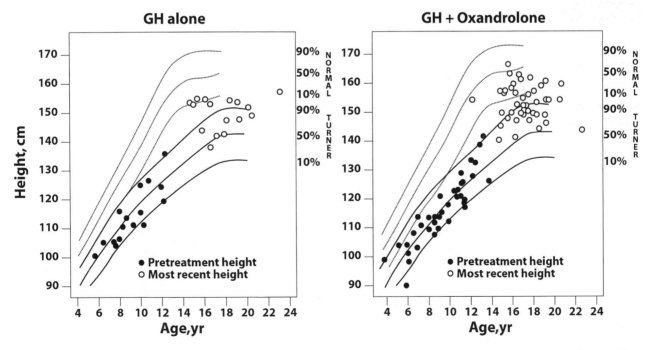

Figure 3 Effect of GH therapy alone and with oxandrolone on last available height in girls with Turner syndrome. (From Ref. 99.)

tors for a successful outcome appear to be GH dosage and the number of years of GH treatment before estrogenization (101).

As a result, initiation of GH therapy is currently recommended as soon as a patient with TS has dropped below the 5th percentile of the normal female growth curve. This may be as early as 2 years of age. For girls below 9–12 years of age, the recommended starting dosage is 0.05 mg/kg/day, although individualization of dosing is appropriate based upon response. In older girls or in girls >8 years of age in whom therapy is started when short stature is extreme, concomitant administration of a steroid that cannot be aromatized to estrogen, such as oxandrolone (0.05 mg/kg/day), should be considered. Girls given oxandrolone should be monitored for potential side effects including clitoral enlargement and glucose intolerance. GH + oxandrolone therapy is continued until a satisfactory height is achieved or until bone age is >14 and annual growth rate is <2 cm. Estrogen is not recommended as a growth-promoting agent, and the initiation of estrogen therapy should be timed to minimize negative effects on growth and adult height (102).

Adverse effects of GH therapy in TS patients have been minimal. Although osteopenia is more prevalent in patients with TS, bone mineral status is not impaired (and may be improved) in GH-treated adolescents with TS (103). Autoantibodies to endocrine organs also occur in TS with increased frequency; GH therapy does not alter immune function in TS (104). Glucose tolerance is of particular interest given the increased incidence of diabetes mellitus in adults with TS and the diabetogenic action of GH. Frequency of impaired glucose tolerance is increased over normal in children with TS. Investigations to date have revealed no significant change in glucose tolerance tests or levels of glycosylated hemoglobin during GH therapy (105). However, obese patients or patients with high insulin concentrations before start of GH therapy may be at greater risk for deterioration (106). Elevations in plasma insulin concentrations are more frequent when GH therapy is combined with oxandrolone, which may also impair glucose tolerance by induction of insulin resistance.

Noonan syndrome (NS) is an autosomal dominant disorder that shares clinical features with TS, including growth retardation usually in the absence of GH deficiency. A recent 3 year controlled trial showed a mean increase in growth rate from a baseline of 4.4 cm/year to 8.4, 6.2, and 5.8 cm/year during years 1, 2, and 3 of GH therapy respectively. Mean height SD score increased from −2.7 to −1.9 in GH-treated NS patients compared with a change from −2.7 to −2.4 in nontreated NS children. However, height acceleration was not significant during the second or third years when pubertal subjects were excluded (107). Others report that initial GH-induced growth acceleration is followed by a waning of effect with long-term therapy; in a small group of 10 pa-

tients, a mean increment in final height of only 3.1 cm was observed (108). In both studies, no deleterious effects on myocardial thickness were observed

VII. INTRAUTERINE GROWTH RETARDATION

For approximately 10% of children with intrauterine growth retardation (IUGR), the pattern of growth continues to be abnormal from intrauterine life to full maturity (109). Included in this group are children with dysmorphic features compatible with Russell-Silver syndrome. Even though bone age is often delayed early in childhood, the adolescent growth spurt usually occurs early and is reduced in magnitude (110). Although a minority of children with IUGR display subnormal spontaneous or provoked GH concentrations, results of these tests do not predict their responsiveness to GH.

In a study reported more than 30 years ago, approximately 50% of prepubertal children with IUGR responded to twice- or three times weekly GH injections with significant growth acceleration (111). Studies of daily administration of GH reveal consistent increases in short-term growth velocity (e.g., from 6.7 to 10.4 cm/year) (112); greater increments in growth velocity have been achieved with higher GH dosages (113). Prolonged (3 years) GH treatment of children with IUGR sustains an accelerated growth rate but does not increase height for bone age score, pointing to an unaltered final height outcome (114). Nevertheless a recent report of 5 years of treatment (115) and a separate epianalysis of four randomized studies of 6 years duration (116) both indicate that administration of GH (0.033–0.067 μg/kg/day with both continuous and discontinuous regimens employed) can normalize stature of short, non-GHD IUGR children, at least during childhood and early puberty (Fig. 4).

Growth failure in IUGR children has recently been approved by the FDA as an indication for GH therapy. Furthermore, the successful and novel use of intermittent high-dosage GH therapy in this group of patients is an important observation that could potentially be applied to other GH treatment indications. Whether IUGR children derive substantial psychological benefits from a more rapid tempo of growth during childhood (even without enhanced final stature) remains uncertain. It is noted that difficulty of accurately assessing bone age maturation in dysmorphic syndromes such as Russell-Silver syndrome may reduce validity of predicted heights. Higher-dose GH therapy has also led to hyperinsulinemia in some of these children. Therefore, continuation of these clinical trials until final height will be required to determine the safety and efficacy of GH for IUGR. Given the accelerated tempo of puberty in these patients, concomitant administration of GnRH analog or aromatase inhibitors to permit a longer period of growth may be indicated for severely height-disabled individuals with IUGR.

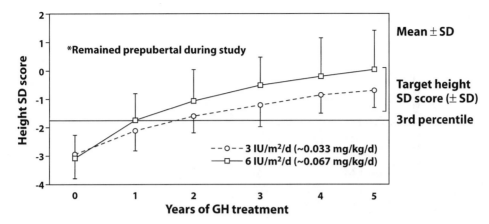

Figure 4   Effect of varying dosages of long-term GH therapy on heights in children with intrauterine growth retardation. (From Ref. 115.)

VIII. CHRONIC RENAL FAILURE AND HYPOPHOSPHATEMIC RICKETS

Poor nutrition, anemia, and chronic metabolic acidosis contribute to the growth failure characteristic of chronic renal failure (CRF). In addition, elevated fasting GH levels, exaggerated responses to provocative stimuli, depressed serum IGF-1 levels, and increased levels of IGF-1 binding protein (in particular IGFBP-1) suggest resistance to the action of GH (117). Pharmacological dosages of GH are able to overcome these growth-retarding influences in some patients with CRF through metabolic effects of GH (e.g., enhanced renal acid excretion [118]), increases in IGFs and ternary complexes that overcome inhibitory effects of excess IGFBPs (119), and direct growth-promoting effects. A randomized, double-blind, placebo-controlled study of 125 prepubertal growth-retarded children with CRF revealed first-year (10.7 ± 3.1 cm/yr) and second-year (7.8 ± 2.1 cm/yr) growth rates in the GH-treated group that were significantly greater than those seen in the placebo group. The beneficial effect on final height potential predicted by this study (Fig. 5) (120) was recently confirmed in one study of 38 GH-treated children with CRF who reached a final height 1.4 SD *above* standardized height at baseline compared with mean final height of 50 nontreated matched control children with CRF that was 0.6 SD *below* standardized height at baseline (121). In general, responsiveness to GH appears to be inversely related to the degree of renal function impairment and metabolic compromise. Growth failure due to CRF is an approved indication for GH therapy.

Growth hormone excess produces hyperfiltration and increases glomerular sclerosis in the setting of uremia, (122), raising a theoretical concern that GH treatment of children with CRF could accelerate deterioration in renal function. However, current information suggests no adverse effect of GH therapy on glomerular filtration rate (GFR); loss of GFR is unchanged during the first year of GH treatment compared to the year before treatment (123). Reports of accelerated rises in serum creatinine may reflect increased body size and creatinine production without a commensurate increase in GFR (124). Thus, growth itself, rather than GH, may place additional metabolic demands upon compromised, but stable, renal function. Hyperinsulinemia, often present before GH therapy due to uremic insulin resistance, may remain stable or worsen during GH therapy. However, glucose homeostasis, assessed by oral glucose tolerance testing and glycosylated hemoglobin levels, has remained stable (125). Transient intracranial hypertension may occur during GH treatment of children with CRF, but is relatively rare and is reversible with temporary cessation of drug or reduction in dosage.

In normal kidneys, GH increases renal phosphate retention. Consequently, GH has been administered to poorly growing children with X-linked hypophosphatemic rickets (XHR). In a recent study reporting final height outcome, GH therapy combined with conventional treatment resulted in a change in height SD score in six children with XHR (mean baseline −3.4, mean post-treatment, −2.4) whereas no change in height SD score was observed in six XHR patients not treated with GH. Phosphate retention, bone markers, and radial bone mineral density increased only in the GH-treated group (126). Additional long-term studies are needed to verify the value of long-term GH therapy for patients with this disorder.

IX. SKELETAL DYSPLASIAS

Numerous forms of skeletal dysplasia may cause significant growth retardation. Detailed descriptions of clinical and radiological features and inheritance patterns belie a lack of understanding of the basic pathophysiology for many of these disorders, although associated genetic mu-

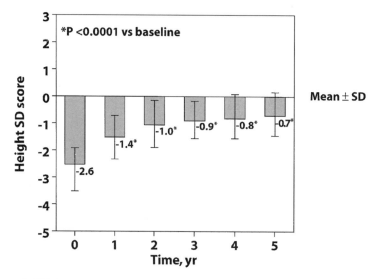

Figure 5 Beneficial effects of GH therapy on long-term growth in children with chronic renal insufficiency. (From Ref. 120.)

tations (e.g., fibroblast growth factor receptor-3 in achondroplasia) are steadily being recognized.

A short-term study of GH therapy in children with hypochondroplasia showed an increase in first year growth rate that was proportionally distributed between limb and spine growth (127). Variation in response to GH with regard to rate and proportionality of growth has also been reported, and may be related to defects in the IGF-1 gene in some patients (128). Growth response to GH is generally less than that observed in children treated for classic GH deficiency and declines after initial acceleration. Thus, modest improvement in adult height might be expected from currently used regimens of GH therapy. Higher GH dosage, concomitant GnRH analog treatment, and use of aromatase inhibitors could conceivably alter this prognosis. Patients with achondroplasia demonstrate normal secretion of GH, IGF-1 levels, and IGF-1 receptor activity (129). Reports of response to GH are variable. Some data indicate little change in growth rate, even when higher than conventional dosages are used (130). More recent studies suggest that GH therapy can increase growth rate and height z-score in a dose-dependent manner without significant side effects (131). Effects on ultimate height remain unknown. Preliminary trials of GH therapy for spondyloepiphyseal dysplasia and multiple epiphyseal dysplasia are in progress.

X. GLUCOCORTICOID-TREATED CHILDREN

Treatment of many chronic disorders (e.g., juvenile rheumatoid arthritis, asthma, renal transplantation, inflammatory bowel disease), which themselves may lead to growth failure, includes glucocorticoid therapy. Glucocorticoids (GC) impede linear growth through several mechanisms,

including promoting protein catabolism, inhibiting collagen synthesis, impairing the action of IGF-1, and suppressing endogenous GH secretion through augmentation of hypothalamic somatostatin tone (132). Thus, these patients could be considered logical candidates to benefit from both the growth-promoting and anabolic effects of GH therapy.

Early studies, implementing relatively low dosage and infrequent administration of GH, demonstrated marginal and inconsistent beneficial effects (133). Subsequent investigations of daily GH therapy for children with stable GC-treated illness (134) or who had undergone renal transplantation (135) show more consistent resumption of normal growth velocity during 1–3 years of treatment. Biochemical markers of growth (e.g., type 1 procollagen levels) are also normalized by GH administration. Responsiveness to GH appears greatest in those on moderate-dosage GC regimens with stable, nonarthritic underlying disease. Persistence of disease activity and higher GC dosage (e.g., prednisone dosage >0.35 mg/kg/day) (136) interfere with GH responsiveness.

Recent analysis of larger numbers of GC-dependent children (n = 83) evaluated over a 12 month period reveal a mean response to GH therapy (mean dosage = 0.3 mg/kg/week) of doubling of baseline growth rate (e.g., 3.0 ± 1.2 cm/year to 6.3 ± 2.6 cm/yr) (Fig. 6) (137). Responsiveness to GH is negatively correlated with the dosage of GC. In 14 severely growth-impaired children with rheumatoid arthritis (mean height SDS = −4.0), GH administered at a dosage of 0.5 mg/kg/week resulted in an increase in mean growth velocity from 1.9 to 4.5 cm/year (138). While difficult to prove, *preservation of height SDS* most likely represents a beneficial therapeutic outcome for these children. Long-term GH-responsiveness and effects of GH therapy on final height in GC-treated children nev-

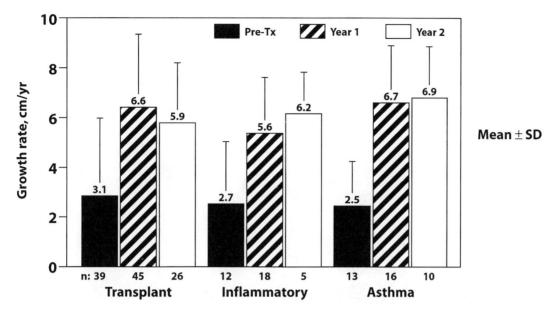

Figure 6   Effect of GH therapy on growth in children treated with glucocorticoids. (From Ref. 137.)

ertheless remain unknown, and GH treatment of GC-dependent children remains experimental.

Salutary effects of GH therapy (0.05 mg/kg/day administered daily) on the growth of children following renal transplantation are also reported. Growth rates of prepubertal children after renal transplantation have generally increased two- to threefold during the first 1–2 years of GH therapy, decline subsequently but remain above baseline growth velocity (139). Gains in height SD scores approximate 1 SD following 2–4 years of therapy, and approximately one-half of the children achieve "normal" heights (i.e., within 2 SD of the mean). Growth stimulation in pubertal children with renal allografts, while less consistent than that observed in younger patients, is still significant (140).

In addition to restoring linear growth, GH therapy may counter some of the catabolic effects of GC. Studies using isotope tracer infusions suggest that GH, directly or through IGF-1, counteracts GC-induced protein catabolism through independent stimulation of protein synthesis without altering protein breakdown (141). Alternatively, accompanying hyperinsulinemia might contribute substantially to the observed protein anabolic effect by decreasing proteolysis. GH may also counteract the antianabolic effects of GC on bone. In a group of adults receiving chronic GC treatment, in whom GHRH-stimulated GH levels were suppressed, levels of osteocalcin and carboxy-terminal propeptide of type I procollagen rose with short-term GH therapy (142). Detailed studies of the metabolic effects of GH administration in children receiving long-term GC therapy have not yet been done.

Potential adverse effects of combined GH/GC therapy in children with GC-dependent disorders include altered

carbohydrate metabolism, stimulation of autoimmune disease activity, increased cancer risk, and, in transplant recipients, graft dysfunction or rejection. Elevated fasting and stimulated insulin levels have been observed in renal allograft patients receiving GH; however, these changes frequently predate institution of GH therapy, correlate with prednisone dosage, and are not affected by the addition of GH. Among all GH-treated GC-dependent children, detectable elevations in blood glucose concentrations have been rare. GH-induced exacerbations of chronic disease activity also appear to be very unusual, but the number of patient-years available for study of this question remains small. With regard to renal allograft function and survival, actions of GH on glomerular hemodynamics, glomerular morphology, and immune stimulation are theoretical reasons for concern. Nevertheless, most investigators report no difference between GH-treated and control renal allograft patients with regard to changes in GFR, effective plasma flow, other measures of renal function, and rates of allograft rejection. Although preliminary analysis of one randomized prospective study suggested that GH might slightly increase allograft rejection rates, final analysis indicated that biopsy-proven acute rejection episodes were not significantly more frequent in the group receiving GH (143). Long-term and careful follow-up of children with renal transplants receiving GH therapy is still needed to resolve this important issue.

XI. PRADER-WILLI SYNDROME

Growth of children with Prader-Willi syndrome (PWS) is characterized by moderate intrauterine and postnatal growth retardation, followed by near-normal growth rates as caloric intake increases and obesity typically develops. Substantial evidence now supports a true GH deficient state in PWS: lack of nutrition-induced growth acceleration, relatively low IGF1 levels, diminished GH responses to GH provocation, and body composition abnormalities (i.e., reduced muscle mass, increased fat mass) resembling states of GH deficiency. Administration of GH to children with PWS results in growth rate increases equivalent to those observed in severely GH-deficient children (Fig. 7). In addition, GH therapy increases lean body mass, decreases fat mass, and increases bone mineral density (144, 145). Reductions in fat mass result from increases in total body energy expenditure and preference for fat oxidation as an energy source (confirmed reductions in respiratory quotient). In addition to cognitive and behavioral disabilities, profound hypotonia severely limits the physical function of individuals with PWS. Treatment with growth hormone improves measures of strength and agility in children with PWS, substantiating claims of so-called real-life benefits of GH for these children. These changes in body composition and physical function are dose-dependent and attenuate, but do not regress, during prolonged GH therapy (146). Growth failure related to PWS is a recent approved indication for GH treatment.

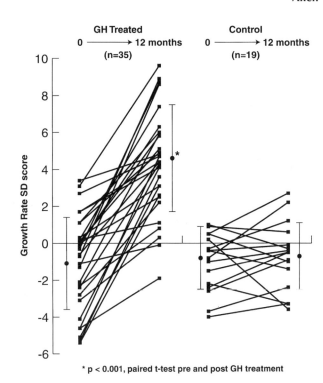

Figure 7 Growth rates of children with Prader-Willi syndrome treated with GH compared to untreated control subjects with PWS. (from Ref. 144.)

XII. OTHER SYNDROMES AND DEFECTS ASSOCIATED WITH SHORT STATURE

Short stature is a component of more than 100 syndromes. Subnormal secretion of GH has been reported in some children with Down syndrome (147). Preliminary treatment trials of these children show short-term responses to GH similar to those of Russell-Silver syndrome and Turner syndrome. Short stature is also a common problem in children with neural tube defects such as spina bifida or myelomeningocele, who may have spinal and/or lower skeletal abnormalities. Secretion of GH is normal unless accompanying hydrocephalus impairs hypothalamic–pituitary function. In a small group of patients with neural tube defects and subnormal GH secretion, GH treatment over 36 months significantly improved growth rates of body length and arm span. However, the increase in length SD score was not significant (148).

The expansion of GH therapy into populations affected by mental disability or with limited ambulatory capability raises complex ethical questions by focusing attention on the expectation that successful GH therapy ought to improve the quality of life, rather than merely the height, of treated individuals (149). For each of these groups of patients, analysis of larger, longer prospective trials, conducted within a GH investigational protocol, are needed before recommendations about efficacy can be made. When this information is available, treatment decisions can be made for individual patients (rather than

diagnostic groups) based upon degree of disability and likelihood of long-term enhancement in quality of life.

XIII. ADULTS WITH GH DEFICIENCY AND THE ELDERLY

The availability of unlimited supplies of human GH has been accompanied by a wealth of new information regarding the consequences of GH deficiency in adults and the benefits of replacement treatment. Lack of GH in adulthood can lead to contraction of lean body mass and water, expansion of fat mass (particularly central abdominal fat), diminution of bone mineral content, increased concentrations of total and low-density lipoprotein (LDL) cholesterol, increased atherothrombotic propensity, impaired cardiac function, impaired psychological well-being, and decreased life expectancy (150). Placebo-controlled studies of GH therapy in adults with *complete* GH deficiency have revealed a marked increase in muscle mass, decrease in fat mass (151, 152), and improvements in exercise performance (153). Subjective improvements in quality of life indicators such as vigor, ambition, and sense of well-being are also reported (154). Consequently, adult GHD is now an FDA-approved indication for GH therapy.

Adverse effects due to fluid retention (e.g., edema, carpal tunnel syndrome) are fairly common, but reverse with dosage reduction or continuation of the same dosage. Dosages used are markedly lower than those used per kilogram during childhood: the Growth Hormone Research Society recommends that dosage not be weight-based. Patients are to be commenced on a low-dosage (0.15–0.3 mg/day) regimen, which is then gradually increased in accordance with clinical and biochemical responses. Maintenance dosages varies considerably, and is influenced by gender and age, but rarely exceed 1 mg/day. Women usually require higher dosages than men, while the elderly require lower dosages (155).

The normal decline in the activity of the GH-IGF-1 axis that occurs with advancing age appears to contribute to the decrease in lean body mass, increase in adipose tissue mass, and possibe loss of energy. Administration of GH to non-GH-deficient men over 60 years old caused significant increases in lean body mass, bone density, and skin thickness, with concomitant reductions in fat mass (156). Following GH therapy, deterioration of these parameters resume in age-appropriate fashion. Although the implications of such therapy are enticing, the risk–benefit ratio and cost-effectiveness of GH therapy in the general aging but healthy population have not been established. Administration of GH has also been used by younger adults in conjunction with heavy resistance exercise training in an effort to maximize skeletal muscle protein anabolism and strength. However, in a placebo-controlled study of young normal men, resistance training supplemented with GH did not further enhance muscle anabolism and function (157). These results suggest that increased fat-free mass seen with GH supplementation was probably due to an increase in lean tissue other than skeletal muscle.

XIV. CATABOLIC STATES

Well-documented salutary effects of GH on nitrogen retention and protein synthesis rates have prompted investigation of GH therapy in various catabolic, regenerative, or reparative states. Nitrogen balance is improved by GH in postoperative patients under hypocaloric conditions (158) and GH partially reverses nitrogen wasting in obese humans made catabolic by dietary restriction (159). Growth hormone also improves the efficiency of parenteral nutrient utilization in patients requiring total parenteral nutrition. Improvements in weight and lean tissue mass have also been documented in pediatric burn patients (160). However, results of controlled trials of GH treatment in acute-care settings have not all been favorable. One placebo-controlled trial in normal adults showed that full-thickness wound healing was significantly *delayed* by GH therapy (161). A large randomized controlled trial of high-dosage GH treatment of adult patients during a severe catabolic illness in the intensive care setting showed higher mortality in GH-treated patients (162). Although perhaps influenced substantially by the high dosages of GH administered, these data have nevertheless created substantial concern about use of GH in the critical care setting. Most physicians currently discontinue GH in acutely ill patients in the hospital who are taking GH chronically. Whether GH treatment of overwhelmingly ill patients induces the release or potentiates the action of harmful cytokines is currently under investigation.

Anabolic effects of GH therapy have also created interest in its use as ancillary therapy for several chronic illnesses. GH has been shown to improve the body composition of patients with acquired immunodeficiency syndrome's (AIDS) wasting syndrome (another FDA-approved use of GH). Improved lean tissue mass, height and weight gain, and decreased protein catabolism have been reported in children with Crohn's disease and chronic ulcerative colitis (163). In children with cystic fibrosis, a randomized controlled trial showed significant improvements in height and weight gain, lean tissue mass, and pulmonary function, accompanied by decreased hospitalization time (164). During the next decade, we can look forward to considerable new knowledge about the anabolic effects of GH in these and related settings.

XV. ADVERSE EFFECTS OF GH TREATMENT

Recombinant biosynthetic GH preparations are highly purified and free of contaminants. The possibility of viral transmission through GH has been virtually eliminated. However, surveillance of patients who received pituitary-derived GH for development of Creutzfeld-Jakob remains important. Antigenicity of GH preparations is also low (165), although GH antibodies can be detected in 10–30% of treated children. With rare exceptions (less than 0.1%), these antibodies do not impede effects of GH.

GH administration to healthy subjects acutely increases serum T3 and reciprocally decreases free T4. Laboratory indications of hypothyroidism may likewise be seen in as many as 25% of GH-deficient children treated with GH, with declines in serum T4 levels reflecting increased peripheral conversion of T4 to T3 (166). GHD patients who display subnormal nocturnal TSH surges, signifying a pre-existing central hypothyroidism, are more likely to display subnormal T4 and free T4 levels during GH therapy, and to benefit from thyroid replacement (167). Most studies, however, indicate that children with normal thyroid function before treatment do not develop significant perturbations in thyroid hormone metabolism during GH therapy.

GH deficiency is associated with reductions in lean body mass and total body water, with accompanying reductions in renal plasma flow and glomerular filtration rates. Edema and sodium retention rarely occurs early in the course of GH therapy (particularly in older, heavier children and adolescents), attributable to an antinatriuretic effect on the renal tubule of GH and/or IGF-1. Minor elevations in plasma renin activity and aldosterone observed in the first 3 days of treatment resolve within a week or 2 (168). Occasionally, fluid shifts within the central nervous system are sufficient to cause benign intracranial hypertension (pseudotumor cerebri) and its symptoms of headache, visual loss, vomiting, and papilledema. It is speculated that direct fluid-retaining properties of GH and/or action of locally produced IGF-1 on cerebrospinal fluid (CSF) production are causative. Most instances have occurred during early (although not invariably) treatment of patients with severe GHD or other risk factors for this condition (e.g., chronic renal insufficiency, Prader-Willi syndrome). Cessation of GH therapy has reversed the symptoms in reported cases, and some patients experience spontaneous resolution of symptoms in spite of continued GH treatment (169). Resumption of GH treatment has been successfully accomplished with reinitiation at a lower dosage and gradual return to the initial dosage. It is recommended that fundoscopic examination be performed on all patients before initiation of GH therapy and periodically thereafter (170).

Until recently, GH had been used primarily as replacement therapy for GH deficiency. Adverse effects of GH therapy become more likely as higher dosages are used for pharmacological GH *augmentation* therapy. Recommendations for GH dosage, derived largely from growth response data, are in excess of calculated estimates of normal GH production in a prepubertal child, and dosing guidelines for adolescents are increasing further. IGF-1 levels in some GH-treated girls with Turner's syndrome approach those found in acromegaly (171), and anecdotal reports of development of acromegaloid features (e.g., large hands and feet) during higher than conventional dosage GH therapy have appeared. GH excess reduces insulin sensitivity, and given the trend toward higher dosages, it is important to assess a GH dosage's effect on carbohydrate metabolism. Nearly all studies of GH therapy in children and adults show an increase in fasting and postprandial insulin levels. However, glucose homeostasis is generally not impaired (172). Furthermore, normal levels of blood glucose and glycosylated hemoglobin may be preserved by hyperinsulinemia, which when persistent can be associated with atherosclerosis and hypertension. One study of long-term high-dosage GH therapy found normal glucose metabolism and higher levels of insulin (which did not correlate closely with dosage) that returned to normal when GH therapy was discontinued (173). Given these reassuring data, a recent report of an increased frequency of type 2 diabetes in childhood GH recipients was surprising. Fewer than half of affected subjects were obese or had other risk factors for diabetes, two-thirds were in puberty, and diabetes persisted in all patients after GH discontinuation (174). Other pharmacoepidemiological databases have not reported an increase in diabetes incidence. Careful prospective follow-up of individuals during and after GH therapy is needed to resolve this issue.

Perhaps the greatest concern regarding GH therapy is the theoretical possibility that GH could facilitate the de-

velopment of cancers. Growth hormone is mitogenic, and there is evidence in animals of a cause and effect relation between supraphysiological doses of GH and development of leukemia (175). Three clinical settings have raised concern: GH-treatment-induced new malignancy; GH-treatment-induced recurrent malignancy; GH-treatment-induced second malignancy in those already treated for one tumor. In 1988, reports from Japan describing leukemia in GH-treated children raised concern about new malignancy (176). An extended follow-up study of 6284 recipients of pituitary-derived GH revealed a relative risk of leukemia in recipients of GH of 2.6 (90% confidence interval, 1.2–5.2). Five of six subjects had antecedent cranial tumors as the cause of GH deficiency, and four had received radiotherapy (177). Subsequent analyses, based on much larger total patient-years of GH treatment, indicate that the rates of new leukemia in (non-Japanese) patients without pre-existing risk factors who are treated with GH is no greater than expected for the general population (178). This lack of increased risk in children without pre-existing risk factors was recently confirmed in the Japanese population (179). Any possible increased incidence of leukemia appears limited to those patients with known risk factors, and due to the small numbers of events in such patients, it remains impossible to determine any contribution of GH therapy. With regard to nonleukemia cancers, a retrospective analysis of large postmarketing database found no evidence of an increased risk of developing an extracranial, nonleukemia neoplasm in GH-treated patients (180).

With regard to recurrent malignancy, no report has associated GH therapy with an increased incidence of tumor recurrence. A lack of reliable knowledge about the natural history of recurrence of these tumors, however, supports a cautious interpretation of such data. Most recurrences occur within the first 2 years of treatment, and most endocrinologists defer institution of treatment until a year of stable remission has passed. While this may result in some lost growth for the child, it also avoids the inevitable association of GH therapy and tumor recurrence during this high-risk period. With regard to second malignancy, no study to date has directly compared the incidence of new second tumors in those receiving GH and those not.

In humans, GH and IGF-1 have been shown to affect numerous immune functions, but these effects do not appear to translate into clinically relevant problems in GH-treated children. The possibility that GH might influence the growth rate of melanocytic nevi has been raised. However, a recent study failed to show any relationship between melanocytic nevi count and duration of GH therapy in girls with TS, and the melanocyte count in children with GHD was not different from controls and was not influenced by GH therapy (181). GH treatment causes an increase in both the proliferative and hypertrophied zones of the growth plate that may reduce the force needed to shear it. An increased frequency of slipped capital femoral epiphysis has been reported during treatment with GH (182). This rare complication is more common in children with organic causes of severe GHD, who require close monitoring for limp and hip or knee pain (183). Progression of scoliosis may be more rapid during GH therapy, but available data do not suggest an increased frequency of scoliosis as a result of GH exposure. Nevertheless, some children more likely to receive GH therapy (e.g., those with Turner syndrome, Prader-Willi syndrome) already have an increased frequency of scoliosis, and require close monitoring. Concerns raised regarding other potential adverse effects of GH therapy (e.g., reduced testicular volume, gynecomastia, deterioration of renal function in patients with CRF, cardiac ventricular hypertrophy in those with Turner and Noonan syndromes) have, to date, either not been realized or considered not to be of sufficient clinical significance to alter prescribing (184).

In summary, nearly two decades of experience with recombinant GH has proven this therapy to be remarkably safe when used in conventional substitution dosages for GH deficiency. Higher-dosage therapy for other causes of growth retardation also appear to be safe, but continued surveillance of its metabolic effects is indicated. There appear to be very few medical contraindications to GH therapy. Nevertheless, the experience of transmission of Creutzfeldt-Jakob syndrome via pituitary GH is a poignant reminder that a farsighted view must be taken of the potential ramifications of long-term hormonal therapy.

XVI. ETHICAL ISSUES IN GH TREATMENT

Limited availability of GH once provided a barrier to expanding its use beyond children who were unequivocally GH deficient. Today, increased supply of GH has been matched by increased demand. Ten years ago in the United States, there was one approved indication for GH, two GH manufacturers, and approximately 10,000 children receiving treatment at a cost ranging between $5000 and $40,000 per year. Today, there are six FDA-approved indications for GH (Table 1), multiple US and international manufacturers, and well over 30,000 patients treated. Nevertheless, GH therapy remains expensive. Relaxed diagnostic criteria have obliterated any clear boundary between GH deficiency and sufficiency, allowing many partially affected children access to treatment. Future goals of GH therapy appear likely to shift further toward supplementing and enhancing individuals' well being rather than merely returning them to some physiological baseline. Careful longitudinal studies, many of which are already in progress, will be required to determine the efficacy of GH in accomplishing these goals.

But what *can* be done with GH is not necessarily what *should* be done. Ethical justification for these goals, not merely the efficacy of GH therapy in accomplishing them, also deserves careful scrutiny. New uses of GH raise complex philosophical, psychological, and economic, as well as medical questions that physician–scientists alone cannot answer (185). Even if GH is shown to increase effectively the growth of non-GH-deficient children and even if treatment can be accomplished without toxicity, additional considerations are needed to assess responsibly the long-term *value* of the added height increment, and to balance expected benefit with issues of resource allocation and fairness.

Widespread distribution of GH has been partially deterred by high drug costs. It is a paradox that although the source of GH is no longer limited, the resources with which to pay for it are becoming increasingly so. Prescribing GH requires a difficult and often uncomfortable balancing of responsible use of medical resources with an obligation to do the best for each individual patient. But is taller really better for each patient (186)? Concern about psychological harm is invoked as a primary rationale for treating short stature, yet data confirming the efficacy of GH therapy in alleviating the psychosocial consequences of short stature are scarce. If the ultimate goal of GH therapy is not tall stature but, rather, an improved quality of life, documentation of psychosocial impairment due to stature prior to therapy and improvement following GH therapy ought to play an important role in the initiation of GH therapy and evaluation of its efficacy (187). To date, however, growth rate and final adult height remain the measures by which therapeutic success is judged.

Responsiveness to GH, described above in many groups of short-statured individuals, is a necessary but not sufficient indication for treatment. Because of enormous expense and concerns that such widespread access would not ameliorate disadvantages of short stature, it seems appropriate to restrict access within this group based upon the presence of significant functional or psychological disability related to stature and the likelihood of improvement with treatment. Most short children will not satisfy these additional criteria. Children with severe GH deficiency are likely to be both more disabled and more responsive than non-GH-deficient children, justifying the former's preferential treatment. Is it justified to restrict access of others to GH based on the laboratory diagnosis of GH deficiency? Some have argued that equally short children share a similar disability, regardless of whether stimulated GH levels fall just above or just below an arbitrary threshold. If both are GH responsive and truly disabled by height, there appears to be little ethical justification for treating only the child with lower GH test results (188).

Alleviating the disability of short stature, rather than normalization of GH levels, has traditionally been the primary goal of GH therapy. Determining an appropriate end-point for GH therapy remains controversial. Attainment of genetic potential for height, which is a realistic possibility with optimal diagnosis and treatment, remains a goal for many (189). Consistent adherence to the goal of alleviating disabling short stature, on the other hand, implies that GH therapy be discontinued when *each* treated child reaches an adult height no longer considered a disability. No policy regarding GH therapy will ever eliminate the first percentile on the growth curve, but the second strategy has as its goal bringing children into the *normal opportunity range for height* without further enhancing those who have achieved a height within the normal adult distribution. By adhering to the *treatment* of disabling short stature, and resisting the *enhancement* of normal stature, physicians treating children with GH would minimize their contribution to society's heightist perception that to be taller is to be better (190).

REFERENCES

1. Raben MS. Treatment of a pituitary dwarf with human growth hormone [letter]. J Clin Endocrinol 1958; 18:901.
2. Burns EC, Tanner JM, Preece MA, Cameron N. Final height and pubertal development in 55 children with idiopathic growth hormone deficiency, treated for between 2 and 15 years with human growth hormone. Eur J Pediatr 1981; 137:155–164.
3. Bundak R, Hindmarsh PC, Smith PJ, Brook CGD. Long term auxologic effects of human growth hormone. J Pediatr 1988; 112:875–879.
4. Joss E, Juppinger K, Schwarz HP, Roten G. Final height of patients with pituitary growth failure and changes in growth variables after long-term hormonal therapy. Pediatr Res 1983; 17:676–679.
5. Fradkin JE, Schonberger LB, Mills JL, et al. Creutzfeldt-Jakob disease in pituitary growth hormone recipients in the United States. JAMA 1991; 265:880–884.
6. Underwood LE, Fisher DA, Frasier SD, et al. Degenerative neurologic disease in patients formerly treated with human growth hormone—Report of the Committee on Growth Hormone Use of the Lawson Wilkins Pediatric Endocrine Society, May 1985. J Pediatr 1985; 107:10.
7. Goeddel DV, Heyneker JL, Hozumi T, et al. Direct expression in Escherichia coli of a DNA sequence coding for human growth hormone. Nature 1979; 281:544.
8. Frasier SD, Rudlin CR, Zeisel HJ, Liu HH, Long PC, Senior M, Finegold D, Bercu B, Marks J, Redmond G. Effect of somatotropin of mammalian cell origin in growth hormone deficiency. Am J Dis Child 1992; 146:582–587.
9. Stabler B, Clopper RR, Siegel PT, Stoppani C, Compton PG, Underwood LE, the National Cooperative Growth Study. Academic achievement and psychological adjustment in short children. J Develop Behav Pediatr 1994; 15(1):1–6.
10. Stabler B, Siegel PT, Clopper RR. Growth hormone deficiency in children has psychological and educational comorbidity. Clin Pediatr 1991; 30(3):156–160.
11. Sandberg DE, MacGillivray MH. Growth hormone therapy in childhood-onset growth hormone deficiency; adult anthropometric and psychological outcomes. Endocrine 2000; 12(2):173–182.
12. Root AW, Diamond FB. Regulation and clinical assessment of growth hormone secretion. Endocrine 2000; 12(2):137–145.
13. Hunter WM, Rigal WM. The diurnal pattern of plasma growth hormone concentration in children and adolescents. J Endocrinol 1966; 34:147–153.
14. Leung DW, Spencer SA, Cachianes G, et al. Growth hormone receptor and serum binding protein: Purification, cloning and expression. Nature 1987; 330:537–543.
15. Guevara-Aguirre J, Rosenbloom AL, Fielder PJ, Diamond FB, Rosenfeld RG. Growth hormone receptor deficiency in Ecuador: clinical and biochemical phenotype in two populations. J Clin Endocrinol Metab 1993; 76:417–423.
16. Ho KKY, Valiontis E, Waters MJ, Rajkovic IA. Regulation of growth hormone binding protein in man: comparison of gel chromatography and immunoprecipitation methods. J Clin Endocrinol Metab 1993; 76:302–308.
17. Miller MD, Esparza A, Wright NM, Garimella V, Lai J, Lester SE, Mosier ED. Spontaneous growth hormone release in term infants: changes during the first four days of life. J Clin Endocrinol Metab 1993; 76:1058–1062.
18. Martha PM, Rogol AD, Veldhuis JD, Kerrigan JR, Goodman DW, Blizzard RM. Alterations in the pulsatile properties of circulating growth hormone concentrations during puberty in boys. J Clin Endocrinol Metab 1989; 69:563–570.
19. Kerrigan JR, Rogol AD. The impact of gonadal steroid hormone action on growth hormone secretion during childhood and adolescence. Endocr Rev 1992; 13:281.
20. Keenan BS, Richards GE, Ponder SW, Dallas JS, Nagamani M, Smith ER. Androgen-stimulated pubertal growth: the effects of testosterone and dihydrotestosterone on growth hormone and insulin-like growth factor-1 in the treatment of short stature and delayed puberty. J Clin Endocrinol Metab 1993; 76:996–1001.
21. Weissberger AJ, Ho KKY. Activation of the somatotropic axis by testosterone in adult males: evidence for the role of aromatization. J Clin Endocrinol Metab 1993; 76:1407–1412.
22. Albertsson-Wiklund K, Rosberg S. Analysis of 24-hour growth hormone profiles in children: Relationship to growth. J Clin Endocrinol Metab 1988; 67:493–500.
23. Hindmarsh P, Smith PJ, Brook CGD, Matthews DR. The relationship between height velocity and growth hormone secretion in short prepubertal children. Clin Endocrinol 1987; 27:581–591.
24. Collett-Solberg PF, Cohen P. Genetics, chemistry, and function of the IGF/IGFBP system. Endocrine 2000; 12(2):121–136.
25. Isaksson OGP, Lindahl A, Nilsson A, Isgaard J. Mechanism of the stimulatory effect of growth hormone on longitudinal bone growth. End Rev 1987; 8(4):426–438.
26. Guler HP, Zapf J, Scheiwiller E, et al. Recombinant human insulin-like growth factor I stimulates growth and has distinct effects on organ size in hypophysectomized rats. Proc Natl Acad Sci USA 1988; 85:4889–4893.
27. Berelowitz M, Szabo M, Frohman LA. Somatomedin-C mediates growth hormone negative feedback by effects on both the hypothalamus and the pituitary. Science 1981; 212:1279–1281.
28. Yamashita S, Melmed A. Insulin-like growth factor I action on rat anterior pituitary cells: suppression of growth hormone secretion and messenger ribonucleic acid levels. Endocrinology 1986; 18:176–182.
29. Rubin KR, Lichtenfels JM, Ratzan SK. Relationship of somatomedin-C concentration to bone age in boys with constitutional growth delay. Am J Dis Child 1986; 140:555–558.

30. Ziegler TR, Rombeau JL, Young LS, Fong Y, Marano M, Lowry SF, Wilmore DW. Recombinant human growth hormone enhances the metabolic efficacy of parenteral nutrition: a double-blind randomized controlled study. J Clin Endocrinol Metab 1992; 74(4):865–873.

31. Chipman JJ, Zerwekh J, Nicar M, Marks J, Pak CJC. Effect of growth hormone administration: reciprocal changes in serum 1-alpha,25-dihydroxyvitamin D and calcium metabolism. J Clin Endocrinol Metab 1980; 51: 321–324.

32. Saggese G, Baroncelli BI, Bertelloni S, Cinquanta L, DiNero G. Effects of long-term treatment with growth hormone on bone and mineral metabolism in children with growth hormone deficiency. J Pediatr 1993; 122: 37–45.

33. Carrel A, Allen DB. Effects of growth hormone on body composition and bone metabolism. Endocrine 2000; 12(2):163–172.

34. Goodman HM, Grichting G. Growth hormone and lipolysis: a reevaluation. Endocrinology 1983; 113:1697.

35. Argyropoulou M, Perignon F, Brauner R, Brunelle F. Magnetic resonance imaging in the diagnosis of growth hormone deficiency. J Pediatr 1992; 120:886–891.

36. Rimoin DL, Merimee TJ, McKusick VA. Growth hormone deficiency in man: an isolated, recessively inherited defect. Science 1966; 152:1635.

37. Vimpani CV, et al. Prevalence of severe growth hormone deficiency. Br Med J 1977; 2:427.

38. Pankin JM. Incidence of growth hormone deficiency. Arch Dis Child 1974; 49:905.

39. Stanhope R. Is growth hormone deficiency a discrete entity? Against the notion. Growth Genet Horm 1992; 8(suppl 1):6–9.

40. Veldhuis JD, Blizzard RM, Rogol AD, Martha PM, Kirkland JL, Sherman BM. Properties of spontaneous growth hormone secretory bursts and half-life of endogenous growth hormone in boys with idiopathic short stature. J Clin Endocrinol Metab 1992; 74:766–773.

41. Goodman HG, Grumbach MM, Kaplan SL. Growth and growth hormone. II. A comparison of isolated growth hormone deficiency and multiple pituitary hormone deficiencies in 35 patients with idiopathic hypopituitary dwarfism. N Engl J Med 1968; 278:57.

42. Duck S, Schwarz HP, Costin G, et al. Subcutaneous growth hormone-releasing hormone therapy in growth hormone deficient children: first year of therapy. J Clin Endocrinol Metab 1992; 75:1115.

43. Brasel JA, Wright JC, Wilkins L, et al. An evaluation of 75 patients with hypopituitarism beginning in childhood. Am J Med 1965; 38:484.

44. Thomsett MJ, Conte FA, Kaplan SL, et al. Endocrine and neurologic outcome in childhood craniopharyngioma. Review of effect of treatment in 42 patients. J Pediatr 1980; 97:728.

45. Blatt J, Bercu BB, Gillin JC, et al. Reduced pulsatile growth hormone secretion in children after therapy for acute lymphoblastic leukemia. J Pediatr 1984; 104:182–186.

46. Shalet SM. The effects of irradiation on endocrine function in children. Growth Genet Horm 1992; 8(3):7–11.

47. Littley MD. Radiation and the hypothalamic–pituitary axis. Radiation Injury to the Nervous System. New York: Raven Press, 1991:311.

48. Root AW. Methods of assessing growth hormone secretion and determining growth hormone deficiency. Growth Genet Horm 1992; 8(suppl 1):1–6.

49. Marin G, Barnes KM, Domene H. Failure of normal prepubertal children to respond to growth hormone stimulation tests. Endocrinology 1991; 128:82A.

50. Brauner F, Rappaport R, Prevot C, et al. A prospective study of the development of growth hormone deficiency in children given cranial irradiation, and its relation to statural growth. J Clin Endocrinol Metab 1989; 68(2): 346–351.

51. Rose SR, Ross JL, Uriarte M, Barnes KM, Cassorla FG, Cutler GB Jr. The advantage of measuring stimulated as compared with spontaneous growth hormone levels in the diagnosis of growth hormone deficiency. N Engl J Med 1988; 319:201–208.

52. Tauber M, Moulin P, Pienkowski C, Jouret B, Rochiccioli P. Growth hormone (GH) retesting and auxologicaldata in 131 GH-deficient patients after completion of treatment. J Clin Endocrinol Metab 1997; 82:352–356.

53. Hedin L, Olsson B, Diczfalusy M, Flyg C, Petersson A, Rosberg S, Albertsson-Wikland K. Intranasal administration of human growth hormone in combination with a membrane permeation enhancer in patients with GH deficiency: a pharmacokinetic study. J Clin Endocrinol Metab 1993; 76:962–967.

54. Vanderschueren-Lodeweyckx M, Van den Broeck J, Wolter R, Malvaux P. Early initiation of growth hormone treatment: influence on final height. Act Paediatr Scand 1987; 337(suppl):4–11.

55. Frasier SD, Costin G, Lippe BM, Aceto T, Bunge PF. A dose–response curve for human growth hormone. J Clin Endocrinol Metab 1981; 53:1213.

56. Keizer-Schrama SMPF, Rikken B, Wynne HJ, Hokken-Koelega ACS, Wit JM, Bot A, Drop S. Dose–response study of biosynthetic human growth hormone (GH) in GH-deficient children: effects on auxological and biochemical parameters. J Clin Endocrinol Metab 1992; 74: 898–905.

57. Cohen P, Bright GM, Rogol AD, Kappelgaard AM, Rosenfeld RG. Effects of dose and gender on the growth and growth factor response to GH in GH-deficient children. J Clin Endocrinol Metab 2002;87:90–98.

58. Jorgensen JOL, Flyvbjerg A, Lauritzen T, Alberti KGMM, Orskov H, Christiansen JS. Dose-response studies with biosynthetic human growth hormone (GH) in GH-deficient patients. J Clin Endocrinol Metab 1988; 67:36.

59. MacGillivray MH, Baptista J, Johanson A. Outcome of a four-year randomized study of daily versus three times weekly somatropin treatment in prepubertal naïve growth hormone deficient children. J Clin Endocrinol Metab 1996; 81:1806–1809.

60. Reiter EO, Attie KM, Neuwirth R, Ford KM. Efficacy and safety of sustained-release GH given once or twice monthly in children with GH deficiency. Proceedings of the 81st meeting of the Endocrine Society, San Diego, (abstract) R14-2, 1999.

61. Smith PJ, Hindmarsh PC, Brook CGD. Contribution of dose and frequency of administration to the therapeutic effect of growth hormone. Arch Dis Child 1988; 63:491–494.

62. Gertner JM, Tamborlane WV, Gianfredi SP, Genel M. Renewed catch-up growth with increase replacement doses of human growth hormone. J Pediatr 1987; 110(3):425–428.

63. Tiwary C. Seasonal and latitudinal effects on growth in patients on Protropin growth hormone in the US and Can-

ada. Genentech National Cooperative Growth Study Summary Report 15. June, 1993.

64. Costin G, Kogut MD, Phillips LS, Daughaday WH. Craniopharyngioma: the role of insulin in promoting postoperative growth. J Clin Endocrinol Metab 1976; 42:370.

65. Geffner ME. The growth without growth hormone syndrome. Endocrinol Metab Clin of North Am 1996; 25(3): 649–663.

66. Van der Werff ten Bosch JJ, Bot A. Growth of males with idiopathic hypopituitarism without growth hormone treatment. Clin Endocrinol 1990; 32:707–717.

67. Stanhope R, Uruena M, Hindmarsh P, Leiper AD, Brook CGD. Management of growth hormone deficiency through puberty. Acta Paediatr Scand 1991; 372:47–52.

68. Mauras N, Attie K, Reiter E, Saenger P, Baptista J. High dose recombinant human growth hormone (GH) treatment of GH-deficient patients in puberty increases near final height: a randomized, multicenter trial. J Clin Endocrinol Metab 2000; 85:3653–3660.

69. Allen DB. Childhood growth hormone deficiency: statural and psychological effects of long-term GH replacement. Endocrinologist 1998; 8:3S–7S.

70. Dean HJ. Demographic outcome of growth hormone deficient individuals. In Holmes CS, ed. Psychoneuroendocrinology: Brain, Behavior, and Hormonal Interactions. New York: Springer-Verlag, 1990:79–91.

71. Bjork S, Jonsson B, Westphal O, Levin JE. Quality of life of adults with growth hormone deficiency: a controlled study. Acta Paediatr Scand 1989; 356(suppl):55–59.

72. Allen DB. Issues in the transition from childhood to adult growth hormone therapy. Pediatrics 1999; 104:1004–1009.

73. Feldman SD. The presentation of shortness in everyday life: height and heightism in American society—toward a sociology of stature. In: Feldman SD, ed. Life-Styles: Diversity in American Society. Boston: Little, Brown, 1975:437–452.

74. Lippe BM. Growth hormone treatment: does ascertainment bias determine treatment practices? Growth Genet Horm 1992; 8(suppl 1):31–35.

75. Rotnem D, Benel M, Hintz RL, et al. Personality development in children with growth hormone deficiency. J Am Acad Child Psychiatry 1977; 16:412–426.

76. Penny R, Blizzard RM. The possible influence of puberty on the release of growth hormone in three males with apparent isolated growth hormone deficiency. J Clin Endocrinol 1972; 34:82–84.

77. Hindmarsh PL, Brook CGD. Effect of growth hormone on short normal children. Br Med J 1987; 295:573–577.

78. Albertsson-Wikland K. Growth hormone treatment in short children: short-term and long-term effects on growth. Acta Paediatr Scand 1988; (suppl) 343:77–84.

79. Hopwood NJ, Hintz RL, Gertner JM, Attie KM, Johanson AJ, Baptista M, Kuntze J, Blizzard RM, Cara JF, Chernausek SD, Kaplan SL, Lippe BM, Plotnick LP, Saenger P. Growth response of children with non-growth-hormone deficiency and marked short stature during three years of growth hormone therapy. J Pediatr 1993; 123:215–222.

80. Moore WV, Moore KC, Gifford R, Hollowell JG, Donaldson DL. Long-term treatment with growth hormone of children with short stature and normal growth hormone secretion. J Pediatr 1992; 120:702–708.

81. Attie KM, Hintz RL, Hopwood NJ, Johanson AJ, and the Genentech Collaborative Study Group. Growth hormone treatment of idiopathic short stature and its effect on the onset and tempo of puberty. Pediatr Res 1992; 31:72A.

82. Rekers-Mombarg LT, Kamp GA, Massa GG, Wit JM. Influence of growth hormone treatment on pubertal timing and pubertal growth in children with idiopathic short stature. J Pediatr Endocrinol Metab 1999; 12(5 Suppl 2): 611–622.

83. Kaplan SL, Grumbach MM. Long-term treatment with growth hormone of children with non-growth hormone deficient short stature. In Isaksson O, Binder C, Hall K, et al., eds. Growth Hormone: Basic and Clinical Aspects. Amsterdam: Excerpta Medica, 1987:197–204.

84. Lesage C, Walker M, Landier F, Chatelain P, Chaussain JL, Bougneres PF. Near normalization of adolescent height with growth hormone therapy in very short children without growth hormone deficiency. J Pediatr 1991; 119:29–34.

85. Bareille P, Azcona C, Matthews DR, Conway GS, Stanhope R. Lipid profile, glucose tolerance and insulin sensitivity after more than four years of growth hormone therapy in non-growth hormone deficient adolescents. Clin Endocrinol 1999; 51(3):347–353.

86. Buchlish JG, Irizarry L, Crotzer B, Shine BJ, Allen L, Macgillivray M. Comparison of final heights of growth hormone treated vs. untreated children with idiopathic growth failure. J Clin Endocrinol Metab 1998; 83:1075–1079.

87. Hintz RL, Attie KM. Baptista J, Roche A. Effect of growth hormone treatment on adult height of children with idiopathic short stature. N Engl J Med 1999; 340: 502–507.

88. Kamp GA, Mul D, Waelkens JJ, et al. A randomized controlled trial of three years growth hormone and gonadotropin-releasing hormone agonist treatment in children with idiopathic short stature and intrauterine growth retardation. J Clin Endocrinol Metab 2001; 86: 2969–2975.

89. Faglia B, Arosia M, Porretti S. Delayed closure of epiphyseal cartilage induced by the aromatase inhibitor anastrozole: would it help short children grow up? J Endocrinol Invest 2000; 23:721–723.

90. Lyon AL, Preece MA, Grant DB. Growth curve for girls with Turner syndrome. Arch Dis Child 1985; 60:932–935.

91. Lippe BM, Frane J, Attie K, the Genentech National Collaborative Group. Growth in Turner syndrome. Updating the United States experience (abstract). Proceedings, 3rd International Symposium on Turner's Syndrome, 1992: 32.

92. Rappaport R, Sauvion S. Possible mechanism for the growth retardation in Turner syndrome. Acta Paediatr Scand 1989; 356(suppl):82–86.

93. Ranke MG, Blum WF, Haug F, et al. Growth hormone somatomedin levels and growth regulation in Turner's syndrome. Acta Endocrinol (Copenh) 1987; 116:305–313.

94. Ross JL, Meyerson L, Loriaux DL, et al. Growth hormone secretory dynamics in Turner syndrome. J Pediatr 1985; 106:202–205.

95. Kohno H, Honda S. Low urinary growth hormone values in patients with Turner's syndrome. J Clin Endocrinol Metab 1992; 74:619–622.

96. Rosenfeld RG. Update on growth hormone therapy for Turner's syndrome. Acta Paediatr Scand 1989; (suppl.) 356:103–108.

97. Takano K, Shizume K, Hibi I. Turner's syndrome: treatment of 203 patients with recombinant human growth

hormone for one year. Acta Endocrinol 1989; 120:559–568.

98. Lin TH, Kirkland JS, Kirkland RT. Growth hormone assessment and short term treatment with growth hormone in Turner syndrome. J Pediatr 1988; 112:919–921.

99. Rosenfeld RG, Frane J, Attie KM, et al. Growth hormone therapy of Turner's syndrome: beneficial effects on final height. J Pediatr 1998; 132:319–324.

100. Schweizer R, Ranke MB, Binder G, Herdach F, Zapadlo M, Grauer ML, Schwarze CP, Wollman HA. Experience with growth hormone therapy in Turner syndrome in a single center: low total height gain, no further gains after puberty onset and unchanged body proportions. Horm Res 2000; 53(5):228–238.

101. Chernausek SD, Attie KM, Cara JF, Rosenfeld RG, Frane J. Growth hormone therapy of Turner syndrome: the impact of estrogen replacement on final height. J Clin Endocrinol Metab 2000; 85(7):2439–2445.

102. Saenger P, Albertsson-Wikland K, Conway GS, et al. Recommendations for the diagnosis and management of Turner syndrome. J Clin Endocrinol Metab 2001; 86:3061–3069.

103. Neely EK, Marcus R, Rosenfeld RG, Bachrach LK. Turner syndrome adolescents receiving growth hormone are not osteopenic. J Clin Endocrinol Metab 1993; 76:861–866.

104. Rongen-Weserlaken C, Rijkers GT, Scholtens EJ, van Es A, Wit JM, van den Brande JL, Zegers BJ. Immunologic studies in Turner syndrome before and during treatment with growth hormone. J Pediatr 1991; 119:268–272.

105. Stahnke N, Stubbe P, Keller E, et al. Effects and side effects of GH plus oxandrolone. In: Ranke MB, Rosenfeld RG, eds. Turner Syndrome: Growth Promoting Therapies. Amsterdam: Elsevier, 1991:241–249.

106. Haeusler G., Frisch H. Growth hormone treatment in Turner's syndrome: short and long-term effects on metabolic parameters. Clin Endocrinol 1992; 36:247–254.

107. MacFarlane CE, Brown DC, Johnston LB, Patton MA, Dunger DB, Savage MO, McKenna WJ, Kelnar CJ. Growth hormone therapy and growth in children with Noonan's syndrome: results of 3 years followup. J Clin Endocrinol Metab 2001; 86(5):1953–1956.

108. Kirk JM, Betts PR, Butler GE, Donaldson MD, Dunger DB, Johnston DI, Kelnar CJ, Price DA, Wilton P. Short stature in Noonan syndrome: response to growth hormone therapy. Arch Dis Child 2001; 84(5):440–443.

109. Karlberg J, Albertsson-Wikland K. Growth in full-term small-for-gestational-age infants: from birth to final height. Pediatr Res 1995; 38:733–739.

110. Davies PSW, Valley R, Preece MA. Adolescent growth and pubertal progression in the Silver-Russell syndrome. Arch Dis Child 1988; 63:130–135.

111. Tanner JM, Whitehouse RH, Hughes PCR, Vince FP. Effect of human growth hormone treatment for 1 to 7 years on growth of 100 children with growth hormone deficiency, low birth weight, inherited smallness, Turner's syndrome and other complaints. Arch Dis Child 1971; 46:745–782.

112. Albertsson-Wikland K. Growth hormone secretion and growth hormone treatment in children with intrauterine growth retardation. Acta Paediatr Scand 1989; 349:35–41.

113. Stanhope R, Ackland F, Hamill G, Clayton J, Jones J, Preece MA. Physiological growth hormone secretion and response to growth hormone treatment in children with

short stature and intrauterine growth retardation. Acta Paediatr Scand 1989; (suppl) 349:47–52.

114. Stanhope R, Preece MA, Hamill G. Does growth hormone treatment improve final height attainment of children with intrauterine growth retardation? Arch Dis Child 1991; 66:1180–1181.

115. Sas T, Waal W, Mulder P, et al. Growth hormone treatment in children with short stature born small for gestational age: 5-year results of a randomized, double-blind, dose-response trial. J Clin Endocrinol Metab 1999; 84:3064–3070.

116. De Zegher F, Albertsson-Wikland K, Wollman H, et al. Growth hormone treatment of short children born small for gestational age: growth responses with continuous and discontinous regimens over 6 years. J Clin Endocrinol Metab 2000; 85:2816–2821.

117. Mehls O, Ritz E, Hunziker EB, Tonshoff B, Heinrich U. Role of growth hormone in growth failure of uremia: perspectives for application of recombinant growth hormone. Acta Paediatr Scand 1989; 343(suppl):118–126.

118. Allen DB, El-Hayek R, Friedman AL, Chobanian MC. Growth hormone stimulated urinary ammonia excretion in normal and 75% nephrectomized rats. Pediatr Res 1991; 29(4):2202.

119. Powell DR, Liu F, Baker BK, Hintz RS, Kale A, Suwanichkul A, Durham SK. Effect of chronic renal failure and growth hormone therapy on the insulin-like growth factors and their binding proteins. Pediatr Nephrol 2000; 14(7):579–583.

120. Fine RN, Kohaut EC, Brown D, Kuntze J, Attie KM. Long-term treatment of growth retarded children with chronic renal insufficiency with recombinant human growth hormone. Kidney Int 1996; 49:781–785.

121. Haffner D, Schaefer F, Nissel R, Wuhl E, Tonshoff B, Mehls O. Effect of growth hormone treatment on the adult height of children with chronic renal failure. N Engl J Med 2000; 343(13):923–930.

122. Allen DB, El-Hayek R, Friedman AL. Effects of prolonged growth hormone administration on growth, renal function, and renal histology in 75% nephrectomized rats. Pediatr Res 1992; 31:406–410.

123. Tonshoff B, Tonshoff C, Mehls O, Pinkowski J, Blum WF, Heinrich U, Stover B, Gretz N. Growth hormone treatment in children with preterminal chronic renal failure: no adverse effect on glomerular filtration rate. Eur J Pediatr 1992; 151:601–607.

124. Andersson HC, Markello T, Schneider JA, Gahl WA. Effect of growth hormone treatment on serum creatinine concentration in patients with cystinosis and chronic renal disease. J Pediatr 1992; 120:716–720.

125. Koch VH, Lippe BM, Nelson PA, Boechat MI, Sherman BM, Fine RN. Accelerated growth after recombinant human growth hormone treatment of children with chronic renal failure. J Pediatr 1989; 115:365–371.

126. Baroncelli GI, Bertelloni S, Ceccarelli C, Saggese G. Effect of growth hormone treatment on final height, phosphate metabolism, and bone mineral density in children with X-linked hypophosphatemic rickets. J Pediatr 2001; 138(2):236–243.

127. Appan S, Laurent S, Chapman M, Hindmarsh PC, Brook CGD. Growth and growth hormone (GH) therapy in hypochondroplasia. Horm Res 1989; 31(suppl. 1):170A.

128. Mullis PE, Patel MS, Brickell PM, Hindmarsh PC, Brook CGD. Growth characteristics and response to growth hormone therapy in patients with hypochondroplasia: genetic

linkage of the insulin-like growth factor 1 gene at chromosome 12q23 to the disease in a subgroup of these patients. Clin Endocrinol 1991; 34:265–274.

129. Rosenfeld RG, Hintz RL. Normal somatomedin and somatomedin receptors in achondroplastic dwarfism. Horm Metabol Res 1980; 12:76–77.

130. Butenandt O. Growth hormone therapy in children with bone disease. Pediatr Adolesc Endocrinol 1987; 16:118–120.

131. Seino Y, Yamanaka Y, Shinohara M, Ikegami S, Koike M, Miyazawa M, Inoue M, Moriwake T, Tanaka H. Growth hormone therapy in achondroplasia. Horm Res 2000; 53(suppl 3):53–56.

132. Wehrenberg WB, Janowski BA, Piering AW, Culler F, Jones KL. Glucocorticoids: potent inhibitors and stimulators of growth hormone secretion. Endocrinology 1990; 126:3200–3203.

133. Butenandt O, Eder R, Clados-Kelch A. Growth hormone studies in patients with rheumatoid arthritis and Still syndrome. Verh Dtsch Ges Rheumatol 1976; 4:68–77.

134. Allen DB, Goldberg BD. Stimulation of collagen synthesis and linear growth by growth hormone in glucocorticoid-treated children. Pediatrics 1992; 89(3):416–421.

135. Van Dop CV, Jabs KL, Donohoue PA, Bock GH, Fivush BA, Harmon WE. Accelerated growth rates in children treated with growth hormone after renal transplantation. J Pediatr 1992; 120:244–250.

136. Rivkees SA, Danon M, Herrin J. Prednisone dose limitation of growth hormone treatment of steroid-induced growth failure. J Pediatr 1994; 125:322–325.

137. Allen DB, Julius J, Breen T, Attie K. Treatment of glucocorticoid-induced growth suppression with growth hormone. J Clin Endocrinol Metab 1998; 83:2824–2829.

138. Touati G, Prieur AM, Ruiz JC, Noel M, Czernichow P. Beneficial effects of one-year growth hormone administration to children with juvenile chronic arthritis on chronic steroid therapy. J Clin Endocrinol Metab 1998; 83:403–409.

139. Hokken-Koelega ACS, VanZaal MAI, deRidder MAJ, Wolff ED, DeJong MCJW, Donckerwolcke RA. Growth after renal transplantation in prepubertal children; impact of various treatment modalities. Pediatr Res 1994; 35:367–371.

140. Fine RN, Sullivan EK, Kuntze J, Blethen S, Kohaut E. The impact of recombinant human growth hormone treatment during chronic renal insufficiency on renal transplant recipients. J Pediatr 2000; 136:376–382.

141. Bennet WM, Haymond MW. Growth hormone and lean tissue catabolism during long-term glucocorticoid treatment. Clin Endocrinol 1992; 36:161–164.

142. Guistina A, Bussie AR, Jacobello C, Wehrenberg WB. Effects of recombinant human growth hormone on bone and intermediary metabolism in patients receiving chronic glucocorticoid treatment with suppressed endogenous response to GH-releasing hormone. J Clin Endocrinol Metab 1995; 80:122–129.

143. Guest B, Berard E, Crosnier H, Chevalier T, Rappaport R, Broyer M. Effects of growth hormone in short children after renal transplantation. Pediatr Nephrol 1998; 12:437–446.

144. Carrel AL, Myers SE, Whitman BY, Allen DB. Growth hormone improves body composition, fat utilization, physical strength and agility, and growth in Prader-Willi syndrome. J Pediatr 1998; 134:215–221.

145. Lindgren AC, Hagenas L, Muller J, Blichfeldt S, Rosenborg M, Brismar M, Ritzen EM. Growth hormone treat-

ment of children with Prader-Willi syndrome affects linear growth and body composition favourably. Acta Paediatr Scand 1998; 87:28–31.

146. Myers S, Carrel AL, Whitman BY, Allen DB. Sustained benefit after 2 years of growth hormone upon body composition, fat utilization, physical strength and agility in children with Prader-Willi syndrome. J Pediatr 2000; 137:42–49.

147. Castells S, Torrado C, Bastian W, Wisniewski KE. Growth hormone deficiency in Down's syndrome children. J Intell Disabil Res 1992; 36:29–43.

148. Trollmann R, Strehl E, Wenzel D, Dorr HG. Does growth hormone enhance growth in GH-deficient children with myelomeningocele. J Clin Endocrinol Metab 2000; 85(8):2740–2743.

149. Allen DB, Pescowitz O, Frasier SD, Foley T. Growth hormone for children with Down syndrome. J Pediatr 1993; 123:742–743.

150. Ho KKY. Diagnosis and management of adult growth hormone deficiency. Endocrine 2000; 12(2):189–196.

151. Salomon F, Cuneo RC, Hesp R, Sonksen PH. The effects of treatment with recombinant human growth hormone on body composition and metabolism in adults with growth hormone deficiency. N Engl J Med 1989; 321:1797–1803.

152. Bengtsson G, Eden S, Lonn L, Kvist H, Stokland A, Lindstedt G, Bosaeus I, Tolli J, Sjostrom L, Isaksson OGP. Treatment of adults with growth hormone deficiency with recombinant human GH. J Clin Endocrinol Metab 1993; 76:309–317.

153. Cuneo RC, Salomon R, Wiles CM, Hesp R, Sonksen PH. Growth hormone treatment in growth-hormone deficient adults. II. Effects on exercise performance. J Appl Physiol 1991; 70(2):695–700.

154. McGaulley GA. Quality of life assessment before and after growth hormone treatment in adults with growth hormone deficiency. Acta Paediatr Scand 1989; 356(suppl):70–72.

155. Growth Hormone Research Society. Consensus guidelines for the diagnosis and treatment of adults with growth hormone deficiency: summary statement of the growth hormone research society workshop on adult growth hormone deficiency. J Clin Endocrinol Metab 1998; 83:379–381.

156. Rudman D, Feller AG, Hagraj HS, Gergans GA, Lalitha PY, Goldberg AF, Schlenker RA, Cohn L, Rudman IW, Mattson DE. Effects of growth hormone in men over 60 years old. N Engl J Med 1990; 323:1–6.

157. Yarasheski KE, Campbell JA, Smith K, Rennie MJ, Holloszy JO, Bier DM. Effect of growth hormone and resistance exercise on muscle growth in young men. Am J Physiol 1992; 262 (Endocrinol Metab 25):E261–E267.

158. Ponting GA, Halliday D, Teale JD, Sim AW. Post-operative positive nitrogen balance with intravenous hyponutrition and growth hormone. Lancet 1988: 1438–439.

159. Snyder DK, Clemmons DR, Underwood LE. Treatment of obese, diet-restricted subjects with growth hormone for 11 weeks: effects on anabolism, lipolysis, and body composition. J Clin Endocrinol Metab 1988; 67:54–61.

160. Ramirez RJ, Wolfe SE, Barrow RE. Growth hormone is safe and efficacious in the treatment of severe pediatric burns. Ann Surg 1998; 228:439–446.

161. Welsh K, Lamit M, Morhenn V. The effect of recombinant human growth hormone on wound healing in normal individuals. J Dermatol Surg Oncol 1991; 17:942–945.

162. Takala J, Ruokonen E, Webster NR, Nielsen MS, Zandstra DF, Vundelinckx G, Hinds CJ. Increased mortality associated with growth hormone treatment in critically ill adults. N Engl J Med 1999; 341:785–792.

163. Mauras N. Treatment of chronic bowel disease with growth hormone. Metabolism 2001.

164. Hardin DS, Ellis K, Dyson M, et al. Growth hormone improves clinical status in children with cystic fibrosis: results of a randomized controlled trial. J Pediatr 2001; 139(5):636–642.

165. Buzi F, Buchanan C, Morrell DJ, Preece MA. Antigenicity and efficacy of authentic sequence recombinant human growth hormone (somatropin): first year experience in the United Kingdom. Clin Endocrinol 1989; 30:531–538.

166. Sato T, Suzuki Y, Taketani T. Enhanced peripheral conversion of thyroxine to triiodothyronine during GH therapy in GH deficient children. J Clin Endocrinol Metab 1977; 45:324–329.

167. Municchi G, Malozowski S, Nisula BC, Cristiano A, Rose SR. Nocturnal thyrotropin surge in growth hormone-deficient children. J Pediatr 1992; 121:214–220.

168. Lampit M, Nave T, Hochberg Z. Water and sodium retention during short-term administration of growth hormone to short normal children. Horm Res 1998; 50: 83–88.

169. Otten BJ, Rotteveel JJ, Cruysberg JRM. Pseudotumor cerebri following treatment with growth hormone. Horm Res 1992; 37(suppl 4):16.

170. Maneatis T, Baptista J, Connelly K, Blethen S. Growth hormone safety update from the national cooperative growth study. J Pediatr Endocrinol 2000; 13:1035–1044.

171. Van Vliet G. Use of growth hormone in the management of growth disorders. In: Sizonenko PC, Aubert M, eds. Developmental Endocrinology. New York: Raven Press, 1990:195–202.

172. Saenger P, Attie K, DiMartinao-Nardi J, Fine RN. Carbohydrate metabolism in children receiving growth hormone therapy for 5 years. Pediatr Nephrol 1996; 10:261–263.

173. Sas TC, Cromme-Dijkhuis AH, de Muinck Keizer-Schrama, Stijnen T, van Tenunenbroek A, Drop SL. Carbohydrate metabolism during long-term GH treatment. J Clin Endocrinol Metab 2000, 85:769–775.

174. Cutfield WS, Wilton P, Bennmarker H, et al. Incidence of diabetes mellitus and impaired glucose tolerance in children and adolescents receiving growth hormone treatment. Lancet 2000; 355:610–613.

175. Estrov Z, Meir R, Barak Y, Zaizov R, Zadik Z. Human growth hormone and insulin-like growth factor-1 enhance the proliferation of human leukemic cells. J Clin Oncol 1991; 9:394–399.

176. Watanabe S, Tsunematsu Y, Fujimoto J, Komiyama A. Leukemia in patients treated with growth hormone. Lancet 1988; 2:1159.

177. Fradkin JE, Mills JL, Schonberger LB, Wysowski DK, Thomson R, Durako SJ, Robison LL. Risk of leukemia after treatment with pituitary growth hormone. JAMA 1993; 270:2829–2832.

178. Allen DB, Rundle AC, Graves DA, Blethen SL. Risk of leukemia in children treated with growth hormone: review and reanalysis. J Pediatr 1997; 131:S32–S36.

179. Nishi Y, Tanaka T, Takano K, et al. Recent status in the occurrence of leukemia in growth hormone-treated patients in Japan. J Clin Endocrinol Metab 1999; 84:1961–1968.

180. Tuffli GA, Johanson A, Rundle AC, Allen DB. Lack of increased risk for extracranial, nonleukemic neoplasms in recipients of recombinant growth hormone. J Clin Endocrinol Metab 1995; 80:1416–1422.

181. Zvulunov A, Wyatt DT, Laud PW, Esterly NB. Lack of effect of growth hormone therapy on the count and density of melanocytic nevi in children. Br J Dermatol 1997; 137:545–548.

182. Prassad B, Greig F, Bastian W, Castells S, Juan C, AvRuskin TW. Slipped capital femoral epiphysis during treatment with recombinant growth hormone for isolated partial growth hormone deficiency. J Pediatr 1990; 116:397–399.

183. Blethen SL, Rundle AC. Slipped capital femoral epiphysis in children treated with growth hormone. Horm Res 1996; 46:113–116.

184. Clayton PE, Cowell CT. Safety issues in children and adolescents during growth hormone therapy—a review. Growth Horm IGF-1 Res 2000; 10:306–317.

185. Allen DB, Fost NC, eds. Ethical issues in growth hormone therapy: where are we now? Endocrinologist 2001; 11(4):1S–89S (suppl 1).

186. Diekema DS. Is maximizing height good parenting? Endocrinologist 2001; 11(4):67S–71S.

187. Sandberg DE. The quality of life benefits of growth hormone-increased final height: what do we know? Endocrinologist 2001; 11(4):8S–14S(suppl 1).

188. Allen DB, Fost NC. Growth hormone for short stature: panacea or Pandora's box? J Pediatr 1990; 117:16–21.

189. Kappy MS. Growth hormone treatment until genetic potential is reached. Endocrinologist 2001; 11(4):60S–66S (suppl 1).

190. Allen DB. Terminating growth-promoting growth hormone therapy: in favor of the normal opportunity range. Endocrinologist 2001; 11(4):56S–59S (suppl 1).

4

Skeletal Dysplasias

Mordechai Shohat
Rabin Medical Center–Beilinson Campus, Petah Tikva, Israel

David L. Rimoin
Cedars–Sinai Medical Center and UCLA School of Medicine, Los Angeles, California, U.S.A.

I. INTRODUCTION

The human skeletal dysplasias are a heterogeneous group of disorders that result in disproportionate short stature. Although most are rare, these developmental defects of the skeleton cause a significant proportion of the cases of moderate to severe short stature (1).

Before 1970, the diagnosis for most patients with disproportionate shortening of the limbs was achondroplasia, and those with short trunks were thought to have Morquio syndrome. The understanding and appreciation of the heterogeneity within the skeletal dysplasias led to a systematic description of over 100 different forms, which have been primarily classified on the basis of clinical and radiographic changes. With the recent explosion of knowledge in the biochemistry and molecular biology of connective tissue, rapid progress has occurred in the delineation of the basic defect in these disorders. It is important to make a specific diagnosis in each case so that an accurate prognosis can be given and proper genetic counseling provided. Furthermore, each of these disorders is associated with a variety of skeletal or nonskeletal complications, which an accurate diagnosis allows one to anticipate, treat promptly, or prevent.

II. DIFFERENTIATION

The current nomenclature for these disorders is confusing. The specific name for a given condition usually describes the skeletal segment involved (e.g., the epiphyseal dysplasias and the metaphyseal dysplasias), or uses a descriptive Greek term (e.g., thanatophoric [death-bringing] dysplasia, metatropic [changing] dysplasia, and diastrophic [twisted] dysplasia). Some disorders are eponyms (e.g.,

Kniest dysplasia and Ellis–van Creveld syndrome). Occasionally, the name was derived to describe the pathogenesis (osteogenesis imperfecta), but usually inaccurately (e.g., achondroplasia and achondrogenesis).

The extent of the heterogeneity in these disorders and the variety of methods used for their classification have resulted in further confusion. Clinical classifications have organized the skeletal dysplasias into those with short-limbed dwarfism and those with short-trunk dwarfism. Age of onset of the disease and associated clinical abnormalities have also been used in subclassifying these disorders. Still other disorders have been classified on the basis of their apparent mode of inheritance, for example the dominant and X-linked varieties of spondyloepiphyseal dysplasia.

The most widely used method for differentiating the skeletal dysplasias has been the detection of skeletal radiographic abnormalities. Radiographic classifications are based on the different parts of the long bones that are abnormal (epiphyses, metaphyses, or diaphyses; Figs. 1, 2). Thus, there are epiphyseal and metaphyseal dysplasias, which can be further classified depending on whether the spine is also involved (spondyloepiphyseal dysplasias and spondylometaphyseal dysplasias). Furthermore, each of these classes can be subclassified into several distinct disorders based on a variety of other clinical and radiographic differences.

As the morphology, pathogenesis, and especially the basic biochemical and molecular defect in each of these disorders are unraveled, this nomenclature is being changed to refer to the specific pathogenetic or metabolic defect. The etiological or pathogenetic nomenclature is now being used for certain skeletal dysplasias, such as the mucopolysaccharidoses, mucolipidoses (e.g., β-glucuron-

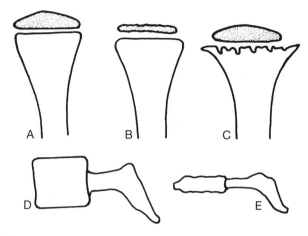

Figure 1 Classification of chondrodysplasias based on radiological involvement of long bones (A–C) and vertebrae (D and E).

Involvement	Disease category
A + D	Normal
B + D	Epiphyseal dysplasia
C + D	Metaphyseal dysplasia
B + E	Spondyloepiphyseal dysplasia
B + C + E	Spondyloepimetaphyseal dysplasia

idase deficiency, fucosidosis), type II collagenopathies, and disorders of mineralization (hypophosphatasia).

III. INTERNATIONAL CLASSIFICATION AND NOMENCLATURE

In an attempt to develop a uniform nomenclature for these syndromes, an international nomenclature and classification for the skeletal dysplasias were proposed in 1969 and updated in 1977, 1983, 1991, and 1997 (6). The most recently updated classification can be found on the World Wide Web at www.csmc.edu/genetics/skeldys.

The term "dwarfism" is no longer used and the disorders have been referred to as "dysplasias" or "dysostoses." The international classification, originally organized the skeletal dysplasias into five major groups:

1. Osteochondrodysplasias: abnormalities of cartilage or bone growth and development
2. Dysostoses: malformation of individual bones, singly or in combination (does not reflect a generalized disorder of the skeleton)
3. Idiopathic osteolyses: a group of disorders associated with multifocal resorption of bone
4. Skeletal disorders associated with chromosomal aberrations
5. Skeletal disorders associated with primary metabolic disorders

In the differential diagnosis of short stature, osteochondrodysplasias are of major importance. These are a complex group of diseases caused by primary abnormalities of cartilage or of bone growth or development. This group was organized following classifications:

1. Defects of growth of tubular bones or spine, or both (further referred to as chondrodysplasias)
2. Abnormalities in the amount, density, and remodeling of bone (includes disorders with a decrease or increase in bone and disorders of mineralization and mineral metabolism)
3. Disorders involving disorganized development of cartilage and fibrous connective tissue

Recent advances in molecular genetics have made possible the identification of the basic defects in many common skeletal disorders. The Fifth International Nomenclature committee, which met in Los Angeles in 1997, not only updated the nomenclature with the addition of a number of newly described syndromes but also completely revised the organization of these disorders into a clinically and pathogenetically based classification (Table 1). Thus, disorders that share clinical, radiographic, morphological, or biochemical features, suggesting that they share common pathogenetic mechanisms, were grouped together. This classification will certainly undergo constant revision as the basic defect in each of these disorders is discovered.

IV. DIAGNOSIS AND ASSESSMENT

The diagnosis of skeletal dysplasias is based on the clinical, radiographic, pathological, and, increasingly, biochemical and molecular studies. Table 1 summarizes the clinical, genetic, and radiographic features of the common chondrodysplasias and those with abnormalities in the amount, density, and remodeling of bone.

A. History

An accurate medical and family history may be of major importance in arriving at a diagnosis. A complete family history, details of stillborn children, and parental consanguinity should be obtained. Parents should always be closely examined, looking for evidence of a dysplasia in a partially expressed form. Because each of the skeletal dysplasias most frequently appears as a sporadic case in the family, an isolated instance of a skeletal dysplasia in a family cannot provide information on the mode of inheritance of the particular disorder. However, the type of familial aggregation, when it occurs, can be helpful. For example, if two dwarfed siblings are born to normal parents, then achondroplasia, which is an autosomal dominant trait, is unlikely, and one should suspect an autosomal recessive disorder. If two achondroplastic parents produce a severely affected offspring, it is most likely homozygous achondroplasia, rather than thanatophoric dysplasia. However, different modes of inheritance have been observed in disorders that resemble each other clinically, such as the X-linked and certain autosomal forms of spondyloepiphyseal dysplasia. On the other hand, in some dominant disorders, a high incidence of gonadal mosaicism has been shown to account for recurrent cases in the same family. For example, in osteogenesis imperfecta

type II, gonadal mosaicism may result in a recurrence risk of 6%.

Because the skeletal dysplasias become apparent at various ages, it is helpful to obtain accurate measurements from infancy onward and, especially, to know whether the shortening was evident at birth. Although in certain disorders marked variability in expression is seen with both prenatal and postnatal onset of the disease in the same

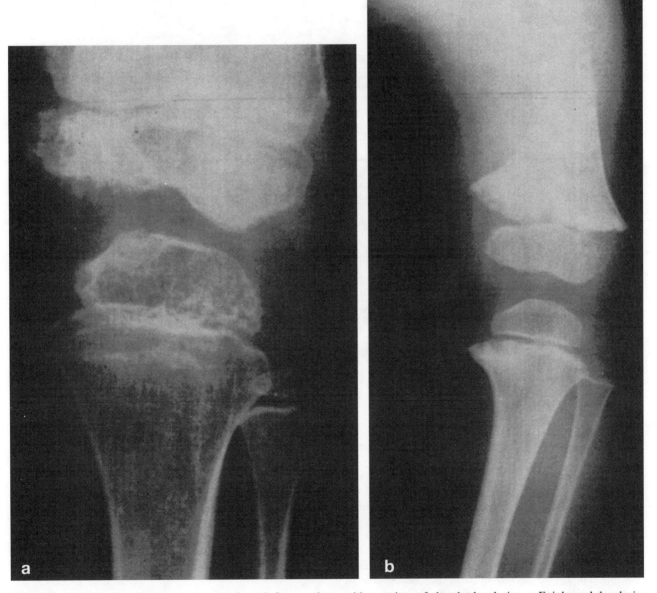

Figure 2 Radiographs of knee (a–c) and spine (d) from patients with a variety of chondrodysplasias. a. Epiphyseal dysplasia: note the small irregular epiphyses and normal metaphyses from a patient with spondyloepiphyseal dysplasia congenita. b. Metaphyseal dysplasia: note the irregular and widened metaphyses with normal epiphyses from a patient with metaphyseal dysplasia, Schmid type.

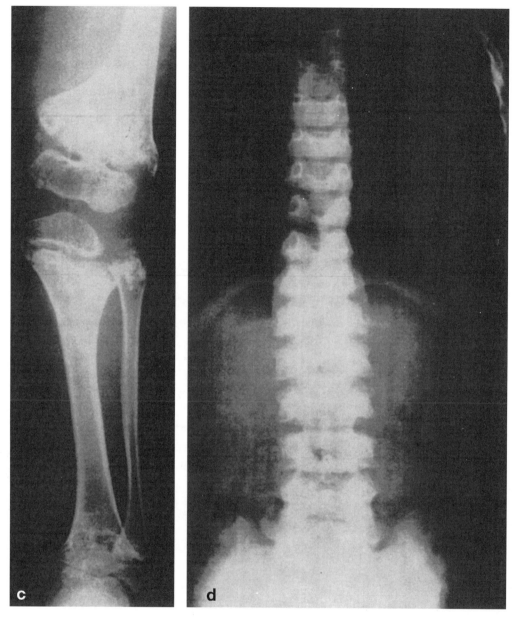

Figure 2 Continued. c. Epimetaphyseal dysplasia: note the abnormal epiphyses and metaphyses from a patient with spondyloepimetaphyseal dysplasia, Strudwick type. d. Platyspondyly: note the flat and irregular vertebrae from a patient with spondylometaphyseal dysplasia, Kozlowski type.

family (e.g., osteogenesis imperfecta type I), this information may help limit the diagnosis to a small number of disorders. Thus, a child who was normal until 2 years of age and then developed disproportionate short-limbed dwarfism is more likely to have pseudoachondroplasia or multiple epiphyseal dysplasia than achondroplasia or spondyloepiphyseal dysplasia congenita. In some disorders, growth may be normal for several years. For instance, in the X-linked form of spondyloepiphyseal dysplasia tarda, growth retardation is not apparent until

between 5 and 10 years of age. Relative body proportions may change with age in some disorders, such as metatropic dysplasia, in which only the limbs are short at birth; because of progressive kyphoscoliosis, such patients become short-trunked during childhood.

B. Physical Examination

A detailed physical examination may disclose the correct diagnosis or point to the likely diagnostic category. It is

Table 1 Clinical, Genetic, and Radiographic Features in the Chondrodysplasias

Dysplasias	Clinical features	Radiographic features
Achondroplasia group (the disorders in this group have similar radiographic changes but range from severe neonatally lethal thanatophoric dysplasia through achondroplasia to mild hypochondroplasia).		
Achondroplasia	AD; 80% represent new mutation; the most common skeletal dysplasia (1:25,000 births); rhizomelic shortening of limbs (recognizable at birth); final height averages 135 cm in men and 125 cm in women, with wide variability; hands are short and broad, wedge-shaped gap between third and fourth fingers (trident); lumbar gibbus in infancy usually replaced by prominent lumbar lordosis; limbs with skin folds in children; the mean head circumference follows a curve above the 97th percentile for normal individuals; achondroplasia specific curves are valuable to recognize hydrocephalus; prominent frontal bossing, hypoplasia of maxilla, mandibular prognathism; hypotonia is frequent during infancy; mental development is normal; except for patients with severe complications or sudden infant death, life span is normal; recurrent otitis media and chronic serous otitis are common and lead to conductive hearing loss in adults; overgrowth of fibula and joint laxity cause progressive genu varum; nerve root compression and spinal claudication are common complications in adults; (FGFR3 mutation)	Large calvaria, short base of skull, small foramen magnum (computed tomographic scan norms are available); ribs are short, cupped anteriorly; decreased lumbosacral interpedicular distance, squared off ilia, small sacrosciatic notches; limbs are short and broad; oval radiolucency in proximal femur and humerus in infancy; overgrowth of fibula
Hypochondroplasia	AD; recognized from 2 to 3 years of age; short-limbed (rhizomelic) short stature; there is wide variability in severity and much overlap in appearance with achondroplasia; this type of skeletal dysplasia is probably very common and easily undiagnosed in mildly short individuals; head is normal; patients are stocky and muscular; hands and feet are short and broad; mild genu varum and mild lumbar lordosis; mild mental retardation has been reported in some cases	Mild achondroplastic changes: skull normal or mildly enlarged; ribs are normal or slightly flared; distal lumbosacral interpedicular narrowing; long bones: rhizomelia; short wide bones; elongated fibula; prominent deltoid tubercles
Thanatophoric dysplasia	AD; the most common lethal type; markedly short limbs; large bulging forehead ± cloverleaf skull; prominent eyes; small, narrowed, pear-shaped thorax; ±congenital heart and CNS defects (FGFR3 mutation)	The long bones are short and bowed; metaphyseal flaring with medial spikes; severe platyspondyly; the vertebrae are hypoplastic, U-shaped on AP view; cupped and short ribs; large calvaria

Table 1 Continued

Dysplasias	Clinical features	Radiographic features
Spondylodysplasic and other perinatally lethal conditions group (distinct lethal types of skeletal dysplasia)		
Achondrogenesis type IA	AR; lethal; very short limbs; short and barrel-shaped chest; extremely soft skull; round or oval face	Characterized by poor ossification of the spine, more extreme shortening of femora and other long bones; long bones have concave ends and spurs in the middle shaft; type IA (Houston-Harris) is differentiated from Achondregenesis IB (Fraccaro) by the lack of rib fractures, appearance of the long bone, and cartilage histology
Metatropic dysplasia group		
Metatropic dysplasia	AD; normal to long in length at birth, short-limbed in infancy, becoming short trunked later with progressive kyphoscoliosis; prominent joints; tail-like sacral appendage, large head with ventriculomegaly may be present; C1/C2 subluxation is frequent and requires surgical fusion; severe cases die in infancy of RDS	Extreme platyspondyly with flattening of vertebrae and relatively large intervertebral spaces; long bones: irregularly expanded metaphyses giving barbell-like appearance; flattened and irregular epiphyses; short and broad tubular bones in hands; marked flaring of iliac crests (halberd appearance)
Short rib dysplasia (SRD) group with or without polydactyly		
Short-rib polydactyly syndrome (I, II, III)	AR; lethal, hydropic appearance, narrow thorax, severe RDS, polydactyly; in type I (Saldino Noonan) high frequency of cloacal abnormalities and postaxial polydactyly; type III is probably the mild end of type I disease; type II (Majewski) has high frequency of cleft lip and palate, multiple internal anomalies, and pre- and postaxial polydactyly	Extremely short horizontal ribs; the pelvis is small and hypoplastic in type I, whereas in II the pelvis is normal; in type I the long bones are very short with metaphyseal spurs; in type II the long bones have a more rounded appearance, especially the middle segment
Asphyxiating thoracic dysplasia (ATD) (Jeune)	AR; long narrow thorax and RDS with variable severity; ±postaxial polydactyly; progressive nephropathy; cystic changes in kidney, liver and pancreas	Ribs are short, cupped anteriorly; square short ilia; flat acetabulum with spurs at ends (trident appearance)
Chondroectodermal dysplasia (Ellis van Creveld)	AR; narrowed thorax, short limbs, and polydactyly; often with congenital cardiac anomalies (ASD, single atrium, PDA) and ectodermal abnormalities; hypoplastic nails, natal teeth, multiple frenula, cleft lip and palate, epispadias	Ribs and pelvis are similar to ATD; acromesomelic shortening of limbs; hamate–capitate fusion
Atelosteogenesis and omodysplasia group (characterized by hypoplastic humeri or femora, absence of ossification of several bones, or ossification of what should remain cartilage)		

Table 1 Continued

Dysplasias	Clinical features	Radiographic features
Otopalatodigital syndrome type II	X-linked; characterized by distinct facies, short and broad distal segments of thumbs and toes; proportional short stature and sometimes mental retardation; facies have prominent forehead, flat nasal root, flattening of the midface and small jaw; ±hearing defect (conductive); dislocation of radial heads and/or hips may be present	Small ilia; hypoplastic distal radius results in dislocations; wide lumbar interpedicular distance; small mandible; radiographic changes may not become apparent until later in infancy
Diastrophic dysplasia group		
Diastrophic dysplasia	AR; acute swelling of pinnae of ears in infancy; cauliflower ears; laryngomalacia; short limbed (rhizomelic), severe clubfeet, joint contractures, proximally placed abducted thumb; progressive scoliosis; there is wide variability in expression even within the same family; sulfate transporter defect (DTDST). More severe DTDST deficiency in atelosteogenesis 2 and achondrogenesis IB	Hypoplasia of epiphyses and flaring metaphyses in long bones; extracarpal bones; short and wide metacarpals and phalanges; lumbar interpedicular narrowing; C2/C3 dislocation; peritracheal, ear pinnae, and precocious costal cartilage ossification
Type II collagenopathies group (all the disorders in this group share defects in type II collagen secondary to mutations in the COL2A1 gene)		
Kniest dysplasia	AD; short trunk, progressive kyphoscoliosis; joint limitation; face is flat and round; myopia and cleft palate are common; Swiss cheese cartilage	Coronal clefts in flattened vertebrae, small ilia, increased acetabular angles; barbell-like femora as a result of broad metaphyses, delayed ossification of femoral heads, cloud effect in epiphyseal region; squared-off metacarpals and phalanges
Stickler syndrome	AD; marfanoid habitus, myopia, retinal detachment, conductive hearing loss, hyperextension of joints, may lead to joint pains and morning stiffness; cleft palate and mandibular hypoplasia. In some families, a type XI collagen defect has been found, and in a few, the disorders does not segregate with either COL2 or COL11	Mild epiphyseal dysplasia (especially proximal femur and distal tibia), degenerative arthrosis (hips), wedging of thoracic vertebrae, and Schmorl's disease of spine
Spondyloepiphyseal dysplasia (SED) congenita (Spranger-Wiedeman)	AD; evident at birth; variable severity; rhizomelic shortening of limbs, but these appear long relative to trunk; hands and feet are normal in size; clubfeet; neck is extremely short; it is important to rule out C1/C2 subluxation, which may lead to dislocation; broad barrel chest, lordosis; severe myopia, joint laxity, cleft palate, genu valgum or varum, waddling gait	Platyspondyly and epiphyseal dysplasia; delayed ossification of epiphyseal centers and the epiphyses appear irregular, fragmented, and flattened (especially femoral); coxa vara; vertebrae are ovoid in childhood but later become flat, irregular, with narrowed disk space; odontoid hypoplasia with C1/C2 subluxation

Table 1 Continued

Dysplasias	Clinical features	Radiographic features
Achondrogenesis II (Langer-Saldino) and hypochondrogenesis	AD; lethal; very short limbs; short and barrel-shaped chest; extremely soft skull; round or oval face; deficient type II and the presence of type I collagen in cartilage	In contrast to achondrogenesis type I, the long bones are straighter, relatively longer with cupping of their ends, with milder cases known as hypochondrogenesis
Spondyloepimetaphyseal dysplasias (SEMD; Strudwick type)	AD; resembles SED congenita at birth; SEMD is differentiated from SED by radiologic evidence of metaphyseal changes; Strudwick type is characterized by specific radiological changes such as peripheral "popcornlike" ossification of the femoral epiphyses, pectus carinatum, and genu valgum; type II collagen abnormalities have been documented	Delayed epiphyseal ossification, club shaped femora (first year), metaphyseal changes (>3 years), multiple epiphyseal centers in femoral heads, greater involvement of fibular and ulna than tibia and radius; platyspondyly; pear-shaped vertebrae; C1/C2 subluxation
Other spondyloepiphyseal (meta) physeal dysplasias group		
SED tarda	X-linked recessive; short stature develops in midchildhood; short limbs and short trunk; mild to severe kyphoscoliosis; large chest capacity; hands and feet are normal in size; early onset osteoarthritis in back and hips mutations in sedlin	Flat vertebrae with hump-shaped center; hypoplastic iliac wings; epiphyseal hypoplasia of large bones; premature osteoarthrosis of hips
Dyggve-Melchior-Clausen dysplasia	AR; short trunk, short stature with barrel chest, lumbar lordosis, restricted joint mobility, and waddling gait; mental retardation in most cases	Changes similar to those in SED; anterior beaking of vertebral bodies; a fine lacelike ossification above the iliac crest and irregular small carpal and metacarpal bones
Multiple epiphyseal dysplasia and pseudoachondroplasia group		
Pseudoachondroplastic dysplasia	AD; short limbs, short stature usually not apparent until 2–3 years; in some patients the limb shortening is predominantly rhizomelic, in others mesomelic; hyperlaxity of joints is associated with severe varus or valgus or as a combined ("windswept") deformity; the facies are characteristically attractive; all cases have been found to have mutations in COMP	Epiphyses and metaphyses of the tubular bones are involved, with platyspondyly and anterior tonguing of the vertebral bodies; acetabular irregularity, hypoplastic ischium and pubis; striking hand involvement with shortening of tubular bones, irregular metaphyses, and small round epiphyses
Multiple epiphyseal dysplasias (Fairbanks and Ribbing types)	AD; mild short stature; pain and stiffness in knees, hips, and ankles; waddling gait is common in severe Fairbanks type; osteoarthropathy of hips in mild Ribbing type—Mutations in COMP, COL9A2, and COL9A3 have been described to date	Characterized by flattened, fragmented, or irregular epiphyses (all areas, including hands and feet in Fairbanks; primarily the hips in Ribbing); earliest features may be delay in epiphyseal ossification; no metaphyseal or vertebral changes are seen; Schmorl's nodes are common

Table 1 Continued

Dysplasias	Clinical features	Radiographic features
Chondrodysplasia punctata group (stippled epiphyses)		
Chondrodysplasia punctata (punctate epiphyseal dysplasia)	Several dysplasias (AR, rhizomelic type; XLD, Conradi-Hunerman; and XLR forms); laryngomalacia and upper airway obstruction; limbs are proximally shortened in the rhizomelic type and asymmetrically shortened in the XLD types; cataract, ichthyosis, and contractures are common; rhizomelic type is caused by a peroxisomal defect, whereas the Conradi-Hunerman form is due to a sterol metabolic defect	Stippled calcification of epiphyses, periarticular tissues, and growth plate zones; stippling of laryngeal cartilage; coronal clefts of vertebrae
Metaphyseal dysplasia group		
Metaphyseal dysplasias		
Jansen	AD; severe short stature; recognizable in early infancy; rhizomelic shortening; severe leg bowing, mandibular hypoplasia; joints are large with contractures; arms less affected than legs. Mutations in PTHRP receptor	All types are characterized by metaphyseal involvement; all metaphyses including hands and feet are severely affected but improve with age
Schmid	AD; mild to moderate short stature (130–160 cm) and bowing of legs; enlarged wrists and flaring of rib cage; coxa vara; mutations in type X collagen	Most prominent changes are in hips, shoulders, knees, ankles, and wrists
McKusick type (cartilage–hair hypoplasia)	AR; severe to moderate postnatal growth deficiency, short broad hands and loose joints; genu varum; fine, light, sparse hair and light complexion; increased susceptibility to severe varicella infection	Knees especially are involved, in contrast to Schmid; proximal femoral metaphyses are normal to mildly involved; fibula is long relative to tibia; ribs are short with anterior cupping
Others	Combination of metaphyseal abnormalities and immune deficiency can also be found in Schwachman syndrome (AR), associated with pancreatic insufficiency and chronic neutropenia; metaphyseal chondrodysplasia—thymic alymphopenia syndrome (AR); and in adenosine deaminase deficiency (AR)	
Spondylometaphyseal dysplasia group (association of vertebral changes along with metaphyseal abnormalities in the long bones		
Spondylometaphyseal dysplasia (SMD) Kozlowski type	AD; growth retardation is usually apparent after 1–2 years; short trunk, short stature, and waddling gait develop; pectus carinatum, kyphoscoliosis, and precocious osteoarthritis; numerous other less well defined types of SMD have been described	Platyspondyly and general metaphyseal irregularities in the tubular bones; "open staircase" appearance to vertebrae on AP films; marked retardation of carpal ossification

Table 1 Continued

Dysplasias	Clinical features	Radiographic features
Mesomelic dysplasia group	Heterogeneous group characterized predominantly by shortening of the middle segments of the limbs	In all types, the bones of the forearms and shins are disproportionately shortened
Dyschondrosteosis	AD, the common type; mesomelic short stature (mild to moderate); Madelung deformity of the wrist; heterozygous mutations in SHOX gene	Hypoplasia of the distal ulna; ±radial head dislocation (Madelung deformity)
Langer type	AR, rare, represents the homozygous form of dyschondrosteosis; severe short stature, mandibular hypoplasia; homozygous for SHOX mutation	Limb bones are short and thick; hypoplastic fibula and distal ulna
Robinow	AD; flat facial profile, mesomelic shortening, and genital hypoplasia; hypoplastic mandible and hypertelorism, flat nose, and hypoplastic nails	Madelung deformity; posterior osseous fusion of vertebrae; hemivertebrae
Nievergelt type	AD; brachydactyly and clubfeet	Rhomboid-shaped radius, ulna, tibia, fibula; radioulnar and tarsal synostosis
Rheinhardt	AD; radial bowing of hands and lateral bowing of legs	Short radius and ulna; hypoplasia of distal ulna and proximal fibula
Acromelic and acromesomelic dysplasia group (shortening of the limbs, primarily affecting the hands and feet)		
Acromesomelic dysplasia	AR; several distinct skeletal dysplasias characterized by disproportionate shortening, predominantly affecting forearms, hands, feet, and legs; recognizable at birth; trunk slightly shortened	Mild epiphyseal ossification delay; brachydactyly with cone epiphyses; hypoplasia of iliac base and irregular acetabulum; wedging of vertebrae in adults
Trichorhinophalangeal 1 (TRP) dysplasia	AD; mild disproportionate short stature, sparse hair, pear-shaped nose, medial accentuation of the eyebrows; short stubby hands; multiple joint contractures; severe genu valgum or varum; a small chromosomal deletion in 8q24.12 was shown to be the cause for all types; TRP type 1 involves a smaller deletion than in the Langer–Giedion syndrome	Numerous phalangeal cone-shaped epiphyses of the hands; Legg-Perthes-like changes occasionally occur in the hips
Pseudohypoparathyroidism (type E brachydactyly)	AD, mild short stature, marked short IV metacarpal in hand (±feet); ±hypocalcemia; ±parathyroid hormone unresponsiveness	Short IV metacarpals and metatarsals
Dysplasia with significant membranous bone involvement group		
Cleidocranial dysplasia	AD; variable expressivity; large prominent forehead, wide persistent open fontanelles, drooping shoulders, narrow chest, abnormal dentition, coxa vara and joint laxity, short and squared fingers; proportionate short stature may occur. Transcription factor defect (CFBAI)	Varying degree of hypoplasia of membranous bones; absent or hypoplastic clavicles; narrowed and high pelvis; delayed closure of the anterior fontanelle with wormian bones are characteristic

Table 1   Continued

Dysplasias	Clinical features	Radiographic features
Bent-bone dysplasia group		
Campomelic dysplasia	AR; bending of long bones; cutaneous dimples at the site of bend; large head, 46 XY sex reversal in phenotypic females is common; some with severe RDS because of small thorax, hypoplastic tracheal rings, and other anomalies; Sox 9 mutations. Various types of short-limb bent bone dysplasias have been described (kyphomelic dysplasia) that must be differentiated	Slender bent femur and tibia; enlarged dolichocephalic skull with shallow orbits; pelvis is tall and narrow; hypoplastic ischiopubic rami, hypoplastic scapulae
Multiple dislocations with dysplasia group		
Larsen syndrome	AD (AR?); marked hyperlaxity and multiple dislocations (especially hips, knees, elbows) are characteristic; prominent forehead, low nasal bridge, hypertelorism, and cleft uvula are common features; disproportionate short stature; the associated skeletal abnormalities and craniofacial features help to differentiate Larsen syndrome from Ehlers-Danlos syndrome	Multiple joint dislocations with secondary epiphyseal deformities; supernumerary carpal and tarsal ossification centers develop; premature fusion of the epiphyses and shaft of the first distal phalanges

Dysplasias	Clinical features	Radiographic features	Inheritance
Dysplasias with decreased bone density group			
Osteogenesis imperfecta (defects in type I collagen as a result of mutations in either COL2A1 gene or COL1A2 gene)			
Type 1	Excessive bone fragility, blue sclerae, conductive hearing loss in adolescence, hyperlaxity of ligaments, nonprogressive aortic root dilatation (12%), most have late-onset short stature, some families with opalescent teeth	General osteopenia (especially vertebral bodies), angulation at site of previous fractures, wormian bones in skull	AD
Type 2	Lethal, low birth weight and short birth length, soft skull, beaking of the nose, hypotelorism, short and deformed limbs, thin and fragile skin; prenatal diagnosis by ultrasound, biochemical and molecular genetic studies	Extreme beading of ribs, crumpled appearance of long bones (femora), diffuse osteopenia of skull	Almost all are AD; gonadal mosaicism
Type 3	Nonlethal severe bone fragility leading to progressive deformity and marked short stature, sclerae may be blue at birth but become less blue with age, most with opalescent dentin, cardiorespiratory complications may lead to death	General osteopenia and marked deformity of bones; fractures may be present at birth, bowed long bones, progressive platyspondyly (codfish vertebrae) and kyphoscoliosis, wormian bones in skull	AD

Table 1 Continued

Dysplasias	Clinical features	Radiographic features	Inheritance
Type 4	As type 1 but with white sclerae (may be blue at birth), some families with opalescent teeth	Osteopenia, variability in severity and age of onset of fractures, multiple wormian bones of skull	AD
Disorders with defective mineralization			
Hyperphosphatasemia with osteoectasia	Onset 2–3 years, progressive painful skeletal deformity, fractures, short stature, large skull; elevation of alkaline phosphatase	Dense areas interspersed with lucent areas, generalized demineralization (juvenile Paget's disease)	AR
Hypophosphatasia congenital lethal	Disproportionate short stature at birth, bowing deformity, thin skull vault, death from respiratory distress; low serum alkaline phosphatase	Generalized poor ossification, thin ribs, hypoplastic vertebrae, splayed and frayed metaphyses	AR
Tarda	Milder, onset in childhood, bowing of legs, premature loss of teeth; reduced serum alkaline phosphatase, elevated phosphoethanolamine in the urine	As in congenital type but milder changes	AD
Hypophosphatemic rickets	X-linked hypophosphatemic rickets; bowing of legs and short stature, late dentition; low serum phosphate	Radiographic changes are those of rickets	X-linked dominant
Pseudo vitamin D deficiency rickets (VDD)			
Type 1	Defective 1α-hydroxylation of 25-hydroxyvitamin D	As in rickets	AR
Type 2	Impaired target organ responsiveness to vitamin D	As in rickets	AR
Increased bone volume or density **Osteopetrosis**			
Precocious form	Onset in early infancy, failure to thrive, malignant hypocalcemia, anemia, thrombocytopenia, hepatosplenomegaly, optic atrophy leading to blindness, impaired bone resorption as a result of defect in maturation of osteoclasts; early bone marrow transplantation may be successful	Generalized hyperostosis at birth, "bone in bone" appearance (vertebrae), crowded marrow cavity, dense base of skull	AR
Tarda	Onset in childhood; may go undetected until adulthood; excessive fractures, mild craniofacial disproportion, mild anemia, osteonecrosis of bones (especially mandible) may develop; a distinct form with renal tubular acidosis and mental retardation has been found to be caused by a deficiency of carbonic anhydrase type 2; chromosome location: 8q22	Generalized increased density, defective metaphyseal modeling, dense base of skull	AD or AR

Table 1   Continued

Dysplasias	Clinical features	Radiographic features	Inheritance
Pycnodysostosis	Short limbs, short stature from infancy; wide anterior fontanelle, large cranium with open fontanelle, small chin, short hands and feet, increased fractures, sclerae may be blue, mutation in cathepsin K	General hyperostosis, hypoplasia of distal phalanges in hands, wide sutures, and wormian bones	AR
Dysosteosclerosis	Postnatal onset of short stature, severe hypodontia and early loss of teeth, fractures, visual and hearing loss	General hyperostosis, platyspondyly	AR
Osteopoikilosis	Commonly asymptomatic, joint pains	Numerous small osteodense foci in epiphyses and carpal centers or tubular bones	AD
Craniotubular dysplasias			
Craniometaphyseal dysplasia	Broad osseous prominence of nasal root, bony encroachment on cranial foramina and nasal passages	Hyperostosis of skull, mandible, nasal and maxillary bones; lack of modeling of metaphyses of long bones (Ehrlenmeyer flask appearance)	AD and AR
Diaphyseal dysplasia (Camurati Engelmann)	Failure to thrive and fatigability, onset at age 4–10 years, progressive increased pain in the legs, encroachment on cranial nerves; syndactyly, enamel hypoplasia	Symmetrical fusiform enlargement of the diaphyses, normal metaphyses and epiphyses, sclerosis of anterior base of skull	AD
Craniodiaphyseal dysplasia	Flattening of nasal root in early infancy, with increasing hypertelorism, marked encroachment of cranial nerves in foramina, normal stature	Massive hyperostosis and sclerosis of the skull and face with widened shafts of tubular bones	AR
Endosteal hyperostosis and sclerosteosis	Progressive mandibular enlargement from childhood; in adults sclerotic encroachment of optic and acoustic nerves	Marked accretion of osseous tissue at the endosteal surface, fusion between carpal bones	AR and AD
Tubular stenosis (medullary stenosis)	Hypocalcemia, delayed closure of fontanelle, and early-onset myopia	Narrowing of medullary cavity caused by widening diaphyseal cortex	AD
Pachydermoperiostosis	Progressive thickening of the skin, clubbing of fingers, easy fatiguability, joint pain, blepharitis, sensory hearing loss	Subperiosteal thickening of tubular bones	AD
Frontometaphyseal dysplasia	Pronounced supraorbital ridge	Prominent frontum, ±large frontal sinuses; no hyperostosis of rest of skull; mild metaphyseal changes in long bones	X-linked dominant
Osteodysplasty (Melnick-Needles)	Abnormal gait and bowing of extremities, dislocation of hip, delayed closure of fontanelle, usually normal stature, exophthalmos, protruding cheeks, micrognathia, incurving of the distal segment of the thumbs	Uneven thickening of cortex bones, metaphyseal modeling defect, wavy ribs, narrowed iliac wings	AD (AR rare)

AR, autosomal recessive; AD, autosomal dominant; XLR, X-linked recessive; XLD, X-linked dominant; ASD, atrial septal defect; PDA, patent ductus arteriosus; CNS, central nervous system; AP, anteroposterior. RDS, respiratory distress syndrome.
For a complete listing of Skeletal Dysplasias, see The International Nomenclature of Constitutional Disorders of Bone, 1998; www.csmc.edu/genetics/skeldys/nomenclature.

essential to determine whether the shortening is proportional. In general, patients with disproportionate short stature have skeletal dysplasias, whereas those with relatively normal body proportions have endocrine, nutritional, prenatal, or other nonskeletal defects. There are exceptions to these rules: cretinism can lead to disproportionate short stature, and a variety of skeletal dysplasias, such as osteogenesis imperfecta and hypophosphatasia, may result in normal body proportions.

A disproportionate body habitus may not be readily apparent on casual physical examination. Measurements that are essential for determining whether an abnormally short individual is disproportionate include the following:

1. Upper/lower segment ratio (U/L ratio): Although sitting height is a more accurate measure of the head and trunk length, it requires special equipment for consistent accuracy. U/L segment ratio, on the other hand, provides a fairly accurate measure of body proportions and can be easily obtained. The lower segment measure is taken from the symphysis pubis to the floor at the inside of the heel, and the upper segment is obtained by subtracting the lower segment value from the total height. McKusick has published standard U/L curves for both white and black Americans that are quite useful for rapid assessment of proportion (1). For example, a normal white infant has an upper/lower segment ratio of approximately 1.7; it decreases to 1.0 at 7–10 years and then falls to an average U/L of 0.95 as an adult. Blacks, on the other hand, have relatively long limbs and have an U/L of approximately 0.85 as adults.
2. Arm span: Another index of limb versus trunk length, this measurement usually falls within a few centimeters of total height.

These measurements must be obtained before the possibility of a mild skeletal dysplasia, such as hypochondroplasia or multiple epiphyseal dysplasia, can be excluded. Short-limbed dwarfs have an abnormally high U/L ratio and an arm span that is considerably shorter than their height.

If a child has short-limbed dwarfism, it is important to determine whether all segments of the limb are equally shortened or whether the shortening primarily affects the proximal (rhizomelic), middle (mesomelic), or distal (acromelic) segment (Fig. 3).

The presence or absence of extraskeletal manifestations may be helpful in making a diagnosis. During the examination, attention should be given to the head size, facial appearance, and specific physical findings, such as myopia, cleft palate, clubfoot, hearing, joint laxity, and bone deformity. In the older child or adult, the complications associated with specific disorders may provide ad-

ditional information for making the diagnosis. For example, spinal stenosis with spinal cord claudication is characteristic of achondroplasia; odontoid hypoplasia and C1/C2 subluxation are frequently found in Morquio syndrome, spondyloepiphyseal dysplasia, and metatropic dysplasia; fibular overgrowth (and genu varum) is seen in achondroplasia and cartilage hair hypoplasia.

C. Skeletal Radiographs

A full series of skeletal views is usually required (2). These views include anteroposterior (AP), lateral, and Towne views of the skull, AP and lateral views of the spine, and AP views of the pelvis and extremities, with separate AP views of hands and feet. Lateral views of the foot are particularly helpful in identifying punctate calcifications of the calcaneus, which may be a clue to the diagnosis of the milder forms of chondrodysplasia punctata, confirming the delayed ossification of the calcaneus and talus in newborns with spondyloepiphyseal dysplasia congenita, and in delineating the double ossification centers of the calcaneus in Larsen syndrome.

Attention should be paid to the specific parts of the skeleton involved (spine, limbs, pelvis, and skull) and, within each, where the abnormality is located (epiphysis, metaphysis, diaphysis, or combination). Because the skeletal radiographic features in many of these disorders change with age, reviewing radiographs taken at different ages is helpful. Moreover, epiphyseal closure, which occurs after puberty, frequently obliterates the specific abnormalities that would have permitted a specific diagnosis to be made had the films been taken before puberty. Nevertheless, skeletal radiographs alone are often sufficient to make the diagnosis because the classification of these disorders has been based primarily on their radiographic features.

Apart from the changes in the epiphyses, diaphyses, and metaphyses, some radiographic features characterize certain disorders:

So-called Dumbbell-shaped femur in the newborn period: metatropic dysplasia and Kniest dysplasia

Bending of long bones (campomelia): common in campomelic dysplasia, kyphomelic dysplasias, osteogenesis imperfecta, congenital hypophosphatasia, and thanatophoric dysplasia.

Calcified projections or spikes on lateral borders of the metaphyses of the femur: thanatophoric dysplasia, achondrogenesis, and short-rib polydactyly syndrome type I/III

Fractures of long bones in the newborn: osteogenesis imperfecta, congenital osteopetrosis, and severe hypophosphatasia. In the older individual, fractures may also be seen in a variety of osteopetrotic syndromes, including dysosteosclerosis and pyknodysostosis.

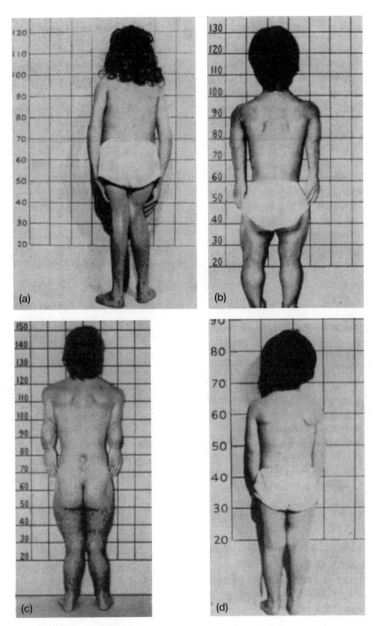

Figure 3 Different forms of disproportionate dwarfism. a. Short-trunk dwarfism in a girl with Dyggve-Melchior-Clausen syndrome. b. Short-limb dwarfism of the rhizomelic type in a boy with achondroplasia. c. Short-limb dwarfism of the mesomelic type in a boy with mesomelic dysplasia, Langer type. d. Short-limb dwarfism of the acromelic type in a girl with peripheral dysostosis.

Marked delay in epiphyseal center ossification: spondyloepiphyseal dysplasia (SED) congenita, Kniest dysplasia, and other SED and multiple epiphyseal dysplasias.

Stippled epiphyses: the chondrodysplasia punctatas, cerebrohepatorenal syndrome, warfarin-related embryopathy, and, occasionally, with chromosomal trisomy, lysosomal storage diseases, diphenylhydantoin-induced embryopathy, the Smith-Lemli-Opitz syndrome, and congenital infections.

Severely shortened ribs: short-rib polydactyly syndromes, asphyxiating thoracic dysplasia, chondroectodermal dysplasia, thanatophoric dysplasias, and metatropic dysplasia.

Decreased ossification of the vertebral bodies: most severe in the achondrogenesis syndromes.

Severe platyspondyly: metatropic dysplasia, thanatophoric dysplasia (U-shaped in thoracic spine and
inverted U shape in the lumbar spine), osteogenesis imperfecta type II, congenital hypophosphatasia Morquio syndrome, spondylometaphyseal dysplasia, brachyolmia, and others.

Coronal clefts of the vertebra: Kniest dysplasia, Rol-
land-Desbuquois syndrome, Weisenbach-Zwey-
muller syndrome, chondrodysplasia punctata,
and atelosteogenesis.

Oval translucent appearance of the proximal femora
and humeri in infants: achondroplasia, thanatophoric dysplasia and hypochondroplasia.

These examples are representative of only a few of
the many typical radiographic features seen in the skeletal
dysplasias (see Table 1). Other radiographic differences
within what is now considered a given skeletal dysplasia
may be found as the complete heterogeneity of this group
of disorders is delineated by results of the molecular and
biochemical studies.

D. Microscopic Evaluation

Histological examination of the chondroosseous tissue can
be useful in making an accurate diagnosis of several specific skeletal disorders, especially the lethal neonatal
types. In certain other conditions, the pathological examination is useful in ruling out a diagnosis. (A protocol for
the collection of skeletal tissues can be found in Sec. VII.)

On morphological grounds, the chondrodysplasias
can be broadly classified into the following disorders:

1. Minimal or no qualitative abnormality in endo-
chondral ossification: achondroplasia and hypochondroplasia (in which abnormalities in the
height and arrangement of proliferative columns,
particularly in the center of the large growth
plates, are the only changes).

2. Abnormalities mainly in cellular morphology:
large chondrocytes, containing prominent inclusions; for example, achondrogenesis IA, pseudoachondroplasia, and certain SEDs; sparse matrix with collagen rings around the chondrocytes
as in diastrophic dysplasia and achondrogenesis
IB. Dilatation of the chondrocyte rough endoplasmic reticulum (RER): for example, the SEDs,
pseudoachondroplasia, and Kniest dysplasia.
Thus dilatation of the RER is not a diagnostic
finding, although it suggests defective synthesis
or abnormal processing of a matrix protein in
these conditions.

3. Abnormalities in matrix morphology: areas of
cell degeneration with wide collagen fibrils,
scar formation, and intracartilaginous ossification: diastrophic dysplasia. So-called Swiss-
cheese appearance of cartilage: Kniest dysplasia.
Large la-cunae containing numerous chondro-

cytes: Dyggve-Melchior-Clausen syndrome. Areas of dystrophic ossification, fibrous dysplasia,
and fat deposition in the reserve zone cartilage
of the matrix: chondrodysplasia punctata. Wide
interwoven connective septa in epiphyseal cartilage and basal zone: fibrochondrogenesis.

4. Abnormalities primarily localized to the area of
chondroosseous transformation: reduced and disorganized columnization: thanatophoric dysplasia, short-rib polydactyly syndromes. Broad matrix septa surrounding clusters of hypertrophic
cells: the metaphyseal dysplasias, opsismodys-
plasia.

E. Biochemical Studies

Great progress has been made in recent years in our
knowledge about the biochemical defect involved in certain of the skeletal dysplasias. These findings may help us
to understand the basic biology of the normal bone and
provide us with new means for prenatal diagnosis and
treatment.

F. Molecular Studies

Significant developments in the field of molecular genetics have allowed mapping and identification of the genes
causing many of the skeletal dysplasias (3–5). The specific gene defects that produce skeletal dysplasias can be
classified into several distinct pathogenetic categories: *Abnormalities in the structural proteins of cartilage*, including collagens type II, IX, X and XI and cartilage oligomeric matrix protein (COMP); *inborn errors of cartilage
metabolism*, including the diastrophic dysplasia sulfate
transport (DTDST) disorders, arylsulfatase E, lysomsomal
enzymes, and cathespin K; *local regulators of cartilage
growth*, such as fibroblast growth factor receptor (FGFR3)
and parathyroid hormone receptor protein; *systemic defects influencing cartilage*, including adenosine deaminase
deficiency, peroxisomal enzyme deficiencies, and phos-
phoadenosine-phosphosulfate synthetase (PAPS); *transcription factor mutations*, such as CBFA1, CDMP1,
SoX9, LMxaB, SHOX; *tumor suppressor* genes, as in the
multiple exostoses; and *signal protein inactivators*, such
as Noggin.

The emerging data of the last few years outlining the
molecular basis of skeletal dysplasias has been instructive
in several respects. For example, phenotypically distinct
entities have been found to be allelic variants, with mutations in the same gene (e.g., achondroplasia, hypochondroplasia, thanatophoric dysplasia, and certain cranio-
synostotic syndromes). On the other hand, certain
dysplasias have been found to be due to mutations in different genes (e.g., multiple epiphyseal dysplasia with mutations in cartilage oligomeric matrix protein or type IX
collagen); and Stickler syndrome, with mutations in type
II and type XI collagen. In most of the conditions in

which the molecular basis has been defined, numerous different mutations are described. Consequently, diagnosis by DNA analysis is difficult, unless the distinct mutation in the family has been defined, or expensive sequencing of the entire gene is performed. Chip technology will eventually solve this problem. Achondroplasia is unusual in that over 98% of the cases are due to a single mutation, making an inexpensive molecular diagnostic test possible.

V. PRENATAL DIAGNOSIS

Many of the skeletal dysplasias manifest in the prenatal period and can be identified by prenatal ultrasound. The great majority of cases, however, occur for the first time in a family and are thus unsuspected and picked up by routine ultrasonography by measurement of femur length. This is true for both dominant disorders such as thanatophoric dysplasia and spondyloepiphyseal dysplasia congenita and for recessive disorders such as diastrophic dysplasia and cartilage hair hypoplasia. Many of these disorders will manifest shortening of the extremities by as early as 13–16 weeks, but in achondroplasia femoral shortening may not be evident until the late second trimester (2). Of course, disorders that do not present in the newborn period cannot be detected by prenatal ultrasound.

Retrospective analysis (7) in 250 cases revealed that the accuracy in diagnosis in 250 cases referred to the International Skeletal Dysplasia Registry at Cedars–Sinai Medical Center (*www.csmc.edu/genetics/skeldys*) was approximately 30%. Further retrospective analysis of accuracy of prenatal diagnosis in 1000 cases referred to the Registry (1990–2000) indicated that a correct referring diagnosis was made in 37% of the cases, but in over 60% of the cases either an incorrect diagnosis or no diagnosis was made (8). Analysis of this 1000 case cohort showed that the most common diagnoses were osteogenesis imperfecta type II (20%), thanatophoria (11%), and achondrogenesis II (8.2%). The other 37% of cases were specific skeletal dysplasias, 12% were syndromes, and 5% were nonskeletal dysplasias and probably represented early-onset intrauterine growth retardation. In 4.5% of the referred cases, radiographs or histological examination could not make a specific diagnosis. With the increasing use of prenatal ultrasound, increasing numbers of skeletal dysplasia cases are recognized by ultrasound. However, the above data show that prenatal ultrasound parameters need to be defined for a more accurate prenatal diagnosis of the skeletal dysplasias.

With the explosion of knowledge concerning the basic molecular defect in the skeletal dysplasias, prenatal diagnosis by mutation detection in amniocytes or chorionic villous cells can be accomplished if the exact mutation is known in a previously affected child, since most of these disorders are due to private mutations in the same gene. Linkage analysis can be used in families with multiple affected members, even if the specific mutation is

not known. In achondroplasia, in which almost all cases share the same mutation, molecular diagnosis can be readily accomplished by sequence analysis or restriction fragment polymorphism. This is especially valuable when both parents are achondroplasts and want to rule out the 25% possibility of the fetus being a lethal homozygote.

VI. MANAGEMENT

Effective management requires precise diagnosis, prompt recognition of specific skeletal and nonskeletal complications, appropriate orthopedic and rehabilitative care, emotional support and psychosocial counseling, and genetic counseling. There is no specific cure for any of these conditions.

Orthopedic management aims at maximizing mobility and correcting deformity; if deformities in the lower limbs are left uncorrected beyond puberty, early onset of osteoarthritis may lead to mechanically unsound joints. Early recognition of spinal deformity and its early treatment with bracing or surgical intervention may reduce morbidity (from scoliosis) in adult life.

VII. EXTENDED LIMB LENGTHENING

Extended limb lengthening was first developed for the treatment of leg length discrepancy and later became utilized bilaterally for increasing the height of dwarfed individuals. The original techniques involved osteotomies involving the periosteum and distraction of the broken ends, the gap being filled in with bone grafts and stabilized with hardware, which was subsequently removed. Serious complications including osteomyelitis, hypertension, nerve and vascular damage frequently followed. The Siberian orthopedist Ilizarov developed a new technique, which involved percutaneous breaks in the bone with the periosteum remaining intact. He developed a new circular fixator–distractor, but the secret to his success was the subperiosteal break, leaving nerve and blood supply intact and the extremely slow rate of distraction. Up to 6 inches of new bone could be achieved in each of the limb segments, allowing many dwarfs to enter normal growth curves.

Over the last 20 years a number of other techniques have been developed, which all involve percutaneous osteotomies of the metaphases or diaphyses of the long bones, the insertion of screws and wires above and below the fracture line, and the attachment of an external telescoping fixator. The device is then turned several times a day, extending the fracture gap by about 1 cm/day. When the desired increase in length is attained, the distraction is stopped and the callus allowed to consolidate. When consolidation is complete, the device and pins are removed. There is a substantial recovery time requiring active physical therapy, as the muscles become stretched and weak. The different techniques vary in the type of distractor, whether pins or wires are used, and which bones are extended simultaneously and in what sequence. If using the large circular Ilizarov distractors, both femurs cannot be done simultaneously, and either both segments of one leg or a contralateral femur and tibia are done simultaneously. If one has to stop before the entire process is completed, significant asymmetry will result. If one uses a linear fixator and pins, both tibias can be done simultaneously, followed by both femurs. The humeri are frequently lengthened by 4 inches between doing the two leg segments.

All patients experience one or more complications during this prolonged lengthening process, including pin tract infections; malunion; delayed consolidation; varus or valgus deviations; joint contractures or dislocations; and muscle, nerve, and vascular damage. We have used the Vilarrubias technique, which utilizes a linear Wagner fixator with two large screws on each side of the break and simultaneous lengthening of the tibias followed by the humeri and then the femurs. Tendonotomies of the Achilles tendon and flexors and the hips are also performed, allowing plantar flexion of the foot and a marked decrease in the lumbar lordosis. We believe that the latter will significantly increase spinal canal volume, and thereby, we hope, prevent or decrease the spinal claudication that most achondroplastic dwarfs experience.

By using a team approach of orthopedists, geneticists, psychologists, physical therapists, and other specialists, and carefully monitoring nerve conduction and blood flow, one can minimize the complications. We do not start limb lengthening in dwarfed children until they are at least 13 years of age. We believe that it should be the child and not the parents who make the decision to undergo this prolonged, inconvenient, and complication-ridden procedure. Achondroplastic dwarfs are excellent candidates for ELL since only their limbs are short and they have excessive soft tissues, with joint laxity and tortuous vessels and nerves. The procedure has also been done in a variety of other forms of short limb dwarfism and the tibias alone have been modified in patients with Turner's syndrome. It is not recommended for patients with short trunks or proportionate short stature.

VIII. GROWTH HORMONE THERAPY IN ACHONDROPLASIA

The use of recombinant growth hormone therapy for achondroplasia has been evaluated by several centers in relatively short-term trials. In most of the trials, there is a statistically significant increase in predicted growth rate in the first year of treatment (9). However, this trend of increased growth velocity decreases in the second year of treatment and thereafter. If the data are extrapolated for a prolonged period of treatment, it appears that the increase in final height in these patients will be only a few centimeters above predicted, and will not result in a significant increase in final height. No studies have pursued multiyear trials. Furthermore, several studies have shown great individual variability in responsiveness in these patients. This data is not dissimilar to the data describing human growth hormone (hGH) treatment in Turner syndrome. Some Turner syndrome patients have had a statistically significant increase in growth velocity with prolonged treatment, while others do not respond. We have conducted a long-term follow-up on our 2 year hGH-treated achondroplasia patients, who were then left untreated for up to 8 years. Although these patients demonstrated an increase in growth velocity during treatment during the first year of therapy, long-term evaluation showed no significant change in height from pretreatment predicted height. Multiyear trials must be conducted to document whether any long-term benefits could take place. The data suggesting a decrease in responsiveness to hGH over time bring up the question of whether performing pulsatile therapy (e.g., treatment for 2 years, off for a year) and whether continuation of this cycle will replicate the increase in growth velocity seen in the first year of treatment. The pertinent issue is whether this treatment can produce a clinically relevant increase in height. Only a few studies with a limited number of patients have been performed in hypochondroplasia with variable results. Furthermore, these studies were not performed on patients with a documented molecular defect in FGFR3, which may complicate the interpretation of the responsiveness, since hypochondroplasia is genetically heterogeneous. Growth hormone trials on only a few patients with other less common skeletal dysplasias have been conducted, and there are not sufficient available data to conclude whether there is a treatment benefit. However, in view of the increased predisposition to malignancy in cartilage–hair hypoplasia, we believe that growth hormone therapy should not be attempted in this condition.

IX. COLLECTION OF SKELETAL TISSUES

A variety of histological, histochemical, immunohistochemical, ultrastructural, and biochemical studies of chondroosseous tissue and skin can be performed. Specimens can be sent to one of the laboratories that specialize in processing and interpreting tissue from the skeletal dysplasias (e.g., The International Skeletal Dysplasia Registry, Cedars–Sinai Medical Center, Los Angeles, CA). Protocols for collection of samples and discretions for obtaining informed consent and shipping can be found on its website: www.csmc.edu/genetics/skeldys.

ACKNOWLEDGMENTS

We thank Drs. Deborah Krakow, Bill Wilcox, and Dan Cohn for their helpful comments. This work was supported by an NIH Program Project Grant (HD 22657). The International Skeletal Dysplasia Registry can be accessed at www.csmc.edu/genetics/skeldys.

REFERENCES

1. Rimoin DL, Lachman RS. Genetic disorders of the osseous skeleton. In: Beighton P, ed. McKusick's Heritable Disorders of Connective Tissue. St. Louis: C.V. Mosby, 1992:557.
2. Ornoy A, Borochowitz Z, Lachman R, Rimoin DL. Atlas of Fetal Skeletal Radiology. Chicago: Year Book Medical Publishers, 1988.
3. Horton WA. Molecular genetics of the human chondrodysplasias. Eur J Hum Genet 1995;3:357–373.
4. Reardon W. Skeletal dysplasias detectable by DNA analysis. Prenatal Diagnosis 1996;16:1221–1236.
5. Rimoin DL: Molecular Defects in the Chondrodysplasias. Clinical Courier. Vol 16, No. 27, 24–25. November 1997.
6. Rimoin DL et al. International Nomenclature and Classification of the Osteochondroplasias (1997). Am Journal of Medical Genetics 1998;79:376–382.
7. Sharony R, Browne C, Lachman RS, Rimoin DL. Prenatal diagnosis of the skeletal dysplasias. Am J Obstet Gynecol 1993;169:668–675.
8. Rimoin D, Krakow D. Skeletal dysplasias. In: New M, ed. Diagnosis and Treatment of the Unborn Child. Reddick, FL: Idelson-Gnocchi, 1999.
9. Shohat M, Tick D, Barakat S, Bu X, Melmed S, Rimoin, DL. Short-term recombinant human growth hormone treatment increases growth in achondroplasia. J Clin Endocr 1996;81:11.

5

Tall Stature and Excessive Growth Syndromes

S. Douglas Frasier
UCLA School of Medicine, Los Angeles, California, U.S.A.

Tall stature and excessive growth syndromes are relatively rare concerns in pediatric and pediatric endocrine practice. Nevertheless, an important group of pathological conditions and variants in the pattern of normal growth and development is first brought to the physician's attention by these complaints. The causes of excessive growth that are important in children and adolescents are shown in Table 1. This chapter considers growth syndromes and disorders of importance to pediatric endocrinclogists, including constitutional tall stature. However, disorders of sexual maturation are discussed elsewhere in this book.

I. DEFINITION AND CLASSIFICATION OF OVERGROWTH SYNDROMES

Overgrowth syndromes can be classified into three categories:

1. Generalized overgrowth syndromes
2. Regional overgrowth snyndromes
3. Parameter-specific growth overgrowth disorders

Generalized overgrowth syndromes, which include the classic overgrowth conditions, are those in which all or most parameters of growth and physical development are in excess of 2 standard deviations above the mean for the person's age and gender. Some of the classic conditions in this category are listed in Table 1 and are discussed in detail in this chapter. The regional overgrowth disorders include those in which excessive growth is confined to one or a few regions of the body. An example is benign familial macrocephaly and hemihyperplasia or hemihypertrophy, among others. There are also parameter-specific overgrowth disorders in which a single or at most several growth parameters are in excess of normal. For example, familial idiopathic obesity and Prader-Willi Syndrome are examples in this category.

The incidence of each overgrowth syndrome or disorder varies greatly, from being as common as 1:1000–

1500 as occurs with the fragile x syndrome, to less than 1:1,000,000 births in other more rare syndromes such as Elejalde syndrome, a striking prenatal overgrowth syndrome that has been reported in only three siblings. The reader is referred to volume 1, number 10 of *Growth, Genetics and Hormones* (March, 1994) which published two very good reviews of overgrowth syndromes, including their causes and diagnosis.

II. GROWTH HORMONE EXCESS

As recently reviewed (1, 2) and as exemplified by several representative reports (3–10), growth hormone excess, although rare, must be considered as a cause of tall stature and rapid growth in all patients with this clinical picture.

A. Causes and Pathogenesis

Excessive growth hormone secretion is most often a primary disorder and is associated with a functioning pituitary adenoma. If growth hormone excess is present, the pituitary tumor, regardless of its staining characteristics, contains typical growth-hormone-secretory granules. Occasionally, the tumor secretes excess prolactin in addition to growth hormone (11–13) and prolactin-secretory granules are also demonstrated. Growth hormone excess is usually present as an isolated abnormality, but associations occur with McCune-Albright syndrome (14–17), tuberous sclerosis (18) neurofibromatosis (19, 20), and optic chiasm glioma (20, 21).

As with all functioning endocrine tumors, the specific pathogenesis of growth-hormone-secreting adenomas is not completely understood. In some patients, the excess growth hormone (GH) secretion and ademoma formation may be secondary to unrestrained stimulation of the somatotrophs by growth-hormone-releasing hormone (22–24). Impaired somatostatin (somatotropin release-inhibiting factor; SRIF) secretion is also a theoretical pathogenic

Table 1 Causes of Tall Stature and Excessive Growth

Endocrine disorders
   Growth hormone excess
   Disorders of sexual maturation
      Precocious puberty
      Virilization
      Feminization
      Hypogonadism
Nonendocrine disorders
   Cerebral gigantism (Sotos syndrome)
   Klinefelters syndrome
   XYY males
   Marfan syndrome
   Homocystinuria
Normal variants: Constitutional tall stature

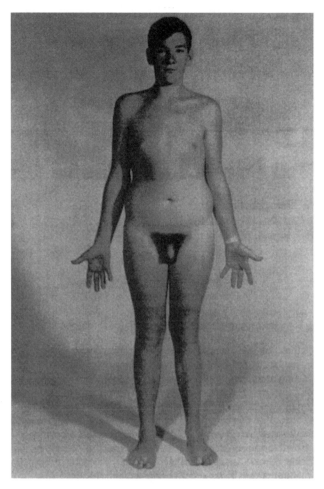

Figure 1 A 17-6/12-year-old boy with growth hormone excess due to a pituitary adenoma. Height was 193 cm and weight was 108.3 kg. (From Frasier SD, Pediatric Endocrinology. New York: Grune and Stratton Inc., 1980.)

consideration (19–21). Various mutations in the gene for the alpha subunit of the stimulatory G protein, which increases cyclic AMP formation, have been demonstrated in growth-hormone-secreting pituitary adenomas (25–27). These putative oncogenes may cause somatotropin hyperplasia and the development of an adenoma through the unrestrained production of cyclic AMP, which leads to an increase in both cell growth and cell function. Specific constitutive G protein alpha gene mutations have been demonstrated in patients with McCune-Albright syndrome and pituitary adenoma (28, 29). Recently, a loss in heterozygosity for a tumor suppressor gene at the 11q13 locus has been described in both isolated familial GH-secreting pituitary adenomas and in similar tumors in families with the multiple endocrine neoplasia (MEN type 1) syndrome (30, 31).

B. Clinical Manifestations

Growth hormone excess leads to either gigantism or acromegaly, depending on whether the epiphyses are open or closed. Typically, gigantism occurs in young children and acromegaly is seen in adults. The adolescent who still has open epiphyses shows a mixed picture of rapid growth and acromegalic features, termed acromegalic gigantism (Fig. 1).

Young patients with excess growth hormone secretion are both tall and grow at a rate greater than normal for their age. Their growth curve progressively deviates away from normal. When growth hormone excess begins during adolescence, there is enlargement of the lower jaw, hands, and feet in addition to the rapid increase in height.

In rare cases, this clinical picture may be imitated by the syndrome of pseudoacromegaly or acromegaloidism, in which growth hormone secretion is normal but other non-growth-hormone-dependent growth factors may be present in excess (32).

Expanding adenomas may interfere with the secretion of one or more pituitary trophic hormones. Thus, a growth-hormone-secreting adenoma may be associated with gonadotropin deficiency leading to delayed or arrested puberty and, less often, adrenocorticotropin (ACTH) and/or thyroid-stimulating hormone (TSH) deficiency. When there is combined growth hormone excess and gonadotropin deficiency, patients may show both excessive growth and eunuchoid body proportions.

Impaired vision and visual field abnormalities may accompany growth hormone excess. The characteristic abnormality is bitemporal homonymous hemianopsia (so-called tunnel vision) because of midline compression of the optic chiasm. However, a wide variety of visual field defects may be produced depending on the size and location of the tumor. Expanding intrasellar tumors may also lead to increased intracranial pressure and/or symptoms of hypothalamic dysfunction.

C. Diagnosis

The clinical diagnosis of growth hormone excess is confirmed by demonstrating an elevated serum concentration of growth hormone that is not suppressed by raising the concentration of blood glucose during performance of a standard glucose tolerance test. The administration of glucose by mouth in a dosage of 1.75 g/kg, up to a maximum of 100 g, will raise the blood glucose concentration to a level that will suppress the serum GH concentration to less than 5 ng/ml in normal persons. The lowest concentration of GH is seen between 60 and 120 min after the ingestion of glucose. Failure to suppress the serum concentration of GH supports the diagnosis of growth hormone excess due to hypothalamic or pituitary dysfunction (4). Confirmation of the diagnosis is also aided by demonstrating an elevated serum somatomedin-C (IGF-1) concentration (33). The level of growth hormone activity may be better correlated with the somatomedin-C concentration than with the concentration of growth hormone after glucose suppression.

In at least 25% of patients there is glucose intolerance and hyperinsulinism. Failure to increase the serum concentration of growth hormone above the already elevated levels in response to hypoglycemia and relative resistance to the hypoglycemic effects of exogenous insulin are also present.

When growth hormone excess is confirmed, the possibility of pituitary trophic hormone deficiencies should be investigated by performing standard tests of pituitary function.

Complete neuroradiological studies aimed at demonstrating the size and location of the pituitary adenoma are essential in planning therapy. A number of studies have been recommended in the past: these have included skull films, cone-down views of the sella turcica, sellar polytomography, computed tomography (CT), and magnetic resonance imaging (MRI). MRI with and without gadolinium contrast is the preferred modern technology.

D. Treatment

Treatment is directed at eliminating excess growth hormone secretion (34). In the past, this has meant destruction of the tumor, and a number of ablative techniques have been employed. Radiation from an external source is the least effective. Transsphenoidal microsurgery appears to offer the best possibility of complete removal of the tumor with preservation of remaining pituitary function. This technique is particularly useful when small tumors without extrasellar extension are the source of excess GH secretion (35). When the tumor is too large for this approach, a craniotomy with direct visualization and removal of the tumor must be performed.

There has been significant progress in the pharmacological management of growth hormone excess with the dopamine receptor agonist, bromocriptine, and with analogs of somatostatin, octreotide, and lantreotide. Bromocriptine inhibits the secretion of both growth hormone and prolactin through direct effects on the pituitary. There is also evidence indicating an inhibitory effect on cell growth leading to a decrease in the size of some pituitary tumors. This agent has been used successfully in several children with growth hormone excess (36, 37). In these patients excess growth hormone secretion was partially inhibited and associated excess prolactin secretion was abolished. There was significant clinical improvement, even though the suppresion of GH secretion was incomplete. Between 10 and 20 mg/day of bromocriptine was therapeutic and no significant side effects were observed.

Somatostatin is a potent inhibitor of growth hormone secretion initially isolated from the hypothalamus. Although native somatostatin inhibits GH secretion in acromegaly, its effect is very short lived and somatostatin administration has variable undesirable effects on glucose metabolism. The somatostatin analog octreotide, which may be given every 6–8 h and has relatively little effect on insulin secretion, has been found useful in the management of GH excess. This agent has now been administered to pediatric patients with growth-hormone-producing tumors (38–40). Effective dosages were 50–100 μg given every 6–8 h. Side effects have been minimal and both growth hormone secretion and pituitary tumor size have decreased significantly in response to octreotide administration.

Recent studies in adults with acromegaly have indicated that lantreotide, a long-acting somatostatin analog that can be given every 10–14 days (41), and a very-long-acting formulation of octreotide that can be given every 4 weeks (42) are both effective and safe as treatment for growth hormone excess. Studies in pediatric patients have not yet been reported.

E. PROGNOSIS

The rarity of growth hormone excess and the relatively recent application of transsphenoidal surgery and medical suppression of growth hormone secretion make generalizations regarding the prognosis of GH excess in children and adolescents difficult. However, a report from Manchester, England (43), describes the serious physical and psychological disability observed in 10 untreated or partially treated patients. Marked skeletal deformity and psychological problems were common. More aggressive therapy and current methods of management may improve this poor outcome.

III. CEREBRAL GIGANTISM (SOTOS SYNDROME)

Cerebral gigantism is a clinical syndrome of rapid growth in infancy, dysmorphic features, and a nonprogressive neurological disorder first described by Sotos and others in 1964 (44). Since this initial description more than 250 patients have been reported in numerous case reports and in several reviews (45–48).

A. Causes and Pathogenesis

The underlying cause(s) of cerebral gigantism are not understood. Although most instances of this syndrome are sporadic, there have been reports of familial occurence and dominant inheritance has been suggested in several families (48). In addition, here have been reports of the syndrome in first cousins, siblings in a highly inbred family, and monozygotic twins (46), suggesting the possibility of recessive inheritance. One report identified fragile X chromosomes in two affected patients (49), but this appears to be a fortuitous association. These data clearly suggest genetic heterogeneity as well as clinical heterogeneity in cerebral gigantism and make a single cause unlikely.

The constellation of abnormalities suggests hypothalamic dysfunction, but no specific neuropathological lesions have been identified (50). Extensive investigation has not shown any consistent abnormality of growth hormone secretion or IGF-I or IGF-II concentrations. Other abnormal growth factors may be present, but they have not yet been identified.

B. Clinical Manifestations

The major clinical manifestations of cerebral gigantism are listed in Table 2. Patients are large at birth, both in weight and length (47), and growth is rapid during the first year. By 1 year of age most patients are above the 97th percentile height for age and gender. Growth velocity also exceeds the 97th percentile. Rapid growth continues for the first 3–4 years (Fig. 2). Body proportions are abnormal, with arm span exceeding height by as much as 5 cm. This difference is normally negative up to age 12 and only exceeds 2 cm in young men older than 13 or 14 years (45).

Fine motor control is impaired in infancy and early childhood and developmental milestones are delayed. Intellectual impairment is mild to moderate and median IQ score is 70–75 (45, 51). The neonatal period is characterized by irritability and feeding problems in addition to large size.

The bone age is generally advanced between 1 and 2 years. Mildly dilated cerebral ventricles are present in the majority of patients when they are studied by pneumoencephalography or CT scanning.

C. Diagnosis

The diagnosis depends on the characteristic clinical picture. There are no definitive physical findings and no specific laboratory results. As yet no characteristic mutations have been described in this group of patients. Other causes

Table 2 Clinical Manifestations of Cerebral Gigantism

Clinical sign/symptom	% of cases
Gigantism	100
Rapid growth in infancy	100
Prominent forehead	96
High-arched palate	96
Hyperteleorism	91
Long head	84
Pointed chin	83
Developmental retardation	83
Advanced bone age	74
Impaired fine motor control	52
Neonatal irritability	44
Feeding problems	44

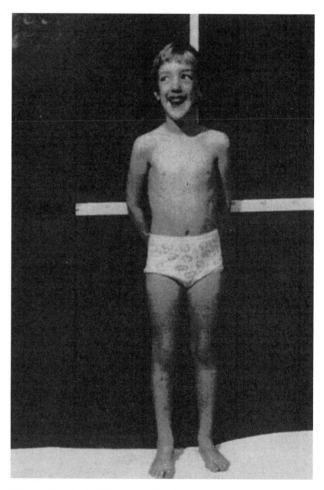

Figure 2 A 4-9/12-year-old girl with cerebral gigantism. Height was 55.7 cm (height age, 11-9/12) and weight was 33.7 kg (weight age, 10-10/12). Developmental level was 3–3-6/12 years. (Courtesy of Juan F. Sotos M.D., Children's Hospital, Columbus, Ohio.)

of overgrowth and mental retardation, such as fragile X syndrome and Marfan syndrome, need to be excluded.

D. Treatment

Treatment is directed at improving the level of motor and intellectual function, as with any child who manifests developmental delay and intellectual handicap. Modification of ultimate height might be considered under very unusual circumstances (see below).

E. Prognosis

The prognosis for normal adult intellectual function is poor even in the best of circumstances. A recent study evaluated 20 male and 20 female patients with Sotos syndrome to their ultimate height (52). The mean adult height in men was 183.4 (standard deviation [SD] 6.0) cm and the mean adult height in women was 172 (SD 5.7) cm. The average height achieved was not excessive and these data would point away from any need to attempt modification of height with hormonal therapy.

Concern has been expressed that patients with cerebral gigantism may be particularly susceptible to the development of tumors (48, 53). This may represent another facet of growth without proper control that may be the basic mechanism underlying this and other overgrowth syndromes.

IV. KLINEFELTER SYNDROME

Klinefelter syndrome is a relatively common abnormality in phenotypic males, occurring in 1:500–1000 live male births (54–56). Although it may present in a variety of different ways, tall stature is a frequent finding in both children and adolescents.

A. Causes and Pathogenesis

Klinefelter syndrome is due to an abnormality in chromosome number in which two or more X chromosomes are present in male patients. By far the most usual abnormal karyotype is 47 XXY. However, mosaic karyotypes such as XY/XXY have also been described, as have other aneuploid karyotypes such as 48 XXXY or 49 XXXXY. The presence of one or more extra X chromosomes is associated with testicular failure, which results in infertility and impaired testosterone production. The testes show hyalinization and fibrosis of the seminiferous tubules with histologically intact interstitial cells.

B. Clinical Manifestations

Klinefelter syndrome is infrequently diagnosed in prepubertal children. However, the increased frequency of amniocentesis has led to a number of fetal diagnoses. Several clinical clues point to this diagnosis in childhood and

should lead to appropriate laboratory evaluation (54). Prepubertal boys with an extra X chromosome are often tall for their age. Body proportions are often abnormal, with relatively long legs reflected in a low upper/lower segment ratio. Patients tend to be thin and underweight for their height and age. Genital abnormalities such as small phallus, hypospadias, and cryptorchidism may be present. Although the testes are often normal in size prior to puberty, they are abnormally small (<2 ml in volume) in a few patients. The major means of revealing Klinefelter syndrome before puberty is studying boys with mental retardation or school and/or behavior difficulties. Learning and psychological problems are common in this group of children.

Adolescent patients with Klinefelter syndrome are usually taller than expected for their age and have abnormal proportions with persistent increased leg length (57). The testes are disproportionally small for the level of pubertal development. Testicular maturation begins with the onset of puberty but regresses by midadolescence and testicular volume rarely exceeds 2–3 ml. Testicular length is generally below 2.0 cm. The testes are usually firm and show diminished sensitivity to pressure. Androgen function is initially preserved and almost all boys enter puberty. Penile and pubic hair development are generally satisfactory. However, oligospermia or aspermia is uniformly present. Adolescent development may be delayed and impotence or other problems of sexual function may develop (57–59).

Gynecomastia is common. This begins as simple adolescent breast enlargement but is often marked and persistent. It is frequently the reason that patients seek medical advice and is very distressing to most.

As a group, patients with Klinefelter syndrome have lower than expected verbal IQ scores and a significant increase in learning, behavioral, and psychosocial problems (60, 61).

C. Diagnosis

The clinical picture of tall stature, gynecomastia, and small testes in a male with adequate secondary sex characteristics is often diagnostic. The clinical diagnosis of Klinefelter syndrome is confirmed by the demonstration of one or more extra X chromosomes in the karyotype. Primary gonadal failure is reflected in elevated serum concentrations of pituitary gonadotropins. Although levels of both luteinizing hormone (LH) and follicle-stimulating hormone (FSH) are elevated, the major increase is in FSH (58, 59). Testosterone concentrations are variable but usually in the low–normal adult male range (58). Average concentrations are clearly below those seen in normal adolescent boys (57).

D. Treatment

The administration of testosterone may be helpful when adolescent development is delayed or when sexual function is impaired. Full replacement therapy with 200–400 mg long-acting, intramuscular testosterone every 3 or 4 weeks should be given to restore serum testosterone concentrations to the normal range. Gynecomastia may require surgical therapy with simple mammoplasty using a circumareolar incision.

E. Prognosis

Although some patients function normally, impaired intellectual function and psychosocial difficulties persist in a significant number (62). Sexual function may be impaired. A recent study of cancer risk in patients with Klinefelter syndrome found an increased incidence of mediastinal germ cell tumors during adolescence and young adulthood (63). Impaired fertility has been managed by the use of donor sperm and artificial insemination of wives of Klinefelter syndrome patients (62), and by the ingenious in-vitro fertilization technique of intracytoplasmic injection into the wife's ova of sperm extracted from the testes of affected men (64).

V. XYY SYNDROME

The presence of an extra Y chromosome also predisposes to tall stature (60, 65). Males with the XYY syndrome are relatively common in the general population. Newborn screening studies indicate an incidence of between 1:500 and 1:1000 live male birth (55, 56). There is no uniform phenotypic expression of this abnormal karyotype, but the incidence is much higher when males whose height exceeds 183 cm (72″) are screened.

In addition to tall stature there appear to be few phenotypic expressions of the XYY syndrome. Those described include severe acne, hypospadias and/or cryptorchidism, radioulnar synostosis, and mild or moderate mental retardation (60, 61, 66, 67). The finding of an XYY karyotype in a newborn does not necessarily predict intellectual function or behavior. Generalizations cannot be made regarding the correlation between karyotype and behavioral phenotype (60, 62).

VI. MARFAN SYNDROME

Marfan syndrome is a heritable disorder of connective tissue in which tall stature is one of a spectrum of abnormalities that lead to significant morbidity and early mortality.

A. Causes and Pathogenesis

Marfan syndrome is an autosomal dominant disorder. In 65–75% of patients one parent is affected and sporadic new mutations account for 25–35% of patients. There is a 50% recurrence risk in the offspring of affected individuals. Although the degree of expression and severity of

clinical features may vary from family to family, involvement in a particular individual cannot be predicted from knowledge of the family history.

Marfan syndrome is caused by mutations in the fibrillin gene located on chromosome 15 (68–71). The affected gene product, fibrillin, a 350 kD glycoprotein, is a structural component of a microfibril, the elastin-associated microfibril, found in the extracellular matrix of connective tissue. Patients with Marfan syndrome have a deficiency of elastin-associated microfibrils, which leads to the syndrome's clinical manifestations (72, 73).

B. Clinical Manifestations

A complex constellation of abnormalities characterize Marfan syndrome. As shown in Table 3, skeletal, ocular, and cardiovascular systems are involved (48, 74, 75).

Height is increased and body proportions are abnormal. Both arm and leg length are greater than normal so that arm span is significantly greater than height and the upper/lower segment ratio is diminished. Arachnodactyly (long fingers and toes) is seen in the majority of patients. There is often a pectus excavatum chest deformity and scoliosis is common. The joints are hyperextensible and lax.

Ocular abnormalities are extremely common. The cornea is flat and congenital subluxation of the lens with upward displacement is frequently present. The ability to accommodate is retained. Refractive errors, particularly myopia, are present in many patients. Retinal detachment is a common complication.

The shortened life span of patients with Marfan syndrome is due to its cardiovascular manifestations. The combination of physical examination and echocardiography shows some abnormality in almost all patients. Both aortic and mitral regurgitation are present. Aortic

Table 3 Clinical Manifestations of Marfan Syndrome

Skeletal
    Tall stature
    Long, thin extremities
    Long fingers (arachnodactyly)
    Loose joints
    Scoliosis
    Pectus deformity
Ocular
    Flat cornea
    Dislocated lens
    Myopia
    Retinal detachment
Cardiovascular
    Diffuse aortic aneurysm
    Dissecting aortic aneurysm
    Mitral regurgitation

root dilatation is seen relatively early when sophisticated diagnostic tools are employed. Aortic regurgitation, dissection, and rupture are major life-threatening complications (76).

C. Diagnosis

The characteristic familial, musculoskeletal, ocular, and cardiovascular manifestations of Marfan syndrome are usually diagnostic. Specific molecular diagnosis, while possible, is not yet generally available. Careful measurements including assessment of body proportions, ocular examination including slit lamp evaluation, and cardiovascular studies including echocardiography should allow the clinician to make the correct diagnosis once it is considered to be a possibility.

D. Treatment

There is no specific treatment, but several approaches may reduce the morbidity and perhaps even the mortality of patients with Marfan syndrome (75). Early recognition and correction of a refractive error will prevent the amblyopia that often limits vision. Prevention or correction of scoliosis and repair of the pectus deformity may be very helpful.

When significant aortic regurgitation is noted, an aortic valve prosthesis may be utilized. Progressive aortic dilatation may be managed by graft placement. Attempts have been made to limit progression of aortic dilatation by administering propranolol or other beta-adrenergic blocking agent. Theoretically, this will decrease left ventricular ejection impulse and protect the aortic root from a maximal exposure to left ventricular pressure. It remains to be seen whether such therapy is effective.

E. Prognosis

The life expectancy of patients with Marfan syndrome is about half that of the general population. Half of the affected male patients are dead by age 40–45 and half of affected female patients die by age 50–55. In more than 95% of patients death is due to cardiovascular complications (76). Newer therapeutic approaches may be improving these figures. In a recent study from the United Kingdom (77), the median total survival was 53 years for men and 72 years for women.

VII. HOMOCYSTINURIA

Homocystinuria due to a deficiency of cystathionine beta-synthase (CBS) is an unusual disorder of amino acid metabolism (78) in which the phenotype has a significant resemblance to that of Marfan syndrome. It also carries a significant morbidity and mortality (79–81).

A. Causes and Pathogenesis

Cystathionine B-synthase deficiency is inherited as an autosomal recessive inborn metabolic error. It is caused by a large number of mutations in the CBS gene (82). The recurrence rate is 25% for each pregnancy when both parents are carriers. This enzyme is active in the pathway through which methionine is converted to cystine. It catalyzes the metabolic step at which homocystine and serine combine to form cystathionine. When the enzyme is deficient, homocystine and methionine accumulate in plasma and homocystinuria is seen. The plasma concentrations of cystathionine and cystine are markedly reduced. There is a significant quantitive, and probably qualitative, heterogeneity in the enzyme deficiency. The best example of this is the dichotomy between patients in whom the administration of pyridoxine (vitamin B6) leads to correction of the chemical abnormality and those in whom it does not. There is apparent segregation of these two types of abnormality among affected families (80, 81).

B. Clinical Manifestations

The clinical manifestations of homocystinuria are reviewed by Sotos (48) and are shown in Table 4. In addition to tall stature and marfanoid habitus, patients with homocystinuria show abnormalities involving multiple organ systems. The eye, nervous system, skeleton, and vascular system are all affected. Patients are usually normal at birth and the clinical manifestations come to the physician's attention in the first few years of life.

Mental retardation occurs very frequently and is often the presenting abnormality. The original patients were found by screening a population of retarded children for aminoaciduria. Convulsions are seen in 10–20% of patients.

The optic lens is dislocated in the majority of patients. Displacement is usually downward and the eyes lose their ability to accommodate. There is marked myopia and astigmatism. Osteoporosis, scoliosis, and vertebral collapse may be seen.

Thromboembolic phenomenon, especially in the postoperative period, is a life-threatening complication. Both arterial and venous occlusion are seen and sudden death may result. Heterozygotes develop premature thrombotic

Table 4 Clinical Manifestations of Homocystinuria

Tall stature
Marfanoid habitus
Mental retardation
Dislocated lens
Osteoporosis
Thrombosis

disease affecting coronary, cerebral, and peripheral arteries (83).

C. Diagnosis

Cystathionine B-synthase deficiency may be suspected on the basis of homocystinuria and elevated plasma concentrations of homocystine and methionine. Plasma cystine concentrations are low. Confirmation depends on demonstrating a deficiency of cystathionine B-synthase in a liver biopsy specimen, cultured phytohemagglutinin-stimulated lymphocytes, or skin fibroblasts. Newborn screening is available in populations at increased risk (84).

D. Treatment

Dietary methionine is restricted and dietary cystine is supplemented. Special synthetic diets that are virtually methionine-free are generally used.

All patients should be given a trial of therapy with pyridoxine. Patients should not be considered to be unresponsive to pyridoxine until 500–1000 mg daily for 3–4 weeks is shown to be ineffective. Responsive patients can usually be managed with 150–250 mg pyridoxine daily.

E. Prognosis

Methionine restriction ameliorates mental retardation when it is begun after diagnosis on the basis of newborn screening. When patients are not diagnosed in the newborn period, a significant number are mentally retarded and have other complications by age 15. The prognosis also depends significantly on whether or not the patient is pyridoxine-responsive (80). Lens dislocation, osteoporosis, and late thromboembolic phenomenon are less frequent in B6-responsive patients. However, there is an increase in mortality due to thromboembolism in both responsive and nonresponsive patients. Almost 25% of nonresponsive patients and 5% of responsive patients die by age 30.

VIII. BECKWITH-WIEDEMANN SYNDROME

Beckwith-Wiedemann syndrome (BWS), (85, 86) which is also termed exomphalos–macroglossia–gigantism (EMG) syndrome, is generally recognized in the neonatal period on the basis of a characteristic phenotype, which includes somatic overgrowth and hypoglycemia (87).

A. Causes and Pathogenesis

Beckwith-Wiedemann syndrome is a genetically determined set of phenotypic features in which there are abnormalities of a region of the short arm of chromosome 11, 11p15.5 (88–90). This disorder is an example of chromosomal imprinting in which the abnormality is derived from only the male or female parent. In the case of BWS the abnormality is paternal (91–94) and affected patients show either trisomy for this region with the duplication arising in the father, or paternal disomy for this region with loss of the maternal chromosome contribution. The specific gene or genes that are duplicated have not yet been determined, but the IGF-II gene is the putative candidate. The IGF-II gene, or some other growth promoter, appears to be the probable cause of the characteristic phenotype of this disorder (95).

B. Clinical Manifestations

The typical clinical appearance of patients with Beckwith-Wiedemann syndrome (Table 5) includes macroglossia; umbilical abnormalities, such as ompholocele, umbilical hernia, and diastasis recti; craniofacial anomalies such as midface hypoplasia, prominent occiput, flat nasal bridge, and high-arched palate; increased birthweight and postnatal gigantism; earlobe anomalies that include grooves, pits, and notches; enlarged liver, kidneys, and other organs; facial flame nevus; and hyperinsulinemic hypoglycemia. A significant number of patients have somatic assymetry that may be associated with the development of various cancers, particularly nephroblastoma (Wilms' tumor), adrenocortical carcinoma, hepatoblastoma, and rhabdomyosarcoma (96, 97).

Hypoglycemia, if it is present, usually occurs in the first few days of life. It is extremely important to recognize and manage this feature of BWS as soon as possible to prevent subsequent brain damage, developmental delay, and microcephaly that may result from an unrecognized chronic low blood glucose concentration. Blood glucose should be monitored frequently during the first 72 h of life in all neonates showing the clinical features of this disorder.

C. Diagnosis

As with other dysmorphic syndromes, the diagnosis of BWS depends on a characteristic clinical picture rather

Table 5 Major Clinical Manifestations of Beckwith-Wiedemann Syndrome

Clinical sign/symptom	Percentage of cases
Macroglossia	95
Craniofacial anomalies	80
Visceromegaly	80
Umbilical anomalies	75
Earlobe anomalies	70
Increased birthweight	60
Postnatal gigantism	60
Facial flame nevus	60
Hypoglycemia	55
Cardiac defects	35

than any specific diagnostic test. Demonstration of the underlying genetic abnormalities requires extremely sophisticated methodology beyond the scope of a standard clinical or genetics laboratory. The major features (Table 5) should be present before a diagnosis of BWS is assigned to an individual patient.

D. Treatment

Treatment is directed at specific features of this syndrome. Surgical repair of umbilical abnormalities is sometimes necessary. Management of associated cardiac anomalies depends on the nature of the defect and on whether or not cardiac failure is present. Associated tumors require a specific management plans.

Since the pathogenesis of the neonatal hypoglycemia of BWS is hyperinsulinism, treatment is directed at reducing the excess insulin secretion. A number of agents, such as glucocorticoids, Susphrine®, and zinc glucagon have been employed, but most effective medical management has been with diazoxide. Subtotal pancreatectomy is reserved for patients who are not made normoglycemic with diazoxide therapy.

E. Prognosis

There is a very high mortality rate in infancy among BWS patients: 20–25% die by age 1 year (85). The causes of death are not well documented but associated heart disease and unrecognized hypoglycemia are significant contributors. Patients generally continue to grow excessively and the majority remain above the 95th percentile for height and weight through adolescence. Intellectual function is variable and delayed development is often seen when hypoglycemia has been recognized late or when its management has been suboptimal. When malignancies develop in BWS patients, the prognosis becomes that of the associated cancer. Children who survive infancy with good control of their hypoglycemia appear to have a reasonable prognosis for growth and intellectual function (98).

IX. HEMIHYPERTROPHY

Hemihypertrophy or assymetrical overgrowth is of particular significance because of its association with malignancy. By far the most common associated cancer is Wilms' tumor (99). Other tumors that occur in patients with hemihypertrophy are adrenocortical carcinoma and adenoma, rhabdomyosarcoma, and hepatoblastoma. These cancers are the same as those noted in patients with Beckwith-Wiedemann syndrome. As in BWS, abnormalities of chromosome 11 at the 11 15p site are found in these tumors (100). By far the most significant aspect of hemihypertrophy is not the overgrowth itself but the development of malignancy. All such patients require close

follow-up to discover these tumors at the earliest possible time.

X. CONSTITUTIONAL TALL STATURE

Constitutional tall stature is a variant of the normal pattern of childhood growth and development (101). Its incidence varies with the sociocultural definition of normal and the level of parental concern regarding height. In the past, pediatric endocrinologists were often asked to see tall girls whose tall mothers were concerned about their daughters' ultimate height. A great deal of the initial concern over the patient's height reflected whatever social and psychological problems the mother may have had as a tall adolescent and young adult and anticipated that her daughter would have. Over the past 20–30 years, as the role of women in American society has expanded and as it has become first permitted and then fashionable for girls to be athletic and to concentrate on physical training, the frequency of this complaint has declined significantly. It has always been extremely unusual for American families to consider that their sons were too tall. Nevertheless, there remains considerable interest in constitutional tall stature and its treatment, particularly in Western Europe (102).

A. Causes and Pathogenesis

The growth pattern of patients with constitutional tall stature follows that of one or both parents who are also tall. Thus, genetic and familial factors appear to play the most important role in the condition's cause and pathogenesis.

Endocrinological studies of tall children have yielded variable results. An increased serum concentration of growth hormone in response to both glucose loading (103, 104) and the administration of thyrotropin-releasing hormone (TRH) (104) has been demonstrated, but similar observations have been made in normal pubertal children (105). This apparent paradoxical growth hormone response may be a phenomenon of normal adolescence (105, 106) and have no significance relative to tall stature.

B. Clinical Manifestations

Patients with constitutional tall stature are between 2 and 4 standard deviations above the average height for their age. Length is normal at birth and tall stature is evident by age 3 or 4 years. Growth velocity is accelerated in early childhood but slows after 4 or 5 years of age when the growth curve is parallel to the normal curve (107). Body proportions are normal. There is the same variability in the timing of adolescent development, as in children of average height, and the age of onset of puberty tends to follow the pattern characteristic for the patient's family.

C. Diagnosis

The diagnosis is generally clear from the family history, record of growth, and results of physical examination.

Specific laboratory studies of endocrine function are rarely indicated. Bone age determination as part of the initial evaluation is essential so that the most accurate prediction of adult height can be given to the patient and family. The bone age shows the same variability as that of the general population of children. Advanced bone age is not associated with constitutional tall stature in the same way that delayed bone age is associated with constitutional short stature.

D. Treatment

Management of tall children and adolescents remains among the more controversial topics in pediatric endocrinology. Generally, therapy has been aimed at inducing incomplete precocious puberty and accelerating the rate of development of secondary sex characteristics through the pharmacological administration of gonadal steroids. In theory, the acceleration of epiphyseal maturation that accompanies gonadal steroid administration should lead to early closure of the epiphyses. Somatomedin generation may also be inhibited by pharmacological dosages of estrogen (108).

A large number of reports have appeared describing the administration of estrogens in tall girls. A variety of preparations and dose schedules have been employed. These include injectable estradiol valerate (109, 110), implanted estradiol pellets (111), and oral stilbestrol 3 mg/day (112), diethylstilbestrol 5 mg/day (113), ethinyl estradiol 0.1 mg/day (114, 115), 0.25 mg/day (113, 115), 0.3 mg/day (114–116), or 0.5 mg/day (114–116), and conjugated estrogens 2.5–10.0 mg/day (108, 118–121).

There is general agreement that a favorable effect on ultimate height results from such pharmacological therapy (122). The overall average decrease in ultimate height has varied from 2.3 to 7.3 cm, with the mean effect in most studies being between 3.0 and 5.0 cm. Much greater effects have been claimed in selected patients. Most investigators consider that the effects are greatest when therapy is begun at a bone age below 12–13 years and/or a chronological age below 11 to 12 years. Treatment should be continued until the epiphyses have fused. The exact age at which estrogen treatment should be started and the predicted mature height that would serve as an indication for treatment remain in question.

Short-term side effects of estrogen administration include nausea, weight gain, pigmentation, leg cramps, and transient hypertension (108–119, 121). There may be the induction of hyperlipidemia, glucose intolerance, or cholelithiasis (120). Thromboembolism is a potential hazard (123). During treatment the gonadotropin response to gonadotropin-releasing hormone is uniformly suppressed (108, 124). However, menstrual function generally returns promptly after discontinuing estrogen administration. There appear to be no deleterious long-term effects on reproductive function in treated women studied 10 years after receiving estrogen for tall stature (115). The overall late effects of pharmacological estrogen administration on gonadal function and both genital tract and breast neoplasia are unknown.

There remains considerable disagreement about whether the benefits of the effect on ultimate height outweigh the risks of high-dosage estrogen administration in young girls. I believe that too much is unknown about the late effects of such therapy on reproductive function and the development of neoplasms of the breast and female genital tract. In my opinion, the potential risks outweigh the benefits. Girls with Marfan syndrome and with the potential for development of scoliosis may be a special case (125). The difficulties that a patient's tall stature present to her and, more often, to her mother, can usually be dealt with through sympathetic support. Occasionally, more intensive individual or family psychotherapy is necessary.

Although tall stature has not been a complaint among adolescent boys in the United States, it has been a sufficient cause of concern in Europe to lead to gonadal steroid therapy (116, 126). The administration of a long-acting intramuscular testosterone preparation, 500 mg every 2 or 3 weeks (mean dosage 500 mg/m^2/month), has produced a significant reduction in predicted mature height (116). Short-term treatment of 6 months' duration was ineffective (127). Long-term gonadal function appears to be normal in treated boys (128, 129). The same questions regarding benefits and risks as well as the same psychological considerations apply to the treatment of tall boys as to tall girls.

Bromocriptine has also been used to treat tall patients. If growth hormone secretion were suppressed in tall adolescents while pubertal epiphyseal maturation progressed at a normal rate, ultimate height might be reduced. There are conflicting reports of the efficacy of bromocriptine in limiting adult height. An initial report suggested a significant effect (130), but subsequent studies have reported equivocal (131) or negative (132) results.

Octreotide has recently been used in small groups of tall children to inhibit growth hormone secretion and growth velocity (133, 134). Preliminary results suggest a role for this agent in the management of tall stature. However, a great deal of additional data must accumulate before the administration of somatostatin analogs can be considered other than experimental therapy.

E. Prognosis

The long-term prognosis for mature height in a patient with constitutional tall stature is consistent with the height attained by the rest of their family. An accurate prognosis for ultimate height obtained as part of the initial evaluation often indicates that the patient will not be nearly as tall as his parents fear. In these instances, the prognosis becomes part of the supportive therapy given to the family. However, height predictions often prove to be inaccurate when final height is attained (135).

REFERENCES

1. Sotos JF. Overgrowth. Section II. Hormonal causes. Clin Pediatr 1996; 35:579–590.
2. Eugster EA, Pescovitz OH. Commentary: gigantism. J Clin Endocrinol Metab 1999; 84:4379–4384.
3. Lopis S, Rubenstein AH. Measurements of serum growth hormone and insulin in gigantism. J Clin Endocrinol Metab 1967; 28:393–398.
4. Frasier SD, Kogut MD. Adolescent acromegaly: studies of growth hormone and insulin metabolism. J Pediatr 1967; 71:832–839.
5. Spence HJ, Trias EP, Raiti S. Acromegaly in a 9 1/2 year old boy. Am J Dis Child 1972; 123:504–506.
6. AvRuskin TW, Say K, Tang S, Juan C. Childhood acromegaly: successful therapy with conventional radiation and effects of chlorpromazine on growth hormone and prolactin secretion. J Clin Endocrinol Metab 1973; 37: 380–388.
7. Haigler Jr ED, Hershman JM, Meador CK. Pituitary gigantism. Arch Intern Med 1973; 132:588–594.
8. Blumberg DK, Sklar CA, David R, Rothenberg S, Bell J. Acromegaly in an infant. Pediatr 1989; 83:998–1002.
9. Gelber SJ, Heffez DS, Donohoue PA. Pituitary gigantism caused by growth hormone excess from infancy. J Pediatr 1992; 120:931–934.
10. Lu PW, Silnik M, Johnston I, Cowell CT, Jimenez M. Pituitary gigantism. Arch Dis Child 1992; 667:1039–1041.
11. Guyda H, Robert F, Colle E, Hardy J. Histologic, ultrastructural, and hormonal characterization of a pituitary tumor secreting both hGH and prolactin. J Clin Endocrinol Metab 1973; 36:531–547.
12. Moran A, Asa SL, Kovacs K, Hovarth E, Singer W. Sagman U, Reubi JC, Wilson CB, Larson R, Pescovitz OH. Gigantism due to pituitary mammosomatotroph hyperplasia. N Engl J Med 1990; 323:322–327.
13. Dubuis JM, Deal CL, Drews RT, Goodyer CG, Lagacae G, Asa SL, Van Vliet G, Collu R. Mammosomatotroph adenoma causing gigantism in an 8-year old boy: a possible pathogenetic mechanism. Clin Endocrinol 1995; 42: 530–549.
14. Joishy SK, Morrow LB. McCune-Albright syndrome associated with a functioning chromophobe adenoma. J Pediatr 1976; 83:73–75.
15. Lighther, ES, Penny R, Frasier SD. Pituitary adenoma in McCune-Albright syndrome: follow-up information. J Pediatr 1976; 89:159.
16. Nakagawa H, Nagasaka A, Sugiura T, Nakagawa K, Yabe Y, Nehei N, Hirooka M, Itoh M, Ohyama T, Asono T, Gerich JE. Gigantism associated with McCune-Albright syndrome. Horm Metab Res 17:522–527.
17. Tinschert S, Gerl H, Gewies A, Jung HP, Neurnberg P. McCune Albright syndrome: clinical and molegular evidence of mosaicism in an unusual giant patient. Am J Med Genet 1999; 83:100–108.
18. Hoffman WH, Perrin JCS, Halac E, Gala RR, England BG. Acromegalic gigantism and tuberous sclerosis. J Pediatr 1978; 93:478–480.
19. Douchowny MD, Katz R, Bejar RL. Hypothalamic mass and gigantism in neurofibromatosis: treatment with bromocriptine. Ann Neurol 1984; 15:302–304.
20. Fuqua JS, Berkovitz GD. Growth hormone excess in a child with neurofibromatosis type I and optic pathway tumor: a patient report. Clin Pediatr 1998; 37:749–752.

21. Manski TJ, Haworth CS, Duval-Arnould BJ, Rushing EJ. Optic pathway glioma infiltrating into somatostatinergic pathways in a young boy with gigantism. J Neurosurg 1994; 81:595–600.
22. Zimmerman D, Young Jr WF, Ebersold MJ, Scheithauer BS, Kovaks K, Horvath E, Whitaker MD, Eberhardt NL, Downs TR, Frohman LA. Congenital gigantism due to growth hormone releasing hormone excess and pituitary hyperplasia with adenomatous transformation. J Clin Endocrinol Metab 1993; 76:216–221.
23. Asa SL, Scheithauer BS, Bilbao JM, Horvath E, Ryan N, Kovaks K, Randal RV, Laws Jr ER, Singer W, Linfoot JA, Thorner MO, Vale W. A case for hypothalamic acromegaly: a clinicopathological study of six patients with hypothalamic gangliocytoma containing gastrin and growth hormone-releasing factor. J Clin Endocrinol Metab 1984; 58:796–803.
24. Bevin JS, Asa SL, Rossi ML, Esiri MM, Adams CB, Burke CW. Intrasellar gangliocytoma containing gastrin and growth hormone-releasing hormone associated with a growth hormone-secreting pituitary adenoma. Clin Endocrinol 1989; 30:213–224.
25. Landis CA, Masters SB, Spada A, Pace AM, Bourne HR, Valler L. GTPase inhibiting mutations activate the a chain of Gs and stimulate adenylyl cyclase in human pituitary tumors. Nature 1989; 340:692–696.
26. Lyons J, Landis CA, Harsh G, Vallar L, Gruenwald, K, Feichtinger H, Duh Q-Y, Clark OH, Kawasaki E, Bourne HR, McCormick F. Two G protein oncogenes in human endocrine tumors. Science 1990; 249:655–659.
27. Shimon I, Melmed S. Genetic basis of endocrine disease. Pituitary tumor pathogenesis. J Clin Endocrinol Metab 1997; 82:1675–1681.
28. Weinstein LS, Shenker A, Gejman PV, Merino MJ, Friedman E, Spiegel AM. Activating mutations of stimulatory G protein in the McCune Albright syndrome. N Engl J Med 1991; 325:1688–1695.
29. Shenker A, Weinstein LS, Moran A, Peskovitz OH, Charest NJ, Boney CM, Van Wyk JJ, Merino MJ, Feuillan PP, Spiegel AM. Severe endocrine and nonendocrine manifestations of the McCune-Albright syndrome associated with activating mutations of stimulatory G protein Gs alpha. J Pediatr 1993; 123:509–518.
30. Yamada S, Yoshiomoto K, Sano T, Takada K, Itakura M, Usui M, Teramoto A. Inactivation of the tumor suppressor gene on 11q13 in brothers with familial acrogigantism without multiple endocrine neolasia type 1. J Clin Endocrinol Metab 1997; 82:239–242.
31. Gadelha MR, Prezant TR, Une KN, Glick RP, Moskal II SF, Vaisman S, Kineman RD, Frohman LA. Loss of heterozygosity on chromosome 11q13 in two families with acromegaly/gigantism is independent of mutations of the multiple endocrine neoplasia type 1 gene. J Clin Endocrinol Metab 1999; 84:249–256.
32. Ashcroft NW, Hartzband PI, Van Herle AJ, Bersch N, Golde DW. A unique growth factor in patients with acromegaloidism. J Clin Endocrinol Metab 1983; 57:272–276.
33. Clemmons DR, Van Wyk JJ, Ridgway EC, Kliman B, Kjellberg RN, Underwood LE. Evaluation of acromegaly by radioimmunoassay of somatomedin-C. N Engl J Med 1979; 301:1138–1142.
34. Frohman LA. Clinical review: therapeutic options in acromegaly. J Clin Endocrinol Metab 1991; 72:1175–1181.
35. Abe T, Tara LA, Ludecke DK. Growth hormone-secreting pituitary adenomas in childhood and adolescence: fea-

tures and results of transnasal surgery. Neurosurgery 1999; 45:1–10.

36. Lightner ES, Winder JD. Treatment of juvenile acromegaly with bromocriptine. J Pediatr 1981; 98:494–496.

37. Ritzen EM, Wetterell G, Davies G, Grand DM. Management of pituitary gigantism: the role of bromocriptine and radiotherapy. Acta Paediatr Scand 1985; 74:807–814.

38. Geffner, ME, Nagel RA, Dietrich RB, Kaplan SA. Treatment of acromegaly with a somatostatin analog in a patient with McCune-Albright syndrome. J Pediatr 1987; 111:740–743.

39. Barkan AL, Kelch RP, Hopwood NJ, Beitins IZ. Treatment of acromegaly with a long acting somatostatin analog SMS 201-995. J Clin Endocrinol 1988; 66:16–23.

40. Moran A, Peskovitz OH. Long-term treatment of gigantism with combination octreotide and bromocriptine in a child with McCune Albright syndrome. Endocrin J 1994; 2:111–113.

41. Caron P, Morange-Ramos I, Cogne M, Jaquet P. Three year follow-up of acromegalic patients treated with intramuscular slow-release lantreotide. J Clin Endocrinol Metab 1997; 82:18–22.

42. Flogstad AK, Halse J, Bakke S, Lancranjan I, Marbach P, Bruns C, Jervell J. Sandostatin LAR in acromegalic patients: long term treatment. J Clin Endocrinol Metab 1997; 82:23–28.

43. Whitehead EM, Shalet SM, Davies D, Enoch BA, Price DA, Beardwell CG. Pituitary gigantism: a disabling condition. Clin Endocrinol 1982; 17:271–277.

44. Sotos JF, Dodge PR, Muirhead D, Crawford JD, Talbot NB. Cerebral gigantism in childhood: a syndrome of excessively rapid growth with acromegalic features and a nonprogressive neurologic disorder. N Engl J Med 1964; 271:109–116.

45. Jaeken J, Van Der Scheren-Lodeweyckx M, Eeckels R. Cerebral gigantism syndrome. A report of 4 cases and a review of the literature. Z Kinderheilkd 1972; 112:332–346.

46. Sotos JF. Cerebral gigantism. Am J Dis Child 1977; 131: 625–627.

47. Wit JM, Beemer FA, Barth PG, Oorthuys JWE, Dijkstra PF, Van den Brande JL, Leschot NJ. Cerebra gigantism (Sotos syndrome). Compiled data of 22 cases. Analysis of clinical features, growth and plasma somatomedine. Eur J Pediatr 1985; 144:131–140.

48. Sotos JF. Overgrowth. Section V. Syndromes and other disorders associated with overgrowth. Clin Pediatr 1997; 37:91–103.

49. Beemer FA, Veenema H, de Pater JM. Cerebral gigantism (Sotos syndrome) in two patients with fra(X) chromosome. Am J Med Genet 1986; 23:221–226.

50. Whitaker MD, Scheithauer BW, Hayles AB, Okazaki H. The hypothalamus and pituitary in cerebral gigantism: a clinicopathologic and immunocytochemical study. Am J Dis Child 1985; 139:682–697.

51. Rutter SC, Cole TRP. Psychological characteristics of Sotos syndrome. Dev Med Child Neurol 1991; 33:898–902.

52. Agwu JC, Shaw NJ, Kirk J, Chapman S, Ravine D, Cole TRP. Growth in Sotos syndrome. Arch Dis Child 1999; 80:339–342.

53. Hersh JH, Cole TRP, Bloom AS, Bertolone SJ, Hughes HE. Risk of malignancy in Sotos syndrome. J Pediatr 1992; 80:250–258.

54. Caldwell PD, Smith DW. The XXY (Klinefelter's) syndrome in childhood: detection and treatment. J Pediatr 1972; 80:250–258.

55. Nielsen J, Wohlert M. Chromosome abnormalities found among 34910 newborn children: results from a 13 year incidence study in Arhus, Denmark. Hum Genet 1991; 87:81–81.

56. Sotos JF. Overgrowth. Section IV. Genetic disorders associated with overgrowth. Clin Pediatr 1997; 36:39–49.

57. Ratcliffe SG, Bancroft J, Axworthy D, McLaren W. Klinefelter's syndrome in adolescence. Arch Dis Child 1982; 57:6–12.

58. Ratcliffe SG. The sexual development of boys with the chromosome constitution 47,XXK (Klinefelter's syndrome). Clin Endocrinol Metab 1982; 11:703–716.

59. Salbenblatt JA, Bender BG, Puck MH, Robinson A, Faiman C, Winter JSD. Pituitary–gonadal function in Klinefelter syndrome before and during puberty. Pediar Res 1985; 19:82–86.

60. Ratcliffe SG, Butler GE, Jones M. Edinburgh study of growth and development of children with sex chromosome abnormalities IV. Birth Defects 1991; 26:1–44.

61. Walzer S, Bashir AS, Silbert AR. Cognitive and behavioral factors in the learning disabilities of 47,XXY and 47,XYY boys. Birth Defects 1991; 26:45–58.

62. Ratcliffe S. Long term outcome in children of sex chromosome abnormalities. Arch Dis Child 1999; 80:192–194.

63. Hasle H, Mellemgaard A, Nielsen J, Hansen J. Cancer incidence in men with Klinefelter syndrome. Br J Cancer 1995; 71:416–420.

64. Palermo GD, Schlegel PN, Sills ES, Veeck LL, Zaninovic N, Menendez S, Rosenwaks Z. Births after intracytoplasmic injection of sperm obtained by testicular extraction from men with nonmosaic Klinefelter's syndrome. N Engl J Med 1998; 338:588–590.

65. Ratcliffe SG, Pah H, McKie M. Growth during puberty in the XYY boy. Ann Hum Biol 1992; 19:579–587.

66. Court-Brown WM. Males with an XYY chromosome complement. J Med Genet 1968; 5:341–359.

67. Valentine GH, McClelland MA, Sergovich FR. The growth and development of four XYY infants. Pediatrics 1971; 48:583–594.

68. Dietz HC, Cutting GR, Pyeritz RE, Maslen CL, Sakai LY, Corson GM, Puffenberger EG, Hamosh A, Nanthakumar EJ, Curristin SM, Stetten G, Meyers DA, Francomano CA. Marfan syndrome caused by a recurrent de novo missense mutation in the fibrillin gene. Nature 1991; 352: 337–339.

69. Dietz HC, Pyeritz REA, Puffenberger EG, Kendzior RJ, Jr., Corson GM, Maslen CL, Sakai LY, Francomano CA, Cutting GR. Marfan phenotype variability in a family segregating a missense mutation in the epidermal growth factor-like motif of the fibrillin gene. J Clin Invest 1992; 89:1674–1680.

70. Kainulainen K, Pulkkinen L, Savolainen A, Kaitila I, Peltonen L. Location on chromosome 15 of the gene defect causing Marfan syndrome. New Engl J Med 1990; 323: 935–939.

71. Robinson PN, Godfrey M. The molecular genetics of Marfan syndrome and related microfibrillopathies. J Med Genet 2000; 37:9–25.

72. Milewicz D McG, Pyeritz RE, Crawford ES, Crawfore ES, Byers PH. Marfan syndrome: defective synthesis, secretion and extracellular matrix formation of fibrillin by cultured dermal fibroblasts. J Clin Invest 1992; 89:79–86.

73. Aoyama T, Francke U, Gasner C, Furthmyr H. Fibrillin

abnormalities and prognosis in Marfan syndrome and related disorders. Am J Med Genet 1995; 58:169–176.

74. Pyeritz RE, McKusick VA. The Marfan syndrome: diagnosis and management. N Engl J Med 1979; 300:772–777.

75. Pyeritz RE. The Marfan syndrome. Am Fam Physician 1986; 34:83–94.

76. Roberts WC, Honig HS. The spectrum of cardiovascular disease in the Marfan syndrome: a clinico-morphologic study of 18 necropsy patients and comparison to 151 previously reported necropsy patients. Am Heart J 1981; 104:115–135.

77. Gray JR, Bridges AB, West RR, McLeish L Stuart AG, Dean JCS, Proteous MEM, Boxer M, Davies SJ. Life expectancy in British Marfan syndrome populations. Clin Genet 1998; 54:124–128.

78. Carson NAJ, Cusworth DC, Dent CE, Field MB, Neill DW, Westall RG. Homocystinuria: a new inborn error of metabolism associated with mental deficiency. Arch Dis Child 1963; 38:425–436.

79. Mudd SH, Levy HL. Disorders of transsulfuraton. In Stanbury JB, Wyngaarden JB, Fredickson DS, Goldstein JL, Brown MS, eds.: The Metabolic Basis of Inherited Disease, 5th ed. New York: McGraw-Hill, 1983: 522–559.

80. Mudd SH, Skovby F, Levy HL, Pettigrew KD, Wilcken B, Pyeritz RE, Andria G, Boers GHJ, Bromberg IL, Cerone R, Fowler B, Grobe H, Schmidt H, Schweitzer L. The natural history of homocystinuria due to cystathionine B-synthase deficiency. Am J Hum Genet 1985; 37:1–31.

81. Skovby F. Homocystinuria: clinical, biochemical and genetic aspects of cystathionine B-synthase and its deficiency in man. Acta Paediatr Scand Suppl 1985; 321:1–21.

82. Kraus JP. Biochemisty and molecular genetics of cystathionine B-synthase deficiency. Eur J Pediatr 1998; 157 Suppl 2:S50–S53.

83. Rodgers GM, Chandler WL. Laboratory and clinical aspects of inherited thrombotic disorders. Am J Hematol 1992; 41:113–122.

84. Yap S, Naughten E. Homocystinuria due to cystathionine B-synthase deficiency in Ireland: 25 years' experience of a newborn screened and treated population with reference to clinical outcome and biochemical control. J Inher Metab Dis 1998; 21:738–747.

85. Pattenati MJ, Haines JL, Higgins RR, Wappner RS, Palmer CG, Weaver DD. Wiedemann-Beckwith syndrome: presentation of clinical and cytogenetic data on 22 new cases and review of the literature. Hum Genet 1986; 74:143–154.

86. Engstrom W, Lindham S, Schofield P. Wiedemann-Beckwith syndrome. Eur J Pediatr 1988; 147:450–457.

87. Sotos JF. Overgrowth. Section VI. Genetic syndromes and other disorders associated with overgrowth. Clin Pediatr 1997; 37:157–170.

88. Koufos A, Grundy P, Morgan K, Aleck KA, Hadro T, Lampkin BC, Kalbakji A, Cavenee WK. Familial Wiedemann-Beckwith syndrome and a second tumor locus both map to 11p15.5. Am J Hum Genet 1989; 44:711–719.

89. Ping AJ, Reeve AE, Law DJ, Young MR, Boehnke M, Feinberg AP. Genetic linkage of Beckwith-Wiedemann syndrome to 11p15.5. Am J Hum Genet 1989; 44:720–723.

90. Li M, Squire JA, Weksberg R. Molecular genetics of Wiedemann-Beckwith syndrome. Am J Med Genet 1998; 79:253–259.

91. Little M, Van Heyningen V, Hastie N. Dads, disomy and disease. Nature 1991; 351:609–610.

92. Henry I, Bonaiti-Pellie C, Chehensse V, Beldjord C, Schwartz C, Untermann G, Junien C. Uniparental paternal disomy in a genetic cancer-predisposing syndrome. Nature 1991; 351:665–667.

93. Viljoen D, Ramesar R. Evidence for paternal imprinting in familial Beckwith-Wiedemann syndrome. J Med Genet 1992; 29:221–225.

94. Li M, Squire JA, Weksberg R. Overgrowth syndromes and genomic imprinting: from mouse to man. Clin Genet 1998; 53:165–170.

95. Morison IM, Becroft, DM, Taniguchi T, Woods CG, Reeve AE. Somatic overgrowth associated with overexpression of insulin-like growth factor II. Nature Med 1996; 2:311–316.

96. Wiedemann HR. Tumours and hemihypertrophy associated with Wiedemann-Beckwith syndrome. J Med Genet 1992; 29:221–225.

97. Sotelo-Avila C, Gonzalez-Crussi F, Fowler JW. Complete and incomplete forms of Beckwith-Wiedemann syndrome: their oncogenic potential. J Pediatr 1980; 96:47–50.

98. Weng EY, Moeschler JB, Graham JM Jr. Longitudinal observations on 15 children with Wiedemann-Beckwith syndrome. Am J Med Genet 1995; 56:366–373.

99. Fraumeni JF Jr, Geiser CF, Manning MD. Wilms' tumor and congenital hemihypertrophy: report of five new cases and review of the literature. Pediatrics 1967; 40:886–899.

100. Stalens JP, Maton P, Gosseye S, Clapuyt P, Ninane J. Hemihypertrophy, bilateral Wilms' tumor, and clear-cell adenocarcinoma of the uterine cervix in a young girl. Med Pediatr Oncol 1993; 21:671–675.

101. Sotos JF. Overgrowth. Section I. Overgrowth disorders. Clin Pediatr 1996; 36:517–529.

102. Drop SLS, de Waal WJ, de Muinck Keizer-Sharama SMPF. Sex steroid treatment of constitutionally tall stature. Endocrinol Rev 1998; 19:540–558.

103. Pieters GFFM, Smals AGH, Kloppenborg PWC. Defective suppression of growth hormone after oral glucose loading in adolescence. J Clin Endocrinol Metab 1980; 51:265–270.

104. Evain-Brion D, Garnier P, Schimpff RM, Chaussain JL, Job JC. Growth hormone response to thyrotropin-releasing hormone and oral glucose loading in adolescents. J Clin Endocrinol Metab 1983; 56:429–432.

105. Eiholzer U, Torresani T, Bucher H, Prader A, Illig R. Paradoxical rise of growth hormone after oral glucose load in tall girls: a physiological finding in puberty? Pediatr Res 1985; 19:633.

106. Hindmarsh PC, Stanhope R, Kendall BE, Brook CGD. Tall stature: a clinical, endocrinological and radiological study. Clin Endocrinol 1986; 25:223–231.

107. Dickerman Z, Lowewinger J, Laron Z. The pattern of growth in children with constitutional tall stature from birth to age 9 years. Acta Paediatr Scand 1984; 73:530–536.

108. Bierich JR. Estrogen treatment of girls with constitutional tall stature. Pediatrics 1968; 62:1196–1201.

109. Whitelaw MJ. Experiences in treating excessive height in girls with cyclic oestradiol valerate: a ten year survey. Acta Endocrinol 1967; 54:473–484.

110. Andersen H, Jacobsen BB, Kastrup KW, Krabbe S, Peitersen B, Petersen KE, Thamdrup E, Wichmann R. Treatment of girls with excessive height prediction. Acta Paediatr Scand 1980; 59:293–297.

111. Colle ML, Alperin H, Greenblatt RB. The tall girl: prediction of mature height and management. Arch Dis Child 1977; 52:118–120.

112. Wettenhall HNB, Cahill C, Roche AF. Tall girls: a survey of 15 years of management and treatment. J Pediatr 1975; 86:602–610.

113. Crawford JD. Treatment of tall girls with estrogen. Pediatr 1968; 62:1189–1197.

114. Gruters A, Heidemann P, Schlugter H, Stubbe P, Weber B, Helge H. Effect of different oestrogen doses on final height reduction in girls with constitutional tall stature. Eur J Pediatr 1989; 149:11–13.

115. de Waal WJ, Torn M, de Muinck Keizer-Schrama SMPF, Aarsen RSR, Drop SLS. Long term sequelae of sex steroid treatment in the management of constitutionaly tall stature. Arch Dis Child 1995; 73:311–315.

116. Prader A, Zachmann M. Treatment of excessively tall girls and boys with sex hormones. Pediatrics 1978; 62:1202–1210.

117. Kuhn B, Blunck W, Stanhnke N, Weibel J, Willig RP. Estrogen treatment in tall girls. Acta Paediatr Scand 1977; 66:161–167.

118. Frasier SD, Smith FG Jr. Effect of estrogens on mature height in tall girls: a controlled study. J Clin Endocrinol Metab 1968; 28:416–419.

119. Schoen EJ, Solomon IL, Warner O, Wingerd J. Estrogen treatment of tall girls. Am J Dis Child 1973; 125:71–74.

120. Binder G, Grauer ML, Wehner AV, Wehner F, Ranke MB. Outcome in tall stature. Final height and psychological aspects in 220 patients with and without treatment. Eur J Pediatr 1997; 156:905–910.

121. Weimann E, Bergmann S, Bohles HJ. Oestrogen treatment of constitutional tall stature: a risk–benefit ratio. Arch Dis Child 1998; 78:148–151.

122. Sorgo W, Scholler K, Heinze F, Heinze E, Teller WM. Critical analysis of height reduction in estrogen-treated tall girls. Eur J Pediatr 1984; 142:260–265.

123. Werder EA, Waibel P, Sege D, Flury R. Severe thrombosis during oestrogen treatment for tall stature. Eur J Pediatr 1990; 149:389–390.

124. Hanker JP, Schellong G, Schneider HPG. The functional state of the hypothalmo-pituitary axis after high-dose estrogen therapy in excessively tall girls. Acta Endocrinol (Kbh) 1979; 91:19–29.

125. Skovby F, McKusick VA. Estrogen treatment of tall stature in girls with the Marfan syndrome. Birth Defect Orig Art Ser 1977; 13:155–161.

126. Zachmann M, Ferrandez A, Murset G, Gnehm HE, Prader A. Testosterone treatment of excessively tall boys. J Pediatr 1976; 88:116–123.

127. Bettendorf M, Heinrich UE, Schonberg DK, Grulich-Henn J. Short-term, high-dose testosterone treatment fails to reduce adult height in boys with constitutional tall stature. Eur J Pediatr 1997; 156:911–915.

128. de Wall WJ, Vreeburg JTM, Bekkering F, de Jong FH, de Muinck Keizer-Schrama MPF, Drop SLS, Weber RFA. High dose testosterone therapy for reduction of final height in constitutionally tall boys: does it influence testicular function in adulthood? Clin Endocrinol 1995; 43:87–95.

129. Lemcke B, Zentgraf J, Behre HM, Kliesch S, Branswig JH, Nieschlag E. Long-term effects on testicular function of high-dose testosterone treatment for excessively tall stature. J Clin Endocrinol Metab 1996; 81:296–301.

130. Evain-Brion D, Garnier P, Blanco-Garcia M, Job J. Studies in constitutionally tall adolescents. II Effects of bromocriptine on growth hormone secretion and adult height prediction. J Clin Endocrinol Metab 1984; 58:1022–1026.

131. Schwarz HP, Joss EE, Zuppinger KA. Bromocriptine treatment in adolescent boys with familial tall stature: a pair-matched controlled study. J Clin Endocrinol Metab 1987; 65:136–140.

132. Schoenle EJ, Theintz G, Torresani T, Prader A, Illig R, Sizonenko PC. Lack of bromocriptine-induced reduction of predicted height in tall adolescents. J Clin Endocrinol Metab 1987; 65:355–358.

133. Hindmarsh PC, Pringle PJ, di Silvio L, Brook CGD. A preliminary report on the role of somatostatin analogue (SMS 201-995) in the management of children with tall stature. Clin Endocrinol 1990; 32:83–91.

134. Tauber MT, Tauber JP, Vigoni F, Harris AG, Rochicchioli P. Effect of the long-acting somatostatin analogue SMS 201-995 on growth rate and reduction of predicted adult height in ten tall adolescents. Acta Paediatr Scand 1990; 79:176–181.

135. de Waal WJ, Greyn-Fokker MH, Stijnen TH, van Gurp EAFJ, Toolens AMP, de Muinck Keizer-Schrama SMPF, Aarsen RSR, Drop SLS. Accuracy of final height prediction and effect of growth-reductive therapy in 362 constitutionally tall children. J Clin Endocrinol Metab 1996; 81:1206–1216.

6

Adrenal Cortex: Hypo- and Hyperfunction

Claude J. Migeon
Johns Hopkins University School of Medicine and Johns Hopkins Hospital, Baltimore, Maryland, U.S.A.

Roberto L. Lanes
Hospital de Clinicas Caracas and Universidad Central de Venezuela, Caracas, Venezuela

I. INTRODUCTION

The adrenal gland is made of two parts, the cortex and the medulla, which have different embryonic origins. By 4–5 weeks of fetal life, cells from the mesoderm aggregate to form a primitive cortex between the posterior part of the dorsal mesentery and the gonadal ridge (1). Shortly thereafter, this primitive cortex becomes surrounded by a narrow band of cells termed permanent cortex. By 7–8 weeks of fetal life, the primitive cortex is invaded by chromaffin cells that develop rapidly and eventually replace most of the primitive cortical cells, forming the medulla (1). At that time, the adrenal gland is in close relation with the cranial part of the primitive kidney and not far from the genital ridge.

The adrenal medulla, which originates from ectodermal cells, has an entirely different function from the mesodermal adrenal cortex. In this chapter only the latter is discussed.

In the adult, the adrenal cortex is made of three distinctive zones. The outer zona glomerulosa secretes aldosterone; the middle zona fasciculata and the inner zona reticularis together are involved in the secretion of the cortisol and adrenal androgens (1). We first discuss the physiological function of the adrenal cortex. Then we consider the disorders related to the hyposecretion and hypersecretion of adrenal cortical hormones.

II. PHYSIOLOGY

A. Biosynthesis of Adrenocortical Steroids

1. The Enzymes

Cholesterol is the precursor of all steroids of both gonadal and adrenocortical origin (2). The biosynthetic pathway of adrenal steroids is shown in Figure 1. The conversion of cholesterol to the various hormones requires the sequential action of a series of six enzymes, as listed in Table 1. All but 3β-hydroxysteroid dehydrogenase are members of a family of enzymes termed cytochromes P450. They are heme-containing proteins that act as mixed-function oxidases (3). Three of these enzymes have a very similar structure: cholesterol side-chain cleavage enzyme encoded by the gene CYP11A, 11β-hydroxylase encoded by CYP11B1, and aldosterone synthetase encoded by CYP11B2. The last two genes are contiguous on the long arm of chromosome 8q22. The gene CYP11A is located on chromosome 15q23–24; this enzyme requires the activity of another gene product, the steroidogenic acute regulatory protein (StAR).

The cholesterol side-chain cleavage enzyme has the ability to add a hydroxyl group on carbons 20 and 22 of the cholesterol molecule as well as to remove a side chain between carbons 20 and 22 (4). The 3β-hydroxysteroid dehydrogenase (3β-HSD) converts pregnenolone to progesterone as well as 17α-hydroxypregnenolone to 17α-hydroxyprogesterone; this is accomplished by reduction of the 3,β-hydroxyl group into a 3-ketone and isomerization of the 5,6 double bond to a 3,4 double bond. Its gene is located in chromosome 1p13.1 The 17α-hydroxylase enzyme (chromosome 10 q24–25) has the ability of both 17α-hydroxylation and 17,20-lyase. The latter activity transforms steroids with 21 carbons into steroids with 19 carbons. 21-Hydroxylase (CYP21) and 11β-hydroxylase (CYP11B1) are specific for the function of adding a hydroxyl group in carbons 21 and 11, respectively. Aldosterone synthetase (CYP11B2) adds an 11β-hydroxyl group and an 18-hydroxyl group and is also capable of 18-oxidation (5). Whereas the CYP11A, 3β-HSD, and CYP21 genes are expressed in all the zones of the adrenal

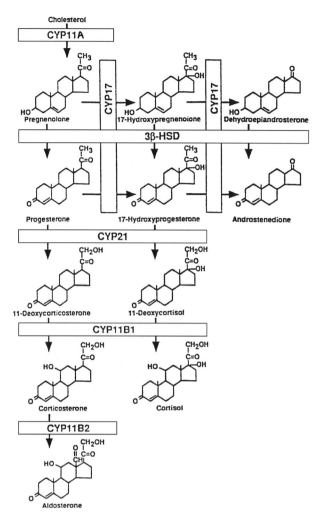

Figure 1 Biosynthesis of adrenocortical steroids. The pathway from cholesterol to cortisol, aldosterone, and adrenal androgens requires the action of five cytochrome P450 (CYP11A, CYP17, CYP21, CYP11B1, and CYP11B2) and one dehydrogenase (3β-hydroxysteroid dehydrogenase). (From Ref. 2.)

Table 1 Nomenclature for the Various Steroid Biosynthetic Enzymes and the Respective Genes

Enzyme activity	Gene	Chromosomal locus
Cholesterol side-chain cleavage enzyme (20-hydroxylase, 22-hydroxylase, 20,22-lyase)	*CYP11A*	15223–q24
3β-Hydroxysteroid dehydrogenase	*3β-HSD*	1p13.1
17α-Hydroxylase and 17,20-lyase	*CYP17*	10q24–q25
21-Hydroxylase	*CYP21*	6p21
11β-Hydroxylase (some 18-hydroxylation)	*CYP11B1*	8q22
Aldosterone synthetase (11β-hydroxylation, 18-hydroxylation, and 18-oxidation)	*CYP11B2*	8q22

resulting steroids include 11-deoxycorticosterone (DOC) and 11-deoxycortisol as well as two C-19 carbon steroids, androstenedione and dehydroepiandrosterone (DHA). At that point, DOC and 11-deoxycortisol return to the mitochondria, where they are converted into corticosterone and cortisol, respectively. This is basically the end of the biosynthetic process in the cells of the zona fasciculata.

In the cells of the zona glomerulosa, there is no 17-hydroxylase activity and, therefore, no formation of cortisol or androgens. However, the mitochondria of these cells include CYP11B2 enzyme, which transforms DOC into corticosterone, 18-hydroxycorticosterone, and aldosterone.

Finally, it must be noted that the activity of all cytochrome P450 enzymes requires a gain of electrons. These electrons are transferred from NADPH. In the mitochondria this transfer is made via two intermediaries, adrenodoxin and adrenodoxin reductase, whereas in the microsomes the transfer requires only the presence of an adrenodoxin (2).

3. The Placental–Fetal Adrenal Unit

Early in fetal life, the adrenal cortex is capable of secreting steroids. It lacks 3β-hydroxysteroid dehydrogenase, however, and the major hormones secreted include pregnenolone, 17α-hydroxypregnenolone, DHA, and 16α-hydroxy-DHA. All these steroids circulate mainly as sulfate conjugates, which are then transferred to the placenta (Fig. 3) (1). This organ is rich in sulfatase, which makes the native steroids available to the greatly active placental 3β-hydroxysteroid dehydrogenase. The resulting progesterone and 17α-hydroxyprogesterone are returned in part to the fetus and are used by the fetal adrenal to make aldosterone and cortisol and by the fetal gonad to make testosterone.

cortex, the CYP17 and CYP11B1 genes are expressed only in the zona fasciculata–reticularis and the CYP11B2 gene is expressed only in the zona glomerulosa. This accounts for the specificity of steroid production by the various zones of the cortex.

2. Subcellular Location of the Various Enzymes

As shown in Figure 2, cholesterol is stored in the adrenal cell as cholesterol esters. Under the influence of an esterase, cholesterol becomes available and is transported to the mitochondria, where it is converted to pregnenolone (2). This steroid then moves into the endoplasmic reticulum, where 3β-hydroxysteroid dehydrogenase, 21-hydroxylase, and 17-hydroxylase enzymes are located. The

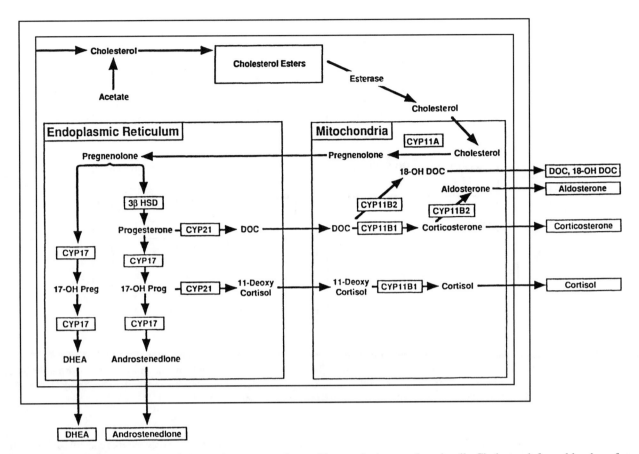

Figure 2 Subcellular location of the various steps of steroidogenesis in an adrenal cell. Cholesterol from blood or from intracellular synthesis is stored as cholesterol esters. An esterase makes cholesterol available when needed. CYP11A is located in the mitochondria. The pregnenolone formed moves to the endoplastic reticulum where it is submitted to the effects of 3β-HSD, CYP17, and CYP21. The resulting 11-deoxycorticosterone (DOC) and 11-deoxycortisol return to the mitochondria where the CYP11B1 and CYP11B2 cytochromes are located. The main steroids secreted by the adrenal cortex are shown outside of the adrenal cell. (From Ref. 2.)

The placental 3β-hydroxysteroid dehydrogenase also transforms DHA and its 16α-hydroxylated derivative into androstenedione and its 16α-hydroxylated derivative. In the next step, placental aromatase transforms androstenedione into estrone and estradiol, whereas 16α-hydroxyandrostenedione is metabolized into estriol. Most of these estrogens are excreted by the mother. The large amounts of estriol excreted by the mother are related to the large amounts of 16α-OH-DHA secreted by the adrenal cortex of the fetus.

B. Control of Adrenal Steroid Secretion

1. Regulation of Cortisol Secretion

The ability of the adrenal gland to synthesize cortisol is dependent upon the secretion by the hypothalamus of corticotropin-releasing hormone (CRH). By the use of the short loop of the portal vessel system from the hypothalamus to the anterior pituitary, CRH reaches the cortico-

trophs and triggers the secretion of adrenocorticotropic hormone (ACTH).

a. CRH and ACTH. CRH is a 41 amino acid straight-chain peptide (6). It is secreted mainly by the median eminence. However, it has also been detected in the cortical part of the brain. CRH binds with high affinity to receptors located on the membrane of the corticotrophs of the anterior pituitary. This in turn activates the formation of cyclic AMP, which then activates a series of protein kinases, resulting in increased transcription of the pro-opiomelanocortin gene; appropriate processing of this mRNA results in ACTH formation. ACTH has a half-life in blood of a few minutes. Although the native hormone has 39 amino acid residues, the first 1–24 amino-acid sequence has as much activity as the ACTH itself (7). Like other peptide hormones, ACTH binds to specific membrane receptors of the adrenocortical cells to increase the formation of cyclic AMP and activation of various protein kinases. The ACTH stimulation of cortisol secretion in-

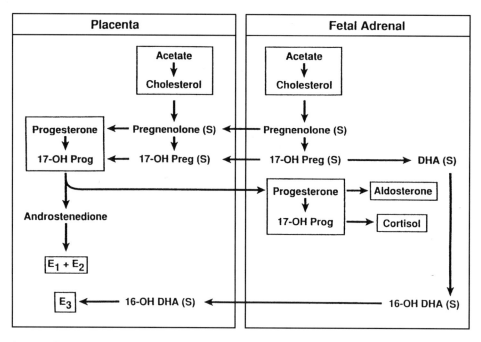

Figure 3 The placenta–fetal adrenal unit. The fetal adrenal can readily synthesize pregnenolone, 17-hydroxypregnenolone, and 16-hydroxy-DHA. However, it has little or no 3β-HSD. The placenta, which is rich in this enzyme, transforms the fetal steroids into progesterone, 17-hydroxyprogesterone, and estriol. In the next step, progesterone and 17-hydroxyprogesterone are returned to the fetal adrenal, which can then synthesize aldosterone and cortisol. (From Ref. 1.)

cludes an acute and chronic phase (2). In the acute phase, which takes only a few minutes, cholesterol is made available for steroidogenesis by activating the effect of an esterase on stored cholesterol esters. The more chronic phase is related to a stimulation of transcription of the various cytochrome P450 genes. A so-called steroidogenetic factor 1 (SF-1) appears to be responsible for this stimulation (8). Of great interest is the recent finding that SF-1 is also a transcription factor. Along with DAX-1, it plays a major role in the formation of steroidogenic tissues, specifically the adrenal glands and the gonads (9).

b. Mechanisms Regulating Cortisol Secretion. Three physiological mechanisms play an important role in the secretion of cortisol: pulsatile secretion and diurnal variation, stress, and negative feedback.

Pulsatile secretion and diurnal variation in cortisol. The collection of blood samples at frequent intervals has shown that cortisol is secreted in a pulsatile manner (10). Previously (11) it was observed that the plasma concentration of cortisol showed a specific diurnal variation, the highest peak taking place between 4 and 6 a.m. The concentrations then tend to decrease for the rest of the day, being at their lowest in the evening and during the night (Fig. 4).

Stress. Surgical stress, such as trauma and tissue destruction; medical stress, such as acute illness, fever, and hypoglycemia; and emotional stress related to psychological upset result in most cases in an important increase in

cortisol secretion. How these various types of stress influence steroid output is not clear. However, studies of the immune system have shown that leukocytes secrete a series of peptide hormones, the interleukins (12). Their formation is markedly increased during stress, and two of them, interleukin-1 and interleukin-6, have been shown to stimulate CRH secretion and therefore to increase cortisol secretion (13).

Negative feedback. Another important physiological mechanism controlling cortisol secretion is negative feedback. Under normal conditions, there is equilibrium between the rate of secretion of ACTH and that of cortisol. When the plasma concentration of cortisol increases markedly, it has a negative effect on the secretion of CRH and ACTH. By this mechanism, cortisol levels in blood regulate the rate of output of CRH and ACTH.

c. Cortisol Secretion Rate. In normal children of various ages and in adult subjects, the rate of cortisol secretion increases with body size (14). When the values are corrected for body surface area, the rates are similar at various ages; the average ± standard deviation (SD) was 12 ± 2 (Fig. 5) with a range of 8–16 mg/m^2/24 h. However, the circadian variation of the clearance rate of cortisol resulted in an overestimation. An appropriate correction gave a lower normal range of 6–14 mg/m^2/24 h. Using stable isotope dilution/mass spectometry Esteban et al. (15) reported a cortisol secretion rate for 12 normal subjects of 5.7 ± 1.5 mg/m^2/24 h. Kerrigan et al. (16),

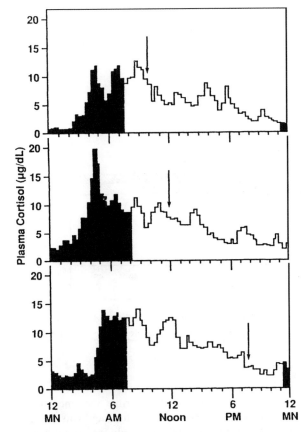

Figure 4 Diurnal variation of plasma cortisol in three normal adult subjects. Black areas represent periods of sleep. (From Ref. 105.)

using deconvolution analysis, found a similar value in 18 normal male children.

2. Regulation of Aldosterone Secretion

Aldosterone is secreted by the cells of the zona glomerulosa of the adrenal cortex. It is mainly under the control of angiotensin II. As shown in Figure 6, the liver produces a large protein, angiotensinogen, which is cleaved by a proteolytic enzyme, renin, which is secreted by the juxtaglomerular cells of the kidney. A converting enzyme then transforms angiotensin I into angiotensin II.

Potassium concentration in plasma and ACTH also play a role in the control of aldosterone secretion. The effect of ACTH is an acute stimulation related to the rapid increase in availability of cholesterol from the cholesterol ester reserve (17). As shown in Figure 7, an intravenous (IV) injection of ACTH very quickly raises plasma aldopchsterone levels, but after 60 min the levels tend to decrease.

3. Regulation of Adrenal Androgen Secretion

Adrenal androgens are secreted in large amounts during fetal life. Their production decreases rapidly after birth

and is not resumed until puberty. The factor that triggers the pubertal secretion of adrenal androgens is not ACTH because its levels are not different before and after puberty. However, large amounts of ACTH given chronically markedly increase the secretion of adrenal androgens. It has been postulated that a pituitary peptide other than ACTH but not yet characterized is responsible for this stimulation, and it has been named adrenal androgen-stimulating hormone (18).

C. General Metabolism

As shown in Figure 8, adrenal steroids are transported by blood to reach their target tissues. The liver is one of the target tissues as well as an important site for the catabolism of the steroids. The main glucocorticoid is cortisol. Between 80 and 90% is bound to a specific glycosylated α-globulin known as corticosteroid-binding globulin (CBG), also called transcortin (19). Transcortin has a very high affinity for cortisol, but it can also bind progesterone, prednisolone, and, with less affinity, aldosterone (20). Another 7% of the total circulating cortisol is loosely bound to albumin, and 2–3% is not bound to protein. This unbound cortisol is the fraction of the total available to target cells. In these cells, cortisol binds to a specific glucocorticoid receptor. The receptor–steroid complex binds to the glucocorticoid receptor elements located in the promoter area of responsive genes. By activating the transcription of such genes, glucocorticoids express their biological activity.

The main mechanism of catabolism is a reduction of the steroid molecule and eventually conjugation with glucuronic or sulfuric acid to make products that are water soluble and readily excreted by the kidney as urinary metabolites.

Although aldosterone can bind to CBG, most of the binding sites of this protein are occupied by cortisol. For this reason, aldosterone is physiologically mainly bound to albumin. Its half-life in blood is 20–30 min, compared with 60–80 min for cortisol. In target cells, aldosterone binds to its own specific receptor, the mineralocorticoid receptor. The mode of action of this steroid–receptor complex is similar to that described for cortisol.

D. Tests of Adrenocortical Function

Many types of tests have been proposed for the determination of adrenocortical function. We outline here only the tests considered important and practical for diagnostic purposes.

1. Tests Related to Glucocorticoid Function

a. 8 a.m. Plasma Cortisol Concentrations. It is necessary to obtain plasma levels of cortisol at a specific time of the day (8 a.m.) because of the diurnal variation discussed earlier. However, even this precaution may not

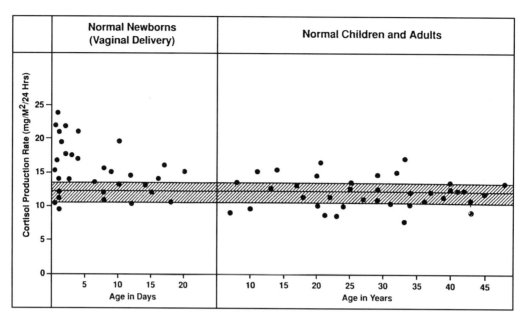

Figure 5 Cortisol secretion rate in newborn infants, children and adults. The values have been corrected for body surface area. The rates expressed in mg/m²/24 h, were fairly constant throughout life except in the first few days when they were somewhat higher. (From Ref. 1.)

be sufficient because of the episodic secretion of the steroid. In general, a single plasma value is of limited clinical significance. There are conditions for which one must determine the plasma concentrations of cortisone and corticosterone. Normally, their concentrations are approximately one-tenth that of cortisol at 8 a.m. Changes in the ratios of these steroids to cortisol in a single blood sample may therefore be indicative of a specific abnormality of adrenal secretion.

b. Urinary 17-Hydroxycorticosteroids. About 30% of secreted cortisol is excreted as urinary 17-hydroxycorticosteroids (17-OHCS). For this reason, determination of 24 h urine excretion gives a good indication of the 24 h cortisol secretion. Indeed, this test is of interest in ruling out Cushing's disease. In normal subjects, the mean ± SD urinary 17-OHCS is 2.5 ± 1.0 mg/m²/24 h (14).

c. Urinary Free Cortisol. Approximately 0.25–0.5% of secreted cortisol is excreted as cortisol itself. Because urinary free cortisol reflects the amount of unbound cortisol available to target cells (ie, non-protein-bound cortisol), this test is considered of greater biological importance than that of urinary 17-OHCS. In our opinion, however, both tests should be obtained in a single 24 h urine specimen when screening for Cushing syndrome.

d. ACTH Test. At present, the standard technique involves the IV bolus administration of 0.25 mg 1,24-ACTH (Cortrosyn). Blood samples are obtained at 0, 60, and 120 min after ACTH injection. As seen in Figure 7, plasma cortisol increases to about 30 μg/dl (17).

A normal baseline and a normal increment by 120 min rule out primary adrenal insufficiency. This test is also useful when determining the mineralocorticoid function of the adrenals. Recent studies have shown that administration of a very low amount of ACTH (1 μg) may be more sensitive than the standard 250 μg test in the detection of dysfunction of the hypothalamopituitary–adrenal axis. This would be particularly true in mild adrenal insufficiency, as can be seen in the case of pituitary disease or with the use of inhaled steroids as reported by Mayenknecht et al. (21) and Nye et al. (22).

e. Metyrapone (Metopirone) Test. Given acutely, Metopirone has the property of blocking 11β-hydroxylation. This results in decreased secretion of cortisol and corticosterone with a decrease in negative feedback on the hypothalamic–pituitary axis. As a consequence, there is an increase in ACTH secretion with an increased secretion of 11-deoxysteroid, specifically 11-deoxycortisol (compound S), and 11-deoxycorticosterone. The present standardized test consists of the administration of a single oral dose of Metopirone (300 mg/m²/per dose) at midnight and measurement the next day at 8 a.m. of plasma 11-deoxycortisol. If adrenocortical function is normal and if the pituitary is capable of increasing its ACTH secretion, the plasma concentration of 11-deoxycortisol rises to values of 7–22 μg/dl (23).

There is the possibility that Metopirone may not be available commercially in the near future. If this occurs, the acute ACTH test described earlier can give similar information.

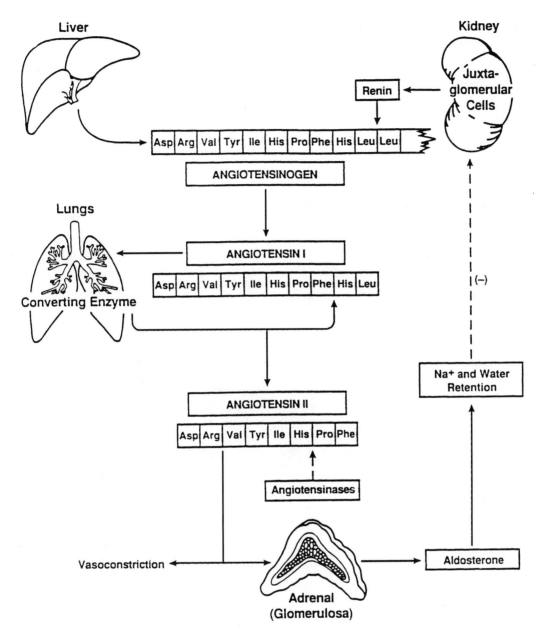

Figure 6   Control of aldosterone secretion. Angiotensinogen of hepatic origin is cleaved by renin from the kidney. The resulting angiotensin I is further cleaved into angiotensin II, an 8 amino-acid peptide that has properties of vasoconstriction on vessels and of activating secretion of aldosterone by the cells of the glomerulosa. (From Ref. 1.)

f. Dexamethasone Suppression Test. Dexamethasone is a potent glucocorticoid that, given in small amounts, suppresses ACTH secretion and secondarily decreases cortisol secretion. The suppressing effects of the test are measured by the determination of either plasma ACTH and cortisol or urinary excretion of free cortisol and total 17-OHCS. In the low-dose or single-dexamethasone suppression test, 1.25 mg dexamethasone/m^2/24 h is

administered for 2 days. In the high-dose or triple-dexamethasone suppression test, 3.75 mg dexamethasone/m^2/24 h is administered for an additional 2 days.

g. The CRH Test. Following the IV administration of CRH (100 μg/dose), there is a moderate but significant increase in both plasma cortisol and ACTH, the maximum response being about 60 min after injection. In Cushing's

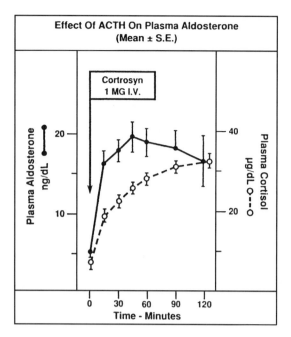

Figure 7 Effects of 1,24-ACTH on the plasma concentration of cortisol and aldosterone in 16 normal subjects. (From Ref. 15.)

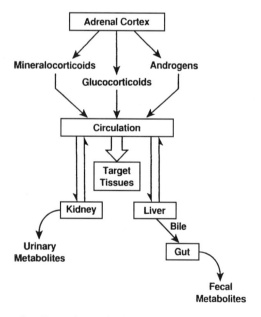

Figure 8 General metabolism of adrenal steroids. In the blood circulation, the steroids are mainly bound to specific proteins. The small unbound fraction is available to target tissues where the steroids express their biological effects. At the same time, steroids are metabolized and conjugated by the liver. The conjugates are returned to the circulation and excreted in bile by the kidney as urinary metabolites. (From Ref. 1.)

disease, there is a greatly exaggerated response of both plasma cortisol and ACTH, whereas in ectopic ACTH syndrome there is no change, as shown in Figure 9 (24).

2. Tests Related to Mineralocorticoid Secretion

a. Plasma Aldosterone and 11-Deoxycorticosterone. Concentrations of plasma aldosterone are quite variable, changing rapidly in relation to body posture, the standing values being greater than those while supine (17). Plasma concentrations of aldosterone are also influenced by chronic changes in sodium intake, the concentration being 15–30 ng/dl on a low-sodium diet (less than 17 mEq/24 h) and 2–12 ng/dl on a normal-sodium diet (150–200 mEq/24 h in adults).

The plasma concentrations of DOC, like those of aldosterone, tend to be higher in early infancy (from 8 to 5 ng/dl) than later in childhood (5–10 ng/dl), as reported by Lashansky et al. (25).

As shown in Figure 7, ACTH acutely increases aldosterone concentration. There is also a three- to fivefold increase in DOC.

b. Urinary Excretion of Aldosterone and DOC. A small fraction of secreted aldosterone is excreted as a 21-oxoglucuronide conjugate. Following hydrolysis at pH 1.0, aldosterone is freed and is measured by radioimmunoassay. Under normal sodium intake, the values are 3–10 μg/24 h and, on a low-sodium diet, they are 20–50 μg/24 h.

III. HYPOADRENOCORTICISM

Adrenal insufficiency can be caused by an abnormality of the adrenal glands (primary adrenocortical insufficiency) or by a decreased secretion of hypothalamic CRH and pituitary ACTH (hypoadrenocorticism secondary to deficient CRH and/or ACTH secretion). In rare cases the insufficiency is related to an inability of the target organs to respond to adrenal steroids (hypoadrenocorticism related to end-organ unresponsiveness). The classification of these various disorders is outlined in Table 2.

IV. HYPOADRENOCORTICISM: PRIMARY ADRENOCORTICAL INSUFFICIENCY

There are many causes of primary adrenal insufficiency (Table 2). In some cases, there has been a lack of differentiation of the glands (congenital adrenal aplasia) or inappropriate development (X-linked adrenal hypoplasia). In other cases, a mutation of the ACTH receptor on the membrane of the adrenocortical cells does not permit adequate stimulation of adrenal secretion (adrenocortical unresponsiveness to ACTH). Another group of abnormalities involves a mutation of one of the enzymes necessary for steroid biosynthesis (congenital adrenal hyperplasia, adrenoleukodystrophy, acid lipase deficiency, steroid sulfa-

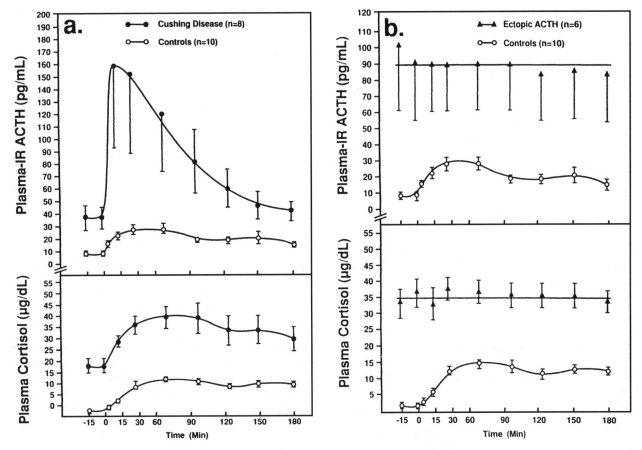

Figure 9   The CRH stimulation test. The figure shows the response of plasma cortisol and ACTH to IV administration of 100 μg CRH (a) in adult controls and in patients with Cushing's disease and (b) in patients with Cushing's due to ectopic ACTH. (From Ref. 20.)

tase deficiency, and mineralocorticoid deficiency). Finally, there can be postnatal destruction of the adrenal cortex, either acute (adrenal hemorrhage) or chronic (Addison's disease).

A.   Congenital Adrenal Aplasia

This is believed to be caused by a developmental disorder of the adrenal anlage during fetal life. Symptoms occur shortly after birth and are characterized by acute shock with tachycardia, hyperpyrexia, cyanosis, and rapid respiration. Untreated, it evolves to total vascular collapse and death. The symptoms of congenital adrenal aplasia are similar to those present in other conditions, such as septicemia and intracranial hemorrhage. The rapid evolution of adrenal aplasia to death is the reason it is often diagnosed at autopsy.

B.   X-Linked Adrenal Hypoplasia Congenita

Among families presenting multiple cases of adrenal insufficiency, several suggested the possibility of an X-

linked trait. In 1980, Guggenheim et al. (26) reported an association of glycerol kinase deficiency (GKD) with Duchenne muscular dystrophy (DMD) and adrenal hypoplasia congenita (AHC). Later, these disorders were reported to be associated with Xp21 interstitial deletion (27).

1.   Pathophysiology

The deletions of the X chromosome associated with AHC, GKD, and DMD have permitted mapping the locus of these three disorders, as well as the locus of chronic granulomatous disease, retinitis pigmentosa, and ornithine transcarbamylase deficiency, the last being the closest to the centromere, and AHC being the closest to the end of Xp (28). However, it is not clear how the deletion of the AHC locus results in hypoplastic adrenals. The adrenal cortex in patients studied at autopsy shows a small number of large adrenocortical cells, hence the name cytomegalic adrenal hypoplasia given by pathologists.

Table 2 Classification of Syndromes of Hypoadrenocorticism

Primary adrenocortical insufficiency
  Congenital adrenal aplasia
  X-linked adrenal hypoplasia
  Adrenocortical unresponsiveness to ACTH (deficient
    ACTH receptor)
  Congenital adrenal hyperplasia (CAH)
  Adrenoleukodystrophy/adrenomyeloneuropathy
  Wolman disease (acid lipase deficiency)
  Steroid sulfatase deficiency (X-linked ichthyosis)
  Mineralocorticoid CMOI or CMOII (CYP11B2)
    deficiency
  Adrenal hemorrhage of the newborn
  Adrenal hemorrhage of acute infection
  Chronic hypoadrenocorticism (Addison's disease)
Secondary to deficiency CRH and/or ACTH secretion
  Hypopituitarism
  Cessation of glucocorticoid therapy
  Removal of a unilateral cortisol-producing tumor
  Infants born to steroid-treated mothers
  Respiratory distress syndrome
  Anencephaly
Related to end-organ unresponsiveness
  Cortisol resistance (deficient glucocorticoid receptor)
  Aldosterone resistance (deficient mineralocorticoid
    receptor)

2. Clinical Manifestations and Mapping of Xp2l

AHC appears early in infancy with signs of acute adrenal insufficiency. However, the signs may occur later in childhood and be somewhat milder. Growth failure with short stature is often observed. In AHC caused by a deletion involving other genetic loci, such as GKD and DMD, signs of glycerol kinase deficiency and myopathy are also present.

In a series of patients presenting with the association of AHC, GKD, and DMD, mental retardation was reported in most of the cases, suggesting the existence of a contiguous locus involved in mental function (29). However, it must be considered that subjects with adrenal insufficiency may have intrinsic reasons for mental retardation in relation to hypoglycemic episodes and abnormal electrolyte imbalance. It is believed that the gene locus of adrenal hypoplasia congenita is the DAX-1 gene (30). As previously noted, DAX-1 plays a major role in the differentiation of fetal cells into both adrenal glands and gonads. In addition, it is necessary for the formation of the hypothalamus, in cooperation with the SF-1 transcription factor. This explains why abnormalities of the DAX-1 gene result in hypogonadotropic hypogonadism (HH) in addition to AHC. Finally, it is of interest to note that a duplication of DAX-1 locus results in testicular abnormalities in 46, XY subjects (31). This is related to the

complex relationships of DAX-1 with the SRY and SF-1 proteins during male sex differentiation.

3. Laboratory

Hormonal and electrolyte studies are characteristic of adrenocortical insufficiency: low basal cortisol and aldosterone levels responding poorly to an ACTH test, elevated ACTH concentrations, and hyponatremic, hyperkalemic acidosis. GKD association is demonstrated by elevated serum and urine glycerol levels. Because glycerol is measured in the triglyceride assay, there is pseudohypertriglyceridemia. Muscle biopsy showing elevated serum creatine kinase confirms Duchenne muscular dystrophy. Results of a luteinizing hormone-releasing hormone (LHRH) test helps in determining hypogonadotropic hypogonadism (32).

4. Genetics

The clinical abnormalities of AHC and associated disorders in patients with Xp2ldel most probably demonstrate a relation of cause to effects between the chromosomal deletion and the specific symptoms.

All cases of AHC, GKD, and DMD associated with an X deletion occurred in male subjects, suggesting X-linked recessive traits. Unaffected mothers of patients have been shown to be heterozygous for the deletion Xp2i del (27). However, one case in a female patient has been reported (29).

5. Treatment

Steroid replacement for both glucocorticoids and mineralocorticoids is necessary. If GKD is present, appropriate therapy must be given. Unfortunately, Duchenne muscular dystrophy is not treatable at this time.

C. Adrenocortical Unresponsiveness to ACTH (Deficient ACTH Receptor)

1. Pathogenesis

This disorder is caused by an inability of the adrenal cells of the zona fasciculata and reticularis to respond to ACTH. The lack of ACTH response is caused by a genetic abnormality of the ACTH receptor (33).

2. Clinical Manifestations

It is characterized by feeding problems in early life, failure to thrive, hypoglycemia, and hyperpigmentation of the skin (34). In some cases, the symptoms seem to occur later in infancy, perhaps because the frequent feedings of the neonatal period prevented major hypoglycemic episodes.

3. Laboratory

As already noted, glucose levels are quite low but there is no electrolyte abnormality. During a hypoglycemic episode, a blood sample demonstrates high growth hormone and low insulin concentrations with low cortisol levels. ACTH measurement shows elevated values, even when cortisol values are low.

4. Genetics

Recently the gene for the ACTH receptor was isolated and sequenced (35). The coding sequence does not contain an intron. The product of this gene is a 297 amino acid protein with seven transmembranic domains, a cytosolic COOH terminus that can react with a G protein to activate adenyl cyclase activity, and an extracellular NH_2 terminus with two possible glycosylation sites.

The disorder is an autosomal recessive trait. In one family, both parents were heterozygous for the same mutation, the proband being hemozygous for this mutation (36), whereas in another family the parents had different mutations, the patient being an allelic compound (37). A postreceptor mutation has also been reported (38).

5. Treatment

Patients require only glucocorticoid replacement therapy, the mineralocorticoid function being normal.

6. Other Disorders

Although more than 30 cases of adrenocortical unresponsiveness to ACTH have been reported in the literature, it is probable that some of these patients presented with a different disorder. Some patients who presented with neurological symptoms (39) probably had unrecognized cases of adrenoleukodystrophy. Other patients presented with sodium loss (40). Several cases of an association of adrenal insufficiency, achalasia, and alacrima (triple A syndrome) have been reported (41, 42). This syndrome usually appears in the first decade of life, a severe hypoglycemia being often the early sign. Aldosterone deficiency is associated to cortisol deficiency in only 10–15% of cases. Some patients present only two of the triad signs, but in some cases multiple additional abnormalities have been observed. The triple A syndrome is an autosomal recessive trait and its locus is on chromosomes 12q13 (43).

D. Congenital Adrenal Hyperplasia

There are five major forms of congenital adrenal hyperplasia (CAH), each caused by a mutation of one of the five enzymes required for the biosynthesis of cortisol. In each of these forms, the decrease in cortisol secretion results in a decrease in negative feedback at the level of the hypothalamus–pituitary (1, 2). The resulting increase in ACTH output attempts to return the cortisol secretion to normal if the mutation permits some degree of enzymatic activity. At the same time, the increased ACTH secretion results in a markedly elevated production of the cortisol precursors before the mutant block.

The five forms of CAH are 21-hydroxylase deficiency (salt-losing form, simple virilizing form, and attenuated form), 11β-hydroxylase deficiency related to a mutation of CYP11B1, 17-hydroxylase deficiency (hypertensive form) related to CYP17, 3β-HSD deficiency, and lipoid adrenal hyperplasia related to a mutation of CYP11A. These disorders arediscussed in a separate chapter of this book.

E. Adrenoleukodystrophy and Adrenomyeloneuropathy

These two disorders have also been called diffused cerebral sclerosis associated with adrenal insufficiency.

1. Pathophysiology

Also known as Siemerling-Creutzfeldt or Schilder's disease, the basic biochemical abnormality is an elevation in plasma and various tissues of the concentration of the very-long-chain fatty acids (VLCFA), C24, C25, and C26. They probably accumulate because of a defect in their normal breakdown in cellular organelles known as peroxisomes. On pathological examination, the adrenal cortex at first shows cytoplasmic striations containing cholesterol esterified with VLCFA. Later the adrenal cells appear to be filled with the abnormal cholesterol esters, and in the final stage the cells tend to atrophy and die (44).

2. Clinical Manifestations

This is a progressive disease of the brain that manifests in its early stage by mild symptoms, such as unusual behavior, a mild decrease in visual acuity, and a loss of muscle strength in some limbs. Over a period of a few years, the symptoms progress to dementia, blindness, and quadriparesis, and end in death. At various times during this degenerative process, symptoms of adrenal insufficiency may occur, involving both cortisol and aldosterone function.

3. Genetics

The locus of adrenoleukodystrophy maps to the long arm of the X chromosome (Xq28) (45, 46). Because of the location of the gene on the X chromosome, the disorder is expressed only in male subjects. Recently the adrenoleukodystrophy (ALD) gene was identified (47). It encodes a 745 amino acid protein that includes six membrane-spanning segments and an ATP-binding domain. The role of the ALD protein may be to transport the VLCFA-COA synthetase. Different mutations have been reported in different families, including six detectable deletions, nine point mutations, three frameshift mutations, and one splicing mutation (48).

4. Various Clinical Forms

Most commonly, the symptoms of adrenoleukodystrophy appear at around 7 years of age. In such patients the neurological deterioration is somewhat rapid, leading to a bedridden state in 2–3 years. There is also a group of boys in whom the illness appears between 12 and 20 years of age: in these subjects, the neurological deterioration is usually slower. Finally, the neurological symptoms may occur after 21 years of age (49). This form of the disorder is called adrenomyeloneuropathy (AMN) because the neurological manifestations involve the peripheral nerves rather than the brain. However, some patients with AMN may have early symptoms of mild adrenal insufficiency. These men also present with primary gonadal failure (50). It must also be noted that some cases present with either only neurological manifestations or only addisonian symptoms. A few subjects with the biochemical abnormality of ALD present no clinical features of the disorder, at least for a long period of time. All the forms mentioned earlier are considered allelic and are all X-linked recessive traits. Except in the rare cases of de novo mutation, the mothers of ALD patients are obligate heterozygotes. These women are free of symptoms, but some may present with neurological abnormalities late in life, usually between 40 and 50 years of age.

5. Autosomal Recessive Forms

Whereas ALD is an X-linked trait, there are also autosomal recessive forms that express themselves in the neonatal period. The biochemical defect appears to be similar to that seen in X-linked ALD, but the symptoms of adrenal insufficiency and central nervous system manifestation are more acute. The neonatal ALD is caused by a marked decrease in peroxisomes, in contrast to X-linked ALD, which presents with a normal number of peroxisomes. In Zellweger syndrome (cerebrohepatorenal form), the peroxisomes are almost completely absent. Normal peroxisomes are seen in pseudoneonatal ALD, and such a case has been reported to present with a deletion of the peroxisomal acyl-CoA oxidase gene (51).

The treatment of ALD has been very disappointing. Efforts have been made to change the diet by decreasing the amount of very-long-chain fatty acids. There have also been attempts at supplementation with glycerol trioleate oil as well as addition of glycerol trierucate oil. Although such drugs appear to improve the condition temporarily, the amelioration is not sustained. Attempts have also been made to treat by bone marrow transplantation but without clear success.

F. Wolman Disease (Acid Lipase Deficiency)

Wolman disease is caused by a deficiency of lysosomal acid lipase (52). This enzyme is an esterase that hydrolyzes cholesterol esters and triglycerides. In such patients the normal esterified lipids accumulate in various cells. It is also called generalized xanthomatosis with calcified adrenals. Symptoms occur in the first month of life as failure to thrive, anemia, hepatomegaly, and splenomegaly. There is also vomiting and diarrhea as well as jaundice. Shortly thereafter, one can notice the calcified, enlarged adrenal gland and decreased cortisol secretion. The locus for lysosomal acid lipase deficiency has been mapped to chromosome 10 (53). This is an autosomal recessive trait. There is no treatment for this extremely rare disorder, which ends in death rapidly.

G. Steroid Sulfatase Deficiency (X-Linked Ichthyosis)

A deficiency of steroid sulfatase results in the accumulation of sulfated products, such as $3,\beta$-hydroxysteroids (particularly DHA-S) and cholesterol sulfate. The ichthyosis is thought to be related to the accumulation in the skin of a large amount of cholesterol sulfate (54). This syndrome is not an adrenocortical insufficiency because cortisol and aldosterone secretion is normal. The normal fetus has low steroid sulfatase activity and relies on the placenta to accomplish this function. Because the placenta is made of maternal cells and at least one of the maternal X chromosomes is normal, the steroid sulfatase activity is adequate during pregnancy.

The steroid sulfatase gene has been mapped to the X chromosome (Xp22.3) near the pseudoautosomal region of the terminal part of the short arm. Large deletions of the X chromosome in the area of the steroid sulfatase gene have been associated with hypogonadotropic hypogonadism and anosmia (Kallmann's syndrome).

H. Mineralocorticoid Deficiency Caused by Mutations of CYP11B2 Gene

As previously discussed, the cytochrome P450 encoded by the CYP11B2 gene is capable of making the conversion of DOC to aldosterone by a series of three enzymatic steps: addition of the 11β-hydroxyl group to form corticosterone, 18-hydroxylation (also called corticosterone methyloxidase type I) to form 18-hydroxycorticosterone, and 18-dehydrogenation (also called corticosterone methyloxidase type II) to form aldosterone. Although the same enzyme appears to be involved, two types of aldosterone deficiency, 18-hydroxylase and 18-dehydrogenase, have been reported in the literature.

1. 18α-Hydroxylase Deficiency

These patients present with a general failure to thrive related to mild salt wasting. Laboratory studies show decreased aldosterone and 18-hydroxycorticosterone with a concomitantly elevated secretion of corticosterone and DOC (55, 56). Mineralocorticoid replacement therapy results in the resumption of normal growth in infancy and early childhood. Later in life, treatment becomes unnecessary. Only a few patients have been reported with this disorder.

2. 18-Dehydrogenase Deficiency

The onset of this disorder is also in infancy or early childhood. It is characterized by a failure to thrive and symptoms of mineralocorticoid deficiency, including hyponatremia, hyperkalemia, and acidosis. However, these patients rarely present in acute adrenal crisis. This is probably because some of the precursors of aldosterone that have some sodium-retaining activity are produced in increased amount. Hormonal study shows an increase in plasma renin activity as well as an increase in DOC, corticosterone, and 18-hydroxycorticosterone, along with low aldosterone (57). It is of interest that these patients present with an increased excretion of urinary 17-OHCS; this is because the urinary metabolites of 18-hydroxycorticosterone give the Porter-Silber reaction (58). A very large Iranian Jewish pedigree has been reported with this salt-wasting disorder (59, 60). Recently, mutations in the CYP11B2 gene were reported by Pascoe et al. (61). Treatment consists of mineralocorticoid replacement therapy. It is of interest to note that later in life many of these patients have successfully withdrawn from treatment.

I. Adrenal Hemorrhage of the Newborn

Adrenal hemorrhage occurs more often after prolonged labor and a traumatic delivery, usually of a large male infant. The normal adrenal has a rich network of small vessels between the capsule and the cortex. This is the site of bleeding in adrenal hemorrhage.

Children with massive bilateral adrenal hemorrhage appear in acute shock caused by adrenal insufficiency and incipient blood loss. On the other hand, if the hemorrhage is unilateral, there are usually no adrenal symptoms. The typical laboratory finding is hypoglycemia with hyponatremic, hyperkalemic acidosis. On physical examination a mass can be felt in the flanks. Sonography reveals a mass that tends to displace the kidney downward (62). Residual calcification may be visible on x-ray of the abdomen 3–6 weeks after the bleeding occurred and as the hemorrhage resolves. With time, the calcifications themselves disappear. The differential diagnosis includes renal vein thrombosis. An ACTH test is useful in differentiating this condition from bilateral adrenal hemorrhage.

J. Adrenal Hemorrhage of Acute Infection

An adrenal crisis may occur during an acute infection, such as fulminating meningococcemia, pneumococcal, streptococcal, *Haemophilus*, and diphtheria infections. The acute adrenal insufficiency occurring with meningococcemia has also been called Waterhouse-Friderichsen syndrome. The subcapsular hemorrhage is thought to be related to the effects of arterioantitoxin.

Such an acute adrenal crisis occurring at the time of a fulminating infection has an extremely poor prognosis. It is clear that rapid and energetic treatment of the infection, as well as therapy with adrenal steroids in stress doses (IV Solucortef), is necessary.

V. ADDISON'S DISEASE (CHRONIC HYPOADRENOCORTICISM)

In the days of Thomas Addison, tuberculosis was the most common pathogenesis of this condition. Other infections have been reported, such as fungal infections (histoplasmosis and coccidiomycosis). Recently, it was also reported associated with human immunodeficiency virus infection (63). At present, the most important mechanism of destruction of the adrenals is an autoimmune disorder (64). Addison's disease is much less frequent in children than in adult subjects. The clinical features are directly related to the decreased production of adrenal steroids. All or some of the symptoms of adrenal insufficiency outlined in Table 3 may appear. Initially, there is usually general fatigue, muscle pain, weight loss, gastrointestinal symptoms, and hypotension related to salt loss. An acute adrenal crisis may occur at the time of a minor infection or febrile illness. The skin hyperpigmentation is distributed mainly in pressure areas (axillae and groin), as well as in the buccal and vaginal mucosa, the creases of the hand, and the nipples. This hyperpigmentation is related to the increased pituitary secretion of β-lipotropin, which occurs concomitantly with the increased ACTH secretion.

Depending on the cause of Addison's disease, some other specific symptoms can be expected. In cases involv-

Table 3 Signs and Symptoms of Adrenal Insufficiency

Glucocorticoid deficiency
    Fasting hypoglycemia
    Increased insulin sensitivity
    Decreased gastric acidity
    Gastrointestinal symptoms (nausea, vomiting)
    Fatigue
Mineralocorticoid deficiency
    Muscle weakness
    Weight loss
    Fatigue
    Nausea, vomiting, anorexia
    Salt craving
    Hypotension
    Hyperkalemia, hyponatremia, acidosis
Adrenal androgen deficiency
    Decreased pubic and axillary hair
    Decreased libido
Increased β-lipotropin levels
    Hyperpigmentation

ing an infectious agent, there are also signs of this infection in other sites. If the cause is an autoimmune syndrome, one usually finds positive adrenal antibodies. In this latter case, the pathology is a progressive lymphocytic infiltration of the adrenal cortex. In such cases, Addison's disease is often associated with other autoimmune disorders, resulting in a polyglandular syndrome (64). Two types of autoimmune disease associations have been described. Type I includes mucocutaneous candidiasis, hypoparathyroidism, and Addison's disease. In addition, one can also observe pernicious anemia, alopecia, vitiligo, and chronic progressive hepatitis. In type II the association includes Addison's disease and chronic lymphocytic thyroiditis. This association has also been called Schmidt's syndrome. If insulin-dependent diabetes also occurs, it is then called Carpenter syndrome. The diagnosis of Addison's disease is made based on the demonstration of a low cortisol concentration in plasma concomitantly with elevated ACTH levels. Early in the development of the disorder, the cortisol levels may be normal because of adrenal hyperstimulation by high levels of ACTH. The short ACTH test described earlier shows a low or normal cortisol baseline but no increase on ACTH stimulation. Because of the consequences of establishing a diagnosis of Addison's disease, we usually advise also carrying out an intramuscular (IM) ACTH test (25 mg/m² every 8 h for 2–3 days). Urine samples are collected before and on the third day of stimulation for the determination of urinary 17-OHCS and free cortisol.

The typical treatment is replacement of the missing hormone, specifically glucocorticoids and mineralocorticoids. In children, the glucocorticoids are replaced by oral cortisol or prednisone (see Table 4), whereas mineralocorticoids are replaced with Florinef (fludrocortisone). In

adolescent and adult women, the lack of adrenal androgens may need to be compensated for by administration of a mild androgenic preparation to improve the libido and the growth of pubic hair.

VI. HYPOADRENOCORTICISM SECONDARY TO DEFICIENT CRH AND/OR ACTH SECRETION

Unless there is an organic abnormality of the hypothalamus or the anterior pituitary, it is often difficult to determine whether a deficient ACTH secretion is related to a deficient output of CRH.

A. Hypopituitarism

Hypopituitarism is characterized by a deficient secretion of one, some, or all pituitary hormones (65). In infancy and childhood the main deficiencies are those of growth hormone, thyroid-stimulating hormone, and ACTH. A deficiency of gonadotropins and prolactin is detected only at puberty. In this chapter we consider ACTH deficiency.

1. Pathophysiology

Various congenital malformations of the brain, particularly midline defects, can result in a deficiency of secretion of hypothalamic hormones, including CRH. The most frequently recognized malformation is the septo-optic dysplasia as originally described by de Morsier. This condition includes agenesis of the septum pellucidum, hypoplasia or aplasia of optic nerves and chiasma resulting in various degrees of visual impairment, and abnormality of the hypothalamus causing secondary hypopituitarism. The midline defects may be mild, with partial hypopituitarism and no eye disorder. It may also be extensive and associated with cleft palate and cleft lip. An absence of gonadotropin secretion during fetal life may result in micropenis in male infants. Congenital malformation of the pituitary gland can also occur and may be the cause of empty sella turcica. Head trauma either at delivery or later in life may result in hemorrhage in the area of the hypothalamus or pituitary gland. This in turn may cause hypopituitarism with ACTH deficiency. Disorders that result in the destruction of normal tissues (hemochromatosis, sarcoidosis, and histiocytosis) can cause hypothalamic and/or pituitary dysfunction. A similar situation can occur following various types of infections, such as meningitis or encephalitis. Tumors arising in the sella (craniopharyngioma) or the hypothalamus likewise result in hypopituitarism. Radiation of a brain tumor may have the same effect. In some patients, no specific cause for the hypopituitarism can be detected. Such cases can involve several hormones of the anterior pituitary (idiopathic panhypopituitarism) or, on rare occasions, only ACTH secretion (idiopathic isolated ACTH deficiency).

Table 4 Maintenance and Stress Dosage of Glucocorticoid and Mineralocorticoid in Treatment of Adrenal Insufficiency

Therapy	Maintenance mean (range)		Stress
Glucocorticoid replacement (mg/m²/24 h)			
Oral cortisol (one-third dose every 8 h)	20	(12–24)	60
Oral cortisone acetate (one-third dose every 8 h)	25	(15–30)	75
Oral prednisolone (one-half dose every 12 h)	3	(2–4)	9
Oral prednisone (one-half dose every 12 h)	3.5	(2–4)	10
Mineralocorticoid replacement (mg/day)			
Oral fludrocortisone acetate (Florinef)	0.1	(0.05–0.125)	0.1

2. Clinical Manifestations

The congenital malformations described earlier can be manifested by hypoglycemia if ACTH and cortisol secretion are deficient. The hypoglycemia may be more marked if there is concomitant growth hormone secretion deficiency. Persistent hypoglycemia in a newborn requires the collection of a blood sample for the determination of true glucose, cortisol, growth hormone, and insulin concentrations. In hypopituitarism the concentration of all these hormones is very low. In contrast, in nesidioblastosis, the concentration of insulin, growth hormone, and cortisol is markedly elevated concomitantly with low glucose levels. When the diagnosis of hypopituitarism is established, magnetic resonance imaging (MRI) of the head may show some of the characteristics of septo-optic dysplasia or other brain malformation or injury. In head trauma, the MRI shows evidence of hemorrhage. Brain tumors can also be visualized by MRI studies. Various degrees of impairment of mental development can be present, particularly in hypopituitarism secondary to meningitis or encephalitis. Because hypopituitarism can involve various combinations of tropic hormones, the clinical manifestations in childhood may include symptoms of growth hormone deficiency and hypothyroidism.

Aldosterone secretion is controlled by the renin–angiotensin system, so that there are usually no electrolyte or water abnormalities in hypopituitarism. When a destructive process has taken place, however, there can be involvement of the neuronal cells that secrete antidiuretic hormone (ADH), resulting in a disturbance of electrolytes and water balance characteristic of diabetes insipidus. In addition, following neurosurgery, inappropriate ADH secretion can occur that results in electrolyte abnormalities.

By definition, patients with idiopathic isolated ACTH deficiency have normal thyroid function as well as normal growth and normal sexual maturation at puberty (66). Because females rely on adrenal androgens for the development of pubic hair at puberty, women with idiopathic isolated ACTH deficiency present with scant pubic hair.

3. Laboratory Diagnosis

It is expected that a decreased cortisol secretion would result in hypoglycemia. Indeed, hypoglycemia is marked in patients who have a combined deficiency of ACTH and growth hormone but is usually mild in the absence of growth hormone deficiency. A low cortisol concentration in an 8 a.m. blood sample may be observed, but values are often low–normal to normal.

A single oral dose of Metopirone (metyrapone) given at midnight and an 8 a.m. plasma sample obtained the next morning show a decreased response of plasma 11-deoxycortisol (compound S) in subjects with ACTH deficiency. However, most subjects can respond to the marked stress resulting from the administration of IV Metopirone or IV pyrogen (67, 68). When reviewing a large group of patients with hypopituitarism, Brasel et al. (69) found that about 50% of the patients had normal adrenocortical function; most of the others had normal basal cortisol but a poor response to the regular Metopirone test. Among the latter subjects, only those who had an organic lesion could not respond to the IV Metopirone test. The 1 μg ACTH test is particularly helpful in detecting the mild adrenal insufficiency characteristic of panhypopituitarism. Finally, in hypopituitarism, it is important to check the function of all pituitary hormones.

4. Treatment

Treatment consists of appropriate replacement of the deficient hormones. If basal cortisol levels are abnormally low, maintenance as well as stress therapy is required. When basal levels are normal but the oral Metopirone test is inappropriate, then stress therapy only is needed. In addition, patients who have thyroid-stimulating hormone and/or growth hormone deficiency need appropriate replacement. Finally, in ADH deficiency, treatment with intranasal desmopressin (DDAVP) is necessary.

B. Cessation of Glucocorticoid Therapy

It is well established that the administration of glucocorticoids suppresses the secretion of CRH by the hypothalamus and of ACTH by the pituitary gland, resulting in secondary adrenal cortex atrophy. When the dosage is less than the replacement level, however, for whatever period of time, or if the dosage is greater than replacement but for a duration of less than 4 weeks, no adrenocortical atrophy is expected. By contrast, if the dosage is greater than replacement and the duration of treatment is greater than 4 weeks, suppression is expected. Experience has shown that recovery occurs within 6 weeks in about half of patients and within 6 months in all subjects (70).

1. Clinical Features

Hypoglycemia may be observed in some patients. Growth delay is mainly related to the duration of glucocorticoid therapy rather than its cessation (65). The greatest problem may occur at the time of a major medical or surgical stress.

2. Laboratory Tests

A Metopirone test is necessary to determine whether the patient has recovered normal adrenocortical function. As mentioned for hypopituitarism, a 1 μg ACTH test is simpler and as informative.

3. Treatment

Clearly there is no need for treatment in subjects who have been treated for less than 4 weeks or for those who have received less than replacement therapy for any period of time. For other patients, treatment is required only at times of stress using a dosage equivalent to two to four times replacement and only for the period of stress. Because more than 90% of subjects recover adrenocortical function after 6 months of cessation of therapy, additional stress doses of steroid are not required after this period of time.

C. Removal of a Unilateral Adrenal Tumor

Tumors that produce excessive amounts of cortisol usually secrete steroids independently of ACTH stimulation. For this reason, such a subject usually presents with suppressed CRH/ACTH secretion and an atrophic contralateral adrenal. During the surgical removal of such tumors, the patient should receive stress dosages of glucocorticoids. After surgery, the dosage should be decreased progressively and the patient should then be considered as are those discussed earlier for cessation of glucocorticoid therapy.

D. Infants Born to Mothers Treated with Glucocorticoids

Cortisol administered during pregnancy can cross the placenta, but the fetal concentration is only about 10% of maternal levels. This is in part because the placenta is rich in the enzyme that transforms cortisol into cortisone. This same enzyme transforms prednisolone into prednisone. Experience has shown that pregnant women treated with prednisone at a dosage of two to five times replacement therapy gave birth to infants whose cortisol secretion rate was normal shortly after birth (71). Nevertheless, such infants should be evaluated for the possible development of hypoglycemia. Because of the physiology of the control of aldosterone secretion, no electrolyte abnormality is expected in infants born of mothers treated with glucocorticoids. In contrast to cortisol or prednisone, dexamethasone readily crosses from the mother to the fetus and is used for fetal therapy.

E. Respiratory Distress Syndrome

There are some differences of opinion on the optimal use of surfactant and glucocorticoids in the treatment of respiratory distress syndrome (RDS). If steroids are used, dexamethasone is the choice because it readily crosses the placenta. Therapy may be continued for a period of time in the neonatal period and may therefore result in suppressed adrenocortical function when treatment is stopped (72). In such cases, therapy might be needed at times of stress.

F. Anencephaly

Adrenal glands are very small in patients with anencephaly, probably secondary to the absence of pituitary tissue, leading to adrenal insufficiency.

VII. HYPOADRENOCORTICISM SECONDARY TO END-ORGAN UNRESPONSIVENESS

Cortisol and aldosterone, like all other steroids, express their effects by binding to a protein specific for each steroid, called a receptor. Receptor abnormalities can cause steroid resistance.

A. Cortisol Resistance

This is a rare disorder that has been discovered in a small number of families (73, 74). In all cases the resistance appeared partial: none of the affected subjects completely lacked glucocorticoid activity. The main laboratory characteristics of cortisol resistance are markedly increased plasma concentrations of cortisol and ACTH, as well as elevated excretion of urinary free cortisol and total 17-hydroxycorticosteroids. In addition, a standard dexamethasone suppression test is partially negative. Such laboratory findings are typical of patients with Cushing's disease, yet subjects with cortisol resistance do not present with any of the symptoms of this disorder. The elevated levels of ACTH result in increased secretion not only of cortisol but also of deoxycorticosterone and corticosterone. These two steroids are responsible for the signs of mineralocorticoid excess, including hypertension, hypokalemia, and metabolic alkalosis. As previously mentioned, the genesis of the resistance syndrome is related to an abnormal glucocorticoid receptor. The gene for this receptor has been mapped to chromosome 5q31-q32 (75). In one family, a point mutation was found in the receptor gene. In all the families reported with this condition, the mode of inheritance has been found to be autosomal dominant.

B. Aldosterone Resistance

Aldosterone resistance is most probably a heterogeneous group of disorders that express themselves clinically as an unresponsiveness of the kidney to aldosterone. One of the first patients described in 1958 by Cheek and Perry (76) presented with a salt-losing syndrome that responded poorly to mineralocorticoid therapy but was adequately corrected by sodium chloride supplementation. A large number of these patients have shown an improvement with age and often did not require further therapy after 1 or 2 years of age. In other affected subjects, however, therapy had to be continued.

Aldosterone resistance represents at least two different entities since autosomal dominant and autosomal recessive modes of inheritance have been reported (77, 78). The gene encoding the mineralocorticoid receptor was cloned recently and mapped to chromosome 4q31 (79). This new knowledge should help us in understanding better the various forms of this disorder.

VIII. TREATMENT OF HYPOADRENOCORTICISM

A. Acute Adrenal Insufficiency

In the acute adrenal crisis, a deficiency of cortisol and aldosterone as well as dehydration must be considered. Fluid and electrolyte replacement to expand blood volume and increase blood pressure must be instituted immediately, particularly in the neonate or small child, who otherwise may decompensate rapidly. During the first hour of therapy, the patient should receive 20 ml/kg 0.9% sodium chloride in 5% glucose solution. The intravenous solution should then be continued to deliver 60 ml/kg over the following 24 h. In general, serum electrolytes improve, with plasma concentrations of sodium and chloride returning to normal but serum potassium often remaining elevated. At some time during the period of fluid replacement therapy, steroid replacement is instituted. Cortisol sodium succinate (Solucortef) is given as a IV bolus at a dosage of 25 mg/m^2 and is followed by a similar dose added to the 24 h IV maintenance fluid solution. Note that 20–35 mg Solucortef has a mineralocorticoid activity equivalent to 0.1 mg Florinef. After the acute crisis, maintenance therapy is instituted.

B. Maintenance Therapy

1. Glucocorticoid Replacement

Cortisol is the drug of choice because it is the major glucocorticoid secreted physiologically by the adrenal cortex. In infants and children, synthetic preparations with high potency are not recommended for replacement treatment because their proper dosage is difficult to adjust. Furthermore, cortisol has some mineralocorticoid activity, whereas the synthetic preparations have little or none. On the basis of a cortisol secretion rate of 6–14 mg/m^2/24 h, a dosage similar to this secretion given over a 24 h infusion should be a maintenance dose. The oral dosage is approximately twice the physiological secretion rate, because some oral cortisol is destroyed by the gastric acidity. Because of the short half-life of cortisol, the total 24 h dose must be given in thirds every 8 h.

Experience has shown that children of school age and adolescents have problems remembering to take the midday dose. Prednisone, which has a longer half-life than cortisol, can be used, half of the daily dose being given every 12 h (see Table 4). Prednisolone is the only glucocorticoid available presently in liquid form. It is about seven times more potent than cortisol. There are two commercial preparations: Pediapred contains 1 mg prednisolone per 1 ml; Prelone contains 5 mg prednisolone per 1 ml.

2. Mineralocorticoid Replacement

As previously noted, the secretion rate of aldosterone in human subjects is similar from 2 weeks of age to adulthood. Therefore, replacement therapy remains constant regardless of the age of the patient. The only preparation available is 9α-fluorocortisol acetate (fludrocortisone, Florinef). It is given orally as a single dose of 0.05–0.150 mg/24 h. Mineralocorticoid therapy is effective only if salt is ingested simultaneously. Infant formulas are very low in salt (8–10 mEq/day), and such patients may require a modest sodium chloride supplement (15–30 mEq/day), particularly when they show serum electrolyte abnormalities and elevated plasma renin levels. When the infants start eating regular table food, the additional salt becomes unnecessary.

C. Therapy During Stress

Subjects who receive glucocorticoid therapy for more than 1 month have an unresponsive hypothalamic–pituitary–adrenal axis. As a result, they require additional glucocorticoids during stress. For minor infection with low-grade fever, increased medication may not be required. In moderate stress the dosage is increased to twice maintenance, and in more severe stress to three to four times replacement (see Table 4). If a patient is unable to retain oral therapy during an acute illness, the parents must administer an IM injection of Solucortef (50 mg/m^2). Following the IM injection, the parents are advised to discuss the problem with their physician or to attend the hospital emergency room. If this cannot be done within 8 h following the first injection, another IM Solucortef is required every 8 h.

D. Treatment at Time of Surgery

At present we recommend using Solucortef. A dose of 25 mg/m^2 is given IV just before the start of anesthesia. This is followed by a second dose of 50 mg/m^2 administered as a constant infusion throughout the surgical procedure. A third 50 mg/m^2 dose of Solucortef is then given at a constant rate for the rest of the first 24 h period. During the time that the patient is unable to take oral treatment, constant infusions of Solucortef are continued at 50–75 mg/m^2/24 h.

In both medical and surgical stress it is important to limit the time of increased glucocorticoid dosage to the period of acute stress and to return to maintenance therapy as soon as improvement occurs. Otherwise, the patient may be overtreated and will then present with symptoms of Cushing's disease.

IX. HYPERADRENOCORTICISM

The syndromes of hyperadrenocorticism can be classified into four subgroups, depending on the predominance of a specific type of adrenocortical steroid. In each of these entities, however, levels of other steroids can also be elevated.

1. Hypercortisolism, characterized by elevated cortisol secretion
2. Adrenogenital syndrome, characterized by abnormal secretion of adrenocortical androgens
3. Feminizing syndrome, related to increased estrogen secretion
4. Hyperaldosteronism, caused by excessive aldosterone secretion

X. HYPERCORTISOLISM

A. Pathophysiology

Except for the iatrogenic hypercortisolism related to glucocorticoid therapy given in pharmacological dosages, this disorder is rare in the newborn period and in childhood. Its frequency increases in adolescence. Harvey Cushing described patients with hypercortisolism related to a pituitary adenoma (80), and the condition has been termed Cushing's disease. When the hypercortisolism is related to an adrenal tumor, it is termed Cushing's syndrome. In adults and, rarely, in children, malignant tumors not necessarily related to an endocrine gland can produce an excessive amount of ACTH, in which case the disorder is called ectopic ACTH syndrome. On occasion, the tumor may produce CRH, which in turn results in increased ACTH secretion and cortisol secretion. Also in adults, chronic alcoholism has been shown to result in increased CRH secretion, which in turn increases ACTH and cortisol output.

B. Clinical Manifestations

The symptoms of hypercortisolism are similar whatever its cause. Because of the ubiquitous effects of glucocorticoid on general metabolism, the symptoms are multiple and varied (81). In muscle cells, cortisol increases the breakdown of proteins into amino acids but decreases glucose uptake, resulting in decreased glycogen storage and muscle wasting. In fat cells, cortisol increases lipolytic enzymes, resulting in hyperlipidemia, hypercholesterolemia, and redistribution of fat with truncal obesity and moon facies. In liver cells, cortisol increases gluconeogenetic enzymes and aminotransferases, resulting in hyperglycemia, glycosuria, and what is termed insulin-resistant diabetes. In bone cells, cortisol increases the reabsorption of the protein matrix, Simultaneously, cortisol decreases the synthesis of a specific calcium-binding protein, resulting in the inhibition of vitamin D-mediated calcium absorption from the gut; this, in turn, produces hypocalcemia, osteomalacia, and growth retardation. These effects of cortisol on bone are further aggravated by an increased renal calcium excretion. Because cortisol has some mineralocorticoid activity, hypercortisolism increases sodium retention and potassium loss along with water retention, resulting in often marked hypokalemia but only slight hypernatremia and mild hypertension. In addition to increasing cortisol secretion, ACTH increases androgen secretion. Hence, when the hypercortisolism is caused by elevated ACTH secretion, the patients present with signs of virilism.

Hypercortisolism increases gastric acidity, which in turn may result in peptic ulcers. However, this is seen more frequently in adults than in children. Also note that hypercortisolism can affect the central nervous system, resulting in emotional instability that alternates between depression and euphoria.

C. Laboratory Diagnosis

1. Demonstrate the Presence of Hypercortisolism

This is reliably done by obtaining a 24 h urine specimen and determining both total urinary 17-hydroxycorticosteroids and free cortisol. In children and adults, the urinary excretion of 17-OHCS is similar when the values are corrected for body size. The normal value is 2.9 ± 1.2 mg/m^2/24 h (mean $\pm$ SD), as shown by the shaded area in Figure 10. Therefore, values of the urinary 17-OHCS below 5.5 mg/m^2/24 h and urinary free cortisol of less than 70 μg/m^2/24 h rule out hypercortisolism. Among obese subjects, about 30% (Fig. 10) have urinary 17-OHCS values above 5.5 mg/m^2/24 h (14). Such subjects require a low-dosage dexamethasone suppression test (1.25 mg dexamethasone/m^2/24 h for 2 days). A good suppression suggests obesity and lack of it suggests hypercortisolism.

2. Determine the Cause of the Disorder

This is done by carrying out a CRH stimulation test (24) and/or a high-dosage dexamethasone suppression test (3.75 mg/m^2/24 h for 2 days). The response of plasma ACTH and cortisol to CRH administration is presented in Figure 9. A marked response in the CRH stimulation test and a good suppression in the high-dosage dexamethasone suppression test suggest an hypercortisolism that is pituitary dependent, that is, Cushing's disease. In contrast, a lack of response to the CRH stimulation and a lack of suppression (24) to the high-dosage dexamethasone suppression test strongly favor hypercortisolism being caused by an adrenal tumor or possibly a tumor producing ectopic ACTH.

3. MRI of the Head and Abdomen

In theory, MRI of the head will demonstrate the presence of a pituitary adenoma. Unfortunately, the adenoma can be very small and is visualized in about only one-third to one-half of cases. MRI of the abdomen visualizes adrenal tumors 1 cm or more in diameter. In hypersecretion of ACTH, bilateral adrenal hyperplasia is observed by MRI in some cases.

4. Bilateral Petrosal Sinus Sampling

This has been proposed as a means to localize a small pituitary adenoma that is not visible on the MRI scan.

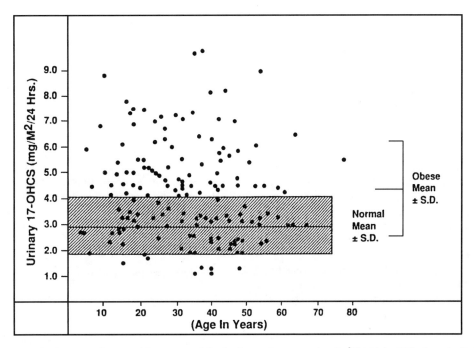

Figure 10 Urinary 17-hydroxycorticosteroids corrected for body surface area (mg/m²/24 h) in 160 obese individuals of various age. Their values are compared to the mean ± SD of control subjects (shaded area). About 30% of obese subjects had excretions above the control mean +2 SD. (From Ref. 14.)

Catheters are placed in the left and right inferior petrosal sinuses and blood samples are obtained before and 10 and 30 min after administration of CRH (100 μg/m²). High baseline concentrations of ACTH are expected. The differential in ACTH increase following CRH should help to determine the location of the microadenoma on the left or right side of the pituitary gland. Although this technique has been reported by some investigators to be successful (82), others have found it to be traumatic for the patient, resulting in a fair amount of body radiation, and not always accurate.

D. Treatment

Clearly, the treatment is dictated by the cause of the hypercortisolism. The treatment of Cushing's syndrome caused by an adrenal tumor is surgical. An adenoma or well-encapsulated carcinoma without metastasis offers the best opportunity for a complete cure. By contrast, the prognosis of malignant adrenal tumors that produce glucocorticoids is generally poor.

If the adrenal tumor is localized before surgery, a transthoracic approach affords excellent exposure and ease of removal. If the tumor is not well localized, a transperitoneal approach is indicated. Patients with metastasis can be treated with the drug rnitotane (o,p'-DDD), but results have been disappointing and the drug is not always well tolerated. Cisplatin has also been used with limited success.

Autonomous adrenal tumors secrete cortisol in high concentrations and suppress ACTH secretion, resulting in atrophy of the contralateral adrenal gland. Therefore, we advise the following therapy at the time of surgery: an IV dose of 25 mg/m² of Solucortef administered immediately before the start of anesthesia; this is followed by a constant-rate infusion of 50 mg/m² of Solucortef throughout surgery; after surgery, an additional IV constant-rate infusion of 50 mg/m² is given for the rest of the first 24 h. On postsurgical days, a constant infusion of Solucortef is continued at 50 mg/m²/24 h until oral therapy can be given at three to four times replacement dosage. After the acute period, it may be necessary to continue oral therapy at three-fourths to one-fourth replacement therapy for a few months.

In Cushing's disease with bilateral adrenal hyperplasia, several forms of therapy have been used. In the past, bilateral adrenalectomy was widely employed, resulting in immediate cure of hypercortisolism but also in adrenal insufficiency that required glucocorticoid and mineral corticoid replacement for life and the possibility of development of a pituitary tumor (83). Radiation of the sella turcica has also been used extensively in adults but not in children because it often results in destruction of growth hormone-secreting cells; however, newer stereotactic techniques of delivery of radiation have given good results (84).

Transsphenoidal microsurgery is now used to remove pituitary microadenomas and has been successful in bringing about complete cures in many patients (85, 86). This form of therapy requires an experienced neurosurgical team to obtain the best chances of success (87). In a few patients, surgery has resulted in panhypopituitarism. Recurrence of the pituitary adenoma can also occur (88).

Several drugs have been used in the treatment of Cushing's disease. Cyproheptadine, a serotonin antagonist, can suppress ACTH secretion but it is generally not recommended as long-term medical management of the disease and it often does not return the cortisol secretion rate to normal. Bromocriptine, a dopamine agonist, although useful for the treatment of prolactin and growth-hormone-secreting pituitary adenomas, has not been of value in treating ACTH-secreting pituitary tumors. Metopirone and aminoglutethimide, which suppress adrenal secretion, have been recommended for the short-term, presurgical treatment of Cushing's disease.

Treatment of ectopic ACTH syndrome consists of the removal of the ACTH-secreting tumor. In cases of iatrogenic Cushing's syndrome, stopping the excessive glucocorticoid therapy is recommended.

XI. ADRENOGENITAL SYNDROME

The adrenogenital syndrome is characterized by an abnormally elevated secretion of adrenal androgens. Hence, the virilizing forms of congenital adrenal hyperplasia, mainly 21-hydroxylase and 11-hydroxylase deficiency, are part of the syndrome. However, the excessive androgen secretion of CAH is secondary to an increased ACTH secretion, itself secondary to a deficiency of one of the enzymes required for cortisol biosynthesis. For this reason, CAH is considered a form of hypoadrenocorticism, and the only cause of adrenogenital syndrome is a virilizing adrenal tumor, which is a rare condition in childhood.

A. Clinical Manifestations

These tumors result in masculinization of prepubertal children. In boys, it produces a pseudoprecocious puberty (89, 90). Sexual hair (pubic, axillary, and sometimes facial hair) develops and the penis is enlarged to adult size, with frequent erections. However, the testes remain prepubertal or slightly enlarged. In girls, this masculinizing syndrome is characterized by pubic and axillary hair with an enlarged and erectile clitoris (Fig. 11).

In both boys and girls, the excessive secretion of androgens accelerates growth, with an advancement of height age and bone age along with an increase in muscle mass.

An association of such a tumor with body hemihypertrophy and congenital malformations of the urogenital tract has been reported (91). If the clinical picture includes signs of hypercortisolism caused by increased cortisol secretion, the patient should be considered as presenting with Cushing syndrome. This distinction is important be-

cause the prognosis of purely virilizing tumors and mixed tumors is different.

B. Pathology

Virilizing adrenal tumors are usually carcinomas containing malignant cells. Experience shows that the degree of malignancy is low, however, and it is rare to observe metastasis at the time of surgery. In cases of long standing, the tumor may invade the capsule of the adrenal and may metastasize to the kidneys, liver, lungs, and bones. On occasion, an adrenal adenoma may also be virilizing. However, it is often difficult to determine microscopically whether the tumor is malignant or benign. Moreover, the clinical evolution does not always parallel the pathological appearance.

C. Laboratory Studies

These tumors secrete large amounts of androgens, as demonstrated by the elevated urinary excretion of total 17-ketosteroids and of dehydroepiandrosterone, along with abnormally high plasma concentrations of DHA and DHA sulfate (92). The latter two steroids are typical markers of virilizing adrenal tumors. There is also hypersecretion of androstenedione. The peripheral metabolism of DHA and androstenedione to testosterone is the cause of the virilism.

In contrast with congenital adrenal hyperplasia, the excessive androgen secretion of virilizing adrenal tumors is not suppressed by dexamethasone administration. In premature adrenarche, the increase in DHA, DHA sulfate, and androstenedione is at or below adult values and can also be suppressed by dexamethasone.

The differential diagnosis also includes virilizing gonadal tumors. In boys, Leydig cell tumors produce mainly testosterone with minimal amounts of DHA and DHA sulfate. In girls, virilizing ovarian tumors occur only after puberty and include the various types of tumors seen in adult women (adrenal rest tumor, hilar cell tumor, and arrhenoblastoma).

Although ultrasound study of the abdomen is usually excellent for the detection of ovarian tumors, it is not very sensitive as far as adrenal tumors are concerned. A computed tomographic (CT) scan or MRI without and with contrast is necessary to localize an adrenal mass.

D. Treatment

The tumor should be excised carefully, without damaging its capsule. Every effort should be made to remove the tumor en bloc. If present, metastases should be removed as completely as possible. In such cases, radiotherapy or chemotherapy with o,p'-DDD can be attempted.

Glucocorticoid therapy should be used during and after surgery until the status of the contralateral adrenal gland is determined. Theoretically, such treatment should

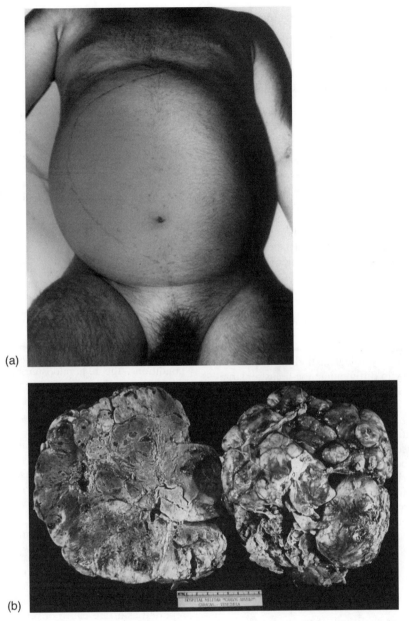

(a)

(b)

Figure 11   (a) Abdomen of a 4-year-old girl with virilizing adrenocorticol carcinoma. (b) Surgical specimen. (From Ref. 106.)

not be needed if the tumor does not secrete excessive cortisol. Practically, it is easy and safer to administer glucocorticoid. As previously noted, the prognosis of purely virilizing tumors that are well encapsulated is usually excellent, whereas that of tumors that also secrete excessive amounts of cortisol is generally poor.

XII.   FEMINIZING ADRENAL TUMORS

These tumors are even rarer than virilizing adrenal tumors in infants and children. Extrapolating from experience in

adults, approximately half of feminizing adrenal tumors are malignant (93).

A.   Clinical Manifestations

In boys, the major sign is gynecomastia; the testes are prepubertal in size, but pubic hair is often present, being related to the concomitant secretion of androgens and estrogens by the tumor. In girls, there is breast development, as seen in precocious puberty; pubic hair can be present, and breakthrough vaginal bleeding may occur. In children of both sexes, there is rapid statural and osseous development, height age and bone age being significantly advanced.

B. Pathology

For virilizing adrenal tumors, the diagnosis of malignancy is often difficult.

C. Laboratory Diagnosis

Urinary and plasma estrogen levels are usually elevated. Most of the tumors also secrete an excess of androgens, resulting in increased urinary 17-ketosteroids and plasma DHA, DHA sulfate, androstenedione, and, to some extent, testosterone. This excessive secretion of steroids is not dexamethasone suppressible. Often the laboratory results are not characteristic. CT scan and/or MRI is needed to make the definitive diagnosis of adrenal tumor.

D. Differential Diagnosis

Because of the lack of specificity of the clinical signs and hormone assays, the diagnosis of feminizing adrenal tumor is usually difficult.

Gynecomastia is a physiological finding in pubertal boys, and it is not easy to differentiate the breast enlargement that accompanies precocious puberty in a young boy from that of a feminizing adrenal tumor. A modest increase in testicular size in precocious puberty may not be differentiated from infantile testes in feminizing tumor. An LHRH test may be useful, showing a pubertal increase in LH in precocious puberty.

In prepubertal girls, a feminizing adrenal tumor must be differentiated from premature telarche and idiopathic sexual precocity. Estrogens are markedly increased in an adrenal tumor but not in premature telarche. A positive LHRH test should be helpful in determining sexual precocity.

E. Treatment

The tumor should be removed surgically promptly after the diagnosis has been established. If the tumor did not secrete excessive amounts of cortisol or 11-deoxycortisol, the prognosis is usually good.

XIII. HYPERALDOSTERONISM

The various syndromes of hyperaldosteronism are outlined in Table 5.

A. Secondary Hyperaldosteronism

An increase in plasma renin activity with increased aldosterone secretion is a physiological mechanism for the maintenance of serum electrolyte concentrations and fluid volume. It occurs with sodium loss, potassium retention,

Table 5 Syndromes of Hyperaldosteronism

Secondary hyperaldosteronism
    Physiological attempts to maintain serum
      electrolytes and fluid volumes
Primary hyperreninemia
    Renal ischemia
    Juxtaglomerular cell tumor
Primary hyperaldosteronism
    Adrenocortical adenoma
    Bilateral glomerular hyperplasia
Bartter's syndrome
Dexamethasone-suppressible hyperaldosteronism
Apparent mineralocorticoid excess: Familial
    11β-dehydrogenase deficiency

or decreased intravascular volume. Sodium loss occurs during diarrhea or excessive sweating. It also happens with administration of diuretics, in patients with renal tubular acidosis or salt-losing nephritis. The edema of the nephrotic syndrome or the ascites of cirrhosis of the liver causes a decrease in blood volume that results in compensatory increased aldosterone secretion. In all these conditions, the hyperaldosteronism is an attempt to reestablish an electrolyte–water balance, and this is termed secondary hyperaldosteronism. It may also occur in hypertension related to a unilateral renal disease with increased plasma renin activity. The increased aldosterone secretion characteristic of the non-salt-losing form of 21-hydroxylase deficiency can also be considered a secondary hyperaldosteronism because it occurs in response to the salt-losing tendency created by excessive secretion of 17-hydroxyprogesterone and progesterone.

B. Primary Hyperreninemia

The most common cause is renal ischemia, whether unilateral or bilateral. Such ischemia results in excessive secretion of renin by the juxtaglomerular apparatus. Tumors of the juxtaglomerular apparatus have also been reported as a rare cause of renin excess (94).

C. Primary Hyperaldosteronism

In 1955, Conn (95) described a disorder termed primary aldosteronism that was caused by an aldosterone-producing tumor of an adrenal gland. The symptoms included arterial hypertension, hypokalemic alkalosis, muscle weakness, and polyuria. Subsequently it was demonstrated that the plasma renin activity was markedly decreased. This syndrome is encountered mainly in adults, and only a very few cases have been reported in children.

1. Clinical Manifestations

The full clinical picture of this disorder is directly related to the hyperaldosteronism. Aldosterone increases potassium excretion, resulting in hypokalemia. This in turn results in muscle weakness with various types of paresthesias and sometimes unusual types of periodic paralysis. It is thought that the chronic hypokalemia is also responsible for the polyuria and resulting polydipsia. Aldosterone increases the retention of sodium, but the hypernatremia is largely compensated for by increased water retention. The increase in blood volume in turn results in hypertension, both systolic and diastolic.

2. Laboratory Diagnosis

The typical finding is a high aldosterone secretion with low plasma renin activity. Administration of a high-sodium diet or of DOCA fails to suppress aldosterone secretion. The low plasma renin activity differentiates the syndrome from the high renin levels seen in secondary hyperaldosteronism. A CT scan or MRI is necessary to demonstrate the presence of a mass in one of the adrenals. Because the adrenocortical tumor may be quite small, it may not be seen by MRI. Catheterization of the renal veins and selective adrenal vein sampling for measurement of aldosterone may demonstrate a very large secretion on one side and a lack of aldosterone on the other.

3. Pathology

In most cases, the tumor is an adenoma, but on occasion it can be a carcinoma (96). There can also be bilateral nodular hyperplasia of the adrenal cortex or focal hyperplasia of normal glomerular cells arranged in a nodular fashion.

4. Treatment

The adrenal tumor should be removed. Because it does not secrete cortisol, there is usually no need for glucocorticoid therapy during surgery.

In bilateral nodular hyperplasia, bilateral adrenectomy may be considered. In such cases, however, medical treatment with spironolactone, an inhibitor of aldosterone biosynthesis, is preferable if it can control the hypertension.

D. Bartter's Syndrome

This disorder is thought to be related to a renal tubular defect of chloride reabsorption. This results in passive loss of sodium, which in turn activates the renin–angiotensin–aldosterone system. In addition, the hyperaldosteronism results in hypokalemic alkalosis.

Patients usually present in infancy with failure to thrive, vomiting, weakness, and dehydration. Blood pressure is normal. There is hypochloremic metabolic alkalosis with hypokalemia and usually normal blood sodium. Plasma renin activity and aldosterone are elevated. One finds an increased urinary excretion of chloride and potassium with elevated excretion of prostaglandin. Renal biopsy shows hyperplasia of the juxtaglomerular apparatus (97).

There is no specific therapy, and an attempt is made to correct the electrolyte abnormalities. In some patients, the use of prostaglandin synthetase inhibitors, such as indomethacin or salicylates, can be beneficial.

E. Dexamethasone-Suppressible Hyperaldosteronism (Glucocorticoid-Remediable Aldosteronism)

In 1966, Sutherland et al. (98) reported a clinical condition characterized by hypertension, increased aldosterone secretion, and low plasma renin activity that was fully relieved by administration of dexamethasone (93, 94). Most recent progress in the molecular biology of steroid biosynthesis has been able to demonstrate that this disorder was related to a chimeric gene encoding for a cytochrome P450 possessing aldosterone synthetase activity but capable of responding to ACTH stimulation (Fig. 12). It is inherited as an autosomal dominant trait.

1. Clinical Manifestations

Symptoms and laboratory abnormalities in this disorder are identical to those found in primary hyperaldosteronism caused by an adrenal adenoma (98, 99). They include hypertension, hypokalemia, elevated plasma aldosterone concentrations, and low plasma renin activity. However, and in contrast to primary hyperaldosteronism, the hypertension, hypokalemia, increased aldosterone secretion, and low plasma renin activity can be returned to normal by the administration of dexamethasone. It has been noted that affected subjects always present with hypertension, but the degree of hypokalemia is variable.

2. Pathogenesis

Two genes, CYP11B1 and CYP11B2, encode for a cytochrome P450 possessing 11β-hydroxylase activity. However, CYP11B1 is mainly expressed in the zona fasciculata, under ACTH control, and CYP11B2 is mainly expressed in the zona glomerulosa, under angiotensin II control. The product of the CYP11B2 gene is also called aldosterone synthetase, which is capable of activating 18-hydroxylation and 18-oxidation in addition to 11β-hydroxylation. Both genes are located on chromosome 8q22.

It was recently proposed that a hybrid gene, CYP11B1/CYP11B2, as shown in Figure 12, is the cause of the disorder (101–103). The promoter of the hybrid gene is derived from the CYP11B1 and is therefore responsive to ACTH, but the chimeric protein encoded by this gene has the function of the aldosterone synthetase, hence the reason for the ACTH-dependent hyperaldosteronism. Because the chimeric gene is expressed in the zone fasciculata, which also expresses the CYP17 gene, there can be secretion of cortisol, which has also been hydroxylated in the carbon 18. Indeed, the secretion of 18-hydroxy and 18-oxocortisol is characteristic of dexamethasone-suppressible hyperaldosteronism. A series of

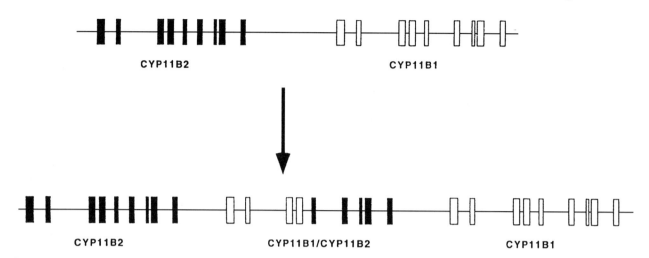

Figure 12 Gene organization of *CYP11B1* and *CYP11B2* genes (upper part of the figure) and organization of the hybrid *CYP11B1/CYP11B2* gene resulting from unequal crossing over (lower part of the figure). The resulting hybrid gene can be stimulated by ACTH as it includes the promotor of the B1 gene and can form aldosterone as it includes the 3' end of the B2 gene. (From Ref. 2.)

recent reports has identified such a chimeric gene, which includes the 5' sequences of the CYP11B1 gene and the 3' sequences from the CYP11B2 gene.

3. Treatment

As expressed by the name of the syndrome, dexamethasone or other glucocorticoid administration in replacement dosages turns off ACTH secretion, which in turn blocks aldosterone secretion as well as cortisol output. Although glucosteroid-remediable aldosteronism remains rare as a cause of hypertension in children, a recent report (100) suggested that it should be considered in severe cases with a positive family history of early-onset hypertension.

F. Familial Deficiency of 11β-Dehydrogenase

This congenital disorder is characterized by an apparent mineralocorticoid excess (104, 105). A gene encoding 11β-dehydrogenase has been cloned and mapped to chromosome 1 (106). This enzyme has the property of metabolizing cortisol into cortisone. In blood, the ratio of cortisol to cortisone is 5:1–10:1. In contrast, the kidney is rich in 11β-dehydrogenase, and only cortisone is found in this organ (107, 108). Under physiological conditions the receptor protein for mineralocorticoids has equal affinity for cortisol and aldosterone, but cortisone does not bind.

1. Pathophysiology

In this syndrome, a deficiency of 11β-hydroxysteroid dehydrogenase in the kidneys results in binding of cortisol to the mineralocorticoid receptor. In view of the large concentration of cortisol relative to aldosterone, there is sodium retention and water retention. The increased blood volume results in hypertension, and the increased mineralocorticoid activity generates hypokalemia. Under such conditions, plasma concentrations of aldosterone and renin activity are low.

2. Treatment

The severe hypertension in this disorder is generally resistant to any medical therapy. Dexamethasone binds to the glucocorticoid receptor with high activity but does not interact with the mineralocorticoid receptor. The full suppression of cortisol secretion by dexamethasone does not improve the hypertension, however, suggesting that the increased mineralocorticoid activity of the syndrome is mediated by both the renal glucocorticoid receptor and the mineralocorticoid receptor (109).

It has been reported that subjects who ingest large amounts of licorice develop hypertension and hypokalemia, with low levels of plasma aldosterone and plasma renin activity. It has been shown (110) that licorice contains glycyrrhizic acid, which has the property of inhibiting 11β-hydroxysteroid dehydrogenase activity.

REFERENCES

1. Migeon CJ, Donohoue PA. Adrenal disorders In: Kappy MS, Blizzard RM, Migeon CJ, eds. Wilkins Diagnosis and Treatment of Endocrine Disorders in Childhood and Adolescence. Springfield, IL: Charles C. Thomas, 1994: 717–856.
2. Donohoue PA, Parker K, Migeon CJ. Congenital adrenal hyperplasia. In: Scriver CR, et al., eds. The Metabolic Basis of Inherited Disease. New York: McGraw-Hill, 2001:4077–4115.
3. Gotoh O, Tagashira Y, Iizuka T, Fujii-Kuriyarnan Y. Structural characteristics of cytochrome P-450. Possible

location of the heme-binding cysteine is determined amino-acid sequences. J Biochem 1983; 93:807.

4. Miller WL. Structure of genes encoding steroidogenic enzymes. J Steroid Biochem 1987; 27:759.

5. Cumow KM, Tusie-Luna MT, Pascoe L, et al. The product of the CYPI IB2 gene is required for aldosterone biosynthesis in the human adrenal cortex. Mol Endocrinol 1991; 5:1513.

6. Vale W, Spiess J, Rivier C, Rivier J. Characterization of a 41-residue ovine hypothalamic peptide that stimulates secretion of corticotropin and A-endorphin. Science 1981; 213:1394.

7. Li CH, Geschwind 11, Cole RD, Raacke ID, Harris Ji, Dixon JS. Amino acid sequence of alpha corticotropin. Nature 1955; 176:687.

8. Lala DS, Rice DA, Parker KL. Steroidogenic factor 1, a key regulator of steroidogenic enzyme expression, is the mouse homolog of Fushi-Tarazu-factor 1. Mol Endocrinol 1992; 6:1249.

9. Luo X, Ikeda Y, Parker KL. A cell-specific nuclear receptor is essential for adrenal and gonadal development and sexual differentiation. Cell 1994; 77:481.

10. Weitzman ED, Fukushima D, Nogeire C, Roffwarg H, Gallagher TF, Hellman L. Twenty-four hour pattern of the episodic secretion of cortisol in normal subjects. J Clin Endocrinol Metab 1971; 33:14–22.

11. Migeon CJ, Tyler FH, Mahoney JP, et al. The diurnal variation of plasma levels and urinary excretion of 17-hydroxycorticosteroids in normal subjects, night workers and blind subjects. J Clin Endocrinol Metab 1956; 16: 622–633.

12. Dinarello CA, Mier JW. Current concepts. Lymphokines. N Engl J Med 1987; 317:940.

13. Sapolsky R, Rivier C, Yamamoto G, et al. Interleukin I stimulates the secretion of hypothalamic corticotropin releasing factor. Science 1987; 238:522.

14. Migeon CJ, Green OC, Eckert JP. Study of adrenocortical function in obesity. Metabolism 1963; 12:718.

15. Esteban NV, Longhlin T, Yergey AL, et al. Daily cortisol production rate in man determined by stable isotope dilution/mass spectometry. J Clin Endocrinol Metab 1991; 72:39–45.

16. Kerrigan, JR, Veldhuis JD, Leyo SA, et al. Estimation of daily cortisol production and clearance rates in normal pubertal males by deconvolution analysis. J Clin Endocrinol Metab 1993; 76:1505–1510.

17. Kowarski A, Lacerda L, Migeon CJ. Integrated concentration of plasma aldosterone in normal subjects: correlation with cortisol. J Clin Endocrinol Metab 1975; 40: 205.

18. Sklar CA, Kaplan SL, Grumbach MD. Evidence for dissociation between adrenarche and gonadarche. Studies in patients with idiopathic precocious puberty, gonadal dysgenesis, isolated gonadotropin deficiency and constitutionally delayed growth and adolescence. J Clin Endocrinol Metab 1980; 53:548.

19. Dunn JF, Nisula BC, Rodbard D. Transport of steroid hormones. J Clin Endocrinol Metab 1981; 53:58–68.

20. Orth DN, Kovacs WJ, DeBold CR. The adrenal cortex. In: Wilson JD, Foster DW, eds. Williams Textbook of Endocrinology, 8th ed. Philadelphia: WB Saunders, 1992: 489.

21. Mayenknecht J, Diederich S, Bahr V, et al. Comparison of low and high dose Corticotropin stimulation test in patients with pituitary disease. J Clin Endocrinol Metab 1998; 83:1558–1562.

22. Nye E, Grice JE, Hockings GI, et al. Comparison of adrenocorticotropin (ACTH) stimulation test and insulin hypoglycemia in normal humans: low dose, high dose, and 18 hour (ACTH (1–24) infusion tests. J Clin Endocrinol Metab 1999; 84:3648–3655.

23. Aron, DC. Diagnostic implications of adrenal physiology and clinical Epidemiology for evaluation of glucocorticoid excess and deficiency. In DeGroot LJ, Jamerson JL, eds. Endocrinology, 4th ed. Philadelphia: WB Saunders, 2001:1655–1670.

24. Chrousos GP, Schulte HM, Oldfield EH, et al. The corticotropin-releasing factor stimulation test. N Engl J Med 1984; 310:622.

25. Lashansky G, Saenger P, Fishman K, et al. Normative data for adrenal steroidogenesis in a healthy pediatric population: age- and sex-related changes after adrenocorticotropin stimulation. J Clin Endocrinol Metab 1991; 73: 674–686.

26. Guggenheim MA, McCabe ERB, Roig M, et al. Glycerol kinase deficiency with neuromuscular, skeletal, and adrenal abnormalities. Ann Neurol 1980; 7:441.

27. Bartley JA, Patil S, Davenport S, et al. Duchenne muscular dystrophy, glycerol kinase deficiency, and adrenal insufficiency associated with Xp2i interstitial deletion. J Pediatr 1986; 108:189.

28. Franke U, Ochs HD, DeMartinville B, et al. Minor Xp2l chromosome deletion in a male associated with expression of Duchenne muscular dystrophy, chronic granulomatous disease, retinitis pigmentosa and McLeod syndrome. Am J Human Genet 1985; 37:250.

29. Wise JE, Matalon R, Morgan AM, McCabe ERB. Phenotypic features of patients with congenital adrenal hypoplasia and glycerol kinase deficiency. Am J Dis Child 1987; 141:744.

30. Goonewardena P, Dahl N, Ritzen M, et al. Molecular Xp deletion in a male: suggestion of a locus for hypogonadotropic hypogonadism distal to the glycerol kinase and adrenal hypoplasia loci. Clin Genet 1989 (1):5–12.

31. Bardoni B, Zanaria E, Guioli S, et al. A dosage sensitive locus at chromosome Xp2l is involved in male to female sex reversal. Nature Genet 1994; 7:497–501.

32. Prader A, Zachmann M, Illig R. Luteinizing hormone deficiency in hereditary congenital adrenal hypoplasia. J Pediatr 1975; 86:421.

33. Migeon CJ, Kenny FM, Kowarski A, et al. The syndrome of congenital adrenocortical unresponsiveness to ACTH. Report of six cases. Pediatr Res 1968; 2:501–513.

34. Shepherd TH, Landing BH, Mason DG. Familial Addison's disease. Am J Dis Child 1959; 97:154–162.

35. Mountjoy KG, Robbins LS, Mortrud MT, Cone RD. The cloning of a family of genes that encode the melanocortin receptors. Science 1992; 257:1248–1251.

36. Clark AJL, McLoughlin L, Grossman A. Familial glucocorticoid deficiency associated with point mutation in the adrenocorticotropin receptor. Lancet 1993; 341:461–462.

37. Tsigos C, Arai K, Hung W, Chrousos GP. Hereditary isolated glucocorticoid deficiency is associated with abnormalities of the adrenocorticotropin receptor gene. J Clin Invest 1993; 92:2458–2461.

38. Yamaoka T, Kudo T, Takuwa Y, et al. Hereditary adrenocortical unresponsiveness to adrenocorticotropin with post-receptor defect. J Clin Endocrinol Metab 1992; 75: 270–274.

39. Franks RC, Nance WE. Hereditary adrenocortical unresponsiveness to ACTH. Pediatrics 1970; 45:43.

40. Stempfel RS Jr, Engel FL. A congenital familial syndrome of adrenocortical insufficiency without hypoaldosteronism. J Pediatr 1960; 57:443.

41. Allgrove J, Clayden GS, Grant DB, Macaulay JC. Familial glucocorticoid deficiency with achalasia of the cardia and deficient tear production. Lancet 1978; 1:1284–1286.

42. Lanes R, Plotnick L, Bynum TE, et al. Glucocorticoid and partial mineralocorticoid deficiency associated with achalasia. J Clin Endocrinol Metab 1980; 50:268–271.

43. Weber A, Wienker TF, Jung M, et al. Linkage of the gene for the triple A syndrome to chromsome 12q13 near the type II keratin gene cluster. Hum Mol Genet 1999; 5:2021–2066.

44. Powers JM, Schaumburg HH, Johnson AB, et al. A correlative study of the adrenal cortex in adrenoleukodystrophy—evidence for a fatal intoxication with very long chain saturated fatty acids. Invest Cell Pathol 1980; 3:353.

45. Fanconi A, Prader A, Isler W, et al. Morbus Addison mit Hirnskierose in Kindersaiter. Ein hereditares Syndrom mit X-chromosomaler Verebung? Helv Paediatr Acta 1964; 18:480.

46. Migeon BR, Moser HW, Moser AB, et al. Adrenoleukodystrophy: evidence for x-linkage inactivation, and selection favoring the mutant allele in heterozygous cells. Proc Natl Acad Sci USA 1981; 78:5066.

47. Mosser J, Douar AM, Sarde C-O, et al. Putative X-linked adrenoleukodystrophy gene shares unexpected homology with ABC transporters. Nature (London) 1993; 361:726–730.

48. Fanen P, Guidoux S, Sarde C-O, et al. Identification of mutations in the putative ATP-binding domain of the adrenoleukodystrophy gene. J Clin Invest 1994; 94:516–520.

49. Griffen JW, Goren E, Schaurnberg H, et al. Adrenomyeloneuropathy: a probable variant of adrenoleukodystrophy. Neurology 1977; 27:1107.

50. Libber SM, Migeon CJ, Brown FR III, Moser, HW. Adrenal and testicular function in 14 patients with adrenoleukodystrophy or adrenomyeloneuropathy. Hormone Res 1986; 24:1–8.

51. Fournier B, Saudubray J-M, Benichou B, et al. Large deletion of the peroxisomal Acyl-CoA oxidase gene in pseudoneonatal adrenoleukodystrophy. J Clin Invest 1994; 94:526–531.

52. Patrick AD, Lake BD. Deficiency of an acid lipase in Wolman syndrome. Nature 1969; 222:1067.

53. Koch GA, Lalley PA, McAvoy M, et al. Assignment of LIPA, associated with human acid lipase deficiency to chromosome 10 and comparative assignment to mouse chromosome 19. Somat Cell Genet 1981; 7:345.

54. Ballabio A, Shapiro LJ. Steroid sulfatase deficiency and X-linked ichthyosis. In: Scriver CR, et al., eds. The Metabolic Basis of Inherited Disease. New York: McGraw-Hill, 2001, p. 4241–4262.

55. Visser HKA and Cost WS. A new hereditary defect in the biosynthesis of aldosterone: urinary C2t-corticosteroid pattern in three related patients with a salt-losing syndrome, suggesting an 18-oxidation defect. Acta Endocrinol 1964; 47:589.

56. Degenhart HJ, Frankena L, Visser HKA, Cost WS, Van Setters AP. Further investigation of a new hereditary defect in the biosynthesis of aldosterone: evidence for a defect in the 18-hydroxylation of corticosterone. Acta Physiol Pharmacol Neerl 1966; 14:88.

57. Ulick S, Gautier E, Vetter KK, et al. An aldosterone biosynthesis defect in a salt-losing disorder. J Clin Endocrinol Metab 1964; 24:669.

58. David R, Golan S, Drucker W. Familial aldosterone deficiency: enzyme defect, diagnosis and clinical course. Pediatrics 1968; 41:403.

59. Rösler A, Rabinowitz D, Theodor R, Ramirez LC, Ulick S. The nature of the defect n in a salt-wasting disorder in Jews of Iran. J Clin Endocrinol Metab 1977; 44:279–291.

60. Globerman H, Rösler A, Theodor R, New MI, White PC. An inherited defect in aldosterone biosynthesis caused by a mutation in or near the gene for steroid 11-hydroxylase. N Engl J Med 1988; 319:1193.

61. Pascoe L, Curnow KM, Slutsker L, Rösler A, White PC. Mutations in the human CYP 11 B2 (aldosterone synthetase) gene causing corticosterone methyloxidase 11 deficiency. Proc Natl Acad Sci USA 1992; 89:4996–5000.

62. Ferran JL, Couture A, Cabissole MA, et al. Hematome de la glande surrenale chez un noveau-né: diagnostic et surveillance par echographie. Ann Pediatr (Paris) 1980; 27:391.

63. Dobs AS, Dempsey MA, Ladenson PW, et al. Endocrine disorders in men infected with human immunodeficiency virus. Am J Med 1987; 84:611.

64. Winter WE. Autoimmune endocrinopathies. In: Kappy MS, Blizzard RM, Migeon CJ, eds. Wilkins Diagnosis and Treatment of Endocrine Disorders in Childhood and Adolescence. Springfield, IL: Charles C. Thomas, 1994:317–382.

65. Blizzard RM, Johanson A. Disorders of Growth. In: Kappy MS, Blizzard RM, Migeon CJ, eds. Wilkins Diagnosis and Treatment of Endocrine Disorders in Childhood and Adolescence. Springfield, IL: Charles C. Thomas, 1994:383–455.

66. Cleveland WW, Green OC, Migeon CJ. A case of proved adrenocorticotropin deficiency. J Pediatr 1960; 57:376.

67. Aarskog D, Blizzard RM, Migeon CJ. Response to methopyrapone (Su4885) and pyrogen test in idiopathic hypopituitary dwarfism. J Clin Endocrinol 1965; 25:439–444.

68. Keenan BS, Beitins IZ, Lee PA, Kowarski AA, Blizzard RM, Migeon CJ. Estimation of ACTH reserve on normal and hypopituitary subjects. Comparison of oral and intravenous metyrapone with insulin hypoglycemia. J Clin Endocrinol Metab 1973; 37:540–549.

69. Brasel JA, Wright JC, Wilkins L, et al. An evaluation of seventy-five patients with hypopituitarism beginning in childhood. Am J Med 1965; 38:484.

70. Migeon CJ, Weldon VV, Guild HG. Adolescent Endocrinology. New York: Appleton-Century-Crofts, 1970:149.

71. Kenny FM, Preeyasombat C, Spaulding JS, Migeon CJ. Cortisol production rate. IV. Infants born of steroid-treated mothers and of diabetic infants with trisomy syndrome and with anencephaly. Pediatrics 1966; 37:34.

72. Alkalay AL, Pomerance JJ, Puri AR, et al. Hypothalamic–pituitary–adrenal axis function in very low birth weight infants treated with dexamethasone. Pediatrics 1990; 86:204–210.

73. Vingerhoeds ACM, Thijssen JH, Schwarz F. Spontaneous hypercortisolism without Cushing syndrome. J Clin Endocrinol Metab 1976; 43:1128–1133.

74. Chrousos GP, Vingerhoeds AMC, Loriaux DL, Lipsett MB. Primary cortisol resistance: a family study. J Clin Endocrinol Metab 1983; 56:1243–1245.

75. Francke U, Foellmer BE. The glucocorticoid receptor gene is in 5q3l-q32. Genomics 1989; 4:610–612.

76. Cheek DB, Perry JW. A salt-wasting syndrome in infancy. Arch Dis Child 1958; 33:252.

77. Kuhnle U, Nielsen MD, Tietze HU, et al. Pseudohypoaldosteronism in eight families: different forms of inheritance are evidence for various genetic defects. J Clin Endocrinol Metab 1990, 70:638.

78. Hanukoglu A. Type I pseudohypoaldosteronism includes two clinically and genetically distinct entities with either renal or multiple target organ defects. J Clin Endocrinol Metab 1991; 73:936–944.

79. Morrison N, Harrap SB, Arriza JL, et al. Regional chromosomal assignment of the human mineralocorticoid receptor gene to 4q3 1.1. Hum Genet 1990; 85:130.

80. Cushing H. Basophil adenoma of the pituitary body. Bull Johns Hopkins Hosp 1932; 50:137.

81. Liddle GW, Shute AM. The evolution of Cushing syndrome as a clinical entity. Adv Intern Med 1969; 15:155.

82. Oldfield EH, Schulte HM, Chrousos GP, et al. CRH stimulation in Nelson's syndrome: response of ACTH secretion to pulse injection and continuous infusion of CRH. J Clin Endocrinol Metab 1986; 62:1020–1026.

83. Grua JR, Nelson DH. ACTH-producing tumors. Endocrinol Metab Clin North Am 1991; 20:319–369.

84. Jennings AS, Liddle GW, Orth DN. Results of treating childhood Cushing's disease with pituitary irradiation. N Engl J Med 1977; 297:957–962.

85. Tyrrell JB, Brooks RM, Fitzgerald PA, et al: Cushing's disease: selective transsphenoidal resection of pituitary micro-adenomas. N Engl J Med 1978; 298:753–758.

86. Mampalam TJ, Tyrrell JB, Wilson CB. Transsphenoidal microsurgery for Cushing's disease: a report of 216 cases. Ann Intern Med 1988; 109:487–493.

87. Styne DM, Grumbach MM, Kaplan SL, et al. Treatment of Cushing's disease in childhood and adolescence by trans-sphenoidal microsurgery. N Engl J Med 1984; 310: 889–893.

88. Tindall OT, Herring CJ, Clark RV, et al. Cushing's disease: results of transsphenoidal microsurgery with emphasis on surgical failures. J Neurosurg 1990; 72:363–369.

89. Kenny FM, Haskida Y, Askari A, et al. Virilizing tumors of the adrenal cortex. Am J Dis Child 1968; 115:445.

90. Ribeiro RC, Sandrini-Neto RS, Schell MJ, et al. Adrenocortical carcinoma in children: a study of 40 cases. J Clin Oncol 1990; 8:67.

91. Fraumeni JE, Miller RW. Adrenocortical neoplasms with hemihypertrophy, brain tumors and other disorders. J Pediatr 1967; 70:129.

92. Saez JM, Rivarola MA, Migeon CJ. Studies in patients with adrenocortical tumors. J Clin Endocrinol Metab 1967; 27:615.

93. Gabrilove JL, Sharma DC, Wotiz HH, et al. Feminizing adrenocortical tumors in male: a review of 52 cases including a case report. Medicine (Baltimore) 1965; 44:37.

94. Conn JW, Cohen EL, Lucas CP, et al. Primary reninism: hypertension, hyperreninemia, and secondary aldosteronism due to renin-producing juxtaglomerular cell tumors. Arch Intern Med 1972; 130:682.

95. Conn JW. Primary aldosteronism, a new clinical syndrome. J Lab Clin Med 1955; 45:3.

96. Melby JC. Diagnosis of hyperaldosteronism. Endocrinol Metab Clin North Am 1991; 20:247–255.

97. Bartter FC, Pronove P, Gill JR Jr, et al. Hyperplasia of the juxtaglomerular apparatus with hyperaldosteronism and hypokalemic alkalosis: a new syndrome. Am J Med 1962; 33:811.

98. Sutherland DJ, Ruse JL, Laidlaw JC. Hypertension, increased aldosterone secretion and low plasma renin activity relieved by dexamethasone. Can Med Assoc J 1966; 95:1109.

99. New MI, Peterson RE. A new form of congenital adrenal hyperplasia. J Clin Endocrinol Metab 1967; 27:300.

100. Dluhy RG, Andeson B, Harlin B et al. Glucocorticoid remediable aldosteronism is associated with severe hypertension in early childhood. J Pediatr 2001; 138:715–720.

101. Pascoe L, Curnow KM, Slutsker L, et al. Glucocorticoid-suppressible hyperaldosteronism results from hybrid genes created by unequal crossovers between CYP11B1 and CYP11B2. Proc Natl Acad Sci USA 1992; 89:8327.

102. Lifton RP, Dluhy RG, Powers M, et al. Hereditary hypertension caused by chimaeric gene duplications and ectopic expression of aldosterone synthase. Nature Genet 1992; 2:66.

103. Miyahara K, Kawamoto T, Mitsuuchi Y, et al. The chimeric gene linked to glucocorticoid suppressible hyperaldosteronism encodes a fused P-450 protein possessing aldosterone synthase activity. Biochem Biophys Res Commun 1992; 189:885.

104. Ulick S, Levine LS, Gunczler P, et al. A new syndrome of acquired mineralocorticoid excess associated with defects in the peripheral metabolism of cortisol. J Clin Endocrinol 1979; 44:757.

105. Stewart PM, Corrie JET, Shackleton CHL. Syndrome of apparent mineralocorticoid excess. A defect in the cortisol–cortisone shuttle. J Clin Invest 1988; 82:340.

106. Tannin GM. The human gene for 11β-hydroxysteroid dehydrogenase, structure, tissue distribution, and chromosomal localization. J Biol Chem 1991; 266:16653.

107. Monder C. Corticosteroids, receptors, and the organ-specific function of 11β-hydroxysteroid dehydrogenase. FASEB J 1991; 5:3047.

108. Walker BR, Campbell JC, Williams BC, Edwards CR. Tissue-specific distribution of the NAD(+)-dependent isoform of 11 beta-hydroxysteroid dehydrogenase. Endocrinology 1992; 131:970.

109. Funder JW, Pearce PT, Myles K, et al. Apparent mineralocorticoid excess, pseudohypoaldosteronism, and urinary electrolyte excretion: toward a redefinition of mineralocorticoid action. FASEB J 1990; 4:3234.

110. Farese RV Jr, Biglieri EG, Shackleton CHL, Irony 1, Gomez-Fontex R. Licorice-induced hypermineralocorticoidism. N Engl J Med 1991; 325:1223.

111. DeLacera L, Kowarski A, Migeon CJ. Integrated concentration and diurnal variation of plasma cortisol. J Clin Endocrinol Metab 1993; 36:227.

112. Lanes R, Gonzalez S, Obregon O. Adrenal cortical carcinoma in a 4 year old child. Clin Pediatr 1982; 21:164–166.

7
Congenital Adrenal Hyperplasia

Maria I. New
Weill Medical College of Cornell University, New York Presbyterian Hospital, New York, New York, U.S.A.

Lucia Ghizzoni
University of Parma, Parma, Italy

I. INTRODUCTION

Congenital adrenal hyperplasia (CAH) is a family of inherited disorders of adrenal steroidogenesis. With only one exception, each disorder results from a deficiency in one of the several enzymatic steps necessary for normal steroid synthesis. Since the earliest case of CAH documented in 1865 by the Neapolitan anatomist De Crecchio (1), numerous investigators have unraveled the mechanisms of adrenal steroid synthesis and the associated enzyme defects responsible for the clinical syndromes. This report includes recent advances in the investigation and understanding of these disorders.

II. PATHOPHYSIOLOGY

The adrenal glands synthesize three main classes of hormones: mineralocorticoids, glucocorticoids, and sex steroids. Figure 1 shows a simplified scheme of the adrenal synthesis of these steroids from the cholesterol precursor molecule. Each enzymatic step is indicated.

The pituitary regulates adrenal steroidogenesis via adrenocorticotropic hormone (ACTH). ACTH stimulates steroid synthesis by acting on the adrenals to increase the conversion of cholesterol to pregnenolone, which is the principal substrate for the steroidogenic pathways. The central nervous system controls the secretion of ACTH, its diurnal variation, and its increase in stress via corticotropin-releasing factor (2, 3). The hypothalamic–pituitary–adrenal feedback system is mediated through the circulating level of plasma cortisol; any condition that decreases cortisol secretion results in increased ACTH secretion. Cortisol therefore exerts a negative feedback effect on ACTH secretion.

In most forms of congenital adrenal hyperplasia, an enzyme defect blocks cortisol synthesis, thus impairing cortisol-mediated negative feedback control of ACTH secretion (Fig. 2). Oversecretion of ACTH ensues, which stimulates excessive synthesis of the adrenal products of those pathways unimpaired by an enzyme deficiency and causes an accumulation of precursor molecules in pathways blocked by an enzyme deficiency.

The clinical symptoms of the different forms of congenital adrenal hyperplasia result from the particular hormones that are deficient and those produced in excess. In the most common case, that of 21-hydroxylase deficiency, the aldosterone and cortisol pathways are blocked and the androgen pathway, which does not involve 21-hydroxylation, is overstimulated. The characteristic virilization caused by 21-hydroxylase deficiency is due to excessive secretion of adrenal androgens.

An enzymatic deficiency of 11β-hydroxylase also results in decreased cortisol synthesis with consequent overproduction of cortisol precursors and sex steroids, as seen in 21-hydroxylase deficiency. Thus, 11β-hydroxylase deficiency shares the clinical feature of virilization with the 21-hydroxylase disorder. An additional finding in many, but not all, patients with 11β-hydroxylase deficiency is hypertension. The hypertension is thought to derive from the excess accumulation of the aldosterone precursor, deoxycorticosterone (DOC), a steroid with salt-retaining activity.

Disorders of adrenal steroidogenesis have also been described in association with deficiencies of 3β-hydroxysteroid dehydrogenase, 17α-hydroxylase/17, 20-lyase, and steroidogenic acute regulatory protein. A summary of the biochemical features of these disorders is presented in Table 1. The enzyme deficiency of 21-hydroxylase is the most common type of CAH, accounting for 90–95% of

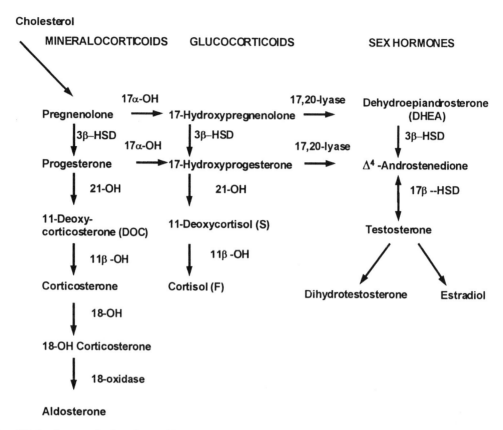

Figure 1 Simplified scheme of adrenal steroidogenesis shows abnormal secretion of hormones in congenital adrenal hyperplasia resulting from 21-hydroxylase deficiency. OH, hydroxylase; HSD, hydroxysteroid dehydrogenase.

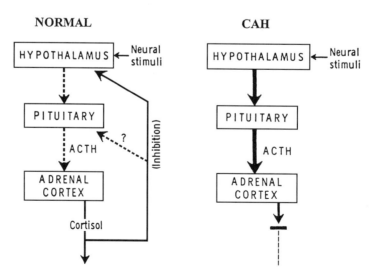

Figure 2 Regulation of cortisol secretion in normal subjects and in patients with congenital adrenal hyperplasia. (From Ref. 133.)

Table 1 Clinical and Laboratory Features of Various Disorders of Adrenal Steroidogenesis

Deficiency (syndrome)	Genital ambiguity	Postnatal virilization	Salt metabolism	Diagnostic hormones	Treatment
21-Hydroxylase					
Classic					
Salt wasting (SW)	F	Yes	Salt wasting	17-Hydroxyprogesterone (17OHP) Δ^4-Androstenedione (Δ^4-A) Aldosterone	Hydrocortisone (HC), 15–20 mg/m^2/day orally (PO), and fludrocortisone acetate (9αFF), 0.05–0.2 mg/day orally
Simple virilizing (SV)	F	Yes	Normal (elevated renin)	17-OHP, Δ^4-A	HC (same); addition of 9αFF (same) if elevated renin
Nonclassic (symptomatic and asymptomatic)	No	Yes	Normal	17-OHP, Δ^4-A	HC, 10–15 mg/m^2/day or dexamethasone, 0.25–0.5 mg/day or prednisone 5–10 mg/day
3β-Hydroxysteroid dehydrogenase					
Classic	M($\pm$F)	Yes	Salt wasting	17-OHP 17-hydroxypregnenolone (Δ^5 17-OHP) Dehydroepiandrosterone (DHEA) Δ^4-A	HC and 9αFF as for SW 21-hydroxylase deficiency
Nonclassic	No	Yes	Normal	17-OHP DHEA	HC as for nonclassic 21-hydroxylase deficiency
11β-Hydroxylase					
Classic (hypertensive CAH)	F	Yes	Salt retention (lowered PRA)	Deoxycorticosterone (DOC) 11-Deoxycortisol (S) Δ^4-A Plasma renin activity	HC, 15–20 mg/m^2/day
Nonclassic	No	Yes	Normal	S DOC	HC, dexamethasone, or prednisone as for nonclassic 21-hydroxylase deficiency
17α-Hydroxylase/17,20-lyase	M	No	Salt retention (lowered PRA)	DOC, Corticosterone (B)	HC, 15–20 mg/m^2/day[a]
Steroidogenic acute regulatory protein (StAR; congenital lipoid hyperplasia)	M	No	Salt wasting	None	HC, 15–20 mg/m^2/day 9αFF, 0.05–0.2 mg/day[a]

[a]With addition of sex steroid replacement at puberty.

all cases, with 11β-hydroxylase deficiency the second most common, occurring in 5–8% of cases.

III. CLINICAL FEATURES

The most prominent clinical feature of 21- and 11β-hydroxylase deficiency is virilization. Because adrenocortical function begins by month 3 of gestation, a fetus with 21- or 11β-hydroxylase deficiency is exposed to oversecreted adrenal androgens at the critical time of sexual differentiation. In a female fetus, the excessive adrenal androgens masculinize the external genitalia and female pseudohermaphroditism results. In rare cases, the masculinization is so profound that the urethra is penile (4). The internal genitalia (i.e., uterus and fallopian tubes), which arise from the müllerian ducts, are normal because the female fetus does not possess Sertoli's cells of the testes, the source of müllerian-inhibiting factor. The female genital abnormalities are present only in the androgen-responsive external genitalia. Males with 21- or 11β-hydroxylase deficiency do not manifest genital abnormalities at birth but may demonstrate hyperpigmentation.

The simple virilizing form of 21-hydroxylase deficiency is characterized by excess adrenal androgen secretion, which causes prenatal virilization of the genetic female and postnatal virilization of both boys and girls. In the salt-wasting form, in addition to the excess adrenal androgens, there is aldosterone deficiency causing low serum sodium, high serum potassium, and vascular collapse. In the more severe salt-wasting form, both newborn boys and girls are subject to early, life-threatening, salt-wasting crises within the first few weeks of life.

The various clinical and biochemical features associated with the different forms of congenital adrenal hyperplasia are indicated in Table 1. Continued oversecretion of adrenal androgens as a result of untreated 21- or 11β-hydroxylase deficiency results in progressive penile or clitoral enlargement; advanced bone age and tall stature in early childhood with ultimate short stature caused by premature epiphyseal closure; early appearance of facial, axillary, and pubic hair; and acne. In 11β-hydroxylase deficiency hypertension is frequently, although not necessarily, an additional finding. Girls with congenital adrenal hyperplasia who remain untreated do not develop breasts or menstruate and are further virilized. In untreated boys, the testes may remain small and there may be infertility, although some untreated men have been fertile (5).

In 3β-hydroxysteroid dehydrogenase deficiency (3β-HSD), steroid synthesis in both the adrenal cortex and in the gonads is affected, and only Δ^5 steroid precursors are formed and secreted. Circulating Δ^5 precursors undergo conversion peripherally to active Δ^4 steroids and are believed to cause virilization of the external genitalia in genetic females with 3β-HSD. Genetic males have incomplete external genital development due to deficient Δ^4 androgen production in the gonads (6, 7). Thus, genital ambiguity results in children of both sexes. Similar to 21-

and 11β-hydroxylase deficiency, the appearance of the external genitalia at birth does not predict the severity of the enzyme defect. There have been reports of a milder, nonclassic form of 3β-HSD deficiency; however, mutations in the gene for 3β-HSD have yet to be identified in these patients (8, 9).

Steroid 17α-hydroxylase/17,20-lyase deficiency, which accounts for approximately 1% of all CAH cases, affects steroid synthesis in the adrenals and gonads (10). Patients have impaired cortisol synthesis, leading to elevated ACTH that increases serum levels of deoxycorticosterone and especially corticosterone, resulting in low-renin hypertension, hypokalemia, and metabolic alkalosis. Affected females are born with normal external genitalia. Affected males are also born with undervirilized genitalia due to their deficient gonadal testosterone production. 17α-Hydroxylase/17,20-lyase deficiency is often recognized at puberty in girls who fail to develop secondary sex characteristics.

Congenital lipoid hyperplasia is an extremely rare and severe form of CAH in which cholesterol is not converted to pregnenolone. Synthesis of all adrenal and gonadal steroids is deficient and results in accumulations of cholesterol and cholesterol esters in the newborn. Recent studies have revealed that abnormalities of the steroidogenic acute regulatory protein (StAR) are responsible for this disorder (11, 12). StAR is involved in the transfer of cholesterol from the outer to the inner mitochondrial membrane, which is the rate-limiting step in steroidogenesis. Males with congenital lipoid hyperplasia are born with female-appearing external genitalia. Females have a normal genital phenotype at birth but remain sexually infantile without treatment, and all patients present with salt wasting. If not detected and treated, lipoid CAH is usually fatal (13).

IV. CLINICAL FORMS OF ADRENAL HYPERPLASIA CAUSED BY 21-HYDROXYLASE DEFICIENCY

Two major phenotypes are recognized in 21-hydroxylase deficiency: classic and nonclassic (late onset; Fig. 3). Within the latter class of patients are those who demonstrate the biochemical defect but lack any overt stigmata of hyperandrogenism. Table 2 delineates the differences between classic and nonclassic 21-hydroxylase deficiency.

A. Classic

Classic congenital adrenal hyperplasia is a well-known genetic disorder transmitted by an autosomal recessive gene. The biochemical and clinical abnormalities of this form of CAH are clearly present in patients both prenatally and postnatally. Progesterone, 17-OH-progesterone, androstenedione, and testosterone are secreted in excess, consequent to increased ACTH stimulation resulting from an inherited 21-hydroxylase deficiency that impairs cor-

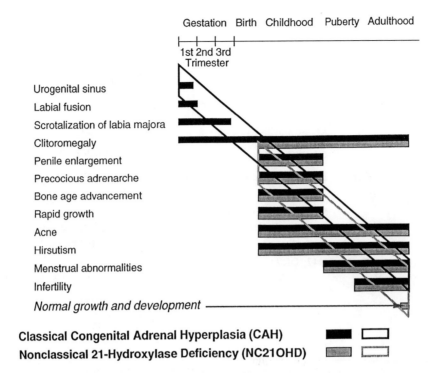

Figure 3 There is a wide spectrum of clinical presentation in 21-hydroxylase deficiency, ranging from prenatal virilization with labial fusion to precocious adrenarche, to pubertal or postpubertal virilization. During their lifetimes, patients' conditions may change from symptomatic to asymptomatic. (From New MI, Dupont B. Grumbach K, Levine LS. The adrenal hyperplasias. In: Stanbury JB, Wyngaarden JB, et al., eds. The Metabolic Basis of Inherited Disease, 5th ed. New York: McGraw-Hill, 1983: 973–1000.)

tisol synthesis (14–21). As expected, the urinary excretion of the metabolites of these steroids is also increased (22, 23). Abnormalities in cortisol secretion are also associated with alterations in the secretion of other pituitary hormones such as GH and TSH (24, 25).

In genetic females with congenital 21-hydroxylase deficiency, the developing fetus is exposed to the excessive adrenal androgens, equivalent to the male fetal level, secreted by the hyperplastic adrenal cortex. External genitalia in the genetic female range from mildly ambiguous to completely virilized. The internal genitalia (uterus and fallopian tubes) are not affected by the excess androgens. Boys with 21-hydroxylase deficiency do not manifest genital abnormalities at birth. Postnatally, in untreated boys and girls, continued excessive androgen production results in rapid somatic growth; advanced epiphyseal maturation; progressive penile or clitoral enlargement; early appearance of facial, axillary, and pubic hair; and acne. Without treatment, early epiphyseal closure and short stature result (26).

In three-quarters of cases with classic 21-hydroxylase deficiency, salt wasting occurs, as defined by hyponatremia, hyperkalemia, inappropriate natriuresis, and low serum and urinary aldosterone levels with concomitant high plasma renin activity (PRA). The increase in the propor-

tion of salt-wasting cases in recent years may be attributed in part to enhanced ascertainment because of advancements in diagnostic capabilities, as well as increased survival because of the availability of exogenous mineralocorticoid supplements. Salt wasting results from inadequate secretion of salt-retaining steroids, especially aldosterone. In addition, hormonal precursors of 21-hydroxylase may act as mineralocorticoid antagonists in the marginally competent sodium-conserving mechanism of the immature newborn renal tubule (27–29). It has been observed that an aldosterone biosynthetic defect apparent in infancy may be ameliorated with age (30, 31) and a spontaneous partial recovery from salt wasting in adulthood was described in a patient with severe salt wasting in infancy. This variation in the ability to produce mineralocorticoids may be attributable to another adrenal enzyme with 21-hydroxylase activity (32). Therefore, it is desirable to evaluate the sodium and mineralocorticoid requirements carefully by measuring plasma renin activity in patients who have been labeled neonatally as salt wasters.

Although it has been claimed that salt wasting correlates with severe virilism (33), it is important to recognize that the extent of virilism may be the same in simple virilizing and salt-wasting CAH. Thus, even a mildly

Table 2 Comparison of Classic and Nonclassic 21-Hydroxylase Deficiency

Feature	Classic	Nonclassic
Disease frequency	1:14,000	1:100 all white patients 1:27 Ashkenazi Jews
Prenatal virilization	Females	No
Postnatal virilization	Males and females	Variable
Salt wasting	60–75% cases	No
17-Hydroxyprogesterone levels after ACTH challenge	Extreme elevation (>20,000 ng/dl)	Moderate elevation (2000–15,000 ng/dl)
Genotype of CYP21	Severely affected allele/severely affected allele	Mildly affected allele/mildly affected allele; or severely affected allele/mildly affected allele
Associated HLA haplotype	B47; DR7	B14; DR1
Common mutations		
Simple virilizing	I172N Intron 2, A → G	V281L P30L P453S
Salt-wasting	Deletion Lg. conversion Intron 2, A → G Exon 3, −8 bp Codons 234–238 Q318 → Stop codon R356W	

virilized newborn with 21-hydroxylase deficiency should be observed carefully for signs of a potentially life-threatening crisis within the first few weeks of life.

B. Nonclassic 21-Hydroxylase Deficiency

An attenuated, late-onset form of adrenal hyperplasia was first suspected by gynecologists in clinical practice who used glucocorticoids for the treatment of women with physical signs of hyperandrogenism, including infertility (34, 35). The first documentation of suppression of 21-hydroxylase precursors in the urine of such patients after glucocorticoid therapy was by Baulieu and co-workers in 1957 (36). The precise diagnosis of a mild 21-hydroxylase defect was made possible when a radioimmunoassay for 17-hydroxyprogesterone (17-OHP) the direct precursor of the enzyme in the adrenal zona fasciculata, was developed (37). The autosomal recessive mode of genetic transmission of the nonclassic form of 21-hydroxylase deficiency (NC21-OHD) became apparent through family studies of classic 21-OHD (38–40). The establishment of linkage to HLA (41, 42) confirmed the existence of this disorder as an allele of classic 21-OHD (38, 43). The HLA associations for nonclassic 21-OHD (41, 44, 45) are distinct from

those found in classic 21-OHD and differ according to ethnicity (42, 46, 47).

The clinical symptoms of NC21-OHD are variable and may present at any age. NC21-OHD can result in premature development of pubic hair in children; to our knowledge, the youngest such patient was noted to have pubic hair at 6 months of age (39). In a review of 23 patients presenting for evaluation of premature pubarche, 7 children demonstrated a 17-OHP response to ACTH stimulation consistent with the diagnosis of nonclassic 21-hydroxylase deficiency, a prevalence of 30% in this preselected group of pediatric patients at high risk (48). Other investigators found that 7 of 46 children (15%) with premature pubarche demonstrated an ACTH-stimulated 17-OHP response greater than that of obligate heterozygote carriers of the 21-hydroxylase deficiency gene (49). Elevated adrenal androgens promote the early fusion of epiphyseal growth plates. It is common, but not universally found, that children with the disorder have advanced bone age and accelerated linear growth velocity, and ultimately are shorter than the height that might be predicted based on midparental height and on linear growth percentiles before the apparent onset of excess androgen secretion (50).

Severe cystic acne refractory to oral antibiotics and retinoic acid has been attributed to NC21-OHD. In one study of 31 young female patients with acne and/or hirsutism tested with low-dose ACTH stimulation after overnight dexamethasone suppression, no cases of 21-hydroxylase deficiency were found (51). In another study comparing the responses of 11 female patients with acne and 8 female control subjects to a 24 h infusion of ACTH, elevated urinary excretion of pregnanetriol in 6 patients was suggestive of a partial 21-hydroxylase deficiency (52).

Male pattern baldness in young women with this disorder has been noted as the sole presenting symptom. Severe androgenic alopecia in association with marked virilization has also been reported in an undiagnosed and therefore untreated 59-year-old woman with the simple virilizing form of the disease (53). Menarche may be normal or delayed, and secondary amenorrhea is a frequent occurrence. The syndrome of polycystic ovarian disease includes a subgroup of women with NC21-OHD. The pathophysiology of this phenomenon probably relates to adrenal sex steroid excess disrupting the usual cyclicity of gonadotropin release and/or the direct effects of adrenal androgens upon the ovary, leading ultimately to the formation of ovarian cysts, which then may autonomously produce androgens.

Retrospective analysis of the causes of hirsutism and oligomenorrhea revealed that 16 of 108 (14%) of young women presenting to this institution for endocrinological evaluation of these complaints had nonclassic 21-hydroxylase deficiency (54). In other published series the prevalence of nonclassic 21-hydroxylase deficiency in hirsute, oligomenorrheic women ranges from 1.2 to 30% (55–59). The disparity in frequency of nonclassic 21-hydroxylase deficiency reported by different authors may be attributed to differences in the ethnic groups studied because the disease frequency is ethnic-specific (Table 3).

In boys, early beard growth, acne, and growth spurt may be detected. A highly reliable constellation of physical signs of adrenal (as opposed to testicular) androgen excess in boys is the presence of pubic hair, enlarged phallus, and relatively small testes. In men, signs of androgen excess are difficult to appreciate and may theoretically be manifest only by short stature and/or adrenal sex steroid-induced suppression of the hypothalamic–pituitary–gonadal axis, resulting in diminished fertility.

Oligospermia and subfertility have been reported in men with nonclassic 21-hydroxylase deficiency (60, 61). Reversal of infertility with glucocorticoid treatment in three men has been observed (61–63).

The presence of 21-hydroxylase deficiency can be discovered during the evaluation of incidental adrenal masses (64). An increased incidence of adrenal incidentalomas has in fact been found in male and female patients with homozygous congenital adrenal hyperplasia (82%) and also in heterozygote subjects (45%), probably arising from hyperplastic tissue areas and not requiring surgical intervention (65).

A subset of NC-21OHD individuals is overtly asymptomatic when detected (usually as part of a family study), but it is thought, based on longitudinal follow-up of such patients, that symptoms of hyperandrogenism may wax and wane with time. The gene defect in these so-called cryptic 21-hydroxylase deficient subjects is the same as that found in symptomatic patients with the nonclassic disease.

V. PUBERTAL MATURATION IN CLASSIC CONGENITAL ADRENAL HYPERPLASIA

A. Onset of Puberty

In most patients treated satisfactorily from early life, the onset of puberty in both girls and boys with classic CAH occurs at the expected chronological age (66–69). The pattern of gonadotropin response to luteinizing hormone-releasing hormone (LHRH) is appropriate for age in prepubertal and pubertal girls with well-controlled CAH (70, 71). Physiologic secretion of gonadotropins, however, may not be entirely normal (72, 73).

True precocious puberty may occur in some well-treated children with CAH, perhaps correlated with bone age. Another setting in which central puberty sometimes occurs in CAH is after initiation of glucocorticoid therapy, producing a sudden decrease in sex steroid levels and leading to hypothalamic activation. LHRH analogs may be employed as an adjunct to therapy with hydrocortisone in such children (74). Long-term data on final height in a small number of CAH patients suggest that LHRH analogs (75, 76), along with growth hormone treatment (77), are not only effective in arresting the pubertal process but also improve final height.

In most untreated or poorly treated adolescent girls, and in some adolescent boys, spontaneous true pubertal development does not occur until proper treatment is instituted (Table 4) (67, 68, 78–80). Studies suggest that excess adrenal androgens (aromatized to estrogens) inhibit the pubertal pattern of gonadotropin secretion by the hypothalamic–pituitary axis (67). The inhibition probably occurs via a negative feedback effect; whether it is pri-

Table 3 Frequency of Nonclassic 21-Hydroxylase Deficiency

Ethnic group	Frequency
Ashkenazi Jewish	1:27
Hispanic	1:53
Slavic	1:63
Italian	1:333
General white population	1:100

Source: Data from Ref. 46.

Table 4   Pubertal Disorders in 21-Hydroxylase Deficiency CAH

	Classic: abnormal (poorly treated or untreated)	Classic: normal	Nonclassic: abnormal	Cryptic: normal
Girls	No thelarche; no menarche; secondary amenorrhea or menstrual irregularity; cystic ovaries, anovulation, infertility	None reported	Precocious adrenarche, hirsutism, cystic acne; amenorrhea or menstrual irregularity; anovulation, infertility, cystic ovaries	No abnormalities
Boys	Small testes[a] Decreased spermatogenesis	Normal testicular size Spermatogenesis	Precocious adrenarche Cystic acne	No abnormalities

[a]Adolescent males may have nodular testes as a result of adrenal rest tumor.

marily at the hypothalamus or pituitary is not known. This inhibition is reversible by suppression of the adrenal hormone production with glucocorticoid treatment.

Following gonadarche, in a majority of successfully treated patients, the milestones of further development of secondary sex characteristics in general appear to be normal (66, 69), although a somewhat delayed sequence of pubertal events was present in girls (66).

B.   Menstrual Disorders

Many patients with treated classic CAH have regular menses after menarche (67, 68, 81). However, expected age at menarche of treated CAH patients from various clinics as shown in Table 4, suggests that menarche was significantly delayed, especially when those patients who were not menstruating after 16 years of age were included. Menarche was not observed in untreated patients, but only in patients who had received suppressive glucocorticoid treatment (66–69, 82, 83).

Menstrual irregularity and secondary amenorrhea with or without hirsutism are not uncommon complications in postmenarchal girls (5, 68, 69, 82, 84, 85). These menstrual abnormalities have been found frequently in patients with inadequately controlled disease (Table 4) (66, 67, 69, 81, 82, 85). Several studies subsequently reported menarche or the normalization of the menstrual cycle following adequate suppression of adrenal sex steroids with long-acting and more potent glucocorticoid treatment (82, 85, 86). Delayed menarche or even primary amenorrhea may result from poor treatment or overtreatment. In poorly treated patients, the mechanism for delayed menarche may be interference by adrenal sex steroids in the cyclicity of the hypothalamic–pituitary–ovarian axis (66, 67). Delayed menarche in patients who are overtreated may be related to the delay in bone age and general maturation known to occur with excessive glucocorticoid treatment (66).

Many treated women have had successful pregnancies with the delivery of a normal, healthy, full-term infant (67, 87, 88). A recent study reports successful pregnancy outcomes in four women with classic CAH (1 with simple virilizing and 3 with salt-wasting) (89). All four gluco-

corticoid-treated mothers delivered unaffected and non-virilized baby girls. A retrospective survey of fertility rates in a large group of women with 21-hydroxylase deficiency showed that simple virilizers were more likely than salt wasters to become pregnant and carry the pregnancy to term (90). Adequacy of glucocorticoid therapy is probably an important variable with respect to fertility outcome (91). Among all patients questioned, only 50% reported that the vaginal introitus was adequate for intercourse; 5% reported homosexual preference, and 38% had no sexual experience. Based on these data, it seems prudent to perform early surgical correction of clitoromegaly but to delay vaginoplasty until adolescence (when the patient can be expected to assume responsibility for vaginal dilatation and strict adherence to medical therapy).

The clinical observation of gonadal function as described earlier clearly suggests that excess adrenal sex steroid production is the major contributing factor to gonadal dysfunction, menstrual disorders, anovulation, and infertility in girls with classic CAH. The generally accepted theory is that the excessive adrenal androgens may disrupt gonadotropin secretion, leading ultimately to hypogonadism (69, 72, 79, 83).

C.   Male Reproductive Function

Several long-term studies indicate that in a majority of successfully treated male patients with CAH, pubertal development, normal testicular function, and normal spermatogenesis and fertility occur (5, 68, 69, 92–94). However, complications of small testes and aspermia have been reported in some patients with inadequately controlled disease (5, 68, 80, 95). In contrast to this observation, some investigators have reported normal testicular maturation and normal spermatogenesis and fertility in patients who had never received glucocorticoid treatment (5, 78, 93, 96, 97) or in those whose glucocorticoid therapy was discontinued for several years (5, 93). Thus, male patients with CAH and excessive adrenal androgens may have either normal gonadal function or hypogonadism. The factors resulting in such a disparity in puberty among patients with the same disorder are not known. Some patients with normal gonadal function may have nonclassic rather than classic CAH (see later). Hormonal studies in untreated classic patients with normal sexual maturation have shown either normal or increased gonadotropin production (98) or concentrations and follicle-stimulating hormone excretion (5, 93, 98). Of great interest is that in these male patients, excess adrenal sex steroids or their precursor steroids did not seem to affect gonadotropin secretion. Adrenal androgen levels in untreated boys with normal gonadal function did not appear to be lower than those patients with gonadal dysfunction in poor control (5, 68, 95). This suggests that adrenal androgens alone have no effect on gonadotropin secretion via a negative feedback mechanism in male patients.

Another frequently reported complication in postpubertal boys with inadequate control of CAH is hyperplastic nodular testes. Almost all patients with such complications were found to have adenomatous adrenal rests within the testicular tissue, as indicated by the presence of specific 11β-hydroxylated steroids in the blood from gonadal veins (99). These tumors have been reported to be ACTH dependent and to regress following adequate steroid therapy (100–106).

VI. GENETICS

Studies of families carrying 21-hydroxylase deficiency have demonstrated that the disease locus is situated in the HLA major histocompatibility complex on the short arm of the sixth chromosome (107, 108). Both classic and nonclassic 21-hydroxylase deficiency are transmitted as recessive traits. Characteristic combinations of HLA alleles, or HLA haplotypes, are associated with different forms of 21-hydroxylase deficiency. The genotype for classic 21-hydroxylase deficiency results from the presence of two severely affected alleles. Nonclassic 21-hydroxylase deficiency results from the presence of either two mild 21-hydroxylase deficiency alleles or one severe and one mild allele (109).

Based on estimates of its frequency among Ashkenazi Jews (3%) and all ethnic whites (individuals of mainly European descent) (1%) (46), it is apparent that nonclassic 21-hydroxylase deficiency is among the most frequent human autosomal recessive disorders. Molecular genetic studies have demonstrated that the gene encoding the cytochrome P$_{450}$ enzyme specific for 21-hydroxylation (P450c21) is located in the HLA complex between the genes encoding the transplantation antigens, HLA-B and HLA-DR. This gene, *CYP21*, and an inactive homolog or

pseudogene, *CYP21P*, are immediately adjacent to the *C4B* and *C4A* genes encoding the fourth component of serum complement (110, 111) (Fig. 4). The protein-encoding sequence of *CYP21P* is 98% homologous to that of *CYP21*. The high degree of homology permits two types of mutation-causing recombination events: unequal crossing over during meiosis that results in complementary deletions/duplications of *CYP21* (112, 113), and noncorrespondences between the pseudogene and the coding gene that, if transferred by gene conversion, result in deleterious mutations (114).

Approximately 25% of classic 21-hydroxylase deficiency alleles result from deletions of *CYP21* (115–117). The remaining three-quarters of classic alleles are caused by smaller mutations in *CYP21*, some of which are *de novo* point mutations resulting in amino acid substitutions (118–121) that significantly disrupt synthesis of the protein. Nonclassic 21-OHD is associated with conservative (or mild) amino acid substitutions in highly conserved portions of the gene encoding the active 21-hydroxylase (122–124).

In studies evaluating the phenotype–genotype relationship, there is generally a good correlation between the severity of the clinical disease and the discrete mutations observed (118, 125). Recent studies, however, have demonstrated that there is often a divergence in phenotypes within mutation-identical groups, the reason for which requires further investigation (126, 127).

VII. EPIDEMIOLOGY

Screening studies indicate that the worldwide incidence of classic 21-OHD is 1:14,199 live births (128), of which approximately 75% are salt wasters. The frequency of nonclassic 21-OHD is considerably higher; based on population genetic studies this allelic variant occurs in 1:100 persons in the general white population and in higher frequency among selected ethnic groups, most notably Ashkenazi Jews (46). The frequency of 11β-OHD is approximately 1:100,000 live births (129); however, among Sephardic Jews of northern Morocco the incidence is estimated to be between 1:5000 and 1:6000 births (130).

VIII. DIAGNOSIS

Congenital adrenal hyperplasia must be suspected in infants born with ambiguous genitalia. The physician is

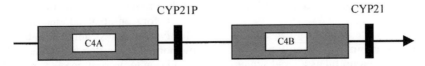

Figure 4   Diagram of *CYP21* region on chromosome 6p21.3. *CYP21P*, 21-hydroxylase pseudogene; *C4A* and *C4B*, genes encoding fourth component of serum complement. The arrow indicates the direction of transcription.

obliged to make the diagnosis as quickly as possible, to initiate therapy, and to arrest the effects of the enzyme disorders. The diagnosis and a rational decision of sex assignment must rely on the determination of genetic sex, the hormonal determination of the specific deficient enzyme, and an assessment of the patient's potential for future sexual activity and fertility. Physicians are urged to recognize the physical findings of ambiguous genitalia characteristic of congenital adrenal hyperplasia in newborns and to refer such cases to appropriate clinics for full endocrine evaluation.

As indicated in Table 1, each form of congenital adrenal hyperplasia has its own unique hormonal profile, consisting of elevated levels of precursors and elevated or diminished levels of adrenal steroid products (20, 21). Traditionally, laboratory tests have measured the urinary excretion of adrenal hormones or their urinary metabolites (e.g., 17-ketosteroids). Collection of 24 h urine excretion may be difficult, however, and the results in neonates may often be misleading (21). The development of simple and reliable radioimmunoassays for circulating serum levels of adrenal steroids is a significant advance in the laboratory diagnostic technique (20). The direct serum measurement of accumulated precursors and oversecreted adrenal steroids, such as 17-hydroxyprogesterone, Δ4-androstenedione, and dehydroepiandrosterone is now possible, and more exact hormonal profiles of the different forms of congenital adrenal hyperplasia have been established (Table 1).

A. Hormonal Standards for Genotyping 21-Hydroxylase Deficiency

In our experience, the best diagnostic hormonal test for 21-hydroxylase deficiency has proven to be an ACTH (Cortrosyn, 0.25 mg) stimulation test measuring the serum concentration of 17-OHP at 0 and 60 min after intravenous bolus ACTH administration (131). The nomogram (Fig. 5) provides hormonal standards for assignment of the 21-hydroxylase genotype: patients whose hormonal values fall on the regression line within a defined group are assigned to this group. Because of the diurnal variation in 17-OHP, an early morning serum concentration of 17-OHP may be useful as a screening test for genotyping 21-OHD. In addition, early morning salivary 17-OHP has proven to be an excellent screening test for the nonclassic form (132). ACTH stimulation, however, remains the most definitive diagnostic test (59, 132, 133). It is important to note that the ACTH stimulation test should not be performed during the initial 24 h of life: samples from this period are typically elevated in all infants and may yield false-positive results.

Diagnosis of 21-hydroxylase deficiency can also be made by microfilter paper radioimmunoassay for 17-hydroxyprogesterone; this has been useful as a rapid screening test for congenital adrenal hyperplasia in newborns (19). This convenient test requires only 20 μl blood, obtained by heel prick and blotted on microfilter paper, to provide a reliable diagnostic measurement of 17-hydroxyprogesterone, which is a cortisol precursor that accumulates in elevated concentrations in 21-hydroxylase deficiency. The simplicity of the test and the ease of transporting microfilter paper specimens through the mail has facilitated the implementation of many congenital adrenal hyperplasia newborn screening programs in the United States and worldwide.

B. Prenatal Diagnosis and Prenatal Treatment

1. Prenatal Diagnosis

Since the report by Jeffcoate et al. of the successful identification of an affected fetus by elevated concentrations of 17-ketosteroids and pregnanetriol in the amniotic fluid, investigators have undertaken prenatal diagnosis for congenital adrenal hyperplasia by similar measurements of hormone levels in pregnancy (134–136). The most specific hormonal diagnostic test for 21-hydroxylase deficiency is amniotic fluid 17-OHP (37, 137–140). Δ4-Androstenedione may be employed as an adjunctive diagnostic assay (139). It has been suggested that elevated amniotic fluid 21-deoxycortisol may also be a marker for 21-hydroxylase deficiency (141). Amniotic fluid testosterone levels may not be outside the normal range in an affected male (142).

HLA genotyping of amniotic fluid cells is a possible means of diagnosis but has now been superseded by direct molecular analysis of the 21-hydroxylase locus. With the advent of chorionic villus sampling (CVS), evaluation of the fetus at risk is now possible in the first trimester (9–11 weeks' gestation). The fetal DNA is used for specific amplification of the *CYP21* gene utilizing polymerase chain reaction (PCR) and Southern blotting, which has the advantage of requiring only small amounts of DNA (126).

2. Prenatal Treatment

Prenatal treatment with dexamethasone can be administered in pregnancies at risk for 21-hydroxylase deficiency (143–147). When properly administered, dexamethasone is effective in preventing ambiguous genitalia in the affected female. An algorithm for the diagnostic management of potentially affected pregnancies is given in Figure 6. The current recommendation is to treat the mother with a pregnancy at risk for 21-hydroxylase deficiency with dexamethasone at a dosage of 20 μg/kg divided into three doses daily (147).

Institution of such therapy prior to 10 weeks gestation, before onset of adrenal androgen secretion, would effectively suppress adrenal androgen production and allow normal separation of the vaginal and urethral orifices, in addition to preventing clitoromegaly. Obviously, if dexamethasone is to be administered at such an early date, treatment is blind to the status of the fetus. If the fetus is

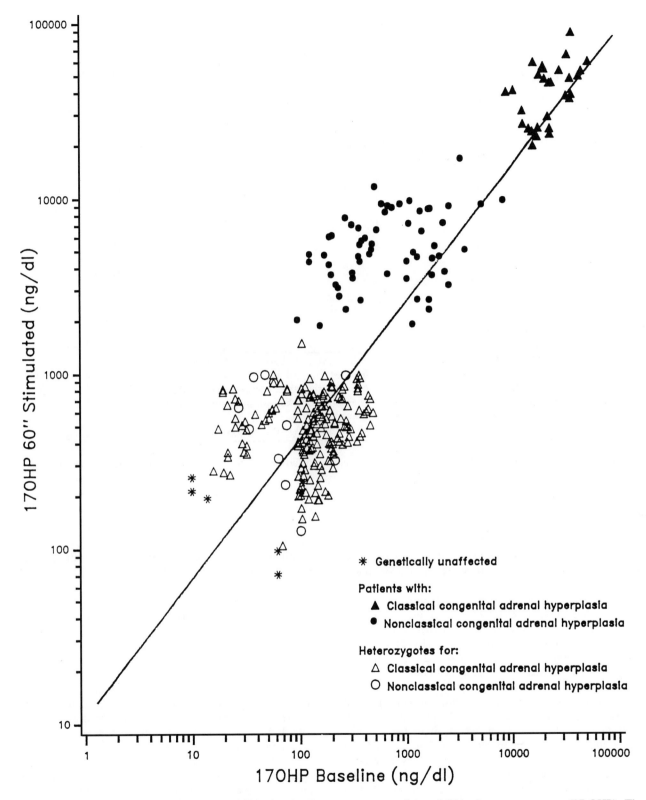

Figure 5 Nomogram relates baseline to ACTH-stimulated serum concentrations of 17-hydroxyprogesterone (17-OHP). The scales are logarithmic. A regression line for all data points is shown. (Data from Department of Pediatrics, New York Hospital–Cornell Medical Center, 1982–1991.)

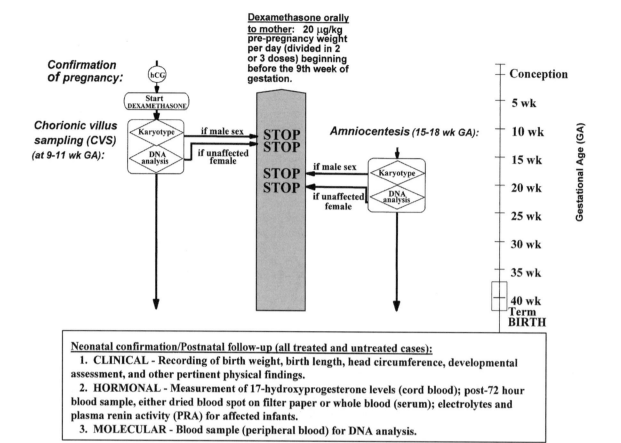

Figure 6   Algorithm depicts prenatal management of pregnancy in families at risk for a fetus with 21-hydroxylase deficiency. (From Ref. 147.)

determined to be a male upon karyotype or an unaffected female upon DNA analysis, treatment is discontinued. Otherwise, treatment is continued to term.

Between 1986 and 1999 prenatal diagnosis and treatment of CAH due to 21-OHD was carried out in over 400 pregnancies in The New York Presbyterian Hospital– Weill Medical College of Cornell University, of which 84 babies had classic 21-OHD. Of these, 52 were females, 36 of whom were treated prenatally with dexamethasone. Dexamethasone administered at or before 10 weeks of gestation was effective in reducing virilization thus, avoiding postnatal genitoplasty (148). No significant or enduring side effects were noted in either the mothers (other than weight gain greater than that in untreated mothers) or the fetuses. Specifically, no cases have been reported of cleft palate, placental degeneration, or fetal death, which have been observed in a rodent model of *in utero* exposure to high-dosage glucocorticoids (149). Another study, in contrast, noted significant maternal side effects in a few cases including excessive weight gain,

cushingoid facial features, severe striae resulting in permanent scarring, and hyperglycemic response to oral glucose administration (150).

A long term follow-up study of 44 children treated prenatally in Scandinavia demonstrated normal pre- and postnatal growth compared to matched controls (151). In the experience of the Weill Medical College of Cornell University–New York Presbyterian Hospital, prenatally treated newborns also did not differ in weight, length, or head circumference from untreated, unaffected newborns. Therefore, we believe that proper prenatal treatment of fetuses at risk for CAH can be considered effective and safe. Long-term studies on the psychological development of patients treated prenatally are currently underway.

A recent study has shown the efficacy of prenatal treatment in 11β-OHD CAH. In 1999, Cerame et al. reported the first prenatal diagnosis and treatment of an affected female with 11β-OHD CAH (152). The treatment was successful, as the newborn had normal female external genitalia.

IX. TREATMENT

In cases of ambiguous genitalia caused by congenital adrenal hyperplasia, appropriate surgical repair may be made once a sex assignment has been made based on a reliable diagnosis of the underlying enzyme disorder. In female pseudohermaphroditism caused by 21- or 11β-hydroxylase deficiency, the aim of surgical repair should be to remove the redundant erectile tissue, preserve the sexually sensitive glans clitoris, and provide a normal vaginal orifice that functions adequately for menstruation, intromission, and delivery (153). Because of the normal internal genitalia in these patients, normal puberty, fertility, and childbearing are possible when there is early therapeutic intervention.

The aim of endocrine therapy is to replace the deficient hormones. In 21- and 11β-hydroxylase deficiencies, replacing cortisol both corrects the deficiency in cortisol secretion and suppresses ACTH overproduction. Proper replacement prevents excessive stimulation of the androgen pathway, preventing further virilization and allowing normal growth and a normal onset of puberty.

Better understanding of the role of the renin–angiotensin system in congenital adrenal hyperplasia has made better therapeutic control of this condition possible. In addition to hypothalamic–pituitary regulation of adrenal steroidogenesis, the renin–angiotensin system exerts a primary influence on the adrenal secretion of aldosterone. The juxtaglomerular apparatus of the kidney secretes the enzyme renin in response to the state of electrolyte balance and plasma volume. Renin initiates a series of reactions that produce angiotensin II, which is a potent stimulator of aldosterone secretion (154).

Although aldosterone levels are not deficient in the simple virilizing form of 21-hydroxylase deficiency, plasma renin activity is commonly elevated in the simple virilizing as well as in the salt-wasting forms (155). Despite elevated plasma renin activity, it has not been customary to supplement conventional glucocorticoid replacement therapy with the administration of salt-retaining steroids in cases of simple virilizing 21-hydroxylase deficiency. However, Rosler et al. have demonstrated that adding salt-retaining hormone to glucocorticoid therapy in patients with classic simple virilizing CAH with elevated plasma renin activity in fact improves hormonal control of the disease (156). When plasma renin activity was normalized by the addition of 9-fludrocortisone acetate, a salt-retaining steroid, the ACTH level also fell and excessive androgen secretion decreased. The addition of salt-retaining steroids to the therapeutic regimen often made possible a decrease in the glucocorticoid dosage. Normalization of plasma renin activity also resulted in improved statural growth.

Steroid radioimmunoassay methods have been an asset not only for the initial diagnosis of congenital adrenal hyperplasia but also for improved monitoring of hormonal control once therapy has been instituted. Studies indicate that serum 17-hydroxyprogesterone and androstenedione levels provide the most sensitive index of biochemical control. In girls and prepubertal boys (but not in newborn and pubertal boys), the serum testosterone level is also a useful index (20). The combined determination of plasma renin activity, 17-hydroxyprogesterone, and serum androgens, as well as the clinical assessment of growth and pubertal development, must all be considered in adjusting the dosage of glucocorticoid and salt-retaining steroid. Recently, 3α-androstenediol (3AG) has been proposed as a useful serum metabolic marker of integrated adrenal androgen secretion in CAH patients. However, whether serum 3AG determinations would be useful for therapeutic monitoring of CAH requires further long-term study (157). Both in our clinic and in others, combinations of hydrocortisone and 9α-fludrocortisone acetate have proven to be highly effective treatment modalities (158). Monitoring of plasma renin activity is also a useful index of hormonal control in other forms of congenital adrenal hyperplasia.

X. CONCLUSION

Abnormalities of sexual differentiation and development, often in combination with hypertension (as in 11β-hydroxylase deficiency) or severe salt wasting (associated with 21-hydroxylase and 3β-hydroxysteroid dehydrogenase deficiency), are clinical hallmarks of congenital adrenal hyperplasia. The pathophysiology can be traced to discrete, inherited defects in the genes encoding enzymes for adrenal steroidogenesis. Treatment of CAH is targeted to replace the hormones produced in insufficient quantity. With proper hormone replacement therapy, normal and healthy development may often be expected. Radioimmunoassay of serum and urinary steroid levels permits reliable diagnosis of the various forms of congenital adrenal hyperplasia. Prenatal diagnosis and therapy are possible in 21-hydroxylase deficiency, and recently has been shown to be successful in the treatment of 11β-hydroxylase deficiency as well.

The most common form of CAH, 21-hydroxylase deficiency, has served as a prototype for examination of the molecular genetic basis of phenotypic diversity. Similar studies in other enzymatic defects are now in progress.

REFERENCES

1. De Crecchio L. Sopra un caso di apparenzi virili in una donna. Morgagni 1865;7:154–188.
2. Ganong W. The central nervous system and the synthesis and release of adrenocorticotrophic hormone. In: Nalbandov A, ed. Advances in Neuroendocrinology. Urbana, IL: University of Illinois Press, 1963:92.
3. Guillemin R, Schally A. Recent advances in the chemistry of neuroendocrine mediators originating in the central nervous system. In: Nalbandov A, ed. Advances in Neu-

roendocrinology. Urbana, IL: University of Illinois Press, 1963:314.

4. Wilkins L. Adrenal disorders. II. Congenital virilizing adrenal hyperplasia. Arch Dis Child 1962;37:231.

5. Prader A, Zachmann M, Illig R. Normal spermatogenesis in adult males with congenital adrenal hyperplasia after discontinuation of therapy. In: Lee P, Platnick L, Kowarski A, Migeon C, eds. Congenital Adrenal Hyperplasia. Baltimore, MD: University Park Press, 1977:397.

6. Simard J, Rheaume E, Mebarki F, et al. Molecular basis of human 3 beta-hydroxysteroid dehydrogenase deficiency. J Steroid Biochem Mol Biol 1995;53:127–138.

7. Moisan A, Ricketts M, Tardy V, et al. New insight into the molecular basis of 3 beta-hydroxysteroid dehydrogenase deficiency: identification of eight mutations in the HSD3B2 gene eleven patients from seven new families and comparison of the functional properties of twenty-five mutant enzymes. J Clin Endocrinol Metab 1999;84: 4410–4425.

8. Zerah M, Rheaume E, Mani P, et al. No evidence of mutations in the genes for type I and type II 3 beta-hydroxysteroid dehydrogenase (3 beta HSD) in nonclassical 3 beta HSD deficiency. J Clin Endocrinol Metab 1994;79: 1811–1817.

9. Tajima T, Nishi Y, Takase A, Nakae J, Murashita M, Fujieda K. No genetic mutation in type II 3 beta-hydroxysteroid dehydrogenase gene in patients with biochemical evidence of enzyme deficiency. Horm Res 1997;47:49–53.

10. Yanase T, Simpson E, Waterman M. 17 Alpha-hydroxylase/17,20-lyase deficiency: from clinical investigation to molecular definition. Endocr Rev 1991;12:91–108.

11. Lin D, Sugawara T, Strauss JF, et al. Role of steroidogenic acute regulatory protein in adrenal and gonadal steroidogenesis. Science 1995;267:1821–1831.

12. Bose H, Sugawara T, Strauss JF, Miller W. The pathophysiology and genetics of congenital lipoid adrenal hyperplasia. International Congenital Lipoid Adrenal Hyperplasia Consortium. N Engl J Med 1996;335:1870–1878.

13. Stocco D, Clark B. The role of the steroidogenic acute regulatory protein in steroidogenesis. Steroids 1997;62: 29–36.

14. Levine LS, New MI, Pitt P, Peterson RE. Androgen production in boys with sexual precocity and congenital adrenal hyperplasia. Metabolism 1972;21:457–464.

15. Lippe B, La FS, Lavin N, Parlow A, Coyotupa J, Kaplan S. Serum 17-alpha-hydroxyprogesterone, progesterone, estradiol, and testosterone in the diagnosis and management of congenital adrenal hyperplasia. J Pediatr 1974; 85:782–787.

16. Janne O, Perheentupa J, Viinikka L, Vihko R. Plasma pregnenolone, progesterone, 17-hydroxyprogesterone, testosterone and 5alpha-dihydrotestosterone in different types of congenital adrenal hyperplasia. Clin Endocrinol (Oxf) 1975;4:39–48.

17. Solomon I, Schoen E, Donelan L, Brandt-Erichsen D. Blood testosterone values in patients with congenital virilizing adrenal hyperplasia. J Clin Endocrinol Metab 1975;40:355–362.

18. Hughes I, Winter J. The application of a serum 17OH-progesterone radioimmunoassay to the diagnosis and management of congenital adrenal hyperplasia. J Pediatr 1976;88:766–773.

19. Pang S, Hotchkiss J, Drash AL, Levine LS, New MI. Microfilter paper method for 17-hydroxyprogesterone ra-

dioimmunassay. J Clin Endocrinol Metab 1977;45:1003–1008.

20. Korth-Schutz S, Virdis R, Saenger P, Chow DM, Levine LS, New MI. Serum androgens as a continuing index of adequacy of treatment of congenital adrenal hyperplasia. J Clin Endocrinol Metab 1978;46:452–458.

21. Pang S, Levine LS, Chow DM, Faiman C, New MI. Serum androgen concentrations in neonates and young infants with congenital adrenal hyperplasia due to 21-hydroxylase deficiency. Clin Endocrinol (Oxf) 1979;11: 575–584.

22. Bongiovanni AM, Eberlein WR, Cara J. Studies on metabolism of adrenal steroids in adrenogenital syndrome. J Clin Endocrinol Metab 1954;14:409.

23. Butler GC, Marrian GF. The isolation of pregnane-3,17,20-triol from the urine of women showing the adrenogenital syndrome. J Biol Chem 1937;119:565.

24. Ghizzoni L, Mastorakos G, Vottero A, Magiakou M, Chrousos G, Bernasconi S. Spontaneous cortisol and growth hormone secretion interactions in patients with nonclassic 21-hydroxylase deficiency (NCCAH) and control children. J Clin Endocrinol Metab 1996;81:482–487.

25. Ghizzoni L, Mastorakos G, Street M, et al. Spontaneous thyrotropin and cortisol secretion interactions in patients with nonclassical 21-hydroxylase deficiency and control children. J Clin Endocrinol Metab 1997;82:3677–3683.

26. New M, Levine L. Adrenal hyperplasia in intersex states. In: Laron Z, Tikva P, eds. Pediatric and Adolescent Endocrinology, vol 8. Basel: S Karger, 1981:51.

27. Klein R. Evidence for and evidence against the existence of a salt-losing hormone. J Pediatr 1960;57:452.

28. Kowarski A, Finkelstein J, Spaulding J, Holman G, Migeon C. Aldosterone secretion rate in congenital adrenal hyperplasia. A discussion of the theories on the pathogenesis of the salt-losing form of the syndrome. J Clin Invest 1965;44:1505.

29. Kuhnle U, Land M, Ulick S. Evidence for the secretion of an antimineralocorticoid in congenital adrenal hyperplasia. J Clin Endocrinol Metab 1986;62:934–940.

30. Stoner E, Dimartino-Nardi J, Kuhnle U, Levine LS, Oberfield SE, New MI. Is salt-wasting in congenital adrenal hyperplasia due to the same gene as the fasciculata defect? Clin Endocrinol (Oxf) 1986;24:9–20.

31. Luetscher JA. Studies of aldosterone in relation to water and electrolyte balance in man. Recent Prog Horm Res 1956;12:175.

32. Speiser PW, Agdere L, Ueshiba H, White PC, New MI. Aldosterone synthesis in salt-wasting congenital adrenal hyperplasia with complete absence of adrenal 21-hydroxylase. N Engl J Med 1991;324:145–149.

33. Verkauf B, Jones HJ. Masculinization of the female genitalia in congenital adrenal hyperplasia: relationship to the salt losing variety of the disease. South Med J 1970;63: 634–638.

34. Jones H, Jones G. The gynecological aspects of adrenal hyperplasia and allied disorders. Am J Obstet Gynecol 1954;68:1330.

35. Jefferies W, Weir W, Weir D, Prouty R. The use of cortisone and related steroids in infertility. Fertil Steril 1958; 9:145.

36. Decourt MJ, Jayle MF, Baulieu E. Virilisme cliniquement tardif avec excretion de pregnanetriol et insuffisance de la production du cortisol. Ann Endocrinol (Paris) 1957; 18:416.

37. Frasier S, Thorneycroft I, Weiss B, Horton R. Letter: Elevated amniotic fluid concentration of 17 alpha-hydroxy-

progesterone in congenital adrenal hyperplasia. J Pediatr 1975;86:310–312.

38. Levine LS, Dupont B, Lorenzen F, et al. Cryptic 21-hydroxylase deficiency in families of patients with classical congenital adrenal hyperplasia. J Clin Endocrinol Metab 1980;51:1316–1324.

39. Kohn B, Levine LS, Pollack MS, et al. Late-onset steroid 21-hydroxylase deficiency: a variant of classical congenital adrenal hyperplasia. J Clin Endocrinol Metab 1982; 55:817–827.

40. Rosenwaks Z, Lee PA, Jones GS, Migeon CJ, Wentz AC. An attenuated form of congenital virilizing adrenal hyperplasia. J Clin Endocrinol Metab 1979;49:335.

41. Pollack MS, Levine LS, O'Neill GJ, et al. HLA linkage and B14, DR1. BfS haplotype assocation with the genes for late onset and cryptic 21-hydroxylase deficiency. Am J Hum Genet 1981;33:540–550.

42. Laron Z, Pollack MS, Zamir R, et al. Late-onset 21-hydroxylase deficiency and HLA in the Ashkenazi population: a new allele at the 21-hydroxylase locus. Hum Immunol 1980;1:55–66.

43. Levine LS, Dupont B, Lorenzen F, et al. Genetic and hormonal characterization of cryptic 21-hydroxylase deficiency. J Clin Endocrinol Metab 1981;53:1193–1198.

44. Blankstein J, Faiman C, Reues FI, Schroeder ML, Winter JSD. Adult-onset familial adrenal 21-hydroxylase deficiency. Am J Med 1980;68:441.

45. Migeon CJ, Rosenwaks Z, Lee PA, Urban MD, Bias WB. The attenuated form of congenital adrenal hyperplasia as an allelic form of 21-hydroxylase deficiency. J Clin Endocrinol Metab 1980;51:647.

46. Speiser PW, Dupont B, Rubinstein P, Piazza A, Kastelan A, New IM. High frequency of nonclassical steroid 21-hydroxylase deficiency. Am J Hum Genet 1985;37:650–667.

47. Dumic M, Brkljacic L, Speiser PW, et al. An update on the frequency of nonclassical deficiency of adrenal 21-hydroxylase in the Yugoslav population. Acta Endocrinol 1990;122:703–710.

48. Temeck JW, Pang SY, Nelson C, New MI. Genetic defects of steroidogenesis in premature pubarche. J Clin Endocrinol Metab 1987;64:609–617.

49. Hawkins L, Chasalow F, Blethen S. The role of adrenocorticotropin testing in evaluating girls with premature adrenarche and hirsutism/oligomenorrhea. J Clin Endocrinol Metab 1992;74:248–253.

50. New MI, Gertner JM, Speiser PW, del Balzo P. Growth and final height in congenital adrenal hyperplasia (classical 21-hydroxylase deficiency) and in nonclassical 21-hydroxylase deficiency. In: Cavallo L, Job JC, New MI, eds. Growth Disorders: The State of the Art, vol 81. New York: Raven Press, 1991:105–110.

51. Lucky A, Rosenfield R, McGuire J, Rudy S, Helke J. Adrenal androgen hyperresponsiveness to adrenocorticotropin in women with acne and/or hirsutism: adrenal enzyme defects and exaggerated adrenarche. J Clin Endocrinol Metab 1986;62:840–848.

52. Rose L, Newmark S, Strauss J, Pochi P. Adrenocortical hydroxylase deficiencies in acne vulgaris. J Invest Dermatol 1976;66:324–326.

53. Odriscoll J, Anderson D. Untreated congenital adrenal hyperplasia. J R Soc Med 1993;86:229.

54. Pang SY, Lerner AJ, Stoner E, et al. Late-onset adrenal steroid 3 beta-hydroxysteroid dehydrogenase deficiency. I. A cause of hirsutism in pubertal and postpubertal women. J Clin Endocrinol Metab 1985;60:428–439.

55. Child D, Bu'lock D, Anderson D. Adrenal steroidogenesis in hirsute women. Clin Endocrinol (Oxf) 1980;12:595–601.

56. Gibson M, Lackritz R, Schiff I, Tulchinsky D. Abnormal adrenal responses to adrenocorticotropic hormone in hyperandrogenic women. Fertil Steril 1980;33:43–48.

57. Lobo R, Goebelsmann U. Adult manifestation of congenital adrenal hyperplasia due to incomplete 21-hydroxylase deficiency mimicking polycystic ovarian disease. Am J Obstet Gynecol 1980;138:720–726.

58. Chrousos G, Loriaux D, Mann D, Cutler GJ. Late-onset 21-hydroxylase deficiency is an allelic variant of congenital adrenal hyperplasia characterized by attenuated clinical expression and different HLA haplotype associations. Horm Res 1982;16:193–200.

59. Kuttenn F, Couillin P, Girard F, et al. Late-onset adrenal hyperplasia in hirsutism. N Engl J Med 1985;313:224–231.

60. Chrousos GP, Loriaux DL, Sherines RJ, Cutler GB. Unilateral testicular enlargement resulting from inapparent 21-hydroxylase deficiency. J Urol 1981;126:127.

61. Wischusen J, Baker HWG, Hudson B. Reversible male infertility due to congenital adrenal hyperplasia. Clin Endocrinol 1981;14:571.

62. Bonaccorsi AC, Adler I, Figueiredo JG. Male infertility due to congenital adrenal hyperplasia: testicular biopsy findings, hormonal evaluation, and therapeutic results in three patients. Fertil Steril 1987;47:664–670.

63. Augartan A, Weissenberg R, Pariente C, Sack J. Reversible male infertility in late onset congenital adrenal hyperplasia. J Endocrinol Invest 1991;14:237–240.

64. Mokshagundam S, Surks M. Congenital adrenal hyperplasia diagnosed in a man during workup for bilateral adrenal masses. Arch Intern Med 1993;153:1389–1391.

65. Jaresch S, Kornely E, Kley H, Schlaghecke R. Adrenal incidentaloma and patients with homozygous or heterozygous congenital adrenal hyperplasia. J Clin Endocrinol Metab 1992;74:685–689.

66. Jones H, Verkauf B. Congenital adrenal hyperplasia: age at menarche and related events at puberty. Am J Obstet Gynecol 1971;109:292.

67. Klingensmith G, Garcia S, Jones H, Migeon C, Blizzard R. Glucocorticoid treatment of girls with congenital adrenal hyperplasia: effects on height, sexual maturation, and fertility. J Pediatr 1977;90:996–1004.

68. Pang S, et al. Growth and sexual maturation and elevated progesterone levels in women treated for congenital virilizing 21-hydroxylase deficiency. In: Lee P, et al., eds. Congenital Adrenal Hyperplasia. Baltimore, MD: University Park Press, 1977:233–246.

69. Ghali I, David M, David L. Linear growth and pubertal development in treated congenital adrenal hyperplasia due to 21-hydroxylase deficiency. Clin Endocrinol (Oxf) 1977;6:425–436.

70. Reiter E, Grumbach M, Kaplan S, Conte F. The response of pituitary gonadotropes to synthetic LRF in children with glucocorticoid-treated congenital adrenal hyperplasia: lack of effect of intrauterine and neonatal androgen excess. J Clin Endocrinol Metab 1975;40:318–325.

71. Kirkland J, Kirkland R, Librik L, Clayton G. Serum gonadotropin levels in female adolescents with congenital adrenal hyperplasia. J Pediatr 1974;84:411–414.

72. Wentz A, Garcia S, Klingensmith G, Migeon C, Jones G. Hypothalamic maturation in congenital adrenal hyperplasia. In: Lee P, Plotnick L, Kowarski A, Migeon C, eds.

Congenital Adrenal Hyperplasia. Baltimore, MD: University Park Press, 1977:379.

73. Levin J, Carmina E, Lobo R. Is the inappropriate gonadotropin secretion of patients with polycystic ovary syndrome similar to that of patients with adult-onset congenital adrenal hyperplasia? Fertil Steril 1991;56:635–640.

74. Pescovitz O, Comite F, Cassorla F, et al. True precocious puberty complicating congenital adrenal hyperplasia: treatment with a luteinizing hormone-releasing hormone analog. J Clin Endocrinol Metab 1984;58:857–861.

75. Dacou-Voutetakis C, Karidis N. Congenital adrenal hyperplasia complicated by central precocious puberty: treatment with LHRH-agonist analogue. Ann NY Acad Sci 1993;687:250–254.

76. Soliman AT, Al Lamki M, Al Salmi I, Asfour M. Congenital adrenal hyperplasia complicated by central precocious puberty: linear growth during infancy and treatment with gonadotropin-releasing hormone analog. Metabolism 1997;46:513–517.

77. Quintos J, Vogiatzi M, Harbison M, New M. Growth hormone and depot leuprolide therapy for short stature in children with congenital adrenal hyperplasia. San Diego, CA: 81st Annual Meeting of the Endocrine Society. 1999.

78. Wilkins L, Crigler J, Silverman S, Gardner L, Migeon C. Further studies on the treatment of congenital adrenal hyperplasia with cortisone. II. The effects of cortisone on sexual and somatic development, with an hypothesis concerning the mechanism of feminization. J Clin Endocrinol Metab 1952;12:277.

79. Klingensmith G, Wentz A, Meyer W, Migeon C. Gonadotropin output in congenital adrenal hyperplasia. J Clin Endocrinol Metab 1976;43:933.

80. Kiesslin G, Schwarz G. Zur genese des hypogonadismus beim kongenitalen adrenogenitalen syndrome. Arch Klin Dermatol 1966;228:684.

81. Kirkland R, Keenan B, Clayton G. Long-term follow-up of patients with congenital adrenal hyperplasia in Houston. In: Lee P, Plotnick L, Kowarski A, Migeon C, eds. Congenital Adrenal Hyperplasia. Baltimore, MD: University Park Press, 1977:273.

82. Richards G, Grumbach M, Kaplan S, Conte F. The effect of long acting glucocorticoids on menstrual abnormalities in patients with virilizing congenital adrenal hyperplasia. J Clin Endocrinol Metab 1978;47:1208–1215.

83. Richards G, Styne D, Conte F, Kaplan S, Grumbach M. Plasma sex steroids and gonadotropins in pubertal girls with congenital adrenal hyperplasia: relationship to menstrual disorders. In: Lee P, Plotnick L, Kowarski A, Migeon C, eds. Congenital Adrenal Hyperplasia. Baltimore, MD: University Park Press, 1977:233.

84. Grayzel E. Postpubertal adrenogenital syndrome. Treatable cause of infertility. NY State J Med 1974;74:1038–1039.

85. Granoff A. Treatment of menstrual irregularities with dexamethasone in congenital adrenal hyperplasia. J Adolesc Health Care 1981;2:23–27.

86. Rosenfield R, Bickel S, Razdan A. Amenorrhea related to progestin excess in congenital adrenal hyperplasia. Obstet Gynecol 1980;56:208–215.

87. Riddick D, Hammond C. Adrenal virilism due to 21-hydroxylase deficiency in the postmenarchial female. Obstet Gynecol 1975;45:21–24.

88. Mori M. Congenital adrenogenital syndrome and successful pregnancy: report of a case. J Obstet Gynecol 1970;35:394.

89. Lo J, Schwitzgebel V, Tyrrell J, et al. Normal female infants born of mothers with classic congenital adrenal hyperplasia due to 21-hydroxylase deficiency. J Clin Endocrinol Metab 1999;84: 930–936.

90. Mulaikal RM, Migeon CJ, Rock JA. Fertility rates in female patients with congenital adrenal hyperplasia due to 21-hydroxylase deficiency. N Engl J Med 1987;316:178–182.

91. Premawardhana L, Hughes I, Read G, Scanlon M. Longer term outcome in females with congenital adrenal hyperplasia (CAH): the Cardiff experience. Clin Endocrinol (Oxf) 1997;46:327–332.

92. Stewart J. A fertile male with untreated congenital adrenal hyperplasia. Acta Endocrinol Suppl 1960;51:661.

93. Urban M, Lee P, Migeon C. Adult height and fertility in men with congenital virilizing adrenal hyperplasia. N Engl J Med 1978;299:1392.

94. Valentino R, Savastano S, Tommaselli A, et al. Success of glucocorticoid replacement therapy on fertility in two adult males with 21-CAH homozygote classic form. J Endocrinol Invest 1997;20:690–694.

95. Molitor J, Chertow B, Fariss B. Long-term follow-up of a patient with congenital adrenal hyperplasia and failure of testicular development. Fertil Steril 1973;24:319.

96. Bahner F, Schwarz G. Congenitale nebennierenrinden hyperplasie beim mann mit normaler keimdrusenfunktion und fertilitat. Acta Endocrinol 1961;38:236.

97. Wilkins L. The Diagnosis and Treatment of Endocrine Disorders. Springfield, IL: Charles C. Thomas, 1965: 368–381.

98. Raiti S, Maclaren N, Akesode F. Gonadotropin–adrenal–testicular axis in males with congenital adrenal hyperplasia and idiopathic sexual precocity. In: Lee P, Plotnick L, Kowarski A, Migeon C, eds. Congenital Adrenal Hyperplasia. Baltimore, MD: University Park Press, 1977:403.

99. Blumberg-Tick J, Boudou P, Nahoul K, Schaison G. Testicular tumors in congenital adrenal hyperplasia: steroid measurements from adrenal and spermatic veins. J Clin Endocrinol Metab 1991;73:1129–1133.

100. Schoen E, DiRaimondo V, Dominguez O. Bilateral testicular tumors complicating congenital adrenocortical hyperplasia. J Clin Endocrinol Metab 1961;21:518.

101. Miller E, Murray H. Congenital adrenocortical hyperplasia: case previously reported as bilateral interstitial cell tumor of the testicle. J Clin Endocrinol Metab 1962;22:655.

102. Glenn J, Boyce W. Adrenogenitalism with testicular adrenal rests simulating interstitial cell tumor. J Urol 1963; 89:456.

103. Radfar N, Bartter F, Easley R, Kolins J, Javadpour N, Sherins R. Evidence for endogenous LH suppression in a man with bilateral testicular tumors and congenital adrenal hyperplasia. J Clin Endocrinol Metab 1977;45:1194–1204.

104. Srikanth M, West B, Ishitani M, Isaacs HJ, Applebaum H, Costin G. Benign testicular tumors in children with congenital adrenal hyperplasia. J Pediatr Surg 1992;27:639–641.

105. Rutgers J, Young R, Scully R. The testicular "tumor" of the adrenogenital syndrome. A report of six cases and review of the literature on testicular masses in patients with adrenocortical disorders. Am J Surg Pathol 1988;12:503–513.

106. Chakraborty J, Franco-Saenz R, Kropp K. Electron microscopic study of testicular tumor in congenital adrenal hyperplasia. Hum Pathol 1983;14:151–157.

107. Dupont B, Oberfield SE, Smithwick EM, Lee TD, Levine LS. Close genetic linkage between HLA and congenital adrenal hyperplasia (21-hydroxylase deficiency). Lancet 1977;2:1309–1312.

108. Levine LS, Zachmann M, New MI, et al. Genetic mapping of the 21-hydroxylase-deficiency gene within the HLA linkage group. N Engl J Med 1978;299:911–915.

109. Speiser P, New M. Genotype and hormonal phenotype in nonclassical 21-hydroxylase deficiency. J Clin Endocrinol Metab 1987;64:86–91.

110. White PC, Grossberger D, Onufer BJ, et al. Two genes encoding steroid 21-hydroxylase are located near the genes encoding the fourth component of complement in man. Proc Natl Acad Sci USA 1985;82:1089–1093.

111. Carroll MC, Campbell RD, Porter RR. The mapping of 21-hydroxylase genes adjacent to complement component C4 genes in HLA, the major histocompatibility complex in man. Proc Natl Acad Sci USA 1985;82:521–525.

112. Higashi Y, Yoshioka H, Yamane M, Gotoh O, Fujii-Kuriyama Y. Complete nucleotide sequence of two steroid 21-hydroxylase genes tandemly arranged in human chromosome: a pseudogene and a genuine gene. Proc Natl Acad Sci USA 1986;83:2841–2845.

113. White PC, New MI, Dupont B. Structure of the human steroid 21-hydroxylase genes. Proc Natl Acad Sci USA 1986;83:5111–5115.

114. Tusie-Luna M, White P. Gene conversions and unequal crossovers between CYP21 (steroid 21-hydroxylase gene) and CYP21P involve different mechanisms. Proc Natl Acad Sci USA 1995;92:10796–10800.

115. Werkmeister JW, New MI, Dupont B, White PC. Frequent deletion and duplication of the steroid 21-hydroxylase genes. Am J Hum Genet 1986;39:461–469.

116. White PC, Vitek A, Dupont B, New MI. Characterization of frequent deletions causing steroid 21-hydroxylase deficiency. Proc Natl Acad Sci USA 1988;85:4436–4440.

117. Rumsby G, Carroll M, Porter R, Grant D, Hjelm M. Deletion of the steroid 21-hydroxylase and complement C4 genes in congenital adrenal hyperplasia. J Med Genet 1986;23:204–209.

118. Wedell A, Ritzen EM, Haglund SB, Luthman H. Steroid 21-hydroxylase deficiency: three additional mutated alleles and establishment of phenotype-genotype relationships of common mutations. Proc Natl Acad Sci USA 1992;89:7232–7236.

119. Rodrigues NR, Dunham I, Yu CY. Molecular characterization of the HLA-linked steroid 21-hydroxylase B gene from an individual with congenital adrenal hyperplasia. EMBO J 1987;6:1653–1661.

120. Owerbach D, Ballard A, Draznin M. Salt-wasting congenital adrenal hyperplasia: detection and characterization of mutations in the steroid 21-hydroxylase gene, CYP21, using the polymerase chain reaction. J Clin Endocrinol Metab 1992;74:553–558.

121. Tajima T, Fujieda K, Fujii-Kuriyama Y. de novo mutation causes steroid 21-hydroxylase deficiency in one family of HLA-identical affected and unaffected siblings. J Clin Endocrinol Metab 1993;77:86–89.

122. Speiser PW, New MI, White PC. Molecular genetic analysis of nonclassic steroid 21-hydroxylase deficiency associated with HLA-B14,DR1. N Engl J Med 1988;319:19–23.

123. Tusie-Luna MT, Speiser PW, Dumic M, New MI, White PC. A mutation (Pro-30 to Leu) in CYP21 represents a potential nonclassic steroid 21-hydroxylase deficiency allele. Mol Endocrinol 1991;5:685–692.

124. Owerbach D, Sherman L, Ballard AL, Azziz R. Pro-453 to ser mutation in CYP21 is associated with nonclassic steroid 21-hydroxylase deficiency. Mol Endocrinol 1992;6:1211–1215.

125. Speiser PW, Dupont J, Zhu D, et al. Disease expression and molecular genotype in congenital adrenal hyperplasia due to 21-hydroxylase deficiency. J Clin Invest 1992;90:584–595.

126. Wilson RC, Mercado AB, Cheng KC, New MI. Steroid 21-hydroxylase deficiency: genotype may not predict phenotype. J Clin Endocrinol Metab 1995;80:2322–2329.

127. Krone N, Braun A, Roscher A, Knorr D, Schwarz H. Predicting phenotype in steroid 21-hydroxylase deficiency? Comprehensive genotyping in 155 unrelated, well defined patients from southern Germany. J Clin Endocrinol Metab 2000;85:1059–1065.

128. Pang SY, Wallace MA, Hofman L, et al. Worldwide experience in newborn screening for classical congenital adrenal hyperplasia due to 21-hydroxylase deficiency. Pediatrics 1988;81:866–874.

129. Zachmann M, Tassinari D, Prader A. Clinical and biochemical variability of congenital adrenal hyperplasia due to 11beta-hydroxylase deficiency. J Endocrinol Metab 1983;56:222–229.

130. Rosler A, Leiberman E, Cohen T. High frequency of congenital adrenal hyperplasia (classic 11 beta-hydroxylase deficiency) among Jews from Morocco. Am J Med Genet 1992;42:827–834.

131. New M, Lorenzen F, Lerner A, et al. Genotyping steroid 21-hydroxylase deficiency: hormonal reference data. J Clin Endocrinol Metab 1983;57:320–326.

132. Zerah M, Pang SY, New MI. Morning salivary 17-hydroxyprogesterone is a useful screening test for nonclassical 21-hydroxylase deficiency. J Clin Endocrinol Metab 1987;65:227–232.

133. Kutten F. Late-onset adrenal hyperplasia (letter). N Engl J Med 1986;314:450.

134. Jeffcoate T, Fleigner J, Russell S, Davis J, Wade A. Diagnosis of the adrenogenital syndrome before birth. Lancet 1965;2:553.

135. New MI, Levine LS. Congenital adrenal hyperplasia. Adv Hum Genet 1973;4:251–326.

136. Levine L. Prenatal detection of congenital adrenal hyperplasia. In: Milunsky A, ed. Genetic Disorders and the Fetus. New York: Plenum Press, 1986:369–385.

137. Nagamani M, McDonough P, Ellegood J, Mahesh V. Maternal and amniotic fluid 17 alpha-hydroxyprogesterone levels during pregnancy: diagnosis of congenital adrenal hyperplasia in utero. Am J Obstet Gynecol 1978;130:791–794.

138. Hughes I, Laurence K. Antenatal diagnosis of congenital adrenal hyperplasia. Lancet 1979;2:7–9.

139. Pang S, Levine LS, Cederqvist LL, et al. Amniotic fluid concentrations of delta 5 and delta 4 steroids in fetuses with congenital adrenal hyperplasia due to 21 hydroxylase deficiency and in anencephalic fetuses. J Clin Endocrinol Metab 1980;51:223–229.

140. Hughes I, Laurence K. Prenatal diagnosis of congenital adrenal hyperplasia due to 21-hydroxylase deficiency by amniotic fluid steroid analysis. Prenat Diagn 1982;2:97–102.

141. Blankstein J, Fujieda K, Reyes F, Faiman C, Winter J. Cortisol, 11-desoxycortisol, and 21-desoxycortisol concentrations in amniotic fluid during normal pregnancy. Am J Obstet Gynecol 1980;137:781–784.

142. Frasier S, Weiss B, Horton R. Amniotic fluid testosterone: implications for the prenatal diagnosis of congenital adrenal hyperplasia. J Pediatr 1974;84:738–741.

143. Speiser PW, Laforgia N, Kato K, et al. First trimester prenatal treatment and molecular genetic diagnosis of congenital adrenal hyperplasia (21-hydroxylase deficiency). J Clin Endocrinol Metab 1990;70:838–848.

144. Forest M, David M. [Antenatal diagnosis and treatment of congenital adrenal hyperplasia due to 21-hydroxylase deficiency.] Rev Prat 1991;41:1183–1187.

145. Dorr H, Sippell W, Haack D, Bidlingmaier F, Knorr D. Pitfalls of prenatal treatment of congenital adrenal hyperplasia (CAH) due to 21-hydroxylase deficiency. Program and Abstract. Zurich: 25th Annual Meeting of the European Society for Paediatric Endocrinology, 1986

146. Evans M, Chrousos G, Mann D, et al. Pharmacologic suppression of the fetal adrenal gland in utero. Attempted prevention of abnormal external genital masculinization in suspected congenital adrenal hyperplasia. JAMA 1985;253:1015–1020.

147. Mercado AB, Wilson RC, Cheng KC, Wei JQ, New MI. Extensive personal experience: prenatal treatment and diagnosis of congenital adrenal hyperplasia owing to steroid 21-hydroxylase deficiency. J Clin Endocrinol Metab 1995;80:2014–2020.

148. Carlson AD, Obeid JS, Kanellopoulou N, Wilson RC, New MI. Prenatal treatment and diagnosis of congenital adrenal hyperplasia owing to steroid 21-hydroxylase deficiency. In: New MI, ed. Diagnosis and Treatment of the Unborn Child. Reddick, FL: Idelson-Gnocchi, 1999:75–84.

149. Goldman A, Sharpior B, Katsumata M. Human foetal palatal corticoid receptors and teratogens for cleft palate. Nature 1978;272:464–466.

150. Pang S, Clark AT, Freeman LO, et al. Maternal side-effects of prenatal dexamethasone therapy for fetal congenital adrenal hyperplasia. J Clin Endocrinol Metab 1992;76:249–253.

151. Lajic S, Wedell A, Bui T, Ritzen E, Holst M. Long-term somatic follow-up of prenatally treated children with congenital adrenal hyperplasia. J Clin Endocrinol Metab 1998;83:3872–3880.

152. Cerame BI, Newfield RS, Wilson RC, New MI. Prenatal diagnosis and treatment of 11beta-hydroxylase deficiency congenital adrenal hyperplasia. In: New MI, ed. Diagnosis and Treatment of the Unborn Child. Reddick, FL: Idelson-Gnocchi, 1999:175–178.

153. Mininberg DT, Levine LS, New MI. Current concepts in congenital adrenal hyperplasia. Invest Urol 1979;17:169–175.

154. Laragh J. Aldosteronism in man: factors controlling secretion of the hormone. In: Christy N, ed. The Human Adrenal Cortex. New York: Harper and Row, 1971:483.

155. Bartter F. Adrenogenital syndromes from physiology to chemistry. In: Lee P, Lotnick LP, Kowaraski A, Migeon C, eds. Congenital Adrenal Hyperplasia. Baltimore, MD: University Park Press, 1977:9.

156. Rosler A, Levine LS, Schneider B, Novogroder M, New MI. The interrelationship of sodium balance, plasma renin activity and ACTH in congenital adrenal hyperplasia. J Clin Endocrinol Metab 1977;45:500–512.

157. Pang S, MacGillivray M, Wang M, et al. 3 alpha-androstanediol glucuronide in virilizing congenital adrenal hyperplasia: a useful serum metabolic marker of integrated adrenal androgen secretion. J Clin Endocrinol Metab 1991;73:166–174.

158. Winter J. Current approaches to the treatment of congenital adrenal hyperplasia [editorial]. J Pediatr 1980;97:81–82.

8

Disorders of the Adrenal Medulla: Catecholamine-Producing Tumors in Childhood

Karel Pacak, Graeme Eisenhofer, Frederieke M. Brouwers, and Christian A. Koch
National Institutes of Health, Bethesda, Maryland, U.S.A.

Martina Weise
Institute for Drugs and Medical Devices, Bonn, Germany

I. THE CATECHOLAMINES

Catecholamines are produced by various neuroendocrine tumors mainly by pheochromocytoma, neuroblastoma, ganglioneuroma, and ganglioneuroblastoma. The catecholamines, norepinephrine and epinephrine, are produced by the sympathoneuronal and adrenomedullary systems. Levels of both catecholamines can be nonspecifically elevated during a variety of physiological conditions or pathological states that reflect activation of sympathoneuronal and sympathomedullary systems (e.g., emotional stress, physical activity, eating, fever). Also, pheochromocytomas or other chromaffin cell tumors secrete catecholamines episodically; between episodes, plasma levels or urinary excretion of catecholamines may be normal. Thus, commonly utilized tests of plasma or urinary catecholamines and their urinary metabolites do not always exclude or confirm the presence of a tumor (1–3). A more recently developed biochemical test in our laboratory involving high-performance liquid chromatographic (HPLC) measurements of plasma free metanephrines, the O-methylated metabolites of catecholamines, offers advantages over other tests for diagnosis of pheochromocytoma (4, 5). Plasma levels of the adrenomedullary hormones epinephrine and metanephrine are higher in children than in adults and higher in boys than in girls (75), possibly due to the suppressive effect of sex steroids, particularly estrogen, on adrenomedullary function (6–8, 75). Therefore, age- and gender-specific reference ranges

should be used for evaluation of sympathoadrenal function or catecholamine-producing tumors.

A. Pathways of Catecholamine Synthesis and Metabolism

Tyrosine hydroxylase is the rate-limiting enzyme in catecholamine biosynthesis and catalyzes the conversion of tyrosine to 3,4-dihydroxyphenylalanine (DOPA) (Fig. 1) (9). DOPA is converted to dopamine by L-aromatic amino acid decarboxylase. The presence of the intravesicular enzyme, dopamine β-hydroxylase, leads to conversion of dopamine to norepinephrine. In the presence of the enzyme, phenylethanolamine N-methyltransferase (PNMT); (localized in adrenomedullary chromaffin cells, or pheochromocytoma cells producing epinephrine) epinephrine is generated (10, 11).

Norepinephrine and epinephrine are metabolized by multiple enzymes, including monoamine oxidase (MAO), catechol-O-methyltransferase (COMT), and sulfotransferase (12–14). From a diagnostic point of view, the most important pathway of catecholamine metabolism involves COMT-catalyzed O-methylation of norepinephrine to normetanephrine and epinephrine to metanephrine (15–18). Another metabolite, vanillylmandelic acid (VMA), is the principal end-product of norepinephrine and epinephrine metabolism in humans. VMA is formed in the liver, mainly from hepatic extraction of circulating dihydroxyphenylglycol and 3-methoxy-4-hydroxyphenylglycol. All catecholamines and their metabolites (with the exception of VMA) are converted to sulfate conjugates, which represent other end-products of catecholamine metabolism.

B. Production of Metanephrines Within Chromaffin Tissue

In contrast to catecholamines, the metanephrines are relatively poor markers of sympathoadrenal activation (16, 18). This makes the metanephrines less prone to false-positive results in physiological and pathological states associated with sympathoadrenomedullary activation. Furthermore, plasma free metanephrines are constantly produced by the actions of COMT on catecholamines leaking from storage vesicles within tumors and are relatively independent of catecholamine secretion. Therefore, measurements of plasma metanephrines show larger and more consistent increases above normal than plasma catecholamines in patients with pheochromocytoma, and appear to exclude reliably the presence of all but the smallest of pheochromocytomas.

II. PHEOCHROMOCYTOMA

Pheochromocytomas arise in about 90% of cases from adrenomedullary tissue and in about 10% of cases from extra-adrenal chromaffin tissue (paragangliomas). Paragangliomas arise from chromaffin tissue in the abdomen along great vessels, most commonly around the aorta below the diaphragm and at the origin of the inferior mesenteric artery (organ of Zuckerkandl) (19).

Although pheochromocytomas are the most common endocrine tumors in children, they account for only 5–10% of all pheochromocytomas with an incidence of 2 per million (20, 21). In children, pheochromocytomas are frequently familial (9–50%), extra-adrenal (8–43%), bilateral adrenal (7–53%), and multifocal (22, 23). Childhood pheochromocytomas peak at 10–13 years with a male predominance before puberty (22–24). Less than 10% of pediatric pheochromocytomas are malignant (22, 23, 25, 26) with reported mean survival rates of 73% at 3 years and 40–50% at 5 years after diagnosis (27, 28). Recurrent pheochromocytomas are rare in children but recurrent tumors may appear years after initial diagnosis, emphasizing the importance of close long-term follow up (26).

A. Clinical Presentations

The presence of pheochromocytoma in children is characterized by clinical signs and symptoms that result from various actions of circulating catecholamines, including

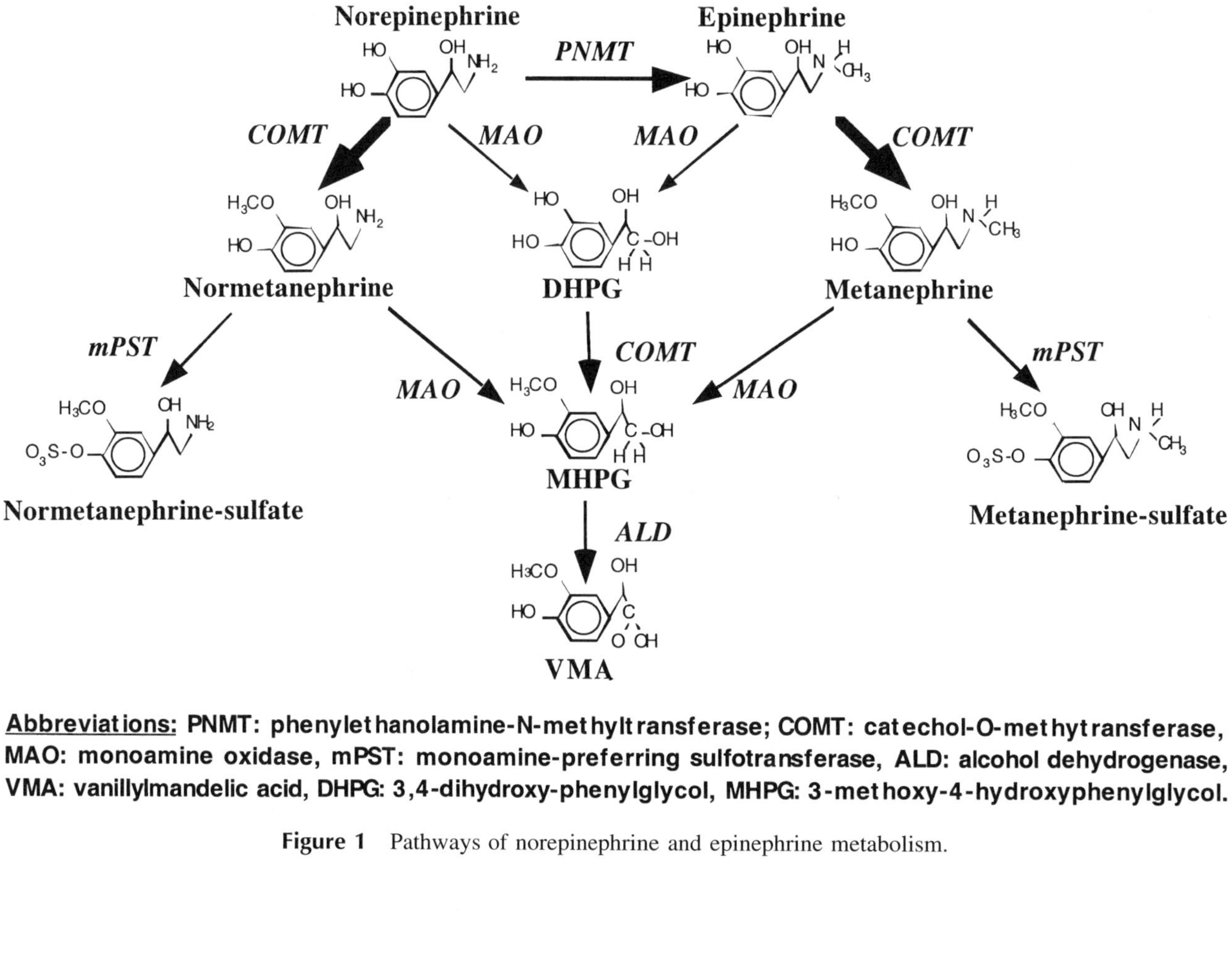

Abbreviations: PNMT: phenylethanolamine-N-methyltransferase; COMT: catechol-O-methytransferase, MAO: monoamine oxidase, mPST: monoamine-preferring sulfotransferase, ALD: alcohol dehydrogenase, VMA: vanillylmandelic acid, DHPG: 3,4-dihydroxy-phenylglycol, MHPG: 3-methoxy-4-hydroxyphenylglycol.

Figure 1 Pathways of norepinephrine and epinephrine metabolism.

norepinephrine, epinephrine, and dopamine (Table 1). In contrast to adult patients in whom sustained hypertension is found in only 50% of cases, more than 70–90% of children present with sustained hypertension (21, 22, 26). Pheochromocytoma is the underlying cause in 1–2% of cases of pediatric hypertension and should be considered after exclusion of the more common causes such as renal diseases and renal artery stenosis (23). Pheochromocytomas secreting epinephrine may also present with hypotension, particularly postural hypotension (29). Sweating, visual problems, weight loss, nausea, and vomiting are more common in children than in adults (30) as are polyuria and polydypsia. In addition, children commonly present with palpitations, anxiety, and hyperglycemia (31). Other signs of catecholamine excess are pallor and flushing (31). As summarized by Manger and Gifford (31) occasionally some children present with a reddish blue mottling of the skin and a puffy red and cyanotic appearance of the hands. Less frequent clinical manifestations include fever and constipation. As with adult patients, the presence of the triad of headache, palpitations, and sweating in children in combination with hypertension should arouse immediate suspicion of a pheochromocytoma. Pheochromocytoma spells may last from a few seconds to several hours, with intervals between attacks varying widely and occurring as infrequently as once every few weeks or months. The occurrence of attacks is unpredictable since they often occur at rest. However, some are always associated with physical activity, trauma, by direct stimulation of tumor (e.g., urinary bladder distention), or after using certain drugs or taking food (e.g., tyramine in chocolate). Unusual symptoms related to paroxysmal blood pressure elevation or sudden arrhythmia during diagnostic procedures (e.g., endoscopy, catheterization), or anesthesia should promptly arouse a suspicion of pheochromocytoma. Malignant pheochromocytoma may present with pain due to bone metastatic lesions. In children, the differential diagnosis includes renal diseases, renal artery stenosis, coarctation of the aorta, and, less commonly, panic/ anxiety disorders, "autonomic epilepsy," cluster or migraine headache, hyperthyroidism, and side effects of medications or dietary supplements (32–34).

B. Biochemical Diagnosis of Pheochromocytoma

Biochemical diagnosis of different types of pheochromocytomas is based on measurements of plasma and urine catecholamines and metanephrines. Plasma free metanephrines have been shown to be the single most reliable biochemical test for the detection or exclusion of pheochromocytoma in adults (35) and children (75) with a sensitivity of 97–100% and specificity of 80–96%. Measurements of 24 h urinary excretion of fractionated metanephrines performed by modern HPLC methods is another sensitive tool for detection of pheochromocytoma although this test is less specific than measurement of plasma free metanephrines. Reliable 24 h urine collections may be difficult to obtain in children and the commonly used attempt to correct urinary results for creatinine excretion adds another confounder due to creatinine's dependence on diet (36), muscle mass (37), physical activity (38), and diurnal variation (39). Therefore, measurements of plasma free metanephrines under standardized conditions with the use of age- and gender-specific reference ranges appear to be the biochemical test of choice for detecting childhood pheochromocytoma. Patients should be instructed to abstain from caffeinated foods and drinks for at least 24 h and to avoid acetaminophen, which interferes with the normetanephrine assay, for at least 5 days prior to the blood draw. After an overnight fast (water permitted), the blood sample should be drawn through an indwelling intravenous cannula with the subjects rested in supine position for at least 20 min after insertion of the cannula.

Metastatic pheochromocytomas are often characterized by high tissue, plasma, and urinary levels of DOPA and dopamine (40–45). Elevations in plasma or urinary DOPA and dopamine are not in themselves particularly sensitive or specific markers of benign or metastatic pheochromocytoma. However, when accompanied by elevations in plasma norepinephrine or other clinical evidence of pheochromocytoma, such elevations should arouse immediate suspicion of metastatic disease.

Rarely in children, when the diagnosis of pheochromocytoma is questionable (e.g., only slight or moderate elevation of plasma free metanephrines are present) additional tests such as clonidine or glucagon tests may be necessary. If a norepinephrine-producing tumor is suspected, we suggest using the clonidine test coupled with measurements of plasma free normetanephrine. The clinician must be aware of the possibility of a rapid and marked increase in blood pressure and heart rate after glucagon, and hypotension and bradycardia after clonidine administration.

Table 1 Signs and Symptoms of Pheochromocytoma in Children

Sign/symptom	%
Hypertension	82
Headache	81
Sweating	36–68
Palpitations	34–45
Weight loss	44
Pallor/flushing	11–36
Nausea/emesis	27–56
Polyuria	25

Adapted from Refs. 24, 26, and 31.

C.   Localization

A variety of conventional imaging techniques are available for localization of a pheochromocytoma (for review, see [5]). These techniques include computed tomography (CT), magnetic resonance imaging (MRI), and scintigraphy after administration of ^{131}I- or ^{123}I-labeled meta-iodobenzylguanidine (MIBG). In children, more than 90% of pheochromocytomas are localized in the abdomen, therefore, imaging studies should be directed to this part of the body. Although CT localizes about 95% of pheochromocytomas, MRI is the preferred imaging modality in children to avoid radiation exposure. Furthermore, MRI is superior to CT in detecting extra-adrenal tumors and familial adrenal pheochromocytoma due to the tumor's typical appearance on T2-weighted image. Both CT and MRI have poor specificity ranging from 65 to 75%. In some cases, ultrasound is sufficient to locate pheochromocytomas in children.

When pheochromocytoma is highly suspected by either positive biochemical results or by both imaging studies and positive biochemistry, MIBG is used to confirm the presence of pheochromocytoma (in some European medical centers, MIBG is used as the first imaging modality in patients with biochemically proven pheochromocytoma). The specificity of MIBG is 95–100% but this technique is not sensitive (sensitivity: 78–83%). Currently only ^{131}I-MIBG is available at most academic medical centers in the United States (46). ^{123}I-MIBG offers superior image quality and seems to be especially useful for detecting recurrent or metastatic pheochromocytoma, tumors with fibrosis or distorted anatomy, and tumors in unusual locations (47–49). In addition, the biological half-life of ^{123}I is shorter than of ^{131}I, resulting in a favorable decrease in radiation exposure.

Other imaging modalities that can be used in children to locate pheochromocytoma are octreotide scintigraphy (50) and positron emission tomography (PET), using [^{18}F]fluorodeoxyglucose, [^{11}C]hydroxyephedrine, [^{11}C]epinephrine and recently, 6-[^{18}F]fluorodopamine (51–53). Our preliminary results show that 6-[^{18}F]fluorodopamine PET scanning can detect and localize pheochromocytoma, not only as a primary tumor in the adrenal gland but also as a recurrent extra-adrenal or metastatic tumor and that it is superior to MIBG scanning.

D.   Treatment of Pheochromocytoma

The first-line treatment of pheochromocytoma in children is surgical excision of the tumor. To prevent perioperative complications due to massive outpouring of catecholamines from the tumor, preoperative pharmacological blockade of catecholamine effects and synthesis is required (54). Routinely used pharmacological agents include phenoxybenzamine, an α1-adrenoceptor noncompetitive antagonist, that opposes catecholamine-induced vasoconstriction and propranolol, atenolol, or metoprolol

as β-adrenoceptor blockers that oppose catecholamine-induced arrhythmia and the reflex tachycardia (5, 23, 26, 55). Beta-blockade alone is contraindicated because it does not prevent and can actually augment effects of catecholamines at α-adrenoceptors. The average oral dosage of phenoxybenzamine in children is between 20 and 50 mg/day given at 6–8 h intervals. To reach adequate preoperative blockade, phenoxybenzamine may be increased until orthostatic hypotension is present or mean arterial pressure is normalized (56, 57). However, several reports questioned this approach, finding no correlations between duration of preoperative treatment and the dosage of α-blockers and intraoperative cardiovascular instability (58). The average dosage of atenolol in children is 20–60 mg/day divided into two or three doses. Side effects of phenoxybenzamine include postural hypotension, reflex tachycardia, nasal congestion, and sedation. Atenolol can mainly cause bradycardia and sedation. If hypertensive crisis occurs, as with adult patients, an intravenous bolus of 5 mg phentolamine (Regitine) is the treatment of choice. Phentolamine has a very short half-life; if necessary, the same dose can be repeated every 2 min until hypertension is adequately controlled. As an alternative, phentolamine may be given as continuous infusion (100 mg of phentolamine in 500 ml 5% dextrose in water). α-Methyl-*para*-tyrosine (metyrosine, Demser), a competitive inhibitor of tyrosine hydroxylase is routinely administered preoperatively in some institutions (the starting dosage is usually 250 mg twice to four times a day) and may be tried in patients in whom elevated blood pressure and arrhythmia cannot be controlled by using α- and β-blockade. At some other centers, calcium channel blockers are used as a primary drug to control hypertension (1, 23, 29). Significant hypovolemia should be corrected by perioperative administration of intravenous fluids to avoid hypotension. Since children have a higher risk of catecholamine-induced pulmonary edema, fluid replacement should not exceed 10 cc/kg/h (57). Pressor agents are not usually effective in the presence of severe and persistent hypovolemia. Children should also be monitored for hypoglycemia up to 48 h after surgery (catecholamines block insulin release via α-adrenoceptors).

Surgical removal of intra-adrenal pheochromocytomas in children is usually successfully carried out by laparoscopy, a procedure that minimizes catecholamine-induced hemodynamic changes during operation, postoperative morbidity, hospital stay, and expenses compared to conventional transabdominal adrenalectomy (59). In children with familial pheochromocytoma that carries a higher risk for bilateral adrenal involvement, prophylactic adrenalectomy of the contralateral side is not recommended. When metastatic disease is present, medical treatment is the initial treatment of choice.

After surgical removal of a pheochromocytoma, yearly follow-up evaluations for assessment of recurrence are recommended for at least 5 years and should include measurements of plasma free metanephrines. Children with familial pheochromocytoma should undergo annual screening indefinitely. If plasma free metanephrine levels are elevated, urine metanephrines and plasma and urine catecholamines may be measured to confirm the presence of the tumor. If recurrent or metastatic pheochromocytoma is suspected, imaging studies should be initiated. Children with familial pheochromocytoma should undergo at least annual screening.

In the presence of metastatic and therefore incurable disease, drug therapy is the first-line treatment with the goal of controlling cardiovascular effects and complications related to catecholamine excess. Malignant pheochromocytoma requires more aggressive treatment including chemotherapy, MIBG therapy, octreotide therapy, external radiation, and in some cases embolization of the tumor. However, fewer than 40% of patients with metastatic pheochromocytoma respond (mostly partial remission) to these currently used therapeutic modalities such as MIBG or chemotherapy. Therefore, most children are only treated when the quality of their life is affected by catecholamine excess or metastatic lesions that are aggressive and affect local surrounding tissue. Clinicians using the above therapies, particularly chemotherapy, should be aware of potentially fatal complications arising from excessive catecholamine release as tumor cells are destroyed (usually within the first 24 h). With the use of MIBG, a major complication is bone marrow suppression, usually 4 weeks after initiation of therapy.

III. MULTIPLE ENDOCRINE NEOPLASIA SYNDROMES

Multiple endocrine neoplasia (MEN) syndromes are familial disorders inherited in an autosomal dominant pattern with high penetrance but variable expressivity. MEN syndromes are subclassified into MEN 1, MEN 2, and Carney complex. These rare disorders are characterized by hyperplasia or tumor involving more than one endocrine gland.

A. Multiple Endocrine Neoplasia 2A (Sipple Syndrome)

MEN 2A was first described in 1961 by Sipple and is defined by the occurrence of medullary thyroid carcinoma (MTC), pheochromocytoma (affecting about 50% of patients), and hyperparathyroidism caused by parathyroid gland hyperplasia (affecting about 20% of patients) (60–63). There is also familial MTC characterized by hereditary MTC without other associated endocrinopathies (although adrenomedullary hyperplasia secondary to a germline RET mutation may still be present but undiagnosed). Familial MTC belongs genotypically to MEN 2A. Rare variants of MEN 2A represent MEN 2A associated with cutaneous lichen amyloidosis and MEN 2A or

familial medullary thyroid carcinoma associated with Hirschprung's disease (64–67).

MEN 2A accounts for the majority of MEN 2 cases. In general, MEN 2 affects about 1:40,000 individuals, and there are less than 1000 kindreds worldwide. The gene responsible for MEN 2 is a proto-oncogene called RET (68). In contrast to MEN 1, RET is specifically expressed in neural-crest-derived cells, such as the calcitonin-producing C-cells in the thyroid gland and the catecholamine-producing chromaffin cells in the adrenal gland. Whether it is also expressed in the parathyroid glands, remains to be ascertained, especially when considering the low rate of hyperparathyroidism in patients with MEN 2A and the lack of hyperparathyroidism in MEN 2B, although both conditions are caused by mutations in the RET gene. RET plays a role in normal gastrointestinal neuronal and kidney development as exemplified by the RET knockout mouse, which has a Hirschprung-like phenotype and renal dys- or agenesis (69, 70). RET is located on chromosome 10q11.2 and encodes a receptor tyrosine kinase, RET protein. As an oncogene, activation of RET leads to hyperplasia of target cells in vivo. Subsequent secondary events then lead to tumor formation (Fig. 2) (71–74). RET consists of 21 exons with six so-called "hot spot exons" (exons 10, 11, 13–16) in which mutations are identified in 97% of patients with MEN 2. RET germline mutation screening is commercially available (*http://endocrine.mdacc.tmc.edu*; Mayo Clinic, Rochester, MN) and has widely replaced the cumbersome provocative testing of calcitonin stimulation (with calcium and/or pentagastrin). It has been notoriously unreliable in children, since for this population the normal range of basal and stimulated calcitonin is still unknown. The normal range for catecholamines including metanephrines in children with and without pheochromocytoma and/or adrenal medullary hyperplasia has likewise only recently been elucidated (75). Hyperplasia of C-cells

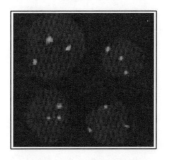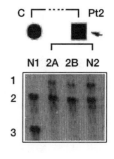

Figure 2 Duplication of mutant RET in trisomy 10 in MEN 2-related pheochromocytoma. Pheochromocytoma tumor cells are shown in **gray** color. The **dot** signals are FISH markers for chromosome 10. Each tumor cell has trisomy 10. C, cousin; Pt2, patient; N, normal tissue; 2A and 2B, pheochromocytoma; 1–3 are alleles with allel 2 being the inherited, mutant RET allele shared by cousin C and patient Pt2. (Modified from Ref. 71.)

in the thyroid gland or the adrenal medulla has been identified as precursor lesion for MTC or pheochromocytoma (76, 77).

The inaccuracy of calcitonin stimulation testing in the diagnosis of MTC has been demonstrated by results of prophylactic thyroidectomy carried out based on positive *RET* germline mutation testing. Fifty percent of patients with a negative pentagastrin test but positive for a *RET* germline mutation had already developed MTC. This led to the recommendation to perform prophylactic thyroidectomy with lymph node dissection around age 5, if mutation testing of *RET* is positive (66, 78–88). Hyperplasia of C-cells has been observed in *RET* gene mutation carriers (MEN 2A) as young as 3 years. In children with MEN 2B, metastatic MTC has been described shortly after birth (89, 90). Therefore, prophylactic thyroidectomy in children with MEN 2B is recommended at an earlier age than in children with MEN 2A *RET* mutations. Although provocative calcitonin testing is nowadays not recommended in children with MEN 2A identified by a *RET* germline mutation, determination of calcitonin plasma levels can be used as a follow-up parameter, as they are indicative of tumor mass. Upon presentation in early childhood, there is usually no abnormal finding on physical examination or ultrasound in patients with MEN 2A. If *RET* germline mutation testing or the family history is positive for MEN 2, a neck computed or magnetic resonance tomogram (baseline) for evaluation of already developed metastases from MTC should be performed.

Before any surgery including prophylactic thyroidectomy in children with MEN 2, a search for pheochromocytoma should be undertaken by measuring plasma free metanephrines. Pheochromocytoma (at least 70% are bilateral) develops on the grounds of adrenomedullary hyperplasia secondary to a *RET* germline mutation, and becomes manifest (e.g., biochemically or on imaging) in about 50% of patients. The peak age is around age 40 but children as young as age 10 can be affected (91, 92). Thus, annual surveillance for plasma and urine catecholamines and metanephrines is recommended after age 6. Based on our recent studies and recommendations, we suggest measuring plasma free metanephrines (93). Patients with MEN 2-related pheochromocytoma are often normatensive (occurs only in about 50%) and have beta-adrenergic symptoms including palpitations and tachycardia. When catecholamine levels are abnormally increased, CT and/or MRI plus MIBG scintigraphy should be performed (5). MEN2-related pheochromocytomas can be located extra-adrenally but are rarely malignant (<25%) (77, 94, 95). If a pheochromocytoma is localized, adrenalectomy should be performed, if possible by laparoscopy (depending on tumor size), after appropriate preoperative blockade as discussed earlier.

Fewer than 25% of patients with MEN 2A develop frank hyperparathyroidism indicated by an inappropriately elevated serum calcium level compared to parathyroid hormone. However, this condition rarely occurs in childhood and nowadays is especially less diagnosed in prophylactically thyroidectomized children [96]. Reasons for this low prevalence and the discrepancy with MEN 2B, which is also caused by mutations in *RET* (more "severe" mutations in exon 16), are unclear. Authorities recommend measurement of the serum calcium concentration every other year after age 10 for early diagnosis (91, 96, 97).

The cutaneous skin lesions in MEN 2A have been observed in fewer than 16 kindreds and occur over the upper part of the back. Pruritus is the first symptom preceding visible lesions with lichenoid–papular appearance for years. In more advanced lesions, amyloid deposits are found (64).

B. Multiple Endocrine Neoplasia 2B

MEN 2B represents about 5% of all MEN 2 cases and is defined by the presence of MTC, pheochromocytoma, and associated abnormalities including mucosal neuromas (within the lips, gastrointestinal tract, on the tongue tip and eyelids), medullated corneal nerve fibers, and marfanoid habitus (61, 98). In contrast to Marfan's syndrome, however, patients with MEN 2B do not have lens or aortic abnormalities. Mucosal neuromas within the lips often give patients a "blubbery/bumpy lip look." Physical examination is remarkable for these associated abnormalities. For instance, slit lamp examination may reveal medullated, hypertrophied corneal nerves. Often, patients have an acromegaloid appearance. Intestinal ganglioneuromatosis may cause diarrhea alternating with constipation or even obstruction.

In contrast to patients with MEN 2A, patients with MEN 2B do not have hyperparathyroidism, although MEN 2B is also caused by germline mutations of *RET* (99). These mutations affect exons 15 and 16, coding for the intracellular tyrosine kinase domain of RET protein. This molecular difference with MEN 2A supposedly leads to autophosphorylation without dimerization and may explain why patients with MEN 2B present at an earlier age with MTC and/or pheochromocytoma. It remains puzzling, however, why hyperparathyroidism only rarely occurs in MEN 2B. Authorities recommend total thyroidectomy and central lymph node dissection within the first 6 months of life for children with MEN 2B (*RET* germline mutations in codons 883, 918, and 922), since metastases from MTC may develop within the first year of life (89, 90). Also, pheochromocytoma in patients with MEN 2B occurs at an earlier age than in MEN 2A. Clinical management of MTC and/or pheochromocytoma is otherwise identical in MEN 2A and MEN 2B. An important finding is that about 7% of patients with apparently sporadic MTC have germline mutations in *RET*, making it reasonable to perform *RET* mutation analysis in all patients with MTC (100–102).

C. Von Hippel-Lindau Syndrome

Von Hippel-Lindau (VHL) is another autosomal dominant inherited tumor syndrome with pheochromocytoma (VHL type II) or without pheochromocytoma (VHL type I) (103, 104) that may occur in children. Apart from pheochromocytoma, major tumors in VHL disease include renal cell carcinoma, hemangioblastoma, neuroendocrine pancreatic tumors, and endolymphatic sac tumors (105, 106). All children with familial, multiple or early onset of pheochromocytoma should be examined for VHL disease, which has variable expression and age and tumor-dependent penetrance. Pheochromocytoma occurs in about 10% of VHL patients and is the presenting manifestation in about 5% of cases (107, 108). However, there are large interfamilial variations, with some families having pheochromocytoma as the most frequent complication of VHL disease (107, 108). Children with VHL syndrome who underwent unilateral adrenalectomy for pheochromocytoma need lifelong follow-up to diagnose recurrence or another pheochromocytoma in a timely fashion on the contralateral side. In contrast to pheochromocytomas of children with MEN 2 (so-called adrenergic), VHL-associated pheochromocytomas have more of a so-called noradrenergic phenotype. MEN-2-related pheochromocytomas frequently possess all the enzymes to synthesize catecholamines from tyrosine to epinephrine, whereas less differentiated pheochromocytomas including those in VHL disease lack the enzymes involved in the final catecholamine biosynthesis pathway (109). Thus, symptoms and signs of patients with VHL-related pheochromocytoma are related to norepinephrine excess, including hypertension. Metastatic pheochromocytoma is more common in patients with VHL disease than MEN 2 and neurofibromatosis type 1 (NF1). The diagnostic algorithm is the same as in other patients with pheochromocytoma and is commented on in other parts of this chapter (5).

The VHL tumor suppressor gene is located on chromosome 3p25-26. The cloned coding sequence comprises three exons. Most patients with VHL-associated pheochromocytoma have missense mutations (110–112). There are genotype-specific VHL phenotypes (106). Founder effects may explain regional prevalence rates, for example, the Black Forest area in southern Germany with the missense mutation tyrosine to histidine at codon 98 (Tyr98His) and subsequent high risk of pheochromocytoma (94, 113, 114). VHL missense mutations may have tissue-specific effects (113). A so-called second hit is required in patients with VHL germline mutations in order to develop pheochromocytoma (115).

The VHL gene product forms a stable complex with the highly conserved transcription elongation factors elongin B and elongin C, which regulate RNA polymerase II elongation. Formation of this heterotrimeric complex with elongin B and C appears to be the tumor-suppressor function of the VHL gene, since the majority of tumor-predisposing mutations of VHL disrupt the formation of this complex (81, 116, 117). Normal VHL protein function leads to degradation of a proteasome complex (118).

D. Neurofibromatosis Type 1

Neurofibromatosis type 1 (NF1) is the most common familial cancer syndrome predisposing to pheochromocytoma and affects about 1:4000 individuals. The risk of pheochromocytoma in NF1, however, is small, about 1% (119, 120). NF1 is inherited in an autosomal dominant manner with variable expression. Fifty percent of patients have new mutations and mutation analysis is cumbersome because of the large gene size (11 kb of coding sequence). Pheochromocytoma in patients with NF1 is rarely seen in children since it usually occurs at a later age (around age 50). Only 12% of NF1 patients are diagnosed with bilateral and multifocal pheochromocytomas and fewer than 6% of patients have metastatic pheochromocytoma (121).

The NF1 gene is a tumor-suppressor gene mapping to chromosome 17q11.2. Patients with NF1-associated pheochromocytoma show loss of the wild type allele (122) following Knudson's two-hit hypothesis. Neurofibromin, the NF1 gene product, bears homology to the ras/GTPase-activating protein (GAP) (73). P21-ras/GAP increases the rate of intrinsic GTP hydrolysis in the small G proteins, the ras genes, thereby mediating the return of the G protein switch to the off GDP-bound form. By this mechanism, signal transduction is controlled via the ras pathways.

E. Familial Pheochromocytoma

Familial pheochromocytoma is usually inherited in an autosomal dominant manner. However, detailed investigation may reveal subclinical evidence of VHL disease or MEN 2 (123, 124). VHL germline mutations in the absence of other features of VHL disease have been detected by molecular genetic screening for VHL and RET mutations in familial pheochromocytoma (81, 110). Recently, germline mutations in the SDHD gene have been found in families with extra-adrenal chromaffin tissue tumors (125).

IV. NEUROBLASTOMA

Neuroblastomas are tumors that derive from primordial neural crest cells of the sympathetic system. They are the most common solid extracranial tumor in children and they account for 7–10% of all tumors diagnosed in children (126–128). Neuroblastomas have been found to have the highest percentage of spontaneous regression among tumors (129).

The annual incidence in the US is 1:100,000 children under the age of 15. It is predominantly a tumor of very young children: in 80% the tumor presents in children younger than 5 years, in 15% in children between the age of 5 and 10, and in 5% in children older than 10 (130).

The median age at diagnosis is found to be between 18 and 24 months (131–133). Often two peaks can be identified in the incidence of neuroblastoma and each is associated with a distinct pattern of clinical behavior. Tumors detected in the first year of life (initial peak) have a more benign course than those diagnosed in older children (second peak in children around 2 years of age) (132, 134). The tumor has a slight predominance in boys (with boys to girls ratio of 1.2:1) and is reportedly more common in white than in black children (127).

Most cases are sporadic; rarely, cases are familial or associated with familial syndromes such as NF, Hirschsprung's disease, and Beckwith-Wiedemann syndrome. However, until now no genetic analyses have been able to link neuroblastomas indisputably with the respective familiar syndromes (135–138).

In recent years, a rise in incidence over time has been noted (127). This rise may reflect increased physician awareness, improved diagnostic procedures, or changes in reporting (139).

A. Pathogenesis

Although the influence of exposure to several environmental factors (such as parental occupation, use of medication, lifestyle) on the risk of developing neuroblastoma has been investigated, no unequivocal relationship has been demonstrated (132, 140). Further investigation of some possible risk factors, such as parental exposure to metals, solvents, or radiation and maternal use of hormones during pregnancy, appears warranted (141).

Numerous studies using a range of experimental techniques have been undertaken to discover the genes involved in neuroblastoma development. It has become apparent that both inactivation of tumor suppressor genes and activation of tumor oncogenes are involved in neuroblastoma tumorigenesis. Chromosomal loci that have been found to show loss of heterozygosity (LOH), indicative of a tumor-suppressor gene, include 1p (19–31%), 2q (30%), 3p (9–25%), 4p (14–19.5%), 9p (19–36%), 11q (5–44%), 14q (10–31%) and 18q (31–81%) (142–156). Although intensive research has been directed towards identifying candidate genes in the regions that show LOH, no indisputable tumor suppressor gene has yet been identified (157, 158).

Amplification of the MYCN tumor oncogene, located on the distal short arm of chromosome 2 (2p24), was first reported in 1983 (159, 160). In recent years it has become apparent that gain of the long arm of chromosome 17q, occurring in 54–83% of primary tumors, is probably the most frequent chromosomal abnormality in neuroblastomas (142, 151, 152, 161, 162). At present, genetic abnormalities found in neuroblastomas seem rather to have prognostic relevance than to provide insight into its pathogenesis.

B. Clinical Presentation

The symptoms and signs at presentation depend largely on the size and the location of the primary tumor, and whether or not the tumor has metastasized (Table 2). Metastases can occur as a result of both lymphatic and hematogenous extension and are most common in lymph nodes, liver, skin, bone, bone marrow, and soft tissues (163). In case of lymph node involvement outside the cavity of origin, a child is considered to have disseminated disease (163). Thus, a patient can present with local, regional, or disseminated disease. The proportion of patients with disseminated disease at diagnosis (about 50%) is age dependent (164). Metastasized disease is more commonly seen in older children. In 35% of patients with apparent localized disease regional lymph node metastases are found.

The most common site of tumor localization is intraabdominal (65%), most commonly in the adrenal gland. Children older than 1 year have a higher incidence of adrenal tumors than infants (40% vs. 25%, respectively). In 20% of cases the tumor is localized in the chest, in 2–3 % in the pelvis, in 1–5% in the neck, and in 6–12% other localizations. In 1% the primary tumor is not found (132, 133, 163–165).

The tumor may mimic other diseases: for instance, bone metastasis may resemble musculoskeletal diseases such as rheumatoid arthritis (166) and paraspinal tumors

Table 2 Presentation

Disease	Tumor site	Possible symptoms
Localized	Abdomen	Abdominal discomfort, fullness, abdominal pain, rarely respiratory distress
	Pelvis	Bladder and bowel disorders as a result of compression
	Neck, Thorax	Dyspnea, dysphagia, Horner syndrome
Disseminated	Nonspecific	General malaise, low-grade fever, weight loss
	Bone	Limp, joint swelling, bone pain
	Paraspinal	Neurological symptoms
	Orbital area	Proptosis, periorbital ecchymoses (raccoon eyes)
Producing	Catecholamines	Hypertension, sweating, flushing, tachycardia, paroxysmal phenomena
	VIP	Chronic secretory diarrhea (Kerner-Morrison syndrome)

compressing nerve roots or extending into vertebral bodies may mimic neurological diseases. Furthermore, the tumor may be accompanied by paraneoplastic phenomena such as opsoclonus–myoclonus syndrome, which occurs in 2–3% of children with neuroblastoma (167), or secretory diarrhea if the tumor is producing vasoactive intestinal peptide (VIP).

In rare cases, production of catecholamines contributes to symptoms and signs seen at presentation. Although 95% of tumors produce catecholamines or catecholamine metabolites such as VMA and HVA, this only rarely causes symptoms of catecholamine excess such as hypertension or paroxysmal phenomena such as tachycardia and flushing (168). Compared to pheochromocytomas, neuroblastomas appear to have a paucity of storage granules and low levels of tissue catecholamines, which is suggestive for an ineffective storage mechanism. Furthermore, in patients with neuroblastoma, catecholamines are effectively metabolized by COMT and MAO to yield nonpressor catecholamine metabolites such as HVA, which are thereafter excreted in the urine. This may explain the absence of symptoms of catecholamine excess (168). No correlation has been found between tumor size and the level of urine catecholamine excretion. A less differentiated tumor may predominantly secrete dopamine instead of VMA or HVA.

At physical examination care should be given to the detection of palpable masses in the abdomen or flank and the presence of hepatomegaly. Skin including scalp and joints should be inspected for lesions, swelling, and tenderness. A neurological examination, including assessment of pupil sizes in both eyes and strength in the lower limbs, should be part of the work-up for neuroblastomas.

Histopathologically, the differential diagnosis includes other small blue round cell neoplasia of childhood such as rhabdomyosarcoma, Ewing's sarcoma, peripheral neuroepithelioma (primitive neuroectodermal tumor [PNET]), lymphoma, and leukemia (169). Wilms' tumor, hydronephrotic kidney, enlarged spleen or liver, lymphoma, germ cell tumor, and mesenteric cysts should also be considered in the differential diagnosis (133, 170).

C. Diagnosis and Localization

In 1988, a set of international criteria was formulated for neuroblastomas with respect to diagnosis, staging and response to treatment (171). In 1993, these criteria were revised (169). Obtaining tumor tissue is critical for diagnosis and staging of neuroblastoma.

According to the International Neuroblastoma Staging System (INSS) criteria a neuroblastoma is confirmed if either an unequivocal pathological diagnosis is made from tumor tissue by light microscopy, or a bone marrow aspirate or trephine biopsy specimen contains unequivocal tumor cells (e.g., syncytia or immunocytologically positive clumps of cells), and increased urine or serum catecholamines or their metabolites. In case of equivocal

histological and immunohistological findings, genetic features characteristic of neuroblastoma, such as 1p deletions or N-*myc* amplification, can support the diagnosis.

Seventy-one to 95% of neuroblastomas excrete abnormally large amounts of dopamine, HVA, norepinephrine, and VMA (132, 172). In patients with suspected neuroblastoma, measurement of urinary catecholamine metabolites is mandatory. In 15% of the tumors urinary VMA is not elevated. In order to be considered elevated VMA or HVA levels normalized to milligrams of creatinine have to be above 3.0 SD for the mean for age (132). With this cut-off approximately 92% of biopsy-proven neuroblastoma patients will have elevations at diagnosis. It is recommended that both VMA and HVA are measured in a patient with suspected neuroblastoma.

For localization of the tumor, several imaging modalities are available. Plain radiographs can detect the tumor if calcifications are present. Ultrasonography may yield good information and is the least expensive imaging technique. Other imaging techniques such as CT and MRI provide better anatomical detail including the tumor's relation to surrounding tissues. This information is important when operability and resectability are discussed. To evaluate the presence of bone metastases, bone scintigraphy with ^{99m}Tc-diphosphates is most sensitive (173). If available ^{131}I-MIBG or ^{123}I-MIBG scintigraphy should be performed routinely in the evaluation of all patients suspected of harboring a neuroblastoma (169). Ninety-one percent of the neuroblastomas concentrate ^{131}I-MIBG, which makes it a specific and very sensitive indicator for neuroblastoma comparable with urine analysis for catecholamine metabolites (173, 174). Addition of single-photon emission computed tomography (SPECT) has been found to be beneficial for the interpretation of the MIBG scan (175).

The recommendations of the INSS for clinical testing include CT and/or MRI scan with three-dimensional measurements for the primary site and abdomen/liver. To assess bone marrow involvement, bone marrow biopsy is required. Bone involvement should be assessed by MIBG scan or ^{99}Tc scan. At physical examination care should be taken to assess lymph node involvement. These findings should be confirmed with histology. Every patient should undergo a chest radiograph; if this is found to be positive a chest CT or MRI should be performed. Imaging modalities are also important for staging and follow-up.

D. Staging

In the INSS classification, four stages are identified (Table 3). In stages 1–3, the disease is localized and the stage depends on the extent of lymph node involvement and the presence of midline extension of the disease. In stage 4, the disease is disseminated (169). Stage 4S is a special subcategory: it consists of infants with a distinct pattern of disseminated disease associated with spontaneous re-

Table 3 International Neuroblastoma Staging System

Stage 1	Complete gross resection of localized tumor. Residual disease may or may not be present microscopically. Identifiable lymph node(s), ipsi- and contralateral, negative for tumor at microscopy.
Stage 2 A	Incomplete gross excision of localized tumor. Identifiable ipsi- and contralateral lymph nodes negative for tumor microscopically.
Stage 2 B	Complete or incomplete gross resection of localized tumor with ipsilateral no adherent lymph nodes positive for tumor. Enlarged contralateral lymph nodes negative for tumor microscopically.
Stage 3	Unresectable unilateral tumor infiltrating across the midline, regional lymph node involvement may be either present or absent; or localized unilateral tumor with contralateral regional lymph node involvement; or midline tumor with bilateral extension by infiltration or by lymph node involvement.
Stage 4	Dissemination of tumor to distant lymph nodes, bone, bone marrow, liver, or other organs except as defined for stage 4S.
Stage 4S	Localized primary tumor (as defined in stage 1 or 2) with dissemination limited to skin, liver and or bone marrow[a] in an infant <1 year of age.

[a]Less than 10% of nucleated cells are tumor cells.
Source: Data from Refs 163, 169, and 171.

gression. With or without nonsurgical treatment, these infants experience a high cure rate (176, 177).

E. Prognosis

Over the years numerous factors have been studied in neuroblastomas for their capability to predict outcome. Stage, age, and site of primary tumor are most important for the prognosis. Biological variables found to be associated with outcome can be organized into several categories: histopathological characteristics, serum markers, and genetic features.

The International Neuroblastoma Pathology Committee developed an age-linked classification system based on morphological features of neuroblastomas in relation to prognosis. Patients are classified in four different categories based on the differentiation grade of the neuroblastomas, their cellular turnover index, and the presence or absence of schwannian stromal development (170, 178). Other factors relating to prognosis taken into account in this classification system are mitosis–karyorrhexis index, mitotic rate, and calcification.

Serum markers known to have a correlation with outcome are serum ferritin, neuron-specific enolase (NSE), circulating ganglioside$_{D2}$ shed from neuroblastoma cell membranes, and serum lactic dehydrogenase (LDH). Increases in ferritin (179), NSE (180), and circulating ganglioside$_{D2}$ (181–183) are all associated with worse prognosis. Increases in LDH are non-specific and may indicate rapid cell turnover or large tumor burden. Increased LDH levels are associated with poor outcome (184).

Genetic features that have been found to correlate with prognosis are tumor cell ploidy, MYCN amplification, chromosome 1 deletion or allelic loss, telomerase activity, and expression of the TRKA-gene. Of these features a hyperdiploid karyotype and a high level of expression of the TRKA-gene, encoding for a primary component of the high-affinity nerve growth factor receptor are associated with a favorable outcome (185–190). In contrast, poor survival is predicted by MYCN amplification, chromosome 1 deletion or allelic loss, and a high telomerase activity [191–197].

F. Treatment

INSS stage, age, and biological features are the most important determinants in the design of a specific management plan for a patient. The intensity of the treatment program depends highly on the assessment of a patient's risk for recurrent disease (198).

Surgery is usually performed in all patients to establish the diagnosis and to procure tumor tissue for biological studies and staging of the tumor. If feasible, the tumor can be excised at initial surgery. Chemotherapy is the principal treatment modality (199). Multiple-agent therapy has proven to be more advantageous than single-agent therapy (132). In many patients, however, multimodality treatment is required. Radiation therapy and autologous bone marrow transplantation are used most frequently to supplement chemotherapy. Other treatment modalities studied for their effectiveness in neuroblastomas include radionuclide therapy with ^{131}I-MIBG, retinoid therapy, and immunotherapy.

The International Neuroblastoma Response Criteria give definitions to assess response (169). Response should be determined based on the best approximation of the volume of both primary tumor and metastatic sites. Six categories are identified: complete response, very good partial response, partial response, mixed response, no response and progressive disease. Complete response is characterized by complete disappearance of tumor at primary and metastatic sites. Partial response is defined by a decrease of over 50% in volume of primary tumor and metastatic sites. If the response of the primary tumor is found to be 90–99% and all metastatic sites have disappeared, it is classified as very good partial response. In mixed response there is a response of 50% or greater at one or more sites and a reduction of 50% or less at one or more other sites. In cases of no response, no new lesions occur and the volume of primary tumor and metastases changes between a reduction of less than 50% and an increase of less than 25%. Progressive disease is defined by a 25% increase in any pre-existing lesion or the occurrence of any new lesion. However, discussion is underway as to whether the number of categories should be decreased.

The 3-year event-free survival for stage 1, 2, 4S lies between 75 and 90%. For stage 3 and 4, age is important: if a child with stage 3 is younger than 1 year, she or he has an 80–90% chance of cure; with an age of over 1 year the 3 year survival rates drop to 50%. For children with stage 4 disease these percentages are 60–75% and 15% for the 3-year survival, respectively.

Late effects of treatment include disturbed linear growth and gonadal function and the occurrence of second malignant neoplasms such as thyroid carcinoma or myelodysplasia/leukemia.

G. Screening

Screening programs for the detection of neuroblastomas have been set up in Japan, North America, and Europe. Studies evaluating the effect of these screening programs are emerging. It is disputed whether these screening programs for neuroblastoma are successful in decreasing the incidence of poor-prognosis disease in neuroblastoma and thereby decreasing mortality and morbidity (200–203).

V. GANGLIONEUROMA

Ganglioneuroma is a rare benign tumor that originates from the sympathetic chain. It is defined by the World Health Organization as "a benign tumour of ganglion cells in various proportions, which may be immature or dysmorphic (e.g., multinucleation and nuclear pyknosis), and Schwann cells" (204). They either occur de novo or are a result of maturation and differentiation of neuroblastomas (129, 205). According to the International Neuroblastoma Pathology Committee it is not a separate entity but should be considered a final stage of matured neuroblastomas (170). In a series of 88 patients described by the Armed Forces Institute of Pathology, the majority of patients were above 10 years of age, only 16% (14 of 88) were younger than 10 years (131). In contrast, in recent studies the median age at presentation was found to be between 5.5 and 7.6 years (206–208). Boys and girls appear to be equally affected.

The posterior mediastinum (38%) is the most frequent site of occurrence and, together with localization in the retroperitoneum, accounts for most of the cases (131, 206, 207, 209). For abdominal tumors a preference was observed for nonadrenal (37.5%) over adrenal ganglioneuromas (21%) (207).

Up to half of the patients are asymptomatic (209–211). If symptoms are present, they are usually unspecific

and related to a mass effect of the tumor or intraspinal tumor extension. Some patients may experience hypertension due to excessive catecholamine secretion of the tumor. The percentage of tumors reported to secrete catecholamines or catecholamine metabolites varies in the literature between 20 and 39% (206, 207, 212). A ganglioneuroma is seldom found to be the cause of watery diarrhea by secreting VIP (213, 214). The tumor can be visualized with ultrasonography, CT, or MRI. Furthermore, 57% of the tumors are positive on ^{123}I-MIBG scintigraphy (207). MRI is superior to CT for studying local and intraspinal extension in retroperitoneal ganglioneuromas (208). Complete excision of the tumor is curative. Usually the prognosis remains excellent even if resection of the ganglioneuroma is incomplete.

VI. NEURAL TUMORS AND CHRONIC DIARRHEA

Chronic diarrhea caused by neuroendocrine or neural tumors often is related to the production of VIP. The most common tumors in this group are VIPomas, which can occur sporadically but also in the context of MEN 1. VIPomas cause secretory, watery diarrhea, which subsequently leads to disturbances in water and electrolyte homeostasis including hypokalemia and metabolic acidosis. Symptomatic treatment concerns replacement of water and electrolyte losses. Definitive treatment consists of tumor removal. For VIPomas, resection of a single and/or multiple tumors is indicated, which may include a pancreatic tail resection. For neuroendocrine or neuroectodermal tumors such as VIP-producing pheochromocytoma, ganglioneuroma, ganglioneuroblastoma, and medullary thyroid carcinoma, definitive therapy also is achieved by surgical tumor removal (213, 215–222). If the diarrhea-causing tumor is composed of chromaffin cells, it may also secrete large amounts of catecholamines. Therefore, measurements of plasma VIP and plasma/urinary catecholamines including metanephrines should be performed in children with watery diarrhea (216, 223). The somatostatin analog octreotide improves diarrhea in the majority of patients, including those with carcinoid syndrome (224, 225). In patients with MTC, nonvoluminous diarrhea may be the initial complaint. The cause of the diarrhea in this setting is unclear (226).

REFERENCES

1. Bravo E. Evolving concepts in the pathophysiology, diagnosis, and treatment of pheochromocytoma. Endocr Rev 1994; 15:356–368.
2. Sinclair D, Shenkin A, Lorimer A. Normal catecholamine production in a patient with a paroxysmally secreting phaeochromocytoma. Ann Clin Biochem 1991; 28:417–419.

3. Stewart M, et al. Biochemical diagnosis of phaeochromocytoma: two instructive case reports. J Clin Pathol 1993; 46:280–282.

4. Lenders J, Keiser H, Goldstein D. Plasma metanephrines in the diagnosis of pheochromocytoma. Ann Intern Med 1995; 123:101–109.

5. Pacak K, et al. Recent advances in genetics, diagnosis, localization, and treatment of pheochromocytoma. Ann Intern Med 2001; 134(4):315–329.

6. Lopez MG, et al. Membrane-mediated effects of the steroid 17-alpha-estradiol on adrenal catecholamine release. J Pharmacol Exp Ther 1991; 259(1):279–285.

7. Del Rio G, et al. Effect of estradiol on the sympathoadrenal response to mental stress in normal men. J Clin Endocrinol Metab 1994; 79(3):836–840.

8. Ceresini G, et al. The effects of transdermal estradiol on the response to mental stress in postmenopausal women: a randomized trial. Am J Med 2000; 109(6):463–468.

9. Eisenhofer G, et al. Plasma metanephrines: a novel and cost-effective test for pheochromocytoma. Braz J Med Biol Res 2000; 33(10):1157–1169.

10. Hillarp NA, Hokfelt B. Evidence of adrenaline and noradrenaline in separate adrenal medullary cells. Acta Physiol Scand 1953; 30:55–68.

11. Livett BG. Adrenal medullary chromaffin cells in vitro. Physiol Rev. 1984; 64(4):1103–1161.

12. Jarrott B, Louis WJ. Abnormalities in enzymes involved in catecholamine synthesis and catabolism in phaeochromocytoma. Clin Sci Mol Med 1977; 53(6):529–535.

13. Nagatsu T, et al. Tyrosine hydroxylase in human adrenal glands and human pheochromocytoma. Clin Chim Acta 1972; 39(2):417–424.

14. Tyce GM, et al. The adrenal gland as a source of dihydroxyphenylalanine and catecholamine metabolites. Adv Pharmacol 1998; 42:370–373.

15. DeQuattro V, et al. Central and regional normetadrenaline in evaluation of neurogenic aspects of hypertension: aid to diagnosis of phaeochromocytoma. Clin Sci (Colch), 1980; 59 Suppl 6:275s–277s.

16. Eisenhofer G, Friberg P, Pacak K, et al. Plasma metadrenalines: do they provide useful information about sympatho-adrenal function and catecholamine metabolism? Clin Sci 1995; 88:533–542.

17. Eisenhofer G, Rundqvist B, Aneman A, et al. Regional release and removal of catecholamines and extraneuronal metabolism to metanephrines. J Clin Endocrinol Metab 1995; 80:3009–3017.

18. Eisenhofer G, et al. Plasma metanephrines are markers of pheochromocytoma produced by catechol-O-methyltransferase within tumors. J Clin Endocrinol Metab 1998; 83(6)2175–2185.

19. Whalen RK, Althausen AF, Daniels GH. Extra-adrenal pheochromocytoma. J Urol 1992; 147(1):1–10.

20. Bloom DA, Fonkalsrud EW. Surgical management of pheochromocytoma in children. J Pediatr Surg 1974; 9(2):179–184.

21. Fonkalsrud EW. Pheochromocytoma in childhood. Prog Pediatr Surg 1991; 26:103–111.

22. Caty MG, et al. Current diagnosis and treatment of pheochromocytoma in children. Experience with 22 consecutive tumors in 14 patients. Arch Surg 1990; 125(8):978–981.

23. Ross JH. Pheochromocytoma. Special considerations in children. Urol Clin North Am 2000; 27(3):393–402.

24. Hume DM. Pheochromocytoma in the adult and in the child. Am J Surg 1960; 99:458–496.

25. Kaufman BH, et al. Pheochromocytoma in the pediatric age group: current status. J Pediatr Surg 1983; 18(6):879–884.

26. Reddy VS, et al. Twenty-five-year surgical experience with pheochromocytoma in children. Am Surg 2000; 66(12):1085–1092.

27. Coutant R, et al. Prognosis of children with malignant pheochromocytoma. Report of two cases and review of the literature. Horm Res 1999; 52(3):145–149.

28. Loh KC, et al. The treatment of malignant pheochromocytoma with iodine-131 metaiodobenzylguanidine (131I-MIBG): a comprehensive review of 116 reported patients. J Endocrinol Invest 1997; 20(11):648–658.

29. Bravo EL, Gifford RW Jr. Pheochromocytoma. Endocrinol Metab Clin North Am 1993; 22(2):329–341.

30. Fonseca V, Bouloux PM. Phaeochromocytoma and paraganglioma. Baillieres Clin Endocrinol Metab 1993; 7(2):509–544.

31. Manger W, Gifford R. Clinical and Experimental Pheochromocytoma. Cambridge, MA: Blackwell Science, 1996.

32. Kuchel O. Increased plasma dopamine in patients presenting with the pseudopheochromocytoma quandary: retrospective analysis of 10 years' experience. J Hypertens 1998; 16(10):1531–1537.

33. Mann SJ. Severe paroxysmal hypertension (pseudopheochromocytoma): understanding the cause and treatment [see comments]. Arch Intern Med 1999; 159(7):670–674.

34. Londe S. Causes of hypertension in the young. Pediatr Clin North Am 1978; 25(1):55–65.

35. Eisenhofer G, et al. Plasma normetanephrine and metanephrine for detecting pheochromocytoma in von Hippel-Lindau disease and multiple endocrine neoplasia type 2. N Engl J Med 1999; 340:1872–1879.

36. Neubert A, Remer T. The impact of dietary protein intake on urinary creatinine excretion in a healthy pediatric population. J Pediatr 1998; 133(5):655–659.

37. Wang ZM, et al. Total-body skeletal muscle mass: evaluation of 24-h urinary creatinine excretion by computerized axial tomography. Am J Clin Nutr 1996; 63(6):863–869.

38. Calles-Escandon J, et al. Influence of exercise on urea, creatinine, and 3-methylhistidine excretion in normal human subjects. Am J Physiol 1984; 246(4 Pt 1):E334–338.

39. Curtis G, Fogel M. Creatinine excretion: diurnal variation and variability of whole and part-day measures. A methodologic issue in psychoendocrine research. Psychosom Med 1970; 32(4):337–350.

40. Anton AH, et al. Dihydroxyphenylalanine secretion in a malignant pheochromocytoma. Am J Med 1967; 42(3):469–475.

41. Fossati P, et al. [Dopamine-secreting phaeochromocytoma. A little known clinical and biochemical entity (author's transl)]. Nouv Presse Med 1982; 11(21):1607–1610.

42. Goldstein DS, et al. Plasma 3,4-dihydroxyphenylalanine (dopa) and catecholamines in neuroblastoma or pheochromocytoma. Ann Intern Med 1986; 105(6):887–888.

43. John H, et al. Pheochromocytomas: can malignant potential be predicted? Urology 1999; 53(4):679–683.

44. McClean DR, et al., Malignant phaeochromocytoma with high circulating DOPA, and clonidine-suppressible noradrenaline. Blood Press 1995; 4(4):215–217.

45. Proye C, et al. [Dopamine-secreting pheochromocytoma. An unrecognized entity?]. Chirurgie 1984; 110(3):304–308.

46. Eisenhofer G, et al. 123I-MIBG scintigraphy of cate-cholamine systems: impediments to applications in clinical medicine. Eur J Nucl Med 2000; 27(5):611–612.

47. Lynn MD, et al. Pheochromocytoma and the normal adrenal medulla: improved visualization with I-123 MIBG scintigraphy. Radiology 1985; 155(3):789–792.

48. Shulkin BL, et al. Primary extra-adrenal pheochromocytoma: positive I-123 MIBG imaging with negative I-131 MIBG imaging. Clin Nucl Med 1986; 11(12):851–854.

49. Tsuchimochi S, et al. Metastatic pulmonary pheochromocytomas: positive I-123 MIBG SPECT with negative I-131 MIBG and equivocal I-123 MIBG planar imaging. Clin Nucl Med 1997; 22(10):687–690.

50. Hofland L, et al. Immunohistochemical detection of somatostatin receptor subtypes sst1 and sst2A in human somatostatin receptor positive tumors. J Clin Endcorinol Metab 1999; 84:775–780.

51. Shulkin B, Wieland D, Schwaiger M, et al. PET scanning with hydroxyephedrine: a new approach to the localization of pheochromocytoma. J Nucl Med 1992; 33:1125–1131.

52. Shulkin B, et al. PET epinephrine studies of pheochromocytoma. J Nucl Med 1995; 36:22–23.

53. Shulkin BL, et al. Pheochromocytomas: imaging with 2-[Fluorine-18]fluoro-2-deoxy-D-glucose PET. Nucl Med 1999; 212:35–41.

54. Walther M, Keiser H, Linehan W. Pheochromocytoma: evaluation, diagnosis, and management. World J Urol 1999; 17:35–39.

55. Ciftci AO, et al. Pheochromocytoma in children. J Pediatr Surg 2001; 36(3):447–452.

56. Ein SH, et al. Pediatric pheochromocytoma. A 36-year review. Pediatr Surg Int 1997; 12(8):595–598.

57. Turner MC, Lieberman E, DeQuattro V. The perioperative management of pheochromocytoma in children. Clin Pediatr (Phila) 1992; 31(10):583–589.

58. Hack HA. The perioperative management of children with phaeochromocytoma. Paediatr Anaesth 2000; 10(5):463–476.

59. Vargas H, et al. Laparoscopic adrenalectomy: a new standard of care. Urology 1997; 49:673–678.

60. Sipple JH. The association of pheochromocytoma with carcinoma of the thyroid gland. Am J Med 1961; 31:163–166.

61. Eng C. Seminars in medicine of the Beth Israel Hospital, Boston. The RET proto-oncogene in multiple endocrine neoplasia type 2 and Hirschsprung's disease. N Engl J Med 1996; 335(13):943–951.

62. Eng C. RET proto-oncogene in the development of human cancer. J Clin Oncol 1999; 17(1):380–393.

63. Hansford JR, Mulligan LM. Multiple endocrine neoplasia type 2 and RET: from neoplasia to neurogenesis. J Med Genet 2000; 37(11):817–827.

64. Gagel RF, et al. Multiple endocrine neoplasia type 2a associated with cutaneous lichen amyloidosis. Ann Intern Med 1989; 111(10):802–806.

65. Borst MJ, et al. Mutational analysis of multiple endocrine neoplasia type 2A associated with Hirschsprung's disease. Surgery 1995; 117(4):386–391.

66. Decker RA, Peacock ML. Occurrence of MEN 2a in familial Hirschsprung's disease: a new indication for genetic testing of the RET proto-oncogene. J Pediatr Surg 1998; 33(2):207–214.

67. Inoue K, et al. Mutational analysis of the RET proto-oncogene in a kindred with multiple endocrine neoplasia type 2A and Hirschsprung's disease. J Pediatr Surg 1999; 34(10):1552–1554.

68. Mulligan L, et al. Germ-line mutations of the RET proto-oncogene in multiple endocrine neoplasia type 2A. Nature 1993; 363:458–460.

69. Schuchardt A, et al. Defects in the kidney and enteric nervous system of mice lacking the tyrosine kinase receptor Ret. Nature 1994; 367(6461):380–383.

70. Lore F, et al. Multiple endocrine neoplasia type 2 syndromes may be associated with renal malformations. J Intern Med 2001; 250(1):37–42.

71. Huang SC, et al. Duplication of the mutant RET allele in trisomy 10 or loss of the wild-type allele in multiple endocrine neoplasia type 2-associated pheochromocytomas. Cancer Res 2000; 60(22):6223–6226.

72. Koch CA, et al. Do somatic RET mutations represent a phenomenon of tumor progression? Curr Opin Clin Exp Res 2001; 3(3):140–145.

73. Koch CA, et al. Genetic aspects of pheochromocytoma (Review). Endocr Regul 2001; 35(1):43–52.

74. Koch CA, et al. Allelic imbalance between mutated and wild-type RET in MEN 2-associated medullary thyroid carcinoma. Oncogene 2001; 20:7809–7811.

75. Weise M, Merke DP, Pacak K, Walther MM, Eisenhofer G. Utility of plasma free metanephrines for detecting childhood pheochromocytoma. J Clin Endocrinol Metab 2002; 87:1955–1960.

76. DeLellis RA, et al. Adrenal medullary hyperplasia. A morphometric analysis in patients with familial medullary thyroid carcinoma. Am J Pathol 1976; 83(1):177–196.

77. Carney JA, Sizemore GW, Tyce GM. Bilateral adrenal medullary hyperplasia in multiple endocrine neoplasia, type 2: the precursor of bilateral pheochromocytoma. Mayo Clin Proc 1975; 50(1):3–10.

78. Graham SM, et al. Provocative testing for occult medullary carcinoma of the thyroid: findings in seven children with multiple endocrine neoplasia type IIa. J Pediatr Surg 1987; 22(6):501–503.

79. Lips CJ, et al. Clinical screening as compared with DNA analysis in families with multiple endocrine neoplasia type 2A. N Engl J Med 1994; 331(13):828–835.

80. Marsh D, et al. Germline and somatic mutations in an oncogene: RET mutations in inherited medullary thyroid carcinoma 1. Adv Brief 1996; 56:1241–1243.

81. Neumann H, et al. Consequences of direct genetic testing for germline mutations in the clinical management of families with multiple endocrine neoplasia, type II. JAMA 1995; 274:1149–1151.

82. Frohnauer MK, Decker RA. Update on the MEN 2A c804 RET mutation: is prophylactic thyroidectomy indicated? Surgery 2000; 128(6):1052–1058.

83. Hassett S, et al. Prophylactic thyroidectomy in the treatment of thyroid medullary carcinoma. Age for surgery? Eur J Pediatr Surg 2000; 10(5):334–336.

84. Iler MA, et al. Multiple endocrine neoplasia type 2A: a 25-year review. J Pediatr Surg 1999; 34(1):92–97.

85. Skinner MA, et al. Medullary thyroid carcinoma in children with multiple endocrine neoplasia types 2A and 2B. J Pediatr Surg 1996; 31(1):177–182

86. van Heurn LW, et al. Predictive DNA testing for multiple endocrine neoplasia 2: a therapeutic challenge of prophylactic thyroidectomy in very young children. J Pediatr Surg 1999; 34(4):568–571.

87. Heptulla RA, et al. Familial medullary thyroid carcinoma: presymptomatic diagnosis and management in children. J Pediatr 1999; 135(3):327–331.

88. Uchino S, et al. Presymptomatic detection and treatment of Japanese carriers of the multiple endocrine neoplasia type 2A gene. Surg Today 1999; 29(9):862–867.

89. Moyes CD, Alexander FW. Mucosal neuroma syndrome presenting in a neonate. Dev Med Child Neurol, 1977; 19(4):518–534.

90. Samaan NA, et al. Multiple endocrine syndrome type IIb in early childhood. Cancer 1991; 68(8):1832–1834.

91. Gagel RF, et al. The clinical outcome of prospective screening for multiple endocrine neoplasia type 2a. An 18-year experience. N Engl J Med 1988; 318(8):478–484.

92. Jadoul M, et al. Pheochromocytoma-induced hypertensive encephalopathy revealing MEN-IIa syndrome in a 13-year old boy. Implications for screening procedures and surgery. Horm Metab Res Suppl 1989; 21:46–49.

93. Pacak K, et al. Pheochromocytoma: progress in diagnosis, therapy, and genetics. In: Margioris A, Chrousos GP, eds. Adrenal Disorders, Totowa: Humana Press, 2001:479–523.

94. Neumann HP, et al. Pheochromocytomas, multiple endocrine neoplasia type 2, and von Hippel-Lindau disease. N Engl J Med 1993; 329(21):1531–1538.

95. Casanova S, et al. Phaeochromocytoma in multiple endocrine neoplasia type 2A: survey of 100 cases. Clin Endocrinol 1993; 38:531–537.

96. Cance WG, Wells SA Jr. Multiple endocrine neoplasia. Type IIa. Curr Probl Surg 1985; 22(5):1–56.

97. Heath H III, Sizemore GW, Carney JA. Preoperative diagnosis of occult parathyroid hyperplasia by calcium infusion in patients with multiple endocrine neoplasia, type 2a. J Clin Endocrinol Metab 1976; 43(2):428–435.

98. Carney JA, et al. Alimentary-tract ganglioneuromatosis. A major component of the syndrome of multiple endocrine neoplasia, type 2b. N Engl J Med 1976; 295(23):1287–1291.

99. Carney JA, et al. The parathyroid glands in multiple endocrine neoplasia type 2b. Am J Pathol 1980; 99(2):387–398.

100. Wohllk N, et al. Relevance of RET proto-oncogene mutations in sporadic medullary thyroid carcinoma. J Clin Endocrinol Metab 1996; 81(10):3740–3745.

101. Decker RA, et al. Progress in genetic screening of multiple endocrine neoplasia type 2A: is calcitonin testing obsolete? Surgery 1995; 118(2):257–264

102. Eng C, et al. Low frequency of germline mutations in the RET proto-oncogene in patients with apparently sporadic medullary thyroid carcinoma. Clin Endocrinol (Oxf) 1995; 43(1):123–127.

103. Zbar B, et al. Germline mutations in the Von Hippel-Lindau disease (VHL) gene in families from North America, Europe, and Japan. Hum Mutat 1996; 8(4):348–357.

104. Chen F, et al. Germline mutations in the von Hippel-Lindau disease tumor suppressor gene: correlation with phenotype. Hum Mutat 1995; 5:66–75.

105. Vortmeyer AO, et al. Somatic von Hippel-Lindau gene mutations detected in sporadic endolymphatic sac tumors. Cancer Res 2000; 60(21):5963–5965.

106. Walther M, Reiter R, Keiser H, et al. Clinical and genetic characterization of pheochromocytoma in von Hippel-Lindau families: comparison with sporadic pheochromocytoma gives insight into natural history of pheochromocytoma. J Urol 1999; 162:659–664.

107. Maher ER, et al. Clinical features and natural history of von Hippel-Lindau disease. Q J Med 1990; 77(283):1151–1163.

108. Richard S, et al. Pheochromocytoma as the first manifestation of von Hippel-Lindau disease. Surgery 1994; 116:1076–1081.

109. Eisenhofer G, et al. Pheochromocytomas in von Hippel-Lindau syndrome and multiple endocrine neoplasia type 2 display distinct biochemical and clinical phenotypes. J Clin Endocrinol Metab 2001; 86(5):1999–2008.

110. Crossey PA, et al. Identification of intragenic mutations in the von Hippel-Lindau disease tumour suppressor gene and correlation with disease phenotype. Hum Mol Genet 1994; 3(8):1303–1308.

111. Ritter MM, et al. Isolated familial pheochromocytoma as a variant of von Hippel-Lindau disease. J Clin Endocrinol Metab 1996; 81(3):1035–1037.

112. van der Harst E, et al. Germline mutations in the vhl gene in patients presenting with phaeochromocytomas. Int J Cancer 1998; 77(3):337–340.

113. Brauch H, et al. Von Hippel Lindau (VHL) disease with pheochromocytoma in the Black Forest region of Germany: evidence for a founder effect. Hum Genet 1995; 95:551 556.

114. Gross D, et al. Familial pheochromocytoma associated with a novel mutation in the von Hippel-Lindau gene. J Clin Endocrinol Metab 1996; 81:147–149.

115. Bender BU, et al. Differential genetic alterations in von Hippel-Lindau syndrome-associated and sporadic pheochromocytomas. J Clin Endocrinol Metab 2000; 85(12):4568–4574.

116. Duan DR, et al. Inhibition of transcription elongation by the VHL tumor suppressor protein. Science 1995; 269(5229):1402–1406.

117. Aso T, et al. Elongin (SIII): a multisubunit regulator of elongation by RNA polymerase II. Science 1995; 269(5229):1439–1443.

118. Kondo K, Kaelin WG Jr. The von Hippel-Lindau tumor suppressor gene. Exp Cell Res 2001; 264(1):117–125.

119. Huson SM, et al. A genetic study of von Recklinghausen neurofibromatosis in south east Wales. I. Prevalence, fitness, mutation rate, and effect of parental transmission on severity. J Med Genet 1989; 26(11):704–711.

120. Riccardi VM. Neurofibromatosis: past, present, and future. N Engl J Med 1991; 324(18):1283–1285.

121. Walther M, et al. von Recklinghausen's disease and pheochromocytomas. J Urol 1999; 162:1582–1586.

122. Xu W, et al. Loss of NF1 alleles in phaeochromocytomas from patients with type I neurofibromatosis. Genes Chromosomes Cancer 1992; 4(4):337–342.

123. Mulvihill JJ, et al. Familial pheochromocytoma due to mutant von Hippel-Lindau disease gene. Arch Intern Med 1997; 157(12):1390–1391.

124. Neumann H, Berger D, Sigmund G, et al. Pheochromocytomas, multiple endocrine neoplasia type 2, and von Hippel-Lindau disease [see comments] [published erratum appears in N Engl J Med 1994; 331(22):1535]. N Engl J Med 1993; 329:1531–1538.

125. Baysal BE, et al. Mutations in SDHD, a mitochondrial complex II gene, in hereditary paraganglioma. Science 2000; 287(5454):848–851.

126. Gurney JG, et al. Trends in cancer incidence among children in the U.S. Cancer 1996; 78(3):532–541.

127. Gurney JG, et al. Infant cancer in the U.S.: histology-specific incidence and trends, 1973 to 1992. J Pediatr Hematol Oncol 1997; 19(5):428–432.

128. Parkin DM, et al. International Incidence of Childhood Cancer, vol. II. Lyon: International Agency for Research on Cancer, 1998.

129. Everson TC. Spontaneous regression of cancer. Ann NY Acad Sci 1964; 114(2):721–735.

130. Stiller CA. Trends in neuroblastoma in Great Britain: incidence and mortality, 1971–1990. Eur J Cancer 1993; 7(12):1008–1012.

131. Enzinger FM, Weiss SW. Soft Tissue Tumors, 3rd ed. 1995, St. Louis: Mosby–Year Book, 1995.

132. Brodeur GM, Castleberry RP. Neuroblastoma. In: Pizzo PA, Poplack DG, eds. Principles and Practice of Pediatric Oncology. Philadelphia: Lippincott–Raven, 1997:761–796.

133. Abeloff MD, et al. Clinical Oncology, 2nd ed. Philadelphia: Churchill Livingstone, 2000.

134. Carlsen NL. Neuroblastomas presenting in the first year of life: epidemiological differences from those presenting at older ages. Cancer Detect Prev 1996; 20(3):251–261.

135. Clausen N, Andersson P, Tommerup N. Familial occurrence of neuroblastoma, von Recklinghausen's neurofibromatosis, Hirschsprung's agangliosis and jaw-winking syndrome. Acta Paediatr Scand 1989; 78(5):736–741.

136. Kushner BH, Hajdu SI, Helson L. Synchronous neuroblastoma and von Recklinghausen's disease: a review of the literature. J Clin Oncol 1985; 3(1):117–120.

137. Hofstra RM, et al. No mutations found by RET mutation scanning in sporadic and hereditary neuroblastoma. Hum Genet 1996; 97(3):362–364.

138. Maris JM, et al. Molecular genetic analysis of familial neuroblastoma. Eur J Cancer 1997; 33(12):1923–1928.

139. Linet MS, et al. Cancer surveillance series: recent trends in childhood cancer incidence and mortality in the United States. J Natl Cancer Inst 1999; 91(12):1051–1058.

140. Little F. Epidemiology of Childhood Cancer. Lyon: International Agency for Research on Cancer, 1999.

141. Olshan AF, et al. Hormone and fertility drug use and the risk of neuroblastoma: a report from the Children's Cancer Group and the Pediatric Oncology Group. Am J Epidemiol 1999; 150(9):930–938.

142. Vandesompele J, et al. Multicentre analysis of patterns of DNA gains and losses in 204 neuroblastoma tumors: how many genetic subgroups are there? Med Pediatr Oncol 2001; 36(1):5–10.

143. Maris JM, et al. Comprehensive analysis of chromosome 1p deletions in neuroblastoma. Med Pediatr Oncol 2001; 36(1):32–36.

144. Vettenranta K, et al. Comparative genomic hybridization reveals changes in DNA-copy number in poor-risk neuroblastoma. Cancer Genet Cytogenet 2001; 125(2):125–130.

145. Maris JM, et al. Significance of chromosome 1p loss of heterozygosity in neuroblastoma. Cancer Res 1995; 55(20):4664–4669.

146. Fong CT, et al. Loss of heterozygosity for chromosomes 1 or 14 defines subsets of advanced neuroblastomas. Cancer Res 1992; 52(7):1780–1785.

147. Caron H, et al. Allelic loss of chromosome 1p36 in neuroblastoma is of preferential maternal origin and correlates with N-myc amplification. Nat Genet 1993; 4(2):187–190.

148. Caron H. Allelic loss of chromosome 1 and additional chromosome 17 material are both unfavourable prognostic markers in neuroblastoma. Med Pediatr Oncol 1995. 24(4):215–221.

149. Caron H, et al. Allelic loss of the short arm of chromosome 4 in neuroblastoma suggests a novel tumour suppressor gene locus. Hum Genet 1996; 97(6):834–837.

150. Srivatsan ES, Murali V, Seeger RC. Loss of heterozygosity for alleles on chromosomes 11q and 14q in neuroblastoma. Prog Clin Biol Res 1991; 366:91–98.

151. Lastowska M, et al. Comparative genomic hybridization study of primary neuroblastoma tumors. United Kingdom Children's Cancer Study Group. Genes Chromosomes Cancer 1997; 18(3):162–169.

152. Altura RA, et al. Novel regions of chromosomal loss in familial neuroblastoma by comparative genomic hybridization. Genes Chromosomes Cancer 1997; 19(3):176–184.

153. Thompson PM, et al. Loss of heterozygosity for chromosome 14q in neuroblastoma. Med Pediatr Oncol 2001; 36(1):28–31.

154. Theobald M, et al. Sublocalization of putative tumor suppressor gene loci on chromosome arm 14q in neuroblastoma. Genes Chromosomes Cancer 1999; 26(1):40–46.

155. Vandesompele J, et al. Genetic heterogeneity of neuroblastoma studied by comparative genomic hybridization. Genes Chromosomes Cancer 1998; 23(2):141–152.

156. Takita J, et al. Allelotype of neuroblastoma. Oncogene 1995; 11(9):1829–1834.

157. Huang S, LU, Pack S, Wang C, Kim AC, Lutchman M, Koch CA, Huang SC, Bez EJ Jr, Christansen H, Dockhorn-Dwornickzak, Poremba C, Vortmeyer AO, Chishti AH, Zhuang Z. Reassignment of the EPB4.1 gene to 1p36 and assessment of its involvement in neuroblastomas. Eur J Clin Invest, 2001; 31:907–914.

158. Bauer A, et al. Smallest region of overlapping deletion in 1p36 in human neuroblastoma: a 1 Mbp cosmid and PAC contig. Genes Chromosomes Cancer 2001; 31(3):228–239.

159. Kohl NE, et al. Transposition and amplification of oncogene-related sequences in human neuroblastomas. Cell 1983; 35(2 Pt 1):359–367.

160. Schwab M, et al. Amplified DNA with limited homology to myc cellular oncogene is shared by human neuroblastoma cell lines and a neuroblastoma tumour. Nature 1983; 305(5931):245–248.

161. Bown N, et al. Gain of chromosome arm 17q and adverse outcome in patients with neuroblastoma. N Engl J Med 1999; 340(25):1954–1961.

162. Plantaz D, et al. Gain of chromosome 17 is the most frequent abnormality detected in neuroblastoma by comparative genomic hybridization. Am J Pathol 1997; 150(1):81–89.

163. Castleberry RP. Biology and treatment of neuroblastoma. Pediatr Clin North Am 1997; 44(4):919–937.

164. Haase GM, Perez C, Atkinson JB. Current aspects of biology, risk assessment, and treatment of neuroblastoma. Semin Surg Oncol 1999; 16(2):91–104.

165. Brossard J, Bernstein ML, Lemieux B. Neuroblastoma: an enigmatic disease. Br Med Bull 1996; 52(4):787–801.

166. Murthi GV, et al. Musculoskeletal manifestations of neuroblastoma at diagnosis. Med Pediatr Oncol 2001; 36(6): 671.

167. Rudnick E, et al. Opsoclonus-myoclonus-ataxia syndrome in neuroblastoma: clinical outcome and antineuronal antibodies-a report from the Children's Cancer Group Study. Med Pediatr Oncol 2001; 36(6):612–622.

168. Voorhess ML. Neuroblastoma-pheochromocytoma: products and pathogenesis. Ann NY Acad Sci 1974; 230:187–194.

169. Brodeur GM, et al. Revisions of the international criteria for neuroblastoma diagnosis, staging, and response to treatment. J Clin Oncol 1993; 11(8):1466–1477.

170. Shimada H, et al. Terminology and morphologic criteria of neuroblastic tumors: recommendations by the International Neuroblastoma Pathology Committee. Cancer 1999; 86(2):349–363.

171. Brodeur GM, et al. International criteria for diagnosis, staging, and response to treatment in patients with neuroblastoma. J Clin Oncol 1988; 6(12):1874–1881.

172. LaBrosse EH, et al. Urinary excretion of 3-methoxy-4-hydroxymandelic acid and 3-methoxy-4-hydroxyphenyl-acetic acid by 288 patients with neuroblastoma and related neural crest tumors. Cancer Res 1980; 40(6):1995–2001.

173. Hoefnagel CA, de Kraker J. Childhood neoplasia. In: Murray IPC, Ell PJ, eds. Nuclear Medicine in Clinical Diagnosis and Treatment. Hong Kong: Churchill Livingstone, 1998:1001–1014.

174. Leung A, et al. Specificity of radioiodinated MIBG for neural crest tumors in childhood. J Nucl Med 1997; 38(9):1352–1357.

175. Petjak M, et al. Diagnostic imaging in abdominal neuroblastoma: is there a complementary role of MIBG-scintigraphy and ultrasonography? Eur J Pediatr 1997; 156(8):610–615.

176. Evans AE, et al. A review of 17 IV-S neuroblastoma patients at the children's hospital of Philadelphia. Cancer 1980; 45(5):833–839.

177. Evans AE, Baum E, Chard R. Do infants with stage IV-S neuroblastoma need treatment? Arch Dis Child 1981; 56(4):271–274.

178. Shimada H, et al. The International Neuroblastoma Pathology Classification (the Shimada system). Cancer 1999; 86(2):364–372.

179. Silber JH, Evans AE, Fridman M. Models to predict outcome from childhood neuroblastoma: the role of serum ferritin and tumor histology. Cancer Res 1991; 51(5):1426–1433.

180. Zeltzer PM, et al. Raised neuron-specific enolase in serum of children with metastatic neuroblastoma. A report from the Children's Cancer Study Group. Lancet 1983; 2(8346):361–363.

181. Schulz G, et al. Detection of ganglioside GD2 in tumor tissues and sera of neuroblastoma patients. Cancer Res 1984; 44(12 Pt 1):5914–5920.

182. Schengrund CL, Repman MA, Shochat SJ. Ganglioside composition of human neuroblastomas. Correlation with prognosis. A Pediatric Oncology Group Study. Cancer 1985; 56(11):2640–2646.

183. Valentino L, et al. Shed tumor gangliosides and progression of human neuroblastoma. Blood 1990; 75(7):1564–1567.

184. Shuster JJ, et al. Serum lactate dehydrogenase in childhood neuroblastoma. A Pediatric Oncology Group recursive partitioning study. Am J Clin Oncol 1992; 15(4):295–303.

185. Christiansen H, Lampert F. Tumour karyotype discriminates between good and bad prognostic outcome in neuroblastoma. Br J Cancer 1988; 57(1):121–126.

186. Gansler T, et al. Flow cytometric DNA analysis of neuroblastoma. Correlation with histology and clinical outcome. Cancer 1986; 58(11):2453–2458.

187. Taylor SR, et al. Flow cytometric DNA analysis of neuroblastoma and ganglioneuroma. A 10-year retrospective study. Cancer 1988; 62(4):749–754.

188. Kaneko Y, et al. Different karyotypic patterns in early and advanced stage neuroblastomas. Cancer Res 1987; 47(1):311–318.

189. Look AT, et al. Cellular DNA content as a predictor of response to chemotherapy in infants with unresectable neuroblastoma. N Engl J Med 1984; 311(4):231–235.

190. Nakagawara A, et al. Association between high levels of expression of the TRK gene and favorable outcome in human neuroblastoma. N Engl J Med 1993; 328(12):847–854.

191. Brodeur GM, et al. Amplification of N-myc in untreated human neuroblastomas correlates with advanced disease stage. Science 1984; 224(4653):1121–1124.

192. Seeger RC, et al. Association of multiple copies of the N-myc oncogene with rapid progression of neuroblastomas. N Engl J Med 1985; 313(18):1111–1116.

193. Cohn SL, et al. Analysis of DNA ploidy and proliferative activity in relation to histology and N-myc amplification in neuroblastoma. Am J Pathol 1990; 136(5):1043–1052.

194. Look AT, et al. Clinical relevance of tumor cell ploidy and N-myc gene amplification in childhood neuroblastoma: a Pediatric Oncology Group study. J Clin Oncol 1991; 9(4):581–591.

195. Brodcur GM, Nakagawara A. Molecular basis of clinical heterogeneity in neuroblastoma. Am J Pediatr Hematol Oncol 1992; 14(2):111–116.

196. Hiyama E, et al. Telomerase activity in neuroblastoma: is it a prognostic indicator of clinical behaviour? Eur J Cancer 1997; 33(12):1932–1936.

197. Hiyama E, et al. Correlating telomerase activity levels with human neuroblastoma outcomes. Nat Med 1995; 1(3):249–255.

198. Bowman LC, et al. Impact of intensified therapy on clinical outcome in infants and children with neuroblastoma: the St Jude Children's Research Hospital experience, 1962 to 1988. J Clin Oncol 1991; 9(9):1599–1608.

199. Rubie H, et al. Localised and unresectable neuroblastoma in infants: excellent outcome with primary chemotherapy. Neuroblastoma Study Group, Societe Francaise d'Oncologie Pediatrique. Med Pediatr Oncol 2001; 36(1):247–250.

200. Brodeur GM, et al. Biological aspects of neuroblastomas identified by mass screening in Quebec. Med Pediatr Oncol 2001; 36(1):157–159.

201. Parker L, Powell J. Screening for neuroblastoma in infants younger than 1 year of age: review of the first 30 years. Med Pediatr Oncol 1998; 31:455–469.

202. Woods WG, et al. Screening for neuroblastoma is ineffective in reducing the incidence of unfavourable advanced stage disease in older children. Eur J Cancer 1997; 33(12):2106–2112.

203. Woods WG, et al. Screening infants for neuroblastoma does not reduce the incidence of poor-prognosis disease. Med Pediatr Oncol 1998; 31:450–454.

204. Solcia E, Klöpel G, Sobin LH. Histological Typing of Endocrine Tumours, 2nd ed. Berlin-Heidelberg: Springer-Verlag, 2000.

205. Hicks MJ, Mackay B. Comparison of ultrastructural features among neuroblastic tumors: maturation from neuroblastoma to ganglioneuroma. Ultrastruct Pathol 1995; 19(4):311–322.

206. Lucas K, et al. Catecholamine metabolites in ganglioneuroma. Med Pediatr Oncol 1994; 22(4):240–243.

207. Geoerger B, et al. Metabolic activity and clinical features of primary ganglioneuromas. Cancer 2001; 91(10):1905–1913.

208. Scherer A, et al. Imaging diagnosis of retroperitoneal ganglioneuroma in childhood. Pediatr Radiol 2001; 31(2):106–110.

209. Stowens D. Neuroblastoma and related tumors. Arch Pathol 1957; 63:451–453.
210. Radin R, et al. Adrenal and extra-adrenal retroperitoneal ganglioneuroma: imaging findings in 13 adults. Radiology 1997; 202(3):703–707.
211. Carpenter WB, Kernohan JW. Retroperitoneal ganglioneuromas and neurofibromas. A clinicopathological study. Cancer 1963; 16(June):788–797.
212. Hamilton JP, Koop CE. Ganglioneuromas in children. Surg Gynecol Obstet 1965; 121(4):803–812.
213. Scheibel E, et al. Vasoactive intestinal polypeptide (VIP) in children with neural crest tumours. Acta Paediatr Scand 1982; 71(5):721–725.
214. Hansen LP, et al. Vasoactive intestinal polypeptide (VIP)-producing ganglioneuroma in a child with chronic diarrhea. Acta Paediatr Scand 1980; 69(3):419–424.
215. Hollenberg CH. Medullary carcinoma of the thyroid. Arch Otolaryngol 1983; 109(2):103–105.
216. Kaplan SJ, et al. Vasoactive intestinal peptide secreting tumors of childhood. Am J Dis Child 1980; 134(1):21–24.
217. Long RG, et al. Clinicopathological study of pancreatic and ganglioneuroblastoma tumours secreting vasoactive intestinal polypeptide (vipomas). Br Med J (Clin Res Ed) 1981; 282(6278):1767–1771.
218. Yagihashi S, et al. Ganglioneuroblastoma containing several kinds of neuronal peptides with watery diarrhea syndrome. Acta Pathol Jpn 1982; 32(5):807–814.
219. Schuman AJ, Alario AJ, Pitel PA. Occult ganglioneuroma with diarrhea: localization by venous catecholamines. Med Pediatr Oncol 1984; 12(2):93–96.
220. Viale G, et al. Vasoactive intestinal polypeptide-, somatostatin-, and calcitonin-producing adrenal pheochromocytoma associated with the watery diarrhea (WDHH) syndrome. First case report with immunohistochemical findings. Cancer 1985; 55(5):1099–1106.
221. Krejs GJ. VIPoma syndrome. Am J Med 1987; 82(5B):37–48.
222. Van Eeckhout P, et al. Acute watery diarrhea as the initial presenting feature of a pheochromocytoma in an 84-year-old female patient. Horm Res 1999; 52(2):101–106.
223. Cooney DR, et al. Vasoactive intestinal peptide producing neuroblastoma. J Pediatr Surg 1982; 17(6):821–825.
224. Kulke MH, Mayer RJ. Carcinoid tumors. N Engl J Med 1999; 340(11):858–868.
225. Koch CA, et al. Carcinoid syndrome caused by an atypical carcinoid of the uterine cervix. J Clin Endocrinol Metab 1999; 84(11):4209–4213.
226. Isaacs P, Whittaker SM, Turnberg LA. Diarrhea associated with medullary carcinoma of the thyroid. Studies of intestinal function in a patient. Gastroenterology 1974; 67(3):521–526.

9

Puberty and Its Disorders

Peter A. Lee

Pennsylvania State College of Medicine, The Milton S. Hershey Medical Center, Hershey, Pennsylvania, U.S.A.

I. NORMAL PUBERTY

A. Definition and Mechanism

Puberty is the stage of human development when sexual maturation and growth are completed, resulting in the capacity for reproduction. Accelerated somatic growth, growth and maturation of the primary sexual characteristics (gonads and genitals), and the appearance of secondary sexual characteristics (e.g., sexual hair, female breast development, and male voice change) occur. Menstruation and spermatogenesis begin. These changes are a consequence of increased gonadotropin and sex steroid secretion. Androgens and estrogens are both involved. Although estrogen (primarily estradiol) stimulates breast and reproductive system maturity in girls and testosterone stimulates pubertal changes in boys, androgen is responsible for certain changes among both boys and girls. Androgen stimulates sexual hair development, increased oiliness of skin related to acne, and apocrine gland secretion causing adult-type body odor. Sex steroids directly and indirectly stimulate overall somatic growth, estradiol appearing to be the key hormone stimulating skeletal maturity among both sexes.

Increased gonadal activity results from increased stimulation by pituitary gonadotropins: luteinizing hormone (LH) and follicle-stimulating hormone (FSH). Increased testicular sex hormone production is stimulated by LH; FSH stimulates primarily maturation of spermatogonia. In the female both LH and FSH are necessary for hormonogenesis, while FSH plays a primary role in ova maturation.

The physiological secretion pattern of gonadotropins is a periodic intermittent release, more dramatically apparent for LH (1–5). Amplitude is low and release infrequent before puberty. At pubertal onset, accentuated episodes of LH first occur during sleep, then progressively increase in frequency and amplitude, extending throughout the 24 h period (6). The intermittent gonadotropin release is a direct response to episodic release of hypothalamic gonadotropin-releasing hormone (GnRH or LHRH) (7). During childhood this system is downregulated since GnRH secretion is minimal. Throughout childhood, the pituitary and gonads are capable of full function at any age after a relatively short period of physiological stimulation. The onset of puberty is a consequence of enhanced GnRH secretion. The mechanisms by which this occurs are incompletely understood, but they appear to involve the stimulatory and inhibitory influences of such neurotransmitters as acetylcholine, catecholamines, γ-aminobutyric acid (GABA), opioid peptides, prostaglandins, and serotonin.

Negative feedback of hypothalamic–pituitary gonadotropin–gonadal control is first acquired in fetal life and is operative thereafter (8). Changes in feedback sensitivity are inadequate to explain differences in fetal, neonatal, childhood, and pubertal physiology. Overriding central nervous system (CNS) control is an obligatory component. Episodic release is present in the neonatal period and childhood, with gonadotropin secretion diminishing during childhood (9). Mean LH and FSH levels are both low in childhood, FSH levels being relatively higher than LH levels, particularly in girls (3, 5, 9). Since the pituitary gland is always capable of response to GnRH stimulation, the characteristic response during childhood is markedly less than at puberty, with a greater response of FSH than LH. The childhood response pattern may not be distinguishable from that typical of hypogonadotropism. With the onset of puberty, the mean LH and FSH levels increase, with a relatively greater rise in the LH levels. Generally, however, for most patients baseline values may overlap the prepubertal and pubertal range. Levels of pubertal individuals may not be discernible from a single sample. GnRH or GnRH analog stimulation is the most useful test to differentiate pubertal and prepubertal status, since LH responses to exogenous GnRH stimulation becomes more pronounced with pubertal maturity (10, 11).

211

The incremental rise of FSH after GnRH stimulation changes less with pubertal maturation and hence is less useful to ascertain differences (10, 11). A marked FSH response is already evident in prepubertal children, and particularly among girls may not increase discernibly with puberty.

Because of the greater rise of LH in relation to FSH with pubertal secretion, LH/FSH ratios, either baseline or stimulated, may be used as an indication of status. A ratio of less than 1 is typical of prepuberty, while a ratio of greater than 1 characteristic of pubertal secretion (12).

B. Normal Female Development

Milestones of female puberty include thelarche (onset of pubertal breast development) and menarche (the onset of menstrual periods). Pubarche is a term used to signify the onset of sexual hair development, a result of adrenarche (the onset of pubertal adrenal androgen secretion), although androgen production by the ovaries also occurs with the increased steroidogenesis during puberty.

1. Age of Puberty

The most common first evidence of puberty in girls is thelarche (Fig. 1), although it may occasionally be preceded by pubarche (13–15). The best available data currently indicate that the mean age for the onset of breast development in girls is between 9.5 and 10 years of age, with 5% of girls having breast development by their eighth birthday. The average age of full pubertal breast development is 14 years (Fig. 1) (15). Based on the most recent data, the average duration of pubertal development is 3–4 years. European data (16) but not U.S. data suggest

that the tempo may be somewhat faster while there may be considerable variation in the tempo. Data suggest that the earlier the onset, the slower the tempo of puberty (17), the pace of pubertal development correlating with the level of sex steroids (18). It is clear that the onset of breast and pubic hair development occurs, on the average, earlier among African-American than among white girls (14).

2. Hormone-Stimulated Changes

Mean LH, FSH, and estradiol levels increase before physical changes begin, but because of fluctuation within and between individuals, this rise may not be discernible in individual instances. A pubertal GnRH-stimulated LH response or elevated estradiol values signify that gonadarche has occurred, the estrogen-stimulated development that follows includes breast, genital, and uterine maturation; increase in body fat content and lean body mass (19); and acquisition of fat distribution in the typical female contours. Breast growth may begin asymmetrically, progresses throughout puberty and may be classified into five Tanner stages (Table 1). Pubic hair growth, which begins in the average girl at age 10 years, can also be staged to follow progression (Table 1).

3. Adrenarche

The increased adrenal androgen production (onset designated as adrenarche) precedes the pubertal rise of gonadotropins and gonadarche. Adrenarche may be detected in girls by age 6 by an elevation in circulating levels of dehydroepiandrosterone (DHEA) and DHEA sulfate (DHEAS). The stimulus of adrenarche is unknown; no stimulating factor has been identified.

4. Growth and Progression

The pubertal growth spurt in girls, occurring early, usually is present at the time of the appearance of the first signs of puberty (Fig. 1). The interval between pubertal onset and menarche is variable, the average being 2 years. The magnitude of sex steroid exposure before menarche inversely correlates with the amount of statural growth after menarche, those with greater exposure being closer to final height at menarche. While the average girl grows 4–6 cm after menarche, those with relatively early menarche may grow as much as 10 cm, whereas those with more prolonged or greater estrogen stimulation before the onset of menses may grow less than 4 cm. Generally earlier menses is correlated with shorter adult height. It is not necessarily atypical for adolescent girls to have irregular menses for a year or longer after menarche; careful attention is warranted until menses become regular. Ovulation may occur before menarche or much later.

C. Normal Male Development

Although pubic hair growth is usually the first evidence of puberty noticed, increased testicular volume is the ear-

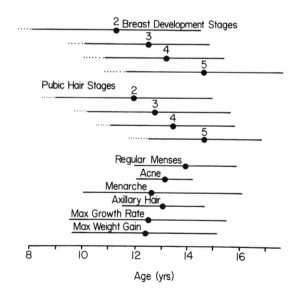

Figure 1 Mean ages (dots) and ranges (horizontal lines) of onset of pubertal development in girls. Dashed lines show early limit for African-Americans.

Table 1 Staging of Pubertal Development (Tanner)

Staging	Pubic hair staging	Concomitant changes	Prader orchidometer (ml)
Girls: breast			
1. Prepubertal, papilla elevation	No pigmented hair		
2. Budding; larger areole; palpable and visible elevated contour	Pigmented hair, mainly labial	Accelerated growth rate	
3. Enlargement of the breast and areola	Coarser, spread of pigmented hair over mons	Peak growth rate, thicker vaginal mucosa, axillary hair	
4. Secondary mound of areola and papilla	Adult type but smaller area	Menarche (stage 3 or 4) Decelerated growth rate	
5. Mature	Adult distribution		
Boys: genital size			
1. Prepubertal	No pigmented hair	Long testis axis <2.5 cm	1, 2, 3
2. Early testicular, penile, and scrotal growth	Minimal pigmented hair at base of penis	Early voice changes; testes length 2.5–3.3 cm	3, 4, 5, 6, 8
3. Increased penile length and width; scrotal and testes growth	Dark, coarse, curly hair extends midline above penis	Light hair on upper lip, acne, maximal growth, testes length 3.3–4.0 cm	10, 12, 15
4. Increased penis size including breadth; pigmented scrotum	Considerable, but less than adult distribution	Early sideburns; testes 4.0–4.5 cm	15, 20
5. Adult size and shape	Adult distribution, spread to medial thighs or beyond	Beard growth; testes >4.5 cm	25

liest physical evidence (20). A testis of 4 cc or 2.5 cm long is evidence of pubertal growth. This occurs, on the average, by 12 years and may occur normally as early as 9.5 years. Pubertal development in boys can be gauged by Tanner staging (Table 1) of genital size and pubic hair (Fig. 2).

1. Age of Puberty

As with girls, there were no large-scale studies of the on-set and progression of male pubertal development until the National Health and Nutrition Examination survey (NHANES). Mean ages and early limits were loosely based upon small studies from the United States and larger studies from the United Kingdom. Data from the NHANES has shown that puberty among African–American boys begins and progresses earlier than among whites and Mexican–Americans (21). These data concerning pubic hair development, the most reliable criteria, indicate that the early limit and mean age of the onset of Tanner stage 2 is similar to that previously used for white boys; about 9.5 years and 12 years, respectively. Among African-Americans, both ages would appear to be about 1 year earlier. The data for Tanner 2 genital staging differs so drastically from older data that one can only conclude that different criteria were used.

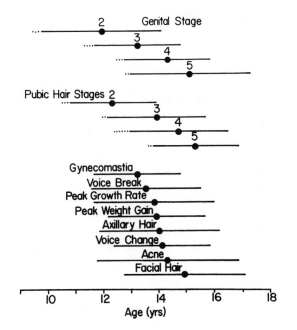

Figure 2 Mean ages (dots) and ranges (horizontal lines) of various pubertal changes in boys. Dashed lines show earlier limit for African-Americans.

Also, similar to the female data, the age of completion of puberty according to NHANES (21) is similar to older data. Thus, if puberty is beginning earlier, it is proceeding at a slower tempo, which is an unlikely phenomenon.

2. Hormonal Changes

As puberty progresses, there is a progressive rise of LH, FSH, and testosterone levels indicative of a continuing upregulation of secretion of the hypothalamic–pituitary–testicular axis (1, 2, 4). Levels of other steroids of adrenal or testicular origin also rise: estrone, estradiol, androstenedione, 17-hydroxyprogesterone, DHEA, and DHEAS (22). The rise of the latter two signifies adrenarche and precede gonadarche. Inhibin B levels, indicative of seminiferous tubule integrity, progressively rise during puberty (23). Mullerian inhibiting hormone levels in boys rise rapidly during the first year of life, are the highest during late infancy, and then gradually decline until puberty, while in girls levels rise minimally through prepubertal years (23, 24). This marker for testicular development has an inverse relationship with testosterone, with levels progressively falling throughout puberty (23, 24).

3. Growth

During midpuberty, the period when testosterone levels are rapidly rising, the peak of the pubertal growth spurt, voice change, and the onset of axillary hair growth occur (25, 26; Fig. 2). There is a progressive increase in total body bone mineral content, lean body mass, and a progressive decrease in body fat (19, 26). The onset of acne and gynecomastia are also typically midpubertal events.

Facial hair growth begins about 3 years after the onset of pubic hair growth. The density and distribution of the beard, chest hair, and abdominal and pubic hair may progress for years after puberty and vary considerably among adult men. These correlate more with familial or genetic factors than with hormonal levels, as do quantity and density of hair on the extremities.

In contrast to girls, the period of accelerated growth occurs during midpuberty rather than generally concomitant with the onset (25). Peak growth velocity is generally at 14–15 years of age and during Tanner stages 3 and 4. Onset of spermarche (first evidence of completed spermatogenesis, usually first observable by presence of sperm in urine, particularly first morning void) is usually at Tanner stage 3, occurring at age 13.5–14 years. It occurs after considerable testosterone stimulation, but before adult levels are reached.

4. Pubertal Gyncecomastia

Gynecomastia, defined as palpable or visible breast tissue, occurs in at least two-thirds of boys some time during puberty. Subareolar breast hyperplasia measuring 0.5 cm or more may be palpable. When a discrete symmetrical disk is palpable, with or without surrounding tissue full-

ness, this can be considered true gynecomastia. This may be difficult to differentiate from pseudogynecomastia resulting from accumulation of fatty tissue, particularly in boys who are heavy. Pubertal gynecomastia is a variant of normal development, which may develop excessively. Onset may coincide with the onset of puberty but primarily begins at ages 13–14, before testosterone levels have reached the adult range. Most commonly it persists for 18–24 months, and then regresses, usually by age 16 years. If the quantity of breast tissue is considerable and regression is not apparent after 2 years, plastic surgical excision should be offered. Drugs blocking estrogen effect may inhibit growth and cause regresssion, no medical therapy has been shown to cause full regression.

Gynecomastia develops at a point when circulating estrogen to testosterone levels are relatively greater than after testosterone levels reach adult values. This is apparently a consequence of extraglandular aromatization of adrenal and testicular androgens. Among boys with significant gynecomastia, this aromatization may occur within breast tissue.

II. PRECOCIOUS PUBERTY

A. Classification

When puberty begins and progresses early, the condition is, by definition, precocious puberty. However, because recent data, particularly for girls, suggest that the onset of puberty is occurring earlier, so one cannot make the diagnosis based simply upon the early limits of age for the normal onset of pubertal changes (27). The traditional early limit for girls was 8 years, the age that was considered to approximately 2 standard deviations below the mean (the lowest 2–3% of the normal population range). Recent data suggest that 5–6% percent of girls have breast development by their 8th birthday, suggesting a slight shift to a younger age.

Since breast development (thelarche) is reported to be occurring earlier, and there are differences among the African-American population, the diagnosis of precocious puberty should not be made in a girl unless, at presentation, she shows pubertal levels of hormones, early onset and inappropriately rapid progression of physical development, with an inappropriate acceleration of skeletal age in relation to growth rate. Since earlier onset of breast development is not being accompanied with the same tempo of puberty (with puberty being completed at the same age), early physical signs alone do not necessarily mean that the hypothalamic–pituitary–ovarian axis is being activated earlier. Thus, if the initial signs first appear earlier, without rapid progression, the diagnosis of precocious puberty should not be made. Early onset of breast development not followed by progressive change may be a variant of normal or constitute nonprogressive precocious puberty (28, 29). A young girl with pubertal breast development may be a variant of normal, have physiologically normal but early puberty, or have an underlying pathological cause of early development. Precocious puberty is diagnosed based on early onset, plus clinical, hormonal, and radiological evidence of excessive progression.

1. Gonadotropin-Dependent and -Independent Precocious Puberty

Precocious puberty is classified as physiologically normal but early and progressive (GnRH-dependent) or GnRH-independent (Table 2). GnRH-dependent or central (true) precocious puberty results from early onset of pubertal hypothalamic–pituitary–gonadal activity; it is (true)

Table 2 Differential Diagnosis of Precocious Puberty

Central (GnRH driven)
  Idiopathic (sporadic or familial)
  Central nervous system abnormalities
    Acquired (abscess, chemotherapy, granulomas, inflammation, radiation, surgical, trauma)
    Congenital anomalies (arachnoid cysts, hydrocephalus, hypothalamic hamartomas, septo-optic dysplasia, suprasellar cyst)
    Tumors (LH-secreting adenoma, astrocytoma, glioma (may be associated with neurofibromatosis), craniopharyngiomas, ependymomas)
    Secondary to chronic exposure to sex steroids (causes of peripheral puberty; CVAH, GIP, tumors)
    Reversible forms: space-occupying or pressure-associated lesions (abscess, hydrocephalus)
Peripheral (GnRH independent)
  Genetic disorders (mutations)
    Congenital virilizing adrenal hyperplasia (CVAH), males
    Gonadotropin-independent puberty
      LH receptor-activating mutations
      DAXI gene mutations
    McCune-Albright syndrome
  Tumors
    Adrenal sex steroid secreting (adenoma, carcinoma)
    Gonadotropin-producing (choriocarcinoma, chorioepithelioma, dysgerminoma, hepatoblastoma, hepatoma, teratoma)
    Ovarian (granulosa cell, may be associated with Peutz-Jeghers syndrome); granulosa, theca cell
    Testicular (Leydig cell)
  Limited or reversible forms
    Chronic primary hypothyroidism
    CVAH
    Exogenous sex steroid or gonadotropins
    Ovarian cysts
Variants of normal development
  Premature pubarche (secondary to premature adrenarche)
  Premature thelarche

physiological gonadotropin stimulation emanating from the GnRH secretion of (central) CNS–hypothalamic origin. Central precocious puberty is in contrast to peripheral (GnRH independent) or precocious pseudopuberty in which the sex steroid stimulating the physical changes of puberty is not produced as a result of physiological pituitary gonadotropin secretion. The source of sex steroid may be exogenous or endogenous, gonadal or extragonadal. The hormone may be autonomously produced, independent of gonadotropin stimulation.

2. General Terminology

The terms complete and incomplete sexual precocity have been used with different meanings. Central precocious puberty has been called complete and peripheral incomplete, but the more common designation has used complete to describe any form of precocious puberty while incomplete designates some partial early pubertal development such as thelarche or pubarche. Because of the confusion with this terminology, the latter changes are more appropriately termed partial development or variations of normal. A further classification designates isosexual precocity (early pubertal development appropriate for sex) and contrasexual or heterosexual precocity (early development inappropriate for sex or appropriate for opposite sex). Such terminology has become cumbersome. Use of feminization among males and masculinization in females should adequately designate those conditions known as contrasexual puberty.

B. Girls

1. Gonadotropin-Dependent (Central) Precocious Puberty

Central precocious puberty (CPP) is diagnosed if physical pubertal changes and laboratory results are consistent with progressive changes of normal puberty. The majority of girls presenting with precocious puberty have the central form, with underlying neurological abnormalities being unusual.

    a. Causes. Central precocious puberty may not be associated with anatomically demonstrable CNS abnormalities that apparently disrupt the restraint typical of childhood. Associated CNS abnormalities in girls are listed in Table 2. Patients surviving CNS tumor involvement who have received radiation and chemotherapy may show central precocious puberty. Precocious puberty is a well-recognized phenomenon among children emigrating from developing countries both in eastern Europe and Asia to western countries. Improved nutrition, environmental stability and psychological support lead to dramatic catch-up growth, weight gain and central precocious puberty. Loss of height potential may be excessive (30, 31). Among patients is a subset who did not have growth retardation at adoption, leading to the hypothesis that early puberty may be a consequence of exposure to estrogenic endocrine disrupters (32).

GnRH-secreting hypothalamic hamartomas contain apparently redundant CNS tissue containing GnRH neurons that function independently of CNS inhibitory influences, an ectopic hypothalamus episodically secreting GnRH (33). The loss of such episodic release after complete removal of a pedunculated hamartoma was early evidence that the pulse generator itself resides within the network of communicating GnRH secreting neurons. Hamartomas, present with CPP at very young ages, more frequently among boys than girls.

b. Hormonal Documentation. Hormone levels and responses consistent with gonadarche principally include basal and GnRH- or GnRH analog stimulated gonadotropin levels within the pubertal range; LH responses increase to a greater degree than FSH with pubertal onset and are hence more useful in diagnosing central precocious puberty. The difference in FSH between prepubertal and pubertal children may be undetectable.

2. Gonadotropin-Independent (Peripheral) Precocious Puberty

Precocious pseudopuberty, defined as early puberty resulting from any other mechanism other than hypotha-

lamic GnRH–pituitary LH and FSH-stimulated gonadal activity, in girls results from excessive estrogen stimulation for age from ovarian, adrenal cortical, or exogenous source. Among girls, this form of precocious puberty is rare (Table 2).

a. McCune-Albright Syndrome. The McCune-Albright syndrome, which occurs in girls far more frequently than boys, includes a unique form of peripheral precocious puberty in which an activating missense mutation occurs in the gene for the alpha subunit of G_s, the G protein that stimulates cyclic adenosine monophosphate formation (34). Abnormalities in this syndrome consist of multicentered localized osseous lesions called polycystic fibrous dysplasia, melanotic cutaneous macules called cafe-au-lait spots, and one or more endocrinopathies. These include precocious puberty (Fig. 3), hyperthyroidism, hyperadrenocorticism, pituitary gigantism or acromegaly, and hypophosphatemia. The mutation has been found in variable abundance in affected tissues, a finding consistent with a mosaic distribution of aberrant cells from a somatic cell mutation (34) and also compatible with variable expression and exacerbations and remissions of disease activity characteristic of this syndrome. Mechanisms usually stimulated by the trophic hormones are activated as a result of this mutation; female patients with

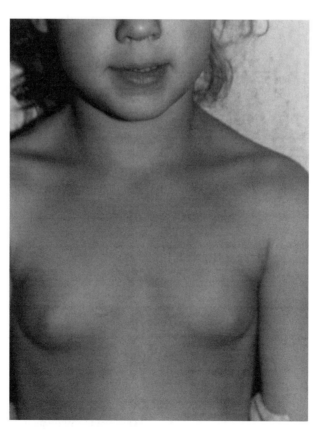

Figure 3   Premature breast development (stage 3) in a 4-year-old girl with McCune-Albright syndrome.

sexual precocity secrete increased ovarian estrogen without gonadotropin stimulation. Mean ovarian volume is increased and ovaries are asymmetrical, primarily as consequences of large ovarian cysts (35). Levels of estrogen fluctuate, with spontaneous regression occurring.

Because ovarian estrogen secretion in patients with the McCune-Albright syndrome is not gonadotropin-driven, such secretion is not suppressed by GnRH analog therapy. Thus, therapy to diminish estrogen secretion or action is indicated (see section on therapy, below).

As with other entities of peripheral precocious puberty, skeletal age and biological maturity become advanced and, eventually, mature hypothalamic–pituitary control of ovarian function commences, even at an early age (secondary central precocious puberty) (36).

After hypothalamic–pituitary maturation, ovarian function is under the usual control mechanisms and GnRH analogs may have a place in therapy for early puberty. Eventually these patients ovulate and true menstrual cycling and pregnancy may occur, in spite of persistent autonomous ovarian activity (37).

b. Ovarian Cysts. Ovarian cysts, readily identified by sonography, may occur with central precocious puberty, as part of normal ovarian development of childhood (38), secondary to intermittent unsustained gonadotropin stimulation and in the McCune-Albright syndrome. An isolated follicular cyst may be present with apparent autonomous estrogen production, presenting as peripheral precocious puberty. Such cysts are usually self-limiting; estrogen levels fall as the cyst spontaneously regresses. A drop in estrogen levels may be accompanied by withdrawal bleeding. Initial treatment of an isolated follicular cyst should be conservative, with careful monitoring and without surgical intervention, unless a surgical emergency such as torsion is likely. Follow-up sonography and measurement of estrogen levels after 1–4 months usually show regression.

c. Chronic Primary Hypothyroidism. Although hypothyroidism is usually accompanied by growth, skeletal, and pubertal delay, in rare cases patients with thyroid gland failure and elevated TSH levels have evidence of advanced pubertal development. The mechanism is likely related to excessive trophic hormone or alpha subunit secretion An excessive secretion of the alpha subunit accompanies the TSH hypersecretion. In such large quantities, TSH or the alpha subunit may compete for and activate gonadotropin receptors (39). Patients present with breast development that may be accompanied by galactorrhea. Marked pituitary enlargement may occur in this syndrome (40). Appropriate thyroid replacement therapy results in normalization of pituitary hormone levels. Pubertal changes regress and no other therapy is necessary.

d. Tumors. Estrogen-secreting tumors of the ovaries and adrenal cortex are rare. They present typically with markedly elevated estrogen levels, rapidly progressing pubertal changes and asymmetry and unilateral en-

largement of the ovarian or adrenal glands. Androgen excess and androgen stimulated changes may also be present.

3. Diagnostic Evaluation

The approach to the assessment of the girl with early pubertal development is outlined in Table 3.

a. History and Physical Findings. A complete history should emphasize the points noted in Table with careful consideration of any possible exposure to exogenous hormone, previous or current CNS abnormalities or symptoms, pubertal history of other family members, and height and growth rates. Gelastic seizures may occur in association with organic causes of central precocious puberty, including hypothalamic hamartomas.

Physical examination should include height, weight, span, upper/lower body segment ratio, skin, hair, thyroid, neurological findings, breast and pubic hair staging, inspection of the genitalia to determine pubertal maturation, and visualization of the vaginal mucosa.

Visual inspection, without palpation, to assess estrogen effect upon the vaginal mucosa should avoid traumatizing the patient. If the patient is positioned prone with knees drawn up and legs spread, the introitus can be visualized without touching the vulva but by gently spreading the labia. A glistening red appearance is consistent with a thin, non-estrogen-stimulated mucosa, whereas a pink mucosa with a mucous covering is indicative of a thicker more cornified mucosa; mucous secretion is suggestive of concomitant estrogen stimulation. However, irritation or infection can also result in the latter appearance. A bimanual abdominal–rectal examination should be avoided unless an abdominal pelvic ultrasound study is inadequate.

b. Hormonal Testing. A plasma estradiol measurement using a sensitive assay and GnRH or GnRH analog stimulation testing is indicated. Gonadotropin responses are pubertal with CPP. The LH response is more helpful than FSH in demonstrating a characteristic pubertal pattern; patients with peripheral precocious puberty (PPP) have a prepubertal or suppressed response. Figure 4 shows the range of responses of 12 prepubertal girls. Most pubertal patients do not have an FSH response outside the prepubertal range; hence FSH responses are seldom discriminatory. Low responses of both LH and FSH, which are normal for prepubertal individuals, cannot be differentiated from a suppressed response found in patients with some forms of PPP.

Prepubertal higher baseline and stimulated FSH levels are greater than LH responses, and pubertal basal and response levels are greater for LH than FSH. Ratios of LH to FSH less than 1.0 are consistent with a prepubertal status while ratios greater than 1.0 suggest a pubertal state (12).

Other laboratory testing may involve thyroid function tests including TSH to rule out primary hypothyroidism,

Table 3 Criteria to Plan Diagnostic Evaluation of Premature Pubertal Development

	Girls	Both sexes	Boys
A Clinical findings of precocious puberty	Breast development Genital maturation Accelerated linear growth ±Sexual hair ±Menstruation		Genital development with testicular growth Sexual hair Accelerated linear growth Increased muscle mass
		Assess the following depending upon particular situation: **History** Exposure to exogenous hormones CNS trauma, anomalies, or infection CNS symptoms Familial history of age of pubertal onset Growth pattern and rates **Physical examination**	Familial forms usually involve males

	Tanner breast and pubic hair stage
	Clitoral size
	Rectal-abdominal bimanual examination
	Inspect for galactorrhea, estrogenized vaginal mucosa
		Pubertal maturational staging (Tanner)
		Body proportions (upper/lower segment ratios)
		Body and skeletal symmetry
		Acne and skin pigmentation
		Fundoscopic and visual field examinations
		Thyroid examination
		Evidence of thyroid dysfunction
		Neurologic examination
		Laboratory evaluation
		Serum or plasma assessment
			Tanner genital size and pubic hair stages
			Penis size
			  Stretched length
			  Description of width
			Testicular examination
			  Size: long axis or volume
			  Symmetry
			  Consistency

	Estradiol	LH, FSH Thyroid function tests DHEA or DHEAS	Testosterone hCG
	Increased LH response	GnRH stimulation **Radiologic assessment** Skeletal age MRI of hypothalamic region (if "peripheral" causes excluded)	Increased LH and FSH rise
	Abdominal-pelvic sonography		Testicular sonography
		Other	
	Vaginal cytology		Morning void for sperm
		History	
B Clinical findings of premature thelarche	Breast development without growth acceleration or other pubertal findings	Exposure to gonadotropins or estrogen Growth pattern **Physical examination:** thorough examination (see earlier) **Laboratory examination** Serum LH, FSH, estradiol Skeletal age x-ray Pelvic sonography	(see Table 4 for contrasexual development)

Table 3 Continued

	Girls	Both sexes	Boys
		Follow-up Reassess growth rate, pubertal progression after 2–6 months Repeat sonography if follicular cysts **History** Exposure to androgens Growth pattern	
C Clinical findings of adrenarche	Sexual hair (pubic or axillary) without growth acceleration or other pubertal changes (Table 4)	**Physical examination** **Laboratory examination** Plasma DHA or DHAS Skeletal age x-ray **Follow-up:** reassess growth rate and pubertal progression in 3–6 months	

plasma DHEAS levels to determine if adrenarche has occurred, and DHEA or androstenedione if excessive adrenal androgen secretion is suspected. In menarcheal patients, a progesterone level may document luteal phase and verify ovulation.

c. Other Testing. A skeletal maturity (bone age) roentgenogram should be obtained to estimate the extent of excessive stimulation and remaining growth potential (41). Pelvic sonography should be done in all patients to determine if ovarian and uterine size is enlarged for age, but appropriate for stage of puberty (consistent with CPP); unilateral or asymmetrical ovarian enlargement may be indicative of a tumor or cysts. All young girls (less than 5 years) with central precocious puberty in whom the cause is not already explained should undergo MRI of the CNS, particularly the hypothalamic region, to investigate lesions (Table 2) even if the neurological examination is normal. Lesions are rarely demonstrated among girls older than 6 years so the need for such a study should be determined individually. An electroencephalogram (EEG) is not generally indicated, even though abnormalities have been reported in cases of central precocious puberty.

C. Boys

1. Gonadotropin-Dependent (Central) Precocious Puberty

a. Causes. Causes of early pubertal development among boys are outlined in Table 2. A larger portion of boys than girls with CPP have CNS lesions than have the idiopathic variety. Therefore, assessment of boys with early unexplained puberty, regardless of age, should include an MRI. The CNS disorders include hamartomas (Fig. 5), subarachnoid cysts, glial cell tumors, and germ cell tumors. CPP occurs consistently in patients with hypothalamic hamartomas and subarachnoid cysts, and in about two-thirds of those with germ cell tumors but only a minority of children with glial cell tumors (42). Rarely astrocytomas and craniopharyngiomas are associated with CPP. Treatment of these lesions is the same, whether or not CPP occurs. Since hamartomas are congenital malformations rather than tumors and rarely have neurological consequences, therapy is directed at the CPP. Medical therapy is indicated except in those rare situations in which the lesion is pedunculated, making surgical removal a treatment option.

As among girls, central precocity occurs as a consequence of CNS radiation therapy, with or without chemotherapy, among patients with cancer. This sequela may occur with growth hormone deficiency, hence without growth acceleration. Other CNS-related causes include trauma, surgery, inflammation, and severe neurological–mental deficits of congenital or acquired origin. Precocity related to hydrocephalus, brain abscesses, or granulomas may be related to pressure changes and, in some instances, is reversible when pressure is decreased.

In children of either gender, secondary central precocity may develop secondary to prolonged sex steroid exposure associated with peripheral precocious puberty. Boys may develop central precocious puberty as a consequence of a prolonged hyperandrogenic state, as in undiagnosed or inadequately treated congenital virilizing adrenal hyperplasia. Patients with known peripheral precocious puberty present with evidence of pubertal maturation of the hypothalamic–pituitary axis including a pubertal response to GnRH or GnRHa stimulation. Secondary CPP tends to occur among patients with advanced biological maturation, as evidenced by bone age matura-

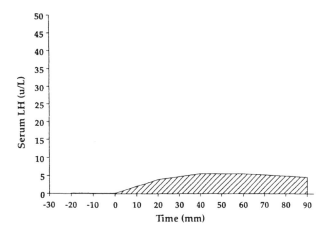

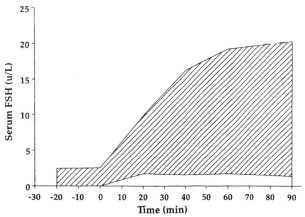

Figure 4 Range of serum LH and FSH responses to GnRH stimulation in 12 pubertal girls shows the wide variation in response, especially FSH. Actual units vary depending upon the gonadotropin assay used, but pubertal individuals have an LH response greater than the prepubertal response, although the rise of the FSH response cannot be expected to be greater. The initial rise in FSH may be more brisk, so that values within the first 40 min may be somewhat greater than the prepubertal range, and maximum incremental rise does not differ. Therefore, to verify central precocious puberty, a rise in LH above the prepubertal range should be demonstrated.

tion advanced to or beyond 12 years among boys or 10 years in girls.

b. Physical and Laboratory Findings. Central precocity in boys is characterized not only by pubertal testosterone levels and basal and GnRH- or GnRHa-stimulated gonadotropin levels (LH > FSH), but also full physical pubertal development. Testicular growth is symmetrical characteristic of gonadotropin stimulation, and hence is found in CPP and unique forms of gonadotropin-independent precocious puberty, which are a consequence of an activating LH-receptor mutation, but not in other forms of PPP.

3. Gonadotropin-Independent (Peripheral) Precocious Puberty

Precocity in boys also results from inappropriate androgen stimulation from either endogenous or exogenous sources, nonpituitary gonadotropin stimulation, and rare activating mutations.

a. Virilizing Adrenal Hyperplasia. A common cause of peripheral precocious puberty in boys is endogenous androgen excess in undiagnosed or inadequately treated congenital adrenal hyperplasia (CAH) caused by 21-hydroxylase deficiency. Fortunately, with neonatal screening for this form of CAH, many boys are being diagnosed now before developing early pubertal changes. Other rare forms of virilizing adrenal hyperplasia, 11β-hydroxylase deficiency and 3β-hydroxysteroid dehydrogenase deficiency, may present in a similar manner.

b. Familial Male-Limited Gonadotropin-Independent Puberty (GIP). A unique entity of male-limited gonadotropin-independent precocious puberty occurs in which gonadal steroidogenesis and spermatogenesis proceed, even though gonadotropin stimulation is age-appropriately low or suppressed, as a consequence of activating mutations of the LH receptor (43). Since these mutations are inherited in a dominant pattern, the child's father may have a history of precocious puberty. Onset is usually but not always at a very young age. The physical findings of boys with this disorder are full pubertal development, including bilateral testicular growth, similar to that of boys with central precocious puberty. Gonadotropin baseline levels and responses to exogenous GnRH are consistent with prepuberty or suppression, while testosterone is elevated and often within the adult male range.

The activating mutations of the LH receptor result in G-protein activation and increased cyclic AMP production with Leydig-cell testosterone secretion. These mutations do not cause precocious puberty or other abnormality among girls, since FSH receptor activation, in addition to LH, is necessary for ovarian steroidogenesis.

Among boys, genital enlargement, including bilateral testicular growth and skeletal age acceleration, are the primary presenting features, usually by age 3 years. Spermatogenesis sufficient to produce mature forms and considerable seminiferous tubular growth occurs. Eventually, a pubertal hypothalamic–pituitary–testicular axis can be demonstrated among affected boys, with normal fertility. Adult height may be compromised. This form of peripheral precocious puberty is commonly followed by central precocity, since there is not adequate therapy to fully suppress androgen production. After maturation of the hypothalamic–pituitary axis has occurred, GnRH analog treatment will result in suppression of LH and FSH response to exogenous GnRH, but testosterone levels will not be full suppressed.

A unique form of gonadotropin-independent precocious puberty has been found to be associated with pri-

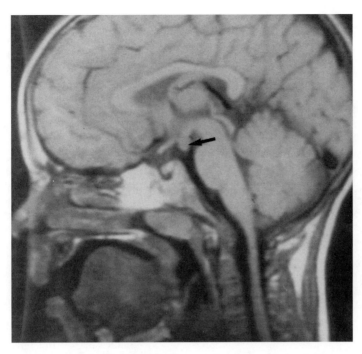

Figure 5   A hypothalamic hamartoma associated with episodic gonadotropin-releasing hormone secretion in a young boy with central precocious puberty. The arrow points to the harmartoma.

mary adrenal insufficiency and a mutation in the DAXI gene (44).

   c. Chronic Primary Hypothyroidism.   Rarely prepubertal-aged boys with chronic primary hypothyroidism present with testicular enlargement. It is most likely the result of occupation of the FSH receptors in the testes by TSH, when TSH occurs in such supraphysiological quantities (39). Hyperprolactemia is present and galactorrhea occurs. Prolactin levels fall and testicular size decreases when TSH levels are suppressed with thyroid replacement therapy.

   d. Androgen-Secreting Tumors.   Testosterone-secreting Leydig-cell tumors are associated with dramatic somatic and genital growth with muscular development. Typical presentation includes rapid onset with unilateral testicular enlargement. Adrenocortical androgen-secreting tumors are rare, are often accompanied by physical and hormonal evidence of other adrenal cortical hormonal excess, and present with prepubertal-sized testes. Hormonal profiles suggest autonomous secretion.

   e. Chorionic Gonadotropins Secreting Tumors.   In rare cases Leydig-cell testosterone secretion as a consequence of abnormal gonadotropins stimulation causes PPP. This occurs in settings that include chorionic gonadotropin-secreting tumors, such as teratomas, embryonal tumors, hepatoblastomas, and CNS germinomas. Often the primary tumor is highly malignant.

3.   Assessment

The evaluation of boys with early puberty should be guided by pertinent aspects of the history, physical ex-

amination, and laboratory assessment outlined in Table 3. A history of growth patterns and pubertal progression can provide clues to cause. Tanner staging and testicular symmetry and volume should be verified. Generally, prepubertal-sized testes (less than 2.0 cm in the longitudinal axis) suggest a cause other than pubertal hypothalamic–pituitary gonadotropin function; pubertal-sized testes (longer than 2.5 cm) suggest central precocious puberty (Fig. 6). Asymmetrical or unilateral enlargement suggests a Leydig-cell tumor or hyperplasia adrenal rest tissue. The latter is seen in inadequately treated CAH and may also be bilateral.

   Gonadotropin response to GnRH or GnRHa stimulation should be documented, with particular attention to whether the LH response is above the prepubertal range, noting the LH:FSH ratio (<1 suggests prepubertal secretion). Testosterone levels above the prepubertal range verify the early pubertal status but do not differentiate the source. Skeletal age documents the extent of advanced maturity and can be used to estimate remaining growth potential. Because of the high incidence of CNS lesions in male sexual precocity, MRI or CT scans should be done unless the cause is otherwise explained.

D.   Natural History

The natural history of gonadotropin-dependent (central) precocious puberty is outlined in Figure 7. All phases of pubertal development are precocious including spermatogenesis, premature pubertal growth, and skeletal age acceleration. Depending upon the rate of progression, early

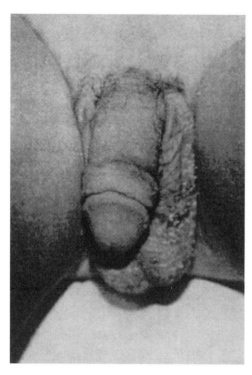

Figure 6 Genitalia of a 25-month-old boy with sexual precocity associated with a hypothalamic hamartoma. Tanner stage 2 pubic hair, Tanner stage 3 genital development, and enlarged testes for age are evident.

skeletal maturity. With a premature growth spurt and skeletal maturation, children with precocity are tall for age during childhood. However, if their skeletal maturity becomes disproportionately advanced for their concomitant growth rate, their projected adult height diminishes, becoming less than expected based upon familial heights (Figure 8). In most situations, the adult height deficit is only a few centimeters (41). With rapidly progressive precocious puberty characterized by skeletal age disproportionately advanced for height, without treatment growth is completed at a younger age and shorter height than if puberty and the pubertal growth spurt had occurred during the usual years. Therefore, the indications for treatment of progressive central precocious puberty are to stop or cause regression of pubertal characteristics and to preclude or reclaim loss of height potential.

Tall stature, advanced pubertal development, and menarche during childhood may cause social and psychological adjustment problems. Psychosocial concerns are an indication for counseling and consideration of medical treatment to suppress excessive growth rate and pubertal advancement.

Whether or not the precocity will be treated medically, the patient and parents need to understand what is happening. If puberty is idiopathic, they should understand that normal things are happening, but at an early age. An explanation, geared to the child's ability to understand is usually satisfactory: that it is normal for the body of a child to change into the body of an adult, but sometimes it starts too soon and happens too fast. The discussion with the patient, often with the parent present, should include age-appropriate sex education. Psychosexual development is generally commensurate with age not physical maturity, hence, inappropriate sexual behavior is seldom a problem. In contrast to being sexually aggressive, patients may be naive and misinterpret sexual advances by older individuals. Both girls and boys are potential victims of sexual encounters with older persons

pubertal development leads to premature attainment of adult height, as well as sexual and reproductive capabilities. The rate of development is determined by the magnitude of androgen secretion, with persistent high levels resulting in the greatest acceleration of changes. Very early or rapidly progressive precocious puberty leads to diminished total height increase for amount of advance of

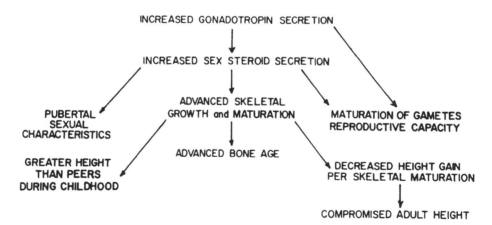

Figure 7 Schematic representation of the natural history of early pubertal development. (Used by permission, Year Book Medical Publishers.)

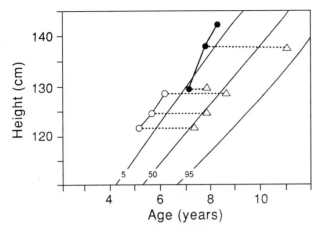

Figure 8 Growth chart for girls shows percentile of height for age. The solid circles represent height for age for a girl presenting with central precocious puberty; the connected triangles depict height for bone age. Note that although growth rate is accelerated, bone age has accelerated considerably more in the same time period, resulting in decrease in projected adult height. In contrast, the patient whose heights are depicted (open circles) with Tanner stage 2 breast and pubic hair development did not have an acceleration in growth rate or bone maturity. Although she was tall for age with early pubertal development, she did not have a decreased adult height potential.

who would take advantage of their childlike concept of, and vulnerability to, intimacy. Once children recognize that they are more mature, they tend to avoid incidents of childhood sex play. Children with early puberty share interests with age peers. Even though boys experience frequent erections and masturbation, and may have the capacity for ejaculation, they are not an increased threat of potential sexual aggression. Children of both sexes become potentially fertile.

III. THERAPY

If there is an underlying treatable cause resulting in early puberty, therapy should be given. Examples include surgery and radiation or chemotherapy for CNS, ectopic gonadotropin-producing, gonadal, or adrenal tumors. Adrenal suppression is indicated in CAH, thyroid replacement in primary hypothyroidism, and cessation of administration for inappropriate steroid or gonadotropin treatments in those instances. If the underlying treatment is completely successful and central pubertal maturation has not occurred, progression of pubertal development should cease, and some regression may follow. In patients with autonomous gonadal steroid production, such as in McCune-Albright syndrome or male familial gonadotropin-independent puberty, therapy is aimed at reducing sex steroid production or effect. Drugs that have been tried

included initially medroxyprogesterone and spironolactone, and, more recently, steroid synthesis inhibitors, (ketoconazole) aromatase inhibitors (testolactone and anastrozole), and the estrogen-receptor antagonist (tamoxifen) (45–49). None of these completely suppress the sex steroid effect in a sustained fashion, and in both of the situations secondary precocious puberty is not unexpected (50). When this occurs, GnRHa therapy can be begun in addition to other therapy in an attempt to retard pubertal development and growth as much as possible. Patients so treated should be carefully monitored for pubertal development, growth rates and skeletal age, sex steroid levels, and side-effects of the agent(s) used.

A. Criteria

Among patients with central precocious puberty, idiopathic or otherwise, marked by a pubertal pattern of gonadotropin response to GnRH or GnRHa stimulation, gonadotropin production can be halted with adequate dosages of GnRH analog (51). The decision for or against treatment should be a joint decision with the parents, with consideration given to all aspects of the child's physical and mental maturity (52). Therapy should not be considered unless the following criteria have been documented: (a) a pubertal response to GnRH or GnPHa stimulation testing or some other documentation of pubertal gonadotropin secretion (basal plasma or urinary levels clearly above the prepubertal range), (b) a sustained accelerated linear growth rate, (c) an accelerated advancement of skeletal age, and (d) physical changes consistent with progressive pubertal development. Even if these criteria are met, therapy may not be chosen unless the child is developing at a rate clearly outside the range for age; the skeletal age maturity rate has exceeded the growth rate so that adult height is becoming compromised; and the parents and child perceive a need to delay further pubertal growth and development.

If therapy is indicated to stop the progression of puberty or menses and to preclude or attempt to reclaim compromised growth potential, GnRH analog therapy is the only effective treatment. The pharmacological basis is the suppression of episodic secretion of gonadotropins by overriding the episodic release of GnRH with continued high levels of GnRH analog. After an initial LH and FSH release in response to GnRH analog, the long-term effect of persistent adequate dosing is downregulation of responsiveness; GnRH receptor numbers decrease, and gonadotropin responses are essentially obliterated. The result of such treatment is first a fall in circulating gonadotropins, followed by a return of sex steroids to prepubertal levels. Adequacy of suppression should be monitored by the demonstration of the lack of gonadotropin response to exogenous GnRH stimulation. With adequate dosing, suppression is demonstrable within the first 8 weeks of therapy.

B. Institution

GnRH analogs are available as depot injection, short-acting injection, and nasal spray. Dosing adequacy and effectiveness can be monitored by lack of progression of clinical indices and results of hormonal testing, including GnRH or GnRHa stimulation. In boys a fall in plasma testosterone levels to a prepubertal range is indicative of adequate dosage. In girls estradiol levels are less helpful because of fluctuating and low levels present in the pubertal state. When suppression is not achieved, the dosage should be increased. Once suppression is verified, patients can be monitored at 4–6 month intervals with GnRH testing, and with skeletal age monitoring at least annually.

C. Monitoring Therapy

Hormonal suppression with GnRH analog treatment results in a deceleration of the puberty growth rate and a cessation of pubertal development.

1. Pubertal Development and Growth Rates

In girls, breasts may regress, vaginal mucosa becomes nonestrogenized, and menses cease. There may be an episode of withdrawal bleeding during the institution of suppression. This can be expected if an endometrial stripe is discernible by ultrasonography before therapy.

In boys, genital, including testicular, growth ceases and regression may occur. Further diminishing of projected adult height should not occur; it may increase among those with compromised predictions before beginning therapy.

Since GnRHa does not influence adrenal androgen secretion, if adrenarche has occurred, it progresses during treatment (53). With sufficient and increasing levels of adrenal androgen, sexual hair will be maintained and progress. This should not be interpreted as evidence of lack of gonadal suppression, although documentation of pubertal levels of adrenal androgens can be used as verification.

Growth rates return to a prepubertal growth rate, although rates may become subnormal, particularly among those with very advanced skeletal ages.

2. Skeletal Maturity

The stimulus for accelerated skeletal maturity is removed once sex steroid levels are suppressed. However, there is a clear lag since the steroid effect upon bone maturity is delayed. Therefore, it is not uncommon not to document deceleration during the first 6 months on therapy. Thereafter, skeletal maturity should slow to normal until the skeletal age is consistent with the age of puberty. Thus, if the bone age is 7.5 years after the first 6 months, it can be expected to be 8.5 years a year later. This progression of a year per year is expected to continue until skeletal age reaches the years of puberty. From this point on, the skeletal age progresses very slowly without sex steroids.

Bone age x-rays with concomitant heights can be used to estimate growth potential and hence predict adult height. During therapy, usually the growth potential gradually increases unless skeletal age was not excessive for height at the onset of therapy.

3. Ancillary Tests

Monitoring of ovarian ultrasound and bone density is not typically indicated. Ovarian and uterine volume both diminish. Bone mineral density can be expected to remain relatively constant. Since density is greater than expected for age, lack of increase in bone density during the hiatus of therapy is not considered detrimental.

4. Additional Medical Therapy

Growth hormone has been used as supplemental therapy among patients who have lost considerable height potential, grown at subnormal rates on GnRHa therapy, still have growth potential, and have evidence of inadequate growth hormone. It is expensive, and even though adult height may be enhanced, it should be used only after careful consideration. Also, since estrogen is the primary hormone stimulating skeletal maturity, the use of drugs that block estrogen synthesis (aromatase inhibitors) or action (estrogen receptor blockers) are being considered for use in CPP. No trials using such therapy have been completed.

D. Discontinuation of Therapy

1. Decision to Discontinue

The age at which to discontinue therapy must be individualized. Characteristically, therapy is discontinued when the child reaches the age when puberty typically is occurring, assuming the child is psychologically prepared. When predicted height is still less than target height, therapy may be continued in an attempt to gain greater height. However, as discussed below, the gain in growth potential diminishes with advancing age and skeletal age, largely because of waning growth rates.

2. Recovery of Hormonal Secretion After Discontinuation

Resumption of pubertal hypothalamic–pituitary–gonadal activity begins promptly, becoming complete within weeks or months (54). LH and FSH responses to GnRH are pubertal within 6 months. Attainment of pubertal milestones including attainment of Tanner stages proceeds at a rate similar to that during normal puberty. Testicular or ovarian volume (55) increase concomitantly. Menses among girls who were postmenarchal before therapy occurs within 12 months. Among premenarchal patients, most experience menarche within 18 months, but among some it may take up to 4.5 years. Ovulatory cycling begins and menstrual regularity is similar to that among other similarly aged girls (56). Among boys, spermatogenesis resumes and normalizes for stage of development.

Outcome data for boys indicate normal postpubertal status (29), including these with hypothalamic hamartomas (57).

E. Long-Term Outcome Data

1. Fertility

Although not yet well documented, both pregnancy with birth of normal infants and normal spermatogenesis have been demonstrated.

2. Growth After Discontinuation of Therapy

Particularly among girls, growth rates and total growth after therapy have uniformly been less than projected based upon height and skeletal age at discontinuation. There is little or no growth spurt among girls, even among those who begin therapy early.

Adult heights after ideal therapy are not yet available, while the results from patients whose treatment was begun late indicate height less than the range of target height. However, those who were well treated generally reach the range but not mean of target height. Overall, adult heights are greater than among untreated patients (58) and the predicted at the onset of therapy (59–63), less that predicted at the end of therapy (60, 63). Changes in height prediction during therapy are directly related to skeletal age at onset of therapy (61). Adult heights are often less than target height (59–62) and below the mean adult height for sex. Improvement of height is greatest among those with early onset of precocity as well as early onset of therapy (before ages 5–6 years) (59, 60, 62, 64).

3. Hyperandrogenism

With the withdrawal of gonadotropin and estrogen during GnRHa therapy, it would not be unexpected if ovarian cysts develop secondary to interruption of the stimuli for follicle growth. However, it has not been verified that a greater portion of patients who were treated with GnRHa have an increased incidence of ovarian cysts or hyperandrogenism. Some girls who were diagnosed with CPP and treated with GnRHa have subsequently been found to have hyperandrogenism (65), but there is no evidence that this is related to GnRHa therapy. However, it is important to verify any evidence of androgen excess at presentation, particularly among patients who present with sexual hair and other androgen-stimulated effects, in addition to estrogen-stimulated effects. Early androgen effect has been associated with later ovarian hyperandrogenism (66).

IV. PARTIAL PUBERTAL DEVELOPMENT: VARIANTS OF NORMAL

A. Premature Thelarche: Girls

Traditionally, premature thelarche (isolated premature breast development) has been diagnosed during two age periods. Significant breast tissue is most commonly noted during the first two years of life. In most instances, the history suggests that this is a persistence or increase of the palpable breast tissue present at birth caused by a persistence of infant gonadotropin secretion. Since ovarian hormone production is greater during infancy than later childhood, breast development may persist or growth may occur as a consequence. Such development almost always regresses before 24 months of age.

The second period when isolated breast growth has long been noted is after age 6 years. As in normal puberty, when breast development is first noticed it may be asymmetrical or unilateral. This may account for the small percentage of children found to have Tanner stage 2 breast development reported in the large population surveys (14, 15), as well as those girls who have been reported to have nonprogressive precocious puberty (27, 52). This development may be a consequence of temporarily increased ovarian steroid secretion, highly sensitive estrogen receptors to low pubertal circulating estrogen levels, or both.

In any instance in which breast development at presentation is not accompanied by other evidence of puberty, careful monitoring of development over subsequent months is mandatory but only a limited assessment is indicated (see Table 3). Some patients may have early menarche, but adult height is not compromised (67). Estrogen levels, height, and bone age may be normal or slightly advanced for age. Rarely, an ovarian follicular cyst, which does not persist, may be identified. Since this condition is benign and may regress, treatment can be limited to education and counseling. However, because there may be episodes of greater gonadotropin secretion during childhood in girls, it may be difficult to ascertain where a given patient lies along the continuum from premature thelarche and central precocity (3, 5, 12). It has been reported that 14% of one group of 100 girls originally presenting with premature thelarche progressed to central precocious puberty (68). Occasionally, what initially appears to be isolated breast development may actually be the first sign of what will eventually become manifest central precocity. However, more commonly there is minimal progression until the usual age of onset of puberty. Without hormonal evidence of pubertal onset, it is inappropriate to interpret Tanner stage 2 breast development as the onset of either normal puberty or as a diagnosis of precocious puberty. The greater proportion of 5-, 6- and 7-year-old girls reported to have pubertal onset in the general population, the entity of nonprogressive precocious puberty, and premature thelarche may all be part of the same clinical entity.

B. Premature Pubarche

Premature pubarche, the early development of sexual hair, is normally the result of premature adrenarche, defined as an early onset of the pubertal increase of adrenal androgen production. Adrenarche usually precedes and is independent at gonadarche, is not accompanied by a mature response to GnRH stimulation, nor is it suppressed with GnRH analog therapy. Premature pubarche is more common in girls than boys and is rare before 6 years of age except in African-American girls. The early pubic hair may be an isolated finding or be accompanied by mild acne, oily skin, onset of adult-type body odor, and axillary hair. If there are no other associated findings or pathological conditions, minimal assessment including measurement of androgen levels to verify that levels are not greater than those consistent with early adrenarche is required (Table 3). Documentation of the status of adrenarche is indicated by demonstrating that circulating levels of DHEA, DHEAS, or androstenedione are within the range of early adrenarche and above the prepubertal range. Height and skeletal age may be normal or transiently advanced (69). Growth and subsequent pubertal development should be expected to occur normally. The degree of advancement should be followed: abnormal progression, excessive virilization, or elevated DHEA and DHEAS levels may indicate pathological causes of excessive androgen. Also, there is evidence that early onset of androgen production may be the first evidence of ovarian hyperandrogenism (70). If so, the mechanism would likely involve not only a defect of control of androgen production, but also involve both the adrenal glands and the ovaries.

V. INAPPROPRIATE SEX-STEROID-STIMULATED CHANGES FOR SEX

Contrasexual (in contrast to isosexual) pubertal development, whether during childhood or puberty, is defined the development of sexual characteristics inappropriate for the sex of the individual (i.e., feminization among boys and virilization among girls). Causes among girls include the differential of androgen excess and for boys that of estrogen excess.

A. Girls

Although premature development of sexual hair (premature pubarche) in girls is not uncommon, excessive virilization of the prepubertal girl is rare and may present with the development of oily skin, acne, clitoromegaly, and hirsutism. Causes are listed in Table 4. The degree of virilization is generally greatest with adrenal and ovarian tumors and less with adrenal hyperplasia. The mildest forms of adrenal hyperplasia may present as premature adrenarche, being diagnosed only after adrenocorticotropic hormone (ACTH) stimulation testing or DNA analysis. Assessment is indicated with significantly advanced skeletal age, growth rate, or degree of virilization. The virilizing adrenal hyperplasias include 21-hydroxylase deficiency, 11β-hydroxylase deficiency, and 3β-hydroxysteroid dehydrogenase deficiency. These usually present with virilization before puberty; mild forms may present at puberty.

Table 4 Causes of Contrasexual Pubertal Development, Prepubertal or Pubertal Onset

Virilization in girls
    Adrenal sources of androgen excess: adenoma, carcinoma, virilizing adrenal hyperplasia
    Exogenous androgen
    Idiopathic hirsutism
    Ovarian sources of androgen excess: arrhenoblastoma, teratoma, polycystic ovarian syndrome
Feminization in boys
    Adolescent, pubertal, or idiopathic gynecomastia
    Drugs (amphetamines, antineoplastics, gonadotropin, isoniazid, ketoconazole, marijuana, sex steroids, tricyclic antidepressants, others)
    Neoplasms (adrenal or testicular steroid-producing tumors, teratomas)
    Primary hypogonadal conditions
        Congenital (anorchia, dysgenetic testes, enzyme biosynthetic defects, Klinefelter syndrome, partial androgen insensitivity syndrome)
        Acquired (cryptorchidism, infection, radiation, torsion, trauma)
    Systematic illness: hepatic, renal, recovery from malnutrition

Most verified mild forms of adrenal hyperplasia are 21-hydroxylase deficiency. Basal 17-hydroxyprogesterone levels may be elevated with 21-hydroxylase deficiency adrenal hyperplasia, while corticotropin (ACTH) stimulated values may be needed to ascertain the mildest cases. Such testing with measurement of adrenal steroid intermediate metabolites may be useful in identifying mild forms of adrenal hyperplasia (71). Adrenal suppression may be necessary to differentiate adrenal hyperplasia from adrenal tumors or ovarian sources. The polycystic ovarian syndrome is a heterogenous disorder presenting with hyperandrogenism, hirsutism, and amenorrhea or oligomenorrhea.

B. Boys

Gynecomastia, either unilateral or bilateral, in a pubertal boy is usually a variation of normal puberty. The most common pathological cause of gynecomastia is hypogonadism, particularly Klinefelter syndrome. Gynecomastia caused by abnormal estrogen production because of increased steroid aromatization (72) (Table 4) is rare, but it should be ruled out in a prepubertal boy, or at any age, when the degree or progression is troublesome. Plasma estrogen levels or total urinary estrogen levels are elevated if there is a persistent source of abnormal endogenous estrogen. Appropriate plasma and urinary levels, an otherwise normal history and physical examination, and a negative history of contact with estrogen-containing medicine or cosmetics is sufficient to delay further work-up with follow-up to watch for progression of gynecomastia. It may be difficult to ascertain gynecomastia from pseudogynecomastia in an overweight boy. The presence of a discernible mass of firmer tissue centered beneath the areolae suggest breast tissue rather than simply adipose tissue.

There are pathological conditions that may be associated with gynecomastia during the pubertal years. Testicular tumors, including Leydig-cell tumors, Sertoli-cell tumors, and germ cell tumors all may rarely secrete estrogen and present with gynecomastia. Gynecomastia may occur in association with gonadal disorders, including primary and secondary hypogonadism, true hermaphroditism, and enzyme defects of testosterone production. Feminizing adrenal cortical tumors are very rare. A patient with an essentially male phenotype and mild partial androgen insensitivity could present with gynecomastia. Ingestion of drugs may be a cause, including androgens, ketoconazole, and illicit drugs including marijuana.

VI. DELAYED PUBERTY AND HYPOGONADISM PRESENTING DURING ADOLESCENCE

A. Definition and General Approach

If the initial physical changes of puberty are not present by age 13 years in girls or age 14 in boys, evaluation should be considered for possible causes of lack of pubertal development. Abnormality may also be present if pubertal development has begun but does not progress appropriately. Therefore evaluation may also be indicated if more than 5 years have elapsed between the first signs of puberty and menarche in girls or completion of genital growth in boys. The aim of the assessment is to determine whether the delay or lack of development is a result of a lag in normal pubertal maturation of the hypothalamic–pituitary–gonadal axis or if it represents an underlying abnormality (Table 5).

If patients have no pertinent findings on medical history and examination, a delay in the onset of puberty is most likely to be so-called constitutional delay of puberty. Such patients are healthy, but generally have a history of delayed growth and development throughout childhood, including short stature but a relatively normal growth rate.

The initial approach to patients of both sexes with delayed or lack of progression of puberty is to determine gonadotropin status (Table 5) and skeletal age. Elevation of gonadotropin levels indicates gonadal failure and redirects further assessment, while low levels of gonadotropins do not differentiate physiological delay from gonadotropin deficiency. Skeletal age, determined by radiographic analysis of the ossification centers of the hands and wrists, compares patterns of growth and ossification with the average for age and sex. When bone age indicates a biological age less than that of the onset of

puberty (10–11 years for girls and 12–13 for boys), it is impossible to determine if gonadotropin secretion is delayed and immature or defective. In either situation gonadotropin levels, both before and after GnRH or gonadotropin-releasing hormone analog (GnRHa) stimulation, are within the prepubertal range, although as patients grow older greater responsiveness is expected. Persistence of low levels or an inadequate response over time suggests a hypothalamic or pituitary deficiency; a progressive rise is consistent with normal, but delayed, puberty.

When bone age, an index of biological age, is at or beyond the age of puberty, gonadotropin (LH and FSH) levels are elevated if gonadal failure is present because of maturation of the hypothalamus–pituitary–gonadotropin (HPG) axis and the absence of negative feedback by sex steroids. GnRH stimulation is unnecessary. If gonadotropin levels are mildly elevated, GnRH stimulation may be used to document partial primary gonadal failure.

Hypogonadism may not become manifest until during or after adolescence. Physical pubertal development may begin with expected physical changes but not progress normally. Among girls, the presentation may be because of primary or secondary amenorrhea. Among boys, growth and development may not be completed, testes may be abnormal, or no abnormalities may be noted unless fertility becomes a problem.

B. Boys

1. Assessment

Most boys who present with the complaint of delayed puberty who have short stature and normal prepubertal genitalia with prepubertal testes of normal size and consistency likely have constitutional delay. A plot of previous heights-for-age on a growth curve show low–normal growth rates. Skeletal maturation documents delay. Body proportions are immature (a greater upper/lower ratio than usual for age; relatively short legs for height). Primary hypogonadism (testicular failure), usually presenting with normal or tall stature, is very unlikely in such a patient.

Except in cases of testicular failure, gonadotropin levels are low for age in delayed puberty, whether due to constitutional delay or gonadotropin deficiency. At presentation, temporary delay or permanent deficiency cannot be absolutely differentiated; there is an overlap of responses to GnRH stimulation, with the rare exception of no response among those with an absent or destroyed pituitary.

The initial work-up should involve an evaluation aimed at the differential diagnosis listed in Table 5. The history should include a review of rates of weight and height gain, testicular descent, any other evidence suggestive of gonadal pathology, including endocrinopathies. Growth rates should be assessed with the knowledge that growth rates are slowest just before the onset of puberty in normal boys and may continue to decelerate until pubertal growth commences. Current or prior illnesses and

Table 5 Causes of Delay or Lack of Pubertal Development

Hypergonadotropic states (primary gonadal failure)
  Chromosomal, genetic disorders, and syndromes: androgen enzymatic synthesis defects, complete and partial androgen
      insensitivity syndrome, 46, XX males, 47, XYY syndromes, galactosemia, Klinefelter syndrome (47, XXY),
      mixed 45, X/46, XY gonadol dysgenesis, multiple X-Y syndromes, multiple Y syndromes, myotonic dystrophy,
      Noonan syndrome, pure 46, XY gonadol dysgenesis, 5α-reductase deficiency, resistant ovary syndrome, Turner
      syndrome, vanishing testes syndrome
  Acquired: autoimmune, chemotherapy, infectious (coxsackie, mumps), irradiation, surgical, torsion, traumatic
Hypogonadotropic states (hypothalamic-pituitary defect or lag)
  Hypothalamic-pituitary deficiencies
    Gonadotropin deficiency
      LH only (fertile eunuch syndrome)
      LH and FSH
        Acquired [autoimmune, cranial irradiation, granulomatous disease, hemosiderosis (thalassemia), sickle cell disease]
        Congenital, genetic, syndromes [Alstrom syndrome, Borjenson-Forssman-Lehmann syndrome, CHARGE syndrome,
            Kallmann syndrome, Laurence-Moon-Bardet-Biedl syndrome, multiple lentigines syndrome, Prader-Willi
            syndrome, prosencephalon defects (associated with central incisor syndrome, cleft-lip palate, midfacial cleft),
            septooptic dysplasia]
      Endocrinopathies (may include gonadotropin deficiency): hypopituitarism [idiopathic or secondary to empty sella
          syndrome, inflammation, pituitary dysgenesis, radiation, Rathke pouch cysts, surgery, trauma, tumors
          (craniopharyngioma, pituitary adenomas, prolactinomas)]
  Delayed or deferred function
    Constitutional delay of growth and/or puberty
    Chronic illness [cardiac, gastrointestinal (regional enteritis), hematologic (sickel cell disease), malignancy, pulmonary
        (cystic fibrosis), renal]
    Drug abuse
    Excessive energy expenditure, exercise
    Exogenous obesity
    Endocrinopathies: diabetes mellitus, growth hormone deficiency, glucocorticoid excess, hyperprolactinemia,
        hypothyroidism
    Malnutrition
    Psychiatric illness (anorexia nervosa, psychosocial dwarfism)

their treatment, including irradiation, surgery, chemotherapy or glucocorticoid therapy, should be considered. A family history of pubertal delay, hypogonadism, or infertility should be sought. Evidence of craniofacial–CNS midline defects, including anosmia or hyposmia, are important and suggestive of Kallmann syndrome, a unique hypogonadotropic syndrome with concomitant defects in the sense of smell (73, 74).

Physical examination must include careful documentation of height, weight, pubertal stage (Table 1), and upper/lower (U/L) segment ratios. This ratio is determined by subtracting, from standing height (U), the vertical distance from the pubic symphysis to the floor (L), or by subtracting the sitting height (U) from standing height (L). A ratio higher than normal suggests immaturity and delay, whereas a ratio lower than normal is suggestive of a defect or prolonged delay. In general, a ratio of less than unity (0.88 in black subjects) results from excessive leg (long-bone) growth characteristic of hypogonadism. Such eunuchoid ratios may be pronounced in patients with primary hypogonadism, such as Klinefelter syndrome. Testicular location (scrotal, inguinal, or nonpalpable), size,

and consistency (firm, soft, nodular) are important. A testis less than 2.0 cm along the longitudinal axis is prepubertal in size; length longer than 2.5 cm suggests pubertal growth. A testis in a pubertal-aged boy of 1.0 cm or less, particularly if unusually firm or soft, is suggestive of a hypogonadal state. A careful neurological examination should be done including assessment of fundi, visual fields, and sense of smell.

Laboratory evaluation should include serum LH and FSH levels, and a hand and wrist x-ray to determine bone age. If growth rate is subnormal, assessment of growth hormone secretion and thyroid function may be indicated. If IGF$_1$ levels are used as a screen for growth hormone, levels should be compared with normal ranges for stage of development and skeletal age, rather than chronological age. Various studies may be indicated to rule out CNS, renal, or gastrointestinal disease, and may include blood and urinary pH, urinary specific gravity, sedimentation rate, blood urea nitrogen, creatinine, and MRI of the head. If testes are small and firm or if there is other evidence suggestive of Klinefelter syndrome or other forms of primary hypogonadism, determination of karyotype is indicated. Human chorionic gonadotropin (HCG) stimulation testing is indicated if testes are nonpalpable or a testicular defect is suspected; only if gonadotropin levels are not elevated. A rise in circulating testosterone levels to higher than 300 ng/dl after 2–5 days of stimulation demonstrates adequate Leydig cell function. Many hCG regimens are used, ranging from 2 to 5 days. To stimulate maximum testosterone response, 5 days of treatment are sufficient. A dosage of 3000 units/m^2 per injection stimulates maximum response. Total dosage should be limited to 3000 units per injection or 15,000 units for the treatment period. To ensure maximum response, a minimum of 5000 units should be given during the treatment period. The drug may be administered two or three times a week. A blood sample for the testosterone should be obtained within 24 h from the last injection.

2. Elevated Gonadotropins: Primary
   Hypogonadism, Testicular Failure

Initial testing will identify patients with elevated gonadotropin levels if bone age is over 12.5 years, indicating inadequate testicular androgen production to suppress the maturing hypothalamic–pituitary axis. Conditions of primary testicular failure listed in Table 5 should be a guide to further evaluation. A karyotype in indicated unless there is a documented history of destruction of normal testes (e.g., torsion or radiation).

a. Klinefelter and Multiple Syndromes. Klinefelter syndrome (47XXY), the most common cause of hypergonadotropic hypogonadism, does not present with delay in the onset of puberty, but puberty may not be completed or progression may be slow. The most persistent physical finding is small, usually firm, testes. Tall stature, disproportionately long limbs, poor muscular development and gynecomastia are characteristic. Hypergonadotropism also occurs with other multiple X and Y syndromes, generally with more severe genital and mental impairment.

Elevation of FSH levels precedes pubertal age followed by LH. Testosterone levels begin to rise at normal ages, may attain adult male levels, but gradually diminish with concomitantly increasing estrogen-testosterone ratios.

b. Other Forms. Other forms of primary hypogonadism in boys include the vanishing testis syndrome (anorchia) and acquired testicular failure secondary to bilateral torsion, trauma, infection, and radiation. Patients with primary hypogonadism and their parents should be informed about therapeutic possibilities. Boys should be counseled appropriately for their level of concern and understanding. The counseling should be based on an understanding of the two basic functions of the testes: male hormone and sperm production.

Patients can be assured that the hormone can be replaced and that they will develop normal physically and function normally sexually. They also need to understand

that their children may be created by fertility-assisted methods available to couples, including sperm donation, or by adoption. They should be given the choice to have saline-filled prosthetic testes placed in the scrotum. If the condition is discovered before pubertal hormonal stimulation is appropriate, the implant should be delayed until the scrotum has matured to accommodate adult-sized prostheses. Having an empty scrotum appears to have minimal psychological effects during boyhood; most adolescent boys choose to have prostheses placed.

Hormonal replacement should begin at the usual age of the onset of puberty (12.5–13 years) or as soon thereafter as the need is recognized. Occasionally, there are reasons to delay treatment, including general growth failure, short stature, emotional or psychological immaturity. The initial dosage may vary depending on whether there has been any pubertal development, and the rapidity of pubertal development desired based on the age, social and intellectual maturation, and psychological needs of the patients (see section on therapy). Although early treatment with androgens accelerates bone age and may ultimately decrease adult height, if replacement therapy is given at the age of usual pubertal development, it does not have a detrimental effect on adult height (75). An initial low dosage is appropriate to avoid excessive genital stimulation, including dramatic reddening and sensitivity in the genital area and frequent, prolonged erections (76). The dosage can then be titered upward over the ensuing months or years.

3. Low Gonadotropin

If gonadotropin levels are low (Table 5), if there are no organic or associated conditions of pituitary malfunction, and if there is no other cause to account for delayed maturation, it usually is not possible to determine whether gonadotropin deficiency or simply delayed maturation exists. Gonadotropin, particularly LH, responses to GnRH stimulation may be helpful if a clear pubertal response is present. A rise consistent with a pubertal response may be discernible before clinical evidence of the onset of puberty, suggesting constitutional delay.

a. Constitutional Delay of Growth and Development. Physiological delay of maturation, including puberty, is characterized by a history of height and growth rate since early childhood along or slightly below 2 standard deviations (SD) for age, normal health, and nutrition. Biological age is usually delayed by about 2 years and development milestones, including pubertal events, are likewise delayed. Skeletal age is useful in estimating the amount of delay, spontaneous puberty being expected when skeletal age reaches 12–13 years in a boy. Such delay occurs more frequently among boys than girls.

Growth rate is characteristically markedly decelerated as the age of usual pubertal development is approached. The lack of sex steroid stimulation of growth hormone secretion results in a relative growth hormone deficiency, contributing to the diminished growth rate (77). Since adult height is foreshortened among those with the greatest delay and shortest stature, timely intervention with temporary treatment using appropriate dosages of testosterone must be considered to stimulate pubertal development and increase growth hormone production.

b. Permanent Gonadotropin Deficiency

Isolated gonadotropin deficiency. This occurs more frequently among boys than girls. Genetic causes include genetic mutations involving the GnRH-receptor, the CNS adhesion protein (KAL, anosmin), and the β-subunits of LH and FSH (73, 74). Isolated gonadotropin deficiency is characterized by normal stature, with the consequence of lack of sex steroid stimulation of skeletal maturity including disproportionally long limbs and delayed skeletal age. CNS and facial developmental abnormalities (midline facial defects), neurosensory hearing loss and synkinesia (mirror movements), anosmia, or hyposmia may be present. The most common form of isolated gonadotropin deficiency is Kallmann syndrome. Defects of Kallmann syndrome involve the association of hypogonadotropism and anosmia, olfactory bulb hypoplasia, and failure of development and migration of GnRH-secreting neurons to the hypothalamus. Not all patients with idiopathic hypogonadotropism (IHH) have Kallmann syndrome, although the latter is usually associated with more profound hypogonadotropism. IHH may present with no pubertal development, or with early but arrested changes. Most cases of Kallmann syndrome are sporadic, although autosomal recessive, autosomal dominant, including (father-to-son transmission), and X-linked modes of inheritance have been described (78). Normal GnRH structure is present in most patients with IHH, although deletion of the KAL1 gene has been described (79, 80), involving an extracellular adhesion molecule involved in the migration of GnRH neurons from the olfactory placode to the hypothalamus. Familial forms appear to be due to mutation at one of several different loci rather than a single gene.

Anatomical abnormalities in the hypothalamic–pituitary region. Intracranial neoplasms, including craniopharyngiomas, germinomas, gliomas, and prolactinomas, may result in GnRH or gonadotropin deficiency.

Syndromes with hypogonadotropism. Laurence-Moon-Biedl syndrome (also with retinitis pigmentosa, polydactyly, obesity, and mental retardation) and its Bardet-Biedl subgroup with dystrophic extremities (polydactyly, syndactyly, brachydactyly), obesity, and retinal disease with several genetic loci identified is associated with hypogonadism, more commonly among boys than girls. Hypogonadotropism may also occur in association with Prader-Willi, Alstrom, Rud, Bloom syndrome and other syndromes listed in Table 5.

c. Pathological Delay of Pubertal Gonadotropin Secretion.

Gonadotropin hyposecretion among those with potential for normal secretion may delay the onset of puberty among boys, or occur during or after puberty secondary to severe physical or mental stressful conditions. Delay occurs with chronic disease associated with malnutrition such as Crohn's disease, other chronic inflammatory disease, cystic fibrosis, hypothyroidism, and poorly controlled diabetes mellitus.

When pubertal delay occurs with low gonadotropin levels, hormonal treatment can be begun, even if delay cannot yet be differentiated from deficiency. Short-term treatment with testosterone (Fig. 9) is appropriate if age and psychosocial development indicate a need for physical pubertal maturation. Such exposure to androgens at a biological age (bone age) of 12–13 years or older has no apparent detrimental effects upon either those with constitutional delay or hypogonadotropic hypogonadism (75). Subsequent development, in the former, is normal, and spermatogenesis in response to exogenous gonadotropin stimulation, in the latter, is not different among those who have received previous testosterone treatment (81).

Androgen treatment administered as an intramuscular (IM) injection, transdermal patch, or gel can be given for an initial course of no longer than 4–6 months. The IM dosage can range from 50 to 100 mg IM every 4 weeks; the lowest available dosages of the dermal patches or gel can be used. The patches can also be used only overnight, rather than for 24 h initially. This avoids the embarrassment that may result from others seeing the patch if worn during other activities. After the initial months of stimulation, no treatment should be given for at least 2 months so that endogenous testosterone levels can be measured. If testosterone levels have risen to the pubertal range (>100 ng/dl), this suggests a diagnosis of delay. Treatment may be continued, if height and development are markedly delayed until endogenous levels are greater than 275 ng/dl. Patients should be evaluated at intervals of 6 months or longer to assess progression of puberty and testosterone levels. Values >300 ng/dl verify normal hypothalamic–pituitary–testicular function. Such a level provides a basis to assume that pubertal growth will proceed without further exogenous therapy.

If testosterone levels are still low, more time, during which a second course of testosterone treatment may be given, may be required to determine if gonadotropin deficiency exists. If this diagnosis is made, based on persistently low LH, FSH, and testosterone levels, androgen replacement therapy should be continued to ensure full physical pubertal development and maintained. Males with hypogonadotropism should be informed that spermatogenesis and fertility is potentially possible among some after exogenous biosynthetic gonadotropin therapy. However, only a portion of patients so treated respond with adequate spermatogenesis; there a correlation between initial testicular volume and response (9). Because of its expense and injection schedules, such treatment is not indicated until fertility is desired. Testosterone replacement is the treatment of choice until that time.

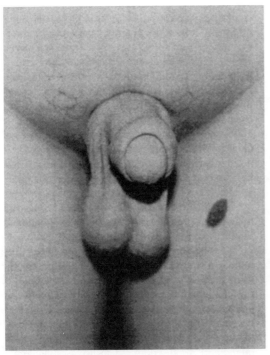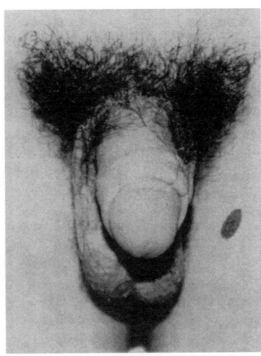

Figure 9 Genitalia of a boy with delayed puberty before (left) and after (right) five monthly injections of 200 mg testosterone enanthate IM. Pubertal development was Tanner 2 before the injections and skeletal age was 12-1/2 years at 14-8/12 years of age. After the injections at 15-2/12 years pubertal development progressed to Tanner 4. A subsequent endogenous testosterone level of 192 ng/dl verified a diagnosis of constitutional delay of puberty.

4. Therapy

Full replacement of androgen is required to attain and maintain an adult male state physically and sexually. This may be given as an injection or transdermally. Adult replacement of the depot injection of testosterone is a dosage up to 100 mg/week, given at intervals of 2 weeks (200 mg) or 3 weeks (300 mg). Injections every 4 weeks of 400 mg are not recommended because they result in supraphysiological levels for 7–10 days and, then, during the fourth week the levels are subnormal. The transdermal patches or gel can be used. The initial dosage depends upon the age and maturity of the patient and the rapidity of pubertal development desired. Optimal dosing may not be available because of packaging limitations. Dosages can be gradually titered upward to full replacement dosages after 3–4 years. Patients can be reassured that others cannot tell that exogenous therapy is stimulating or maintaining their physical development. Pubertal maturity, except testicular growth, and sexual function can be expected to be normal. If accessory sexual glands are appropriately formed, ejaculation, semen volume and appearance are normal.

Other forms of androgen therapy, including oxandrolone, fluoxymesterone, and methyltestosterone buccal or oral tablets do not provide full replacement and have limited usefulness. Oral replacement of methyltestosterone is

associated with hepatocellular malignant changes. Replacement therapy with aqueous testosterone injections requires at least daily administration.

Some hypogonadotropic hypogonadal boys have the potential for spermatogenesis and testosterone production if appropriately stimulated with gonadotropin. Such therapy is limited to adult men at the time they desire paternity.

Because height may be foreshortened among males with marked delay of puberty, and since estrogen stimulates skeletal maturity, aromatase inhibitors are being used to attempt to increase adult height (82).

5. Outcome

While it is assumed that boys with constitutional delay of puberty acquire normal sexual and reproductive function, this has not been carefully studied. With appropriate use of sex steroids, growth is completed without loss of adult height (83, 84). Evaluation has indicated that those who have considerable delay may not reach their genetically expected height, and have a persistence of segmental disproportion of relatively long leg length (85,86). Furthermore, bone mineral density may be diminished, even after full pubertal virilization is complete (87). These data provide evidence for early intervention, with androgen therapy precluding the prolonged period of growth deceleration, increased long bone growth effects upon body proportions, and diminished bone mineral density accrual.

C. Girls

1. Assessment

Delay of onset of pubertal development is a less common complaint among girls than among boys and is more likely to have an underlying pathological cause. Delay should be assessed if breast and pubic hair development has not begun by age 13 years or menarche by 15.5–16 years. Also, lack of completion of pubertal development to Tanner stage 5 within 4 years is considered delay. Categorization of patients as having elevated or low gonadotropin levels (Table 5) should be done initially together with documentation of skeletal age (bone age x-ray). Initial assessment should include a careful history looking for evidence of chronic illness (e.g., occult Crohn's disease), endocrinopathy, prior illnesses and therapy, sense of smell, and a family history of lack of puberty or infertility (Kallmann syndrome). Growth patterns should help differentiate those with short stature who are more likely to have constitutional pubertal delay or chronic illness from those with permanent gonadotropin deficiency and rare forms of primary hypogonadism who are normal or tall. The physical examination should concentrate on body proportions, breast and genital development, neurological examination, and stigmata suggestive of Turner syndrome. Laboratory evaluation should generally be similar to that for boys, although hCG testing is not indicated since hCG alone does not stimulate precocious puberty in girls. Karyotype should be included if the patient has unexplained short stature. Among patients with normal physical pubertal development presenting with amenorrhea, pregnancy must be ruled out.

In an attempt to differentiate patients with a permanent defect from those with delayed or temporary hypogonadotropism, GnRH-stimulated gonadotropin testing may be helpful in the older adolescent. Persistence of low basal or GnRH-stimulated LH and FSH levels in a patient in the late teenage years with a bone age over 11–12 years is indicative of a defect of gonadotropin secretion.

Delayed menarche or secondary amenorrhea may result from lack of gonadotropin or ovarian failure, or may be the consequence of hyperandrogenism, anatomical obstruction (including imperforate hymen) precluding menstrual outflow, or vaginal and uterine agenesis (Mayer-Rokitansky-Kuster-Hauser syndrome).

2. Elevated Gonadotropins

Hypergonadotropism occurs with primary gonadal failure. If elevated gonadotropin levels are found and there is not ample evidence to explain the hypergonadotropic state, such as surgery, radiation, and chemotherapy, a karyotype evaluation should be done.

a. Turner Syndrome. The most common cause of primary amenorrhea associated with primary gonadal failure is Turner syndrome. Ovarian pathology involves early loss of oocytes and accelerated stromal fibrosis. The classic findings of Turner syndrome are short stature, primary hypogonadism, a diversity of congenital anomalies associated with the loss of absence of all or part of an X chromosome (45X- [about 50%-] or 45X/mosaic karyotype). Among the majority, the maternal X is retained. The missing sex chromosome may have been either a paternal X or Y. Sensitive molecular techniques have revealed that some girls with Turner syndrome carry Y chromosomal material (88). The consequences of this are unknown unless Y material associated with malignant degeneration is present. Mosaic karyotypes and structural abnormalities of the X chromosome account for some of the variation of clinical features. Haplo insufficiency of the short stature homeobox (SHOX) gene found on the short end of both sex chromosomes is associated with skeletal anomalies and short stature (89, 90). These involve facial, palatal, and middle ear development. Other stigmata, including low hairline, webbed neck, hand, feet, chest, and nipple configuration, appear to be a consequence of fetal edema. Cardiovascular, renal, and potentially associated autoimmune diseases may require specific therapy. Some aspects of mental and social functioning may be impaired. Rarely, ovarian function persists enough so that spontaneous breast development may occur (91), although endogenous estrogen secretion is usually inadequate for full puberty. Normal ovarian function, with menstruation, ovulation, and successful pregnancy occurs very rarely.

b. 46,XY Gonadal Dysgenesis. Delayed puberty in a phenotypic female is a typical presentation for 46,XY complete gonadal dysgenesis, female genital differentiation being the constitutive result of the complete lack of testicular function. Rarely, mutations of the SRY gene may be present (92, 93). Familial gonadal dysgenesis has been described in which the phenotype and gender of rearing differed between family members despite a common mutation in the SRY gene in all affected family members (94). Duplication of the portions of the short arm of the X chromosome that includes the DAX1 gene is another identified genetic cause of 46,XY sex reversal (95). Ambiguous internal and external genitalia or some pubertal changes may be noted in patients with incomplete or partial forms of 46,XY gonadal dysgenesis. Gonadectomy is generally recommended since dysgenetic gonads have increased risk of developing dysgerminomas or gonadoblastomas.

c. 46,XX Gonadal Dysgenesis. In rare cases, pure ovarian agenesis with a 46,XX karyotype also occurs, being characterized by normal or tall height, no dysmorphic features, normal female external genitalia, and hypoplastic or no ovarian development. Presentation may be with some breast development but amenorrhea. A report of

46,XX and 46,XY sisters with gonadal agenesis provides evidence for an autosomal locus involved in gonadal differentiation (96). Perrault syndrome is XX gonadal dysgenesis and sensorineural deafness (97).

d. Mixed Gonadal Dysgenesis. Individuals with mixed gonadal dysgenesis (98), commonly having a karyotype of 45,X/46,XY, may have somatic features typical of Turner syndrome, including short stature, although genitalia may be masculinized. Genital development reflects in utero testosterone exposure and range from female to ambiguous, to male. The gonads are often asymmetrical, with streak ovaries or dysgenetic testes. External genital development may likewise be asymmetrical. Dysgenetic testes and the Y chromosome increase the risk of gonadoblastoma and virilization at puberty. Based upon physical findings, sex of rearing may have been assigned as male or female. Among females, estrogen replacement is generally required to induce puberty. Spontaneous breast development may occur; however, this may be a consequence of an estrogen-secreting gonadoblastoma.

e. Congenital Adrenal Hyperplasia. Although most enzyme deficiencies present with other complaints at younger ages, 17-hydroxylase-17,20-lyase deficiency (99), characterized by elevated progesterone, pregnenolone 17-hydroxyprogesterone, and 17-hydroxypregnenolone levels, is associated with deficient estrogen synthesis. Female patients are phenotypically normal and present with pubertal delay. Hypergonadotropic hypogonadism becomes evident during adolescence with congenital lipoid adrenal hyperplasia.

f. Acquired, Including Autoimmune, Gonadal Failure. Prepubertal or pubertal gonadal injury may result in hypergonadotropic hypogonadism. The ovary is less vulnerable than seminiferous tubules to injury. Chemotherapy, particularly nitrogen mustard compounds, for malignancies or immunological disorders may damage the gonads. The degree of injury is greater when chemotherapy occurs during rather than before puberty (100). Pelvic irradiation may damage reproductive function, although many girls treated for acute lymphocytic leukemia appear to retain ovarian function (101). Autoimmune oophoritis usually presents after puberty, only rarely during pubertal years (102). It may be associated with type I autoimmune polyglandular syndrome, characterized by hypoparathyroidism, Addison's disease, vitiligo, hypothyroidism, and pernicious anemia. Galactosemia may be associated with ovarian failure (103).

g. Gonadotropin Receptor Mutations. Hypergonadotropic hypogonadism may also be associated with luteinizing hormone receptor mutations. In XX females, the presentation is primary amenorrhea, elevated serum LH and low estradiol levels, rather than delayed puberty (104, 105). XY males with LH receptor mutations have presented with female external genitalia, absence of muller-

ian structures, and lack of breast development. Biopsy of the inguinal gonads shows absence of Leydig cells, but Sertoli cells, spermatogonia and primary spermatocytes. Limited response to hCG administration has been demonstrated. Mutations in the FSH receptor gene have been identified in women presenting with primary amenorrhea, normal breast development, and elevated FSH. Numerous small follicles up to the antral stage are present in the ovaries, but there is disruption of later stages (106, 107).

h. Complete Androgen Insensitivity Syndrome. Patients with androgen insensitivity may present with inadequate progression of female puberty (108, 109). Breast onset typically occurs at an appropriate age; complaints may include amenorrhea or lack of sexual hair.

3. Low Gonadotropin Levels

If gonadotropin levels are low, the search for the cause is also an attempt to determine if the hypogonadotropism represents a delay in maturity or a permanent hypothalamic–pituitary defect.

If there is an underlying chronic illness, prolonged pharmacological glucocorticoid therapy, excessive emotional stress, unusual physical activity, or an inadequate nutritional state, the hypogonadotropism is likely a secondary and potentially reversible condition (110). Chronic conditions related to pubertal delay may include anorexia, inflammatory bowel disease, cystic fibrosis (111), and chronic renal failure. If the underlying problem can be adequately treated, normal gonadotropin secretion should follow. Conversely, while the underlying problem persists, estrogen therapy is relatively ineffective. Noonan's syndrome may be associated with delayed pubertal development; most patients attain normal ovarian function.

a. Permanent Deficiency

Idiopathic hypogonadotropism. Idiopathic hypogonadotropism (IHH) is less common in females than in males. Kallmann syndrome is associated with anosmia. DAX1 mutations result in IHH in association with congenital adrenal hyperplasia (112). Multiple pituitary hormonal deficiencies, including gonadotropism may be congenital or acquired. Congenital defects may be associated with septo-optic dysplasia or midline facial defects. Acquired defects may occur with histiocytosis X, sarcoidosis, radiation therapy, and hemochromatosis (113).

FSH gene mutations. Primary amenorrhea in otherwise normal XX females occurs with FSH β gene mutations. LH levels are elevated and FSH low or undetectable (114). A normal response to exogenous FSH can be elicited in affected patients.

Multiple congenital or acquired pituitary deficiencies. Hypogonadotropic hypogonadism may also occur in association with other anterior pituitary hormone deficiencies. Both congenital and acquired disorders may involve the hypothalamus and/or the pituitary. Midline facial defects, septo-optic dysplasia, or ectopic location of the posterior pituitary at the base of the hypothalamus may coexist with congenital hypopituitarism. Structural abnormalities may result from craniopharyngiomas, hamartomas, gliomas, and hypothalamic cysts. Histiocytosis X, sarcoidosis, infiltration (Wilson's disease and hemochromatosis) and radiation therapy may cause acquired hypopituitarism. Granulomatous infiltrates may interfere with GnRH, LH, and FSH release. Deficiency of more than one pituitary hormone, except in idiopathic hypopituitarism diagnosed in early childhood, strongly suggests an anatomical lesion, particularly if diabetes insipidus or hyperprolactinemia is present.

b. Temporary Hypogonadotropism with Potential of Normal Function. Constitutional delay of puberty is relatively rarer among girls than boys and should be a diagnosis of exclusion. Such children are healthy and have short stature and delayed bone age. Bone age progresses in this condition, in contrast to cases with a persistent chronic disease.

Several conditions associated with functional hypogonadotropic hypogonadism may have similar neuroendocrine dynamics (115). Increases in physical activity, deficiency of calories, and mental disturbances appear to impair hypothalamic–pituitary–ovarian function progressively while correction of energy imbalance is followed by correction

c. Prolactinomas. Prolactinomas may present with delayed puberty or arrested pubertal development, primary or secondary amenorrhea, and low gonadotropins. Galactorrhea may not be present. Treatment includes bromocriptine, transsphenoidal surgery, or pituitary irradiation (116, 117).

Hemochromatosis. Hemochromatosis leading to pituitary infiltration, whether idiopathic or secondary (sickle cell disease or thalassemia), may also result in gonadotropin deficiency because of deposits in the gonadotropin-producing cells and present with delayed puberty (113). Reversal of the pituitary gonadotropin deficiency and recovery of reproductive function may follow aggressive phlebotomy and chelation therapy in patients with the idiopathic and familial forms of the disease (118).

Physical and psychological deprivation. Delayed or arrested puberty may occur in athletes and with chronic illnesses, particularly anorexia nervosa (110). The latter is often associated with delayed puberty, slowing of normal pubertal progression, primary or secondary amenorrhea, and osteopenia (119). Inadequate caloric intake (120) or excessive physical exertion contributes to the temporary physiological delay. Pubertal delay is a consequence of hypothalamic hypofunction resulting from strenuous exercise, stress-related and intentional caloric restriction, especially in activities such as ballet, gymnastics, or track. The GnRH pulsatile pattern is altered, resulting in low gonadotropin levels (121).

Chronic illness. The chronic illnesses frequently associated with delayed puberty (e.g., inflammatory bowel disease, cystic fibrosis, chronic renal disease, and poorly controlled diabetes mellitus) are characterized by undernutrition. Mechanisms resulting in failure of gonadotropin secretion are likely similar to those in the deprivational conditions discussed above.

Hypothyroidism. Untreated primary hypothyroidism during childhood delays maturation, as indicated by delayed skeletal age, most commonly resulting in pubertal delay. Onset during or after pubertal development is associated with menstrual disorders, primary or secondary amenorrhea, and menometrorrhagia.

Cushing Syndrome. Glucocorticoid excess, either endogenous or exogenous, among children or adolescents, may result in pubertal delay, amenorrhea, and low gonadotropin levels.

Syndromes associated with gonadotropin deficiency. Syndromes with hypogonadotropic hypogonadism include the Laurence-Moon-Biedl syndrome. Hypogonadism is less common among females; hirsutism and elevated LH levels appear to be more common (122). Other syndromes are listed under the section on boys.

4. Treatment

Replacement therapy for girls should eventually consist of cyclic estrogen–progesterone therapy. However, initial therapy for young pubertal-aged patients can be daily low-dosage estrogen therapy for 6, to, at most, 12 months. If breakthrough bleeding occurs during this time, cyclic medication should be initiated. The lowest available estrogen dosage preparation (such as Premarin 0.3 mg or ethinyl estradiol 0.02 mg daily), or the transdermal patch (Estraderm 0.025 mg applied once or twice a week) may be used as initial treatment. Cyclic estrogen–progesterone therapy can be given by administering low-estrogen birth control pills. Alternatively, a daily estrogen regimen or the transdermal form can be used for the first 3 weeks (21 days) of the calendar month, regardless of the length of the month, with progesterone added for the last 10 of the 21 days (day 12 to day 21). With this regimen the patient is easily aware, based on the actual date, of what pills she should take. From the 22nd until the end of the month, no matter how many days in the month, she should take no medication. On the first of the month, even if her period has not stopped, she should begin estrogen again. The dosage of estrogen can be varied, based on the rapidity and adequacy of pubertal development. Ethinyl estradiol (0.02–0.10 mg/day), conjugated estrogen (0.3–1.25 mg/day), or transdermal treatment to deliver 0.05 or 0.1 mg daily can be used. Once full pubertal development has been reached, the estrogen dosage should be the minimum that will maintain normal menstrual flow and prevent calcium bone loss, equivalent to 0.625 mg conjugated estrogen. Progesterone in this regimen can be given as medroxyprogesterone (5 or 10 mg/day) or norethindrone (5 mg/day). Various low-dosage oral contraceptives may also be used.

Among girls with a tentative diagnosis of constitutional delay, the therapy should be reassessed at 6 month intervals to determine if pubertal hormonal activity has begun.

It should be recognized that spontaneous pubertal development or menstruation may rarely occur in patients with Turner syndrome; replacement therapy may not be needed in all patients, and fertility may occur (123). Patients with Turner syndrome, and others with ovarian failure but normal mullerian duct differentiation, are candidates for assisted fertility using donated ova (124).

Growth potential and skeletal maturation can be monitored using periodic bone age x-ray films at intervals no more frequently than every 6 months. Growth hormone is an indicated therapy for Turner syndrome. Testing for growth hormone deficiency and possible growth hormone therapy should be considered among those with severe short stature or subnormal growth rates.

Psychosocial aspects of delayed pubertal development may be associated with poor socialization, school performance, and self-esteem. Parents and teachers should be encouraged to relate to the child according to her age rather than appearance and to encourage appropriate responsibilities and independence (125).

REFERENCES

1. Dunkel L, Alfthan H, Stenman U, Tapanainen P, Perheentupa J. Pulsatile secretion of LH and FSH in prepubertal and early pubertal boys revealed by ultrasensitive time-resolved immunofluorometric assays. Pediatr Res 1990; 27:215–219.
2. Goji K, Tanikaze S. Comparison between spontaneous gonadotropin concentration profiles and gonadotropin response to low-dose gonadotropin-releasing hormone in prepubertal and early pubertal boys and patients with hypogonadotropic hypogonadism: assessment by using ultrasensitive, time-resolved immunofluorometric assay. Pediatr Res 1992; 31:535–539.
3. Apter D, Bützow TL, Laughlin GA, Yen SSC. Gonadotropin-releasing hormone pulse generator activity during pubertal transition in girls: pulsatile and diurnal patterns of circulating gonadotropins. J Clin Endocrinol Metab 1993; 76:940–949.
4. Kletter GB, Padmanabhan V, Foster CM, Brown MB, Kelch RP, Beitins IZ. Luteinizing hormone pulse characteristics in early pubertal boys are the same whether measured by radioimmuno- or immunofluorometric assay. J Clin Endocrinol Metab 1993; 76:1173–1176.
5. Goji K. Twenty-four-hour concentration profiles of gonadotropin and estradiol (E2) in prepubertal and early pubertal girls: The diurnal rise of E2 is opposite the nocturnal rise of gonadotropin. J Clin Endocrinol Metab 1993; 77:1629–1635.
6. Delemarre-Van De Waal HA, Wennink JMB, Odink RJH. Gonadotropin and growth hormone secretion throughout puberty. Acta Paediatr Scand 1991; 372:26–31.
7. Knobil E. The neuroendocrine control of the menstrual cycle. Recent Prog Horm Res 1980; 36:53–88.
8. Lee PA. Pubertal neuroendocrine maturation: early differentiation and stages of development. Adolesc Pediatr Gynecol 1988; 1:3–12.
9. Wu FCW, Butler GE, Kelnar CJH, et al. Patterns of pulsatile luteinizing hormone and follicle-stimulating hormone secretion in prepubertal (midchildhood) boys and girls and patients with idiopathic hypogonadotropic hypogonadism (Kallman's syndrome): a study using an ultrasensitive time-resolved immunofluorometric assay. J Clin Endocrinol Metab 1991; 72:1229–1237.
10. Lee PA. Laboratory monitoring of children with precocious puberty. Arch Pediatr Adolesc Med 1994; 148:369–376.
11. Lee PA. Advances in the management of precocious puberty. Clin Pediatr 1994; 33:54–61.
12. Neely EK, Hintz RL, Wilson DM, et al. Normal ranges of immunochemiluminometric gonadotropin assays. J Pediatr 1995; 127:40–46.
13. Roche AF, Wellens R, Attie KM, Siervogel RM. The timing of sexual maturation in a group of US White Youths. J Pediatr Endocrinol Metab 1995; 8:11–18.
14. Herman-Giddens ME, Slora EJ, Wasserman RC, Bourdony CJ, Bhapkar MV, Koch GG, Hasemeier CM. Secondary sexual characteristics and menses in young girls seen in office practice: a study from the Pediatric research in Office Settings Network. Pediatrics 1997; 99:505–512.
15. Lee PA, Shumei SG, Kulin HE. Age of puberty: data from the United States of America APMIS 2001; 109:81–88.
16. de Munick Keizer-Schrama SMP, Mul D. Trends in pubertal development in Europe. Human Reprod Update 2001; 7:287–91.
17. Marti-Henneberg C, Vizmonso B. The duration of puberty in girls is related to the timing of its onset. J Pediatr 1997; 131:618–621.
18. DeRidder CM, Thijssen JHH, Bruning PF, Van Den Brande JL, Zonderland ML, Erich WBM. Body fat mass, body fat distribution, and pubertal development: a longitudinal study of physical and hormonal sexual maturation of girls. J Clin Endocrinol Metab 1992;75:442–446.
19. Rico H, Revilla M, Villa LF, Hernandez ER, Alvarez de Buergo M, Villa M. Body composition in children and Tanner's stages. A study with dual-energy X-ray absorptiometry. Metabolism 1993; 42:967–970.
20. Biro FM, Lucky AW, Huster GA, Morrison JA Pubertal staging in boys. J Pediatr 1995; 127:100–102.
21. Herman-Giddens ME, Wang L, Koch G. Secondary sexual characteristics in boys: Estimates from the National Health and Nutrition Examination Survey III, 1988–91994. Arch Pediatr Adolesc Med 2001; 155:1022–1028.
22. Richards RJ, Svec F, Bao W, Srinivasan SR, Berenson GS. Steroid hormones during puberty: Racial (black-white) differences in androstenedione and estradiol—The Bogalusa Heart Study. J Clin Endocrinol Metab 1992; 75:624–631.
23. Anderson A-M, Jull A, Petersen JH, Muller J, Groome NP, Skakkebaek N. Serum inhibin B in healthy pubertal and adolescent boys: relation to age, stage of Anderson puberty, and follicle-stimulating hormone, luteinizing hormone, testosterone, and estradiol levels. J Clin Endocrinol Metab 1997; 82:3976–3981.
24. Lee MM, Donahoe PK, Hasegawa T, Silverman B, Crist GB, Best D, Hasegawa Y, Noto RA, Schoenfeld D, MacLaughlin DT. Mullerian inhibiting substance in humans: normal levels from infancy to adulthood. J Clin Endocrinol Metab 1996; 81:571–576.

25. Forbes GB, Porta CR, Herr BE, Griggs RC. Sequence of changes in body composition induced by testosterone and reversal of changes after drug is stopped. JAMA 1992; 267:397–399.

26. Nielson CT, Skakkabak NE, Darling JA, Hunter WM, Richardson DW, Jorgenson M, Keiding N. Longitudinal study of testosterone and luteinizing hormone (LH) in relation to spermarche, pubic hair, height and sitting height in normal boys. Acta Endocrinol Suppl 1986; 279: 98–106.

27. Elders MJ, Scott CR, Frinkik JP, et al. Clinical workup for precocious puberty. Lancet 1997; 350:457–458.

28. Fontoura M, Brauner R, Prevot C, et al. Precocious puberty in girls: early diagnosis of a slowly progressing variant. Arch Dis Child 1989; 64:1170–1176.

29. Lazar L, Pertzelan A, Weintrob N, Phillip M, Kauli R, et al. Sexual precocity in boys: Accelerated versus slowly progressive puberty gonadotropin-suppressive therapy and final height. J Clin Endocrinol Metab 2001; 86:4127–4132.

30. Virdis R, Street M, Zampoli M, et al. Precocious puberty in girls adopted from developing countries. Arch Dis Child 1998; 78:152–154.

31. Baron S, Battin J, David A, Limal JM. Precocious puberty in children adopted from foreign countries. Arch Pediatr 2000; 7:809–816

32. Krstevska-Konstatninova M, Charlier C, Craen M, et al. Sexual precocity after immigration from developing countries Belgium: evidence of previous exposure to organochlorine pesticides. Hum Reprod 2001; 16:1020–1026.

33. Mahachoklertwattana P, Kaplan SL, Grumbach MM. The luteinizing hormone-releasing hormone-secreting hypothalamic hamartoma is a congenital malformation. Nat Hist J Clin Endocrinol Metab 1993; 77:118–124.

34. Shenker A, Weinstein LS, Moran A, Pescovitz OH, Charest NJ, Boney CM, Van Wyk JJ, Merino MJ, Feuillan PP, Spiegel AM. Severe endocrine and nonendocrine manifestations of the McCune-Albright syndrome associated with activating mutations of stimulatory G protein GS. J Pediatr 1993; 123:509–518.

35. Foster CM, Feuillan P, Padmanabhan V, et al. Ovarian function in girls with McCune-Albright syndrome. Pediatr Res 1986; 20:859–863.

36. Pasquino AM, Tebaldi L, Cives C, et al. Precocious puberty in the McCune-Albright syndrome. Progression from gonadotropin-independent to gonadotropin-dependent puberty in a girl. Acta Pediatr Scand 1987; 1:841–843.

37. Escobar ME, Gryngarten M, Domene H, et al. Persistence of autonomous ovarian activity after discontinuation therapy for precocious puberty in McCune-Albright syndrome. J Pediatr Adolesc Gynecol, 1997; 10:147–151.

38. Cohen HL, Eisenberg P, Mandel F, Haller JO. Ovarian cysts are common in premenarchal girls: A sonographic study of 101 children 2–12 years old. AJR 1992; 159: 89–91.

39. Anasti JN, Flack MR, Froelich J, et al. A potential novel mechanism for precocious puberty in juvenile hypothroidism. J Clin Endocrinol Metab 1995; 80:276–279.

40. Atchison JA, Lee PA, Albright AL. Reversible suprasellar pituitary mass secondary to hypothyroidism. JAMA 1989; 262:3175–3177.

41. Bar, A, Linder B, Sobel EH, et al. Bayley-Pinneau method of height predication in girls with central precocious puberty: correlation with adult height. J Pediatr 1995; 126:955–958.

42. Rivarola M, Belgorosky A, Mendilaharzu H, Vidal G. Precocious puberty in children with tumours of the suprasellar pineal areas: organic central precocious puberty. Acta Paediatr 2001; 90:751–756.

43. Lactronico AC, Shinozaki H, Guerra G Jr, et al. Gonadotropin-independent precocious puberty due to luteinizing hormone receptor mutations in Brazilian boys: a novel constitutive activating mutation in the first transmembrane helix. J Clin Endocrinol Metab 2000; 85:4799–4805.

44. Domenice S, Latronica AC, Brito VN, et al. Adrenocorticopin-dependent precocious puberty of testicular origin in a boy with X-linked adrenal hypoplasia congenital to a novel mutation in the DAXI Gene. J Clin Endocrinol Metab 2001; 86:4068–4071.

45. Feuillan PP, Foster CM, Pescovitz OH, et al. Treatment of precocious puberty in the McCune-Albright syndrome with the aromatase inhibitor testolactone. N Engl J Med 1986; 315:1115–1119.

46. Feuillan PP, Jones J, Cutler GB. Long-term testolactone therapy for precocious puberty in girls with the McCune-Albright syndrome. J Clin Endocrinol Metab 1993; 77: 647–651.

47. Syed FA, Chalew SA. Ketoconazole treatment of gonadotropin independent precocious puberty in girls with McCune-Albright syndrome: a preliminary report. J Pediatr Endocrinol Metab 1999;12:81–83.

48. Eugster EA, Shankar R, Feezle LK, et al. Tamoxifen treatment of progressive precocious puberty in a patient with McCune-Albright syndrome. J Pediatr Endocrinol Metab 1999; 12:681–686.

49. Feuillan P, Merke D, Leschek, EW, Cutler GB. Use of aromatase inhibitors in precocious puberty. Endocrinol Rel Cancer 1999; 6:303–306.

50. Bertelloni S, Baroncelli GI, Lala R, et al. Long-term outcome of male-limited gonadotropin independent precocious puberty. Horm Res 1997; 48:235–239.

51. Tato L, Savage MO, Antoniazzi F, et al. Optimal therapy of pubertal disorders in precocious/early puberty. J Pediatr Endocrinol Metab 2001; 14:985–995.

52. Shankar RR, Pescovitz OH. Precocious puberty. Adv Endocrinol Metab 1995;6:55–58.

53. Palmert M, Hayden D, Mansfield MJ, et al. The longitudinal study of adrenal maturation during gonadal suppression: evidence that adrenarche is a gradual process, J Clin Endocrinol Metab 2001;86:4536–4542.

54. Manasco PK, Pescovitz OH, Hill SC, et al. Six-year results of luteinizing hormone releasing hormone (LHRH) agonist treatment in children with LHRH-dependent precocious puberty. J Pediatr 1989; 115:105–108.

55. Manasco PK, Pescovitz OH, Feuillan PP, et al. Resumption of puberty after long term luteinizing hormone–releasing hormone agoinst treatment of central precocious puberty. J Clin Endocrinol Metab 1988; 67:368–373.

56. Jay N, Mansfield MJ, Blizzard RM, et al. Ovulation and menstrual function of adolescent girls with central precocious puberty after therapy with gonadotropin-releasing hormone agonists. J Clin Endocrinol Metab 1992; 75: 890–894.

57. Feuillan PP, Jones JV, Barnes KM, et al. Boys with precocious puberty due to hypothalamic hamartoma reproductive axis after discontinuation of gonadotropin-release hormone analog therapy. J Clin Endocrinol Metab 2000; 85:4036–4038.

58. Kauli R, Galatzer A, Korneich L, et al. Final height girls with central precocious puberty, untreated versus treated

with cyproterone acetate or GnRH analogue. Horm Res 1997; 47:54–61.

59. Paul D, Conte FA, Grumbach MM, et al. Long-term effect of gonadotropin-releasing hormone agonist therapy on final and near-final height in 26 children with true precocious puberty treated at a median age of less than 5 years. J Clin Endocrinol Metab 1995; 80:546–551.

60. Oerter KE, Manasco P, Barnes KM, et al. Adult height in precocious puberty after long-term treatment with Deslorelin. J Clin Endocrinol Metab 1991; 73:1235–1240.

61. Cacciari E, Cassio A, Balsamo A, et al. Long-term follow-up and final height in girls with central precocious puberty treated with luteinizing hormone-relating hormone analogue nasal spray. Arch Pediatr Adolesc Med 1994; 148:1194–1199.

62. Kletter GB, Kelch RP. Effects of gonadotropin-releasing hormone analog therapy on adult stature in precocious puberty. J Clin Endocrinol Metabl 1994; 79:331–334.

63. Oostdijk W, Rikken B, Schreuder S, et al. Final height in central precocious puberty after long-term treatment with a slow release GnRH agonist. Arch Dis Child 1996;75: 292–297.

64. Brauner R, Adan L, Malandry F, et al. Adult height in girls with idiopathic true precocious puberty. J Clin Endocrinol Metab 1994; 79:415–420.

65. Lazar L, Kauli R, Bruchis C, et al. Early polycystic ovary-like syndrome in girls with central precocious puberty and exaggerated adrenal response. Eur J Endocrinol 1995; 133:403–406.

66. Ibanez L, Potau N, Zampolli M, et al. Girls diagnosed with premature pubarche show an exaggerated ovarian androgen synthesis from the early stages of puberty: evidence from gonadotropin-releasing agonist testing. Fertil Steril 1997; 67:849–855.

67. Salardi S, Cacciari E, Mainetti B, et al. Outcome of premature thelarche: relation to puberty and final height. Arch Dis Child 1998; 79:173–174.

68. Pasquino AM, Pucarelli I, Passeri F, Segni M, Mancini MA, Municchi G. Progression of premature thelarche to central precocious puberty. J Pediatr 1995; 127:336–337.

69. Ibanez L, Virdis R, Potau N, Zampolli M, Ghizzoni L, Albisu MA, Carrascosa A, Bernasconi S, Vicens-Calvet E. Natural history of premature pubarche: an auxological study. J Clin Endocrinol Metab 1992; 74:254–257.

70. Ibanez L, Potau N, Virdis R, Zampolli M, Terzi C, Gussinye M, Carrascosa A, Vicens-Calvet E. Postpubertal outcome in girls diagnosed of premature pubarche during childhood: increased frequency of functional ovarian hyperandrogenism. J Clin Endocrinol Metab 1993; 76: 1599–1603.

71. Siegel SF, Finegold DN, Urban MD, VcVie R, Lee PA. Premature pubarche: etiological heterogeneity. J Clin Endocrinol Metab 1992; 74:239–247.

72. Leiberman E, Zachmann M, et al. Familial adrenal feminization probably due to increased steroid aromatization. Horm Res 1992; 37:96–102.

73. Themmen APN, Huhtaniemi IT. Mutations of gonadotropins and gonadotropin receptors: elucidating the physiology and pathophysiology of pituitary-gonadal function. Endocr Rev 2000; 21: 551–583.

74. Roux N, Milgrom E. Inherited disorders of GnRH and gonadotropin receptors. Mol Cell Endocrinol 2001; 179: 83–87.

75. Zachmann M, Studer S, Prader A. Short-term testosterone treatment at bone age of 12 to 13 years does not reduce adult height in boys with constitutional delay of growth and adolescence. Helv Paediatr Acta 1987; 42:21–28.

76. Key LL, Myers MC, Kroovand RL, Kelly WS. Priapism following testosterone therapy for delayed puberty. Am J Dis Child 1989; 143:1001–1002.

77. Martha PM Jr, Reiter EO. Pubertal growth and growth hormone secretion. Endocrinol Metab Clin North Am 1991; 20:165–182.

78. Waldstreicher J, Seminara SB, Jameson JL, et al. The genetic and clinical heterogeneity of gonadotropin-releasing hormone deficiency in the human. J Clin Endocrinol Metab 1996; 81:4388–4395.

79. Hardelin JP. Kallmann syndrome: towards molecular pathogenesis. Mol Cell Endocrinol 2001; 179:75–81.

80. Georgopolous NA, Pralong FP, Seidman CE, et al. Genetic heterogeneity evidenced by low incidence of KAL-I gene mutations in sporadic cases of gonadotropin-releasing hormone deficiency. J Clin Endocrinol Metab 1997; 82:213–217.

81. Ley SB, Leonard JM. Male hypogonadotropic hypogonadism; factors influencing response to human chorionic gonadotropin and human menopausal gonadotropin, including prior exogenous androgens. J Clin Endocrinol Metab 1985; 61:746–752.

82. Wickman S, Sipila I, Ankaberg-Lindgren C, Norjavaara E, Dunkel L. A specific aromatase inhibitor and potential increase in adult height in boys with delayed puberty: a randomized controlled trial. Lancet 2001; 357:1743–1748.

83. Richman RA, Kirsch LR. Testosterone treatment of adolescent boys with constitutional delay in growth and development. N Engl J Med 1988; 319:1563–1570.

84. Tse W, Buyukgebiz A, Hindmarch PC, Stanhope R, Preece MA, Brook CGD. Long term outcome of oxandrolone treatment in boys with constitutional delay of growth and puberty. J Pediatr 1990; 117:588–591.

85. Albanese A, Stanhope R. Predictive factors at presentation in the determination of final height in boys with constitutional delay of growth and puberty. J Pediatr 1995; 126:545–550.

86. Albanese A, Stanhope R. Does constitutional delayed puberty cause segmental disproportion and short stature? Eur J Pediatr 1993; 152:293–296.

87. Finkelstein JS, Klibanski A, Neer R. A longitudinal evaluation of bone mineral density in adult men with histories of delayed puberty. J Clin Endocrinol Metab 1996; 81: 1152–1155.

88. Kocova M, Siegel SF, Wenger SL, Lee PA, Trucco M. Detection of Y chromosome sequences in Turner's syndrome by Southern blot analysis of amplified DNA. Lancet 1993: 342:140–143.

89. Kosho T, Muroya K, Nagai T, et al. Skeletal features and growth patterns in 14 patients with haploinsufficiency of SHOX; implications for the development of Turner syndrome. J Clin Endocrinol Metab 1999; 84:4613–4621.

90. Clement-Jones M, Schiller S, Rao E, et al. The short stature homeobox gene SHOX is involved in skeletal abnormalities in Turner syndrome. Hum Mol Genet 2000; 9: 695–702.

91. Pasquino AM, Passeri F, Pucarelli I, Segni M, Municchi G, on behalf of the Italian Study Group of Turner's syndrome. Spontaneous pubertal development in Turner's syndrome. J Clin Endocrinol Metab 1997; 82:1810–1813.

92. Veitia R, Ion A, Barbaux S, Jobling MA, Souleyreau N, Ennis K, Ostrer H, Tosi M, Meo T, Chibani J, Fellous M, McElreavey K. Mutations and sequence variants in the testis-determining region of the Y chromosome in individuals with a 46,XY female phenotype. Hum Genet 1997; 99:648–652.

93. Jager RJ, Anvret M, Hall K, Scherer G. A human XY female with a frame shift mutation in the candidate testis-determining gene SRY. Nature 1990; 348:452–454.

94. Vilain E, McElreavey K, Jaubert F, et al. Familial case with sequence variant in the testis-determining region associated with two sex phenotypes. Am J Hum Genet 1992; 50:1008–1011.

95. Bardoni B, Zanaria E, Guioli S, Floridia G, Worley KC, Tonini G, Ferrante E, Chiumello G, McCabe ER, Fraccaro M, et al. A dosage sensitive locus at chromosome Xp21 is involved in male to female sex reversal. Nat Genet 1994; 7:497–501.

96. Mendonca BB, Barbose AS, Arnhold IJP, et al. Gonadal agenesis in XX and XY sisters: Evidence for the involvement of an autosomal gene. Am J Med Genet 1994; 52:39–43.

97. Bosze P, Skripeczky K, Gaal M, Toth A, Laszlo J. Perrault's syndrome in two sisters. Am J Med Genet 1983; 16:237–241.

98. Fechner PY, Marcantonio SM, Ogata T, et al. Report of a kindred with X-linked (or autosomal dominant sex-limited) 46XY partial gonadal dysgensis. J Clin Endocrinol Metab 1993; 76:1248–1253.

99. Yanase T, Simpson ER, Waterman FR. 17-Alpha-hydroxylase/17,20-lyase deficiency; from clinical investigation to molecular definition. Endocr Rev 1991; 12:91–108.

100. Rivkees SA, Crawford JD. The relationship of gonadal activity and chemotherapy-induced gonadal damage. JAMA 1988; 259:2123–2125.

101. Poplack DG. Acute lymphoblastic leukemia. In: Pizzo PA, Poplack DG, eds. Principles and Practice of Pediatric Oncology. Philadelphia: JB Lippincott, 1989:323.

102. LaBarbera AR, Miller MM, Ober C, et al. Autoimmune etiology in premature ovarian failure. Am J Reprod Immunol Microbiol 1988; 16:115–122.

103. Kaufman FR, Xu YK, Ngo WG, et al. Gonadal function and ovarian galactose metabolism in classic galactosemia. Acta Endocrinol (Copenh) 1989; 120:129–133.

104. Stavrou SS, Zhu YS, Cai LQ, Katz MD, Herrera C, Defillo-Ricart M, Imperato-McGinley J. A novel mutation of the human luteinizing hormone receptor in 46XY and 46XX sisters. J Clin Endocrinol Metab 1998; 83:2091–2098.

105. Latronico AC, Chai Y, Arnhold IJ, et al. A homozygous microdeletion in helix 7 of the luteinizing hormone receptor associated with familial testicular and ovarian resistance is due to both decreased cell surface expression and impaired effector activation by the cell surface receptor. Mol Endocrinol 1998; 12:442–450.

106. Beau I, Touraine P, Meduri G, Gougeon A, Desroches A, Matuchansky C, Milgrom E, Kuttenn F, Misrahi M. A novel phenotype related to partial loss of function mutations of the follicle stimulating hormone receptor. J Clin Invest 1998; 102:1352–1359.

107. Touraine P, Beau I, Gougeon A, Meduri G, Desroches A, Pichard C, Detoeuf M, Paniel B, Prieur M, Zorn JR, Milgrom E, Kuttenn F, Misrahi M. New natural inactivating mutations of the follicle-stimulating hormone receptor: correlations between receptor function and phenotype. Mol Endocrinol 1999; 13:1844–1854.

108. Quigley CA, DeBellis A, Marschke KB, el-Awady MK, Wilson EM, French FS. Androgen receptor defects: historical, clinical, and molecular perspectives. Endocr Rev 1995; 16:271–321.

109. Gottlieb B, Lehvaslaiho H, Beitel LK, et al. The androgen receptor gene mutations database. Nucl Acids Res 1998; 26:234–238.

110. Mansfield MJ, Emans SJ. Anorexia nervosa, athletics, and amenorrhea. Pediatr Clin North Am 1989; 36:533–549.

111. Boas SR, Fulton JA, Koehler AN, Orenstein DM. Nutrition and pulmonary function predictors of delayed puberty in adolescent males with cystic fibrosis. Clin Pediatr 1998; 37:573–576.

112. Habiby RL, Boepple P, Nachtigall L, Sluss PM, Crowley WF Jr, Jameson JL. Adrenal hypoplasia congenita with hypogonadotropic hypogonadism. Evidence that DAX-1 mutations lead to combined hypothlamic and pituitary defects in gonadotropin production. J Clin Invest 1996;98:1055–1062.

113. De Sanctis V, Vullo C, Katz M, et al. Gonadal function in patients with thalassaemia major. J Clin Pathol 1988; 41:133–137.

114. Matthews CH, Borgato S, Beck-Peccoz P, et al. Primary amenorrhoea and infertility due to a mutation in the ßsubunit of follicle-stimulating hormone. Nat Genet 1993; 5:83–86.

115. Berga SL, Mortola JF, Girton L, et al. Neuroendocrine aberrations in women with functional hypothalamic amenorrhea. J Clin Endocrinol Metab 1989; 68:301–308.

116. Cheyne KL, Lightner ES, Comerci GD. Bromocriptine-unresponsive prolactin macroadenoma in a prepubertal female. J Adolesc Health Care 1988; 9:331–334.

117. Howlett TA, Wass JAH, Grossman A, et al. Prolactinomas presenting as primary amenorrhea and delayed or arrested puberty: response to medical therapy. Clin Endocrinol 1989; 30:131–140.

118. Kelly TM, Edwards CO, Meikle AW, Kushner JP. Hypogonadism in hemochromatosis: reversal with iron depletion. Ann Intern Med 1984; 101:629–632.

119. Soyka LA, Grinspoon S, Levitsky LL, Herzog DB, Kllibanksi A. The effects of anorexia nervosa on bone metabolism in female adolescents. J Clin Endocrinol Metab 1999; 84:4489–4496.

120. Pugliese MT, Lifshitz F, Grad G, et al. Fear of obesity. A cause of short stature and delayed puberty. N Engl J Med 1983; 309:513–518.

121. Veldhuis JD, Evans WS, Demers LM, et al. Altered neuroendocrine regulation of gonadotropin secretion in women distance runners. J Clin Enclocrinol Metab 1985; 61:557–563.

122. Green JS, Parfrey PS, Harnett JD, et al. The cardinal manifestations of Bardet-Biedl syndrome, a form of Laurence-Moon-Biedl syndrome. N Engl J Med 1989; 321:1002–1009.

123. Rey R, Lordereau-Richard I, Carel JC, Barbet P, Cate RL, Roger M, Chaussain JL, Josso N. Anti-müllerian hormone and testosterone serum levels are inversely related during normal and precocious pubertal development. J Clin Endocrinol Metab 1993; 77:1220–1226.

124. Navot D, Laufer N, Kopolovic J, Rabinowitz R, Birkenfeld A, Lewin A, Granat M, Margalioth EJ, Schenker JG. Artifically induced endometrial cycles and the establishment of pregnancies in the absence of ovaries. N Engl J Med 1986; 314: 806–811.

125. Mazur T, Clopper RR. Pubertal disorders—psychology and clinical management. Endocrinol Metab Clin North Am 1991; 20:211–230.

10

Turner Syndrome

E. Kirk Neely

Stanford University Medical Center, Stanford Medical School, Stanford, California, U.S.A.

Ron G. Rosenfeld

Oregon Health and Science University and Doernbecher Children's Hospital, Portland, Oregon, U.S.A.

I. INTRODUCTION

Humans need an intact X chromosome to survive. When all (or part) of the second sex chromosome (the X or the Y chromosome) is absent, a characteristic prenatal and postnatal phenotype results. Of the small percentage that survive to term, affected individuals are phenotypic females with dysgenetic ovaries, short stature, and other typical but highly variable dysmorphic features (Fig. 1).

Otto Ullrich first described the syndrome in a case report in the German literature in 1930 and later recognized the neonatal presentation with lymphedema. University of Oklahoma Professor Henry Turner, whose name is inextricably linked with the syndrome, described seven patients with "infantilism, congenital webbed neck, and cubitus valgus" in 1938 (2). Turner became the first physician to use medical therapies in patients with Turner syndrome (TS), administering injections of various pituitary extracts and estrogen-containing preparations to several of his patients. Rudimentary ovaries ("streak gonads") were identified as the cause of Turner's sexual infantilism in 1944 by Wilkins and Fleishman (3), and the term 45,X gonadal dysgenesis is often used to identify TS (4). Other manifestations of the syndrome were catalogued during this period and collectively termed Turner stigmata (5).

TS was associated with X chromosome monosomy in 1959 by Ford et al. (6) in a prepubertal 14-year-old with short stature and typical features. The development of routine cytogenetic analysis in the 1960s led to recognition of the diversity of chromosomal complements associated with TS (7, 8). Most patient series have reported that approximately half of TS patients have a 45,X karyotype, while others have a mosaicism of 45,X cells with normal cells or with structural anomalies of the second X, the

most common being isochromosome (duplication) of the long arm (9). Mosaicism is more common, however, when stringent cytogenetic methods are utilized. The relative proportions of karyotypes found in representative patient series are presented in Table 1 (10, 11).

II. FEATURES OF TURNER SYNDROME

A. Ascertainment Patterns

TS may be detected incidentally during prenatal diagnostic procedures for advanced maternal age, and it appears that the majority of these pregnancies are electively terminated. Unlike trisomies or Klinefelter syndrome, the incidence of TS does not increase with maternal age (12), therefore a relatively small proportion of affected fetuses are ascertained. TS is also suspected, like other aneuploidies, by increased nuchal thickness or other ultrasonographic anomaly, such as aortic coactation, or by elevated maternal α-fetoprotein, estriol, or β-human chorionic gonadotropin (βhCG), leading to confirmation by karyotyping.

Perhaps a third of TS patients are identified at birth by pterygium coli (webbed neck), lymphedema of the hands and feet, or coarctation of the aorta. Most of these infants have 45,X karyotypes (Fig. 2; 13), because these physical findings, in contrast with other stigmata of TS, are more common in patients with complete X monosomy than in patients with mosaicism or structural abnormality of the X.

TS is additionally suspected in many girls in early to midchildhood when growth failure results in a height noticeably below the normal range. Nevertheless, many patients will not be recognized until pubertal failure or short

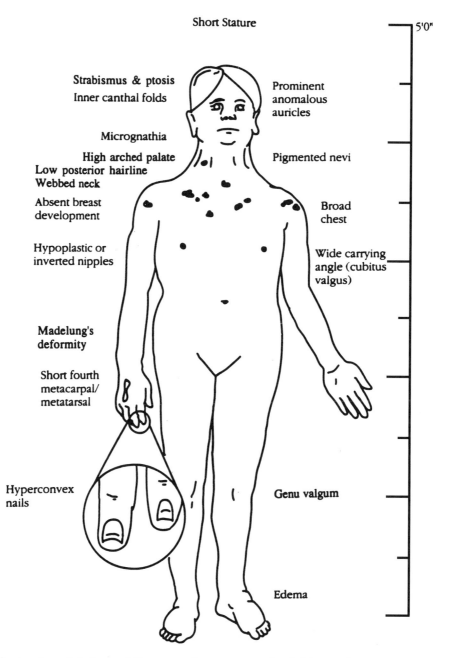

Figure 1 Schematic drawing of features of Turner syndrome commonly visible on physical examination. (Modified from Rosenfeld RG, Turner syndrome: a guide for physicians. Turner syndrome Society, Wayzata, Minnesota, 1989.)

stature in the teenage years leads to medical evaluation. The diagnosis may even be delayed until referral in adulthood for primary or secondary amenorrhea, infertility, or recurrent miscarriage. Patients also are occasionally detected on the basis of one of the less evident features of TS, such as facial or bony abnormalities, learning problems, strabismus, or otitis or hearing loss. It is likely that some patients with mosaicism have manifestations that are mild enough to escape detection altogether.

B. Fetal Demise

X monosomy is the most commonly occurring sex chromosome anomaly, but 90% or more of Turner conceptuses are spontaneously aborted. It is probable that more than 1% of conceptions involve X chromosome loss. As many as 10% of spontaneously aborted fetuses have 45,X karyotypes (14). As a result, TS is common prenatally but occurs with an incidence of only about 1:2000–2500 live

Table 1 Percentages of Karyotypes in Four Series of Patients with Turner Syndrome

Karyotype	Palmer and Reichman (9)	Hall et al. (10)	Park et al. (11)	Held et al. (17)
45,X	58.2	55.0	61.2	20.7
46,XisoXq	7.3	5.5	6.0	5.7
Mosaicism (with 45,X)				
/46,XX	8.2	13.4	11.2	17.2
/46,XisoXq	11.8	4.7	7.8	12.6
/46,XringX	5.5	3.9	1.7	3.5
/46,XY	5.4	3.1	2.6	2.3
/46,XXp-	0.9	0.8	2.6	2.3
/46,XXq-	0	1.6	1.7	3.5
/47,XXX and /46,XX/47,XXX	1.8	0.8	0.9	6.9
/46,X+marker	0	0.8	0	18.4

female births, making the syndrome less common postnatally than either 45,XXY (Klinefelter syndrome) or 45,XXX. Because the peak of fetal deaths occurs at about 12 weeks of gestation, most 45,X fetuses are spontaneously aborted prior to amniocentesis. A smaller proportion of fetuses is aborted in the second trimester, with autopsy findings of massive lymphedema and cystic nuchal hygroma (15).

It has been contended that all fetuses with 45,X karyotypes are spontaneously aborted and that all liveborn individuals with TS, due to early mitotic errors, are X chromosome mosaics, whether cytogenetically detectable or occult (14, 16). Aborted fetuses with X chromosome loss are, indeed, overwhelmingly 45,X, implying a relative fetoprotective effect of mosaicism. By employing techniques such as PCR and FISH, Held et al. (17) were able to document approximately 80% mosaicism in live-

born TS, largely by the detection of small marker chromosomes in some cell populations (Table 1). Mosaicism may be present in multiple tissues without detectability in blood cells, and presence of mosaicism in the trophoblast or in placental tissue might be all that is required to avoid lethality. A recent study uncovered a previously unreported sex chromosome mosaicism in 90% of TS patients, primarily by FISH for X and Y markers (18). It seems clear that mosaicism occurs more commonly that usually reported, but obligate mosaicism in liveborn TS has not been unassailably proven.

C. Cardiac Anomalies

Echocardiography should be performed as soon as the diagnosis of TS is confirmed. Long known to be associated with TS, coarctation of the aorta occurs in 10–15% of TS patients (19–21). Echocardiography has revealed other common left-sided anomalies in TS, including aortic stenosis, aortic insufficiency, and anomalous pulmonary venous return (Table 2). The most frequent anomaly is probably bicuspid aortic valve, either alone or associated with an accompanying lesion such as coarctation (22). Both aortic coarctation and bicuspid aortic valve occur more commonly in association with a 45,X karyotype than with mosaicism or structural abnormality of the X. The spectrum of left-sided cardiac lesions in TS includes the hypoplastic left heart syndrome (23, 24), which, like aortic coarctation, is an indication for chromosomal analysis in a female fetus or infant (25).

In studies of second trimester fetal pathology, a high frequency of these types of heart vessel defects has been noted in association with edema, nuchal cystic hygromas, and lymphatic aberrations at the base of the major vessels, suggesting a causal link between lymphedema and cardiac anomalies (26). However, cardiac anatomy has been normal in many fetuses with severe edema, and the cause of cardiac defects remains conjectural (see discussion of SHOX, below).

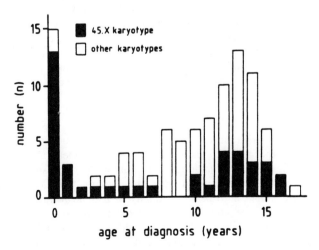

Figure 2 Age of diagnosis in 100 patients with TS. Note the greater percentage of patients with 45,X karyotype diagnosed in infancy. (From Ref. 13.)

Table 2 Prevalence of Cardiac Malformations in Turner Syndrome by Echocardiography in Three Large Series

	Gøtzsche (19)	Sybert (20)	Mazzanti (21)
Total subjects (n)	179	244	594
Subjects with structural abnormalities (%)	46 (26)	96 (40)	136 (23)
Coarctation	18 (10)	34 (14)	41 (7)
Bicuspid valve	25 (14)	28 (11)	74 (13)
Aortic stenosis/insufficiency	5 (3)	11 (5)	19 (3)
Anomalous pulmonary venous drainage	NA	2 (1)	17 (3)
Other (ASD, VSD, hypoplastic left, etc.)	0 (0)	25 (10)	17 (3)

In clinical terms, TS patients are at risk for catastrophic aortic dissection and aneurysmal rupture; more than 50 cases have been reported to date (19, 27, 28). Most aortic ruptures in TS are thoracic. Most of the fatalities have occurred in young women with pre-existing cardiac anomaly or hypertension, but a significant percentage of deaths has occurred in individuals without known risk factors. Cardiac evaluation is mandatory in any TS patient with chest pain or shortness of breath. Mild aortic root dilation (about +1 standard deviation [SD]) by echocardiography or magnetic resonance imaging (MRI) is observed in TS girls matched with controls for body size, but it is not known whether routine follow-up echocardiography is helpful in anticipating aortic dissection. We currently recommend regular cardiological and echocardiographic follow-up for those with a cardiac lesion or hypertension, and repeat echocardiography in all other TS patients at cessation of growth therapy.

D. Renal Anomalies and Hypertension

Renal ultrasound is recommended for all patients at the time of diagnosis. The cause of renal abnormalities in TS is unknown, and cardiac and renal anomalies usually occur independently. Most renal anomalies are silent and do not become clinically significant. Renal dysmorphism was documented by ultrasound in one-third of 141 patients with various karyotypes in the early series of Lippe et al. (29). The most frequent abnormalities were double collecting systems, horseshoe kidney, and rotational abnormalities, each occurring in 5–10% of patients. Abnormalities requiring urological referral included ureteropelvic and ureterovesicle junction obstruction (6%) and absent kidney (3%). In their study, the incidence of renal dysmorphology in girls with 45,X karyotype was 45%, compared with 18% in other karyotypes combined. The greater prevalence of some renal anomalies in 45,X has been confirmed by at least two more recent patient series. A Turkish study of 82 TS patients found the prevalence of horseshoe kidney to be 11%, with eight of nine associated with a 45,X karyotype, whereas collecting duct abnormalities (overall 21%) were as likely with mosaicism or X structural abnormality (30).

Hypertension is common in adolescents and adults with TS. Although elevated pressures secondary to renal causes can occur, hypertension in TS is usually essential. A recent study documented systolic pressures above the 95th percentile in 21% of adolescents with TS (31, 32).

E. Craniofacial and Skeletal Anomalies

The facial appearance of girls with TS may include epicanthal folds, ptosis, downslanting palpebral fissures, maxillary and mandibular hypoplasia, prominent or malformed ears, neck webbing, low hairline, and short neck. Many of these features may represent consequences of fetal edema. However, patients may have few of these phenotypic characteristics, and the features most classically associated with TS, neck webbing and low hairline, are only present in a minority of girls. Reconstructive surgery of the ears or neck is controversial, due to the reported frequency of keloid formation.

Patients may have a high arched palate, which can contribute to the feeding difficulties commonly encountered in infancy or to speech problems. Anatomical anomalies at the cranial base probably alter the angle of the eustachian tube, leading to the high incidence of otitis media. Sinusitis and mastoiditis are also common. Incidence of hearing loss in TS, which can be either conductive or sensorineural, may be as high as 30% in children and 90% in adults (33, 34). The small jaw and high palate are associated with orthodontic problems, such as crowding and malocclusion (35).

Diverse bone abnormalities are found in TS, but they are usually documented only after the diagnosis has been made (36). The most common anomalies are short fourth metacarpal and cubitus valgus. Infrequent skeletal abnormalities include Madelung's deformity of the wrist, sternal deformities, and genu valgum. The common bone abnormalities appear to be seen equally in patients with 45,X monosomy, structural abnormality, or mosaicism. Cubitus valgus and Madelung's wrist deformity are easily seen on physical examination, and short fourth metacarpal is found on examination or on bone age films. Patients should be routinely evaluated for scoliosis, which may worsen as growth therapies are initiated. Congenital dislocation of the hip may be seen in infants with TS. Many investigators have documented short-leggedness and abnormal body segment ratios in TS, and patients tend to exhibit a short, "square" body habitus (37). The appearance of widely spaced nipples (shield chest) may be attributable to this phenomenon.

F. Osteopenia

Osteopenia has been widely reported in adults with TS, but the relative contributions of an underlying bone dysplasia or insufficient acquisition and maintenance of bone mass, due to a presumably avoidable hypoestrogenism, are still unclear. Typical modern assessment of bone mineral is by dual X-ray absorptiometry (DXA) determination of bone mineral content (BMC) and density (BMD). Since both are dependent upon body and bone size, DXA underestimates bone density in TS, unless adjusted volumetrically or interpreted using appropriately matched controls.

In a survey of Swedish TS patients, half of those over 45 years old had osteopenia by DXA (38), and even patients receiving long-term estrogen replacement therapy had deficits in spine and radial bone density. In a report by Stepan (39) mean lumbar BMD was -4.5 SD in untreated subjects and -2.3 SD in those who had received estrogen replacement. Sylven et al. (40), comparing 47 TS women (mean age 47.9 years) with controls matched for age and weight, found a mean whole body BMD of -1.23 SD in the TS subjects; length of hormonal replacement therapy was found to be the significant variable. In another study evaluating BMD and fracture rate in 40 TS patients and 40 subjects with other forms of primary amenorrhea (PA), BMD was low in both TS and PA compared with controls (41). Corrected for height and weight, the TS group had a better bone density measure than the PA group, but fractures were increased in both groups.

Taken together, these studies argue that osteopenia can be a problem in TS, potentially leading to fractures. Nevertheless, there are no convincing reports of increased rates of spinal compression and hip fractures in Turner women. This is surprising given that for each standard deviation that BMD falls below the mean in the normal population, the risk of pathological fracture rises two- to threefold. Furthermore, rather than some intrinsic skeletal factor, the treatable hypoestrogenism is the most important element leading to low bone mineral in adult TS patients.

Reports of osteopenia in children and adolescents with TS are unconvincing and have not always been careful in controlling for body size or delay in estrogenization (42–47). Our group has reported that adolescents with TS receiving growth hormone (hGH) therapy exhibit normal bone mineral properties (44), a finding confirmed by other groups. In another study of 19 TS adolescents receiving hGH and ethinyl estradiol, phalangeal DXA BMD was normal both at baseline and 3 years after discontinuation of growth hormone (45). There is only slight evidence that

hGH contributes to bone mineral other than indirectly by increase in body size, whereas estrogen augments bone density in adolescents and adults independently of growth.

G. Gonadal Dysgenesis

Gonadal dysgenesis is one of the hallmarks of partial or complete X chromosome loss. In most 45,X individuals during childhood, the ovaries are already gonadal streaks consisting of fibrous stroma with diminished numbers of primordial follicles. Histological studies of the gonadal ridge have documented normal densities of primordial germ cells at 12 weeks of gestation, but in the early second trimester oocyte formation and folliculogenesis fail to occur normally and connective tissue proliferates. Oocytes undergo premature atresia in a highly variable manner that may be completed before birth or may continue into adolescence or adulthood (49). The phenotypic manifestations of the declining numbers of functioning ovarian follicles constitute a spectrum from absence of any pubertal development in 70–80% of girls, to midpubertal failure in 10–20%, or to failure to progress to menses, secondary amenorrhea, or early menopause.

Ovarian failure is reflected in reduced steroid feedback on the hypothalamic–pituitary axis and marked elevations in serum follicle-stimulating hormone (FSH) and luteinizing hormone (LH). Most infants and adolescents with TS have markedly elevated FSH values, indicative of ovarian failure. Although not clearly established, it is likely that FSH is moderately elevated throughout the prepubertal period. As many as a third of TS patients may exhibit breast budding, but fewer than 10%, mostly with a 45,X/46, XX karyotype, complete pubertal development and reach menarche spontaneously. Thus, estrogen replacement for secondary sexual development is required in most girls with TS. Pregacy occurs in an occasional TS patient, predominantly but not exclusively in those with mosaic karyotypes. In these cases, miscarriages are common and prenatal diagnosis is advised due to the increased incidence of chromosomal anomalies in the offspring.

Massarano et al. reported the ultrasound appearance of ovaries in 104 TS girls of varying ages (50). The ovaries of two-thirds of the subjects were classified as streak gonads, with ovarian volumes in the remaining one-third of subjects in the lower range of normal. Because the incidence of spontaneous puberty correlates with ovarian volume (51), it is not unreasonable to obtain an ovarian ultrasound concurrently with the initial renal ultrasound, taking care to warn families of the predictive imprecision of the information. Ovaries that are near-normal in size can be most easily detected in infants and toddlers or in girls of pubertal age, matching the temporal pattern of gonadotropin stimulation. Prepubertal uterine volumes are in the normal range, consistent with the anatomically normal, hormonally responsive uterus found in patients with TS. Although the vagina and external genitalia are usually normal in TS, vaginal atresia has been reported, and genital ambiguity can occur in 45,X/46,XY individuals.

From a management point of view, it is important to remember that progressive follicular atresia results in two functional deficits: failure to secrete estrogen and progesterone on the one hand, and loss of germ cells and infertility on the other. For the pediatric endocrinologist, only the former requires medical intervention, as is discussed below. Nevertheless, families appreciate a frank discussion of the probability of infertility and potential options, including adoption and assisted reproductive technologies. Pregnancy in TS following oocyte donation has approximately the same success rate as in the general population (52). Freezing ovarian wedges is theoretically an option; if fertilization and implantation of these oocytes later in life are successful, the issue of chromosomal defects arises.

H. Stature and Body Composition

Manifestation of growth failure in TS begins with mild intrauterine growth retardation. Mean birthweight is about 2800 g, a relatively mild deficit that is ordinarily overlooked. Although growth velocity in the first few years of life has been considered relatively normal, Davenport has

recently emphasized from longitudinal studies that mean height SDS falls from −0.5 at birth to −1.8 at 18 months of age, with a continuing decline during childhood (53). Nevertheless, the 95th percentile of the TS curve does not diverge from the 5th percentile of the normal female curve until 9 years of age (Fig. 3), so that in many girls TS is not diagnosed until late in childhood. Growth failure becomes even more obvious in adolescence, due to the absence of a pubertal growth spurt, and the height nadir in TS relative to normal females occurs at about 14 years of age. In the absence of growth therapy, most TS patients continue to exhibit slow, consistent growth during late adolescence, due to delayed bone maturation and epiphyseal fusion, with typical closure after 17 years old in the absence of hormonal interventions. Historically, this delay has afforded some measure of catch-up growth before complete cessation.

Lyon et al. (54) combined their growth data with those from other European studies to create growth standards for TS in the absence of hormonal therapy. The Lyon curve, as well as other growth standards (55, 56), provides an important means of evaluating growth therapies. These standard curves permit an accurate projection of adult height on the basis of the current height, and a high degree of correlation has been demonstrated between

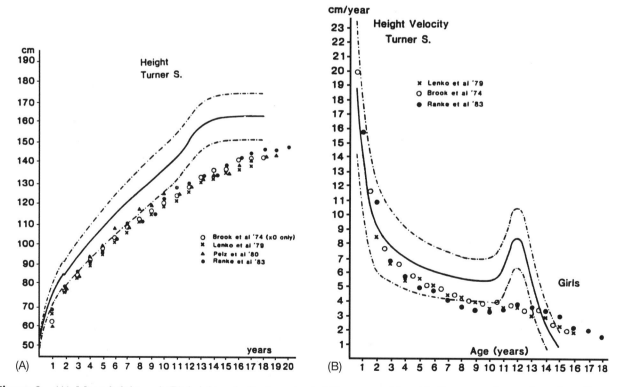

Figure 3 (A) Mean height and (B) height velocity in untreated European girls with Turner syndrome from four European studies, plotted on the growth curve for normal females. Note the steady decline in height velocity beginning in early childhood and the absence of a pubertal growth spurt. (From Ref. 54.)

first measured height in childhood and final adult height (57). Adult heights projected on the basis of standardized curves are as accurate as heights predicted from bone age, which may be difficult to interpret in TS (58). The mean final height of the Lyon curve is 142.9 cm, a figure close to the height reported for the combined European–American experience over the last 20 years. Mean heights of approximately 147 cm are reported in untreated TS populations of Northern European descent (59, 60). Final height in TS is clearly affected by parental height and ethnic group; as a rule of thumb, untreated adults with TS are approximately 20 cm shorter than expected from midparental target height.

The effect of karyotype on the height deficit should generally be minimized. Subjects who are mosaic for ring X and isoXq are just as short as 45,X subjects, whereas those with 46,XX and 46,XY mosaicisms may be on average slightly taller, but there is no consensus in the literature. The influence of spontaneous puberty on adult height also has not been conclusively determined (61, 62). In the minority of patients in whom it occurs, it is generally associated with only a modest pubertal growth spurt, especially if hGH thereapy has already maximized growth velocity, and the pubertal estrogen levels may truncate the duration of growth.

The mean BMI in TS is above age-specific norms except in early childhood, and BMI inceases with age (59, 63). Girls with TS have relatively large trunk, hands, and feet in relation to their height, as well as broad shoulders and pelvis (64), contributing to the short, square appearance. As a group, adults have a higher than expected prevalence of obesity, increased fat mass, and lower lean body mass (65). Consequently, TS adults are vulnerable to comorbidities, such as type 2 diabetes, hypertension, and cardiovascular risk, especially if estrogen deficiency is not adequately treated (66).

I. Causes of Growth Failure

The mechanism of growth failure in TS is poorly understood, but it may be due to the combined effects of aneuploidy (67), a primary skeletal dysplasia, mild growth hormone secretory dysfunction, and estrogen deficiency. Pathological bone development may represent either an intrinsic defect in ossification secondary to loss of critical genes on the X chromosome, such as SHOX (see below), or might be another manifestation of intrauterine edema. However, no consistent histological abnormality has been found in bone tissue of patients with TS. Nevertheless, growth failure is obvious in most girls with TS during childhood, before apparent deficiencies in the growth hormone/insulin-like growth factor (GH/IGF) axis or estrogen production, implying that an intrinsic bone defect, not an endocrine abnormality, is primarily responsible for the short stature of TS.

It is true that a minority of patients with Turner syndrome are GH deficient by provocative GH testing or by

nocturnal GH secretion rates. A recent Italian study reported that 32% did not have GH > 10 μg/L on two provocative tests and 62% had reduced spontaneous GH secretion (68). Diminished GH levels are strongly correlated with high body mass index (69), accounting for much of the variation in GH testing. Furthermore, serum IGF-I levels are generally normal, even in those with diminished GH levels. IGF-I levels do fall below age-related norms in adolescence, probably reflecting estrogen deficiency, a thesis supported by an increase in GH concentrations in response to low-dose estrogen therapy (70–72). GH testing also fails to predict either pretreatment growth rate in TS or responsiveness to exogenous hGH. Accordingly, GH testing and IGF-I (or IGF-binding protein-3 [IGFBP-3]) levels are not needed in the evaluation of TS, although GH deficiency, as well as hypothyroidism and chronic disorder, should be considered in any girl whose height or growth velocity is clearly below normal for TS.

J. Cognition and Behavior

It is essential to remember that individuals with TS are not mentally retarded, as was erroneously reported in some early studies. Later studies have reported an increased prevalence of retardation (full scale IQ less than 80), in addition to aggressiveness and seizure disorder, only in patients carrying a small ring X (73, 74). Paradoxically, this effect is likely not due to loss of X alleles but rather to overexpression of unidentified X genes because of interference with normal expression of the X-inactivating center (XIST) in these small rings (75, 76). There are also occasional reports of autism in 45,X patients (77).

Modern neuropsychological investigations have revealed specific impairments in cognitive functioning in TS. The most commonly reported deficits relate to visual–spatial processing and visual memory, often reported as difficulties on tasks assessing spatial and numerical abilities (78–81). These deficits result in measurable reductions in performance IQ, in contrast with a normal verbal IQ, in TS children and adults. Tests of memory, executive function, and affect recognition may be affected. These deficits are detectable in childhood and into young adulthood. TS subjects also have reduced scores on motor tests. Ross (80, 81) has observed improvement in both motor and nonverbal processing skills during estrogen replacement. Imaging studies have documented various anomalies in brain morphology in TS subjects (82, 83).

Few studies have examined academic outcome in large numbers of subjects, but academic achievement is generally within the mainstream (84), with the exception of mathematics (85). Children with TS are not disruptive in the classroom setting and so may not be referred by the schools for evaluation. Nonetheless, it is crucial that girls with TS receive educational evaluation throughout their school careers. Hearing evaluation is important as an adjunct measure to improve social and academic skills of girls with TS.

Child Behavior Checklist scores from numerous studies in TS children and young adults demonstrate problems in social competence, behavior, and attention. TS girls have reduced self-esteem, more internalizing behavioral problems, and fewer social interactions, and these problems may worsen at the transition to early adolescence (86–90). Physical self-image may be poor, possibly related to peer teasing. Anorexia and clinical depression have been reported. Girls may benefit from psychological counseling during childhood and adolescence.

Skuse et al. (91) compared neuropsychological test results in 80 45,X females aged 6–25 years according to parental origin of the X chromosome. In an initial Achenbach screen, the TS subjects with maternal X (n = 55) had much higher rates of academic failure and social difficulties than those with paternal X (n = 25). On further testing, subjects with an X of paternal origin had superior executive function, better social adjustment, higher verbal IQ, and better verbal memory (92). The authors attributed these findings to maternal imprinting of X chromosome loci, but these putative social and cognitive effects of parental origin of the X need to be confirmed.

K. Autoimmunity

Several types of autoimmunity are found with increased prevalence in TS, including thyroid autoimmunity, inflammatory bowel disease, and rheumatoid arthritis. Although type I diabetes has been reported in TS, it has not been established that the incidence is greater than in controls.

Prevalence in TS of antibodies against thyroid peroxidase and thyroglobulin is 20–30% in several large patient cohorts (93–96). As in a control population, thyroid autoimmunity increases with age from the first to third decade of life. Although occurring in patients with any karyotype, those with long-arm isochromosomes are at highest risk of thyroid autoimmunity (97). Both mothers and fathers of patients with TS have a higher than expected incidence of thyroid autoimmunity (98). This has led to the speculation that familial thyroid autoimmunity might be associated with nondisjunction or related chromosomal defects. As an alternative, maternal thyroid autoimmunity might be associated with a protection against the lethality of X chromsome monosomy in utero (99).

Hypothyroidism (or hyperthyroidism) occurs in 10–20% of TS patients. Individuals should be screened on an annual or biannual basis for thyroid disorder by measurement of TSH, and more frequently if thyroid antibodies have been detected. There does not appear to be an increase in polyglandular autoimmunity associated with thyroid autoimmunity, since islet cell and adrenal antibodies are not elevated.

Both ulcerative colitis and Crohn's disease have a greater than expected prevalence in TS. In a series of 135 TS adults, four had inflammatory bowel disease (100). As with autoimmune thyroid disorders, a disproportionate number of TS patients with inflammatory bowel disease have an X isochromosome (101–102). Intestinal telangiectasia and celiac disease also have been observed in TS. The risk of juvenile rheumatoid arthritis in TS has been estimated to be increased sixfold from a survey of pediatric rheumatology centers (103). The increased risk of these autoimmune disorders in TS mandates that pediatric endocrinologists be attentive to the gastrointestinal and rheumatological complaints of their TS patients.

L. Metabolic Abnormalities

An increased prevalence of diabetes mellitus in TS has been repeatedly cited, but the supportive data are surprisingly weak. An early paper by Forbes and Engel (104) reported from a cohort of 41 TS patients that 6 (15%) had onset of an unspecified type of diabetes after the age of 30. Of interest, all of those with karyotypes reported had an isochromosome X. Since that 1963 paper, there have been no large patient series reporting a meaningful increase in diabetes. However, a hospital records review in all Danish TS patients over a 10 year period (66) reported a higher than expected number of admissions with a diagnosis of either type 1 or type 2 diabetes, clouding the earlier supposition that only the latter might be more common in TS.

Fasting glucose levels have been consistently normal in series of TS subjects. Fasting insulin levels have been reported normal or elevated, with study differences plausibly attributable to the wide normal range. In contrast, an increased frequency of abnormal oral glucose tolerance tests (OGTT) has been compellingly documented in children and adults with TS, including the nonobese (105–110). A review of the literature through 1991 cited a prevalence of abnormal tests of 32.5% in 326 patients, but the reported prevalence in later studies is somewhat lower. The preponderance of evidence points to insulin resistance as the mechanism of carbohydrate intolerance, but earlier papers remarked upon the delayed insulin response to glucose challenge in TS.

Studying 71 TS subjects before and during hGH + oxandrolone therapy, Wilson et al. (106) reported that all girls had normal fasting glucose and insulin levels, both at baseline and during growth therapy. Fifteen percent had an abnormal OGTT at baseline. Integrated glucose and insulin concentrations following oral glucose challenge did not change during hGH treatment, but did rise with the addition of oxandrolone, a finding that was confirmed in other studies. However, other investigators have since demonstrated a rise in both fasting and glucose-stimulated insulin levels during hGH therapy, which may be dose-dependent. The Dutch hGH studies found only a 6% rate of abnormal OGTT that was not increased by hGH, but insulin levels were elevated throughout hGH therapy, albeit reversible at the cessation of treatment (109, 110). Accordingly, it may be prudent to survey patients for carbohydrate intolerance while receiving hormonal therapies in TS.

Mild lipid abnormalities have been reported in TS. Total cholesterol is elevated in adolescents, but not children, and, like insulin resistance, correlates with body mass (111). Growth hormone therapy results in a reduction in low-density lipoprotein and an increase in high density lipoprotein (109). There is no literature to date on the possible physiological benefits of growth hormone therapy in adults with TS. The reported effects of therapeutic estrogen on lipid profiles have been mixed (112, 113).

III. THE GENETIC BASIS OF TS

A. Phenotypic Correlations with Karyotype

The availability of chromosomal analysis in the 1960s allowed for initial attempts to correlate phenotypic manifestations of TS with the variations of X chromosomal loss (114). In his 1965 review, Ferguson-Smith hypothesized that 45,X subjects demonstrated the "complete Turner syndrome" and that the short stature and stigmata of TS were attributable to monosomy of loci on the short arm (7). According to his review of available data, 45,X patients exhibited a higher prevalence of neck webbing, congenital lymphedema, and cardiac malformations than patients with mosaicism or X structural abnormalities. Short stature was a universal feature when the short arm was missing, as in 45,X and karyotypes with long arm isochromosomes. In contrast, normal stature occurred in 20% of 45,X/46,XX, 50% of 45,X/47,XXX, and 63% of long arm deletions. Spontaneous pubertal development and menses, which occurred in only 8% of 45,X patients, were more likely in girls with 45,X/46,XX mosaicism (21%) and deletions of the short arm (25%).

Large patient series since the 1960s have corroborated Ferguson-Smith's summary. Various studies have confirmed the lower incidence of common TS features in certain mosaicisms, although many minor features occur equally in X monosomy and mosaicism. Later improvements in banding techniques and use of X chromosome probes provided a more detailed localization of X chromosome breakpoints, allowing Simpson to provide an updated review of phenotype/karyotype correlations in the late 1970s (115). Location of the breakpoint correlates poorly with the resulting phenotype, and any feature of TS can be seen with major deletion of either Xp or Xq. Nonetheless, there is a crude association of short arm deletions with short stature and of long arm deletions with ovarian dysgenesis. Therman and Susman reviewed the literature on phenotypes of nonmosaic adults with X long or short arm terminal deletions (116). Short stature occurred in 43% and 88% of the Xq and Xp cases, respectively (Table 3). Ovarian failure, including both primary and secondary amenorrhea, occurred in 93% and 65% of

Table 3 Frequency (%) of Phenotypic Features in TS Adults with Complete X Monosomy (45,X), Short Arm Deletion (46,XXp-), or Long Arm Deletion (46,XXq-)

Feature	45,X (n = 332)	46,XXp- (n = 52)	46,XXq- (n = 67)
Short stature	100	88	43
Gonadal dysgenesis	91	65	93
Short neck	77	38	21
Cubitus valgus	77	25	16
"Shield chest"	74	35	13
Low hairline	72	19	9
Delayed bone age	64	17	10
Pigmented nevi	64	27	19
Nail anomaly	57	8	7
Short metacarpal	55	29	12
Renal anomaly	44	8	6
Webbed neck	42	2	1
Hypertension	37	8	7
Cardiac anomaly	23	2	0
Thyroid disease	18	6	3

Source: Adapted from Ref. 117.

Xq and Xp karyotypes, respectively. Essentially the entire pericentromeric region and long arm are involved in ovarian development and maintenance, since deletion breakpoints with apparently identical degrees of ovarian failure are scattered throughout. Lymphedema and cardiovascular anomalies were rare in both short and long arm deletions, compared with 45,X, although lymphedema has resulted from loss of the distal short arm of the Y in XY females.

Identification of parental origin of the remaining X chromosome in TS has been undertaken to look for clues to the causes of X monosomy and to evaluate whether genomic imprinting might explain the phenotypic variation seen with the 45,X karyotype. Different methods have verified that the intact X in 45,X monosomy is maternal (Xm) 70–80% of the time (117). However, there is no difference in the prevalence of maternally or paternally imprinted X in spontaneous abortuses (118), and studies have not discerned any postnatal phenotypic distinctions, other than in the neuropsychological study described above, in 45,X subjects on the basis of parental chromosomal origin.

A model to explain the Turner syndrome phenotype invokes halved expression of a gene or genes on the X chromosome; such a gene must have homologs on the X and the Y and must escape X inactivation. Although many loci on the second X are inactivated throughout all developmental phases and tissues, except in the oocyte and during initial zygotic cell divisions, many other genes that escape X inactivation have been identified in recent years, including the entire pseudoautosomal regions at both termini. Despite sophisticated comprehension of the X chromosome and the rapidly expanding list of genes that escape inactivation (119, 120), there has been relatively slow progress in elucidating the genetic basis of TS since phenotype–karyotype correlations were first drawn 30 years ago.

B. SHOX

The only X chromosome locus to have been convincingly associated with TS is the short-stature homebox-containing (SHOX) gene, located in the pseudoautosomal region of the short arm. Isolated and sequenced independently by two groups of investigators (121, 122), SHOX is highly conserved across species and has two transcripts from alternate splicing: SHOXa is widely expressed, whereas expression of SHOXb is highest in bone marrow fibroblasts. Rao et al. (121) demonstrated deletion of the locus in 36 of 36 short individuals with Xp22 or Yp11.3 breakpoints, and absence of a deletion in normal controls or in subjects with X or Y rearrangements and normal stature. A SHOX mutation was found in 1 of 91 subjects with otherwise unexplained short stature, and other individuals have since been identified.

Belin et al. (123) and Shears et al. (124) reported SHOX deletions in many family members with an autosomal dominant bone dysplasia called Leri-Weill dyschondrosteosis (LWD). Thought to be more severe in females, the syndrome is characterized by a short forearm with Madelung's deformity and limited mobility, tibiofibular shortening, variable metacarpal and metatarsal involvement, and mild short stature (125). In one LWD family, a fetus with Langer mesomelic dysplasia (severe shortening of distal extremities, long considered the homozygous form of LWD) had loss of both SHOX alleles. Thus, loss of one SHOX allele results in LWD, and loss of both results in Langer mesomelic dysplasia.

It was immediately recognized that the SHOX locus meets gene dosage requirements for a Turner gene, being a pseudoautosomal locus, thus not X-inactivated, with a homolog on Yp. Postnatal expression is largely confined to osteogenic cells, such as trabecular cells and bone marrow fibroblasts, correlating with a putative role for the gene in bone physiology. It is also expressed in the pharyngeal arch, suggesting a role in some head and neck anomalies of TS. Although the Turner phenotype is broader and more variable than that of LWD, it seems likely that many of the craniofacial and skeletal features of TS, including cubitus valgus and Madelung's deformity, and some degree of the short stature are due to SHOX haploinsufficiency (126). While other craniofacial and cardiac features may be a consequence of the putative lymphedema locus, SHOX is the first legitimate Turner gene to be identified.

C. Y Chromosome Mosaicism

X chromosomal monosomy occurs in mosaicism with 46,XY cells in 5% or more of patients with Turner syndrome. The phenotype associated with the 45,X/46,XY karyotype, ranging from female to male, provides an interesting story and a cautionary tale about ascertainment bias. The phenotype has historically been described predominantly as ambiguous genitalia and mixed gonadal dysgenesis (streak gonad with dysgenetic testicular elements and possible asymmetry of wolffian and mullerian structures). In an early review, 60% of cases exhibited ambiguous genitalia and mixed gonadal dysgenesis, 25% were phenotypic females with bilateral streak gonads and other features of TS, and the remaining 15% had the appearance of undervirilized males (127). Approximately two-thirds of 45,X/46,XY individuals diagnosed at birth are raised as females. In contrast, 90–95% of the cases diagnosed prenatally have been normal phenotypic males at birth, and features of TS have been rare (128, 129). These data suggest that characteristics of TS are seen less commonly in 45,X/46,XY individuals than in comparable mosaicisms, such as 45,X/46,XX. However, adequate longitudinal studies have not been performed and the incidence of TS features and gonadal dysgenesis may be higher than expected from first reports of normal male external genitalia.

The incidence of gonadal malignancy in 45,X/46,XY mixed gonadal dysgenesis engenders considerable clinical discussion about its translation to the TS patient. In Scully's series of 30 cases of gonadoblastoma, 10 were associated with 45,X/46,XY mosaicism, but most of those individuals had ambiguous genitalia (130). The risk of a patient with this karyotype developing gonadoblastoma/dysgerminoma has been estimated at 15–20%. However, this risk assessment was derived prior to recognition that the postnatal phenotype is usually male, and it undoubtedly overestimates the risk in 45,X/46,XY overall. Nevertheless, gonadoblastomas do occur in unvirilized phenotypic females with this karyotype (TS), and the risk of malignancy, albeit unclear, is greater than in the general population. Based on an increased risk of malignancy and a low likelihood of functional ovarian tissue in the presence of XY mosaicism, gonadectomy should be recommended in these TS patients, at least by adolescence and preferably in early childhood.

This recommendation has consequently raised the question of whether techniques other than routine cytogenetics should be utilized to detect occult Y material in TS. Southern blot, FISH, or PCR analysis of cells from series of TS patients with prior 45,X karyotyping has revealed an incidence of previously undetected Y material ranging from 0 to 15%. Gravholt et al. (131) recently reported Y material in more than 10% of their TS patients, half of them not previously detected by routine cytogenetics. FISH utilizing X- and Y-specific probes can now be performed by most cytogenetics labs and certainly should be utilized to determine the origin of marker chromosomes or small rings (18, 132), either to warn of potential malignancy from Y genetic material or to explain unusual features of TS due to X chromosome fragments. The potential benefit of adjunct FISH studies in all TS patients is not established but warrants further evaluation.

IV. MEDICAL THERAPIES

A. Androgens for Growth

Androgens were utilized for growth promotion in clinical trials in TS prior to the time that human growth hormone (hGH) became widely available (Table 4). Most studies demonstrated short-term efficacy in stimulating growth, and a few reported modest increases in final adult height (133–137). Lenko et al. (134) analyzed growth and final height data in 76 girls treated with fluoxymesterone and/ or conjugated estrogens and found that initial growth velocity was greatest when both were used, but mean final heights were not distinguishable. In a retrospective analysis of 66 TS patients, Sybert (60) reported that the mean adult height of patients given either oxandrolone or fluoxymesterone (148 cm) did not differ significantly from the height of untreated patients (146.3 cm). In contrast, a 3–5 cm increase in final height relative to predicted height was documented in three oxandrolone trials (135–137). As described below, several trials of growth hormone used with and without oxandrolone have shown an improvement in growth and final height from the androgen. Despite this apparent growth benefit and a relatively low cost, androgens are not commonly utilized in the treatment of TS in the United States and only as an adjunct to GH therapy. Oxandrolone has limited androgenic side effects at a dosage of 0.0625 mg/kg per day. As a rule, it

Table 4 Management of Turner Syndrome in Childhood

Medical surveillance
  Karyotype: rule out Y material
  Renal ultrasound
  Echocardiography (repeated in adolescence)
  Regular thyroid screening
  Hypertension monitoring
  Ophthalmology (strabismus, etc.)
  ENT (recurrent otitis) and craniofacial
  Possible orthopedic referral (scoliosis)
  Audiologic evaluation
  Cognitive evaluation
  Psychological counseling
  Dietary advice
  Support groups
Medical therapy
  Begin hGH therapy (0.05 mg/kg per day) by 7–9 years
    old; earlier treatment may be indicated.
  Add oxandrolone (0.0625 mg/kg per day), if hGH is
    started late.
  Initiate estrogen at ±13 years old.
  Cycle with progesterone within 2 years.

can be added to hGH if growth rate is unsatisfactory or if growth therapy has been delayed to a relatively advanced age (>12 years old). In support of the use of androgen in TS is the fact that serum androgens are low in TS adults because of ovarian failure (138).

B. Growth Hormone

Turner himself undertook the first documented administration of growth hormone in TS. His treatment was unsuccessful, presumably utilizing injections of bovine pituitary extract, since human GH from cadavers was not available until the 1950s. In 1960, Escamilla et al. (139) administered pituitary-derived hGH to a patient with TS, resulting in an increase in growth velocity from 3.8 to 7.5 cm/year over several months, a typical degree of first-year growth augmentation from either pituitary-derived or recombinant hGH, which in turn was introduced in the mid-1980s. TS patients constituted the first group after GH deficiency in which clinical trials of recombinant hGH were initiated, principally because of the identifiability and homogeneity of the population and also the lengthy potential treatment period, due to the absence of endogenous puberty.

hGH trials in patients with TS have universally demonstrated an increase in growth velocity. In almost every study, hGH has augmented pretreatment growth velocity by 50–150% in the first year. Many of the early trials combined hGH with estrogens or androgens, both of which had been established as short-term growth stimulants, complicating interpretation of the results. Most early trials used three times a week dosing regimens, and none of the published trials has utilized a randomized control group past the first year. As in hGH treatment of GH deficiency or idiopathic short stature, growth acceleration in girls with TS is sustainable but is most pronounced in the first years of therapy (140).

An early and influential hGH trial in the United States (141) randomized 70 girls at a mean age of 9.3 years to no treatment, oxandrolone, hGH, or both for the first year of therapy. In the second year all subjects except the hGH group were reassigned to a combination group at a reduced oxandrolone dosage (0.0625 mg/kg per day, due to virilization in 30% of subjects at the 0.125 mg dosage). The hGH regimen was switched midstudy to daily (0.05 mg/kg per day) instead of three times weekly. In subjects receiving hGH alone, growth velocity increased from 4.5 cm/year in the pretreatment period to 6.6 and 5.4 cm/year in the first and second year, respectively, whereas growth rates for patients receiving hGH plus oxandrolone were higher at 9.8 and 6.7 cm/year. Compared with a mean adult height of 144.2 cm in historical controls, final heights after hGH and hGH plus oxandrolone were 150.4 and 152.1 cm, respectively, for gains over pretreatment projected height of 8.4 and 10.3 cm, respectively.

The Swedish study (142), also using combination daily hGH and oxandrolone, began at an older mean age of 12.2 years and had no hGH-alone arm. Growth velocity increased from 3.9 cm/year to 9.4 and 6.8 cm/year in the first 2 years of therapy. Final height after combined hGH and oxandrolone therapy was 154.2 cm, which was 8.5 cm greater than the original projected final height. Results of the Swedish, US, and other early studies convinced most investigators that hGH augmented final height in TS, but some doubts persisted because of the lack of long-term randomized controls. This last concern was resolved when preliminary results of a randomized Canadian study using a concurrent untreated control group were presented at the Food and Drug Administration (FDA) hearings prior to approval of hGH for use in TS in 1996. In that study, the mean difference in final height between treatment group and controls was over 6 cm, convincing the remaining doubters that hGH is efficacious in TS.

A significant gain in ultimate height is now beyond controversy, but the expected magnitude of the increase is still being revised as further studies are reported. Key questions of optimal age of initiation and optimal dosage have not been completely resolved. However, it is likely not a coincidence that the greatest height gains have been reported from studies using relatively early starting ages. The TS subjects in the US study gained about 8 cm from hGH alone after beginning therapy at 9 years old, whereas the height gain when age at initiation of hGH is 11–13 years generally has been 6 cm or less, depending upon the use of androgen and estrogen. In the large Genentech hGH database, 622 TS patients treated for a mean 3.7 years beginning at 12.9 years of age had a mean final height of 148.3 cm, for an increase of 6.4 cm over pretreatment projected height (143). Mean height gain was 3.7–4.7 cm in 136 girls with a similar late start in a European Lilly study (144).

In a provocative Dutch study (145), 68 girls were begun on treatment at a dosage of 0.045 mg/kg per day and then randomized to continue receiving that dosage or one increased in subsequent years to 0.0675 or 0.090 mg/kg per day. No estrogens were given until 4 years of hGH therapy had elapsed and the subject reached 12 years of age. Seven year data from all subjects showed that 85% had achieved a height within the normal range for Dutch girls. In the 32 girls who had completed therapy (after a mean 7.3 years), mean heights for the three dose groups were 158.8, 161.0, and 162.3 cm, respectively, with height gains of 12.5, 14.5, and 16.0 cm, respectively. The height gain achieved with hGH alone at the standard dosage, which was far superior to that of any other hGH study in TS, is plausibly attributable to earlier initiation of therapy, averaging 7 years old, plus the standardized delay of estrogen.

Additional height achieved in the Dutch study can be attributed to the higher dosages of hGH in later years of therapy. In a smaller, nonrandomized study, Carel et al. (146) also progressively increased the hGH dosage, to a maximum of 0.1 mg/kg day when growth velocity de-

clined to less than 200% of the pretreatment level. Height gain was 10.6 cm, compared to 5.2 cm in a matched group of 17 patients who had received a fixed dosage of approximately 0.045 mg/kg per day. Thus, it is possible that TS patients could benefit from hGH dosages in later years of therapy in excess of the current standard of 0.05 mg/kg per day.

No studies using dose randomization from the start of hGH therapy have reported completion to final height, but preliminary data from a number of studies suggest that higher dosages do result in faster growth rates in the first year or two of therapy. However, this augmented growth rate may come at the cost of accelerated bone age and diminished growth velocity in later years. In a long-term Japanese study (147), a standard dosage of hGH, as compared with a low dose, stimulated a greater growth velocity for 2 years only, but final heights in the two groups reported to date are not different. Thus, it is unclear whether final height can be significantly improved using higher dosages of hGH from the start.

Several studies have attempted to predict individual response to hGH. In an Australian study, the best response over 2 years occurred in younger, heavier girls with the most delayed bone age and tallest parents (148). In a British study of 52 girls who were prepubertal at the start of therapy, final height gain after 5.8 years averaged 5.2 cm and correlated best with total dose, duration of therapy, and first-year response (149). In a model developed by Ranke et al. from the Pharmacia database (150), hGH dosage was the best predictor of height velocity in year 1 of therapy, with younger age and oxandrolone use associated with higher growth velocities in subsequent years. However, some of these factors may influence only short-term benefit and not result in gain in final height (151). The common theme in these results is the need for a reasonably early initiation of hGH and substantial duration of therapy.

C. Estrogen

Estrogen replacement was also tried historically as a growth therapy in TS. Although estrogen does result in short-term growth acceleration, most studies have failed to document any improvement in final or even predicted adult height, in contrast with androgens or hGH. Indeed, because estrogen is the primary mediator of skeletal maturation, it accelerates short-term growth while abbreviating the duration of growth, as in normal puberty. Not surprisingly, several early TS studies therefore demonstrated that full estrogen replacement during early adolescence resulted in final heights below the expected height in TS (78). Investigators then attempted to identify a reduced dosage of estrogen that might be an effective long-term growth stimulant without causing accelerated skeletal maturation. Significant short-term growth stimulation from low-dosage estrogen was demonstrated, but unfortunately it does not occur without accompanying effects on bone maturation, particularly in younger patients with bone age less than 11 years (152, 153). As a result, there is no perfect dosage of estrogen adequate to achieve a normally timed feminization without inducing an acceleration of bone age and potential reduction in adult height.

Although low or full-dosage estrogen replacement given alone provides a notable growth spurt, little additive growth is observed when estrogen is started during hGH therapy (154, 155). The estrogen-induced advance in skeletal maturation without benefit of substantially greater growth velocity means that early introduction of estrogen therapy can negate gains achieved by hGH therapy. This has now been confirmed in several studies. In the Swedish hGH study mentioned earlier, height gain from the combination of hGH and oxandrolone was 8.5 cm; addition of a relatively low dosage of ethinyl estradiol (100 ng/kg per day) to this regimen at 12 years old resulted in a mean height gain of only 3.2 cm. A second Genentech study (156) randomized 60 girls receiving hGH from a mean of 9.5 years old to begin estrogen at either 12 or 15 years old (Fig. 4). Gains in final height were 5.1 and 8.4 cm in the two groups, respectively. A third cohort of girls who started hGH after 11 years old and began estrogen 1 year later had a mean gain of 4.7 cm. Thus, an effective long-term growth regimen requires reasonably early initiation of hGH, or a lengthy delay in estrogen initiation.

Estrogen therapy is contraindicated in preadolescent patients, plays no legitimate role in growth therapy in TS, and, as a corollary, must be delayed for feminization until certain growth thresholds are achieved. The apparent estrogen-induced acceleration in skeletal age jeopardizes the primary objective of hGH therapy. However, the practice of delaying estrogen replacement until 15 years or older

in an effort to maximize growth, which was the clinical practice prior to introduction of hGH, guarantees significant delays in pubertal development, risks a life-long diminution of bone mineral density, and potentially accentuates the social isolation and stigmatization of girls with TS. A prudent and sympathetic approach is to customize therapy according to the current height, hGH history, and psychological needs of each patient. At a minimum, estrogen should be delayed until 12 years old, but only if a girl has received hGH for 3 years or more. In those with a brief duration of hGH therapy, estrogen may need to be delayed until 13 or even 14 years old.

Balancing the legitimate psychological and physiological need to begin pubertal development against concerns about final height, our typical practice is to begin conjugated estrogens (Premarin) at about 13 years old at an initial dosage of 0.3 mg/day and increasing to 0.625 mg 6–12 months later. Approximately two-thirds of girls will achieve Tanner 3 breast stage after 12 months. After 1–2 years of therapy, estrogens are modified to day 1–26 only and medroxyprogesterone acetate 5–10 mg (Provera) is added on days 17–26, to induce menses and diminish the risk of endometrial hyperplasia or carcinoma. Other estrogen preparations, such as oral ethinyl estradiol (starting at 100 ng/kg per day) or 17β-estradiol, as well as dermal patches, are also effective in feminization (157, 158). Some practitioners believe oral estrogens have more deleterious effects on hepatic metabolism than transdermal preparations. TS patients do have an unexplained baseline elevation in hepatic enzymes, but the relative effects of oral estrogens are unclear (159, 160).

Few direct comparisons of different estrogens for feminization have been made. Indeed, most studies of es-

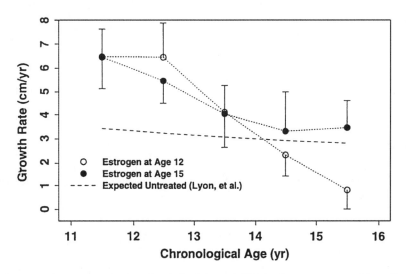

Figure 4 Differences in annual growth velocity after TS girls on hGH begin estrogen at either 12 or 15 years old. (From Ref. 158.)

trogen use in TS have concentrated on the objective of growth stimulation and have failed to provide detailed analysis of the feminizing effects Once progesterones have been added, many TS adolescents and adults prefer oral contraceptive preparations for convenience.

D. Summary

The height deficit in TS is approximately 20 cm. It is tempting to conclude from informal meta-analysis that the portion of the height deficit remediated by hGH depends upon the age therapy is initiated. The expected height gain when hGH is begun at 12 may be only 5 cm, whereas hGH therapy begun at 7 years of age could add in excess of 12 cm. It is therefore prudent to initiate hGH by 7 years old, or earlier if a girl is in the lowest portion of the TS height curve. Better height gains may be achieved by even earlier therapy. Although no data are currently available to prove greater efficacy from an earlier starting age, growth failure is apparent in the first years of life in TS. The standard hGH dosage is 0.05 mg/kg per day, but higher dosages may be justified. We do not routinely attempt to diagnose GH deficiency in TS, unless height is well below that expected from parental height. The optimal time to discontinue hGH has not been established, but convention calls for continued therapy until growth is largely completed, as evidenced by a velocity below 2.5 cm/year.

Oxandrolone increases height by 2–3 cm given alone or combined with hGH , but it is not known if this additive effect occurs when hGH therapy is maximized by an early start or higher doses. Addition of oxandrolone to hGH might allow for earlier termination of therapy and for lower overall medical costs, but its use is customarily limited to adjunct therapy in girls in whom hGH therapy was delayed. Estrogens, in contrast, are not beneficial for growth and may be deleterious for final height if started too early; accordingly, estrogen for feminization should be delayed until 13 years old, preferably after several years of hGH therapy. In tall girls or in those with lengthy duration of hGH treatment, earlier initiation of estrogen may be possible.

REFERENCES

1. Ullrich P. Turner's syndrome and status Bonnevie-Ullrich. Am J Hum Genet 1949; 1:179–202.
2. Turner HH. A syndrome of infantilism, congenital webbed neck, and cubitus valgus. Endocrinology 1938; 23:566–574.
3. Wilkins L, Fleischmann W. Ovarian agenesis: pathology, association with clinical symptoms, and their bearing on the theories of sex differentiation. J Clin Endocrinol Metab 1944; 4:357–368.
4. Grumbach MM, Van Wyk JJ, Wilkins L. Chromosomal sex in gonadal dysgenesis: relationship to male pseudo-hermaphroditism and theories of human sex differentiation. J Clin Endocrinol Metab 1955; 15:1161–1193.
5. Haddad HM, Wilkins L. Congenital anomalies associated with gonadal aplasia. Pediatrics 1959; 23:885.
6. Ford CE, Miller OJ, Polani PE, de Almeida JC, Briggs JH. A sex chromosome anomaly in a case of gonadal dysgenesis (Turner's syndrome). Lancet 1959; 1:711–713.
7. Ferguson-Smith MA. Karyotype–phenotype correlations in gonadal dysgenesis and their bearing on the pathogenesis of malformations. J Med Genet 1965; 2:142–145.
8. Palmer CG, Reichman A. Chromosomal and clinical findings in 110 females with Turner syndrome. Hum Genet 1976; 35:35–42.
9. Otto PG, Vianna-Morgante AM, Otto PA, et al. The Turner phenotype and the different types of human X isochromosome. Hum Genet 1981; 7:159–164.
10. Hall JG, Sybert VP, Williamson RA, Fisher NL, Reed SD. Turner's syndrome. West J Med 1982; 137:32–44.
11. Park E, Bailey JD, Cowell CA. Growth and maturation of patients with Turner's syndrome. Pediatr Res 1983; 17:1–7.
12. Warburton D, Kline J, Stein Z, Susser M. Monosomy X: a chromosomal anomaly associated with young maternal age. Lancet 1980; 1:167.
13. Massa G, Vanderschueren-Lodeweyckx M. Age and height at diagnosis in Turner syndrome: influence of parental height. Pediatrics 1991; 88:1148–1152.
14. Hook EB, Warburton D. The distribution of chromosomal genotypes associated with Turner's syndrome: livebirth prevalence rates and evidence for diminished fetal mortality and severity in genotypes associated with structural X abnormalities or mosaicism Hum Genet 1983; 62:24–27.
15. Canki N, Warburton D, Byrne J. Morphological characteristics of monosomy X in spontaneous abortions. Ann Genet 1988; 31:4–13.
16. Hecht F, Macfarlane JP. Mosaicism in Turner's syndrome reflects the lethality of XO. Lancet 1969; 2:1197–1198.
17. Held KR, Kerber S, Kaminsky E, et al. Mosaicism in 45,X Turner syndrome: does survival in early pregnancy depend on the presence of two sex chromosomes? Hum Genet 1992; 88:288–294.
18. Fernandez-Garcia R, Garcia-Doval S, Costoya S, Pasaro E. Analysis of sex chromosome aneuploidy in 41 patients with Turner syndrome: a study of 'hidden' mosaicism. Clin Genet. 2000; 58:201–208.
19. Gotzsche CO, Krag-Olsen B, Nielsen J, Sorensen KE, Kristensen BO. Prevalence of cardiovascular malformations and association with karyotypes in Turner's syndrome. Arch Dis Child 1994; 71:433–436.
20. Sybert VP. Cardiovascular malformations and complications in Turner syndrome. Pediatr 1998; 101:11.
21. Mazzanti L, Cacciari E. Italian Study Group for Turner Syndrome (ISGTS). Congenital heart disease in patients with Turner's syndrome. J Pediatr 1998; 133:688–692.
22. Miller MJ, Geffner ME, Lippe BM, et al. Echocardiography reveals a high incidence of bicuspid aortic valve in Turner syndrome. J Pediatr 1983; 102:47–50.
23. van Egmond H, Orye E, Praet M, Coppens M, Devloo-Blancquaert A. Hypoplastic left heart syndrome and 45X karyotype. Br Heart J 1988; 60:69–71.
24. Reis PM, Punch MR, Bove EL, van de Ven CJ. Outcome of infants with hypoplastic left heart and Turner syndromes. Obstet Gynecol 1999; 93:532–535.
25. Gembruch U, Baschat AA, Knopfle G, Hansmann M. Results of chromosomal analysis in fetuses with cardiac

anomalies as diagnosed by first- and early second-trimester echocardiography. Ultrasound Obstet Gynecol 1997; 10:391–396.

26. Clarke EB. Web neck and congenital heart defects: a pathogenic association in 45XO Turner syndrome? Teratology 1984; 29:355–361.

27. Allen DB, Hendrich A, Levy JM. Aortic dilation in Turner syndrome. J Pediatr 1986; 109:302–305.

28. Lin AE, Lippe BM, Geffner ME, et al. Aortic dilation, dissection, and rupture in patients with Turner syndrome. J Pediatr 1986; 109:820–822.

29. Lippe B, Geffner ME, Dietrich RB, Boechat MI, Kangarloo H. Renal malformations in patients with Turner syndrome: imaging in 141 patients. Pediatrics 1988; 82: 852–856.

30. Bilge I, Kayserili H, Emre S, Nayir A, Sirin A, Tukel T, Bas F, Kilic G, Basaran S, Gunoz H, Apak M. Frequency of renal malformations in Turner syndrome: analysis of 82 Turkish children. Pediatr Nephrol 2000; 14:1111–1114.

31. Nathwani NC, Unwin R, Brook CG, Hindmarsh PC. Blood pressure and Turner syndrome. Clin Endocrinol 2000; 52:363–370.

32. Nathwani NC, Unwin R, Brook CG, Hindmarsh PC. The influence of renal and cardiovascular abnormalities on blood pressure in Turner syndrome. Clin Endocrinol 2000; 52:371–377.

33. Stenberg AE, Nylen O, Windh M, Hultcrantz M. Otological problems in children with Turner's syndrome. Hear Res 1998; 124:85–90.

34. Barrenasa M, Landin-Wilhelmsenb K, Hansonc C. Ear and hearing in relation to genotype and growth in Turner syndrome. Hear Res 2000; 144:21–28.

35. Simmons KE. Growth hormone and craniofacial changes: preliminary data from studies in Turner's syndrome. Pediatrics 1999; 104:1021–1024.

36. Lubin MB, Gruber HE, Rimoin DL, Lachman RS. Skeletal abnormalities in the Turner syndrome. In: Rosenfeld RG, Grumbach MM, eds. Turner Syndrome. New York: Marcel Dekker, 1990:281–300.

37. Rongen-Westerlaken C, Rikken B, Vastrick P, Jeuken AH, de Lange MY, Wit JM, van der Tweel L, Van den Brande JL. Body proportions in individuals with Turner syndrome. Eur J Pediatr 1993; 152:813–817.

38. Landin-Wilhelmsen K, Bryman I, Windh M, Wilhelmsen L. Osteoporosis and fractures in Turner syndrome—importance of growth promoting and oestrogen therapy. Clin Endocrinol 1999; 51:497–502.

39. Stepan JJ, Musilova J, Pacovsky V. Bone demineralization, biochemical indices of bone remodeling, and estrogen replacement therapy in adults with Turner's syndrome. J Bone Mineral Res 1989; 4:193–198.

40. Sylven L, Hagenfeldt K, Ringertz H. Bone mineral density in middle-aged women with Turner's syndrome. Eur J Endocrinol 1995; 132:47–52.

41. Davies MC, Gulekli B, Jacobs HS. Osteoporosis in Turner's syndrome and other forms of primary amenorrhoea. Clin Endocr 1995; 43:741–746.

42. Rubin K. Turner syndrome and osteoporosis: mechanisms and prognosis. Pediatrics 1998; 102:481–485.

43. Ross JL, Long LM, Feuillan P, Cassorla F, Cutler GB. Normal bone density of the wrist and spine and increased wrist fractures in girls with Turner's syndrome. J Clin Endocrinol Metab 1991; 73:355–359.

44. Neely EK, Marcus R, Rosenfeld RG, Bachrach LK. Bone mineral apparent density is normal in adolescents with

Turner syndrome. J Clin Endocrinol Metab 1993; 76: 861–866.

45. Shaw NJ, Rehan VK, Husain S, Marshall T, Smith CS. Bone mineral density in Turner's syndrome—a longitudinal study. Clin Endocrinol 1997; 47:367–370.

46. Sato N, Nimura A, Horikawa R, Katumata N, Tanae A, Tanaka T. Bone mineral density in Turner syndrome: relation to GH treatment and estrogen treatment. Endocr J 2000; 47 Suppl:S115–S119.

47. Sas TC, De Muinck Keizer-Schrama SM, Stijnen T, Asarfi A, Van Leeuwen WJ, Van Teunenbroek A, Van Rijn RR, Drop SL. A longitudinal study on bone mineral density until adulthood in girls with Turner's syndrome participating in a growth hormone injection frequency-response trial. Clin Endocrinol 2000; 52:531–536.

48. Lanes R, Gunczler P, Esaa S, Martinis R, Villaroel O, Weisinger JR. Decreased bone mass despite long-term estrogen replacement therapy in young women with Turner's syndrome and previously normal bone density. Fertil Steril 1999; 72:896–899.

49. Simpson JL, Rajkovic A. Ovarian differentiation and gonadal failure. Am J Med Genet 1999; 89:186–200.

50. Massarano AA, Adams JA, Preece MA, Brook CGD. Ovarian ultrasound appearances in Turner Syndrome. J Pediatr 1989; 114:568–573.

51. Matarazzo P, Lala R, Artesani L, Franceshini PG, De Sanctis C. Sonographic appearance of ovaries and gonadotropin secretions as prognostic tools of spontaneous puberty in girls with Turner's syndrome. J Pediatr Endocrinol Metab 1995; 8:267–274.

52. Hovatta O. Pregnancies in women with Turner's syndrome. Ann Med 1999; 31:106–110.

53. Davenport ML, Punyasavatsut N, Gunther D, Savendahl L, Stewart PW. Turner syndrome: a pattern of early growth failure. Acta Paediatr Suppl 1999; 88:118–121.

54. Lyon AJ, Preece MA, Grant DB. Growth curve for girls with Turner syndrome. Arch Dis Child 1985; 60:932–935.

55. Ranke MB, Pfluger H, Rosendahl W, et al. Turner syndrome: spontaneous growth in 150 cases and review of the literature. Eur J Pediatr 1983; 141:81–88.

56. Naeraa RW, Nielsen J. Standards for growth and final height in Turner's syndrome. Acta Paediatr 1990; 79: 182–190.

57. Frane JW, Sherman BM, and the Genentech Collaborative Group. Predicted adult height in Turner syndrome. In: Rosenfeld RG, Grumbach MM, eds. Turner Syndrome. New York: Marcel Dekker, 1990:405–419.

58. Schwarze CP, Arens D, Haber HP, Wollmann HA, Binder G, Mayer EI, Ranke MB. Bone age in 116 untreated patients with Turner's syndrome rated by a computer-assisted method (CASAS). Acta Paediatr 1998; 87:1146–1150.

59. Rongen-Westerlaken C, Corel L, van den Broeck J, Massa G, Karlberg J, Albertsson-Wikland K, Naeraa RW, Wit JM. Reference values for height, height velocity and weight in Turner's syndrome. Swedish Study Group for GH treatment. Acta Paediatr 1997; 86:937–942.

60. Sybert VP. Adult height in Turner syndrome with and without androgen therapy. J Pediatr 1984; 104:365–369.

61. Massa G, Vanderschueren-Lodeweyckx M, Malvaux P. Linear growth in patients with Turner syndrome: influence of spontaneous puberty and parental height. Eur J Pediatr 1990; 149:246–250.

62. Page LA. Final heights in 45,X Turner's syndrome with spontaneous sexual development. Review of European

and American reports. J Pediatr Endocrinol 1993; 6:153–158.

63. Blackett PR, Rundle AC, Frane J, Blethen SL. Body mass index (BMI) in turner syndrome before and during growth hormone (GH) therapy. Int J Obesity Rel Metab Disord 2000; 24:232–235.

64. Hojbjerg Gravholt C, Weis Naeraa R. Reference values for body proportions and body composition in adult women with Ullrich-Turner syndrome. Am J Med Genet 1997; 72:403–408.

65. Rongen-Westerlaken C, Rikken B, Vastrick P, et al. Body proportions in individuals with Turner syndrome. Eur J Pediatr 1993; 152:813–817.

66. Gravholt CH, Juul S, Naeraa RW, Hansen JJ. Morbidity in Turner syndrome. Clin Epidemiol 1998; 51:147–158.

67. Haverkamp F, Wolfle J, Zerres K, Butenandt O, Amendt P, Hauffa BP, Weimann E, Bettendorf M, Keller E, Muhlenberg R, Partsch CJ, Sippell WG, Hoppe C. Growth retardation in Turner syndrome: aneuploidy, rather than specific gene loss, may explain growth failure. J Clin Endocrinol Metab 1999; 84:4578–4582.

68. Cavallo L, Gurrado R. Endogenous growth hormone secretion does not correlate with growth in patients with Turner's syndrome. Italian Study Group for Turner Syndrome. J Pediatr Endocrinol Metab 1999; 12:623–627.

69. Pirazzoli P, Mazzanti L, Bergamaschi R, Perri A, Scarano E, Nanni S, Zucchini S, Gualandi S, Cicognani A, Cacciari E. Reduced spontaneous growth hormone secretion in patients with Turner's syndrome. Acta Paediatr 1999; 88:610–613.

70. Cuttler L, Van Vliet G, Conte FA, Kaplan SL, Grumbach MM. Somatomedin-C levels in children and adolescents with gonadal dysgenesis: differences from age-matched normal females and effect of chronic estrogen replacement. J Clin Endocrinol Metab 1985; 60:1087–1092.

71. Massarano AA, Brook CGD, Hindmarsh PC, et al. Growth hormone secretion in Turner's syndrome and influence of oxandrolone and ethinyl estradiol. Arch Dis Child 1989; 64:587–592.

72. Mauras N, Rogol AD, Veldhuis JD. Increased hGH production rate after low-dose estrogen therapy in prepubertal girls with Turner's syndrome. Pediatr Res 1990; 28:626–630.

73. Garron DA. Intelligence among persons with Turner's syndrome. Behav Genet 1977; 7:105–127.

74. Fryns JP, Kleczkowska A, Van Den Berghe H. High incidence of mental retardation in Turner syndrome patients with ring chromosome X formation. Genet Counsel 1990; 38:161–165.

75. Turner C, Dennis NR, Skuse DH, Jacobs PA. Seven ring (X) chromosomes lacking the XIST locus, six with an unexpectedly mild phenotype. Hum Genet 2000; 106:93–100.

76. Matsuo M, Muroya K, Adachi M, Tachibana K, Asakura Y, Nakagomi Y, Hanaki K, Yokoya S, Yoshizawa T. Clinical and molecular studies in 15 females with ring X chromosomes: implications for r(X) formation and mental development. Hum Genet 2000; 107:433–439.

77. Donnelly SL, Wolpert CM, Menold MM, Bass MP, Gilbert JR, Cuccaro ML, Delong GR, Pericak-Vance MA. Female with autistic disorder and monosomy X (Turner syndrome): parent-of-origin effect of the X chromosome. Am J Med Genet 2000; 96:312–316.

78. Rovet J, Netley C. Processing deficits in Turner's syndrome. Dev Psychol 1982; 18:77–94.

79. Bender B, Puck M, Salbenblatt J, Robinson A. Cognitive development of unselected girls with complete and partial x monosomy. Pediatrics 1984; 73:175–182.

80. Ross J, Zinn A, McCauley E. Neurodevelopmental and psychosocial aspects of Turner syndrome. Ment Retard Dev Disabil Res Rev 2000; 6:135–141.

81. Romans SM, Stefanatos G, Roeltgen DP, Kushner H, Ross JL. Transition to young adulthood in Ullrich-Turner syndrome: neurodevelopmental changes. Am J Med Genet 1998; 79:140–147.

82. Reiss AL, Mazzocco MM, Greenlaw R, Freund LS, Ross JL. Neurodevelopmental effects of X monosomy: a volumetric imaging study. Ann Neurol 1995; 38:731–738.

83. Murphy DG, Mentis MJ, Pietrini P, Grady C, Daly E, Haxby JV, De La Granja M, Allen G, Largay K, White BJ, Powell CM, Horwitz B, Rapoport SI, Schapiro MB. A PET study of Turner's syndrome: effects of sex steroids and the X chromosome on brain. Biol Psychiatry 1997; 41:285–298.

84. Swillen A, Fryns JP, Kleczkowska A, Massa G, Vanderschueren-Lodeweyckx M; Van den Berghe H. Intelligence, behaviour and psychosocial development in Turner syndrome. A cross-sectional study of 50 pre-adolescent and adolescent girls (4–20 years). Genet Counsel 1993; 4:7–18.

85. Mazzocco MM. A process approach to describing mathematics difficulties in girls with Turner syndrome. Pediatrics 1998; 102:492–496.

86. Rovet J, Ireland L. Behavioral phenotype in children with Turner syndrome. J Pediatr Psychol 1994; 19:779–790.

87. McCauley E, Ross JL, Kushner H, Cutler G Jr. Self-esteem and behavior in girls with Turner syndrome. J Dev Behav Pediatr 1995; 16:82–88.

88. Pavlidis K, McCauley E, Sybert V. Psychosocial and sexual functioning in women with Turner syndrome. Clin Genet 1995; 47:85–89.

89. Siegel PT, Clopper R, Stabler B. The psychological consequences of Turner syndrome and review of the National Cooperative Growth Study psychological substudy. Pediatrics 1998; 102:488–491.

90. Lagrou K, Xhrouet-Heinrichs D, Heinrichs C, Craen M, Chanoine JP, Malvaux P, Bourguignon JP. Age-related perception of stature, acceptance of therapy, and psychosocial functioning in human growth hormone-treated girls with Turner's syndrome. J Clin Endocrinol Metab 1998; 83:1494–1501.

91. Skuse DH, James RS, Bishop DV, Coppin B, Dalton P, Aamodt-Leeper G, Bacarese-Hamilton M, Creswell C, McGurk R, Jacobs PA. Evidence from Turner's syndrome of an imprinted X-linked locus affecting cognitive function. Nature 1997; 387:705–708.

92. Bishop DV, Canning E, Elgar K, Morris E, Jacobs PA, Skuse DH. Distinctive patterns of memory function in subgroups of females with Turner syndrome: evidence for imprinted loci on the X-chromosome affecting neurodevelopment. Neuropsychologia 2000; 38:712–721.

93. Papendieck LG, Iorcansky S, Coco R, Rivarola MA, Bergada C. High incidence of thyroid disturbances in 49 children with Turner syndrome. J Pediatr 1987; 111:258–261.

94. Radetti G, Mazzanti L, Paganini C, Bernasconi S, Russo G, Rigon F, Cacciari E. Frequency, clinical and laboratory features of thyroiditis in girls with Turner's syndrome. The Italian Study Group for Turner's Syndrome. Acta Paediatr 1995; 84:909–912.

95. Ivarsson SA, Ericsson UB, Nilsson KO, Gustafsson J, Hagenas L, Hager A, Moell C, Tuvemo T, Westphal O,

Albertsson-Wikland K, et al. Thyroid autoantibodies, Turner's syndrome and growth hormone therapy. Acta Paediatr 1995; 84:63–65.

96. Medeiros CC, Marini SH, Baptista MT, Guerra G Jr, Maciel-Guerra AT. Turner's syndrome and thyroid disease: a transverse study of pediatric patients in Brazil. J Pediatr Endocrinol Metab 2000; 13:357–362.

97. de Kerdanet M, Lucas J, Lemee F, Lecornu M. Turner's syndrome with X-isochromosome and Hashimoto's thyroiditis. Clin Endocrinol 1994; 41:673–676.

98. Wilson R, Chu CE, Donaldson MD, Thomson JA, McKillop JH, Connor JM. An increased incidence of thyroid antibodies in patients with Turner's syndrome and their first degree relatives. Autoimmunity 1996; 25:47–52.

99. Schatz R, Maclaren NK, Lippe BM. Autoimmunity in Turner syndrome. In: Rosenfeld RG, Grumbach MM, eds. Turner Syndrome. New York: Marcel Dekker, 1990.

100. Price WH. A high incidence of chronic inflammatory bowel disease in patients with Turner's syndrome. J Med Genet 1979; 16:263–266.

101. Arulanantham K, Kramer MS, Gryboski JD. The association of inflammatory bowel disease and X chromosomal abnormality. Pediatrics 1980; 66:63–67.

102. Hayward PAR, Satsangi J, Jewell DP. Inflammatory bowel disease and the X chromosome. Q J Med 1996; 89:713–718.

103. Zulian F, Schumacher HR, Calore A, Goldsmith DP, Athreya BH. Juvenile arthritis in Turner's syndrome: a multicenter study. Clin Exp Rheumatol 1998; 16:489–494.

104. Forbes AP, Engel E. The high incidence of diabetes mellitus in 41 patients with gonadal dysgenesis, and their close relatives. Metabolism 1963; 12:428–439.

105. Cicognani A, Mazzanti L, Tassinari D, Pellacani A, Forabosco A, Landi L, Pifferi C, Cacciari E. Differences in carbohydrate tolerance in Turner syndrome depending on age and karyotype. Eur J Pediatr 1988; 148:64–68.

106. Wilson DM, Frane JW, Sherman B, et al. Carbohydrate and lipid metabolism in Turner syndrome: effect of therapy with growth hormone, oxandrolone, and a combination of both. J Pediatr 1988; 112:210–217.

107. Weise M, James D, Leitner CH, Hartmann KK, Bohles HJ, Attanasio A. Glucose metabolism in Ullrich Turner syndrome: long-term effects of therapy with human growth hormone. German Lilly UTS Study Group. Horm Res 1993; 39:36–41.

108. Gravholt CH, Naeraa RW, Nyholm B, Gerdes LU, Christiansen E, Schmitz O, Christiansen JS. Glucose metabolism, lipid metabolism, and cardiovascular risk factors in adult Turner's syndrome. The impact of sex hormone replacement. Diabetes Care 1998; 21:1062–1070.

109. van Teunenbroek A, de Muinck Keizer-Schrama SM, Aanstoot HJ, Stijnen T, Hoogerbrugge N, Drop SL. Carbohydrate and lipid metabolism during various growth hormone dosing regimens in girls with Turner syndrome. Dutch Working Group on Growth Hormone. Metabolism 1999; 48:7–14.

110. Sas TC, de Muinck Keizer-Schrama SM, Stijnen T, Aanstoot HJ, Drop SL. Carbohydrate metabolism during long-term growth hormone (GH) treatment and after discontinuation of GH treatment in girls with Turner syndrome participating in a randomized dose-response study. Dutch Advisory Group on Growth Hormone. J Clin Endocrinol Metab 2000; 85:769–775.

111. Ross JL, Feuillan P, Long LM, Kowal K, Kushner H, Cutler GB Jr. Lipid abnormalities in Turner syndrome. J Pediatr 1995; 126:242–245.

112. Lanes R, Gunczler P, Palacios A, Villaroel O. Serum lipids, lipoprotein lp(a), and plasminogen activator inhibitor-1 in patients with Turner's syndrome before and during growth hormone and estrogen therapy. Fertil Steril 1997; 68:473–477.

113. Hojbjerg Gravholt C, Christian Klausen I, Weeke J, Sandahl Christiansen J. Lp(a) and lipids in adult Turner's syndrome: impact of treatment with 17 beta-estradiol and norethisterone. Atherosclerosis 2000; 150:201–208.

114. Neely EK, Rosenfeld RG. Phenotypic correlates of X chromosome loss. In: Wachtel SS, ed. Molecular Genetics of Sex Determination. Orlando, FL: Academic Press, 1993:311–339.

115. Simpson JL. Gonadal dysgenesis and sex chromosome abnormalities: phenotypic-karyotypic correlations. In: Vallet HL, Porter IH, eds. Genetic Mechanisms of Sexual Development. New York: Academic Press, 1979:365–405.

116. Therman E, Susman B. The similarity of phenotypic effects caused by Xp and Xq deletions in the human female: a hypothesis. Hum Genet 1990; 85:175–183.

117. Hassold T, Kumlin E, Takeesu N, et al. Determination of the parenteral origin of sex chromosome monosomy using restriction fragment length polymorphisms. Am J Hum Genet 1985; 37:965–972.

118. Hassold T, Pettay D, Robinson A, Uchida I. Molecular studies of parental origin and mosaicism in 45,X conceptuses. Hum Genet 1992; 89:647–652.

119. Lahn BT, Page DC. Four evolutionary strata on the human X chromosome. Science 1999; 286:964–967.

120. Tsuchiya KD, Willard HF. Chromosomal domains and escape from X inactivation: comparative X inactivation analysis in mouse and human. Mamm Genome 2000; 11:849–854.

121. Rao E, Weiss B, Fukami M, et al. Pseudoautosomal deletions encompassing a novel homeobox gene cause growth failure in idiopathic short stature and Turner syndrome. Nat Genet 1997; 16:54–63.

122. Ellison JW, Wardak Z, Young MF, et al. PHOG, a candidate gene for involvement in the short sature of Turner syndrome. Hum Mol Genet 1997; 6:1341–1347.

123. Belin V, Cusin V, Viot G, et al. SHOX mutations in dyschondrosteosis (Leri-Weill syndrome). Nat Genet 1998; 19:67–69.

124. Shears DJ, Vassal HJ, Goodman FR, et al. Mutation and deletion of the pseudoautosomal gene SHOX cause Leri-Weill dyschondrosteosis. Nat Genet 1998; 19:70–73.

125. Schiller S, Spranger S, Schechinger B, Fukami M, Merker S, Drop SL, Troger J, Knoblauch H, Kunze J, Seidel J, Rappold GA. Phenotypic variation and genetic heterogeneity in Leri-Weill syndrome. Eur J Hum Genet 2000; 8:54–62.

126. Clement-Jones M, Schiller S, Rao E, Blaschke RJ, Zuniga A, Zeller R, Robson SC, Binder G, Glass I, Strachan T, Lindsay S, Rappold GA. The short stature homeobox gene SHOX is involved in skeletal abnormalities in Turner syndrome. Hum Mol Genet 2000; 9:695–702.

127. Hsu LYF. Prenatal diagnosis of 45,X/46,XY mosaicism —a review and update. Prenatal Diagnosis 1989; 9:31–48.

128. Chang HJ, Clark RD, Bachman H. The phenotype of 45,X/46,XY mosaicism: an analysis of 92 prenatally diagnosed cases. Am J Hum Genet 1990; 46:156–168.

129. Wheeler M, Peakman D, Robinson A, et al. 45X/46XY mosaicism: contrast of prenatal and postnatal diagnosis. Am J Med Genet 1988; 29:565–571.

130. Scully RE. Gonadoblastoma: a review of 74 cases. Cancer 1970; 25:1340–1356.

131. Gravholt CH, Fedder J, Naeraa RW, Muller J. Occurrence of gonadoblastoma in females with Turner syndrome and Y chromosome material: a population study. J Clin Endocrinol Metab 2000; 85:3199–3202.

132. Lindgren V, Chen C, Bryke CR, Lichter P, Page DC, Yang-Feng TL. Cytogenetic and molecular characterization of marker chromosomes in patients with mosaic 45,X karyotypes. Hum Genet 1992; 88:393–398.

133. Urban MD, Lee PA, Dorst JP, Plotnick LP, Migeon CJ. Oxandrolone therapy in patients with Turner syndrome. J Pediatr 1979; 94:823–827.

134. Lenko HL, Perheentupa J, Soderholm A. Growth in Turner's syndrome: spontaneous and fluoxymesterone stimulated. Acta Paediatr Scand [Suppl] 1979; 227:57–63.

135. Joss E, Zuppinger K. Oxandrolone in girls with Turner's syndrome. A pair-matched controlled study up to final height. Acta Paediatr 1984; 73:674–679.

136. Naeraa RW, Nielsen J, Pedersen IL, Sorensen K. Effect of oxandrolone on growth and final height in Turner's syndrome. Acta Paediatr 1990; 79:784–789.

137. Crock P, Werther GA, Wettenhall HNB. Oxandrolone increases final height in Turner syndrome. J Paediatr Child Health 1990; 26:221–224.

138. Hojbjerg Gravholt C, Svenstrup B, Bennett P, Sandahl Christiansen J. Reduced androgen levels in adult Turner syndrome: influence of female sex steroids and growth hormone status. Clin Endocrinol 1999; 50:791–800.

139. Escamilla RF, Hutchings JJ, Deamer WC, Li CH. Clinical experiences with human growth hormone (LI) in pituitary infantilism and in gonadal dysgenesis. Acta Endocrinol 1960; 51 suppl:253A.

140. Haeusler G. Growth hormone therapy in patients with Turner syndrome. Horm Res 1998; 49 Suppl 2:62–66.

141. Rosenfeld RG, Attie KM, Frane J, et al. Growth hormone therapy of Turner's syndrome: beneficial effect on adult height. J Pediatr 1998; 132:319–324.

142. Nilsson KO, Albersson-Wikland K, Alm J, et al. Improved final height in girls with Turner's syndrome treated with growth hormone and oxandrolone. J Clin Endocrinol Metab 1996; 81:635–640.

143. Plotnick L, Attie KM, Blethen SL, Sy JP. Growth hormone treatment of girls with Turner syndrome: the National Cooperative Growth Study Experience. Pediatr 1998; 102:479–481.

144. Van den Broeck J, Van Teunenbroek A, Hokken-Koelega A, Wit JM. Efficacy of long-term growth hormone treatment in Turner's syndrome. European Study Group. J Pediatr Endocrinol Metab 1999; 12:673–676.

145. Sas TC, de Muinck Keizer-Schrama SM, Stijnen T, Jansen M, Otten BJ, Hoorweg-Nijman JJ, Vulsma T, Massa GG, Rouwe CW, Reeser HM, Gerver WJ, Gosen JJ, Rongen-Westerlaken C, Drop SL. Normalization of height in girls with Turner syndrome after long-term growth hormone treatment: results of a randomized dose-response trial. J Clin Endocrinol Metab 1999; 84:4607–4612.

146. Carel JC, Mathivon L, Gendrel C, Ducret JP, Chaussain JL. Near normalization of final height with adapted doses of growth hormone in Turner's syndrome. J Clin Endocrinol Metab 1998; 83:1462–1466.

147. Takano K, Ogawa M, Tanaka T, Tachibana K, Fujita K, Hizuka N. Clinical trials of GH treatment in patients with Turner's syndrome in Japan—a consideration of final height. The Committee for the Treatment of Turner's Syndrome. Eur J Endocrinol 1997; 137:138–145.

148. Hofman P, Cutfield WS, Robinson EM, Clavano A, Ambler GR, Cowell C. Factors predictive of response to growth hormone therapy in Turner's syndrome. J Pediatr Endocrinol Metab 1997; 10:27–33.

149. Betts PR, Butler GE, Donaldson MD, Dunger DB, Johnston DI, Kelnar CJ, Kirk J, Price DA, Wilton P. A decade of growth hormone treatment in girls with Turner syndrome in the UK. Arch Dis Child 1999; 80:221–225.

150. Ranke MB, Lindberg A, Chatelain P, Wilton P, Cutfield W, Albertsson-Wikland K, Price DA. Prediction of long-term response to recombinant human growth hormone in Turner syndrome: development and validation of mathematical models. KIGS International Board. J Clin Endocrinol Metab 2000; 85:4212–4218.

151. Joss EE, Mullis PE, Werder EA, Partsch CJ, Sippell WG. Growth promotion and Turner-specific bone age after therapy with growth hormone and in combination with oxandrolone: when should therapy be started in Turner syndrome? Horm Res 1997; 47:102–109.

152. Ross JL, Long LM, Skerda M, et al. Effect of low doses of estradiol on 6-month growth rates and predicted height in patients with Turner syndrome. J Pediatr 1986; 109:950–953.

153. Martinez A, Heinrich JJ, Domene H, et al. Growth in Turner's syndrome: long-term treatment with low dose ethinyl estradiol. J Clin Endocrinol Metab 1987; 65:253–258.

154. Kastrup KW. Oestrogen therapy in Turner's syndrome. Acta Paediatr Suppl 1988; 343:43–46.

155. Vanderschueren-Lodeweyckx M, Massa G, Maes M, Craen M, van Vliet G, Heinrichs C, Malvaux P. Growth-promoting effect of growth hormone and low-dose ethinyl estradiol in girls with Turner's syndrome. J Clin Endocrinol Metab 1990; 70:122–126.

156. Naeraa RW, Nielsen J, Kastrup KW. Growth hormone and 17 beta-oestradiol treatment of Turner girls—2-year results. Eur J Pediatr 1994; 153:72–77.

157. Ross JL, Cassorla F, Carpenter G, et al. The effect of short-term treatment with growth hormone and ethinyl estradiol on lower leg growth rate in girls with Turner's syndrome. J Clin Endocrinol Metab 1988; 67:515–518.

158. Chernausek SD, Attie KM, Cara JF, Rosenfeld RG, Frane J. Growth hormone therapy of Turner syndrome: the impact of age of estrogen replacement on final height. Genentech Collaborative Study Group. J Clin Endocrinol Metab 2000; 85:2439–2445.

159. Wemme H, Pohlenz J, Schonberger W. Effect of oestrogen/gestagen replacement therapy on liver enzymes in patients with Ullrich-Turner syndrome. Eur J Pediatr 1995; 154:807–810.

160. Gravholt CH, Naeraa RW, Fisker S, Christiansen JS. Body composition and physical fitness are major determinants of the growth hormone-insulin-like growth factor axis aberrations in adult Turner's syndrome, with important modulations by treatment with 17 beta-estradiol. J Clin Endocrinol Metab 1997; 82:2570–2577.

11
Nonendocrine Vaginal Bleeding

Albert Altchek

Mount Sinai School of Medicine and Hospital, New York, New York, U.S.A.

I. INTRODUCTION

A. General Considerations

The vast majority of abnormal bleeding in children is a result of local causes, not precocious puberty or other endocrine causes.

Unfortunately, there have been reports from distinguished authorities indicating that the leading cause of bleeding is precocious puberty (for example, Ref. 1). Clearly such reports are a result of case selection bias.

Such distorting of the relative incidence of precocious puberty causing bleeding, combined with the training and interests of pediatricians, causes an immediate reaction that the first thing to rule out if there is bleeding is precocious puberty. Thus it is essential that pediatric endocrinologists recognize and diagnose patients with nonendocrine vaginal bleeding to avoid misdirected investigation that may involve radiation exposure; be wasteful of resources and funds; be prolonged; be stressful to the child, parents, and pediatrician; and delay discovery of the statistically probable local, nonendocrine cause of the bleeding.

Because menstruation may be considered physiological in children age 10 or over, bleeding in girls under age 10 is considered abnormal (1). Ideally, in all cases of vaginal bleeding local nonendocrine causes should be ruled out (Chap. 9).

Even if the presumptive diagnosis is precocious puberty, there should be consideration of the possibility of a nonendocrine, local cause of bleeding. It may even be possible that there is a local cause of bleeding together with precocious puberty. If this occurs, then the bleeding pattern and the lack of response to precocious puberty therapy cause great confusion. Gynecological investigation is relatively brief and inexpensive and, except for the possible need for general anesthesia for vaginoscopy, relatively without danger.

B. Differences Between Endocrine and Nonendocrine Bleeding

Usually with true, constitutional precocious puberty, there is a similarity to the normal puberty sequence of events except that they occur at an earlier age. Therefore, by the time the child has her first episode of vaginal bleeding, she has already had breast development, pubic and axillary hair, and other physical signs of puberty. In addition, the vaginal cytology smear (or urine cytology) shows an estrogenic effect, with superficial and intermediate cells.

By contrast, the child with a local, nonendocrine cause of bleeding does not have the physical changes of puberty, and the vaginal cytology shows an anestrogenic maturation index with mostly parabasal cells, with few if any superficial or intermediate cells. In addition, a local bleeding site is present. Furthermore, the history may give positive clues, such as trauma, symptoms of vulvovaginitis, dysuria, scratching, the presence of a vaginal or vulvar mass, or pain on defecation.

C. Endocrine Bleeding Posing as Nonendocrine Bleeding

Infrequently, an endocrine cause may pose as a local cause because of an absence of physical signs of puberty when bleeding starts as an apparently isolated phenomenon. However, the vaginal smear cytology is usually estrogenic because the vaginal mucosa is the most estrogen sensitive tissue. Specific causes include the following examples.

1. The newborn may have physiological vaginal (uterine estrogen withdrawal bleeding) bleeding and discharge (from the estrogenic vagina).
2. The first clinical sign of McCune-Albright syndrome is often vaginal bleeding. The diagnosis requires the characteristic café-au-lait pigmenta-

tion and radiological bone disease. Eventually secondary sexual development occurs (Chap. 9).

3. Estrogen-secreting ovarian neoplasms, such as granulosa cell tumors, even though small, may also cause bleeding before physical signs of puberty. They may be palpable on rectal examination and can be imaged by ultrasound (Chap. 9, 30).

4. Patients with isolated premature menarche may have isolated or recurrent vaginal bleeding without other signs of precocious puberty (2). Sleep luteinizing hormone (LH) levels may show pulsations; however, follicle-stimulating hormone (FSH) responds more than LH after LH-releasing hormone stimulation, as in prepuberty. There may be transient elevation of estradiol and a later return of LH to a prepubertal pattern. This entity is usually benign and self-limiting and is thought to be the result of a partial, transient activation of true precocious puberty. Careful evaluation and follow-up are required.

5. Prepubertal vaginal bleeding without signs of precocious puberty may be infrequently caused by prolonged, untreated hypothyroidism. In these patients, there may be breast enlargement, galactorrhea, hyperprolactinemia, enlarged sella turcica, ovarian follicular cysts, elevated gonadotropins (mainly FSH), and an estrogenic vaginal smear. There is no androgen excess or pubarche and no pubertal growth spurt. There is a delayed bone age (Chap. 9, 14, 15) (3, 4). Percutaneous aspiration of secondary ovarian cysts added to the standard thyroxin therapy may be helpful (5).

6. Accidental estrogen ingestion may also set off vaginal bleeding without puberty development.

7. Sometimes, precocious puberty caused by a central nervous system lesion may have bleeding before secondary sexual development (1). Brain imaging is necessary for diagnosis.

8. Transient neonatal bleeding with a stimulated uterus and a dominant 3 cm ovarian cyst has been reported with adrenal steroid suppression of congenital adrenal hyperplasia, which resulted in a transient gonadotropin level (6).

9. Prolonged vaginal bleeding is common following long-acting gonadotropin-releasing hormone agonist therapy of central precocious puberty in premenarchal girls (7).

Table 1 Nonhormonal Causes of Bleeding

Severe, usually specific, infections of the vagina, with secondary vulvitis
  Group A β-hemolytic streptococcus
  Candida
  Neisseria gonorrhoeae
  Chlamydia
  Gardnerella (bacterial vaginosis)
  Trichomonas vaginalis
  Rare (geographic endemic) *Shigella*, schistosomiasis, amebiasis
  Pinworm infestation
Trauma
  Management of bleeding
  Types of injury
  Suspicion of sexual abuse
Foreign body in the vagina
  Rolled-up wads of toilet tissue
  "Arrowhead" narrow plastic bottle caps
  Trapped pinworms
Vulva lesions
  Severe nonspecific vulvitis with secondary vaginitis, scratching
  Skin lesions
    General skin disease, seborrheic, atopic, psoriasis, candidiasis
    Hemangioma
    Condylomata acuminata
    Lichen sclerosus
    Diaper rash
    Ulcers: herpetic, syphilis, chancroid
    Systemic infection: chicken pox
    Local infection: bacterial, tinea
    Allergic-irritant: contact
    Scabies
Prolapse of urethra, hematuria, prolapse of bladder, rhabdomyosarcoma, prolapse of ureterocele
Anal fissure, pinworms, perianal dermatitis, condyloma acuminatum, hemorrhoid caused by pelvic cavernous hemagioma, laceration
Hymen polyps
Malignant and benign tumors of the vagina, uterus and ovaries
  Rhabdomyosarcoma
  Midline germ cell endodermal sinus tumor
  Clear cell adenocarcinoma
Rare coagulation defect (in association with skin and mucous membrane bleeding)

II. CAUSES OF LOCAL NONENDOCRINE BLEEDING

A. Causes

The local causes of nonhormonal vaginal bleeding in the child are listed in Table 1. These conditions can also cause abnormal bleeding in the adolescent. The vast majority of adolescent abnormal bleeding is caused by anovulatory dysfunctional uterine bleeding because half of all adolescents do not ovulate at menarche.

B. Incidence and Prevalence

There are no reliable data on the incidence and causes of local bleeding in the child because of case selection factors and age group bias. Adolescent statistics may also reflect pregnancy and its complications (miscarriage, abortion, or ectopic pregnancy), sexually transmitted disease, misuse of oral contraceptives, voluntary sexual activity, and rape.

Among 1300 Viennese children, average age 7.6 years, seen in elective clinic visits for evaluation of gynecological problems, the most frequent conditions were vulvovaginitis (43%), "pathologic vaginal bleeding" (13%), vulva disorders (7%), and suspicion of foreign body (5%) (8). In adolescents, most of the bleeding was anovulatory dysfunctional bleeding.

Emergency rooms tend to report trauma and urethral prolapse as bleeding causes because of the acute and severe presentations. Private pediatric offices and clinics acquire cases with less dramatic bleeding and tend not to report them.

A London referral hospital reported that among 52 girls 10 years of age and under with vaginal bleeding, 28 had a local lesion, of whom 11 had malignant vaginal tumors. These included eight rhabdomyosarcomas, two clear cell adenocarcinomas, and one endodermal sinus tumor. Bleeding from vulvar lesions included lichen sclerosus, warts, and cavernous hemangioma, as well as urethral prolapse, trauma, and vulvovaginitis. Precocious puberty occurred in 11 children: constitutional in two, granuloma cell tumor of the ovary in three, and premature menarche in six. In 13 cases, no cause for bleeding was found (9). I believe that the high incidence of malignancy and precocious puberty and the absence of foreign bodies in the vagina were a result of case selection. The lack of a cause for bleeding may have been a result of a severe vaginitis that cleared by the time of vaginoscopy. In their precocious puberty cases (only 2 of 11 were constitutional), most had bleeding without other signs of secondary sexual development and with normal bone age. Isolated bleeding as the first sign of puberty was also found in another select series (1).

There have been several recent reviews of vaginal bleeding in children (10–21). There is general agreement that the most frequent causes include trauma, vulvovaginitis (especially vaginitis), vulvar lesions, vaginal foreign bodies, and urethral prolapse.

A Japanese hospital reported that of 330 girls referred ages 1–10, 20% had vaginal bleeding. Of these 74% (46 of 62) had local vaginal lesions due to vulvovaginitis (28), urethral prolapse (6), trauma (6), foreign bodies (3), and vaginal tumors (3). Of the latter one was sarcoma botryoides and one was endodermal sinus tumor. Precocious puberty was diagnosed in 16 (20%), of whom 6 had an hormonally active ovarian tumor. There were three cases with idiopathic precocious puberty without secondary sexual development (presumably premature menarche) (16).

Malignant conditions of the vagina are very rare but may present initially as unexplained vaginal bleeding (even only staining for a few days) in an otherwise healthy child. With early discovery, local resection, and contemporary chemotherapy, the dismal prognosis of 30 years ago has been removed from about 85% fatality to apparent cure.

Trauma may result from sexual abuse, which may also be part of general mistreatment of the child. The suspicion of abuse requires reporting to legal authorities. Ideally, sexual abuse should not be overlooked (even though there may not be definite physical findings), and sexual abuse should not be misdiagnosed in conditions that simulate its physical findings (such as lichen sclerosus with bleeding, laceration-like fissures, and ecchymoses).

III. SEVERE VAGINAL INFECTIONS AS A CAUSE OF LOCAL NONENDOCRINE BLEEDING

A. Vulvovaginitis

Vulvovaginitis is the leading gynecological problem of the child, which can cause bleeding. The child is susceptible to infection because of a vulva that

1. Lacks the thick adult labial pads and pubic hair
2. Has delicate skin
3. Is close to the anus

The child is also susceptible because of a vaginal mucosa that

1. Is anestrogenic and thin (about 6 cells thick rather than the approximately five times thicker adult)
2. Lacks glycogen (and lactobacilli) and therefore is of neutral pH rather than the adult acid pH
3. Might lack immune globulin of the adult

In addition, children tend to have poor local hygiene. Most vulvovaginitis is primary vulvitis with secondary vaginitis set off by an episode of poor hygiene.

Primary vaginitis is less common and more deserving of investigation. A culture of the vagina above the hymen is required for diagnosis.

B. Group A β-Hemolytic Streptococcus Vaginitis

Group A β-hemolytic streptococcus is the most frequent cause of a specific vaginal infection causing bleeding, although bleeding does not occur in every case. Q-tip culturing often provokes bleeding. On vaginoscopy, there is a severe inflammation of the upper posterior vaginal wall and fornix with extensive petechial hemorrhages in the anestrogenic atrophic mucosa. Blood comes from a broad area. A single bleeding site cannot be visualized. Although vaginoscopy is recommended, a positive culture with cure after 10 days of antibiotic therapy (similar to a pharyngitis) and observation is a reasonable alternative.

Group A β-hemolytic streptococcus (GAHS) has been reported in 18% of girls who were cultured for clinical vulvovaginitis (actually vaginitis). The incidence is higher in the age group up to 9 years, as opposed to the 10–14-year age group. The younger child is expected to have streptococal vaginitis; the older child, because of an estrogenic thicker vaginal wall, is resistant. It is also increased in the winter months, when streptococcal pharyngitis is increased. The organism is probably transmitted from the pharynx to the vagina (22). This suggests that GAHS is more commonly associated with vulvovaginitis than previously thought. It could indicate a true increase in frequency or better recognition by more liberal use of cultures.

C. *Candida* Vaginitis

Candida may cause a vaginitis with a cottage cheese discharge, a vulvitis with severe excoriation, a perianal dermatitis, a diaper rash, and a secondary infection of any vulvar lesion. The diagnosis is made by inspection, scraping, culture, or microscopic potassium hydroxide wet mount smear.

D. Sexually Transmitted Disease

Any sexually transmitted disease raises the question of sexual molestation (gonorrhea, chlamydia, trichomonads, *Gardnerella,* condyloma, etc.), although it is possible that all of these can be acquired without molestation at the time of vaginal delivery, from a caretaker, or close physical contact with the mother. Trichomonads prefer the estrogenic vagina and tend to be found in the newborn and older child.

E. Unusual Infections

Rare severe vaginal infections usually associated with geographic endemic areas can cause bleeding.

Recurrent vaginal bleeding and bloody discharge may be due to *Shigella* causing a distal localized intense vaginitis. It originates from a previous enteric infection and there may or may not be a residual positive stool culture. Sometimes, prolonged treatment may be required. Contacts should be cultured even if asymptomatic. In the United States, these cases are infrequent. Patients often come from Indian reservations in the Southwest and usually have *Shigella flexneri.* In Peru, the usual cause is *Shigelia sonnei* (13). Other rare causes include *Schistosomiasis* and *Amoebiasis* (24).

IV.   TRAUMA AS A CAUSE OF LOCAL NONENDOCRINE BLEEDING

The physician is faced with two problems: the specific injury (and treatment) and the question of sexual abuse and, with it, sexually transmitted disease (25).

A.   Management of Bleeding

When the child is first seen by the pediatrician, there is the tendency to watch and wait with the hope that the bleeding will spontaneously stop. Unfortunately, if there is persistent active bleeding several hours may be lost, with significant blood loss. A cold compress should be applied to the vulva for about 10 min. If significant bleeding persists, the child should be taken to the operating room for meticulous hemostasis, suturing of lacerations, and reconstruction using fine absorbable nonreactive sutures. The integrity of the bladder and rectum is checked by having the child void, catheterization, and rectal examination. Vaginal lacerations and possible transvaginal peritoneal injury are checked and consideration given to blunt abdominal trauma. Despite fecal contamination, immediate repair of fresh rectal tears gives good results. Antibiotics and tetanus prevention should be considered.

Bleeding as a result of trauma often causes external bleeding. Occasionally, blunt trauma from a fall may result in a deep pelvic hematoma that a number of days later ruptures laterally into the vagina, resulting in the vaginal discharge of old blood.

Genital injury gives rise to anxiety. The little girl is disturbed by pain and bleeding, her parents are worried about serious damage, and the physician is concerned about possible sexual abuse.

Accidental injury is more common than molestation. With the former, there is prompt reporting by the patient and her mother, a clear history, and findings consistent with the history (26).

Most trauma is an accidental fall with a hematoma of the anterior labia majora or perineum. It is usually managed by ice bag pressure and observation. Infrequently a large or enlarging hematoma may require surgery to ligate a bleeding vessel or for packing (21).

Vaginal laceration may result from water slide injury and bleeding may require examinations under anesthesia (27, 28). It may also occur from water-ski douche (29) or jet-ski inquiry (30), high-pressure water jet (31) or sliding down a water chute (32).

Vaginal bleeding may be sign of anorectal injury (33).

Despite denial of trauma and of an intact hymen, profuse vaginal bleeding can occur from a vaginal laceration in the prepubertal child (34).

Compression of the uterus and adnexae as components of a sliding indirect inguinal hernia in an infant apparently may cause vaginal bleeding (35).

B.   Types of Injury

A prospective 33 month study from the accident and emergency department of the Royal Liverpool Children's Hospital revealed 87 girls with genital injuries (26). Of these, 82 had a clear clinical history. Most of the injuries (74) involved straddle or falling onto hard objects, which compresses the vulvar soft tissue against the pubic ramus bone. This resulted in asymmetrical bruising (sometimes severe), abrasion, and (usually superficial) lacerations anteriorly between the labia majora and minora. There may be unilateral medial thigh scraping. With the usual straddle accident, one foot slips and the child falls forward and to one side. Accidents occurred on bicycles, falling on small toys, climbing on furniture, falling astride a fence or bathtub wall, on play or sport apparatus, and from kicking. There were five girls with vaginal-penetrating injuries caused by railing spikes, sticks, and a bath tap. These injuries were severe and required examination under anesthesia and suturing. There were tears of the posterior vestibule and posterior vaginal wall. Stretch injuries ("splits") occurred in three cases, with superficial tears in the perineum and fourchette, especially in those with labial adhesions; two girls had self-inflicted scratch injuries. Of the 87 girls with genital injuries, 80 were considered accidental. Sexual abuse was alleged by only three of the seven girls with suspicion of abuse (26).

C. Sexual Abuse

Suspicion of sexual abuse is raised by an absent or vague history and a delay in presentation in cases of injury to the hymen; (severe) posterior fourchette, perineum, or posterior vaginal wall; and failure to have a return visit. The posterior fourchette is distal to the hymen in the vestibule. The gynecological perineum is between the vagina and anus (the anatomical perineum includes the entire vulva) (26).

Sexual abuse in children involves medical care, emotional support, report to child welfare agencies, collection of evidence, and follow up (36).

Lower abdominal pain and vaginal bleeding may be signs of a posterior vaginal fornix laceration with hematoperitoneum due to initial sexual intercourse (37).

Vaginal digital "fisting" with laceration reported in adults (38) might present in children with a vague history; pain and severe bleeding requiring general anesthesia for assessment; and multiple lacerations of the vagina, rectum, and bladder.

V. FOREIGN BODIES IN THE VAGINA AS A CAUSE OF LOCAL NONENDOCRINE BLEEDING

Foreign bodies in the vagina tend to cause a persistent, foul, bloody vaginal discharge. This is a primary vaginitis and secondary vulvitis. The usual material is rolled-up wads of toilet tissue. These are almost always multiple and of different ages. X-rays usually do not detect them because most foreign bodies are not radiopaque. Also, these wads cannot be detected by rectal examination or ultrasound. Levator muscle action causes these wads to be pulled to the upper posterior vagina, and thus they are usually not visualized by inspection of the vulva. Vaginal cultures may yield any or all of the colon bacteria.

Another frequent foreign body is the hard plastic, narrow bottle cap with an "arrowhead" configuration. It may cause trauma on insertion. It can be palpated on rectal examination.

Almost any small object has been found in the vagina, including rolled-up pieces of cloth and green peas. Rarely, trapped pinworms may be lost on their return migration from the rectum.

The object is usually inserted by the child herself, who forgets or does not wish to remember because she knows that it is not proper. I believe that the child pushes her finger rolled up with toilet tissue into the vagina because of itching, and the tissue remains. Thus, there is usually no history of insertion.

Rolled-up wads of toilet tissue tend to reaccumulate, probably because of habit formation.

On discovery, there is an emotional melodrama as the mother berates the child. Sometimes, the foul odor results in the child being isolated, with secondary psychological reactions occurring before the diagnosis is discovered.

VI. VULVAR LESIONS AS A CAUSE OF LOCAL NONENDOCRINE BLEEDING

A. Trauma

Because of play, abrasions, scratching, and binding clothing combined with an unprotected vulva with delicate skin, children often experience nonspecific abrasions, excoriations, and nonspecific infections of the vulva. These may bleed spontaneously or after rubbing.

B. Skin Disease

1. Condyloma Acuminatum

The incidence of childhood condyloma acuminatum is progressively increasing. It is readily diagnosed by inspection. Scratching or other trauma readily provokes bleeding. The lesions have a characteristic dry, warty, hard, pointed appearance on the skin of the labium majus, perineum, and perianal areas. At the vaginal introitus with mucosa, the lesions are soft, bulky, and rounded, containing 1 mm clear granuloma-like areas suggestive of tapioca pudding. Personal observation suggests that children with sensitive skin (seborrheic or atopic dermatitis) are more susceptible (see Fig. 1).

The presence of vulvar and perianal condyloma acuminatum requires that sexual molestation be ruled out because this is a sexually transmitted disease. Nevertheless, it is possible that in most children anogenital warts are acquired by nonsexual transmission. The sources may be the mother's birth canal, caretakers by direct contact, washcloths, and general body cutaneous verruca vulgaris (39).

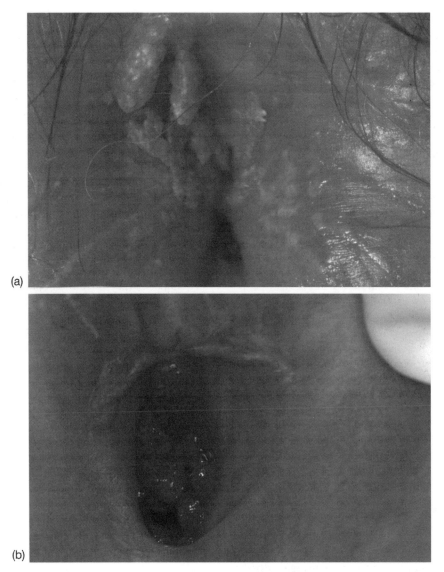

Figure 1   (a) Condylomata acuminata lesions of the skin are dry, hard, and warty, as seen on the perineum and perianal areas. In this case, they are less pointed because of previous podophyllin (podophyllun resin) therapy (b). The lesions of the introitus and periurethral areas (mucosa) are soft and bulky and resemple tapioca pudding

In the differential diagnosis of genital verrucous lesions is Darier's disease (keratosis follicularis), an autosomal dominant acantholytic disorder that may also result from a spontaneous mutation. Initially it resembles a chronic diaper rash or candidiasis, and later, painful infected masses develop (40). A biopsy is necessary for the diagnosis.

2.   Symmetrical Fissures
Seborrheic and atopic dermatitis are frequent childhood skin diseases occurring in more than 5% of all children.

Although not generally recognized, I find a high incidence of vulvar involvement and a frequently underestimated cause of chronic vulvovaginitis. The reason is that the usual diagnosis is made from the vaginal culture and the vulva is overlooked. Both these conditions have characteristic general signs, such as fissures and crusts behind the ears, a prominent lower eyelid fold (Dennie's lines and Morgan's folds), keratosis pilaris of the outer arms, and eczema of the elbow creases. There may be some overlap between these two conditions on purely clinical grounds. Both have a similar, transient subacute appearance of the vulva, with symmetrical fissures between the labia minora and majora and in the midline perineum. There may also be fissures in the midline anterior to the clitoris, radial in the perianal area, and in the midline posterior to the anus (see Fig. 2). When deep, the fissures can bleed. They may be confused with sexual molestation; however, the fine, precise symmetrical lesions and the general body distribution confirm the diagnosis.

Lichen sclerosus et atrophicus, now referred to as lichen sclerosus, in its advanced form has fissures in a similar distribution; however, they are coarser, chronic, and bleed more readily (see Fig. 3). They are often misdiagnosed as sexual molestation. A biopsy confirms the lesion. It begins as white, flat papules that coalesce into atrophic so-called cigarette paper plaques in the anogenital region. The skin becomes thin and fragile, with upper dermal edema and collagen homogenization. It is easily traumatized, causing purpura and bleeding. Mothers may report what appear to be blood blisters after the child goes on long bicycle rides. A biopsy confirms the diagnosis. Whereas in adults topical 2% testosterone in petrolatum has been recommended, topical 1% progesterone may help in children (41).

3. Psoriasis

Psoriasis is not unusual in children. If it first appears on the vulva, it is frustrating because the local heat, humidity, and rubbing modify the typical appearance and it resists therapy. If it appears on the vulva after general body involvement is present, then the diagnosis is simple. Abrasion and chafing can cause bleeding.

4. Diaper Rash, Allergies, and Contact Reactions

The usual diaper rash is an irritant dermatitis related to chemical and bacterial action of the urine and stool. It usually starts on the convex surfaces of the vulva closer to the diaper.

Diaper area rashes also may be caused by candidiasis, atopic eczema dermatitis, seborrheic dermatitis, and psoriasis, and, less often, by dermatophyte fungi or histiocytosis. The last may represent a serious systemic illness and presents as deep intertriginous fissures with severe seborrheic-like dermatitis that resists treatment.

The usual seborrheic dermatitis begins in the intertriginous creases but is less severe and responds to treatment.

The child's sensitive skin is easily irritated by contact or allergic reactions to perfumes, dyes, bubble bath, hot water, excessive soap, and other agents.

5. Hemangiomas

As many as 10% of all infants have hemangiomas, which may grow rapidly in the early months. Slow spontaneous regression usually starts at 6–10 months of age. Vulvar lesions are easy to visualize. Scratching or trauma may cause recurrent bleeding. Vaginal hemangiomas require vaginoscopy for identification. Rare, deep pelvic cavernous hemangiomas may have vulvar extensions, bladder extensions (causing hematuria), and rectal extensions (causing large hemorrhoids). Uncomplicated hemangiomas are observed. Complications are traditionally treated with oral or intralesional glucocorticosteroids (42).

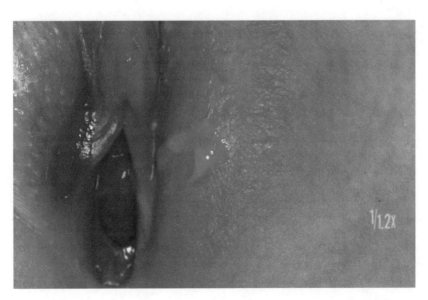

Figure 2 Fissure that caused bleeding on the child's right side between the labium minus and majus

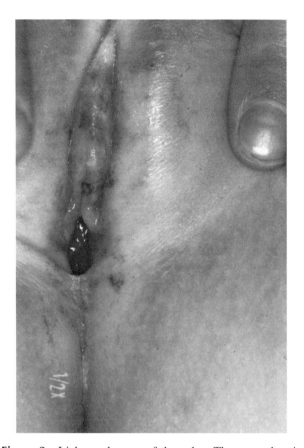

Figure 3 Lichen sclerosus of the vulva. There are chronic coarse deep fissures that readily bleed and white skin. The trauma of bicycle riding can cause ecchymoses.

Dry ice sticks have also been used. Two new modality treatments that seem to be relatively safe and effective are being evaluated: vascular-specific pulsed dye laser and interferon-α2a (43).

Aside from the hemangiomas, the other vascular birthmark is the vascular malformation. It persists throughout life, may involve complex combined vascular malformations, requires evaluation, and is rare (44, 45).

The rare giant hemangioma, which may present as a subcutaneous soft mass, may have a dangerous consumption coagulopathy and thrombocytopenia (Kasabach-Merritt syndrome). Those that do not respond to conventional therapy may respond to systemic subcutaneous interferon-α (46).

There are extremely rare, rapidly growing, congenital hemangiopericytomas that simulate hemangiomas but spontaneously ulcerate with severe bleeding (47).

6. Vulvar Infections

Vulvar candidiasis can cause severe pruritic erythematous lesions with sharp irregular borders and satellite lesions. It suggests diabetes or immune deficiency.

Staphylococcus and *Streptococcus* can cause vulvar and buttock pustules and brawny induration (erysipelas).

Tinea skin infections cause elevated circular lesions.

Chicken pox (varicella) lesions are also present on the vulva, where they are readily infected with bacteria and therefore persist.

The most commnon vulvar ulcers are caused by herpes. Figure 4 shows multiple confluent vulvar ulcers covered with a white exudate of colon-type bacteria. Bacterial culture is misleading. The syphilis lesion may be a primary chancre, secondary congenital condyloma latum, or

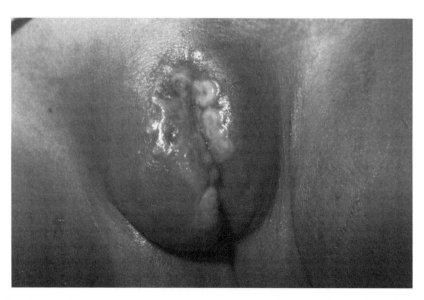

Figure 4   Confluent multiple vulvar ulcers caused by herpes, covered by a white exudate of colon-type bacteria

generalized macular rash. Chancroid ulcers are shaggy, painful, and simulate herpetic ulcers. Tumor chemotherapy can cause vulvar ulcers (48).

In refugee housing with enforced closeness, scabies spreads rapidly and causes intense genital itching. Pediculosis publis occurs in the older child.

There are many rare vulvar lesions. Chronic bullous dermatosis of childhood has subepidermal blisters with the deposition of IgA in a linear pattern along the basement membrane. It may also occur in other areas besides the genitalia, such as the trunk, extremities, and oral and tracheal mucosa (49).

Crohn's disease of the vulva may occur as a direct extension of this granulomatous intestinal disease as ulcerations and fistulas or separately ("metastatic"). On histological appearance, the latter is a sterile, noncaseating, nonspecific granuloma.

Granular cell tumors are slow-growing solitary nodules or plaques with a smooth or hyperkeratotic hyperpigmented verrucous surface that may be confused with squamous cell carcinoma or condyloma (50).

VII. PROLAPSE OF THE URETHRA AS A CAUSE OF LOCAL NONENDOCRINE BLEEDING

In some emergency rooms, urethral prolapse is the leading cause of vaginal bleeding. It presents as acute bleeding with pain and urinary symptoms. On inspection, there is a friable, shaggy, necrotic, bleeding mass suggestive of a malignancy. The diagnosis can be confirmed by passing a urethral catheter. The predisposing factors are an increase in intra-abdominal pressure and trauma. Management op-

tions include conservative therapy (sitz baths and topical estrogen cream), ligation over a Foley indwelling catheter, and excision under general anesthesia. The last gives the best results (51). Milder cases with conservative therapy tend to remain in a subacute condition (see Fig. 5) (52–54).

The differential diagnosis includes hematuria (from bladder or urethral hemangioma), prolapse of ureterocele, and bladder rhabdomyosarcoma.

The most frequent age is 4.9 years. Most cases are initially misdiagnosed by the referring pediatrician or emergency physician (54).

VIII. ANAL LESIONS AS A CAUSE OF LOCAL NONENDOCRINE BLEEDING

A. Fissures

The most common anal lesion causing bleeding is the fissure. It may cause spontaneous bleeding, blood covering the stool, pain, and fear of bowel movement. The usual cause (which is not generally recognized) is seborrheic or atopic dermatitis, in which there are the characteristic symmetrical, interlabial vulvar fissures, midline perineal fissures, and perianal radial fissures. There is often an anterior edematous skin tag.

B. Perianal Dermatitis

Perianal dermatitis on culture usually reveals *Candida*, but *Streptococcus* group A and *Staphylococcus aureus* (55), as well as all the colon bacteria, may be present. A single infecting organism may be predominant and the presumptive cause, but the condition, especially if recurrent, may

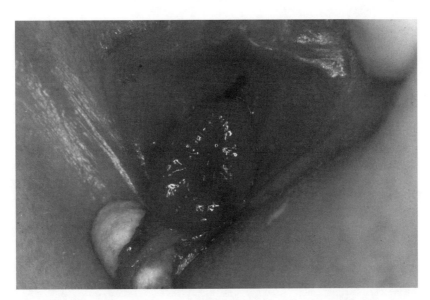

Figure 5 Subacute urethral prolapse. The urethra remained enlarged, simulating the vaginal introitus. A Q-tip is in the actual vagina.

be caused by the predisposing fissures of seborrheic and atopic dermatitis with secondary infection.

C. Pinworm

Pinworm infestation is common in children. About 20% of cases are significantly symptomatic, usually with nocturnal itching and sometimes with abdominal pain. Scratching tears the skin and encourages reinfection. Nocturnal itching may also be the result of blankets that cause an increase in heat and moisture in cases of atopic dermatitis.

D. Condylomata Acuminata

Condylomata acuminata are often perianal in distribution. Their presence requires consideration of molestation. Even without molestation, it occurs in this area especially in children with atopic dermatitis, who are particularly susceptible.

E. Hemorrhoids and Trauma

True hemorrhoids are unusual in children and suggest a large pelvic cavernous hemangioma.

Trauma may be a result of molestation, foreign bodies, or an innocent accident. Prompt evaluation and reconstruction if needed usually result in healing despite contamination.

IX. POLYPS OF THE HYMEN AS A CAUSE OF LOCAL NONENDOCRINE BLEEDING

It is not unusual to find a prominent, fleshy hymen in the newborn, often with a polypoid posterior lip as a result of maternal estrogen. After a week, these recede, with absence of estrogen. Occasionally, true polyps persist and may tear and bleed. Figure 6 shows large true polyps in a 1-week-old child. Even small polyps may persist. Polyps of the hymen are usually benign.

X. MALIGNANT AND BENIGN TUMORS OF THE VAGINA, UTERUS, AND OVARIES

A. Rhabdomyosarcoma

Malignant vaginal tumors are rare but potentially fatal. The victims, when first seen, always look in deceivingly perfect health. The most common is rhabdomyosarcoma (56–58), which gynecologists call sarcoma botryoides. About 30 years ago, it was generally fatal within 2 years, and the only survivors were those whose tumors were discovered early and underwent pelvic exenteration. In recent years, with early discovery, local resection, and contemporary chemotherapy, the prognosis has been reversed, with the expectation of a cure in 85%. The tumor originates in the submucosal mesenchyme of the vagina and initially presents as a protruding polypoid mass and bleeding. Because the tumor surface is normal mucosa, even experienced physicians are misled. In addition, superficial biopsies may be misleading, because aside from the normal surface mucosa, a deep section is necessary. The pathological diagnosis requires more than one cell type and the dermis layer. The tumor usually develops in the upper anterior vaginal wall. The important fact is that although polyps of the hymen are usually benign, polyps that originate above the hymen are considered malignant until proven otherwise. Figure 7 shows a 6-year-old girl (most

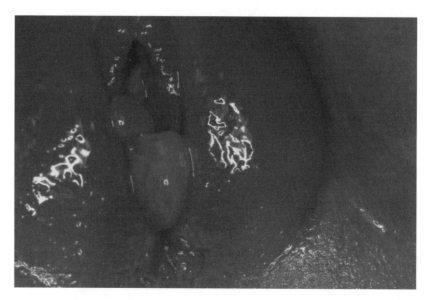

Figure 6   Large true hymen polyps in a 1-week-old child

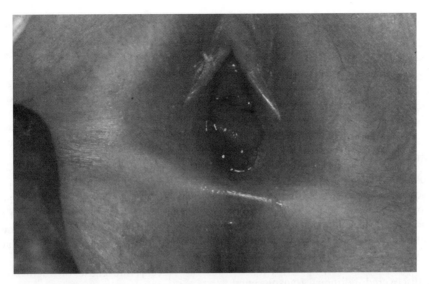

Figure 7 Vaginoscopy showed a polyp. On straining, the polyp protruded as seen here. The surface mucosa is normal vaginal mucosa. Under the normal mucosa of the apparently benign polyp is the very malignant mesenchymal rhabdomyosarcoma. Any vaginal polyp that originates above the hymen is considered malignant until proved otherwise.

are younger) who had staining for 3 days and a normal hymen. Vaginoscopy revealed a polypoid tumor. On straining, a polyp protruded with a normal vaginal mucosal surface whose origin was above the hymen. Early small rhabdomyosarcoma polypoid masses do not prolapse on straining, and this is not a reliable test. Resection of the polyp showed it to be a rhabdomyosarcoma. If the frozen section confirms the diagnosis, then it is advisable

to perform cystoscopy with the same anesthesia to detect possible bladder invasion.

Large vaginal rhabdomyosarcomas may suddenly protrude out of the vagina in grape-like clusters, sometimes after straining at stool. Figure 8 shows this occurrence in an 11-month-old child. Part of the tumor has become necrotic because of a vascular disturbance. Despite the lesion's size, the child was cured.

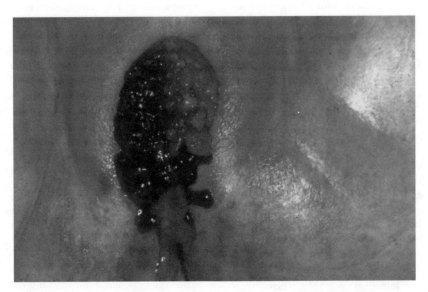

Figure 8 Large vaginal rhabdomyosarcoma protruding from the vagina. The grape-like cluster (so-called sarcoma botryoides) is noted. Part of the tumor is necrotic because of vascular disturbance.

B. Germ Cell Tumors

Endodermal (yolk sac) germ cell tumors (59, 60) are very malignant, midline body neoplasms. They tend to occur in the upper vagina and cervix (61) and cause bleeding but usually do not prolapse to the introitus. In the past 10 years, with contemporary chemotherapy, the previous usually fatal outcome has been reversed.

C. Adenocarcinoma

Clear cell adenocarcinoma (CCA) has been associated with female fetal exposure to maternal ingestion of diethylstilbestrol (DES) (62). Despite this discovery in 1971 and the discontinuation of DES for pregnant women, this cancer still occurs, although at a reduced rate. It is a cause of vaginal bleeding, and the tumor usually is not visible at the vulva.

DES is the first discovered, hormonal transplacental carcinogen. If given in the first trimester to a pregnant woman with a female fetus, DES can cause a CCA of the vagina or cervix at a delayed time, usually at or just after puberty.

DES became popular in the 1940s because it was the first synthetic, inexpensive oral estrogen. It is nonsteroidal.

There were 547 cases of CCA reported as of 1989. In about one-quarter of the cases, there was no history of hormonal exposure. The age range at discovery was 7–34.4 years, with 91% of patients between 15 and 27, and a median age of 19.0. This suggests a stimulation effect of puberty, especially because of a sharp, dramatic rise at age 14.

Before the use of DES, CCA was very rare and tended to occur in older women.

DES was used to treat women with a history of repeated spontaneous abortion. Such women tend to have affected children more than women taking DES without pregnancy losses.

About 60% of CCA are vaginal, usually in the anterior upper third. The remainder are on the ectocervix (portio). They are unifocal. CCA is fatal if untreated.

The risk of CCA in a DES-exposed female is 1:1000.

Benign changes are much more frequent, about 35% having vaginal adenosis (glandular, endocervical-type epithelium). About 25% have cervical structural abnormalities with cervical hoods, ridges, collars, pseudopolyps, or vaginal septa. All the benign changes occur more frequently with higher dosages of DES and with earlier use in pregnancy.

In early embryonic life, the paired müllerian (paramesonephric) ducts (with glandular, columnar, endocervical-type epithelium) form and fuse at about 8 weeks at the urogenital sinus, forming a tubercle or vaginal plate. The latter then grows cephalad as a solid core of squamous epithelium into the fused ducts. Later, the solid core canalizes to become the vagina. Usually, the separation of the two types of epithelium is at the external os of the cervix.

DES, or any stilbene-type estrogen, prevents normal development of the genital epithelium. It can also cause abnormal proliferation of the adjacent connective tissue, resulting in gross structural abnormalities.

DES is considered an incomplete carcinogen, and there may be other unknown predisposing factors.

The benign and malignant changes are not found with steroidal estrogen exposure.

DES-exposed males do not have an increased risk of cancer. There are conflicting reports of possible benign anatomical and seminal abnormalities (62).

My personal speculation is that because DES is still used to fatten chickens and cows for slaughter, this may be a continuing source of ingestion because it can be stored in animal fat.

A very rare cause of vaginal malignancy is mesonephric duct remnant carcinoma.

D. Direct Vaginal Bleeding

Direct vaginal bleeding may also occur due to very rare benign vaginal (63) cervical (64) and vulvar tumors (65). Direct bleeding may result from benign (66) or malignant uterine tumors (67–69) or endometritis. Indirect bleeding may result from benign and malignant ovarian tumors (70–75) by hormone secretion, compression, and disturbance of uterine circulation or unknown mechanisms.

XI. COAGULATION DEFECTS AS A CAUSE OF LOCAL NONHORMONAL BLEEDING

Symptomatic coagulation defects are an unusual cause in children, and any vaginal bleeding is part of the overall body tendency to bleed.

The most common inherited bleeding disorder is von Willebrand's disease (VWD). The prevalence has been estimated to be as high as 1.3% of the general population based on a personal history of bleeding, decreased VW factor (VWF) activity, and a positive family history. It may even be higher especially in subjects with blood group O. Since screening tests (bleeding time) may not be reliable, some recommend that VW factor activity be measured initially in children with mucosal bleeding (76).

Affected children tend to have easy bruising, mucocutaneous bleeding (including epistaxis, oral, rectal, vaginal) and prolonged bleeding after trauma. It usually presents as menorrhagia, which may be significant beginning at menarche (77, 78). About 80% of patients have the mild types 1 and 2 A, 2B. These are autosomal dominant with variable phenotypic penetrance and expressivity. The severe types 2N and 3 are rare and recessive and sometimes occur in clusters in Israel, Sweden, and Iran (79). Type 1 shows a partial quantitive reduction of VWF levels. Type

2 varieties have qualitative mutant VWF protein. Type 3 involves almost complete absence of VWF protein (79). The diagnosis is not simple and repeated tests may be required. There are several confounding problems. Persons with blood group O have a 25% reduced level of VWF and Factor VIII. In addition plasma levels of both increase three- to fivefold with physiological stress, therapeutic estrogen, oral contraceptives, pregnancy, and possibly hyperthyroidism (80, 81). Furthermore, a personal and family bleeding history and low VWF ristocetin cofactor activity, which are the criteria for VWF Type 1, may not cosegregate with genetic markers at the VWF gene locus. The phenotype diagnosis identifies bleeding risk (82). In infancy von Willebrand factor is normally high and therefore the disease "can not be diagnosed with confidence . . ." (81, p. 278). The usual screening test is bleeding time, which may be prolonged and also occurs in cases of platelet dysfunction. There might be a prolonged activated partial thromboplastin time and a mild thrombocytopenia with type 2B VWD (79). Bleeding time has a low sensitivity. High shear system testing is superior (83).

In practice rapid immunoassay screening for von Willebrand disease type 1 had a low yield and limited ability to predict bleeding in surgery (84). More precise standard testing includes the plasma VWF factor protein level (VWF:AG), VWF ristocetin cofactor assay for functional activity (VWF:R Co), VWF ristocetin-induced platelet agglutination (RIPA), factor VIII, and circulating molecular weight profile of VWF (VWF multimeras) (79). Although desmopressin is usually used to treat VWD, about 10% of children fail to achieve an adequate response. Response should be tested measuring VWF:Ag, VWF:Ac, and factor VII:C at the time of diagnosis should there be a need for future surgery (85). Acquired von Willebrand's disease or syndrome (AvWD, AvWS) is rare, may suddenly appear without personal or family bleeding history, and with the same laboratory findings as congenital VWD. There are autoantibodies against von Willebrand factor. It is associated with lymph or myeloproliferative, autoimmune or cardiovascular disease, drugs and solid tumors (86, 87), and may be secondary to hypothyroidism. Childhood embryonal renal adenoma is associated with acquired polycythemia and von Willebrand's disease; preoperative testing is required (88).

Factor XI deficiency has a heterozygous frequency of 8% among Ashkenazi Jews. It has an inherited autosomal pattern. The normal plasma range is 70–150 IU/dl, with heterozygotes showing levels down to 15 IU/dl and homozygotes less than 15 IU/dl. It presents as menorrhagia or bleeding after a hemostatic challenge. Bleeding tendency does not always match plasma levels, and may vary over time. In addition there may be an additional associated von Willebrand's disease (89, 90).

With Glanzmann's thrombasthenia the initial bleeding occurs before 5 years of age. The frequent presentations include epistaxis, gingival bleeding, posttraumatic bruises, menorrhagia (often requiring transfusions), and gastrointestinal and postoperative bleeding (91). It is a rare inherited hematological disorder of glycoprotein IIb–IIIa complex that disturbs platelet function (92). Most cases are discovered at menarche. Uterine packing has been used to stop adolescent bleeding (92).

Rarely there may be severe acute onset of a general tendency to bleed because of hypoprothrombinemia associated with a lupus anticoagulant (93).

Idiopathic thrombocytopenic purpura (ITP) is the most frequent acquired pediatric bleeding disorder. Most cases have only minimal bleeding and usually there is spontaneous recovery in weeks to months. The peak age is 4–8 years. It results from antiplatelet antibodies with the platelet count less than $20,000/m^3$ and a prolonged bleeding time. In apparently healthy children there is the sudden appearance of bruising, petechiae, epistaxis, and sometimes so-called wet purpura with mucus membrane bleeding resulting in uterine, gastrointestinal, and oral bleeding or blood blisters. There is often a preceding viral infection or live virus immunization (94). About 17% have major bleeding including intracranial hemorrhage, epistaxis, or gross hematuria. There is a suspicion that menstruation, infection, and risk factors for systemic lupus erythematosis may predict intracranial hemorrhage in children (95). Death may occur in children from undiagnosed immune thrombocytopenic purpura as an anesthesia complication from profound epistaxis (96). Thrombocytopenia is the most common complication of childhood typhoid fever (97). It may also occur as a congenital limb and bleeding disorder (thrombocytopenia absent radius syndrome) (98, 99). Occasionally with brucellosis there may be severe thrombocytopenia with purpura and mucosal site bleeding (100). The diagnosis of idiopathic thrombocytopenic purpura often overlaps with immune thrombocytopenic purpura. The acute form affects mainly children, whereas the chronic form is usually found in young adults (101). In children generally thrombocytopenia may result from viral infections (varicella, Epstein-Barr virus (EBV), rubella, mumps, measles, cytomegalic virus) by an immune reaction and cause a petechial rash. However, petechial bleeding may occur without thrombocytopenia in both bacterial and viral infections (meningococcus, streptococcus, echovirus, etc.) because of vasculitis or platelet dysfunction (102). Young women with essential thrombocytopenia have a low chronic risk of thrombohemorrhagic complications or acute leukemia (103).

Most vaginal bleeding in the newborn is due to the withdrawal of the maternal estrogen effect on the endometrium and is considered a physiological variant. Most neonatal bleeding problems are due to acquired coagulation disorder. Evaluation may be difficult because coagulation parameters are different from older children and adults and because of rapid changes (104).

Thrombocytopenia is the most common hematological abnormality in the newborn. It may occur in 1–4% of term births and in 40–72% of sick preterm newborns. The leading causes of alloimmune thrombocytopenia and thrombocytopenia are secondary to maternal and uteroplacental factors and pre-eclampsia. It may present as diffuse petechial or mucosal surface bleeding. There may be intracranial bleeding (104–108). Other causes of general and mucous membrane bleeding in the newborn may be coagulation protein disorders due to factors VIII and IX, and vitamin K deficiency; disseminated intravascular coagulation (109); and vascular disorders such as intraventricular hemorrhage in preterm infants and vascular malformations with secondary thrombocytopenia (Kasabach–Merritt syndrome).

In the adolescent most abnormal vaginal bleeding is due to anovulatory dysfunctional uterine bleeding (DUB). About half of all girls at menarche do not ovulate and are at risk (109–111). The characteristic presentation is bleeding for 3–4 weeks due to irregular sloughing of thickened but fragile endometrium followed by 3–4 months of amenorrhea with reaccumulation of flimsy endometrium due to continuous estrogenic stimulation. Another pattern is complete irregularity of bleeding with confusing variations from normal. Ideally the following may be considered: complete blood count (CBC), and other coagulation tests; thyroid function tests; prolactin; human chorionic gonadotropin (hCG); comprehensive metabolic screen; as well as history, physical examination, vaginoscopy, and perhaps pelvic sonography. Annovulatory dysfunctional uterine bleeding is usually managed with oral contraceptives (initially at high dosage) for hemostasis. If unsuccessful, intravenous Premarin is considered for initial hemostasis, especially if there is a thin, raw endometrium and, as a last resort a gentle dilatation and curettage of the uterus and Foley catheter balloon tamponade of the uterine cavity (112). The American College of Obstetricians and Gynecologists (ACOG) Practice Bulletin notes that "Anovulatory bleeding is a normal physiological process in the perimenarchal year of the reproductive cycle" (113). Nevertheless it indicates a 5–20% prevalence of blood dyscrasias in adolescents hospitalized for bleeding. Of course, this is a select group with heavy bleeding. Others consider DUB as abnormal (114). Clinically it is often difficult to decide whether the bleeding is simply DUB or due to significant pathology.

Abnormal vaginal bleeding may be the presenting symptom of a blood dyscrasia such as von Willebrand's disease, factor XI deficiency, thrombocytopenia, platelet dysfunction (112, 115–117), or other factor deficiencies (118). Other causes of adolescent abnormal bleeding include leukemia, pregnancy and its complications, neoplasms (ovary, uterus, vagina), partial ovarian failure, severe liver and renal disease, forgotten tampons, pelvic inflammatory disease, and underlying causes of anovulation (119). Adolescents requiring hospitalization for menorrhagia have significant medical problems including anemia, anovulation, hematological disease (33%), effects of chemotherapy, and infection (120).

The most common malignancy of childhood is leukemia, which accounts for 35%. About 80–85% of leukemias are acute lymphoblastic leukemia (ALL). ALL is the most common specific childhood malignancy (30–35%). The clinical picture is truly acute: two-thirds have symptoms less than 1 month preceding the diagnosis. Initially there is lethargy, exhaustion, and anorexia. Later there is anemia, bleeding tendency (purpura, mucosal bleeding, hematomas), infections, hepatosplenomegaly, generalized lymphadenopathy, and bone–joint discomfort. There is a genetic susceptibility to chromosomal syndromes, DNA fragility, immunodeficiency syndromes, and neurofibromatosis. Nevertheless 99% of cases are of unknown causes. The peak incidence is between ages 2 and 5. Unfortunately there may be an initial normal complete blood count (CBC) and smear and therefore a bone marrow study may be required (121). Acute myeloid (nonlymphoblastic) leukemia causes 17% of cases of childhood leukemia (122, 123).

XII. EVALUATION

For prepubertal vaginal bleeding the history, physical examination and findings on vaginoscopy will give an immediate diagnosis in 80–85% of cases (124).

A. History

It is important to obtain a reliable history from the mother, the child's caretaker, and, if possible, from the child herself. Some suggestions follow.

The bleeding history is detailed: onset, color (bright red or brownish red, mixed with discharge), odor, amount, and continuation: course, pain, and association with scratching, wiping, urination, bowel movement, and tight clothing.

Inquiry is made about vulvovaginitis symptoms: vulvar itching, burning, and pain; vaginal discharge; rubbing; use of bubble baths, perfumed soaps, or deodorants; or wearing of tights, leotards, and ballet outfits. Dysuria caused by vulvitis presents as vulvar dysuria with external pain, a reluctance to void, a distended bladder, and occasionally acute urinary retention. Dysuria caused by cystitis–urethritis causes deep pain, frequency, urgency, and bladder spasms.

Has there been recent antibiotic, drug, aspirin or hormonal therapy or respiratory or skin infection? Does the child have allergies or general chronic skin disturbances, such as atopic or seborrheic dermatitis, eczema, or psoriasis? Does she have diabetes, chronic illnesses (kidney, hepatic, or intestinal), or immunodeficiency defect? Is there a coagulation disturbance?

Was there an acute trauma, such as falling from a play device or from standing on a chair? Could the child have been molested (even by an adult male relative) and have been threatened if she reveals it? Is she left without supervision?

Was the pregnancy uneventful? Did the mother take any unusual medications? The family history includes the health of siblings and such illnesses as diabetes; atopic dermatitis, allergies, asthma, and eczema; bleeding disorders; immunodeficiency states; and malignancies.

B. Physical Examination

Before examination, as an educational device, I indicate to the child in the presence of the mother that only mothers and doctors are allowed to examine, look at, or touch children's "private parts." The mother is kept in the room to reassure the child. Try to communicate in a friendly fashion with the child to help her relax and create a non-threatening environment.

The panties are inspected for blood and discharge.

The physical examination begins with a general examination.

1. Are there signs of precocious puberty? Is there axillary or pubic hair? Is there mammary tissue on palpation, or do the breasts seem enlarged because the child is chubby?
2. Does the child seem irritable? Does she scratch herself generally? Is there white dermatographism? Are there signs of general skin disease, especially seborrheic or atopic dermatitis characterized by erythematous fissures behind the ears with flaking; scalp margins and paranasal erythematous greasy scales; pityriasis alba of the face; prominent lower eyelid skin folds (Morgan's folds) with white edematous edges; keratosis pilaris of the outer arms and thighs, eczema of the elbows, wrists, and popliteal space; and ichthyosis of the legs? Are there signs of psoriasis or chicken pox? Are there skin infections? Is there pharyngitis, rhinitis, or cough? Is there adenopathy (cervical, axillary, or inguinal), abdominal masses, or ecchymosis?
3. Are there petechiae, ecchymoses, hepatosplenomegaly, abdominal masses, cervical, axillary or inguinal adenopathy, anemia or abnormal blood vessels (telangiectasias)?

The frequent local nonhormonal bleeding areas that require attention in the physical examination are listed in Table 2.

As a minimum, the vulva must be visualized. Further office testing must be individualized in accord with the reaction of the child, source of bleeding, experience of the physician, appearance of the vulva, history, and perceived seriousness.

The child may be placed in small stirrups in dorsal lithotomy position or in frog leg position on the exami-

Table 2 Frequent Causes of Nonhormonal Bleeding According to Site

Urethra: prolapse urethra (necrotic, sloughing)
Anus: deep fissure (pain, skin tag edema)
Vulva (inspection with good light and gentle retraction)
　　Trauma
　　Skin disease and lesions
　　Fissures (associated with seborrheic and atopic dermatitis and lichen sclerosus)
　　General ecchymoses (coagulation defect)
　　Hymen polyp
Inspection of distal vagina
　　Vaginal discharge
　　Vaginal bleeding
Vaginal bleeding
　　Severe Streptococcus A vaginitis (usually upper vagina)
　　Foreign body (usually rolled-up wads of toilet tissue causing a foul, bloody discharge)
　　Rhabdomyosarcoma (rare but very malignant with only drops of blood)

nation table or in the lap of the mother, who sits on the table. A good cold light is necessary.

The labia majora are gently held apart and downward to permit adequate inspection. Sometimes, the child's hands can be used by the examiner as retractors to reduce anxiety. Careful inspection requires a trained eye. One method is to start anteriorly and proceed posteriorly, viewing the mons pubis; presence of hair; erythematous fissures in the midline anterior to the clitoris, then between the labia majora and minora symmetrically, in the midline perineum (between vagina and rectum), radially around the anus, and in the midline posterior to the anus; clitoris; urethra; hymen and its orifice; vestibule (just outside the hymen); posterior fourchette; perineum; perianal area; and groin and the adjacent buttocks. Very often the distal vagina can be visualized.

If the site and cause of the bleeding can be identified by visualizing the exposed vulva, then the examination may be discontinued. If these are not apparent, then further investigation is needed and examination under anesthesia may be required to avoid anxiety, thrashing, and resistance by the child.

Placing a Q-tip in the vagina may show blood and indicate the vaginal source of bleeding. Another device is an eye or medicine dropper. Vaginal secretion may be tested for Papanicolaou cytology, bacterial culture, Gram's stain, gonorrhea culture, Chlamydia culture, saline wet mount (for motile trichomonads, white blood cells, lactobacilli, "clue" cells of Gardnerella bacterial vaginosis), and 10% potassium hydroxide wet mount for Candida. Cytology is not reliable to rule out a vaginal malignancy. Cytological maturation index (MI) is helpful in evaluating estrogen activity. The usual anestrogenic prepubertal child has an MI of 0% superficial, 0% intermediate, and 100% parabasal cells. Superficial vaginal cells are large, flat, and polygonal with a small pyknotic nucleus and are indicative of the presence of estrogen. In England and Canada, laboratories often reverse the MI sequence and report parabasal, intermediate, and superficial vaginal cells. The newborn has a temporary estrogenic smear of superficial vaginal epithelial cells because of in utero maternal estrogen exposure.

Although not as reliable as an early morning swab, a clear cellophane type of perianal swab may be made to check for microscopic pinworm ova and to show the mother how to do it at home in the early morning.

Bimanual rectal examination usually cannot detect toilet tissue wads in the vagina but can detect a hard vaginal foreign object, a normal cervix, a firm vaginal tumor mass, and the lower pole of an ovarian neoplasm (the infant's ovary is pelvic). It might "milk out" vaginal discharge or bleeding.

With a cooperative older child, the "knee–chest" position may result in a ballooning out of the vagina to permit visualization of the distal two-thirds of the vagina with a hand-held light (see Fig. 9).

If the bleeding source is not apparent from visualization of the exposed vulva and distal vagina or if a Q-tip inserted into the vagina produces bleeding, then vaginoscopy is appropriate. There may be a specific severe infection (*Streptococcus* A), a foreign body (rolled-up wads of toilet tissue), or a malignant and potentially fatal neoplasm. Vaginoscopy is done generally for the suspicion of significant trauma, foreign body, neoplasm, congenital anomaly, or persistent vaginitis.

Unfortunately, no standard vaginoscope is in use. The vaginoscope instruments that have been used include a simple tube with obturator; a Cameron-Miller tube with obturator, distal light bulb, magnifying glass; a fiberoptic Storz instrument; a hysteroscope; a cystoscope; or a miniature bivalve speculum. Miniature alligator forceps to remove foreign bodies, and long microsurgical instruments should be available for biopsy and local excision of tumors. Experience is required for operative procedures.

Sometimes observation vaginoscopy can be done as an office procedure; however, operative vaginoscopy is best done in an operating room with general anesthesia by an expert pediatric anesthesiologist.

If there is an expectation of a malignant vaginal tumor, then a frozen section is considered and cystoscopy with biopsy may be done with the same anesthesia to check for spread.

Abdominal and pelvic ultrasound are considered for the suspicion of a neoplasm, large or rigid foreign body, and congenital anomaly (therefore the kidneys require imaging). Rolled-up wads of toilet tissue and small vaginal malignant neoplasms may not be able to be imaged. Adrenal enlargements may require computed tomographic

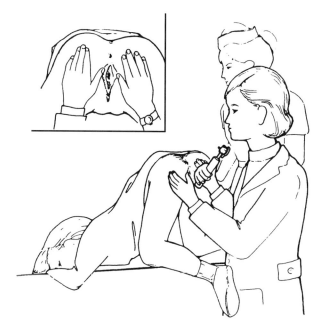

Figure 9 Knee–chest position for visualizing the vagina in the cooperative older child using a hand-held light. (Reproduced with permission from Emans SJ. Section 11. Gynecology. In: Avery ME, First LR, eds. Pediatric Medicine. Baltimore: Williams & Wilkins, 1989:652).

(CT) imaging. The addition of MRI may be helpful for congenital anomalies and neoplasms.

X-rays are to be avoided if possible.

Clinical coagulation defect as a cause of vaginal bleeding is unusual in children but is important in adolescent menorrhagia. For suspicion of coagulation defect consider: CBC, platelet count, prothrombin time, partial thromboplastin time, bleeding time, and von Willebrand tests. For more extensive testing consider platelet function, plasma coagulation factors, circulating anticoagulant, fibrinogen, functional protein C and S, or hematology consultation.

XIII. CONCLUSION

Vaginal bleeding is unusual in children. It creates great anxiety in the child and her parents. The vast majority of bleeding is caused by local, nonhormonal causes. Bleeding requires prompt investigation to determine the site, cause, and management.

The special concerns include precocious puberty, sexual molestation, and malignancy.

If required for the diagnosis of blood coming from the vagina from a site that cannot be visualized externally, vaginoscopy under general anesthesia (if necessary) is appropriate.

REFERENCES

1. Heller ME, Savage MO, Dewhurst J. Vaginal bleeding in childhood: a review of 51 patients. Br J Obstet Gynaecol 1978; 85:721–725.
2. Saggese G, Ghirri P, DelVecchio A, Papini A, Pardi D. Gonadotropin pulsatile secretion in girls with premature menarche. Horm Res 1990; 33:5–10.
3. Rakover Y, Weiner E, Shalev E, Luboshitsky R. Vaginal bleeding: presenting symptom of acquired primary hypothyroidism in a seven year old girl. J Pediatr Endocrinol 1993; 6:197–200.
4. Bajaj S. Primary hypothroidism presenting as vaginal bleeding in a five year old girl. J Assoc Physicians India 2000; 48:930.
5. Gordon CM, Austin DJ, Radovick S, Laufer MR. Primary hypothyroidism presenting as severe vaginal bleeding in a prepubertal girl. J Pediatr Adolesc Gynecol 1997; 10:35–38.
6. Uli N, Chin D, David R, Geneiser N, Roche K, Marino F, Shapiro E, Prasad K, Oberfield S. Menstrual bleeding in a female infant with congential adrenal hyperplasia: altered maturation of the hypothalamic–pituitary–ovarian axis. J Clin Endocrinol Metab 1997; 82:3298–3302.
7. Yeshaya A, Kauschansky A, Orvieto R, Varsano I, Nussinovitch M, Ben-Rafael Z. Prolonged vaginal bleeding during central precocious purberty therapy with a long-acting gonadotropin-releasing hormone agonist. Acta Obstet Gynecol Scand 1998; 77:327–329.
8. Grunberger W. Diagnose und therapie bei gynakologisch erkrankten madchen. Wien Klin Wochenschr 1987; 99:763–767.
9. Hill NC, Oppenheimer LW, Morton KE. The aetiology of vaginal bleeding in children: a 20 year review. Br J Obstet Gynaecol 1989; 96:467–470.
10. Altchek A. Vaginal discharges. In: Stockman JA III, ed. Difficult Diagnosis in Pediatrics. Philadelphia: WB Saunders, 1990:383–389.
11. Emans SJH. Vulvovaginal problems in the prepubertal child. In: Emans SJH, Goldstein DP, eds. Pediatric and Adolescent Gynecology, 3rd ed. Boston: Little, Brown, 1990:67–93.
12. Fishman A, Paidi E. Vaginal bleeding in premenarchal girls: a review. Obstet Gynecol Surv 1991; 46:457–460.
13. Pokorny SF. Prepubertal vulvovaginopathies. Obstet Gynecol Clin North Am 1992; 19:39–58.
14. Wilson MD. Vaginal discharge and vaginal bleeding in childhood. In: Carpenter SEK, Rock JA, eds. Pediatric and Adolescent Gynecology. New York: Raven Press, 1992:139–151.
15. Muram D, Sanfilippo JS, Hertweck SP. Vaginal bleeding in childhood and menstrual disorders in adolescence. In: Sanfilippo JS, Muram D, Lee PA, Dewhurst J, eds. Pediatric and Adolescent Gynecology. Philadelphia: WB Saunders, 1994:222–232.
16. Imai A, Horibe S, Tamaya T. Genital bleeding in premenarcheal children. Int J Gynaecol Obstet 1995; 49:41–45.
17. Merritt DF. Evaluation of vaginal bleeding in the preadolescent child. Semin Pediatr 1998; 7:35–42.
18. Emans SJH. Vulvovaginal problems in the prepubertal child. In: Emans SJH, Laufer MR, Goldstein DP, eds. Pediatric and Adolescent Gynecology, 4th ed. Philadelphia: Lippincott Williams & Wilkins, 1998:75–108.
19. Buckingham K, Fawdry A, Fothergill D. Management of vaginal bleeding presenting to the accident and emergency department. J Accid Emerg Med 1999; 16:130–135.
20. Wilson MD. Vaginal discharge and vaginal bleeding in childhood. In: Carpenter SEK, Rock JA, eds. Pediatric and Adolescent Gynecology, 2nd ed. New York: Lippincott Williams & Wilkins, 2000:122–160.
21. Muram D. Pediatric and adolescent gynecology. In: Ransom SB, ed. Practical Strategies in Obstetics and Gynecology. Philadelphia: WB Saunders, 2000:82–106.
22. Dhar V, Roker K, Adhami MZ, Mckenzie S. Streptococcal vulvovaginitis in girls. Pediatr Dermatol 1993; 10:366–367.
23. Yanovski JA, Nelson LM, Willis ED, Cutler GB Jr. Repeated childhood vaginal bleeding is not always precocious puberty. Pediatrics 1992; 89:149–151.
24. Magana-Garcia M, Arista-Viveros A. Cutaneous amebiasis in children. Pediatr Dermatol 1993; 10:352–355.
25. Dudgeon DL, Grisoni ER. Trauma to the female perineum. In: Carpenter SEK, Rock JA, eds. Pediatric and Adolescent Gynecology, 2nd ed. New York. Lippincott Williams & Wilkins, 2000:114–121.
26. Pierce AM, Robson WJ. Genital injury in girls-accidental or not? Pediatr Surg Int 1993; 8:239–243.
27. Kunkel NC. Vaginal injury from a water slide in a premenarcheal patient. Pediatr Emerg Care 1998; 14:210–211.
28. Mushkat Y. Vaginal evisceration resulting from a water-slide injury. J Trauma 1998; 45:853.
29. Perlman SE, Hertweck SP, Wolfe WM. Water-ski douche in injury in a premenarcheal female. Pediatrics 1995; 96:782–783.
30. Morrison DM, Pasquale MD, Scagliotti CJ. Hydrostatic rectal injury of a jet ski passenger: case report and discussion. J Trauma 1998; 45:816–818.
31. Ramos JP, Carrison D, Phillips DL. Unusual vaginal laceration due to a high-pressure water jet. West J Med 1998; 169:171–172.
32. Muchkat Y, Lessing JB, Jedwab GA, David MP. Vaginal trauma occurring while sliding down a water chute. Br J Obstet Gynaecol 1995;102(11):933–934.
33. Ameh EA. Anorectal injuries in children. Pediatr Surg Int 2000; 16:388–391.
34. Shui LT, Lee CL, Yen CF, Wang CJ, Soong YK. Vaginoscopy using hysteroscope for diagnosis of vaginal bleeding during childhood: case report. Chang Keng I Hsueh Tsa Chih 1999; 22:344–347.
35. Zitsman JL, Cirincione E, Margossiani H. Vaginal bleeding in an infant secondary to sliding inguinal hernia. Obstet Gynecol 1997; 89:840–842.
36. Muram D. Child sexual abuse. In: Goldfarb EF, ed. Atlas of Clinical Gynecology, Vol I. Pediatric and Adolescent Gynecology. Philadelphia: Appleton, 1998:11.2–11.3.
37. Bhagat M. Coital injury presenting in a 13 year old as abdominal pain and vaginal bleeding. Pediatr Emerg Care 1996; 12:354–355.
38. Cerqui AJ, Haylen BT. "Fisting" as a cause of vaginal bleeding. Med J Aust 1998; 169:288.
39. Obalek S, Misiewicz J, Jablonska S, Favre M, Orth G. Childhood condyloma acuminatum: association with genital and cutaneous human papillomaviruses. Pediatr Dermatol 1993; 10:101–106.
40. Salopek TG, Krol A, Jimbo K. Case report of Darier disease localized to the vulva in a 5 year old girl. Pediatr Dermatol 1993; 10:146–148.
41. Serrano G, Millan F, Fortea JM, Grau M, Aliaga A. Topical progesterone as treatment of choice in genital lichen

sclerosis et atrophicus in children (correspondence). Pediatr Dermatol 1993; 10:201.

42. Cook CL, Sanfilippo JS, Verdi GD, Pietsch JP. Capillary hemangioma of the vagina and urethra in a child: response to short term steroid therapy. Obstet Gynecol 1989; 73:883–885.

43. Morelli JG. On the treatment of hemangiomas (commentary). Pediatr Dermatol 1993; 10:84.

44. Pehr K, Moroz B. Cutis marmorata telangiectatica congenita: long term follow-up, review of the literature, and report of a case in conjunction with congenital hypothyroidism. Pediatr Dermatol 1993; 10:6–11.

45. Enjoiras O, Mulliken JB. The current management of vascular birthmarks. Pediatr Dermatol 1993; 10:311–333.

46. Hatley RM, Sabio H, Howell CG, Flickinger F, Parrish RA. Successful management of an infant with a giant hemangioma of the retroperitoneum and Kasabach-Merritt syndrome with alpha-interferon. J Pediatr Surg 1993; 28:1356–1359.

47. Resnick SD, Lacey S, Jones G. Hemorrhagic complications in a rapidly growing, congenital hemangiopericytoma. Pediatr Dermatol 1993; 10:267–270.

48. Muram D, Gold SS. Vulvar ulcerations in girls with myelocytic leukemia. South Med J 1993; 86:293–294.

49. Hruza LL, Mallory SB, Fitzgibbons J, Mallory GB. Linear IgA bullous dermatosis in a neonate. Pediatr Dermatol 1993; 10:171–176.

50. Guenther L, Shum D. Granular cell tumor of the vulva. Pediatr Dermatol 1993; 10:153–155.

51. Fernandes ET, Dekermacher S, Sabadin MA, Vaz F. Urethral prolapse in children. Urology 1993; 41:240–242.

52. Trotman MD, Brewster EM. Prolapse of the urethral mucosa in prepubertal West Indian girls. Br J Urol 1993; 72:503–505.

53. Desai SR, Cohen RC. Urethral prolapse in a premenarchal girl: case report and literature review. Aust NZ J Sur 1997; 67:660–662.

54. Anveden-Hertzberg L, Gauderer MW, Elder JS. Urethral prolapse: an often misdiagnosed cause of urogenital bleeding in girls. Pediatr Emerg Care 1995; 11:212–214

55. Montemarano AD, James WD. *Staphylococcus aureus* as a cause of perianal dermatitis. Pediatr Dermatol 1993; 10:259– 262.

56. Daya DA, Scully RE. Sarcoma botryoides of the uterine cervix in young women: a clinicopathological study of 13 cases. Gynecol Oncol 1988; 29:290–304.

57. Shulman LP. Management quandry. rhabdomyosarcoma botryoid type. J Pediatr Adolesc Gynecol 1999; 12:171–172.

58. Choi CM, Majmudar B, Horowitz, IR. Malignant neoplasms of the vagina and cervix in the neonate, child and adolescent. In: Carpenter SEK, Rock JA, eds. Pediatric and Adolescent Gynecology, 2nd ed., New York: Lippincott Williams & Wilkins, 2000:403–423.

59. Horng, YC, Tsai WY, Lin DT, Huang SF, Lin KH, Li YW, Hsieh FJ, Chen CC. Infantile endodermal sinus tumor presenting with vaginal bleeding: report of a case. J Formos Med Assoc 1994; 93:164–166.

60. de Silva MV, Fernando, MS, Amaratunge K, Hennayake S. Vaginal bleeding in infants caused by endodermal sinus tumors. Ceylon Med J 1997; 42:193–194.

61. Yadav K, Singh G, Budhiraja S, Radhika S. Endodermal sinus tumor of cervix—case report. Indian J Cancer 1996; 33:43–45.

62. Herbst AL, Anderson D. Clear cell adenocarcinoma of cervix and vagina and DES-related abnormalities. In:

Coppleson M, Monaghan JM, Morrow CP, Tattersall MHN, eds. Gynecologic Oncology. Fundamental Principles and Clinical Practice, 2nd ed, Vol 1. New York: Churchill Livingstone, 1992:523–533.

63. Parkes SE, Raafat F, Morland BJ. Paraganglioma of the vagina: the first report of a rare tumor in a child. Pediatr Hematol Oncol 1998; 15:545–551.

64. Terruhn V. Polyps of the uterine cervix during the hormonal resting phase in childhood (German). Geburtshilfe Frauenheilkd 1977; 37:35–38.

65. Brooks GG. Granular cell myoblastoma of the vulva in a 6 year old girl. Am J Obstet Gynecol 1985; 153:897–898.

66. Morad NA, el-Said MM. Cellular uterine myoma causing vaginal bleeding in a 15 year old girl. Aust NZ J Obstet Gynaecol 1993; 33:211–213.

67. Clement PB, Scully RE. Mullerian adenosarcoma of the uterus: a clinicopathologic analysis of 100 cases with a review of the literature. Hum Pathol 1990; 21:363–381.

68. Verschraegen CF, Vasuratna A, Edwards C, Freedman R, Kudelka AP, Tornos C, Kauanagh JJ. Clinicopathologic analysis of mullerian adenosarcoma: the M.D. Anderson Cancer Center experience. Oncol Rep 1998; 5:939–944.

69. Bonita S, Ward, MD, Hitchcock CL, Keyhani S. Primitive neuroectodermal tumor of the uterus: a case report. Acta Cytol 2000; 44:667–672.

70. Lessing JB, Michowitz M, Baratz, M. Granulosa-theca cell tumor in a one-year old infant. Acta Obstet Gynecol Scand 1985; 64:345–347.

71. Aziz MF. Current management of malignant germ cell tumor of the ovary. Gan To Kagaku Ryoho 1995; 22 Suppl 3:262–276.

72. Murthy DP, SenGupta SK, Mola G, R Ageau O, Mathias A. Sclerosing stromal tumor of the ovary. P N G Med J 1996; 39:48–55.

73. Calaminus G, Wessalowski R, Hams D, Gobel U. Juvenile granulosa cell tumors of the ovary in children and adolescents: results from 33 patients registered in a prospective cooperative study. Gynecol Oncol 1997; 65:447–452.

74. Ferrera PC, Whitman MC. Ovarian small cell carcinoma: a rare neoplasm in a 15 year old female. Pediatr Emerg Care 2000; 16:170–172.

75. Horowitz IR, De La Cuesta RS, Majmudar B. Benign and malignant tumors of the ovary. In: Carpenter SEK, Rock JA, eds. Pediatric and Adolescent Gynecology, 2nd ed. New York: Lippincott Williams & Wilkins, 2000:441–462.

76. Werner EJ, Broxson EH, Tucker EL, Giroux DS, Shults J, Abshire TC. Prevalence of von Willebrand disease in children: a multi-ethnic study. J Pediatr 1993; 123:893–898.

77. Sadler JE, Blinder M. von Willebrand disease: diagnosis, classification and treatment. In: Colman RW, Hirsh J, Marder VJ, Clowes AW, George JN, eds. Hemostasis and Thrombosis, 4th ed. Philadelphia: Lippincott Williams and Wilkins, 2001:825–837.

78. Kouides PA, Phatak PD, Burkart P, Braggins C, Cox C, Bernstein Z, Belling L, Holmberg P, MacLaughlin W, Howard F. Gynaecological and obstetrical morbidity in women with type I von Willebrand disease: results of a patient survey. Hemophilia 2000; 6:643–648.

79. Lillicrap D, Dean J, Blanchette VS. von Willebrand disease. In: Lilleyman JS, Hann IM, Blanchette VS, eds. Pediatric Hematology. New York: Churchill Livingstone, 1999:601–609.

80. Dean JA, Blanchette VS, Carcao MD, Stain AM, Sparling CR, Siekmann J, Turecek PL, Lillicrap D, Rand ML. von Willebrand disease in a pediatric-based population—comparison of type 1 diagnostic criteria and use of the PFA-100 and a von Willebrand factor/collagen-binding assay. Thromb Haemost 2000; 84:401–409.

81. Smith H. Diagnosis in Paediatric Haematology. New York: Churchill Livingstone, 1996:278.

82. Castaman G, Eikenboom JC, Bertina RM, Rodeghiero F. Inconsistency of association between type 1 von Willebrand disease phenotype and genotype in families identified in an epidemiological investigation. Thromb Haemost 1999; 82:1065–1070.

83. Schlammadinger A, Kerenyi A, Muszbek L, Boda Z. Comparison of the O'Brien filter test and the PFA-100 platelet analyzer in the laboratory diagnosis of von Willebrand's disease. Thromb Haemost 2000; 84:88–92.

84. Biron C, Mahieu B, Rochette A, Capdevila X, Castex A, Amiral J, D'Athis F, Schved JF. Preoperative screening for von Willebrand disease type 1: low yield and limited ability to predict bleeding. J Lab Clin Med 1999; 134:605–609.

85. Nolan B, White B, Smith J, O'Reily C, Fitzpatrick B, Smith OP. Desmopressin: therapeutic limitations in children and adults with inherited coagulation disorders. Br J Haematol 2000; 109:865–869.

86. van Genderen PJ, Michiels JJ. Acquired von Willebrand disease. Baillieres Clin Haematol 1998; 11:319–330.

87. Federici AB, Rand JH, Bucciarelli P, Budde U, van Genderen PJ, Mohri H, Meyer D, Rodeghiero F, Sadler JE; Subcommittee on von Willebrand Factor. Acquired von Willebrand syndrome: data from an international registry. Thromb Haemost 2000; 84:345–349.

88. Konety BR, Hord JD, Weiner ES, Schneck FX. Embryonal adenoma of the kidney associated with polycythemia and von Willebrand disease. J Urol 1998; 160:2171–2174.

89. Seligshohn U. Factor XI deficiency. Thromb Haemost. 1993; 70:68–71.

90. Kadir RA, Economides DL, Lee CA. Factor XI deficiency in women. Am J Hematol. 1999; 60:48–54.

91. Agarwal MB, Agarwal UM, Viswanathan C, Bhave AA, Bilia V. Glanzmann's thrombasthenia. Indian Pediatr 1992; 29:837–841.

92. Markovitch O, Ellis M, Holzinger M, Goldberger S, Beyth Y. Severe juvenile vaginal bleeding due to Glanzmann's thrombasthenia: case report and review of the literature. Am J Hematol 1998; 57:225–227.

93. Bernini JC, Buchanan GR, Ashcraft J. Hypoprothrombinemia and severe hemorrhage associated with a lupus anticoagulant. J Pediatr 1993; 123:937–939.

94. Medeiros D, Buchanan GR. Idiopathic thrombocytopenic purpura: beyond consensus. Curr Opin Pediatr 2000; 12:4–9.

95. Iyori H., Bessho F, Ookawa H, Konishi S, Shirahata A, Miyazaki S, Fujisana K, Akatsuka J, Japanese Study Group on childhood ITP. Intracranial hemorrhage in children with immune thrombocytopenic purpura. Japanese study group on childhood I TP. Ann Hematol 2000; 79:691–695.

96. Zeller B, Helgestad J, Hellebostad M, Kolmannskog S, Nystad T, Stensvold K, Wesenberg F. Immune thrombocytopenic purpura in childhood in Norway: a prospective, population-based registration. Pediatr Hematol Oncol 2000; 17:551–558.

97. Chiu CH, Tsai JR, Ou JT, Lin TY. Typhoid fever in children: a fourteen-year experience. Acta Paediatr Taiwan 2000; 41:28–32.

98. al-Jefri AH, Dror Y, Bussel JB, Freedman MH. Thrombocytopenia with absent radii: frequency of marrow megakaryoctye progenitors, proliferative characteristics, and megakaryocyte growth and development factor responsiveness. Pediatr Hematol Oncol 2000; 17:299–306.

99. Costelloe CM, De Mouy EH, Neitzschman HR. Radiology case of the month. Congenital limb and bleeding disorder. Thrombocytopenia absent radius syndrome (TAR). J LA State Med Soc 2000; 152:551–552.

100. Young EJ, Tarry A, Genta RM, Ayden N, Gotuzzo E. Thrombocytopenic purpura associated with brucellosis: report of 2 cases and literature review. Clin Infect Dis 2000; 31:904–909.

101. Imbach P. Immune thrombocytopenic purpura. In: Lilleyman JS, Ham IM, Blanchette VS, eds. Pediatric Hematology 2nd ed. New York: Churchill Livingstone, 1999: 437–454.

102. Ritchey AK, Keller FG. Hematologic manifestations of childhood illness. In: Hoffman R, Benz EJ, Jr, Shatil SJ, Furie B, Cohen HJ, Silberstein LE, McGlave P, eds. Hematology Basic Principles and Practice, 3rd ed. New York: Churchill Livingstone, 2000:2391–2410.

103. Tefferi A, Fonseca R, Pereira DL, Hoagland HC. A long term retrospective study of young women with essential thrombocythemia. Mayo Clin Proc 2001; 76:22–28.

104. Chalmers EA, Gibson BES. Hemostatic problems in the neonate. In: Lilleyman VS, Ham IM, Blanchette VS. eds. Pediatric Hematology, 2nd ed. New York: Churchill Livingstone, 1999:651–678.

105. Murphy MF, Manley R, Roberts D. Neonatal alloimmune thrombocytopenia. Haematologica 1999; 84:110–114.

106. Jaegtvik S, Husebekk A, Aune B, Oian P, Dahl LB, Skogen B. Neonatal alloimmune thrombocytopenia due to anti-HPA 1a antibodies; the level of maternal antibodies predicts the severity of thrombocytopenia in the newborn. Br J Obstet Gynaecol 2000; 107:691–694.

107. Sainio S, Jarvenpaa AL, Renlund M, Riikonen S, Teramo K, Kekomaki R. Thrombocytopenia in term infancy: a population based study. Obstet Gynecol 2000; 95:441–446.

108. Edelson M, McKenzie, SE. How to manage bleeding in newborns. Contemporary OB/GYN 2001; 46:441–446.

109. Speroff L, Glass RH, Kase NG. Clinical Gynecologic Endocrinology and Infertility, 6th ed. New York: Lippincott Williams & Wilkins, 1999:580.

110. Edmonds DK. Dysfunctional uterine bleeding in adolescence. Best Pract Res Clin Obstet Gynaecol 1999; 13:239–249.

111. Inglesias EA, Coupey SM. Menstrual cycle abnormalities: diagnosis and management. Adolesc Med 1999; 10:255–273.

112. Quint, EH, Smith YR, Breech LL, Carpenter SE. Management quandary. J Pediatr Adolesc Gynecol 1999; 12:233–235.

113. ACOG Practice Bulletin. Management of anovulatory bleeding. Clinical management guidelines for obstetrician–gynecologists. 14:2000.

114. Bravender T, Emans SJ. Menstrual disorders. Dysfunctional uterine bleeding. Pediatr Clin North Am 1999; 46:545–553.

115. Kadir RA, Sabin CA, Pollard D, Lee CA, Economides DL. Quality of life during menstruation in patients with

inherited bleeding disorders. Haemophilia 1998; 4:836–841.

116. Kadir RA, Economides DL, Sabin CA, Pollard D, Lee CA. Assessment of menstrual blood loss and gynaecological problems in patients with inherited bleeding disorders. Haemophilia 1999; 5:40–48.

117. Ellis MH, Beyth Y. Abnormal vaginal bleeding in adolescence as the presenting symptom of a bleeding diathesis. J Pediatr Adolesc Gynecol 1999; 12:127–131.

118. Bennett K, Daley ML, Pike C. Factor V deficiency and menstruation: a gynecologic challenge. Obstet Gynecol 1997; 89:839–840.

119. Minjarez DA, Bradshaw KD. Abnormal uterine bleeding in adolescents. Obstet Gynecol Clin North Am 2000; 27:63–78.

120. Smith YR, Quint EH, Hertzberg RB. Menorrhagia in adolescents requiring hospitalization. J Pediatr Assoc Gynecol 1998; 11:13–15.

121. Ritter J, Schrappe M. Clinical features and therapy of lymphoblastic leukemia. In: Lilleyman JS, Hann IM, Blanchette VS, eds. Pediatric Hematology. New York: Churchill Livingstone, 1999:537–563.

122. Ching-Hon P, Behm FG. Pathology of acute myeloid leukemia. In: Lilleyman JS, Hann IM, Blanchette VS, eds. Pediatric Hematology. New York: Churchill Livingstone, 1999:369–386.

123. Ching-Hon P, ed. Childhood Leukemias. New York: Cambridge University Press, 1999.

124. David L, Betend B, Berlier P, Evrard A, Guinard A, Francois R. Genital hemorrhage in girls before puberty. Apropos of 13 cases. [French]. 33 cases. Semin Hop 1984; 60:1195–1199.

12

Hirsutism, Polycystic Ovary Syndrome, and Menstrual Disorders

Songya Pang
University of Illinois at Chicago College of Medicine, Chicago, Illinois, U.S.A.

I. INTRODUCTION

Skin, muscle, and the reproductive system are major target sites of excess androgens in adolescent and young women. Androgen excess symptoms in peripubertal and postpubertal girls include hirsutism, acne, virilization or masculinization, and menstrual disorder. Hirsutism is defined as excess body hair growth in females, involving primarily areas of the face, chin, neck, midline chest and abdomen, upper and lower back, buttocks, and inner aspects of the thigh. In general, hirsutism by itself is a mild symptom of androgen overproduction or enhanced androgen metabolism/action in the skin tissue. Increased androgen activity in the sebaceous and apocrine glands is likewise associated with development of acne vulgaris. The androgen activities of hair follicles and sebaceous glands of the skin are not necessarily identical and vary greatly between sites (1). This may explain the heterogeneous expression of cutaneous hyperandrogenic symptoms, such as hirsutism alone, acne alone, or hirsutism and acne together as symptoms of androgen excess or enhanced androgen activity in the skin tissue (2). The clinical expression of androgen excess symptoms does not always correlate with the degree of androgen production or circulating androgen levels. This suggests that androgen metabolic activity in the target tissue is in part governed by a local tissue mechanism

Hypertrichosis is characterized by generalized increased fine body hair with no special preferential sites. This condition is generally not associated with androgen overproduction. Either genetic or ethnic influences on body hair growth may be a contributing factor in hypertrichosis. In some cases, however, hypertrichosis may be the early manifestation of mild androgen excess or is induced by chronic ingestion of drugs that alter hair growth directly or indirectly via the influence on the local or systemic metabolism of certain androgens. Clinically, the more severe androgen excess symptoms involve skin and muscle, as well as the reproductive system, and are termed virilization or masculinization. These include some or all of the following symptoms of hyperandrogenism: clitoral enlargement, masculine body habitus, temporal hair loss, voice changes, breast atrophy, and menstrual disorders (3). Virilization and masculinization are usually manifestations of significant pathology causing androgen overproduction in women.

Excess androgen-producing pathologies in young women are a well-known cause of menstrual disorder. However, many other disorders unrelated to hyperandrogenism cause menstrual disorders in young women. This chapter elaborates the physiology of androgen metabolism in women and disorders of androgen production and action resulting in the manifestation of androgen excess symptoms in young women. In addition, a review of the known causes of menstrual disorders unrelated to excess androgen disorders and their management in adolescents and young women is summarized.

II. PHYSIOLOGY OF ANDROGEN METABOLISM

A. Bioactivity of Androgens

Androgenicity is the term used to describe the bioactivity of a steroid that produces masculine characteristics. The bioactivity of androgens in a laboratory is measured by either determining an exogenous steroidal effect of a known quantity on the weight increase of the seminal vesicle or prostate of castrated male rats or mice, or by measuring the growth of a cock's comb (4). The androgenicity determined by these methods provides its bioactivity only in relation to one end point.

Essentially all androgenic steroids are C-19 steroid compounds and their biopotency is dependent on the presence of a 17-oxygen function of a 17-hydroxyl group in its configuration (4). Naturally occurring C-19 compounds that possess a 17-hydroxyl group are testosterone (T), 5α-dihydrotestosterone (DHT), and 5α-androstanediol (Fig. 1). T and DHT are almost equally biopotent androgens, based on the bioassay described above (5) (Table 1). The bioaction of T and DHT results from the binding of the androgen intracellularly to the androgen receptor protein, which transfers the androgen to the nucleus where the messenger RNA for the androgen becomes expressed. 5α-Androstanediol is significantly less biopotent than T or DHT due to lack of a 3-oxo group in its configuration. T and DHT are the most important androgens, but other clinically significant androgens are androstenedione (Δ^4-A) and dehydroepiandrosterone (DHEA) which are 17-oxo steroids. These steroids by themselves have considerably reduced or smaller androgenic activity than T or DHT due to the lack of a 17-oxygen function and/or 3-oxo configuration (Table 1). These androgens in vivo are required to be metabolized to T and DHT for its androgen action. Nevertheless, these weak androgens are important precursor steroids in androgen biosynthesis and bioaction. Other C-19 steroids like 11β-hydroxy-androstenedione and androstenediol are circulating in the plasma of women. However these steroids are clinically insignificant in androgenic activity due to their low concentration or lack of bioactivity (6).

B. Androgen Metabolism in Normal Females

Both adrenal cortical and ovarian tissue possess $\Delta5$ and $\Delta4$ steroidogenic pathways for androgen biosynthesis (Fig. 1). Thus the adrenal cortex and ovaries are important sources of androgens from an early peripubertal age. Androgens and other C-19 steroids are either directly secreted by the glands or they may arise by extra-adrenal/extra-ovarian conversion of precursor steroids. The rate of androgen production generally influences the circulating levels of androgens.

1. Adrenal Androgen Secretion

A simplified schematic pathway for adrenal androgen biosynthesis is shown in Figure 1. Cholesterol side chain cleavage enzyme (P450 SCC) and steroidogenic acute regulatory (StAR) protein are essential for the transformation and transfer of cholesterol to the intramitochondrial membrane, respectively, for the formation of pregnenolone. Pregnenolone and progesterone are metabolized to androgens by 17-hydroxylation. The 17-side chain cleavage of the 17α-hydroxypregnenolone (Δ^5-17P) leads to the formation of DHEA. DHEA will be converted to Δ^4-A by 3β-hydroxysteroid dehydrogenase/isomerase activity or could be converted to DHEA-sulfate (DHEA-S) by sulfakinase activity. The major androgens secreted by the human adrenals are DHEA, DHEA-S, and Δ^4-A. The

zona reticularis is very active in the 17-side chain cleavage of Δ^5-17P or 17α-hydroxyprogesterone (17-OHP) to form androgens. DHEA and DHEA-S are mainly the products of zona reticularis while Δ^4-A and T are secreted by both zona reticularis and zona fasticulata (7–9). Under normal circumstances, smaller quantities of T and even smaller amounts of androstenediol are secreted by the adrenals (6). Secretion of all adrenal androgens increases from midchildhood onward as the histological development and hormonal biosynthesis of the zona reticularis matures. These then reach a relative plateau toward the completion of pubertal maturation (10) and remain stable throughout young adulthood. At the fourth to sixth decade of life, adrenal androgen secretion normally declines (adrenopause) without significant change in cortisol secretion. This event is independent of menopause event (11).

Corticotropin (ACTH) is the major tropic hormone for adrenal androgen biosynthesis and secretion (7). There are, however, clinical situations in which disparity in adrenal androgen and cortisol secretory patterns suggests the potential for an additional regulatory factor for adrenal androgen synthesis (12, 13). Of several factors proposed in the past as influencing androgen synthesis, prolactin appears to play a role only in its excess state (14, 15) while the role of insulin and insulin-like growth factor I (IGF-I) in adrenal androgen biosynthesis is yet to be proven. However, the role of gonadal sex steroid and growth hormone has been disputed (16, 17). In addition, no tangible evidence for a pituitary tropic factor other than ACTH capable of stimulating adrenal androgen secretion has been adequately demonstrated to date. Recent studies have uncovered intimate contacts between adrenal cortical nerve endings and adrenal steroid-producing cells (18, 19) and interwoven adrenal cortical and medullary cells (18, 20). This suggests that these contacts may mediate paracrine interactions (18). It is further suggested that adrenal androgen secretion may be regulated through an intricate network involving intra-adrenal neuroimmunoregulation (18). Such regulations may involve cytokine-dependent and cytokine-independent mechanisms as well as the so-called cross talk between adrenal androgen-secreting cells of the zona reticularis and the sympathetic adrenal system and between the adrenal gland and the cellular component of the immune system (18). Presently, however, no apparent link or relationship has been demonstrated between the concept of intra-adrenal neuroimmunoregulation and the pathophysiology of the disorder of increased adrenal androgen secretion. Likewise the role of a local corticotropin-releasing hormone and ACTH system reported on DHEA secretion in human adrenals needs further verification at this time (21).

Under ACTH regulation, adrenal androgens are secreted synchronously with that of cortisol in both the episode of secretion and the circadian pattern (22, 23) (Fig. 2). DHEA and Δ^5-17P concentrations are thus normally higher in early morning and decline throughout the day

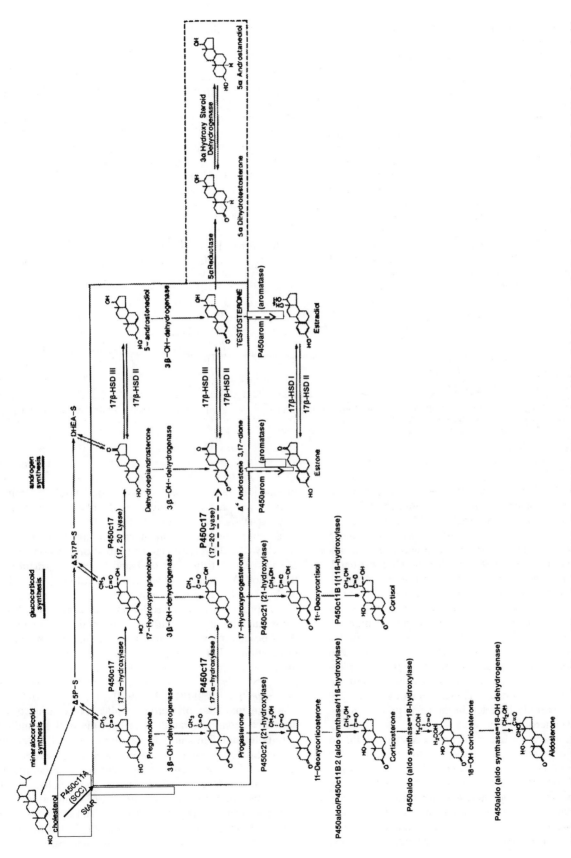

Figure 1 Steroid biosynthetic pathway. The pathway within the solid lined box occurs in both adrenal cortical and ovarian tissue. SCC, P450 cholesterol side chain cleavage enzyme; StAR, steroidogenic acute regulatory protein; 3β-OH-dehydrogenase, 3β-hydroxysteroid dehydrogenase; 17β-HSD, 17β-hydroxysteroid dehydrogenase.

Table 1 Androgen Biopotency, Sources of Androgens in Normal Females, and Plasma Concentrations of Bound and Free Testosterone in Females and Males

Normal females		DHEA	DHEA-S	Δ4-A	T	DHT	5α-Andro	Andro	Etio
Biopotency in a bioassay	In relation to T (%)	10%	—	20%	100%	≈100%	60%	10%	0%
Daily secretion rate (mg/day)		0.8–8	5–7.7	3–3.8	0.35–0.5	—	—	—	—
Adrenal secretion (%)		90%	>99%	40–66%	50–60%	—	—	—	—
Ovarian secretion (%)		10%	<1%	34–60%	34–50%	—	—	—	—
Blood production rate	Secretion + metabolism (mg/day)	6–16	8–16	3.3–3.4	0.23–0.34	—	—	—	—
Contribution to plasma concentration	Adrenals (%)	67%	90%	30–60%	20–26%	—	—	—	—
	Ovaries (%)	8%	0%	30–56%	14–20%	—	—	—	—
	Peripheral (%)	25%	10%	<0.1%	60%	—	—	—	—
Representative total plasma T concentration	Female (ng/dl)				49				
	Male (ng/dl)				810				
SHBG-bound T	Female: ng/dl (%)				39 (80%)				
	Male: ng/dl (%)				486 (60%)				
Albumin-bound T	Female: ng/dl (%)				9.3 (19%)				
	Male: ng/dl (%)				307 (38%)				
Free T concentration	Female: ng/dl (%)				0.7 (1%)				
	Male: ng/dl (%)				22 (2%)				

DHEA, dehydroepiandrosterone; DHEA-S, dehydroepiandrosterone-sulfate; Δ4-A, androstenedione; T, testosterone; DHT, dihydrotestosterone; 5α-Andro, androstanediol; Andro, androsterone; Etio, etiocholanone.
Source: data derived from Refs. 5, 25–31, 35, 47.

(23). 17-OHP and Δ^4-A concentrations in normal women also tend to be higher in the morning hours than thereafter because of the adrenal contribution (23). However, the circadian difference in 17-OHP levels is lessened during the luteal phase of the menstrual cycle when ovarian 17-OHP production is increased. DHEA-S, on the other hand, shows very little circadian or episodic variation in plasma concentration due to the slow rate of clearance of the sulfate (23, 24). Its plasma concentration is 300–400 times greater than that of unconjugated DHEA due to high secretion by the adrenals and low clearance of this conjugate (23). DHEA, DHEA-S, and Δ4-A are further metabolized to etiocholanolone and androsterone. 11β-OH androstenedione and a small amount of cortisol are metabolized to 11-oxy, 17-oxy steroids. These metabolites of C-19 steroids are generally excreted in the urine as 17-ketosteroids (17-oxo-steroids).

The adrenal contribution of androgens in relation to overall androgen production and circulating concentration in women is depicted in Table 1 (25–31). Circulating DHEA and DHEA-S are directly from the adrenal secretion contribution. The adrenals and ovaries from puberty onward secrete approximately equal amounts of Δ4-A. The androgens secreted by the adrenal cortex and ovaries undergo peripheral metabolism and contribute to the blood production rate of androgens. Under normal circumstances, peripheral contribution to the blood production of DHEA, DHEA-S, and Δ4-A is small. The major source of T blood production in women is via peripheral conversion of Δ4-A (27, 28) (Table 1). The blood production rate of Δ4-A is 10–15 times that of T and the rate of fraction of the blood Δ4-A pool conversion to the blood T pool is 5.6% (27, 28). Therefore, approximately 60% of circulating T production is derived from the circulating Δ4-A. Consequently, the conditions associated with increased Δ4-A production would simultaneously increase the blood production of T (Table 1).

2. Ovarian Androgen Secretion

The principal sites of steroid synthesis in ovarian tissue are theca cells, the granulosa cells of the follicle, and the corpus luteum. The pathway involving Δ^5 and Δ^4 steroid biosynthesis process in the ovarian cells is similar to that described for the adrenal cortex (Fig. 1). Ovarian androgen synthesis occurs mainly in the theca cells, stroma cells, and the corpus luteum under LH stimulation (32–34). The ovary further aromatizes the androgens to estrogen in the granulosa cell layers through FSH stimulation. The granulosa cells regulated by FSH and estrogen thus

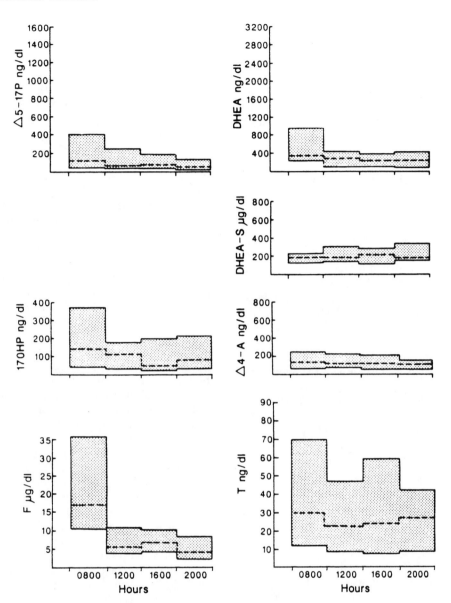

Figure 2 Representative circadian patterns of adrenal and gonadal steroids in normal women. Δ5-17P, 17 hydroxypregneno-lone; Δ4-A, androstenedione; F, cortisol; T, testosterone; 17-OHP, 17α-hydroxyprogesterone. (Modified from Pang S et al. J Clin Endocrinol Metab 1985; 60:434. Reproduced with permission from the Endocrine Society, Bethesda, MD.)

largely produce estrogens. Progesterone is secreted largely from the granulosa cells of the late follicular and midcycle phase and by the corpus luteum derived from granulosa cells (32, 33).

The major androgens secreted by the ovaries are Δ4-A and T (Table 1). The amount of androgen secreted by the ovary is far greater than the amount of estrogens produced. The ovarian source of androgen also increases gradually with the onset of gonadarche. Following menarche, ovarian androgen secretion appears to alter throughout the cycle. The secretion of T and Δ4-A into the ovarian vein is at its highest when estrogens are being

maximally secreted. The effect of variable production of androgen by the ovary on the contribution in plasma is to some extent masked by the adrenal source of androgens and by interconversion that occurs after secretion (35). Peripheral concentration of Δ4-A and T levels was higher at midcycle due to the ovarian contribution (36, 37), although others reported higher Δ4-A and T levels in the luteal phase of normal women (38). Our recent study of steroid concentration throughout the cycle of normally menstruating women, however, revealed no statistically significant changes of most androgens throughout the cycle (39). The ovarian contribution of androgens to the overall blood production rate and circulating androgen concentration in plasma pool is shown in Table 1. In general, the amount of ovarian Δ^4-A and T secretion is similar to that of adrenal secretion, thereby contributing equally in the blood production and concentration of these androgens. In the periovulatory phase, 65% of blood production rate of $\Delta 4$-A is contributed by the increased secretion of the ovarian source of Δ^4-A (6). The ovaries contribute very little to DHEA production and none to DHEA-S. With menopause, ovarian Δ^4-A production declines (40) and aging probably diminishes overall androgen secretion by the ovary (6).

Recent in vitro and in vivo studies indicate insulin action on ovarian steroidogenesis (41, 42). Insulin interacts with gonadotropin in an additive or synergistic manner in both normal and polycystic ovaries (41, 42). Insulin action in the ovaries is mediated by the insulin receptor and not by cross-reaction with the type 1 IGF receptor (41). The mechanism of intraovarian insulin signaling is unknown. Insulin in excess amounts may also enhance LH secretion in addition to modulating LH effect on ovarian androgen synthesis or may potentiate 17α-hydroxylase and 17,20 lyase activity in ovarian steroidogenesis (41, 42). The interaction of excess insulin with LH appears to contribute to premature arrest of follicle growth and also in amplifying thecal cell androgen production (41). Thus, normal ovarian steroidogenesis would require appropriate regulation and interaction between the pituitary tropic factor(s) and systemic metabolic factor(s) at the intra-ovarian cellular level(s) for the appropriate signaling of normal ovarian steroidogenesis.

C. Bioactive Androgens in Blood

The circulating sex steroid hormones are in part present in a protein-bound form and in part in a free form unbound to protein (Table 1). The specific binding protein with a high affinity for sex steroids, (e.g., testosterone/estradiol) are called sex hormone-binding globulin (SHBG). The biologically active T includes both the free and albumin-bound fractions while SHBG-bound androgens are not readily available for bioaction (43). Approximately 1% of the circulating T and DHT in normal females is unbound (Table 1) (44). This unbound T freely diffuses into the target cells to bind to the androgen receptor. At puberty SHBG concentration falls slightly in girls while a greater drop in concentration is noted in boys (35). SHBG concentration is decreased by the androgens and in obesity, and is increased by estrogen (45). Estrogen, by its action of increasing the concentration of SHBG, decreases biologically active free fractions of androgens (35). Thus a hyperandrogenic state further causes availability of the free bioactive form of T. The increased availability of free T or DHT to the target cells by the decrease in SHBG in the presence of normal circulating total T levels may be a pathogenic mechanism of hirsut-

ism in women (46). The binding of DHEA and Δ^4-A to SHBG in circulation is negligible (47).

III. PHYSIOLOGY OF HAIR GROWTH, PROPOSED INTRADERMAL IMMUNOREGULATION, AND SKIN ANDROGEN METABOLISM

Hair growth on the face, neck, trunk, extremities, and pubic and axillary region are androgen dependent. Androgen stimulation in these androgen-dependent areas promotes terminal hair growth, which is thick, long, and dark. The hair follicle undergoes lifelong transformations between telogen (resting), anagen (growth), and catagen (apoptosis-driven regression) (48, 49), which are distinct yet transitional periods (Fig. 3). During anagen, formation of the hair by proliferation and pigmentation of cells occurs from an epidermal matrix of the hair bulb. The catagen stage begins at the termination of anagen, followed by telogen (48). However, substantial metabolic and proliferative activity is noted during telogen, indicating that telogen is not a mere resting stage (49). Generally, in males the duration of anagen for the moustache is 4 months, and for thigh hair it is 2 months. In females, the duration of anagen for thigh hair is less than 1 month (50). The length of the hair is influenced by the length of the anagen phase, which is by comparison more important than the rate of hair growth. The longer thigh hair in men is thus attributed to the longer anagen period. The telogen phase of facial hair is 2–3 months. The growth cycle of the moustache is therefore 6–7 months or more at the very least, and more than 3 months for thigh hair (51). Duration of the hair cycle differs, therefore, depending on location.

Hair follicle development or cycling is controlled by an intrafollicular so-called hair cycle clock of an as yet unknown nature (49), which can be altered by systemic or metabolic (hormones), immunological (cytokines), and nerve-derived (neuropeptides/neurotransmitters) factors in vivo (18, 49). The hair follicles contain stem cells in the bulge or bulb area that migrate to the hair matrix for division and differentiation, which are controlled by a family of cytokines, produced from the dermal papilla cells (52). Androgen-dependent hairs have androgen receptors in the dermal papilla cells and some cells of the inner and center sheaths of the hair follicle (52).

Androgens influence the synthesis and release of cytokines from the dermal papilla cells and control hair growth (52). They also most likely prolong the growth of hair by lengthening the duration of anagen, as evidenced by reduction of the length of hair by antiandrogen treatment in hirsute women (53). Androgen-dependent hair growth is influenced not only by the amount of androgen delivered to the target cells but also by the target cell response to the androgen. In some instances, peripheral target cell response may even be more important in the manifestation of androgen excess symptoms, since no cor-

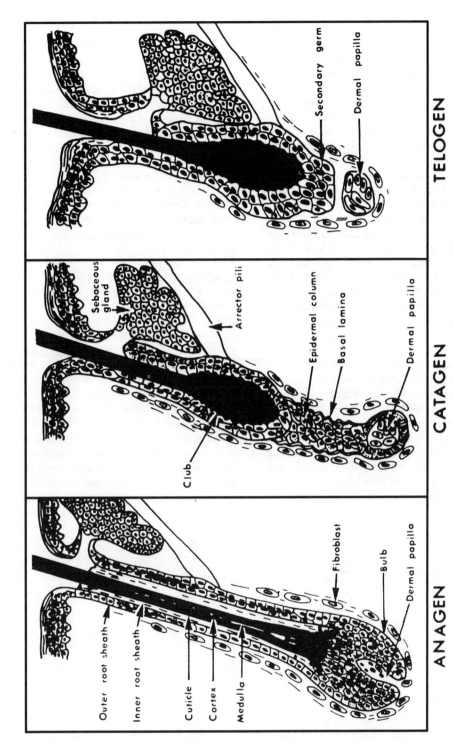

Figure 3 Human hair cycle. (From Ebling FJG. Clinics in Endocrinology and Metabolism 1986:319. Reproduced with permission of WB Saunders Company, Philadelphia, PA.)

relation has been found between the rate of hair growth and circulating total, protein bound, or free T (54).

Androgen bioaction at the cellular level involves the uptake of pre- or active hormone and conversion to DHT, which binds to a specific receptor protein, and then transfers to the nucleus (55) (Fig. 4). All skin structures, including epidermis, sweat and sebaceous glands, hair follicles, and dermis possess 5α-reductase activity and 3β-hydroxysteroid dehydrogenase-$\Delta^{5\rightarrow4}$ isomerase and 17β-, 3β- and 3α-hydroxysteroid dehydrogenase activities (56) (Fig. 4). Immunolocalization study in normal skin and acne skin revealed the predominance of type I 5α-reductase isoenzyme in the sebaceous gland and type 2 5α-reductase in the companion layer of the hair follicle and granular layer of epidermis (57). Human skin thus has the capacity not only to convert T to DHT but also to convert the precursor weak androgens DHEA to Δ^5-androstenediol or to Δ^4-A, which in turn is converted to T and eventually to DHT. DHT is then further reduced to 3α-androstanediol (3α-Adiol) and its glucuronide (gluc) (Fig. 4). The measurement of circulating concentrations of DHT does not reflect the metabolic activities of androgens in peripheral tissue. Only a fraction of this peripherally formed androgen escapes into circulation: most of it is further metabolized *in situ* (58, 59) (Fig. 4).

Glucuronidation is one of the effective disposal mechanisms in skin tissue (60, 61). 3α-Adiol and its gluc have been reported to be a good marker of peripheral skin androgen activity. Circulating concentrations of serum 3α-adiol and its gluc were reported to be increased in hirsute women (62–64). Studies from our laboratory indicate that serum 3α-Adiol gluc levels were significantly correlated with the degree of hirsutism in women with excess ad-

renal androgen production and idiopathic causes, but not in women with excess ovarian androgen production (65). No correlation was found, however, between precursor or circulating androgen levels and the hirsutism scores (65). In addition, 3α-adiol gluc levels in hirsute females correlated significantly with circulating DS and DHEA levels (65), suggesting that in women 3α-adiol gluc is a marker of metabolic activity of largely weak adrenal androgens in the skin tissue.

IV. PATHOPHYSIOLOGY AND CAUSES OF HIRSUTISM AND POLYCYSTIC OVARY SYNDROME

The pathogenesis of hirsutism and other related increased androgen symptoms in the female can be classified as follows: (a) increased glandular secretion of androgens or exogenous androgen administration; (b) increased extraglandular production of active androgens via increased peripheral conversion of precursor steroids; (c) increased availability of circulating bioactive androgens; and (d) increased sensitivity of target cells to androgen in the androgen-dependent skin tissue. One or more of these pathogenic mechanisms may play a role in hirsutism. Approximately 5–8% of the female population is reported to demonstrate hirsutism (66).

Hirsutism associated with virilism and menstrual disorder is caused by a pathology of unequivocal excess adrenal and/or ovarian androgen production. Hirsutism and menstrual disorder alone may result from moderately increased androgen production. Hirsutism and acne, alone

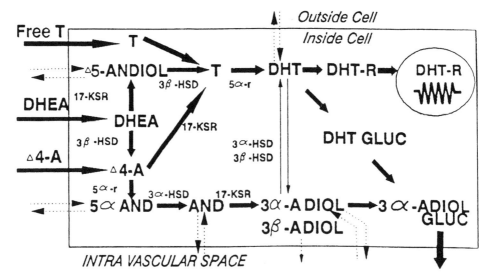

Figure 4 Conversion of androgens in skin tissue. DHT-R, DHT and its receptor complex; AND, androsterone; 5α AND, 5α-androstenedione; Δ^5-ANDIOL, Δ^5 androstenediol; 3α-Adiol, $3\alpha,5\alpha$-androstanediol; GLUC, glucuronide; 3β-HSD, 3β-hydroxysteroid dehydrogenase/$\Delta^{5\rightarrow4}$-isomerase; 17-KSR, 17-ketosteroid reductase; 5α-r, 5α-reductase. (From Pang S et al. J Clin Endocrinol Metab 1992; 72:243. Reproduced with permission from The Endocrine Society, Bethesda, MD.)

or together, coupled with normal menses are generally caused by mildly increased androgen production or normal androgen secretion, in association with mechanisms (b), (c), or (d) described above (67–71).

The most easily clinically identified excess androgen-producing pathologies are those associated with classic manifestations of excess glucocorticoid hormone production (Cushing disease/Cushing syndrome) and those presenting with sudden onset and rapidly advancing androgen excess symptoms caused by adrenal or ovarian androgen producing tumors (Table 2; Fig. 5). These diseases, although rare, usually cause virilization and amenorrhea. The majority of hirsute women, however, present with either peripubertal or postpubertal onset of increased hair growth or acne, with or without menstrual dysfunction, and with no obvious clinical cause for increased androgen symptoms. The causes of clinically indistinguishable hirsutism are many, including those conditions associated with mild to moderately increased adrenal and/or ovarian

sources of androgens (23, 39, 65, 72–76), as well as other conditions associated with apparently normal androgen levels (Table 2). Recent studies of hirsutism have further defined several specific causes of adrenal and ovarian androgen excess production in women (Table 2).

A. Adrenal Causes of Excess Androgen Production

1. Mild Form of Congenital Adrenal Hyperplasia

a. 21-Hydroxylase Deficiency. A partial or mild adrenal 21-hydroxylase deficiency is a well-defined cause of excess adrenal androgen secretion resulting in peripubertal or postpubertal onset of hirsutism and acne, with or without menstrual dysfunction (23, 39, 77–85). This entity has been termed late-onset, attenuated, or symptomatic form of nonclassic congenital adrenal hyperplasia and has been studied in great detail over the two past

Table 2 Causes of Excess Androgen Symptoms in Peripubertal and Postpubertal Females

Adrenals	Ovarian	Others
Nonclassic mild inherited defect in cortisol biosynthesis: 21-hydroxylase deficiency 11β-hydroxylase deficiency 3β-hydroxysteroid dehydrogenase deficiency	Polycystic ovary syndrome with insulin resistance without insulin resistance	Idiopathic hirsutism (normal androgen production)
	Genetic causes of insulin resistance syndrome	Hypothyroidism
Increased adrenal androgen secretion of undefined cause (dysregulation/ functional adrenal hyperandrogenism)	Stromal hyperthecosis Secondary polycystic ovaries excess adrenal or exogenous androgens hyperprolactinemia inherited defect in ovarian steroidogenesis	Ingestion of nonsteroidal drugs diazoxide minoxidil phenytoin
Cushing's syndrome/disease		Ingestion/injection of androgen/anabolic substance
Androgen-producing adrenal tumors (adenoma/carcinoma)	Androgen-producing ovarian tumors lipoma luteoma hilar cell tumor stroma tumor stromal-Leydig cell tumor	
Hyperprolactinemia		
Glucocorticoid receptor gene mutation	Hilar cell hyperplasia	
11β-hydroxysteroid dehydrogenase 1 deficiency (cortisone reductase deficiency)	Inherited defects in ovarian steroidogenesis 17β-hydroxysteroid dehydrogenase deficiency aromatase deficiency Type II 3β-HSD deficiency	
	α-Estrogen receptor defect (?)	

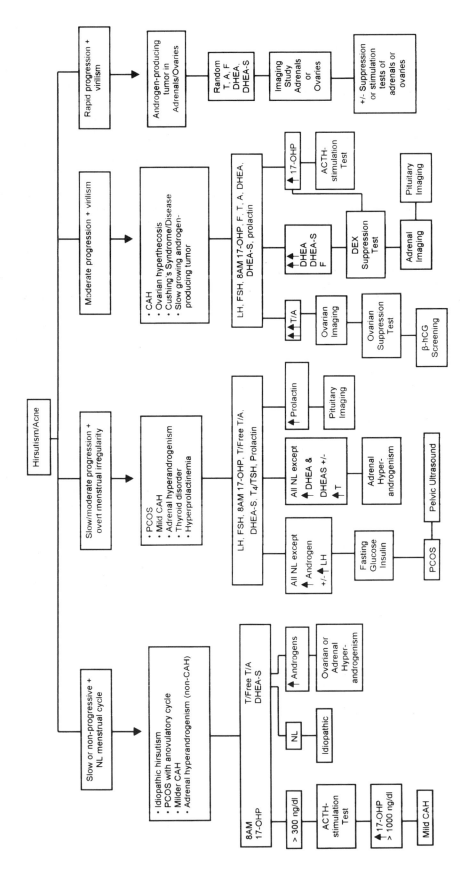

Figure 5   Guideline for evaluation of hirsute patients. 17-OHP, 17-OH progesterone; T, testosterone; A, androstenedione; F, cortisol; CAH, congenital adrenal hyperplasia; NL, normal.

decades (77–98). The mild form of 21-hydroxylase deficiency frequently manifests excess androgen symptoms well before puberty, causing premature pubarche, acne, oily hair, and accelerated skeletal maturation in childhood (77, 80, 83, 99), and is proven to be a progressive disorder (83). In girls over age 10 years with mild 21-hydroxylase deficiency, hirsutism and menstrual irregularity were manifested in 50–55% (77, 83), while virilism and infertility were present in 13% (77, 83). A mildly deleterious missense mutation or a point mutation in the promoter region in one or both alleles of CYP21 gene resulting in a compound heterozygous or homozygous mutation is the basis of the mild phenotype of 21-hydroxylase deficiency (77, 84, 91–96). The V280L allele is in genetic linkage disequilibrium with HLA B14 in Ashkenazi Jews (86–88). A high frequency of this disorder in individuals of mainly eastern European descent (Ashkenazi Jews) has been reported (87, 88). In hirsute females, varying frequencies (0–16%) of this disorder have been reported (23, 39, 77, 82, 85, 97–104). The ethnic and racial background of hirsute females is the likely factor determining the varying incidence rate. In self-referred hirsute females however, the incidence of mild 21-hydroxylase deficiency was low (1–2%) (39, 77, 100, 105).

Characteristic hormonal abnormalities for the mild form of 21-hydroxylase deficiency in women are elevated circulating 17-hydroxyprogesterone (17-OHP), and Δ^4-A. Testosterone levels are also generally mild to moderately elevated. These adrenal sources of hormonal abnormalities can be more accurately detected by early morning blood sampling due to their circadian variations. Confirmative diagnosis of this condition is, however, made by evaluating the adrenal steroid response to exogenous ACTH stimulation regardless of time of day (23, 39, 77, 80, 97–103). Representative 17-OHP and androgen levels in normal and 21-hydroxylase deficient hirsute females are shown in Table 5 (39, 65). 17-OHP response to ACTH stimulation in these women was three standard deviations above the mean 17-OHP response of known carriers for 21-hydroxylase deficiency (23, 65, 80). All other steroid responses, including C-19 steroid levels in response to ACTH stimulation in these women, overlapped with the steroid response of hirsute women with other causes (23, 39, 65, 80). The unequivocally increased 17-OHP levels with or without ACTH stimulation, together with prompt suppression by exogenous glucocorticoid hormone administration, confirm the diagnosis of mild form of 21-hydroxylase deficiency for patients of all ages (77).

b. 11β-Hydroxylase Deficiency. Late-onset 11β-hydroxylase deficiency in women with hirsutism has also been reported (78). In the author's study of over 300 hirsute patients from two different populations, partial 11β-hydroxylase deficiency was not found. Thus, this disorder is an extremely rare cause of hirsutism in women.

c. 3β-Hydroxysteroid Dehydrogenase Deficiency. Early studies reported salt-losing symptoms in early life

as the presenting signs of 3β-hydroxysteroid dehydrogenase deficiency (3β-HSD def.) (106). However, the diagnosis of the non-salt-losing form of 3β-HSD deficiency may be delayed until later in life when either premature pubic hair growth occurs during childhood or hirsutism occurs during puberty as a symptom of 3β-HSD deficiency (106–109). A partial adrenal 3β-HSD deficiency was first described in a woman with pubertal onset of hirsutism and sclerotic ovaries two decades ago (110). Thus partial genetic 3β-HSD deficiency is a cause of pubertal or postpubertal hirsutism and menstrual irregularities in women (108, 109). In the past decade, mild late onset 3β-HSD deficiency was suspected in children with premature pubarche and in women with hirsutism if their ACTH stimulated Δ^5 precursor steroids Δ5-17P and DHEA levels and Δ^5 precursor to Δ^4 product steroid ratios were greater than 2 SD above the age and pubertal stage-matched normal subject's mean value (23, 98, 101, 103, 104, 111, 112). However, our recent genotype and phenotype studies indicate that the published hormonal criteria are not accurate for diagnosing mild inherited 3β-HSD deficiency (77, 113–116). Molecular analysis of the type II 3β-HSD gene in many patients with Δ^5-precursor steroids and Δ^5 precursor to Δ^4 product steroid ratios greater than 2 SD above normal mean value revealed no mutation in the type II 3β-HSD gene (113–115). Thus, a genuine mild late-onset 3β-HSD deficiency would express greater precursor hormonal abnormalities (113–115) than the past published hormonal abnormalities in both hirsute females and children with premature pubarche (23, 98, 101, 103, 104, 111, 112). The hormonal criteria for mild late-onset 3β-HSD deficiency (113–115) are nearly analogous to those of mild late-onset 21-hydroxylase deficiency (i.e., precursor steroid response 21 SD above the genotype-normal population mean) (117–119). It is also apparent that only the values of ACTH-stimulated Δ^5-17P levels and Δ^5-17P to cortisol (F) ratio unequivocally differentiate those with type II genotype-proven 3β-HSD deficiency from genotype-normal patients. DHEA or other hormonal ratios did not consistently differentiate the genotype-proven patients from the genotype-normal patients (113–115). It is now apparent that true mild late-onset 3β-HSD deficiency resulting from the type II 3β-HSD gene mutation is a rare disorder in hirsute females.

2. Type II 3β-HSD Genotype-Normal Mild Defect in Adrenal 3β-HSD Activity

The cause of mildly increased Δ^5 precursor steroid levels and Δ^5 precursor to Δ^4 product steroid ratios (as high as 12 SD above the normal mean) in hirsute females is unknown, but the hormonal abnormalities suggest mildly decreased activity of adrenal 3β-HSD. These hirsute women have clearly increased adrenal androgen secretion and rates of menstrual disorder as high as women with classic polycystic ovary syndrome (PCOS) (39). In addition, in the genotype-normal hirsute females with this mildly decreased adrenal 3β-HSD activity of unknown cause, clinical and/or hormonal findings of PCOS are present (23, 39, 112). The mildly decreased adrenal 3β-HSD activity of unknown cause without the type II 3β-HSD gene mutation is more prevalent than true 3β-HSD deficiency in hirsute females. A recent investigation by the author into the pathogenesis of this disorder strongly suggests that it may be a nonclassic form of PCOS associated with insulin resistance (pediatric research, programs, and abstracts, p 117A, 2002). Further studies will elucidate the nature of this type II 3β-HSD genotype-normal mild defect in adrenal 3β-HSD activity.

3. Increased Adrenal Androgen Producing Condition of Undefined Cause (Idiopathic or Functional Adrenal Hyperandrogenism; Dysregulation of Adrenal Androgen Secretion)

In a study of over 125 hirsute females, 11 patients demonstrated only elevated baseline or ACTH stimulated levels of DHEA and or DHEA-S without other hormonal abnormalities (39, 65). A specific cause for increased adrenal androgen secretion was not found in these patients since they did not meet the criteria of any enzyme deficiency or decreased enzyme activity, and had no hormonal or radiological evidence of adrenal hyperplasia or adrenal tumor (39, 65). This isolated increased adrenal androgen-producing condition has also been labeled as functional adrenal hyperandrogenism (120, 121). The cause of this increased adrenal androgen secretion is not known. A longitudinal study of hirsute adolescent girls with a childhood history of premature pubarche reports that one-third of the premature pubarche cohort had evidence of increased adrenal DHEA and androstenedione secretion (121). This was associated with a history of low birth weight, suggesting the possibility of an endocrine sequence of prenatal onset (121). Adrenal androgen hyperresponsiveness was proposed to be due to dysgeneration of intra-adrenal modulation in androgen secretion (120). Isolated increased adrenal androgen secretion is not a common cause of hirsutism (≈10–12%), but was the most common adrenal cause of hirsutism and was present in a small number of females of all ethnic and racial backgrounds (39). The frequency of menstrual abnormality was lower in this hyperandrogenism than PCOS or genotype-normal defect in 3β-HSD activity (39). The excess adrenal androgen secretion in these females is easily suppressed by a small amount of exogenous glucocorticoid administration (39). However, no long-term data are available to determine whether low-dosage glucocorticoid therapy is efficacious in improving hirsutism in these females.

In some females with adrenal hyperandrogenism, concurrent ovarian hyperandrogenism is also manifested (39, 121). Whether the pathogenic mechanisms of both adrenal and ovarian involvement coexists in these hirsute females or whether one condition results in the other remains unknown.

4. Cushing Disease or Syndrome

Inappropriate adrenocorticotropic hormone (ACTH) secretion by a pituitary tumor or by a disturbed corticotropin-releasing hormone (CRH)–ACTH axis in the CNS (Cushing disease) and ectopic ACTH secretion by the malignant tumor often result in excess adrenal glucocorticoid and androgen secretion simultaneously. Autonomously functioning adrenal cortical tumor (adenoma and carcinoma) may also secrete increased amounts of cortisol and androgen (Cushing syndrome). Thus, the patients with Cushing disease or syndrome would manifest symptoms not only of glucocorticoid excess but also hirsutism or virilism. These conditions are rare causes of hirsutism and are usually clinically more easily recognizable due to the presence of Cushingoid features and muscle-wasting signs. Biochemically abnormal cortisol and/or ACTH dynamics is apparent in these disorders. Classic hormonal abnormalities are nonsuppressed or partially suppressible excess cortisol, DHEA, and DHEA-S levels by dexamethasone administration. Radiological studies are also an essential part of the differential diagnosis of Cushing disease and/or syndrome (Fig. 5). A recent study in 13 females with Cushing disease/syndrome revealed that 70% had menstrual disorders including oligomenorrhea, amenorrhea, and polymenorrhea, while 30% had a normal cycle pattern (122). About one half of the patients had ovarian morphology suggestive of PCO and the patients with higher cortisol secretion had hypogonadotropic hypogonadism (122).

5. Adrenal Androgen-Producing Tumor

An androgen-producing tumor of the adrenal could be adenoma or carcinoma. However rare, it is a cause of virilism. Generally the supraphysiological amount of androgen secreted by these tumors characteristically causes extremely elevated circulating DHEA and DHEA-S levels. Other androgens such as Δ4-A and T or progestin steroid levels may also be elevated by either direct secretion or by peripheral conversion of DHEA and DHEA-S for elevated Δ4-A level. Some androgen-producing tumors may also have the capacity to secrete cortisol but the patient may not present with Cushingoid features. Clinically these diseases are manifested in sudden onset; hormonal symptoms are rapidly progressive. In carcinomas, the metastasis to liver or ovarian tissue may occur, and metastatic tissue often secretes steroids inappropriately. Radiological and hormonal evaluations are essential for the diagnosis; tumor tissue should be removed as soon as possible (123). In rare cases, androgen-producing adrenal adenoma has also been reported in patients with poorly controlled or untreated congenital adrenal hyperplasia (124, 125).

6. Hyperprolactinemia

Elevated adrenal androgen levels (DHEA and DHEA-S) have been found in some hirsute women with high prolactin levels (14, 15, 126) and normal metabolic clearance rate of these steroids (127). Increased plasma Δ4-A and cortisol response to ACTH stimulation and low SHBG in hirsute and hyperprolactinemic patients were also described (128). Controversial data have been reported on the effect of dopamine agonist in lowering serum androgen levels with reduction in serum prolactin levels (14, 129). Recent data suggest a modulation of adrenal androgen production by prolactin based on the observation of dopamine agonist reducing both serum prolactin and androgen levels as well as improving acne and hirsutism (14). Enhanced androgen effect at the target tissue by permissive action of prolactin was also described (130). The associated findings of PCOS in some hyperprolactinemic women suggest an additional cause of hirsutism in the hyperprolactinemic state (131).

7. Glucocorticoid Receptor Gene Mutation

The clinical features of cortisol resistance include fatigue, mild hirsutism, oligomenorrhea, infertility, obesity, hypokalemic hypertension, and precocious puberty (132, 133). Hirsutism is reported as the most common symptom of this disorder (133). Glucocorticoid resistance syndrome is characterized by decreased sensitivity to cortisol signaling, increased cortisol secretion, absence of clinical features of Cushing syndrome, and poor suppression of adrenal steroids. Resistance of adrenal steroids, including cortisol level, is decreased with dexamethasone administration (133). This genetic disorder results from a deleterious mutation in the human glucocorticoid receptor gene. It is an extremely rare cause of hirsutism (134) and menstrual disorders in women, but should be suspected in patients with elevated cortisol levels without the clinical features of Cushing syndrome. The cause of hirsutism is related to increased adrenal androgen secretion due to increased pituitary ACTH secretion, which is due to cortisol resistance.

8. Cortisone Reductase (11β-Hydroxysteroid Dehydrogenase Type 1) Deficiency

This enzyme deficiency is a rare cause of hirsutism without virilization and may be associated with infertility (135, 136). This enzyme catalyzes the reduction of cortisone to cortisol, and its deficiency impairs the metabolism of cortisone to cortisol. The exact mechanism of hirsutism is unknown but may be related to increased adrenal androgen secretion in view of enlarged adrenal size on CT scan in a patient with apparent cortisone reductase deficiency (136).

B. Ovarian Causes of Excess Androgen Production

1. Polycystic Ovary Syndrome

a. Definition. Polycystic ovary syndrome (PCOS) is defined clinically by the presentation of hyperandrogenism (clinical and/or biochemical) and chronic anovulation (regular or irregular anovulatory cycle, amenorrhea, oligomenorrhea, polymenorrhea, or infertility).

Hyperandrogenic symptoms include hirsutism, acne and/or virilism, and menstrual disorders. The hyperandrogenic symptom of PCOS is generally associated with excess androgen production of ovarian or extraovarian source (137–139) and is associated with or without obesity, insulin resistance, or the radiological images of ovaries compatible with PCOS. The morphological changes of ovaries include bilaterally and symmetrically enlarged ovoid ovaries classically, but the ovary may be unilaterally enlarged or normal shaped (140). Characteristic morphological findings of PCOS (140) are an oyster-gray color and smooth glistening surface surrounding a thickened capsule in association with numerous 2–15 mm subcapsular cysts and many ovarian atretic follicles. These findings were initially described as Stein-Leventhal syndrome.

b. Prevalence. Estimated prevalence of PCOS is variable from 2 to 20% in the general population (141). Recent studies described a prevalence of 3.4% in African–Americans, 4.7% in white women aged 18–45 years from a southeastern US region (141), and 6.5% in a white Spanish population (142). A prevalence of PCOS in women seeking electrolysis therapy was conservatively put at 12% (143). A prevalence of PCOS in mothers and sisters of patients with PCOS was 24% and 32%, respectively (144). These data suggest the involvement of a major genetic component for PCOS (144). PCOS is one of the major causes of hirsutism in almost all ethnic populations (39). In New Zealand, white females and Maori females had more hirsutism than other ethnic PCOS females, while white females had less complaint of infertility and Pacific islanders had little or no acne (145). This suggests the influence of ethnic and racial factors on the expression of the hyperandrogenic symptoms of PCOS.

c. Pathophysiology and Causative Factors. Multifactor considerations related to the pathophysiology and causes of PCOS are depicted in Tables 2 and 3. The proposed causative factors of PCOS include defect(s) in the insulin-signaling pathway (146–148) or glucose transporter (149); defect(s) in the metabolic/hormonal regulatory system on body weight control (150); defect(s) in the regulation of steroidogenic biosynthesis (151, 152); or defect(s) in the regulation of gonadotropin secretion (153), as well as secondary adverse effects on one or more of these systems via extraovarian or intraovarian sources of excess androgens or an exogenous source of excess insulin (154) (Table 3). Thus PCOS may be a family of complex genetic and environmental diseases influenced by genetic heterogeneity, fat and carbohydrate consumption, physical exercise level, peripubertal stress, and/or hormonal exposure (155, 156). Of several proposed factors, the peripheral insulin resistance of unknown mechanism with or without obesity, known heritable insulin resistance syndrome, and exogenous insulin treatment for type 1 diabetes mellitus associated with PCOS suggest that hyperinsulinemia is a causative factor related to PCOS mani-

Table 3 Proven or Proposed Pathogenic Causes of Polycystic Ovary Syndrome

Metabolic defect	Other factor	Ovarian	Adrenal

Hyperinsulinemia
Peripheral insulin resistance
  Obesity
    Secondary to post-insulin receptor binding defects
    Secondary to decreased content of adipocyte GLUT-4 glucose transporters
	Dysregulation of gonadotropin secretion
	  Dopamine deficiency
	  Psychological stress
	  Other defect in gonadotropin regulation
	  Increased free estrogen causing increased LH
		Dysregulation of ovarian steroidogenesis
		
		Genetic defect in ovarian E_2 synthesis
		  Aromatase deficiency
		  17β-hydroxysteroid dehydrogenase deficiency
		  Type II 3β-HSD deficiency
			Dysregulation of adrenal steroidogenesis
			
			Detrimental effect of excess adrenal androgens
			
			Classic and nonclassic CAH
			  21-hydroxylase deficiency
			  Type II 3β-HSD deficiency
			  11β-hydroxylase deficiency

Insulin receptor gene mutation
  Leprechaunism
  Type A syndrome
  Rabson-Mendenhall syndrome
	Other hereditary factor (?)
	
	Dysregulation of weight control
	
	Obesity causing a decrease in SHBG/increase in free androgen/estrogen
		Androgen-producing ovarian tumor	Cushing's syndrome/disease
			
			Androgen-producing adrenal tumor

Kahn type B insulin resistance secondary to circulating antibodies for insulin receptor	Exogenous androgens		
Supraphysiological doses of insulin replacement in type 1 diabetes mellitus			

festation. This is further elaborated in the discussion of primary PCOS below.

In excess adrenal androgen-producing conditions, such as 21-hydroxylase deficiency, 11β-hydroxylase deficiency, adrenal androgen-producing tumor, Cushing's disease or syndrome, or with exogenous administration of androgen, the proposed pathogenic mechanism for PCOS is either a direct adverse effect of androgen on the ovarian estrogen synthesis or altering gonadotropin secretion by increased free androgens or estrogens (157–162).

Impaired ovarian estradiol synthesis caused by ovarian 17-ketosteroid reductase deficiency (163), ovarian 3β-HSD deficiency (108, 109), and ovarian aromatase deficiency (164–166) predictably leads to PCOS either as a result of the increased intraovarian androgen effect or because of the increased gonadotropin effect via a feedback regulation. PCOS in ovarian androgen-producing tumor may be caused by either the direct effect of androgen on the process of ovarian estrogen synthesis or by altering gonadotropin secretion via excess androgen or free estrogen converted from excess androgen. It is not certain whether excess androgen production in these adrenal and ovarian conditions alters peripheral insulin sensitivity or some other growth factor action in the modulation of gonadotropin on the ovarian function, thereby leading to the development of PCOS.

d. Primary PCOS

Clinical presentation. Most females with primary PCOS (nonadrenal and nonexogenous excess androgen induced) have normal onset of menarche, although infrequently primary amenorrhea or oligomenorrhea may be present from the beginning (137, 167, 168). Frequently a history of significant weight gain preceding menarche can be obtained in many patients with primary PCOS (169). Hirsutism in primary PCOS generally begins during the late pubertal stage following the menarche (169). Progressive manifestation of hirsutism and menstrual dysfunction correlate with the ovarian androgen production rate (137, 170, 171). Some genetic factors may modify the effects of increased ovarian androgen secreted in some PCOS women who are not hirsute (137). The clinical spectrum of primary PCOS therefore ranges from regular anovulatory withdrawal menstrual cycle, menstrual abnormality, to mild hirsutism with regular anovulatory withdrawal cycle, to severe hirsutism and/or virilism and menstrual abnormalities and/or infertility (137, 139, 171). Approximately 70% of women with PCOS in the United States were reported to be hirsute, and the remaining 30% were not hirsute despite hyperandrogenism (139). In the author's experience with PCOS in young hirsute females, more than 300 of whom were evaluated in the last 20 years, intrinsic primary PCOS defined by clinical presentation of hirsutism with (majority) or without (minority) menstrual disorders and documented increased ovarian Δ^4-A and/or T production in the absence of increased adrenal androgen secretion was diagnosed in one-quarter to one-third of the patients evaluated (23, 39, 65). Primary ovarian hyperthecosis and hyperandrogenism (HA)/insulin resistance (IR)/acanthosis nigricans (AN) (HAIR-AN) syndrome were found in fewer patients.

Hormonal manifestations. An increased ovarian source of Δ^4-A and or T production is frequently present. Elevated basal levels of T and/or Δ^4-A in the absence of elevated adrenal androgens (DHEA, DS) generally signify primary PCOS. However, in some patients, both increased ovarian T and/or Δ^4-A production and increased adrenal androgen levels are present simultaneously in the absence of any known enzyme defect in adrenal and/or ovarian biosynthesis. Thus, PCOS females clinically have elevated serum total and/or free T level or Δ^4-A level, increased free androgen index, and decreased SHBG levels. These hormonal abnormalities may be related in part to obesity in PCOS (172). A mildly elevated random 17-OHP level and 17-OHP response to GnRH analog or hCG administration suggested dysregulation of ovarian 17α-hydroxylase/17–20 lyase activity in PCOS ovaries (120, 173). However CYP17 gene structure is normal in PCOS females. Thus, the mechanism of altered 17α-hydroxylase/17–20 lyase activity in the ovarian steroidogenesis is unknown. Whether hyperinsulinism modifies ovarian enzyme activity in the PCOS female (42) or whether a common defect is the cause of both altered insulin-signaling pathway and some ovarian enzyme gene expression remains to be elucidated.

The increased ovarian androgen production in primary PCOS is associated with inappropriate gonadotropin secretory patterns including elevated basal LH levels (139, 171, 174), elevated basal LH to FSH ratios, high LH amplitude (174–176), or hyperresponse of LH to LHRH stimulations (174). Nonbioactive gonadotropin measurement, such as radioimmunoassay, however, did not demonstrate abnormally elevated LH levels in approximately 25% of primary PCOS patients (177). In the author's experience, the baseline LH levels, LH to FSH ratios, and LH response to LHRH administration in the primary PCOS patients were elevated or apparently appropriate despite increased ovarian androgen secretion. Generally increased ovarian sources of Δ^4-A and/or T in these patients were not significantly suppressible by dexamethasone, although all other adrenal steroid levels were promptly suppressed (39). PCOS associated with both increased ovarian and adrenal androgen secretion of undefined cause was found in about 5% of the patients in the author's study (39).

The inappropriately elevated LH levels in the primary PCOS patients were not related to an alteration in the negative feedback regulation between estradiol and LH secretion, since estradiol infusion effectively suppressed

elevated LH in these patients (174). In addition, the positive feedback mechanism of estrogen on LH release was apparently intact in PCOS patients since the preovulatory elevation of estradiol via clomiphene citrate administration induced an LH surge in patients with primary PCOS (178). The pathogenesis of the inappropriate gonadotropin secretion in the primary PCOS is not yet clearly defined. Inappropriate gonadotropin secretion may be due to abnormal ovarian steroidogenesis of PCOS or primary or secondary hypothalamic–pituitary alteration. The presence of both negative and positive feedback mechanisms of gonadotropin secretion in patients with primary PCOS led to the conclusion that anovulation in primary PCOS is less likely due to an intrinsic hypothalamic abnormality (174, 179). Defective secretion of FSH may play a crucial role in the pathogenesis of PCOS since FSH or clomiphene administration resulted in ovulation in patients with primary PCOS (174, 179, 180). An extraglandular source of estrogen (estrone) via peripheral conversion of Δ^4-A is related to body weight and has been speculated to be of causative importance in the maintenance of chronic anovulation (179, 181). Suppression of gonadotropin secretion by combined treatment of GnRH analog and an oral contraceptive effectively eliminated excess LH and excess ovarian androgen secretion (39, 182). However, a few months following discontinuation of these therapies, ovarian testosterone secretion increased remarkably quickly while LHRH-stimulated LH levels rose only marginally (182). This observation clearly indicates that a systemic or intraovarian factor modulates for the increased ovarian androgen synthesis in the presence of only modest amounts of LH secretion (182). This systemic or intraovarian factor may be insulin or some other yet unidentified factor or mechanism.

Insulin resistance. Many studies indicate that there is a strong relationship between hyperinsulinemia and ovarian hyperandrogenism (139, 183–188). The peripheral insulin resistance is not changed by the suppression in ovarian androgen levels (187, 188). Patients with insulin resistance may or may not be obese, but obesity contributes to a greater degree of insulin resistance and decreasing SHBG levels in women with PCOS. Overt insulin resistance in patients with primary PCOS has been reported in at least 60% or greater based on an elevated insulin to glucose level (189). Also, a high rate (38%) of hyperandrogenic disorder in women treated for type 1 diabetes mellitus has been reported (154). These data indicate that hyperinsulinemia is a causative factor in PCOS.

The mechanism by which hyperinsulinemia results in increased ovarian androgen production in PCOS has been the subject of investigation in the past and current decades. Insulin has a stimulatory effect on steroidogenesis of normal and polycystic ovaries and interacts with LH in a synergistic manner (190, 191). Insulin action in the ovary appears to be mediated by the specific insulin receptor and not by the cross-reaction with the IGF-I receptors (190, 191). Hyperinsulinemia is also suggested to contribute to premature follicular growth arrest and anovulation of PCOS (190). Insulin also appears to have a role in amplifying LH-induced theca cell androgen production in PCOS females (190). A study indicated that lean PCOS females have an equivalent degree of tissue insulin resistance to obese PCOS females (192). Hyperinsulinemia in hyperandrogenic anovulatory females is also often accompanied by an increased amount of abdominal fat (42). This upper-body obesity is a risk factor for development of type 2 diabetes mellitus and ultimately cardiovascular disease (42, 193). Acanthosis nigricans is a cutaneous manifestation of hyperinsulinemia and is commonly noted in PCOS patients with insulin resistance and obesity (193). A retrospective study revealed a rate of 26% of type 2 diabetes occurring among PCOS females (194). However, insulin alone in the absence of gonadotropin secretion in PCOS females did not cause excess ovarian androgen secretion (182, 195). Thus, modulation of ovarian steroidogenesis by both insulin and gonadotropin is a prerequisite for hyperandrogenism in PCOS females with insulin resistance (195). Several studies demonstrated normal insulin receptor-binding capacity and affinity, normal total phosphorylation of the insulin receptor β-subunit (148, 193, 196), and an abnormal dose-dependent effect of insulin on glucose transport, suggesting a postreceptor defect (147, 148). An increased basal phosphorylation of the serine residue of insulin receptor β-subunit in contrast to the tyrosine residue was proposed as a cellular mechanism of insulin resistance of PCOS (148). However equal numbers of PCOS females had a normal receptor tyrosine kinase activity, suggesting a defect beyond insulin receptor phosphorylation (148). A decreased content of GLUT-4 glucose transporter in the adipocyte cell membrane of PCOS patients may also be a mechanism for peripheral insulin resistance (149). Paternally transmitted insulin gene variable number tandem repeat (VNTR) of class III alleles has also been reported to be associated with insulin resistance of PCOS (197). Thus, the cellular and molecular mechanism of insulin resistance of PCOS is yet to be defined.

Other candidate genes or factors. Several recent studies of candidate genes or causative factors of PCOS also uncovered other genetic factors independent of insulin resistance that may play a role in the development of PCOS (Table 4). These include follistatin gene (156), FSH β-subunit gene mutation (198), chromosome II long arm deletion (199), TNF-α-system (200), α-estrogen receptor defect (201), maternal obesity and high birth weight (202), history of premature pubarche (203–205), and a history of central precocious puberty (206). The childhood diagnosis of premature pubarche and central precocious puberty may suggest that either premature ovarian exposure to androgens or sex steroids or a factor

Table 4 Proven or Proposed Positive and Negative Genes/Factors Associated with Hyperandrogenism/Polycystic Ovary Syndrome

	Positive association	Negative findings	Inconsistent findings
PCOS or hyperandrogenism	Serine residue of insulin receptor of β-subunit (148) Paternally transmitted insulin gene variable number tandem repeat (VNTR) class III alleles (197) Follistatin (156) FSH β-subunit gene mutation (198) Chromosome II long arm deletion (199) TNF-alpha system (200) α-estrogen receptor defect (201) Maternal obesity/high birth weight (202) History of premature pubarche (203–205) History of central precocious puberty (206)	StAR gene (207) DAX-I gene (207) Steroidal factor I gene (207) CYP17 gene (208, 209) Insulin receptor binding capacity/affinity (148, 255) CYP21 mutation heterozygosity (211, 212) Androgen receptor gene (156) CYP19 aromatase gene (156) Activin/inhivin genes (156) SHBG gene (156) LH/hCG receptor gene (156) FSH receptor gene (156) Leptin/proleptin receptor gene (156) IGF-I/GR-IR/IGF BP3 genes (156) INSR gene/IRSI gene (1560	CYPIIA gene (156, 207, 213) Hyperprolactinemia (131, 215) VNTR gene (148, 197)
Idiopathic hirsutism	Increase in skin 5α-reductase activity (68, 234–236) Obesity/decreased SHBG (228) Increased free/bioactive androgens (50, 237)	CYPIIA gene (214)	Androgen receptor gene (239–241)

causing this precocity may contribute to the development of PCOS or ovarian hyperandrogenism in later life. On the other hand, many other genes were found not to be linked or associated with PCOS and are not likely candidate genes for PCOS (156, 207–212) (Table 4). There are also inconsistent and conflicting reports with regards to CYPIIA gene (156, 207, 213, 214) and hyperprolactinemia as potential factors for PCOS development (131, 215) (Table 4). The mechanism of altered reproductive function in hyperprolactinemic females is complex (216). An estrogen-stimulatory effect on the pituitary lactotropes has been speculated to cause hyperprolactinemia in patients with this disorder (216).

e. Genetic Causes of Insulin-Resistant Syndrome. A severe degree of excess ovarian androgen production has been found in genetic disorders of severe insulin-resistant syndrome due to point mutation of the gene encoding insulin receptor function (217–220). These patients manifest HAIR-AN syndrome and are usually virilized. Leprechaunism characterized by severe congenital growth retardation appears to be also caused by insulin receptor gene mutation (217) and patients develop PCOS although those with severe cases do not survive long. Other syndromes caused by insulin receptor gene mutation include Rabson-Mendenhall syndrome and type A syndrome (219, 221–223). Kahn type B insulin resistance syndrome due to the presence of circulating antibodies for insulin receptors also causes HAIR-AN syndrome (220). However, fewer than 30% of women with insulin resistance manifest AN (188). The patients with AN, therefore, are at high risk of HAIR-AN syndrome. In patients with HAIR-AN syndrome, ovarian histological study almost always reveals marked stromal hyperthecosis, which results in severe excess ovarian androgen production (188).

f. Hyperthecosis of Stroma. This condition is characterized by the nests of luteinized theca cells within the stroma of bilaterally enlarged ovaries (3, 224, 225). The thickened capsule without subcapsular cysts differentiates hyperthecosis from PCOS (224, 225) and the theca cells produce excess androgen. Patients with stromal hyperthecosis have progressive symptoms of androgen excess and are usually amenorrheic. Serum T levels are generally >150 ng/dl (3, 188). This condition, however, is differentiated from most of the androgen-producing tumors clinically by the nature of slowly progressive symptoms, hormonally by the elevated basal and LHRH-stimulated LH levels, as well as significant presence of acanthosis nigricans in some patients.

g. PCOS Associated with Adrenal Androgen Secretion. In patients with mild 21-hydroxylase deficiency, menstrual disorder was present in about one-half but most of these patients had normal ovarian androgen secretion despite experiencing menstrual problems (77). Previous studies demonstrated that the menstrual disorder in either 21-hydroxylase deficiency or genotype-normal decreased adrenal 3β-HSD activity patients (no longer 3β-HSD deficiency) had PCOS by ultrasound, laparoscopy, or laparotomy study (23). Thus, PCOS in patients with primarily increased adrenal androgen secretion was associated with both normal or mildly increased ovarian androgen production. However, in the poorly controlled severe classic virilizing form of congenital adrenal hyperplasia patients, classic PCOS pathological findings and increased ovarian androgen production were demonstrated (157–161). The pathophysiology of PCOS in these conditions was elaborated in previous sections.

2. Genetic Defects in Ovarian Steroidogenesis

a. Ovarian 17β-HSD Deficiency. This enzyme is also termed as 17β-ketosteroid reductase. Recent molecular studies revealed that 17β-HSD 1 isoenzyme is expressed in the ovary and preferentially reduces estrone to estradiol (226). 17β-HSD 3 is the enzyme that converts Δ^4-A to T and is expressed in the testis. This enzyme deficiency in the testicular tissue due to a mutation in the gene results in male sexual ambiguity (227–230). 17β-HSD 3 isoenzyme expression is either low or undetectable in the ovarian tissue. Thus, the genetic basis of ovarian 17-KSR deficiency resulting in pubertal onset of hirsutism, virilism, menstrual disorder, and PCO reported in females (163) is yet to be characterized.

b. Ovarian Type II 3β-HSD Deficiency. 3β-HSD deficiency has been demonstrated in both adrenal and gonadal tissue in patients with severe 3β-HSD deficiency. To date, two females with proven severe non-salt-losing 3β-HSD deficiency CAH demonstrated a defect in ovarian 3β-HSD activity and both manifested hirsutism, menstrual disorders, and PCO (108, 109). Thus, inherited intra-adrenal and intraovarian genetic type II 3β-HSD deficiency is a rare cause for ovarian dysfunction and PCOS.

c. Ovarian Aromatase (CYP19) Deficiency. Aromatase enzyme deficiency due to a mutation in the aromatase gene (CYP19) is a cause of virilization including clitoromegaly, primary amenorrhea, and multiple ovarian cysts as noted on a pelvic imaging study (164–166). These patients have highly elevated T levels, moderately elevated LH levels, and low estrogen levels (164–166).

3. Ovarian Androgen-Producing Tumors

The clinical presentation of androgen-producing tumors of the ovary is similar to the androgen-producing tumor of the adrenals. Thus, in general marked virilism occurs in short duration in women with ovarian androgen-producing tumors. However, there are exceptional patients whose symptoms of excess androgen production by the ovarian tumor was slowly progressive and long-standing (231). Both clinically rapid or slowly progressive ovarian tumor secreting androgens are associated with extremely high circulating levels of mainly Δ^4-A and T regardless of histopathological classification of the tumors. Serum DHEA and DHEA-S levels may be mildly elevated or normal except in cases of metastasized adrenal carcinoma of the ovary. The tumorous androgen-producing cells arise from lipoid cells, hilus cells, Sertoli-Leydig cells, granulosa-theca cells, and stromal cells.

4.   α-Estrogen Receptor Defect

This is a rare disorder proposed to describe the clinical picture of hirsutism and regular menstrual history associated with extraordinarily elevated serum T and estradiol levels of an ovarian source in the absence of adrenal and ovarian tumor. This abnormality was proposed to be compatible with α-estrogen receptor knockout female mice. The female patient had ovarian imaging findings compatible with classic PCOS (201).

C.   Idiopathic Hirsutism/Acne

By strict definition, idiopathic hirsutism should describe women presenting with hirsutism and/or acne and no other androgen excess symptoms, or other clinical or hormonal causes of hirsutism, normal circulating androgen concentration in the basal state or under dynamic test of adrenal or ovarian steroidogenic function, and normal ovarian function as evidenced by a normal ovulatory cycle or normal reproductive function. In a study of the causes of hirsutism in the author's clinic, idiopathic hirsutism, defined by normal circulating basal and stimulated adrenal and ovarian total steroid levels and normal menstrual cycles, was the most common cause of hirsutism and included 30–50% of hirsute women of various ethnic/racial backgrounds (39). However, idiopathic hirsutism by the strictest definition using absolutely normal circulating total and free androgen levels and documented normal ovulatory menstrual cycles, was identified in only 6% of hirsute females (232) in an Italian study and 17% in an Alabama study (233).

Several pathogenic mechanisms have been speculated for idiopathic hirsutism (Table 4). Increased intracellular conversion of precursor androgens to DHT by the increased intracellular 5α-reductase activity was found in some women with idiopathic hirsutism (68, 234). Increased skin androgen metabolic activity was noted in women with idiopathic hirsutism as evidenced by the increased circulating 3α-adiol gluc levels (62–65, 235) (Fig. 4). Serum 3α-adiol gluc reflects largely 5α-reductase activity (235) and peripheral adrenal androgen metabolism (65). Thus, the increased 5α-reductase activity in the skin of these women could be a causative factor in idiopathic hirsutism (236). Another proposed mechanism for idiopathic hirsutism is the increased availability of bioactive androgens. Free T is a determinant factor in androgen action and was elevated in number of hirsute women with normal total T concentration (50, 237). In obese hirsute females, a reduction in SHBG and an increase in free T are associated with the degree of upper body obesity and may be the cause of hirsutism (238). Thus the decreased

SHBG and increased free T or DHT may be one of the causative factors in idiopathic hirsutism.

The third theory involves increased skin tissue sensitivity to the circulating androgen for idiopathic hirsutism. Although the increased skin 5α-reductase activity may enhance androgen effect at the target cells, the androgen-binding capacity at the receptor protein of the target cell shows no differences between normal and hirsute females (67). Androgen receptor gene polymorphism does not appear to play a significant role in the pathologies of idiopathic hirsutism (239), but this was contradicted by other studies (240, 241). CYPIIA gene was found to have no significant role in the pathology of hirsutism (214). Abnormalities found in some women with idiopathic hirsutism include increased skin androgen metabolizing activity and/or increased bioactive free androgens. Whether these are primary abnormalities or whether they are due to disorders of enzyme and receptor protein regulation or due to increased free component of androgens remains to be elucidated. The mechanism of low SHBG and high free T in nonobese females with idiopathic hirsutism also needs further exploration.

D.   Hirsutism Associated with Thyroid Disorder

Thyroid hormones increase the concentration of SHBG in plasma (25). Thus, high testosterone levels observed in some patients with hyperthyroidism are due to increased protein-bound testosterone levels, with no clinical androgen excess symptoms. On the other hand, hypothyroidism may be associated with hirsutism (242). In the last 20 years, the authors have found only a few women with hirsutism who have hypothyroidism. These women had normal circulating total androgen levels. Thus hypothyroidism seems to be a condition rarely associated with hirsutism and menstrual irregularity. To the best of our knowledge, no studies have been reported of the androgen metabolism, SHBG, or free androgen concentration in hypothyroidism.

V.   DIAGNOSTIC APPROACH AND DIFFERENTIAL DIAGNOSIS

A.   Clinical Assessment of Hirsutism

A detailed history and careful physical examination are essential in evaluating hirsute patients. History of puberty, including adrenarche, thelarche, onset of hirsutism and its progression, menarche, and menstrual history should be obtained. Similar history should be obtained from female family members as well. Evaluation of the severity and progression of terminal hair growth is an essential part of physical examination in hirsute females. A detailed history of cosmetic care, including frequency, method, and the last treatment date of depilation or shaving is necessary to estimate degree of hair growth in a natural state.

The degree of hirsutism on various parts of the body should be examined, including face, chin, neck, chest, areolar, abdomen, pelvic area, upper and lower back, buttocks, intergluteal region, thighs, and other parts of extremities. The best method to determine the degree of hirsutism was described by Ferriman and Gallwey (243). Their original scoring system included 11 areas of the body, using a total of four points for grading each area, with a total score of 44. Further modification of the charts and scoring system of Ferriman and Gallwey has been described by Cooke and Goodal (128) and Hatch et al. (244). The scoring system modified by Cooke and Goodal identifies hirsute scores in nine hormonally more sensitive areas and two hormonally less sensitive areas with a total score of 36 (Fig. 6). We find that this modified scoring system is easy and more informative in evaluating the initial state and for follow-up of treated hirsute patients. Presence or absence and extent of acne, seborrhea, oily hair, masculine body habitus, and clitoral enlargement should also be examined in all hirsute patients.

B. Differential Diagnosis

In the previous section, many of the specific clinical and hormonal abnormalities of each disorder were discussed. In this section, a general approach to the laboratory investigation for differential diagnosis of the hirsutism cause is described. The reference data for basal and ACTH-stimulated steroid levels in normal women and in women who are hirsute due to various causes are depicted in Table 5 (39). In interpreting the patient's hormonal values, it is pertinent to know each laboratory's hormonal reference data due to the variable degrees of purification and specificity of hormonal assay. A guideline for evaluation of hirsutism causes is depicted in Figure 5. Hirsutism/acne with a slow or nonprogressive history and a normal menstrual cycle history is more likely due to an idiopathic cause (no excess androgen production) or a mild spectrum of PCOS with an anovulatory cycle, mild spectrum of CAH, or idiopathic adrenal hyperandrogenism (functional adrenal hyperandrogenism). Thus, a minimal work-up, including measurement of early morning 17-OHP level and a few serum androgen level screenings (total/free T, androstenedione, and DHEA-S) would guide the differential pathway as depicted in Figure 5. Additional 3α-androstenediol glucuronate and SHBG level studies may be helpful for assessing idiopathic hirsutism if circulating androgen levels are unremarkable. Hirsutism/acne with a slow or moderate progression history and overt menstrual irregularity history even in teenaged girls (primary or secondary amenorrhea, polymenorrhea) requires consideration of PCOS, a mild form of CAH, idiopathic adrenal hyperandrogenism, as well as thyroid disorders (hypo-/hyper-), and hyperprolactinemia. Thus, the initial evaluation of 8 am 17-OHP levels, serum androgen levels, LH, FSH, T_4, TSH, and prolactin levels would guide further approaches for a differential pathway, as depicted in Figure 5.

Hirsute patients with menstrual disorders have generally elevated ovarian and/or adrenal androgen levels, although the levels are not as high as in patients with virilism. In those with only elevated total or free T levels

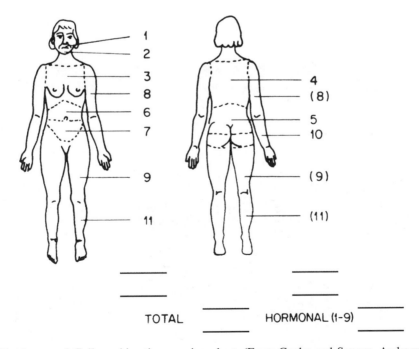

Figure 6 Modified Ferriman and Gallwey hirsutism scoring chart. (From Cooke and Sawers. Androgens and Anti-androgen Therapy 1982:95. Reproduced with permission from John Wiley and Sons, New York, NY.)

Table 5 Baseline and ACTH-Stimulated Adrenal and Ovarian Steroid Levels and Frequency of Various Causes of Hirsutism in 117 Hirsute Females

Hormones	Normal females of all menstrual cycles (n = 33)	Hirsute females					
		21-OH deficiency (n = 2)	Increased adrenal androgens only (n = 14)	Type II genotype-normal mild decrease in adrenal 3β-HSD activity (n = 9)[a]	PCOS only (n = 30)	Increased ovarian/ adrenal androgens (n = 6)	Idiopathic hirsutism (n = 56)
Baseline							
Δ5-17P (nmol/L)	3.2 ± 2.7	4.2, 6	5.7 ± 4.2	12.3 ± 7.2†	5.9 ± 5	8.9 ± 7.4	4.2 ± 3.4
17-OHP (nmol/L)	2.9 ± 2.7	4.7, 26.2	3.3 ± 2.1	2.4 ± 1.4	3.9 ± 2.2†	3.9 ± 2.0	2.5 ± 2.5
DHEA (nmol/L)	13.7 ± 6.7	15.4, 18.5	25 ± 15*	41 ± 25*	18 ± 10	27.4 ± 15.4†	14.5 ± 7.6
DS (μmol/L)	5.1 ± 2.4	5.6, 7.1	9.1 ± 2.3*	12.8 ± 1.6*	5.5 ± 2.0	11 ± 4.5†	5.9 ± 2.4
Δ4-A (nmol/L)	4.3 ± 1.8	6.3, 7.3	5.5 ± 1.5	7.9 ± 3.3†	8.9 ± 3.4†	9.7 ± 3.3*	4.4 ± 1.7
T (nmol/L)	1.0 ± 0.4	1.0, 1.3	1.5 ± 0.5	1.6 ± 0.34*	3.4 ± 1.6*	2.5 ± 0.8*	1.2 ± 0.4
S (nmol/L)	0.6 ± 0.3	0.6, 1.8	1 ± 0.5	0.6 ± 0.3	1.4 ± 1.4	2.3 ± 2.5	0.9 ± 0.5
F (μmol/L)	0.34 ± 0.11	0.3, 0.5	0.35 ± 0.14	0.39 ± 0.11	0.37 ± 0.2	0.39 ± 0.2	0.36 ± 0.2
Δ5-17P/17-OHP	1.8 ± 1.5	0.9, 0.2	2.3 ± 1.3	6.2 ± 3.8†	1.9 ± 2.0	2.7 ± 2.6	2.6 ± 2.1
Δ5-17P/F	8.5 ± 6.1	12.7, 9.1	16 ± 10	23 ± 11*	15 ± 10	19 ± 12†	10.6 ± 8.3
DHEA/Δ4-A	3.5 ± 1.5	2.5, 2.6	4.8 ± 2.8†	6.1 ± 2.5†	2.1 ± 1.0	3.1 ± 1.9	3.6 ± 2.5
ACTH-stimulated							
Δ5-17P (nmol/L)	31.4 ± 11.3	35.1, 27.5	35 ± 11	91 ± 33*	33 ± 14	31.7 ± 5.7	28 ± 12.2
17-OHP (nmol/L)	7.2 ± 4.7	246, 116	6.8 ± 3.3	6.1 ± 3.2	8 ± 7.3	7.3 ± 2.8	6.2 ± 3.8
DHEA (nmol/L)	37.8 ± 13.1	46, 17.7	71 ± 19*	97 ± 29*	39 ± 15	67.1 ± 15.9*	35.1 ± 13.1
DS (μmol/L)	5.6 ± 2.7	3.1, 7.4	9.1 ± 2.5*	12.8 ± 2.1*	5.8 ± 2.3	12.4 ± 5†	6.1 ± 2.6
Δ4-A (nmol/L)	7.1 ± 2.4	12.8, 5.6	5.5 ± 1.5	13.4 ± 3†	11.2 ± 3.9†	11.3 ± 4.1†	3.2 ± 2.2
T (nmol/L)	1.3 ± 0.4	1.4, 1.6	1.5 ± 0.5	1.9 ± 0.7†	3.5 ± 1.4*	2.5 ± 0.6*	1.3 ± 0.4
S (nmol/L)	4.0 ± 1.7	5.6, 4.0	4.9 ± 3	4.9 ± 3.4	6.2 ± 3	6.6 ± 3.4	5.4 ± 2.7
F (μmol/L)	0.9 ± 0.2	0.6, 1.0	0.87 ± 0.23	0.7 ± 0.2	1.0 ± 0.4	0.7 ± 0.2	0.8 ± 0.3
Δ5-17P/17-OHP	5.2 ± 2.3	0.1, 0.2	6.1 ± 2.4	16 ± 7.7†	5.0 ± 3.1	4.9 ± 2	5.4 ± 3.2
Δ5-17-P/F	32.2 ± 11.6	46.2, 23.1	38 ± 13	85 ± 20*	36 ± 20	38.7 ± 12.9	31.3 ± 15.3
DHEA/Δ4-A	5.8 ± 2.2	3.7, 3.3	9.8 ± 4.5†	8.5 ± 2.4†	4.0 ± 2.0	6.6 ± 214	5.9 ± 2.9

Values are given as mean ± SD except for 21-OH deficiency depicting 2 individual values.

*p < 0.001–<0.00001 compared to normal females.

†p < 0.05–0.01 compared to normal females.

To convert the hormonal level to ng/dl: ×33.3 for Δ5-17P and 17-OHP, ×28.6 for DHEA, ×28.64 for Δ4-A, ×28.8 for T, ×34.7 for S. To convert μg/dl: ×36 for F, ×37 for DS.

[a]Type II genotype-normal mild decrease in adrenal 3β-HSD activity is not mild nonclassic 3β-HSD deficiency; etiology of this is uncertain at this time (Luttallah et al. J Clinic Endocrinol Metab 2002.)

Source: data derived from Ref. 39.

with or without elevated LH levels as compared to the normal early follicular phase LH levels, PCOS is a first consideration. Evaluation for insulin resistance and an imaging study of adnexae need to be considered. In those with only elevated DHEA-S levels with or without elevated T, idiopathic adrenal hyperandrogenism and PCOS are equal considerations. The author's experience indicates that the response of LH to LHRH stimulation is variable in patients with primary PCOS and PCOS related to increased adrenal androgen production. The occurrence of menstrual disorders and PCOS in all excess adrenal androgen-producing conditions was discussed earlier. In those with elevated cortisol and adrenal androgen levels and no cushingoid features, glucocorticoid resistance syndrome is a possibility.

Very high basal DHEA (>1500 ng/dl), DHEA-S (>500 μg/dl) levels, and urinary 17-ketosteroid levels, with or without moderately elevated Δ^4-A and T levels, can be seen in women with partial adrenal 3β-HSD deficiency (108, 109) or in type II 3β-HSD genotype-normal but mildly decreased adrenal 3β-HSD activity of unknown cause (no longer 3β-HSD deficiency) (23, 39, 114). The magnitude of Δ^5-17P in true 3β-HSD deficiency, however, is highly abnormal (108, 109) compared to genotype-normal mildly decreased adrenal 3β-HSD activity of unknown cause (23, 114). An adrenal androgen-producing tumor is rare in patients without virilism, but exceptionally higher DHEA and DHEA-S levels would warrant its consideration and a dexamethasone suppression test is warranted, as described below.

In patients with hyperprolactinemia, a causative medication history, such as oral contraceptives or psycholeptic drugs, and CNS symptom history must be obtained. A pituitary imaging study (MRI, CT scan) is essential for evaluation of prolactin-secreting pituitary adenoma. Hirsutism/acne with moderate progression and virilism suggests excess androgen-producing pathologies such as virilizing CAH, stromal hyperthecosis (severely advanced PCOS), a slow-growing androgen-producing tumor, or a clinically recognizable classic or atypical Cushing syndrome or disease. Any apparent clinical and physical stigmata of a disorder such as Cushing syndrome/disease will not be discussed here. In those patients with clinically indistinguishable hirsutism, initial work-up including 8 a.m. 17-OHP, serum F, androgens, LH, FSH, and prolactin levels is warranted. In patients with elevated T and Δ^4-A levels with or without elevated LH levels, an ovarian imaging study, an ovarian suppression test and a β-hCG screening test would be helpful for differentiating among stromal hyperthecosis (or severe PCOS), a slow-growing ovarian androgen-producing tumor, or an hCG-producing tumor. For those with excessively elevated DHEA and DHEA-S levels with or without elevated cortisol levels, an adrenal suppression test by administering dexamethasone and, if indicated, an adrenal imaging study (generally by CT scan) would help to evaluate the nature of excess

adrenal androgen production. In those with any clinical and hormonal data suggesting atypical Cushing syndrome, both dynamic studies of adrenal steroid and ACTH secretion and adrenal and/or pituitary imaging studies need to be considered.

Hirsutism/acne with virilism of a rapidly progressive history generally signifies an androgen-producing tumor of the ovary or adrenal gland. Random androgen and cortisol level determination and, accordingly, an adrenal CT or an abdominal or ovarian imaging study (ultrasound, MRI) are warranted. In those with no obvious anatomical pathology of the adrenal glands or ovaries, endocrine dynamics of the adrenal glands or ovaries need to be evaluated (Fig. 5).

A logical sequence of adrenal and/or ovarian dynamic studies includes an early morning basal hormonal study or circadian basal hormonal study followed by adrenal stimulation/suppression and ovarian suppression/stimulation contiguously. Suppression tests are generally more important than stimulation tests, in evaluating the excess androgen production. For adrenal stimulation, 0.25 mg ACTH is administered by intravenous (IV) bolus and various adrenal steroids and C-19 steroids responses are examined 1 h following ACTH stimulation. The adrenal suppression test is performed by administering a pharmacological dosage of dexamethasone, 2 mg/day in four divided doses/day for 3–5 days. The key circulating adrenal steroids, including C-19 androgens and urinary metabolites of C-19 steroids, may be determined on days 3–5 after dexamethasone administration. While adrenal steroid secretion is suppressed by dexamethasone, ovarian suppression may be evaluated by administering gonadotropin suppressant, such as synthetic estrogen (ethinyl estradiol 50–100 μg orally twice daily), or a progestational compound, such as norethindrone acetate (10 mg orally three times daily) for 3–5 days. The ovarian androgen stimulation test may be performed by administering human chorionic gonadotropin (hCG), 3000–5000 IU/day for 3 days and ovarian steroidal response should be examined 2 to 24–48 hours after the last dose of hCG. An LHRH (GnRH) stimulation test (100–150 μg IV bolus) or LHRH (GnRH) analog stimulation test may also be useful in the differential diagnosis of increased ovarian androgen production. These gonadotropin stimulation tests, however, need to be performed prior to the above-described ovarian suppression or ovarian stimulation test.

With dexamethasone administration, patients with adrenal tumor, DHEA, DHEA-S, and other C-19 steroids and their urinary metabolites may be only slightly or partially decreased. In adrenal 3β-HSD deficiency, genotype-normal mildly decreased adrenal 3β-HSD activity of unknown cause, and idiopathic adrenal hyperandrogenism, these steroid levels are more easily suppressed to a greater degree (39, 65, 108, 109). Clinically, these patients rarely present with virilism. Occasionally patients with partial 21-hydroxylase deficiency present with virilism and menstrual disorder. Serum DHEA and DHEA-S levels may be moderately elevated, but DHEA levels are generally also higher in the early morning hours. These steroidal abnormalities will be more easily suppressed by dexamethasone administration in CAH.

Extremely high basal Δ^4-A (>350 ng/dl) and T (>150–200 ng/dl) levels without concomitantly increased levels of DHEA and DHEA-S are usually seen in patients with long-standing stromal hyperthecosis, ovarian tumor, and ovarian 17-KSR deficiency. These patients generally manifest virilism. The ovarian source of androgen will be suppressed to a greater degree and more easily by administration of ethinyl estradiol or a progesterone compound in ovarian 17-KSR deficiency or PCOS, whereas androgen secretion by the tumor may not change or may only slightly decrease. The LHRH stimulation test results in LH hyperresponse in ovarian hyperthecosis and 17-KSR deficiency (163). In stromal hyperthecosis, suppression of androgens, by administration of estrogen or progestational agents, is not as good as in the patient with PCOS. However, a long-term (>3 month) LHRH analog treatment suppresses ovarian androgen secretion in these patients (182). The definitive differential diagnosis of these three conditions requires ovarian hormonal dynamic studies, radiological evaluation, gynecological examination, and possibly laparoscopic examination in some cases. Laparotomy may also have to be carried out if there is a high suspicion of tumorous lesions in the ovary.

VI. TREATMENT OF HIRSUTISM AND POLYCYSTIC OVARY SYNDROME

The specific and nonspecific therapies for the various causes of hirsutism described here are based partly on the author's experience and a review of the literature (Table 6). The treatment of hirsute symptoms is most effective if aimed at correcting the primary pathogenic mechanism. This is not always straightforward in patients with PCOS, ovarian hyperthecosis, or idiopathic hirsutism. Both specific and nonspecific therapy will be discussed for each disorder.

A. Mild Nonclassic 21-Hydroxylase Deficiency, 3β-HSD Deficiency, and Idiopathic Adrenal Hyperandrogenism

Suppression of excess adrenal androgen production for these conditions can easily be achieved by administration of a relatively low dosage of glucocorticoid hormone. We have used prednisone in a dosage of 2.5 mg twice daily or 5 mg a.m. and 2.5 mg p.m., or dexamethasone 0.25–0.375 mg at bedtime. The dosage of glucocorticoid should be adjusted based on the patient's clinical and hormonal response, as well as side effects of glucocorticoid, such as weight gain, striae, and Cushingoid features. Use of dexamethasone 0.5 mg at bedtime caused Cushingoid fea-

tures in some women with nonclassic CAH within 4–8 weeks in the author's experience as well as in PCOS patients with elevated adrenal androgens (245).

The aim of treatment is to reduce adrenal androgen secretion to a low-normal level, not complete adrenal suppression, thereby minimizing the side effects. Our experience indicates that marginal to significant clinical improvement of hirsutism in a large number of women with these increased adrenal androgen-producing conditions occurred within 8 months to 1 year of treatment. By the second year of treatment, a majority of the patients showed good improvement in hirsutism. In almost all cases recovery of menses occurred in 2–3 months following adequate suppression of excess adrenal androgen secretion. Therapeutic monitoring of 21-hydroxylase deficiency requires periodic follow-up measurement of 17-OHP, Δ4-A, and T levels. Periodic measurement of DHEA, DHEA-S, Δ4-A, and T is necessary to monitor 3β-HSD deficiency and idiopathic adrenal hyperandrogenism. Antiandrogen drug therapy as depicted later in Table 8 may be necessary in those patients whose hirsutism symptoms do not improve significantly despite lowered adrenal androgen levels. Use of spironolactone in nonclassic CAH is, however, not desirable due to its potential salt-wasting effect.

B. Primary PCOS and Stromal Hyperthecosis

Primary PCOS is a more difficult condition to treat successfully for both hirsutism and menstrual disorders (amenorrhea/oligomenorrhea or dysfunctional bleeding). In patients with insulin resistance and/or obesity, additional risk of glucose intolerance or type 2 diabetes and complications of obesity need to be dealt with. In PCOS females with insulin resistance with or without obesity and menstrual disorder, treatment for hyperinsulinemia secondary to insulin resistance is the approach of choice. This is because the pathophysiology of ovarian hyperandrogenism and menstrual disorder is related to a peripheral defect in either the insulin-signaling pathway or glucose metabolic pathway as described earlier. Thus, weight control and weight loss measures in obese patients, including nutritionally healthy eating, controls on both the amount and kinds of food, coupled with a physically active lifestyle in the long term is needed to reduce or prevent ovarian hyperandrogenism, glucose intolerance, type 2 diabetes, hyperlipidemia, and hypertension.

Insulin-sensitizing pharmacological agents used in the past few years and currently available on the market are summarized in Table 6. Metformin hydrochloride (Glucophage) decreases hepatic glucose production, decreases intestinal glucose absorption, increases peripheral glucose uptake/utilization (nonhypoglycemic agent), and has been more widely used than other insulin-sensitizing agents for PCOS females. At a dosage of 1000–2000 mg per day in two to three divided doses, it is effective in improving glycemic parameters, lowering insulin levels, and improv-

Table 6 Reported Effects of Pharmacological Therapies for Hirsutism and Polycystic Ovary Syndrome

Classification of therapy	Drugs and dosage	Hirsutism and androgen levels — Idiopathic	Hirsutism and androgen levels — Hyperandrogenic causes	PCOS Menstrual disorders — Cycle regulation	PCOS Menstrual disorders — Anovulation	Insulin resistance, glucose intolerance	Lipid changes	Ref.	Precautions
Antiandrogens	Spironolactone, 100–200 mg/d ± COC	↓ F-G score ↔ Androgens	↓ F-G score ↓ Free T					257, 267–272	Need of contraception/long-term therapy for efficacy, gradual dose increase from 25 to 100 mg over time, K+ level monitoring, breast tenderness, irregular bleeding, mild volume deletion
	CPA, 50–100 mg/1–10 days of use + COC or 25–50 mg/day + COC	↓ F-G score ↓ Androgens	↓ F-G score ↓ Androgens					257, 263, 270, 272, 275	Same as COC below
	Flutamide, 62.5–250 mg/d, 250 mg bid ± COC	↓ F-G score ↔ T, DHT, 3α-AG	↓ F-G score ↔ T, DHT, 3α-AG					263, 270, 272, 275, 276	Contraception precaution, liver function monitoring a must; fulminant liver failure reported
	Finasteride, 5 mg/d ± COC, 0.25% finasteride cream	↓ F-G score ↔ or ↑ T/E$_2$, ↓ DHT, 3α-AG, DHEA-S	↓ F-G score ↔, ↑ Total T ↓ DHT, 3α-AG					262, 270, 276, 277	Contraception precaution
Glucocorticoids	Dexamethasone, 0.375 mg/d + spironolactone 100 mg/d, Dexamethasone 0.5 mg po qd	↓ F-G score ↓ T/free T ↓ DHEA-S	↓ F-G score ↓ T/free T ↓ DHEA-S ↓ All androgens			No effect		267, 233	Cushingoid side effect/weight gain at 0.5 mg/day dose
COC	Low dose COC, 35 μg EE + progestin Triphasic OC EE, 35 μg + CPA 2 mg/d	↓ F-G score	↓ F-G score only in lean PCOS ↓ T/free T ↓ LH and FSH	Anovulatory cycle regularity		Variable effects No significant changes	↑ TC ↑ HDL ↑ LDL ↑ TG	252, 256–261	↑ risk of venous thrombosis in coagulation factor V cases, ↑ risk of arterial thrombosis in hypertensive patients, smoker and >35 yrs age, weight gain, breakthrough bleeding, GI SYS, breast tenderness, and mood swing
GnRH analog	Leuprolide depot, Triptorelin, decapeptyl 3.75–7.5 mg/q m IM ± COC Goserelin, 3.75 mg/q m IM ± COC	↓ F-G score ↓ T/free T ↓ DHEA, A	↓ F-G score ↓ T/free T/DHEA-S ↓ LH and FSH ↔ Androgen	Anovulatory cycle regularity				262–265 256	Temporary ↑ in LH/FSH, COC Rx to prevent osteoporosis, costly Rx
Insulin-sensitizing agents	Metformin, 1000–2000 mg/d in 2–3 divided doses	↓ F-G score ↔, ↓ F-G score ↓ T/free T index ↔ LH and FSH ↓ or ↔ DHEA/DS	↓ F-G score	Improved menstrual cyclicity/regularity, less for patients with ↑ DHEA-S	Recovery of spontaneous/clomid-induced ovulation	Improved insulin sensitivity ↓ fasting insulin ↓ fasting glucose ↓ insulin response to glucose	↓ free fatty acids	246, 247, 249, 250, 252, 259	Contraindicated for renal/hepatic dysfunction—monitor function yearly, GI side effects, lactic acidosis precaution
	Acarbose, 300 mg/d in 3 divided doses	↓ Acne/seborrhea ↓ Androgen	↓ Androgen	53% normal cycle recovery		↓ insulin to glucose		255	GI side effects, flatulence, pain, diarrhea, do not use in liver disorder, GI disorders, renal failure

F-G, Ferriman-Gallwey hirsutism score; EE, ethinyl estradiol; CPA, cyproterone acetate; A, androstenedione; ↑, increase; ↓, decrease; ↔, no change; 3α-AG, 3α-androstanediol gluconate; COC, combined estrogen/progesterone oral contraceptives.

ing or recovering regular menstrual cyclicity in women with PCOS (246–250) and decreased visceral adiposity (248, 251, 252). The effect of metformin on the Ferriman-Gallwey Hirsutism Score has been inconsistent (247, 250) and appears less effective in patients with elevated DHEA and DHEA-S levels (246). Troglitazone (Rezulin: no longer on the market) is an insulin-sensitizing agent of the thiazolidinedione family. It has the pharmacological action of decreasing hepatic glucose output and increasing insulin-dependent glucose disposal in skeletal muscle via its binding to peroxisome proliferator-activated receptors (253, 254). At a dosage of 400–600 mg per day it improved all glycemic parameters and the ovulatory cycle in PCOS females (253, 254). The drug was removed from the market due to a potential for liver toxicity. Its effect on hirsutism, however, was only slight (253, 254). Rosiglitazone (Avandia) and Pioglitazone (Actos) are potent agonists for peroxisome proliferator-activated receptor-gamma and have pharmacological actions similar to Troglitazone. Both are available on the market, but their use for PCOS females is limited. Acarbose (Precose) is an agent of alpha-glucodase inhibitor that delays digestion of ingested carbohydrates and minimizes glucose use. A dosage of 300 mg per day was reported to be effective in lowering insulin levels and in the recovery of the normal menstrual cycle in 53% of PCOS females. Improved acne has also been reported (255).

If the patient desires mainly hirsutism treatment, as is the case with many adolescent girls with PCOS or hyperandrogenism, the antiandrogen therapies in Table 6 may be considered as well as combined estrogen/progesterone oral contraceptive (COC) therapy. Because all of the antiandrogen agents are potentially teratogenic for the male fetus, women of reproductive age should take contraceptive precautions using either COC or barrier contraceptives during this treatment. Additive effects of an antiandrogen agent and COC are likely to result in a greater degree of improvement in hirsutism. Use of antiandrogen compounds in the treatment of hirsutism is described in greater detail in the section on Idiopathic Hirsutism below. COC treatment alone in PCOS patients is often partially effective in hirsutism improvement and suppression of ovarian androgen secretion and free T levels (252, 256–261). Cyclic COC therapy in PCOS patients, however, has a long-term benefit from the prevention of endometrial hyperplasia to an unopposed effect of increased free estrogen in PCOS. COC has no discernable effect on insulin sensitivity and has variable influence on HDL and LDL, and total cholesterol and triglyceride levels (256–259). Thus, the long-term benefits of COC on lipids are difficult to predict in young women (Table 6).

In women with severe PCOS or stromal ovarian hyperthecosis with a greater degree of elevated ovarian testosterone level associated with increased LH secretion, use of a GnRH analog at a dosage of 3.75–7.5 mg intramuscularly (IM) every 28 days is highly effective in near-total suppression of gonadotropin and ovarian androgen secretion (182, 262–265). GnRH analog therapy is often combined with COC to prevent any undesirable effect on bone mineral density in these patients. The combined therapies of GnRH analog and COC thus have the effect of decreasing ovarian androgen levels, having antiandrogen action in the androgen-sensitive tissue, and increasing SHBG. They were also very effective in the treatment of hirsutism in PCOS and stromal hyperthecosis. The drawback of these therapies, however, is recurrence of ovarian hyperandrogenism and symptoms shortly after the drug therapies are discontinued (182, 260). Although ketoconazole has been reported to be effective in decreasing serum androgen levels and hirsutism (257, 266), this compound has not been widely accepted in the treatment of hirsutism.

C. Idiopathic Hirsutism

In the treatment of idiopathic hirsutism, the antiandrogen agents shown in Table 6 are predicted to be more specific therapeutic agents. However all antiandrogenic agents entail the risk of teratogenic effects. Therefore, absolute contraceptive measures are a must in women receiving antiandrogenic therapy. During the past several years, wider experience with four different antiandrogenic agents for treatment of idiopathic and hyperandrogenic hirsutism have been reported (Table 6), although the Food and Drug Administration has approved of none of these agents for treatment of hirsutism.

Spironolactone (100–400 mg/day) interferes with DHT binding to its receptor and forms inactive complexes at the nuclear level, minimizing the androgen effect on hair growth. Spironolactone treatment has variable results in hirsute females and other cosmetic hair removal care is often necessary. In our experience, spironolactone alone or combined therapy with spironolactone and COC was more effective in women with idiopathic hirsutism defined by normal androgen levels than in women with elevated androgen levels. Recent reports using a lower dosage of spironolactone (at 100–200 mg per day) showed as effective results in decreasing the Ferriman-Gallwey score as COC alone or cyproterone acetate combined with COC or ketoconazole therapy (257, 267–272) or flutamide or finasteride (270).

Cyproterone acetate is a synthetic steroid derivative of 17-OHP and has both antiandrogenic and antigonadotropic action (273). This agent is effective not only in the treatment of idiopathic hirsutism but also in other causes of androgen excess due to its antiandrogenic properties and by reducing androgen production via suppression of gonadotropin secretion (274). Overall, the combination of cyproterone acetate at 50–100 mg from cycle days 1–10, or a daily dose of 25–50 mg together with low-dosage estrogen therapy reduces the production, transport, metabolism, and action of androgens (257, 263, 270, 272, 273, 275). As shown in Table 6, numerous European sources indicate successful treatment of hirsutism of various causes using these combinations.

5α-reductase inhibitor should theoretically be an effective agent in the treatment of hirsutism. The type 1 5α-reductase isoenzyme predominates in peripheral tissue and type 2 isoenzyme in the reproductive system. Recently, type 2 isoenzyme has also been demonstrated in the hair follicle tissue and was described earlier. Of several steroidal and nonsteroidal 5α-reductase inhibitors, only finasteride has been extensively used for the treatment of hirsutism (262, 270, 276, 277). Finasteride at a daily dosage of 5 mg orally has been reported to decrease hirsutism scores in patients with both idiopathic and hyperandrogenic hirsutism (262, 270, 276, 277). Its effect on circulating androgen levels appears variable. The effect of finasteride in decreasing hirsutism has been reported to be either similar to the effect of cyproterone acetate or flutamide (275) or less than the effect of flutamide (276).

Flutamide is a nonsteroidal antiandrogen and prevents androgen from binding to the androgen receptor by its competitive binding without androgenic activity. Variable dosages of flutamide from 62.5 to 500 mg in two divided doses daily have been reported as effective in the treatment of hirsutism in both the idiopathic and hyperandrogenic causes (263, 270, 272, 275, 276, 278). A concern about this drug derives from a few reports of related fulminant hepatic failure (279–281). Thus, close monitoring of liver function is mandatory during the course of flutamide therapy.

COC treatment alone or combined COC and GnRH analog therapy in idiopathic hirsutism decreased the hirsutism score in a few reports (260, 261) (Table 6). The beneficial effects of COC and GnRH were described earlier.

In summary, most of the antiandrogenic drug therapies have been reported as effective in decreasing the amount of hirsutism in patients with either idiopathic or hyperandrogenic cases.

However, the drawbacks of these therapies are their temporary effectiveness during the drug treatment course. Cessation of drug therapies almost invariably results in recurrent hyperandrogenic symptoms with time. In addition, there are known potential side effects with all drug therapies, as summarized in Table 6. Evaluation of renal and hepatic function prior to and during administration of many of these pharmacological compounds and providing precautionary information to the patient with regard to potential side effects of the compounds are prudent measures in clinical practice.

D. Cosmetic Treatment of Hirsutism

Psychological embarrassment as a result of hirsutism and/or acne in adolescents and young adult women is a common observation in clinical practice. Thus, many patients undertake immediate methods of hair elimination prior to seeking medical help. Traditional methods of hair removal include shaving, waxing, tweezing, depilatory creams, and electrolysis. Recently, hair removal methods based on light technology such as lasers or intense pulsed light have been used in darker-skinned patients (282). This was reported to be a useful method when proper patient selection was employed in both darker- and lighter-skinned subjects (282–284). Both cosmetic and medical therapies need to be considered for hirsute females to minimize emotional embarrassment.

VII. MENSTRUAL DISORDERS IN ADOLESCENTS

A. Physiology of the Menstrual Cycle

Maturation of the normal ovulatory menstrual cycle requires intact development and function of the cascade of the system, including maturation of cyclic hypothalamic gonadotropin-releasing hormone secretion in the basal hypothalamus; its effect on the sequence and magnitude of gonadotropin secretion in the anterior pituitary; proper quantity and sequence of ovarian steroidogenesis, which interacts in a positive manner for induction of ovulatory cyclic changes of LH and FSH; evolving spectrum of follicle development, ovulation, and corpus luteum function; and development and cyclic changes of the endometrium in relation to the ovarian steroidogenic and follicular life cycle (Fig. 7). The entire system is regulated by a complex mechanism that integrates biophysical and biochemical information composed of interactive levels of hormonal signals, autocrine and paracrine factors, and target cell reactions (285, 286). In addition, the normal anatomy of menstrual outflow that connects the internal genital source of flow with the outside provides patency and continuity of the endocervix with the uterine cavity, vaginal canal, and orifice.

The average age of menarche in the U.S. is 12.8 years for white girls and 12.6 years for African-American girls, with a range from 9 to 16 years in the normal spectrum. Age of menarche is associated with race, nutritional status, amount of body fat, and maternal age at menarche. Menarche usually occurs 2–2.5 years after thelarche and 1 year after the growth spurt. Normal menstrual cycles vary from 21 to 45 days but remain fairly constant within a given individual. Normal flow lasts 2–7 days with an average blood flow of 30–40 ml. Ovulation may not begin until as late as 2 years after menarche (286, 287).

B. Definition of Menstrual Disorder

Primary amenorrhea is defined by the absence of menarche by age 16 years with normal pubertal development; by 2 years after completed sexual maturation; or without the onset of pubertal development by age 14 years. Secondary amenorrhea is defined by the absence of menstruation for 3 cycle lengths in the setting of oligomenorrhea, for 6 months after establishing regular menses or by 18

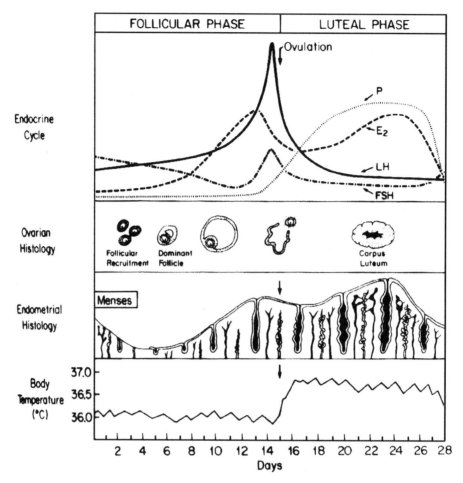

Figure 7   Normal menstrual cycle of hormonal follicular and endometrial changes. (From Carr BR and Wilson JD, Disorders of the Ovary and Female Reproductive Tract in Harrison's Principles of Internal Medicine, 11th Edition, 1987:1818–1837. Reproduced with permission from McGraw-Hill, New York, NY.)

months after menarche (285). Oligomenorrhea is defined by significantly diminished menstrual flow. Polymenorrhea, or intermenorrhea indicates a too frequent menstrual flow cycle (less than 21 days). Menorrhagia indicates excessive uterine bleeding occurring at the regular intervals of menstruation, and menometrorrhagia indicates excessive uterine bleeding occurring at regular or irregular intervals. Table 7 depicts the causes of menstrual disorders/alteration in young women with apparent normal external genitalia.

C.   Causes of Menstrual Disorders

1.   Primary Amenorrhea

Primary amenorrhea may be caused by a congenital or acquired pathology of a significant degree in the CNS–hypothalamic–pituitary–ovarian (H–P–O) axes; in the genital anatomy; as well as other systemic and/or hormonal factors affecting the H–P–O axes; and rarely but not impossibly by pregnancy. Complete absence of sec-

ondary sex characteristic development, including amenorrhea in the absence of hyperandrogenic symptoms or signs, generally signifies complete or near complete failure of either ovarian or hypothalamic–pituitary gonadotrope function of either congenital or inherited causes or causes acquired prior to adolescence. The classification of the causes of primary amenorrhea depicted in Table 7 helps to identify the pathogenic site of this disorder.

a.   Normal Anatomy of the Genital Outflow Tract. Primary ovarian failure results in a hypergonadotropic state with a greater increase in FSH than LH from peripubertal age (288). Congenital causes include gonadal dysgenesis due to an abnormal X chromosome typified by a deletion of an X chromosome during meiosis, resulting in features of classic Turner syndrome including sexual infantilism, short stature, cardiovascular defects, webbed neck, shield chest, short fourth and fifth metacarpals, increased carrying angles of arms, and other associated features. In Turner syndrome, germ cells are absent in the

Table 7 Causes of Menstrual Disorders with Apparent Female External Genitalia in Adolescent Girls

Primary amenorrhea	Secondary amenorrhea	Oligomenorrhea and menometrorrhagia

1. Primary ovarian failure (Hypergonadotropic hypogonadism):
  Congenital
    Gonadal dysgenesis (Turner syndrome/mosaicism, pure 46 XX or XY dysgenesis, other X chromosome abnormalities)
    17α-hydroxylase/17, 20 lyase deficiency
  Other congenital
    FSH receptor gene mutation
    LH receptor gene mutation
  Acquired
    Autoimmune oophoritis
    Mumps oophoritis
    Irradiation
    Chemotherapy
    Galactosemia complication
2. Gonadatropin deficiency:
  Congenital
    GnRH deficiency (Kallman syndrome)
    Hypopituitarism/empty sella syndrome
    GnRH receptor gene mutation
    Prader-Willi syndrome
    Bardet-Biedel syndrome
  Acquired
    CNS trauma
    CNS histiocystosis X
    Suprasella tumors
    Eating disorders
    Rigorous exercise
3. Genital structure abnormalities:
  Congenital in genetic females
    Agenesis of mullerian structure (Mayer-Robitansky-Kuster-Hauser syndrome)
    Agenesis of vagina
    Agenesis of cervix/endometrium
    Hymen imperforation
    Labial agglutination
  Congenital in genetic males
    Complete androgen insensitivity
    17α-hydroxylase/17, 20 lyase deficiency
  Acquired
    Uterine synechia secondary to irradiation/infection
4. Hyperandrogenic disorders:
    Stromal hyperthecosis/PCOS
    Congenital adrenal hyperplasia
    Androgen-producing tumor
5. Pregnancy
	Pregnancy
	Hypothalamic amenorrhea
	PCOS/stromal hyperthecosis
	Hyperprolactinemia
	Hypo/hyperthyroidism
	Turner mosaicism
	Other X chromosome abnormalities
	All acquired causes of hyper/hypogonadotropism
	All acquired virilizing disorders including Cushing syndrome
		Pregnancy
		PCOS
		Hyperprolactinemia
		Functional hypothalamic anovulation
		Thyroid disorder

ovary and are replaced by a fibrous streak. The variants of Turner syndrome are termed Turner mosaicism, with X-chromosome abnormalities such as 45 X/46 XX; and iso or ring X-chromosome. 46 XX/XXX abnormality is also a cause of ovarian failure (289). In subjects with Turner mosaicism, the degree of ovarian failure may be complete or partial, thus development of some secondary sex characteristics may be present despite primary amenorrhea (289). Gonadal dysgenesis is the most common cause of primary amenorrhea. Pure gonadal dysgenesis with a 46 XY karyotype (Swyer syndrome) is a rare cause of primary gonadal failure and is associated with increased risk of gondaoblastoma development from the streak gonads (290). A recent cytogenetic study of adolescent patients with primary amenorrhea revealed a pathologicical or male karyotype in 26.4% (18/68) of patients (289). Pure gonadal dysgenesis with 46 XX karyotype may result from a single gene defect or destruction of germinal tissues in utero by environmental or infectious processes (291, 292). Both genetic females and males with gonadal/adrenal combined 17-α-hydroxylase/17,20 lyase deficiencies of significant degrees are phenotypically feminized and fail to develop female secondary sex characteristics (293, 294). A characteristic clinical clue for this enzyme deficiency is hypertension; biochemical evaluation would verify elevated progesterone and deoxycorticosterone levels and decreased 17-hydroxysteroids, DHEA, other androgens and estrogen levels. Feminized genetic males with this enzyme deficiency do not have the mullerian structure.

Acquired causes of primary ovarian failure include mumps oophoritis; autoimmune oophoritis; destruction of ovarian tissue by trauma, irradiation, or chemotherapeutic complications; or by excessive accumulation of galactose-1-phosphate or deficiency of galactose-containing compounds in the ovary of patients with galactosemia (295); as well as idiopathic cause for primary amenorrhea. Depending on the age at which the disease is acquired, primary amenorrhea may or may not be associated with secondary sex characteristic development. Other rare genetic causes of hypergonadotropic primary amenorrhea include inactivating mutations of the FSH receptor gene in females with normal pubertal development, high plasma FSH level and numerous ovarian follicles (296), and inactivating mutations of the LH receptor gene in females with normal breast development (297, 298).

Gonadotropin deficiency due to a congenital or inherited disorder or acquired cause results in hypogonadotropic hypogonadism and primary amenorrhea. A cause of inherited hypogonadotropic hypogonadism is Kallman syndrome resulting from congenital deficiency of GnRH in the presence or absence of agenesis of olfactory bulbs causing anosmia. This disorder is transmitted by an X-linked gene mutation but may also be transmitted by an autosomal dominant trait (299, 300). Thus, this disorder occurs in both females and males. GnRH receptor

gene mutation has recently been characterized and results in hypogonadotropic hypogonadism and primary amenorrhea in females with normal breast development (301). Other congenital syndromes that have been reported to be associated with hypogonadotropic hypogonadism include Bardet-Biedel syndrome and Prader-Willi syndrome. Other congenital causes of hypogonadotropic hypogonadism are empty sella syndrome, which causes varying degrees of hypopituitarism and idiopathic gonadotropin-deficient hypogonadism. An acquired cause of gonadotropin deficiency causing primary amenorrhea is chronic debilitating systemic disease, which is often associated with overall delayed development of secondary sex characteristics. This delay is seen in patients with congenital hemoglobinopathy, malabsorption, human immunovirus (HIV), chronic nutritional deprivation, malnutrition, or due to eating disorders including anorexia nervosa and bulimia with or without rigorous exercise. Organic and anatomical pathologies in the hypothalamic–pituitary region, including suprasella tumors (craniopharyngioma, germinoma, teratoma, histoliocytosis, etc.); or other inflammatory processes (sarcoidosis, meningitis, tuberculosis, etc.) in the hypothalamic region; pituitary tumors, pituitary infarction or necrosis, or pituitary hemachromatosis or sarcoidosis; or trauma in the pituitary stalk or hypothalamic–pituitary axis region are well-known causes of hypopituitarism and hypogonadism.

Primary amenorrhea may be related to hyperandrogenic disorders including ovarian hyperthecosis and PCOS, CAH, Cushing syndrome, or androgen-producing tumors, as discussed earlier in this chapter. The clinical presentation of these disorders is often associated with hyperandrogenic symptoms. Excess androgens, progesterone, or cyclic production of estrone by extraglandular aromatization of excess androgens is likely to be altering the feedback loop of the H–P–O axis in these disorders. Thyroid disorders including hyper- or hypothyroidism are a cause of amenorrhea of primary and secondary natures and may be associated with estrogen-positive anovulation.

Other gonadal and endocrine disorders to be considered for primary amenorrhea include mixed gonadal dysgenesis, true hermaphroditism, and androgen resistance syndrome in genetic males with complete or near complete female phenotypic presentation. Any slight suspicion of genital ambiguity with or without signs of virilization or palpable gonadal mass in the inguinal or labial region in the female is often a clue for these causes (See Chapter 13 on Ambiguous Genitalia and Sexological Considerations). A varying degree of internal genital abnormality is associated with these causes of sexual ambiguity.

b. Anatomical Defect in the Outflow Genital Tract and Uterus. Characteristically, females with anatomical defects in the genital tract present with normal development of secondary sex characteristics and normal maturation of the H–P–O axis including ovulatory function. Due to an obstruction in the genital tract, menstrual blood accumulates behind the obstruction site. Cyclic and predicted episodes of pain in the absence of menses are a typical presentation and the patient may develop hematocolpos, hematometra, or hematoperitoneum. If undiagnosed, these disorders may lead to endometriosis, adhesion, and eventually infertility. Causes of the obstruction defect in the female tract are many and include agenesis or imperforation at various sites of the anatomy (Table 7). Agenesis of the mullerian structure (Mayer–Rokitansky–Hauser syndrome) is the second most common cause of primary amenorrhea and results in the absence of the vagina and aplasia or hypoplasia of the uterus, such as rudimentary bicornuate cords (302). This syndrome occurs in 1:4000–5000 girls. Renal abnormalities occur in 30–40% of subjects with this syndrome (303) and spinal abnormality has also been reported. Defects in the fusion of the mullerian structure caudally or with the urogenital sinus results in abnormal development of the uterus or uterine septum and failure to discharge outflow. Agenesis of the vagina or cervix, transverse vaginal septum or imperforate hymen, idiopathic labial fusion, and adhesion or secondary labial agglutination are known causes of menstrual outflow obstruction. Endometrial hypoplasia or aplasia is a rare cause of primary amenorrhea.

2. Secondary Amenorrhea

Secondary amenorrhea in otherwise sexually healthy adolescents and young women warrants pregnancy testing. Secondary amenorrhea in patients with hyperandrogenic disorders including PCOS, ovarian hyperthecosis, adrenal causes of excess androgen-producing pathology, hyperprolactinemia, and thyroid disorders were discussed in the previous section. Almost all known causes of hypergonadotropic hypogonadism including Turner mosaicism and other X-chromosome abnormalities and all acquired causes of primary amenorrhea are also causes of secondary amenorrhea. Acquired causes of hypogonadotropic hypogonadism of primary amenorrhea are also causes of secondary amenorrhea. Hypothalamic amenorrhea represents a spectrum of disordered GnRH secretion that can vary over time, from apulsatile to low frequency/amplitude to low amplitude with normal frequency of LH pulses, low frequency and normal amplitude, and normal amplitude and frequency of LH pulses (304). The causes of hypothalamic amenorrhea may be psychological in nature, related to stress, weight loss, eating disorders such as anorexia nervosa and bulimia nervosa (305, 306), chronic, high-intensity physical exercises (307), or idiopathic. The diagnosis of hypothalamic amenorrhea is made by exclusion of other probable causes and normal imaging studies of the hypothalamic–pituitary anatomy.

3. Oligomenorrhea and Menometrarrhagia

Both decreased and increased menstrual volume with regular or irregular cycles may be caused by pregnancy complications or by all of the known causes of endocrine abnormalities for secondary amenorrhea including PCOS, hyperprolactinemia, thyroid disorder, Cushing syndrome, and functional hypothalamic anovulation. Additional causes of menometrorrhagia in adolescent females include bleeding disorders and complications of the genital tract such as trauma, dysplasia, polyps, foreign bodies, and infection.

D. Evaluation of Menstrual Disorder

In all adolescents with menstrual disorders, a detailed history with regard to growth and secondary sex characteristic maturation is helpful in identifying the cause of the abnormality. Careful history of age at thelarche, pubarche, and menarche, menstrual history, flow of menses, presence or absence of excessive weight gain during peripubertal age, dysmenorrhea, cyclic pelvic pain, cyclic breast changes, and the presence or absence of hirsutism/acne are helpful in determining the likely cause of the menstrual disorder. Histories with regard to nutrition, physical training, sexual activity, weight change, dieting, body image, and emotional and family dynamics are also essential in evaluating the patient with primary or secondary amenorrhea or oligomenorrhea. Childhood history of illness, chronic disease, or therapies (chemotherapy/radiation therapy) may determine the causative factor. History-taking should also include vasomotor symptoms (hot flashes), virilizing signs, galactorrhea, symptoms of hypothyroidism, hyperthyroidism, and CNS symptoms including headache, hearing changes, and mood changes. Family history including maternal menstrual history, primary or secondary amenorrhea history in siblings or relatives, and hyperandrogenic history are also useful. Focus on physical examination pertinent to menstrual disorders includes anthropometric data, vital signs, androgen excess, Turner stigmata, acanthosis nigricans in the skin, thyroid gland, sexual maturation stage, breast discharge, presence or absence of sexual hair and genital ambiguity, pelvic mass or fullness in the patient with primary amenorrhea, and a careful gynecological patency examination in those with normal pubertal development despite primary amenorrhea. A guideline for a logical and stepwise approach for evaluation of primary amenorrhea, secondary amenorrhea, oligomenorrhea, and menometrorrhagia is provided in Figure 8.

Excluding those with obvious hyperandrogenic manifestation and sexual ambiguity, the first work-up for both primary and secondary amenorrhea is random gonadotropin level measurements. Those with unquestionably elevated FSH and LH levels have primary ovarian failure (>20 miu/ml). A karyotype study would differentiate gonadal dysgenesis from other causes of primary ovarian failure. A positive antiovarian antibody study with established specificity and sensitivity indicates autoimmune, oophoritis while a negative antiovarian antibody finding cannot rule out the autoimmune disorder unequivocally.

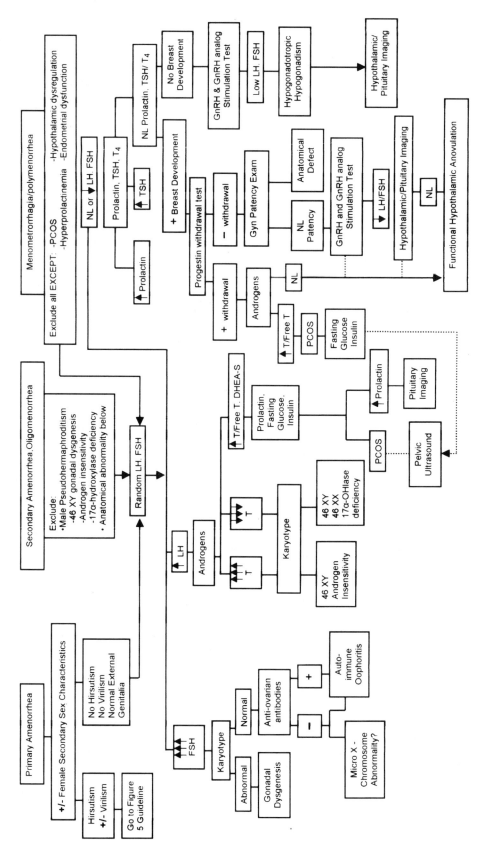

Figure 8 Guideline for evaluation of menstrual disorders. NL, normal; T, testosterone.

Patients with apparently normal karyotypes and a negative antiovarian antibody may have a micro X-chromosome abnormality that cannot be detected by the karyotype study. In amenorrheic patients with mildly elevated LH levels (>10–<20 miu/ml) with normal or low FSH levels (5–10 miu/ml), a serum androgen level study helps to differentiate between those with androgen insensitivity syndrome in genetic males, gonadal/adrenal 17α-hydroxylase/17,20 lyase deficiency in genetic females and males, and PCOS and hyperprolactinemia. Mildly elevated or normal androgen levels would require a serum prolactin level study. Patients with elevated prolactin levels require a further imaging study of the pituitary to look for prolactin-secreting pituitary adenoma. Those with a normal prolactin level are suspected to have PCOS and will need an additional study of fasting glucose and insulin levels to determine insulin resistance. Pelvic ultrasound study may be required to identify imaging of the ovaries compatible with PCOS.

Amenorrheic patients with normal or low random levels of LH and FSH (<10 miu/ml) require prolactin and thyroid function studies to exclude or identify these hormonal disorders as the cause. In patients with normal prolactin and thyroid function, and normal breast development, a careful examination of the genital tract and progestin withdrawal test are necessary. For those with a positive withdrawal response to progestin administration (ie, Provera 5–10 mg orally per day for 5 days), serum androgen level determination helps to differentiate between PCOS and hypothalamic amenorrhea. For those with no withdrawal response to progestin administration, a gynecological examination for genital patency is mandatory in patients with primary amenorrhea. Those with patency of the genital outflow tract require investigation of hypogonadotropic hypogonadism by a GnRH or GnRH analog stimulation test. An imaging examination of the hypothalamic and pituitary region is necessary to exclude an organic cause of hypogonadotropic hypogonadism or hypothalamic amenorrhea. In patients with absent or delayed development of secondary sex characteristics, normal or low random LH and FSH levels, and normal prolactin and thyroid function, hypogonadotropic hypogonadism evaluation is necessary by GnRH or GnRH analog stimulation test. A pituitary imaging study is needed to rule out an organic cause of hypogonadotropism (tumor, empty sella).

E. Medical Treatment of Menstrual Disorders

Table 8 summarizes medical therapy methods commonly used in clinical practice or reported for various menstrual disorders in adolescent girls and young women. Delayed puberty and primary amenorrhea irrespective of primary or central hypogonadism requires incremental estrogen hormone replacement therapy at the appropriate pubertal onset age (≈10–11 years) for the development of secondary sex characteristics. The most commonly used estrogen compound is the natural conjugated estrogen, Premarin, for 1.5–2 years. For menstrual cycle regulation, combined estrogen and progestagen replacement therapy using cyclic Premarin followed by combined Premarin and progestin compound or a low-dose or triphasic COC may be used. Tolerance and efficacy of the cyclic hormone replacement therapy need to be monitored. Providing information to the patient on potential side effects of COC is a prudent measure. Poly- or intermenorrhea is generally treated with cyclic hormonal therapy, as in cases of amenorrhea (308, 309).

Ovulatory menorrhagia may be treated with pharmacological agents that reduce the volume of blood loss during the normal menstrual cycle including tranexahic acids, nonsteroidal anti-inflammatory drugs, cyclic progestin (Norethindrone, Provera, progestin-releasing intrauterine device [IUD]), and Danagel (Table 8). Dysmenorrhea with or without menorrhagia is generally treated with tranexahic acid in countries outside the US and nonsteroidal anti-inflammatory agents as listed in Table 8 (308, 310–312, 315). Any heavy bleeding of a moderate degree is generally treated with a low-dose COC 1/35 every 6–12 hours for 1–2 days with a gradual decrease to 1 pill per day in 5 days (308, 314) followed by cyclic COC therapy. Severe bleeding requires COC 1/50 every 6 h, as in the case of a moderate degree of bleeding if oral treatment is well tolerated. However, hospital admission may be necessary for parenteral administration of conjugated equine estrogen 25 mg every 4 h IV until bleeding stops. Surgical intervention is needed if medicinal therapy is not effective in cessation of severe abnormal uterine bleeding. An iron supplement is also necessary in the patient whose serum hemoglobin is below 12 gm %.

The treatment of menstrual disorders related to PCOS was described in the previous section and in Table 6. With the exception of primary ovarian failure or permanent hypogonadotropic hypogonadism, medical or hormonal replacement therapy may be offered for 6 months or so, with a re-evaluation of menstrual function thereafter. Hypothalamic amenorrhea needs to be dealt with in light of causative factors such as eating disorders, excessive physical exercise, or emotional causes and would require multidisciplinary care including counseling, nutritional help, and hormone replacement therapy if necessary. All other specific organic causes would require treatment for both the underlying organic disease and necessary hormone replacement therapy. For the simple and transient anovulatory cycle, reassurance and follow-up of patients are needed and COC therapy for a short-term period (6 months) may be useful in cases with oligomenorrhea or menometrorrhagia.

ACKNOWLEDGMENTS

The author's recent work described in this chapter was supported by a USPHS grant R01 HD 36399 and by a

Table 8 Medical Therapy Methods Reported/Used for Menstrual Disorders in Adolescent Females

Amenorrhea		Dysfunctional bleeding				PCOS (amenorrhea, oligomenorrhea, polymenorrhea)	
Hypergonadotropic	Hypogonadotropic	Polymenorrhea/ intermenorrhea	Ovulatory menorrhagia	Dysmenorrhea/ovulatory menorrhagia	Acute heavy bleeding	+ Insulin resistance	− Insulin resistance
	For development of secondary sex characteristics	For menstrual cycle regulation	For reduction in volume	For reduction in pain and volume	For moderate bleeding	For cycle recovery	For cycle regulation
	Incremental increase of premarin 0.3 mg to 0.625 mg po qd × 1.5–2 years	Same as amenorrhea	Tranexahic acid 1 gm q 6 h for cycle 1–4 days	Nonsteroidal anti-inflammatory drug:	COC 1/35 q 6–12 h and decrease to 1 dose per day in 5 days. Begin new COC cycle	Insulin sensitizing agents (see Table 6)	Low-dose COC
	For menstrual cycle regulation		Nonsteroidal anti-inflammatory drug	Ibuprofen 600–1200 mg/d in 4 divided doses			Triphasic COC
	Combined cyclic estrogen/progestin		Cyclic progestin	Naproxen 250–500 mg q 6–12 h	For severe bleeding		Combined COC and GnRH analog (see Table 6)
	0.625 mg Premarin days 1–25 and Provera 5–10 mg/d days 16–25		Norethidrone × 10 days/luteal cycle	Mefenamic acid, 250–500 mg q 6–12 h	COC 1/50 q 6 h if tolerating as above		
	low-dose COC 1/35		Provera				
	triphasic COC		Progestin-releasing IUD		Conjugated equine estrogen 25 mg IV q 4 h		
	For ovulatory cycle induction		Donagel				
	Pulsatile GnRH or GnRH analog in only LHRH deficiency						
	(Author's experience, 309)	(308, 309)	(308, 310–312, 315)	(308, 313)	(308, 314)		

USPHS GCRC grant to the University of Illinois at Chicago, College of Medicine. The author is also extremely grateful to Dr. Fuad Ziai in the Department of Pediatric Endocrinology at the University of Illinois and Hope Children's Hospital for his invaluable help and assistance in preparation of this chapter.

REFERENCES

1. Ebling FJG. Hair follicles and associated glands as androgen targets in androgen metabolism in hirsute and normal females. In: Horton R, Lobo RA, eds. Clinics in Endocrinology and Metabolism. Philadelphia: WB Saunders, 1986:319–339.
2. Shuster S. The sebaceous glands and primary cutaneous virilism. In: Jeffcotes SL, ed. Androgens and Anti-androgen Therapy. Chichester: John Wiley & Sons, 1982:1–21.
3. Goebelsman U, Lobo RA. Androgen excess. In: Mischell DR, Davajan V, eds. Infertility, Contraception, and Reproductive Endocrinology. Oradell, NJ: Medical Economics, 1987:303–317.
4. Gower DB, Fotherby K. Biosynthesis of the androgens and oestrogens. In: Makin HLJ, ed. Biochemistry of Steroid Hormones. London: Blackwell Scientific Publications, 1975:77–104.
5. Sommerville IF, Collins WP. Indices of androgen production in women. In: Briggs MH, ed. Advances in Steroid Biochemistry and Pharmacology. New York: Academic Press, 1970:267–307.
6. Longcope C. Adrenal and gonadal androgen secretion in normal females. In: Horton R, Lobo RA, eds. Clinics in Endocrinology and Metabolism. Philadelphia: WB Saunders, 1986:213–228.
7. Pang S, Levine LS, Legido A, New MI. Adrenal androgen response to metyrapone, ACTH and corticotropin releasing factor (CRF) stimulation in children with hypopituitarism. J Clin Endocrinol Metab 1987; 64:282–284.
8. Jones T, Griffith K. Ultramicrochemical studies on the sites of formation of dehydroepiandrosterone sulfate in the adrenal cortex of the guinea pig. J Endocrinol 1968; 42:559–565.
9. McKerns KW. Steroidogenesis and metabolism in the adrenal cortex. In: Steroid Hormones and Metabolism. New York: Appleton-Century-Croft, 1969:9–30.
10. Korth-Schutz S, Levine, LS, New MI. Serum androgens in normal, prepubertal and pubertal children and in children with precocious adrenarche. J Clin Endocrinol Metab 1976; 42:117–124.
11. Parker LN, Odell WD. Control of adrenal androgen secretion. Adrenal Androgens. New York: Raven Press, 1978:27–42.
12. Zumoff BB, Walsh T, Katz JL, Levin J, Rosenfield RS, Kream J, Weimer H. Subnormal plasma dehydroxyandrosterone to cortisol ratio in anorexia nervosa: a second hormonal parameter of ontogenic regression. J Clin Endocrinol Metab 1983; 56:668–672.
13. Cutler GB, Davis SE, Johnsonbaugh RE, Louriaux DL. Dissociation of cortisol and adrenal androgen secretion in patients with secondary adrenal insufficiency. J Clin Endocrinol Metab 1979; 49:604–609.
14. Hagag P, Hetzianu I, Ben-Shlomo A, Weiss M. Androgen suppression and clinical improvement with dopamine agonists in hyperandrogenic–hyperprolactinemia women. J Reprod Med 2001; 46:678–684.
15. Vermeulen A, Ando S. Prolactin and adrenal androgen secretion. Clin Endocrinol (Oxf) 1978; 8:295–303.
16. Azziz R, Rittmaster RS, Fox LM, Bradley EL Jr, Potter HD, Boots LR. Role of the ovary in the adrenal androgen excess of hyperandrogenic women. Fertil Steril 1998; 69:851–859.
17. Escobar-Morreale HF, Serrano-Gotarredona J, Garcia-Robles R, Varela C, Sancho JM. Abnormalities in the serum insulin-like growth factor-1 axis in women with hyperandrogenism. Fertil Steril 1998; 70:1090–1100.
18. Alesci S, Bornstein SR. Neuroimmunoregulation of androgens in the adrenal gland and the skin. Horm Res 2000; 54:281–286.
19. Ehrhart-Bornstein M, Hinson JP, Bornstein SR, Scherbaum WA, Vinson GP. Intra-adrenal interactions in the regulation of adrenocortical steroidogenesis. Endocr Rev 1998; 19:101–143.
20. Bornstein SR, Ehrhart-Bornstein M, Usadel H, Bockmann M, Scherbaum WA. Morphological evidence for a close interaction of chromaffin cells with cortical cells within the adrenal gland. Cell Tissue Res 1991; 265:1–9.
21. Suda T, Tomori N, Tozawa F, Demura H, Shizume K, Mouri T, Mirura Y, Sasano N. Immunoreactive corticotropin and corticotropin-releasing factor in human hypothalamus, adrenal, lung cancer and pheochromocytoma. J Clin Endocrinol Metab 1984; 58:919–924.
22. Rosenfeld RS, Hellman H, Roffwarg H, Weitzman ED, Fukushima DK, Gallagher TF. Dehydroisoandrosterone is secreted episodically and synchronously with cortisol by normal men. J Clin Endocrinol Metab 1971; 33:87–92.
23. Pang S, Lerner A, Stoner E, Oberfield S, Engle I, New MI. Late-onset adrenal steroid 3β-hydroxysteroid dehydrogenase deficiency: a cause of hirsutism in pubertal and post pubertal women. J Clin Endocrinol Metab 1985; 60:428–439.
24. DeJong FH, Van Der Molen HJ. Determination of dehydroepiandrosterone and dehydroepiandrosterone-sulfate in human plasma using electron capture detection of 4-androstene-3,6,-17-trione after gas liquid chromatography. J Endocrinol 1972; 53:461–474.
25. James VHT, Goodal AM. Androgen production in women. In: Jeffcoate SL, ed. Androgens and Anti-androgen Therapy. Chichester: John Wiley & Sons, 1982:23–40.
26. Jeffcoate SL, Brookes RV, Lemi NY, London DR, Prienty FFG, Spathes GS. Androgen production in hypogonadal men. J Endocrinol 1967; 37:401–411.
27. Bardin CW, Lipsett MB. Testosterone and androstenedione blood production rates in normal women and women with idiopathic hirsutism or polycystic ovaries. J Clin Invest 1967; 46:891–902.
28. Horton E, Tait JF. Androstenedione production and interconversion rates measured in peripheral blood and studies on the possible sites of its conversion to testosterone. J Clin Invest 1966; 45:301–313.
29. Lloyd CW, Lobotsky J, Baird DT, McCracken JA, Weisz J, Pupkin M, Zanartu J, Puga J. Concentration of unconjugated estrogens, androgens and gestagens in ovarian and peripheral venous plasma of women: the normal menstrual cycle. N Engl J Med 1971; 32:155–166.
30. Nieschlag E, Loriaux DL, Ruder HJ, Zucker IR, Kirschner MA, Lipsett MB. The secretion of dehydroepiandrosterone and DHEA-S in man. J Endocrinol 1973; 57:123–134.
31. Vande Wiele R, McDonald P, Gurpide E, Lieberman S.

Studies on the secretion and interconversion of the androgens. Rec Prog Horm Res 1963; 19:275–310.

32. Fritz MA, Speroff L. The endocrinology of the menstrual cycle; the interaction of folliculogenesis and neuroendocrine mechanisms. Fertil Steril 1982; 38:509–529.

33. McNatty KP, Makris A, Degrazia C, Osathanondh R, Ryan KJ. Production of progesterone, androgens and estrogens by granulosa cells, thecal tissue and stromal tissue from human ovaries in vitro. J Clin Endocrinol Metab 1979; 49:687–700.

34. Rice BF, Hammerstein J, Savard K. Steroid hormone formation in the human ovary: androstenedione, progesterone and estradiol during the human menstrual cycle. Am J Ob/Gyn 1974; 119:1026–1032.

35. Brooks RV. Androgens: physiology, and pathology In: Makin HLJ, ed. Biochemistry of Steroid Hormones. Oxford: Blackwell Scientific, 1975:289–311.

36. Judd HL, Yen SSC. Serum androstenedione and testosterone levels during the menstrual cycle. J Clin Endocrinol Metab 1973; 36:475–481.

37. Abraham GE. Ovarian and adrenal contribution to peripubertal androgens during the menstrual cycle. J Clin Endocrinol Metab 1974; 39:340–346.

38. Aedo AR, Pederson PH, Pederson SC, Diczfalusy E. Ovarian steroid secretion in normally menstruating women, 1, the contribution of the developing follicles. Acta Endocrinol 1980; 95:212–221.

39. Sakkal-Alkaddour H, Suriano MJ, Riddick L, Chang YT, Ziai F, Pang S. The effect of three menstrual cycle phases on adrenal hormonal dynamics and etiologies of hirsutism in five ethnic/racial female populations. Clin Pediatr Endocrinol 1998; 7:23–34.

40. Judd HL, Judd GE, Lucas WE, Yen SSC. Endocrine function of the post menopausal ovary: concentration of androgens and estrogens in ovarian and peripheral vein blood. J Clin Endocrinol Metab 1974; 39:1020–1024.

41. Franks S, Gilling-Smith C, Watson H, Willis D. Insulin action in the normal and polycystic ovary. Endocrinol Metab Clin North Am 1999; 28:367–378.

42. Goudas VT, Dumesic DA. Polycystic ovary syndrome. Endocrinol Metab Clin North Am 1997; 26:893–912.

43. Cumming DC, Wall SR. Non-sex hormone binding globulin-bound testosterone as a marker for hyperandrogenism. J Clin Endocrinol Metab 1985; 61:873–876.

44. Vermeulen A. The physical state of testosterone in plasma. In: James VHT, Seria MS, Martini L, eds. The Endocrine Function of the Human Testis. New York: Academic Press, 1973:157–170.

45. Burke CW, Anderson DC. Sex-hormone-binding-globulin is an oestrogen amplifier. Nature 1972; 240:38–40.

46. Pentti K, Niklas HS. Changing concepts of active androgens in blood. In: Horton R, Lobo RA, eds. Clinics in Endocrinology and Metabolism. Philadelphia: WB Saunders, 1986:247–258.

47. Rosenfield RL, Maudelonde T, Moll GW. Biologic effects of hyperandrogenism in polycystic ovary syndrome. Semin Reprod Endocrinol 1984; 2:281–295.

48. Kligman AM. The human hair cycle. J Invest Dermtol 1959; 33:307–316.

49. Paus R. Principles of hair cycle control. J Dermatol 1998; 25:793–802.

50. Rosenfield RL. Pilosebaceous physiology in relation to hirsutism and acne. In: Horton R, Lobo RA, eds. Clinics in Endocrinology and Metabolism. Philadelphia: WB Saunders, 1986:341–362.

51. Peereboom-Wynia JDR, Beck CH. The influence of cyproterone-acetate orally on the hair root state in women with idiopathic hirsutism. Arch Dermatol Res 1977; 260:137–142.

52. Jankovic SM, Jankovic SV. The control of hair growth. Dermatol Online J 1998; 4:2.

53. Ebling FJ, Cooke ID, Randall VA, et al. Einfluss Von cyproteronacetat auf die aktivitat der haarfouikel und talgdrüsen beim menschen. In: Hammerstein J, Lachnit-Fixon U, Neumann F, Plewig G, eds. Androgenisierungser Schlinungen bei der Frau. Amsterdam: Excerpta Medica, 1979:243–249.

54. Ebling FJG, Randall VA, Sawers RS. Interrelationship between body hair growth, sebum excretion and endocrine parameters. Prostate 1984; 5:347–348.

55. Fang S, Andersen KM, Liao S. Receptor proteins for androgens; on the role of specific proteins in the retention of 17β-hydroxy-5α-androstan-3-one by the rat ventral prostate in vivo and in vitro. J Biol Chem 1969; 244:6584–6595.

56. Hay JB, Hodgins MB. Distribution of androgen metabolizing enzymes in isolated tissues of human forehead and axillary skin. J Endocrinol 1978; 79:29–39.

57. Thiboutot D, Bayne E, Thorne J, Gilliland K, Flanagan J, Shao Q, Light J, Helm K. Immunolocalization of 5alpha-reductase isoenzymes in acne lesions and normal skin. Arch Dermatol 2000; 136:1125–1129.

58. Mauvais-Jarvi P, Kutten F, Mowszowicz I. Androgen metabolism in human skin: importance of dihydrotestosterone formation in normal and abnormal target cells. In: Molinatti GM, Martini L, James VHT, eds. Androgenization in Women. New York: Raven Press, 1983:47.

59. Toscano V, Petrangeli E, Admo MV, Foli S, Caiola S, Sciarra F. Simultaneous determination of 5α-reduced metabolites of testosterone in human plasma. J Steroid Biochem 1981; 14:572–574.

60. Moghissi E, Ablan F, Horton R. Origin of plasma androstanediol glucuronide in men. J Clin Endocrinol Metab 1984; 59:417–421.

61. Morimoto I, Edmiston A, Hawks D, Horton R. Studies on the origin of androstanediol and androstanediol glucuronide in young and elderly men. J Clin Endocrinol Metab 1981; 52:772–778.

62. Deslyper JP, Sayed A, Punjabi U, Verdonck L, Vermeulen A. Plasma 5α-androstane-3α, 17β-diol and urinary 5α-androstane-3α, 17β-diol glucuronide, parameters of peripheral androgen action: a comparative study. J Clin Endocrinol Metab 1982; 54:386–391.

63. Horton R, Hawks D, Lobo RA. 3α, 17β-androstancdiol glucuronide in plasma. J Clin Invest 1982; 69:1203–1206.

64. Lobo RA, Goebelsmann U, Horton R. Evidence for the importance of peripheral tissue events in the development of hirsutism in polycystic ovary syndrome. J Clin Endocrinol Metab 1983; 57:393–397.

65. Pang S, Wang M, Jeffries S, Riddick L, Clark A, Estrada E. Normal and elevated 3α-androstanediol glucuronide concentrations in women with various causes of hirsutism and its correlation with degree of hirsutism and androgen levels. J Clin Endocrinol Metab 1992; 75:243–248.

66. Hock DL, Seifer DB. New treatments of hyperandrogenism and hirsutism. Obstet Gynecol Clin North Am 2000; 27:567–581.

67. Mowszowicz I, Melinatou E, Doukane A, et al. Androgen binding capacity and 5α-reductase activity in pubic skin

fibroblast from hirsute patients. J Clin Endocrinol Metab 1983; 56:1209–1213.

68. Kuttenn F, Mowszowicz I, Schaison G, Mauvais-Jarvis P. Androgen production and skin metabolism in hirsutism. J Endocrinol 1977; 75:83–91.

69. Thomas JP, Oake RJ. Androgen metabolism in the skin of hirsute women. J Clin Endocrinol Metab 1974; 38:19–122.

70. Glickman SP, Rosenfield RL. Androgen metabolism by isolated hairs from women with idiopathic hirsutism is usually normal. J Invest Dermatol 1984; 82:62–66.

71. Mauvais-Jarvis P, Kuttenn F, Gauthier-Wright F. Testosterone 5α-reductase in human skin as an index of androgenicity. In: James VHT, Serio M, Giusti G, eds. The Endocrine Function of the Human Ovary. London: Academic Press, 1976:481–494.

72. Cruikshak DD, Chapler FK, Yannone ME. Differential adrenal and ovarian suppression. Obs/Gyn 1971; 38:724–733.

73. Abraham GE, Manlimos FS. The role of the adrenal cortex in hirsutism. In: James VHT, Serio M, Giusti G, Martini L, eds. The Endocrine Function of the Human Adrenal Cortex. London: Academic Press, 1976:325–355.

74. Kirshner A, Jacobs J. Combined ovarian and adrenal vein catheterization to determine the site(s) of androgen overproduction in hirsute women. J Clin Endocrinol Metab 1971; 33:199–209.

75. Stahl NL, Teeslink CR, Greenblatt RB. Ovarian adrenal and peripheral testosterone levels in the polycystic ovary syndrome. Am J Obstet Gynecol 1973; 117:194–200.

76. Moltz L, Schwartz U. Gonadal and adrenal androgen secretion in hirsute females. In: Horton R, Lobo RA, eds. Clinics in Endocrinology and Metabolism. Philadelphia: WB Saunders, 1986:229–245.

77. Pang S. Congenital adrenal hyperplasia. In: Rosenfield RL, ed. Bailliere's Clinical Obstetrics and Gynaecology: Hyperandrogenic States and Hirsutism. London: Bailliere Tindall, 1997:281–306.

78. Newmark S, Dluhy RG, Williams GH, Pochi P, Rose LI. Partial 11-β and 21-hydroxylase deficiencies in hirsute women. Am J Obstet Gynecol 1977; 127:594–598.

79. Brooks RV, Mattingly D, Mills IH, Prunty FIG. Postpubertal adrenal virilism with biochemical disturbance of the congenital type of adrenal hyperplasia. Br Med J 1960; 1:1294–1298.

80. Kohn B, Levine LS, Pollack MS, Pang S, Lorenzen F, Levy D, Lerner A, Rondanini GF, Dupont B, New MI. Late-onset steroid 21-hydroxylase deficiency: a variant of classical congenital adrenal hyperplasia. J Clin Endocrinol Metab 1982; 55:817–827.

81. DeWailly D, Vantyghem-Haudiquet MC, Sainsard C, Buvat J, Capoen JP, Ardaens K, Racadot A, Lefebvre J, Fossati P. Clinical and biological phenotypes in late-onset 21-hydroxylase deficiency. J Clin Endocrinol Metab 1986; 63:418–423.

82. Kutten F, Couillin P, Girard F, Billaud L, Vincens M, Boucekkine C, Thalabard JC, Mandelonde T, Spritzer P, Mowszowicz I, Boue A, Mauvais-Jarvis P. Late-onset adrenal hyperplasia in hirsutism. N Engl J Med 1985; 313:224–231.

83. Moran C, Azziz R, Carmina E, Dewailly D, Fruzzetti F, Ibanez L, Knochenhauer ES, Marcondes JA, Mendonca BB, Pingatelli D, Pugeat M, Rohmer V, Speiser PW, Witchel SF. 21-hydroxylase deficient nonclassic adrenal hyperplasia is a progressive disorder: a multicenter study. Am J Obstet Gynecol 2000; 183:1468–1474.

84. Speiser PW, Knochenhauer ES, Dewailly D, Fruzzetti F, Marcondes JA, Azziz R. A multicenter study of women with nonclassical congenital adrenal hyperplasia: relationship between genotype and phenotype. Mol Genet Metab 2000; 71:527–534.

85. Child DF, Builock DE, Anderson DC. Adrenal steroidogenesis in hirsute women. Clin Endocrinol 1980; 12:595–601.

86. Pollack MS, Levine LS, O'Neill GJ, Pang S, Lorenzen F, Kohn B, Rondanini GF, Chiumello G, New MI, Dupont B. HLA linkage and B14,DR1,BfS haplotype association with the genes for late-onset and cryptic 21-hydroxylase deficiency. Am J Hum Genet 1981; 33:540–550.

87. Speiser PW, Dupont B, Rubinstein P, Piazza A, Kastelan A, New MI. High frequency of non-classical steroid 21-hydroxylase deficiency. Am J Hum Genet 1985; 37:650–667.

88. Laron Z, Pollack MS, Zamir R, Roitman A, Dickerman Z, Levine LS, Lorenzen F, O'Neill GJ, Pang S, New MI, Dupont B. Late-onset 21-hydroxylase deficiency and HLA in the Ashkenazi population: new allele at the 21-hydroxylase locus. Human Immunol 1980; 1:55–56.

89. Speiser PW, New MI, White PC. Molecular genetic analysis of non-classic steroid 21-hydroxylase deficiency associated with HLA-B14,DR1. N Engl J Med 1988; 319:19–23.

90. Garlepp MJ, Wilton AN, Dawkins RL, White PC. Rearrangement of 21-hydroxylase gene in disease associated MHC supratypes. Immunogenetics 1986; 23:100–105.

91. Helmberg A, Tusie-Luna MT, Tabarelli M, Kofler R, White PC. R339H and P453S: CYP21 mutations associated with nonclassic steroid 21-hydroxylase deficiency that are not apparent gene conversions. Mol Endocrinol 1992; 6:1318–1322.

92. Higashi Y, Tanae A, Inoue H, Hiromasa T, Fuji-Kuriyama Y. Aberrant splicing and missense mutations cause steroid 21-hydroxylase [P-450(C21)] deficiency in humans: possible gene conversion products. Proc Natl Acad Sci USA 1988; 85:7486–7490.

93. Owerbach D, Sherman L, Ballard AL, Azziz R. Pro 453 to Ser mutation in CYP21 is associated with nonclassic steroid 21-hydroxylase deficiency. Mol Endocrinol 1992; 6:1211–1215.

94. Speiser PW, New MI, White PC. Molecular genetic analysis of nonclassic steroid 21-hydroxylase deficiency associated with HLA-B14,DR1. N Engl J Med 1988; 319:19–23.

95. Wu DA, Chung B. Mutations of P450c21 at Cys[428], Val[281], or Ser[268] result in complete, partial, or no loss of enzymatic activity. J Clin Invest 1991; 88:519–523.

96. White PC, New MI. Genetic basis of endocrine disease 2: congenital adrenal hyperplasia due to 21-hydroxylase deficiency. J Clin Endocrinol Metab 1992; 74:6–11.

97. Azziz R, Zacur HA. 21-Hydroxylase deficiency in female hyperandrogenism: screening and diagnosis. J Clin Endocrinol Metab 1989; 69:577–584

98. Eldar-Geva T, Hurwitz A, Vecsei P, Palti Z, Milwidsky A, Rosler A. Secondary biosynthetic defects in women with late-onset congenital adrenal hyperplasia. N Engl J Med 1990; 323:855–863.

99. Temeck JW, Pang S, Nelson C, New MI. Genetic defects of steroidogenesis in premature adrenarche. J Clin Endocrinol Metab 1987; 64:609–617.

100. Romaguera J, Moran C, Diaz-Montes TP, Hines GA, Cruz RI, Azziz R. Prevalence of 21-hydroxylase deficient non-

classic adrenal hyperplasia and insulin resistance among hirsute women from Puerto Rico. Fertil Steril 2000; 74: 59–62.

101. Siegel S, Finegold DN, Lanes R, Lee PA. ACTH stimulation tests and plasma dehydroepiandrosterone sulfate levels in women with hirsutism. N Engl J Med 1990; 323: 849–854.

102. Killeen AA, Hanson NQ, Eklund R, Cairl CJ, Eckfeldt JH. Prevalence of nonclassical congenital adrenal hyperplasia among women self-referred for electrolytic treatment of hirsutism. Am J Med Genet 1992; 42:197–200.

103. Arnaout MA. Late-onset congenital adrenal hyperplasia in women with hirsutism. Eur J Clin Invest 1992; 22: 651–658.

104. Hawkins LA, Chasalow FI, Blethen SL. The role of adrenocorticotropin testing in evaluating girls with premature adrenarche and hirsutism/oligomenorrhea. J Clin Endocrinol Metab 1992; 74:248–253.

105. Azziz R, Dewailly D, Owerbach D. Nonclassic adrenal hyperplasia: Current concepts. J Clin Endocrinol Metab 1994; 78:810–815.

106. Bongiovanni AM. Unusual steroid pattern in congenital adrenal hyperplasia: deficiency of 3β-hydroxysteroid dehydrogenase. J Clin Endocrinol Metab 1961; 21:860–862.

107. Pang S, Levine LS, Stoner E, Opitz JM, New MI. Non-salt-losing congenital adrenal hyperplasia due to 3β-hydroxysteroid dehydrogenase deficiency with normal glomerulosa function. J. Clin Endocrinol Metab 1983; 56: 808–818.

108. Chang YT, Kulin HE, Garibaldi L, Suriano MJ, Bracki K, Pang S. Hypothalamic-pituitary-gonadal axis function in pubertal male and female siblings with glucocorticoid treated nonsalt-wasting 3β-hydroxysteroid dehydrogenase deficiency congenital adrenal hyperplasia. J Clin Endocrinol Metab 1993; 77:1251–1257.

109. Rosenfield RL, Rich BH, Wolfsdorf JI, Cassorla F, Parks JS, Bongiovanni AM, Wu CH, Shackleton CHL. Pubertal presentation of congenital Δ5-3β-hydroxysteroid dehydrogenase deficiency. J Clin Endocrinol Metab 1980; 51: 345–353.

110. Axelrod LR, Goldzieher JW, Ross SD. Concurrent 3β-hydroxysteroid dehydrogenase deficiency in adrenal and sclerocystic ovary. Acta Endocrinol 1965; 48:392–412.

111. Bongiovanni AM. Acquired adrenal hyperplasia: with special reference to 3β-hydroxysteroid dehydrogenase. Fertil Steril 1981; 35:599–608.

112. Lobo RA, Goebelsman U. Evidence for reduced 3β-ol-hydroxysteroid dehydrogenase activity in some hirsute women thought to have polycystic ovary syndrome. J Clin Endocrinol Metab 1981; 53:394–400.

113. Pang S. Congenital adrenal hyperplasia owing to 3β-hydroxysteroid dehydrogenase deficiency. Endocrinol Metab Clin North Am 2001; 30:81–99.

114. Chang YT, Zhang L, Mason I, Murry B, Wang J, Lin K, Garibaldi LR, Bourdney C, Pang S. Redefining hormonal criteria for mild 3β-hydroxysteroid dehydrogenase (3β-HSD) deficiency (def) congenital adrenal hyperplasia (CAH) by molecular analysis of the type II 3β-HSD gene. Pediatr Res 1994; 35:96A.

115. Sakkal-Alkaddour H, Zhang L, Yang X, et al. Studies of 3β-hydroxysteroid dehydrogenase genes in infants and children manifesting premature pubarche and increased ACTH stimulated Δ5 steroid levels. J Clin Endocrinol Metab 1996; 81:3961–3965.

116. Zerah M, Rheaume E, Mani P, et al. No evidence of mutations in the genes for type I and type II 3β-hydroxysteroid dehydrogenase (3β-HSD) in nonclassical 3β-HSD deficiency. J Clin Endocrinol Metab 1994; 79:1811–1817.

117. Kohn B, Levine LS, Pollack MS, et al. Late-onset steroid 21-hydroxylase deficiency: a variant of classical congenital adrenal hyperplasia. J Clin Endocrinol Metab 1982; 55:817–827.

118. Levine LS, Dupont B, Lorenzen F, et al. Genetic and hormonal characterization of cryptic 21-hydroxylase deficiency. J Clin Endocrinol Metab 1981; 53:1193–1198.

119. New MI, Lorenzen AF, et al. Genotyping steroid 21-hydroxylase deficiency hormonal reference data. J Clin Endocrinol Metab 1983; 57:320–326.

120. Ehrman DA, Barnes RB, Rosenfeld RL. Polycystic ovary syndrome as functional ovarian hyperandrogenism due to dysregulation of androgen secretion. Endocr Rev 1995; 16:322.

121. Ibanez L, Potau N, Marcos MV, De Zegher F. Adrenal hyperandrogenism in adolescent girls with a history of low birthweight and precocious pubarche. Clin Endocrinol 2000; 53:523–527.

122. Kaltsas GA, Korbonitis M, Isidori AM, Webb JA, Trainer PJ, Monson JP, Besser GM, Grossman AB. How common are polycystic ovaries and the polycystic ovarian syndrome in women with Cushing's syndrome? Clin Endocrinol 2000; 53:493–500.

123. Langer P, Bartsch D, Moebius E, Rothmund M, Nies C. Adrenocortical carcinoma—our experience with 11 cases. Langenbeck's Arch Surg 2000; 385:393–397.

124. Pang S, Becker D, Cotelingam J, Foley T, Drash AL. Adrenocortical tumors in a patient with congenital adrenal hyperplasia due to 21-hydroxylase deficiency. Pediatrics 1981; 68:242–246.

125. Forsbach G, Guitron-Cantu A, Vazquez-Lara J, Mota-Morales M, Deai-Mendoza ML. Virilizing adrenal adenoma and primary amenorrhea in a girl with adrenal hyperplasia. Arch Gynecol Obstet 2000; 263:134–136.

126. Kandel FR, Rudd BT, Butt WR, Logan R, Loden DR. Androgen and cortisol response to ACTH stimulation in women with hyperprolactinemia. Clin Endocrinol (Oxf) 1980; 9:123–130.

127. Belisle S, Menard J. Adrenal androgen production in hyperprolactinemic state. Fertil Steril 1986; 33:396–400.

128. Cooke ID, Sawers RS. Investigation of hirsutism and selection of patients for treatment. In: Jeffcoate SL, ed. Androgens and Anti-androgen Therapy. New York: John Wiley and Sons, 1982:95–112.

129. Carter JM, Tyson JE, Warner GL, McNeilly AS, Faiman C, Friesen HG. Adrenalcortical function in hyperprolactinemic women. J Clin Endocrinol Metab 1977; 45:973–980.

130. Ebling FJ, Ebling E, Skinner J. The influence of pituitary hormones on the response of the sebaceous glands of the rat to testosterone. J Endocrinol 1969; 45:245–256.

131. Bracero N, Zacur HA. Polycystic ovary syndrome and hyperprolactinemia. J Clin Endocrinol Metab 2001; 86: 1626–1632.

132. Lamberts SW, Koper JW, Biemond P, den Holder FH, de Jong FH. Cortisol receptor resistance: the variability of its clinical presentation and response to treatment. J Clin Endocrinol Metab 1992; 74:313–321.

133. Ruiz M, Lind U, Gafvels M, Eggertsen G, Carlstedt-Duke J, Lennart N, Holtmann M, Stierna P, Wikstrom AC, Werner S. Characterization of two novel mutations in the glu-

cocorticoid receptor gene in patients with primary cortisol resistance. Clin Endocrinol 2001; 55:363–371.

134. Witchel SF, Smith RR. Glucocorticoid resistance in premature pubarche and adolescent hyperandrogenism. Mol Genet Metab 1999; 66:137–141.

135. Biason-Lauber A, Suter SL, Shackelton CH, Zachmann M. Apparent cortisone reductase deficiency: a rare cause of hyperandrogenemia and hypercortisolism. Horm Res 2000; 53:260–266.

136. Jamieson A, Wallace AM, Andrew R, Nunez BS, Walker BR, Fraser R, White PC, Connell JM. Apparent cortisone reductase deficiency: a functional defect in 11beta-hydroxysteroid dehydrogenase type 1. J Clin Endocrinol Metab 1999; 84:3570–3574.

137. Futterweit W. Clinical features of polycystic ovarian disease. In: Polycystic Ovarian Disease. New York: Springer-Verlag, 1984:83–95.

138. Coney P. Polycystic ovarian disease: current concepts of pathophysiology and therapy. Fertil Steril 1984; 42:667–682.

139. Lobo RA. Hirsutism in polycystic ovary syndrome: current concepts. Clin Obstet Gynecol 1991; 34:817–826.

140. Futterweit W. The pathologic anatomy of polycystic ovarian disease. In: Polycystic Ovarian Disease. New York: Springer-Verlag, 1984:41–46.

141. Knochenhauer ES, Key TJ, Kahsar-Miller M, Waggoner W, Boots LR, Azziz R. Prevalence of the polycystic ovary syndrome in unselected black and white women of the southeastern United States: a prospective study. J Clin Endocrinol Metab 1998; 83:3078–3082.

142. Asuncion M, Calvo RM, San Millan JL, Sancho J, Avila S, Escobar-Morrealle HF. A prospective study of the prevalence of polycystic ovary syndrome in unselected Caucasian women from Spain. J Clin Endocrinol Metab 2000; 85:2434–2438.

143. Farrah L, Lazenby AJ, Boots LR, Azziz R. Prevalence of the polycystic ovary syndrome in women seeking treatment from electrologists. Alabama Professional Electrology Association Study Group. J Reprod Med 1999; 44:870–874.

144. Kahsar-Miller MD, Nixon C, Boots LR, Azziz R. Prevalence of polycystic ovary syndrome (PCOS) in first-degree relatives of patients with PCOS. Fertil Steril 2001; 75:53–58.

145. Williamson K, Gunn AJ, Johnson N, Milsom SR. The impact of ethnicity on the presentation of polycystic ovary syndrome. Aust NZ J Obstet Gynaecol 2001; 41:202–206.

146. Dunaif A, Segal KR, Shelley DR, Green G, Dobrjansky A, Licholai T. Evidence for distinctive and intrinsic defects in insulin action in polycystic ovary syndrome. Diabetes 1992; 41:1257–1266.

147. Dunaif A, Xia J, Book CB, Schneker E, Tang Z. Excessive insulin receptor serine phosphorylation in cultured fibroblasts and in skeletal muscle. A potential mechanism for insulin resistance in the polycystic ovary syndrome. J Clin Invest 1995; 96:801–810.

148. Ciaraldi TP, el-Roeiy A, Madar Z, Reichart D, Olefsky JM, Yen SS. Cellular mechanisms of insulin resistance in polycystic ovarian syndrome. J Clin Endocrinol Metab 1992; 75:577–583.

149. Rosenbaum D, Haber RS, Dunaif A. Insulin resistance in polycystic ovary syndrome: decreased expression of GLUT-4 glucose transporters in adipocytes. Am J Physiol 1993; 264:E197–E202.

150. Kiddy DS, Hamilton-Fairley D, Bush A, Short F, Anyaoku V, Reed MJ, Franks S. Improvement in endocrine and ovarian function during dietary treatment of obese women with polycystic ovary syndrome. Clin Endocrinol 1992; 36:105–111.

151. Gharani N, Waterworth DM, Batty S, White D, Gilling-Smith C, Conway GS, McCarthy M, Franks S, Williamson R. Association of the steroid synthesis gene CYP11a with polycystic ovary syndrome and hyperandrogenism. Hum Mol Genet 1997; 6:397–402.

152. Carey AH, Waterworth D, Patel K, White D, Little J, Novelli P, Franks S, Williamson R. Polycystic ovaries and premature male pattern baldness are associated with one allele of the steroid metabolism gene CYP17. Hum Mol Genet 1994; 3:1873–1876.

153. Franks S. Polycystic ovary syndrome. N Engl J Med 1995; 333:853–861.

154. Escobar-Morrealle HF, Roldan B, Barrio R, Alonso M, Sancho J, de la Calle H, Garcia-Robles R. High prevalence of the polycystic ovary syndrome and hirsutism in women with type 1 diabetes mellitus. J Clin Endocrinol Metab 2000; 85:4182–4187.

155. Kashar-Miller M, Azziz R. Heritability and the risk of developing androgen excess. J Steroid Biochem Mol Biol 1999; 69:261–268.

156. Urbanek M, Legro RS, Driscoll DA, Azziz R, Ehrmann DA, Norman RJ, Strauss III JF, Spielman RS, Dunaif A. Thirty-seven candidate genes for polycystic ovary syndrome: Strongest evidence for linkage is with follistatin. Proc Natl Acad Sci USA 1999; 96:8573–8578.

157. Pang S, Levine LS, New MI. Puberty in congenital adrenal hyperplasia. In: Grumbach MM, Sizonenko PC, Aubert ML, eds. Control of the Onset of Puberty. Baltimore: Williams & Wilkins, 1990:669–687.

158. Levine LS, Korth-Schutz S, Saenger P, Sweeney WJ III, Beling CG, New MI. Disordered puberty in treated congenital adrenal hyperplasia. In: Lee PA, et al., eds. Congenital Adrenal Hyperplasia. Baltimore: University Park Press, 1977:511–526.

159. Sizonenko PC, Schindler AM, Kohlberg IJ, Paunier L. Gonadotropins, testosterone and oestrogen levels in relation to ovarian morphology in 11β-hydroxylase deficiency. Acta Endocrinol (Copenh) 1972; 71:539–550.

160. Bergman P, Siogren B, Hakansson B. Hypertensive form of congenital adrenocortical hyperplasia: analysis of a case with co-existing polycystic ovaries. Acta Endocrinol (Copenh) 1962; 40:555–564.

161. Abu-Haydar N, Laidlaw JC, Nusimovich B, Sturgis S. Hyperadrenocorticism and the Stein-Leventhal syndrome. Abstract of paper presented at 36th Annual Meeting of the Endocrine Society. J Clin Endocrinol Metab 1954; 14:766.

162. Lobo RA. Polycystic ovarian syndrome. In: Mishell DR Jr, Dacajan V, eds. Infertility, Contraception and Reproductive Endocrinology, 2nd. ed. Oradell, NJ: Medical Economics Co, 1985:319–336.

163. Pang S, Softness B, Sweeney WJ III, New MI. Hirsutism, polycystic ovarian disease and ovarian 17-ketosteroid reductase deficiency. N Engl J Med 1987; 316:1295–1301.

164. Simpson ER. Genetic mutations resulting in loss of aromatase activity in humans and mice. J Soc Gynecol Invest 2000; 7: Suppl:S18–S21.

165. Bulun SE. Aromatase deficiency and estrogen resistance: from molecular genetics to clinic. Semin Reprod Med 2000; 18:31–39.

166. Conte FA, Grumbach MM, Ito Y, Fisher CR, Simpson ER. A syndrome of female pseudohermaphroditism, hypergonadotropic hypogonadism, and multicystic ovaries associated with missense mutations in the gene encoding aromatase (P450arom). J Clin Endocrinol Metab 1994; 78:1287–1292.

167. Canales ES, Zarate A, Castelazo-Ayala L. Primary amenorrhea associated with polycystic ovaries: endocrine, cytogenetic and therapeutic considerations. Obstet Gynecol 1971; 37:205–210.

168. Yen SSC, Chaney C, Judd HL. Functional aberrations of the hypothalamic–pituitary system in polycystic ovary syndrome: a consideration of the pathogenesis. In: James VHT, Serio M, Giusti G, eds. The Endocrine Function of the Human Ovary. New York: Academic Press, 1976: 373–385.

169. Yen SSC. The polycystic ovary syndrome. Clin Endocrinol (Oxf) 1980; 12:177–207.

170. Kirschner MA, Zucker IR, Jespersen DL. Ovarian and adrenal vein catheterization studies in women with idiopathic hirsutism. In: James VHT, Serio M, Giusti G, cds. The Endocrine Function of the Human Ovary. New York: Academic Press, 1976:443–456.

171. Takai I, Taii S, Takakura K, Mori T. Three types of polycystic ovarian syndrome in relation to androgenic function. Fertil Steril 1990; 56:856–862.

172. Penttila TL, Koskinen P, Penttila TA, Anttila L, Irjala K. Obesity regulates bioavailable testosterone levels in women with or without polycystic ovary syndrome. Fertil Steril 1999; 71:457–461.

173. Gilling-Smith C, Story H, Rogers V, Franks S. Evidence for a primary abnormality of thecal cell steroidogenesis in the polycystic ovary syndrome. Clin Endocrinol 1997; 47:93–99.

174. Rebar R, Judd HL, Yen SSC, Rakoff J, Vadenberg G, Naftolin F. Characterization of the inappropriate gonadotropin secretion in polycystic ovarian syndrome. J Clin Invest 1976; 57:1320–1329.

175. Burger CW, Korsen T, van Kessel H, van Dop PA, Caron FJM, Schoemaker J. Pulsatile luteinizing hormone patterns in the follicular phase of the menstrual cycle, polycystic ovarian disease (PCOSD) and non-PCOSD secondary amenorrhea. J Clin Endocrinol Metab 1985; 61:1126–1132.

176. Minanni SL, Marcondes JA, Wajchenberg BL, Caveleiro AM, Fortes MA, Rego MA, Vezozzo DP, Robard D, Giannella-Neto D. Analysis of gonadotropin pulsatility in hirsute women with normal menstrual cycles and in women with polycystic ovary syndrome. Fertil Steril 1999; 71:675–683.

177. Lobo RA, Kletzky OA, Campeau JD, et al. Elevated bioactive luteinizing hormone in women in polycystic ovary syndrome. Fertil Steril 1983; 39:674.

178. Rebar RW. Gonadotropin secretion in polycystic ovarian disease. Semin Reprod Endocrinol 1984; 2:223.

179. Futterweit W. Pathophysiology of polycystic ovarian disease. In: Polycystic Ovarian Disease. New York: Springer-Verlag, 1984:49–82.

180. Schoemaker J, Wentz AC, Jones GS, et al. Stimulation of follicular growth with "pure" FSH in patients with anovulation and elevated LH levels. Obstet Gynecol 1978; 51:270–277.

181. Siiteri PK, MacDonald PC. Role of extraglandular estrogen in human endocrinology. In: Greep RO, Astwood EB, eds. Handbook of Physiology: Endocrinology, Vol II, Section 7. Washington DC: American Physiological Society, 1973:615–629.

182. Chang YT, Suriano MJ, Garibaldi L, Riddick L, Pang S. Clinical, hormonal, and radiological studies at baseline, during and after long-term GnRH analog (leuprolide) treatment in adolescent hirsute females with increased ovarian androgen production due to polycystic ovary syndrome. Clin Pediatr Endocrinol 1999; 8:77–84.

183. Shoupe D, Kumar DD, Lobo RA. Insulin resistance in polycystic ovarian syndrome. Am J Obstet Gynecol 1983; 147:588–592.

184. Stuart CA, Peters EJ, Prince MJ, Richards G, Cavallo A, Meyer WJI. Insulin resistance with acanthosis nigricans: the role of obesity and androgen excess. Metabolism 1986; 35:197–205.

185. Jialal I, Naiker P, Reddi K, Moodley J, Joubert SM. Evidence for insulin resistance in nonobese patients with polycystic ovarian disease. J Clin Endocrinol Metab 1987; 64:1066–1069.

186. Geffner ME, Kaplan SA, Bersch N, Golde DW, Landaw EM, Chang RJ. Persistence of insulin resistance in polycystic ovarian disease after inhibition of ovarian steroid secretion. Fertil Steril 1986; 45:327–333.

187. Dunaif A, Green G, Futterweit W, Doberjansky A. Suppression of hyperandrogenism does not improve peripheral or hepatic insulin resistance in the polycystic ovary syndrome. J Clin Endocrinol Metab 1990; 70:699–704.

188. Barbieri RL. Hyperandrogenic disorders. Clin Obstet Gynecol 1990; 33:640–654.

189. Falsetti L, Eleftheriou G. Hyperinsulinemia in the polycystic ovary syndrome: a clinical, endocrine and echographic study in 240 patients. Gynecol Endocrinol 1996; 10:319–326.

190. Franks S, Gilling-Smith C, Watson H, Willis D. Insulin action in the normal and polycystic ovary. Endocrinol Metab Clin North Am 1999; 28:361–378.

191. Nestler JE, Jakubowicz DJ, de Vargas AF, et al. Insulin stimulates testosterone biosynthesis by human theca cells from women with polycystic ovary syndrome by activating its own receptor and using inositolglycan mediators as the signal transduction system. J Clin Endocrinol Metab 1998; 83:2001–2005.

192. Marsden PJ, Murdoch AP, Taylor R. Tissue insulin sensitivity and body weight in polycystic ovary syndrome. Clin Endocrinol 2001; 55:191–199.

193. Pugeat M, Ducluzeau PH, Mallion-Donadieu M. Association of insulin resistance with hyperandrogenia in women. Horm Res 2000; 54:322–326.

194. Peppard HR, Marfori J, Iuomo MJ, Nestler JE. Prevalence of polycystic ovary syndrome among premenopausal women with type 2 diabetes. Diabetes Care 2001; 24: 1050–1052.

195. Motta EL, Baracat EC, Haidar MA, Juliano I, Lima GR. Ovarian activity before and after gonadal suppression by GnRH-a in patients with polycystic ovary syndrome, hyperandrogenism, hyperinsulinemia, and acanthosis nigricans. Rev Assoc Med Bras 1998; 44:94–98.

196. Prelevic GM. Insulin resistance in polycystic ovary syndrome. Curr Opin Obstet Gynecol 1997; 9:193–201.

197. Michelmore K, Ong K, Mason S, Bennett S, Perry L, Vessey M, Balen A, Dunger D. Clinical features in women with polycystic ovaries: relationships to insulin sensitivity, insulin gene VNTR and birth weight. Clin Endocrinol (Oxf) 2001; 55:439–446.

198. Tong Y, Liao WX, Roy AC, Ng SC. Association of Acci polymorphism in the follicle-stimulating hormone beta

gene with polycystic ovary syndrome. Fertil Steril 2000; 74:1233–1236.

199. Meyer MF, Gerresheim F, Pfeiffer A, Epplen JT, Schatz H. Association of polycystic ovary syndrome with an interstitial deletion of the long arm of chromosome 11. Exp Clin Endocrinol Diabetes 2000; 108:519–523.

200. Escobar-Morrealle HF, Calvo RM, Sancho J, San Millan JL. TNF-alpha and hyperandrogenism: a clinical, biochemical and molecular genetic study. J Clin Endocrinol Metab. 2001; 86:3761–3767.

201. Bartolone L, Smedile G, Arcoraci V, Trimarchi F, Benvenga S. Extremely high levels of estradiol and testosterone in a case of polycystic ovary syndrome. Hormone and clinical similarities with the phenotype of the alpha estrogen receptor null mice. J Endocrinol Invest 2000; 23: 467–472.

202. Cresswell JL, Barker DJ, Osmond C, Egger P, Phillips DI, Fraser RB. Fetal growth, length of gestation and polycystic ovaries in adult life. Lancet 1997; 350:1131–1135.

203. Ibanez L, Potau N, Marcos MV, de Zegher F. Corticotropin-releasing hormone: a potent androgen secretagogue in girls with hyperandrogenism after precocious pubarche. J Clin Endocrinol Metab 1999; 84:4602–4606.

204. DiMartino-Nardi J. Pre- and postpubertal findings in premature adrenarche. J Pediatr Endocrinol Metab 2000; 13 Suppl 5:1265–1269.

205. Toscano V, Balducci R, Mangiantini A, Falasca P, Sciarra F. Hyperandrogenism in the adolescent female. Steroids 1998; 63:308–313.

206. Lazar L, Kauli R, Bruchis C, Nordenberg J, Glatzer A, Pertzelan A. Early polycystic ovary-like syndrome in girls with central precocious puberty and exaggerated adrenal response. Eur J Endocrinol 1995; 133:403–406.

207. Calvo RM, Asuncion M, Telleria D, Sancho J, San Millan JL, Escobar-Morrealle HF. Screening for mutations in the steroidogenic acute regulatory protein and steroidogenic factor-1 genes, and in CYP11A and dosage-sensitive sex reversal-adrenal hypoplasia gene on the X chromosome, gene-1 (DAX-1) in hyperandrogenism hirsute women. J Clin Endocrinol Metab 2001; 86:1746–1749.

208. Marszalek B, Lacinski M, Babych N, Capla E, Biernacka-Lukanthy J, Warenik-Szymankiewicz A, Trzeciak WH. Investigations on the genetic polymorphism in the region of CYP17 gene encoding 5'-UTR in patients with polycystic ovary syndrome. Gynecol Endocrinol 2001; 15: 123–128.

209. Witchel SF, Lee PA, Suda-Hartman M, Smith R, Hoffman EP. 17 alpha-hydroxylase/17,20-lyase dysregulation is not caused by mutations in the coding regions of CYP17. J Pediatr Adolesc Gynecol 1998; 11:133–137.

210. Witchel SF, Fageril J, Siegel J, Smith R, Mitwally MF, Lewy V, Arslanian S, Lee PA. No association between body mass index and beta(3)-adrenergic receptor variant (W64R) in children with premature pubarche and adolescent girls with hyperandrogenism. Fertil Steril 2000; 73: 509–515.

211. Knochenhauer ES, Cortet-Rudelli C, Cunningham RD, Conway-Myers BA, Dewailly D, Azziz R. Carriers of 21-hydroxylase deficiency are not at increased risk for hyperandrogenism. J Clin Endocrinol Metab 1997; 82:479–485.

212. Escobar-Morrealle HF, San Millan JL, Smith RR, Sancho J, Witchel SF. The presence of the 21-hydroxylase deficiency carrier status in hirsute women: phenotype–genotype correlations. Fertil Steril 1999; 72:629–638.

213. Gharani N, Waterworth DM, Batty S, White D, Gilling-Smith C, Conway GS, McCarthy M, Franks S, Williamson R. Association of the steroid synthesis gene CYP11A with polycystic ovary syndrome and hyperandrogenism. Hum Mol Genet 1997; 6:397–402.

214. San Millan JL, Sancho J, Calvo RM, Escobar-Morrealle HF. Role of the pentanucleotide (tttta)(n) polymorphism in the promoter of the CYP11A gene in the pathogenesis of hirsutism. Fertil Steril 2001; 75:797–802.

215. Isik AZ, Gulekli B, Zorlu CG, Ergin T, Gokmen O. Endocrinological and clinical analysis of hyperprolactinemic patients with and without ultrasonically diagnosed polycystic ovarian changes. Gynecol Obstet Invest 1997; 43: 183–185.

216. Futterweit W. Hyperprolactinemia and polycystic ovarian disease. In: Polycystic Ovarian Disease. New York: Springer-Verlag, 1984:97–111, 149.

217. Kadawaki T, Berins C, Cama A, et al. Two mutant alleles of the insulin receptor gene in a patient with extreme insulin resistance. Science 1988; 240:787.

218. Yoshimas Y, Seino S, Whittaker J, et al. Insulin resistant diabetes due to a point mutation that prevents insulin pro-receptor processing. Science 1988; 240:784.

219. Moller DE, Flier JS. Detection of an alternation in the insulin-receptor gene in a patient with insulin resistance, acanthosis nigricans and the polycystic ovary syndrome (type A insulin resistance). N Engl J Med 1988; 319:1526.

220. Kahn CR, White MF. The insulin receptor and the molecular mechanism of insulin action. J Clin Invest 1988; 82:1151.

221. Krook A, Kumar S, Laing I, Boulton AJ, Wass JA, O'Rahilly S. Molecular scanning of the insulin receptor gene in syndromes of insulin resistance. Diabetes 1994; 43:357–368.

222. O'Rahilly S, Choi WH, Patel P, Turner RC, Flier JS, Moller DE. Detection of mutations in insulin-receptor gene in NIDDM patients by analysis of single-stranded conformation polymorphisms. Diabetes 1991; 40:777–782.

223. Taylor SI, Cama A, Accili D, Barbetti F, Quon MJ, de la Luz Sierra M, Suzuki Y, Koller E, Levy-Toledano R, Wertheimer E, et al. Mutations in the insulin receptor gene. Endocr Rev 1992; 13:566–595.

224. Judd HL, Scully RE, Herbst AI, et al. Familial hyperthecosis: comparison of endocrinologic and historical findings with polycystic ovarian disease. Am J Obstet Gynecol 1973; 117:976–982.

225. Behrman SJ, Scully RE. Case records of the Massachusetts General Hospital; infertility and irregular menses in a 27 year old woman. N Engl J Med 1972; 217:1192–1195.

226. Zhang Y, Word RA, Fesmire S, Carr BR, Rainey WE. Human ovarian expression of 17 beta-hydroxysteroid dehydrogenase types 1, 2 and 3. J Clin Endocrinol Metab 1996; 81:2594–2598.

227. Saez JM, de Peretti E, Morera AM, David M, Bertrand J. Familial male pseudohermaphroditism with gynecomastia due to a testicular 17-ketosteroid reductase defect. I. Studies in vivo. J Clin Endocrinol Metab 1971; 32: 604–610.

228. Saez JM, Morera AM, de Peretti E, Bertrans J. Further in vivo studies in male pseudohermaphroditism with gynecomastia due to a testicular 17-ketosteroid reductase defect (compared to a case of testicular feminization). J Clin Endocrinol Metab 1972; 34:598–600.

229. Virdis R, Saengerm P. 17β-hydroxysteroid dehydrogenase deficiency. Pediatric and Adolescent Endocrinology. In: Laron Z, New MI, Levine LS, eds. Adrenal Disease in Childhood. Basel: Karger, 1984:110–124.

230. Anderssom S, Geissler WM, Wu L, Grumbach MM, New MI, Schwarz HP, Blethen SL, Mendonca BB, Bloise W, Witchel SF, Cutler GB Jr, Griffin JE, Wilson JD, Russel DW. Molecular genetics and pathophysiology of 17-hydroxysteroid dehydrogenase deficiency. J Clin Endocrinol Metab 1996; 81:130–136.

231. Pang S, Leibel RL, Sweeney WJ III, New MI. Hirsutism due to gonadotropin-dependent androgen secreting lipoid cell ovarian tumor. In: 7th International Congress of Endocrinology. Amsterdam: Excerpta Medical, 1984:1254.

232. Carmina E. Prevalence of idiopathic hirsutism. Eur J Endocrinol 1998; 139:421–423.

233. Azziz R, Waggoner WT, Ochoa T, Knochenhauer ES, Boots LR. Idiopathic hirsutism: an uncommon cause of hirsutism in Alabama. Fertil Steril 1998; 70:274–278.

234. Wright F, Mowszowicz I, Mauvais-Jarvis P. Urinary 5α-androstane 3, 17β-diol radioimmunoassay: a new clinical evaluation. J Clin Endocrinol Metab 1978; 47:850–854.

235. Horton R, Lobo RA. Peripheral androgens and the role of androstanediol glucoronide. In: Horton R, Lobo RA, eds. Clinics in Endocrinology and Metabolism. Philadelphia: WB Saunders, 1986:293–300.

236. Azziz R, Carmina E, Sawaya ME. Idiopathic hirsutism. Endocr Rev 2000; 21:347–362.

237. Rosefield RL, Moll CW Jr. The role of proteins in the distribution of plasma androgens and estradiol. In: Molinatti GM, Martini L, James VHT, eds. Androgenization in Women. New York: Raven Press, 1983:25.

238. Bernasconi D, Del Monte P, Meozzi M, Randazzo M, Marugo A, Badaracco B, Marugo M. The impact of obesity on hormonal parameters in hirsute and nonhirsute women. Metabolism 1996; 45:72–75.

239. Calvo RM, Asuncion M, Sancho J, San Millan JI, Escobar-Morreale HF. The role of the CAG repeat polymorphism in the androgen receptor gene and of skewed X-chromosome inactivation, in the pathogenesis of hirsutism. J Clin Endocrinol Metab 2000; 85:1735–1740.

240. Voterro A, Stratakis CA, Ghizzoni L, Longui CA, Karl M, Chrousos GP. Androgen receptor-mediated hypersensitivity to androgens in women with nonhyperandrogenic hirsutism: skewing of X-chromosome inactivation. J Clin Endocrinol Metab 1999; 84:1091–1095.

241. Sawaya ME, Shalita AR. Androgen receptor polymorphism (CAG repeat lengths) in androgenic alopecia, hirsutism, and acne. J Cutan Med Surg 1998; 3:9–15.

242. Niepomniszcze H, Arnad RH. Skin disorders and thyroid diseases. J Endocrinol Invest 2001; 24:628–638.

243. Ferriman D, Gallwey JD. Clinical assessment of body hair growth in women. J Clin Endocrinol Metab 1961; 21:1440–1447.

244. Hatch R, Rosenfield RL, Kim MH, Tredway D. Hirsutism: implication etiology and management. Am J Obstet Gynecol 1981; 150:825–830.

245. Azziz R, Black VY, Knochenhauer ES, Hines GA, Boots LR. Ovulation after glucocorticoid suppression of adrenal androgens in the polycystic ovary syndrome is not predicted by the basal dehydroepiandrosterone sulfate level. J Clin Endocrinol Metab 1999; 84:946–950.

246. Kolodziejczyk B, Duleba AJ, Spaczynski RZ, Pawelczyk L. Metformin therapy decreases hyperandrogenism and hyperinsulinemia in women with polycystic ovary syndrome. Fertil Steril 2000; 73:1149–1154.

247. Ibanez L, Vallas C, Patau N, Marcos MV, de Zegher F. Sensitization to insulin in adolescent girls to normalize hirsutism, hyperandrogenism, oligomenorrhea, dyslipidemia, and hyperinsulinism after precocious pubarche. J Clin Endocrinol Metab 2000; 85:3526–3530.

248. Pasquali R, Gambineri A, Biscotti D, Vicennati V, Gagliardi L, Colitta D, Fiorini S, Cognigni GE, Filicori M, Morselli-Labate AM. Effect of long-term treatment with metformin added to hypocaloric diet on body composition, fat distribution, and androgen and insulin levels in abdominally obese women with and without the polycystic ovary syndrome. J Clin Endocrinol Metab 2000; 85: 2767–2774.

249. Pugeat M, Ducluzeau PH. Insulin resistance, polycystic ovary syndrome and metformin. Drugs 1999; 58: Suppl 1:41–46.

250. Morin-Papunen LC, Koivunen RM, Ruokonen A, Martikainen HK. Metformin therapy improves the menstrual pattern with minimal endocrine and metabolic effects in women with polycystic ovary syndrome. Fertil Steril 1998; 69(4):691–696.

251. Norman RJ, Kidson WJ, Cuneo RC, Zacharin MR. Metformin and intervention in polycystic ovary syndrome. Endocrine Society of Australia, the Australian Diabetes Society and the Australian Pediatric Endocrine Group. Med J Aust 2001; 17:580–583.

252. Morin-Papunen LC, Vauhkonen I, Koivunen RM, Ruokonen A, Martikainen HK, Tapanainen JS. Endocrine and metabolic effects of metformin versus ethinyl estradiol-cyproterone acetate in obese women with polycystic ovary syndrome: a randomized study. J Clin Endocrinol Metab 2000; 85:3161–3168.

253. Ehrman DA, Schneider DJ, Sobel BE, Cavaghan MK, Imperial J, Rosenfield RI, Polonsky KS. Troglitazone improves defects in insulin action, insulin secretion, ovarian, steroidogenesis, and fibrinolysis in women with polycystic ovary syndrome. J Clin Endocrinol Metab 1997; 82: 2108–2116.

254. Azziz R, Ehrman D, Legro RS, Whitcomb RW, Hanley R, Fereshetian AG, O'Keefe M, Ghazzi MN. PCOS/Troglitazone Study Group. Troglitazone improves ovulation and hirsutism in the polycystic ovary syndrome: a multicenter, double blind, placebo-controlled trial. J Clin Endocrinol Metab 2001; 86:1626–1632.

255. Ciotta L, Calogero AE, Farina M, De Leo V, La Marca A, Cianci A. Clinical, endocrine and metabolic effects of acarbose, an alpha-glucosidase inhibitor, in PCOS patients with increased insulin response and normal glucose tolerance. Hum Reprod 2001; 16:2066–2072.

256. Dahlgren E, Landin K, Krotkiewski M, Holm G, Janson PO. Effects of two antiandrogen treatments on hirsutism and insulin sensitivity in women with polycystic ovary syndrome. Hum Reprod 1998; 13:2706–2711.

257. Gokmen O, Senoz S, Guleki B, Isik AZ. Comparison of four different treatment regimes in hirsutism related to polycystic ovary syndrome. Gynecol Endcrinol 1996; 10: 249–255.

258. Escobar-Morreale HF, Lasuncion MA, Sancho J. Treatment of hirsutism with ethinyl estradiol-desogestrel contraceptive pills has beneficial effects on the lipid profile and improves insulin sensitivity. Fertil Steril 2000; 74: 816–819.

259. Pasquali R, Gambineri A, Anconetani B, Vicennati V, Colitta D, Caramelli E, Casimirri F, Morselli-Labate AM. The natural history of the metabolic syndrome in young

women with the polycystic ovary syndrome and the effect of long-term oestrogen-progestagen treatment. Clin Endocrinol 1999; 50:517–527.

260. Kokaly W, McKenna TJ. Relapse of hirsutism following long-term successful treatment with oestrogen-proestogen combination. Clin Endocrinol 2000; 52:379–382.

261. Venturoli S, Ravaioli B, Bagnoli A, Colombo FM, Marcrelli S, Iadarola I, Vianello F, Mancini F, Flamigni C. Contraceptive and therapeutic effectiveness of two low-dose ethinyl estradiol and cyproterone acetate regiments in the treatment of hirsute patients. Eur J Contracept Reprod Healthcare 1998; 3:29–33.

262. Bayhan G, Bahceci M, Demirkol T, Ertem M, Yalinkaya A, Erden AC. A comparative study of a gonadotropin-releasing hormone agonist and finasteride on idiopathic hirsutism. Clin Exp Obstet Gynecol 2000; 27:203–206.

263. Pazos F, Escobar-Morreale HF, Balsa J, Sancho JM, Varela C. Prospective randomized study comparing the long-acting gonadotropin-releasing hormone agonist triptorelin, flutamide, and cyproterone acetate, used in combination with an oral contraceptive, in the treatment of hirsutism. Fertil Steril 1999; 71:122–128.

264. DeLeo V, Fulghesu AM, la Marca A, Morgante G, Pasqui L, Talluri B, Torrivelli M, Caruso A. Hormonal and clinical effects of GnRH agonist alone, or in combination with a combined oral contraceptive or flutamide in women with severe hirsutism. Gynecol Endocrinol 2000; 14:411–416.

265. Carmina E, Lobo RA. Gonadotropin-releasing hormone agonist therapy for hirsutism is as effective as high dose cyproterone acetate but results in a longer remission. Hum Reprod 1997; 12:663–666.

266. Martikainen H, Heikkinen J, Roukonen A, Kaupila A. Hormonal and clinical effects of ketoconazole on hirsute women. J Clin Endocrinol Metab 1988; 66:987–991.

267. Carmine E, Lobo RA. The addition of dexamethasone to antiandrogen therapy for hirsutism prolongs the duration of remission. Fertil Steril 1998; 69:1075–1079.

268. Farguhar C, Lee O, Toomath R, Jepson R. Spironolactone versus placebo or in combination with steroids for hirsutism and/or acne (Cochrane Review). Cochrane Database 2001; 4:CD000194.

269. Moghetti P, Castello R, Zamberlan N, Rossini M, Gatti D, Negri D, Tosi F, Muggeo M, Adami S. Spironolactone, but not flutamide, administration prevents bone loss in hyperandrogenic women treated with gonadotropin-releasing agonist. J Clin Endocrinol Metab 1999; 84:1250–1254.

270. Moghetti P, Tosi F, Tosti A, Negri C, Misciali C, Perrone F, Caputo M, Muggeo M, Castello R. Comparison of spironolactone, flutamide, and finasteride efficacy in the treatment of hirsutism: a randomized, double blind, placebo-controlled trial. J Clin Endocrinol Metab 2000; 85:89–94.

271. Spritzer PM, Lisboa KO, Mattiello S, Lhullier F. Spironolactone as a single agent for a long-term therapy of hirsute patients. Clin Endocrinol 2000; 52:587–594.

272. Yucelten D, Erenus M, Gurbuz O, Durmusoglu F. Recurrence rate of hirsutism after 3 different antiandrogen therapies. J Am Acad Dermatol 1999; 41:64–68.

273. Miller JA, Jacobs HS. Treatment of hirsutism and acne with cyproterone acetate. In: Horton R, Lobo RA, eds. Clinics in Endocrinology and Metabolism. Philadelphia: WB Saunders, 1986:373–390.

274. Mneumann F, Schleusner A. Pharmacology of cyproterone acetate. In: Horton R, Lobo, RA, eds. Proceedings of the Diane symposium. Brussels: Excerpta Medica: 19–51.

275. Fruzetti F, Bersi C, Parrini D, Ricci C, Genazzani AR. Treatment of hirsutism: comparisons between different antiandrogens with central and peripheral effects. Fertil Steril 1999; 71:445–451.

276. Mudderis II, Bayram F, Guven M. A prospective, randomized trial comparing flutamide (25 mg/d) and finasteride (5 mg/d) in the treatment of hirsutism. Fertil Steril 2000; 73:984–987.

277. Lucas KJ. Finasteride cream in hirsutism. Endocr Pract 2001; 7:5–10.

278. Muderris II, Bayram F, Sahin Y, Kelestimur F. A comparison between two doses of flutamide (250 mg/d and 500 mg/d) in the treatment of hirsutism. Fertil Steril 1997; 68:644–647.

279. Andrade RJ, Lucena MI, Fernandez MC, Suarez F, et al. Fulminant liver failure associated with flutamide therapy for hirsutism. Lancet 1999; 353:983.

280. Wysowski DK, Freiman JP, Tourtelot JB, Horton ML III. Fatal and nonfatal hepatoxiticty associated with flutamide. Ann Intern Med 1993; 118:860–864.

281. Wallace C, Lalor EA, Chik CL. Hepatoxiticity complicating flutamide treatment of hirsutism. Ann Intern Med 1993; 119:1150.

282. Johnson F, Dovale M. Intense pulsed light treatment of hirsutism: case reports of skin phototypes V and VI. J Cutan Laser 1999; 1:233–237.

283. Lask G, Eckhouse S, Slatkine M, Waldman A, Kreindel M, Gottfried V. The role of laser and intense light sources in photo-epilation: a comparative evaluation. J Cutan Laser 1999; 1:3–13.

284. Sadicks NS, Weiss RA, Shea CR, Nagel H, Nicholson J, Prieto VG. Long-term photoepilation using a broad-spectrum intense pulsed light source. Arch Dermatol 2000; 136:1136–1140.

285. Sperof L. Hirsutism. In: Clinical Gynecologic Endocrinology and Infertility, 6th ed. Baltimore: Williams & Wilkins, 1999:421–476.

286. Pletcher JR, Slap GB. Menstrual disorders in adolescent gynecology. Part I—Common disorders. Pediatr Clin North Am 1999; 46:505–518.

287. Polaneczky MM, Slap GB. Menstrual disorders in the adolescent: amenorrhea. Pediatr Rev 1992; 13:43–48.

288. Conte FA, Grumbach MM, Kaplan SL. A diphasic pattern of gonadotropin secretion in patients with the syndrome of gonadal dysgenesis. J Clin Endocrinol Metab 1975; 40:670–675.

289. Temocin K, Vardar MA, Suleymanova D, Ozer E, Tanriverdi N, Demirhan O, Kadayifci O. Results of cytogenetic investigation in adolescent patients with primary or secondary amenorrhea. J Pediatr Adolesc Gynecol 1997; 10:86–88.

290. Simpson JL, Rajkovic A. Ovarian differentiation and gonadal failure. Am J Med Genet 1999; 89:186–200.

291. Levinson G, Zarate A, Guzman-Toledano R, et al. An XX female with sexual infantilism, absent gonads and lack of Mullerian ducts. J Med Genet 1976; 13:68–69.

292. Simpson JL. Gonadal dysgenesis and abnormalities of the human sex chromosomes: current status of phenotypic-karyotypic correlations. Birth Defects 1975; 11:23–59.

293. Auchus RJ. The genetics, pathophysiology and management of human deficiencies of P450c17. Endocrinol Metab Clin North Am 2001 30:101–119.

294. Nagai T, Imamura M, Honma M, Murakami M, Mori M. 17 alpha-hydroxylase deficiency accompanied by adrenal myelolipoma. Intern Med 2001; 40:920–923.

295. Kaufman FR, Kogut MD, Donnell GN, et al. Hypergonadotropic hypogonadism in female patients with galactosemia. N Engl J Med 1981; 304:994–998.

296. Touraine P, Beau I, Gougeon A, Meduri G, Desroches A, Pichard C, Detoeuf M, Paniel B, Prieur M, Zorn JR, Milgrom E, Kuttenn F, Misrahi M. New natural inactivating mutations of the follicle-stimulating hormone receptor: correlations between receptor function and phenotype. Mol Endocrinol 1999; 13:1844–1854.

297. Arnhold IJ, Latronico AC, Batista MC, Mendonca BB. Menstrual disorders and infertility caused by inactivating mutations of the luteinizing hormone receptor gene. Fertil Steril 1999; 71:591–601.

298. Wu SM, Leschek EW, Rennert OM, Chan WY. Luteinizing hormone receptor mutations in disorders of sexual development and cancer. Front Biosci 2000; 5:D343–D352.

299. Van Dop C, Burstein S, Conte FA, et al. Isolated gonadotropin deficiency in boys: clinical characteristics and growth. J Pediatr 1987; 111:684–692.

300. Job JC, Chaussain JL, Toublanc JE. Delayed puberty. In: Grumbach MM, Sizonenke PC, Aubert ML, eds. Control of the Onset of Puberty. Baltimore: Williams & Wilkins, 1990:588–619.

301. de Roux N, Young J, Brailly-Tabard S, Misrahi M, Milgrom E, Schaison G. The same molecular defects of the gonadotropin-releasing hormone receptor determine a variable degree of hypogonadism in affected kindred. J Clin Endocrinol Metab 1999; 84:567–572.

302. Carranza-Lira S, Forbin K, Martinez-Chequer JC. Rokitansky syndrome and MURCS association—clinical features and basis for diagnosis. Int J Fertil Womens Med 1999; 44:250–255.

303. Basile C, De Michele V. Renal abnormalities in Mayer-Rokitansky-Kuster–Hauser syndrome. J Nephrol 2001; 14:316–318.

304. Perkins RB, Hall JE, Martin KA. Neuroendocrine abnormalities in hypothalamic amenorrhea: spectrum, stability, and response to neurotransmitter modulation. J Clin Endocrinol Metab 1999; 84:1905–1911.

305. Stving RK, Hangaard J, Hansen-Nord M, Hagen C. A review of endocrine changes in anorexia nervosa. J Psychiatr Res 1999; 33:139–152.

306. Hasegawa K. Endocrine and reproductive disturbances in anorexia nervosa and bulimia nervosa. Nippom Rinsho 2001; 59:549–553.

307. Dusek T. Influence of high intensity training on menstrual cycles disorders in athletes. Croat Med J 2001; 42:79–82.

308. Munro MG. Dysfunctional uterine bleeding: advances in diagnosis and treatment. Curr Opin Obstet Gynecol 2001; 13:475–489.

309. Thorneycroft IH. Cycle control with oral contraceptives: a review of the literature. Am J Obstet Gynecol 1999; 180:280S–287S.

310. Callender ST, Warner GT, Cope E. Treatment of menorrhagia with trancxahic acid. A double-blind trial. Br Med J 1970; 24:214–216.

311. Preston JT, Cameron IT, Adams EJ, Smith SK. Comparative study of tranexahic acid and norethisterone in the treatment of ovulatory menorrhagia. Br J Obstet Gynecol 1995; 102:401–406.

312. Bonnar J, Sheepars BL. Treatment of menorrhagia during menstruation: randomized controlled trial of ethamsylate, mefenamic acid, and tranexahic acid. Br Med J 1996; 313:579–582.

313. Lethaby A, Augood C, Duckitt K. Nonsteriodal anti-inflammatory drugs for heavy menstrual bleeding (Cochrane Review). In: The Cochrane Library, issue 2. Oxford: Update Software, 2001.

314. Mitan LAP, Slap GB. Adolescent menstrual disorders. MD Consult 2000; 84:1–16.

315. Irvine GA, Cameron IT. Medical management of dysfunctional uterine bleeding. Baillier's Best Pract Res Clin Obstet Gynaecol 1999; 13:189–202.

13

Disorders of Sexual Differentiation

Adriana A. Carrillo and Gary D. Berkovitz
University of Miami School of Medicine, Miami, Florida, U.S.A.

Marco Danon
Miami Children's Hospital, Miami, Florida, and State University of New York, Brooklyn, New York, U.S.A.

The establishment of chromosomal sex (46,XY or 46,XX) is considered the first step in normal sexual differentiation. However, the first sexual structures that form may be considered as either primordial or neutral. These structures have the capacity to develop along male or female lines following the expression of specific genes at approximately $1\frac{1}{2}$ months after conception.

The term sex determination refers to the process in which the primordial gonad is committed to development as a testis or as an ovary. Sex differentiation refers to the process in which the internal accessory duct structures and external genitalia determination following differentiation of testis and ovary (1–5).

I. GONADAL DIFFERENTIATION

A. Embryology

1. Bipotential Gonad

The bipotential gonad develops from an outpouching of tissue on the posterior aspect of the celomic cavity on either side of the aorta. This structure is termed the urogenital ridge. It consists of three regions: the pronephros, the mesonephros, and the metanephros. The central region, the mesonephros, gives rise to the bipotential gonad and the first renal system. The primitive gonad forms on the medial portion of the urogenital ridge and is apparent at about 4 weeks of gestation. It consists of cells from the underlying mesonephric mesenchyme, cells that arise in the celomic epithelium, cells that migrate to the gonad

from the lateral portion of the mesonephros, and germ cells. Germ cells migrate from the yolk sac and enter the gonadal ridge during the 5th and 6th week of gestation. They undergo mitotic division during migration and continue to divide after arriving in the gonadal ridge (4, 6).

2. Testis Determination

Testis determination occurs at about 6 weeks of gestation. The first histological evidence of this is the appearance of Sertoli cells. These cells develop from progenitor cells contributed by the celomic epithelium. Sertoli cells encircle germ cells, form the testicular tubules, and cause mitotic arrest of germ cells. Sertoli cells secrete AMH and inhibin. Leydig cells, which develop later than Sertoli cells, are derived from cells that migrate from the mesonephros before testis determination occurs (7). They begin to secrete testosterone at 7–8 weeks of gestation. Peak serum levels of testosterone are reached by the 16th week of gestation. After testis determination, a second migration of cells from the mesonephros occurs. This migration is necessary to ensure the normal formation of testicular tubules (8, 9).

3. Ovarian Determination

Ovarian determination takes place at about 7 weeks of gestation. It involves formation of follicular cells, which are thought to arise from the same progenitor cells that give rise to Sertoli cells. Follicular cells surround germ cells in a loose configuration and form primordial follicles. This process is associated with arrest of germ cells in meiotic prophase (9).

B. Genetic Control of Gonadal Differentiation

1. Genes Involved in Formation of the Gonadal Ridge

The homeobox gene *LIM-1* plays an important role in formation of the gonadal ridge (10, 11). Mice homozygous for deletions in *Lim-1* lack development of the head, gonadal ridge, and the ureteric bud of the metanephros. The human *LIM1* gene has been identified, but no mutations have been reported. A related gene termed *Lhx9* is expressed in the urogenital ridge in mice and the absence of *Lhx9* causes gonadal agenesis (12). Nonetheless, no mutations in *LHX-9* have been found in humans with abnormal gonadal differentiation (13).

The steroidogenic factor 1 (*SF1*) gene located on chromosome 9p33 is a member of the orphan nuclear receptor family. *SF-1* was first identified as an activator of genes involved in steroid biosynthesis in the adrenals. Later it was found that mice missing *SF-1* lack adrenal glands and gonads and have impaired development of the ventromedial hypothalamus (14). Another gene termed Wilms tumor repressor (*WT-1*) is located on chromosome 11p13 and encodes a transcription factor expressed in the urogenital ridge, mesonephros, kidney, and gonad. It influences in the development of all three structures (15).

2. Genes Involved in Testis Determination

Evidence from early karyotype studies indicated a key role for the Y chromosome in male sex determination. The Y chromosomal gene implicated in this process was called the testis-determining factor (TDF). The gene termed sex-determining region Y (SRY) was isolated in 1990 and has been shown to be identical to TDF (16). SRY is located on chromosome Yp11.3, close to the pseudoautosomal boundary. It belongs to the family of high-mobility group (HMG) proteins, which contain a related DNA-binding motif termed the HMG box. The SRY gene product bends DNA, and the change in configuration of chromatin results in increased transcription of target genes. SRY expression is tightly controlled and appears to be induced by the WT-1 gene product (15). The primary role of SRY in male sex determination was established by the demonstration that XX mice transgenic for the Sry transcript developed as males, by the observation that sex reversal occurred following site-directed mutagenesis of the Sry gene, and by the identification of SRY mutations in women with 46,XY gonadal dysgenesis.

The *SOX-9* gene, located on chromosome 17q 24.3–25.1 encodes an SRY-like protein. The *SOX-9* gene belongs to a family that derives its name from the term *SRY*-related HMG-B*ox* gene. An increase in expression of *SOX-9* follows expression of SRY and *SOX-9* may be a target gene of SRY. Both WT-1 and SF-1 continue to be expressed on the developing testes. *SOX-9* interacts with SF-1 in regulating the expression of antimüllerian hormone (AMH) gene, and mutation of *SOX-9* binding sites in the AMH promoter results in the absence of AMH secretion (17, 18).

DAX-1 is a member of the nuclear hormone receptor superfamily. Like SF-1, DAX-1 is expressed in the bipotential gonad, the embryonic adrenal cortex, pituitary gonadotropes, and in the ventromedial nucleus of the hypothalamus. Expression of DAX-1 is repressed in testis but continues in the ovary after gonadal determination. Duplication of DAX-1 in males causes sex reversal. Hence, DAX-1 has been termed an antitestis gene (19). Mutations of DAX-1 result in X-linked adrenal hypoplasia congenita (AHC), but do not cause abnormalities in gonadal differentiation (20).

In summary, various genes such as *LIM-1*, *LHX-9*, *SF-1*, and *WT-1* are involved in the formation of the gonadal ridge of testis determination. SRY is the trigger of testis determination. Subsequent steps involve the expression of *SOX-9* as well as continued expression of SF-1 and WT-1 (21, 22).

3. Genes Involved in Ovarian Determination

Genetic control of ovarian determination is not well understood. However, the gene termed *WNT4* appears to play a role this process and is also expressed in the mesenchyme surrounding müllerian ducts. Lack of *WNT4* gene impairs ovarian development, and the resulting gonad expresses testis-specific markers such as AMH and testosterone. Moreover, expression of *WNT4* is suppressed in the developing testis (23).

II. ANATOMICAL SEX DIFFERENTIATION OF THE REPRODUCTIVE TRACT

A. Undifferentiated Stage

1. Müllerian and Wolffian Ducts

The reproductive tracts of the male and female fetus are identical until 8 weeks of gestation. They consist of bilateral wolffian and müllerian ducts and neutral external genitalia (Figs. 1, 2). The wolffian, or mesonephric, ducts are the primordia of the epididymis, vas deferens, and seminal vesicles. Wolffian ducts form initially as the excretory canals of the primitive kidney or mesonephros, and are incorporated into the genital system when renal function is taken over by the definitive kidney or metanephros. The müllerian, or paramesonephric, ducts are the primordia of the fallopian tubes, uterus, and upper two-thirds of the vagina. They originate from a cleft between the gonadal ridge and the mesonephros, and grow parallel to the wolffian ducts, crossing them ventrally to form a single structure. By week 8 of gestation, the ducts reach the dorsal wall of the urogenital sinus, where they form

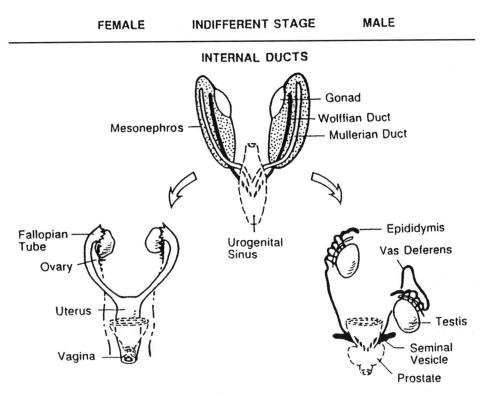

FEMALE   INDIFFERENT STAGE   MALE

INTERNAL DUCTS

Figure 1   Phenotypic differentiation of internal ducts in male and female embryos.

the müllerian tubercle, which separates the cranial vesicourethral canal from the caudal urogenital sinus. The fused tips of the müllerian ducts are separated from the dorsal wall of the urogenital sinus by a solid mass, termed the vaginal cord (Figs. 1, 2) (24).

Several transcription factors are involved in the differentiation of intermediate mesenchyme to form the sex ducts. *Lim1*, which plays a role in formation of the gonadal ridge, is also necessary for expression of transcription factors such as *Pax-2* and *Hox-6* that mediate formation of the accessory sex ducts. *Pax-2* is expressed in the epithelium of the wolffian ducts. *Hox-6*, and other members of the Hox gene family, is expressed in the fallopian tubes (*Hoxa9*), uterus (*Hoxa 10,11*), cervix (*Hoxa11*), and upper vagina (*Hoxa 13*) (25).

The gene termed *WnT4*, which is involved in ovarian development, is also necessary for development of müllerian structures and kidney. Lethal renal agenesis occurs as a result of *WnT4* mutations in both males and females. Mutations of *WnT4* interrupt müllerian duct development, although they do not interfere with wolffian duct formation. In addition, mutations of *WnT-7a* in mice result in poorly developed müllerian ducts (26).

2.   External Genitalia

Early development of external genitalia involves formation of the genital membrane, which closes the ventral part of the cloaca. The cloacal membrane forms the urogenital and anal membranes at week 6 of gestation. By week 8 the cloaca is divided into an anterior urogenital sinus and a posterior anorectal canal. The genital tubercle is located ventrally, the urethral folds are located medially, whereas the genital folds or labioscrotal swellings are located laterally.

B.   Male Differentiation

Regression of müllerian ducts begins at 8 weeks of gestation and depends on secretion of AMH. Regression of the müllerian ducts represents an unusual pattern of cell loss. Few cells actually die. Instead, they lose their polarity and orientation and cease to divide. The basement membrane dissolves, and a tight ring of connective tissue forms around the cells (27). Müllerian ducts have nearly completely disappeared by 10 weeks of gestation. Wolffian ducts are stabilized and subsequently differentiate into epididymis, vas deferens, and seminal vesicles. Mucous epididymal secretion is demonstrable from 25 weeks of gestation.

With respect to differentiation of the urogenital sinus, prostatic buds appear at approximately 10 weeks of gestation at the site of the müllerian tubercle and grow into solid branching cords. Maturation of the prostatic gland is accompanied by development of the prostatic utricle,

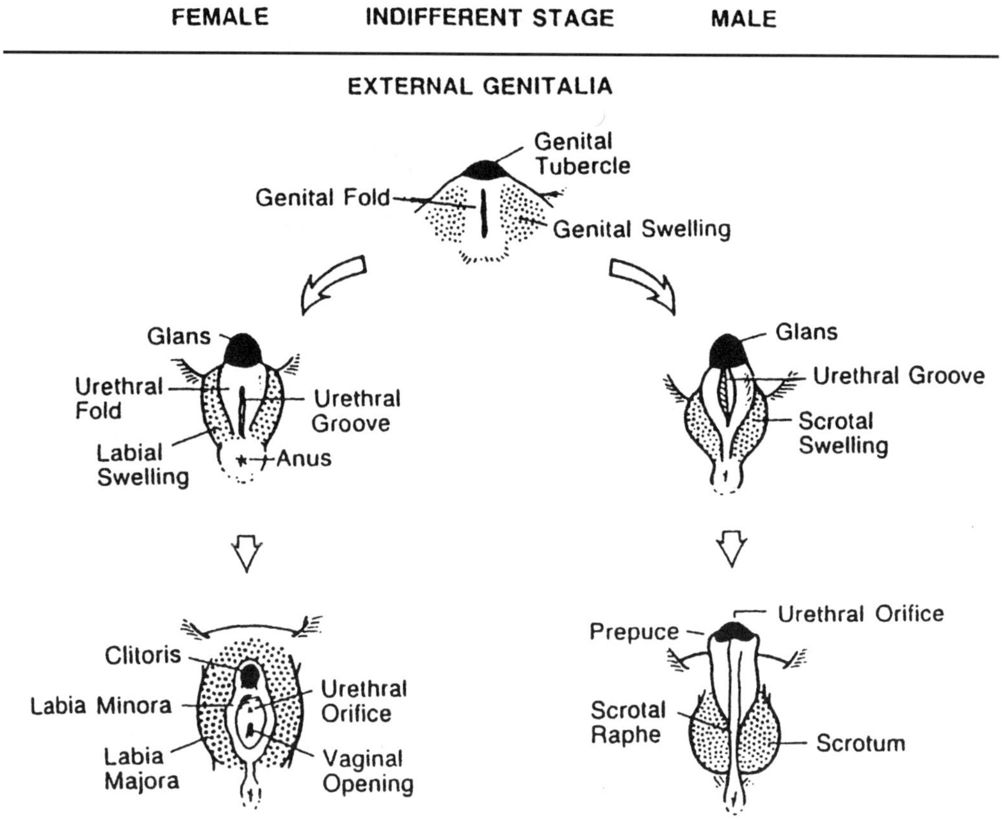

FEMALE   INDIFFERENT STAGE   MALE

EXTERNAL GENITALIA

Figure 2   Phenotypic differentiation of external genitalia in male and female embryos.

which is the male remnant of the vaginal pouch. Two buds of epithelial cells, the sinoutricular bulbs, develop from the urogenital sinus close to the opening of the wolffian ducts and grow inward, fusing with the medial müllerian tubercle to form the sinoutricular cord. This structure makes contact with the caudal tip of the fused müllerian ducts and cannnulizes at 18 weeks of gestation to form the prostatic utricle (28).

Masculinization of the male external genitalia begins in the 9-week-old fetus with lengthening of the anogenital distance, fusion of the labioscrotal folds, and closure of the rims of the urethral groove. This results in formation of a perineal and penile urethra. Penile organogenesis is completed by 11 weeks of gestation. The male and female phallus is the same size until week 16 of gestation (29).

The migration of testis from the lower pole of the kidney to the scrotum is a complex process that involves transabdominal migration and inguinoscrotal descent. The process starts at 12 weeks of gestation. The cranial suspensory ligament connects the testis to the abdominal wall, and the genitoinguinal ligament known as gubernaculum connects the testis to the inguinal canal. Caudal enlargement of the gubernaculum together with shortening of its proximal part and regression of the cranial suspensory ligament are part of the testis descent mechanism.

Transabdominal movement brings the testis to the internal inguinal ring at midgestation, around 22 weeks. The actual passage of the testis through the inguinal canal into the scrotum does not occur until after week 28, and may be delayed until the immediate postnatal period. The mechanism of testicular descent is not fully understood and probably results from a combination of mechanical, genetic, and hormonal factors. Increase in intra-abdominal pressure is an important factor in transit through the inguinal canal. This passage requires development of the processus vaginalis and increased intra-abdominal pressure. Factors controlling growth and differentiation of the gubernaculum are not completely understood, and the mechanism controlling direction of migration remains unknown (30).

C. Female Differentiation

As mentioned previously, müllerian ducts give rise to the fallopian tubes, uterus, and upper two-thirds of the vagina. Beginning at 10 weeks of gestation, the wolffian ducts are incorporated into the wall of müllerian derivatives.

In the female, the genital tubercle becomes the clitoris, the labioscrotal folds become the labia majora, and the urethral folds become the labia minora. At 15 weeks, the lower pole of the müllerian ducts fuses with the upper portion of the vaginal pouch to form the vagina. Later the urogenital sinus is divided by a tissue plane that results in a separate urethral and vaginal opening on the perineum (Fig. 3).

III. HORMONAL CONTROL OF SEX DIFFERENTIATION

A. Jost's Hypothesis

Early experiments conducted by Alfred Jost have contributed greatly to our understanding of sex differentiation. In these studies, castration of fetal rabbits at the undifferentiated stages resulted in female differentiation. Unilateral implantation of testosterone crystal at the site of the testis in a castrated rabbit resulted in development of wolffian structures but not müllerian structures regression. By contrast, unilateral reimplantation of testis resulted in both development of wolffian structures and regression of müllerian structures. These observations led to the conclusion that at least two important factors are nec-

essary in the development of male reproductive sex ducts: testosterone for wolffian duct development and so-called müllerian inhibiting factor for regression of female ducts (31).

B. Antimüllerian Hormone

The müllerian-inhibiting factor that Jost proposed was later identified and named AMH. It produces the cranial–caudal regression of müllerian ducts during weeks 8–10 of gestation. It is a dimeric glycoprotein secreted by Sertoli cells. Granulosa cells also secrete AMH, but not until the critical period for müllerian regression has passed. AMH is a member of the transforming growth factor β (TGF-β) family, which includes inhibin, activins, and other factors. Members of this family control growth, differentiation, and the death of many tissues. Hormones in TGF-β family are usually produced as large precursors, which require cleavage to release the active hormone. AMH is cleaved by plasmin at a site located 109 amino acids away from the carboxyl terminus, generating the TGF-β-like carboxyl-terminal fragment that is thought to contain the biologically active site of AMH. The human AMH gene has been cloned and has been mapped to the short arm of chromosome 19 (5, 32).

The AMH receptor is a complex transmembrane serine/threonine kinase, and it is a heterodimer made up of a type I and type II receptors. Ligand binding to the receptor results in phosphorylation and activation of the type I receptor. The gene for the type I receptor is termed ALK2 and the gene product signals through the bone morphogenic protein (BMP) pathway (33). WnT-7a plays a role in development of the type II receptor. Hence the mutation of WnT-7a in male mice results in the persistence of müllerian ducts (34). The gene for the type II receptor has been cloned and has been mapped to chromosome 12. This gene is expressed in the mesenchyme surrounding the müllerian structures (35).

Serum AMH is also a marker of testicular function in infancy, and serum levels are useful in the diagnosis and management of patients with a variety of intersex and gonadal abnormalities (36). Granulosa cells of the postnatal ovary also produce AMH, and elevated serum levels have been reported in a case of granulosa cell tumor. Although AMH is produced by Sertoli cells until puberty and is also secreted by postnatal granulosa cells, its effects in both sexes after birth has not been confirmed.

The effect of AMH on ovarian function is controversial. AMH has been reported to inhibit progression of meiosis in oocytes and to result in masculinization of the fetal ovary. In a freemartin, a bovine female united to a male twin by placental anastomoses, ovaries are either reduced to fibrous streaks or have evidence of testicular determination. When ovaries grown in a culture are exposed to AMH or when fetal mice overexpressed AMH, ovaries are masculinized. AMH also sex-reverses the pattern of steroidogenesis in the fetal ovary by inhibiting aromatase

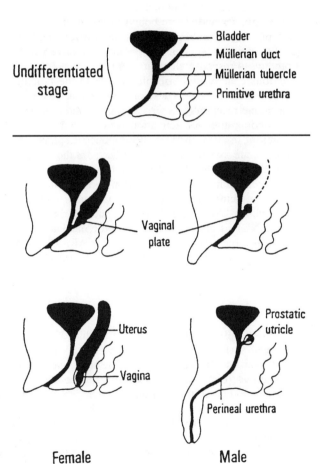

Figure 3 Sex differentiation of the urogenital sinus and external genitalia.

activity (5). Despite the masculinizing effect on fetal ovaries, AMH is not required for testicular development because mutations impairing AMH production do not affect testicular organogenesis.

C. Testosterone

Leydig cells appear between weeks 7 and 8 in the human fetus and proliferate until the 18th week of gestation. Human chorionic gonadotropic (hCG) receptors are present on fetal cells by at least 12 weeks of gestation. Gonadal steroidogenesis in the fetal gonads involves five enzymatic steps: steroidogenic acute regulatory protein (StAR), side chain cleavage (P450scc), 3β-hydroxydehydrogenase (3βHDS), 17-hydroxylase/17-20 desmolase (P45017), and 17β-hydroxysteroid dehydrogenase. The number of Leydig cells decreases after 18 weeks of gestation and, indeed, few Leydig cells are visible by that time. Serum and testicular testosterone concentrations increase to a peak of about 300 ng/dl (range, 200–600) at 15–18 weeks of gestation. After 15 weeks, a low level of testosterone is maintained by hCG. A decrease in testosterone synthesis later in gestation is correlated with a decrease in LH/hCG receptors. During the second half of pregnancy, LH becomes the principal regulator of testosterone secretion. LH secretion is regulated in part by testosterone through a negative feedback at the level of the hypothalamus. In male infants, serum testosterone levels rise again during the first 2 days of life, decline until the end of the first week, and then peak at 2 months of age. By 6 months, testosterone levels reach typical prepubertal levels (37).

D. Mechanism of Testosterone and Dihydrotestosterone Action in the Reproductive Tract

Testosterone enters most cells by passive diffusion, although it has been suggested that the wolffian duct takes up testosterone by pinocytosis. In target tissues, testosterone is converted to dihydrotestosterone (DHT) by steroid 5 α-reductase. The conversion of testosterone to DHT is necessary for sex differentiation of male external genitalia. There are two explanations for this. First, DHT binds to the androgen receptor with greater affinity than does testosterone. Second, DHT cannot be aromatized, and thus its action is purely androgenic. Although masculinization of prostate, urogenital sinus, and external genitalia depends on DHT, proliferation of wolffian ducts occurs in the presence of testosterone alone. This may happen because the internal ducts are exposed to high local concentrations of testosterone.

There are two forms of steroid 5α-reductase, one having optimal activity at pH 5.5 and the other at pH 8. The former enzyme, which is the predominant form in the prostate, is called steroid 5α-reductase 2. The steroid 5α-reductase 2 mediates conversion of testosterone to DHT

in the external genitalia. The gene has been mapped to chromosome 2. By contrast, the enzyme termed steroid 5α-reductase 1 does not appear to play a role in differentiation of the reproductive tract. This gene has been mapped to the short arm of chromosome 5, band 15.

Binding of DHT to the androgen receptor is necessary for androgen effect (38). The androgen receptor has been cloned and is located on the long arm of the X chromosome near the centromere (Xq11-q12) (39). The androgen receptor is a member of a superfamily of nuclear receptors that includes the progesterone, glucocorticoid, mineralocorticoid, estrogen, thyroid hormone, vitamin D, vitamin A, and v-Erb receptors. The androgen receptor consists of eight exons encoding a protein of approximately 919 amino acids. Exon 1 encodes the N-terminal transcription activation domain. Exons 2 and 3 encode the DNA-binding domain, exons 4–8 the steroid binding domain (15). The DNA-binding domain consists of two cysteine-rich zinc fingers, and also encodes sequences for dimerization and translocation of the receptor to the nucleus. The transcriptional activation domain contains variable trimeric repeats. GGN repeats encode 16–27 glycine residues, CAG repeats encode 11–31 glutamine repeats. Heat shock proteins HSP 56, 70, and 90 are bound to the inactive receptor and binding of androgen results in their release. Subsequent conformational changes permit homodimerization and binding to response elements in target genes (40, 41).

Various coactivators also play a role in the function of the androgen receptor. These proteins interact with steroid hormone receptors to increase transcription of target genes. Binding sites for activation factors AF-1 and AF-2 are present in all of the steroid hormone receptors. AF-1 and AF-2 are synergistic in their effects on the receptor (42). Members of the steroid receptor coactivator (SRC) family appear to increase transcription by recruiting other coactivators factors to the receptor coactivator complex. Factors such as AP-1 and the small nuclear ring finger protein (SNURF) also influence receptor mediated transcription of target genes (43). Coactivator ARA-24 binds to the transactivation domain and increases transcription of target genes (44).

E. Estrogen

The biological effects of estrogens are mediated by estrogen receptors (ER). Estrogen diffuses freely into cells where it binds to ER in the nucleus. The ER–ligand complex dimerizes, binds to the estrogen response elements, and hence modulates transcription of estrogen-regulated genes. Two estrogen receptors, α and β, have similar affinity and specificity. The human estrogen receptor β has been detected as early as 13–20 weeks of gestation with highest levels being found in the adrenals, and in the male reproductive tract (45). Expression of the ER α and β has been identified in the uterus at the beginning of the second trimester and plays a role in uterine development.

Estrogen has also been implicated in several pathological states of male sexual differentiation. For example, prenatal exposure to estrogens can result in cryptorchidism possibly by inhibiting the insulin-like factor 3. Hypospadias, epididymal cysts, persistent Müllerian ducts, and prostatic disease have also been related to prenatal exposure to estrogen in males. ER α is essential for fluid reabsorption in the efferent ductulus and its absence results in infertility (46). In the female embryo, ER α and β are detected on epithelium of the oviduct and may modulate oviduct development. ER gene expression has also been identified in the uterus beginning in the early second trimester of fetal development, suggesting a role for ER in differentiation of primitive uterine mesenchyme in stromal and myometrial compartments.

F. Environmental Factors

A recent increase in incidence of developmental abnormalities of the reproductive tract has been noted and has raised great concern. For example, there has been increase in prevalence of cryptorchidism, hypospadias, and micropenis over the past 20–30 years. This has been attributed in part to fetal exposure to environmental compounds with estrogenic effects (xenoestrogens), such as herbicides, pesticides, polychlorinated biphenyls (PCBs), plasticizers, and polysterenes, as well as exposure to antiandrogens such as polyaromatic hydrocarbons, linuron, vinclozolin, and pp′-dichlorodiphenyl ethylene (pp′DDE). Such environmental agents are generally referred to as endocrine disruptors (47).

Xenoestrogens and antiandrogens can disrupt androgen effect by different mechanisms. Various explanations have been proposed, including competition for binding to the androgen receptor, diminished conformational change, as well as suboptimal nuclear transfer, DNA binding, and transcriptional activation. Most antiandrogens interact directly with the androgen receptor. Environmental antiandrogens such as the fungicide vinclozilin disrupt male sex differentiation by blocking androgen receptor (AR) binding to androgen response elements. DDE, a DDT metabolite that accumulates in the environment, inhibits human androgen receptor transcriptional activation (48). Exposure of male fetus to antiandrogens results in diminished masculinization. Xenoestrogens influence male differentiation by interacting indirectly with either ER α or ER β. Hypospadias has been related to estrogen exposure during the first trimester and the occurrence of genital abnormalities in sons of women exposed to diethylstilbestrol (DES) is well documented. At least 20% of these men had epididymal cysts, hypospadias, and cryptorchidism (49).

IV. AMBIGUOUS GENITALIA

Conditions with ambiguous genitalia are classified into three major categories: abnormalities of gonadal differentiation, male pseudohermaphroditism, and female pseudohermaphroditism.

A. Genetic Abnormalities of Gonadal Differentiation

1. 46,XY Gonadal Dysgenesis

Abnormalities of gonadal differentiation in individuals with a 46,XY karyotype can be subdivided into 46,XY complete gonadal dysgenesis, 46,XY partial gonadal dysgenesis, and 46,XY true hermaphroditism. Although each of these conditions has a distinct phenotype, there is considerable overlap. Another condition, termed testicular regression sequence, has various causes, but some evidence suggest that the condition is also related to 46,XY partial gonadal dysgenesis (see Table 1).

a. Complete. The 46,XY complete gonadal dysgenesis is defined by absence of testis determination despite nonmosaic male karyotype. The condition is characterized by normal female external genitalia and streak gonads. The terms Swyer syndrome and 46,XY pure gonadal dysgenesis have also been used to describe this condition.

Clinical presentation. Most subjects with 46,XY complete gonadal dysgenesis present for evaluation of delayed puberty or amenorrhea. Subjects are usually normal in appearance and most have normal height, although some have stigmata of Turner syndrome.

Breast development is present in a few subjects. Presentation of breast tissue and/or menses in subjects with 46,XY complete gonadal dysgenesis is of concern as it may signal the presence of an estrogen-secreting tumor. There is normal development of pubic hair in women with 46,XY complete gonadal dysgenesis, but in some individuals the clitoris may be slightly enlarged (50). Physical examination and ultrasonography indicate normal vagina, uterus, and fallopian tubes. There is an absence of wolffian structures. When subjects present as adolescents or adults, serum levels of luteinizing hormone (LH) and follicle-stimulating hormone (FSH) are abnormally elevated. Serum estradiol levels are usually low, but may be elevated in the presence of an estrogen-secreting tumor. Plasma levels of testosterone are normal or slightly elevated due to the effect of abnormally elevated serum LH on residual theca cells in the streak gonad. The latter ob-

Table 1 Classification of Genetic Abnormalities of Gonadal Differentiation

46,XY gonadal dysgenesis
  46,XY complete gonadal dysgenesis
  46,XY partial gonadal dysgenesis
  46,XY true hermaphroditism
  Embryonic Testicular Regression Sequence
Mosaicism and chimerism involving the Y chromosome
46,XX sex reversal
  46,XX maleness
  46,XX true hermaphroditism.

servation provides an explanation for the clitoromegaly in some subjects (51).

Gonadal histology. This is usually characterized by a wavy fibrous connective tissue, which in part resembles ovarian stroma. Some evidence indicates that the streak gonad of 46,XY complete gonadal dysgenesis was an ovary in utero, which then degenerated into a streak later in gestation (50).

Gonadal tumors occur in 30% of subjects with 46,XY complete gonadal dysgenesis. Although tumors usually develop after puberty, they may be present earlier. The most common tumor is gonadoblastoma. About half of subjects with gonadoblastoma have coincidental dysgerminoma. Although gonadoblastoma is generally considered a carcinoma in situ, dysgerminoma is a malignant tumor. Other malignant tumors also occur but are unusual. They include embryonal carcinoma, endodermal sinu tumor, choriocarcinoma, and immature teratoma (52).

Management. Management of women with 46,XY gonadal dysgenesis involves gonadectomy to prevent malignancy followed by cyclical hormonal therapy to promote normal pubertal development and normal maturation of bones. Since the uterus is normal, pregnancy can be achieved following in vitro fertilization of a donor egg and implantation of the embryo.

b. Partial. 46,XY partial gonadal dysgenesis is defined by incomplete testis determination in an individual with a nonmosaic 46,XY karyotype. This condition has also been referred to as dysgenetic male pseudohermaphroditism and 46,XY mixed gonadal dysgenesis. It is differentiated from 45,X/46,XY mixed gonadal dysgenesis, in which condition the pathology is related to mosaicism.

Clinical presentation. Individuals with this condition usually present ambiguous genitalia in the newborn period, with variable degree of masculinization. A utriculovaginal pouch is present in a large number of subjects. Proliferation of wolffian ducts depends on the extent of embryonic testosterone secretion, whereas the extent of müllerian duct development depends on the secretion of AMH. Gonads are usually intra-abdominal, but in some individuals they may be found in the inguinal canal or in the scrotum. Serum levels of plasma testosterone are low in the newborn period, as are levels following hCG stimulation. If the diagnosis is made after puberty, serum levels of LH and FSH are abnormally high, whereas plasma levels of testosterone are normal or low (50).

Stigmata of Turner syndrome are present in approximately one-quarter of subjects with 46,XY partial gonadal dysgenesis. The explanation for this physical finding is unknown, but many of these cases may have hidden mosaicism with a 45,X cell line.

In some subjects, 46,XY gonadal dysgenesis is associated with specific syndromes. One example is the condition termed WAGR, which has *W*ilms' tumor, *a*niridia, *g*onadal dysgenesis, and mental *r*etardation. Other conditions associated with Wilms tumor and gonadal dysgenesis include Denys-Drash and Frasier syndromes, both of which are characterized by progressive nephropathy. Another syndrome, termed campomelic dysplasia, is an autosomal dominant condition characterized by abnormal growth of long bones and abnormal testis determination. Subjects with complex rearrangement of chromosome 9 can also present 46,XY partial gonadal dysgenesis in association with multiple congenital anomalies (53).

Gonadal histology. Gonadal abnormalities in 46,XY partial gonadal dysgenesis include formation of streak gonads and dysgenetic testes. Streak gonads are similar to those found in subjects with 46,XY complete gonadal dysgenesis, except that they may be more fibrotic. The dysgenetic testes in these individuals are characterized by disordered, poorly formed seminiferous tubules and incomplete formation of the tunica albuginea (50).

Gonadal tumors. The risk of gonadal tumor in subjects with 46,XY partial gonadal dysgenesis is 16–30%. The types of tumors are like those of 46,XY complete gonadal dysgenesis. However, caution is necessary in management of these patients, since tumors have occurred as early as 15 months of life (54).

Management. Surgical correction of the external genitalia should be performed. There is also need to remove internal ducts structures that correspond to those of the opposite sex of rearing. If the child is raised as a boy, streak gonads should be removed, and dysgenetic gonads should be brought into the scrotum or, if this is not possible, they should be removed. Although the risk of malignancy remains even if the gonads are in the scrotum, the development of tumors can be ascertained by careful and regular physical examination. Dysgenetic testes may produce testosterone at puberty, but testosterone therapy is often necessary. If the individual is raised as a female, gonadal tissue should be removed to avoid the possibility of malignancy and to prevent virilization later in life.

Subjects raised as females will require cyclical hormonal therapy at puberty for development of secondary sexual characteristics. Menses can be achieved by hormonal supplementation if the uterus is intact.

c. 46,XY True Hermaphroditism

Clinical presentation. The 46,XY true hermaphroditism is characterized by the presence of gonadal tissue that contains both ovarian follicles and normal-appearing seminiferous tubules in a patient with a male karyotype. Patients usually have ambiguous genitalia, although genitalia range in appearance from completely female to completely male. There is a mix of wolffian and müllerian duct structures depending on development of testicular tissue. Management is the same as that of subjects with 46,XY gonadal dysgenesis (55).

Gonadal histology. The presence of an ovary on one side of the abdomen and a testis on the other side is found in about 50% of patients. In other cases, one or both of the gonads can be ovotestis. The risk of gonadal tumors in subjects with 46,XY true hermaphroditism is approximately 10% (52).

d. Embryonic Testicular Regression Sequence. This condition is characterized by loss of testicular tissue on one or both sides of the abdomen in an individual with 46,XY karyotype. Patients have ambiguous or female genitalia with abnormal differentiation of internal sex ducts. It is thought that loss of the testicular tissue in this syndrome occurs during the critical period of sex differentiation. Early loss of testicular tissue may be associated with female external genitalia, whereas ambiguous genitalia implies loss of testis at a slightly later stage (56).

Some evidence suggests that the cause of the testicular regression sequence is related to 46,XY partial gonadal dysgenesis. This is based on cases in which there is testicular loss on one side and evidence of dysgenesis on the opposite side. Other causes of embryonic testicular regression sequence include teratogenic effect and vascular accidents (54, 57, 58).

Embryonic testicular regression sequence is differentiated from the vanishing testis syndrome in which there is normal sex differentiation in an individual with 46,XY and loss of testicular tissue on one or both sides. In this condition the loss of testicular tissue is likely to have occurred in later part of gestation and may be related to fetal testicular torsion (54).

e. Causes of 46,XY Gonadal Dysgenesis. Deletions of the distal region of the short arm of the Y chromosome including *SRY* have been associated with 46,XY complete gonadal dysgenesis. Physical findings of Turner syndrome are present in most of these patients (59).

Mutations of *SRY* account for approximately 15% of patients with 46,XY complete gonadal dysgenesis. Most of these mutations are in the HMG box and some of them have been shown to reduce binding of *SRY* to DNA or to reduce the *SRY*-induced bending of DNA (15). Two mutations of *SRY* outside of the HMG box have been reported in association with 46,XY complete gonadal dysgenesis. In addition, large deletions 5' and 3' to the *SRY* gene have been detected (60, 61).

With respect to 46,XY partial gonadal dysgenesis, a point mutation outside of the HMG box was reported in one patient (62). In another case, a large deletion 3' to the *SRY* gene was implicated (61). However, for the most part, *SRY* mutations in this condition are rare.

46,XY true hermaphroditism has been attributed to a point mutation of SRY in one subject. In addition, 46,XY true hermaphroditism has also been related to a postzygotic somatic point mutation in the *SRY* gene (63). These observations underscore the possible relationship between 46,XY partial gonadal dysgenesis and 46,XY true hermaphroditism.

Mutations of *WT-1*, *SF-1*, and *SOX-9* have also been implicated in 46,XY gonadal dysgenesis. Large deletions of DNA involving the *WT-1* gene can result in the WAGR syndrome. Mutations in a coding region of *WT-1* can result in syndromes characterized by Wilms tumor and 46,XY gonadal dysgenesis or syndromes with Wilms tumor, 46,XY gonadal dysgenesis, and progressive nephropathy. Recent studies have indicated that there are two splice variants of the *WT-1* gene. Mutation in alternate transcripts has been proposed as the explanation for the presence of these two presentations (64).

A mutation in the *SF-1* gene was reported in an individual with complete gonadal dysgenesis and adrenal failure. Individuals with duplication of the short arm of the X chromosome that include DAX-1 also have 46,XY gonadal dysgenesis. However, mutations of DAX-1 result in adrenal hypoplasia and hypogonadotropic hypogonadism but no abnormality of sex differentiation (65).

Mutations of the *SOX-9* gene can result in campomelic dysplasia and 46,XY gonadal dysgenesis (66). Various missense mutations have been reported. Both 46,XY complete and 46,XY partial gonadal dysgenesis have been associated with these mutations. In addition, rearrangements of the locus encoding the *SOX-9* gene have also been reported. There are no patients to date with 46,XY gonadal dysgenesis who have *SOX-9* mutations who do not also have campomelic dysplasia.

2. Mosaicism and Chimerism Involving the Y Chromosome

Mosaicism and chimerism occur when cells with two or more karyotypes are found in the same individual. In the case of mosaicism, cells are all derived from the same zygote, and the various karyotypes usually result from nondisjunction. By contrast, chimerism occurs when cells are derived from two zygotes. The cause may be double fertilization or fusion of two embryos.

The most common form of mosaicism involving the Y chromosome is that in which there is a 45,X/46,XY karyotype, a condition often referred to as mixed gonadal dysgenesis. It was originally thought that most subjects with 45,X/46,XY mixed gonadal dysgenesis had ambiguous genitalia. More recently, it has been recognized that 90–95% of subjects with 45,X/46,XY karyotypes have normal male external genitalia. However, many subjects have abnormal testicular histological findings.

Subjects with abnormal sex differentiation usually present in the newborn period and many of them have stigmata of Turner syndrome. Gonadal tumors occur in 10–20% of subjects with 45,X/46,XY karyotypes and abnormal sex differentiation. The management of these patients is similar to that of subjects with 46,XY partial gonadal dysgenesis. Complications associated with the Turner phenotype need to be addressed. In particular, therapy with growth hormone should be considered for patients with subnormal growth. Other forms of mosaicism involving the Y chromosome, such as 45,X/47, XYY and 45,X/ 46,XY/47, XYY, are extremely uncommon (54, 67).

Chimerism may be the cause of a 46,XX/46,XY karyotype in some individuals. The most common presentation of these subjects is true hermaphroditism, although some present a clinical picture similar to 46,XY partial gonadal dysgenesis (54, 68).

3. 46,XX Sex Reversal

The term 46,XX sex reversal comprises two conditions: 46,XX maleness and 46,XX true hermaphroditism. In addition, 45,X sex reversal has been reported.

The 46,XX maleness is a condition in which individuals have testis determination despite a nonmosaic 46,XX karyotype. The phenotype of 46,XX males is very similar to that of Klinefelter syndrome. In particular, most affected subjects have normal male phenotype, although about 15% have hypospadias or ambiguous genitalia. Like subjects with Klinefelter syndrome, the majority of individuals present for evaluation of delayed puberty and gynecomastia. Hormonal evaluation indicates abnormally elevated serum levels of LH and FSH. Plasma testosterone concentration may be normal or somewhat low. Management may involve supplementation with testosterone and surgical correction of gynecomastia (69).

The 46,XX true hermaphroditism is characterized by the presence of both ovarian and testicular tissue in an individual with nonmosaic 46,XX karyotype. Although the clinical phenotype is variable, most affected subjects have ambiguous genitalia and a mix of müllerian and wolffian structures. Surgical correction of external genitalia and subsequent hormonal supplementation depend upon sex of rearing. Only about 4% of subjects with 46,XX true hermaphroditism develop gonadal tumors.

Subjects with 45,X maleness have normal testicular determination but frequently have micropenis, cryptorchidism, and azoospermia. There are also may be other associated problems such as developmental delay, short stature, and congenital anomalies. This condition is extremely unusual. Some individuals with apparent 45,X sex reversal may have hidden mosaicism with the Y-bearing cell line.

More than two-thirds of 46,XX males have a translocation of SRY from the paternal Y to the paternal X chromosome and inheritance of the translocated X. By contrast, most subjects with 46,XX true hermaphroditism and one-third of 46,XX males lack SRY. In these patients, it is necessary to exclude mosaicism. An explanation for 46,XX sex reversal in the absence of SRY has been proposed (70). It is based on the hypothesis that male sex determination is repressed and that testes determination involves derepression. This theory invokes the existence of a repressor of testis determination. In this model mutation of the putative repressor could permit male sex determination in the absence of SRY. However, such a repressor has not been identified.

Recent studies of a single individual with SRY-negative 46,XX maleness implicated a duplication of the locus containing the SOX-9 as the cause of 46,XX sex reversal. Several other reports also described duplication of chromosome 22 in 46,XX in true hermaphroditism (71, 72).

B. Male Pseudohermaphroditism

Male pseudohermaphroditism is a condition in which individuals have a 46,XY karyotype, normal testis determination, but incompletely masculinized external genitalia. The appearance of the genitalia ranges from completely female to slightly feminized external genitalia with only hypospadias and cryptorchidism (see Table 2). Male pseudohermaphroditism includes Leydig cell aplasia/hypoplasia, defects of testosterone biosynthesis, steroid 5-α reductase type 2 deficiency, and androgen insensitivity. Defects in synthesis or function of the antimüllerian hormone can also be considered part of this group.

1. Leydig Cell Aplasia/Hypoplasia: Abnormalities of hCG/LH Receptor

Subjects with Leydig cell aplasia have normal female-appearing genitalia. By contrast, subjects with Leydig cell hypoplasia have a wide range in clinical presentation from micropenis to severe hypospadias. In both severe and mild form, there is absence of müllerian structures due to the secretion of AMH. Testes may be located in the abdomen, inguinal canals, or labia majora. Testosterone production is in the normal to low range depending on the severity of the condition. Sertoli cells are normal, but there is hyalinization of the seminiferous tubules and incomplete spermatogenesis.

Leydig cell aplasia and hypoplasia may be caused by mutations of the hCG/LH receptor. Deletions, nonsense mutations, or frame shift mutations diminish binding of

---

Table 2 Classification of Male Pseudohermaphroditism

hCG/LH receptor dysfunction (Leydig cell aplasia/
  hypoplasia)
Testosterone biosynthesis defects
  StAR deficiency (congenital lipoid adrenal hyperplasia)
  3 β-hydroxysteroid dehydrogenase/Δ^5 isomerase type 2
    deficiency
  CYP17 (17 α-hydroxylase/17,20 lyase) deficiency
  CYP17 (17,20lyase) deficiency
  17β-HSD deficiency
Peripheral unresponsiveness to androgens
  Steroid 5 α-reductase type 2 deficiency
  Androgen insensitivity syndrome
    Complete androgen insensitivity syndrome
    Partial androgen insensitivity syndrome
    Infertile men
    Kennedy syndrome
Persistent müllerian duct syndrome

hCG/LH or adversely affect signal transduction. Most patients with these autosomal recessive mutations are homozygotes or compound heterozygotes (73).

2. Defects of Testosterone Biosynthesis

Five enzymatic defects in testosterone biosynthesis have been described. Three of the defects—StAR deficiency, 3β-hydroxysteroid dehydrogenase deficiency (3β HSD), and P-450 c_{17} hydroxylase deficiency—are associated with decreased secretion of cortisol and aldosterone as well as gonadal steroids. Specific guidelines for evaluation and management of adrenal insufficiency and salt-losing crisis are described in Chapter 7. The other two enzymes, 17,20-desmolase and 17-ketoreductase, are only required for androgen secretion, and only manifest sexual ambiguity. The pattern of inheritance in each of these defects is autosomal recessive.

The phenotype of affected individuals depends on the extent of testosterone secretion and ranges from completely female to almost male. Hence it is impossible to differentiate these conditions on the basis of the external genitalia. The testis may be situated within the labioscrotal folds, inguinal canals, and abdomen. The wolffian derivatives are normally developed or hypoplastic, depending on the severity of the testosterone biosynthetic block. Müllerian structures are absent because the secretion of AMH by Sertoli cells is unaffected.

Subjects raised as males may require surgical correction of the external genitalia and surgery for cryptorchidism. Individuals raised as females will require removal of gonads and wolffian structures and may require revision of external genitalia.

a. Steroidogenic Acute Regulatory Protein Deficiency (Congenital Lipoid Adrenal Hyperplasia). Phenotypic presentation varies, but external genitalia are female in most cases and wolffian ducts are hypoplastic. Computed tomography (CT) or magnetic resonance imaging (MRI) of the abdomen demonstrates large adrenal glands secondary to the accumulation of cholesterol and cholesterol esters. Its incidence is greater in people of Japanese, Korean, and Palestinian descent (51).

Lack of glucocorticoid, mineralocorticoid, and androgen secretion occurs because the StAR protein is defective. This enzyme is responsible for the transfer of cholesterol from outer to inner mitochondria membrane and is the first rate-limiting step in acute steroid synthesis. This condition is associated with the most profound defect of steroidogenesis, and subjects with the complete form of the defect have salt-losing crisis early. The majority of mutations causing congenital lipoid adrenal hyperplasia (CLAH) are in the exons 5–7 of the StAR gene (74).

Earlier studies suggested that defects in *CYP11A*, the gene for the P450 side chain cleavage (*CYP450scc*), was responsible for this disorder. However, genetic analysis of this gene proved normal in patients with lipoid CAH. Homozygous *P450scc* mutations can cause spontaneous

abortions through lack of progesterone synthesis. However, haploinsufficiency of *P450scc* may resemble a late onset of congenital lipoid adrenal hyperplasia (75).

b. 3β-Hydroxysteroid Dehydrogenase Deficiency. 3β-hydroxysteroid (HSD) dehydrogenase catalyzes the conversion of 3β-hydroxy-, Δ^5-steroids to Δ^4-3-keto-steroids (pregnenolone to progesterone, 17-hydroxypregnenolone to 17-hydroxyprogesterone, and dehydroepiandrosterone [DHEA] to androstenedione). Hormonal abnormalities are characterized by increased plasma levels of pregnenolone, 17-hydroxypregnenolone, and DHEA.

Deficiency of 3,βHSD II impairs both adrenal and gonadal steroidogenesis. Genotypic males with the complete form have female genitalia, and salt-losing crisis shortly after birth. Subjects with the partial form have ambiguous genitalia and no salt wasting.

Two genes encode 3,βHSD: type I for placental, skin and breast tissues, and type II gene for adrenal and gonads. Type I and II are 93.5% homologous. These genes belong to the aldo-keto-reductase family rather than the cytochrome P450 family. At least 31 mutations of 3,βHSD type II have been identified in this disorder, including splicing, frame deletions, nonsense, frameshift, and 22 missense mutations. The salt-losing form generally results from severe mutations and is associated with absence of functional 3,βHSD. By contrast, the non-salt-losing form usually results from missense mutation (76).

c. CYP17 (17α-hydroxylase/17,20-lyase) Deficiency. Affected individuals with a 46,XY karyotype have phenotypes ranging from normal-appearing female external genitalia with short vagina in the complete form to ambiguous genitalia in the partial form. The testes are located intra-abdominally, in the inguinal canal, and in the labioscrotal folds. Although cortisol production is subnormal, accumulation of corticosterone results in normal glucocorticoid effect. However, an abnormally high level of desoxycorticosterone (DOC) results in hypertension. In the partial form there is subnormal virilization at puberty. Gynecomastia occurs in some subject. Serum levels of FSH and LH, 11-deoxycorticosterone, corticosterone, and progesterone are elevated. Levels of plasma renin activity, aldosterone, and cortisol are decreased. Glucocorticoid supplementation is indicated to reduce abnormally elevated levels of DOC. Hypertension, hypokalemia, and hyporeninemia normalize with glucocorticoid treatment. At puberty gonadal steroid hormone replacement may be necessary (77, 78).

Although 17α-hydroxylase and 17,20 lyase are encoded by the same gene and both activities are mediated by the same protein, there are situations in which 17α-hydroxylase activity is preserved but 17,20 lyase is defective. Cases of CYP17 deficiency have been related to mutations resulting from deletions, premature truncation, frameshift, and splicing errors. Enzymatic activity of the mutant protein correlates with phenotype. If the 17α-hydroxylase activity is less than 25% of normal, affected

46,XY subjects have feminized external genitalia. Hence, enzymatic activity greater than 25% results in normal fetal masculinization (79).

d. P-450c17 (17,20 Lyase) Deficiency. Affected 46,XY subjects present a range in the appearance of external genitalia according to the severity of the defect. Plasma levels of 17-hydroxysteroids are normal. Plasma levels of DHEA and androgens are decreased, as are levels of 24-hour urinary 17-ketosteroids. The ratio of 17-hydroxyprogesterone/androstenedione after human chorionic gonadotropin stimulation is abnormally elevated (>10). At puberty, proper gonadal steroid replacement is required for development of secondary sexual characteristics. CYP17 mutations that cause isolated 17,20 lyase deficiency in 46,XY subjects have been reported. Mutations in the redox partner-binding site of CYP17 can also cause selective loss of 17, 20 lyase activity (80).

e. 17,β-Hydroxysteroid Dehydrogenase Deficiency. This condition is characterized by failure to convert androstendione to testosterone. Subjects usually present female external genitalia but some have ambiguous genitalia with a minimal degree of masculinization. Marked virilization occurs at puberty with muscular development, enlargement of the phallus, and development of pubic hair. However, gynecomastia is almost always present. Subjects have an increased ratio of androstenedione to testosterone in baseline samples or following hCG stimulation. Baseline serum levels of LH and FSH are markedly elevated at puberty.

Five isoenzymes of 17βHSD catalyze the reduction of androstenedione to testosterone, DHEA to androstenedione, and estrone to estradiol. The type 3 isoenzyme is expressed in the testis, where it catalyzes the reduction of androstenedione to testosterone. Its gene is located on chromosome 9q22. To date, at least 20 clinically significant mutations in the HSD17 β3 have been found including missense, so-called splice junction abnormal-like, and frame-shift mutations. Variation in phenotype has been observed among members of the same kindred (81, 82).

3. Peripheral Unresponsiveness to Androgens

Absent or diminished androgen action in target cells can also result in male pseudohermaphroditism. Two forms have been described: an error in conversion of testosterone to DHT, and insensitivity to androgens.

a. Steroid 5α-Reductase Deficiency. Deficiency of the enzyme steroid 5α-reductase is a rare disorder that results in low plasma levels of DHT and abnormal differentiation of male external genitalia. In the newborn period, affected subjects present with feminized external genitalia with small phallus, chordee, bifid scrotum, and a urogenital sinus that opens onto the perineum. Testes are found in the inguinal canal or labioscrotal folds. Müllerian ducts are absent but wolffian ducts are well differentiated except for the ejaculatory ducts, which end in

a blind vaginal pouch or in the perineum, close to the urethra.

At puberty, spontaneous virilization occurs and the body habitus becomes very muscular. The phallus enlarges up to 8 cm in length, and the labioscrotal folds become rugated and pigmented. Testes enlarge and descend into the labioscrotal folds. Acne, facial hair, and enlargement of the prostate do not occur, indicating that these changes are dependent on DHT. There is no gynecomastia. In a study of affected individuals in the Dominican Republic, almost all individuals initially raised as females adopted male gender identity during puberty. Although the majority of patients are infertile, paternity has been reported in subjects with the mild form of the condition (83).

In adult males, the plasma concentration of DHT is low despite normal or slightly elevated levels of testosterone (T). The T/DHT ratio is >36 (normal, 8–16). Serum plasma LH levels are elevated, suggesting a role for DHT in negative feedback at the level of the hypothalamus. FSH levels are normal or high, reflecting damage to seminiferous tubules. In the newborn period, the T/DHT ratio is high. During infancy and childhood, hCG stimulation also results in normal serum levels of testosterone, but subnormal serum levels of DHT. In the first few months of life, when plasma levels of testosterone and DHT are detectable, the normal T/DHT ratio is a value less than 12. Following hCG stimulation, normal boys from 17 days to 6 months have a T/DHT ratio of 5.2±1.5. T/DHT ratio of 11±4.4 is considered normal in boys from 6 months to 14 years. Abnormally high T/DHT ratios indicate 5α reductase deficiency (84).

46,XX subjects with 5α-reductase deficiency have a normal female phenotype and normal puberty, but decreased axillary and pubic hair. Although menarche is delayed, fertility is normal (83).

The pattern of inheritance in 5α-reductase deficiency is autosomal recessive involving homozygous or compound heterozygous mutations. However, paternal uniparental disomy was found in one patient (85). All cases of steroid 5α-reductase deficiency are related to mutations in the coding region of the 5α-reductase 2 gene. Mutations are found in all five exons of the gene. The majority of subjects have missense mutations (86). Other individuals have deletions, splice-junction, and nonsense mutations. The end product is a nonfunctional or subfunctional protein with decreased affinity of the enzyme to NADPH or decreased binding to testosterone.

If affected babies are raised as males, surgical correction of the external genitalia and cryptorchidism should be performed. Prior to surgery, administration of androgens is recommended to increase phallic length and facilitate hypospadias repair. Normal levels of DHT have been achieved in adults following pharmacological doses of testosterone, presumably though activity of 5α-reductase 1. If the child is raised as a female, surgical correction of external genitalia should be performed and gonadal tissue removed before puberty. Cyclic hormonal therapy at puberty for development of secondary sexual characteristics is required (83).

b. Androgen Insensitivity Syndrome. Androgen insensitivity syndrome (AIS) is comprised of four conditions with distinct phenotypes: complete AIS (CAIS), partial AIS (PAIS), androgen insensitivity associated with the infertile man syndrome, and Kennedy syndrome.

Clinical phenotype

1. Complete Androgen Insensitivity (CAIS) is an X-linked trait with an incidence of 1:20.000–1:64000 male births (87). This condition has also been referred to as the testicular feminization syndrome (88). CAIS is characterized by a normal 46,XY karyotype, female external genitalia with short vagina, absence of müllerian structures, and absent or vestigial wolffian structures. Gonads may be located in the inguinal canal or may be intra-abdominal. Some subjects with CAIS present in infancy or childhood when surgery for inguinal hernia reveals testis in the hernia sack. If gonadectomy is not performed in infancy or childhood, affected subjects have breast development at puberty but little or no axillary hair. Although the clitoris or labia majora are normal, the labia minora may be underdeveloped. Patients usually present in their teens or early 20s because of amenorrhea. Serum levels of LH and testosterone are abnormally elevated. Estradiol, which comes from peripheral conversion of testosterone and from testicular secretion, tends to be in the normal female range. Serum AMH is abnormally high in women with CAIS because the physiological suppression of AMH by testosterone does not occur (89). Women with CAIS have a greater incidence of testicular tumor, with risk increasing significantly after puberty. Management of adult women with CAIS involves gonadectomy and sex hormone supplementation. In some women vaginoplasty may be necessary to improve the length of the vagina.

Wisniewski et al. (90) examined long-term outcome of women with CAIS. Fourteen women were studied using questionnaires and follow-up physical examination. These women considered their development of secondary sexual characteristics to be satisfactory. Furthermore, most patients were satisfied with sexual function. All of the women studied were satisfied with sex of rearing. Nonetheless, the study indicated that more two-thirds of the women had incomplete understanding of their condition.

2. Subjects with Partial Androgen Insensitivity (PAIS) usually present in the newborn period with ambiguous genitalia. Müllerian structures are absent and development of wolffian ducts is usually abnormal. The diagnosis is suspected if there are normal levels of testosterone and a normal testosterone/DHT ratio. Several approaches have been suggested to differentiate PAIS from other conditions with a similar hormonal profile. Some authors have suggested that the extent of penile growth after administration of testosterone or hCG provides an indicator

of responsiveness to androgens. Others have advocated determination of sex hormone-binding globulin (SHBG) levels in blood to identify subjects with PAIS. This is based on the fact that androgen secretion typically results in a diminution of SHBG levels. Hence, higher than normal levels of SHBG in an individual with normal male testosterone and DHT concentration might indicate androgen insensitivity (91). Blood levels of AMH are also suppressed by androgens. Hence the combination of male levels of testosterone and DHT in the face of unsuppressed AMH might indicate PAIS (92).

At puberty, serum levels of LH and testosterone are abnormally elevated, although the T/DTH ratio remains normal. There is enlargement of the penis at puberty, but the penis usually remains small. Serum levels of estradiol are abnormally elevated and gynecomastia is almost always present. Testes are small and there is azoospermia.

3. Subjects with androgen insensitivity associated with infertile men present various phenotypes. Some subjects have mild hypospadias, although many have normal male external genitalia. Like subjects with other forms of AIS, these men have elevated levels of serum LH and testosterone. Subjects are typically ascertained during evaluation for infertility (93).

4. Kennedy syndrome is an X-linked from of spinal and bulbar atrophy, which appears in mid to late adulthood. The association of gynecomastia and the variable presence of impotence and infertility suggest a form of androgen insensitivity and subsequent studies identified a defect in the AR gene (94).

Genetic abnormalities related to AIS. Most cases of CAIS and PAIS are related to mutations in the AR gene and the majority of them are point mutations. Relatively few mutations have been detected in the amino terminal domain. Mutations that result in stop codons in this region are typically associated with CAIS. Deletions of polyglutamine repeats are associated with PAIS. Kennedy syndrome results from expansion of polyglutamine repeats to a number greater than 42 (95).

Within the DNA-binding domain, mutations that result in stop codons or in the deletion of the second zinc finger are associated with CAIS (96). Mutations in the phosphorylation site are associated with both CAIS and PAIS.

Mutations in the hormone-binding domain can result in both complete and partial AIS. Frame shift or point mutations that result in premature termination are associated with CAIS. By contrast, mutations causing less severe defects in hormone binding are more likely to be found in patients with PAIS. Splicing mutations in the AR gene have also been reported in PAIS. They result in transcription of mRNA encoding mutant AR as well as lower levels of mRNA encoding normal AR (97).

AR gene mutations have been identified in some subjects with the androgen insensitivity of infertile men. In a group of nearly 200 infertile men, three unrelated subjects had mutations of AR gene. Two of these mutations were in the transactivation domain and one was in the DNA-binding domain (93). In another study, a subject with this condition had a point mutation in the hormone-binding domain that did not diminish steroid binding but resulted in defective transactivation (98). In additional studies Giwercman identified an unusual subject with mutation in the AR gene and phenotypic features of AIS, but normal fertility (99).

Despite correlations between phenotype and genotype that have been made in the AIS, many cases indicate that these relationships do not always apply. For example, most mutations that result in absence of androgen-receptor binding in cultured cells result in CAIS. However, some of these mutations are also associated with PAIS. Most mutations that are associated with intact AR binding in cultured cells are likewise associated with PAIS. Nonetheless, some of them are associated also with CAIS. More surprising is the observation that CAIS and PAIS have been associated with the same mutation in the AR, suggesting that other factors play a role in AR function (95).

Recent reports explain the lack of phenotype–genotype correlation in some patients. In 1997, Holterhus described a patient with PAIS who had a mutation in the AR that resulted in a premature stop codon. Such mutations are usually associated with CAIS. The unexpected mild phenotype in this report was the result of somatic mosaicism (100). The AR was also studied in another family who had AIS and a range of phenotypic appearance among affected members. Studies of this kindred indicated that transactivation of the AR varied over a range of DHT concentrations, suggesting that the range in phenotype might have resulted from variable levels of DHT in each of the individuals in utero (101). More recently Boehmer et al. described a kindred in which one sibling had CAIS and another had PAIS. The differences in phenotype were correlated with differences in 5-reductase activity in the two siblings (102).

AIS has also been attributed to abnormalities in the interaction of coactivators with the AR. In one study CAIS was associated with inability of the AR to interact with AF1 (103). Expansion of the polyglutamine repeats results in decreased binding of ARA 24 and subsequent decreased coactivation, providing a possible explanation for the AIS associated with Kennedy syndrome (44, 94).

4. Male Pseudohermaphroditism Associated with Multiple Congenital Anomalies

Some subjects have well-described syndromes in which there is abnormal sex differentiation in association with other congenital anomalies, but no obvious defect in gonadal differentiation, testosterone biosynthesis, or androgen effect (53). Some examples include Opitz-Frias syndrome, Rieger's syndrome, Rapp-Hodgkin ectodermal dysplasia, the CHARGE association and VATER syn-

drome. Many cases of male pseudohermaphroditism and multiple congenital anomalies are sporadic, but they frequently involve other defects in the genitourinary system. In addition, maternal exposure to certain drugs, such as dilantin, trimethadione, and progesterone, have been implicated in abnormal sex differentiation.

5. Timing Defect and Idiopathic Male Pseudohermaphroditism

Several patients have been reported who had a 46,XY karyotype and ambiguous genitalia, but normal production of testosterone and DHT at puberty and normal responsiveness to androgens. It was suggested that these subjects had delayed differentiation of Leydig cells and the term timing defect was applied to this condition (104). It is possible that subjects with so-called idiopathic male pseudohermaphroditism have such a timing defect.

6. Persistent Müllerian Duct Syndrome

The persistent müllerian duct syndrome (PMDS) is defined by the presence of müllerian derivatives (uterus, fallopian tubes, and superior two-thirds of the vagina) in otherwise normal 46,XY subjects (105). This rare form of male pseudohermaphroditism has been reported in approximately 150 subjects. Patients with PMDS present with cryptorchidism, inguinal hernias, or both. Herniation of the müllerian structures through the inguinal ring and transverse testicular ectopia are frequent associations.

Persistent müllerian duct syndrome occurs in two different anatomical forms. The form characterized by partially descended testes (80–90% of reported cases) occurs with unilateral cryptorchidism and contralateral inguinal hernia. Typically, the undescended testis is in the inguinal canal. This condition is termed hernia uteri inguinalis. Sometimes the opposite testis is in the hemiscrotum with hernia (transverse testicular ectopia). The second form is characterized by undescended testes. The gonads are located in a high position, the uterus is fixed in the pelvis, and both testes are embedded in the round ligament. The round ligament is usually distended in PMDS, leading to abnormal mobility of müllerian derivatives. Furthermore, the testis itself is abnormally mobile because it is not connected to the base of the scrotum. The testes of these males contain germ cells, but are not properly connected to male excretory ducts. Aplasia of the epididymis, as well as aplasia of the upper part of the vas deferens, has been reported. The müllerian segment of the vagina contacts the posterior urethra at the veru montanum, but communication is usually not patent and retrograde urethrography shows a normal male urethra (105).

Affected subjects frequently present for evaluation of undescended testes or inguinal hernia. The diagnosis can be made by sonogram during the evaluation of newborns or infants with cryptorchidism and during surgical exploration. In subjects with bilateral nonpalpable gonads, congenital adrenal hyperplasia in a female must also be excluded. Serum levels of testosterone are typically normal in these patients, but should be assessed. The level of AMH should be measured to help determine the specific problem (abnormality of AMH or receptor) (36). Although pelvic ultrasonography may be useful to detect müllerian structures, false-negative results can occur.

PMDS is inherited either as a sex-limited autosomal recessive trait (the most common) or as a sex-linked recessive trait. Mutations in either the gene for AMH or its receptor are responsible for the lack of regression of the müllerian ducts. Patients with a serum level of AMH in the upper limit of normal are referred to as being AMH-positive. Patients with very low AMH levels, are called AMH-negative. The most common genetic anomaly causing PMDS is a 27 base-pair deletion in exon 10 of the antimüllerian type II receptor gene. This deletion is implicated in approximately 25% of patients presenting with PMDS (106).

The surgical management of patients with PMDS is controversial due to the potential morbidity associated with both the retention and the removal of the müllerian structures. Controversy also exists regarding the malignant potential of the PMDS testes. Surgical excision of persistent müllerian duct structures may result in ischemic and/or traumatic damage to the vas deferens and testes. Optimal management is orchiopexy, leaving the uterus and fallopian tubes in situ. Orchiectomy is indicated for testes that cannot be mobilized to a palpable location. Careful identification of the vas deferens with meticulous dissection of the müllerian structures facilitates intrascrotal placement of the testes. There is an increased risk of malignancy associated with the cryptorchidism (3% to 18%), but not with the retained müllerian structures. These structures remain infantile, and neither cyclic hematuria nor endometrial malignancy occurs. Most of these patients are infertile.

C. Female Pseudohermaphroditism

Female pseudohermaphroditism describes one-third to one-half of patients with ambiguous genitalia. Subjects have 46,XX karyotype, normal müllerian ducts, and masculinization of the external genitalia and urogenital sinus (see Table 3). Wolffian ducts (epididymis, vas deferens, and seminal vesicles) are absent. The degree of masculinization of external genitalia is determined by the extent of androgen secretion and the timing of androgen production. Once female sex differentiation is complete, androgen exposure causes clitoral hypertrophy but no other masculinization of genitalia.

1. Congenital Adrenal Hyperplasia

The most common cause of female pseudohermaphroditism is congenital adrenal hyperplasia (CAH). In these conditions there is an abnormality in the biosynthesis of cortisol and aldosterone. Diminished secretion of cortisol

Table 3 Classification of Female Pseudohermaphroditism

Congenital adrenal hyperplasia
CYP21 (21-hydroxylase) deficiency
CYP11 (11β-hydroxylase) deficiency
3βHSD II deficiency
Exposure to maternal androgens excess
Iatrogenic: androgens and progestins
Virilizing ovarian or adrenal tumor
Luteoma of pregnancy
CYP19 (aromatase) deficiency
Congenital abnormalities

results in marked elevation of plasma ACTH that subsequently stimulates increased production of adrenal androgens and hence masculinization of external genitalia. CYP21 (21 hydroxylase) deficiency is the most common cause of CAH. Two other virilizing forms of CAH are 11βhydroxylase and 3-β hydroxysteroid dehydrogenase deficiencies. (These conditions are discussed at greater length in Chapter 7). A brief summary is presented below.

a. CYP21 (21 Hydroxylase) Deficiency. CYP21 is required for conversion of 17-hydroxyprogesterone to 11-deoxycortisol and progesterone to deoxycorticosterone. Hence CYP21 deficiency decreases both mineralocorticoid and glucocorticoid production. Females with this condition present ambiguous genitalia, or, later in life, virilization. Salt-losing crisis is a potentially life-threatening complication of the severe form of this disorder. Serum levels of 17-hydroxyprogesterone are markedly elevated (3000–40,000 ng/dl), the level depending upon age and severity of the enzyme defect. Androstenedione levels are abnormally high (107, 108).

b. CYP11 (11 Hydroxylase) Deficiency. This condition is characterized by lack of conversion of 11-deoxycortisol to cortisol and conversion of DOC to corticosterone. High blood pressure occurs due to increased levels of DOC (107, 108).

c. 3β-Hydroxysteroid Dehydrogenase/Δ⁴⁻⁵ Isomerase Deficiency. This is characterized by lack of conversion of Δ^5 3βhydroxysteroids to 3 ketosteroids. The synthesis of both aldosterone and cortisol is impaired. Salt-wasting and adrenal crisis can occur in severe forms of this condition. Serum levels of 17-hydroxypregnenolone may be increased due to impaired conversion of 17-hydroxypregnelonone to 17-hydroxyprogesterone. In addition, the ratio of 17-hydroxypregenelonone to 17-hydroxyprogesterone is elevated in these patients (107, 108).

2. Maternal Androgens

a. Iatrogenic. Several drugs have been associated in the past with female pseudohermaphroditism. Progestins such as norethindrone and ethisterone can cause some degree of masculinization of external genitalia. Danazol, used for treatment of endometriosis, has also been implicated as a cause of female pseudohermaphroditism. Stilbestrol and its metabolites are also related to masculinization of female external genitalia through inhibition of 3-β hydroxysteroid dehydrogenase (47).

    b. Androgen-Secreting Tumors. These occurring in the mother can also cause masculinization of the female fetus. Luteoma of pregnancy is a rare tumorlike mass that emerges during pregnancy and regresses spontaneously after delivery. Absence of maternal virilization does not exclude the diagnosis of luteoma of pregnancy. Other androgen-secreting tumors of both the ovary and adrenal have also been reported. Ovarian tumors include Brenner tumor and thecoma, among others. Adrenal tumors causing female pseudohermaphroditism are extremely rare (109).

3. Placental Aromatase Deficiency

Human CYP450 aromatase is expressed in placental syncytiothrophoblast and many other fetal tissues. After the 9th week of gestation, the placenta provides the primary source of circulating estrogens. Lack of placental aromatase exposes the fetus to androgen excess and can result in ambiguous genitalia in females. Diagnosis should be suspected in an infant with female pseudohermaphroditism in whom CAH has been excluded. The diagnosis is suggested by maternal virilization during pregnancy, and abnormally high serum levels of Δ^4 androstenedione, testosterone, and DHT. Low plasma levels of estriol, as well as low urinary estriol concentration, are present. Amniotic fluid concentrations of Δ^4 androstenedione and testosterone are high, while estrone, estradiol, and estriol levels are low (110).

4. Syndromes of Multiple Congenital Abnormalities

Association of female pseudohermaphroditism with cloacal anomalies, renal agenesis or dysplasia, and gastrointestinal and urinary tract anomalies has been reported. The müllerian structures in these patients may be poorly developed and dysplastic. The cause of this defect is uncertain. There is a disorganized differentiation of the caudal development including perineum, genital tubercle, and genital folds (111). Maternal alcohol use during pregnancy has been associated with clitoral hypertrophy.

V. DIAGNOSTIC EVALUATION FOR AMBIGUOUS GENITALIA

When a child is born with ambiguous genitalia, a specialized care team should be convened. A rapid and organized evaluation should be initiated to garner infor-

mation about karyotype, gonadal function, androgen biosynthesis, and internal anatomy.

A. Diagnostic Evaluation

1. History

A thorough family history is important with respect to previous perinatal or neonatal deaths, infertility, consanguinity, or history of infants with ambiguous genitalia. The patterns of inheritance in the various intersex disorders must be considered. A maternal history should focus on complications of pregnancy, especially during the first trimester, and should include information regarding drug and alcohol use as well as hormone administration.

2. Physical Examination

The physical examination should determine whether the infant has dysmorphic features, since many syndromes are associated with ambiguous genitalia. Intrauterine growth retardation suggests a chromosomal anomaly. Abnormal body proportions suggest an associated syndrome of bone dysplasia. Stigmata, such as webbed neck and edematous hands and feet, may be present in mixed gonadal dysgenesis (45,X/46,XY). Table 4 includes some of the conditions associated with genital ambiguity.

    The stretched phallic length should be measured along the dorsum from the pubic ramus to the tip of the glans. The degree of development of the corpora may be assessed by palpation of the shaft. Normal values for stretched penile length in neonates and preterm infants are available, as are normal values for clitoral length (Chap. 42). It is important to note that premature female infants may appear to have clitoromegaly because they have a larger clitoral breadth compared to body size.

    Urethral opening is assessed by careful examination of the ventral area of the phallus for grooves and chordees. The urethral meatus may be anywhere from the tip of the phallus to the perineum. A single opening on the perineum indicates the presence of a urogenital sinus. Fusion of the labia majora should also be assessed. The labioscrotal folds are examined for degree of fusion, development of rugae, and pigmentation. The presence of gonadal tissue must be carefully assessed. Each gonad is evaluated for size, texture, and presence of an epididymis.

    Minimal enlargement of the phallus and only mild posterior fusion may be associated with a mild form of masculinization in an XX individual or a severe form of undermasculinization in an individual with an XY karyotype. Phallic enlargement with nearly complete fusion of the labioscrotal folds may likewise be associated with a minimal defect of masculinization in an individual with a XY karyotype or a very severe abnormality of sexual differentiation in an individual with an XX karyotype. Hence, the extent of masculinization of the external genitalia does not provide information about the underlying diagnosis but merely provides information about the extent of the abnormality once the karyotype is known.

Table 4 Syndromes and Chromosomal Abnormalities Associated with Ambiguous Genitalia

Abnormalities	Clinical findings
Chromosomal	
Trisomy 13	Holoprosencephalia, polydactyly, cleft lip, hypospadias, cryptorchidism
Trisomy 18	Clenched hand, short sternum, malformed auricles, male cryptorchidism, virilized females
Triploidy syndrome	Prenatal growth failure, microphtalmia, congenital heart defects, hypospadias, micropenis
4p$^-$	Supreorbital ridges, synophrys, large ears, incomplete masculinization
13q$^-$	Mycrocephaly, coloboma, thumb hypoplasia, incomplete masculinization
Syndromes	
Aaskog	Hypertelorism, brachydactyly, shawl scrotum, cryptorchidism
Campomelic Dysplasia	Flat facies, bowed tibiae, hypoplastic scapulae, 46, XY partial gonadal dysgenesis
Carpenter	Acrocephaly, polydactyly, and syndactyly of the feet, lateral displacement of inner canthi, mental retardation, hypogonadism
CHARGE	Colobomata, heart defect, choanal atresia, retarded growth, genital hypoplasia, ear anomalies
Curradino	Partial sacral agenesis with intact first sacral vertebra ("sickle-shaped sacrum"), a presacral mass, and anorectal malformation (Currarino triad)
Ellis-Van Crevel	Mesomelic dwarfism, polydactyly, cardiac anomalies, cryptorchidism
Fraser	Cryptophthalmos (eye hidden, fused lids, absence of palpebral fissure), defect of auricle, males with cryptorchidism and hypospadias, females with vaginal atresia
SCARF	Lax skin, joint hyperextensibility, umbilical and inguinal hernias, craniosynostosis, pectus carinatum, abnormally shaped vertebrae, enamel hypoplasia with hypocalcification of the teeth, facial abnormalities, wide webbed neck, ambiguous genitalia, multiple nodular liver tumors, and mild psychomotor retardation
Lissencephaly X-linked	Lissencephaly with ambiguous genitalia
Meckel-Gruber	Encephalocele, polydactyly, renal cystic dysplasia, ambiguous genitalia
Oral–facial–digital	Polydactyly, campomelia, ambiguous genitalia, cystic dysplastic kidneys, and cerebral malformation
Rieger's	Iris dysplasia, maxillar hypoplasia, hypospadias
Robinow	Short stature, mesomelic and acromelic brachymelia, hypertelorism, wide palpebral fissures, midface hypoplasia and large mouth, and hypogenitalism
Short rib polydactylia	Cleft lip, malformed larynx with hypoplastic epiglottis, pulmonary hypoplasia, renal cysts, ambiguous genitalia, pachygyria, and small cerebellar vermis
Smith-Lemli-Opitz, type II	Mutations in the delta-7-dehydrocholesterol reductase gene in chromosome Failure to thrive, facial dysmorphism, ambiguous genitalia, syndactyly, postaxial polydactyly, and internal developmental anomalies (Hirschsprung's disease and cardiac and renal malformations)
Smith-Lemli-Opitz, type I	Failure of masculinization, intra-abdominal testes, a normally shaped uterus and vagina, polydactyly, cleft palate, blepharoptosis, and abnormalities of the kidneys, liver, and lungs
VACTER	*V*ertebral anomalies, *A*nal atresia, *T*racheo-*E*sophageal fistula, *R*adial and *R*enal dysplasia, bifid scrotum
WAGR	Contiguous gene syndrome: *W*ilms tumor, *A*niridia, cataract, ambiguous *G*enitalia, gonadoblastoma, genitourinary abnormalities, mental *R*etardation

3. Etiologic Evaluation

Adrenal hyperplasia is always a possibility in an infant who presents with ambiguous genitalia. Therefore, throughout the period in which diagnostic tests are performed, careful attention must be paid to blood chemistry and vital signs to ensure that early and appropriate treatment is started if clinical presentation suggests congenital adrenal hyperplasia.

Migeon et al. have described a program for the evaluation of the ambiguous genitalia in the first week (54). A karyotype is obtained on the first day of life and is usually done using peripheral lymphocytes. Occasionally chromosome analysis from other tissues may be necessary to exclude mosaicism. Plasma levels of testosterone and dihydrotestosterone are determined on day 1–2 since there is a physiological peak of testosterone secretion in normal boys at this time. Occasionally, assay of other plasma steroids precursors of testosterone synthesis may be indicated. Plasma levels of 17-hydroxyprogesterone and 17-hydroxypregnelonone should be determined on day 3–4. It is necessary to obtain the blood sample until day 3–4, because contaminating plasma steroids result in spuriously high levels. Assays of both testosterone and 17-hydroxyprogesterone require a chromatographic step prior to assay to prevent additional artifacts (112).

If the baby is clinically stable, imaging studies should de performed on day 5 of life. A genitogram with retrograde injection of contrast media into the urogenital sinus should be performed to detect the presence of müllerian structures, as well as to outline the anatomy of the urethra. Sonography may also be performed to detect müllerian structures. In some instances sonography may be useful to identify abdominal or inguinal gonads. Occasionally an MRI of the pelvis may also be needed.

4. Diagnosis of Ambiguous Genitalia

Migeon and Berkovitz have proposed an algorithm for the diagnosis of ambiguous genitalia in the newborn period (54). If the karyotype indicates mosaicism or possible chimerism involving a Y chromosome, the abnormality of sex differentiation is considered to be a function of the cloning of the various cell types in the gonad. If the karyotype is 46,XX or 46,XY the diagnosis will be established by the hormonal profile, the presence of specific internal duct structures, and, in some cases, by gonadal histological results.

In patients with a 46,XY karyotype and a subnormal plasma level of testosterone, abnormally low levels of steroid precursors of testosterone indicate the possibility of 46,XY gonadal dysgenesis, 46,XY true hermaphroditism, and Leydig cell aplasia hypoplasia. Subnormal levels of plasma testosterone, but abnormal elevation of plasma precursors of testosterone, indicate a defect in the biosynthesis of testosterone. If levels of plasma testosterone and DHT are normal or elevated but the ratio of T to DHT is abnormally elevated, a diagnosis of 5α-reductase deficiency is made. If plasma concentration of T and DHT is both normal the differential diagnosis includes androgen insensitivity, syndromes of multiple congenital anomalies, and idiopathic or timing defects.

In subjects with a 46,XX karyotype, diagnostic considerations include abnormalities of gonadal differentiation and those resulting from exposure of the fetus to excess androgen. The former group comprises 46,XX true hermaphroditism and the XX maleness. When normal ovarian differentiation has occurred, masculinization may have resulted from congenital adrenal hyperplasia (deficiency of 21-hydroxylase, 3β HSD, and 11-hydroxylase), androgen-secreting tumors in the mother, placental aromatase deficiency, various drugs, and syndromes of multiple congenital anomalies.

VI. MANAGEMENT OF INTERSEX

A. Introduction

The management of children born with ambiguous genitalia has been guided by the traditional policy developed by psychologists in collaboration with pediatric endocrinologists and other health care professionals (113). This management has been based on assessment of the anatomy of sex organs, on likely cosmetic appearance of the reconstructed genitalia, on the potential for normal sex steroid secretion at puberty, the potential for normal sexual intercourse, and on the potential for fertility. It has also been referred to as the optimal-gender policy.

Gender assignment has been recommended as early as possible to minimize the period of gender uncertainty. Surgery of the external genitalia has been recommended to facilitate consistent gender-typical rearing by the family. As an example, female gender has been considered appropriate for girls with the masculinized form of CAH. This has been based on the consideration that adequate replacement therapy will permit ovarian sex hormone secretion and normal fertility and because reconstructive surgery will allow for sexual intercourse later in life.

Over the past few years, patient activists have questioned aspects of the traditional policy for gender assignment at the earliest age possible and have emphasized the risk of early genital surgery. The Intersex Society of North America was established to involve the public in an open discussion about management of intersex patients. They have objected to early genital surgery on the grounds that the patient is too young to provide informed consent (114).

Another critique of the traditional approach to intersex management comes from biological determinists who claim that prenatal androgens play a critical role in the masculinization of the fetal brain, and therefore influence behavior and gender identity later in life. Improved understanding regarding the long-term outcome of intersex patient management is helping to guide changes in the traditional policy (90, 115).

B. Gender Assignment at Birth

Gender assignment of infants with ambiguous genitalia at birth requires open and intense communication between the medical team and the family. Counseling requires avoidance of oversimplification. However, complete information must be provided and presented in a way that can be assimilated by the family. The physician must be open to new information. For example, recent data show that penile growth potential in newborns with micropenis is greater than previously thought. As a consequence, reassignment in the baby with full male differentiation and micropenis is no longer recommended (116).

The American Academy of Pediatrics has published a statement concerning evaluation of the newborn with developmental anomalies of the external genitalia. It emphasizes that sex of rearing be based on the potential for fertility, capacity for normal sexual function, endocrine function, potential malignant change, and testosterone imprinting. It is useful for health care professionals to develop a sex-assignment team where a multidisciplinary approach that includes parental involvement can be provided for the management of the intersex patient (117). Pediatric endocrine societies are also in the process of developing consensus guidelines for gender assignment. Such guidelines should be revised at regular intervals or whenever major new evidence comes to light.

C. Gender Reassignment in Childhood

Gender reassignment must take into consideration the child's development, the family's beliefs, and the cultural environment. Uncertainty exists regarding the latest time for gender reassignment without an increased risk of conflict in the child's emerging sense of gender identity. Early studies suggested a cut-off age of 18 months. Newer data suggest an earlier cut-off date, perhaps around 9 months of age. After that age, the child's emerging habitual gender-role behavior and identity must be carefully evaluated for compatibility with the recommended gender. Such an evaluation can be an arduous task because of the child's cognitive limitations at this stage of development and because of the potential for emotional sensitivity (118). In addition to considering the child's gender development, the clinician must evaluate the family's expectations, the family's flexibility, and the societal context. The child and the family must be able to cope with the gender reassignment. Clinicians should be careful not to superimpose their own cultural values.

D. Gender Assignment and Reassignment in CAH

Almost all female CAH patients, when appropriately diagnosed, are raised as girls. However, some patients who are born with markedly masculinized external genitalia have been inadvertently assigned to the male gender. In cases in which the diagnosis was made later, many physicians have recommended reassignment to the female gender after appropriate parental consent. Most 46,XX patients with CAH who have been assigned or reassigned to the female gender at an early age remain females lifelong. A small group of patients self-initiate gender reassignment at around puberty or later, and sometimes even as late as in midadulthood. Patients with CAH and 46,XX karyotype who have been reared in the male gender until late childhood or early adolescence usually elect to remain boys even after CAH is diagnosed. However, occasional patient-initiated reassignments to the female gender have been reported. Thus, an apparently stable gender identity in childhood does not necessarily preclude gender change

at a later age, nor does a successful gender reassignment in childhood exclude gender problems later in life (118).

Assigning newborns with CAH and penile urethra to the male gender has also been discussed but remains extremely controversial. Arguments in favor of male gender assignment include the consideration that a well-formed penis with a penile urethra does not require surgery, whereas reconstruction along female lines may not produce a vagina adequate for sexual intercourse, and may damage neuronal connection and vascular supply to the clitoris. Arguments against male gender assignment include the observation that the obligatory gonadectomy will be accompanied by loss of fertility and that there may be a need for sex hormone therapy at puberty. Studies involving large numbers of patients are needed before a change in policy can be made regarding gender assignment in patients with CAH with marked genital masculinization.

E. Gender Identity

Gender identity refers to the sense of belonging to or fitting into the male or female gender. Gender-role behavior denotes the behavior typical of one gender or the other in a given historical time and place.

Considerable information on the influence of prenatal androgen exposure on gender role behavior comes from studies of CAH. Various categories of sexually dimorphic behaviors are affected in girls with CAH. They include toy preferences, rough-and-tumble play, aggressiveness, interest in sports, maternal behavior, and vocational preferences. It has been suggested that the most important factor accounting for the difference in sexually dimorphic behavior between CAH girls and controls appears to be the effect of the prenatal androgens on sexual differentiation of the brain. Several researchers have indicated that the degree of genital masculinization is an indicator of the degree of masculinization of the brain. Indeed masculinized behavior is more prevalent among girls with salt-wasting CAH than it is in the simple virilizing form (119). If, as expected, much of the shift toward increased masculinization of behavior in CAH is due to the atypical prenatal androgen milieu, a reduction in prenatal androgen levels by prenatal dexamethasone treatment should reduce the degree of masculinization on the brain. However, concerns about the potential behavioral side effects of this treatment have been raised and are being addressed in continuing studies (120).

Many parents become anxious and uncomfortable when their daughter with CAH shows markedly gender-atypical behavior. Children with CAH should be monitored regularly and assessed unobtrusively for the degree of gender-atypical behavior. In addition, family milieu should be evaluated for acceptance of such behavior. In this regard appropriate psychological/psychiatric counseling promoting the acceptance of the behavior can be undertaken. Girls with CAH with markedly gender-atypical behavior persisting into late childhood and early to mid-adolescence may become alienated from their gender-typical peer group. The alienation can lead to isolation, self-doubts, and depressive features. Such girls may profit from individual counseling and from contact with other girls in support groups. There is a published counseling guide in the intersex area, which is strongly recommended to patients and health care providers. Women with salt-losing CAH have an increased rate of bisexual or homosexual orientation, as demonstrated in sexual imagery such as erotic and romantic fantasies and dreams and sexual attractions; many of these women consider themselves lesbians.

Long-term studies of outcome in large numbers of subjects with 46,XY karyotypes and ambiguous genitalia are now being performed. Physical and psychological aspects are being explored. Such studies will provide additional perspective on the relative influence of prenatal androgens and environment.

F. Surgery During Infancy and Childhood

The timing of genital surgery in the course of a child's development is likely to have important psychological implications. In infancy, the decision must be made by the parents in consultation with physicians. Parents must have unequivocal commitment to the decision. Comprehensive genital surgery in infancy without any need for later procedures is intuitively beneficial, but no systematic data are available on the differences in psychological consequences of early vs. late surgery. Parents of newborns not only want to reach a decision about sex of rearing as soon as possible but also want the genitalia to appear similar to other children of the same sex and age.

Surgical techniques have advanced dramatically and skillful surgeons have achieved satisfactory outcomes in the majority of intersex patients. In particular, advances in techniques for reconstruction of male external genitalia have allowed definitive repair in infancy and early childhood. Timing of genital reconstruction in female subjects is more problematic. For example, it is not clear whether it is easier for an adolescent woman to undergo vaginal reconstruction just before she is ready to become sexually active or whether is preferable to perform surgery earlier, with the obligation to use dilators until the patient starts engaging in regular sexual intercourse. Prescribing vaginal dilatation during middle childhood presents difficulties. Cessation of early surgical intervention has been advised in several cases because of the emotional effect on the child. However, no systematic data on psychosocial acceptability and outcome are available. Individuals vary widely in the timing and pattern of sexual socialization. However, it is likely that an inadequate vagina and a reduction in erotic sensitivity, orgasmic capacity, and sexual satisfaction will inhibit courtship and perhaps reduce interest in sexual activity altogether.

Esthetic and gender-typical appearance continue to be useful criteria for surgical outcome, although attention must also be paid to long-term sexual functioning. Quality-of-life considerations, including sexual life in adolescence and adulthood, must be considered. In this regard as well, there is a major need for pediatric societies to develop consensus guidelines.

The performance of genital surgery without the child's fully informed consent has been severely criticized by the Intersex Society of North America. This point of view must be weighed against the complexities regarding the need for sex definition (121).

G. Examination of the Genitalia

Examination of the genitalia is crucial in evaluating the need for surgery, the outcome of surgery, and the impact of lapses in hormonal treatment. The physician must be aware of the potentially adverse psychological consequences of such examinations, even if the child seems overtly compliant. Genital examinations have more significant psychological implications than examinations of other body parts. Many patients become oversensitized by frequent examination. Hence, such examinations must be performed with psychological sensitivity. Their repetition by multiple trainees should be avoided. Alternative training strategies should be developed that do not adversely affect the patient.

H. Psychological Counseling

Most authors recommend an annual visit particularly during adolescence, with a mental health professional who is familiar with the psychosocial and sexual problems of intersex patients. It can be beneficial to have the same person involved in this capacity over the years, provided that the rapport with the patient is generally good. In addition, meeting one or more patients with the same or similar condition can be extremely helpful for patients with an uncommon disorder. The creation of clinic-affiliated support groups is recommended. Patient support groups on the Internet can also be useful. When recommending support-group affiliation, one should always make the patient aware of the risks, including biases, of these groups. The patient should be encouraged to discuss novel information acquired from support groups with his or her physician or mental health specialist. Patients with specific sexual dysfunction may need to be evaluated by a specialist who can review all endocrine, anatomical, surgical, and psychological factors that may be involved and who can plan an intervention in consultation with the respective specialists. Given the scarcity of mental health personnel familiar with intersex problems, physicians and patient organizations should press for appropriate training of mental health liaison personnel and for third-party coverage of the respective services.

Table 5 Stretched Penile Length in Normal Males

Age	Mean ± SD (cm)	Mean ± SD (cm)
Newborn, 30 wk	2.5 ± 0.4	1.5
Newborn, 34 wk	3.0 ± 0.4	2.0
Newborn, term	3.5 ± 0.4	2.4
0–5 months	3.9 ± 0.8	1.9
6–12 months	4.3 ± 0.8	2.3
1–2 yr	4.7 ± 0.8	2.6
2–3 yr	5.1 ± 0.9	2.9
3–4 yr	5.5 ± 0.9	3.3
4–5 yr	5.7 ± 0.9	3.5
5–6 yr	6.0 ± 0.9	3.8
6–7 yr	6.1 ± 0.9	3.9
7–8 yr	6.2 ± 1.0	3.7
8–9 yr	6.3 ± 1.0	3.8
9–10 yr	6.3 ± 1.0	3.8
10–11 yr	6.4 ± 1.1	3.7
Adult	13.3 ± 1.6	9.3

Source: Adapted from Ref. 29.

VII. MICROPENIS

Micropenis is characterized by a normally formed penis with a stretched penile length more than 2.5 standard deviations below the mean for age. Normative data are provided in Table 5 and in Chapter 42 (29). The mean stretched penile length in newborns is 3.5 cm (minus 2.5 standard deviation: 1.9 cm). Ethnic differences have been reported, with a smaller mean penile length in newborns of Chinese origin than in newborns of White and East-Indian origins (122).

Measurement of penile length should be made on the fully stretched rather than flaccid penis. A ruler should be pressed against the pubic ramus, depressing the suprapubic fat pad as completely as possible. The penis should be stretched by grasping the glans between the thumb and forefinger. The measurement is made along the dorsum to the tip of the glans without including the foreskin, if present. Accurate examination and measurement are essential in determining the presence of micropenis. Micropenis must be differentiated from so-called hidden penis, defined as a normal penis obscured by excessive suprapubic fat, and from a penis held down by marked chordee, in which it has a downward bowing as a result of a congenital anomaly (123).

Patients with micropenis may be classified in four major groups:

1. Hypogonadotropic hypogonadism is characterized by an abnormality in the hypothalamic–pituitary axis, resulting in inadequate androgen production. Syndromes in this category include Kallmann syndrome, Prader-Willi syndrome, Laurence-Moon syndrome, Rud syndrome, and conditions with multiple pituitary hormone deficiency.

2. Hypergonadotropic hypogonadism is characterized by primary gonadal failure. Conditions included in this category are Klinefelter syndrome, other X polysomies, Robinow syndrome, trisomy 21, Noonan syndrome, and Laurence-Moon syndrome.

3. Failure of androgens' action includes subjects with mild partial androgen insensitivity.

4. Idiopathic micropenis: Subjects in this category have normal hypothalamic–pituitary–gonadal function. Very rarely the entire penis is absent, a condition named aphallia (124).

The work-up of patients with micropenis should be directed toward early diagnosis and therapy. Other potential dangerous conditions that may be associated with gonadotropin deficiency, such as hypothyroidism, hypocortisolemia, growth hormone deficiency, and diabetes insipidus should be excluded and treated. In particular, infants should be carefully monitored. Plasma levels of FSH, LH, and testosterone should be determined. A gonadotropin-releasing hormone stimulation test and/or an hCG stimulation test may also be helpful in establishing the cause of the micropenis.

The ability of the penis to respond to androgens can be assessed following administration of testosterone or hCG in the newborn period. Treatment with intramuscular testosterone in infancy and childhood has been recommended to improve the appearance of the penis and to facilitate toilet training. The side effects of this treatment are minimal, and include temporary acceleration in growth and advancement of bone age, in addition to some others. Replacement therapy at puberty may be necessary in some individuals.

Wisniewski et al. examined long-term outcome among subjects with congenital micropenis (13 raised as males and 5 raised as females). Subjects were studied with questionnaires and physical examination. Penile length in individuals raised male was below the mean in all subjects. Many men reported dissatisfaction with the appearance of their genitalia. Both males and females were satisfied with their sex of rearing. Nonetheless, subjects raised female required several surgical procedures for reconstruction of their genitalia (115).

VIII. HYPOSPADIAS

Hypospadias is defined as abnormal placement of the urethral meatus. Isolated hypospadias is the most common congenital malformation in males, with an estimated incidence of 1:300 live male births. In the United States, the incidence of hypospadias has increased over the past years (125). There is a familial tendency with an increased risk among certain ethnic groups. It has been reported that 21% of subjects with isolated hypospadias had another family member with hypospadias: 14% having an affected brother and 7% having an affected father (126).

Formation of the ventral foreskin of the penis is related to normal urethral development. Failure of the urethra to reach the tip of the glans is accompanied by absence of the ventral foreskin. This absence causes ventral curvature of the penis known as chordee, which frequently accompanies hypospadias. If normal development of the urethra is arrested and the urethral folds fail to fuse, the meatus may be found anywhere along the course of the penis from the perineum to the glans.

Hypospadias is classified based on the location of the urethral meatus after ventral curve has been surgically corrected. The most common form is the anterior hypospadias (glandular or coronal types), which accounts for 50% of all cases of hypospadias. The distal penile, midshaft, and proximal penile forms make up 30%. The remaining 20% are posterior forms (penoscrotal and perineal) (127).

The cause of hypopadias is multifactorial. In the majority of cases of isolated hypopadias the cause remains unknown. Hypospadias has been also associated with disorders of male sexual differentiation (127, 128). Environmental estrogens and antiandrogens have also been associated with isolated hypospadias. Hypospadias may be associated with syndromes of human malformation, such as Smith-Lemli-Opitz syndrome and cerebrohepatorenal syndrome. Subjects with severe hypospadias with and without cryptorchidism required a complete evaluation of ambiguous genitalia (see above).

Surgical reconstruction of hypospadias requires correction of chordee when present. It is recommended that boys with hypospadias not be circumcised, because the foreskin may be used in the urethroplasty. If hypospadias is associated with micropenis, treatment with testosterone is usually performed before surgery.

IX. CRYPTORCHIDISM

A. Definition

Cryptorchidism, defined as failure of the testis to descend into the scrotum, is another common disorder in boys. Undescended testis has a prevalence of 4–5% in full-term boys and 9–30% in premature boys (30). Spontaneous testicular descent usually occurs by the first year of life, when the prevalence of cryptorchidism declines to 1%. Undescended testis is usually unilateral (90%) and most often right-sided. The undescended testis can be located along of the inguinal canal (72%), just distal to the external ring (20%), or intra-abdominally (8%). In rare instances, the testis deviates from the normal pathway, a condition referred to as ectopic testis. The ectopic testis may be located in the superficial inguinal pouch, perineum, femoral canal, prepenile scrotum, or contralateral scrotum.

The true undescended testis must be differentiated from conditions such as the so-called retractile testis: a normal testis that has an active cremasteric reflex that pulls it back into the groin. In this condition, the testis can be brought into the scrotum without the testis being under tension. A retractile testis can often be more easily brought into the scrotum when the child assumes a squatting position. Alternatively, it may be seen in the scrotum when the child is in a warm bath.

B. Etiology

Undescended testis results from a disruption in physiological testicular descent. Decreased androgen production as a consequence of abnormalities of the hypothalamic–pituitary axis, such as anencephaly, pituitary aplasia, and Kallmann syndrome, is associated with the occurrence of undescended testis. Defects of androgen synthesis and androgen-receptor insensitivity are also associated with the presence of undescended testis (129, 130). Mechanical anomalies related to urogenital obstruction including prune belly syndrome, posterior urethral valves, and defects of the abdominal wall such as gastrochisis and omphalocele cause undescended testis (131). Several syndromes with different chromosomal abnormalities (deletions, duplications, trisomies) include undescended testis among their features. Genetic factors may play a role, this being suggested by the occurrence of undescended testis in 1.5–4% of fathers and 6.2% of brothers of patients with cryptorchidism (30).

Insulin-like hormone-3 (INSL-3), also known as Leydig insulin-like protein, is involved in testicular descent. Mice with mutations of INSL-3 have bilateral undescended testis with abnormal development of the gubernaculums (132). Tomboc et al. reported the presence of two mutations in the connecting peptide region of the protein in 2 of 145 patients with undescended testis (133).

C. Evaluation of Undescended Testes

In newborns with male external genitalia and bilateral undescended testis, salt-losing congenital adrenal hyperplasia in a female infant must be excluded. If the karyotype is 46,XY, the presence of dysmorphic features may indicate a specific syndrome. Radiological studies may be warranted in the diagnosis of undescended testis. Testes located in the external inguinal canal or just adjacent to the external inguinal ring are easily detected by a high-resolution ultrasound scan (134). In a 46,XY subject with unilateral undescended testis, evaluation is advised at 1 year of age. In older children with undescended testis, hormonal evaluation, including evaluation of LH, FSH, and AMH is recommended. In children with hypogonadotropic hypogonadism, complete hormonal evaluation is indicated as discussed in the section on micropenis.

D. Consequences of Cryptorchidism

Testicular neoplasm, infertility, testicular torsion, and inguinal hernia are the most common complications of undescended testis. The risk of testicular malignancy in the general population is 1 in 45,000 males. However, 10% of adult testicular tumors occur in men with a history of undescended testis. The risk of testicular tumor in subjects with unilateral and bilateral undescended testis is 15 and 33 times greater, respectively, than that of subjects with normal testes. Intra-abdominal testes are five times more likely to develop a tumor. Germ-cell degeneration and dysplasia are considered the causes of malignancy. Seminomas are the most common type of malignancy, followed by embryonal cell carcinoma. Most studies indicate that bringing the testis down into the scrotum does not reduce the risk of subsequent malignancy. Malignancy may occur after orchiopexy or in the contralateral normally descended testis (30).

Infertility is due to lack of or decrease in the number of germ cells as a consequence of temperature-induced degeneration. Histological abnormalities with decreased number of the spermatogonia in undescended testis are reported as early as 3 months of age (135). By 2 years of age the germ cells have decreased to 40% of normal. There is also an increase in interstitial fibrosis and collagenization in peritubular connective tissue. There is indirect evidence that the abnormality in the contralateral descended testis occurs at an early age. Autoantibodies to the undescended testis may be produced and can cause degenerative changes in the descended testis. Paternity rates are lower in men with history of bilateral cryptorchidism than in men with a history of unilateral cryptorchidism. Sudden painful inguinal swelling in association with cryptorchidism can represent testicular torsion or hernia with incarceration, both of which indicate the need for urgent intervention.

E. Treatment

The therapeutic goals in treating cryptorchidism are to prevent infertility, avoid malignancy, correct an associated hernia, if present, and alleviate psychological stress caused by the empty scrotum.

1. Hormonal Therapy

Different protocols with hCG and/or pharmacological preparation of gonadotropin-releasing hormone (GnRH) have been used with a range of success. The World Health Organization recommends hCG 250 IU twice a week for 5 weeks in boys up to 1 year of age. From 1 to 5 years of age, 500 IU is recommended twice weekly for 5 weeks. In older boys, 1000 IU twice weekly is suggested for 5 weeks. Nonetheless, published dosages and treatment schedules have varied from 100 to 4000 IU per injection given 2–3 days per week for 1–5 weeks. Combined treatment using hCG and GnRH analogs for a total of 4 weeks has been reported to improve response in nonpalpable testis (136).

Successful treatment of the true undescended testis with hCG has varied from 6 to 65%. Hormonal treatment is more effective in the treatment of testis located immediately prescrotally. However, some reports suggest that hormonal therapy is only successful for those testes that would have ultimately descended without surgery.

2. Surgical Therapy

The optimal time to operate is unknown, considering that evidence that histological changes in the testis occur early as 2–3 months of age. However, the recommendation of the Action Committee on Surgery of the Genitalia is to perform orchiopexy at 12 months of age. Numerous studies have reported that 75% of testes descend spontaneously by this age without further chance of descent thereafter. Anesthesia risk by this age is minimal when administered by experienced pediatric anesthesiologists. Most orchiopexies are performed as outpatient procedures. Ectopic testes and testes in the inguinal canal are brought into the scrotum by a small inguinal crease incision. The gubernaculum and cremasteric muscle are separated from the testis, and the lateral Prentiss fibers are divided, thereby allowing the testis a more direct route into the scrotum. The testis is then fixed in place with a suture. There is a 90% incidence of inguinal hernia with undescended testis, which is usually repaired simultaneously. The success rate of this operation is reported to be over 95%. Bilateral inguinal testes can be operated on at the same time. Nonpalpable undescended testis can now be located by laparoscopy to inspect the peritoneal cavity. Of nonpalpable testes, 20% are atrophic, and blind-ending spermatic vessels and vas deferens are noted intra-abdominally. Numerous radiological investigations have been performed, including sonograms, CT scans, venography of the spermatic vessels, and, recently, MRI. If, at the time of laparoscopy, the testis is located, an orchiopexy can be performed.

Most testes can be placed within the scrotal sac by one procedure. However, when the spermatic vessels are extremely short, a two-stage orchiopexy can be performed. The spermatic vessels are ligated or divided during the first stage, allowing collateral blood supply via the vasal artery to develop. Then, 4–6 months later, the testis can be brought into the scrotal sac and nourished with the vasal blood supply with a success rate of 90%. In bilateral nonpalpable testis, hCG stimulation tests should be performed before laparoscopy to rule out testicular agenesis. Laparoscopy in children has been shown to be safe by the age of 1 year and can be done as an outpatient procedure (30).

ACKNOWLEDGMENTS

We gratefully acknowledge the excellent editorial assistance of Kaitlin K. Blazejack.

REFERENCES

1. Drews U. Local mechanisms in sex specific morphogenesis. Cytogenet Cell Genet 2000; 91:72–80.
2. Hughes IA. Minireview: sex differention. Endocrinology 2001; 142(8):3281–3287.
3. Ostrer H. Sexual differentiation. Semin Reprod Med 2000; 18:41–49.
4. Swain A, Lovell-Badge R. Mammalian sex determination: a molecular drama. Genes Dev 1999; 13:755–767.
5. Teixeira J, et al. Mullerian-inhibiting substance regulates androgen synthesis at the transcriptional level. Endocrinology 1999; 140:4732–4738.
6. McLaren A. Gonad development. Curr Biol 1998; 8(5):R175–R177.
7. Lejeune H, Habert R, Saez JM. Origin, proliferation and differentiation of Leydig cells. J Mol Endocrinol 1998; 20:1–25.
8. Martineau J, et al. Male-specific cell migration into the developing gonad. Curr Biol 1997; 7:958–968.
9. Jirasek JE. Germ cells and the indifferent gonad (genital ridge). In Polin RA, ed. Fetal and Neonatal Physiology. Philadelphia: WB Saunders 1992:1854–1864.
10. Greenfield A. Genes, cells and organs: recent developments in the molecular genetics of mammalian sex determination. Mammal Genome 1998; 9:683–687.
11. Capel B. The battle of sexes. Mechanisms Dev 2000; 92:89–103.
12. Birk OS, et al. The LIM homebox gene Lhx9 is essential for mouse gonad formation. Nature 2000; 403:909–913.
13. Ottolenghi C, et al. Absence of mutations involving the Lim homeobox domain gene LHX9 in 46,XY gonadal agenesis and dysgenesis. J Clin Endocrinol Metab 2001; 86:2465–2469.
14. Hammer GD, Ingraham HA. Steroidogenic factor-1: its role in endocrine organ development and differentiation. Front Neuroendocrinol 1999; 20:199–223.
15. Berkovitz GD, Seeherunvong T. Molecular basis of sexual differentiation. In Handwerger S, ed. Molecular and Cellular Pediatric Endocrinology. Towota, NJ: Humana Press 1997:1–8.
16. Sinclair AH, et al. A gene from the human sex-determining region encodes a protein with homology to a conserved DNA-binding motif. Nature 1990; 346:240–244.
17. Marshall OJ, Harley VR. Molecular mechanisms of SOX9 action. Mol Gen Metabol 2000; 71:455–462.
18. De Santa B, et al. Direct interaction of SRY-related protein SOX9 and steroidogenic factor 1 regulates transcription of the human anti-Mullerian hormone gene. Mol Cell Biol 1998; 18(11):6653–6655.
19. Goodfellow PN, Camerino G. DAX-1, an "anti-testis" gene. EXS 2001; 91:57–69.
20. Nachtigal MW, et al. Wilms' tumor 1 and DAX-1 modulate the orphan nuclear receptor SF-1 in sex-specific gene expression. Cell 1998; 93:445–454.
21. Parker KL, Schimmer BP, Schedl A. Genes essential for early events in gonadal development. Cell Mol Life Sci 1999; 55:831–838.
22. Veitia RA, et al. Testis determination in mammals: more questions than answers. Mol Cell Endocrinol 2001; 179:3–16.
23. Vainio S, et al. Female development in mammals is regulated by the Wnt-4 signaling. Nature 1999; 397:405–409.
24. MacLaughlin DT, Teixeira J, Donahoe PK. Perspective: reproductive tract development-New discoveries and future directions. Endocrinology 2001; 142:2167–2172.
25. Kuschert S, et al. Characterization of Pax-2 regulatory sequences that direct transgene expression in the Wolffian duct and its derivatives. Devel Biol 2001; 229:128–140.
26. Parr B, McMahon A. Sexually dimorphic development of the mammalian reproductive tract requires Wnt-7a. Nature 1998; 395:707–710.
27. Trelstad RL, et al. The epithelial mesenchyme interface of the male rate Mullerian duct: loss of membrane integrity and ductal regression. Dev Biol 1982; 92:27–40.
28. Gleinster TW. The development of the utricle and the so-called "middle" or "median" lobe of the human prostate. J Ant 1962; 96:443–445.
29. Feldman KW, Smith DW. Fetal phallic growth and penile standards for newborn male infants. J Pediatr 1975; 86:395–398.
30. Hutson JM, Hasthorpe S, Heyns CF. Anatomical and functional aspects of testicular descent and cryptorchidism. Endocr Rev 1997; 18(2):259–280.
31. Jost A, Magre S. Control mechanisms of testicular differentiation. Phil Trans R Soc Lond 1988; 322:55–61.
32. Joss N, di Clemente N. TGF-β family members and gonadal development. Trends Endocrinol Metab 1999; 10:216–222.
33. Gouedard L, et al. Engagement of bone morphogenetic protein type IB receptor and Smad1 signaling by anti-Mullerian hormone and its type II receptor. J Biol Chem 2000; 36:27973–27978.
34. Parr BA, McMahon AP. Sexually dimorphic development of the mammalian reproductive tract requires Wnt-7a. Nature 1998; 395:707–710.
35. Josso N, di Clemente N, Gouedard L. Anti-Mullerian hormone and its receptors. Mol Cell Endocrinol 2001; 179:25–32.
36. Lane AH, Lee MM. Clinical applications of Mullerian inhibiting substance in patients with gonadal disorders. Endocrinologist 1999; 9:208–215.
37. Prince FP. The triphasic nature of Leydig cell development in humans, and comments on nomenclature. J Endocrinol 2001; 168:213–216.
38. Jenkins EP, et al. Genetic and pharmacological evidence for more than one human steroid 5 alpha-reductase. J Clin Invest 1992; 89:293–300.
39. Kuiper GG, et al. Structural organization of the human androgen receptor gene. J Mol Endocrinol 1989; 2(3):R1–4.
40. McKenna NJ, O'Malley BW. From ligand to response: generating diversity in nuclear receptor coregulator function. J Steroid Biochem Mol 2000; 74:351–356.
41. Brinkmann AO, et al. Mechanisms of androgen receptor activation and function. J Steroid Mol Biol 1999; 69:307–313.
42. Brinkmann AO. Lessons to be learned from the androgen receptor. Eur J Dermatol 2001; 11(4):301–303.
43. Poukka H, et al. Coregulator small nuclear RING finger protein (SNURF) enhances Sp1- and steroid receptor-mediated transcription by different mechanisms. J Biol Chem 2000; 275:571–579.
44. Mongan NP, Lim HN, Hughes IA. Genetic evidence to exclude the androgen receptor-polyglutamine associated coactivator, ARA-24, as a cause of male undermasculinization. Eur J Endocrinol 2001; 145:809–811.
45. Cooke PS, et al. Mechanism of estrogen action: lessons from the estrogen receptor-alpha knockout mouse. Biol Reprod 1998; 59:470–475.
46. Hess RA, Bunick D, Bahr J. Oestrogen, its receptors and function in the male reproductive tract—a review. Mol Cell Endocrinol 2001; 178:29–38.

47. McLahlan JA. Environmental signaling: what embryos and evolution teach us about endocrine disrupting chemicals. Endocr Rev 2001; 22:319–341.

48. Kelce WR, Wilson EM. Environmental antiandrogens: developmental effects, molecular mechanisms, and clinical implications. J Mol Med 1997; 75:198–207.

49. Sultan C, et al. Environmental xenoestrogens, antiandrogens and disorders of male sexual differentiation. Mol Cel Endocrinol 2001; 178:99–105.

50. Berkovitz GD, et al. Clinical and pathologic spectrum of 46,XY gonadal dysgenesis: its relevance to the understanding of sex differentiation. Medicine 1991; 70(8): 375–383.

51. Grumbach MM, Conte FA. Disorders of sex differentiation. In Wilson JD, et al., eds. Williams textbook of Endocrinology. Philadelphia: WB Saunders 1998:1303–1425.

52. Verp MS, Simpson JL. Abnormal sexual differentiation and neoplasia. Cancer Genet Cytogenet 1987; 25:191.

53. Neri G, Opitz J. Syndromal (and nonsyndromal) forms of male pseudohermaphroditism. Am J Med Genet 1999; 89: 201–209.

54. Migeon CJ, Berkovitz GD. Sexual differentiation and ambiguity. In Kappy MS, Blizzard RM, Migeon CJ, eds. Wilkins the Diagnosis and Treatment of Endocrine Disorders in Childhood and Adolescence. Springfield: Charles C Thomas, 1994:573–715.

55. Berkovitz GD, Rock JA, Urban MD. True hermaphroditism. Johns Hopkins Med J 1982; 151:290.

56. Marcantonio SM, et al. Embryonic testicular regression sequence: a part of the clinical spectrum of 46, XY gonadal dysgenesis. Am J Med Genet 1994; 49:1–5.

57. Josso N, Briard ML. Embryonic testicular regression syndrome: variable phenotypic expression in siblings. J Pediatr 1980; 97:200–2004.

58. Corrado F, Stella NC, Triolo O. Testicular regression syndrome. A case report. J Reprod Med 1991; 36:549–50.

59. Hawkins JR, et al. Evidence of increased prevalence of SRY mutations in XY females with complete rather than partial gonadal dysgenesis. Am J Hum Genet 1992; 51(5): 979–984.

60. Canto P, et al. A mutation in the 5′ non-high mobility group box region of the SRY gene in patients with Turner syndrome and Y mosaicism. J Clin Endocrinol Metab 2000; 85:1908–1911.

61. McElreavey K, et al. Loss of sequences 3′ to the testis-determining gene, SRY, including the Y pseudoautosomal boundary associated with partial testicular determination. Proc Natl Acad Sci USA 1996; 93(16):8590–8594.

62. Domenice S, et al. A novel missense mutation (S18N) in the 5′ non-HMG box region of the SRY gene in a patient with partial gonadal dysgenesis and his normal relatives. Hum Genet 1998; 102:213–215.

63. Braun A, et al. True hermaphroditism in a 46,XY individual, caused by a postzygotic somatic point mutation in the male gonadal sex-determining locus (SRY): molecular genetic and histologic findings in a sporadic case. Am J Hum Genet 1993; 52:578–585.

64. Hammes A, et al. Two splice variants of the Wilms tumor 1 gene have distinct functions during sex determination and nephron formation. Cell 2001; 106:319–329.

65. Achermann JC, Meeks JJ, Jameson LJ. Phenotypic spectrum of mutations in DAX-1 and SF-1. Mol Cell Endocrinol 2000; 185:17–25.

66. Preiss S, et al. Compound effects of point mutations causing campomelic dysplasia/autosomal sex reversal upon SOX9 structure, nuclear transport, DNA binding, and transcriptional activation. J Biol Chem 2001; 276:27864–27872.

67. Telvi L, et al. 45,X/46,XY mosaicism: report of 27 cases. Pediatrics 1999; 104:304–308.

68. Reindollar RH, et al. A cytogenetic and endocrinologic study of a set of monozygotic isokaryotic 45,X/46,XY twins discordant for phenotypic sex: mosaicism versus chimerism. Fertil Steril 1987; 47:626–633.

69. Zenteno-Ruiz JC, Kofman-Alfaro S, Mendez JP. 46,XX sex reversal. Arch Med Res 2001; (32):559–566.

70. McElreavey K, et al. A regulatory cascade hypothesis for mammalian sex determination: SRY represses a negative regulator of male development. Proc Natl Acad Sci USA 1993; 90:3368–3372.

71. Seeherunvong T, et al. 46, XX sex reversal with duplications of chromosome 22q. In Endocrine Society's 82nd Annual Meeting, June 21–24, 2000, Toronto, Canada.

72. Somkuti S, et al. 46,XY monozygotic twins with discordant sex phenotype. Fertil Steril 2000; 74:1254–1256.

73. Themmen APN, Huhtaniemi IT. Mutations of gonadotropins and gonadotropin receptors: elucidating the physiology and patophysiology of pituitary-gonadal function. Endocr Rev 2000; 21:551–583.

74. Bose HS, et al. Mutations in the steroidogenic acute regulatory protein (StAR) in six patients with congenital lipoid adrenal hyperplasia. J Clin Endocrinol Metab 2000; 85(10):3636–3639.

75. Tajima T, et al. Heterozygous mutation in the cholesterol side chain cleavage enzyme (p450scc) gene in a patient with 46,XY sex reversal and adrenal insufficiency. J Clin Endocrinol Metab 2001; 86:3820–3825.

76. Pang S. Congenital adrenal hyperplasia owing to 3 beta-hydroxysteroid dehydrogenase deficiency. Endocrinol Metab Clin North 2001; 30:81–99.

77. Auchus RJ. The genetics, pathophysiology, and management of human deficiencies of P450c17. Endocrinol Metab Clin North Am 2001; 30:101–119.

78. Miller WL, Geller DH, Auchus RJ. The molecular basis of isolated 17,20 lyase deficiency. Endocr Res 1998; 24: 817–825.

79. Auchus RJ. Congenital adrenal hyperplasia: The genetics, pathophysiology, and management of human deficiencies of P450c17. Endocrinol Metabol Clin North Am 2001; 30:101–119.

80. Gupta MK, Geller DH, Auchus RJ. Pitfallas in characterizing P450c17 mutations associated with isolated 17,20-lyase deficiency. J Clin Endocrinol Metab 2001; 86: 4416–4423.

81. Boehmer ALM, et al. 17Beta-hydroxy dehydrogenase-3 deficiency: diagnosis, phenotypic variability, population genetics, and worldwide distribution of ancient and de novo mutations. J Clinic Endocrinol Metab 1999; 84: 4713–4721.

82. Lindqvist A, Hughes IA, Andersson S. Substitution mutation C268Y causes 17Beta-hydroxysteroid dehydrogenase 3 deficiency. J Clin Endocrinol Metab 2001; 86: 921–923.

83. Fratianni CM, J I-M. The syndrome of 5 alpha-reductase deficiency. Endocrinologist 1994; 4:302–314.

84. Imperato-McGinley J, Peterson RE, Gautier T. Primary and secondary 5 alpha-reductase deficiency. In Serio M, et al., eds. Sexual Differentiation: Basic and Clinical Aspects. New York: Raven Press, 1984:233.

85. Chavez B, VE, Vilchis F. Uniparental disomy in steroid 5alpha-reductase 2 deficiency. J Clin Endocrinol Metab 2000; 85:3147–3150.

86. Vilchis F, et al. Identification of missense mutations in the SRD5A2 gene from patients with steroid 5alpha-reductase 2 deficiency. Clin Endocrinol (Oxf) 2000; 52: 383–387.

87. Ahmed SF, et al. Phenotypic features, androgen receptor binding, and mutational analysis in 278 clinical cases reported as androgen insensitivity syndrome. J Clin Endocrinol Metab 2000; 85:658–665.

88. Morris JM. The syndrome of testicular feminization in male pseudohermaphroditism. Am J Obstet Gynecol 1953; 65:1192–1953.

89. Rey R, et al. Anti-Mullerian hormone in children with androgen insensitivity. J Clin Endocrinol Metab 1994; 79: 960–964.

90. Wisniewski AB, et al. Complete androgen insensitivity syndrome: Long-term medical, surgical, and psychosexual outcome. J Clin Endocrinol Metab 2000; 85:2664–2669.

91. Bertclloni S, et al. Biochemical selection of prepubertal patients with androgen insensitivity syndrome by sex hormone-binding globulin response to the human chorionic gonadotropin test. Pediatr Res 1997; 41:266–271.

92. Rey RA, et al. Evaluation of gonadal function in 107 intersex patients by means of serum anti-Müllerian hormone measurement. J Clin Endocrinol Metab 1999; 84: 627–631.

93. Hiort O, et al. Significance of mutations in the androgen receptor gene in males with idiopathic infertility. J Clin Endocrinol Metab 2000; 85:2810–2815.

94. Hsiao PW, et al. The linkage of Kennedy's neuron disease to ARA24, the first identified androgen receptor polyglutamine region-associated coactivator. J Biol Chem 1999; 274(29):20229–20234.

95. Brinkmann AO. Molecular basis of androgen insensitivity. Mol Cell Endocrinol 2001; 179:105–109.

96. Matias PM, et al. Structural evidence for ligand specificity in the binding domain of the human androgen receptor. Implications for pathogenic gene mutations. J Biol Chem 2000; 275(34):26164–26171.

97. Hellwinkel OJ, et al. A unique exonic splicing mutation in the human androgen receptor gene indicates a physiologic relevance of regular androgen receptor transcript variants. J Clin Endocrinol Metab 2001; 86:2569–2575.

98. Wang Q, et al. Azoospermia associated with a mutation in the ligand-binding domain of an androgen receptor displaying normal ligand binding, but defective trans-activation. J Clin Endocrinol Metab 1998; 83:4303–4309.

99. Giwercman A, et al. Preserved male fertility despite decreased androgen sensitivity caused by a mutation in the ligand-binding domain of the androgen receptor gene. J Clin Endocrinol Metab 2000; 85:2253–2259.

100. Holterhus PM, et al. Mosaicism due to a somatic mutation of the androgen receptor gene determines phenotype in androgen insensitivity syndrome. J Clin Endocrinol Metab 1997; 82:3584–3589.

101. Hellwinkel OJ, Bassler J, Hiort O. Transcription of androgen receptor and 5 alpha reductase II in genital fibroblasts from patients with androgen insensitivity syndrome. J Steroid Biochem Mol 2000; 75:213–218.

102. Boehmer AL, et al. Phenotypic variation in a family with partial androgen insensitivity syndrome explained by differences in 5alpha dihydrotestosterone availability. J Clin Endocrinol Metab 2001; 86:1240–1246.

103. Adachi M, et al. Androgen-insensitivity syndrome as a possible coactivator disease. N Engl J Med 2000; 343(12):856–862.

104. Walsh PC, Migeon CJ. The phenotypic expression of selective disorders of male sexual differentiation. J Urol 1978; 119:627–629.

105. Diaz A, et al. Persistent Müllerian duct syndrome in an infant with initial bilateral cryptorchidism. Int Pediatr 2000; 15:41–43.

106. Lee MM, et al. Measurements of serum Müllerian inhibiting substance in the evaluation of children with nonpalpable gonads. N Engl J Med 1997; 336:1480–1486.

107. Collett-Solberg PF. Congenital adrenal hyperplasia: from genetics and biochemistry to clinical practice, part 2. Clin Pediatr (Phila) 2001; 40:125–132.

108. Collett-Solberg PF. Congenital adrenal hyperplasia: from genetics and biochemistry to clinical practice, part 1. Clin Pediatr (Phila) 2001; 40:1–16.

109. Mazza V, et al. Prenatal diagnosis of female pseudohermaphroditism associated with bilateral luteoma of pregnancy: case report. Hum Reprod 2002; 17:821–824.

110. Bulun SE. Clinical review 78: Aromatase deficiency in women and men: would you have predicted the phenotypes? J Clin Endocrinol Metab 1996; 81:867–871.

111. Chadha R, et al. Female pseudohermaphroditism associated with cloacal anomalies: faulty differentiation in the caudal developmental field. J Pediatr Surg 2001; 36(7): E9.

112. Fuqua JS, et al. Assay of plasma testosterone during the first six months of life: importance of chromatographic purification of steroids. Clin Chem 1995; 41: 1146–1149.

113. Money J, Danon M. Sexological considerations in patients with history of ambisexual birth defects. In Lifshitz F, ed. Pediatric Endocrinology. New York: Marcel Dekker, Inc, 1996:347–353.

114. Intersex Society of North America (ISNA). http:// www.isna.org.

115. Wisniewski AB, et al. Congenital micropenis: long-term medical, surgical and psychosexual follow-up of individuals raised male or female. Horm Res 2001; 56:3–11.

116. Bin-Abbas B, et al. Congenital hypogonadotropic hypogonadism and micropenis: effects of testosterone treatment on adult penile size—why sex reversal id not indicated. J Pediatr 1999; 134:579–583.

117. American Academy of Pediatrics Committee of Genetics. Evaluation of the newborn with developmental anomalies of the external genitalia. Pediatrics 2000; 106: 138–142.

118. Meyer-Bahlburg HF. Gender and sexuality in classic congenital adrenal hyperplasia. Endocrinol Metab Clin North Am 2001; 30.

119. Berenbaum SA, Duck SC, Bryk K. Behavioral effects of prenatal versus postnatal androgen excess in children with 21-hydroxylase-deficient congenital adrenal hyperplasia. J Clin Endocrinol Metab 2000; 85:727–733.

120. Carlson AD, et al. Congenital adrenal hyperplasia: update on prenatal diagnosis and treatment. J Steroid Biochem Mol Biol 1999; 19–29.

121. Lee PA. Should we change our approach to ambiguous genitalia? The Endocrinologist 2001; 11:118–123.

122. Cheng PS, Chanoine J-P. Should the definition of micropenis vary according top ethnicity? Horm Res 2001; 55: 278–281.

123. Bergeson PS, et al. The inconspicuous penis. Pediatrics 1993; 92:794–799.

124. Skoog SJ, Belman AB. Aphallia: its classification and management. J Urol 1989; 141:589.

125. Baskin LS, Himes K, Colborn T. Hypospadias and endocrine disruption: is there a connection? Environ Health Perspect 2001; 109:1175–1183.
126. Boehmer ALM, et al. Etiological studies of severe or familial hypospadias. J Urology 2001; 165:1246–1254.
127. Albers N, et al. Etiologic classification of severe hypospadias: implications for prognosis and management. J Pediatr 1997; 131:386–392.
128. Nordenskjold A, et al. Screening mutations in candidate genes for hypospadias. Urol Res 1999; 27:49–55.
129. Timohiro I, et al. Micropenis and the AR gene: mutation and CAG repeat-length analysis. J Clin Endocrinol Metab 2001; 86:5372–5378.
130. Lim HN, Hughes IA, Hawkins JR. Clinical and molecular evidence for the role of androgens and WT1 in testis descent. Mol Cel Endocrinol 2001; 185:43–50.
131. Koivusalo A, Taskinen S, Rintala RJ. Cryptorchidism in boys with congenital abdominal wall defects. Pediatr Surg Int 1998; 13:143–145.
132. Adham IM, Emmen JMA, Engel W. The role of testicular factor INSL3 in establishing the gonadal position. Mol Cell Endocrinol 2000; 160:11–16.
133. Tomboc M, et al. Insulin-like 3/relaxin-like factor gene mutations are associated with cryptorchidism. J Clin Endocrinol Metab 2000; 85:4013–4018.
134. Nguyen HT, Coakley F, Hricak H. Cryptorchidism: strategies in detection. Eur Radiol 1999; 9:336–343.
135. Huff DS, et al. Abnormal germ cell development in cryptorchidism. Horm Res 2001; 55:11–17.
136. Giannopoulus MF, Viachakis IG, Charissis GC. 13 years' experience with the combined hormonal therapy of cryptorchidism. Horm Res 2001; 55:33–37.

14
Thyroid Disorders in Infancy

Guy Van Vliet
University of Montreal and Sainte-Justine Hospital, Montreal, Quebec, Canada

I. INTRODUCTION

Around the time of birth and during the first few years of life, thyroid hormone economy undergoes major changes that need to be understood for the proper investigation and treatment of thyroid dysfunction. The dramatic consequences of congenital hypothyroidism (CH) that is not diagnosed during the neonatal period for later brain development underline the importance of prompt recognition of abnormal thyroid function test results. Although congenital *hyper*thyroidism is a much less common and usually self-limited entity, it may also lead to dramatic consequences. Heart failure and even death from this condition have been reported in hyperthyroid newborns, and later developmental problems may occur as well.

The most striking changes in plasma thyroid-stimulating hormone (TSH) and thyroid hormone levels occur immediately after birth. It is therefore important to know about the neonatal TSH surge, which reaches its maximum in the first few hours of life, and is followed by a peak in plasma thyroxine (T_4) approximately 24 h later. An isolated TSH measurement in the first 24 h of life may therefore lead to an erroneous diagnosis of primary hypothyroidism, while an isolated measurement of T_4 on the second day of life may lead to an incorrect diagnosis of hyperthyroidism.

However, it is also important to recognize that several parameters of thyroid function, such as the normal ranges of free T_4 and of total T_3, extend to much higher levels in infancy than in older children or adults. The mechanisms underlying these age-related changes in thyroid hormone levels are briefly reviewed in the following section, and the clinical problems are discussed next in order of frequency and importance. The vast majority of these problems present as abnormalities of thyroid function, but some structural thyroid problems may also present in infancy.

II. CHANGES IN THYROID HORMONE ECONOMY FROM CONCEPTION TO 3 YEARS OF AGE

A. Embryonic Period

The median anlage of the thyroid migrates from the lingual area to its normal location in the neck between the 5th and 7th week of embryonic life. Once migration is complete, the median anlage connects with the lateral lobes that are derived from the fourth and fifth pharyngeal pouches. However, from the functional standpoint, the capacity to concentrate iodine only appears at about 12 weeks and control of thyroid function by the hypothalamopituitary axis is only established at 18 weeks. Because of this, the low amount of T_4 that can be measured in amniotic cavities in the first trimester must be of maternal origin, suggesting that some transplacental passage of T_4 already occurs at that stage (1). This may explain the deleterious effects of *maternal* hypothyroidism (which has been most dramatically illustrated in severe iodine deficiency) on the intellectual development of the offspring. This may justify biochemical screening of women who have a personal or family history of thyroid disease and who are contemplating becoming pregnant (2).

B. Fetal Period

In fetal blood, T_3 is low because of the presence of the placenta, with its very rich content in type III deiodinase (which transforms the prohormone T_4 in the inactive hormone reverse T_3 [(rT_3)] and T_3 itself into the inactive T_2). The low T_3 milieu may be responsible for the maintenance of a low level of *in utero* thermogenesis. TSH is high, probably because of extrahypothalamic sources of TRH, such as the pancreas and the placenta. Between 20 weeks and term, fetal plasma free T_4 increases progressively because of increased secretion by the fetal thyroid (3). However, even in the complete absence of fetal thyroid function, cord blood T_4 is 20–50% of the mean value of euthyroid neonates (4). This suggests that the transplacental passage of T_4 alluded to above may become substantial in the third trimester and allow some protection of the fetal brain against defective function of the fetal thyroid. The fetal brain is also protected against hypothyroidism by its rich content of type II deiodinase, the enzyme that converts T_4 into the active hormone T_3, which is upregulated in hypothyroidism. These two protective mechanisms provide the framework supporting the concept that complete salvage of intellectual potential is possible even in cases of severe congenital hypothyroidism provided effective treatment is administered soon after birth (see below).

Another important consideration deriving from the above is that prenatal screening of all pregnant women for *fetal* hypothyroidism is probably not justified. At present, it would require amniocentesis, and the risks of this procedure would outweigh the possible benefits of diagnosing hypothyroidism in the fetus. However, *in utero* diagnosis of hypothyroidism by cordocentesis and treatment of the fetus by intraamniotic injections of levothyroxine have been reported (5). The major indication is to determine the cause of a fetal goiter discovered by ultrasonography (if it cannot be reasonably guessed from the clinical context), so as to choose the most appropriate treatment to decrease its size. Indeed, a large goiter in the fetus entails potential risks during labor (face presentation) or after birth (respiratory distress).

C. Neonatal Period

Presumably as a consequence of the precipitous drop in ambient temperature, plasma TSH increases markedly in normal newborns, with a peak in the first 24 h of life. This is followed by a more shallow increase in plasma T_4, peaking during the second day of life. Thus, screening for congenital hypothyroidism using TSH as the primary method should be delayed until after 24 h of life, otherwise the number of false positive tests would become unacceptably high. In premature newborns, the postnatal peaks of TSH and of T_4 occur within the same time frame, but their amplitude is somewhat lower than that observed in term newborns.

D. Infancy

The relative dosage (in μg/kg/day) of thyroxine needed to maintain euthyroidism in hypothyroid subjects decreases exponentially during the first 2 years of life from about 10 to about 5 μg/kg/day (6). In absolute terms, the ~50 μg thyroxine needed by a newborn correspond to about 15% of the neonatal intrathyroidal iodine pool, whereas the 150 μg needed by an adult correspond to only 1% of the mature intrathyroidal iodine pool. A higher iodine turnover is in general associated with higher plasma T_3 (7) and, accordingly, the normal range of plasma T_3

extends to higher values in infancy than in adulthood (8) (Table 1).

III. CONGENITAL HYPOTHYROIDISM

A. Nomenclature

As is the case at later ages, hypothyroidism in infancy can be congenital or acquired, peripheral (primary) or central (secondary or tertiary), and permanent or transient in nature (Table 2). Because the most common and most potentially deleterious for long-term intellectual outcome is permanent primary congenital hypothyroidism (PPCH), PPCH will be the focus of this section. On the other hand, transient hypothyroxinemia without elevation of plasma TSH is very common in premature infants. Yet there is still controversy as to whether this is a disease entity requiring treatment or whether it is one of the many mechanisms by which the premature infant adjusts to extrauterine life. Transient hypothyroxinemia is therefore the subject of a section separate from congenital hypothyroidism. Likewise, newborns are very sensitive to iodine deficiency and this remains a major cause of congenital hypothyroidism worldwide. The distribution of neonatal TSH levels and the percentage of newborns with TSH > 5 mIU/l on neonatal blood spot samples has been proposed as a means to evaluate the extent of iodine deficiency in a population (9). This major public health problem is beyond the scope of the present chapter.

The prevalence of *permanent* primary CH is not increased in preterm infants (10). However, an increased prevalence of *transient* primary CH has been reported in some studies of premature newborns. The best characterized is due to the Wolff-Chaikoff effect: the induction of hypothyroidism by acute iodine overload (most often from iodine-containing antiseptic agents) (11). This condition has been mostly reported from areas of Europe where there is mild iodine deficiency and does not appear to occur in North America (12), presumably because the iodine intake of pregnant women in this area remains, on average, above a critical threshold.

Finally, the hypothyroidism resulting from dominantly inherited mutations that inactivate the T_3 receptor can sometimes be severe enough to be recognized in the neonatal period. Molecular confirmation of this diagnosis has now been obtained in over 200 pedigrees, but this condition will not be discussed further in this chapter and the reader is referred elsewhere (13).

B. Epidemiology and Causes of PPCH

PPCH affects 1:2500–4000 newborns. On the basis of newborn screening programs, its worldwide incidence is relatively similar over a wide range of ethnic groups and geographical areas. The only possible exception to this rule is a lower prevalence among black populations (14).

Table 1 Pediatric Reference Intervals for T_4, T_3, TSH, and Free T_4

Analyte	Age	Females			Males		
		Mean	Reference interval	n	Mean	Reference interval	n
T_4, nmol/L[a]	1–11 months	122	82–162	116	120	79–161	135
	1–5 years	120	79–160	471	116	75–158	589
	6–10 years	115	75–154	462	111	69–152	600
	11–15 years	109	69–149	799	106	63–147	614
	16–20 years	104	64–144	565	99	58–142	200
	Total			2413			2138
T_3, nmol/L[b]	1–11 months	2.46	1.52–3.39	70	2.46	1.58–3.35	93
	1–5 years	2.37	1.43–3.30	262	2.38	1.54–3.27	340
	6–10 years	2.20	1.62–3.12	255	2.26	1.37–3.13	362
	11–15 years	2.03	1.09–2.95	483	2.12	1.24–3.00	341
	16–20 years	1.84	0.92–2.78	346	1.98	1.11–2.86	131
	Total			1416			1267
TSH, mIU/L	1–11 months	2.2	0.8–6.3	131	2.2	0.8–6.3	158
	1–5 years	2.0	0.7–5.9	523	2.1	0.7–6.0	659
	6–10 years	1.8	0.6–5.1	562	1.9	0.7–5.4	698
	11–15 years	1.5	0.5–4.4	1057	1.7	0.6–4.9	738
	16–20 years	1.3	0.5–3.9	809	1.6	0.5–4.4	223
	Total			3082			2476
		Females and Males					
Free T_4, pmol/L[c]	1–11 months	19.5	9.5–39.5	47			
	1–5 years	18.4	9.0–37.2	91			
	6–10 years	16.9	8.3–34.1	57			
	11–15 years	15.5	7.6–31.5	88			
	16–20 years	14.1	7.0–28.7	70			
	Total			353			

[a]To convert nmol/L to μg/dl, divide by 12.87.
[b]To convert nmol/L to ng/dl, multiply by 65.1.
[c]To convert pmol/L to ng/dl, divide by 12.87.
Source: From Ref. 8. Reference values were obtained with the AutoDelfia analyzer (Wallac, Finland); different values may be expected with other methods.

Eighty to 90% of PPCH cases are due to developmental defects of the thyroid gland (thyroid dysgenesis), such as arrested migration of the embryonic thyroid in the sublingual area (ectopic thyroid) or an apparently complete absence of thyroid tissue on scan with sodium pertechnetate (athyreosis). Renewed interest in thyroid development has stemmed from the identification of transcription factors that are relatively thyroid-specific and from the generation of knock-out mice for these transcription factors. In humans, a few single gene defects have been shown to account for some cases of familial thyroid dysgenesis, but the vast majority of cases are sporadic and result from as yet unknown mechanisms (15). The remaining 10–20% of PPCH cases have functional defects in one of the steps involved in thyroid hormone biosynthesis (thyroid dyshormonogenesis), which follow an autosomal recessive mode of inheritance.

Recent studies have reevaluated whether genetic factors are involved in thyroid dysgenesis. Thus, a nationwide study of cases diagnosed by neonatal screening in France identified 48 familial cases out of 2472 (2%), which is 15-fold more than expected by chance. Analysis of the most typical pedigrees suggested autosomal dominant inheritance with incomplete penetrance, although there was also evidence for genetic heterogeneity (16).

Ectopy and athyreosis are generally considered as part of a spectrum. Recent arguments in favor of this view are that athyreosis and ectopy can coexist in the same pedigree (16) and that *ttf2 -/-* mice can have either ectopy or athyreosis, with a 50/50 distribution between the two phenotypes (17). On the other hand, the female preponderance classically described for thyroid dysgenesis as a whole is in fact only significant for ectopy, according to the results of two large recent surveys (15,18) (Table 3).

Table 2 Classification of Causes of Congenital Hypothyroidism

Central: Rare
  Mutation of the TRH receptor
  Mutation of beta-TSH
  Mutation of (PROP)PIT-1
  So-called idiopathic hypopituitarism (usually with classic triad on MRI, see text)
Peripheral: Frequent (1:2500–4000 newborns)
  Ectopic thyroid (most often sublingual): ~70% of cases
    Mutations inactivating *PAX-8*
    Other mechanisms (postzygotic stochastic events)
  Athyreosis ~15% of cases
    True (undetectable plasma thyroglobulin)
      Mutations inactivating *TTF-2*
      Other mechanisms
    Apparent
      Permanent
        Mutations inactivating *TSHR* or *NIS*
        Other mechanisms
      Transient: maternal TSH-receptor blocking antibodies
  Dyshormonogenesis (leading to goiter): ~10–20% of cases
  Thyroid of normal shape, position and size: ~5% of cases

Source: See Refs. 15 and 25 for discussion.

This may suggest distinct molecular mechanisms for the two forms of thyroid dysgenesis, or sex-specific modifiers of a common initial event (15). The fetal sex ratio in studies of various embryopathies is seldom reported (19), and indeed was not reported for the *ttf2* -/- mice.

It should also be kept in mind that athyreosis itself may be heterogeneous (Table 2). Undetectable uptake on scan may represent so-called true athyreosis (a diagnosis that should be validated by an undetectable plasma thyroglobulin) or apparent athyreosis from transplacental transfer of TSH-receptor blocking antibodies; Na/I sym-

Table 3 Proportion of Girls with Ectopy or Athyreosis from Quebec and Toronto

	Quebec	Toronto
Ectopy:		
Proportion of girls	0.74	0.78
95% confidence interval	0.67–0.81	0.67–0.89
Number of subjects	141	54
Athyreosis:		
Proportion of girls	0.58	0.61
95% confidence interval	0.42–0.74	0.44–0.78
Number of subjects	36	31

Source: Adapted from Refs. 15 and 18

porter mutations; or ectopic tissue too small for the limit of detection of nuclear medicine scans.

The differentiation between athyreosis and ectopy is of more than academic interest. Apparent athyreosis from transplacental transfer of TSH-receptor blocking antibodies leads to transient CH but has a very high risk of recurrence in subsequent pregnancies (20). The observation that PPCH from athyreosis does not have a sex ratio that is significantly different from 0.5 (Table 3) suggests that autosomal recessive mechanisms may be involved in a significant proportion of cases. Indeed, several pedigrees have been described in which apparent athyreosis was due to either compound heterozygosity (21) or homozygosity (22) for mutations that result in complete inactivation of the TSH receptor. Anatomically, the absent uptake was due to the fact that the gland was severely hypofunctional, but careful ultrasonography demonstrated that a hypoplastic gland was present and was of normal shape and position. This is consistent with the concept that TSH and its receptor are necessary for growth and function of the thyroid, but not involved in the initial differentiation of thyroid cells or in the migration of the thyroid anlage.

A milder form of TSH resistance can be seen in pseudohypoparathyroidism, in which an increased level of TSH at neonatal screening or during infancy may be the presenting sign (23), before obvious phenotypic features are recognized; and in non-TSH-receptor-related TSH resistance, with a consistently normal plasma T$_4$, a normal orthotopic gland on ^{99m}Tc imaging, and a dominant pattern of inheritance (24). Permanent or transient hyperthyrotropinemia of infancy, with normal plasma T$_4$ and normal thyroid anatomy, can also be seen without a family history and its mechanisms remain to be elucidated. It may occur in otherwise normal children or in children with other phenotypic abnormalities, such as respiratory distress and developmental delay (as in patients with mutations in TTF-1; see Table 4). It can also be seen in Down syndrome (see below).

Aside from TSH receptor mutations in athyreosis, a search for mutations in the genes coding for thyroid transcription factor-1 (TTF-1), for TTF-2 or for the paired domain factor PAX 8 has so far yielded only a handful of positive results. The careful description of the phenotypes of these naturally occurring mutation in humans and of the corresponding knock-out experiments in mice is of great importance for our understanding of thyroid gland development, but is beyond the scope of this chapter. The reader is referred elsewhere for this aspect (25). For clinical purposes, Table 4 proposes guidelines for when a specific gene should be examined.

C. Clinical Aspects and Rationale for Biochemical Screening

Signs and symptoms of hypothyroidism in the newborn period are almost always overlooked, yet this is when irreversible brain damage occurs. In the experience of the

Table 4 Transcription Factor Mutations and Congenital Hypothyroidism

Thyroid phenotype	Other features	Gene	Type of genetic lesion	Transmission
Mildly ↑ TSH	RDS	*TTF-1*	Chromosomal deletion	*de novo* or inherited
Gland normal in shape, size, and position	Developmental delay		Missense	*de novo*
	Ataxia			
Athyreosis	Cleft palate	*TTF-2*	Missense	AR
	Choanal atresia			
	Kinky hair			
Ectopy or orthotopic hypoplasia	Cysts within thyroid remnants	*PAX-8*	Missense	AD or *de novo*

RDS, respiratory distress syndrome; TTF, thyroid transcription factor; AR, autosomal recessive; AD, autosomal dominant.

last 12 years at the author's institution, the diagnosis was suspected clinically in only 2 of more than 150 newborns.

For this reason, systematic biochemical screening of newborns was undertaken in the 1970s and is becoming the standard of care in an ever-increasing number of countries. The screening strategy is based on primary TSH measurements in most countries, followed by T_4 measurement if TSH is raised above a certain cutoff. As an alternative, the so-called primary T_4 strategy is still used in most American states. The time at which the sample is taken may also vary between centers, with some taking cord blood, but the majority take blood from a heel prick after 24 h of age, to avoid an unacceptable percentage of recall due to the neonatal TSH surge alluded to above. Therefore, the practice of discharging newborns on the day of birth represents an organizational challenge to screening for CH.

Knowledge of the specific technique and cutoff levels used by the screening program is not as important as the clinician's awareness that a positive screening result should prompt immediate action and that continuous auditing of the turnaround time of the screening program is essential. Many individuals are involved between the time the sample is taken and sent to the screening laboratory and when the laboratory technician reports an abnormal result to the clinician. Human errors are the single most important factor in delayed or missed diagnoses of CH. The current guidelines used by the Quebec screening program are given in Table 5.

Aside from human errors, truly normal screening TSH and T_4 values have been found in infants who developed severe hypothyroidism during infancy. Thus, for unknown reasons, children with thyroid dyshormonogenesis can have normal TSH and T_4 as newborns and yet

Table 5 Screening and Evaluation Strategies for CH: Quebec Guidelines, 2001

Heel prick after 24 h of life except if
    Transfer to another hospital (sample should be taken at hospital of birth)
    Exchange blood transfusion
    Death within 24 h
Note: entire surface of the spot should be filled (avoid soiling)
Samples should be sent to screening laboratory every weekday
Assay for TSH by time-resolved fluorometric assay technique
    If TSH is less than 15 mIU/L: normal
    If TSH between 15 and 29 mIU/L, total T_4 is measured on blood spot:
        If total T_4 is less than 87 mmol/l,[a] immediate referral
        If total T_4 is greater than 87 nmol/l,[a] a second blood spot is requested and the infant is referred if TSH is still 15 mIU/l
        or above
    If TSH is greater than 30 mIU/l, *immediate referral*
Upon referral:
    History and physical examination
    Anteroposterior x-ray of knee
    ^{99m}Tc scintigraphy of cervical, lingual, and mediastinal area
    blood for TSH, free T_4, T_3, antithyroperoxidase antibodies in mother and baby
    plasma thyroglobulin in baby if apparent athyreosis on scan
    Start treatment without waiting for results of blood tests

[a] 65 nmol/l if birthweight less than 2.5 kg.

present in the first 2 years of life with clinical and biochemical evidence of severe hypothyroidism (10, 26). The second situation arises from the fact that monozygotic twins are generally discordant for thyroid dysgenesis and that the affected twin may have normal screening values because of subtle blood mixing between the euthyroid and the hypothyroid fetus (27). Lastly, dopamine infusions may lead to a false-normal plasma TSH result in spite of primary hypothyroidism (28). Thus, in spite of normal neonatal screening results, the appearance of signs and symptoms suggestive of hypothyroidism in an infant justifies repeating the determination of TSH and T_4.

D. Diagnostic Evaluation of the Hypothyroid Newborn

As stated above, a clinical diagnosis is almost never made in the newborn period. However, when a baby is referred for evaluation of a positive test, it is sometimes possible to elicit a history of increased sleepiness, poor feeding, or constipation. The family history should focus on whether there are other cases of CH or whether the mother is known to have autoimmune thyroid disease. On physical examination, prolonged icterus and large fontanelles are the most frequently encountered signs. A careful inspection of the cervical area, with the neck hyperextended, is important to detect a goiter. However, even obvious goiters on nuclear medicine scanning can be missed by experienced clinicians and imaging studies are almost always necessary. Extrathyroid abnormalities should be noted: congenital hypothyroidism can be part of a polymalformative syndrome (Table 4) and a fivefold increase in the prevalence of minor defects in septation of the embryonic heart has been reported in children with thyroid dysgenesis (15).

Blood is taken to confirm the positive screening results. In addition to TSH, we routinely measure free T_4, total T_3, and thyroglobulin from this sample. Although the prevalence of transient CH from transplacental transfer of TSH receptor-blocking antibodies is low (29), this possibility should be investigated in cases with apparent athyreosis or with a gland of normal shape and size but decreased uptake.

Because of the importance of a precise diagnosis in establishing that CH is permanent (as in true athyreosis and ectopy) or that it has a 25% recurrence risk in subsequent siblings (as in dyshormonogenesis), a nuclear medicine scan should be obtained. This should ideally be carried out on the day of the initial diagnostic evaluation, but can be performed during the first few days of thyroxine treatment because, as long as plasma TSH is still elevated, there will be uptake of the tracer by thyroid tissue. The isotope of choice is sodium pertechnetate (^{99m}Tc), which is available daily in most nuclear medicine services. However, difficulties in arranging for imaging studies should never be taken as an excuse for not initiating treatment on the first visit. A nuclear medicine scan can always be obtained after withdrawing treatment for a month at 3 years of age (when hypothyroidism no longer has permanent consequences for brain development); however, obtaining good imaging is easier in a newborn than in a toddler. Lastly, one should *not* wait for the results of confirmatory blood tests before starting treatment.

The technical quality of nuclear medicine scans is important (30). The unequivocal demonstration of ectopic sublingual tissue requires that the salivary glands be empty (which can easily be achieved in newborns by feeding them between the intravenous [IV] injection of technetium and scanning, and in toddlers by giving them a piece of candy). Ascertaining that the technetium has been injected in the vein is also essential. Because of these pitfalls of nuclear medicine imaging (and the radiation involved, although the dosage is minimal), ultrasound scanning has been evaluated for the etiological diagnosis of CH. The differentiation between normal thyroid lobes and the hyperechogenic structures (likely the ultimobranchial bodies) in the same location when there is no orthotopic thyroid is difficult and requires a highly skilled pediatric radiologist (31). Ultrasound scanning has therefore not replaced nuclear medicine imaging at most centers.

E. Treatment and Outcome of Congenital Hypothyroidism

Before systematic biochemical screening of newborns, the mean IQ of CH children was 76 (32) and 40% required special education (33). Even in those with normal IQs, specific cognitive deficits were common (34). These numbers provide the historical background against which to gauge the success of biochemical screening and different treatment regimens.

In the first generation of screened CH newborns, treatment was started at a mean age of 23–30 days and the starting dosage of levothyroxine was 5–6 μg/kg·day. While it was recognized that such a dosage did not normalize plasma TSH for weeks or even months, this was thought to reflect resistance to the normal feedback control mechanisms. However, such a resistance occurs only in a minority of CH newborns (35). The first report of developmental outcome of screened CH children suggested that intellectual impairment had been completely eliminated (36). This first report also found no impact of the initial severity of hypothyroidism at diagnosis. However, a meta-analysis published 15 years later and including 675 children with CH and 570 controls from 7 studies clearly showed that initial disease severity was an important determinant of outcome. Specifically, the subgroup of children with severe CH had a mean loss of six IQ points compared to controls, and in some studies the difference was in the range of 10–20 IQ points, which is not only statistically but also clinically significant (37).

Severity of CH at diagnosis can be evaluated in a number of different ways (38). Most commonly, this has been done on the basis of the plasma level of T_4, of the bone maturation, or of the cause (athyreosis vs. ectopy). An important concept is that the impact of severity of CH on developmental outcome does not appear linear: rather, there seems to be a threshold below which an infant with CH was at greater risk of developmental problems. This has been most convincingly demonstrated by Tillotson et al. (33), who defined a plasma total T_4 at diagnosis of 43 nmol/l as the critical point below which the IQ became affected by CH.

A more detailed description of these studies mostly carried out in the eighties does not seem necessary, because age at starting treatment and initial dosage of levothyroxine have changed substantially since then. In the last decade, most centers have been able to start treatment at a mean age of 9–14 days. Also in the last decade, because several lines of evidence suggested that the dosage used was suboptimal (not only persistent elevation of TSH, but also persistent delay in bone maturation at 3 years were observed [39]), the starting dosage of levothyroxine has been increased at many centers to 10–15 μg/kg·day. This regimen promptly normalizes plasma TSH, but is associated with plasma free T_4 levels above the reference range of most laboratories. However, as reviewed above, the normal range of plasma free T_4 extends to much higher levels in infants than in older children or adults (Table 1). In addition, the mean plasma level of T_3 remains within the normal range and objective signs of hyperthyroidism have not been documented. Frequent monitoring of thyroid function (i.e., every 1–3 months) was recommended by the American Academy of Pediatrics in 1993 (40). With frequent monitoring, the dosage of levothyroxine will be titrated upwards in a timely fashion when the starting dosage is low (41) and may be titrated downwards if TSH is consistently below the normal range and/or if T_3 is high. Infants with dyshormonogenesis appear to need less levothyroxine than those with dysgenesis (18). Thus, further studies on the biochemical endpoints of treatment and the development of guidelines for change in dosage are needed with the high initial dosages currently used at many centers.

However, the most important aspect of outcome is developmental and several recent studies have shown that the developmental gap that existed between severe CH children and controls has now been closed (6). *Both* early and high-dosage treatment appear necessary (42). Detailed studies of neurophysiological functions that may be more sensitive to the effects of both over- and undertreatment than the measurement of IQ may lead to greater individualization of initial dosage recommendations. In the meantime, starting as early as possible with 10–15 μg/kg·day appears safe and effective in achieving the major goal of neonatal screening: to allow all CH children, including those with a severe form of the disease, to achieve their full intellectual potential (43).

IV. HYPOTHYROXINEMIA OF THE NEWBORN

It is essential to define whether one is discussing decreased *total* or decreased *free* T_4. The first condition that needs to be ruled out in a newborn with low total T_4 concentrations associated with normal plasma TSH is thyroxin-binding globulin (TBG) deficiency. This X-linked condition is discovered only by screening programs using a primary T_4 approach (for technical reasons, total and not free T_4 is measured on the neonatal blood spot). It does not require treatment, since the plasma levels of free thyroid hormones are normal and the subjects are euthyroid. Loss of protein from nephrotic syndrome may also lead to low total T_4. With the generalization of free T_4 assays, unnecessary investigation and treatment of TBG deficiency has become rarer.

In a term neonate with a low free T_4 but normal TSH level, true central hypothyroidism needs to be ruled out. Isolated central hypothyroidism is exceedingly rare but may also have profound long-term deleterious effects on later development: it can be caused by mutations that inactivate the gene coding for the beta-subunit of TSH (44) or the gene coding for the TRH receptor (45). More commonly, central hypothyroidism occurs in association with other anterior pituitary hormone deficiencies: hypoglycemia, prolonged conjugated hyperbilirubinemia, and microphallus and/or cryptorchidism will suggest associated deficiencies in growth hormone, adrenocorticotropin (ACTH) and luteinizing hormone (LH), respectively. Clinical clues to a midline defect include cleft lip and palate and optic nerve hypoplasia. Magnetic resonance imaging reveals the classic triad of ectopic posterior pituitary; thin, interrupted, or absent stalk; and hypoplastic anterior pituitary in most cases of congenital hypopituitarism. A normal pituitary anatomy should lead to consideration of mutations in *PIT-1* or in *PROP-1* (46).

On the other hand, hypothyroxinemia relative to term values, but with normal TSH, is a very common finding in premature newborns (10). It does not only reflect low TBG levels because free T_4 levels are low as well. This should probably be considered as a situation akin to that seen at later ages in the presence of severe nonthyroidal illness. Indeed, numerous studies have shown that there is a correlation between the degree of lowering of T_4 and negative outcomes, both short-term (mortality) and long-term (developmental problems). However, correlation does not imply causation: indeed, randomized, double-blind, placebo-controlled studies of thyroxin supplementation have not shown an overall benefit in terms of morbidity, mortality, or developmental outcome. In fact, *lower* IQs were observed in levothyroxine-treated infants born after 27 weeks of gestation. Further research is underway to determine if the apparent benefit from thyroxin supplementation in extremely premature (<26 weeks) infants is confirmed (47). Systematic supplementation of all low-birthweight babies is not recommended at this time.

V. CONGENITAL HYPERTHYROIDISM

As is the case later in life, a high plasma T_4 level does not necessarily indicate hyperthyroidism. As noted above, there is a physiological, transient peak of plasma T_4 on the second day of life. Aside from the precise postnatal age, the next most important thing to know is whether the laboratory reports total or free T_4. A high T_4 in the face of a normal free T_4 suggests TBG excess, a condition that, like TBG deficiency, should not be treated. TBG excess may be genetically determined or may be due to liver disease. In the syndrome of generalized resistance to thyroid hormone mentioned above, high circulating levels of thyroid hormones are in fact associated with *hypo*thyroidism and plasma TSH is high.

On the other hand, and as is also true in later life, a low or undetectable plasma TSH level, even with ultrasensitive third-generation assays, is not sufficient to establish a diagnosis of hyperthyroidism: it can be seen in central hypothyroidism or in severe nonthyroidal illness. To make a diagnosis of true hyperthyroidism, the combination of a low or undetectable TSH with high T_4 and/or T_3 is required.

A. Transient Graves' Disease

Most commonly, hyperthyroidism in infancy occurs during the early neonatal period and is due to the transplacental transfer of TSH receptor-stimulating antibodies from a mother with either a current or a past history of Graves' disease. Given the high prevalence of Graves' disease in the population of women of childbearing age, it is surprising that clinically significant hyperthyroidism occurs so seldom in newborns: estimates of 1:25,000 births, or of 1–3% of the offspring of mothers with Graves' disease, are quoted in the literature. The measurement of TSH receptor-stimulating antibodies in the plasma of pregnant women with past or current Graves' disease has been advocated as a means to detect the fetuses more at risk, but is not universally practiced (48). In spite of its rarity, the serious nature of the condition justifies careful clinical screening. The mother should be warned of the potential risk; fetal growth and heart rate should be monitored; the newborn should be examined for the presence of a goiter, of exophthalmia, or of tachycardia without underlying heart disease; and weight gain during the first 3 months of life should be meticulously monitored.

The recommendations about antithyroid drug treatment in pregnancy are that it should be aimed at maintaining the patient slightly hyperthyroid so as to avoid fetal hypothyroidism from transplacental transfer of the drug. However, a woman may occasionally be treated with dosages of antithyroid drugs that are high enough to make the fetus hypothyroid. This may even lead to the development of a large goiter in the fetus and newborn, which may become apparent on prenatal ultrasound or because of the development of respiratory distress from tracheal compression in the immediate neonatal period. This transient drug-induced hypothyroidism may be followed after a few days (i.e., after the drug is cleared from the newborn's circulation) by a period of a few weeks of hyperthyroidism from the maternally derived TSH-receptor-stimulating antibodies.

TSH-receptor stimulating antibodies may remain present long after definitive cure of hyperthyroidism has been achieved by the therapeutic administration of radioactive iodine to an adolescent or adult with Graves' disease. Therefore, it is important to enquire from the great many women receiving thyroxine replacement for hypothyroidism who become pregnant whether their hypothyroidism results from radioiodine treatment, even if this has occurred years earlier.

Once this transient type of hyperthyroidism is recognized in a newborn, it should be treated vigorously to prevent the development of heart failure. Hospital admission is usually required initially, and tachycardia may be severe enough to justify continuous electrocardiographic monitoring. Beta-blockers such as propranolol should be administered at a dosage of 2 mg/kg. day in four divided doses. Lugol's solution, at a dosage of 1 drop every 8 h, will block the release of the thyroid hormone stored in the gland and can be given for a few days. The short-acting propylthiouracyl is the preferred antithyroid drug for the following reasons: in a newborn who is fed four to six times a day, the need to give a drug four times a day does not pose problems of compliance, as it does in older children and adolescents; and compared to methimazole, it has the extra benefit of decreasing the conversion of T_4 into T_3. The starting dosage of propylthiouracyl is 5–10 mg/kg. day, divided in four doses, and should be carefully tapered over the first few weeks of life so as to avoid the development of drug-induced hypothyroidism once the TSH-receptor stimulating antibodies are cleared. Pharmacological dosages of glucocorticoids have also been used, because they block the conversion of T_4 to T_3. More heroic treatments such as exchange blood transfusions (49) or less traditional ones such as the administration of sodium ipodate (50) have been proposed. Although their use is logical on the basis of the pathophysiology of neonatal Graves' disease, they have not gained wide acceptance and, in our experience, have not been necessary.

With prompt recognition and early, vigorous treatment, the classically reported high death rate of neonates with Graves' disease should be a thing of the past. Likewise, the classically described intellectual impairment and development of craniosynostosis (51) has no longer been reported in recent series.

B. TSH Receptor-Activating Mutations

A familial form of nonautoimmune, persistent hyperthyroidism with dominant inheritance had been described 20 years ago in Nancy, France. The authors had hypothesized that this phenotype resulted from intrinsic activation of TSH receptor function (52). The cloning of the human TSH receptor has allowed to confirm this hypothesis (53). Inherited mutations leading to constitutive activation of the TSH receptor have now been described in several pedigrees from France and have begun to be recognized in other areas of the world as well. Some of these pedigrees had been considered as having familial Graves' disease. However, the neonates recognized as having hyperthyroidism from a mutation that constitutively activates the TSH-receptor typically experience an unrelenting course, in contrast to those with congenital hyperthyroidism from maternal antibodies. Thus, definitive treatment is required in these patients. Given the fact that there is no experience with radioiodine in the very young, thyroidectomy has been most commonly performed.

A handful of cases with *de novo* germline mutations activating the TSH receptor have also been described (54). Clinically, their phenotype has been uniformly severe and early thyroidectomy is therefore advised. From the molecular standpoint, it is interesting to note that these *de novo* mutations are "private", that is, they are different from the ones that have so far been found in the pedigrees with the dominantly inherited form (and are, in fact, only seen also as somatic mutations in so-called hot nodules): it has been suggested that the phenotypic consequences of these *de novo* mutations are so severe that they became extinguished because the affected individuals could not reach the age of reproduction before modern medicine led to recognition and definitive treatment of this condition (55).

Lastly, *somatic* mutations activating the TSH receptor have now been recognized as the most common mechanism underlying the development of "hot" nodules (56). This entity is predominantly a disease of adults and older children, but a single case of a somatic mutation leading to the formation of a hot nodule and to hyperthyroidism of fetal onset has been reported (57).

VI. ACQUIRED HYPO- AND HYPERTHYROIDISM IN INFANCY

The most common causes of acquired hypo- and hyperthyroidism are Hashimoto's thyroiditis and Graves' disease, respectively. These two entities are exceptional in infancy. Specifically, Hashimoto's thyroiditis has been reported in only a handful of patients below the age of 3 years (58); the youngest patient we have observed with Graves' disease was 3 years and 8 months. The principles of diagnostic evaluation are the same as in older children. Prompt treatment of hypothyroidism is important, since infancy is still a period during which the brain may undergo irreversible alterations from hypothyroidism. Treatment of hyperthyroidism is restricted to the use of antithyroid drugs (with thyroidectomy as a second line), since

there is no experience of radioiodine use in patients under the age of 6 years (59).

A category of infants who present often with mild hyperthyrotropinemia with or without detectable antibodies to thyroperoxidase are those with Down syndrome. These children are known to have a higher prevalence of autoimmune thyroid disease. However, even in the absence of antibodies, Down syndrome infants often present with mild hyperthyrotropinemia. A study of of CH screening in *all* newborns with Down syndrome born in the Netherlands over a 2-year period showed that, compared to normal newborns, the distribution of T_4 was shifted downwards and that of TSH was shifted upwards (60). Furthermore, the elevated TSH is biologically active, suggesting that there is a mild primary thyroid defect in all children with Down syndrome (61). However, the clinical relevance of these biochemical findings is difficult to assess: the abnormalities are mild and the Québec TSH screening program has not identified a single case of permanent primary CH associated with Down syndrome (15). Furthermore, signs of hypothyroidism are particularly difficult to document objectively in these children. While it is reasonable to treat with thyroxine, on the basis of the concept that a high TSH level implies that pituitary (and, by inference, brain) receptors are perceiving an insufficient amount of intracellular T_3, there is no evidence of clinical benefit (62).

VII. STRUCTURAL THYROID PROBLEMS

A. Thyroglossal Duct Cysts

The migration of the median thyroid anlage described above occurs along a path that is paved by epithelial cells. This path, which is called the thyroglossal duct, usually closes after migration is complete. However, when it remains patent, fluid may collect at its more caudal end and constitute a thyroglossal duct cyst. These cysts typically present as a midline, soft, regular mass in the lower neck of an asymptomatic infant (or older child). However, they may also present with acute swelling, pain, and redness secondary to an acute infection.

Elective surgical removal of thyroglossal duct cysts is therefore advised, because surgery after an acute infection has occurred is more difficult (63). Before elective surgery, we still recommended performing a ^{99m}Tc scan (rather than an echogram, for the technical reasons discussed above), to ascertain that the midline neck mass does not represent ectopic thyroid tissue, which usually will be the only thyroid tissue present in the patient and removal of which will lead to severe and irreversible hypothyroidism.

B. Suppurative Thyroiditis

Because of its rich content in iodine, a potent disinfectant, the thyroid gland is seldom the site of bacterial infections.

In infancy (and even later), bacterial infection of the thyroid in a host with normal immune function is often associated with a fistula arising from the pyriform sinus. Although thyroid abscesses can present at any age, the fact that they are causally linked to a congenital malformation (which is usually present on the left side) explains their relatively high frequency in young children. Thus, in an infant presenting with a rapidly growing mass in the left thyroid lobe, thyroid abscess is the first diagnosis. The mass is very tender, but redness of the overlying skin may be absent. Increased leukocytosis and sedimentation rate are further clues to the diagnosis. Fine needle aspiration has been used and allows identification of the germs causing the abscess (which are most often from the flora of the oropharynx). The aspiration, coupled with antibiotic treatment, may also contribute to curing the abscess (64). However, a careful search for a fistula from the pyriform sinus should be carried out. This is best achieved with the use of barium swallow studies and/or laryngoscopy. If such a fistula is found, definitive surgical treatment is required to prevent recurrent abscess formation.

C. Subacute Thyroiditis

In contrast to bacterial thyroiditis, subacute thyroiditis (also known as de Quervain's thyroiditis) occurs very rarely in children. However, cases have been reported in children as young as 2 years (65).

D. Thyroid Cancer

This entity is described in great detail in another section. In infants, it is important to remember that medullary thyroid cancer can occur very early in life in the familial syndrome of multiple endocrine neoplasia type IIB. In such a family, we have observed a boy in whom we performed thyroidectomy at 1.5 years of age because of high plasma calcitonin concentrations, and in whom pathological examination revealed definite medullary thyroid cancer (66).

VIII. CONCLUSION

Thyroid disorders during infancy are as varied, if not more so, than any other period of the lifespan. Their importance is that, if not promptly recognized and treated, they can lead to irreversible short- or long term sequelae, as exemplified by congenital hyper- and hypothyroidism, respectively. Hence all clinicians must always bear these diagnoses in mind whenever suggestive clinical clues are present.

REFERENCES

1. Contempre B, Jauniaux E, Calvo R, Jurkovic D, Campbell S, de Escobar GM. Detection of thyroid hormones in human embryonic cavities during the first trimester of pregnancy. J Clin Endocrinol Metab 1993; 77:1719–1722.
2. Glinoer D, Delange F. The potential repercussions of maternal, fetal, and neonatal hypothyroxinemia on the progeny. Thyroid 2000; 10:871–887.
3. Fisher DA. Thyroid function in premature infants. The hypothyroxinemia of prematurity. Clin Perinatol 1998; 25: 999–1014.
4. Vulsma T, Gons MH, de Vijlder JJ. Maternal–fetal transfer of thyroxine in congenital hypothyroidism due to a total organification defect or thyroid agenesis. N Engl J Med 1989; 321:13–16.
5. Guibourdenche J, Noel M, Chevenne D, Vuillard E, Volumenie JL, Polak M, Boissinot C, Porquet D, Luton D. Biochemical investigation of foetal and neonatal thyroid function using the ACS-180SE analyser: clinical application. Ann Clin Biochem 2001; 38:520–526.
6. Dubuis JM, Glorieux J, Richer F, Deal CL, Dussault JH, Van Vliet G. Outcome of severe congenital hypothyroidism: closing the developmental gap with early high dose levothyroxine treatment. J Clin Endocrinol Metab 1996; 81:222–227.
7. Delange F. Thyroid hormones: Biochemistry and Physiology. In: Bertrand J, Rappaport R, Sizonenko PC, eds. Pediatric Endocrinology. Baltimore: Williams & Wilkins, 1993:242–251.
8. Zurakowski D, Di Canzio J, Majzoub JA. Pediatric reference intervals for serum thyroxine, triiodothyronine, thyrotropin, and free thyroxine. Clin Chem 1999; 45:1087–1091.
9. Delange F. Screening for congenital hypothyroidism used as an indicator of the degree of iodine deficiency and of its control. Thyroid 1998; 8:1185–1192.
10. Vincent MA, Rodd C, Dussault JH, Van Vliet G. Very low birth weight newborns do not need repeat screening for congenital hypothyroidism. J Pediatr 2002; 140:311–314.
11. Chanoine JP, Pardou A, Bourdoux P, Delange F. Withdrawal of iodinated disinfectants at delivery decreases the recall rate at neonatal screening for congenital hypothyroidism. Arch Dis Child 1988; 63:1297–1298.
12. Brown RS, Bloomfield S, Bednarek FJ, Mitchell ML, Braverman LE. Routine skin cleansing with povidone–iodine is not a common cause of transient neonatal hypothyroidism in North America: a prospective controlled study. Thyroid 1997; 7:395–400.
13. Refetoff S, Dumont JE, Vassart G. Thyroid Disorders. In: Scriver CR, Beaudet AL, Sly WS, Valle D, eds. The Metabolic and Molecular Basis of Inherited Disease. New York: McGraw-Hill, 2001:4029–4076.
14. Grant DB, Smith I. Survey of neonatal screening for primary hypothyroidism in England, Wales, and Northern Ireland 1982–4. Br Med J 1988; 296:1355–1358.
15. Devos H, Rodd C, Gagne N, Laframboise R, Van Vliet G. A search for the possible molecular mechanisms of thyroid dysgenesis: sex ratios and associated malformations. J Clin Endocrinol Metab 1999; 84: 2502–2506.
16. Castanet M, Polak M, Bonaiti-Pellie C, Lyonnet S, Czernichow P, Leger J. Nineteen years of national screening for congenital hypothyroidism: familial cases with thyroid dysgenesis suggest the involvement of genetic factors. J Clin Endocrinol Metab 2001; 86:2009–2014.
17. De Felice M, Ovitt C, Biffali E, Rodriguez-Mallon A, Arra C, Anastassiadis K, Macchia PE, Mattei MG, Mariano A, Scholer H, Macchia V, Di Lauro R. A mouse model for hereditary thyroid dysgenesis and cleft palate. Nat Genet 1998; 19:395–398.

18. Hanukoglu A, Perlman K, Shamis I, Brnjac L, Rovet J, Daneman D. Relationship of etiology to treatment in congenital hypothyroidism. J Clin Endocrinol Metab 2001; 86: 186–191.

19. Machado AF, Zimmerman EF, Hovland DN Jr, Weiss R, Collins MD. Diabetic embryopathy in C57BL/6J mice. Altered fetal sex ratio and impact of the splotch allele. Diabetes 2001; 50:1193–1199.

20. Pacaud D, Huot C, Gattereau A, Brown RS, Glorieux J, Dussault JH, Van Vliet G. Outcome in three siblings with antibody-mediated transient congenital hypothyroidism. J Pediatr 1995; 127:275–277.

21. Gagne N, Parma J, Deal C, Vassart G, Van Vliet G. Apparent congenital athyreosis contrasting with normal plasma thyroglobulin levels and associated with inactivating mutations in the thyrotropin receptor gene: are athyreosis and ectopic thyroid distinct entities? J Clin Endocrinol Metab 1999; 83:1771–1775.

22. Abramowicz MJ, Duprez L, Parma J, Vassart G, Heinrichs C. Familial congenital hypothyroidism due to inactivating mutation of the thyrotropin receptor causing profound hypoplasia of the thyroid gland. J Clin Invest 1997; 99:3018–3024.

23. Heinrichs C, Toppet M, Perlmutter N, Keutgen H, Loveridge N, Mallet E, Herens C, Bergmann P. Infant primary hypothyroidism as the first manifestation of pseudohypoparathyroidism. Clin Pediatr Endocrinol 1995; 4:47–53.

24. Xie J, Pannain S, Pohlenz J, Weiss RE, Moltz K, Morlot M, Asteria C, Persani L, Beck-Peccoz P, Parma J, Vassart G, Refetoff S. Resistance to thyrotropin (TSH) in three families is not associated with mutations in the TSH receptor or TSH. J Clin Endocrinol Metab 1997; 82:3933–3940.

25. Van Vliet G. Molecular mechanisms of thyroid gland development : insights from clinical studies and from mutant mice. In: Eugster EA and Pescovitz OH, eds. Developmental Endocrinology: From Research to Clinical Practice. Totowa, NJ: Humana Press, 2002:123–134.

26. de Zegher F, Vanderschueren-Lodeweyckx M, Heinrichs C, Van Vliet G, Malvaux P. Thyroid dyshormonogenesis: severe hypothyroidism after normal neonatal thyroid stimulating hormone screening. Acta Paediatr 1992; 81:274–276.

27. Perry RJ, Heinrichs C, Bourdoux P, Khoury K, Szöts F, Dussault JH, Vassart G, Van Vliet G. Discordance of monozygotic twins for thyroid dysgenesis: implications for screening and for molecular pathophysiology. Clin Endocrinol Metab 2002 (in press).

28. de Zegher F, Van den Berghe G, Dumoulin M, Gewillig M, Daenen W, Devlieger H. Dopamine suppresses thyroid-stimulating hormone secretion in neonatal hypothyroidism. Acta Paediatr 1995; 84:213–214.

29. Brown RS, Bellisario RL, Botero D, Fournier L, Abrams CA, Cowger ML, David R, Fort P, Richman RA. Incidence of transient congenital hypothyroidism due to maternal thyrotropin receptor-blocking antibodies in over one million babies. J Clin Endocrinol Metab 1996; 81:1147–1151.

30. Verelst J, Chanoine JP, Delange F. Radionuclide imaging in primary permanent congenital hypothyroidism. Clin Nucl Med 1991; 16:652–655.

31. Chanoine JP, Toppet V, Body JJ, Van Vliet G, Lagasse R, Bourdoux P, Spehl M, Delange F. Contribution of thyroid ultrasound and serum calcitonin to the diagnosis of congenital hypothyroidism. J Endocrinol Invest 1990; 13:103–109.

32. Klein RZ, Mitchell ML. Neonatal screening. In: Braverman LE, Utiger RD, eds. Werner and Ingbar's The Thyroid. Philadelphia: Lippincott Williams & Wilkins, 2000: 973–977.

33. Tillotson SL, Fuggle PW, Smith I, Ades AE, Grant DB. Relation between biochemical severity and intelligence in early treated congenital hypothyroidism: a threshold effect. Br Med J 1994; 309:440–445.

34. Wolter R, Noel P, De Cock P, Craen M, Ernould C, Malvaux P, Verstraeten F, Simons J, Mertens S, Van Broeck N, Vanderschueren-Lodeweyckx M. Neuropsychological study in treated thyroid dysgenesis. Acta Paediatr Scand Suppl 1979; 277:41–46.

35. Fisher DA, Schoen EJ, La Franchi S, Mandel SH, Nelson JC, Carlton EI, Goshi JH. The hypothalamic–pituitary–thyroid negative feedback control axis in children with treated congenital hypothyroidism. J Clin Endocrinol Metab 2000; 85:2722–2727.

36. New England congenital hypothyroidism collaborative. Effects of neonatal screening for hypothyroidism: prevention of mental retardation by treatment before clinical manifestations. Lancet 1981; 2:1095–1098.

37. Derksen-Lubsen G, Verkerk PH. Neuropsychologic development in early treated congenital hypothyroidism: analysis of literature data. Pediatr Res 1996; 39:561–566.

38. Van Vliet G. Neonatal hypothyroidism: treatment and outcome. Thyroid 1999; 9:79–84.

39. Van Vliet G, Barboni Th, Klees M, Cantraine F, Wolter R. Treatment strategy and long-term follow-up of congenital hypothyroidism. In: Delange F, Glinoer D, Fisher DA, eds. Proceedings of the NATO Advanced Research Workshop on Congenital Hypothyroidism. New York: Plenum Press, 1989:245–252.

40. American Academy of Pediatrics AAP Section on Endocrinology and Committee on Genetics, and American Thyroid Association Committee on Public Health: Newborn screening for congenital hypothyroidism: recommended guidelines. Pediatrics 1993; 91:1203–1209.

41. Vogiatzi MG, Kirkland JL. Frequency and necessity of thyroid function tests in neonates and infants with congenital hypothyroidism. Pediatrics 1997; 100:E6.

42. Bongers-Schokking JJ, Koot HM, Wiersma D, Verkerk PH, de Muinck Keizer-Schrama SM. Influence of timing and dose of thyroid hormone replacement on development in infants with congenital hypothyroidism. J Pediatr 2000; 136:292–297.

43. Van Vliet G Treatment of congenital hypothyroidism. Lancet 2001; 358:86–87.

44. Heinrichs C, Parma J, Scherberg NH, Delange F, Van Vliet G, Duprez L, Bourdoux P, Bergmann P, Vassart G, Refetoff S. Congenital central isolated hypothyroidism caused by a homozygous mutation in the TSH-beta subunit gene. Thyroid 2000; 10:387–391

45. Collu R, Tang J, Castagne J, Lagace G, Masson N, Huot C, Deal C, Delvin E, Faccenda E, Eidne KA, Van Vliet G. A novel mechanism for isolated central hypothyroidism: inactivating mutations in the thyrotropin-releasing hormone receptor gene. J Clin Endocrinol Metab 1997; 82: 1561–1565.

46. Ward L, Chavez M, Huot C, Lecocq P, Collu R, Decarie JC, Martial JA, Van Vliet G. Severe congenital hypopituitarism with low prolactin levels and age-dependent anterior pituitary hypoplasia: a clue to a PIT-1 mutation. J Pediatr 1998; 132:1036–1038.

47. Briet JM, van Wassenaer AG, Dekker FW, de Vijlder JJ, van Baar A, Kok JH. Neonatal thyroxine supplementation

in very preterm children: developmental outcome evaluated at early school age. Pediatrics 2001; 107:712–718.

48. Smith C, Thomsett M, Choong C, Rodda C, McIntyre HD, Cotterill AM. Congenital thyrotoxicosis in premature infants. Clin Endocrinol (Oxf) 2001; 54:371–376.

49. Wit JM, Gerards LJ, Vermeulen-Meiners C, Bruinse HW. Neonatal thyrotoxicosis treated with exchange transfusion and Lugol's iodine. Eur J Pediatr 1985; 143:317–319.

50. Transue D, Chan J, Kaplan M. Management of neonatal Graves disease with iopanoic acid. J Pediatr 1992; 121:472–474.

51. Daneman D, Howard NJ. Neonatal thyrotoxicosis: intellectual impairment and craniosynostosis in later years. J Pediatr 1980; 97:257–259.

52. Thomas JS, Leclere J, Hartemann P, Duheille J, Orgiazzi J, Petersen M, Janot C, Guedenet JC. Familial hyperthyroidism without evidence of autoimmunity. Acta Endocrinol (Copenh) 1982; 100:512–518.

53. Duprez L, Parma J, Van Sande J, Allgeier A, Leclere J, Schvartz C, Delisle MJ, Decoulx M, Orgiazzi J, Dumont J, Vassart G. Germline mutations in the thyrotropin receptor gene cause non-autoimmune autosomal dominant hyperthyroidism. Nat Genet 1994; 7:396–401.

54. Kopp P, van Sande J, Parma J, Duprez L, Gerber H, Joss E, Jameson JL, Dumont JE, Vassart G. Brief report: congenital hyperthyroidism caused by a mutation in the thyrotropin-receptor gene. N Engl J Med 1995; 332:150–154.

55. Duprez L, Parma J, Van Sande J, Rodien P, Sabine C, Abramowicz M, Dumont JE, Vassart G. Pathology of the TSH receptor. J Pediatr Endocrinol Metab 1999; 12:295–302.

56. Parma J, Duprez L, Van Sande J, Hermans J, Rocmans P, Van Vliet G, Costagliola S, Rodien P, Dumont JE, Vassart G. Diversity and prevalence of somatic mutations in the thyrotropin receptor and Gs alpha genes as a cause of toxic thyroid adenomas. J Clin Endocrinol Metab 1997; 82:2695–2701.

57. Kopp P, Muirhead S, Jourdain N, Gu WX, Jameson JL, Rodd C. Congenital hyperthyroidism caused by a solitary toxic adenoma harboring a novel somatic mutation (serine281—>isoleucine) in the extracellular domain of the thyrotropin receptor. J Clin Invest 1997; 100:1634–1639.

58. Foley TP Jr, Abbassi V, Copeland KC, Draznin MB. Hypothyroidism caused by chronic autoimmune thyroiditis in very young infants. N Engl J Med 1994; 330:466–468.

59. Ward L, Huot C, Lambert R, Deal C, Collu R, Van Vliet G. Outcome of pediatric Graves' disease after treatment with antithyroid medication and radioiodine. Clin Invest Med. 1999; 22:132–139.

60. van Trotsenburg AS, Vulsma T, van Santen HM, de Vijlder JJM. Are young Down syndrome infants hypothyroid? Horm Res 2000; 53(suppl 2):115.

61. Konings CH, van Trotsenburg AS, Ris-Stalpers C, Vulsma T, Wiedijk BM, de Vijlder JJ. Plasma thyrotropin bioactivity in Down's syndrome children with subclinical hypothyroidism. Eur J Endocrinol. 2001; 144:1–4.

62. Tirosh E, Taub Y, Scher A, Jaffe M, Hochberg Z. Short-term efficacy of thyroid hormone supplementation for patients with Down syndrome and low-borderline thyroid function. Am J Ment Retard 1989; 93:652–656.

63. Sprinzl GM, Koebke J, Wimmers-Klick J, Eckel HE, Thumfart WF. Morphology of the human thyroglossal tract: a histologic and macroscopic study in infants and children. Ann Otol Rhinol Laryngol 2000; 109:1135–1139.

64. Van Vliet G, Glinoer D, Verelst J, Spehl M, Gompel C, Delange F. Cold thyroid nodules in childhood: is surgery always necessary? Eur J Pediatr 1987; 146:378–382.

65. Geva T, Theodor R. Atypical presentation of subacute thyroiditis. Arch Dis Child 1988; 63:845–846.

66. Lallier M, St-Vil D, Giroux M, Huot C, Gaboury L, Oligny L, Desjardins JG. Prophylactic thyroidectomy for medullary thyroid carcinoma in gene carriers of MEN2 syndrome. J Pediatr Surg 1998; 33:846–848.

15

Hypothyroidism

John S. Dallas
University of Texas Medical Branch–Galveston, Galveston, Texas, U.S.A.

Thomas P. Foley, Jr.
University of Pittsburgh and Children's Hospital of Pittsburgh, Pittsburgh, Pennsylvania, U.S.A.

I. HISTORICAL BACKGROUND

For more than 2000 years, endemic goiter and cretinism have been prevalent in iodine-deficient regions of the world, as evidenced by Andean sculptures of goitrous dwarfs dating from the 4th century BCE (1) and by descriptions recorded in Europe during the 1st century BCE (2, 3). Nonendemic cretinism, however, was not reported until 1850 when Curling described two children who had no detectable thyroid tissue at autopsy (4). In 1871, Fagge used the term "sporadic cretinism" to describe four children with cretinism, one being a 16-year-old girl with classic symptoms and signs of hypothyroidism, absence of thyromegaly, and "mental faculties unimpaired" (5). In 1878, W.M. Ord associated the term "myxoedema" with his descriptions of the supraclavicular "fatty tumours" found in hypothyroid middle-aged women (6). The Committee of the Clinical Society of London was nominated in 1883 to study hypothyroidism and presented its report in 1888 describing lymphocytic infiltration and atrophy of the thyroid gland (7) (Fig. 1). This first description of chronic lymphocytic thyroiditis preceded Hashimoto's classic description of asymptomatic goiter (8) by 24 years.

During the last decade of the 19th century several reports of successful treatment of hypothyroidism with thyroid gland extracts were reported. These therapeutic achievements were summarized in 1898 so elegantly by Sir William Osler:

"That we can to-day rescue children otherwise doomed to helpless idiocy—that we can restore to life the hopeless victims of myxoedema—is a triumph of experimental medicine for which we are indebted very largely to Victor Horsley and to his pupil Murray. Transplantation of the gland was first tried; then Murray used an extract subcutaneously. Hector Mackenzie in London and Howitz in Copenhagen introduced the method of feeding. We now know that the gland, taken either fresh, or as the watery or glycerin extract, or dried and powdered, is equally efficacious in a majority of all the cases of myxoedema in infants or adults . . . The results, as a rule, are most astounding—Unparalleled by anything in the whole range of curative measures. Within 6 weeks a poor, feeble-minded, toad-like caricature of humanity may be restored to mental and bodily health" (9).

Photographs depicting hypothyroid children before and after the initiation of thyroid extract therapy began to appear in textbooks soon thereafter (10) (Fig. 2).

During the 20th century our understanding of the biochemical and physiological functions of the thyroid gland expanded considerably. The discovery of the structures of the iodothyronines, the need for adequate dietary intake of iodine, and the identity of the types of familial goiter and their causes have improved our ability to diagnose and treat hypothyroidism more accurately. The pathogenesis of autoimmunity, which is the most common cause of hypothyroidism in nonendemic goiter regions of the world, has been elucidated with the pioneering serological studies of Roitt and Doniach (11) and the experimental studies of Rose and Witebsky (12). More recently, competitive binding assays, thyroid epithelial cell culture systems, and advances in molecular biology have provided improved methods to study thyroid hormone secretion and action. They have also expanded our knowledge into the causes and pathogenesis of autoimmunity, inborn errors of thyroid hormone synthesis, regulation and metabolism, and other causes of hypothyroidism.

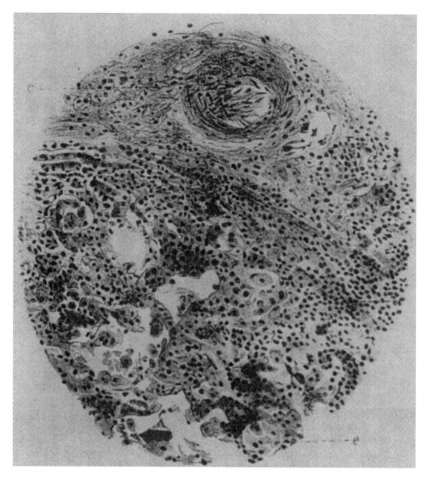

Figure 1 Lymphocytic infiltration of the thyroid gland of an adult with myxedema reported in 1888, or 24 years before the description by Hashimoto. (From Refs. 7, 8).

II. CLASSIFICATION AND CAUSES

A. Classification

Normal thyroid hormone secretion depends on an intact hypothalamic–pituitary–thyroid axis. In normals, thyrotropin-releasing hormone (TRH) modulates the release of thyrotropin (TSH) from the pituitary gland. TSH then binds to plasma membrane receptors on the thyrocyte and stimulates a cascade of biochemical processes that result in the production and release of primarily L-thyroxine (T_4) and, in smaller molar concentrations, 3, 3′, 5-L-triiodothyronine (T_3). An abnormality at any point within this axis can lead to decreased thyroid hormone secretion and result in hypothyroidism. By convention, hypothyroidism is classified according to the anatomical location within this axis where the abnormality occurs (13). For example, hypothyroidism resulting from thyroid gland failure, such as occurs with autoimmune destruction in Hashimoto's thyroiditis, is referred to as primary hypothyroidism. Likewise, secondary and tertiary hypothyroidism refer to hypothyroidism resulting from disorders at the level of the pituitary and hypothalamus, respectively. These diseases also are referred to as pituitary and hypothalamic hypothyroidism, and, in patients at all ages, they are much less common than primary hypothyroidism.

Selective peripheral resistance to thyroid hormone is a very rare cause of hypothyroidism (14). In this syndrome, the hypothalamic–pituitary–thyroid axis is normal, but nuclear thyroid hormone receptors in peripheral tissues do not respond adequately to T_3. Affected patients have symptoms and signs of hypothyroidism from an early age. Basal serum TSH, thyroid hormone levels, and TSH responses to TRH are normal. Why the resistance to thyroid hormone is present only in the peripheral tissues, and not also in the pituitary, remains to be fully elucidated.

B. Causes

Hypothyroidism during childhood and adolescence can result from a variety of congenital or acquired defects (Table

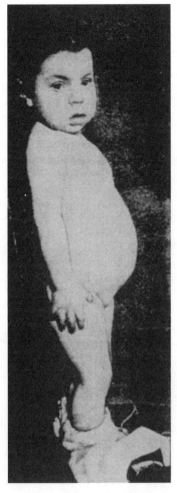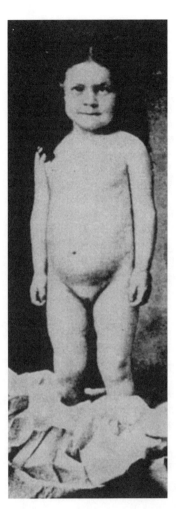

Figure 2 An early example of the effects of thyroid hormone therapy in a 7-year-old girl with the onset of hypothyroidism around age 3 years.

1). In economically advantaged countries, the majority of children with congenital primary hypothyroidism will be detected through neonatal thyroid screening programs. Rarely, however, patients with hypothyroidism caused by ectopic or hypoplastic thyroid glands, or with inborn errors of thyroid hormone synthesis (Fig. 3), may not be recognized until later in infancy or childhood. In general, ectopic and hypoplastic glands occur sporadically, whereas the inborn errors of hormone synthesis (thyroid dyshormonogenesis) are inherited as autosomal recessive disorders (15). Specific mutations have been identified in the genes that regulate the synthesis of proteins (usually enzymes) involved in the specific steps of hormonogenesis (16).

Autoimmune chronic lymphocytic thyroiditis is the most common cause of acquired primary hypothyroidism in nonendemic goiter regions of the world. The disease occurs most often during childhood or adolescence and more frequently in girls than boys. However, it may pre-

sent during infancy (as early as 6–9 months of age) with subtle symptoms and signs of hypothyroidism of short duration (17). The disease also occurs with increased frequency in patients with other autoimmune-mediated diseases, especially insulin-dependent diabetes mellitus and the polyglandular autoimmune syndromes and in Down, Turner, and Klinefelter syndromes. In a recent study, serum thyroid antibodies were found in 52% of girls with Turner syndrome compared to 17% in age-matched normal girls (18). Thyroid autoimmune disease is most commonly associated with an X-isochromosome karyotype, but is also common with a 45,X karyotype (19). This association suggests that the loss of one or more genes, known as haploinsufficiency, on the short arm of the X or Y chromosome that normally are not inactivated play an important role in the pathogenesis of autoimmune thyroid disease.

Other causes of primary hypothyroidism include irradiation of the thyroid, surgical removal of thyroid tissue,

Table 1 Causes of Juvenile Primary Hypothyroidism

Congenital hypothyroidism: mild, late-onset
   Ectopic thyroid dysgenesis
   Familial thyroid dyshormonogenesis
   Peripheral resistance to thyroid hormone action
Acquired primary hypothyroidism
   Chronic autoimmune thyroiditis
      Lymphocytic thyroiditis of childhood and adolescence
         with thyromegaly
      Hashimoto's thyroiditis with thyromegaly (struma
         lymphomatosa)
      Chronic fibrous variant
   Drug-induced hypothyroidism
   Endemic goiter
      Iodine deficiency
      Environmental goitrogens
   Irradiation of the thyroid
      Therapeutic radioiodine
      External irradiation of nonthyroid tumors
   Surgical excision
   Nephropathic cystinosis
   Subacute thyroiditis: transient phase

goitrogen ingestion, iodine deficiency, and nephropathic cystinosis (Table 1). Transient primary hypothyroidism may occur during the recovery phase from subacute and toxic thyroiditis.

Secondary and tertiary hypothyroidism result from deficiencies in TSH and TRH, respectively. Most children with secondary or tertiary (also known as central) hypothyroidism will have other pituitary or hypothalamic hormone deficiencies, but an isolated deficiency of either TSH or TRH secretion can occur as familial or sporadic diseases (20), and mutations have been found in the genes that control the synthesis of the TSH beta chain and the TSH and TRH receptors (21). Malformation syndromes, such as septo-optic dysplasia, or midline facial anomalies, such as cleft lip or palate, can be associated with central hypothyroidism. Trauma, neoplasms, infectious or inflammatory processes, irradiation, and surgery can damage the hypothalamus or pituitary and cause TRH, TSH, and other hormone deficiencies. These diseases are discussed in further detail elsewhere. In very low birth weight (VLBW) preterm infants less than 27 weeks of gestation, and in critically ill infants and children, hypothalamic hypothyroidism may occur as a progression of the nonthyroidal illness state and inhibition by certain therapeutic modalities.

III. PATHOPHYSIOLOGY

In primary hypothyroidism, abnormalities of the thyroid gland or of thyroid gland function impair thyroid hormone production and/or release. Early in the course of thyroid

gland failure, a slight decrease in the serum free T_4 (FT_4) concentration occurs, but in most cases the level usually remains within the normal range for age. A decrease in FT_4 leads to minor reductions in pituitary FT_4 concentrations and the intrapituitary conversion of T_4 to T_3 (22). With a decrease in the pituitary free T_3 (FT_3) concentration, TSH production and release increase. The subsequent increase in serum TSH that causes further stimulation of the TSH receptor results in an increase in thyroid hormone synthesis and release in an attempt to maintain normal serum FT_4 and FT_3 levels. However, as thyroid gland failure progresses, increased TSH secretion no longer is able to maintain normal thyroid hormone synthesis, and serum FT_4 and FT_3 levels decrease to abnormal levels. Since serum TSH rises before serum thyroid hormone levels decrease below the normal range, the measurement of serum TSH is the most sensitive test for the early detection of primary hypothyroidism.

Pituitary TSH synthesis and secretion are directly controlled by serum levels of free or unbound T_4 (FT_4) and FT_3. This control occurs by negative feedback; that is, rising serum levels of FT_4 and FT_3 inhibit, whereas decreasing FT_4 and FT_3 levels enhance, TSH synthesis and secretion. Through TRH and somatostatin secretion, the hypothalamus modulates this negative feedback system, and the so-called set point of the molar concentrations of FT_4/FT_3 for TSH secretion is fine-tuned (23). TRH secretion enhances and somatostatin inhibits TSH release. Thus, patients with TRH deficiency have a decreased release of TSH causing a decrease in thyroid hormone production. However, TRH deficiency is associated with increased pituitary stores of TSH because low intrapituitary FT_4 and FT_3 concentrations continue to stimulate TSH synthesis. Therefore, TSH responses to TRH in experimental animals and patients often are exaggerated and the TSH rise is usually delayed, a pattern that is diagnostic of hypothalamic TRH deficiency (see below) (24).

IV. CLINICAL PRESENTATION

Children with hypothyroidism may have a variety of clinical presentations (Table 2) and often a family history of thyroid or pituitary disease. Some children present with an asymptomatic goiter, whereas others may present with mild tenderness or a sensation of fullness in the anterior neck. Other presenting symptoms are often nonspecific and include weakness, lethargy, decreased appetite, cold intolerance, constipation, and dry skin. Although children with hypothyroidism may have mild obesity, hypothyroidism generally does not cause morbid obesity. The course of hypothyroidism is often so insidious that neither the child nor his or her parents are aware of the physical changes that have occurred. These children often experience marked growth retardation before the disease is recognized, and this expected effect on linear growth emphasizes the importance of serial growth measurements in

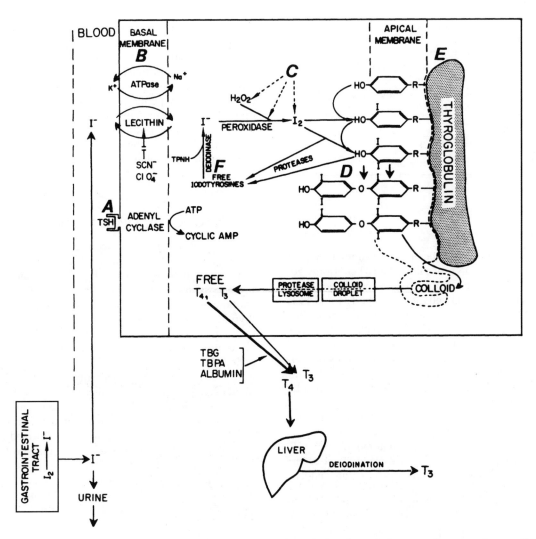

Figure 3 Schematic representation of thyroid hormone synthesis and the sites of the most frequent abnormalities seen in patients with familial dyshormonogenesis (15, 16). A. Impaired thyroid response to TSH. B. Iodide transport defect. C. Iodide oxidation and tyrosyl iodination defects, including Pendred syndrome. D. Iodotyrosine coupling defect. E. Thyroglobulin synthetic defects. F. Iodotyrosine deiodinase defect. Each defect is associated with thyromegaly, except A. An increase in ^{123}I-iodide uptake occurs in each defect, except A and B. A rapid discharge of ^{123}I-iodide from the thyroid after oral perchlorate occurs in the iodide oxidation and tyrosyl iodination defects.

all children. Whereas children who develop hypothyroidism before age 2 years may suffer some irreversible central nervous system damage and developmental delay, the onset of hypothyroidism after age 2 years does not cause mental retardation.

Infants with acquired autoimmune-mediated infantile hypothyroidism present between 6 and 24 months of age with symptoms and signs similar to those in infants with congenital hypothyroidism (17). Deceleration of linear growth is an important sign that is helpful in the early recognition of this disease.

Most adolescents with untreated primary hypothyroidism will have delayed pubertal development, although an occasional patient will present with precocious puberty. Girls may have galactorrhea that usually is associated with an elevated serum prolactin level; boys may have macroorchidism. The cause of precocious puberty in primary hypothyroidism originally was postulated to occur as a result of increased LH and FSH secretion through an overlap in the pituitary regulation of TSH secretion (25). Other studies suggest that hyperprolactinemia, which presumably results from chronic TRH stimulation of the pituitary, may play a role in this syndrome through an inhibition of gonadal stimulation by luteinizing hormone (LH), but not follicle-stimulating hormone (FSH), thereby resulting in sustained stimulation of the gonad by FSH (26). More

Table 2 Clinical Features Unique to
Juvenile Hypothyroidism

Growth retardation with delayed skeletal maturation
Delayed dental development and tooth eruption
Onset of puberty usually delayed; rarely precocious
Galactorrhea: elevated prolactin
Increased skin pigmentation
Sellar enlargement
Pseudotumor cerebri
Myopathy and muscular hypertrophy

recently, studies involving the use of mammalian cells transfected with the cDNA of either the LH/chorionic gonadotropin (CG) receptor or the FSH receptor have shown that TSH can bind to and activate both the LH and FSH receptors (27, 28). Based on these studies, elevated TSH levels associated with severe primary hypothyroidism may result in stimulation of both LH and FSH receptors and contribute to the development of precocious puberty (27, 28). The adolescent girl who acquires hypothyroidism after menarche often experiences excessive and irregular menstrual bleeding.

The child with severe primary hypothyroidism may develop enlargement of the sella turcica. When this is identified by skull x-rays, computed tomographic (CT) scan, or magnetic resonance image (MRI) of the head, the child may be referred to a neurosurgeon or an endocrinologist for evaluation of suspected pituitary tumor. This pituitary mass represents hypertrophy and hyperplasia of thyrotrophs in response to the lack of negative feedback by thyroid hormones (29). Therefore, these patients with primary hypothyroidism usually have markedly elevated serum TSH levels and low serum levels of thyroid hormones; patients with hypothalamic and pituitary hypothyroidism usually have normal or very mildly elevated serum TSH levels (30) and low serum FT_4 values. Pituitary enlargement usually resolves with adequate thyroid hormone replacement therapy. Primary hypothyroidism with enlargement of the sella and pituitary gland was reported in a boy in whom an empty sella and hypopituitarism occurred after thyroid hormone replacement (31). Visual field defects also may be detected in these patients (32).

Children with hypothalamic and pituitary hypothyroidism can present with the same nonspecific symptoms found in primary hypothyroidism, as well as with symptoms suggestive of other hormone deficiencies. Patients with organic defects also may present with symptoms of increased intracranial pressure, such as headaches, morning vomiting, and decreased visual acuity.

Features of hypothyroidism on physical examination include bradycardia, decreased pulse pressure, short stature with an increased upper-to-lower body ratio, delayed

dentition, mild obesity, facial puffiness and dull facial expression, coarse hair, cool and dry carotenemic skin, and delayed relaxation of deep tendon reflexes. The majority of patients with primary hypothyroidism will have thyromegaly, but some patients with autoimmune thyroiditis and ectopic or hypoplastic glands will not have detectable thyroid enlargement. Thyromegaly is not associated with hypothalamic and pituitary hypothyroidism. These children may have an abnormal optic fundus examination (i.e., papilledema), and visual field defects may be found.

V. DIAGNOSTIC EVALUATION

Patients with nongoitrous, acquired primary hypothyroidism require very few diagnostic tests prior to therapy. Serum determinations of TSH, FT_4 and thyroid antibodies, thyroperoxidase antibodies (TPOAb), and thyroglobulin antibodies (TGAb), should be obtained. The presence of thyroid antibodies permits a presumptive diagnosis of autoimmune thyroiditis. Some patients with autoimmune thyroiditis have negative thyroid antibodies on initial evaluation, but, on repeat determinations 3–6 months later, have elevated thyroid antibody titers (11, 33). Thyroid antibodies may be positive in other forms of thyroiditis (34), although the levels tend to be lower and not as persistently elevated as in patients with autoimmune thyroiditis. Similar thyroid function tests should be performed in patients with goitrous hypothyroidism since the most common cause is autoimmune thyroiditis. However, if thyroid antibodies are negative on repeated determinations in a child with persistent thyromegaly, these additional tests may be useful to determine the cause of hypothyroidism:

1. Radioiodide uptake test with perchlorate discharge at 2–4 h after dose, salivary-to-plasma ratio of radioiodide 2 h after the dose, and serum thyroglobulin (to identify inborn errors of thyroid hormone synthesis)
2. Urinary iodine excretion (to identify iodine deficiency)
3. Fine-needle aspiration (FNA) biopsy of the thyroid nodule(s) or tissue, if progressive asymptomatic enlargement of the thyroid occurs despite treatment with full replacement or suppressive dosages of L-thyroxine (to identify rare malignant infiltrative diseases).

In addition to serum thyroid function tests, a TRH test often is indicated for patients with suspected hypothalamic or pituitary hypothyroidism. In children with hypothalamic hypothyroidism the peak serum TSH response to TRH often is delayed beyond 30 min, and the TSH response may be prolonged with serum TSH values that remain elevated for 2–3 h. The TSH response to TRH is low or absent in patients with pituitary thyrotroph deficiency (24, 35).

The nonthyroidal illness (NTI) syndrome refers to the various alterations in thyroid function often seen in preterm and VLBW infants, as well as in older children in association with a variety of conditions such as acute or chronic illnesses, surgery, trauma, malnutrition, and starvation. The magnitude of change in thyroid function tends to correlate directly with the severity of systemic illness or tissue injury. Although there are exceptions, the typical pattern of serum thyroid function tests that allows the diagnosis of this syndrome includes low total and free T_3, low to normal T_4, normal to high 3,3′,5′-L-triiodothyronine [known as reverse T_3 (rT_3)], increased T_3 resin uptake, and normal TSH (36). The serum FT_4 is usually normal and often in the high–normal range. Low serum FT_4 values have been reported, especially in the most severely ill patients (37). The direct dialysis method to measure FT_4 in serum is the most accurate determination and rarely is associated with false-positive or false-negative results (38). However, heparin use in infants and children, such as occurs with heparin-supplemented total parenteral nutrition, can cause spurious elevations in FT_4 levels measured by direct dialysis methods (39).

Various factors contribute to the changes in thyroid hormone economy that occur in patients with this syndrome. In the normal state, peripheral tissue conversion of T_4 to T_3 is the major source of circulating T_3, and conversion occurs through monodeiodination via the 5′-deiodinase pathway. This pathway also converts rT_3 to T_2. In the NTI syndrome, 5′-deiodinase activity is decreased in peripheral tissues, causing a decreased production of T_3 and decreased clearance of rT_3. Therefore, decreased 5′-deiodinase activity accounts for the low serum T_3 and elevated serum rT_3 levels in these patients. The increased T_3 resin uptake indicates a reduction in available serum thyroid hormone binding sites. The concentrations of thyroxin-binding globulin (TBG) and transthyretin (TTR), and the binding capacity of TBG, are decreased. These changes are largely responsible for the reduction in available binding sites. Nondialyzable substances, shown to be specific lipoproteins, inhibit thyroid hormone binding to TBG and TTR, and are detectable in serum during severe illness (40). Decreased T_4 binding to serum proteins leads to an increased percentage of FT_4 in serum and accounts for normal FT_4 levels even when TT_4 levels are low. The factors responsible for low TT_4 levels are less well understood. Although decreased serum binding of T_4 and inhibitors of binding to serum proteins may contribute, accelerated disposal of T_4 and decreased TSH secretion are factors that contribute to the low T_4 levels. Accelerated disposal of T_4 occurs through the 5-deiodinase pathway, which converts T_4 to rT_3, and through nondeiodinative pathways (36). Inhibition of TSH release occurs when patients become severely ill. Abnormal hypothalamic–pituitary function during severe illness results in hypo-thalamic hypothyroidism that is evident when FT_4 levels become low (41).

Thyroid function tests are often obtained in severely ill infants and children who are evaluated for such clinical findings as hypothermia, weakness, lethargy, and growth failure. Not only can the underlying illness or injury produce alterations in thyroid function, but the severely ill child may also be receiving medications such as dopamine, glucocorticoids, and phenytoin that can alter thyroid hormone economy (36). Cytokines also may interfere with TSH synthesis and release.

Whereas the ill child with low serum T_3 but normal serum TT_4 and FT_4 levels usually does not pose a diagnostic problem, the question of hypothyroidism frequently arises in the ill child with low serum levels of T_3 and T_4. In this situation a normal serum FT_4 level is used as evidence against central hypothyroidism, especially when measured by direct dialysis methods (38). In the child with a low serum T_4, an elevated rT_3, and normal TSH, the diagnosis of the NTI syndrome is very likely, and is differentiated from hypothyroidism by normal FT_4 and TSH levels. An elevated serum TSH level in a severely ill patient usually indicates primary hypothyroidism, especially when FT_4 levels by direct dialysis are low (36, 37). However, modest elevations of TSH may occur during recovery from illness (36), and serial TSH measurements may be required to establish the correct diagnosis (37, 41).

Children with hypothalamic or pituitary hypothyroidism generally have normal TSH and low serum FT_4 and rT_3 levels. These children may develop severe systemic illness, and it may be difficult to differentiate them from severely ill patients with the NTI syndrome. The history and physical examination may help to differentiate between the two disorders, but a more extensive evaluation including a MRI study of the hypothalamic–pituitary region and pituitary function testing may be necessary. The TSH response to TRH in the NTI syndrome can be normal, delayed, or blunted, and may not be useful in differentiating the NTI syndrome from hypothalamic or pituitary hypothyroidism (36, 37). Determination of rT_3 is not always helpful because the level may be normal in sick hypothyroid children (36, 37).

Thyroid hormone replacement is not recommended in the treatment of the NTI syndrome unless the FT_4, preferably measured by direct dialysis, is low, and especially when the serum TSH is elevated. Management should be directed towards supportive or specific treatment of the underlying illness. To date, studies that have evaluated the effects of T_4 or T_3 replacement in patients with this syndrome have not demonstrated increased survival with replacement therapy (42–44). However, controversy still exists as to whether the NTI syndrome represents an adaptive and beneficial response to severe illness or whether, in its most advanced stage, it represents a functional type of secondary hypothyroidism as a result of a prolonged, severe illness that responds to thyroxine replacement therapy (36, 44).

VI. CLINICAL COURSE AND MANAGEMENT

A. Primary Hypothyroidism

L-thyroxine is the safest and most efficacious thyroid medication for treatment of hypothyroidism in children and adolescents (35, 37, 45, 46). Other thyroid preparations, such as thyroid extract, desiccated thyroid, and T_4–T_3 combination drugs, offer no advantage over L-thyroxine and may have some disadvantages when therapy is monitored by thyroid function tests. Recent claims that T_3 therapy is clinically efficacious in the treatment of an entity described on a web site as Wilson's syndrome, caused by a reduced T_4 to T_3 conversion disorder, cannot be substantiated by studies reported in the literature. In these patients, any perceived benefits of T_3 replacement likely result from mild hyperthyroidism induced by the T_3 therapy. Approximately 20% of patients who are prescribed L-thyroxine after total thyroidectomy for thyroid cancer report symptoms of hypothyroidism despite normal results of thyroid function tests. These symptoms improve with higher dosages of L-thyroxine and mildly elevated T_4 values and suppressed TSH; it is yet to be determined if instances of reduced T_4 to T_3 conversion occur in these patients. Generic preparations of L-thyroxine should be prescribed cautiously as some may have variable potencies and, therefore, may provide inconsistent replacement therapy (46). The importance of prescribing reliable L-

thyroxine preparations for treatment of hypothyroidism is essential for restoration of the euthyroid state. L-thyroxine is prescribed orally as a single daily dose and should be taken at least 30 min before food intake to maximize absorption. The estimated dosage for children and adolescents is based on age and body weight (Table 3).

To minimize central nervous system damage, children who are less than 2 years of age require prompt treatment with L-thyroxine in full replacement dosages. Rapid achievement of euthyroidism is not as essential in the older child and adolescent; in fact, children with chronic or severe hypothyroidism often experience undesirable side effects, such as irritability, restlessness, decreased attention span, and restless sleep or insomnia when L-thyroxine is prescribed in full replacement dosages at diagnosis. For these children it is preferable to restore euthyroidism gradually by initiating treatment with 25 μg daily for 2 weeks, and thereafter increasing the dose by 25 μg daily every 2–4 weeks until the desired dosage is achieved. This regimen is not necessary for children with mild hypothyroidism, or those with clinical symptoms of short duration. On initiation of therapy in older children and adolescents, it is important, however, to avoid excessive replacement and prudent to begin with the lower dosage per kilogram body weight for age.

In patients with compensated, or subclinical, hypothyroidism, defined as an elevated serum TSH level (47), but normal concentrations of TT_4 and FT_4, it is worthwhile to confirm that the process is persistent by repeating the serum TSH evaluation before initiating long-term therapy. This is especially important in patients with negative thyroid antibodies and no apparent cause for the elevated

Table 3 Guidelines for Maintenance Sodium L-Thyroxine Therapy

Age	Daily dosage (μg/kg)	Daily dosage range (μg/day)	Weight range (kg)
<6 months[a]	6–10	25–50	3–9
6–12 months	5–8	37.5–75	6–12
1–5 years	4–6	50–100	9–23
5–12 years	3–5	50–125	15–55
12–18 years	2–3	75–175	30–90
Adult	1–2	100–200	50–100

The dosage of L-thyroxine must be determined for each patient, since the rate of absorption and metabolism will vary among patients of the same body weight. These dosages approximate 100 μg/m²/day. In general, patients with hypothalamic hypothyroidism seem to require a lower dosage per kg than patients with primary hypothyroidism.

L-thyroxine usually is usually manufactured in 25, 50, 75, 88, 100, 112, 125, 137, 150, 175, and 200 μg tablets. Tablets should be given at least 30–60 min before a meal.

[a] The dosage of L-thyroxine in the initial treatment of newborn infants with congenital hypothyroidism is 10–15 μg/kg once daily for the initial 1–2 weeks. The appropriate maintenance dosage is determined by the results of serial measurements of serum TSH and FT_4, and, on rare occasions when the results of the two tests do not agree, serum T_3 should be measured.

TSH value. Some children have persistent hyperthyrotropinemia of unknown cause without symptoms or signs of hypothyroidism. Thyroxine therapy is indicated in patients with compensated hypothyroidism in whom there is a known cause for hypothyroidism, or serial TSH measurements steadily increase, especially if FT_4 concentrations steadily decline (48).

Subclinical hypothyroidism is commonly observed in patients with Down syndrome (49). Recent studies have shown that elevated TSH levels in some patients with Down syndrome are associated with zinc and selenium deficiencies (50, 51); elevated TSH levels in Down syndrome patients with zinc deficiency can normalize following adequate zinc replacement (50). However, patients with Down syndrome have an increased risk of autoimmune thyroiditis compared to the general population. Therefore, the measurement of thyroid antibodies is important in Down syndrome patients with subclinical hypothyroidism. A recent study revealed that Down syndrome patients with subclinical hypothyroidism and positive thyroid antibody levels are at increased risk of clinically overt thyroid disease compared to Down syndrome patients with subclinical hypothyroidism but negative thyroid antibody levels (49).

Serum thyroid function tests should be monitored at regular intervals to determine adequacy of therapy, anytime symptoms of hypothyroidism or hyperthyroidism occur, and 6–8 weeks after a dosage change. In young children, thyroid function should be monitored every 2–4 months, whereas in older children and adolescents thyroid function can be monitored every 6–12 months to determine adequacy of therapy. Serum TSH is the most useful test to monitor primary hypothyroidism, and levels should be maintained between 0.1 and 5 mU/l using sensitive TSH methods that can accurately differentiate normal and suppressed levels; the TSH assay should have a sensitivity of 0.05 mU/l or lower. Serum FT_4 levels are usually adequate to determine whether the patient is receiving excessive L-thyroxine therapy; however, for some children, particularly those with congenital hypothyroidism, measurement of serum T_3 and, rarely, rT_3 levels may help to determine if the L-thyroxine dose is excessive.

Generally, the child with primary nongoitrous hypothyroidism who has had elevated serum TSH levels (>20 mU/l) on at least two separate occasions and requires an increase in his/her L-thyroxine replacement does not have transient hypothyroidism that will recover spontaneously. Therefore, this child should be treated with L-thyroxine indefinitely. On the other hand, reports indicate that approximately 20% of patients with autoimmune goitrous hypothyroidism may revert to the euthyroid state (52, 53). These children may be given a 2–3 month trial off L-thyroxine treatment if the thyroid size and consistency become normal during treatment. The serum TSH level should be determined at the end of this trial, or sooner if symptoms of hypothyroidism develop. If the serum TSH

level is normal, the child should be monitored every 3 months for a year and then annually thereafter if thyroid antibody titers remain abnormal. If the TSH level becomes abnormal, L-thyroxine therapy should be resumed indefinitely.

Serum TSH should be monitored in children receiving lithium carbonate or similar drugs that block thyroid function (54). If these children also have autoimmune thyroiditis, they very likely will develop primary hypothyroidism during lithium treatment (55). Patients should not take iron-containing (56) or calcium-containing (57) medications at the same time as thyroxine tablets. These and other medications, like certain soy-based infant formulas and high-fiber diets, very effectively block the absorption of thyroxine from the intestine (58). Other drugs, such as phenobarbital, phenytoin, carbamazepine, and rifampin, induce accelerated hepatic metabolism of L-thyroxine and can increase dosage requirements in hypothyroid patients (59).

Some adolescent girls and young women with hypothyroidism receiving estrogen replacement therapy have an increase requirement for thyroxine and need to increase their dosages of thyroxine if serum TSH becomes elevated (60). During pregnancy, women with hypothyroidism require an average of 45% more thyroxine to maintain serum TSH values in the normal range (60) as a result of an increase in thyroxine-binding globulin levels (61). Estrogen stimulates glycosylation of TBG and this reduces the metabolic clearance of thyroxine (61). Maintenance of euthyroidism in the mother during early pregnancy is necessary to protect the fetus from the adverse effects of maternal hypothyroxinemia on fetal thyroxine levels that are necessary for normal central nervous system maturation (61, 62).

Prepubertal children with severe hypothyroidism and short stature usually experience a period of catch-up growth after initiation of L-thyroxine replacement therapy, but, despite adequate treatment, some have incomplete catch-up and never reach their full genetic growth potential (63). The mechanisms responsible for this incomplete catch-up growth have not been clearly defined, but delay in treatment of hypothyroidism may be a critical factor (63).

B. Disorders of Thyrotropin Secretion

Hypothyroidism, either hypothalamic or pituitary, may be present at the time of an initial diagnosis of hypopituitarism, or hypothyroidism may occur at a later time during growth hormone replacement therapy. To avoid any confusion in the differential diagnosis between hypothalamic or pituitary hypothyroidism and the NTI syndrome that occurs during severe illnesses or severe caloric/carbohydrate deprivation states, serum FT_4 and, if possible, rT_3 levels should be measured. The FT_4 and rT_3 levels are low in hypothyroidism whereas the FT_4 is usually normal (37) and the rT_3 is normal or elevated (36) in the NTI syndrome. These measurements may be extremely helpful in patients with CNS tumors who are in a catabolic state following surgery. In general, patients with the NTI syndrome do not require L-thyroxine replacement, whereas patients with hypothyroidism do. As previously mentioned, results of TRH tests may differentiate between hypothalamic and pituitary hypothyroidism (35).

Children with hypothalamic or pituitary hypothyroidism usually require lower dosages of L-thyroxine than children with congenital and acquired primary hypothyroidism. Serum levels of FT_4 should be monitored during L-thyroxine therapy. It is unnecessary to monitor TSH levels, however, since patients with hypothalamic or pituitary hypothyroidism will have normal or low TSH values on thyroxine therapy. Once the dosage has been established and the patient is clinically and biochemically euthyroid, further serum thyroid function tests only need to be obtained annually to ensure compliance and reliability of the medication.

Although children with hypothalamic or pituitary hypothyroidism and short stature may exhibit a period of catch-up growth after initiation of L-thyroxine therapy, their course is often complicated by deficiencies of growth hormone, gonadotropins, and sex hormones, and many fail to reach their full genetic height potential. Further discussion of the treatment of hypopituitarism may be found in Chapter 3. Because L-thyroxine therapy increases the metabolic clearance rate of cortisol, patients with deficiencies of hypothalamic–pituitary–adrenal and thyroid function should begin cortisol replacement with initiation of L-thyroxine replacement to avoid the precipitation of hypocortisolism and an adrenal crisis.

REFERENCES

1. Gaitan E. Iodine deficiency and toxicity. In: White PL, Selvey N, eds. Proceedings, Western Hemisphere Nutrition Congress-IV. Acton, MA: Publishing Sciences Group, 1975:56–63.
2. Cranefield PF. The discovery of cretinism. Bull Hist Med 1962; 36:489.
3. Thompson J. Historical Notes. In: Smithers D, ed. Tumours of the Thyroid, vol. 6, Neoplastic Diseases at Various Sites. Edinburgh: Livingstone, 1970.
4. Curling TB. Two cases of absence of the thyroid body. Med Chir Trans 1850;33:303.
5. Fagge CH. On sporadic cretinism, occurring in England. R Med Chir Soc London 1871;54:155.
6. Ord WM. On myxedema, a term proposed to be applied to an essential condition in the "cretinoid" affection occasionally observed in middle-aged women. Med Chir Trans 1878;61:57.
7. Report of a Committee of the Clinical Society of London, nominated December 14, 1883, to investigate the subject of myxedema. Trans Clin Soc London (suppl) 1888;21:1–202.
8. Hashimoto H. Zur Kenntniss der lymphomatösen Veränderung der Schilddrüse (struma lymphomatosa). Arch Klin Chir 1912;97:219.
9. Osler W. The Principles and Practice of Medicine, 3rd Ed. D. Appleton and Co, 1898:843.
10. Sajous CE de M. The Internal Secretions and the Principles of Medicine, 8th Ed. London: F. A. Davis, 1919:198–201.
11. Roitt IM, Doniach D, Campbell RN, Hudson RV. Autoantibodies in Hashimoto's disease. Lancet 1956;2:820.
12. Rose NR, Witebsky E. Studies on organ-specificity. V. Changes in the thyroid glands of rabbits following active immunization with rabbit thyroid extract. J Immunol 1956; 76:417.
13. Braverman LE, Utiger RD. Introduction to hypothyroidism. In: Braverman LE, Utiger RD, eds. Werner and Ingbar's The Thyroid, 8th ed. Philadelphia: Lippincott Williams & Wilkins, 2000:719–720.
14. Kaplan MM, Swartz SL, Larsen PR. Partial peripheral resistance to thyroid hormone. Am J Med 1981;70:1115.
15. Refetoff S, Dumont JE, Vassart G. Thyroid disorders. In: Scriver CR, Beaudet AL, Sly WS, Valle D, eds. The Metabolic and Molecular Bases of Inherited Disease, 8th ed. New York: McGraw-Hill, 2001:4029–4075.
16. Medeiros-Neto GA, Billerbeck AEC, Wajchenberg BL, Targovnik HM. Defective organification of iodide causing hereditary goitrous hypothyroidism. Thyroid 1993;3:143.
17. Foley TP Jr, Abbassi V, Copeland KC, Draznin MB. Acquired autoimmune mediated infantile hypothyroidism: a pathologic entity distinct from congenital hypothyroidism. N Engl J Med 1994;330:466.
18. Ivarrson SA, Ericsson UB, Nilsson KO, et al. Thyroid autoantibodies, Turner's syndrome and growth hormone therapy. Acta Pediatr 1995;84:63.
19. Elsheikh M, Wass JAH, Conway GS. Autoimmune thyroid syndrome in women with Turner's syndrome—the association with karyotype. Clin Endocrinol 2001;55:223.
20. Foley TP Jr. Congenital hypopituitarism. In: Dussault JH, Walker P, eds. Congenital Hypothyroidism. New York: Marcel Dekker, 1983:331–348.
21. Tatsumi K-I, Miyai K, Tsugunori N, et al. Cretinism with combined hormone deficiency caused by a mutation in the PIT1 gene. Nat Genet 1992;1:56.
22. Larsen PR. Thyroid–pituitary interaction. N Engl J Med 1982;306:23.
23. Scanlon MF, Toft AD. Regulation of thyrotropin secretion. In: Braverman LE, Utiger RD, eds. Werner and Ingbar's The Thyroid, 8th ed. Philadelphia: Lippincott Williams & Wilkins, 2000:234–253.
24. Foley TP Jr, Owings J, Hayford JR, Blizzard RM. Serum thyrotropin (TSH) responses to synthetic thyrotropin releasing hormone (TRH) in normal children and hypopituitary patients: a new test to distinguish primary pituitary hormone deficiency. J Clin Invest 1972;51:431.
25. Van Wyk JJ, Grumbach MM. Syndrome of precocious menstruation and galactorrhea in juvenile hypothyroidism: an example of hormonal overlap in pituitary feedback. J Pediatr 1960;59:416.
26. Castro-Magana M, Angulo M, Canas A, et al. Hypothalamic-pituitary-gonadal axis in boys with primary hypothyroidism and macroorchidism. J Pediatr 1988;112:397.
27. Hidaka A, Minegishi T, Kohn LD. Thyrotropin, like luteinizing hormone (LH) and chorionic gonadotropin (CG) increases cAMP and inositol phosphate levels in cells with recombinant human LH/CG receptor. Biochem Biophys Res Commun 1993;196:187.
28. Anasti JN, Flack MR, Froehlich J, et al. A potential novel mechanism for precocious puberty in juvenile hypothyroidism. J Clin Endocrinol Metab 1995;80:2543.

29. Yamada T, Tsukaii T, Ikejiri K, et al. Volume of sella turcica in normal subjects and in patients with primary hypothyroidism and hyperthyroidism. J Clin Endocrinol Metab 1976;42:817.

30. Illig R, Krawczy'nska H, Torresani T, Prader, A. Elevated plasma TSH and hypothyroidism in children with hypothalamic hypopituitarism. J Clin Endocrinol Metab 1975; 41:722.

31. LaFranchi SH, Hanna CE, Krainz PL. Primary hypothyroidism, empty sella, and hypothyroidism. J Pediatr 1986; 108:571.

32. Yamamoto K, Saito K, Takai T, et al. Visual field defects and pituitary enlargement in primary hypothyroidism. J Clin Endocrinol Metab 1983;57:283.

33. Foley TP Jr. Acute, subacute, and chronic thyroiditis. In: Kaplan SA, ed. Clinical Pediatric and Adolescent Endocrinology. Philadelphia: WB Saunders, 1982:96–109.

34. Emerson CH, Farwell AP. Sporadic silent thyroiditis, postpartum thyroiditis, and subacute thyroiditis. In: Braverman LE, Utiger RD, eds. Werner and Ingbar's The Thyroid, 8th ed. Philadelphia: Lippincott Williams & Wilkins, 2000: 578–589.

35. Foley TP Jr. Acquired hypothyroidism during infancy, childhood, and adolescence. In: Braverman LE, Utiger RD, eds. Werner and Ingbar's The Thyroid, 8th ed. Philadelphia: Lippincott Williams & Wilkins, 2000:983–988.

36. Fisher DA. Euthyroid low thyroxine (T_4) and triiodothyronine states in prematures and sick neonates. Pediatr Clin North Am 1990;37:1297.

37. Foley TP Jr, Malvaux P, Blizzard RM. Thyroid Disease. In: Kappy MS, Blizzard RM, Migeon CJ, eds. Wilkins The Diagnosis and Treatment of Endocrine Disorders in Childhood and Adolescence, 4th ed. Springfield: Charles C Thomas, 1994:513–515.

38. Nelson JC, Wilcox RB, Pandian MR. Dependence of free thyroxine estimates obtained with equilibrium tracer dialysis on the concentration of thyroxine-binding globulin. Clin Chem 1992;38:1294.

39. Dallas JS, Dallas DV, Frost PH, et al. Measurement of free T_4 levels in preterm infants receiving heparin-supplemented parenteral nutrition: comparison between equilibrium dialysis and a two-step RIA method. Program and Abstracts, 73rd Annual Meeting of the American Thyroid Association, Washington, D.C., 2001:167.

40. Oppenheimer JH, Schwartz HL, Mariash CN, Kaiser FE. Evidence for a factor in the sera of patients with nonthyroidal disease which inhibits iodothyronine binding by solid matrices, serum proteins, and rat hepatocytes. J Clin Endocrinol Metab 1982;54:757.

41. Wehmann RE, Gregerman RI, Burns WH, et al. Suppression of thyrotropin in the low-thyroxine state of severe nonthyroidal illness. N Engl J Med 1985;312:546.

42. Becker RA, Vaughan GM, Ziegler MG, et al. Hypermetabolic low triiodothyronine syndrome of burn injury. Crit Care Med 1982;10:870.

43. Rapaport R, Rose SR, Freemark M. Hypothyroxinemia in the preterm infant: the benefits and risks of thyroxine treatment. J Pediatr 2001;139:182.

44. Wiersinga WM. Nonthyroidal illness. In: Braverman LE, Utiger RD, eds. Werner and Ingbar's The Thyroid, 8th ed. Philadelphia: Lippincott Williams & Wilkins, 2000:281–295.

45. Foley TP Jr. Pediatric thyroid disorders. In: Cooper DS, ed. Medical Management of Thyroid Disease. New York: Marcel Dekker, 2001:313–344.

46. Rees-Jones RW, Rolla AR, Larsen PR. Hormone content of thyroid replacement preparations. JAMA 1980;243:549.

47. Cooper DS. Subclinical hypothyroidism. N Engl J Med 2001;345:260.

48. LaFranchi S. Thyroiditis and acquired hypothyroidism. Pediatr Ann 1992;21:29.

49. Rubello D, Pozzan GB, Casara D, et al. Natural course of subclinical hypothyroidism in Down's syndrome: prospective study results and therapeutic considerations. J Endocrinol Invest 1995;18:35.

50. Bucci I, Napolitano G, Giuliani C, et al. Zinc sulfate supplementation improves thyroid function in hypozincemic Down children. Biol Trace Elem Res 1999;73:93.

51. Kanavin OJ, Aaseth J, Birketvedt GS. Thyroid hypofunction in Down's syndrome: is it related to oxidative stress? Biol Trace Elem Res 2000;78:35.

52. Sklar CA, Qazi R, David R. Juvenile autoimmune thyroiditis: hormonal status at presentation and after long-term follow-up. Am J Dis Child 1986;140:877.

53. Maenpaa J, Raatikka M, Rasanen J, et al. Natural course of juvenile autoimmune thyroiditis. J Pediatr 1985;107:898.

54. Levy RP, Jensen JB, Laus VG, et al. Serum thyroid hormone abnormalities in psychiatric disease. Metabolism 1981;38:1060.

55. Bocchetta A, Bernardi F, Burrai C, et al. The course of thyroid abnormalities during lithium treatment: a two-year follow-up study. Acta Psychiatr Scand 1992;86:38.

56. Shakir KMM, Chute JP, Aprill BS, Lazarus AA. Ferrous sulfate-induced increase in requirement for thyroxine in a patient with primary hypothyroidism. South Med J 1997; 90:637.

57. Singh N, Weisler SL, Hershman JM. The acute effect of calcium carbonate on the intestinal absorption of levothyroxine. Thyroid 2001;11:967.

58. Chiu AC, Sherman SI. Effects of pharmacological fiber supplements on levothyroxine absorption. Thyroid 1998;8:667.

59. Surks MI, Sievert R. Drugs and thyroid function. N Engl J Med 1995;333:1688.

60. Arafah BM. Increased need for thyroxine in women with hypothyroidism during estrogen therapy. N Engl J Med 2001;344:1743.

61. Utiger RD. Estrogen, thyroxine binding in serum, and thyroxine therapy. N Engl J Med 2001;344:1784.

62. Smallridge RC, Ladenson PW. Hypothyroidism in pregnancy: consequences to neonatal health. J Clin Endocrinol Metab 2001;86:2349.

63. Rivkees SA, Bode HH, Crawford JD. Long-term growth in juvenile acquired hypothyroidism: the failure to achieve normal adult stature. N Engl J Med 1988;318:599.

16
Hyperthyroidism

John S. Dallas
University of Texas Medical Branch–Galveston, Galveston, Texas, U.S.A.

Thomas P. Foley, Jr.
University of Pittsburgh and Children's Hospital of Pittsburgh, Pittsburgh, Pennsylvania, U.S.A.

I. PATHOGENESIS AND ETIOLOGY

Thyrotoxicosis is an uncommon disorder of childhood characterized by accelerated metabolism of body tissues resulting from excessive levels of unbound circulating thyroid hormones. Graves' disease accounts for at least 95% of cases in children (1). Other causes are rare and are listed in Table 1.

Mechanisms that can produce thyrotoxicosis include thyroid follicular cell hyperfunction with increased synthesis and secretion of T_4 and T_3, thyroid follicular cell destruction with release of preformed T_4 and T_3, and ingestion or administration of thyroid hormone or iodide preparations.

Hyperfunction of thyroid follicular cells can either be autonomous or mediated through stimulation of thyrotropin receptors by substances such as thyrotropin (TSH) or thyrotropin receptor antibodies (TSHrAb). Autonomous hyperfunction of thyroid follicular cells is rarely seen during childhood and is represented by toxic adenoma, familial nonautoimmune hyperthyroidism, hyperfunctioning thyroid carcinoma, and the hyperthyroidism of the Mc-Cune-Albright syndrome.

Stimulation of thyrotropin receptors by TSHrAb produces the diffuse toxic goiter of Graves' disease and accounts for the majority of childhood thyrotoxicosis. In rare cases, increased TSH secretion resulting either from a TSH-producing pituitary adenoma or from pituitary resistance to thyroid hormone can produce thyrotoxicosis. Another glycoprotein hormone, human chorionic gonadotropin (hCG), also binds to the TSH receptor and stimulates thyroid cell function (2, 3). The thyrotropic potency of hCG is much less than that of TSH, but extremely high serum levels of hCG, such as those seen in individuals with hydatidiform moles or other trophoblastic tumors,

can lead to hyperthyroidism (4, 5). Although extremely rare, the possibility of a molar pregnancy should be considered in adolescent girls with thyrotoxicosis.

Inflammation of thyroid follicular cells can be associated with viral or autoimmune processes, and extensive destruction can release large amounts of preformed T_4 and T_3 into the circulation. The resultant thyrotoxicosis tends to be mild and transient, usually only lasting a few weeks to a few months. Examples include the toxic thyroiditis of Hashimoto's disease and subacute thyroiditis.

Acute or chronic ingestion of thyroid hormone preparations such as L-thyroxine or desiccated thyroid can produce excessive levels of circulating thyroid hormones. Ingestion may be surreptitious, iatrogenic, or accidental. Ingestion or parenteral administration of iodides may also result in thyrotoxicosis. This phenomenon, known as jodbasedow, most frequently occurs in iodine-deficient areas when supplemental iodides are added to the diet. Iodine-induced hyperthyroidism generally occurs in thyroid glands that are functioning independently of TSH stimulation (6, 7). However, iodine-induced hyperthyroidism has also been described both in adults (6, 7) and in a neonate (8) with apparently normal thyroid glands who were exposed to high concentrations of iodine over prolonged periods.

II. GRAVES' DISEASE

A. Introduction

Graves' disease is an immunogenetic disorder characterized clinically by thyromegaly, hyperthyroidism, and infiltrative ophthalmopathy. A family history of autoimmune thyroid disease is present in up to 60% of patients (9).

Table 1 Causes of Thyrotoxicosis in Childhood and Adolescence

---

Graves' disease
Autonomous functioning nodule(s)
    Toxic adenoma
    Hyperfunctioning papillary or follicular carcinoma
    McCune-Albright syndrome
Familial nonautoimmune hyperthyroidism
TSH-induced hyperthyroidism
    TSH-producing pituitary adenoma
    Pituitary resistance to thyroid hormone
Thyroiditis
    Subacute thyroiditis
    Toxic thyroiditis of Hashimoto's disease
Exogenous thyroid hormone
Iodine-induced hyperthyroidism (jodbasedow)
Tumor-produced thyroid stimulators
    Hydatidiform mole
    Choriocarcinoma

Genetic studies have shown it to be a polygenic disorder, and most of the genes that have been implicated appear to be involved in immunoregulation (10). Human leukocyte antigens (HLA) and the CTLA-4 gene region have been established as susceptibility loci, although the magnitude of their contributions seems to vary depending on age of onset and racial background (11, 12). Recent reports indicate that HLA-DRB1*03 and -DRB1*08 are positively associated with Graves' disease in White children, whereas the DRB1*07 haplotype is protective (13, 14). For the Japanese population, HLA-DPB1*0501 is significantly increased in children with Graves' disease (15). Recently, genome-wide linkage analysis studies have identified regions on chromosomes 14q31, 18q21, 20q11.2, and Xq21.33–22 that appear to represent susceptibility loci for Graves' disease (12, 16).

The concordance rate between monozygotic twins has been reported to range between 20 and 60% (11–13), thus implying that environmental factors play a significant role in the development of the disease. The extent to which chemicals, drugs, infections, and psychological stress can alter immunoregulatory genes is unknown. However, the existence of a two-way interaction between the immune and neuroendocrine systems may provide a mechanism by which biological and psychological stresses can affect lymphocyte subpopulations and immunoregulation (17).

The exact incidence of Graves' disease during childhood in North America is unknown, but it is uncommon and has been reported to account for fewer than 5% of cases seen in most thyroid clinics (18). A recent study has estimated the incidence of childhood thyrotoxicosis in Denmark to be 0.1:100,000 in the very young increasing with age to 3:100,000 by 14 years old (19). Just as in North America, the vast majority (>95%) of childhood thyrotoxicosis in Denmark is due to Graves' disease (19).

More than two-thirds of childhood cases in North America occur between the ages of 10 and 15 years (1), and it occurs more frequently in girls in a ratio of 3:1 to 5:1 (9).

B. Pathogenesis: Thyrotropin Receptor and Thyrotropin Receptor Antibodies

The thyrotropin (TSH) receptor is a member of the large family of guanine-nucleotide-binding (G) protein-coupled receptors and represents the primary target antigen for autoantibodies that mediate the hyperthyroidism and thyromegaly of Graves' disease. The cDNA encoding the human TSH receptor has been cloned and characterized (20, 21). As deduced from the cDNA sequence, the mature receptor is a glycoprotein with a single polypeptide chain of 744 amino acids. Like all other G-protein-coupled receptors, the TSH receptor has an extracellular domain, seven transmembrane domains, and an intracellular domain. The TSH and other glycoprotein hormone (i.e., luteinizing hormone [LH]/chorionic gonadotropin [CG] and follicle-stimulating hormone [FSH]) receptors each have relatively large extracellular domains, and this characteristic differentiates them from the other G-protein-coupled receptors. The TSH, LH/CG, and FSH receptors are closely related structurally and share about 70% and 45% homology in their transmembrane and extracellular domains, respectively (22).

The extracellular domain of the TSH receptor (398 amino acids) represents the amino-terminal end, and the transmembrane and intracellular domains (346 amino acids) represent the carboxyl-terminal end of the protein. The extracellular domain contains six potential N-glycosylation sites and nine leucine-rich repeats of a loosely conserved 25 amino acid residue motif. Proper glycosylation appears to be important both for normal expression of the receptor on the thyroid cell membrane and for normal hormone–receptor interactions (20, 21). The leucine-rich repeats, which have the potential to form amphipathic α-helices, are believed to be involved in protein–protein or protein–membrane interactions. Recent studies have confirmed that both TSH and autoantibodies to the TSH receptor (TSHrAb) bind to the extracellular domain (20, 21). The transmembrane and intracellular domains are involved in signal transduction, acting through G-protein to stimulate the production of cyclic AMP by adenylyl cyclase (20, 21).

The hyperthyroidism and thyromegaly of Graves' disease are mediated through immunoglobulin G (IgG) that binds to the extracellular domain of the TSH receptor and stimulates follicular cell function and growth. In addition to the stimulating TSHrAbs, sera from patients with Graves' disease may also contain other IgG to the TSH receptor that block thyroid cell function and growth. Stimulating TSHrAbs are restricted to the IgG1 subclass, suggesting that they are either oligo- or monoclonal in origin (23). On the other hand, blocking TSHrAbs appear to be polyclonal in origin and may be of IgG1, IgG2, IgG3, or

IgG4 subclass (24). Current evidence suggests that disease caused by the immune system (i.e., autoimmune disease) appears to result from a restricted immune response involving B and/or T lymphocytes against one or a few epitopes of the target antigen (25). These observations, therefore, support the importance of stimulating TSHrAbs in the cause of Graves' disease and imply that blocking TSHrAbs, much like antithyroglobulin and antithyroid peroxidase, arise as a result of thyroid tissue damage. Nevertheless, blocking TSHrAbs can still modulate the biological effects of stimulating TSHrAbs. Therefore, a patient's clinical presentation and course may be determined by the net biological effect of the simultaneous interaction of various stimulating and blocking TSHrAbs with the TSH receptor.

Several investigators have proposed that the functional effect(s) a particular TSHrAb exhibits is determined by the specific region to which the antibody binds on the TSH receptor (26, 27). Following the successful cloning of the TSH receptor, numerous studies have attempted to identify binding sites for the various TSHrAbs. To date, the major experimental approaches to defining TSHrAb epitopes have included transfecting mammalian cells with mutant cDNA of the TSH receptor and using synthetic peptides derived from the predicted amino acid sequence of the TSH receptor (reviewed in 21, 28–30). Although some of these studies have localized functional epitopes to a few relatively narrow regions of the extracellular domain (31), others have identified multiple regions throughout the entire extracellular domain that appear to be involved in TSHrAb binding (32). Although controversy still exists regarding the specific sites that compose TSHrAb epitopes, current evidence supports the concept that the antibodies bind to conformational epitopes made up of discontinuous segments across the extracellular domain (11). The amino acid region 55–254 contains residues important for the binding of at least some stimulating TSHrAbs (33–35), whereas the amino acid region 370–400 contains residues important for the binding of some inhibitory TSHrAbs (20, 31, 36). Despite these recent advances, the exact mechanisms by which stimulating and blocking TSHrAbs exert their biological effects remain unknown. The precise determination of TSHrAb epitopes, as well as the study of molecular mechanisms, will require the development of human, disease-associated monoclonal antibodies.

The major source of TSHrAb production appears to be intrathyroidal lymphocytes (27), but lymphocytes in the spleen, lymph nodes, bone marrow, and peripheral blood may also produce these antibodies (37, 38). The mechanisms and control of stimulating TSHrAb production are uncertain, but several hypotheses have been proposed. One hypothesis suggests that a deficiency of specific suppressor T-cell function accounts for TSHrAb production (39); a second hypothesis suggests that a breakdown in the idiotype–anti-idiotype network of B

lymphocyte immunoregulation may be responsible (40). An increased frequency of antibodies to certain serotypes of *Yersinia enterocolitica* has been reported in patients with Graves' disease (41), and infection with this bacterium has been proposed as an important initiating event in the development of the disease (42). *Y. enterocolitica* has a specific, saturable binding site for TSH, and antibodies produced against this site may cross react with the TSH receptor on the thyroid follicular cell membrane (41). A fourth hypothesis relies on the fact that thyroid follicular cells can express HLA-DR antigens and are, therefore, endowed with the capacity to present other antigenic material to primed T lymphocytes. Through this mechanism, the follicular cell could present the TSH receptor as antigen and direct the synthesis of TSHrAb (43). Although experimental evidence exists for each of the above hypotheses, none can fully account for all aspects of TSHrAb production; further studies will be necessary to identify the responsible mechanisms.

Currently, two major types of assays are used to measure TSHrAbs (44). Receptor assays assess the ability of Graves' IgG to inhibit labeled TSH from binding to the TSH receptor, and antibodies detected by this method have been designated thyrotropin-binding inhibitory immunoglobulins (TBII). It should be emphasized that receptor assays do not differentiate TSHrAb that stimulate thyroid cell function from TSHrAb that inhibit thyroid cell function; both types of TSHrAbs can be detected as long as they inhibit TSH from binding to its receptor. Receptor assays that employ a combination of detergent-solubilized porcine TSH receptors and receptor-purified [^{125}I]-labeled bovine TSH (referred to as first-generation TSH receptor assays) are both sensitive and specific, and they provide a reproducible, inexpensive means of measuring TSHrAb in unextracted serum (27, 45). Studies using these receptor assays have detected TSHrAb in 82–100% of adults (27) and 93% of children (46) with untreated active Graves' disease. TSHrAb can also be detected by receptor assays in small numbers (10–20%) of patients with Hashimoto's thyroiditis (27, 46, 47). A newer second-generation TSH receptor antibody assay is now commercially available (48) that utilizes purified labeled bovine TSH and an immobilized recombinant human TSH receptor protein (48). Recent reports show that this assay retains very high specificity and is more sensitive than the first-generation receptor assay (48, 49). In one report (49), the second-generation assay detected TSHrAb in 41 of 46 patients with Graves' disease who had negative results with the standard first-generation assay.

Bioassay methods constitute the other major type of assay currently used to measure TSHrAb. Most commonly, these assays employ isolated thyroid cells in culture to assess the ability of immunoglobulin concentrates from patient sera to stimulate thyroid cell production of cAMP. Antibodies detected by these assays have been designated thyroid-stimulating immunoglobulins (TSI).

These assays can be performed using cells taken from human or porcine thyroid tissue as well as from the immortal rat thyroid line: the FRTL-5 cells. More recently, transfected mammalian cells (e.g., Cos-7 and CHO cells) expressing the recombinant human TSH receptor have been used to detect stimulating TSHrAbs (20, 50). Recently, a bioassay method utilizing CHO cells transfected with the human TSH receptor was found to detect TSI in 10 of 11 (91%) children with active Graves' disease, whereas TSI were not detected by this assay in 13 normal children, 2 children in remission from Graves' disease, and 11 children with chronic lymphocytic thyroiditis (51). Although the bioassays possess high sensitivity and specificity, they are less precise and are more expensive and time-consuming to perform than the receptor assays (26, 27, 44, 51).

Although some reports have demonstrated highly positive correlations between TSHrAb levels detected by the receptor and bioassay methods (52), most have demonstrated no such correlation (26). Some investigators suggest that the lack of correlation between TBII and TSI levels in patient sera is due to the presence of different populations of TSHrAbs that exhibit different degrees of TSH agonist activity (53). Others suggest that the poor correlation results from the coexistence of both stimulating and blocking TSHrAb in some patients' sera (54).

C. Clinical Manifestations

During childhood and adolescence most patients with Graves' disease present with the classic symptoms and signs (9). Early during the course of the disease the symptoms and signs specific to children (Table 2) may be minimal since the disease usually develops insidiously over several months (9). Often the initial awareness of any problem is in school, where teachers notice changes in behavior and academic performance. Insomnia, restless sleep, and nocturia are common and often are associated

Table 2 Common Symptoms and Signs of Graves' Disease in 290 Children and Adolescents

	Percentage affected
Goiter	98
Tachycardia	82
Nervousness	82
Increased pulse pressure	80
Proptosis	65
Increased appetite	60
Tremor	52
Weight loss	50
Heat intolerance	30

Source: Ref. 9.

with easy fatigability and lethargy during the day. Other clinical manifestations include palpitations, increased stool frequency, increased sweating, and proximal muscle weakness. Children who develop Graves' disease before the age of 3–4 years can experience transitory speech and language delays, mental retardation, and craniosynostosis (55). The symptoms of hyperthyroidism in Graves' disease, although variable, tend to be more severe than in other causes of hyperthyroidism.

Ophthalmic abnormalities are present in over one-half of patients (refer to Chapter 16, Sec. X), and thyromegaly is almost invariably present. In fact, the absence of goiter raises serious doubt about the diagnosis of Graves' disease, and other causes of hyperthyroidism should be sought. The thyroid gland usually is symmetrically enlarged, smooth, soft, and nontender. A palpable thrill or an audible bruit may be present and reflects increased blood flow through the gland. Less often, and usually in association with coexisting Hashimoto's thyroiditis, the gland may be firm, bosselated, and asymmetrically enlarged. Although pretibial myxedema is observed in 1–2% of adults with Graves' disease (11), it rarely, if ever, occurs in children. Other diseases have been observed in association with Graves' disease and include Hashimoto's thyroiditis, vitiligo, systemic lupus erythematosus, rheumatoid arthritis, Addison's disease, insulin-dependent diabetes mellitus, myasthenia gravis, and pernicious anemia (1).

Although their occurrence is extremely rare, thyroid storm and thyrotoxic periodic paralysis (TPP) are two endocrine emergencies that have been reported in children/adolescents with hyperthyroidism. Although most reported patients have had Graves' disease, these situations can also occur with other causes of hyperthyroidism (56–59). Thyroid storm is a life-threatening manifestation of thyrotoxicosis characterized by fever (generally greater than 38.5°C), tachycardia out of proportion to the fever, high-output cardiac failure, gastrointestinal dysfunction (such as vomiting, diarrhea, and jaundice), and neurological changes (such as confusion, obtundation, seizures, and coma). The diagnosis of thyroid storm requires a high index of suspicion. The syndrome complex may occur either in previously undiagnosed patients or in patients with poorly controlled hyperthyroidism. If left untreated, mortality rates of up to 90% have been reported (60). The exact mechanisms underlying the clinical progression from uncomplicated thyrotoxicosis to storm have not been determined. A number of precipitating factors have been identified and include infection, trauma, surgery, concomitant ingestion of sympathomimetic agents (e.g., pseudoephedrine), withdrawal of antithyroid medication, and radioactive iodine therapy (56, 61–65). Therapeutic intervention includes emergency and supportive care to maintain adequate respiratory and cardiovascular functions and to control body temperature; management of precipitating factors, if indicated; and limiting the amount of thyroid hormones available to the peripheral body tissues, by using propylthiouracil (PTU), iodide, β-adrenergic blockers, and glucocorticoids (64, 65). PTU inhibits production of new thyroid hormone and blocks conversion of T_4 to T_3 in peripheral tissues. During the first 24–48 h of management, PTU can be administered orally, rectally, or by nasogastric tube in dosages ranging from 100 to 200 mg every 4–6 h (66). Once initial control of thyrotoxicosis has been achieved, PTU dosages can be reduced to 5–10 mg/kg/day in divided oral doses every 6–8 h. Iodides (SSKI, 5–6 drops orally every 8 h) inhibit release of preformed hormones from the thyroid, acutely impair organification of T_4, and inhibit T_4 to T_3 conversion. Preferably, iodides should be used only after PTU has been administered to avoid an increase in new thyroid hormone production. Propranolol (2 mg/kg/day in divided oral doses every 6–8 h) and hydrocortisone (2 mg/kg as an intravenous [IV] bolus, then 36–45 mg/m^2/day in divided IV doses every 6 h) are used to treat the exaggerated adrenergic effects and possible relative glucocorticoid insufficiency, respectively, that accompany thyroid storm. Both also inhibit conversion of T_4 to T_3.

TPP is a reversible cause of sudden-onset weakness that most commonly affects hyperthyroid patients of Asian descent. However, TPP has also been observed in susceptible White, African-American, Hispanic, and Native American persons (59). The disorder affects 1–2% of hyperthyroid patients in Asian populations, but only 0.1–0.2% of hyperthyroid patients in North America (67, 68). A very strong male preponderance has been observed, but the mode of inheritance is unknown and the majority of affected individuals do not have a family history of periodic paralysis. Most patients present between the ages of 20 and 39 years, but older adolescents with TPP have been reported (69). At presentation, the clinical signs and symptoms of thyrotoxicosis are often subtle and may be overlooked. In the majority of patients, episodes of weakness usually occur precipitously and vary from mild weakness to total paralysis of affected muscle groups. Weakness usually involves the limbs, with proximal muscles being more severely affected than distal muscles. Mental function, sensory function, respiratory, ocular, and bulbar muscle groups are not affected. However, cardiac rhythm disturbances and electrocardiographic (ECG) abnormalities (e.g., U waves, ST segment abnormalities, prolongation of QT interval) are common (70).

TPP typically occurs in the early morning hours, following a day of strenuous exercise. Other apparent precipitating factors include high carbohydrate intake, trauma, infection, menses, emotional stress, and alcohol ingestion (59, 71). The frequency of attacks is variable, and individual episodes typically last from 3 to 36 h. Laboratory evaluation during episodes reveals biochemical evidence of thyrotoxicosis (e.g., elevated serum levels of total and free thyroid hormones with suppressed TSH), and, in the vast majority of cases, significant hypokalemia.

Body stores of potassium are normal, and hypokalemia is the result of intracellular shifts of potassium. Neuromuscular symptoms appear to resolve as potassium moves back out of the cells and may be hastened with supplemental potassium administration. Although the severity of muscle weakness/paralysis tends to reflect the degree of hypokalemia, episodes have occurred in a few patients with normal potassium levels (68, 71).

Although the exact mechanisms responsible for this disorder remain unclear, patients experience TPP only while they are thyrotoxic. Thyrotoxicosis alters plasma membrane permeability to sodium and potassium, a function linked to Na^+-K^+ ATPase activity. Thyrotoxicosis also enhances tissue responsiveness to β-adrenergic stimulation and this further increases Na^+-K^+ ATPase activity. Na^+-K^+ ATPase is also activated by insulin, and this may explain the relationship between attacks and large carbohydrate loads. In addition, a defect in the muscles themselves has been proposed, since they fail to respond to direct electrical stimulation during the period of paralysis (72). Medical management includes hospital admission for the acute paralysis, cardiac monitoring, and close observation of serum potassium levels. Potassium supplements should be used to correct hypokalemia, and antithyroid therapy should be started. Episodes of TPP always cease once thyrotoxicosis is corrected, and permanent treatment for the overactive thyroid is imperative. While awaiting normalization of thyroid status, patients should avoid precipitating factors such as strenuous exercise and high carbohydrate intake. β-Adrenergic-blocking agents and pharmacological glucocorticoid therapy can be useful adjunctive treatments for TPP (67, 68).

III. AUTONOMOUS THYROID NODULE

The autonomously functioning thyroid nodule is a discrete thyroid nodule that functions independently of normal pituitary control. The pathogenesis has not yet been established in all cases, but recent evidence suggests that somatic mutations of the α-subunit of G-protein ($G_{s\alpha}$; see below) and the third intracellular loop of the TSH receptor are probably responsible for the development of some cases (73, 74). In both situations, the mutations result in constitutive activation of adenylyl cyclase and unregulated production of cAMP. The unregulated cAMP production is responsible for the subsequent tissue hyperplasia and hyperthyroidism.

This disorder predominantly occurs in adults, is rare during childhood, but has been reported in a child as young as 22 months (75). Most children with a thyroid nodule come to the attention of a physician because of a mass in the region of the thyroid gland. The majority of patients with autonomous thyroid nodules are clinically euthyroid, and in contrast to adults, clinical hyperthyroidism occurs very rarely in children. Autonomously functioning nodules that cause hyperthyroidism are almost invariably benign adenomas (toxic adenoma), but very rarely hyperthyroidism caused by hyperfunctioning papillary or follicular carcinoma has been reported (76). In these cases, the patients usually have extensive metastatic disease and the diagnosis of carcinoma has been established prior to onset of hyperthyroidism.

The hyperthyroidism of the McCune-Albright syndrome (MAS) is also associated with single or multiple hyperfunctioning adenomatous nodules. This syndrome is characterized by polyostotic fibrous dysplasia, multiple café-au-lait spots, and endocrine hyperfunction. The most common endocrinopathy is isosexual precocious puberty, but hyperthyroidism, acromegaly, Cushing syndrome, and hyperparathyroidism have been reported (77). In contrast to polyostotic fibrous dysplasia and precocious puberty that occur more commonly in girls with the syndrome, hyperthyroidism occurs with equal frequency in boys and girls. The age of onset of hyperthyroidism tends to be between 3 and 12 years (78), which is somewhat younger than the usual age of onset of hyperthyroidism caused by hyperfunctioning nodules in other individuals. The hyperthyroidism is clearly due to autonomous function of the thyroid gland; basal TSH levels are suppressed and the TSH response to TRH is blunted, thyroid-stimulating antibodies are undetectable, and T_3 treatment fails to suppress radioactive iodide uptake by the thyroid.

Current evidence indicates that the receptors for each of the hormones (i.e., LH, FSH, TSH, growth-hormone-releasing hormone [GHRH], adrenocorticotropic hormone [ACTH], and parathyroid hormone [PTH]) that might otherwise be implicated in the observed endocrinopathies of MAS are all coupled to G-proteins. The G-proteins are hetereotrimers composed of an α-subunit and a tightly coupled $\beta\gamma$-dimer (79). The α-subunit contains the guanine-nucleotide-binding site and has intrinsic GTPase activity. In the normal situation, the binding of one of these stimulatory hormones to its receptor facilitates the exchange of GTP for GDP in the guanine-nucleotide-binding site of the α-subunit ($G_{s\alpha}$). This results in the release of the G-protein from the receptor and its dissociation into free $G_{s\alpha}$-GTP and free $\beta\gamma$-dimer. Free $G_{s\alpha}$-GTP stimulates adenylyl cyclase activity, with the subsequent production of intracellular cAMP. After a preset time, the intrinsic GTPase of $G_{s\alpha}$ hydrolyses GTP to GDP, and the $G_{s\alpha}$-GDP reassociates with the $\beta\gamma$-dimer. The G-protein is thus returned to its inactive state and can now reassociate with its receptor and participate in another cycle (79). Recent studies have identified mutations in the $G_{s\alpha}$ gene in endocrine organs, bone, and skin from patients with MAS (79–81). These mutations involve the amino acid residue Arg^{201} that is critical for the intrinsic GTPase activity of $G_{s\alpha}$. Therefore, certain substitution mutations involving this amino acid residue result in the constitutive activation of adenylyl cyclase and unregulated production of intracellular cAMP. In some cases, the mutation has been

found in abnormal sections of tissue but not in histologically normal sections from the same tissue (79). This observation would tend to explain the development of hyperfunctioning nodules within the thyroid gland.

The amount of thyroid hormone that an autonomously functioning nodule produces appears to be related to its size. In adults with single autonomous nodules, hyperthyroidism usually occurs only when the nodule measures more than 2.5–3 cm in diameter (82). Both T_4 and T_3 can be produced in excess, but an elevated serum T_3 level is frequently the only biochemical abnormality. In some patients, the T_3 level may be elevated enough to inhibit the TSH response to TRH, but not enough to cause clinical hyperthyroidism (83).

A radionuclide image, preferably using [^{123}I]-iodine, should be included in the evaluation of the hyperthyroid child with a thyroid nodule. The radioiodine image allows one to study both trapping and organification by the nodule. Technetium images only demonstrate trapping by the nodule, and images are not always identical to those obtained with iodine. The diagnosis of a hyperfunctioning or "hot" nodule is established when the image reveals increased accumulation of the radioisotope in the nodule and decreased or absent uptake in the surrounding thyroid tissues.

Surgical removal is the preferred method of treatment for the toxic thyroid nodule and usually is accomplished by partial thyroidectomy. Significant surgical complications are not expected, and postoperative hypothyroidism seldom occurs. With complete surgical removal of the autonomous nodule, hyperthyroidism should not recur postoperatively. Since the hyperthyroidism produced by the autonomous nodule is usually mild, a long preoperative preparation with antithyroid drugs is seldom necessary. Propranolol may be used to decrease the symptoms of hyperthyroidism. The administration of iodides is not indicated in the preoperative treatment of the autonomous nodule. Percutaneous intranodular ethanol injection under ultrasound guidance has been employed for the ablation of autonomous thyroid nodules (84). This approach appears to be safe and effective in adults and may prove to be a practical alternative to surgical treatment in children.

IV. FAMILIAL NONAUTOIMMUNE HYPERTHYROIDISM

Familial nonautoimmune hyperthyroidism (FNH) is a rare condition that clinically can be confused with Graves' disease. It has been estimated that FNH (also referred to as nonautoimmune hereditary hyperthyroidism) may account for 2–5% of all cases of diffuse hyperthyroidism (85). The disorder occurs because of a germline mutation in the TSH receptor gene. These so-called gain of function mutations result in the constitutive activation of the TSH receptor–G protein–effector system complex that ultimately leads to increased thyroid follicular cell growth and function. The first family recognized to have this disorder was described in 1982 (86); as of this writing, approximately 10 kindreds with FNH have been identified (87, 88). Except for amino acid 281 (Ser^{281}) in the extracellular domain, all the other identified mutation sites are located in transmembrane domains 1, 2, 3, 5, 6, and 7 of the TSH receptor (87).

The disease is transmitted in an autosomal dominant fashion. Therefore, unlike in Graves' disease, males and females can be affected equally. In described families, hyperthyroid individuals are spread over three to four generations. The onset of clinical hyperthyroidism is highly variable, with some patients presenting before the age of 1 year and others presenting in adolescence or early adulthood. However, clinically asymptomatic individuals can exhibit suppressed serum TSH levels for years prior to the clinical appearance of goiter or thyrotoxicosis (85).

In affected individuals, both thyroid gland size and structure tend to change over time. In the youngest patients, the gland tends to be normal to slightly enlarged. In older patients, the thyroid is symmetrically enlarged and bruits may be audible over the lobes. Eventually, the diffusely enlarged gland may evolve into a multinodular goiter (85). Although eye signs of thyrotoxicosis (e.g., stare, lid lag, widened palpebral fissures, mild proptosis) may be present, infiltrative ophthalmopathy has not been observed in FNH. Laboratory evaluation reveals elevated serum levels of both total and free thyroid hormones and suppressed TSH. TSH receptor antibodies are not present. In general, serum antibodies to thyroid peroxidase and thyroglobulin also are not present, but these autoantibodies have been detected in a few patients with confirmed FNH (88). In the research setting, DNA from peripheral blood leukocytes can be used to sequence the TSH receptor gene for identification of point mutations associated with FNH.

The recognition of FNH is of great importance for its management. The diagnosis should be considered in cases of apparent Graves' disease when extrathyroidal signs and thyroid antibodies are absent and in patients with an extensive family history of hyperthyroidism. As in Graves' disease, antithyroid drug therapy can control the hyperthyroidism; but, due to the persistent functional effects of the TSH receptor mutation, remission does not occur. While subtotal thyroidectomy may restore euthyroidism in some patients (87), significant regrowth of thyroid tissue may likewise occur with subsequent recurrence of clinical hyperthyroidism (85). Therefore, total ablation of the gland, either surgically or with radioiodine, should be considered in patients with FNH. Regular systematic screening for either clinical symptoms or early biochemical evidence of hyperthyroidism (i.e., suppressed serum TSH levels) should be undertaken to identify other affected family members. In addition, genetic counseling should be offered to affected families.

V. TSH-INDUCED HYPERTHYROIDISM

Hyperthyroidism from increased TSH secretion can occur as the result of either a TSH-secreting pituitary adenoma or selective pituitary resistance to thyroid hormone. Although both are rare, each has been reported in childhood and adolescence (89). Unlike Graves' disease, the gender ratio in patients with TSH-induced hyperthyroidism is 1:1. Most cases of TSH-producing pituitary adenoma occur sporadically, but familial cases have been reported (90). Pituitary resistance to thyroid hormone appears to be familial with an autosomal dominant pattern of inheritance (89). The cause of pituitary resistance to thyroid hormone has not been established for all cases, but most represent forms of the syndrome of generalized resistance to thyroid hormone (GRTH; see below) (91, 92). The syndrome of GRTH is caused by a mutation in TRβ, one of the thyroid hormone receptor genes (92). Approximately 60 different mutations have been identified in patients from over 100 families (92). Although the reasons remain unclear, affected members within a family can exhibit different degrees of resistance to thyroid hormone, and various tissues (e.g., heart, liver, bone, and pituitary) can be affected to a greater or lesser degree (92, 93). Therefore, the pituitary gland in such individuals would be relatively more resistant to thyroid hormones than other tissues in the body. Pituitary thyrotroph resistance in these individuals is selective for thyroid hormones, since there is normal inhibition of pituitary TSH secretion by glucocorticoids and dopaminergic agents (89). Criteria essential for the diagnosis of this disorder include evidence of increased peripheral metabolism, diffuse thyromegaly, elevated free thyroid hormone levels, and inappropriately elevated serum levels of TSH (90). Although the TSH level may not be elevated above the normal range, it is always detectable, even in highly sensitive and specific immunoassays. In all other causes of hyperthyroidism, sensitive immunoassays will reveal very suppressed or undetectable serum levels of TSH.

The clinical presentation is often very similar to Graves' disease, and a high degree of suspicion is needed to make the diagnosis. The patient with pituitary adenoma, however, may present with visual complaints due to compression of optic nerve tracts by the adenoma. Increased pituitary secretion of growth hormone and prolactin has also been reported in patients with TSH-secreting tumors (90).

Once the diagnosis of TSH-induced hyperthyroidism has been established, the clinician needs to determine if the increased TSH secretion results from a pituitary tumor or from pituitary resistance to thyroid hormone in order to determine the proper course of therapy. The TRH and T$_3$ suppression tests may help differentiate these two disorders. In general, serum TSH levels do not increase in response to TRH when a pituitary tumor is the cause of hyperthyroidism. In contrast, the TSH response to TRH tends to be normal or exaggerated in pituitary resistance to thyroid hormone (89). Pharmacological dosages of T_3 cause significant TSH suppression in patients with pituitary resistance but fail to reduce TSH levels in patients with TSH-secreting pituitary adenomas.

Determination of serum levels of the free α-subunit of the glycoproteins, including TSH, also can aid in differentiating these conditions; patients with TSH-secreting pituitary tumors generally have elevated (greater than 1) molar α-subunit/TSH ratios. This ratio tends to be less than 1 in patients with pituitary resistance to thyroid hormone (90). The measured α-subunit is usually expressed in ng/ml, whereas TSH is usually expressed in μU/ml. In order to determine the molar α-subunit/TSH ratio, one assumes a molecular weight for TSH of 28,000 D, a molecular weight for α-subunit of 13,600 D, and a specific activity for human TSH of 5 μU/ng (94). This results in a conversion factor of (28,000/13,600)/0.2 or approximately 10 (95). Therefore, [α-subunit (ng/ml)/TSH (μU/ml)] $\times$ 10 = molar α-subunit/TSH ratio. CT scan and MRI studies of the pituitary region also can help to establish the diagnosis and to guide treatment.

Treatment for TSH-secreting adenomas consists of selective adenonectomy or radiotherapy, or a combination of the two (93, 96). In the past, a brief course of antithyroid drugs was used to render the patient euthyroid prior to surgery. More recently, the somatostatin analog, octreotide, has proven useful in the management of TSH-producing pituitary tumors (93, 96). This drug normalizes thyroid hormone levels in most patients and causes a decrease in tumor size in some. However, because of tachyphylaxis, octreotide cannot be considered definitive treatment. The current approach to managing the TSH-producing pituitary tumor consists of achieving a euthyroid state with octreotide, followed by surgical resection of the tumor.

Treatment of patients with pituitary resistance to thyroid hormone is more difficult. Ideally, treatment should be aimed at reducing TSH secretion by the pituitary. A number of agents including L-T_3, D-T_4, bromocriptine, and triiodothyroacetic acid (Triac) have been advocated (90, 93, 97–99). To date, each agent has been used in a limited number of patients, and the overall efficacy of each has not been determined. Octreotide has not been useful in the long-term treatment of these patients (93). Atenolol, a β-adrenergic-blocking agent that does not impair the peripheral conversion of T_4 to T_3, can be used to decrease the symptoms of hyperthyroidism (100). Although antithyroid drugs will reduce serum thyroid hormone levels, they will also increase TSH secretion and goiter size. Since prolonged TSH hypersecretion may lead to thyrotroph hyperplasia and potentially to the development of a TSH-secreting pituitary adenoma (101), prolonged treatment with antithyroid drugs is discouraged. Likewise, subtotal thyroidectomy and radioiodine therapy should not be used in patients with pituitary resistance to thyroid hormone.

VI. SUBACUTE AND HASHIMOTO'S THYROIDITIS

Subacute or granulomatous thyroiditis is a self-limited, presumably viral, inflammation of the thyroid gland. This entity is rarely seen in children, occurring more frequently between the third and fifth decades of life. Mild symptoms of thyrotoxicosis may occur, but they are often overshadowed by malaise, fever, and tenderness of the thyroid gland. The erythrocyte sedimentation rate is consistently elevated. Thyroid antibodies are usually negative early in the disease, but titers may rise transiently to abnormal levels during recovery. The thyrotoxic phase of this disease probably results from destruction of thyroid follicular cells with release of large amounts of preformed thyroid hormones.

The toxic thyroiditis of Hashimoto's disease occurs early in the course of chronic lymphocytic thyroiditis and probably results from extensive autoimmune destruction of thyroid follicular cells. The child may present with mild symptoms of thyrotoxicosis and a slightly enlarged, sometimes tender, thyroid gland. Thyroid antibodies are usually positive.

Laboratory evaluation of both disorders reveals elevated serum T_4, free T_4, and T_3 levels and undetectable TSH levels. The TSH response to TRH is either blunted or absent. The radioiodine uptake is typically low or absent during the thyrotoxic phase of these disorders and helps to differentiate toxic thyroiditis from Graves' disease.

Treatment of these disorders is symptomatic. Antithyroid drugs are not indicated in the treatment, but propranolol can be used to relieve the symptoms of thyrotoxicosis in both. The pain and tenderness of the thyroid gland may be relieved by therapeutic dosages of salicylates, but on occasion glucocorticoids may be required. These disorders have been discussed in detail in Chapters 15 and 17.

VII. EXOGENOUS THYROID HORMONE

Thyrotoxicosis may result from the ingestion, usually chronic, of excessive quantities of thyroid hormone preparations (102). The term thyrotoxicosis factitia has been used to describe this situation. In children and adolescents, this ingestion may be surreptitious, iatrogenic, or accidental. Although therapeutic thyroid hormone preparations are the most obvious source, the clinician should keep in mind that ground meats and diet pills have reportedly been contaminated with large amounts of thyroid hormones and implicated in some patients with thyrotoxicosis factitia (102).

Although acute accidental or intentional overdoses of thyroid hormones can produce marked elevations in serum T_4 levels, the majority of children who take as much as 5–10 mg L-T_4 in a single dose have few or no symptoms of thyrotoxicosis (103). When symptoms of thyrotoxicosis occur in these cases, they are usually mild and consist of fever, tachycardia, irritability, vomiting, diarrhea, and hyperactive behavior. Although more serious reactions such as seizures have been reported, these occur very infrequently and several hours to days after the acute overdose (104). When preparations containing significant levels of T_3 have been ingested, the onset of symptoms is within 6–12 h. The onset of symptoms following acute ingestion of L-T_4 is generally within 12–48 h, but may be as late as 7–10 days after ingestion. The delayed onset of symptoms may be explained by the conversion of T_4 to its biologically more active metabolite, T_3. Serum levels of T_4 and/or T_3 following acute ingestion correlate poorly with development of toxicity (105). Because the majority of these cases are relatively benign and symptoms are absent or delayed, initial therapy should be limited to gastric decontamination with syrup of ipecac followed by activated charcoal and/or a cathartic (106). Some authorities also recommend cholestyramine as an initial adjunctive therapy because this agent binds thyroid hormones and reduces their enterohepatic circulation (105). Patients who have ingested thyroid hormone accidentally can then be evaluated closely at home pending the onset of symptoms. As in other accidental poisonings, the parents should be counseled on child safety measures. Only when symptoms occur should hospitalization or further treatment be considered. Propranolol is helpful in controlling tachycardia as well as improving symptoms of nervousness, diaphoresis, or tremor. Acetaminophen may be useful for control of fever. In the rare situation when a massive ingestion results in a life-threatening situation, exchange transfusion has been shown to reduce serum thyroid hormone concentrations effectively (105). Psychiatric evaluation may be indicated for patients with acute intentional overdoses.

Chronic ingestion of thyroid hormone preparations can produce symptoms similar to hyperthyroidism of thyroid origin. However, thyromegaly is not present unless the patient also has a coincident thyroid disease such as Hashimoto's thyroiditis. Likewise, infiltrative ophthalmopathy is absent; however, as in other causes of thyrotoxicosis, lid lag and stare may be present. The diagnosis of this disorder is not difficult if the clinician is able to obtain a history of thyroid hormone ingestion. However, this history may be difficult to obtain, especially in cases of surreptitious ingestion. Nevertheless, the clinician should still be able to diagnose this disorder using a limited number of tests. Thyroid function test results will depend on the type of preparation responsible for the thyrotoxicosis. If the preparation is composed mainly of T_4, the patient will have elevated serum T_4 and free T_4 levels. If the preparation is T_3 or has a high T_3/T_4 ratio, the patient will have a low to normal serum T_4 level. In both cases the serum T_3 level is elevated. The radioiodine uptake is low to reflect the suppression of thyroid gland activity induced by exogenous thyroid hormone. Unlike all other causes of thyrotoxicosis, the plasma thyroglob-

ulin level in this disorder is undetectable or extremely low. Therefore, the plasma thyroglobulin level may be extremely helpful in differentiating this disorder from other causes of thyrotoxicosis.

Treatment of thyrotoxicosis resulting from chronic ingestion of thyroid hormone preparations should be guided by the circumstances surrounding ingestion. For example, patients receiving excessive replacement for treatment of hypothyroidism should have their dosage reduced. The patient who is taking thyroid hormone surreptitiously should be advised to discontinue the medication; in some cases, psychotherapy may be necessary.

VIII. EUTHYROID HYPERTHYROXINEMIA

The term euthyroid hyperthyroxinemia is used to describe the various conditions in which the serum T_4 level, either total or free, is elevated in the absence of thyrotoxicosis. The causes are listed in Table 3 and can be classified into four major categories: increased T_4 binding by serum proteins, generalized resistance to thyroid hormones, impaired peripheral conversion of T_4 to T_3, and changes in thyroid stimulation associated with psychiatric illness.

Alterations in any of the serum thyroid hormone-binding proteins can produce elevations of the total T_4 level, but the free T_4 level remains normal. Increased thyroxine-binding globulin (TBG) concentration results from a variety of causes (Table 4) and produces concurrent elevations of the serum total T_4 and T_3 levels. Familial dysalbuminemic hyperthyroxinemia (FDH) is due to the presence of significant amounts of serum albumin with an unusually high affinity for T_4. Since this albumin typically binds T_3 only weakly, the serum T_3 level remains normal. FDH is inherited in an autosomal dominant fashion and is expressed equally in males and females. Increased serum concentration or binding affinity of thyroxine-binding

Table 3 Conditions Causing Hyperthyroxinemia in the Absence of Thyrotoxicosis

Increased T_4-binding by serum proteins
    Increased concentration of TBG
    Familial dysalbuminemic hyperthyroxinemia
    Increased T_4-binding by transthyretin
    Anti-T_4 antibodies
Generalized (pituitary and peripheral tissues) resistance to thyroid hormone
Impaired conversion of T_4 to T_3
    Pathophysiological conditions (e.g., type I deiodinase deficiency and certain nonthyroidal illnesses)
    Pharmacological agents (e.g., amiodarone, propranolol, heparin, iodine contrast agents, amphetamines, L-thyroxine)
Changes in thyroid stimulation associated with psychiatric illness

Table 4 Factors Associated with
Increased TBG Concentration

Pregnancy
Neonatal state
Estrogens
Oral contraceptives
Acute intermittent porphyria
Infectious and chronic active hepatitis
Perphenazine
Genetic determination

prealbumin (TBPA) or transthyretin can produce elevated serum total T_4 levels but, as in FDH, the serum T_3 level remains normal. The presence of endogenous antibodies directed against T_4 can produce either true or spurious elevations in serum total T_4 levels.

The serum free T_4 level is normal in the disorders of protein binding when it is determined by equilibrium dialysis or the two-step coated tube method. Determination of the free T_4 by an analog-based free T_4 method gives falsely high results in patients with FDH and endogenous anti-T_4 antibodies. This occurs because the variant albumin or anti-T_4 antibody in the serum readily binds the analog tracer used in these competitive immunoassays, and, thereby decreases the amount of tracer available to compete for the assay antibody. The low binding of tracer by the assay antibody gives the false impression of a high free T_4 concentration.

The FT$_4$ index, as usually calculated from the resin T_3 uptake test, accurately reflects the FT$_4$ level only when increased T_4 binding is due to TBG excess. T_4 and T_3 share the same binding site on TBG. When the concentration of TBG is increased, the available binding sites for both T_4 and T_3 are increased. The resin T_3 uptake is inversely proportional to the number of available binding sites for T_3; that is, when the available serum binding sites for T_3 are increased, the resin T_3 uptake is decreased. The FT$_4$ index, when calculated as the product of the T_4 and the resin T_3 uptake, is usually normal in TBG excess because the elevated T_4 is offset by the decreased resin T_3 uptake. However, when increased serum T_4 binding results because of FDH or increased T_4-binding by TBPA or anti-T_4 antibodies, the resin T_3 uptake remains normal because none of these proteins binds significant amounts of T_3. Consequently, the FT$_4$ index values are spuriously elevated. Therefore, one should always consider the possibility of an abnormal T_4-binding protein when serum T_3 and resin T_3 uptake results are normal in the face of an elevated serum T_4 level. It should be emphasized that patients with elevated serum T_4 levels resulting from abnormal serum binding proteins are euthyroid; no antithyroid treatment is indicated.

Generalized (pituitary and peripheral tissues) resistance to thyroid hormone (GRTH) is a rare disorder char-

acterized by thyromegaly, elevated serum total and free T_4 and T_3 levels, a preserved TSH response to TRH, and absence of the usual symptoms and signs of thyrotoxicosis. Although this syndrome is probably congenital, it is rarely diagnosed at birth and more often recognized during childhood and adult life (107). In the majority of affected individuals, it is inherited in an autosomal dominant fashion, but recessive transmission has also been reported (107). The male to female ratio in GRTH is close to 1. The tissue resistance to thyroid hormones is selective, and studies have shown that the pituitary thyrotrophs and peripheral tissue fibroblasts respond normally to dopaminergic drugs and/or glucocorticoids (108, 109). Pituitary secretion of TSH is responsible for thyromegaly, increased thyroid gland activity, and excessive thyroid hormone synthesis and secretion seen in this syndrome. Although the serum TSH level may not always be elevated, it is always detectable; administration of TRH produces a further increase in TSH levels. On the other hand, administration of supraphysiological dosages of exogenous T_3 suppresses pituitary secretion of TSH in virtually all affected patients.

The syndrome of GRTH results from mutations in one of the thyroid hormone receptor genes (92). Two thyroid hormone receptor genes, TRβ and TRα, are located on chromosomes 3 and 17, respectively (92). By alternative splicing of primary transcripts, these two genes code for four main isoforms of the thyroid hormone receptor (TRα-1 and c-erbA α-2; TRβ-1 and TRβ-2). With the exception of the c-erbA α-2 isoform, each of these proteins has both T_3-binding and DNA-binding domains and functions as a thyroid hormone receptor (92). All molecular genetic studies on patients with GRTH have revealed mutations in the T_3-binding domain of the TRβ gene. About 60 different mutations in TRβ have now been identified in patients from over 100 families; the mutations consist of single amino acid substitutions at a single codon, single amino acid deletions, frameshift mutations, or truncations due to premature termination of translation from a mutation-generated stop codon (92). These mutations result in thyroid hormone receptors with defective T_3 binding. In some cases, the same mutations have been described in different families. The clinical phenotype can vary among the families that have the same mutation and also within a family. This suggests that there may be other genetic modifiers that determine the clinical phenotype (92). Patients who inherit this disorder in an autosomal recessive fashion have mutations in both alleles of the TRβ gene. On the other hand, patients who inherit GRTH in an autosomal dominant fashion have a wild-type allele, as well as a mutant allele for the receptor. These mutations are dominant negative in that the mutant receptors inhibit the function of the normal β-receptor (from wild-type allele) and the normal α-receptor (92). Recently, families with GRTH have been identified that have neither TRβ nor TRα mutations (110). It has been proposed that abnormal intracellular thyroid hormone transport, mutations in thyroid hormone receptor cofactors, or dysregulation of cofactor expression may be responsible for the GRTH phenotype in these families. Thus far, no defects have been identified in any of the several thyroid hormone cofactor genes that have been studied in these patients (111). To date, no germline $TR\alpha$-1 mutants have been described in humans (92). It is possible that $TR\alpha$-1 mutations are either lethal in utero, silent, and/or extremely rare.

Despite the elevated levels of circulating thyroid hormones, most patients with GRTH are clinically euthyroid. Although symptoms and signs of hypo- or hyperthyroidism are generally absent, a few patients have been reported with retarded bone age, mental retardation, stunted growth, and hearing defects (112). Persistent tachycardia, tremor, anxiety, and hyperactivity have likewise been observed in some patients (113). These findings suggest that the degree of resistance to thyroid hormone may not be the same in all tissues.

The diagnosis of GRTH requires elevated serum levels of T_4 and free T_4. Serum T_3 and reverse T_3 levels are also elevated. The TBG level is normal and the resin T_3 uptake is elevated. As mentioned above, serum TSH is always detectable, and the TSH response is either normal or exaggerated (89). The radioiodine uptake is increased. Laboratory tests of metabolic status such as basal metabolic rate, serum cholesterol and triglycerides, and carotene are usually normal. Most patients with GRTH require no treatment, but resistance to thyroid hormone may vary from tissue to tissue. Some patients may benefit from treatment with pharmacological dosages of T_4 or T_3; this is especially true in cases where the peripheral tissues are more resistant than the pituitary thyrotrophs. Affected children should be monitored closely for growth deceleration, delayed bone maturation, and impaired mental development. Thyroid hormone treatment should be instituted as necessary. Any therapeutic maneuvers that may reduce the elevated circulating thyroid hormone levels are contraindicated in patients with GRTH and should be avoided.

Peripheral conversion of T_4 to T_3 occurs through the activity of 5'-deiodinase. A variety of pathophysiological conditions and pharmacological agents have been associated with impaired T_4 to T_3 conversion. The clinical syndrome of type I iodothyronine-deiodinase deficiency has been reported but appears to be extremely rare (114). The reported patient was clinically euthyroid and had elevated serum levels of T_4 and reverse T_3, along with normal serum T_3 and TSH levels (115).

Alterations in serum thyroid hormone levels often accompany nonthyroidal illnesses. Although the T_4 level is typically low or normal, on occasion it may be elevated. The euthyroid sick or nonthyroidal illness syndrome is discussed in Chapter 15. Various drugs have been found to cause an elevation of serum T_4 levels in adults, but the majority of these agents are not commonly used in chil-

dren and adolescents. Examples include amiodarone, propranolol, heparin, oral cholecystographic agents, and amphetamines.

Elevated serum T_4 levels are sometimes seen in clinically euthyroid children who are receiving replacement or suppressive therapy with L-T_4. In these children the serum T_3 level is normal. The mechanism responsible for normal T_3 levels despite increased T_4 concentrations has not been completely defined, but may be explained by the fact that 5'-deiodinase activity in peripheral tissues appears to be autoregulated by the levels of circulating T_4. Thus, as the serum T_4 concentration increases from low to elevated levels, the peripheral generation of T_3 from T_4 decreases, as reflected in the steady decline in the serum T_3/T_4 ratio (102). Therefore, in patients receiving L-T_4 therapy, the serum T_3 level is better than the serum T_4 level as an indicator of metabolic status.

Mild elevations in serum T_4 levels are observed in about 20% of patients hospitalized for acute psychiatric disorders (116). This situation is most commonly observed in patients with mania, schizophrenia, and other major affective disorders, but is also occasionally seen in patients with alcoholism or personality disorder. Both total and free T_4 levels are elevated, and, in an occasional patient, serum T_3 is also mildly elevated (116). The serum TSH is usually normal to mildly increased at baseline, and this finding helps to differentiate this condition from the most common forms of thyrotoxicosis. Often, the TSH response to TRH is blunted. These biochemical findings do not appear to represent thyrotoxicosis, and they usually resolve spontaneously within a few weeks without specific therapy. It has been proposed that a decrease in central nervous system (CNS) dopaminergic inhibition results in activation of the hypothalamic–pituitary axis with enhanced TSH secretion and consequent elevations in serum T_4 levels (117).

IX. T₃ AND T₄ TOXICOSIS

Increased serum concentrations of both T_4 and T_3 are observed in the majority of children presenting with hyperthyroidism. However, some thyrotoxic children may present with an increased serum T_3 concentration but a normal or occasionally low serum T4 concentration (i.e., T_3 toxicosis), while others may present with an elevated serum T_4 concentration and a normal or slightly decreased T_3 level (i.e., T_4 toxicosis). Just as in the usual presentation of thyrotoxicosis, the serum TSH level is suppressed in both these situations.

T_3 toxicosis can occur in the course of any disorder that causes hyperthyroidism. Most patients have elevations in both total and free T_3 concentrations, but some will present with elevated free T_3 levels while total T_3 levels are still within the normal range (118, 119). During childhood, T_3 toxicosis is most often encountered early in the course of either initial or relapsing Graves' disease or in association with an autonomous nodule. In these situations, T_3 toxicosis reflects a predominant hypersecretion of T_3 by the thyroid gland, rather than an increase in the peripheral conversion of T_4 to T_3 (120). If left untreated, some patients with T_3 toxicosis due to true hyperthyroidism, over time, will develop elevated serum concentrations of both T_3 and T_4. T_3 toxicosis is also seen in thyrotoxicosis factitia related to ingestion of liothyronine (L-T_3).

T_4 toxicosis occurs in two circumstances: iodine-induced thyrotoxicosis and thyrotoxicosis accompanied by severe intercurrent illness. With iodine-induced thyrotoxicosis, about one-third of patients have elevated serum T_4 but normal serum T_3 levels, and the remainder have proportionate elevations of serum T_3 and T_4 levels (120). In severe illness, peripheral conversion of T_4 to T_3 is impaired because of marked reductions in 5′-deiodinase activity. This accounts for the normal or low serum T_3 levels in the presence of abnormally elevated serum T_4 levels. Furthermore, serum reverse T_3 (rT_3) levels are also increased because of the impaired 5′-deiodinase activity. With resolution of the intercurrent illness, 5′-deiodinase activity normalizes with subsequent declines in serum rT_3 levels and increases of serum T_3 levels into the thyrotoxic range. On a clinical level, T_4 toxicosis of this type needs to be differentiated from the low serum T_3/elevated serum T_4 levels occasionally observed in the euthyroid sick syndrome. The serum TSH level will be suppressed in T_4 toxicosis, and it may also be very low or suppressed in the euthyroid sick syndrome. Therefore, serum TSH measurement may not be helpful initially in differentiating between these two conditions.

X. GRAVES' OPHTHALMOPATHY

Ophthalmic abnormalities are clinically evident in over half of the children and adolescents with Graves' disease. In most of these patients, the signs and symptoms are relatively mild and include lid lag, lid retraction, stare, proptosis, conjunctival injection, chemosis, and periorbital and eyelid edema. Less commonly, patients may complain of eye discomfort, pain, or diplopia. Severe ophthalmopathy, associated with marked chemosis, severe proptosis, periorbital ecchymosis, corneal ulceration, eye muscle paralysis, and optic atrophy, is extremely rare during childhood and adolescence. The clinical onset of eye disease usually coincides with that of thyroid dysfunction, but it can precede or follow it by several months to years (121).

Lid lag, lid retraction, and stare most commonly result directly from thyrotoxicosis with enhanced sympathetic stimulation of Müller's muscle of the upper lid. These features can be found in patients with thyrotoxicosis of any cause and generally improve with normalization of thyroid hormone levels. The other signs and symptoms, however, are characteristic of Graves' ophthal-

mopathy and can be explained by the mechanical effects of an increase in tissue volume within the bony orbit. Histological examination reveals accumulation of glycosaminoglycans (GAGs) in the connective tissue components of the orbital fat and muscles, as well as lymphocytic infiltration of the orbital tissues. The GAGs are hydrophilic macromolecules produced by orbital fibroblasts, and their accumulation results in enlargement of the extraocular muscles and surrounding fat (122). Enlargement of these tissues within the fixed space of the bony orbit leads to forward displacement of the globe (proptosis or exophthalmos). Chemosis and periorbital edema result from decreased venous drainage from the orbit and intraorbital inflammation. Extraocular muscle dysfunction results from accumulation of GAGs, edema, inflammation, and fibrosis of the endomysial connective tissues investing the muscle fibers (122).

Although information regarding its pathogenesis is limited, Graves' ophthalmopathy (GO) is generally considered to represent an organ-specific autoimmune disorder. Current evidence supports the contention that orbital fibroblasts are the primary targets of the autoimmune attack (123). However, the nature of the autoimmune reaction is unclear, and a target orbital autoantigen has not been conclusively identified. The close association of GO with autoimmune thyroid disease strongly suggests that the orbital antigen(s) may share unique structural characteristics with antigens of the thyroid gland. Recent studies support that two such candidate antigens, the TSH receptor (124) and thyroglobulin (125), are present in orbital tissues from patients with GO. Therefore, it is possible that either of these two proteins could be the primary target antigen in GO, thus providing a common link between the thyroid and eye diseases. Because the TSH receptor is the primary target antigen in Graves' hyperthyroidism, most investigators currently consider it to be the leading candidate target antigen in GO. Several human and animal studies have provided compelling, although not yet definitive, evidence (reviewed in 123, 126) to support this role for the TSH receptor in GO. However, more studies are needed to determine which, if either, of these two proteins is the target autoantigen in GO. Thus far, thyroid peroxidase has not been detected in orbital tissues (121).

Cell-mediated immunity appears to play a major role in the pathogenesis of GO. The extraocular muscles and orbital connective tissues are infiltrated by lymphocytes and macrophages. The lymphocytes are predominantly CD4$^+$ and CD8$^+$ T cells with a few B cells. Regardless of the target antigen that causes the lymphocytic infiltration, the proximal events in the pathogenesis of GO appear to be cytokine-mediated activation of orbital fibroblasts, secretion of GAGs by these cells, and ultimately, fibrosis. Immunohistochemical studies have demonstrated the presence of the cytokines, interferon-gamma (IFN-γ), tumor necrosis factor-α (TNF-α), and interleukin-1α (IL-1α), in the cytoplasm of orbital-infiltrating mononuclear cells and in adjacent orbital connective tissue from patients with early active GO (127). These findings support that T cells and antigen-presenting cells within these tissues are activated. Because transplacental passage of maternal thyroid-stimulating antibodies does not appear to cause infiltrative ophthalmopathy in neonates, and the presence of antibodies to orbital antigens is inconsistently related to eye disease, humoral autoimmunity appears to play at most a secondary role in the pathogenesis of GO (11).

Because ophthalmopathy is relatively mild and self-limited in the vast majority of affected children and adolescents, specific treatment is usually not necessary. In general, eye findings improve in association with control of the hyperthyroidism. Occasionally, local measures may be used to treat symptoms. For example, eye drop or ointment preparations containing methylcellulose may be necessary to prevent corneal drying. Sleeping with the head elevated may help to reduce chemosis and periorbital edema. Other forms of treatment, such as oral corticosteroids, orbital irradiation, and surgical decompression, are rarely indicated in children and should be reserved for those with severe ophthalmopathy.

XI. LABORATORY EVALUATION

The laboratory evaluation of thyrotoxicosis should be guided by the patient's clinical presentation as determined by the medical history and physical examination. In all causes of thyrotoxicosis, except for TSH-induced hyperthyroidism, the serum TSH level will be undetectable or very suppressed using modern second- or third- generation TSH assays. For the child or adolescent presenting with obvious signs and symptoms of Graves' disease, including a soft, diffusely enlarged, smooth goiter and proptosis, only a few laboratory tests are needed. In addition to the undetectable serum TSH, an elevated free T_4 (or free T_4 index) and the presence of TSHrAb (either TBII or TSI) substantiate the clinical diagnosis. When antithyroid drugs are selected as therapy, a baseline complete blood cell count with differential white blood count should be obtained: leukopenia occurs in untreated thyrotoxicosis and granulocytopenia is an occasional toxic reaction to antithyroid drugs.

In less severe presentations, however, further laboratory tests may be necessary. Serum T_3 levels will be elevated in nearly all patients with Graves' disease. Measurement of serum total and/or free T_3 levels can be useful in the occasional patient with early Graves' disease who presents with an undetectable TSH but a normal serum free T_4 level.

For the patient who presents with symptoms of thyrotoxicosis and a firm, mildly tender, asymmetric goiter, the radioiodine uptake (RAI-U; Table 5) can differentiate Graves' disease from either the toxic thyroiditis of Hashimoto's disease or subacute thyroiditis (128, 129). Fur-

Table 5 Classification of Thyrotoxicosis by Radioiodine Uptake (RAI-U)

RAI-U usually elevated:
  Graves' disease
  Toxic adenoma
  Toxic multinodular goiter
  Familial nonautoimmune hyperthyroidism
  TSH-induced hyperthyroidism
  Trophoblastic disease
RAI-U typically low:
  Subacute thyroiditis
  Toxic thyroiditis of Hashimoto's disease
  Thyrotoxicosis factitia
  Iodine-induced hyperthyroidism
  Metastatic thyroid carcinoma

thermore, the RAI-U also can help to differentiate Graves' disease from thyrotoxicosis factitia.

Graves' disease is the most common cause of thyrotoxicosis during pregnancy (4). However in the pregnant adolescent with mild symptoms of thyrotoxicosis and a normal to slightly enlarged thyroid gland, the possibility of hCG-mediated hyperthyroidism should be considered. Biochemical and clinical hyperthyroidism can occur when serum hCG levels exceed 100,000–300,000 IU/l (4).

TSHrAb and autoantibodies to thyroglobulin and/or thyroid peroxidase are present in the majority of patients with Graves' disease and reflect the autoimmune nature of the disorder. However, none of these autoantibodies is specific to Graves' disease. Although almost all hyperthyroid patients with serum TSHrAb will have Graves' disease, these antibodies also can be detected in patients with Hashimoto's thyroiditis (27, 46, 47) and in patients with subacute thyroiditis (130). Thyroglobulin and/or thyroid peroxidase antibodies are present in the majority of patients with Hashimoto's thyroiditis (131) and have been reported in several patients with subacute thyroiditis (130, 132) and a few patients with familial nonautoimmune hyperthyroidism (88). Therefore, by themselves, none of these antibodies should be considered as absolute proof of Graves' disease in patients with thyrotoxicosis.

Several studies have suggested that the recently cloned and characterized Na^+/I^- symporter (NIS) may represent an important autoantigen in Graves' disease (133). Although earlier studies (based on relatively small sample sizes) suggested that NIS autoantibodies might be present in up to 60–80% of Graves' sera (133), a more recent study evaluating 177 Graves' sera found these antibodies in only 5–10% of the samples (134). Furthermore, NIS antibodies also are present in 15–20% of sera from patients with Hashimoto's thyroiditis (133, 134). At present, the functional roles, if any, that these antibodies play in either Graves' disease or Hashimoto's disease remain unclear. Although assays are not yet available for routine clinical use, based on current data, the measurement of NIS antibodies does not appear to offer any additional diagnostic benefit for patients with Graves' disease.

More detailed discussions of clinical features and laboratory studies that can be used to evaluate patients with other causes of thyrotoxicosis and to differentiate these disorders from Graves' disease are presented in the appropriate subsections of this chapter.

XII. PROGNOSIS AND TREATMENT

A. Introduction and Overview

The clinical course of Graves' disease is variable and unpredictable. However, the hyperthyroidism in untreated Graves' disease usually persists and progresses unless the thyroid gland has limited responsiveness as a result of coexisting chronic lymphocytic thyroiditis. Therefore, therapeutic intervention is recommended for all patients with active Graves' disease. Despite recent advances in our knowledge of the TSH receptor and TSHrAbs, none of the currently available treatments is specifically directed against the underlying immunological abnormality that causes Graves' disease. The three acceptable methods of therapy (antithyroid drugs, radioiodine ablation, and subtotal/total thyroidectomy) merely interrupt the disease process at the level of the thyroid gland, although treatment with thioureas has been reported to reduce levels of TSHrAb (135).

The treatment of Graves' disease in children and adolescents remains controversial. Although all three therapeutic modalities represent effective treatments for Graves' hyperthyroidism, each has specific advantages and disadvantages that should be addressed when individual treatment plans are developed for affected individuals. The antithyroid drugs are generally well tolerated, their inhibitory effects on the thyroid are completely reversible, and some patients treated with them will achieve long-term or permanent remission (136). Therefore, antithyroid drug treatment will allow some children to avoid surgery or exposure to radioiodine. However, antithyroid drugs usually take 4–8 weeks initially to control hyperthyroidism, and a treatment period of several years is typically required to achieve a long-term remission. During this prolonged treatment period, noncompliance and drug toxicity (Table 6) can complicate patient management. Furthermore, relapse of hyperthyroidism frequently occurs following discontinuation of therapy (136). As yet, no reliable clinical, biochemical, immunological or genetic factors have been identified that allow absolute prediction of those patients likely to do well, or poorly, in achieving long-term remission with antithyroid drug therapy (137).

Radioiodine (RAI) represents the easiest form of treatment, and the majority of patients can be successfully treated with a single oral dose (136). However, RAI ther-

Table 6 Toxic Side Effects of Antithyroid Drug Therapy

Elevated liver enzymes	Nausea, abdominal discomfort
Granulocytopenia	Edema
Dermatitis, urticaria	Conjunctivitis
Arthralgia, arthritis	Thrombocytopenia
Lupus-like syndrome	Hypoprothrombinemia
Lymphadenopathy	Toxic psychosis
Peripheral neuritis	Sensorineural hearing loss
Fever	Loss of taste sensation
Hepatitis	Disseminated intravascular coagulation

apy is absolutely contraindicated during pregnancy and breastfeeding (137). Although hospitalization is not required, patients receiving RAI are usually advised to limit close contact with others and properly dispose of their urine for several days following treatment. RAI therapy is also slow to control hyperthyroidism; it usually takes 6–18 weeks to have its full effects on the thyroid. Some patients may require multiple doses of RAI to treat their disease adequately. Although RAI is generally well tolerated, radiation thyroiditis may occur. This is characterized by a transient increase in serum thyroid hormone levels with, occasionally, a worsening of hyperthyroid symptoms and thyroid gland tenderness. With ablative dosages, the thyroid gland will shrink and hypothyroidism will occur in the majority of patients. In rare cases parathyroid dysfunction may develop after RAI therapy (138). Concerns regarding the potential long-term carcinogenic and genetic risks of RAI in children/adolescents continue to linger (136).

Surgical therapy represents the most rapidly effective form of treatment. Following at least 10–14 days of preoperative preparation with antithyroid drugs, stable iodine (e.g., SSKI or Lugol's solution), and β-adrenergic blockers, either subtotal or total thyroidectomy can be performed. Both are complicated procedures, and the long-term cure rates and the incidence of complications depend in large part on the skill and experience of the surgeon. Due to the continued reliance on antithyroid drugs and the increasing acceptance of RAI as primary therapies for juvenile Graves' disease, clinicians now infrequently recommend surgery for children with Graves' disease. However, clinical indications for surgical therapy still exist. These include the patient with a very large goiter; the patient who fails to respond to medical treatment and refuses RAI; the very young patient (i.e., <5 years old) who fails to respond to medical management; the pregnant patient with moderate to severe hyperthyroidism uncontrolled by medical treatment; and the patient with Graves' disease who develops a solid cold thyroid nodule that raises the suspicion of thyroid carcinoma (11, 136–139). Hypothyroidism occurs in 60–~100% of children undergoing subtotal and total thyroidectomy, respectively (136).

Hyperthyroidism recurs in 10–15% of patients following subtotal thyroidectomy, but in fewer than 3% of children who undergo total thyroidectomy (136). Potential surgical complications include pain, hemorrhage/hematoma, transient hypocalcemia, transient hoarseness, temporary tracheostomy, permanent hypoparathyroidism, vocal cord paralysis, keloid formation, and death (136).

Regardless of the modality ultimately used for the treatment of Graves' hyperthyroidism, patients will require long-term regular medical follow-up. Thyroid function studies will need to be monitored on a regular basis to aid in maintenance of the euthyroid state. Patients will need to be treated and/or observed for other associated autoimmune disorders that may potentially accompany Graves' disease. Patients will also need to be monitored for the potential occurrence of thyroid tumors and any long-term consequences that may be associated with the preceding treatment(s) for hyperthyroidism.

A recent study in adults showed that despite successful treatment of Graves' hyperthyroidism and a return to the euthyroid state, some patients will continue to exhibit symptoms of physical, emotional, and neuropsychological illness (140). Anxiety, depression, lack of energy, sleep disturbance, emotional lability, impaired memory, and forgetfulness are some of the difficulties experienced by patients who had remained euthyroid for more than a year (140). Other studies have demonstrated cognitive deficits in hyperthyroid adults in remission (141, 142). It has been proposed that these impairments represent residual sequelae of elevated thyroid hormone levels on the brain (140). Although similar studies involving children or adolescents have not been published, it is highly likely that some previously hyperthyroid children and adolescents, despite a return to euthyroidism, also suffer from these or similar problems. Therefore, as part of the regular medical follow-up, previously hyperthyroid children and adolescents should be monitored for behavioral, emotional, and learning or other neuropsychological problems. Appropriate counseling and support services should be offered as necessary.

Discussions regarding specific treatments for other causes of thyrotoxicosis are presented in the appropriate subsections of this chapter.

B. β-Adrenergic Blocking Agents

From the preceding discussion, it is clear that each of the currently acceptable treatment options carries a lag time between the onset of therapy and the control of hyperthyroidism. This lag time ranges from as short as 10–14 days for surgery to as long as several weeks to months for both antithyroid drug and radioiodine treatments. β-Adrenergic blockade with either propranolol or atenolol represents an important and very effective adjunctive therapy for the rapid control of adrenergic symptoms during the thyrotoxic course of the disease. These drugs should not be used alone for long-term management of hyperthyroidism

in children, because they do not significantly affect thyroid hormone secretion or correct the abnormal increases in metabolic rate and oxygen consumption (143). However, both propranolol (10–20 mg every 6–8 h) and atenolol (25–50 mg once or twice daily) are effective in controlling the distressing symptoms and signs of restlessness, tachycardia, heat intolerance, tremor, hyperhidrosis, diarrhea, and myopathy. In addition, propranolol (but not atenolol) reduces conversion of T_4 to T_3 by inhibiting the 5'-deiodination pathway, thus producing some decrease in serum T_3 levels (143). The dosages of these medicines should be adjusted over time to return the pulse rate to normal. β-Adrenergic blocking agents should be avoided or used very cautiously in patients with a history of asthma, hypoglycemia (including patients with insulin-dependent diabetes mellitus), heart block, or heart failure (144). Atenolol, in relatively small dosages, represents the safer choice in hyperthyroid patients with a history of asthma and hypoglycemia, because it is more cardioselective (i.e., β_1-adrenergic receptor specific) than propranolol (144). Neither drug should be discontinued abruptly, since symptoms and signs of hyperthyroidism may acutely worsen. Instead, the dosage should be decreased gradually over several days before being stopped.

C. Antithyroid Drug Therapy

The antithyroid drugs for long-term therapy of children in the United States include propylthiouracil (PTU) and methimazole (MMI). In addition to these two agents, a methimazole derivative, carbimazole, is available in Europe (145). These drugs block the incorporation of oxidized iodide into tyrosine residues of thyroglobulin by serving as substrates for thyroid peroxidase. The drugs are iodinated and degraded within the gland, thus diverting oxidized iodide away from thyroglobulin (146). Furthermore, they block the coupling of iodotyrosyl residues in thyroglobulin to form T_4 and T_3. They do not interfere with the thyroid gland's ability to concentrate iodide, nor do they block the release of stored thyroid hormone into the circulation (146). Because they do not block the release of preformed, stored thyroid hormones, most patients will require 4–8 weeks of antithyroid drug therapy before a euthyroid state is achieved. PTU, but not methimazole or carbimazole, also inhibits the peripheral conversion of T_4 to T_3 (146). Because of this, many clinicians tend to use PTU initially in patients with more severe hyperthyroidism.

In addition to their direct effects on thyroid hormone synthesis, the thioureas also may have immunosuppressive activity. Several investigators have reported significant reductions in circulating TSHrAbs during antithyroid drug treatment (135, 147). Some studies suggest that thioureas have direct effects on thyroid autoantibody-producing lymphocytes, whereas others suggest that these drugs primarily act by reducing the antigenicity of thyrocytes (147).

MMI has a longer half-life (12–16 h vs. 4–6 h), and, on a weight basis, is about 10-fold more potent than PTU (136). To control hyperthyroidism initially, PTU is given every 6–8 h, whereas MMI can be given every 8–12 h; after 3–4 weeks of therapy, dosing of MMI usually can be changed to once or twice a day (136, 137). For patients with moderate to severe hyperthyroidism, the recommended starting dosages for PTU and MMI are 5–10 mg/kg/day and 0.5–1.0 mg/kg/day, respectively. In patients with mild hyperthyroidism, lower dosages of antithyroid drugs may be effective. Once clinical and biochemical euthyroidism have been achieved, maintenance therapy may proceed by either of two methods: reduce the dosage by one-third to one-half to maintain thyroid hormone levels in the normal range; or continue the initial therapeutic dosage to induce hypothyroidism, and initiate replacement L-thyroxine therapy. The latter method is preferred by many clinicians for children because euthyroidism seems easier to maintain, and it involves fewer clinic visits for monitoring of thyroid function. Although a study from Japan demonstrated that the combined use of antithyroid drugs and L-thyroxine decreased the incidence of relapse in adult patients (148), several recent studies from around the world have been unable to reproduce this finding (149–151).

After 1–3 years of therapy, the medication is either slowly tapered or a T_3 suppression of serum T_4 using exogenous doses of oral T_3 (1.5 μg/kg/day in three divided doses) can be performed (46). The administration of exogenous T_3 for 3 weeks to normal children or patients in remission with Graves' disease will cause a decrease in the serum T_4 concentration to values below the normal range. The test is performed as follows:

1. While the patient is still receiving the antithyroid drug, T_3 is started at the dosage listed above. L-thyroxine therapy must be discontinued in those patients on combined therapy.
2. Three weeks later, serum T_4 and free T_4 levels are evaluated.
   a. If the results are normal or elevated, antithyroid drug therapy is continued.
   b. If the results are below normal, discontinue the antithyroid drug and exogenous T_3 therapy.
3. One or two weeks later, repeat the serum T_4 values.
   a. If normal or elevated, resume antithyroid drug therapy.
   b. If the serum T_4 values are low, discontinue T_3 therapy and monitor serum T_4 and T_3 levels at 3 month intervals for the next year and annually thereafter. If relapse occurs, antithyroid therapy may be resumed, or the patient may be offered the choice of surgical or radioiodine therapy (9).

In adults, the presence of TSHrAb during antithyroid drug therapy may be associated with clinical relapse of disease on termination of therapy (40). Studies have shown that patients (adults and children) with negative TSHrAb values during antithyroid drug therapy remain in remission after cessation of therapy (46, 152). One study in children with Graves' disease compared TSHrAb values and the clinical course with results of the T_3 suppression tests (46). TSHrAb values correctly predicted the subsequent clinical course in 72%, and the T_3 suppression tests accurately predicted the course in 64% of patients. Furthermore, the TSHrAb values and the T_3 suppression tests were in agreement 75% of the time. This study suggests that TSHrAb values are as effective as T_3 suppression tests in determining when antithyroid drug therapy can be discontinued. However, both tests are limited in their ability to predict accurately the clinical course of the disease, and patients will continue to require periodic clinical evaluations and laboratory assessment after discontinuation of antithyroid drug therapy.

The major disadvantages of antithyroid drug therapy are prolonged duration of therapy required to achieve a long-term remission, high relapse rate following cessation of therapy, and the risk of toxic side effects (9, 136, 146). In children, long-term remission rates are at best 50–60% after several years of drug therapy and are usually less than 20–40% (136, 153). Furthermore, remission rates following antithyroid drug therapy are considerably less in prepubertal than in pubertal children (154). A recent study has demonstrated that the severity of hyperthyroidism at diagnosis, as determined by multiple clinical and laboratory variables, is important in predicting remission within two years of therapy (155). Specifically, this study found that within 2 years of treatment, patients with a minimal/small goiter and a body mass index score above −0.5 SD at time of initial diagnosis had a probability of 86% of achieving remission for at least 6 months, compared with only 13% for those with a moderate/large goiter and BMI below −0.5 SD (155). Other studies have shown that high levels of TSI at the time of diagnosis are associated with decreased long-term remission rates (156, 157). A recent study showed that elevated serum IgE levels following 18 months of MMI therapy are associated with lower rates of remission (158). Although none of these factors can predict with absolute certainty which patients will achieve long-term remission with antithyroid drugs, they may be helpful in selecting specific treatment plans for individual patients.

Side effects of antithyroid drugs occur in up to 20–30% of treated children and may be either idiosyncratic or dose related (136). The majority of side effects are mild and include elevated liver enzyme levels, mild leukopenia, skin rashes, and mild gastrointestinal symptoms such as nausea. In the case of mild side effects, complications may resolve after switching to an alternative antithyroid drug. Fortunately, more serious side effects are either uncommon or rare. When a patient reports any serious toxic effect with antithyroid drugs, therapy must be stopped immediately, and the patient should be evaluated. The occurrence of serious side effects necessitates discontinuation of all antithyroid drugs, and an alternative mode of therapy (i.e., radioiodine or surgery) must be selected for subsequent treatment. Although very rare, the most serious complication of antithyroid drug treatment is agranulocytosis. Patients should have a complete blood count performed if sore throat, fever, or mouth ulcers occur. Treatment of agranulocytosis consists of complete discontinuation of the antithyroid drug, hospitalization for monitoring, and treatment with a broad-spectrum antibiotic (11). A recent randomized trial in adults found no benefit of granulocyte colony-stimulating factor (159). Another rare complication is drug-induced hepatitis; cholestatic hepatitis is typically associated with MMI use, whereas cytotoxic hepatitis tends to occur with PTU. In either case, antithyroid drugs must be stopped immediately, and administration of glucocorticoids may hasten recovery (136).

D. Radioiodine Therapy

Although still controversial, RAI therapy is becoming more acceptable for the treatment of juvenile Graves' disease as long-term experience with its use accumulates (136, 139, 149, 160, 161). RAI is administered as an oral solution or capsule containing Na ^{131}I. After absorption through the gastrointestinal tract, it is concentrated into the thyroid gland and organified. β-Emissions from the ^{131}I result in extensive tissue damage; histological findings after RAI therapy are consistent with acute inflammation and include epithelial swelling and necrosis, edema, and leukocyte infiltration (136). Within 4–10 days after RAI administration, serum levels of thyroid hormones may rise as a result of thyroid hormone release from degenerating follicular cells (162). The acute inflammatory phase is subsequently followed by extensive fibrosis and ablation of the thyroid gland within 6–18 weeks (145).

RAI may be used as either first- or second-line therapy in children/adolescents with Graves' disease. Because RAI is absolutely contraindicated during pregnancy, a pregnancy test must be obtained in the adolescent before proceeding with RAI therapy. The authors consider RAI therapy to represent a definitive method for control of Graves' hyperthyroidism, and, therefore, recommend that it be used in ablative dosages. When used as first-line therapy in patients with mild to moderate hyperthyroidism, a preceding course of antithyroid drugs is generally not necessary. β-Adrenergic-blocking agents can be used both before and after RAI administration to relieve thyrotoxic symptoms until the gland has been ablated. However, for the patient with severe hyperthyroidism, some clinicians recommend a 4–8 week course of antithyroid drugs to reduce the severity of hyperthyroidism before RAI is administered (11). In these patients, and in those

who have been receiving antithyroid drugs as first-line therapy prior to RAI ablation, the antithyroid drugs should be stopped at least 4–7 days before RAI is administered (136, 139).

Prior treatment with PTU, even when discontinued for several days before RAI dosing, reduces the effectiveness of RAI therapy (163); this should be considered when determining the therapeutic dosage of RAI (163). Conversely, MMI appears to have very little or no effect on the success of RAI therapy when discontinued at least 3–4 days prior to RAI dosing (163, 164). Again, β-adrenergic blocking agents are used both before and after RAI administration to control symptoms of hyperthyroidism. Occasionally after RAI therapy, thyrotoxic symptoms cannot be adequately controlled with β-adrenergic blockers alone. In this situation, either antithyroid drugs or concentrated iodide solutions (SSKI or Lugol's solution) may be used until RAI takes effect (136). The use of a concentrated iodide solution (e.g., SSKI, 5–6 drops by mouth daily) beginning 7 days after administration of RAI has been shown to treat thyrotoxicosis effectively more rapidly than ^{131}I alone without adversely affecting the outcome of RAI therapy (165). A single ablative dose of RAI (i.e., 150–200 μCi ^{131}I/g thyroid tissue) will successfully treat hyperthyroidism in the majority of patients within 6–18 weeks (136, 145). Some patients will require more than one dose of RAI to treat their hyperthyroidism. Repeat doses of RAI can be given at intervals of 2–6 months if hyperthyroidism persists beyond the first treatment (136).

Acute complications following RAI therapy are uncommon and tend to be mild. Radiation thyroiditis with mild pain over the gland may occur within the first 3–5 days and can generally be relieved with nonsteroidal anti-inflammatory agents. Symptoms of hyperthyroidism may worsen temporarily during the first 2 weeks due to the release of preformed thyroid hormones from degenerating follicular cells. Typically, these symptoms can be controlled with the β-adrenergic blocking drugs. In rare cases, thyroid storm can occur after RAI treatment (62, 63, 136).

Although there is some concern in adult patients regarding progression of ophthalmopathy following RAI, there is currently no evidence to support that RAI promotes progression of eye disease in children (136, 139). Current studies suggest that eye disease may worsen in 3–5% of children with Graves' ophthalmopathy after RAI. However, this rate of progression is very similar to the rates observed in children undergoing either antithyroid drug or surgical therapy (136). Parathyroid dysfunction may occur in rare cases after RAI therapy (136, 138). Up to 90% or more of patients who receive ablative doses of RAI will eventually develop primary hypothyroidism (136, 139). Thyroid function tests should be monitored every 2–3 months after RAI, so that thyroid hormone replacement can be started before the onset of clinical symptoms.

The reluctance of clinicians to recommend RAI as first-line therapy has traditionally stemmed from the theoretical possibility of increased risk for subsequent thyroid tumors (both malignant and benign), other nonthyroid malignancies, infertility, and genetic defects among progeny (160). Patients with Graves' disease have a higher incidence of thyroid tumors than the general population (136). However, Graves' patients receiving RAI appear to have lower rates of thyroid cancer than those receiving long-term antithyroid drug therapy; this most likely is explained by the presence of more thyroid tissue in patients treated with drugs than in those treated with RAI (136). Currently available studies involving the long-term follow-up (from <5 years to about 20 years) of ~1000 children and adolescents who received RAI therapy for hyperthyroidism have not revealed an increased risk of thyroid malignancy (136). Although an increased incidence of benign thyroid adenoma has been observed in children treated with low-dosage RAI (50 μCi ^{131}I/g thyroid tissue) (166), the incidence of thyroid adenoma is not increased when higher dosages (100–200 μCi/g) are used (166). There is currently no evidence for an increased risk of leukemia. With the possible exception of a small increase in the incidence of stomach cancer, there is currently no evidence for an increased risk of other nonthyroid malignancies in adults who have received RAI (136). However, a comprehensive follow-up study of nonthyroid cancer risks has not yet been performed for children treated with RAI. There is no evidence for decreased fertility in patients who have received RAI, and the incidence of congenital anomalies among the offspring of patients treated with RAI is not different from that observed in the general population (136).

Based on current experience and knowledge, RAI represents a convenient, effective, and apparently relatively safe therapeutic option for childhood Graves' disease. After considering that antithyroid drug therapy is associated with disappointingly low long-term remission rates despite prolonged therapy and relatively high rates of adverse side effects, it is easy to understand why RAI is becoming more acceptable for the treatment of childhood Graves' disease. However, RAI is absolutely contraindicated during pregnancy and breastfeeding. ^{131}I readily crosses the placenta, and if administered to a pregnant female after 10–12 weeks' gestation, it will be concentrated by the fetal thyroid gland. This can result in ablation of the fetal thyroid and subsequent fetal hypothyroidism (139). RAI should probably be avoided in children less than 5 years old because experience with RAI is currently quite limited in this age group, and the risks of thyroid cancer after external irradiation are highest in children less than 5 years of age (136).

REFERENCES

1. Hayles AB, Zimmerman D. Graves' disease in childhood. In: Ingbar SH, Braverman LE, eds. Werner's The Thyroid, 5th ed. Philadelphia: JB Lippincott, 1986:1412–1428.

2. Tomer Y, Huber GK, Davies TF. Human chorionic gonadotropin (hCG) interacts directly with recombinant human TSH receptors. J Clin Endocrinol Metab 1992;74:1477.

3. Hershman JM. Human chorionic gonadotropin and the thyroid: hyperemesis gravidarum and trophoblastic tumors. Thyroid 1999;9:653.

4. Seely BL, Burrow GN. Thyrotoxicosis in pregnancy. Endocrinologist 1991;1:409.

5. Ngowngarmratana S, Sunthornthepvarakul T, Kanchanawat S. Thyroid function and human chorionic gonadotropin in patients with hydatidiform mole. J Med Assoc Thai 1997;80:693.

6. Roti E, Colzani R, Braverman LE. Adverse effects of iodine on the thyroid. Endocrinologist 1997;7:245.

7. Roti E, Uberti ED. Iodine excess and hyperthyroidism. Thyroid 2001;11:493.

8. Bryant WP, Zimmerman D. Iodine induced hyperthyroidism in a newborn. Pediatrics 1995;95:434.

9. Clayton GW. Thyrotoxicosis in children. In: Kaplan SA, ed. Clinical Pediatric and Adolescent Endocrinology, Philadelphia: WB Saunders, 1982:110–117.

10. Farid NR. Immunogenetics of autoimmune thyroid disorders. Endocrinol Metab Clin North Am 1987;16:229.

11. Weetman AP. Graves' disease. N Engl J Med 2000;343:1236.

12. Gough SCL. The genetics of Graves' disease. Endocrinol Metab Clin North Am 2000;29:255.

13. Chen Q-Y, Huang W, She J-X, et al. HLA-DRB1*08, DRB1*03/DRB3*0101, and DRB3*0202 are susceptibility genes for Graves' disease in North American Caucasians, whereas DRB1*07 is protective. J Clin Endocrinol Metab 1999;84:3182.

14. Lavard L, Madsen HO, Perrild H, et al. HLA class II associations in juvenile Graves' disease: indication of a strong protective role of the RBI*0701, DQA1*0201 haplotype. Tissue Antigens 1997;50:639.

15. Onuma H, Ota M, Sugenoya A, Inoko H. Association of HLA-DPB1*0501 with early onset Graves' disease in Japanese. Hum Immunol 1994;39:195.

16. Vaidya B, Imrie H, Perros P, et al. Evidence for a new Graves disease susceptibility locus at chromosome 18q21. Am J Hum Genet 2000;66:1710.

17. Smith EM, Morrill AC, Meyer WJ III, et al. Corticotropin releasing factor induction of leukocyte-derived immunoreactive ACTH and endorphins. Nature 1986;32:881.

18. Hayles AB, Chaves-Carballo E. Diagnosis and treatment of exophthalmic goiter in children. Clin Pediatr (Phila) 1967;6:681.

19. Lavard L, Perrild H, Ranlov I, et al. Incidence of juvenile thyrotoxicosis in Denmark 1982–88. Eur J Endocrinol 1994;130:565.

20. Nagayama Y, Rapoport B. The thyrotropin receptor 25 years after its discovery: new insight after its molecular cloning. Mol Endocrinol 1992;6:145.

21. Vassart G, Dumont JE. The thyrotropin receptor and the regulation of thyrocyte function and growth. Endocrin Rev 1992;13:596.

22. Vassart G, Parmentier M, Libert F, Dumont J. Molecular genetics of the thyrotropin receptor. Trends Endocrinol Metab 1991;2:151.

23. Weetman AP, Yateman ME, Ealey PA, et al. Thyroid-stimulating antibody activity between different immunoglobulin G subclasses. J Clin Invest 1990;86:723.

24. Kraiem Z, Cho BY, Sadeh O, et al. The IgG subclass

distribution of TSH receptor blocking antibodies in primary hypothyroidism. Clin Endocrinol 1992;37:135.

25. Davies TF. New thinking on the immunology of Graves' disease. Thyroid Today 1992;15(4):1–11.

26. Gupta MK. Thyrotropin receptor antibodies: advances and importance of detection techniques in thyroid diseases. Clin Biochem 1992;25:193.

27. Rees Smith B, McLachlan SM, Furmaniak J. Autoantibodies to the thyrotropin receptor. Endocrinol Rev 1988; 9:106.

28. Rapoport B, Chazenbalk GD, Jaume JC, McLachlan SM. The thyrotropin receptor: interaction with thyrotropin and autoantibodies. Endocrinol Rev 1998;19:673.

29. Kohn LD, Shimura H, Shimura Y, et al. The thyrotropin receptor. Vitam Horm 1995;50:287.

30. Prabhakar BS, Fan JL, Seetharamaiah GS. Thyrotropin-receptor-mediated disease: a paradigm for receptor autoimmunity. Immunol Today 1997;18:437.

31. Kosugi S, Ban T, Akamizu T, Kohn LD. Identification of separate determinants on the thyrotropin receptor reactive with Graves' thyroid-stimulating antibodies and with thyroid-stimulating blocking antibodies in idiopathic myxedema; these determinants have no homologous sequence on gonadotropin receptors. Mol Endocrinol 1992; 6:168.

32. Nagayama Y, Wadsworth HL, Russo D, et al. Binding domains of stimulatory and inhibitory thyrotropin (TSH) receptor auto- antibodies determined with chimeric TSH-lutropin/chorionic gonadotropin receptors. J Clin Invest 1991;88:336.

33. Cundiff JG, Kaithamana S, Seetharamaiah GS, et al. Studies using recombinant fragments of human TSH receptor reveal apparent diversity in the binding specificities of antibodies that block TSH binding to its receptor or stimulate thyroid hormone production. J Clin Endocrinol Metab 2001;86:4254.

34. Nagayama Y, Wadsworth HL, Russo D, et al. Binding domains of stimulatory and inhibitory thyrotropin (TSH) receptor autoantibodies determined with chimeric TSH-lutropin/chorionic gonadotropin receptors. J Clin Invest 1991;88:336.

35. Tahara K, Ishikawa N, Yamamoto K, et al. Epitopes for thyroid stimulatory and blocking autoantibodies on the extracellular domain of the human thyrotropin receptor. Thyroid 1997;7:867.

36. Dallas JS, Desai RK, Cunningham SJ, et al. TSH interacts with multiple discrete regions of the TSH receptor: polyclonal rabbit antibodies to one or more of these regions can inhibit TSH binding and function. Endocrinology 1994;134:1437.

37. Weetman AP, McGregor AM. Autoimmune thyroid disease: developments in our understanding. Endocrinol Rev 1984;5:209.

38. Valente WA, Vitti P, Yavin Z, et al. Monoclonal antibodies to the thyrotropin receptor: stimulating and blocking antibodies derived from the lymphocytes of patients with Graves' disease. Proc Natl Acad Sci USA 1982;79:6680.

39. Volpe R. Suppressor T lymphocyte dysfunction is important in the pathogenesis of autoimmune thyroid disease: a perspective. Thyroid 1993;3:345.

40. Zakarija M, McKenzie JM, Banovac K. Clinical significance of assay of thyroid-stimulating antibody in Graves' disease. Ann Intern Med 1980;93:28.

41. Weiss M, Ingbar SH, Windblad S, et al. Demonstration of a saturable binding site for thyrotropin in Yersinia enterocolitica. Science 1983;219:131.

42. Tomer Y, Davies TF. Infection, thyroid disease, and autoimmunity. Endocrinol Rev 1993;14:107.

43. Londei M, Lamb JR, Botazzo GF, et al. Epithelial cells expressing aberrant MHC class II determinants can present antigen to cloned human T cells. Nature 1984;312: 639.

44. Dallas JS, Prabhakar BS. Detection of autoantibodies to the thyrotropin receptor. In: Thomas JA, ed. Endocrine Methods. San Diego, CA: Academic Press, 1996:299–318.

45. Southgate K, Creagh FM, Teece M, et al. A receptor assay for the measurement of TSH receptor antibodies in unextracted serum. Clin Endocrinol (Oxf) 1984;20:539.

46. Foley TP Jr, White C, New A. Juvenile Graves' disease: Usefulness and limitations of thyrotropin receptor antibody determinations. J Pediatr 1987;110:378.

47. Takasu N, Yamada T, Katakura M, et al. Evidence for thyrotropin (TSH)-blocking activity in goitrous Hashimoto's thyroiditis with assays measuring inhibition of TSH receptor binding and TSH-stimulated thyroid adenosine $3',5'$-monophosphate responses/cell growth by immunoglobulins. J Clin Endocrinol Metab 1987;64:239.

48. Costagliola S, Morgenthaler NG, Hoermann R. Second generation assay for thyrotropin receptor antibodies has superior diagnostic sensitivity for Graves' disease. J Clin Endocrinol Metab 1999;84:90.

49. Giovanella L, Ceriani L, Garancini S. Clinical applications of the 2nd generation assay for anti-TSH receptor antibodies in Graves' disease: evaluation in patients with negative 1st generation test. Clin Chem Lab Med 2001; 39:25.

50. Vitti P, Elisei R, Tonacchera M, et al. Detection of thyroid-stimulating antibody using Chinese hamster ovary cells transfected with cloned human thyrotropin receptor. J Clin Endocrinol Metab 1993;76:499.

51. Botero D, Brown RS. Bioassay of thyrotropin receptor antibodies with Chinese hamster ovary cells transfected with recombinant human thyrotropin receptor: clinical utility in children and adolescents with Graves' disease. J Pediatr 1998;132:612.

52. Creagh F, Teece M, Williams S, et al. An analysis of thyrotropin receptor binding and thyroid stimulating activities in a series of Graves' sera. Clin Endocrinol (Oxf) 1985;23:395.

53. Ginsberg J, Shewring G, Rees Smith B. TSH receptor binding and thyroid stimulation by sera from patients with Graves' disease. Clin Endocrinol (Oxf) 1983;19:305.

54. Zakarija M, McKenzie JM. The spectrum and significance of autoantibodies reacting with the thyrotropin receptor. Endocrinol Metab Clin North Am 1987;16:343.

55. Segni M, Leonardi E, Mazzoncini B, et al. Special features of Graves' disease in early childhood. Thyroid 1999; 9:871.

56. Lawless ST, Reeves G, Bowen JR. The development of thyroid storm in a child with McCune-Albright syndrome after orthopedic surgery. Am J Dis Child 1992;146:1099.

57. Minegishi Y, Kumada S, Suzuki H, et al. Repetitive monomorphic ventricular tachycardia in a 4 year old boy with toxic multi-nodular goiter. Acta Paediatr Scand 1991;80:726.

58. Layzer RB, Goldfield E. Periodic paralysis caused by abuse of thyroid hormone. Neurology 1982;24:949.

59. Ober KP. Thyrotoxic periodic paralysis in the United States: report of 7 cases and review of the literature. Medicine 1992;71:109.

60. Graves L. Thyroid storm and other endocrine emergencies. Emerg Med 1990;22:61.
61. Wilson BE, Hobb WN. Case report: pseudoephedrine-associated thyroid storm: thyroid hormone-catecholamine interactions. Am J Med Sci 1993;306:317.
62. Kadmon PM, Noto RB, Boney CM, et al. Thyroid storm in a child following radioactive iodine (RAI) therapy: a consequence of RAI versus withdrawal of antithyroid medication. J Clin Endocrinol Metab 2001;86:1865.
63. Hayeck A. Thyroid storm following radioiodine for thyrotoxicosis. J Pediatr 1978;93:978.
64. Aiello DP, Du Plessis AJ, Pattishall III EG, Kulin HE. Thyroid storm: presenting with coma and seizures. Clin Pediatr 1989;28:571.
65. Ureta-Raroque SS, Abramo TJ. Adolescent female patient with shock unresponsive to usual resuscitative therapy. Ped Emerg Care 1997;13:274.
66. Hung, W. Graves' disease in children. Curr Ther Endocrinol Metab 1997;6:77.
67. Akhter J, Weide LG. Thyrotoxic periodic paralysis; a reversible cause of paralysis to remember. South Dakota J Medicine 1997;50:357.
68. Kodali VRR, Jeffcote B, Clague RB. Thyrotoxic periodic paralysis: a case report and review of the literature. J Emerg Med 1999;17:43.
69. Kelley DE, Gharib H, Kennedy FP, et al. Thyrotoxic periodic paralysis: report of 10 cases and review of electromyographic findings. Arch Intern Med 1989;149:2597.
70. Ee B, Cheah JS. Electrocardiographic changes in thyrotoxic periodic paralysis. J Electrocardiol 1979;12:263.
71. Gonzalez-Trevino O, Rosas-Guzman J. Normokalemic thyrotoxic periodic paralysis: a new therapeutic strategy. Thyroid 1999;9:61.
72. DeGrandia D, Fiaschi A, Tomelleri G, Orrico D. Hypokalemic periodic paralysis: a single fiber electromyographic study. J Neurol Sci 1978;37:107.
73. Lyons J, Landis CA, Harsh G, et al. Two G protein oncogenes in human endocrine tumors. Science 1990;249:655.
74. Parma J, Duprez L, Van Sande J, et al. Somatic mutations in the thyrotropin receptor gene cause hyperfunctioning thyroid adenomas. Nature 1993;365:649.
75. Namba H, Ross JL, Goodman D, Fagin JA. Solitary polyclonal autonomous thyroid nodule: a rare cause of childhood hyperthyroidism. J Clin Endocrinol Metab 1991;72:1108.
76. Hamilton CR, Maloof F. Unusual types of hyperthyroidism. Medicine 1973;52:195.
77. DiGeorge AM. Albright syndrome: is it coming of age? J Pediatr 1975;87:1018.
78. Samuel S, Gilman S, Maurer HS, Rosenthal IM. Hyperthyroidism in an infant with McCune-Albright syndrome: report of a case with myeloid metaplasia. J Pediatr 1972;80:275.
79. Schwindinger WF, Levine MA. McCune-Albright syndrome. Trends Endocrinol Metab 1993;4:238.
80. Spada A, Vallar L, Faglia G. G protein oncogenes in pituitary tumors. Trends Endocrinol Metab 1992;3:355.
81. Weinstein LS, Yu S, Warner DR, Liu J. Endocrine manifestations of stimulatory G-protein α-subunit mutations and the role of genomic imprinting. Endocrinol Rev 2001;22:675.
82. Molnar GD, Wilber RD, Lee RE, et al. On the hyperfunctioning solitary thyroid nodule. Mayo Clin Proc 1965;40:665.
83. Ridgeway EC, Weintraub BD, Cevallos JL, et al. Suppression of pituitary TSH secretion in the patient with a hyperfunctioning thyroid nodule. J Clin Invest 1973;52:2783.
84. Monzani F, Caraccio N, Goletti O, et al. Five-year followup of percutaneous ethanol injection for the treatment of hyperfunctioning thyroid nodules: a study of 117 patients. Clin Endocrinol (Oxf) 1997;46:9.
85. Leclere J, Bene MC, Aubert V, et al. Clinical consequences of activating germline mutations of TSH receptor, the concept of toxic hyperplasia. Horm Res 1997;47:158.
86. Thomas JL, Leclere J, Hartemann P, et al. Familial hyperthyroidism without evidence of autoimmunity. Acta Endocrinol (Copenh) 1982;100:512.
87. Biebermann H, Schoneberg T, Hess C, et al. The first activating TSH receptor mutation in transmembrane domain 1 identified in a family with non-autoimmune hyperthyroidism. J Clin Endocrinol Metab 2001;86:4429.
88. Fuhrer D, Warner J, Sequeira M, et al. Novel TSHR germline mutation (Met463Val) masquerading as Graves' disease in a large Welsh kindred with hyperthyroidism. Thyroid 2000;10:1035.
89. Weintraub BD, Gershengorn MC, Kourides IA, Fein H. Inappropriate secretion of thyroid-stimulating hormone. Ann Intern Med 1981;95:339.
90. Kourides IA. TSH-induced hyperthyroidism. In: Ingbar SH, Braverman LE, eds. Werner's The Thyroid, 5th ed. Philadelphia: JB Lippincott, 1986:1064–1071.
91. Beck-Peccoz P, Forloni F, Cortelazzi, et al. Pituitary resistance to thyroid hormones. Horm Res 1992;38:66.
92. Yen P. Physiological and molecular basis of thyroid hormone action. Physiol Rev 2001;81:1097.
93. Magner JA. TSH-mediated hyperthyroidism. Endocrinologist 1993;3:289.
94. Kourides IA, Ridgway C, Weintraub BD, et al. Thyrotropin-induced hyperthyroidism: use of alpha and beta subunit levels to identify patients with pituitary tumors. J Clin Endocrinol Metab 1977;45:534.
95. Oppenheim DS. TSH- and other glycoprotein-producing pituitary adenomas: alpha-subunit as a tumor marker. Thyroid Today 1991;14(3):1–11.
96. Shomali ME, Katznelson L. Medical therapy for gonadotroph and thyrotroph tumors. Endocrinol Metab Clin North Am 1999;28:223.
97. Rosler A, Litvin Y, Hage C, et al. Familial hyperthyroidism due to inappropriate thyrotropin secretion successfully treated with triiodothyronine. J Clin Endocrinol Metab 1982;54:76.
98. Klett M, Schonberg D. Congenital hyperthyroidism due to inappropriate secretion of thyroid stimulating hormone. Proceedings of the 26th Annual Meeting of the European Society for Paediatric Endocrinology, Toulouse 6–8 September 1987, abstract 178.
99. Beck-Peccoz P, Piscitelli G, Cattaneo MG, Faglia G. Successful treatment of hyperthyroidism due to non-neoplastic pituitary TSH hypersecretion with 3,5,3'-triiodothyroacetic acid (TRIAC). J Endocrinol Invest 1983;6:217.
100. Weiss RE, Refetoff S. Treatment of resistance to thyroid hormone—primum non nocere. J Clin Endocrinol Metab 1999;84:401.
101. Furth J, Moy P, Hershman JM, Ueda G. Thyrotropic tumor syndrome. Arch Pathol 1973;96:217.
102. Cohen JH III, Ingbar SH, Braverman LE. Thyrotoxicosis due to ingestion of excess thyroid hormone. Endocrinol Rev 1989;10:113.

103. Litovitz TL, White JD. Levothyroxine ingestions in children: an analysis of 78 cases. Am J Emerg Med 1985;3: 297.

104. Kulig K, Golightly LK, Rumack BH. Levothyroxine overdose associated with seizures in a young child. JAMA 1985;254:2109.

105. Lehrner LM, Weir MR. Acute ingestions of thyroid hormones. Pediatrics 1984;73:313.

106. Golightly LK, Smolinske SC, Kulig KW, et al. Clinical effects of accidental levothyroxine ingestion in children. Am J Dis Child 1987;141:1025.

107. Jaffiol C, de Boisvilliers F, Baldet L, Torresani J. Thyroid hormone generalized resistance. Horm Res 1992;38:62.

108. Cooper DS, Ladenson PW, Nisula BC, et al. Familial thyroid hormone resistance. Metabolism 1982;31:504.

109. Murata Y, Refetoff S, Horowitz AL, Smith TJ. Hormonal regulation of glycosaminoglycan accumulation in fibroblasts from patients with resistance to thyroid hormone. J Clin Endocrinol Metab 1983;57:1233.

110. Pohlenz J, Weiss RE, Macchia PE, et al. Five new families with resistance to thyroid hormone not caused by mutations in the thyroid hormone receptor beta gene. J Clin Endocrinol Metab 1999;84:3919.

111. Reutrakul S, Sadow PM, Pannain S, et al. Search for abnormalities of nuclear corepressors, coactivators and a coregulator in families with resistance to thyroid hormone without mutations in thyroid hormone receptor beta or alpha genes. J Clin Endocrinol Metab 2000;85:3609.

112. Refetoff S, Salazar A, Smith TJ, Scherberg NH. The consequences of inappropriate treatment due to failure to recognize the syndrome of pituitary and peripheral tissue resistance to thyroid hormone. Metabolism 1983;32:822.

113. Bode HH, Danon M, Weintraub BD, et al. Partial target organ resistance to thyroid hormone. J Clin Invest 1973; 52:776.

114. St. Germain DL. Iodothyronine deiodinases. Trends Endocrinol Metab 1994;5:36.

115. Kleinhaus N, Faber J, Kahana L, et al. Euthyroid hyperthyroxinemia due to generalized 5'-deiodinase defect. J Clin Endocrinol Metab 1988;66:684.

116. Hennessey JV, Jackson MD. The interface between thyroid hormones and psychiatry. Endocrinologist 1996;6: 214.

117. Stockigt JR. Hyperthyroxinemia secondary to drugs and acute illness. Endocrinologist 1993;3:67.

118. Root AW. Free triiodothyronine toxicosis in two adolescents. J Pediatr 1994;124:276.

119. Arisaka O, Hosaka A, Yabuta K. Free triiodothyronine toxicosis. J Pediatr 1994;125:304.

120. Larsen PR, Davies TF, Hay ID. Special aspects of thyrotoxicosis. In: Wilson JD, Foster DW, Kronenberg HM, Larsen PR, eds. Williams Textbook of Endocrinology, 9th ed. Philadelphia: WB Saunders, 1998:459–460.

121. Perros P, Kendall-Taylor P. Pathogenesis of thyroid associated ophthalmopathy. Trends Endocrinol Metab 1993; 4:270.

122. Bahn RS, Heufelder AE. Pathogenesis of Graves' ophthalmopathy. N Engl J Med 1993;329:1468.

123. Wiersinga WM, Prummel MF. Pathogenesis of Graves' ophthalmopathy—current understanding. J Clin Endocrinol Metab 2001;86:501.

124. Bahn RS, Dutton CM, Natt N, et al. Thyrotropin receptor expression in Graves' orbital adipose/connective tissues: potential autoantigen in Graves' ophthalmopathy. J Clin Endocrinol Metab 1998;83:998.

125. Marino M, Lisi S, Pinchera A, et al. Identification of thyroglobulin in orbital tissues of patients with thyroid-associated ophthalmopathy. Thyroid 2001;11:177.

126. Bahn RS. Understanding the immunology of Graves' ophthalmopathy: is it an autoimmune disease? Endocrinol Metab Clin North Am 2000;29:287.

127. Heufelder AE, Bahn RS. Detection and localization of cytokine immunoreactivity in retro-ocular connective tissue in Graves' ophthalmopathy. Eur J Clin Invest 1993; 23:10.

128. Cavalieri RR. Thyroid radioiodine uptake: indications and interpretation. Endocrinologist 1992;2:341.

129. Ross DS. Syndrome of thyrotoxicosis with low radioactive iodine uptake. Endocrinol Metab Clin North Am 1998;27:169.

130. Bliddal H, Bech K, Feldt-Rasmussen U, et al. Humoral autoimmune manifestation in subacute thyroiditis. Allergy 1985;40:599.

131. Weetman AP. Autoimmune thyroiditis: predisposition and pathogenesis. Clin Endocrinol 1992;36:307.

132. Hwang SC, Tap TS, Ho LT, Ching KN. Subacute thyroiditis: 61 cases review. Chung Hua I Hsueh Tsu Chih (Taipei) 1989;43:113.

133. Spitzweg C, Morris JC. The immune response to the iodide transporter. Endocrinol Metab Clin North Am 2000; 29:389.

134. Seissler J, Wagner S, Schott M, et al. Low frequency of autoantibodies to the human Na^+/I^- symporter in patients with autoimmune thyroid disease. J Clin Endocrinol Metab 2000;85:4630.

135. Franklyn JA. The management of hyperthyroidism. N Engl J Med 1994;330:1731.

136. Rivkees SA, Sklar C, Freemark M. The management of Graves' disease in children, with special emphasis on radioiodine treatment. J Clin Endocrinol Metab 1998;83: 3767.

137. Gittoes NJL, Franklyn JA. Hyperthyroidism: current treatment guidelines. Drugs 1998;55:543.

138. Zimmerman D, Lteif AN. Thyrotoxicosis in children. Endocrinol Metab Clin North Am 1998;27:109.

139. Foley TP Jr, Charron M. Radioiodine treatment of juvenile Graves disease. Exp Clin Endocrinol Diabetes 1997; 105 (suppl 4):61.

140. Fahrenfort JJ, Wilterdink AML, van der Veen EA. Long-term residual complaints and psychosocial sequelae after remission of hyperthyroidism. Psychoneuroendocrinology 2000;25:201.

141. Bommer M, Eversman T, Pickardt A, et al. Psychopathological and neuropsychological symptoms in patients with subclinical and remitted hyperthyroidism. Klin Wochenschr 1990;68:552.

142. Perrild H, Hansen JM, Arnung K, et al. Intellectual impairment after hyperthyroidism. Acta Endocrinol 1986; 112:185.

143. Wiersinga WM. Propranolol and thyroid hormone metabolism. Thyroid 1991;1:273.

144. Hoffman BB, Lefkowitz RJ. Catecholamines, sympathomimetic drugs, and adrenergic receptor antagonists. In: Hardman JG, Limbird LE, Molinoff PB, Ruddon RW, Gilman AG, eds. Goodman and Gilman's The Pharmacological Basis of Therapeutics, 9th ed. New York: McGraw-Hill, 1996:199–248.

145. Ross DS. Current therapeutic approaches to hyperthyroidism. Trends Endocrinol Metab 1993;4:281.

146. Cooper DS. Antithyroid drugs. N Engl J Med 1984;311: 1353.

147. Wartofsky L. Has the use of antithyroid drugs for Graves' disease become obsolete? Thyroid 1993;3:335.

148. Hashizume K, Ichikawa K, Sakurai A, et al. Administration of thyroxine in treated Graves' disease. N Engl J Med 1991;324:947.

149. Raza J, Hindmarsh PC, Brook CGD. Thyrotoxicosis in children: thirty years' experience. Acta Paediatr 1999;88: 937.

150. Rittmaster RS, Abbott EC, Douglas R, et al. Effect of methimazole, with or without L-thyroxine, on remission rates in Graves' disease. J Clin Endocrinol Metab 1998; 83:814.

151. Tamai H, Hayaki I, Kawai I, et al. Lack of effect of thyroxine administration on elevated thyroid stimulating hormone receptor antibody levels in treated Graves' disease patients. J Clin Endocrinol Metab 1995;80:1481.

152. Allannic H, Fauchet R, Lorcy Y, et al. A prospective study of the relationship between relapse of hyperthyroid Graves' disease after antithyroid drugs and HLA haplotype. J Clin Endocrinol Metab 1983;57:719.

153. Karlsson FA, Tuvemo T, Akerstrom G. Childhood Graves' disease—remission rate and risk factors. J Clin Endocrinol Metab 1998;83:1398.

154. Shulman DI, Muhar I, Jorgensen EV, et al. Autoimmune hyperthyroidism in prepubertal children and adolescents: comparison of clinical and biochemical features at diagnosis and responses to medical therapy. Thyroid 1997;7: 369.

155. Glaser NS, Styne DM. Predictors of early remission of hyperthyroidism in children. J Clin Endocrinol Metab 1997;82:1719.

156. Vitti P, Rago T, Chiovato L, et al. Clinical features of patients with Graves' disease undergoing remission after antithyroid drug treatment. Thyroid 1997;7:755.

157. Mussa GC, Corrias A, Silvestro L, et al. Factors at onset predictive of lasting remission in pediatric patients with Graves' disease followed for at least three years. J Pediatr Endocrinol Metab 1999;12:537.

158. Komiya I, Yamada T, Sato A, et al. Remission and recurrence of hyperthyroid Graves' disease during and after methimazole treatment when assessed by IgE and interleukin 13. J Clin Endocrinol Metab 2001;86:3540.

159. Fukata S, Kuma K, Sugawara M. Granulocyte colony-stimulating factor (G-CSF) does not improve recovery from antithyroid drug-induced agranulocytosis: a prospective study. Thyroid 1999;9:29.

160. Ward L, Huot C, Lambert R, et al. Outcome of pediatric Graves' disease after treatment with antithyroid medication and radioiodine. Clin Invest Med 1999;22:132.

161. Clark JD, Gelfand MJ, Elgazzar AH. Iodine-131 therapy of hyperthyroidism in pediatric patients. J Nucl Med 1995;36:442.

162. Becker DV, Hurley JR. Complications of radioiodine treatment of hyperthyroidism. Semin Nucl Med 1971;1: 442.

163. Tuttle MR. Effect of pretreatment with antithyroidal drugs on the failure rate of radioiodine therapy in Graves' disease. Endocrinologist 2000;10:403.

164. Andrade VA, Gross JL, Maia AL. The effect of methimazole pretreatment on the efficacy of radioactive iodine therapy in Graves' hyperthyroidism: one-year follow-up of a prospective, randomized study. J Clin Endocrinol Metab 2001;86:3488.

165. Ross DS, Daniels GH, De Stefano P, et al. Use of adjunctive potassium iodide after radioactive iodine (^{131}I) treatment of Graves' hyperthyroidism. J Clin Endocrinol Metab 1983;57:250.

166. Dobyns BM, Sheline GE, Workman JB, et al. Malignant and benign neoplasms of the thyroid in patients treated for hyperthyroidism: a report of the cooperative thyrotoxicosis therapy follow-up study. J Clin Endocrinol Metab 1974;38:976.

17

Thyromegaly

John S. Dallas
University of Texas Medical Branch–Galveston, Galveston, Texas, U.S.A.

Thomas P. Foley, Jr.
University of Pittsburgh and Children's Hospital of Pittsburgh, Pittsburgh, Pennsylvania, U.S.A.

I. INTRODUCTION

Thyromegaly, or goiter, is a common clinical disorder during childhood and adolescence. Prospective studies in the United States and Japan have shown that thyromegaly may occur in up to 6% of school-aged children (1–3). A child may present with either diffuse or nodular thyromegaly, and the enlargement can be either symmetrical or asymmetrical. In 1960, the World Health Organization (WHO) established criteria for determining goiter prevalence. According to these criteria, diffuse thyromegaly was present in a child if the lateral lobes of the gland were larger than the terminal phalanx of the child's thumb (4). In 1994, WHO revised and simplified its classification criteria and defined goiter as any enlarged thyroid that is palpable and/or visible (5). A nodular thyroid contains at least one solid or cystic mass that has a consistency different from the remainder of the gland. Thyromegaly usually occurs during adolescence with a female to male predominance (6).

II. PATHOGENESIS

Enlargement of the thyroid gland may occur as a result of stimulation, infiltration, and/or inflammation of the gland (6) (Table 1). Stimulation of follicular cell growth, either hyperplasia or hypertrophy, can be mediated by thyroid-stimulating hormone (TSH), various thyrotropin receptor antibodies (TSHrAb), and other growth factors (7–10). Increased TSH secretion is usually the result of an alteration in the production, release, or the metabolism of the major thyroid hormones, T_4 and T_3. In rare cases, increased TSH secretion results from a TSH-producing pituitary adenoma or from pituitary resistance to thyroid hormone; in these conditions, the patient presents with mild to moderate thyromegaly, normal to elevated serum levels of TSH, and elevated serum levels of total and free T_4 and T_3.

A variety of TSHrAbs have been identified in patients with autoimmune thyroid disease, and some of these antibodies stimulate both thyroid function and growth through interaction with TSH receptors on the follicular cell membrane (7–9). Several reports have provided evidence for IgG antibodies, referred to as thyroid growth-stimulating antibodies (TGAb), that may be found in sera from patients with a variety of thyroid disorders, including Graves' disease, Hashimoto's thyroiditis, sporadic nontoxic (simple) goiter, and endemic goiter due to iodine deficiency (10–14). It is assumed that these IgG bind to either the TSH receptor or some other follicular cell membrane structure to promote thyroid cell growth without affecting thyroid cell function. However, other reports either have failed to demonstrate the presence of TGAb in patients with some of these thyroid disorders or have challenged the concept of specific IgG that bind to the TSH receptor and stimulate cellular growth without affecting thyroid cell function (13, 15, 16). Therefore, further studies will be required to define fully the specific nature of these so-called TGAbs and their exact role in goitrogenesis.

Infiltration of the thyroid gland may occur from a neoplastic (i.e., adenoma or carcinoma) or a nonneoplastic (i.e., cyst) process. During childhood, a thyroid neoplasm, whether benign or malignant, usually presents as an isolated nodule in the thyroid gland. In rare cases, thyromegaly is found in patients with histiocytosis X or lymphoma because of cellular infiltration of the gland (17).

Although a variety of infectious agents (bacterial, viral, fungal) can cause acute or subacute inflammation and

Table 1 Pathogenesis of Thyromegaly

Stimulation
  Thyrotropin
    Inhibition of thyroidal hormonogenesis
    Excessive hypothalamic and pituitary secretion
  Thyrotropin receptor antibodies
    Thyroid-stimulating antibodies
    Thyroid growth-stimulating antibodies
Infiltration
  Neoplasia
    Adenoma
    Carcinoma
    Lymphoma
    Histiocytosis
  Nonneoplasia: cysts
Inflammation
  Infection
    Bacterial
    Viral
    Other pathogens
  Noninfection: lymphocytic (autoimmune)

Table 2 Causes of Thyromegaly

Diffuse thyromegaly
  Autoimmune (Hashimoto's) thyroiditis
  Thyrotoxicosis
    Graves' disease
    Toxic thyroiditis
    TSH-secreting pituitary adenoma
    Pituitary resistance to thyroid hormone
  Acute and subacute thyroiditis
  Iodine deficiency
  Goitrogen ingestion
    Antithyroid drugs
    Antithyroid agents and foods
  Familial thyroid dyshormonogenesis
  Idiopathic (simple) thyromegaly
Nodular thyromegaly
  Autoimmune (Hashimoto's) thyroiditis
  Thyroid cyst
  Thyroid tumors
  Adenoma
    Hyperfunctioning (hot): hyperthyroid or euthyroid
    Nonfunctioning (cold)
  Carcinoma
  Other tumors
Nonthyroidal masses
  Lymphadenopathy
  Brachial cleft cyst
  Thyroglossal duct cyst

enlargement of the thyroid gland, infectious thyroiditis rarely occurs during childhood (6). However, Hashimoto's disease, the goitrous form of chronic autoimmune thyroiditis, is the most common cause of thyromegaly during childhood in nonendemic goiter regions of the world (1–3, 10). In this disease, lymphocytic infiltration of the thyroid may be diffuse and cause generalized enlargement of one or both lobes, or may be localized and cause nodular enlargement of the gland (6). The latter entity may be difficult to differentiate from tumors of the thyroid gland.

Disorders associated with thyromegaly during childhood can be classified depending on whether thyromegaly is diffuse or nodular (Table 2). Since the child initially presents for evaluation based upon the physical examination of the thyroid gland, the differential diagnosis and laboratory investigation should be considered according to clinical symptoms and physical characteristics of the gland and the surrounding structures in the neck.

III. AUTOIMMUNE THYROID DISEASE: THYROIDITIS

A. Pathogenesis

Recent advances in immunology have led to a greater understanding of the basic abnormalities in the cellular and humoral immune systems that result in autoimmune thyroid diseases. In patients with Graves' disease the immune defect results in the production of immunoglobulin G (IgG) antibodies to the TSH receptor. These antibodies bind to and stimulate the TSH receptor to cause an increase in function and size of the thyroid gland. These effects are responsible for the clinical findings of thyro-

toxicosis and goiter in patients with Graves' disease (9). The pathogenesis of Graves' disease is discussed in detail in Chapter 16.

In chronic lymphocytic thyroiditis, the autoimmune process is believed to begin with activation of CD4$^+$ (helper) T lymphocytes specific for thyroid antigens (18). The mechanisms responsible for T-lymphocyte activation remain unclear. One hypothesis, based on the immunological concept of molecular mimicry, proposes that infection with a virus or bacterium that contains a protein similar to a thyroid protein may lead to activation of thyroid-specific T cells (18). An alternative hypothesis states that thyroid follicular cells present their own intracellular proteins through major histocompatibility complex (MHC) class II proteins to helper T cells (18). These MHC class II proteins (human leukocyte antigen [HLA]-DR, -DP, and -DQ) are required for antigen presentation to CD4$^+$ T cells. Studies have demonstrated that thyroid cells from patients with autoimmune thyroiditis, but not normal cells, express MHC class II proteins (19). In addition, certain cytokine products of activated T cells, such as interferon gamma, can induce the expression of MHC class II molecules by thyroid cells (20). At present, there is evidence to support each of these hypotheses. However, neither appears to explain fully the mechanisms involved

Table 3 Spectrum of Thyroid Function in Autoimmune Thyroid Diseases

Clinical thyroid function	Free T$_4$	T$_3$	TSH	TSH response to TRH
Primary hypothyroidism	Low	Low or normal	Increased	Exaggerated
Compensated hypothyroidism	Normal	Normal	Increased	Exaggerated
Euthyroidism with decreased thyroid reserve	Normal	Normal	Normal	Exaggerated
Goitrous and nongoitrous euthyroidism	Normal	Normal	Normal	Normal
Nonsuppressible euthyroidism	Normal	Normal	Normal	Blunted
Thyrotoxicosis with limited thyroid reserve	Mildly increased	Increased	Undetectable	Absent
Thyrotoxic phase of thyroiditis	Increased	Increased	Undetectable	Absent
T$_3$ thyrotoxicosis	Normal	Increased	Undetectable	Absent
Thyrotoxicosis	Increased	Increased	Undetectable	Absent

in initial T-lymphocyte activation; further studies will be required to define better the exact mechanisms involved.

Following activation, self-reactive CD4$^+$ T cells recruit B lymphocytes as well as cytotoxic (CD8$^+$) T lymphocytes into the thyroid gland. The B cells are stimulated by activated helper T cells to produce and secrete antibodies against various thyroid proteins. The three major target antigens for thyroid antibodies are thyroglobulin, thyroid peroxidase, and the TSH receptor.

Autoimmune destruction of thyroid follicular cells is characteristic of Hashimoto's thyroiditis. Current evidence supports that thyroid cell destruction primarily occurs through the process of apoptosis, or programmed cell death (21–23). Cytotoxic T lymphocytes (CTL) mediate thyroid cell destruction through two different mechanisms: CD4$^+$ CTLs express so-called death ligands that bind to death receptors on target cells, thereby activating apoptotic pathways; and CD8$^+$ CTLs release exocytotic granules that contain perforin (which perforates target cell membranes) and Granzyme B (which directly initiates the apoptosis cascade system at a postreceptor level) (21). Activated CD4$^+$ CTLs have been shown to express functionally the death ligands referred to as tumor necrosis factor-α (TNF-α), Fas ligand (FasL), and TNF-related apoptosis-inducing ligand (TRAIL) (21–23). Furthermore, the Fas and TRAIL apoptotic pathways are present and functional in thyroid cells (21–23). In addition to these cellular mechanisms, complement-fixing cytotoxic antibodies and antibody dependent, cell-mediated cytotoxicity involving natural killer cells may also contribute to thyroid cell destruction (24). Although TSH receptor-blocking antibodies and cytokines may contribute to thyroid cell dysfunction, autoimmune destruction of follicular cells appears to be the primary cause of hypothyroidism in Hashimoto's thyroiditis (25).

Thyroid autoimmunity is familial. Up to 50% of the first-degree relatives of patients with chronic autoimmune thyroiditis have thyroid antibodies, apparently inherited as a dominant trait (18). Clinical Hashimoto's disease occurs in up to 33% of siblings of affected patients (26). The prevalence of clinical Hashimoto's thyroiditis in the general population ranges from 1 to 4% (18, 26). Therefore, familial clustering of this disorder indicates that a significant genetic component exists in its origin. However, the genetic predisposition appears to be complex, possibly caused by a number of genes. At present, no conclusions regarding the number of involved genes can be made. The association of Hashimoto's thyroiditis with Down and Turner syndromes suggests that part of the genetic susceptibility to this disease may reside on chromosomes 21 and X (18, 26). Association studies have revealed weak associations between Hashimoto's thyroiditis and HLA (e.g., DR3, DR4, DR5 and DQ7) and the cytotoxic T lymphocyte antigen 4 (CTLA-4) genes (18, 26). Although these associations provide evidence that HLA and CTLA-4 gene variations increase the risk for Hashimoto's thyroiditis, they are not the sole determinants of the genetic predisposition. Linkage analysis studies have identified regions on chromosomes 6p (marker D6S257), 12q11–12, and 13q32–34 that may represent susceptibility loci for Hashimoto's thyroiditis (26). More recently, strong evidence has been reported showing that chromosome 8q24 represents a susceptibility gene for autoimmune thyroid disease (27). This locus contains the thyroglobulin gene and has been linked and associated with autoimmune thyroid disease. Therefore, polymorphisms in the thyroglobulin gene may be involved in the causes of autoimmune thyroid disease. Unlike other potential susceptibility loci (e.g., CLTA-4) involved in immune regulation, thyroglobulin is a thyroid-specific gene, and this may help to explain why the thyroid gland becomes the target of an autoimmune response (27). Further studies are needed to confirm these preliminary findings and to identify other susceptibility loci within the human genome.

Environmental factors also play a role in the development of chronic autoimmune thyroiditis. Recent studies have suggested that the prevalence of autoimmune thyroiditis in children has been increasing over the past 25–30 years (28, 29). The reason(s) for this increasing prevalence remains unclear. Some have hypothesized that a decrease in exposure to infection in early life may play a role (28). Excessive iodine intake also appears to be involved. The prevalence of chronic autoimmune thyroiditis is correlated with iodine intake, with the highest prevalences in the countries with the highest intake of iodine, such as the United States and Japan (18). Furthermore, iodine supplementation in areas of iodine deficiency increases the prevalence of lymphocytic infiltration of the thyroid threefold (30). An association has been reported between feeding soy formulas to infants and the development of autoimmune thyroid disease in later childhood (31). The potential role(s) that other chemicals and dietary goitrogens may play in autoimmune thyroid disease remains to be determined.

B. Chronic Lymphocytic Thyroiditis of Childhood and Adolescence

1. Classification

The autoimmune-mediated mechanisms cause histological changes in the thyroid that are the basis for the classification of the disease during childhood. These mechanisms result in the characteristic histological abnormalities of lymphocytic infiltration and lymphoid follicles of juvenile Hashimoto's disease. However, the usual histological appearance during childhood and adolescence is follicular cell hyperplasia and minimal fibrosis (6). The fibrous variant of the disease is characterized by epithelial destruction and fibrosis (6).

2. Clinical Manifestations

Most patients with Hashimoto's thyroiditis present with an asymptomatic enlargement of the thyroid gland, but an occasional patient may complain of pain or a sensation of fullness in the area of the thyroid. Less often the disease manifests clinically with deceleration of linear growth and other clinical features associated with hypothyroidism during childhood (see Chap. 15). In rare cases, the child with thyroiditis presents initially with symptoms and signs of thyrotoxicosis; this transient phase of thyrotoxicosis occurs early in the course of autoimmune thyroiditis (toxic thyroiditis) and presents as a mild disease without exophthalmos. Whereas thyrotoxicosis of Graves' disease results from overproduction and secretion of thyroid hormones due to TSHrAb stimulation of TSH receptors, the thyrotoxicosis of toxic thyroiditis results from release of excessive amounts of preformed thyroid hormones due to inflammatory destruction of thyroid follicular cells. These two disorders may be difficult to differentiate based on clinical criteria alone unless the exophthalmos of Graves' disease is present, or thyroid-stimulating antibodies are detected in serum.

On examination, the thyroid gland is either symmetrically or asymmetrically enlarged and usually nontender and firm in consistency. The surface texture may be finely granular (seedy) or discretely nodular (pebbly, crenated).

Lymphoid follicles may be palpable as single or multiple nodules within one or both lobes of the gland. The gland should move freely with swallowing and should not be affixed to adjacent tissues. Nontender regional lymphadenopathy may be present (6).

Autoimmune thyroiditis frequently occurs in patients with other autoimmune diseases, particularly insulin-dependent diabetes mellitus (IDDM) (32, 33), but also Addison's disease, alopecia, vitiligo, myasthenia gravis, ulcerative colitis, pernicious anemia and the collagen vascular diseases (18, 34, 35). Chronic urticaria with or without angioedema (CUA) and Hashimoto's encephalopathy (HE) represent two additional presumed autoimmune conditions associated with chronic autoimmune thyroiditis (36–38). The majority of reported patients have had Hashimoto's thyroiditis, but both conditions can also occur in association with Graves' disease (39, 40). Both represent potentially life-threatening illnesses that can occur in adults and children. The pathogenic mechanisms linking these disorders to autoimmune thyroid disease remain unclear. Abnormal thyroid hormone levels do not account for either condition. Although some reported patients have had either hypo- or hyperthyroidism, the majority of affected individuals have been euthyroid. Usually these conditions occur in patients with existing serological or clinical evidence of autoimmune thyroid disease. However, a few patients have been described in whom thyroid antibody levels were negative at initial presentation, but then became positive several months to a few years later (39, 41). Both conditions exhibit a strong female to male preponderance.

Urticaria is a well-demarcated skin reaction characterized by edema involving the superficial portion of the dermis (42). Lesions are raised and erythematous and usually pruritic. Angioedema differs from urticaria in that the edematous process is located in the deep dermis and subcutaneous or submucosal tissues (42). Lesions tend to be more painful than pruritic. The involvement of the upper respiratory tract may result in severe and sometimes fatal complications. Chronic urticaria, defined as recurrent episodes of hives with or without angioedema of at least 6 weeks duration, is a relatively common disorder for which the cause is rarely determined (36).

Clinical studies have demonstrated that 10–15% of patients with idiopathic CUA have serological and/or clinical evidence of autoimmune thyroid disease (36, 37). These patients have been as young as 8 years old (range, 8–72 years), and 80–90% have been female (36, 37). Almost all patients have had elevated levels of thyroid antibodies at presentation; thyroid peroxidase or microsomal antibodies have been detected more commonly than thyroglobulin antibodies. Current evidence supports the finding that thyroid antibodies are not directly responsible for the skin lesions, since their levels do not correlate with disease activity (43). The antibodies are most likely to serve as evidence for the underlying autoimmune process in the affected patient. In some cases, L-thyroxine treatment in hypo- or euthyroid patients with autoimmune thyroiditis and refractory idiopathic CUA has resulted in full remission or marked improvement of CUA (36, 43, 44).

A recent study comparing two distinct groups of patients with CU, one group with CU of known cause and the other with idiopathic CU found the prevalence of elevated serum thyroid antibodies (33% vs. 23%, respectively) and of clinical thyroid disease in seropositive patients (39% vs 42%, respectively) to be similar for the groups (45). Therefore, it is recommended that thyroid function and thyroid antibody tests be performed in all patients with CUA. This will result in the diagnosis of existing or potential thyroid disease in some patients and will identify patients whose CUA may benefit from thyroid hormone therapy. Despite a euthyroid state, suppressive L-thyroxine therapy should be considered in all patients with severe CUA and evidence of autoimmune thyroid disease (43).

Hashimoto's encephalopathy represents a progressive or relapsing encephalopathy associated with autoimmune thyroid disease. It is a rare, but also underdiagnosed, condition (38). Since the diagnosis of autoimmune thyroid disease may not be realized or suspected in affected patients at presentation, a high degree of suspicion is required to make the diagnosis of HE. Many of the reported patients initially have been misdiagnosed as having a psychiatric disorder, such as depression, anxiety, or psychosis. HE should be considered and thyroid antibody levels checked in children and adults exhibiting unexplained neuropsychiatric deterioration. HE is a treatable form of encephalopathy; therefore, timely diagnosis will allow for appropriate intervention that can rapidly reverse clinical symptoms and prevent additional morbidity resulting from undiagnosed HE.

Most reported patients with HE have been adults, but children as young as 9 years of age have been described (46). Some 85–90% percent of reported patients have been female (38, 47, 48). Although there is some symptom overlap, two types of clinical presentation are observed: a vasculitic type, involving stroke-like episodes (e.g., hemiparesis, aphasia, and ataxia), and only mild cognitive impairment; and a diffuse progressive type, with insidious onset of dementia, seizures, hallucinations, psychotic episodes, or lethargy and coma (38). Myoclonus, tremors, and seizures may occur in both types (38). The majority of reported children/adolescents have presented with the diffuse progressive form, and most have had seizures (48). Generalized tonic–clonic followed by complex partial seizures, with or without secondary generalization, are the most common types of seizures associated with HE in children (48).

The pathogenesis of this encephalopathy remains unknown. Abnormal thyroid function does not appear to be responsible, since most reported patients have had normal results of thyroid function studies at presentation (38).

Current evidence supports an autoimmune basis for the disease, but the exact mechanism has not been determined. Some findings suggest an acute disseminated encephalomyelitis, while others favor a cerebral angiitis (49, 50). Although the vast majority of patients have elevated serum thyroid antibody levels at initial presentation, these antibodies are unlikely to be the cause of encephalopathy. There is no obvious correlation between the thyroid antibody levels and the type or severity of clinical presentation (38). The most likely explanation if that the thyroid antibodies serve as markers of an underlying autoimmune process.

No clinical, laboratory, or neuroimaging findings are specific for HE; therefore, other more common causes of encephalopathy (e.g., inflammatory, infectious, metabolic, toxic, vascular, neoplastic, and paraneoplastic) first must be considered and reasonably excluded (38). Elevated serum thyroid antibody (thyroid peroxidase and/or thyroglobulin antibodies) levels are necessary, but not sufficient, for making the diagnosis. The erythrocyte sedimentation rate may be mildly elevated. Cerebrospinal fluid (CSF) protein levels are elevated in the majority of patients, but CSF glucose levels are normal. A CSF mononuclear pleocytosis and oligoclonal bands may be present. Electroencephalography (EEG) is abnormal in more than 90% of cases (47). EEG findings can vary considerably over the course of the illness, and abnormalities are maximal during episodes of encephalopathy. The typical EEG shows generalized slowing or frontal rhythmic slowing followed by triphasic waves and periodic sharp waves; patients also can have focal temporal slowing (51, 52). Following successful treatment, the EEG shows improvement or normalizes (38). Neuroimaging studies are often normal but can reveal nonspecific findings. Mild cerebral atrophy and ventricular dilatation have been seen with CT. Magnetic resonance imaging (MRI) abnormalities include increased T_2 signals in the subcortical region, and, occasionally, more diffuse white matter abnormalities or a focal mesiotemporal abnormality may be seen (47, 52).

Most patients with HE respond dramatically to pharmacological glucocorticoid therapy. Daily prednisone therapy should be started at a high dosage (2–3 mg/kg/day in 2–3 divided doses) for 1 month and maintained at least at 1 mg/kg/day for another 2–4 months or until remission of symptoms, and then tapered slowly (38). Rapid improvement can occur over a few days, but the average time from start of therapy to significant clinical improvement is usually 4–6 weeks (38). Patients with hypothyroidism should also receive L-thyroxine replacement therapy; the potential role of L-thyroxine therapy in clinically euthyroid patients with HE is unknown. Although some patients with HE have experienced improvement with L-thyroxine treatment (50, 53), several case reports have demonstrated that L-thyroxine therapy, by itself, usually fails to correct the encephalopathy or prevent relapses (38). Anticonvulsants should be used to control status epilepticus or recurrent episodes of myoclonus. Despite clinical improvement, thyroid antibody levels may remain elevated. Serial EEGs and neuropsychological testing can be used to monitor the response and length of therapy. The prognosis of HE when treated appears to be good; however, some children or adolescents may be left with long-term sequelae (e.g., residual cognitive deficits, recurrent seizures, progressive brain atrophy) despite early recognition and appropriate therapy (48).

3. Laboratory Evaluation

An elevated serum level of thyroid antibodies is the characteristic abnormality that permits a presumptive diagnosis of Hashimoto's thyroiditis. Thyroid peroxidase (formerly known as microsomal) and thyroglobulin antibodies are the two generally available thyroid antibody tests. Autoantibodies against thyroid peroxidase and thyroglobulin can be detected in 80–95% and in 30–60%, respectively, of patients with Hashimoto's thyroiditis (18, 54). Occasionally, a child with Hashimoto's thyroiditis will present with low or absent titers of thyroid antibodies, but, on repeat determinations 3–6 months later, the titers will be distinctly abnormal. Transient elevations of thyroid antibodies may occur during the course of other thyroid disorders (e.g., subacute thyroiditis), so a positive titer may not be indicative of chronic thyroiditis.

Although most children with autoimmune thyroiditis are clinically euthyroid, serum levels of TSH should be determined to exclude primary hypothyroidism. Additional studies may be needed for patients with an atypical clinical presentation. For the child with mild symptoms of hyperthyroidism, important initial tests include serum T_3 and TSHrAb determinations (6). In the child with hyperthyroidism, serum T_3 should be elevated unless the patient either is severely ill or has experienced very poor nutritional intake for several days prior to testing. Further diagnostic tests are needed infrequently. The $[^{123}I]$-iodide uptake test can be used to differentiate toxic thyroiditis from early Graves' disease and other causes of hyperthyroidism (55).

Ultrasonographic features in children with Hashimoto's thyroiditis are variable. In a recent report (56), the most common finding was thyromegaly with an increase in reflectivity compared to the adjacent muscle and widespread coarse echopenic areas. Another frequently observed pattern consists of an enlarged thyroid that is isoreflective to muscle and coarse echo-poor lesions. Nodular areas larger than 5 mm in diameter are often observed and some of the nodules have small echogenic centers. The patchiness of the echo-poor regions tends to be a useful sign when differentiating diseased glands from normal. Another recent study found that reduced thyroid echogenicity is a valid predictor of autoimmune thyroid disease (both Hashimoto's thyroiditis and Graves' disease), with corresponding positive and negative predictive values of 88% and 93% (57).

In the early stages of Hashimoto's thyroiditis, the 24 h radioactive iodine uptake (RAIU) is typically normal or mildly elevated (58). However, as the disease progresses and more thyroid parenchyma are replaced by fibrous tissue, the RAIU decreases (58). An abnormal release of accumulated thyroidal $[^{123}I]$-iodide following either oral or intravenous administration of potassium perchlorate can also be observed in adults and children with Hashimoto's thyroiditis (2, 59). This positive perchlorate discharge test indicates a defect in the intrathyroidal oxidation of iodide to iodine. This test usually is not required unless the patient has persistent clinical features of thyroiditis and negative thyroid antibodies on repeated determinations.

A thyroid biopsy in children with diffuse thyromegaly very rarely is necessary unless coexisting malignancy of the thyroid gland is suspected, such as in a child with negative serum thyroid antibodies and an asymptomatic, enlarging nonfunctional nodule within a diffusely enlarged thyroid gland.

4. Clinical Course and Management

a. Toxic Thyroiditis. The rare patient who presents with autoimmune toxic thyroiditis may gradually return to a euthyroid state within 1–2 months or may experience mild hypothyroidism before recovery. The duration of the hypothyroid phase of toxic thyroiditis is variable; it may last for a few weeks to several months or may be permanent. Patients who experience only mild symptoms during the thyrotoxic phase usually require no treatment, but low dosages of propranolol (10–20 mg three or four times daily) can relieve symptoms in patients with more severe thyrotoxicosis. Antithyroid drugs are not indicated in the treatment of toxic thyroiditis. It is important to monitor serum thyroid function tests during the recovery phase of toxic thyroiditis. If hypothyroidism develops, the child should be treated with L-thyroxine. Since this phase usually is transient, the child can be given a trial off medication after 3–6 months of treatment and reevaluated 4–6 weeks later. If serum TSH levels are elevated, L-thyroxine replacement therapy should be resumed indefinitely. However, if the child is clinically and biochemically euthyroid, he or she should be reassessed at 6–12 month intervals with serum TSH to monitor for hypothyroidism that may occur during the course of chronic lymphocytic thyroiditis.

b. Chronic Lymphocytic Thyroiditis. Autoimmune thyroiditis is a dynamic disease. A study that examined the natural history of thyroid abnormalities over a 20 year period found that autoimmune thyroiditis persisted in approximately two-thirds (34 of 50), and apparently remitted in 28%, of patients originally diagnosed during adolescence (60). Of the 34 individuals with persistent disease, 17 (50%) had become hypothyroid over the 20 year interval. For these reasons, clinical evaluation and assessment of serum TSH values are advised at 6–12 month intervals to follow the course of disease and to identify the development of hypothyroidism (6). Treatment with L-thyroxine may lead to reduction in goiter size in both euthyroid and hypothyroid patients (29). However, L-thyroxine treatment probably does not influence the long-term progression of thyroiditis (60). Once hypothyroidism occurs in a child with Hashimoto's thyroiditis, it typically is permanent and requires long-term treatment (29). Further discussion of the management of primary hypothyroidism may be found in Chapter 15.

C. Autoimmune Thyrotoxicosis: Graves' Disease

For further review of Graves' disease, see Chapter 16.

IV. ACUTE AND SUBACUTE THYROIDITIS

Acute thyroiditis, which is a rare disease, is easy to recognize but difficult to manage. In classic cases the child presents with an acute onset of pain in the area of the thyroid gland associated with fever, chills, dysphagia, hoarseness, and sore throat. The onset is usually preceded by an upper respiratory infection. On examination, the skin over the thyroid may be warm and red, and there may be regional lymphadenopathy. The thyroid is enlarged (locally or diffusely) and extremely tender, and the child resists efforts to extend the neck. Although the child may appear "toxic" from the infections process, he or she is not thyrotoxic. Laboratory investigation reveals leukocytosis and an elevated erythrocyte sedimentation rate. Serum thyroid function tests are usually normal at presentation and remain normal throughout the course of the disease. Antimicrobial therapy should be instituted promptly once appropriate cultures are obtained. A variety of aerobic and anaerobic organisms have been identified on culture of thyroid aspirates (61), and a Gram's stain of the aspirate may help to determine initial antibiotic therapy pending culture results. Serial ultrasonography of the gland can be used to detect abscess formation, at which time surgical intervention becomes indicated. Most of the recently reported cases of acute thyroiditis have been associated with an internal fistulous tract between the left pyriform sinus and the corresponding thyroid lobe (62, 63). Therefore, any child who presents with acute thyroiditis primarily involving the left lobe or who experiences recurrent acute thyroiditis should undergo a barium esophagram once he or she has recovered from the acute infectious process. If a fistula is identified, operative excision of the entire epithelial tract and adjacent thyroid tissue is essential to prevent recurrent thyroiditis and abscess (63).

Subacute thyroiditis is also rare during childhood and adolescence. The two major forms are subacute granulomatous thyroiditis (de Quervain's thyroiditis) and subacute lymphocytic thyroiditis (painless or silent thyroiditis). Both of these conditions are most commonly seen in

women between 30 and 50 years of age (64). Subacute granulomatous thyroiditis presumably results from a viral infection of the thyroid gland; the patient often has a history of a recent upper respiratory infection. Mumps, Coxsackie, echo, Epstein-Barr, influenza, and adenovirus are among the viruses implicated as causative (55, 64); there is also an association with HLA-B35 (55). An affected patient may have low-grade fever with flulike symptoms; generally, the chief complaint is neck pain in the region of the thyroid that may radiate to the jaws or ears. The patient may be clinically euthyroid or have symptoms suggestive of hyperthyroidism. The thyroid gland is usually enlarged, quite firm or tense, and tender. Thyroid enlargement may be localized or diffuse, and tenderness varies from mild to severe. The patient may resist efforts either to extend the neck or palpate the thyroid gland. The erythrocyte sedimentation rate (ESR) is characteristically elevated, usually above 50 mm/h (55).

Subacute lymphocytic thyroiditis is considered an autoimmune thyroid disease. It may occur either sporadically or during the post-partum period. On pathological examination it resembles Hashimoto's thyroiditis, but there is generally less lymphocytic infiltration and fibrosis. Thyroid peroxidase antibodies can be detected in about 60% of patients, and TSHrAb (either blocking or stimulating) can be found in about 20% of patients (55). Subacute lymphocytic thyroiditis has been associated with HLA-DR3 and HLA-DR5 (55). Some 50–60% of affected patients present with symptoms of mild thyrotoxicosis and a small, nontender goiter (55). The ESR tends to be normal (64). In the early stages, this disorder may be difficult to differentiate clinically from Graves' disease.

The expected results of laboratory tests during the early phase of these diseases include normal to elevated levels of total and free T_4 and T_3, a normal or suppressed TSH level, negative or low levels of thyroid antibodies, and a low or absent uptake of radioactive iodine (55).

The clinical course of subacute thyroiditis is variable, but it often progresses through three phases (toxic thyroiditis, euthyroid goiter, and mild hypothyroidism) before the patient returns to normal thyroid function. The transient phase of hypothyroidism during recovery will vary in length and severity. Although most will recover completely, between 5 and 10% of affected patients will remain permanently hypothyroid (64, 65). After recovery, late recurrences are uncommon in patients with subacute granulomatous thyroiditis, but it is not uncommon for the painless variety to recur after months or even years (55).

Symptomatic therapy may be necessary during the initial phase of the disease. This includes propranolol if symptoms of hyperthyroidism are present, and therapeutic dosages of salicylates or other nonsteroidal anti-inflammatory agents if local pain and tenderness of the thyroid gland persist. Prednisone therapy is necessary infrequently to control symptoms. Antithyroid drugs, which inhibit the production of new thyroid hormone, are not indicated for the management of thyrotoxicosis in subacute thyroiditis, because symptoms are caused by release of preformed thyroid hormones from the damaged gland. Should hypothyroidism eventually occur, the patient can be treated with L-thyroxine (50–100 μg daily) for 3–6 months, after which time the dosage can be discontinued. Thyroid function should be checked 4–6 weeks later; if the serum TSH level is elevated, L-thyroxine therapy should be resumed indefinitely.

V. IODINE DEFICIENCY

Iodine deficiency remains the most common cause of thyromegaly worldwide (66). Although iodine deficiency is still prevalent in various regions of the Americas, Africa, Europe, and Asia (66), it has been virtually eradicated in the United States since the introduction of iodized salt in the 1920s. Iodine deficiency can, however, occur in patients with chronic renal and nutritional diseases, or in patients consuming iodine-deficient diets. The currently recommended daily iodine intakes are 90 μg, 120 μg, and 150 μg for children ≤5 years old, 6–12 years old, and >12 years old, respectively (66). A diagnosis of iodine deficiency is supported if urinary iodine excretion is less than 100 μg/l, with values <20 μg/l, 20–49 μg/l, and 50–99 μg/l indicating severe, moderate, and mild iodine deficiency, respectively (66).

Multiple nutritional and environmental influences contribute to the prevalence and severity of iodine deficiency disorders (IDD) in iodine-deficient areas. General malnutrition, water-borne goitrogens (e.g., resorcinol and polyhydroxyphenols), and a variety of goitrogenic foods (e.g., millet, soy, and cassava) can aggravate goiter (67, 68). Deficiencies of selenium, vitamin A, or iron can modify thyroid hormone synthesis and/or metabolism, and thereby contribute to goitrogenesis and limit the effectiveness of iodine intervention programs (67).

VI. GOITROGENS

A variety of chemicals, drugs, and foods can interfere with thyroid hormone synthesis, secretion, and/or metabolism. This interference can lead to a reduction in serum thyroid hormone levels followed by a compensatory increase in TSH secretion and thyromegaly. Although chronic ingestion of these substances alone can lead to goiter formation, patients with pre-existing thyroid disease or iodine deficiency are more susceptible to the antithyroid effects of these agents (69). Therefore, complete dietary and medication histories should be included in the clinical evaluation of patients with thyromegaly.

Drugs that can interfere with thyroid gland function include the thionamides (e.g., propylthiouracil, methimazole, and carbimazole), sulfonamides (e.g., sulfisoxazole and sulfamethoxazole), and lithium. Both the thionamides and sulfonamides inhibit the actions of thyroid peroxidase

(i.e., oxidation and organification of iodine and the coupling of iodotyrosyl residues to form iodothyronines). The sulfonamides are less potent than the thionamides, and, in the dosages generally used in clinical practice, they have little to no antithyroid effects (68). Lithium interferes with thyroid function by inhibiting the release of thyroid hormone (69).

Phenobarbital, phenytoin, carbamazepine, and rifampin are examples of medications that induce hepatic mixed-function oxygenases that increase the metabolic clearance rate of T_4 (69). These drugs have little effect on the metabolic clearance of T_3. As a result, serum T4 concentrations decrease, but serum T3 levels remain unchanged or increase slightly. Basal serum TSH levels increase slightly, but not significantly (69). Therefore, most patients taking these drugs have no clinical signs of hypothyroidism and have normal TSH levels. However, hypothyroidism may occur or worsen in patients with underlying primary thyroid disease who receive these medications chronically (69).

Foods of the genus *Brassica* (e.g., cabbage, broccoli, cauliflower, brussels sprouts, turnips) contain goitrin, a naturally occurring thionamide compound (68). Cassava, maize, and lima beans contain cyanoglucosides that, following ingestion, release cyanide (70). Cyanide is detoxified to thiocyanate, a powerful goitrogenic agent that inhibits thyroid iodide transport and the organification of iodine (70). Millet and soybeans contain goitrogenic compounds known as flavonoids (e.g., glycosides of apigenin and luteolin) and isoflavonoids (e.g., genistein and daidzein), respectively (71). Although these compounds may possess diverse antithyroid properties, their goitrogenic activity is commonly expressed in terms of their ability to inhibit thyroid peroxidase activity (71). In these terms, apigenin and genistein are more potent than either methimazole or PTU. In recent years, soy consumption and the use of soy isoflavone supplements (also referred to as phytoestrogens) have increased due to the belief that isoflavones may be protective against a variety of hormone-dependent diseases, including breast and prostate cancers (71). It is important to recognize that these isoflavone compounds are also present in infant soy formulas (71). Studies have demonstrated a greater incidence of thyroid antibodies in children who received soy formulas during infancy than in children who were breastfed (72), as well as an association between feeding soy formulas and the development of autoimmune thyroid disease in later childhood (31).

VII. FAMILIAL THYROID DYSHORMONOGENESIS

Inborn errors in thyroid hormone synthesis, secretion, or recycling account for about 10–15% of all cases of permanent primary congenital hypothyroidism. The molecular mechanisms in most of these forms have been characterized; mutations of the individual genes encoding the TSH receptor, the $G_{s\alpha}$ protein, the sodium/iodide symporter, thyroid peroxidase, and thyroglobulin have all been identified as causes of thyroid dyshormonogenesis (73, 74). Although the majority are inherited as autosomal recessive disorders, some forms of resistance to TSH, not linked to mutations of the TSH receptor, are inherited in an autosomal dominant fashion (74). Except for mutations in the TSH receptor–G-protein complex, these cases are characterized clinically by the presence of goiter. However, the limited, but substantial, maternal to fetal transfer of thyroid hormone is usually sufficient to protect the affected fetus from mental retardation and goitrogenesis (75). Therefore, these infants rarely show overt goiter at birth. After birth, if these infants are not treated with thyroid hormone, goiter will develop in most because of the thyroid growth-stimulating actions of TSH. In regions of the world with screening programs for congenital hypothyroidism, the vast majority of infants with thyroid dyshormonogenesis will be identified in the newborn period. However, for reasons that remain unclear, some patients with thyroid dyshormonogenesis can have both normal screening results (T_4 and/or TSH) and normal laboratory determinations for serum T_4 and TSH in the neonatal period, only to present months to years later with marked goitrous hypothyroidism (76). Therefore, physicians evaluating children, particularly those in families with a history of thyroid dyshormonogenesis, need to be aware that normal neonatal thyroid screening results do not exclude the possibility that severe hypothyroidism will occur later in infancy or childhood (76).

Pendred syndrome is an autosomal recessive disease characterized by goiter and congenital sensorineural deafness. The disease gene has been mapped to chromosome 7q22-q31.1 and is named PDS (77, 78). The predicted protein of this gene has been named pendrin and consists of 780 amino acids (86 kD); pendrin is a transmembrane glycoprotein containing 11 or 12 transmembrane domains (77). It belongs to a family of proteins, all of which appear to be anion transporters; pendrin has significant structural homology with proteins known to function as sulfate transporters (77). However, expression of pendrin in eukaryotic cells demonstrates that it does not transport sulfate but functions as a sodium-independent transporter of chloride and iodide (77). PDS is highly expressed in the thyroid and, to lesser extents, in fetal kidney, brain, and cochlea (77, 78). Pendrin is localized exclusively at the apical membrane of the thyroid cell; it has been hypothesized that pendrin promotes the transport of iodide from the cytoplasm to the colloid space, delivering iodide to the thyroid peroxidase region involved in iodide organification (77). Although its role in the inner ear remains obscure, pendrin may function as an anion transporter, maintaining the appropriate ionic balance within the endolymph of the inner ear, which is known to play a crucial role in the hearing process (77).

The exact incidence of Pendred syndrome is not known but has been estimated to be as high as 7.5–10: 100,000 individuals (78). It may account for about 10% of cases of hereditary deafness and may be the most common form of syndromic deafness (78). Males and females appear to be equally affected. More than 40 different PDS mutations have been reported in either homozygosity or compound heterozygosity in families with Pendred syndrome (77). Individuals with disease-causing mutations in PDS can present with at least two distinct phenotypes. Most commonly, individuals have a so-called classic Pendred syndrome phenotype of sensorineural hearing loss and goiter. Other affected individuals have sensorineural hearing loss with inner ear malformations (e.g., Mondini cochlea, enlargement of the vestibular aqueduct, alterations of the membranous labyrinth, and enlargement of the endolymphatic duct and sac) in the absence of goiter (77). Although some authors have advocated that a Mondini malformation of the cochlea (i.e., the two-and-a-half turns of the cochlea are replaced by a single cavity in the apical region due to an absence of the interscalar septum) be included as an essential prerequisite to the diagnosis (79), this defect is not specific for Pendred syndrome and is not found in all patients (78). The hearing loss is of moderate to severe degree, being more pronounced in the higher frequencies. The deafness is thought to be congenital and is certainly prelingual in most cases (79). Vestibular function may also be abnormal (77).

In classic cases the goiter appears in midchildhood, but is often postpubertal, especially in affected boys (79). There are rare reports of congenital goiter (79). The goiter tends to be diffuse initially but may become nodular later. An enlarged thyroid gland is present in 50–70% of patients with Pendred syndrome, and there is distinct intrafamilial variability in the presence and extent of goiter among affected individuals (77). Goiter size can range from marginal to marked enlargement (78, 79). The majority of affected individuals are clinically and biochemically euthyroid, but both subclinical and overt hypothyroidism can occur (77–79). It has been postulated that these phenotypic differences may be due to differences in iodine intake (77). Whether a goiter is present or not, a positive perchlorate discharge test is found in the majority of patients with Pendred syndrome (77–79). This reflects the fact that disrupted transport of iodide by pendrin results in decreased iodide flux into the colloid and pooling of unbound iodide within thyrocyte cytoplasm (77). However, PDS mutations have been found in some patients with sensorineural deafness without either goiters or positive perchlorate discharge tests (78).

Further discussion regarding thyroid dyshormonogenesis can be found in Chapter 14.

VIII. IDIOPATHIC GOITER

This form of goiter, also referred to as simple, colloid, or nonspecific goiter, usually occurs in adolescent girls. The patient presents with an asymptomatic diffuse enlargement of the thyroid and is clinically and biochemically euthyroid. The causes of simple goiter are incompletely understood; the condition is generally believed to be multifactorial in origin. The patient's history is negative for iodine deficiency or known goitrogen ingestion. Tests for serum thyroid antibodies are negative. A recent study involving female twin pairs in Denmark supports that genetic factors play a major causative role in some female populations, but environmental factors are also of importance (80). The genes that may represent susceptibility loci for simple goiter have not yet been determined. A number of reports have suggested that TGAbs may produce simple goiter in 40–70% of affected patients (10–12). Mutations in the thyroglobulin gene have recently been identified as uncommon causes of simple goiter. Patients who carry either a heterozygous point mutation within exon 10 or a monoallelic deletion in the 5′ region of the thyroglobulin gene have been described (81, 82). It has been proposed that these heterozygous mutations lead to insufficient thyroglobulin production. As a result, thyroid hormone production is inadequate. Increased stimulation of the thyroid gland by TSH might induce a higher level of transcription from the normal allele and also cause thyroid enlargement. In this way, euthyroidism can be maintained, but at the expense of goiter development (82).

Longitudinal studies have shown that simple goiter may regress over time (60, 83). A study that examined the natural history of thyroid abnormalities over a 20 year period found that simple goiter regressed in 60%, and persisted in 20%, of patients originally diagnosed during childhood (60). However, these longitudinal studies also showed that 5–10% of children initially diagnosed with simple goiter eventually showed clinical evidence of autoimmune thyroiditis (60, 83). Both hypo- and hyperthyroidism were also reported to occur in a few of the patients in these series (60, 83). Therefore, it seems likely that some children diagnosed with simple goiter have atypical or unrecognized autoimmune thyroid disease. For this reason, children with simple goiter should be evaluated at least annually, and the minimal laboratory evaluation at these visits should include serum TSH and thyroid antibody levels.

IX. NODULAR THYROMEGALY

Most children with a solitary thyroid nodule will present with an asymptomatic neck mass discovered either by the child (or his or her parent) or by the physician during a physical examination. The nodule may be present either in one of the lobes or in the isthmus of the gland. There is an increase in frequency of thyroid nodules as age advances. For children and young adults, the reported prevalence rates for thyroid nodules are about 0.22% and 1.5–2.2%, respectively (60).

Although a localized enlargement (i.e., nodule) of the gland may be seen in patients with Hashimoto's thyroiditis or in idiopathic goiter, a mass in the thyroid must be evaluated to determine if it represents a benign or a malignant lesion. To accomplish this, the evaluation of a child with a thyroid nodule should begin with a thorough history and physical examination. The history should inquire about goitrogen exposure, prior irradiation to the head or neck, and a family history of thyroid disease or malignancy. In addition, symptoms of hypo- or hyperthyroidism should be sought. The history should elucidate recent growth and physical characteristics of the nodule; for example, a rapidly enlarging, painless firm, or hard nodule in an otherwise normal thyroid gland is highly suggestive of a malignant process. Likewise, a rapidly enlarging mass in the region of the thyroid associated with hoarseness and/or dysphagia is suggestive of a malignant process. A history of transient pain and tenderness in a nodule may be indicative of an inflammatory process, hemorrhage into a cyst, or a degenerating adenoma. Physical findings that suggest a malignant lesion include a hard nodule, fixation of the thyroid to surrounding tissues, and regional lymphadenopathy. A medullary thyroid carcinoma should be suspected in the child with a thyroid nodule and physical features of multiple endocrine neoplasia IIb syndrome (i.e., marfanoid body habitus, multiple mucosal neuromas, and skeletal defects such as dorsal kyphosis, pectus excavatum, and pes cavus).

Most malignant lesions of the thyroid are carcinomas, but other malignant tumors, such as lymphoma and sarcoma, may occur. There are a number of benign lesions, both thyroidal and nonthyroidal, which may present as a thyroid nodule. Thyroidal lesions include cysts and papillary or follicular adenomas. Nonthyroidal masses that may appear to represent thyroid nodules include teratomas, branchial cleft and thyroglossal duct cysts, lymph nodes, hemangiomas, lymphangiomas, and neurofibromas. Hemiagenesis of the thyroid may also present as a nodular goiter (84).

Although its occurrence is rare, an ectopic thyroid gland can reside off the midline of the neck as far laterally as the submandibular and carotid sheath region (85). Affected patients may present during childhood with either congenital or acquired primary hypothyroidism, or later in life as clinically euthyroid individuals with an asymptomatic or enlarging lateral neck mass (85–89). Because so-called classic teaching dictates that any thyroid tissue ectopically located in the lateral neck represents a lymph node metastasis from a thyroid cancer (86–88), these latter patients often undergo extensive evaluation for suspected thyroid malignancy. The ectopic thyroid gland can also be mistaken for an abnormal submandibular gland that is discovered to be thyroid tissue only after surgical excision (86, 89). Lateral ectopic thyroid glands may occur in association with thyroid tissue in the normal pretracheal location (87) or with other midline ectopic thyroid tissue (e.g., lingual or sublingual glands) (86), or may represent the only thyroid tissue in the body (86, 89). Because the lateral ectopic gland may be the only functional thyroid tissue in the body, it is important to realize that surgical excision can lead to irreversible primary hypothyroidism (86, 89). It is also important to recognize that ectopic thyroid glands may undergo any pathological change that can occur in a normal thyroid gland and may be the site of colloid goiters, hyperthyroidism, adenomas, or even carcinomas (89).

Laboratory evaluation in the child with a thyroid nodule should include serum free T_4, T_3, TSH, and thyroid antibody levels. These studies are obtained to establish the diagnosis of hypothyroidism, most likely due to chronic lymphocytic thyroiditis, or hyperthyroidism due to a hyperfunctioning nodule. The majority of hyperfunctioning nodules are adenomas; hyperfunctioning thyroid carcinomas are exceedingly rare. High serum thyroid antibody levels strongly suggest the presence of chronic lymphocytic thyroiditis. However, some patients originally assumed to have chronic lymphocytic thyroiditis (based on clinical and laboratory findings) as the cause of a thyroid nodule later were found to have papillary thyroid cancer (90). In addition, several studies have reported a significant association between chronic lymphocytic thyroiditis and thyroid cancers (especially papillary carcinoma) and suggest an increased risk of thyroid cancer in patients with chronic lymphocytic thyroiditis (91–93). Therefore, the clinician must still consider the possibility of thyroid malignancy in patients with presumed autoimmune thyroiditis, especially if the gland contains a single dominant nodule and/or there is associated firm cervical lymphadenopathy.

Important studies for the patient with a thyroid nodule are those designed to determine its structure and consistency: ultrasonography and the radionuclide (^{123}I-iodide or Technetium-99m) scan. Ultrasonography will rule out the presence of thyroid anomalies (e.g., thyroid hemiagenesis), confirm that the clinically detected mass represents a solitary thyroid nodule, and determine if the nodule is solid or cystic. Almost all malignant thyroid tumors will appear as a solid mass or a solid mass with a cystic component (94). On the other hand, small cystic lesions (less than 2 cm in diameter) without a solid component are usually benign. The radionuclide scan will determine if the nodule is functioning (warm or hot nodule) or nonfunctioning (cold). Almost all malignant thyroid tumors will appear as nonfunctioning masses, although hyperfunctioning thyroid carcinomas have been described in children (95).

In adults, fine-needle aspiration (FNA) is currently considered the most reliable diagnostic method in the clinical evaluation of thyroid nodules (96). Recent studies have shown that FNA is not only safe in children but is a better diagnostic tool than either ultrasonography or radionuclide scanning in the evaluation of thyroid nodules (97–99). However, proper use of FNA requires individuals who are experienced in performing needle aspirations and cytopathologists who are experienced in interpreting FNA specimens. Even when these requirements are met, false-negative results may be reported. Because of the possibility of a false-negative result and the relatively high incidence (~10–25%) in children of thyroid cancer in nodules (90, 100), some authors have urged caution in the use of FNA in children (90). Instead, they recommend surgical biopsy of all solitary solid thyroid nodules or goiters associated with lymphadenopathy (90). Surgical biopsy without FNA has also been recommended for the child with a thyroid nodule if there is a history of exposure to ionizing radiation, family history of thyroid cancer, or if clinical findings are suspicious of malignancy, such as rapid growth of a firm nodule or if a large nodule (>1.5 cm) is present (100).

Further discussion of the evaluation, management, and prognosis of thyroid nodules and thyroid malignancies can be found in Chapter 18.

X. EVALUATION OF PATIENTS WITH THYROMEGALY

Evaluation of the patient with thyromegaly (Table 4) depends upon the initial history and results of an examination of the thyroid gland. The child with a symmetrical, diffusely enlarged, smooth thyroid gland should be investigated for hyperthyroidism and primary hypothyroidism. The determination of serum thyroid antibodies is important to identify autoimmune thyroid disease. The serum TSH level, determined with a second- or third-generation assay method, is the most sensitive test for thyrotoxicosis. Total and free T_4 and T_3 levels will be elevated in the majority of patients. Only in the presence of mild, equivocal thyrotoxicosis of undetermined cause are additional tests indicated. For the patient with a firm, irregular thyroid gland, the evaluation should be directed toward the diagnosis of autoimmune thyroiditis by determining serum thyroid antibodies and thyroid function.

Most children with autoimmune thyroiditis are clinically and biochemically euthyroid. Although the patient infrequently may present with toxic thyroiditis, the most common abnormality of thyroid function in autoimmune thyroiditis is hypothyroidism, which may develop any time during the course of the disease and can be best detected by the measurement of serum TSH every 6–12 months. When a serum TSH value is slightly elevated, a second specimen should be tested, and, if elevated again, the patient should be started on L-thyroxine therapy. Mild primary hypothyroidism in patients with autoimmune thyroiditis may be transient or permanent, particularly if the disease presents with toxic thyroiditis.

Table 4 Evaluation of the Patient with Thyromegaly

Clinical presentation	Causes	Thyroid function tests	Additional diagnostic tests
Diffuse, smooth symmetrical enlargement	Family history Goitrogen and drug history Serum thyroid antibodies Serum TBII, TSAb, and TGAb	Serum T_3 (thyrotoxicosis) Serum T_4 (hypo- and hyperthyroidism) Serum free T_4 Serum TSH (hypo- and hyperthyroidism)	$[^{123}I]$-iodide uptake at 4–6 and 24 h TRH test Perchlorate discharge Urinary iodide excretion Serum thyroglobulin
Firm, irregular enlargement	Family history Serum thyroid antibodies	Serum TSH (hypo- and hyperthyroidism) Serum T_4 (hypo- and hyperthyroidism) T_3 (thyrotoxicosis)	$[^{123}I]$-iodide uptake at 24 h with image Ultrasonography of neck Perchlorate discharge
Thyroid nodule	Radiation exposure Ultrasonography of neck Thyroid image with $[^{123}I]$-iodide or Technetium-99m Scrum thyroid antibodies Fine needle aspiration Thyroid excisional biopsy	Serum T_3 (thyrotoxicosis) Serum T_4 (hypo- and hyperthyroidism) Serum TSH (hypo- and hyperthyroidism)	T_3 suppression test to evaluate autonomous hypersecretion Serum thyroglobulin Serum calcitonin response to pentagastrin and calcium infusions

REFERENCES

1. Rallison M, Dobyns B, Keating F, et al. Occurrence and natural history of chronic lymphocytic thyroiditis in children. J Pediatr 1975;86:675.
2. Inoue M, Taketani N, Sato T, Nakjima H. High incidences of chronic lymphocytic thyroiditis in apparently healthy school children: epidemiological and clinical study. Endocrinol Jpn 1975;22:483.
3. Trowbridge FL, Matovinovic J, McLaren GD, Nichaman MZ. Iodine and goiter in children. Pediatrics 1975;56:82.
4. Stanbury JB, Hetzel BS, eds. Endemic goiter and endemic cretinism. In: Iodine Nutrition in Health and Disease. New York: John Wiley and Sons, 1980:164.
5. WHO, UNICEF, ICCIDD. Indicators for assessing iodine deficiency disorders and their control through salt iodization. WHO/NUT/94.6. Geneva:WHO, 1994.
6. Foley TP Jr. Goiters in adolescents. Endocrinol Metab Clin North Am 1993;22:593.
7. Foley TP Jr, White C, New A. Juvenile Graves' disease: usefulness and limitations of thyrotropin receptor antibody determinations. J Pediatr 1987;110:378.
8. DeGroot LJ, Quintans J. The causes of autoimmune thyroid disease. Endocr Rev 1989;10:537.
9. Smith BR, McLachlan SM, Furmaniak J. Autoantibodies to the thyrotropin receptor. Endocr Rev 1988;9:106.
10. Fisher DA, Pandian MR, Carlton E. Autoimmune thyroid disease: an expanding spectrum. Pediatr Clin North Am 1987;34:907.
11. Valente WA, Vitti P, Rotella CM, et al. Antibodies that promote thyroid growth: a distinct population of thyroid stimulating autoantibodies. N Engl J Med 1983;309:1028.
12. Van de Gaag RD, Drexhage HA, Wiersinga WM, et al. Further studies on thyroid growth-stimulating immunoglobulins in euthyroid nonendemic goiter. J Clin Endocrinol Metab 1985;60:972.
13. Dumont JE, Roger PP, Ludgate M. Assays for thyroid growth immunoglobulins and their clinical implications: methods, concepts, and misconceptions. Endocr Rev 1987;8:448.
14. Miyamoto S, Kasagi K, Alam MS, et al. Assessment of thyroid growth stimulating activity of immunoglobulins from patients with autoimmune thyroid diseases by cytokinesis arrest assay. Eur J Endocrinol 1997;136:499.
15. Zakarija M, Shixin J, McKenzie JM. Evidence supporting the identity in Graves' disease of thyroid-stimulating antibody and thyroid growth-promoting immunoglobulin G as assayed in FRTL-5 cells. J Clin Invest 1988;81:879.
16. Davies R, Lawry J, Bhatia V, Weetman AP. Growth stimulating antibodies in endemic goiter: a reappraisal. Clin Endocrinol 1995;43:189.
17. Foley TP Jr. Acute, subacute and chronic thyroiditis. In: Kaplan SA, ed. Clinical Pediatric and Adolescent Endocrinology. Philadelphia: WB Saunders, 1982:96–109.
18. Dayan CM, Daniels GH. Chronic autoimmune thyroiditis. N Engl J Med 1996;335:99.
19. Hanafusa T, Pujol-Borrell R, Chiovato L, et al. Aberrant expression of HLA-DR antigen on thyrocytes in Graves' disease: relevance for autoimmunity. Lancet 1983;2:1111.
20. Todd I, Pujol-Borrell R, Hammond LJ, et al. Interferon-gamma induces HLA-DR expression by thyroid epithelium. Clin Exp Immunol 1985;61:265.
21. Phelps E, Wu P, Bretz J, Baker JR Jr. Thyroid cell apoptosis: a new understanding of thyroid autoimmunity. Endocrinol Metab Clin North Am 2000;29:375.
22. Palazzo FF, Hammond LJ, Goode AW, Mirakian R. Death of the autoimmune thyrocyte: is it pushed or does it jump? Thyroid 2000;10:561.
23. Eguchi K. Apoptosis in autoimmune diseases. Intern Med 2001;40:275.
24. Bogner U, Wall JR, Schleusener H. Cellular and antibody mediated cytotoxicity in autoimmune thyroid disease. Acta Endocrinol (Copenh) Suppl 1987;281:133.
25. Bretz JD, Baker JR Jr. Apoptosis and autoimmune thyroid disease: following a TRAIL to thyroid destruction? Clin Endocrinol 2001;55:1.

26. Barbesino G, Chiovato L. The genetics of Hashimoto's disease. Endocrinol Metab Clin North Am 2000;29:357.

27. Tomer Y, Greenberg DA, Concepcion E, et al. Thyroglobulin is a thyroid specific gene for the familial autoimmune thyroid diseases. J Clin Endocrinol Metab 2002; 87:404.

28. Hunter I, Greene SA, MacDonald TM, Morris AD. Prevalence and etiology of hypothyroidism in the young. Arch Dis Child 2000;83:207.

29. Roth C, Scortea M, Stubbe P, et al. Autoimmune thyroiditis in childhood—epidemiology, clinical and laboratory findings in 61 patients. Exp Clin Endocrinol Diabetes 1997;105(Suppl 4):66.

30. Harach HR, Escalante DA, Onativia A, et al. Thyroid carcinoma and thyroiditis in an endemic goitre region before and after iodine prophylaxis. Acta Endocrinol (Copenh) 1985;108:55.

31. Fort P, Lanes R, Dahlem S, et al. Breast and soy-formula feeding in early infancy and the prevalence of autoimmune thyroid disease in children. J Am Coll Nutr 1990; 9:164.

32. Drash AL, Becker DJ, Villapando S, et al. The incidence of clinical and subclinical thyroid and adrenal disease and their association with antibodies to endocrine tissues in children with juvenile diabetes mellitus. J Pediatr 1978; 93:310.

33. Neufeld M, Maclaren NK, Riley WJ, et al. Islet cell and other organ-specific antibodies in U.S. Caucasians and Blacks with insulin-dependent diabetes mellitus. Diabetes 1980;29:589.

34. Neufeld M, Maclaren N, Blizzard R. Autoimmune polyglandular syndromes. Pediatr Ann 1980;9:154.

35. Becker RL, Titus JL, Woolner LB, McConahey WM. Significance of morphologic thyroiditis. Ann Intern Med 1965;62:1134.

36. Leznoff A, Sussman GL. Syndrome of idiopathic chronic urticaria and angioedema with thyroid autoimmunity: a study of 90 patients. J Allergy Clin Immunol 1989;84:66.

37. Turktas I, Gokcora N, Demirsy S, et al. The association of chronic urticaria and angioedema with autoimmune thyroiditis. Int J Dermatol 1997;36:187.

38. Kothbauer-Margreiter I, Sturzenegger M, Komor J, et al. Encephalopathy associated with Hashimoto thyroiditis: diagnosis and treatment. J Neurol 1996;243:585.

39. Altus P, Blandon R, Wallach PM, Flannery MT. Case report: the spectrum of autoimmune thyroid disease with urticaria. Am J Med Sci 1993;306:379.

40. Canton A, de Fabregas O, Tintore M, et al. Encephalopathy associated to autoimmune thyroid disease: a more appropriate term for an underestimated condition? J Neurol Sci 2000;176:65.

41. Peschen-Rosin R, Schabet M, Dichgans J. Manifestation of Hashimoto's encephalopathy years before onset of thyroid disease. Eur Neurol 1999;41:79.

42. Amoroso A, Garzia P, Pasquarelli C, et al. Hashimoto's thyroiditis associated with urticaria and angio-oedema: disappearance of cutaneous and mucosal manifestations after thyroidectomy. J Clin Pathol 1997;50:254.

43. Rumbyrt JS, Katz JL, Schocket AL. Resolution of chronic urticaria in patients with thyroid autoimmunity. J Allergy Clin Immunol 1995;96:901.

44. Dreyfus DH, Schocket Al, Milgrom H. Steroid-resistant chronic urticaria associated with anti-thyroid microsomal antibodies in a nine-year-old boy. J Pediatr 1996; 128:576.

45. Zauli D, Deleonardi G, Foderaro S, et al. Thyroid autoimmunity in chronic urticaria. Allergy Asthma Proc 2001; 22:93.

46. Watemberg N, Willis D, Pellock JM. Encephalopathy as the presenting symptom of Hashimoto's thyroiditis. J Child Neurol 2000;15:66.

47. Chen HC, Masharani U. Hashimoto's encephalopathy. South Med J 2000;93:504.

48. Vasconcelos E, Pina-Garza JE, Fakhoury T, Fenichel GM. Pediatric manifestations of Hashimoto's encephalopathy. Pediatr Neurol 1999;20:394.

49. Takahashi S, Mitamura R, Itoh Y, et al. Hashimoto encephalopathy: etiologic considerations. Pediatr Neurol 1994;11:328.

50. Forchetti CM, Katsamakis G, Garron DC. Autoimmune thyroiditis and a rapidly progressive dementia: global hypoperfusion on SPECT scanning suggests a possible mechanism. Neurology 1997;49:623.

51. Henchey R, Cibula J, Helvston W, et al. Electroencephalographic findings in Hashimoto's encephalopathy. Neurology 1995;45:977.

52. Isik U, Tennison M, D'Cruz O. Recurrent encephalopathy and seizures in an adolescent girl. Clin Pediatr 2001;40: 273.

53. Garrard P, Hodges JR, DeVries PJ, et al. Hashimoto's encephalopathy presenting as "myxoedematous madness." J Neurol Neurosurg Psychiatry 2000;68:100.

54. Saravanan P, Dayan CM. Thyroid autoantibodies. Endocrinol Metab Clin North Am 2001;30:315.

55. Ross DS. Syndromes of thyrotoxicosis with low radioactive iodine uptake. Endocrinol Metab Clin North Am 1998;27:169.

56. Set PAK, Oleszczuk-Raschke K, Von Lengerke JH, Bramswig J. Sonographic features of Hashimoto's thyroiditis in childhood. Clin Radiol 1996;51:167.

57. Pederson OM, Aardal NP, Larssen TB, et al. The value of ultrasonography in predicting autoimmune thyroid disease. Thyroid 2000;10:251.

58. Intenzo CM, Capuzzi DM, Jabbour S, et al. Scintigraphic features of autoimmune thyroiditis. Radiographics 2001; 21:957.

59. Gray HW, Hooper LA, Greig WR. An evaluation of the twenty minute perchlorate discharge test. J Clin Endocrinol Metab 1973;37:351.

60. Rallison ML, Dobyns BM, Meilke AW, et al. Natural history of thyroid abnormalities: prevalence, incidence, and regression of thyroid diseases in adolescents and young adults. Am J Med 1991;91:363.

61. Abe K, Taguchi T, Okuno A, et al. Acute suppurative thyroiditis in children. J Pediatr 1979;94:912.

62. Abe K, Fujita H, Matsuura N, et al. A fistula from pyriform sinus in recurrent acute suppurative thyroiditis. Am J Dis Child 1981;135:178.

63. Miller D, Hill JL, Sun CC, et al. The diagnosis and management of pyriform sinus fistulae in infants and young children. J Pediatr Surg 1983;18:377.

64. Slatosky J, Shipton B, Wahba H. Thyroiditis: differential diagnosis and management. Am Fam Physician 2000; 1047.

65. Schubert MF, Kountz DS. Thyroiditis: a disease with many faces. Postgraduate Med 1995;98:101.

66. Delange F, de Benoist B, Pretell E, Dunn JT. Iodine deficiency in the world: where do we stand at the turn of the century? Thyroid 2001;11:437.

67. Zimmermann M, Adou P, Torresani T, et al. Persistence of goiter despite oral iodine supplementation in goitrous

children with iron deficiency anemia in Cote d'Ivoire. Am J Clin Nutr 2000;71:88.

68. Salabe GB. Pathogenesis of thyroid nodules: histological classification? Biomed Pharmacother 2001;55:39.

69. Meier CA, Burger AG. Extrinsic and intrinsic variables: effects of drugs and other substances on thyroid hormone synthesis and metabolism. In: Braverman LE, Utiger RD, eds. Werner and Ingbar's The Thyroid: A Fundamental and Clinical Text. 8th ed. Philadelphia: Lippincott, Williams & Wilkins, 2000:265–280.

70. Delange FM. Extrinsic and intrinsic variables: effects of drugs and other substances on thyroid hormone synthesis and metabolism. In: Braverman LE, Utiger RD, eds. Werner and Ingbar's The Thyroid: A Fundamental and Clinical Text. 8th ed. Philadelphia: Lippincott, Williams & Wilkins, 2000:295–316.

71. Fitzpatrick M. Soy formulas and the effects of isoflavones on the thyroid. NZ Med J 2000;113(1103):24.

72. Fort P, Moses N, Fasano M, et al. Breast feeding and insulin-dependent diabetes mellitus in children. J Am Coll Nutr 1986;5:439.

73. Krude H, Biebermann H, Schnabel D, et al. Molecular pathogenesis of neonatal hypothyroidism. Horm Res 2000;53(Suppl 1):12.

74. Macchia P. Recent advances in understanding the molecular basis of primary congenital hypothyroidism. Mol Med Today 2000;6:36.

75. de Vijlder JJM, Ris-Stalpers C, Vulsma T. Inborn errors of thyroid hormone biosynthesis. Exp Clin Endocrinol Diabetes 1997;105(Suppl 4):32.

76. de Zegher F, Vanderschueren-Lodeweyckx M, Heinrichs C, et al. Thyroid dyshormonogenesis: severe hypothyroidism after normal neonatal thyroid stimulating hormone screening. Acta Paediatr 1992;81:274.

77. Fugazzola L, Cerutti N, Mannavola D, et al. The role of pendrin in iodide regulation. Exp Clin Endocrinol Diabetes 2001;109:18.

78. Kopp P. Pendred's syndrome: identification of the genetic defect a century after its recognition. Thyroid 1999;9:65.

79. Reardon W, Trembath RC. Pendred syndrome. J Med Genet 1996;33:1037.

80. Brix TH, Kyvik KO, Hegedus L. Major role of genes in the etiology of simple goiter in females: a population-based twin study. J Clin Endocrinol Metab 1999;84:3071.

81. Corral J, Martin C, Perez R, et al. Thyroglobulin gene point mutation associated with non-endemic simple goiter. Lancet 1993;341:462.

82. Gonzalez-Sarmiento R, Corral J, Mories MT, et al. Monoallelic deletion in the 5' region of the thyroglobulin gene as a cause of sporadic nonendemic simple goiter. Thyroid 2001;11:789.

83. Jaruratanasirikul S, Leethanaporn K, Suchat K. The natural clinical course of children with an initial diagnosis of simple goiter: a 5-year longitudinal follow-up. J Pediatr Endocrinol Metab 2000;13:1109.

84. Hopwood NJ, Carroll RG, Kenny FM, Foley TP. Functioning thyroid nodules in childhood and adolescence. J Pediatr 1976;89:710.

85. Okstad S, Mair IWS, Sundsfjord JA, et al. Ectopic thyroid tissue in the head and neck. J Otolaryngol 1986;15:52.

86. Kumar R, Sharma S, Marwah A, et al. Ectopic goiter masquerading as submandibular gland swelling: a case report and review of the literature. Clin Nucl Med 2001;306.

87. Block MA, Wylie JH, Patton RB, Miller JM. Does benign thyroid tissue occur in the lateral part of the neck? Am J Surg 1966;112:476.

88. Clopp CT, Kirson SM. Therapeutic problems with ectopic non-cancerous follicular thyroid tissue in the neck: 18 case reports according to etiologic factors. Ann Surg 1965;163:653.

89. Helidonis E, Dokianakis G, Papazoglou G, et al. Ectopic thyroid gland in the submandibular region. J Laryngol Otol 1980;94:219.

90. Flannery TK, Kirkland JL, Copeland KC, et al. Papillary thyroid cancer: a pediatric perspective. Pediatrics 1996;98:464.

91. Holm LE, Blomgren H, Lowhagen T. Cancer risks in patients with chronic lymphocytic thyroiditis. N Engl J Med 1985;312:601.

92. Okayasu I, Fujiwara M, Hara Y, et al. Association of chronic lymphocytic thyroiditis and thyroid papillary carcinoma: a study of surgical cases among Japanese, and White and African Americans. Cancer 1995;76:2312.

93. Singh B, Shaha AR, Trivedi H, et al. Coexistent Hashimoto's thyroiditis with papillary thyroid carcinoma: impact on presentation, management, and outcome. Surgery 1999;126:1070.

94. Desjardins JG, Khan AH, Montupet P, et al. Management of thyroid nodules in children: a 20-year-experience. J Pediatr Surg 1987;22:736.

95. Mircescu H, Parma J, Huot C, et al. Hyperfunctioning malignant thyroid nodule in an 11-year-old girl: pathologic and molecular studies. J Pediatr 2000;137:585.

96. Gharib H. Changing concepts in the diagnosis and management of thyroid nodules. Endocrinol Metab Clin North Am 1997;26:777.

97. Khurana KK, Labrador E, Izquierdo R, et al. The role of fine-needle aspiration biopsy in the management of thyroid nodules in children, adolescents, and young adults: a multi-institutional study. Thyroid 1999;9:383.

98. Arda IS, Yildirim S, Demirhan B, Firat S. Fine needle aspiration biopsy of thyroid nodules. Arch Dis Child 2001;85:313.

99. Corrias A, Einaudi S, Chiorboli E, et al. Accuracy of fine needle aspiration biopsy of thyroid nodules in detecting malignancy in childhood: comparison with conventional clinical, laboratory, and imaging approaches. J Clin Endocrinol Metab 2001;86:4644.

100. Hung W. Solitary thyroid nodules in 93 children and adolescents: a 35-years experience. Horm Res 1999;52:15.

18

Thyroid Tumors in Children

Donald Zimmerman

Mayo Medical School and Mayo Medical Clinic, Rochester, Minnesota, U.S.A.

I. EPIDEMIOLOGY

Thyroid cancers, particularly papillary cancers, are found at autopsy in a large minority of individuals dying of other causes. The prevalence varies from 5.6% in Colombia (1) to 35.6% in Finland (2). Autopsy prevalence of thyroid cancers is relatively low in children and adolescents. The prevalence in Finnish youth 20 years of age or less is 13.6%; no cases were detected in Finnish children 10 years of age or younger (3).

In light of the high autopsy prevalence of thyroid cancer, the annual incidence of clinical thyroid cancer is remarkably low. The incidence of thyroid cancer in children and adolescents has been estimated to be between 0.2 and 3.0 cases per million per year (4, 5). Clinical thyroid cancers in childhood and adolescents form only approximately 5% of such tumors (6, 7).

Thyroid cancer in adults in (two to four times more frequent in women than in men (8). This female predominance is less evident in children and is not observed in children less than 11 years of age (5, 9).

The best-established environmental risk factor promoting thyroid cancer is radiation exposure (10–14). Residence in a volcanic area, particularly Hawaii or Iceland, appears to increase the risk of thyroid cancer (15).

The vast majority of medullary thyroid cancers detected in childhood form one component of a genetic syndrome: either familial medullary thyroid cancer or multiple endocrine neoplasia type 2 (MEN 2). MEN 2a comprises medullary thyroid carcinoma, pheochromocytoma, and hyperparathyroidism. MEN 2b includes medullary carcinoma of the thyroid, pheochromocytoma, and ganglioneuromatosis of the gastrointestinal tract in association with a marfanoid habitus (16; Fig. 1). Medullary thyroid carcinoma occurring in all age groups is inherited in approximately 25% of cases (17).

Nonmedullary thyroid carcinoma is heritable less frequently than is medullary carcinoma. Recent estimates of familial occurrence in patients of all ages have been in the range of 5% (18). Heritable nonmedullary thyroid cancers include oxyphilic papillary cancers (19). Classic papillary thyroid carcinoma may be heritable without other abnormality (20) or in association with nontoxic multinodular goiter (21).

Papillary thyroid carcinoma, or a thyroid carcinoma somewhat different from typical papillary cancer, occurs in approximately 1% of patients with familial adenomatous polyposis (FAP) (22–24). Approximately 85% of FAP patients with thyroid carcinoma are women, and most thyroid cancers in these patients are diagnosed before 35 years of age (25–27).

Another hereditary setting for nonmedullary thyroid cancers is in patients with Cowden disease, a condition similar to FAP that is transmitted with an autosomal dominant pattern of inheritance. This condition consists of hamartomas arising in ectoderm, mesoderm, and endoderm. The most characteristic features are facial papules (trichilemmomas and verrucae), oral papillomatosis, and palmoplantar keratoses (Fig. 2). Other features include fibrocystic disease of the breast, nodular goiter, gastrointestinal polyposis, and ovarian cysts. Malignancies associated with Cowden disease include papillary and follicular thyroid cancer in 7% of patients as well as breast carcinoma, non-Hodgkin's lymphoma, melanoma, colon and uterine adenocarcinoma, squamous and basal cell skin carcinoma, and acute myelogenous leukemia (28, 29).

Another multiple neoplasia syndrome transmitted with an autosomal dominant pattern of inheritance is the Carney complex of spotty skin pigmentation, myxomas, endocrine overactivity, and schwannomas. Pigmented skin lesions include pinpoint brown to black macules (also present on mucosal membranes), café au lait spots, and blue nevi (Fig. 3). Myxomas occur in heart, skin, breast, and in other tissues. Endocrine abnormalities include primary adrenal Cushing's syndrome associated with pigmented adrenal nodules, growth hormone-producing pi-

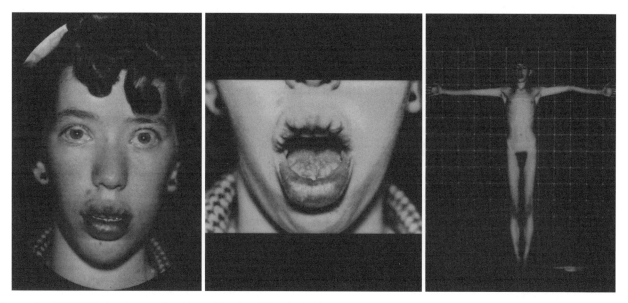

Figure 1 MEN 2B is characterized by a Marfanoid body habitus (right) and by characteristic facies (left and center). The facies include thickened lips with nodules due to ganglioneuromas. The tongue has nodular ganglioneuromas as do the eyelids.

tuitary adenomas, and testicular Sertoli and Leydig cell tumors. Some 3.8% of patients have either papillary or follicular thyroid carcinoma. Nodular thyroid disease is present in 60 to 67% of patients (30).

II. PATHOLOGY

Some thyroid tumors arise from the thyroid follicular epithelium. This epithelium produces thyroglobulin, thyroxine, and triiodothyronine. Other thyroid tumors arise from C cells that derive from the most caudal branchial pouches (ultimobranchial bodies). These cells are located between the basal lamina and the follicular epithelial cells. Unlike follicular epithelial cells, C cells do not extend into the

colloid-containing follicular lumen. They produce calcitonin in addition to a number of other peptides such as somatostatin and calcitonin gene-related peptide. They do not produce thyroglobulin. Thyroid lymphomas arise from intrathyroidal lymphocytes.

The most common benign thyroid tumors arise from thyroid follicular cells and include adenomas and adenomatous nodules. Adenomas are solitary. They are encapsulated and have a uniform internal structure. They may have follicular or solid architecture (Fig. 4). Adenomatous nodules have more varied internal structure. They are commonly multiple rather than solitary (Fig. 5). Thyroid teratomas are found most commonly in the newborn. Large teratomas may be associated with polyhydramnios

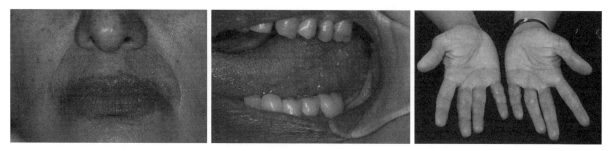

Figure 2 Cowden disease has a number of skin and mucous membrane hamartomas. Facial trichilemmomas are seen on the left. Cobble-stone-like papules are seen in the buccal mucosa at the base of the tongue (center). Verrucous lesions (palmoplantar keratosas) are seen on the palms (right).

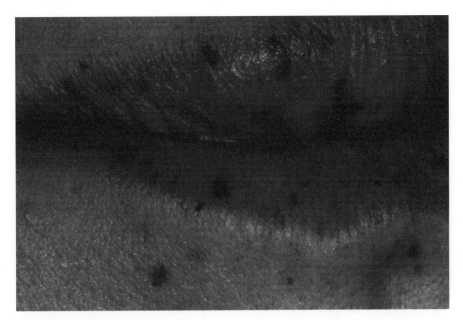

Figure 3 Principal skin findings in Carney complex (myxoma, spotty pigmentation, and endocrine overactivity) include ephelides or melanin spots in and around the lips.

since they may interfere with fetal swallowing of amniotic fluid.

Malignant tumors of the thyroid follicular epithelium may be classified into papillary carcinomas, follicular carcinomas, and poorly differentiated carcinomas (31).

Papillary carcinomas make up approximately 72% of childhood thyroid cancers (32). These tumors often infiltrate surrounding tissue and are only infrequently encap-

sulated. Most contain papillae with a fibrovascular core and a single layer of typical epithelial cells (Fig. 6). Often this pattern forms only a small proportion of the tumor. Other patterns found in papillary cancer include follicular, trabecular, cribriform, and diffuse. The epithelial cells contain large irregular nuclei that are folded and indented with cytoplasmic inclusions. Since the nuclear heterochromatin is concentrated near the nuclear membrane, the cen-

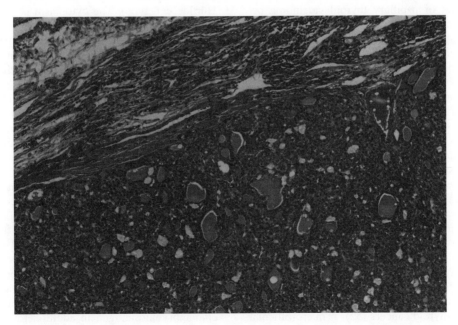

Figure 4 Follicular adenomas of the thyroid are encapsulated and have uniform structure.

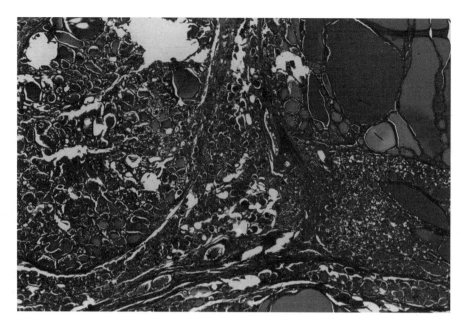

Figure 5   Benign adenomatous nodules have more varied internal structures than follicular adenomas.

tral portion has a pale ground-glass appearance. The nuclei are often aligned similarly on the basal or apical part of the cell and therefore overlap one another.

Children less than 10 years of age appear to have a distinctive so-called childhood type of papillary thyroid cancer in which the nuclei are more rounded rather than elongated, smooth rather than grooved, and not crowded or overlapping. The predominant pattern of this type of papillary cancer is solid rather than pure papillary or a mixture of papillary and follicular (5).

Another variant of papillary thyroid carcinoma occurring most commonly in younger patients is the diffuse sclerosing type (Fig. 7). The tumor involves all lymphatics of one or both thyroid lobes and is associated with severe lymphocytic thyroiditis or interstitial fibrosis. Lymph nodes and pulmonary metastases are frequent (33).

The thyroid cancer occurring in association with familial adenomatous polyposis has been described as atypical papillary carcinoma. Tumors have mixed patterns including cribriform, papillary, glandular, and solid. The nuclei most commonly lack the central ground-glass appearance. Cytoplasmic inclusions and nuclear membrane grooving tend to be less prominent than they are in classic papillary tumors (22, 26).

Papillary thyroid cancers are frequently multifocal and are bilateral in up to 80% of cases (34). Papillary thyroid carcinoma metastasizes to cervical lymph nodes in 90% of affected children and to lungs in approximately 7% (6). Only rarely does the tumor invade blood vessels or metastasize to distant sites other than to lung.

Follicular thyroid carcinoma makes up approximately 18% of childhood thyroid cancers (32). A microfollicular pattern is usually predominant in follicular tumors (Fig.

8). Other less frequent tumor patterns include trabecular and solid. Nearly all follicular carcinomas are encapsulated, and the vast majority are unifocal and unilateral. Characteristically, follicular carcinomas invade blood vessels and, not rarely, also invade the tumor capsule. Thus, this tumor spreads hematogenously to lungs, bone, liver, and brain. Lymphatic invasion by follicular cancer is relatively infrequent.

One important variant of follicular thyroid cancer is the oncocytic cell type (also called the oxyphilic or Hürthle cell type). The cytoplasm is granular and eosinophilic because of the presence of a large number of mitochondria (Fig. 9). These tumors exhibit extrathyroidal extension and lymph node and distant metastases more frequently than do other follicular carcinomas.

Anaplastic carcinoma is extremely aggressive and has been described as forming 2.6% of childhood thyroid cancers (32). Insular carcinomas have islands of small, dense cells that aggregate in solid, follicular, or papillary patterns. This tumor appears to be intermediate in aggressiveness between differentiated cancers (follicular and papillary) and anaplastic cancer (35).

Medullary thyroid carcinoma makes up approximately 2.6% of childhood thyroid cancers (32). These tumors arise most frequently at the junction of the upper third and the lower two-thirds of the thyroid gland: the thyroid region most densely populated with C cells. The cells in this tumor may be round, spindle-shaped, or polygonal and form sheets separated by fibrous stroma. Sixty to 80% of tumors contained amyloid (Fig. 10). The C cells forming medullary carcinoma produce calcitonin and carcinoembryonic antigen in addition to a number of other substances. Hereditary medullary tumors are multicentric

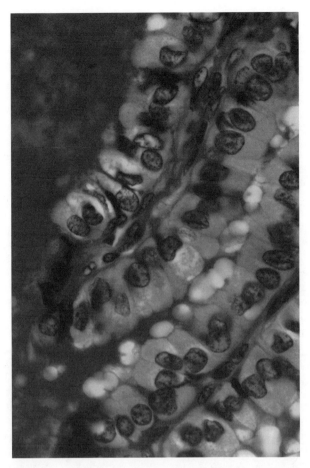

Figure 6 The finger-like projections, or papillary thyroid carcinoma have a fibrovascular core and single layer of epithelial cells located basally. The nuclei appear to overlap.

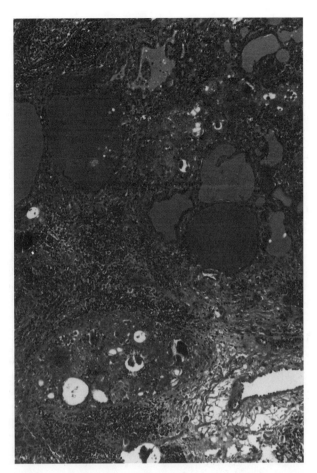

Figure 7 Diffuse sclerosing papillary carcinoma is associated with lymphocytic infiltration and interstitial fibrosis. It tends to diffusely involve one or both thyroid lobes.

and bilateral. Nonhereditary tumors are most frequently solitary.

III. PATHOGENESIS

Two classes of mutated genes contribute to tumorigenesis. The first is the class of proto-oncogenes, which code for protein products that regulate cell growth. Many of these gene products contribute to the biochemical cascade involving cellular response to growth factors. An important example of a proto-oncogene contributing to thyroid carcinogenesis is RET (rearranged during transfection). The RET gene product is a transmembrane protein anchored in the plasma membrane. It is part of a receptor complex binding a family of ligands including glial cell line-derived neurotrophic factor, neurturin, persephin, and artemin. These ligands are members of the transforming growth factor β superfamily (36–38). The RET ligands form head-to-tail dimers; this structure facilitates dimeri-

zation of adjacent RET molecules, which in turn triggers activation of tyrosine kinase and receptor autophosphorylation (39; Fig. 11).

RET mutations have been found in medullary carcinoma of the thyroid (40–42). RET gene mutations in MEN 2A and in familial medullary thyroid carcinoma (FMTC) most frequently produce a change from cysteine (which in the unmutated molecule participates with another cysteine in an intramolecular disulfide bond) to another amino acid. This transversion frees the other usually intramolecularly coupled cysteine to couple with the corresponding uncoupled cysteine in a neighboring mutated RET molecule. This intermolecular cysteine coupling dimerizes RET and results in constitutive activation (43; Fig. 12).

RET mutations in MEN 2B occur in the intracellular tyrosine kinase domain rather than in the cysteine-rich extracellular domain of the RET molecule (44). These tyrosine kinase mutations activate RET without need of dimerization (Fig. 13). This nondimeric structure of acti-

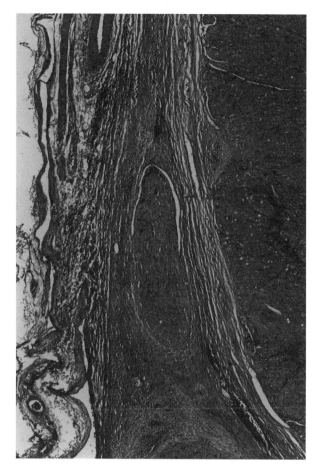

Figure 8 Follicular thyroid carcinoma frequently invades blood vessel walls.

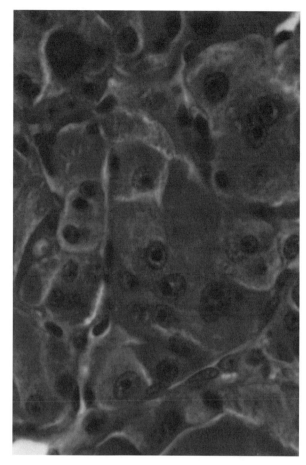

Figure 9 Oncocytic cell thyroid carcinoma has granular cytoplasm that is intensely eosinophilic.

vated RET in MEN 2B alters the substrate specificity of tyrosine kinase. In addition, unlike MEN 2A RET mutations, MEN 2B mutations allow persistence of RET ligand responsiveness (45). Perhaps these differences contribute to phenotype differences between MEN 2A and 2B.

Intestinal ganglioneuromatosis, characteristic of MEN 2B, reflects the embryologic role of RET in development of the enteric nervous system (46). Inactivating RET mutations are found in 23 to 33% of patients with Hirschsprung's disease, a condition characterized by absence of ganglia within a portion of the distal colonic wall (47). Some kindreds have RET mutations that predispose to both MEN 2A (or FMTC) and Hirschsprung's disease. Such mutations may produce constitutively active RET molecules that are numerically limited, causing constitutively active C-cells but numerically insufficient RET signals to effect gangliogenesis (48).

In addition to its role in MCT tumorigenesis, RET has been implicated as one of the most frequent oncogenes contributing to production of papillary thyroid carcinomas. Since RET is not ordinarily expressed in thyroid follicular cells (unlike thyroid C cells), the very expression of RET in follicular cells is dependent on chromosomal rearrangement, which apposes regulatory subunits of other genes to the tyrosine kinase domain of the RET gene. In addition, these oncogenes code for protein coiled coil domains that predispose to constitutive dimerization of the proteins with one another and in this manner activate the tyrosine kinase (49). At least eight chromosomal rearrangements involving RET have been found in papillary thyroid carcinoma (50–56). Although most of the chromosomal rearrangements involving RET include inversion of a segment of chromosome 10 containing the RET gene (Fig. 14), some involve translocation of a fragment of chromosome 10 to a different chromosome such as chromosome 17 (53, 56).

At least one mechanism of thyroid tumorigenesis due to radiation is radiation induction of RET rearrangements (57). The Chernobyl thyroid cancer experience suggests that a particular RET rearrangement (PTC-3) is associated with short latency between radiation exposure and clinical cancer (58, 59).

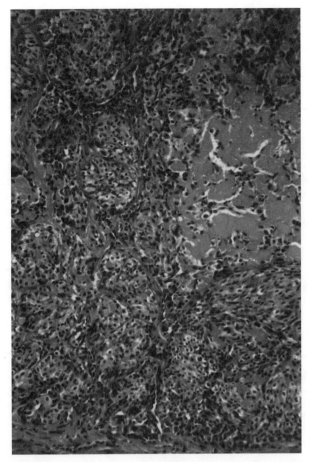

Figure 10 The C cells that make up medullary thyroid carcinoma may be round, spindle-shaped, or polygonal. They form sheets separated by fibrous stoma and may produce amyloid.

C-met is a transmembrane, high-affinity receptor for hepatic growth factor. This growth factor receptor is over-expressed in 96% of papillary thyroid carcinomas and may contribute to lymph node metastases and to advanced pathological stage (60).

NTRK-1 is a component of the high-affinity receptor for nerve growth factor. The gene for this proto-oncogene is on chromosome 1q22, and a number of chromosomal rearrangements including the NTRK-1 gene are found in papillary thyroid cancers. NTRK-1 rearrangements are less frequent in papillary thyroid carcinoma (12%) than are RET mutations (46%). Both are more common in younger patients than in older ones (61).

A number of studies have suggested that lymphocytic infiltration of thyroid neoplasms is associated with a favorable prognosis (62, 63). Recent evidence suggests that thyroid cancers may be able to evade immunological attack mediated by lymphocytic infiltration by expressing FAS ligand, a transmembrane protein of the TNF family

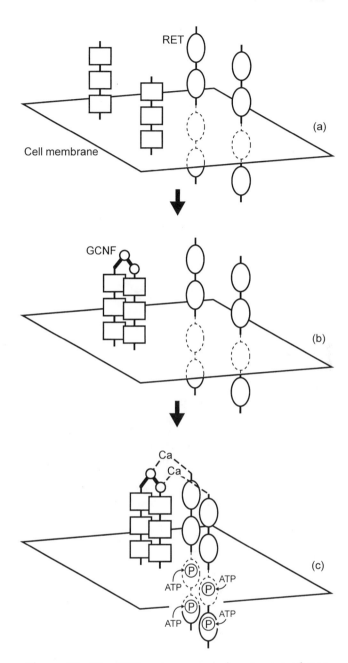

Figure 11 The RET proto-oncogene is a transmembrane molecule. It collaborates with specific receptors for each of the members of the glial cell line-derived neurotrophic factor family (e.g., the GCNF receptor depicted by a line with square domains) in transducing signals to the interior of the cell.

that binds to a specific receptor on activated T cells and induces apoptosis (64, 65).

Tumor-suppressor gene mutations contributing to thyroid tumorigenesis include mutations in P53. Although P53 mutations are found in up to 40% of undifferentiated

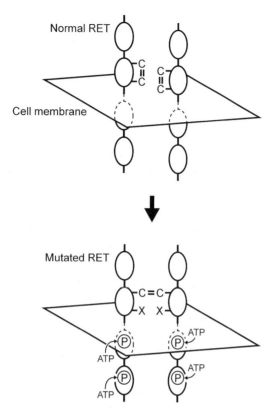

Figure 12 In MEN 2A, most of the RET mutations involve a nucleic acid transversion resulting in a change in the cysteine-rich portion of the extracellular portion of RET. Since one of the *intra*molecular disulfide bonds does not form, a "spare" cysteine is available for *inter*molecular disulfide bonding. This bonding results in dimerization of RET molecules. This dimerization, in turn, constitutively activates RET.

thyroid cancers, they are observed in less than 10% of differentiated thyroid cancers. These mutations are more common in aggressive tumors (66). P53 mutations are observed with greater frequency in radiation-induced thyroid cancers (67).

Angiogenesis stimulators and inhibitors appear to facilitate tumor growth. Overexpression of vascular endothelial growth factor C (an angiogenesis stimulator) is increased in lymph node invasive thyroid tumor such as papillary cancer. Thrombospondin-1 (an angiogenesis inhibitor) is underexpressed in hematogenously spreading thyroid tumors such as follicular cancer (68–70).

Genes associated with heritable, nonmedullary thyroid cancer contribute in various ways to the development of thyroid cancers. Patients with familial adenomatous polyposis have mutations in the adenomatous polyposis (APC) gene located on chromosome 5q21. Individuals with mutations between codons 463 and 1387 are at greater risk for thyroid carcinoma and for congenital hy-

pertrophy of the retinal pigment epithelium. Some studies of loss of heterozygosity for the APC gene in thyroid tumors have been negative in the setting of familial adenomatous polyposis. Although there was no observable loss of heterozygosity for the APC gene, three of four patients had RET-PTC rearrangements (71). In other studies of APC and thyroid cancer, the thyroid cancers in this setting did manifest loss of heterozygosity (72).

Cowden disease results from mutations in PTEN, a tumor suppressor gene with protein tyrosine phosphatase activity located on chromosome 10q23 (73). Thyroid tumors and other tumors associated with Cowden disease are associated with loss of heterozygosity in tumor tissue (74). Although PTEN mutations are infrequent in sporadic thyroid carcinomas, PTEN expression is decreased at the RNA and protein level in 40% of these carcinomas (75).

The Carney complex results from mutations of the gene on chromosome 17q23–24, which encodes the protein kinase A type 1-alpha regulatory subunit. This gene has not yet been studied in thyroid tumor tissue (76).

IV. DIAGNOSIS

Thyroid cancer presents as a thyroid nodule in approximately 54% of patients. Twelve percent have both a thyroid nodule and enlarged cervical lymph nodes, and 36% have enlarged cervical lymph nodes without a palpable thyroid mass (77). Between 18% and 25% of solitary thyroid nodules in children are found to be cancerous (78–80). Since only 5% of thyroid nodules in adults are malignant, fine-needle aspiration of such nodules is generally favored to avoid unnecessary surgery in adults (81). Fine-needle aspiration of childhood thyroid nodules is recommended by investigators (82), but others caution that aspiration biopsy results may be misleading. These individuals favor surgery in all children with thyroid nodules (83). False-negative results of aspiration cytology may be obtained in 2.3–3.6% of thyroid nodules (80, 82).

Evaluation of thyroid nodules by ultrasonography and radionuclide scanning has been largely replaced by fine-needle aspiration (FNA) because of the latter's superior sensitivity and specificity (81). In general, FNA cytology that is positive or suspicious for malignancy should prompt thyroid surgery. Nondiagnostic cytology should prompt repeat aspiration perhaps performed under ultrasound guidance (Fig. 15). Ultrasound guidance may be particularly useful if there is a cystic component of the lesion since sampling of the wall of the lesion is most likely to give a meaningful cytologic result (84).

V. TREATMENT

The surgical procedure most frequently advocated for treatment of papillary thyroid carcinoma is bilateral near-total or total thyroidectomy. Unilateral procedures are associated with a higher incidence of local tumor recurrence

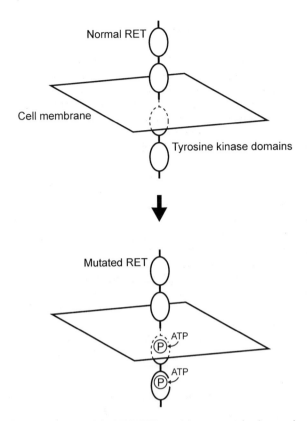

Normal RET

Cell membrane

Tyrosine kinase domains

Mutated RET

ATP

ATP

Figure 13 In MEN 2B, RET mutations occur in the portion of the gene coding for the portion of the RET protein containing tyrosine kinase activity. These mutations are constitutively active despite absence of dimerization of the RET proteins.

in low-risk as well as in high-risk patients (85). Unilateral surgeries are associated with higher mortality only in high-risk patients (advanced patient age, large tumor size, local invasion, and/or distant metastases, and high tumor grade) (86, 87). Bilateral thyroid surgery significantly decreased the rate of tumor recurrence in a study of 1685 patients of all ages evaluated for a mean of 18 years (87). Study of a subset of this patient group including the 90 children less than 17 years of age also demonstrated decreased tumor recurrence in patients undergoing bilateral surgical procedures (88). A more recent study of a different patient population has also confirmed these results (89). Another study of 329 patients younger than 21 years of age evaluated for a mean of 11.3 years did not report a difference between unilateral and bilateral surgeries. This study demonstrated a higher frequency of permanent hypoparathyroidism in bilateral operations than in unilateral ones (90). In addition to the probable advantage in preventing tumor recurrence offered by bilateral surgery, this surgical approach facilitates the usefulness of thyroglobulin measurement and of radioiodine scanning in evaluating thyroid cancer patients postoperatively for re-

currence of tumor (91). The role of the surgical procedure in bolstering the sensitivity of the postoperative management techniques is particularly important in evaluating patients with follicular thyroid carcinoma, which not infrequently metastasizes by the hematogenous route. The recurrence rate of follicular thyroid carcinoma may not be significantly affected, however, by bilateral rather than by unilateral surgical procedures (92).

During the surgical procedure the lymph nodes of the tracheoesophageal groove are palpated. Those on the side of the tumor are biopsied. If these nodes are positive, then a modified neck dissection is performed. In addition, lymph nodes in the supraclavicular area are palpated and, if enlarged, these are also biopsied.

Another controversial aspect of the treatment of papillary thyroid carcinoma is the use of radioiodine ablation of the postoperative normal thyroid remnant. There appears to be substantial agreement that [131]-iodine treatment of tumors smaller than 1.5 cm does not reduce the rate of tumor recurrence (93). One large series strongly suggests decreased tumor recurrence and decreased mortality in [131]-iodine treated patients (94); another does not demonstrate such benefits. The results of a number of studies seem to support the view that total or near-total thyroidectomy reduces the apparent benefit of [131]-iodine ablation (93).

Measurement of serum thyroglobulin levels is a cornerstone of postoperative monitoring. Presently, thyroglobulin is usually measured with immunoradiometric assays. Approximately 15% of patients with thyroid cancer have antibodies directed against thyroglobulin. These antibodies may interfere with thyroglobulin measurement, often resulting in underestimation of thyroglobulin levels (95). Patients with thyroglobulin antibodies might be studied using a PCR-based assay for thyroglobulin mRNA. This assay is not subject to erroneous readings as a result of antibodies being present in the circulation (96).

Withdrawal of thyroid hormone replacement allows detection of thyroglobulin in almost all patients with tumor in lymph nodes and in distant sites (95). Measurement of thyroglobulin postoperatively or following withdrawal of thyroid hormone replacement is frequently preceded by 1-T_3 replacement (in doses of approximately 25 μg/1.73 m^2 body surface area three times daily) for 4 weeks. Thereafter, 1-T_3 is withdrawn for a period of 2 weeks. This practice allows 1-T_4 levels to decline gradually (in light of the long T_4 half-life of 1 week) while prolonging TSH suppression by T_3. T_3 has a much shorter half-life (approximately 24 h), allowing robust TSH release over a presumably safer and shorter period of time.

Instead of withdrawing thyroid hormone, patients may be given recombinant TSH by intramuscular injection prior to measurement of thyroglobulin levels. This method obviates the need to produce hypothyroidism (97, 98).

In addition to thyroglobulin measurement, thyroid cancer is monitored by total body scanning employing 1–

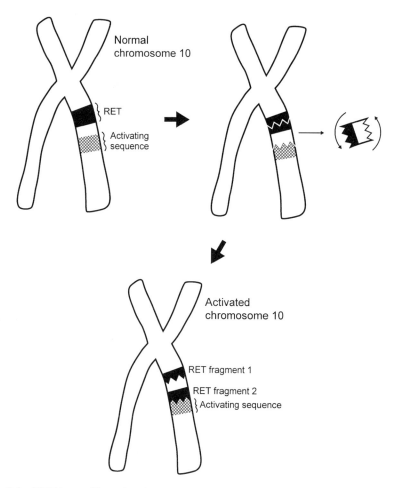

Figure 14 Activation of the RET in papillary thyroid carcinoma results from chromosomal rearrangements involving the 10th chromosome (which contains the RET gene). This diagram shows an inversion of a segment of chromosome 10 resulting in RET activation.

5 mCi [131]-iodine. For adequate scanning sensitivity, TSH levels should be greater than 35 mIU/l. This can be accomplished either by withdrawing patients from thyroid hormone or by injecting them with recombinant TSH. Tumor detected by [131]-iodine scanning and inaccessible to neck surgery may be treatable with radioiodine (99). At times, administration of [131]-iodine for diagnostic scans stuns thyroid tissue, thereby interfering with tumor uptake of therapeutic radioiodine (100). In the future, use of [123]-iodine for diagnostic scanning may be able to avoid this effect. Treatment of tumor detected by thyroglobulin but not by diagnostic scan remains controversial (101, 102).

High-resolution real-time ultrasonography is useful in monitoring patients for tumor recurrence in the neck. Suspicious masses may be aspirated under ultrasound guidance for cytological study. Confirmed tumor may then be surgically removed (84).

Thyroid hormone replacement should be adjusted to suppress TSH (103). Low-risk patients may not require

marked suppression (104). It has therefore, been recommended that high-risk patients have suppression of TSH below 0.1 mIU/l while low risk patients should have TSH levels between 0.1 and 0.4 mIU/l (105).

The outcome of treatment of papillary and follicular thyroid carcinoma in children is generally favorable. Mortality tends to be in the range of 1% at 10 years (6, 106). With more prolonged follow-up, 5–7% of patients may die from thyroid cancer and another group of similar size may die from conditions resulting from treatment of their cancer (106). The patients most likely to die from thyroid cancer seem to be those younger than 10 years of age at the time of diagnosis (5, 107).

Management of medullary thyroid carcinoma in children focuses on detection of inherited disease before appearance of symptoms or signs. In the past, affected family members were detected by provocative tests stimulating calcitonin secretions. Pentagastrin (currently unavailable) and calcium infusion have been used in this

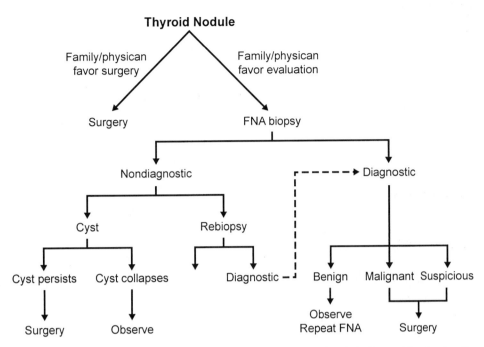

Figure 15 Thyroid nodules in children may be removed surgically if this approach is favored by the family or the physician. Otherwise, fine-needle aspiration (FNA) is the most cost-effective test to guide further evaluation and treatment.

setting (15, 108). Formed medullary thyroid carcinoma may be detected in children with MEN 2 as early as 2 to 3 years of age (15, 109). The need to perform surgery early in these patients is highlighted by the finding of lymph node metastases of medullary thyroid cancer in children as young as 5 years of age (110, 111). These reports suggest that thyroid surgery should be performed in RET-positive children by 5 years of age and perhaps as early as 2 years of age.

Because of the possibility of pheochromocytoma in MEN 2 patients, all should undergo appropriate measurement of serum and urine catecholamines and catecholamine metabolite studies. Additionally, patients who may have MEN 2A should have studies of calcium since hyperparathyroidism can be treated at the same time that thyroidectomy is being performed. Preoperative calcitonin levels should be measured.

There is general agreement that patients with medullary thyroid carcinoma should undergo total thyroidectomy. Patients with familial disease have bilateral multifocal tumors. Similar multifocal disease may be found in 5–30% of patients with apparently sporadic medullary thyroid cancer (110, 112).

If serum calcitonin levels remain elevated postoperatively, physical examination and neck ultrasonography may reveal persistent cervical lymph node metastases that should be surgically excised. Aggressive surgical therapy of patients without obvious disease in the neck, mediastinum, liver, or lungs may render approximately 30% of postoperation hypercalcitonemic patients normocalcito-

nemic with a follow-up of approximately 6 years (113). A more conservative approach to such patients has been advocated by others in view of their 10-year survival rate of 86% (114).

REFERENCES

1. Fukunaga FH, Yatani R. Geographical pathology of occult thyroid carcinomas. Cancer 1975;36:1095–1099.
2. Harach HR, Franssila KO, Wasenius V-M. Occult papillary carcinoma of the thyroid: a "normal" findings in Finland. A systematic autopsy study. Cancer 1985;558:715–719.
3. Franssila KO, Harach H. Occult papillary carcinoma of the thyroid in children and young adults: a systematic autopsy study in Finland. Cancer 1985;56:531–538.
4. Parkin DM, Muir C, Whelan SL, Gao Y-T, Ferhy J, Powell J. Cancer incidence in five continents. IARC Sci Publ 1992;1(120).
5. Harach HR, Williams ED. Childhood thyroid cancer in England and Wales. Br J Cancer 1995;72:777–783.
6. Zimmerman D, Hay IH, Gough IR, Goellner JR, et al. Papillary thyroid carcinoma in children and adults: long-term follow-up of 1039 patients conservatively treated at one institution during three decades. Surgery 1988;104:1157–1166.
7. Ezaki H, Ebihara S, Fujimoto Y, et al. Analysis of thyroid carcinoma based on material registered in Japan during 1977–1986 with special reference to predominance of papillary type. Cancer 1992;70:808–814.
8. Franceschi S, Boyle P, Maisonneuve P, et al. The epidemiology of thyroid carcinoma. Crit Rev Oncogen 1993;4:25–52.

9. Zimmerman D, Lo CY, Hay ID, van Heerden JA, Thompson GB, et al. Thyroid carcinoma in childhood: long-term follow-up of 90 patients treated over 5 decades (submitted).

10. Duffy BJ, Fitzgerald PJ. Thyroid cancer in childhood and adolescence: a report on 28 cases. Cancer 1950;3:1018–1032.

11. Socolow EL, Hashizume A, Nerishi S, Nitani R. Thyroid carcinoma in man after exposure to ionizing radiation. A summary of the findings in Hiroshima and Nagasaki. N Engl J Med 1963;268:406–410.

12. Hamilton TE, van Belle G, LoGerto JP. Thyroid neoplasia in Marshall Islanders exposed to nuclear fallout. JAMA 1987;258:629–636.

13. Ron E, Lubin JH, Shore RE, et al. Thyroid cancer after exposure to external radiation: a pooled analysis of seven studies. Radiat Res 1995;141:259–277.

14. Bauerstock K, Egloff B, Pinchera A, Ruchti C, Williams D. Thyroid cancer after Chernobyl. Nature 1992;359:21–22.

15. Langsteger W, Koltringer P, Wolf G, et al. The impact of geographical, clinical, dietary and radiation-induced features in epidemiology of thyroid cancer. Eur J Cancer 1993;29A:1547–1553.

16. Telander RL, Zimmerman D, Sizemore GW, et al. Medullary carcinoma in children. Arch Surg 1989;124:841–843.

17. Ponder BAJ, Finer N, Coffey R, et al. Family screening in medullary thyroid carcinoma presenting without a family history. QJ Med 1988;67:299–308.

18. Malchoff CD, Malchoff DM. Familial non-medullary thyroid carcinoma. Semin Surg Oncol 1999;16:16–18.

19. Canzlan F, Amati P, Harach R, et al. A gene predisposing to familial thyroid tumors with cell oxyphilia maps to chromosome 19p 13.2. Am J Hum Genet 1998;63:1743–1748.

20. LeSueur F, Stark M, Toreo T, et al: Genetic heterogeneity in familial non-medullary thyroid carcinoma: exclusion of linkage to RET, MNG1, and TCO in 56 families. J Clin Endocrinol Metab 1999;84:2157–2162.

21. Bignell GR, Canzian F, Shayeshi M, et al. Familial non-toxic multinodular goiter locus maps to chromosome 14q, but does not account for familial non-medullary thyroid cancer. Am J Hum Genet 1997;61:1123–1130.

22. Harach HR, Williams GT, Williams ED. Familial adenomatous polyposis associated thyroid carcinoma: a distinct type of follicular cell neoplasm. Histopathology 1994;25:549–561.

23. Bulow S. Papillary thyroid carcinoma in Danish patients with familial adenomatous polyposis. Int J Colorect Dis 1988;3:29–31.

24. Cetta F, Toti P, Petracci M, et al. Thyroid carcinoma associated with familial adenomatous polyposis. Histopathology 1997;31:231–236.

25. van der Linde K, Vasen HFA, van Vliet ACM. Occurrence of thyroid carcinoma in Dutch patients with familial adenomatous polyposis. An epidemiologic study and report of new cases. Eur J Gastroenterol Hepatol 1998;10:777–781.

26. Giardiello FM, Offerhaus GJA, Lee DH, et al. Increased risk of thyroid and pancreatic carcinoma in familial adenomatous polyposis. Gut 1993;217:101–108.

27. Perrier ND, van Heerden JA, Goellner JR, et al. Thyroid cancer in patients with familial adenomatous polyposis. World J Surg 1998;22:738–742.

28. Marsh DJ, Coulon V, Lunetta KL, et al. Mutation spectrum and genotype-phenotype analyses in Cowden Disease and Bannayan-Zonana syndrome, two hamartoma syndromes with germline PTEN mutation. Hum Mol Genet 1998;7:507–515.

29. Perriard J, Saurat J-H, Harms M. An overlap of Cowden's Disease and Bannayan-Riley-Ruvalcaba syndrome in the same family. J Am Acad Dermatol 2000;42:348–350.

30. Stratakis CA, Courcoutsakis NA, Abati A, et al. Thyroid gland abnormalities in patients with the syndrome of spotty skin pigmentation, myxomas, endocrine overactivity, and Schwannomas (Carney complex). J Clin Endocrinol Metab 1997;82:2037–2043.

31. Oertel JE, LiVolsi VA. Pathology of thyroid diseases. In: Ingvar FH, Braverman LE, eds. Werner's The thyroid. A Fundamental and Clinical Text, 5th ed. Philadelphia: J. B. Lippincott, 1986:651–686.

32. Winship T, Rosvoll RV. Thyroid carcinoma in childhood: final report on a 20-year study. Clin Proc Child Hosp DC 1970;26:327–349.

33. Carcangiu ML, Bianci S. Diffuse sclerosing variant of papillary thyroid carcinoma: clinico-pathologic study of 15 cases. Am J Surg Pathol 1989;13:1041.

34. Katoh R, Sasaki J, Kurihara N, Suzuki K, Iida Y, Kawaoi A. Multiple thyroid involvement (intraglandular metastasis) in papillary thyroid carcinoma: a clinico-pathologic study of 105 consecutive patients. Cancer 1992;70:1585–1590.

35. Carcangiu ML, Zampi G, Rosai J. Poorly differentiated "insular" thyroid carcinoma. A reinterpretation of Langhans "wuchernde struma." Am J Surg Pathol 1984;8:655–668.

36. Durbec P, Marcos-Guitierrez CV, Kilkomy C, et al. Glial cell line-derived neurotrophic factor signaling through the RET receptor tyrosine kinase. Nature 1995;381:789–793.

37. Buj-Bello A, Adu J, Pinon LGP, et al. Neurturin responsiveness requires a GP1-linked receptor and the RET receptor tyrosine kinase. Nature 1997;387:721–724.

38. Enokido Y, de Sauvage F, Hongo J-A, et al. GFα4 and the tyrosine kinase RET form a functional receptor complex for persephin. Curr Biol 1998;8:1019–1022.

39. van Weering DHJ, Bos JL. Signal transduction by the receptor tyrosine kinase RET. Rec Results Cancer Res 1998;154:271–281.

40. Mulligan LM, Kwot JB, Healy CS, et al. Germ-line mutations of the RET proto-oncogene in multiple endocrine neoplasia type 2A. Nature 1993;363:458–460.

41. Donis-Keller H, Dou S, Chi D, et al. Mutations in the RET proto-oncogene are associated with MEN 2A and FMTC. Hum Mol Genet 1993;2:851–856.

42. Eng C, Smith DP, Mulligan LM, et al. Point mutation within the tyrosine kinase domain of the RET proto-oncogene in multiple endocrine neoplasias type 2B and related sporadic tumors. Hum Mol Genet 1994;3:237–241.

43. Asai N, Iwashita T, Matsuyama M, et al. Mechanism of activation of the RET proto-oncogene by multiple endocrine neoplasia 2A mutations. Mol Cell Biol 1995;3:1613–1619.

44. Santoro M, Carlomagno F, Romano A, et al. Germ-line mutations of MEN 2A and MEN 2B activate RET as a dominant transforming gene by different molecular mechanisms. Science 1995;267:381–383.

45. Carlomagno F, Melillo RM, Visconti R, et al. GDNF differentially stimulates RET mutants associated with the multiple endocrine neoplasia type 2 syndrome and Hirschsprung's disease. Endocrinol 1998;139:3613–3619.

46. Taraviras S, Marcos-Guiterrez CV, Durbec P, et al. Signaling by the RET receptor tyrosine kinase and its role in the development of the mammalian enteric nervous system. Development 1999;126:2785–2797.

47. Eng C. The RET proto-oncogene in multiple endocrine neoplasia type 2 and Hirschsprung disease. N Engl J Med 1996;335:943–951.

48. Borst MJ, van Camp JM, Peacock, et al. Mutational analysis of multiple endocrine neoplasia type 2A associated with Hirschsprung disease. Surgery 1995;117:386–389.

49. Lanzi C, Borrello MG, Bongarzone I, et al. Identification of the product of five oncogenic rearranged forms of the RET proto-oncogene in papillary thyroid carcinomas. Oncogene 1992;7:2189–2194.

50. Grieco M, Santoro M, Berlingiori MT, et al. PTC is a novel rearranged form of the RET proto-oncogene and is frequently detected in vivo in human thyroid papillary carcinomas. Cell 1990;60:557–563.

51. Sozzi G, Bongarzone I, Miozzo M, et al. At(10;17) translocation creates the RET/PTC2 chimeric transforming sequence in papillary thyroid carcinoma. Genes Chromosomes Cancer 1994;9:244–250.

52. Santoro M, Dathan NA, Berligiere MT, et al. Molecular characterization of RET/PTC3; a novel rearranged version of the RET proto-oncogene in a human thyroid papillary carcinoma. Oncogene 1994;9:509–516.

53. Fugazzola L, Pierotti MA, Vigano E, et al. Molecular and biochemical analysis of RET/PTC4; a novel oncogenic rearrangement between RET and ELE1 genes in a post-Chernobyl papillary thyroid cancer. Oncogene 1996;13:1093–1097.

54. Klugbauer S, Bemidchik EP, Lengfelder E, Rabes HM. Detection of the novel type of RET rearrangement (PTC5) in thyroid carcinomas after Chernobyl and analysis of the involved RET-fused gene RFG5. Cancer Res 1998;58:198–203.

55. Klugbauer S, Rabes HM. The transcription co-activator HTIF1 and a related protein are fused to the RET receptor tyrosine kinase in childhood papillary thyroid carcinomas. Oncogene 1999;18:4388–4393.

56. Nakata T, Kitamura Y, Shimizu K. Fusion of a novel gene, ELKS to RET due to translocation of t(10;12(q11;p13)) in a papillary thyroid carcinoma. Genes Chromosomes Cancer 1999;25:97–103.

57. Ito T, Seyama T, Iwamoto KS, et al. In vitro irradiation is able to cause RET oncogene rearrangement. Cancer Res 1993;53:2940–2943.

58. Bournacer A, Wicker R, Caillou B, et al. High prevalence of activating RET proto-oncogene rearrangements in thyroid tumor from patients who had received external radiation. Oncogene 1997;15:1263–1273.

59. Pisarchik AV, Ermak G, Demidchik EP, et al. Low prevalence of the RET/PTC3rl rearrangement in a series of papillary thyroid carcinomas presenting in Belarus ten years post-Chernobyl. Thyroid 1998;8:1003–1008.

60. Chen BK, Ohtsuki Y, Furihata M, et al. Overexpression of C-met protein in human thyroid tumors correlated with lymph node metastasis and clinical pathological stage. Pathol Res Pract 1999;195:427–433.

61. Pierotti MA, Vigneri P, Bongarzone I. Rearrangements of RET and NTRK-1 tyrosine kinase receptors in papillary thyroid carcinomas. Rec Results Cancer Res 1998;154:237–247.

62. Mancini A, Rabitti C, Conte G, et al. Lymphocytic infiltration in thyroid neoplasms. Preliminary prognostic assessments. Minerva Chir 1993;48:1283–1288.

63. Kashima K, Yokoyama S, Noguchi S, et al. Chronic thyroiditis as a favorable prognostic factor in papillary thyroid carcinoma. Thyroid 1998;8:197–202.

64. Ju ST, Panka DJ, Cui H, et al. Fas (CD95)/FasL interactions required for programmed cell death after T cell activation. Nature 1995;373:444–448.

65. Mitsiades N, Vassiliki P, Mastorakas G, et al. Fas ligand expression in thyroid carcinomas: a potential mechanism of immune evasion. J Clin Endocrinol Metab 1999;84:2924–2932.

66. Herrmann M, Baunoch DA, Maliarik M, et al. p53 gene alterations in differentiated thyroid cancers. Oncol Res 1995;2:741.

67. Fogelfeld L, Bauer TK, Schneider AB, et al. p53 gene mutations in radiation-induced thyroid cancer. J Clin Endocrinol Metab 1996;81:3039.

68. Bunone G, Vigneri P, Mariani L, et al. Expression of angiogenesis stimulators and inhibitors in human thyroid tumors and correlation with clinical pathologic features. Am J Pathol 1999;155:1967–1976.

69. Fenton C, Patel A, Dinauer C, et al. The expression of vascular endothelial growth factor and the type 1 vascular endothelial growth factor receptor correlate with the size of papillary thyroid carcinoma in children and young adults. Thyroid 2000;10:349–357.

70. Belletti B, Ferraro P, Arra C, et al. Modulation of in vivo growth of thyroid tumor-derived cell lines by sense and antisense vascular endothelial growth factor gene. Oncogene 1999;18:4860–4869.

71. Cetta F, Olschwang S, Petracci M, et al. Genetic alterations in thyroid carcinoma associated with familial adenomatous polyposis: clinical implications and suggestions for early detection. World J Surg 1998;22:1231–1236.

72. Iwama T, Konishi M, Iijima T, et al. Somatic mutation of the APC gene in thyroid carcinoma associated with familial adenomatous polyposis. Jpn J Cancer Res 1999;90:372–376.

73. Liau D, Marsh DJ, Li J, et al. Germ line mutations of the PTEN gene in Cowden disease, an inherited breast and thyroid cancer syndrome. Nat Genet 1997;16:64–67.

74. Marsh DJ, Dahia PL, Coulon V, et al. Allelic imbalance including deletion of PTEN/MMAC1 at the Cowden disease locus on 10q22-23 in hamartomas from patients with Cowden syndrome and germ line PTEN mutation. Genes Chromosomes Cancer 1998;21:61–69.

75. Bruni P, Boccia A, Baldassarra G, et al. PTEN expression is reduced in a subset of sporadic thyroid carcinomas: evidence that PTEN-growth suppressing activity in thyroid cancer cells mediated by p27kip1. Oncogene 2000;19:3146–3155.

76. Kirschner LS, Carney JA, Pack SD, et al. Mutations of the gene encoding the protein kinase A type 1-alpha regulatory subunit in patients with the Carney complex. Nat Genet 2000;26:89–99.

77. Samuel AM, Sharma SM. Differentiated thyroid carcinomas in children and adolescents. Cancer 1991;67:2186–2190.

78. Raab SS, Silverman JF, Elsheikh TM, et al. Pediatric thyroid nodule: disease demographics and clinical management as determined by fine-needle aspiration biopsy. Pediatrics 1995;95:46–49.

79. Hung W, Anderson KD, Chandra RS, et al. Solitary thyroid nodules in 71 children and adolescents. J Pediatr Surg 1992;27:1407–1409.

80. Khurana KK, Labrador E, Izquierd R, et al. The role of fine-needle aspiration biopsy in the management of thy-

roid nodules in children, adolescents, and young adults: a multi-institutional study. Thyroid 1999;9:383–386.

81. Gharib H. Changing concepts in the diagnosis and management of thyroid nodules. Endocrinol Metab Clin North Am 1997;26:777–800.

82. Gharib H, Zimmerman D, Goellner JR, et al. Fine-needle aspiration biopsy: use in diagnosis and management of pediatric thyroid diseases. Endocrine Pract 1995;1:9–13.

83. Flannery TK, Kirkland JL, Copeland KC, et al. Papillary thyroid cancer: a pediatric perspective. Pediatrics 1996; 96:464–466.

84. Haber RS. Role of ultrasonography in the diagnosis and management of thyroid cancer. Endocr Prac 2000;6:396–400.

85. Grant CS, Hay ID, Gough IR, et al. Local recurrence in papillary thyroid carcinoma: is extent of surgical resection important? Surgery 1988;104:954–962.

86. Hay ID, Grant CS, Taylor WF, McConahey WM. Ipsilateral lobectomy versus bilateral lobar resection in papillary thyroid carcinoma: a retrospective analysis of surgical outcome using a novel prognostic scoring system. Surgery 1987;102:1088–1095.

87. Hay ID, Grant CS, Bergstralh EJ, et al. Unilateral total lobectomy: is it sufficient surgical treatment for patients with AMES low-risk papillary thyroid carcinoma? Surgery 1998;124:958–964.

88. Zimmerman D, Hay ID, Bergstralh EJ. Papillary thyroid carcinoma in children. In: Robbins J, ed. Treatment of Thyroid Cancer in Childhood. Washington, D.C.: U.S. Department of Energy, 1994:3–10.

89. Welch-Dinauer CA, Tuttle RM, Robie DK, McClellan DR, Francis GL. Extensive surgery improves recurrence-free survival for children and young patients with class 1 papillary thyroid carcinoma. Pediatr Surg 1999;34:1799–1804.

90. Newman KD, Black T, Heller G, et al. Differentiated thyroid cancer: determinants of disease progression in patients less than 21 years of age at diagnosis. A report from the surgical discipline committee of the children's cancer group. Ann Surg 1998;227:533–541.

91. Patwardhan N, Cataldo T, Braverman LE. Surgical management of the patient with papillary cancer. Surg Clin North Am 1995;75:449–464.

92. Taylor T, Specker B, Robbins J, et al. Outcome after treatment of high-risk papillary and non-Hürthlecell follicular thyroid carcinoma. Ann Intern Med 1998;129:622–627.

93. Schlumberger M, Hay ID. Use of radioactive iodine in patients with papillary and follicular thyroid cancer: towards an elective approach. J Clin Endocrinol Metab 1998;83:4201–4203.

94. Mazzaferri EL, Jhiang SM. Long-term impact of initial surgical and medical therapy on papillary and follicular thyroid cancer. Am J Med 1994;97:418–428.

95. Schlumberger M, Baudin E. Serum thyroglobulin determination in the follow-up of patients with differentiated thyroid carcinoma. Eur J Endocrinol 1998;138:249–252.

96. Ditkoff BA, Marvin MR, Yemul S, et al. Detection of circulating thyroid cells in peripheral blood. Surgery 1996;120:959–965.

97. Haugen Pacini F, Reiners C, et al. A comparison of recombinant human thyrotropin and thyroid hormone withdrawal for the detection of thyroid remnant or cancer. J Clin Endocrinol Metab 1999;84:3877–3885.

98. Davies TF. Analysis of the results of phase III controlled clinical trials with recombinant human thyrotropin: developing a clinical guide. Endocr Prac 2000;6:391–395.

99. Samuel AM, Rajashekharrao B, Shah DH. Pulmonary metastases in children and adolescents with well-differentiated thyroid cancer. Radiother Oncol 1994;31:207–212.

100. Park HM, Perkins OW, Edmonson JW, Schaute RB, Manatunga A. Influence of diagnostic radioiodine on the uptake of ablative doses of iodine-131. Thyroid 1994;4:49–54.

101. Wartofsky L, Sherman SI, Gopal J, et al. Management of patients with scan-negative, thyroglobulin-positive thyroid carcinoma. J Clin Endocrinol Metab 1998;83:4195–4200.

102. Hurley JR. Management of thyroid cancer: radioiodine ablation, "stunning," and treatment of thyroglobulin-positive, ^{131}I scan-negative patients. Endocr Prac 6:401–406.

103. Pujol P, Daunes JP, Nsalaka N, et al. Degree of thyrotropin suppression as a prognostic determinant in differentiated thyroid cancer. J Clin Endocrinol Metab 1996;81:4318–4323.

104. Cooper DS, Specker B, Ho M, et al. Thyrotropin suppression and disease progression in patients with differentiated thyroid cancer: results from the National Thyroid Cancer Treatment Cooperative Registry. Thyroid 1998;8:737–744.

105. Hay ID, Feld S, Garcia M, et al. AACE clinical practice guidelines for the management of thyroid carcinoma. Endo Pract 1997;3:60–71.

106. Vassilipoulov-Sellin R, Goepfert H, Schultz RB. Differentiated thyroid cancer in children and adolescents: clinical outcome and mortality after long-term follow-up. Head Neck 1998;20:549–555.

107. Travagli JP, Schlumberger M, de Vathaire F, Francese C, Parmentier C. Differentiated thyroid carcinoma in children. J Endocrinol Invest 1995;18:161–164.

108. Giuffrida D, Gharib H. Current diagnosis and management of medullary thyroid carcinoma. Ann Oncol 1998; 9:695–701.

109. van Heurn LWE, Schaap C, Sie G, et al. Predictive DNA testing for multiple endocrine neoplasia 2: a therapeutic challenge of prophylactic thyroidectomy in very young children. J Pediatr Surg 1999;34:568–571.

110. Jones BA, Sisson JC. Early diagnosis and thyroidectomy in multiple endocrine neoplasia type 2b. J Pediatr 1983; 102:219–223.

111. Gill JR, Reyes Mugica M, Iyongar S, et al. Early presentation of metastatic medullary carcinoma in multiple endocrine neoplasia type 2A: implications of therapy. J Pediatr 1996;129:459–464.

112. Evans DB, Fleming JB, Lee JE, Cote G, Gagel RF. The surgical treatment of medullary thyroid carcinoma. Semin Surg Oncol 1999;16:50–63.

113. Tissell LE, Dilley WG, Wells SA Jr. Progression of postoperative residual medullary thyroid carcinoma as monitored by plasma calcitonin levels. Surgery 1996;119:34–39.

114. van Heerden JA, Grant CS, Gharib H, et al. Long-term course of patients with persistent hypercalcitonemia after apparent curative primary surgery for medullary thyroid carcinoma. Ann Surg 1990;212:395–400.

19

Hypoparathyroidism and Mineral Homeostasis

Jaakko Perheentupa

University of Helsinki, Helsinki, Finland

I. INTRODUCTION

Starting with an outline of the basic physiology of mineral homeostasis, this chapter discusses the disease states involving deficient parathyroid hormone (PTH) effect, hypoparathyroidism in the wide sense of the word. Commonly, the name hypoparathyroidism (HP) is limited to meaning deficient secretion of PTH, while defects in the effector mechanism of PTH are collectively called pseudo-HP (PHP). Causes are many, both inborn and acquired, and several of them are not well understood. Delay in the recognition of these disorders may lead to permanent brain damage or even death. Effective therapy is available. It is not, however, a real substitution therapy but employs calciferol sterols, which lack the renal effects of PTH and are potentially toxic. Hence, the therapy needs to be carefully monitored.

II. PHYSIOLOGICAL BACKGROUND: THE PARATHYROID GLANDS AND HORMONES

The homeostasis of calcium (Ca^{2+}) and inorganic phosphate (Pi) ion concentrations in the extracellular fluid (1) is maintained by an integrated regulation of their absorption from the intestine, reabsorption from the glomerular filtrate, and movement into and out of the skeleton. The parathyroid glands (PTG) are the regulatory center that controls tightly the concentration of Ca^{2+} in the extracellular fluid (Fig. 1); its function is adjusted by the Ca^{2+}-sensing receptors present on the surface of its cells. The action of PTG is directly mediated by PTH and indirectly via the steroid hormone calcitriol. Also, extracellular concentrations of the minerals exert direct short-loop feedback effects on the rate of their reabsorption in the kidney tubules and the production of calcitriol.

Most people have four PTGs, with an average total weight of 120 mg in the adult. The lower pair arise in association with thymus from the third branchial pouch and migrate caudally to separate from the thymus at the 18 mm embryo stage. They assume a variable final location, commonly at the lower pole of the thyroid gland but sometimes mediastinally even at the level of the pericardium. The upper pair derive from the more caudal fourth branchial pouch and remain stationary with final location at the upper pole of the thyroid. Chief cells, the major cells of the glands, are arranged in cords and sheets. These cells regulate plasma Ca^{2+} concentration on a minute-to-minute basis by rapidly adjusting their secretion of stored PTH in response to changes in that concentration; synthesize, process, and store large amounts of PTH in a regulated manner; and replicate in response to a chronic hypocalcemia.

The actions of the PTH are stimulation of renal production of calcitriol, which increases intestinal absorption of Ca and Pi; stimulation of Ca reabsorption and inhibition of Pi reabsorption from renal tubules; and stimulation of osteoclastic bone resorption and release of Ca and Pi ions from the skeleton (Fig. 1).

The gene for PTH, located in chromosome 11p15, consists of three exons and two introns encoding pre-pro-PTH of 115 amino acids including a 25-residue signal so-called pre sequence, and a 6-residue pro sequence (2–3). These sequences direct the protein into the secretory pathway. The prehormone is cleaved during posttranslational processing to a 90 amino acid pro-PTH and then to the 84 amino acid mature PTH (1). This PTH is stored in secretory granules. It is secreted with chromogranin A, which may behave as autocrine or paracrine regulator of PTH release (1). As a regulatory mechanism, a portion of the PTH is inactivated by proteases within the secretory granules and secreted as carboxy-terminal fragments (4). Several polymorphisms of the PTH gene have been reported, which allow linkage studies (5–7).

PTH_{1-34} possesses the full adenylyl cyclase stimulating activity of the hormone, residues 1 and 2 being nec-

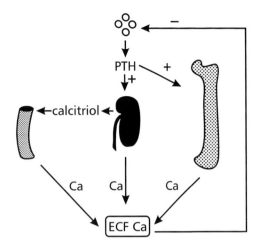

Figure 1 Calcium homeostasis. The parathyroid glands control the extracellular fluid Ca^{2+} concentration by regulating the flux of Ca from the kidneys and skeleton and, through adjusting the production of calcitriol by the kidneys, from the intestine. This control is mediated by PTH; its secretion is regulated trough feedback by ECF Ca^{2+} concentration.

essary for this potency, and residues 10–34 for binding to a specific cell membrane receptor (8). A PTH molecule lacking residues 1 and 2 is a competitive inhibitor of the hormone in vitro, lacking the biological potency but retaining the full receptor-binding activity.

PTH-related peptide (PTHrP), a polyhormone produced by PTG, is similar to PTH in its amino terminus, which in both peptides comprises the receptor-activating domain, accounting for the binding of both peptides to the receptor shared by them, the PTH/PTHrP receptor. PTHrP is the precursor of multiple biologically active peptides, which are of vital importance during the organogenesis. An amino-terminal peptide PTHrP$_{1-36}$ with its PTH-like domain can activate the PTH/PTHrP receptor fully and produce all the classic actions of PTH. Midregion PTHrP peptides stimulate placental Ca transport, presumably through a specific receptor. Carboxy-terminal fragments inhibit bone resorption and stimulate osteoblast growth. PTHrP acts as a calciotropic hormone during fetal life and lactation. PTHrP secreted by fetal PTG stimulates placental transport of Ca in the sheep (9), whereas PTH has no such effect. PTHrP may be the signal responsible for the adaptation of maternal Ca metabolism to the stress of lactation (10). Hypoparathyroid mothers can maintain normocalcemia during lactation. Large amounts of PTHrP are secreted in milk, but its role in milk is unknown. Also, PTHrP may delay the differentiation of growth plate chondrocytes and allow them to proliferate and form orderly columns of cells (11). Various PTHrP peptides are responsible for many different local functions in diverse tissues and through several receptors, while PTH uses the shared receptor to regulate the systemic homeostasis of

Ca^{2+}. Otherwise, only in hypercalcemia of malignancy enough of PTHrP reaches circulation to produce systemic effects (12).

A. The Ca^{2+}-Sensing Receptor

At normal extracellular Ca^{2+} levels PTH is synthesized at a nearly maximal rate, and changing Ca^{2+} concentration has no rapid effects on PTH mRNA expression. The primary control of availability of PTH probably works via the effect of Ca^{2+} on PTH secretion and degradation. At high Ca^{2+} levels a smaller proportion of the secretion of PTG is intact PTH and a larger proportion PTH fragments.

Both positive and negative regulatory elements exist in the 5' flanking region of the PTH gene (3). Cytoplasmic levels of prepro-PTH mRNA may be directly regulated by Ca^{2+}; probably Ca^{2+} modifies the PTH gene transcription. Calcitriol is also a potent downregulator of the expression of the gene. Normal extracellular concentration of Mg^{2+} (8) is a prerequisite of normal PTH secretion: both hypermagnesemia and hypomagnesemia inhibit it. Persons with low borderline plasma Mg^{2+} concentration recover slower from induced reduction of plasma Ca^{2+} than persons with high normal plasma Mg^{2+} (13).

The extracellular Ca^{2+} concentration is monitored by Ca^{2+}-sensing receptors (CaRs) that are plentiful on the surface of the chief cells of the parathyroid glands, and are also present in the kidneys in the juxtaglomerular apparatus, along the luminal surface of the proximal convoluted tubule, the basolateral surface of the cortical thick ascending limb of the loop of Henle, and the apical and luminal membrane of the inner medullary collecting duct (14), in the intestine (15), parts of the brain (16), the thyroid C cells, breast, and the adrenal glands (17). The human 1078 amino acid protein, encoded by CaR gene in chromosome 3q13, consists of three structural regions: a large amino terminal extracellular domain that contains clusters of acidic amino acids thought to be involved in binding of Ca^{2+}, seven transmembrane helices characteristic of the G protein-coupled receptors, and a cytoplasmic carboxy terminal domain. Once activated by Ca^{2+}, the CaR activates phospholipase C through a G protein. Through intracellular accumulation of inositol triphosphate and, secondarily, Ca^{2+}, this activation leads to inhibition of the secretion and synthesis of PTH, and activation of its proteolysis. The receptor lacks specificity: it is also stimulated by other divalent cations, most importantly Mg^{2+}.

B. Regulation of PTH Synthesis and Secretion

There is an inverse sigmoidal relationship between extracellular Ca^{2+} concentration and the release of intact PTH, with the normal set point (the 50% response) at approximately 1.25 mmol/l (Fig. 2). The chief cells of the PTG are exquisitely sensitive to small fluctuations in extracel-

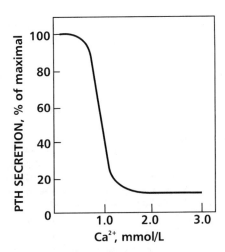

Figure 2 ECF Ca^{2+} concentration determines the secretory rate of PTH following a sigmoidal dose–response curve. The normal level of the ECF Ca^{2+} concentration corresponds approximately to the midpoint of the slope. The minimum secretory rate is not zero. (From Ref. 19.)

lular Ca^{2+} concentration (18, 19) signaled by their CaRs (17). When extracellular Ca^{2+} concentration decreases below the system set point, the secretion of preformed PTH is stimulated in seconds to minutes. In addition to decreases in the intracellular concentrations of inositol triphosphate and Ca^{2+}, increased production of cAMP is also involved. PTG adenylyl cyclase has an absolute requirement for Mg^{2+}, is stimulated by low Ca^{2+} concentration, and has a sensitivity to inhibition by high Ca^{2+} concentrations some 100–200-fold higher than this enzyme in other cell types. If the extracellular Ca^{2+} concentration is not corrected, the PTH gene expression increases in hours. Chronic hypocalcemia leads to an increase in the number of the chief cells and the size of PTG. Conversely, increased extracellular Ca^{2+} concentration inhibits the secretion and synthesis of PTH, and activates the proteolysis of PTH. These cause a rapid decrease in the release of intact PTH. A Ca^{2+} independent, nonsuppressible baseline component of PTH secretion is also present.

Newborn infants under 3 days of postnatal age have poorer PTH secretory responses to hypocalcemia than older infants. Postnatal age here has a dominant effect over gestational age (20).

C. Parathyroid Hormone in the Circulation

After being released from the PTG, PTH has a half-life in the circulation of 2 min. This means that the plasma level is determined by the rate of secretion, and responds rapidly to changes in it. PTH is cleared by the hepatic Kupffer's cells and the kidneys. Its carboxy-terminal fragments released circulate longer, mainly because they are cleared exclusively by glomerular filtration. Hence, most of the immunoreactive PTH in the plasma is a mixture of

carboxyterminal fragments. In normocalcemia, the proportions of the intact PTH, its active aminoterminal fragment, and its inactive carboxyterminal fragments in plasma are approximately 10%, 10%, and 80% (1). At low extracellular Ca^{2+} levels large quantities of the intact hormone are secreted, and at high levels more of the carboxyterminal fragments are secreted.

D. Cellular Mechanism of Parathyroid Hormone Action

The regulation of mineral ion homeostasis by PTH is mediated mainly through the PTH/PTHrP receptor present in the kidney, intestine, skeleton and cartilage, aorta, adrenal gland, urinary bladder, brain, and the skeletal muscles. It acts through three distinct second messenger pathways (Fig. 3).

The PTH/PTHrP receptor gene is located in chromosome 3p22–p21.1. The receptor is a 585-amino acid membrane-bound protein with seven transmembrane domains (27, 28). It has a striking homology with the receptors of calcitonin and secretin, and lacks homology with the other G protein-linked receptors. A PTH-sensitive adenylyl cyclase has been identified in skin fibroblasts, cardiac cells, and vascular smooth muscle. PTH may regulate cytosolic Ca^{2+} in those cells (26).

The $G_s\alpha$ subunit is coded for by the *GNAS1* gene located in chromosome 20q13.2. It is a complex gene, comprising at least 17 exons, including three alternative first exons. The $G_s\alpha$ is produced by one of the four major splice variants derived from this gene (21). Two of the splice variants are expressed only from the paternal allele, and one only from the maternal allele (cf. Sec. XV.C.).

A second PTH receptor has been identified (29, 30). It is not expressed in the skeleton and the kidney, and its role remains unclear. PTH_{1-84} binds to a cell surface receptor distinct from the PTH/PTHrP receptor. Such carboxy-terminal fragments stimulate osteoclast formation and activity (31).

III. CALCITRIOL (1,25-DIHYDROXYCALCIFEROL)

Calcitriol increases the intestinal absorption of Ca and Pi and thereby their concentrations in the extracellular fluid; increases bone reabsorption; enhances the capacity of PTH to promote Ca reabsorption in the renal tubuli; is a powerful differentiation factor for committed osteoclast precursors, causing their maturation to form multinucleated cells capable of resorbing bone; suppresses the expression of the PTH gene; and has profound effects unrelated to mineral homeostasis, on the hematopoetic tissues, immune system, skin, and muscles (32).

The inactive prohormone vitamin D_3 or cholecalciferol is formed in sun-exposed skin. A byproduct in the synthesis of cholesterol, 7-dehydrocholesterol, undergoes

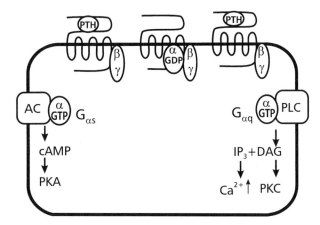

Figure 3 Binding of PTH to the PTH/PTHrP receptor activates three distinct second-messenger pathways (cAMP, inositol 1,4,5-trisphosphate, diacyl glycerol), varyingly in different target cells. Different heterotrimeric (α, β, γ) guanine nucleotide-binding proteins (G proteins) couple the receptor to the effectors. Binding of PTH to the receptor facilitates activation of the G protein, a process in which the α subunit exchanges bound GDP for GTP and dissociates from the $\beta\gamma$ dimer and the receptor. The free, GTP-bound α subunit is the primary modulator of the effector molecules. An intrinsic GTPase activity of the α subunit acts as a molecular timing mechanism: after a predetermined interval, GTP is hydrolyzed to GDP (21). G_s activates adenylyl cyclase leading to production of cAMP, which activates protein kinase A. G_q activates phopholipase C, which hydrolyzes phosphatidyl-inositol 1,4,5-trisphosphate to diacyl glycerol (DAG) and inositol 1,4,5-trisphosphate (IP_3). The DAG activates protein kinase C, and the IP_3 activates a receptor on microsomal vesicles that directs the movement of Ca^{2+} from microsomal vesicles into the cytosol. Also, an inhibitory G protein (G_i) complex, mediating inhibitory signals to the adenylyl cyclase, is present in the epithelial cells of proximal renal tubules (22). The phospholipase C/protein kinase C cascade may be predominant (23) in the actions of PTH on bone remodeling and the Ca reabsorption in the distal renal tubuli (24–26).

photochemical cleavage of the bond between carbons 9 and 10 of the sterol B ring. The resulting previtamin D undergoes a temperature-dependent rearrangement producing the vitamin. In prolonged sunlight alternative inert products are formed, and excessive production of the vitamin is avoided. Both vitamins D_2, from plant sources, and D_3 are also components of food. They are hydroxylated in the liver to 25-(OH)D, a partially active compound, and in the mitochondria of the proximal tubules of the kidney and placenta further to the hormone calcitriol (1,25-$(OH)_2$D) or, alternatively, to 24,25-$(OH)_2$D, which is a less active compound of unclear significance. These hydroxylations in the kidney are the key points in the regulation of the synthesis of calcitriol. Vitamins D_2 and D_3, and their corresponding metabolites, are potent in

humans. Calcitriol acts on the kidneys, skeleton, intestine, and PTG. Also, it regulates the activity of T lymphocytes, and is a growth factor for many types of cells, both normal and tumoral (33).

A. The Production of Calcitriol and Its Regulation

Vitamins D_2 and D_3 are absorbed from the duodenum and jejunum into the lymphatic channels. In states of fat malabsorption this absorption may fail (34–36). Both prohormones are stored in adipose tissue and muscle in amounts depending simply on their intake. Their hydroxylated metabolites are less fat-soluble and less likely to be stored in amounts that may be harmful. Conversion to 25-(OH)D depends directly on the quantity of circulating vitamin D.

The synthesis of the 1- and 24-hydroxylases is regulated reciprocally so that conditions favoring the synthesis of one inhibit the synthesis of the other (37, 38). High PTH concentration, low concentration of calcitriol, and low extracellular concentrations of Pi and/or Ca^{2+} increase the synthesis of 1-hydroxylase, and vice versa. Manipulation of Ca intake within the normal range has a pronounced effect on circulating calcitriol levels by modifying the secretion of PTH (39). Low extracellular concentrations of Pi promote the synthesis of calcitriol, and high concentrations inhibit it. These effects are independent of PTH. In turn, calcitriol stimulates mobilization of Pi from bone and its absorption from the intestine. Thus a plasma phosphate–calcitriol feedback loop exists regulating plasma Pi concentration independently of the Ca^{2+}–PTH–calcitrol loop.

B. Calciferols in Plasma

Normally, the total concentration of D_2 and D_3 in plasma is 2.6–26 nmol/l (1–10 ng/ml), and their half-lives in the circulation are about 24 h. The major circulating form is the 25-(OH)D, with an average plasma concentration of 75 nmol/l and a circulating half-life of about 15 days. Its concentration reflects accurately the vitamin D reserve of the body. Calcitriol circulates at almost 1000-fold lower concentrations (Table 1) with a half-life of 6–8 h (40); 15% is excreted as urinary metabolites and 50% as fecal metabolites. However, the ratio of the active free concentrations of calcitriol and 25-(OH)D is only 1 to 100.

These sterols are bound to albumin and a specific α-globulin, vitamin-D-binding protein (DBP), of which only about 5% is saturated at physiological levels of the sterols. The protein appears also to have a storage function. When bound to this carrier, calcitriol is the most freely dissociable of the group. However, less than 1% of it is unbound, freely diffusible, constituting the active fraction. In general, its concentration remains constant when the DBP levels change.

Table 1 Reference Values for Parameters of Mineral Metabolism

Parameter	mmol/l	mg/dl	Conversion factor
Ca, serum, ionized	1.18–1.30	4.7–5.2	0.25
total	2.20–2.65	8.8–10.6	
Calcitriol, plasma	50–150 pmol/l	20–60 pg/ml	2.40
25(OH)-D, plasma	25–125	10–50 ng/ml	2.50
Mg, serum, newborn	0.75–1.15	1.82–2.80	0.41
child and adult	0.70–1.00	1.70–2.40	
PTH intact, serum (IRMA)	1.1–5.8 pmol/l	10–55 pg/ml	
Pi (as P) serum, newborn	1.40–3.05	4.3–9.4	0.32
1 to 5 months	1.55–2.60	4.8–8.1	
6 to 24 months	1.30–2.20	4.0–6.8	
2 to 3 years	1.16–2.10	3.6–6.5	
prepubertal child	1.16–1.80	3.6–5.6	
puberty	1.07–1.95	3.3–6.0	
after puberty	0.80–1.40	2.5–4.3	
TmP/GFR, newborn	1.30–3.46	4.0–10.7	0.32
3 months	1.30–3.07	4.0–9.5	
6 months	1.30–2.62	4.0–8.2	
child	1.30–2.58	4.0–8.0	
puberty: gradual decrease to adult values			
adult	0.71–1.45	2.2–4.5	

Source: Values for TmP/GRF are from Refs. 52 and 53.

C. Cellular Mechanism of Calcitriol Action

Like other steroid hormones, calcitriol binds in its target cells to a specific cytoplasmic receptor, vitamin D receptor (VDR) (41). It has a high affinity for calcitriol, and lesser affinities for the other homologs such as 25-(OH)D and vitamin D_3. The sterol–receptor complex is translocated to the nucleus where it binds to response elements on specific DNA and activates or suppresses gene transcription. Heterodimerization of the VDR with the retinoid X receptor is essential for its transactivating function (42). The synthesis of several proteins is increased: calbindins, the 25-(OH)D 24-hydroxylase, the VDR itself, the plasma membrane Ca pump, osteocalcin, osteopontin, and others. The synthesis of some other proteins such as PTH, PTHrP, collagen type I and IL-2 is reduced. In addition to genomic actions, calcitriol has rapid nongenomic activities. It increases cytosolic Ca in a number of cell types, including osteoblasts, parathyroid cells, enterocytes and myocytes within seconds to minutes. These are probably carried out by a distinct receptor (32).

The VDR gene, located in chromosome 12q13–14 (43), is a member of the steroid receptor supergene family. The human VDR is a 50 kD protein consisting of 427 aminoacids; its amino terminal 110 residues constitute the DNA-binding domain with two Zn-fingers, and amino acids 150–410 the steroid-binding domain. The receptor is present in a great variety of cells (32).

D. Synthetic Analogs

Two synthetic vitamin D analogs are therapeutically important, 1 α-(OH)D$_3$ and dihydrotachysterol (DHT). These do not need the 1-hydroxylation for activation and are therefore potent in states of reduced 1-hydroxylation activity such as HP. DHT is rapidly hydroxylated to 25-(OH)DHT. 1α-(OH)D$_3$ is similar in potency to the hormone, presumably after 25-hydroxylation in the liver.

IV. THE KIDNEYS

Regulation of urinary excretion plays an important role in the homeostasis of minerals, especially Pi (1). This regulation is mediated by PTH. Also, plasma concentrations of the divalent cations influence their own excretion. The PTG–kidney axis regulates the intestinal absorption of Ca^{2+} and Pi, by determining the rate of synthesis of calcitriol.

A. Mineral Reabsorption and Effects of the Parathyroid Hormone

The mRNA encoding the PTH/PTHrP receptor is expressed in the convoluted and straight proximal tubules, the cortical portion of the thick ascending limb, and the distal convoluted tubules (44, 45). All these segments show cAMP accumulation in response to PTH (46). The responses of other second messengers in the cells of the proximal and distal tubules seem to differ strikingly. The increase in intracellular free Ca^{2+} depends entirely on its release from intracellular stores in the proximal cells, but largely on extracellular Ca^{2+} in the distal cells (47). PTH-dependent renal actions that require the second messengers cAMP, and increases in intracellular free Ca^{2+} and inositol 1,4,5-triphosphate, include the inhibition of the reabsorption of Pi, the stimulation of the 25-(OH)D-1α-hydroxylase, and the reabsorption of Ca^{2+} from the distal convoluted tubules (47, 48) (Fig. 4).

The total rate of Pi excretion is always less than its filtered load, normally 5–20%. Pi is reabsorbed in the proximal tubules by a pH- and Na^+-dependent, active, saturable mechanism involving types I and II Na^+/Pi cotransporter (49, 50). Hence this reabsorption has a maximum rate (TmP). If other factors remain unaltered, increased plasma PTH concentration reduces TmP and decreased concentration enhances it. TmP in turn determines the fasting plasma Pi concentration, which is maintained close to the value of the quotient of TmP and the glomerular filtration rate (TmP/GFR, Fig. 5, Table 1). This quotient is also called the Pi threshold. TmP/GFR is the best laboratory indicator of renal PTH action (51–53). In response to an injection of PTH, an abrupt increase in Pi

excretion occurs within minutes. PTH induces a rapid endocytosis of the type II Na^+/Pi cotransporters, resulting in a reduction of their number at the apical membrane of the proximal tubules, and their degradation (54). Calcitriol may have a permissive role for this effect (55). Lack of PTH results in an increased TmP/GFR and thus an elevated plasma Pi level. PTH likewise reduces the reabsorption of bicarbonate, and in HP plasma bicarbonate levels are often elevated.

The tubular reabsorption of Ca^{2+} and Mg^{2+} is in normal circumstances extremely efficient: only 1–3% of the filtered load is excreted. Reabsorption takes place at multiple sites. Of Ca^{2+} approximately 60–70% is reabsorbed in the proximal tubule, 20% within the thick ascending limb of Henle, 5% in the distal tubule, and 10–15% in the collecting duct. Of Mg^{2+}, only some 20% appears to be reabsorbed in the proximal tubule and 70% within the thick ascending limb of Henle (56). The reabsorption mechanisms are different in the various sections (Fig. 4) (57).

The proximal process is mostly passive, unsaturable, and strongly linked to Na^+ reabsorption. The majority is absorbed through the paracellular pathway by diffusion and solvent drag. A smaller part presumably enters the cells via Ca^{2+} channels of the apical membrane. Most of it is extruded into the extracellular fluid (ECF) through the basolateral membrane by an Na^+/Ca^{2+} exchanger, a carrier protein, that derives its energy from the inwardly directed Na^+ gradient generated by the continuous activity of the Na^+, K^+-ATPase. A small part may be extruded by plasma membrane Ca^{2+}-ATPase pump (58). Factors that enhance the delivery of Na^+ to the distal tubule (high Na^+ intake, furosemide) lead to a decrease in the fractional reabsorption of Ca^{2+} in the proximal tubule. For Mg^{2+}, the proximal reabsorption mechanism is unknown (56).

In the thick ascending limbs of Henle's loop, reabsorption of Ca^{2+} and Mg^{2+} proceeds through both an active, transcellular pathway, and by passive mechanisms through the paracellular pathway. The high transtubular voltage gradient generated by the luminal Na^+/K^+/$2Cl^-$ transporter is important for the reabsorption of Ca^{2+} and Mg^{2+}. Their resting absorption is passive and is driven by the ambient electrochemical gradient for the divalent cations. PTH stimulates their active transcellular absorption in the cortical thick ascending limbs. Vasopressin, through stimulating Na^+ absorption by the Na^+/K^+/$2Cl^-$ cotransporter, causes parallel increases in the absorption of Ca^{2+} and Mg^{2+} by elevating the transepithelial voltage and the driving force for passive absorption. Loop diuretics bumetadine and furosemide, by inhibiting the Na^+/K^+/$2Cl^-$ cotransport, decrease the transpithelial voltage and diminish the absorption of Ca^{2+} and Mg^{2+} with a consequent increase in their excretion (58).

In the distal convoluted tubules Ca^{2+} enters the cells through the Ca^{2+} channels of the apical membrane. Its efflux is presumably mediated by the plasma membrane

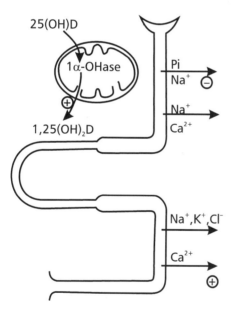

Figure 4 Effects of PTH in the kidney. The three effects are marked + (stimulation) and − (inhibition): inhibition of the reabsorption of phosphate and Na^+ in the proximal tubule; stimulation of the synthesis of 1-hydroxylase in the proximal tubule, and, thereby production of calcitriol (1,25(OH)₂D); and stimulation of reabsorption of Ca^{2+} in the distal tubule. The proximal tubule has a different mechanism for reabsorption of Ca^{2+}; this is associated with the absorption of Na^+ and is not affected by PTH.

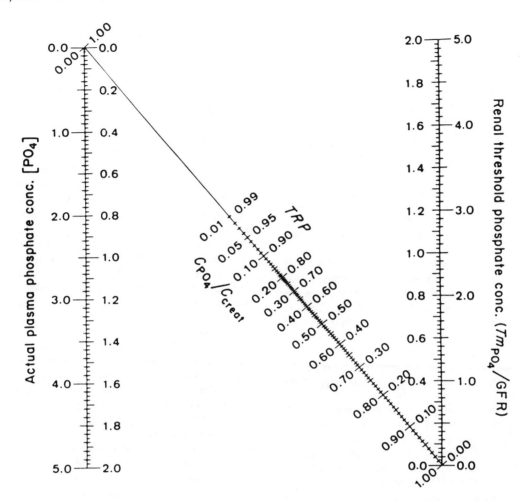

Figure 5 Nomogram for determination of renal threshold Pi concentration, TmP/GFR. TmP/GFR is obtained by drawing a straight line from the serum Pi concentration on the left vertical scale through the value on the lower diagonal scale of the quotient of Pi and creatinine clearances (C_{PO4}/C_{creat}) [calculated as (U-P × S-Cr)/(S-P × U-Cr), where U stands for urine, P for Pi, S for serum, and Cr for creatinine]. The point of intersection of that line and the right vertical scale indicates the value of TmP/GFR. On the vertical scales the outer scales are in mg/100 ml and the inner scales in mmol/l. For reference values see Table 1. (From Ref. 51.)

Ca^{2+}-ATPase pump and an Na^+–Ca^{2+} exchanger. There is no paracellular absorption. This is the major site of the Ca^{2+}-retaining action of PTH. It stimulates the apical entry of Ca^{2+} through the Ca^{2+} channels. This action hyperpolarizes the membrane voltage. These effects of PTH require the activation of both protein kinases A and C . The thiazide diuretics and amiloride stimulate the Ca^{2+} transport and membrane voltage in the distal convoluted tubules similarly to the effects PTH (58).

The distal Ca^{2+} reabsorption mechanism is saturable, independent of Na^+ transport, but dependent on the Ca^{2+}-sensing receptors that are abundant there (59). Saline diuresis (except when induced by thiazide diuretics) is accompanied by an increase in Ca^{2+} excretion, because the distal reabsorptive capacity is overwhelmed by the increased distal delivery of Ca^{2+}. Only the distal reabsorp-

tion is adjusted by PTH (23, 25). Patients with HP, when normocalcemic while taking calciferol medication, excrete about threefold more Ca^+ than normal subjects (25, 64).

B. Effects of Extracellular Ca^{2+} and Mg^{2+}

Extracellular homeostasis of Ca^{2+} is also maintained by a short-loop feedback mechanism involving a direct effect of Ca^{2+} on the nephrons. Ca^{2+}-sensing receptors are present in the basolateral membrane of the tubular cells in the thick ascending limb of the loop of Henle. Activation of these receptors by elevated concentrations of Ca^{2+} (or Mg^{2+}) in the peritubular compartment inhibit the reabsorption of Ca^{2+} and Mg^{2+}, thus increasing the urinary excretion of Ca^{2+}, Mg^{2+}, Na^+, and Cl^- (59). The high transtubular voltage gradient generated by the luminal

$Na^+/K^+/2Cl^-$ transporter is important for the reabsorption of Ca^{2+} and Mg^{2+}. Activation of the apical CaR stimulates phospholipase C, leading to release of arachidonic acid, metabolites of which inhibit the apical K^+ channel and may also inhibit the $Na^+/K^+/2Cl^-$ transporter. This results in a marked reduction of the transluminal voltage, leading to a decrease in the paracellular transport of Ca^{2+} and Mg^{2+}. Activation of the CaRs also inhibits the PTH-stimulated adenylyl cyclase, reducing the cAMP-mediated transport of Ca^{2+} and Mg^{2+}. These actions explain the steep relationship between extracellular Ca^{2+} and urinary Ca excretion. Increased extracellular Ca^{2+} thus leads directly to increased urinary excretion of Ca^{2+}, and vice versa (60). Because CaR is activated by Mg^{2+}, hypermagnesemia leads to a renal loss of Ca^{2+} even during hypocalcemia (61).

The CaRs are also present on the apical and luminal membranes of the inner medullary collecting ducts, where their activation inhibits the vasopressin-mediated increase in water permeability (62). The inhibition of the $Na^+K^+2Cl^-$ cotransporter in the thick ascending limb reduces the medullary hypertonicity and hence the effectiveness of the countercurrent mechanism, thus further reducing the urine concentrating ability (60). This results in dilution of urine, which helps to prevent nephrolithiasis.

The CaRs are also activated by polycationic compounds such as neomycin and gentamicin. This may account for the effects of these drugs on the kidney, including nonoliguric renal failure, perhaps due to impairment of the vasopressin-sensitive renal concentrating mechanism via activation of the CaR of the collecting ducts.

Also, extracellular Ca^{2+} participates in the control of the production of calcitriol by the proximal tubule, independent of PTH. Hypercalcemia reduces this production. This effect is probably mediated by the CaRs.

C. Effects of Calcitriol

Calcitriol suppresses the synthesis of the 1-hydroxylase and induces the synthesis of 24-hydroxylase in the cells of the proximal tubules.

Both PTH and calcitriol are needed for the normal control of the fractional Ca^{2+} excretion (63). Calcitriol seems to have no role in the proximal mechanism of Ca^{2+} absorption. In contrast, all the components of the transport of Ca^{2+} that are genomically regulated by calcitriol are located within the distal segments of the nephron. Their roles appear to be identical here and in the intestine (Sec. VI.).

Calcitriol does not appear to exert a direct influence on TmP, but it has a permissive role in the phosphaturic effect of PTH. When used in the treatment of HP, vitamin D sterols reduce Pi reabsorption from elevated to normal levels. This results largely from an increase in plasma Ca^{2+}, which directly reduces proximal tubular Pi reabsorption. Calcitriol may be involved in the inherent ability

of the nephrons to adapt to altered plasma Pi levels. This adaptability is independent of PTH, but appears to be more efficient in the presence of calcitriol than in its absence (49).

V. THE SKELETON

The skeleton serves as a store of the Ca and Pi ions through two metabolic systems: the homeostatic and the remodeling system. The main regulators of both systems are PTH and calcitriol. Both PTH and calcitriol exert dual actions, which provide a basis for coupling of the bone formation and the bone resorption processes. In the homeostatic system the surface osteocytes alter on a minute-to-minute basis the flux of mineral between the skeletal surface compartment and the extracellular fluid. The remodeling system consists of osteoclasts resorbing old bone and osteoblasts laying down new bone.

PTH activates the adenylyl cyclase and stimulates proliferation in the chondrocytes and chondroprogenitor cells. It stimulates bone formation and increases bone mass. This effect is mediated by the insulin-like growth factors IGF-I and IGF-II, and by TGF β, which are released during osteoclastic bone resorption. PTH binds to osteoblasts that are actively laying down bone matrix, and inhibits synthesis of collagen type I. Also, it inhibits maturation of osteoblast precursors. On the other hand, PTH stimulates bone resorption by increasing the activity and number of osteoclasts. These cells lack receptors of both PTH and calcitriol, and their response to these hormones depends on contact with osteoblasts. In vitro, PTH_{53-84} stimulates glucocorticoid-primed osteoblast alkaline phosphatase activity, and inhibits the mitogenic effect of PTH_{1-34} on mouse cartilage explants. PTH regulates both these systems with calcitriol in a permissive role, especially in the homeostatic system (64). During sustained hypocalcemia these hormones inhibit the osteoblastic bone formation while activating the osteoclasts and increasing their number.

Calcitriol is essential for the development and maintenance of mineralized skeleton. Its major targets are osteoblasts and their precursors: stromal cells and preosteoblasts. It regulates the genes associated with osteoblast proliferation and differentiation, and enhances the expression of the genes that are specific markers of mature osteoblasts. Induction of interleukin-11 by calcitriol appears to mediate its effect on the osteoblastogenesis (65). On the other hand, calcitriol mobilizes Ca stores by inducing the dissolution of bone mineral and matrix (66). It induces bone resorption by enhancing osteoclastogenesis and osteoclast activity. It recruits undifferentiated stem cells in the bone marrow to become osteoclasts. Calcitriol appears to induce release of osteoblast-derived resorption factors that stimulate osteoclast activity (67). For that, osteoclast–osteoblast cell contact is required. Calcitriol apparently induces mineralization simply by maintaining the circulating concentrations of Ca^{2+} and Pi.

The role of 24,25-(OH)2D3 in bone metabolism is controversial.

Modest elevations of plasma concentrations of calcitriol (e.g., to 70 pg/ml) are not associated with hypercalcemia, which only develops with elevations to the range of 125 pg/ml (1).

VI. THE INTESTINE

One of the main functions of calcitriol is to enhance the efficiency of the small intestinal Ca and Pi ion absorption (32, 68). These are absorbed along the entire small intestine, but calcitriol primarily stimulates the Ca^{2+} transport in the duodenum, and the Pi absorption in the jejunum and ileum. The absorption of Ca^{2+} is precisely regulated according to the needs of the body, and calcitriol is the only hormone known to stimulate it directly. PTH is involved only as the regulator of the synthesis of calcitriol. Calcitriol enhances the entry of Ca^{2+} through the plasma membrane into the absorptive cell, its movement through the cytoplasm, and its transfer across the basolateral membrane into the circulation.

Calcitriol regulates the absorption at the brush-border membrane by rapid nongenomic mechanisms. It is presumed to increase the fluidity of the microvillus membrane, which allows Ca^{2+} channels to move to the cell surface and enhance the Ca^{2+} uptake at the membrane. A VDR-mediated induction of various brush-border proteins follows. These include the Ca^{2+}-binding calmodulin, calbindin D_9K, brush-border bound calbindin $D_{28}K$, an integral brush-border protein, and alkaline phosphatase. The calbindins bind Ca^{2+}, because they possess a much greater affinity than the brush-border membrane to the Ca^{2+}. They facilitate the entry of Ca^{2+} by decreasing its concentration adjacent to the brush-border. The calbindins also function as intracellular Ca^{2+} translocators and Ca^{2+}-buffering agents, thus facilitating the intracellular diffusional transfer of Ca^{2+} to the basolateral membrane. When the Ca^{2+}-bound calbindin reaches the basolateral membrane, it releases the Ca^{2+} to the plasma membrane Ca^{2+} pump, which has an even greater affinity to the Ca^{2+}. The Ca^{2+} must be pumped into the extracellular fluid against an electrochemical gradient by an energy-requiring, Na^+-dependent process. Calcitriol stimulates the expression of the plasma membrane Ca^{2+} pump and the Na^+/Ca^{2+} exchanger. Calmodulin and calbindin stimulate the activity of the Ca^{2+} pump. Also, activation of the Ca^{2+}-channels appears to be important for the extrusion of the Ca^{2+} from the basolateral membrane into the general circulation.

Calcitriol also increases active Pi transport. This is independent of the Ca^{2+} transport and less dependent on calcitriol. In the absence of calcitriol, Pi is absorbed at half-normal rate. Na^+ is required at the brush-border surface, and an Na^+/Pi cotransporter moves luminal Pi uphill into the cell, using the energy from the downhill Na^+ gradient. Calcitriol appears to stimulate Pi transport by inducing the synthesis of additional cotransporter units and by decreasing the permeability of the brush-border membrane to Na^+, thus helping to maintain the gradient required for the uphill Pi transport.

Net Ca^{2+} absorption normally averages about 20% of the Ca^{2+} intake, but can vary over the range of 15–75%, depending on the calcitriol status. The absorption of Pi and Mg^{2+} is a linear function of their dietary intake (69). Both are absorbed predominantly by (separate) active carrier-mediated transport mechanisms, and by passive diffusion. The proportion absorbed is about 3fold larger for Pi than for Ca^{2+}.

VII. CALCIUM, PHOSPHATE, AND MAGNESIUM IN PLASMA

A. Calcium

The total content of Ca in normal human plasma (Table 1) consists of three fractions: approximately 47% is free Ca^{2+}, another 47% is protein-bound (70% of it being bound to albumin), and 6% is complexed to phosphate, citrate, and bicarbonate, and freely diffusible through membranes. The free Ca^{2+} is the regulated, physiologically important fraction.

The regulation of the plasma Ca^{2+} concentration is so precise that it normally fluctuates by less than 0.025 mmol/l (0.1 mg/dl) in either direction from its so-called set value. The skeletal and renal effects of PTH make up a fast-acting short-loop feedback system. The renal–intestinal effect provides a slower (12–24 h) long-loop feedback system (1).

The binding to albumin is pH-dependent: the concentration of Ca^{2+} decreases in acute alkalosis and increases in acute acidosis. If plasma albumin concentration decreases by 50%, the total Ca concentration is reduced by about 20%. Also, for every 10 g/l (g/dl) reduction in plasma albumin, the total Ca decreases by approximately 0.25 mmol/l (1.0 mg/dl). These changes as such do not alter the Ca^{2+} concentration. Total Ca varies little with age, the actual extent depending on the protein concentration.

A decrease in the concentration of Ca^{2+} increases Na^+ permeability and enhances the excitability of all excitable cells. An increased concentration has the reverse effect.

Hypocalcemic challenges are of varying severity. A 12–15 h fast is a mild challenge. Because of continued loss of Ca^{2+} loss via the urine, its plasma concentration decreases slightly and is rapidly corrected by increased entry from the kidneys and skeleton, induced by a minor increase in PTH secretion (Fig. 6). A stronger challenge, such as an extra urinary loss of Ca^{2+} after administration of a high dosage of furosemide, calls for a moderate increase in PTH secretion; part of the response is an in-

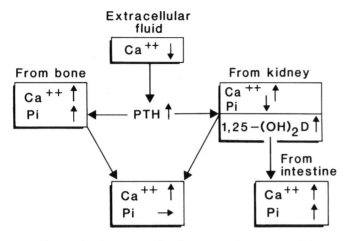

Figure 6 Sequence of adjustments (long arrows) in response to hypocalcemia. The short arrows indicate directions of changes in concentrations in the extracellular fluid (middle), in release from the skeleton (left), in retrieval in the kidneys, and in absorption from the intestine (right).

crease in the synthesis of calcitriol. The increased PTH activity also decreases the renal reabsorption of Pi and this rids the extracellular fluid of the extra Pi. The plasma levels of Ca^{2+} and Pi are thus normalized, but a mild secondary hyperparathyroidism persists, with the improved intestinal absorption of minerals replacing what was initially mobilized from the skeleton.

Hypercalcemia, even a slight rise in plasma Ca^{2+}, is combatted by suppression of the PTH secretion. This leads to an increased urinary loss of Ca^{2+}, and a reduced entry of minerals from the skeleton and, with prolonged hypercalcemia, through suppression of the synthesis of calcitriol, from the intestine. The hypercalcemia raises the concentration of calcitonin in plasma. Calcitonin directly, in minutes, inhibits osteoclastic bone resorption. However, it does not appear to contribute in an important way to the protection against hypercalcemia. A limit to the protection against hypercalcemia is set by the excretory capacity of the kidneys. This may be impaired by a vicious cycle based on the fact that hypercalcemia leads to excessive urinary loss of water and hence tends to cause dehydration.

B. Phosphate

Plasma Pi concentration is more variable than the Ca concentration. It is influenced by age (Table 1), diet, and some hormones. No known endocrine factor protects it as a primary function. An adequate ion-product of Ca^{2+} and Pi is required for normal mineralization of the skeleton. Of the total plasma Pi about 52% is ionized; 35% is complexed to Na^+, Ca^{2+}, and Mg^{2+}; and 13% is protein-bound. The role of the kidneys is paramount in the main-

tenance of a normal plasma Pi level, which tends to be close to TmP/GFR (Sec. IV.A.; Fig. 5).

A decrease in plasma Pi leads to an activation of the renal synthesis of calcitriol and thereby to an increased intestinal absorption of Ca and a slight rise in its plasma level. Suppression of PTH secretion follows, leading to a reduction of the renal Pi clearance and an enhancement of Ca clearance. Within 3–4 days of phosphate withdrawal, its excretion may be virtually abolished and even the phosphaturic response to exogenous PTH becomes blunted. An excess of plasma Pi is cleared rapidly by normal kidneys, because the filtered Pi load exceeds the renal threshold.

C. Magnesium

The plasma concentration is less narrowly regulated for Mg^{2+} than Ca^{2+}. It is determined principally by the renal threshold for Mg excretion. Roughly one-third is protein bound, 15% is loosely complexed with Pi and other anions, and 55% is free Mg^{++}. Extracellular Mg is critical for normal neuromuscular excitability and nerve conduction. The mechanisms of Mg homeostasis are poorly understood. PTG responds similarly to changes in plasma Mg^{++} than to changes in plasma Ca^{2+}, but less sensitively.

VIII. MANIFESTATIONS OF DEFICIENT PARATHYROID HORMONE ACTION

A. Chemical Effects

Deficiency of PTH action leads to a decrease in the production of calcitriol, resulting in a bihormonal deficiency. Hypocalcemia and hyperphosphatemia are pathognomonic to frankly deficient PTH action. The hypocalcemia results from reduced osteocytic Ca transfer due to both deficiencies, a decrease in PTH-dependent osteoclastic bone resorption and distal tubular Ca reabsorption, and impaired intestinal Ca absorption due to calcitriol deficiency. The hyperphosphatemia is caused by increased renal tubular Pi reabsorption due to the absence of its adequate inhibition by PTH. The hyperphosphatemia further lowers calcemia by physicochemical means and by further reducing calcitriol synthesis.

1. Hypocalcemia

Severity of deficiency of PTH action varies. Consequently, plasma Ca concentration in different patients ranges from 1.25 mmol/l (5 mg/dl) to normal (70). In all cases the stability of the plasma Ca level is impaired. It fluctuates with changes in Ca intake and reciprocally with changes in plasma Pi concentration (71). Even in the mildest cases the reserve capacity of the calcemia homeostatic system is limited, but normocalcemia is maintained by its maximal activity. In the next degree of severity normocalcemia is maintained in normal situations, but periodic hypocalcemia ensues with fasting or an otherwise unusually low Ca intake, and with excessive phosphate influx from the intestine, or breakdown of intracellular organic phosphate compounds during febrile illness. With more severe failure, hypocalcemia is continuous and minor hypocalcemic factors evoke symptoms.

Hypocalcemic patients are hypocalciuric, although their Ca excretion is high relative to their plasma Ca level.

2. Hyperphosphatemia

This is a much less constant feature than hypocalcemia, because less PTH effect is needed to maintain a normal renal Pi threshold (Sec. IV.A.) than to maintain normocalcemia (70), and because Pi flow from the skeleton and intestine is subnormal owing to the deficiency of PTH effect.

3. Other

Because deficiency of PTH effect also causes increased renal reabsorption of bicarbonate, plasma bicarbonate levels and blood pH may be elevated (72). Bone remodeling is reduced and this is reflected by decreased urinary excretion of hydroxyproline in a majority of patients (73). Subnormal levels are usual for plasma osteocalcin but uncommon for alkaline phosphatase (73–75).

B. Clinical Manifestations

The main cause of clinical manifestations (76) of deficient PTH effect is hypocalcemia, largely as a result of increased irritability of the central and peripheral nervous systems. Manifestations are more likely to appear when plasma Ca level is falling rapidly than during steady hypocalcemia. Low concentrations of Mg^{2+} and H^+ (alkalosis), and high concentrations of Pi and K^+ predispose to tetany. Moderately longstanding hypocalcemia may be symptomless.

1. Tetany

Tetany refers to a spectrum of manifestations of increased neural excitability. It ranges from signs evocable by testing (latent tetany), and minor tingling sensations and numbness of the hands to abdominal pain and major convulsive seizures with loss of consciousness. A typical attack of tetany (2) begins with increasing tingling starting in the fingertips, around the mouth and sometimes in the feet, and spreading proximally and over the face. Numbness may follow. The muscles then feel tense and go into spasm in the same pattern as the sensory symptoms. The hands and forearms are the parts of the body most commonly involved. First, the thumbs become adducted, followed in order by flexion of the metacarpophalangeal joints, extension of the interphalangeal joints, and flexion of the wrist and elbow: the classic "obstetrician's hand" posture. The muscle spasm causes pain, which may be severe. A similar spasm in the feet is less common, with

plantar flexion of the toes, arching of the feet, and contraction of the calf muscles. With a severe attack the face may become involved, with wrinkling of the forehead, a staring gaze, and pursed lips. Hypocapnia and increased epinephrine secretion (due to panicking) worsen the tetany. Hyperventilation is a common feature of hypocalcemic tetany, and hysteria is often incorrectly diagnosed.

a. Atypical Tetany. Patients may experience cramps, stiffness, or clumsiness. With longstanding hypocalcemia they may have frequent mild paresthesias and cramps instead of clearly defined attacks of tetany, or may have carpal spasm only during prolonged use of the hand and forearm. Symptoms may be provoked by hyperventilation due to emotional stress or exercise. The symptoms may be exclusively sensory. Limping and falling may occur as a result of leg spasms. The symptoms may be unilateral. Laryngeal spasm may occur, causing stridor, crowing respiration, and cyanosis. Minor difficulties in vocalization are not uncommon. Smooth muscle spasms may cause dysphagia, abdominal pain, biliary colic, and wheezing with shortness of breath. Persistent diarrhea may occur (77). Infants are unlikely to develop carpopedal spasms, but are prone to tremors and twitches.

b. Signs of Latent Tetany. Signs of latent tetany remain useful in diagnosis and in adjusting therapy. Chvostek's sign is elicited by tapping the facial nerve with a fingertip as a hammer, 1–2 cm anterior to the earlobe just below the zygomatic process. The response consists of twitching of the muscles innervated by the facial nerve, and is graded as level 1 with twitching of upper lip at the corner of mouth only, level 2 as twitching of the alae nasi also, level 3 as contraction of the orbicularis oculi also, and level 4 as contraction of all the muscles of that side. The relative sensitivity with which these signs are elicited varies individually. A grade 1 sign is said to be found in >25% of normal children (76). Trousseau's sign is evoked by a sphygmomanometer cuff on the upper arm when inflated to above the systolic pressure for up to 3 min. The sensory and motor manifestations of tetany develop to a typical carpal spasm within 2 min. In the mildest cases the patient can overcome the spasm. In the severest, not even the examiner can overcome it. Only the severe grade of the sign is abnormal with certainty, since the milder grade occurs in a small percentage of normal subjects. The sign depends on induction of ischemia of the ulnar nerve.

c. Seizures. Seizures resembling epilepsy occur. These are of two distinct types. First, as hypocalcemia lowers the threshold for pre-existing subclinical epilepsy, epileptic seizures of any type may occur (78). The other type consists of generalized tetany followed by prolonged tonic spasms. It may be preceded by the sensory symptoms of tetany. During the seizure there may be tongue biting, loss of consciousness, incontinence, and postictal confusion. Hypocalcemia is frequently associated with characteristic changes in the EEG (79); in severe hypocalcemia irregular, sharp spike-and-wave patterns may appear. These changes may not disappear for some days after restoration of normocalcemia, and abnormal background activity may continue for several weeks.

2. Other

   a. *Basal Ganglion Calcification and Extrapyramidal Signs.* In patients with HP or, especially, PHP untreated for many years, small irregular calcifications may be seen in the basal ganglia in skull radiographs, and particularly on computed tomographic scans (80). These lesions may cause various extrapyramidal signs, including choreoathetosis, dystonic spasms, and classic parkinsonism.

   b. *Papilledema and Raised Intracranial Pressure.* In longstanding untreated HP there may be swelling of the optic discs. This may occur within as little as 2 weeks after the onset of HP as seen following thyroid surgery. It is moderate in degree (<4 diopters) and unaccompanied by hemorrhage or impaired vision. It may lead to suspicion of an intracranial tumor. The papilledema usually begins to subside within a few days of normocalcemia, but may take several weeks to disappear.

   c. *Psychic Disorders.* Impaired mental functioning occurs in patients with longstanding HP or PHP. Psychiatric disorders of many kinds have also been described.

   d. *Dermal and Dental Changes.* The skin may be dry and scaling, the nails brittle and fissured, and the hair coarse, dry, fractured, and easily shed. Eruption of teeth may be delayed and their roots may be blunted. These nail and tooth changes are distinct from the ectodermal dystrophy of autoimmune polyendocrinopathy–candidiasis–ectodermal dystrophy (APECED; Sec. XI.A.).

   e. *Cataracts.* Lenticular cataracts are a common complication of chronic hypocalcemia. They first appear as discrete punctate or lamellar opacities in the cortex, separated by a clear zone from the capsule (81). They may occur in distinct layers, more in the posterior pole than the anterior, and within 5–10 years they become confluent, with total opacification of the lens. Control of hypocalcemia arrests their progression.

   f. *Cardiovascular and Muscle Disorders.* Hypocalcemia delays ventricular depolarization and prolongs the Q-T$_c$ and ST intervals on the electrocardiogram. A 2:1 heart block may occur. Ca^{2+} exerts a positive ionotropic effect on the myocardium, but hypocalcemia rarely causes clinical cardiac problems. However, congestive heart failure does occur in children with HP (82) and sudden death due to ventricular arrhythmia is possible.

   Myopathy, in the mildest cases reflected by markedly supranormal plasma creatine kinase levels, has been reported in several hypocalcemic patients (83, 84).

IX. CAUSES OF HYPOPARATHYROIDISM

Congenital HP may be due to hyperfunction of the CaR, a specific defect in the synthesis or processing of PTH,

and aplasia or hypoplasia of PTG. PTG aplasia and hypoplasia occur as isolated defects and as part of malformation syndromes. Depending on its severity, congenital HP may manifest neonatally or only (even several years) later. Late manifestation may be due to failure of growth of hypoplastic PTG. Hence it may be difficult to differentiate between inborn and acquired forms of HP, and the inborn defects should be considered in cases of HP manifesting at any age (77). Acquired HP may be due to autoimmune destruction or other kinds of damage to PTG, and transient disturbances of the function of PTG (Table 2).

X. FAMILIAL ISOLATED HYPOPARATHYROIDISM

The criteria of this heterogeneous group include no demonstrable anatomical cause, no evidence of APECED, no developmental defects that might indicate an embryological disorder such as familial branchial pouch dysgenesis, and undetectable or subnormal plasma levels of immunoreactive PTH. Age at manifestation varies even

Table 2 Causes of Postneonatal Hypoparathyroidism

Familial isolated PTH deficiency
  Autosomal dominant
    HP due to constitutionally activated CaR
      (hypercalciuric hypocalcemia)
    HP due to mutant preproPTH gene
  Autosomal recessive
  X-linked
APECED
PTH deficiency of dysmorphic syndromes
  DiGeorge malformation complex
    Monosomy 22q11.2
    Partial monosomy 10p
  Autosomal recessive syndromes of Kenny-Caffey and
    Sanjad-Sakati
  Autosomal dominant syndrome of Kenny-Caffey
  Other syndromes
Other congenital isolated PTH deficiency
Transient PTH deficiency
  Critical illness
  Transient congenital hypoparathyroidism
  Maternal hyperparathyroidism
  Magnesium depletion
  Toxic influence
Other acquired PTH deficiency
  Surgical removal or lesion of PTG
  Radiation damage
  Infiltration of PTG
Pseudohypoparathyroidism
  Type Ia
  Type Ib
  Type Ic
  Type II

within pedigrees, often from newborn to adult (85, 86), or there may be no manifestation at all (87).

A. Autosomal Dominant Isolated Hypoparathyroidism

1. Hypercalciuric Hypocalcemia (MIM 146200)

This, apparently the commonest entity of autosomal dominant isolated HP, is caused by mutations leading to constitutionally activated CaR (Sec. II.A.) (88–90). Severity of the phenotype varies depending on the mutation, and even within families. Several patients have had seizures already in the first week of life, others show symptoms only in adulthood or no symptoms at all. At least 12 activating mutations have been observed, most of them in the extracellular domain of the CaR (89–91), and at least five in the transmembrane domains or the intervening extracellular loops (92). These mutant CaRs show a leftward shift and higher maximum in the dose–response curve for extracellular Ca^{2+}-activated accumulation of IP_3, indicating that these mutant receptors have increased activity and probably increased activity per receptor than the wild-type receptor (93). The setpoint for maintenance of plasma Ca^{2+} levels is subnormal and plasma PTH levels are maintained subnormal for the level of Ca^{2+}. Besides familial occurrence, at least five sporadic cases have been reported, with de novo mutations (91, 94, 95).

In a series of six kindreds, 11 of a total of 20 affected members had carpopedal spasms or childhood seizures (90). Two of them had calcifications of the basal ganglia, and in one of those the seizures continued to adult life. The other nine affected subjects had asymptomatic hypocalcemia; 16 subjects also had hypomagnesemia. Most of them (84%) were hyperphosphatemic. Serum PTH concentration was within normal range, but low for the hypocalcemia. Urinary Ca excretion was either inappropriately within the normal range or supranormal at the time of the initial diagnosis. In all the patients it was supranormal for the level of calcemia, and higher than in untreated subjects with idiopathic or postoperative HP and similar levels of hypocalcemia. Conventional treatment with vitamin D preparations frequently led to overt hypercalcemia, with renal calcification and impairment. This was probably due to presence of the abnormally active CaRs in their distal tubules, with reduced reabsorption of Ca^{2+}. Some of the patients even developed polyuria and polydipsia during normocalcemia, probably due to the presence of the abnormal CaRs in the collecting ducts leading to subnormal water permeablity. Some of the patients experience hypercalcemic symptoms, polydipsia, polyuria, and weakness at serum Ca^{2+} levels approaching the lower limit of normal (92).

2. HP Due to Mutant PreproPTH Gene (MIM 2212001)

A point mutation in the preproPTH gene has been observed in a father and two of his (six) children with au-

tosomal dominant HP, resulting in disruption of the hydrophobic signal sequence. It is presumed to impair translocation of the preproPTH molecule across the endoplasmic reticulum (86, 96). The children had hypocalcemic seizures in infancy. The father had no history of hypocalcemic symptoms, and his failing Ca^{2+} homeostasis appeared only as a subnormal plasma PTH response to hypocalcemia induced by an EDTA infusion test.

B. Autosomal Recessive Isolated Hypoparathyroidism (MIM 241400)

Two kindreds with autosomal recessive isolated HP have been published, each with a mutation in the PTH gene. In one kindred, each of the three affected members experienced hypocalcemic seizures in the neonatal period and had undetectable circulating PTH concentrations with normal renal response to PTH_{1-38}. A donor splice mutation was detected at the exon 2–intron 2 boundary, resulting in loss of exon 2 in the PTH mRNA. As exon 2 encodes the initiation codon and the signal peptide, loss of this exon presumably prevents translation of the PTH mRNA and translocation of the peptide. Affected members of the kindred were homozygous for this mutation (97).

In another large pedigree, HP manifested with seizures in the neonatal period or infancy. It was associated with a homozygous point mutation in exon 2 of the PTH gene, located at the first nucleotide of position 23 in the 25-amino acid signal peptide. Since this is the -3 position in the signal peptide, the resulting prepro-PTH mutant is presumably not cleaved by signal peptidase at the normal position, and it might be degraded in the rough endoplasmic reticulum (98).

C. X-Linked Isolated Hypoparathyroidism (MIM 307700)

Two large kindreds with X-linked recessive isolated HP have been reported from eastern Missouri (99, 100). Only male subjects were affected; they had hypocalcemic seizures starting in the neonatal or early infantile period. Circulating immunoreactive concentrations of PTH were undetectable, and renal response to bovine PTH was normal. In a careful search at autopsy of one of the patients who died accidentally as a teenager, no PTH tissue could be identified (101). The mutant gene, which thus appears to cause defective development of PTG, was localized to Xq26–27 (102).

XI. AUTOIMMUNE POLYENDOCRINOPATHY–CANDIDIASIS–ECTODERMAL DYSTROPHY (APECED) (MIM 240300)

This condition has been given many names, most commonly type I autoimmune polyglandular disease/syndrome (103). I prefer the term APECED (73), because it includes the two identifying features and does not include specific endocrinopathies (none is constant) (104). This autosomal recessive disease (105, 106) manifests as a widely variable combination of three groups of components (104, 107): autoimmune destruction of tissues, predominantly endocrine glands; consequences of a partial defect of cell-mediated immunity, most commonly chronic superficial candidiasis; and ectodermal dystrophy.

A.   Clinical Picture

The commonest components are mucocutaneous candidiasis, HP, and adrenocortical insufficiency, but more than 10 other components may occur. The following description is mainly based on my experience with 89 Finnish patients (104, 120, 120a).

1.   Endocrinopathies

HP appeared at an age varying from the 1st year to the 5th decade of life, with peak incidence at 2–11 years. Its prevalence gradually reaches 86% (Table 3). It remained the only endocrinopathy in 20% of our patients at the age 20 years and in 18% at 30. Several patients had experienced vague tetany for a few years before the diagnosis. In some patients we observed progression of HP from latent to severe over a few months. Addison's disease appeared from the 4th year to the 5th decade, with peak incidence at 4–12 years. Its prevalence reaches 79% (Table 3). It remained the only endocrinopathy in 8% of our patients at the age of 20.0 years and 11% at 30.0. Deficiencies of cortisol and aldosterone appeared even 5 years apart. Type I diabetes mellitus appeared at the age of 4–58 years, with highest incidences in the second, fourth, and fifth decades. Hypogonadism develops eventually in more than two-thirds of female patients and in one-quarter of males. It was due to autoimmune gonadal atrophy in all except one male patient, who had gonadotropin deficiency. Male infertility due to antisperm antibodies does also occur. Hypothyroidism rises eventually in prevalence to 18%. Parietal cell atrophy appears to reach one-third prevalence by the age of 40 years, with peak incidence at around 15 years. Pituitary hormone deficiencies occur, mostly singly. Growth hormone deficiency occurred in 4% of our patients (in one with adrenocorticotropic hormone [ACTH] deficiency), and several others are on record. Three patients have been reported with central diabetes insipidus (108–109), and two patients with ACTH deficiency (110).

2.   Other Autoimmune/Possibly Autoimmune Components

Alopecia was present in 33% of our patients, by the age of 2.5–30 years, being the first or part of the initial manifestation in 2%. Vitiligo of highly variable extent appeared in 21% of our patients at the age of 1.7–47 years.

In a few patients the spots faded, but in most patients they grew larger with time.

Gastrointestinal disorders are common. Autoimmune hepatitis is the most dangerous of all the common components of APECED. It was evident at the ages of 0.7–16 years in 17% of our 89 patients. Of them three died of fulminant hepatitis within 2 months, despite intensive therapy. Six other patients had clearly elevated serum levels of alanine aminotransferase, which subsided without immunosuppressive medication. Cholelithiasis may occur (112).

Sjögren syndrome was reported in 12% of a series of 41 patients and scleroderma in one patient (108). One of our patients died of complications of rapidly advancing rheumatoid arthritis. Eight (9%) of our pediatric patients experienced over several months a flashing rash, often associated with peaks of fever. Several cases of autoimmune hemolytic anemia are on the record (108), including one of our patients. Several patients with acquired splenic atrophy have been reported (108, 112, 113, 120a). Interstitial nephritis occurred in 7% of our patients; two of them needed a donor kidney.

Of our patients 16% had prolonged periods of watery or fatty diarrhea. Specific diagnosis was reached only in a few of them. Most of the patients with watery diarrhea had HP and they experienced periods of a vicious cycle of diarrhea and hypocalcemia. Of note, a patient's intractable diarrhea and therapy-resistant hypocalcemia responded to high dosage intravenous methylprednisolone and maintenance oral methotrexate (114). Atrophy of the exocrine pancreas with insulin deficiency occurred in one patient. Two other such cases are on record (115, 116); in one fat excretion responded to immunosuppressive medication (116). The chronic diarrhea of a 12-year-old patient of ours was caused by defective bile acid reabsorption and controlled with cholestyramin therapy. Intestinal lymphangiectasia was reported as a cause of diarrhea in one patient (117).

3.   Ocular Disease

Keratopathy may be a serious problem and calls for intensive local medication with glucocorticoid and often antimicrobials. Of our patients 22% showed keratopathy at the ages of 1.0–16 years. Five of them became blind. The early symptoms are intense photophobia, blepharospasm, and lacrimation (Fig. 7). In 10% of our patients keratopathy was the first or part of the initial manifestation of APECED, or the second only to oral candidiasis. Less common eye manifestations include recurring irodocyclitis, optic atrophy, retinal detachment, and severe dry eye (111).

4.   Nonautoimmune Components

Candidiasis involves the mouth first, appearing in the mildest cases as intermittent soreness of mouth corners

Table 3 Prevalences (%) of the Common Components[a] of APECED, Estimated[b] from Finnish Series of 89 Patients (45 males)

Component	\multicolumn{8}{c}{Age (years)}								Age range at appearance
	1	2	5	10	15	20	30	40	
Hypoparathyroidism	0	6	33	64	78	84	85	86	1st year to 5th decade
Hypoadrenocorticism	0	0	8	39	63	71	77	79	3 years to 5th decade
Diabetes mellitus	0	0	2	3	6	10	14	23	4 years to 6th decade
Hypothyroidism	0	0	0.6	1.5	2.4	5	11	18	4 to 32 years
Ovarian atrophy[c]					39	57	64	72	up to 36 years
Male hypogonadism[d]						9	18	26	15 to 37 years
Pernicious anemia[e]	0	0	0	2	10	17	20	31	6 years to 5th decade
Hepatitis[f]	1	2	4	11	15	17	17	17	1st year to 16 years
Candidiasis[g]	24	41	63	79	93	95	98	100	1st year to 3rd decade
Keratitis[h]	0	4	9	16	21	22	22	22	1st year to 16 years
Alopecia	0	0	4	15	29	34	40	40	2 to 30 years
Vitiligo	0.5	1	2	8	15	19	22	26	1st year to 5th decade
Diarrhea[i]	0	0	6	11	12	12	18	18	2 years to 3rd decade
Severe obstipation[i]	1	1	5	6	10	15	15	21	1st year to 4th decade

[a]Prevalences of the components of ectodermal dystrophy are only known for a subgroup of 68 patients of various ages: enamel hypoplasia of permanent teeth 77%, pitted nail dystrophy 52%, and calcium salt deposits of the tympanic membranes 33% with no history of middle ear disease (Ahonen et al., 1990).
[b]Estimated from the observed incidence rates over the age intervals, assuming that all the patients live until the age of 40 years.
[c]Primary amenorrhea in 52%, secondary in 48%, prevalence known from age 15 only.
[d]Prevalance known only from age 20.
[e]Includes (2 of 21) patients without clinical disease but with circulating antibodies against parietal cells and/or intrinsic factor.
[f]Includes three patients who died of fulminant hepatitis.
[g]The early oral candidiasis may easily be unnoticed, the earliest figures are hence probably too low.
[h]One third of these patients developed blindness or severely impaired vision.
[i]Chronic or periodic diarrhea/obstipation. Three of 89 patients had alternating periods of both.
Source: Perheentupa, unpublished.

(angular cheilosis) (Fig. 7). Its peak incidence is over the first year of life. In some patients it appears late, and in our series the prevalence of 100%, intermittent cases included, was not reached until the fifth decade of life (Table 3). Mild oral candidiasis may remain unnoticed, hence its prevalence figures at early ages, as reported in the literature, are probably erroneously low. More severe forms include an acute inflammation of most of the oral mucosa, hyperplastic chronic candidiasis with thick white coating of the tongue, and atrophic disease with scant coatings and a scarred thin mucosa with leukoplakia-like areas (118). This chronic condition is carcinogenic; four of our patients had evidence of epithelial carcinoma of the oral mucosa at the age of 27–45 years, and three of them died of it. Hence, candidiasis should be carefully evaluated and suppressed by good dental care and oral hygiene, and local and systemic antimycotics. Candidal esophagitis is painful and may cause strictures. Intestinal mucosal candidiasis may manifest as abdominal pain, meteorism and diarrhea. The infection may spread to the skin of the face and hands, and to the nails. Postpubertal female patients often experience candidal vulvovaginitis.

5. Ectodermal Dystrophy

The most frequent component of ectodermal dystrophy (Fig. 7) is enamel hypoplasia of permanent teeth (118, 119), which affects three-quarters of our patients (104). Pitted nail dystrophy is present in one-half and tympanic membrane calcium salt deposits in one-third of our patients.

6. Individual Variation

The clinical picture varies also very widely in aspects other than age at appearance of the individual disease components. In our series the total number of component diseases varies from 2 to 10 (median 4), and the number of endocrine components from 1 to 5 (median 2). The so-called classic triad of candidiasis, HP, and adrenal insufficiency was present in 50% of the patients at the age of 20.0 years, in 55% at 30.0, and 40% at 40.0 years.

The first components to appear as part of the initial clinical picture were candidiasis in 54%, HP in 31%, adrenal insufficiency in 6%, keratopathy in 7%, chronic diarrhea in 7%, alopecia in 2%, flashing rash with fever in

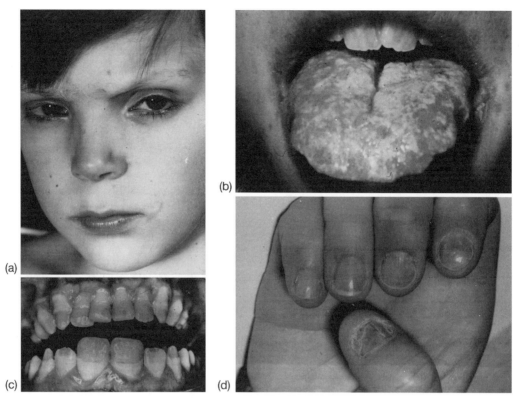

Figure 7 Ectodermal manifestations of APECED. a. Keratopathy and angular cheilosis. b. Hyperplastic chronic candidiasis of the tongue with angular cheilosis. c. Enamel hypoplasia in permanent teeth. d. Pitted nail dystrophy of second, fourth, and fifth fingers with eroding nail candidiasis of the thumb.

2%, hepatitis in 1%, and vitiligo in 1%. Of the endocrinopathies the first one was HP alone in 64% and adrenal insufficiency alone in 27%, HP and adrenal insufficiency together in 6%, GH deficiency in 1%, and hypothyroidism in 1%.

B. Follow-Up

For a review of the follow-up for HP, see Sec. XVII.B.7. Patients with the diagnosis of APECED should receive written information about the possibility and symptoms of further disease components with instructions on where to turn in case they appear. Later, it is necessary to check repeatedly that the patient has adopted this information. The patient should be examined at least once or twice annually for the possibility of new disease components: thorough anamnestic details and physical examination including search for oral candidiasis, search for antibodies, and determination of serum levels of Ca, Pi, Na, K, alanine aminotransferase, ACTH, TSH and the GnHs, plasma renin activity, and blood glycohemoglobin, as appropriate in the patient's situation.

C. Immunology

A limited T-cell defect appears to be part of APECED (120). It is reflected by cutaneous anergy or weak delayed-type hypersensitivity reactions to PPD and *Candida* antigens, and the high prevalence of mucocutaneous *Candida* infections. No consistent abnormality of T cells has been demonstrated in laboratory studies. The destructive autoimmune attack of endocrine glands appears initially as infiltration by lymphocytes and macrophages. The process is presumed to be T-cell-mediated. Antibodies to certain antigens of the gland commonly appear in blood, most frequently antibodies against intracellular enzymes. The role of such autoantibodies in the destructive process remains unclear, but they are important as diagnostic messengers from the process and appear commonly before clinical hormone deficiency is evident. No antiparathyroid autoantibodies are recognized. Association with HP of autoantibodies against the Ca^{2+}-sensing receptor has been reported (121), but this finding has not been confirmed. Such antibodies were not found in any patient of a large series of our Finnish patients with HP of APECED (Spiegel AM, Perheentupa J, unpublished).

The most frequently found antiadrenocortical antibodies are directed against 21-hydroxylase (P450c21). Although positive results do not always predict Addison's disease, this disease is almost always preceded by their appearance in blood. Anti-P450c21 antibodies are equivalent to antiadrenal antibodies demonstrated by indirect immunofluorescence (122, 123). Of the other enzymes of adrenal steroid hormone synthesis, cholesterol side chain cleavage enzyme (P450scc), 3βOH-steroid dehydrogenase (3βHSD), and 17α-hydroxylase (P450c17) are also present in the ovarian granulosa and theca cells, and the testicular Leydig cells (124–129). Circulating antibodies against them predict development of premature ovarian failure (130). Sera positive by immunofluorescence against those steroid-producing cells contain antibodies specific to P450scc, P450c17, and/or (rarely) 3βHSD (128).

Patients with autoimmune vitamin B_{12} malabsorption or so-called pernicious anemia have autoantibodies against the intrinsic factor or the gastric H^+/K^+-ATPase. The latter is the specific antigen to the parietal cell antibody detected by indirect immunofluorescence (131, 132). In the chronic autoimmune hepatitis of APS-1, P450 1A2 may be the specific hepatic autoantigen (133–135).

In alopecia, immunoreactivity has been observed against differentiating keratinocytes in hair follicle (136). Antibodies against tyrosine hydroxylase correlated with presence of alopecia in patients with APS-1 (137, 138), and antibodies against transcription factors SOX9 and SOX10 with presence of vitiligo in various patients (137). Antibodies against tryptophan hydroxylase of intestinal mucosa correlate with intestinal dysfunction in patients with APS-1 (139).

D. Genetics

APECED is caused by loss-of-function mutations in both copies of the *AIRE* (for AutoImmune REgulator) gene on chromosome 21q22.3 (140, 141). *AIRE* contains 14 exons. It is mainly expressed in subsets of epithelial and monocyte lineage cells in thymus medulla; in rare cells in lymph node paracortex and medulla, spleen, and fetal liver; and in very few blood leukocytes. These all are antigen-presenting cells. Wider expression is disputed, but it has been also reported in the respiratory system, central nervous system, endocrine glands, urinary system, and genitals (142). Human and mouse *AIRE* promoters include conserved sites for several transcription factors, which are thymus-specific or important in hematopoesis (143).

The *AIRE* protein consists of 545 amino acids. At its amino terminal is a highly conserved ASS domain necessary for subnuclear targeting and dimerization, which appears to be essential for its transcription activating action (144). The SAND domain is needed for DNA binding, two plant homeodomain type Zn fingers presumably serve protein–protein interaction, and two nuclear localization signals and four LXXLL motifs act in nuclear re-

ceptor binding. Human and mouse *AIRE* proteins are 71% identical (143, 145). They exist in nucleoplasmic granules, and occasionally along the cytoplasmic microtubular cytoskeleton (146, 147). The protein is an activator of gene transcription (144, 148), but its exact physiological role is unknown. It may be involved in determination of thymic stromal organization and thus in the induction of self-tolerance (149, 150).

To date, some 35 mutations of *AIRE* have been described in patients with APECED, most of them in four mutational hotspots (116, 141, 144, 151–153). Many are either missense mutations in the ASS region (presumably preventing the dimerization of the protein) or nonsense mutations leading to its truncation. The internationally most common mutation, C889T, covers almost 90% of the Finnish APECED genes (140, 144). It leads to a deletion of both Zn fingers and most of the SAND domain. The second most common mutation (140, 144), predominant in the United States (152) and United Kingdom (153), is a 13 nucleotide deletion, which leads to a protein lacking the C-terminal third. The predominant Sardinian mutant protein (154) consists only of the N-terminal fourth. All the reported Iranian Jewish patients are homozygous for a missense mutation in a single nucleotide, which disrupts the dimerization domain (144). In some 10% of the *AIRE* genes of clinically ascertained patients, identification of a mutation has failed (144). These may be mutations of the promoter region or the introns.

Determinants of the wide variability of the APECED phenotype are unknown. The Iranian Jewish patients have been reported to have much less candidiasis and adrenocortical insufficiency than other patients (155), which could depend on their unique mutation. Otherwise the phenotype variation seems not to depend on nature of the mutation. The HLA appears not to be a determinant of the variation, and there are no gender-specific differences.

XII. HYPOPARATHYROIDISM OF DYSMORPHIC SYNDROMES

A. DiGeorge Malformation Complex (MIM 188400; DiGeorge Syndrome, Dysbranchiogenesis, Shprintzen Velocardiofacial Syndrome, Conotruncal Anomaly Face Syndrome)

According to the traditional definition, DiGeorge malformation complex (DMC) is a causally heterogeneous developmental field defect of the third and fourth pharyngeal pouches (99). Its main components are hypoplasia of the PTG, which may present as neonatal tetany or seizures; a deficit of T cells with susceptibility to infection, due to hypoplasia or aplasia of the thymus; congenital defect of the heart or the great arteries, particularly affecting the outflow tract; and a characteristic facial dysmorphism. At least three of these four components are required for the clinical diagnosis of DMC (156). However, the prevalence of these components has probably been overestimated, because DMC has been delineated by studying series of thus clinically diagnosed patients. Cases are often labeled as complete (with thymus aplasia) or partial DMC (thymus hypoplasia). This division does not correlate with presence or absence of other anomalies, save the fact that PTG aplasia is commonly associated with thymus aplasia (157). Patients with complete DMC die early (158). Reliable diagnosis of thymic aplasia can only be made at autopsy.

There is disagreement about the names and definitions of this malformation complex. Because approximately 90% of the patients with the clinical diagnosis of DMC have monosomy of the DiGeorge chromosome region (DGCR) of chromosome 22q11.2, some authors consider that this majority should be termed monosomy 22q11.2 syndrome and separated from other causative groups, particularly that caused by hemizygosity of DGS2 of chromosome 10p (see below). Because most large series of patients published were selected according to the clinical diagnosis of DiGeorge syndrome, that is discussed next. Then the available information specific to the chromosomal deletion syndromes will be presented.

1. Incidence and Age at Manifestation

Hundreds of patients have been reported. A neonatal manifestation occurred in 83% of cases, mostly cardiac problems, and in one-third of cases convulsions (157, 159). Sometimes the first symptoms only appeared at school age, and in several cases DMC was diagnosed in an asymptomatic adult patient because of symptomatic disease of his or her offspring (160). In the 1960s and 1970s some 80% of recognized patients died within a year of birth, a majority from cardiac causes and one-fifth from infection (157).

2. Endocrine Disorders

Hypocalcemic convulsions occurred in 61% and hypocalcemia in 85% of the reported cases (157, 159). The hypocalcemia resolved in early childhood in a majority of patients (26 of 40) (159). However, deficient function of the parathyroids may still manifest in adulthood during a hypocalcemic stress, such as an infusion of disodium edetate (161–163). It may even evolve again to frank symptomatic HP (162). PTGs were searched for at autopsy in 85 patients; a hypoplastic PTG was observed in 30, and none could be found in 41 even by careful serial sectioning (157). A malformation of the thyroid gland is also common (157) and at least two of 44 patients were hypothyroid (159). Calcitonin-producing C cells of the thyroid gland, belonging to the derivatives of the third and fourth branchial pouches (cephalic neural crest cells) are deficient in numbers (164, 165).

3. Cardiac Defects

Approximately 90% of recorded patients have had a cardiac defect, half of them an anomaly of the aortic arch,

most commonly type B interrupted arch or right aortic arch. One fifth have truncus arteriosus communis (157–159). Hypoplastic left heart and coarctation of the aorta also occur. The right outflow tract is affected in some 12% of the patients, predominantly by obstructive anomalies, and a similar proportion has Fallot's tetralogy. An associated ventricular septal defect is present in a majority of the patients, and associated valve anomalies are common. In contrast, isolated septum defects and valve anomalies are infrequent, but ventricular septal defect alone may be present in late manifesting cases. One fourth of the patients have an aberrant right subclavian artery that may cause dysphagia. The spectrum of circulatory anomalies ranges from left heart hypoplasia to an harmless abnormality of the subclavian artery.

4. Immune Defect

Although infections are relatively rare causes of early death of patients with DMC, susceptibility to infections becomes more prominent with increasing age. Half of the 20 patients who died at the ages of 3–12 months succumbed in pneumonia or sepsis (157). Bacteria and *Candida albicans* were the common agents. However, patients have a predominantly mild cell-mediated immunodeficiency, usually associated with infections characteristic of humoral immunodeficiencies (166). Comparison between 19 newborns with chromosome 22q11.2 deletion detected because of a cardiac defect and comparable newborn cardiac patients without deletion showed that the deletion group had significantly lower peripheral blood T-cell numbers, although the function of their T cells was largely preserved. A subgroup with markedly diminished T-cell numbers showed an increase in these cells over the first year of life (167). Only two cases of malignant neoplasm seem to be on record (157). Failure of the descent of thymus is very common, but immunodeficiency requiring correction occurs only in approximately 25% of the cases. Such patients can be identified by CD4+ T cell enumeration, and by in vitro proliferation response to phytohemagglutinin (159, 168, 169). Approximately three-quarters of patients have frankly subnormal T-cell counts or evidence of thymus hypoplasia. Of 85 patients tested only five had a completely normal immune function. In the others findings varied greatly. The total blood lymphocyte count was normal in 71%. B lymphocyte counts were supranormal in half the patients, but antibody production capacity was subnormal in one-third. IgG responses to immunization with bacterial polysaccharides may be particularly impaired (170). Diversification of the immunoglobulin VH gene repertoire is restricted (171). Many patients have hypergammaglobulinemia (171). Transplantation with fetal thymus tissue or bone marrow has given promising results (157, 172). There may be a specific predisposition to autoimmune diseases: several cases of Graves' disease and idiopathic thrombocytopenia have been reported, as well as two patients with juvenile rheumatoid arthritis (173).

5. Dysmorphic Features

All patients have some facial dysmorphism, but the features that are most helpful for the diagnosis are ear shape, prominence of nasal root, and, in the younger child, small mouth (159). The ears are low set and posteriorly rotated with deficient upper helices and an increase in anteroposterior diameter, giving a relatively circular shape (Fig. 8). At least one-fourth of the patients have a hearing deficit. The root and bridge of the nose are wide and prominent (Fig. 8), and there is a marked indentation on either side of the nasal tip above the midpoint of each nostril. Most patients have micrognathia, and about one-fourth have palatal clefts. The lips are often prominent and U-shaped, and the philtrum is short and poorly modeled. Lateral displacement of the inner canthi is frequent. Telecanthus with short palpebral fissures is common. The eyes may slant upward or downward (Fig. 8).

A great number of variable other malformations have been reported. Among these, different renal and urinary tract anomalies are most common. Other frequent sites are the pharynx, gastrointestinal tract, lungs, spleen, skeleton, brain, and genitals (157, 159).

In the older child the features overlap with Shprintzen velocardiofacial syndrome (MIM 192430) with a bulbous nose, square nasal tip, and hypernasal speech associated with submucous or overt palatal clefting (174).

6. Development and Growth

Of surviving patients, at least one-half have had moderate to severe developmental delay, in some series all have (158). Hypoxic episodes may have contributed to this (159), and management of hypocalcemia and avoidance of hypoxia are important in prevention of developmental problems. Growth is said to be retarded, with stature often below the third percentile (157). Mild to moderate learning difficulties are frequent.

7. Causes

Approximately 90% of the patients have a deletion within chromosome 22q11.2 (segmental monosomy) identifiable with fluorescent in situ hybridization (175–181). A minority have a microscopic deletion, and some patients have monosomy of the whole chromosome 22. The DGCR contains several genes (see MIM 188400). Most of the cases are sporadic with a de novo deletion. In many families multiple members carry the deletion with the variable phenotype behaving as an autosomal dominant trait (182). In approximately 25% of the cases one of the parents has the deletion (159), and for such couples the risk of any child being affected is 50%.

Other established causes of DMC include monosomy of a section (DMC2) of chromosome 10 p, or fetal exposure to alcohol, retinoic acid, or maternal diabetes mellitus. There is evidence for a common denominator of these conditions, namely existence of a dysmorphogenetically reactive unit; a population of cephalic neural crest cells (183).

8. Monosomy 22q11.2 (22q11.Deletion Syndrome)

A spectrum of phenotypes, often collectively called CATCH22 (for *c*ardiac defect, *a*nomaly of face, *t*hymic hypoplasia, *c*left *p*alate, *H*P), is associated with heterozygous deletions of chromosome 22q.11.2 (monosomy 22q.11.2, the DiGeorge critical region I [DGCR-I]). This spectrum includes the overlapping entities DMC, the Shprintzen velocardiofacial syndrome (174, 184), so-called conotruncal anomaly face, and isolated outflow tract defects of the heart (conotruncal heart defects: tetralogy of Fallot, truncus arteriosus, and interrupted aortic arch) (159, 185, 186). Most of the cases are sporadic, but many families show autosomal dominant transmission. The same deletion may cause phenotypes that vary within families from normal to syndromic (187–189) and differ even between identical twins (190). In fact, over 90% of patients have the same deletion breakpoints (191).

In a European collaborative study of 558 patients with deletions of 22q11 (192), in 204 cases of the 285 patients with known parental deletion status neither parent had the deletion. Of the 79 cases with known gender of the parent with the deletion, it was maternal in 61 and paternal in 18. Growth data were available for 131 of the 158 patients whose heights and/or weights were below the median; 57 of 158 were below the third percentile for either height or weight. Forty-four patients had died, and of the 29 for whom age at death was available, 16 had died within the first month of life and 25 within the first 6 months consequent to congenital heart disease. There was only one death from severe immune deficiency. Of 338 patients 107 were developmentally normal; 37 of the 107 had speech delay. Of the 231 patients with abnormal development, 102 had a mild delay and 60 had either moderate or severe learning difficulties. Of 252 children in the study 22 had behavioral or psychiatric problems, including two with episodes of psychosis; 11 of 61 adults had a psychiatric disorder, and four of the 11 had had at least one episode of psychosis. Of the 545 patients who underwent cardiac studies, 409 had significant cardiac pathology, most commonly tetralogy of Fallot, ventricular septal defect, interrupted aortic arch, pulmonary atresia/ventricular septal defect, or truncus arteriosus. Of the 496 patients examined, 242 had otolaryngeal abnormalities, 72 either an overt cleft palate or submucous cleft; 161 patients had velopharyngeal insufficiency without clefting. Of 159 patients with hearing data available, 52 had abnormal hearing, which was of conductive type in all the 17 patients appropriately examined. A total of 49 of 136 patients had renal abnormalities, with absent, dysplastic, or multicystic kidneys in 23; obstructive abnormalities in

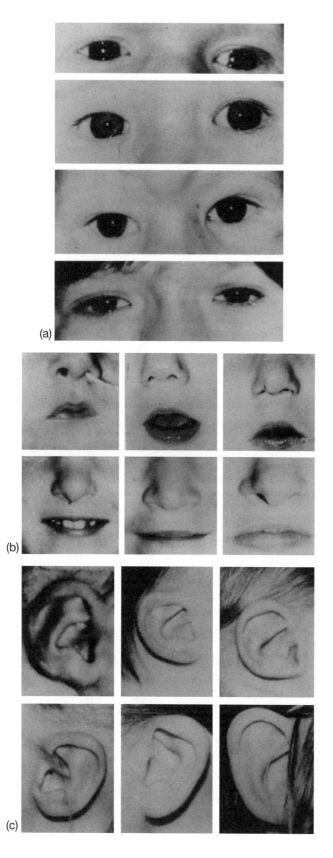

(a)

(b)

(c)

14; and vesicoureteric reflux in six. A total of 203 of 340 had recorded hypocalcemia, 108 of them with a history of seizures, and 42 of these seizures secondary to hypocalcemia. Most cases of hypocalcemia were reported in the neonatal period, but one patient presented at 18 years of age. Of 218 patients with laboratory and clinical evaluation of immune function and thymus status, only four were classified as having a major immune function abnormality. Two of these had died, one of them consequent to severe immunodeficiency. Of 548 patients 94 had minor abnormalities of the skeletal system, and 39 had ocular anomalies. Of the patients' offspring, 27 of 35 had more severe congenital heart disease than the parent and eight the same degree of severity. Developmental status was worse in nine of 17 and the same in seven of 17. Palatal abnormalities were better in 10 of 22 children and similar to the parent's in 12 of 22 children. Of the families 12 had a total of 26 affected siblings; they showed considerable variation in heart abnormalities between the siblings; development status was similar in most cases.

The phenotype varies widely. What has been discussed above with regard to the DMC is probably valid for monosomy 22q11.2. Several patients have been described with HP, facial abnormality, and intellectual impairment (173). The deletion appears to predispose to schizophrenia (193).

In northern England the minimum birth prevalence of the 22q.11.2 deletions was 13:100,000 live births, making it the second most common cause of congenital heart disease after Down's syndrome (194).

9. Partial Monosomy 10p

Monosomy of the tip of the short arm of chromosome 10 (p13-pter) is a rare anomaly (1:27,500 consecutive births in Tokyo; 195), and another cause of a spectrum of phenotypes that includes among others DMC (196), velocardiofacial syndrome, and the syndrome of HP, deafness, and renal dysplasia (HDR syndrome; MIM 146255). It is a contiguous gene spectrum. More than 50 patients have been reported (197). Two nonoverlapping regions have been defined that contribute to this complex phenotype. The proximal one is DiGeorge critical region II (DGCR-

Figure 8 Characteristic facial features in patients with the DiGeorge malformation complex. a. Nasal root and eyes (from the top) of a baby, an infant, a young child, and a teenager. b. The tip of the nose, philtrum, and mouth. Age increases from neonate to young child on the top row and on into teenage years on the bottom row. The length of the philtrum, the size of the mouth, and the thickness of the lips are variable. c. Abnormalities of the ear, from neonate (top left) to adult (bottom right). (From Ref. 159.)

II) on 10p13–14. Hemizygocity for it may cause cardiac defects and T-cell deficiency. Hemizygocity for the distal one on 10p14–10pter may cause the HDR syndrome: HP, sensorineural deafness, renal dysplasia and, perhaps, T-cell deficiency (197–199). Patients with cardiac defect and HP have haploinsuffiency of both these chromosome regions (197). The HDR syndrome appears to be caused by haploinsufficiency of the *GATA3* gene (MIM 131320; 200), which belongs to a family of zinc-finger transcription factors involved in vertebrate embryonic development. It is abundantly expressed in T-lymphocyte lineage and is thought to participate in T-cell receptor gene activation through binding to enhancers (201). Investigation for *GATA3* mutations in three HDR probands identified one nonsense mutation and two intragenic deletions that predicted a loss of function, as confirmed by absence of DNA binding by the mutant *GATA3* protein (200). *GATA3* is thus essential in the embryonic development of the parathyroids, the auditory system and the kidneys.

Phenotypic external characteristics include an abnormally shaped, usually microcephalic skull, prominent forehead, epicanthic folds, downward slanting palpebral fissures, hypertelorism, ptosis, flat nasal bridge, everted nostrils, micrognathia, prominent upper lip, low-set dysplastic ears, high-arched or cleft palate, short neck, and hand and foot abnormalities. Most patients have been retarded in intellectual and motor functions. The deafness is of the sensorineural type, bilateral, nonprogressive, and more severe at the higher frequencies. At least one patient had conductive hearing loss. Prenatal- or postnatal-onset growth deficiency is common. Eye abnormalities are frequent: fundus anomalies, arteria hyaloidea persistens, microphthalmus, strabismus, exudative maculopathy, astigmatism, cataract, and amblyopia. Half the patients have genital and/or urinary tract abnormalities, which may include kidney aplasia, hypoplasia or dysplasia, hydronephrosis, ureter duplex, ureteral stenosis, cystic kidneys with normal filtration rate (202), steroid-resistant nephrotic syndrome due to fetal glomeruli (203), hypoplastic penis and scrotum with cryptorchidism, and hypospadias. Limb anomalies include syndactyly, clinodactyly, clubbed hands and feet, short terminal phalanges, short upper limbs, proximally implanted or broad thumbs, and pre-axial polydactyly. Half the patients have heart defects: septum defects, patent ductus arteriosus, pulmonary stenosis, coarctation of aorta, or truncus arteriosus. Many patients died neonatally of cardiac failure. Postmortem observations included hypoplasia or aplasia of the olfactory bulbs and tracts, and hypoplasia of the cerebellum and brainstem (204). Two patients had hypothyroidism. Probably several patients previously thought to present different entities should be classified as belonging to this group (202, 203, 205). A boy with the hypoparathyroidism/sensorineural deafness/renal dysplasia (HDR) syndrome had recurrent cerebral infarctions of the basal ganglia with hemipegia, the first one at the age of 7 months (206).

Approximately 80% of cases have been due to a de novo mutation. In the others a parent carries a balanced translocation (207).

B. Autosomal Recessive Syndromes of Kenny-Caffey and Sanjad-Sakati

The autosomal recessive syndromes of Kenny-Caffey (KCS1, *MIM 244460*) and Sanjad-Sakati (HP/retardation/dysmorphism [HRD], *MIM 241410*) are very rare. They have the same mutant gene locus in chromosome 1q42–q43 and appear to be allelic or perhaps even caused by the same mutation (208–209). The KCS1 is characterized by extreme growth failure, congenital HP, abnormal physiognomy, and mental retardation, which is mostly severe but sometimes mild (210–211). The physical findings have included microcephaly, prominent forehead, deep-set eyes often with microphthalmos, and esotropia, depressed nasal bridge with beaked nose, long philtrum, thin upper lip, micrognathia, large and low-set and/or posteriorly rotated ears, often with floppy ear lobes, small hands and feet, cryptorchidism, and micropenis. All patients in the first series had cortical thickening of long bones with medullary stenosis. In the original series of patients with HRD (210) all had tetany or convulsions, nine of 12 neonatally. Immune system abnormalities were not observed. What appeared to differentiate HRD from KCS1 was that none of the patients had medullary stenosis. With the next series of patients with the HRD (212) this difference disappeared; seven of eight patients had medullary stenosis. Also, all the patients presented with hypocalcemia neonatally, three patients had neonatal septicemia, and there were three probable additional cases in the families who had died of neonatal sepsis; all four patients tested had subnormal T-lymphocyte counts. All the reported patients with HRD were of Middle Eastern origin (210, 212–214), and so is a large series of patients diagnosed the KCS1 (215).

C. Autosomal Dominant Syndrome of Kenny-Caffey

Characteristics of the autosomal dominant type 2 syndrome of Kenny and Caffey (*KCS2*, MIM 127000) were originally (216) described as markedly stunted stature with slender dense tubular bones and narrow marrow cavities. Congenital HP is a frequent (>70%) component. In 23 of 24 patients serum PTH levels were inappropriately low or undetectable, but in one levels were high as measured by N-terminal assay but undetectable by carboxy-terminal assay (217). No PTG was found at the one autopsy that has been reported (217). Other frequent features are macrocephaly, absent diploid space in calvarium, delayed closure of the anterior fontanelle, dysmorphic face, and eye abnormalities (microphthalmia, hyperopia, papillary pseudoedema) (217–220). Micro-orchidism is common, with suspected subfertility. The short stature was short-limbed in three families and proportional in the others.

D.   Other Syndromes

Among 212 cases collected from literature of the Kearns-Sayre syndrome associated with a distinct defect of the mitochondrial genome, 14 had HP. Four of these patients were hypomagnesemic, five had hypogonadism, four had diabetes mellitus, and two had hypothyroidism. These associated endocrinopathies were not more prevalent than in the non-HP patients (221).

Two brothers have been described with a probable X-linked recessive syndrome with congenital lymphedema of all limbs and pulmonary lymphangiectasia, HP, nephropathy, dysmorphism (medial flare of eyebrows, broad nasal bridge with lateral displacement of the inner canthi, hypertrichosis of the face and forehead, short nail beds, brachydactyly, and an increased carrying angle), prolapsing mitral valve, and brachytelephalangy. One of them had cataracts and the other dry itchy skin (222).

In one family six members in three generations had autosomal dominant HP associated with short stature and premature osteoarthritis; in at least two of them HP appeared in childhood (223).

Single cases with HP have been observed in association with the Dubowitz syndrome (MIM 223370; 224, 225), Hallermann-Streif syndrome (226, 227), Mulibrey nanism (MIM 253250; 228), and Silver-Russel syndrome (MIM 180860; 229).

E.   Other Congenital Isolated PTH Deficiency

Isolated PTG hypoplasia (also termed transient congenital HP or transient congenital PTG dysplasia; 230, 231) may become manifest as late neonatal tetany, or may not appear until the age of several weeks. Calcemia is then usually normalized within weeks or months. However, these patients may have permanent latent HP. Tetany may recur during a hypocalcemic stress, and permanent HP may occur after several years (161, 224, 232, 233).

XIII.   TRANSIENT HYPOPARATHYROIDISM

HP limited to the neonatal period is discussed in Chapter 21.

A.   Critical Illness

Hypocalcemia is frequently associated with critical illness in children (153–155), and some of these children have PTH deficiency (234, 235). Of 145 patients admitted to a pediatric intensive care unit (53 after major surgery, 92 for acute medical problems) 71 had subnormal total serum Ca. Subnormal serum Ca^{2+} was observed in 26 of them; but many others presumably had it because Ca^{2+} could

not be predicted from total Ca. As a group, these 26 patients were more critically ill than the rest; 17 had inappropriately low plasma PTH level (234). No information was given on magnesemia, although hypomagnesemia is very common in critically ill patients (236).

According to others, hypocalcemia in critically ill children was often associated with hypercalcitoninemia (237) or hypermagnesemia (238). These dysmineralemias seem to predict high mortality (234, 238) and their correction may improve the outcome.

Children with severe burns may develop hypocalcemia, Mg depletion, HP, and renal resistance to PTH infusion. Fourteen sequentially recruited children with a burn of at least 40% of total body surface area were given a urinary Mg retention test a median of 20 days after the burn. Seven of them remained Mg depleted, which was not attributable to the burn size or to time from burn to study, or combined enteral and parenteral Mg intake. Both the Mg-depleted and the nondepleted group had low intact serum PTH levels in relation to serum Ca^{2+} concentration, indicating persistent HP. Thus, not the Mg depletion but rather a reduced set point for Ca suppression of PTH secretion was concluded to be the chief cause of the persistent HP (239).

In an experiment, sheep were subjected to a 40% total body surface area burn or sham burn receiving anesthesia and fluid resuscitation only. The burned sheep were hypocalcemic and hypomagnesemic compared with the sham-burned controls. In their PTGs and kidneys the CaR mRNA was increased by 50% with a corresponding increase in the intensity of CaR immunoreactivity associated with the cell surface in the PTGs. These findings are consistent with upregulation of the parathyroid CaR and a related decrease in the set point for Ca suppression of PTH secretion that may contribute to the reported postburn HP and hypocalcemia (240).

B.   Maternal Hyperparathyroidism

HP is common in infants born to hyperparathyroid mothers; the maternal disease is often undiagnosed. Symptoms usually appear within the first 2 weeks, but may be delayed (241). Complete recovery is the rule, but the condition may be prolonged, and even permanent (242). It is presumed that this HP develops because of suppression of the fetal PTG by fetal hypercalcemia maintained by excessive placental transfer of Ca from the hypercalcemic mother.

C.   Magnesium Depletion

HP is a frequent manifestation of Mg depletion. The mechanism involves impaired secretion of PTH (243, 244), target cell resistance to PTH, and independent disturbance of the blood–bone equilibrium. Mg depletion may be due to an inborn error of metabolism, a specific defect in the intestinal absorption of Mg, called primary congenital hypomagnesemia (MIM 248250; 245, 246). It usually manifests as tetany at the age of 1–4 months. Serum Mg levels are <0.4 mmol/l (<1.0 mg/dl), distinct from the less severe hypomagnesemia frequently encountered in late neonatal hypocalcemia (247). The hypocalcemia can only be controlled by continuous Mg substitution. Mg deficiency may also occur as an acquired condition caused by nonspecific intestinal malabsorption (chronic diarrhea, Crohn's disease, large resection of small bowel) (248) and renal wasting of Mg^{2+} due to loop di-

uretics, aminoglycosides, pentamidine, cyclosporine, and diabetic ketoacidosis, transplanted kidney, urinary tract obstruction, or the diuretic phase of acute renal failure. This type of HP is resistant to the calciferols, and can only be corrected by Mg repletion (Fig. 9).

D. Toxic Influence

Transient HP may occur during cytotoxic therapy with asparaginase (249), adriamycin, cisplatinum, cytarabine,

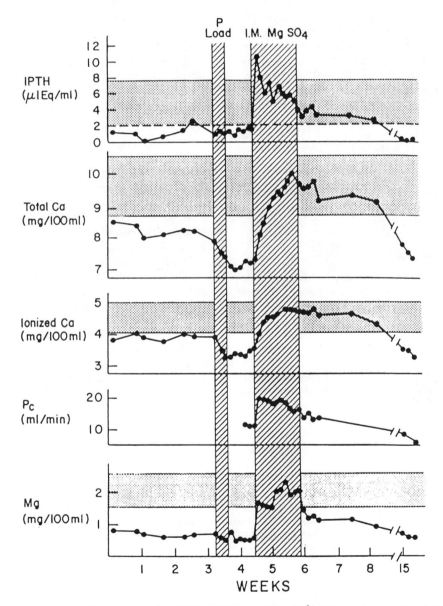

Figure 9 Plasma concentrations of immunoreactive PTH (IPTH), total Ca, Ca^{2+}, Mg, and renal phosphate clearance (P_C) in a patient with HP caused by severe hypomagnesemia. First, hypocalcemia was made more severe by an oral phosphate challenge; this did not result in increased secretion of PTH. Then Mg was replenished by intramuscular injections of Mg sulfate. The shaded areas indicate the normal ranges. (From Ref. 243.)

or amphotericin B (250). The condition may be complicated by acute renal failure and hypomagnesemia. The role of drugs and various metabolic derangements in the causation of the HP is unclear. L-asparaginase leads to necrosis of chief cells in rabbit PTG, with ensuing HP (251). (See also Sec. XII.A.)

XIV. OTHER ACQUIRED HYPOPARATHYROIDISM

A. Surgical Removal or Lesion of PTG

This condition, which is the most common variety of HP in adults (76, 251), is rare in children. After thyroid surgery hypocalcemia is relatively frequent and must not be equated with HP. A sudden transition from the hyperthyroid to the euthyroid state, with reversal of negative bone Ca balance, is often associated with so-called hungry bone phenomenon. Such hypocalcemia disappears spontaneously within 24–48 h and is unlikely to cause tetany.

Postoperative HP may be caused by PTG injury due to ischemia, depending on the extent of dissection and hemostasis (76). Patients recovering from postoperative HP usually do so within a few weeks to 6 months, but occasionally only after years. Latent HP may persist with intermittent relapses during hypocalcemic stress. This is inevitable after delayed recovery (76).

B. Irradiation Damage

Permanent combined HP and hypothyroidism has occurred in the infant after ^{131}I treatment of the hyperthyroid pregnant mother (252). Otherwise, irradiation HP is rare because the PTGs are relatively resistant to radiation.

C. Infiltration

Iron storage in the PTG is a rare cause of HP; it is usually associated with similar destruction induced by hemosiderosis of the thyroid gland, gonads, pancreatic islets, liver, myocardium, and, occasionally, pituitary gland. This condition may complicate any disease in which blood transfusions are frequently required, such as thalassemia major and hypoplastic anemia. In β-thalassemia major, HP commonly manifests in the second decade of life, but latent HP may occur much earlier (253, 254).

HP may also develop in Wilson's disease (MIM 277900), presumably due to deposition of copper in the PTG (255).

Destructive infiltration by a metastasizing neoplasm or by amyloid is rare in children.

XV. PSEUDOHYPOPARATHYROIDISM

Pseudohypoparathyroidism (PHP; 21, 256) is a group of diseases with supranormal plasma levels but deficient action of PTH, indicating end-organ resistance. The resistance can be further proven by giving a test intravenous injection of PTH: phosphaturic, calcemic, and calcitriolemic responses are absent or markedly blunted.

A. Types of Pseudohypoparathyroidism

Because of the complexity of the signal transduction cascade of PTH (Sec. II.D.; Fig. 3), there are many possible sites for failure. Several kinds of basic defects have been identified in PHP, and others will certainly follow (Table 4; 256). The primary basis for classification is location of the defect proximal or distal to the generation of cAMP. Proximal defects are identified by absence or markedly blunted response of plasma and urinary cAMP to exogenous PTH stimulation; this is the criterion for PHP type I. In this type the renal mechanism of response to cAMP is intact as evidenced by responsiveness to injected (dibutyryl) cAMP (257). In patients with distal defects, plasma and urinary cAMP responses to exogenous PTH are normal and basal urinary cAMP exretion may even be supranormal; such patients have type II PHP.

The second basis for classification is the extent of the consequences of the defect. Although PTH shares the G_s protein complex and the adenylyl cyclase of the cellular signal transduction cascade with other hormones (258), a part of the cascade is specific to PTH (and PTHrP) by structure (PTH receptor) or cell type (effector phosphoproteins of the cascade). Defects of the shared components may cause resistance to several hormones. Most of the

Table 4 Clinical and Laboratory Findings in Patients with Different Types of PHP

	Serum Ca	Serum Pi	Serum PTH	Urinary cAMP	Pi-uric response	Serum TSH	AHO	Gsα activity	Gsα mutation
PHP-Ia	↓	↑	↑	↓	↓	(↑)	+	↓	+
pPHP	→	→	→	→	→	→	+	↓	+
PHP-Ib	↓	↑	↑	↓	↓	→	−	→	−(?)
PHP-Ic	↓	↑	↑	↓	↓	(↑)	+	−	−
PHP-II	↓	↑	↑	→	↓	→	−	→	−(?)

PHP, pseudohypoparathyroidism; pPHP, pseudo-PHP; Pi, inorganic phosphate; AHO, Albright's hereditary osteodystrophy; Gsα, α subunit of guanyl-nucleotide binding protein.

known cases are due to inactivating mutations in the gene *GNAS1* encoding the α subunit of the stimulatory G protein (Gsα, Sec. II.D.). Such mutations are the cause of PHP-Ia and pseudo-PHP (pPHP). All patients are heterozygous and have one normal *GNAS1* allele and one defective allele. Mutations of *GNAS1* may also be involved in PHP-Ib. In kindreds with PHP-Ia and pPHP, at least 25 heterozygous nucleotide exchanges in *GNAS1* gene have been identified causing variable mutations of Gsα (21, 256). Gsα is ubiquitously expressed, but appears to have tissue-specific roles, and its heterozygous mutations may cause autosomal dominant diseases with resistance only to a few hormones. In some type I patients normal quantity of G$_s$α has been observed; in one such patient a mutation of the adenylyl cyclase was identified (259).

In addition to the entities mentioned, there are at least two others: PHP-Ic and PHP-II. Patients with PHP-Ic have no detectable defect in the Gsα protein, despite clinical and laboratory features similar to patients with PHP-Ia.

Patients with PHP-Ia, PHP-Ic, and pPHP share an abnormal habitus called Albright's hereditary osteodystrophy (AHO, Fig. 10). Patients with PHP-II are similar to those with PHP-Ib in having no skeletal and developmental defects, but differ by having normal urinary cAMP excretion but blunted phosphaturic response to exogenous PTH. PHP-Ic and PHP-II are poorly characterized compared with the other types.

B. Albright's Hereditary Osteodystrophy

Albright's hereditary osteodystrophy (AHO) is the collective name of the abnormal features of habitus that patients with PHP-Ia, PHP-Ic and pPHP have (Fig. 10; 260): short stature, round or moon-shaped face, depressed nasal bridge, thick-set stocky or obese body, and bone anomalies. The latter include selective shortness and stubbiness of metacarpals (brachymetacarpia of, in decreasing order of prevalence, metacarpals IV, V, I, III, and, rarely and

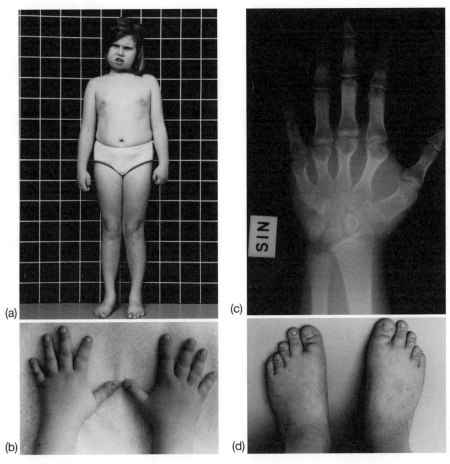

Figure 10 Abnormal features of habitus in the Albright hereditary osteodystrophy (AHO) in an 11-year old girl. a. Short stocky habitus with round face. b,c. Plump hands. d. Feet with short metatarsals. A bone was excised from this girl's upper eyelid.

never alone, II), metatarsals (brachymetatarsia IV, V, III, I), and phalanges (brachyphalangia, most often of distal phalanx I leading to a thumb nail width to length ratio of >2.0), radius curvus, cubitus valgus, coxa vara, and genu valgum (261). Short digits arise from early closure of the epiphyses, preceded by decrease in longitudinal growth. Cone-shaped epiphyses may be formed, and phalangeal rudimentary or pseudo epiphyses occur (251). Hand and foot abnormalities generally are not apparent before the age of 4 years, and AHO habitus may only appear slowly to be clear by school age. It may become more pronounced in successive generations (262). Selective brachymetacarpia or brachymetatarsia and/or heterotopic soft tissue ossifications, and absence of tall stature, have often been used as the minimum criteria of AHO (263).

Dental abnormalities are common: enamel hypoplasia, small crowns, enlarged pulp chambers, root canals with open apices, pulp stones, blunted roots, delayed eruption of deciduous and permanent teeth, hypodentia, thickening of the lamina dura, and early tooth loss due to caries (264).

Height SD score correlates with the activity of the G_s protein (265). Bone age is often advanced rather than retarded, unless hypothyroidism is present.

A mild to moderate mental retardation occurs in 50–75% of patients; it is also associated with the deficiency of the Gs activity (266). Subnormal senses of smell (elevated detection and recognition thresholds for all vapors) and taste (detection and recognition thresholds supranormal for sour and bitter, normal for salt and sweet) are part of the picture (251, 267). Olfaction is known to be mediated by $G_{olf}\alpha$ protein, which shows 88% amino acid identity to $G_s\alpha$ (268, 269).

Hypothenar dermatoglyphic patterns and distally located triradii are frequent (270). Degenerative changes occur in the hip joints, even necrosis of the femoral head (271). Spinal cord compression has occurred as a result of combination of abnormal vertebral fusion, shortened vertebral lamina, and soft tissue calcifications within the spinal canal (272). Hypertension is common in adult patients (273).

C. Genetics: Important Role of Imprinting

Both PHP-Ia and pPHP are caused by the same $G_s\alpha$-affecting mutations of the GNAS1 gene in chromosome 20q13.2, as evidenced by common occurrence of both diseases in the same kindreds. In such kindreds, all patients with pPHP are offspring of healthy women with men affected with either PHP-Ia or pPHP, whereas all patients with PHP-Ia are offspring of healthy men with women affected with either of the two disorders (274). This results from paternal imprinting of the hormonal resistance: PHP-Ia occurs only if the defective gene is inherited from a mother affected by either PHP-Ia or pPHP (275).

The pattern of imprinting is complex. Although $G_s\alpha$ expression may derive in only the maternal allele in some

tissues, it may derive from both alleles in other tissues (276). Hence, there may be no $G_s\alpha$ in some tissues but 50% of the normal level in other tissues. This may explain why there is resistance to some of the hormones using $G_s\alpha$-coupled receptors, while the resistance is partial or absent to some others (21). In contrast, the mode of inheritance of AHO is dominant; this remains to be explained. AHO is presumed to be caused by the same heterozygous GNAS1 mutations responsible for the decrease in the activity of the $G_s\alpha$ protein. The PTH/PTHrP receptor also has an important role in chondrocyte proliferation and differentiation and thus in skeletal growth (277). Reduced concentrations of Gsα in the proliferative layer of the growth plate chondrocytes might result in an insufficient PTHrP-dependent inhibition of chondrocyte maturation, and hence to the abnormally short bones of AHO (256).

PHP-Ib, in all four kindreds studied, was also invariably inherited from an obligate female carrier, indicating paternal imprinting. DNA study of these kindreds showed that the genetic defect of PHP-Ib maps to an approximately 8 cM region on chromosome 20q13.3, the region that includes the GNAS1 gene (278). In the equivalent region of the mouse, gnas is the only known imprinted gene. Several different splice variants of it are known that are specific to parent-of-origin in expression, and the same is true for the human GNAS1. Hence the current data indicate that mutations of GNAS1 (other than those affecting the $G_s\alpha$ protein) are also responsible for at least some forms of PHP-Ib (256).

D. Pseudohypoparathyroidism Type-Ia (MIM 139320)

In addition to resistance to the actions of PTH, PHP type Ia (PHP-Ia) includes AHO and partial resistance to other hormones.

1. Renal Resistance

The PTH resistance in patients with PHP-Ia (and particularly those with PHP-Ib) is clearest in the proximal tubules. All responses to PTH are impaired: production of cAMP and calcitriol, and excretion of Pi and bicarbonate. The lack of phosphaturic response to PTH causes hyperphosphatemia, which probably further inhibits the production of calcitriol, aggravating its deficiency. The calcitriol response to an acute lowering of plasma Pi level is also subnormal, in clear contrast to patients with PTH deficiency. There is no such difference in calcitriol response to dibutyryl cAMP injection. This suggests that there may be an abnormality in the 1α-hydroxylase system. Indeed, many features of the disease appear to be secondary to the calcitriol deficiency. One such secondary defect is in the distal tubular Ca reabsorption response to PTH; it is normalized by correction of the hypocalcemia and the calcitriol deficiency (25; Fig. 11). The primary

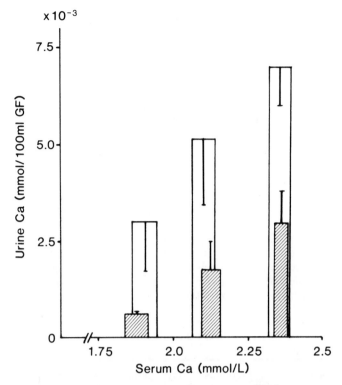

Figure 11 Comparison of urinary Ca excretion (vertical scale) at three different concentration ranges of calcemia (horizontal scale; the width of each column represents the mean ± SD of the individual concentrations) between patients with PHP (shaded columns) and HP (nonshaded columns) during therapy with different dosages of $1\alpha(OH)D_3$. Normal controls had the same mean values as the normocalcemic patients with PHP. The patients with HP (in contrast to the patients with PHP) have marked hypercalciuria at all levels of plasma Ca. (From Ref. 25.)

renal resistance thus seems to be confined to the proximal tubular actions of PTH.

Significantly stronger calciuria and lower plasma PTH levels have been observed in type I PHP patients without AHO than in those with AHO, despite similar calcemia levels (279). This observation is consistent with normal PTH responsiveness of the distal tubules.

2. Skeletal Resistance

Whether skeletal resistance to PTH is an innate part of PHP has been a matter of dispute. The remodeling system appears active; there is even evidence for its acceleration due to the supranormal levels of PTH. In contrast to patients with HP and similar degrees of hypocalcemia and hypocalcitriolemia, patients with PHP as a group have subnormal bone density (280), and more than doubled urinary excretion of hydroxyproline (an index of osteoclastic bone degradation) (73, 280). They respond to exogenous

PTH by an increase in hydroxyproline excretion similarly to patients with HP (280). During substitution therapy, an inverse correlation appears between plasma Ca level and hydroxyproline excretion, and this excretion is normalized in most patients during normocalcemia (73). However, plasma alkaline phosphatase activity and osteocalcin concentration (markers of osteoblastic bone formation) are normal in patients with PHP in contrast to supranormal levels in patients with primary hyperparathyroidism, although plasma PTH levels are more elevated in patients with PHP (73). In patients with HP, osteocalcin levels are subnormal. Despite the higher plasma PTH levels in patients with PHP than patients with hyperparathyroidism, none of the three markers of bone turnover was different between these patient groups, suggesting that the remodeling system does have some degree of resistance to PTH in PHP (73). Radiological evidence of hyperparathyroidism, subperiosteal resorption, and/or cysts have been reported in PHP, but are rare (251, 260, 280–283). Seven of 18 patients with such changes had slipped capital femoral epiphysis (283). Histological hyperparathyroid changes (osteitis fibrosa) are much more common; they disappear during adequate therapy (283).

The increased bone turnover in response to high PTH levels may contribute to the maintenance of calcemia. Estrogen, which blocks PTH-mediated bone resorption, has induced hypocalcemia in women with normocalcemic PHP (284). The other skeletal metabolic system, the mineral homeostatic system, is unresponsive to PTH, but this may be secondary to the calcitriol deficiency (285, 286). Prolonged treatment with pharmacological dosages of vitamin D has restored the calcemic responsiveness to PTH in some patients to normal (285, 286), and physiological amounts of calcitriol normalize calcemia (287, 288). In fact, PTH resistance of this system is part of the pathophysiology in vitamin D-deficiency rickets (289). It is assumed that this osteocytic system is more calcitriol-dependent than the osteoclastic–osteoblastic remodeling system (280).

In conclusion, if there is skeletal resistance to PTH in PHP, it is only partial in contrast to the complete resistance of the proximal renal tubules.

3. Clinical and Metabolic Picture and Their Variability

Most patients maintain normocalcemia for the first several years of life: hypocalcemia and hyperphosphatemia occur at an average age of 8 years, and rarely before the age of 3 years (260). Plasma PTH levels may be elevated much earlier, and sometimes this is associated with mild hypercalcemia. Clinical manifestation may occur only at an adult age. Often, the hypocalcemia or the hyperphosphatemia has been noted incidentally. The hypocalcemia may alternate with normocalcemia. Hence, the resistance may be acquired and depend on factors other than the primary defect (260). Deficiency of calcitriol is a possibility, as described above for the skeletal homeostatic system and the distal tubular Ca reabsorption. The response of cAMP to exogenous PTH is defective from early infancy (271); it is further impaired with the development of hypocalcemia and improves during spontaneous remissions (290). However, the spontaneous normocalcemia recovery periods seem not to be associated with an increase in calcitriolemia (290). Pregnancy, despite its high estrogen levels, has temporarily improved PHP patients' Ca homeostasis. This may be due to production of calcitriol by the fetally derived trophoblastic portion of placenta.

The regulation of PTH secretion is qualitatively normal, and persistent hypocalcemia maintains supranormal secretion of HPT. Plasma levels of PTH and Ca show an inverse correlation (73). Spontaneously normocalcemic patients may also have supranormal plasma PTH (73, 271). During therapy with an active vitamin D analog, plasma PTH is normalized only when plasma Ca^{2+} levels are brought to the upper normal range; this indicates an elevated set point for suppression of the PTH secretion (74), presumably due to an involvement of the G_s protein–cAMP system in PTG. In some patients the secretion of PTH may be suppressed secondary to calcitriol deficiency (271).

In addition to the hypocalcemia, often associated with grand mal seizures, the first manifestation may be either primary nongoitrous hypothyroidism, which may be congenital (291–293), or features of ovarian hypofunction, subcutaneous ossifications, bone pain (294), or slipped capital femoral epiphysis (283) caused by cystic bone disease. Convulsions seem to be more prevalent in PHP than HP, occurring in as many as 60% of the patients, and mostly resembling grand mal seizures.

Ossified plaques and nodules, also called osteomas, occur frequently in subcutaneous tissues, brain, and heart; they may be present at birth and years before hypocalcemia develops (262, 295). Calcifications of the basal ganglia have been observed in up to 100% of adult patients (80), and have often given the first clue to the diagnosis of PHP (80).

Hypertension may be common in adult patients (273).

4. Other Endocrine Abnormalities

Resistance to other hormones is frequent, but variable even between affected siblings (260, 264, 271, 296–298). Clinical hypothyroidism due to thyroidal resistance to TSH is quite common, and it frequently precedes the clinical HP. It was observed in 15 of 26 patients (299), and TSH response to TRH was exaggerated in nearly all the patients. Hypothyroidism may even be the first and congenital manifestation; it is often detected by neonatal screening (291, 292).

Clinical hypogonadism is common in female patients, due to ovarian gonadotropin resistance. It may result in incomplete development of secondary sexual characteristics, primary amenorrhea or delayed menarche, and infertility. Menstrual function ranges from amenorrheic to normal (298). Plasma levels of the gonadotropins are generally not elevated. Fertility may be subnormal in male patients, because few of them seem to have reproduced (260).

As a group, the patients have a significantly subnormal plasma cAMP response to glucagon test, indicating subnormal hepatic cAMP (although normal glucose) response to glucagon (298). Prolactin deficiency is less common (300, 301). GH secretion has usually been reported as normal, but there are exceptions (293, 302). Single cases of resistance to ADH (303) and ACTH (304) have been reported.

Two unrelated males have been observed with both precocious puberty and PHP Ia. They had identical mutations of *GNAS1*, which resulted in a temperature-sensitive $G_s\alpha$ that is rapidly degraded at the normal body temperature but constitutively activated in the cooler environment of the testis, resulting in so-called testotoxicosis (MIM 176410) (305).

E. Pseudopseudohypoparathyroidism (MIM 300800)

Patients with pseudopseudohypoparathyroidism (pPHP) have the AHO habitus and the approximately 50% subnormal level of $G_s\alpha$ activity similarly to patients with PHP-Ia, but no endocrine abnormality and a normal cAMP response to PTH. The latter feature differentiates pPHP from the normocalcemic phase of or incompletely expressed PHP-Ia. Pedigrees with G_s protein deficiency commonly include both members with P-PHP and those with PHP, and the level of G_s is similarly deficient in the cell membranes of both kinds of patients (306, 307).

F. Pseudohypoparathyroidism Type Ib (MIM 603233)

Patients with PHP type Ib (PHP-Ib) have normal appearance and intelligence with hormone resistance limited to PTH. Symptomatic hypocalcemia appears, as in PHP-Ia, usually within the first decade of life but in some patients only much later (308). The disturbance appears to be produced predominantly by renal resistance to PTH, which results in impaired excretion of Pi and production of calcitriol. The skeleton appears to respond normally to PTH, releasing continuously Ca^{2+} and Pi (308a). The inevitable secondary hyperparathyroidism may lead to hyperparathyroid skeletal disease, sometimes called pseudohypohyperparathyroidism. Short stature is common (298). Although this bone resorption helps to maintain relatively normal calcemia, it also maintains a flux of Pi into blood. Because of renal PTH resistance, the excretion of Pi is inefficient and results in hyperphosphatemia. The acitivity of $G_s\alpha$ is normal. Mutations in the genes coding for PTH and the PTH/PTHrP receptor seem to be excluded (309).

PHP-Ib may vary considerably in severity, even within kindreds, from seizure-causing disease to absence of even the laboratory abnormalities at adult age (278). Seasonal variation can also be significant. Although most cases have been considered to be sporadic, it may just be that other cases in the family have been asymptomatic.

One patient had severe osteitis fibrosa cystica with bone pain, which only resolved after parathyroidectomy. Osteoblastlike cells cultured from her trabecular bone responded normally to PTH and calcitriol (294).

G. Pseudohypoparathyroidism Type II (PHP-II; MIM 203330)

At least 20 patients of PHP type II (PHP-II) have been reported (260). It appears heterogeneous and, in at least some cases, acquired. Hence, all reported features may not be universally true. In contrast to patients with type I, patients with type II have normal Na^+ and bicarbonate excretory responses to PTH. After prolonged normalcemia has been maintained by Ca infusion or vitamin D administration, some of these patients have shown a normal phosphaturic response to PTH (263, 310). This suggests that the primary defect may be absence of a response to PTH in the renal cell membrane permeability to Ca^{2+}. Age at onset of this disease varied from 1.8 to 70 years (260). In one patient clinical manifestation occurred only during the hypocalcemic stress of the second half of her pregnancies (311). This is in contrast to the improvement of Ca homeostasis experienced during pregnancy by patients with PHP-I. Hyperparathyroid bone disease has been reported in some patients (260).

PHP-II may occur with vitamin D deficiency (312, 313). Sjögren syndrome may include PHP-II, presumably by an autoimmune mechanism (314).

XVI. DIAGNOSIS

A. Diagnosis of Hypocalcemia

The Chvostek test (Sec. VIII.B.1.b.) is very useful for obtaining immediate evidence pointing to or ruling out hypocalcemia. A grade 2 sign suggests, and higher grades indicate, hypocalcemia; the more severe, the stronger the sign. Absence of the sign argues against hypocalcemia, but does not exclude it.

In a convulsing patient with some evidence of hypocalcemia, it may be advisable to give a Ca-gluconate injection (Sec. XVII.A.) after inserting a venous catheter and taking adequate samples of blood to allow definite studies in case of hypocalcemia or hypoglycemia. Cessation of the convulsion during or immediately after the injection provides strong evidence for hypocalcemia, but continuation of the conculsion may not exclude it. In case of hypocalcemia, determinations must also be obtained of serum Mg, Pi, total protein, urea, or creatinine, and, preferably, Ca^{2+}.

B. Diagnosis of Deficient Parathyroid Hormone Effect and Latent Hypoparathyroidism

Manifestly deficient PTH effect is recognizable from the coexistence of hypocalcemia and hyperphosphatemia, provided that primary renal failure is excluded by determination of serum creatinine or urea (Fig. 12). In mild cases of HP the serum Pi concentration may be normal.

To identify persons at risk of hypocalcemia during periods of hypocalcemic stress due to fasting, exceptionally low Ca intake or high Pi intake, or therapy with loop diuretics, reserve capacity of PTG should be evaluated with the EDTA infusion test (Table 5) in normocalcemic patients with components of the syndromes that often include HP, especially the DiGeorge malformation complex (Sec. XII.A.), or with a history of so-called transient HP in the neonatal period of later (161, 162, 225, 232, 233).

C. Differentiation of Hypoparathyroidism and Pseudohypoparathyroidism

Features of AHO in the habitus and radiographic evidence of hyperparathyroidism strongly suggest PHP. Characteristics of a specific form of HP (APECED, the DiGeorge malformation complex, the Kenny–Caffey syndromes, hypomagnesemia, surgical HP) may suggest or even give a definite diagnosis. HP and PHP are differentiated by simultaneous measurements of serum Ca and intact PTH (315) or PTH_{1-32}. In unclear cases, those measurements should be obtained during hypocalcemia (before therapy, or induced by cessation of therapy, or by an EDTA infusion; Table 5), because that increases plasma PTH in PHP, accentuating the contrast between subnormal levels in HP and supranormal levels in PHP. Subnormal levels include levels within the so-called normal range during hypocalcemia.

A determination of serum 25-hydroxyvitamin D may be needed to exclude vitamin D deficiency, which may cause PTH resistance (313) and suppress the supranormal levels of PTH in PHP. Some patients with PHP may show the characteristic supranormal plasma PTH levels only after repletion of calcitriol (271). Hypomagnesemia may likewise have to be corrected to reveal the supranormal PTH levels of PHP (316).

The PTH test (Fig. 13) may help to confirm or exclude PHP, in addition to being the key to the diagnosis of the specific type of PHP. This test may not differentiate between HP and PHP-II, however, because the cAMP response is normal in both. The phosphaturic response should differentiate between these two conditions but is not quite reliable but may give both false-positive and false-negative results even when the ideal response index, the relative decrement in TmP/GFR (Sec. IV.A.), is used (317, 318).

An alternative approach is to test whether the kidneys respond to a PTH test dose by an increase in plasma cal-

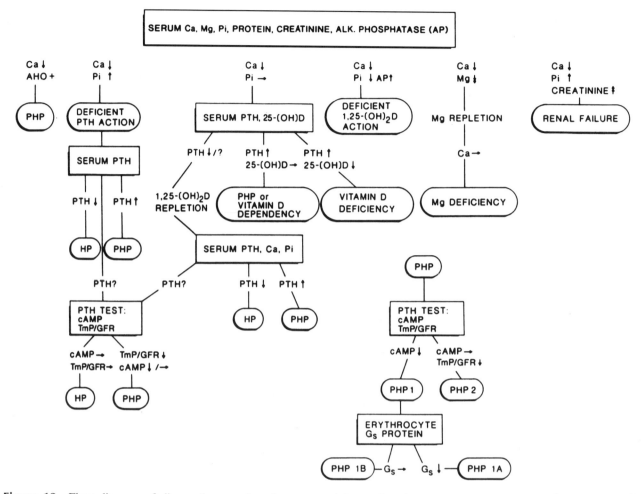

Figure 12 Flow diagram of diagnostic procedure for suspected hypocalcemia. Pi, inorganic phosphate; ↓, subnormal; ↑, supranormal; →, normal; AHO, the Albright hereditary osteodystrophy; TmP/GFR, quotient of maximum rate of tubular phosphate reabsorption and glomerular filtration rate (relative decrement of this quotient is the best index of PTH effect on tubular reabsorption of phosphate [Sec. IV.A.; Fig. 5]). Plasma cAMP measurement may be preferable to urine cAMP in the PTH test (Fig. 13). In a normocalcemic patient with suspicion of latent HP, perform EDTA test (Table 5).

citriol. In a small series of mostly adult patients, all 14 patients with HP showed a 24 h increment in plasma calcitriol of at least 24 pmol/l (10 pg/ml), whereas the responses all four patients with PHP were below this limit (319). Another method is to observe whether the skeleton responds to a trial treatment with PTH over some days by an increase in calcemia.

D. Diagnosis of Specific Forms of Hypoparathyroidism

Patients with APECED should be identified, because of their risk of developing new, possibly dangerous, components of the disease. A firm clinical diagnosis of APECED requires the presence of at least two of the following: chronic or recurring mucocutaneous candidiasis, HP, and adrenocortical failure (or antiadrenal or 21-hy-

doxylase autoantibodies). If a sibling fulfills this criterion, one of any of the autoimmune or clear ectodermal components of APECED (Sec. XI) suffices for the diagnosis. The two-out-of-three-criterion became fulfilled within the first 5 years of life in only 22% of our patients, in the next 5 year period in another 45%, in the second decade of life in a further 22%, in the third decade in 4.5%, and only later in 2%. It was not fulfilled in a male patient by the time of his death at the age of 45 years from oral cancer, a consequence of APECED; his *postmortem* diagnosis depended on his sister's diagnosis. Thus the criterion gives no false-positive diagnoses, but false-negative results are common, especially at a young age.

Hence, for appropriate clinical diagnosis, knowledge of the disease components other than the above-named three most common ones should be utilized. When a person under the age of 50 years has a disease that belongs

Table 5 EDTA Infusion Test of PTG Reserve

Procedure

After an overnight fast infuse over 2 h disodium EDTA intravenously 75 mg/kg (not exceeding 3 g) in 200–500 ml (depending on the size of the patient) 5% glucose solution containing 0.1 mg/kg lidocaine.

Obtain blood samples for determinations of serum Ca^{2+} and PTH just before the infusion and at 30, 60, 120, 180, and 240 min.

Assessment

Normal PTG reserve is indicated by a clear rise in serum PTH already at 30 min, and full recovery of serum Ca^{2+} by 240 min. Defective reserve is reflected by absent or subnormal rise of serum PTH and delayed recovery of serum Ca^{2+} levels.

Source: Refs. 163, 251.

to the components of APECED, he or she should be evaluated for the ectodermal, oral, and ophthalmic components. If two components of APECED are present without any other definite explanation, the patient should be evaluated for development of further components, or a search for *AIRE* mutations should be considered. Mutation diagnosis (Sec. XI.D.) is available from several specialized laboratories internationally. The relatively large number of mutations, and the fact that many others remain unrecognized, causes problems in the mutation approach to the diagnosis. Hence, APECED cannot be thus excluded.

It is also important to identify patients with hypocalcemic hypercalciuria among subjects with HP, to avoid renal complications. A finding of hypocalcemia not associated with an undetectable or very low serum PTH concentration (but not supranormal as in PHP) and normal or supranormal calciuria should suggest that diagnosis. However, it is not possible to detect all cases by those measurements. Family screening for hypocalcemia, especially of the patient's parents, is advisable and may indicate dominant inheritance. The single-strand conformational polymorphism (SSCP) technique may be helpful for rapid molecular genetic screening for mutations of the Ca-R (90), but the same limitations are valid for the DNA diagnosis of hypocalcemic hypercalciuria as for APECED.

DiGeorge malformation complex-type dysmorphic facial appearance in an individual with a major outflow tract defect of the heart or a history of susceptibility to infections should raise suspicion of this condition. In infancy, hypocalcemia is a characteristic feature, although it may be intermittent and has a tendency to resolve during the first year. Immunological assessment relies on chest radiography to detect a thymic shadow (a notoriously unreliable investigation, particularly in a stressed infant) and measurement of the CD4-positive subset of lymphocytes. The investigations of choice are a standard karyotype to

exclude major rearrangements, and search for the 22q11.2 and 10p monosomies by the fluorescence *in situ* hybridization techniques (178, 181). Parents should be screened for carrier status (320). The possibility of HP and an immune defect should be kept in mind in apparently isolated cases of conotruncal defects, particularly truncus arteriosus communis, D-transposition of the great vessels, Fallot's tetralogy (321), and supracristal ventricular septal defect.

Phenotypic differences between DiGeorge malformation complex as associated with monosomy of 22q11 and monosomy 10p, involve a higher frequency of renal abnormality and deafness, and more heterogeneous cardiac defects in the latter. The type of deafness differs: about one-third of the patients with monosomy of 22q11 have a conductive hearing loss owing to recurrent otitis media or palatal abnormality or both, while the deafness in patients with monosomy 10p is sensorineural.

To diagnose the transient nature of neonatal and surgical HP, substitution therapy should be interrupted in the young infant with HP (the first time at 6 weeks after its introduction) and in surgical HP (the first time 3 weeks after its introduction), with close observation of the patient for recurrence of hypocalcemia. Absence of recurrence proves the transient nature of the disorder. However, PTH reserves should be tested for permanent subnormal levels (Sec. XVI.B.).

HP secondary to maternal hyperparathyroidism is confirmed by definite diagnosis of the mother's disease and the transient nature of the infant's HP. HP secondary to Mg depletion (XIII.C) is confirmed if hypomagnesemia is severe and Mg repletion corrects the HP. Mg deficiency appears to be a more frequent secondary feature of HP than commonly recognized. It may be particularly prevalent in patients with hypocalcemic hypercalciuria (322).

Isolated idiopathic HP can be positively differentiated from APECED only if the patient belongs to a kindred with definite case(s) of isolated idiopathic HP.

E. Type Diagnosis of Pseudohypoparathyroidism; Diagnosis of Pseudopseudohypoparathyroidism

The type of PHP should be determined for assessing the risk of hypothyroidism and hypogonadism and for purposes of genetic counseling. Presence of AHO points to types Ia and Ic, and its absence to Ib and II. Firm diagnosis requires that the PTH test be performed with biosynthetic fragments of human PTH, such as PTH_{1-34} or PTH_{1-38}, with determination of plasma and/or urinary cAMP response (Fig. 13) (317, 318). The patient should have a steady water diuresis during the test (323). Deficient cAMP response identifies type I and normal response identifies type II. PHP-Ia is recognized from evidence of other hormone resistance, most readily by a supranormal TSH response to TRH test. Deficient activity

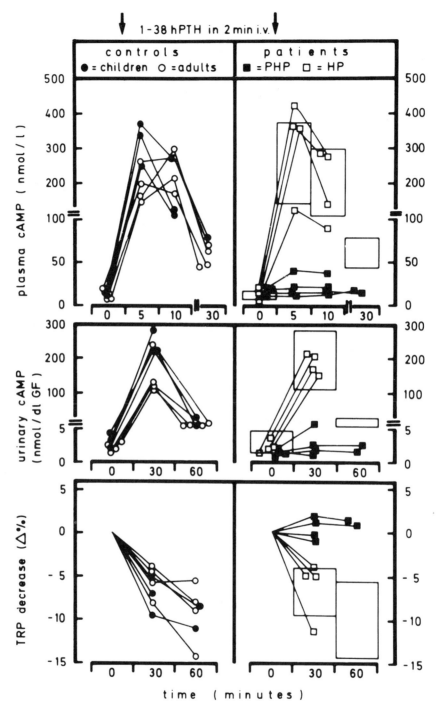

Figure 13 PTH test: effect of an intravenous injection of human PTH (0.5 μg/kg of PTH$_{1\text{-}38}$ over 2 min) on cAMP concentration in plasma (upper panels, nmol/l) and urine (middle panels, nmol/dL glomerular filtrate), and on tubular reabsorption of phosphate (TRP, lower panels, decrease in %) in controls (left) and in patients with PHP and HP (right). The rectangles in the right panels indicate the ranges of controls. (From Ref. 318.)

of the Gs protein may be demonstrated or excluded by studying erythrocyte membranes (324), and specialized laboratories can search for $G_s\alpha$-affecting mutations of the *GNAS1* gene (324a).

The definition of P-PHP is the presence of AHO with a normal cAMP response to the PTH test (Fig. 13).

XVII. THERAPY

A. Therapy of Tetany

A patient who is convulsing or has laryngeal stridor or severe tetany should promptly be given an intravenous injection of 10% Ca–gluconate solution. This solution contains 0.22 mmol/ml (8.8 mg/ml) Ca. The most rapid effect can be attained by injection of 0.25 ml/kg (0.055 mmol or 2.2 mg/kg) over not less than 2 min. This may ameliorate the tetany for 15 min to several hours; if not, the injection may be repeated in case of confirmed hypocalcemia. A continuous infusion should then follow: 1.8 ml/kg (0.4 mmol; 16 mg Ca/kg) of the 10% solution over 6–12 h (325). Extravasation of the solution should be strictly avoided, because of the risk of tissue necrosis. It should preferably be given diluted (e.g., 1:10 in 5% glucose solution). Oral administration of Ca salts is efficient for the control of hypocalcemia and is preferable to prolonged infusion. Liberal amounts should be given orally; for example, 50 mg Ca/kg/24 h in four or five divided doses. To sequestrate Pi in the intestine, dosages may be 4fold higher. The Ca content of oral preparations varies: carbonate 40%, chloride 36%, lactate 13%, gluconate 8.8%, and glucobionate 6.5%. Thus, 2.5 g, 2.8 g, 7.7 g, and 11.0 g are required, respectively, to provide 1.0 g Ca. Chloride can only be given in dilute (2%) solution (preferably in fruit juice) because it irritates the gastric mucosa. During fat malabsorption, the effect of oral administration may be poor.

B. Long-Term Therapy

1. General Aspects

The aim of therapy for patients with HP is to maintain plasma Ca at around the lower limit of the normal concentration range (2.0–2.2 mmol/l [8.0–8.8 mg/dl], Ca^{2+} 0.98–1.08 mmol/l) so that hypocalcemic manifestations are limited to the mildest symptoms and harmful hypercalciuria is avoided. Plasma Pi levels should also be normal. If therapy is successful, HP does not disturb the patient's life, and long-term complications will be avoided. The most serious risk to be most carefully avoided is hypercalcemia. It easily remains unnoticed, yet may cause irreparable kidney damage in a few weeks. In addition to drugs, therapy includes regular intake of relatively large amounts of fluid (to avoid low urine flow) and normal nutrition, with particular avoidance of fasting and high phosphate intake.

Treatment of patients with hypercalciuric hypocalcemia (Sec. X.A.) must be undertaken particularly carefully because of their higher level of hypercalciuria. Asymptomatic patients should not be given any medication for their hypocalcemia, and even symptomatic patients should be given only enough to alleviate their symptoms, not to make them normocalcemic.

In patients with PHP, in contrast to those with HP, therapy should aim at maintaining plasma Ca at a high-normal level (73). The basic differences between these two conditions dictating this difference in therapy are that normocalcemia causes hypercalciuria in HP but not in PHP, and that in PHP even low normal calcemia is associated with secondary hyperparathyroidism, which may harm the skeleton.

Two principles of long-term drug therapy apply: (a) PTH replacement with a calciferol sterol is a necessity; and (b) oral Ca supplementation is a recommendable adjunct therapy, and oral Mg should be added to avoid Mg depletion. The dosage of the sterol has to be carefully adjusted and frequently readjusted, because the need may fluctuate even after long periods of steady normocalcemia. Serum Ca and Pi levels, and urinary Ca excretion, must be regularly monitored. Responsibility for control of calcemia lies with the family. The patients should carry a physician-alert sign identifying that he or she has the disease.

The patient and family should be well informed about the patient's lack of normal tolerance of varying Ca intake. Once the substitution therapy has been adjusted to a level of Ca intake, this should be maintained. An extra intake of Ca, such as an unusually large amount of milk or a tablet containing 1 g Ca, which would be well tolerated by a normal person by means of a prompt reduction of PTH secretion, may produce a period of hypercalcemia in the patient. A reduction of Ca intake due to fast or a change in diet may likewise lead to hypocalcemia, because of the absence of a normal ability to increase promptly the secretion of PTH.

PTH1-34, should it become available affordably, would offer the benefits of physiological replacement therapy. Two daily subcutaneous injections seem to provide for normocalcemia without the risk of hypercalciuria (322).

2. Sterol Therapy

Calciferol sterols (Table 6) are the only drugs generally available for long-term replacement therapy. Hypocalcemia can be effectively controlled with them and the desired level of calcemia can be maintained, because they increase the flow of Ca^{2+} from the intestine and skeleton (Fig. 14). Normocalcemia will, in itself, restore the inherent ability of the kidneys to adjust the excretion of Pi to phosphatemia. Reaching a sustained decrease in plasma Pi levels requires, on average, 2 months (326). However, the sterols lack one important renal action of PTH: stimulation of the distal tubular reabsorption of Ca^{2+}. Hence,

Table 6 Calciferol Sterols Used in the Therapy of
Patients with HP and PHP

Sterol	Average dosage[a] (μ/kg/day)	Average half-life (days)	Comments
Calcitriol	0.03	1	Good, limited experience
1α(OH)D	0.06	2	Good, limited experience
DHT	20	7	Highly recommended
25(OH)D	4	15	Questionable value
D$_2$ and D$_3$	50	30	Risk of cumulative action

[a]Individual variation in requirement is great, and may fluctuate. Therapy should be initiated with about half this dosage, and the dosage carefully adjusted according to response. Frequent monitoring of serum Ca and Pi levels and 24 h urinary Ca is mandatory, even in patients with stable response (see text). Clear onset of action is usually evident approximately at half-life, a plateau in 2–4 half-lives, and after discontinuation of the drug, its action continues for 2–3 half-lives, but this may be much longer for the D vitamins.

normocalcemic patients with HP excrete on average three-fold more Ca in urine than normal persons (Fig. 11). This poses a risk of Ca sedimentation in the kidneys. To avoid this danger plasma Ca levels should be maintained no higher than the lower border of the normal range, and measurements of urinary Ca excretion are a part of the routine monitoring of therapy. In contrast, patients with

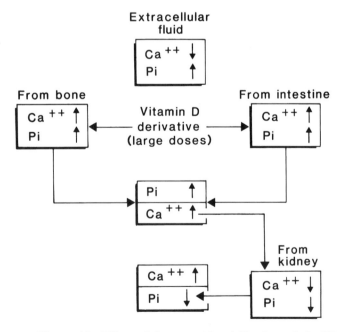

Figure 14 Effect of therapy with calciferol sterols in HP. For explanations and comparison, see Figure 6; this therapy is not complete replacement of PTH because the calciferols lack the renal effects of PTH.

PHP normalize calciuria with therapy (Fig. 11). It is assumed that their endogenous PTH stimulates the distal tubular absorption of Ca^{2+} as soon as their calcitriol levels are normalized. Even optimized sterol therapy does not substitute for normal PTH secretion, which varies greatly according to mineral balance.

The D vitamins (D$_2$ and D$_3$ are identically efficient) have a slow, prolonged, and cumulative action. They involve a risk of severe prolonged hypercalcemia, even after years of stable maintenance of normocalcemia, because they are stored in the adipose tissue. The stores may become large enough to maintain replacement therapy for as much as 6 months (77). Therefore, vitamin D is not recommended for routine replacement therapy, especially not for labile patients, and when regular laboratory monitoring cannot be guaranteed. The effect of vitamin D is probably based on the generation of large amounts of 25-(OH)D, which has a low affinity for the VDR. 25-(OH)D$_3$ is available in the Unites States and some other countries. It has little to recommend it, particularly if its cost is high.

Calcitriol and 1α-(OH)D are the fastest- and shortest-acting derivatives, and probably good alternatives for therapy. Two very favorable reports have appeared on the long-term use of calcitriol in children with HP. None of them had APECED (in which HP may be very labile and the longer-acting DHT may therefore be the drug of choice). In a report on 10 children (326) the dosage, initially 0.25 μg/day, was raised in increments of 0.25 μg until normocalcemia was achieved, over a minimum of 3 days. The final dosage was 0.50–1.25 μg/day, given in two or three divided doses. It was neither weight- nor age-related. Hypercalcemia was observed eight times during a total of 35 patient years; it was controlled by an interruption of therapy for 3 days. Hypocalcemia was registered 10 times, half of them transient and related to intercurrent febrile illness. In a report on four children (327), the dosage required to maintain plasma Ca at levels above 2.0 mmol/l (8.0 mg/dl) was 0.75–1.00 μg/day. Only two hypercalcemic and two hypocalcemic periods were observed during a total of 21 patient years.

In a comparative study of therapy in adults with HP or PHP (328), the mean daily doses required were similar with calcitriol (1.5 μg) and DHT (450 μg). In contrast, consistently in several studies (25, 328, 329) of 1α(OH)D, more was required in patients with HP (4 μg) than with PHP (2 μg). This may reflect a pathophysiological difference between these two diseases. Long-term safety of 1α(OH)D has been established (330).

Crystalline DHT is an intermediate-acting derivative, and an excellent drug for long-term therapy. This vitamin D derivative has multiple advantages for use in patients requiring pharmacological dosages, as in HP (331). The crystalline form of this drug has an ideal duration of action.

It is important to become well acquainted with the use of one drug, and establish clear rules for it, which must also be given to the patient and parents. The author's rules for DHT therapy are provided as an example. The full effect of a dose of DHT is reached in 10–20 days. In regular therapy, one daily dose is given or, in the case of a very small dose (<0.05 mg), one dose every second day. Therapy is started with a dose likely to be too small rather than too large. The dose is increased at intervals of 10–14 days as necessary to maintain the ideal serum Ca level. For fine adjustment, the increments/decrements of the dose should be around 10%. At the start of therapy and whenever the dose is increased, an extra dose is given that is sevenfold the increment. Whenever the dose needs to be adjusted slightly downward, a similar omission (sevenfold the decrement) is made at once. In moderate hypercalcemia (at or above 2.6 mmol/l, 10.4 mg/dl; Ca^{2+} 1.27 mmol/l) the DHT intake is discontinued for a few days and restarted only when a repeat serum Ca determination shows a decrease to close the ideal level.

3. Refractoriness to Sterol Therapy

Some patients become refractory to oral sterol therapy. This is not uncommon in patients with APECED, and another kind of case is on record (331, 332). In APECED one frequent contributing factor is fat malabsorption. Patients with this condition need to be monitored very carefully. Usually, however, maintenance of the recommended level of calcemia will keep the malabsorption under control. Fat malabsorption leads to a vicious cycle: like other lipids the sterol is poorly absorbed and this causes impairment of the hypocalcemia, which makes the fat malabsorption more severe. The cycle might be broken by increasing the oral doses of the sterol and Ca, and by decreasing fat intake or replacing ordinary fat by medium-chain triglycerides, which are more completely absorbed in this situation than are ordinary fats (77).

It is important to use the shorter-acting derivatives in the oral therapy of these patients, because very high doses (even 20-fold the regular dose) may be needed. In these situations serum Ca needs to be monitored several times weekly so that the dose may be immediately reduced when the calcemia starts to improve. Parenteral administration of calcitriol or 1α-(OH)D may help to break the cycle, if daily injections can be arranged. An attempt to decrease the malabsorption by intravenous Ca infusion failed, since the large amount of Ca passed rapidly into the urine.

Mg deficiency may sometimes be a factor in the resistance (77), and magnesemia reflects the Mg nutrition poorly. $MgCl_2$, in dosages up to 2 mmol/kg day orally, has reduced the sterol requirements of some refractory patients (77, 331).

Other factors may be involved. One patients of ours, who has had no clear steatorrhea, has been resistant to oral therapy with both DHT and 9α-fluorocortisol.

4. Calcium and Magnesium Supplementation

The ideal long-term therapy of HP probably includes a supplement of approximately 20 mg elementary Ca/kg daily (up to the total dose of 1.0 g) given as one of the oral preparations (Sec. XVII.A.), the most palatable of which may be the effervescent tablets. It must be divided in three to four doses to avoid single doses in excess of 7 mg/kg, and undue fluctuation of plasma Ca level (Sec. XVII.B.1.). This supplementation may help to control the hyperphosphatemia, and it offers the possibility of rapid correction of intervening hypercalcemia by stopping the substitution. However, if taking the supplement regularly would be uncertain, or if the supplementation is thought to be too stressful, it should not be prescribed at all. A good balance can usually be achieved without it.

The supplementation should be used at the beginning of therapy at least as long as the patient is expected to be hypocalcemic. In intervening situations of hypocalcemic stress (Sec. VII.A.) or hypocalcemia, a temporary substitution may be restarted, or the dosage of continuing substitution may be increased. However, single dosages should not exceed 7 mg/kg.

A daily oral supplement of 50 to 200 mg Mg is also recommended.

5. Therapy of Hyperphosphatemia

In the beginning of therapy for HP or PHP, it is advisable to restrict ingestion of milk and cheese for 2 months to reduce phosphate intake. The corresponding amount of Ca should be replaced with one of the oral Ca preparations. The described therapy commonly leads (within approximately 2 months) to normalization of phosphatemia, because the correction of hypocalcemia directly reduces the supranormal tubular Pi reabsorption. Furthermore, normalization of calcitriol activity may partially restore the inherent tubular ability to adapt to phosphatemia (Sec. IV.C.).

In some patients, however, the normalization of phosphatemia fails. In such patients, the dietary phosphate restriction should be continued. Aluminum hydroxide and carbonate, a dose with each meal, have been used for intestinal binding of Pi in patients with chronic uremia. These chemicals carry a risk of aluminum toxicity. Furthermore, my personal experiences with this therapy in HP have not been successful.

6. Therapy of Magnesium Deficiency

Secondary Mg deficit should be eliminated with oral administration of Mg chloride, citrate or lactate, which may need to be continuous. Often, 2 mmol/kg Mg daily divided in three or four doses is adequate (77).

In HP secondary to Mg depletion, the initial therapy consists of an intravenous infusion of a solution of Mg chloride or gluconate; 1–2 mmol/1.7 m^2/h is generally required to reach and maintain normal plasma level of Mg^{2+}. In a convulsing patient, the replacement may be started by giving slowly a bolus of 5–10 mmol/1.7 m^2, and continued at a rate of 5–7.5 mmol/1.7 m^2/h for the first 1–2 h. The use of intramuscular MgSO$_4$ is not recommended, because the injections are painful.

Deficits of Ca, K, and Pi should simultaneously be corrected. Oral calciferol should be given for vitamin D efficiency; calcitriol should not be used because it may worsen the hypomagnesemia (333). The intracellular deficit of Mg is only slowly corrected and most of the infused Mg^{2+} may be excreted, hence the infusion may have to be continued for 3–5 days. The therapy can then be continued with oral Mg salts, 2 mmol/kg daily (up to a total daily dose of 1.0 g Mg or 40 mmol) divided in four doses (77).

7.   Laboratory Follow-Up

Serum Ca and Pi determinations should routinely be done together. The accuracy and precision of Ca determinations are often less than excellent, and an unexpected value should be promptly confirmed before being taken as a basis for adjustment of therapy. Measurements of plasma Ca^{2+} are preferable to measurements of total Ca (326). Plasma total Ca may change postprandially, depending on the nature of the meal. Therefore, measurements after an overnight fast are preferable to random measurements. Also, prolonged application of a tourniquet leads to spurious elevation of plasma Ca. Normal plasma Pi levels depend on age (Table 1). Increments and decrements of 0.4 mmol/l (1.0 mg/dl) may occur after phosphate- or carbohydrate-rich meals, respectively. Therefore samples for routine determinations should be taken after an appropriate fast (overnight for all but infants).

It is our rule to have these determinations done at the maximum intervals of 6 weeks even in patients with stable levels. During labile periods, repeats may be needed even twice weekly. Frequent determinations of 24 h urinary Ca are recommended to check that the kidneys are not at risk for hypercalciuria, which is not reliably reflected by calcemia (77). Shorter collection periods are not recommended, because of the inconsistent diurnal variation of calciuria. The 24 h excretion should remain below 0.1 mmol/kg (4 mg/kg). If this rate is exceeded, calcemia should be maintained at a lower level. We do most of the laboratory checking by having the laboratory closest to the patient's home take the blood samples and mail the serum and a sample of urine to our laboratory. The 24 h urine specimens are likewise collected at home and, with a few milliliters of glacial acetic acid added, a sample from the measured total mixed volume is mailed to the laboratory. This is clearly more reliable than the use of unknown laboratories.

Serum Mg levels should also be checked at least twice annually for the development of secondary Mg deficiency. Serum creatinine levels should likewise be checked even in patients with no known hypercalcemic periods.

8.   Control by the Patient or the Parents

Parents and cooperative patients must be familiar with the symptoms of hypocalcemia and, especially, hypercalcemia (headache, increased nocturnal urine flow, thirst, anorexia, nausea, vomiting, constipation, lethargy, weakness, alterations of mental status) to be able to react to these without delay. They need detailed written information about the disease and these symptoms, including the immediate steps to be taken if they should appear. These steps include having a blood sample taken without delay to check serum Ca and Pi levels, contacting the physician, and, should this fail, first-aid adjustment of the drug therapy according to rules that are provided.

The parents and cooperative patients should be taught to perform the Chvostek test (Sect. VIII.B.1.b.). The value of this test needs to be established individually: in some cases, even the grade 1 sign may be significant. Some patients have discovered personal methods for recognizing hypocalcemia.

9.   Patients with Associated Addison's Disease

In patients with HP who also have Addison's disease, it is important to anticipate a decrease in Ca absorption and, consequently, hypocalcemia whenever the cortisol substitution dosage is increased even slightly, and the opposite may occur after a decrease in dosage.

Unexpected hypercalcemia may be the first signal of Addison's disease.

10.   Special Aspects of Pseudohypoparathyroidism

In patients with PHP, maintenance of normocalcemia is likely to improve endogenous Ca mobilization, and bring about a decrease in the sterol requirement. In contrast to patients with HP, patients with PHP during adequate sterol therapy have normal calciuria (Fig. 11). Hence, they should not need continuous Ca supplementation.

It is essential that hypothyroidism, which is frequently associated with PHP-Ia, be diagnosed and treated.

11.   Therapy of Complicating Hypercalcemia

Intervening hypercalcemia should be prevented through adequate monitoring, even during prolonged periods of stable normocalcemia, through an anticipatory decrease in replacement therapy in hypercalcemic risk situations (reduced mobility during illness, unusually high intake of milk products), and familiarity of the patients and parents with symptoms of hypercalcemia.

In hypercalcemia it is particularly important to maintain a relatively large fluid intake. Ca supplementation must be interrupted and foods with a high Ca content must be eliminated: milk, cheese, fish with bones (canned salmon, sardines etc.), leafy greens, and almonds. Mild hypercalcemia in a patient receiving a short- or intermediate-acting sterol may be controlled by a break of one-half to a complete half-life of the sterol in taking the sterol therapy followed by a decreased dose. In moderate hypercalcemia (serum Ca at or above 2.6 mmol/l, 10.4 mg/dl, Ca^{2+} 1.27 mmol/l) it is advisable to delay reintroduction of the sterol until serum Ca has returned to the target level. This is mandatory during therapy with vitamin D. During this therapy, and even during therapy with DHT, the patient may be unusually sensitive to reintroduction of the drug after a hypercalcemic period.

Some patients enter a vicious cycle in which hypercalcemia causes increased urine flow and a hyponatremic dehydration, which in turn aggravates the hypercalcemia. In these situations, rapid rehydration with a physiological Na^+ solution is mandatory. The rehydration with the ensuing natriuresis will usually rapidly alleviate the hypercalcemia.

In severe hypercalcemia (at or above 3.0 mmol/l, 12.0 mg/dl, Ca^{2+} 1.47 mmol/l) stronger measures are needed. Available alternatives are therapies with calcitonin and glucocorticoids (20–40 mg/m^2/24 h prednisolone in four daily doses, to inhibit the intestinal absorption of Ca), maintaining natriuresis with an intravenous infusion of physiological Na^+ solution, and furosemide (which increases calciuria in contrast to thiazide diuretics).

12. Risk Situations

Febrile illness and fasting predispose to hypocalcemia. The stress of a febrile illness may cause breakdown of intracellular organic phosphate compounds, with an increase in extracellular Pi leading to a decrease in Ca^{2+} level (77). Fasting reduces the inflow of Ca. Immobility, because of bed rest for illness, predisposes the patients to hypercalcemia. If motility is markedly reduced, as in transition from a normally moving to a motionless state, a preventive reduction of the sterol dosage should be considered, and plasma Ca and Pi levels should be evaluated closely.

Introduction of therapy with thiazide diuretics or anticonvulsants is another hypercalcemogenic intervention; these drugs reduce calciuria. The opposite is true of furosemide. A decrease in the glucocorticoid dosage also elevates calcemia, and an increase does the reverse.

REFERENCES

1. Kronenberg HM, Bringhurst FR, Nussbaum S, Jüppner H, Abou-Samra AB, Segre GV, Potts Jr JT. Parathyroid hormone: biosynthesis, secretion, chemistry, and action. In: Mundy GR, Martin TJ, eds. Handbook of Experimental Pharmacology, Heidelberg: Springer, 1993:185–201.
2. Vasicek TJ, McDevitt BE, Freeman MW, Fennick BJ, Hendy GH, Potts JT, Rich A, Kronenberg HM. Nucleotide sequence of the human parathyroid hormone gene. Proc Natl Acad Sci USA 1983;80:2127–2131.
3. Reis A, Hecht W, Gröger R, Böhm I, Cooper DN, Lindenmaier W, Mayer H, Schmidtke J. Cloning and sequence analysis of the human parathyroid hormone gene region. Human Genet 1990;84:119–124.
4. Hashizume Y, Waguri S, Watanabe T, Kominami E, Uchiyama Y. Cysteine proteinases in rat parathyroid cells with special reference to their correlation with

5. Miric A, Levine MA. Analysis of the preproPTH gene by denaturing gradient gel electrophoresis in familial isolated hypoparathyroidism. J Clin Endocrinol Metab 1992;74:509–516.
6. Mullersman JE, Shields JJ, Saha BK. Characterization of two novel polymorphisms at the human parathyroid hormone gene locus. Hum Genet 1992;88:589–592.
7. Parkinson DB, Shaw NJ, Himsworth RL, Thakker RV. Parathyroid hormone gene analysis in autosomal hypoparathyroidism using an intragenic tetranucleotide (AAAT)$_n$ polymorphism. Hum Genet 1993;91:281–284.
8. Habener JF, Rosenblatt M, Potts JT. Parathyroid hormone: biochemical aspects of biosynthesis, secretion, action, and metabolism. Physiol Rev 1984;64:985–1053.
9. Mallette LE. The parathyroid polyhormones: new concepts in the spectrum of peptide hormone action. Endocr Rev 1991;12:110–117.
10. Kovacs CS, Lanske B. Hunzelman JL, Guo J, Karaplis AC, Kronenberg HM. Parathyroid hormone-related protein regulates fetal-placental calcium transport through a receptor distinct from the PTH/PTHrP receptor. Proc Natl Acad Sci USA 1996;93:15233–15238.
11. Karaplis AC, Luz A, Glowacki J Bronson RT, Tybulewicz VL, Kronenberg HM, Mulligan RC. Lethal skeletal dysplasia from targeted disruption of the parathyroid-related peptide gene. Genes Dev 1994;8:277–289.
12. Strewler GJ. The parathyroid hormone-related protein. Endocrinol Metab Clin North Am 2000;29:629–645.
13. Ratzmann GW, Zöllner H. Relative Nebenschilddruseninsuffizienz bei Hypomagnesiämie. Kinderärztl Praxis 1991;59:380–383.
14. Riccardi D, Hall AE, Chattopadhyay N, Xu JZ, Brown EM, Hebert SC. Localization of the extracellular Ca^{2+}/polyvalent cation-sensing protein in rat kidney. Am J Physiol 1998;274:F611–F622.
15. Chattopadhyay N, Cheng I, Rogers K, Riccardi D, Hall A, Diaz R, Hebert SC, Soybel DI, Brown EM. Identification and localization of extracellular Ca^{2+}-sensing receptor in rat intestine. Am J Physiol 1998;274:G122–G130.
16. Rogers KV, Dunn CK, Hebert SC, Brown EM. Localization of calcium receptor mRNA in the rat central nervous system by in situ hybridization. Brain Res 1997;744:47–56.
17. DeLuca F, Baron J. Molecular biology and clinical importance of the Ca^{2+}-sensing receptor. Curr Opin Pediatr 1998;10:435–440.
18. Copp DH. Parathyroids, calcitonin and control of plasma calcium. Recent Prog Horm Res 1964;20:59–88.
19. Brown EM. Four-parameter model of the sigmoidal relationship between parathyroid hormone release and extracellular calcium concentration in normal and abnormal parathyroid tissue. J. Clin Endocrinol Metab 1983;56:572–581.
20. Dincsoy MY, Tsang RC, Laskarzewski P, Chen MH, Chen IW, Lo D, Donovan EF. The role of postnatal age and magnesium on parathyroid hormone response during "exchange" blood transfusion in the newborn period. J Pediatr 1992;100:277–283.
21. Levine MA. Pseudohypoparathyroidism: from bedside to bench and back. J Bone Miner Res 1999;14:1255–1260.

parathyroid hormone in storage granules. J Histochem Cytochem 1993;41:273–282.

22. Reed RR. G protein diversity and the regulation of signaling pathways. New Biologist 1990;2:957–960.
23. Rasmussen H. Ca and cAMP as Synarchic Messengers. New York: John Wiley & Sons, 1981.
24. Radeke HH, Auf'Mkolk B, Jüppner H, Krohn H-P, Keck E, Hesch R-D. Multiple pre- and postreceptor defects in pseudohypoparathyroidism (a multicenter study with twenty four patients). J Clin Endocrinol Metab 1986; 162:393–401.
25. Yamamoto M, Takuwa Y, Masuko S, Ogata E. Effects of endogenous and exogenous parathyroid hormone on tubular reabsorption of calcium in pseudohypoparathyroidism. J Clin Endocrinol Metab 1988;66:618–624.
26. Gupta A, Martin KJ, Miyauchi A, Hruska KA. Regulation of cytosolic calcium by parathyroid hormone and oscillations of cytosolic calcium in fibroblasts from normal and pseudohypoparathyroid patients. Endocrinology 1991;128:2825–2836.
27. Jüppner H, Abou-Samra AB, Freeman M, Kong XF, Schipani E, Richards J, Kolakowski LF Jr, Hock J, Potts JT Jr, Kronenberg HM, Segre GV. A G-protein-linked receptor for parathyroid hormone and parathyropid hormone-related peptide. Science 1991;254:1024–1026.
28. Jüppner H, Schipani E, Bringhurst FR, McLure I, Keutmann HT, Potts JT, Kronenberg HM, Abou-Samra AB, Segre GV, Gardella TJ. The extracellular amino-terminal region of the parathyroid hormone (PTH)/PTH-related peptide receptor determines the binding affinity for carboxy-terminal fragments of PTH-(1–34). Endocrinology 1994;134:879–884.
29. Usdin TB, Gruber C, Bonner TI. Identification and functional expression of a receptor selectively recognizing parathyroid hormone, the PTH2 receptor. J Biol Chem 1995;270:15455–15458.
30. Behar V, Pines M, Nakamoto C, Yang QM, Rashti-Behar V, Adams AE, Chin KR, Stueckle SM, Rosenblatt M. The human PTH-2 receptor: binding and signal transduction properties of the stably expressed recombinant receptor. Endocrinology 1996;137:2748–2757.
31. Kaji H. Sugimoto T, Kanatani M, Fukase M, Chihara K. Carboxy-terminal parathyroid hormone fragments stimulate osteoclast-like cell formation and osteoclastic activity. Endocrinology 1994;134:1897–1904.
32. Brown A, Dusso A, Slatopolsky E. Vitamin D. In: Seldin DW, Giebisch G, eds. The Kidney, Physiology and Pathophysiology. Philadelphia: Lippincott, 1999:1047–1090.
33. Reichel H, Koeffler HP, Norman AW. The role of the vitamin D endocrine system in health and disease. N Engl J Med 1989;320:980–981.
34. DeLuca HF, Schnoes HK. Vitamin D: Recent advances. Annu Rev Biochem 1983;52:411–439.
35. Bell NH. Vitamin D-endocrine system. J Clin Invest 1985;76:1–6.
36. Norman AW, Roth J, Orci L. The vitamin D endocrine system: steroid metabolism, hormone receptors, and biological response. Endocr Rev 1982;3:331–366.
37. Breslau NA. Normal and abnormal regulation of 1,25-(OH)$_2$D synthesis. Am J Med Sci 1988;296:417–425.
38. Henry HL, Dutta C, Cunningham N, Blanchard R, Penny R, Tang C, Marchetto G, Chou S. The cellular and molecular regulation of 1,25(OH)$_2$D$_3$ production. J Steroid Biochem Mol Biol 1992;41:401.
39. Adams ND, Gray RW, Lemann J. The effects of oral CaCO$_3$ loading and dietary calcium deprivation on plasma 1,25-dihydroxyvitamin D concentrations in

healthy adults. J Clin Endocrinol Metab 1979;1008–1016.
40. Kumar R. Metabolism of 1,25-dihydroxyvitamin D3. Physiol Rev 1984;64:478–504.
41. Pike JW. Vitamin D$_3$ receptors: structure and function in transcription. Annu Rev Nutr 1991;11:189–216.
42. Haussler MR, Haussler CA, Jurutka PW, Thompson PD, Hsieh JC, Remus LS, Selznick SH, Whitfield GK. The vitamin D hormone and its nuclear receptor: molecular actions and disease states. J Endocrinol 1997;154:S57–S73.
43. Labuda M, Fujiwara TM, Ross MV, Morgan K, Garcia-Heras J, Ledbetter DH, Hughes MR, Glorieux FH. Two hereditary diseases related to vitamin D metabolism map to the same region of chromosome 12q13-14. J Bone Miner Res 1992;7:1447–1453.
44. Lee K, Brown D, Urena P, Ardaillou N, Ardaillou R, Deeds J, Segre GV. Localization of parathyroid hormone/parathyroid hormone-related peptide receptor mRNA in kidney. Am J Physiol 1996;270:F186–F191.
45. Yang T, Hassan S, Huang YG, Smart AM, Briggs JP, Schnermann JB. Expression of PTHrP, PTH/PTHrP receptor, and Ca(2+)-sensing receptor mRNAs along the rat nephron. Am J Physiol 1997;272:F751–F758.
46. Chabardes D, Gagnan-Brunette M, Imbert-Teboul M, Gontcharevskaia O, Montegut M, Clique A, Morel F. Adenylate cyclase responsiveness to hormones in various portions of human nephron. J Clin Invest 1980;65:439–448.
47. Friedman PA, Gesek FA, Morley P, Whitfield JF, Willick GE. Cell-specific signaling and structure-activity relations of parathyroid hormone analogs in mouse kidney cells. Endocrinology 1999;140:301–309.
48. Friedman PA, Coutermarsh BA, Kennedy SM, Gesek FA. Parathyroid hormone stimulation of calcium transport is mediated by dual signaling mechanisms involving protein kinase A and protein kinase C. Endocrinology 1996;137:13–20.
49. Mizgala CL, Quamme GA. Renal handling of phosphate. Physiol Rev 1985;65:431–466.
50. Murer H. Cellular mechanisms in proximal tubular Pi reabsorption: some answers and more questions. J Am Soc Nephrol 1992;2:1649–1695.
51. Walton RJ, Bijvoet OLM. Nomogram for derivation of renal threshold phosphate concentration. Lancet 1975;2:309–310.
52. Kruse K, Kracht U, Göpfert G. Renal threshold phosphate concentration (TmPO$_4$/GFR). Arch Dis Child 1982;57:217–223.
53. Bistarakis L, Voskaki I, Lambadaridis J, Sereti H, Sbyrakis S. Renal handling of phosphate in the first six months of life. Arch Dis Child 1986;61:677–681.
54. Pfister MF, Ruf I, Stange G, Ziegler U, Lederer E, Biber J, Murer H. Parathyroid hormone leads to the lysosomal degradation of the renal type II Na/Pi cotransporter. Proc Natl Acad Sci USA 1998;95:1909–1914.
55. Silve C, Friedlander G. Renal regulation of phosphate excretion. In: Seldin DW, Giebisch G, eds. The Kidney, Physiology and Pathophysiology. Philadelphia: Lippincott, 1999:1885–1904.
56. Quamme GA, Rouffignac C de. Renal magnesium handling. In: Seldin DW, Giebisch G, eds. The Kidney, Physiology and Pathophysiology. Philadelphia: Lippincott, 1999:1711–1729.
57. Ng RCK, Rouse D, Suki WN. Calcium transport in the

rabbit superficial proximal convoluted tubule. J Clin Invest 1984;74:834–842.

58. Friedman PA. Renal calcium metabolism. In: Seldin DW, Giebisch G, eds. The Kidney, Physiology and Pathophysiology. Philadelphia: Lippincott, 1999:1749–1789.
59. Brown EM, Hebert SC. A cloned extracellular Ca^{2+}-sensing receptor: a mediator of direct effects of extracellular Ca^{2+} on renal function? J Am Soc Nephrol 1995; 6:1530–1540.
60. Coburn JW, Elangovan L, Goodman WG, Frazaõ JM. Calcium-sensing receptor and calcimimetic agents. Kidney Int 1999;56 Suppl 73:S52–S58.
61. Cholst IN, Steinberg SF, Tropper PJ, Fox HE, Segre GV, Bilezikian JP. The influence of hypermagnesemia on serum calcium and parathyroid hormone levels in human subjects. N Engl J Med 1984;310:1221–1225.
62. Sands J, Naruse M, Baum M, Hebert SC, Brown EM, Harris W. An apical extracellular calcium/polyvalent cations-sensing receptor (CaR) regulates vasopressin-elicited water permeability in rat kidney inner medullary collecting duct. J Clin Invest 1997;99:1399–1405.
63. Yamamoto M, Kawanobe Y, Takahashi H, Shimazawa E, Kimura S, Ogata E. Vitamin D deficiency and renal calcium transport in the rat. J Clin Invest 1984;74:507–513.
64. Rasmussen H, Bordier P. Vitamin D and bone. Metab Bone Dis Rel Res 1978;1:7–17.
65. Romas E, Udagawa N, Zhou H, Tamura T, Saito M, Taga T, Hilton DJ, Suda T, Ng KW, Martin TJ. The role of gp130-mediated signals in osteoclast development: regulation of interleukin 11 production by osteoblasts and distribution of its receptor in bone marrow cultures. J Exp Med 1996;183:2581–2591.
66. Holick MF. Vitamin D and bone health. J Nutr 1996; 126:1159S–1164S.
67. Rodan GA, Martin TJ. Role of osteoblasts in hormonal control of bone resorption—a hypothesis. Calcif Tissue Int 1981;33:349–351.
68. Veenstra TD, Kumar R. Hormonal regulation of calcium metabolism. In: Seldin DW, Giebisch G, eds. The Kidney, Physiology and Pathophysiology. Philadelphia: Lippincott, 1999: 1795–1809.
69. Wasserman RH. Intestinal absorption of calcium and phosphorus. Fed Proc 1981;40:68–72.
70. Parfitt AM. The spectrum of hypoparathyroidism. J Clin Endocrinol Metab 1972;34:152–158.
71. Parfitt AM. The actions of parathyroid hormone on bone: relation to bone remodeling and turnover, calcium homeostasis and metabolic bone disease. Part 2, PTH and bone cells: bone turnover and plasma calcium regulation. Metabolism 1976;25:909–955.
72. Barzel US. Systemic alkalosis in hypoparathyroidism. J Clin Endocrinol Metab 1969;29:917–918.
73. Kruse K, Kracht U, Wohlfart K, Kruse U. Biochemical markers of bone turnover, intact serum parathyroid hormone and renal calcium excretion in patients with pseudohypoparathyroidism and hypoparathyroidism before and during vitamin D treatment. Eur J Pediatr 1989;148: 535–939.
74. Kruse K, Kracht U. Evaluation of serum osteocalin as an index of altered bone metabolism. Eur J Pediatr 1986; 145:27–33.
75. Price PA, Parthemore JG, Deftos LJ. New biochemical marker of bone metabolism. Measurement by radioimmunoassay of bone Gla protein in the plasma of normal subjects and patients with bone disease. J Clin Invest 1980;66:878–883.
76. Parfitt AM. Surgical, idiopathic, and other varieties of parathyroid hormone-deficient hypoparathyroidism. In: DeGroot, LJ, Besser GM, Marshall JC, Nelson DH, Odell WD, Potts JT Jr, Rubenstein AH, Steinberger E, eds. Endocrinology, 2nd ed. Philadelphia: WB Saunders, 1989;1049–1064.
77. Harrison HE, Harrison HC. Disorders of Calcium and Phosphate Metabolism in Childhood and Adolescence. Philadelphia: WB Saunders, 1979.
78. Frame B. Neuromuscular manifestations of parathyroid disease. In: Vinken PB, Bruyn GW, eds. Handbook of Clinical Neurology. Vol. 27. Amsterdam: North-Holland, 1976.
79. Swash M, Rowan AJ. Electroencephalographic criteria for hypocalcemia and hypercalcemia. Arch Neurol 1972; 26:218–228.
80. Illum F, Dupont E. Prevalences of CT-detected calcification in the basal ganglia in idiopathic hypoparathyroidism and pseudohypoparathyroidism. Neuroradiology 1985;27:32–37.
81. Ireland AW, Hornbrook JN, Neale FC, et al. The crystalline lens in chronic surgical hypoparathyroidism. Arch Intern Med 1968;122:408–411.
82. Aryanpur I, Farhoudi A, Zangeneh F. Congestive heart failure secondary to idiopathic hypoparathyroidism. Am J Dis Child 1974;127:738–739.
83. Kruse K, Scheunemann W, Baier W, Schaub J. Hypocalcemic myopathy in idiopathic hypoparathyroidism. Eur J Pediatr 1982;138:280–282.
84. Battistella PA, Pozzan GB, Rigon F, Zancan L, Zacchello F. Autoimmune hypoparathyroidism and hyper-CK-emia [letter]. Brain Dev 1991;13:61.
85. Ahn TG, Antonarakis SE, Kronenberg HM, Igarashi T, Levine MA. Familial isolated hypoparathyroidism: a molecular genetic analysis of 8 families with 23 affected persons. Medicine 1986;65:73–81.
86. Arnold A, Horst SA, Gardella TJ, Baba H, Levine MA, Kronenberg HM. Mutation of the signal peptide-encoding region of the preproparathyroid hormone gene in familial isolated hypoparathyroidism. J Clin Invest 1990; 86:1084–1087.
87. De Campo C, Piscopello L, Noacco C, Da Col P, Englaro GC, Benedetti A. Primary familial hypoparathyroidism with an autosomal dominant mode of inheritance. J Endocr 1988;11:91–96.
88. Finegold DN, Armitage MM, Galiani M, Matise TC, Pandian MRT, Perry YM, Deka R, Ferrel RE. Preliminary localization of a gene for autosomal dominant hypoparathyroidism to chromosome 3q13. Pediatr Res 1994;36:414–417.
89. Pollak MR, Brown EM, Estep HL, McLane PN, Kifor O, Park J, Hebert SC, Seidman CE, Seidman JG. Autosomal dominant hypocalcemia caused by Ca^{2+}-sensing receptor gene mutation. Nat Genet 1994;8:303–307.
90. Pearce SHS, Williamson C, Kifor O, Baio M, Coulthard M, Davies M, Lewis Barned N, Powell H, Kendall-Taylor P, Brown EM, Thakker RV. A familial syndrome of hypocalcemia with hypercalciuria due to mutations in the calcium-sensing receptor. N Engl J Med 1996;335: 1115–1122.
91. Baron J, Winer K, Yanovski JA, Cunningham AW, Laue L, Zimmerman D, Cutler G. Mutations in the Ca^{2+}-sensing receptor gene causing autosomal dominant and spo-

radic hypoparathyroidism. Hum Mol Genet 1996;5:601–606.

92. Watanabe T, Bai M, Lane CR, Matsumoto S, Minamitani K, Minagawa M, Niimi H, Brown EM, Yasuda T. Familial hypoparathyroidism: identification of a novel gain of function mutation in transmembrane domain 5 of the calcium-sensing receptor. J Clin Endocrinol Metab 1998;83:2497–2502.

93. Mancilla EE, De Luca F, Ray K, Winer K, Fan GF, Baron J. A Ca^{2+}-sensing receptor mutation causes hypoparathyroidism by increasing receptor activity to Ca^{2+}-sensing receptor and maximal signal transduction. Pediatr Res 1997;42443–42447

94. De Luca F, Ray K, Mancilla EE, Fan GF, Winer KK, Gore P, Spiegel AM, Baron J. Sporadic hypoparathyroidism caused by de novo gain-of-function mutations of the Ca^{2+}-sensing receptor. J Clin Endocrinol Metab 1997;82:2710–2715.

95. Nakae J, Shonohara N, Tanahashi Y, Murashita M, Abe S, Hasegawa T, Hasegava Y, Fujieda K. New mutation of the Ca^{2+}-sensing receptor gene in two Japanese patients with sporadic hypoparathyroidism and hypercalciuria. Horm Res 1997;48:Suppl 2 P 179, Abs 798.

96. Karaplis AC, Lim S-K, Baba H, Arnold A, Kronenberg HM. Inefficient membrane targeting, translocation, and proteolytic processing by signal peptidase of a mutant preproparathyroid hormone protein. J Biol Chem 1995; 270:1629–1635.

97. Parkinson DB, Thakker RV. A donor splice site mutation in the parathyroid hormone gene is associated with autosomal recessive hypoparathyroidism. Nature Genet 1992;1:149–152.

98. Sunthornthepvarakul T, Churesigaew S, Ngowngarmratana S. A novel mutation of the signal peptide of the preproparathyroid hormone gene associated with autosomal recessive familial isolated hypoparathyroidism. J Clin Endocrinol Metab 1999;84:3792–3796.

99. Peden VH. True idiopathic hypoparathyroidism as a sex-linked recessive trait. Am J Hum Genet 1960;12:323–337.

100. Whyte MP, Weldon VV. Idiopathic hypoparathyroidism presenting with seizures during infancy: X-linked recessive inheritance in a large Missouri kindred. J Pediatr 1981;99:608–11.

101. Whyte MP, Kim GS, Kosanovich M. Absence of parathyroid tissue in sex-linked recessive hypoparathyroidism. J Pediatr 1986;109:915.

102. Thakker RV, Davies KE, Whyte MP, Wooding C, O'Riordan JLH. Mapping the gene causing X-linked recessive idiopathic hypoparathyroidism to Xq26-Xq27 by linkage studies. J Clin Invest 1990;86:40–45.

103. Neufeld M, Maclaren NK, Blizzard RM. Two types of autoimmune Addison's disease associated with different polyglandular autoimmune syndromes. Medicine 1981; 60:355–362.

104. Ahonen P, Myllärniemi S, Sipilä I, Perheentupa J. Clinical variation of autoimmune polyendocrinopathy-candidiasis-ectodermal dystrophy (APECED) in a series of 68 patients. N Engl J Med 1990;322:1829–1836.

105. Spinner MW, Blizzard RM, Childs B. Clinical and genetical heterogeneity in idiopathic Addison's disease and hypoparathyroidism. J Clin Endocrinol Metab 1968;28: 795–804.

106. Ahonen P. Autoimmune polyendocrinopathy-candidosis-ectodermal dystropy (APECED): autosomal recessive inheritance. Clin Genet 1985;27:535–542.

107. Myhre AG, Halonen M, Eskelin P, Ekwall O, Hedstrand H, Rorsman F, Kämpe O, Husebye E. Autoimmune polyendocrine syndrome type 1 in Norway. Clin Endcrinol 2001;54:211–217.

108. Betterle C, Greggio NA, Volpato MJ. Autoimmune polyglandular syndrome type I. Clin Endocrinol Metab 1998; 83:1049–1055.

108a. Clifton-Bligh P, Lee C, Smith H, Posen S. The association of diabetes insipidus with hypoparathyroidism, Addison's disease and mucocutaneous candidiasis. Aust NZ J Med 1980;10:548–551

109. Scherbaum WA, Bottazzo GF. Autoantibodies to vasopressin cells in idiopathic diabetes insipidus. Lancet 1983;1:897–901.

110. Arvanitakis C, Knouss RF. Selective hypopituitarism, impaired cell-mediated immunity and chronic mucocutaneous candidiasis. JAMA 1973;225:1492–1495.

111. Merenmies L, Tarkkanen A. Chronic bilateral keratitis in autoimmune polyendocrinopathy–candidiasis-ectodermal dystrophy. Acta Ophthalmol Scand 2000;78:532–535.

112. Friedman TC, Thomas PM, Fleischer TA, Feuillan P, Parker RI, Cassorla F. Frequent occurrence of asplenism and cholelithiasis in patients with autoimmune polyendocrine disease type I. Am J Med 1991;91:625–630.

113. Parker RI, O'Shea P, Forman EN. Acquired splenic atrophy in a sibship with the autoimmune polyendocrinopathy-candidiasis syndrome. J Pediatr 1990;117:591–593.

114. Padeh S, Theodor R, Jonas A, Passwell JH. Severe malabsorption in autoimmune polyendocrinopathy-candidosis-ectodermal dystrophy syndrome successfully treated with immunosuppression. Arch Dis Child 1997; 76:532–534.

115. Scirè G, Magliocca FM, Cianfarani S, Scalamandrè A, Petrozza V, Bonamico M. Autoimmune polyendocrine candidiasis syndrome with associated chronic diarrhea caused by intestinal infection and pancreas insufficiency. J Pediatr Gastroenterol Nutr 1991;13:224–227.

116. Ward L, Paquette J, Seidman E, Huot C, Alvarez F, Crock P, Delvin E, Kämpe O, Deal C. Severe autoimmune polyendocrinopathy-candidiasis-ectodermal dystrophy in an adolescent girl with a novel *AIRE* mutation: response to immunosuppressive therapy. J Clin Endocrinol Metab 1999;84:844–852.

117. Bereket A, Lowenheim M, Blethen SL, Kane P, Ichyama AJ. Intestinal lymphangiectasia in a patient with autoimmune polyglandular disease type I and steatorrhea. Clin Endocrinol Metab 1995;80:933–935.

118. Myllärniemi S, Perheentupa J. Oral findings in the autoimmune polyendocrinopathy–candidosis syndrome (APECED) and other forms of hypoparathyroidism. Oral Surg 1978;45:721–729.

119. Lukinmaa P-L, Waltimo J, Pirinen S. Microanatomy of the dental enamel in autoimmune polyendocrinopathy–candidiasisis–ectodermal dystrophy: report of three cases. J Craniofac Genet Dev Biol 1996;16:174–181.

120. Perheentupa J, Miettinen A. Autoimmune polyendocrine syndrome type I. In: Eisenbarth GS, ed. Molecular Mechanisms of Endocrine and Organ Specific Autoimmunity. Austin: Landes, 1999:19–40.

120a. Perheentupa J. APS-I/APECED: the clinical disease and therapy. In: Eisenbarth GS, ed. Autoimmune Polyendocrine Syndromes. Endocrinol Metab Clin North Am 2002;31:295–320.

121. Li Y, Song YH, Rais N, Connor E, Schatz D, Muir A, Maclaren N. Autoantibodies to the extracellular domain

of the calcium sensing receptor in patients with acquired hypoparathyroidism. J Clin Invest 1996;97:910–914.

122. Bednarek J, Furmaniak J, Wedlock N. Steroid 21-hydroxylase is a major autoantigen in idiopathic Addison's disease. FEBS Lett 1992;309:51–55.

123. Winqvist O, Karlsson FA, Kämpe O. 21-hydroxylase, a major autoantigen in idiopathic Addison's disease. Lancet 1992;339:1559–1562.

124. Uibo R, Aavik E, Peterson P, Perheentupa J, Aranko S, Pelkonen R, Krohn KJE. Autoantibodies to cytochrome P450 enzymes P450scc, P450c17, and P450c21 in autoimmune polyglandular disease types I and II and in isolated Addison's disease. J Clin Endocrinol Metab 1994;78:323–328.

125. Uibo R, Perheentupa J, Ovod V, Krohn KJE. Characterization of adrenal autoantigens recognized by sera from patients with autoimmune polyglandular syndrome type I. J Autoimm 7: 399–411.

126. Winqvist O, Gustafsson J, Rorsman F, Karlsson FA, Kämpe O. Two different cytochrome P450 enzymes are the adrenal antigens in autoimmune polyendocrine syndrome type I and Addison's disease. J Clin Invest 1993; 92:2377–2385.

127. Winqvist O, Gebre-Medhin G, Gustafsson J, Ritzén EM, Lundkvist Ö, Karlsson FA, Kämpe O. Identification of the main gonadal autoantigens in patients with adrenal insufficiency and associated ovarian failure. J Clin Endocrinol Metab 1995;80:1717–1723.

128. Arif S, Vallian S, Farzaneh F, Zanone MM, James SL, Pietropaolo M, Hettiarachchi MM, Vergani D, Conway G, Peakman M. Identification of 3β-hydroxysteroid dehydrogenase as a novel target of steroid cell autoantibodies: association of autoantibodies with endocrine autoimmune disease. J Clin Endocrinol Metab 1996;81: 4439–4445.

129. Krohn K, Uibo R, Aavik E, Peterson P, Savilahti K. Identification by molecular cloning of an autoantigen associated with Addison's disease as steroid 17alpha-hydroxylase. Lancet 1992;339:770–773.

130. Ahonen P, Miettinen A, Perheentupa, J. Adrenal and steroidal cell antibodies in patients with autoimmune polyglandular disease type I and risk of adrenocortical and ovarian failure. J Clin Endocrinol Metab 1987;64: 494–500.

131. Burman P, Mardh S, Norberg, Karlsson FA. Parietal cell antibodies in pernicious anemia inhibit H^+, K^+-adenosine triphosphatase, the proton pump of the stomach. Gastroenterology 1989;96:1434–1438.

132. Toh BH, van Driel IR, Gleeson PA. Pernicious anemia. New Engl J Med 1996;337:1441–1448.

133. Manns MP, Griffin KJ, Quattrochi L, Sacher M, Thaler H, Tukery RH, Johnson EF. Identification of cytochrome P450IA2 as a human autoantigen. Arch Biochem Biophys 1990;280:229–232.

134. Clemente MG, Obermayer-Straub P, Meloni A, Strassburg CP, Arangino V, Tukey RH, Virgiliis SD, Manns MP. Cytochrome P450 1A2 is a hepatic autoantigen in autoimmune polyglandular syndrome type 1. J Clin Endocrinol Metab 1997;82:1353–1361.

135. Obermayer-Straub, P, Perheentupa J, Braun S, Kayser A, Barut A, Loges S, Harms A, Dalekos G, Strassburg CP, Manns MP. Hepatic autoantigens in patients with autoimmune polyendocrinopathy-candidiasis-ectodermal dystrophy. Gastroenterology 2001;121:668–677.

136. Hedstrand H, Perheentupa J, Ekwall O, Gustafsson, J, Michaëlsson G, Husebye E, Rorsman F, Kämpe O. Antibodies against hair follicles are associated with alopecia totalis in autoimmune polyendocrine syndrome type I. J Invest Dermatol 1999;113:1054–1058.

137. Hedstrand H, Ekwall O, Haavik J, Landgren E, Betterle C, Perheentupa J, Gustafsson J, Husebye E, Rorsman F, Kämpe O. Identification of tyrosine hydroxylase as an autoantigen in autoimmune polyendocrine syndrome type 1. Biochem Biophys Res Commun 2000;267:456–461.

138. Song Y-H, Conner E, Li Y, Zorovich B, Balducci P, Maclaren N. The role of tyrosinase in autoimmune vitiligo. Lancet 1994;344:1049–1052.

139. Ekwall O, Hedstrand H, Grimelius L, Haavik J, Perheentupa J, Gustafsson J, Husebye E, Kämpe O, Rorsman F. Identification of tryptophan hydroxylase as an intestinal autoantigen. Lancet 1998;352:279–283.

140. The Finnish-German APECED Consortium. An autoimmune disease, APECED, caused by mutations in a novel gene featuring two PHD-type zinc-finger domains. Nature Genet 1997;17:399–403.

141. Nagamine K, Peterson P, Scott HS, Kudoh J, Minoshima S, Heino M, Krohn KJE, Lalioti MD, Mullis PE, Antonorakis SE, Kawasaki K, Asakawa S, Ito F, Shimizu N. Positional cloning of the APECED gene. Nature Genet 1997;17:393–398.

142. Halonen M, Pelto-Huikko M, Eskelin P, Peltonen L, Ulmanen I, Kolmer M. Subcellular location and expression pattern of autoimmune regulator (Aire), the mouse orthologue of human gene defective in autoimmune polyendocrinopathy candidiasis ectodermal dystrophy. J Histochem Cytochem 2001;49:197–208.

143. Mittaz L, Rossier C, Heino M, Peterson P, Krohn KJ, Gos A, Morris MA, Kudoh J, Smimizu N, Antonorakis SE, Scott HS. Isolation and characterization of the mouse Aire gene. Biochem Biophys Res Commun 1999; 255:483–490.

144. Björses P, Halonen M, Palvimo JJ, Kolmer M, Aaltonen J, Ellonen P, Perheentupa J, Ulmanen I, Peltonen L. Mutations in the AIRE gene: effects on subcellular location and transactivation function of the autoimmune polyendocrinopathy-candidiasis-ectodermal dystrophy protein. Am J Hum Genet 2000;66:378–392.

145. Blechschmidt K, Schweiger M, Wertz K, Poulson R, Christensen HM, Rosenthal A, Lehrach H, Yaspo ML. The mouse *Aire* gene: comparative genomic sequencing, gene organization, and expression. Genome Res 1999;9: 158–166.

146. Björses P, Pelto-Huikko M, Kaukonen J, Aaltonen J, Peltonen L, Ulmanen I. Localization of the APECED protein in distinct nuclear structures. Hum Mol Genet 1999;8:259–266.

147. Rinderle C, Christensen HM, Schweiger S, Lehrach H, Yaspo ML. AIRE encodes a nuclear protein co-localizing with cytoskeletal filaments: altered sub-cellular distribution of mutants lacking the PHD zinc fingers. Hum Mol Genet 1999;8:277–290.

148. Pitkänen J, Doucas V, Sternsdorf T, Nakajima T, Aratani S, Jensen K, Will H, Vähämurto P, Ollila J, Vihinen M, Scott HS, Antonorakis SE, Kudoh J, Shimizu N, Krohn K, Peterson P. The autoimmune regulator protein has transcriptional transactivating properties and interacts with the common coactivator CREB-binding protein. J Biol Chem 2000;275:16802–16809.

149. Zuklys S, Balciunaite G, Agarwal A, Fasler-Kan E, Palmer E, Holländer GA. Normal thymic architecture and

negative selection are associated with *Aire* expression, the gene defective in autoimmune polyendocrinopathy–candidiasis–ectodermal dystrophy (APECED). J Immunol 2000;165:1976–1983.

150. Heino M, Peterson P, Kudoh J, Nagamine K, Lagerstedt A, Ovod V, Ranki A, Rantala I, Nieminen M, Tuukkanen J, Scott HS, Antonorakis SE, Shimizu N, Krohn K. Autoimmune regulator is expressed in the cells regulating immune tolerance in thymus medulla. Biochem Biophys Res Commun 1999;257:821–825.

151. Scott HS, Heino M, Peterson P, Mittaz L, Lalioti MD, Betterle C, Cohen A, Seri M, Lerone M, Romeo G, Collin P, Salo M, Metcalfe R, Weetman A, Papasavvas MP, Rossier C, Nagamine K, Kudoh J, Shimizu N, Krohn KJE, Antonorakis SE. Common mutations in autoimmune polyendocrinopathy–candidiasis–ectodermal dystrophy patients of different origins. Mol Endocrinol 1998;12:1112–1119.

152. Heino M, Scott HS, Chen Q, Peterson P, Mäenpää U, Papasavvas MP, Mittaz L, Barras C, Rossier C, Chrousos GP, Stratakis CA, Nagamine K, Kudoh J, Shimizu N, Maclaren N, Antonorakis SE, Krohn K. Mutation analyses of North American APS-1 patients. Hum Mutat 1999;13:69–74.

153. Pearce SH, Cheetham T, Imrie H, Vaidya B, Barnes ND, Bilous RW, Carr D, Meeran K, Shaw NJ, Smith CS, Toft AD, Williams G, Kendall-Taylor P. A common and recurrent 13-bp deletion in the autoimmune regulator gene in British kindreds with autoimmune polyendocrinopathy type 1. Am J Hum Genet 1998;63:1675–1684.

154. Rosatelli MC, Meloni A, Meloni A, Devoto M, Cao A, Scott HS, Peterson P, Heino M, Krohn KJE, Nagamine K, Kudoh J, Shimizu N, Antonorakis SE. A common mutation in Sardinian autoimmune polyendocrinopathy–candidasis–ectodermal dystrophy patients. Hum Gen 1998;103:428–434.

155. Zlotogora J, Shapiro MS. Polyglandular autoimmune syndrome type I among Iranian Jews. J Med Genet 1992;29:824–826.

156. Carey JC. Spectrum of the DiGeorge "syndrome"(letter). J Pediatr 1980;96:955.

157. Belohradsky BH. Thymusaplasie und -hypoplasie mit Hypoparathyreoidismus, Herz- un Gefässmissbildungen (DiGeorge-Syndrom). Ergeb Inn Med Kinderheilkd 1985;54:36–105.

158. Müller W, Peter HH, Wilken M, Jüppner H, Kallfelz HC, Krohn HP, Miller K, Rieger CH. The DiGeorge syndrome. I. Clinical evaluation and course of partial and complete forms of the syndrome. Eur J Pediatr 1988;147:496–502.

159. Wilson DI, Burn J, Scambler P, Goodship J. DiGeorge syndrome: part of CATCH 22. J Med Genet 1993;30:852–856.

160. Maaswinkel-Mooij PD, Papapoulos SE, Gerritse EJ, Mudde AH, Van de Kamp JJ. Facial dysmorphia, parathyroid and thymic dysfunction in the father of a newborn with the DiGeorge complex. Eur J Pediatr 1989;149:179–183.

161. Bainbridge R, Mughal Z, Mimouni F, Tsang RC. Transient congenital hypoparathyroidism: how transient is it? J Pediatr 1987;111:866–868.

162. Gidding SS, Minciotti AL, Langman CB. Unmasking of hypoparathyroidism in familial partial DiGeorge syndrome by challenge with disodium edetate. N Engl J Med 1988;319:1589–1591.

163. Hasegawa T, Hasegawa Y, Yokoyama T, Koto S, Asamura S, Tsuchiya Y. Unmasking of latent hypoparathyroidism in a child with partial DiGeorge syndrome by ethylenediaminetetraacetic acid infusion. Eur J Pediatr 1993;152:316–318.

164. Palacios J, Gamallo C, Garcia M, Rodriguez JI. Decrease in thyrocalcitonin-containing cells and analysis of other congenital anomalies in 11 patients with DiGeorge anomaly. Am J Med Genet 1993;46:641–646.

165. Pueblitz S, Weinberg AG, Albores-Saavedra J. Thyroid C cells in the DiGeorge anomaly: a quantitative study. Pediatr Pathol 1993;13:463–473.

166. Kornfeld SJ, Zeffren B, Christodoulou CS, Noorbibi K, Cawkwell G, Good RA. DiGeorge anomaly: a comparative stude of the clinical and immunologic characteristics of patients positive and negative by fluorescence in situ hybridization. J Allergy Clin Immunol 2000;105:983–987.

167. Sullivan KE, McDonald-McGinn D, Driscoll DA, Emanuel BS, Zackhai EH, Jawad AF. Longitudinal analysis of lymphocyte function and numbers in the first year of life in chromosome 22q11.2 deletion syndrome. Clin Diagn Lab Immunol 1999;6:906–911.

168. Bastian J, Law S, Vogler L, Lawton A, Herrod H, Anderson S, Horowitz S, Hong R. Prediction of persistent immunodeficiency in the DiGeorge anomaly. J Pediatr 1989;115:391–396.

169. Hong R. The DiGeorge anomaly. Immunodefic Rev 1991;3:1–14.

170. Schubert MS, Moss RB. Selective polysaccharide antibody deficiency in familial DiGeorge syndrome. Ann Allergy 1992;69:231–238.

171. Haire RN, Buell RD, Litman RT, Ohta Y, Fu SM, Honjo T, Matsuda F, de la Morena M, Carro J, Good RA, et al. Diversification, not use, of the immunoglobulin VH gene repertoire is restricted in DiGeorge syndrome. J Exp Med 1993;178:825–834.

172. Markert ML, Boeck A, Hale LP, Kloster AL, McLaughlin TM, Batchvarova MN, Douek DC, Koup RA, Kostyu DD, Ward FE, Rice HE, Mahaffey SM. Transplantation of thymus tissue in complete DiGeorge syndrome. N Engl J Med. 1999;341:1180–1189.

173. Adachi M, Tachibana K, Masuno M, Makita Y, Maesaka H, Okada T, Hizukuri K, Imaizumi K, Kuroki Y, Kurahashi H, Suwa S. Clinical characteristics of children with hypoparathyroidism due to 22q11.1 microdeletion. Eur J Pediatr 1998;157:34–38.

174. Motzkin B, Marion R, Goldberg R, Shprintzen R, Saenger P. Variable phenotypes in velocardiofacial syndrome with chromosomal deletion. J Pediatr 1993;123:406–410.

175. De la Chapelle A, Herva R, Koivisto M, Aula P. A deletion in chromosome 22 can cause DiGeorge syndrome. Hum Genet 1981;57:253–256.

176. Scambler PJ, Carey AH, Wyse RKH, Roach S, Dumanski JP, Nordenskjöld M, Williamson R. Microdeletions within 22q11 associated with sporadic and familial DiGeorge syndrome. Genomics 1991;7:201–206.

177. Carey AH, Clausen U, Ludecke HJ, Horsthemke B, Ellis D, Oakey H, Wilson D, Burn J Williamson R, Scambler PJ. Investigation of deletion in DiGeorge syndrome detected from microclones from 22q11. Mammalian Genome 1992;3:101–105.

178. Desmaze C, Scambler P, Prieur M, Halford S, Sidi D, Le Deist F, Aurias A. Routine diagnosis of DiGeorge

syndrome by fluorescent in situ hybridization. Hum Genet 1993;90:663–665.

179. Driscoll DA, Salvin J, Sellinegr B, Budarf ML, McDonald-McGinn DM, Zackai EH, Emanuel BS. Prevalence of 22q11 microdeletions in DiGeorge and velocardiofacial syndromes: implications for genetic counselling and prenatal diagnosis. J Med Genet 1993; 30:813–817.

180. Lindsay EA, Halford S, Wadey R, Scambler PJ, Baldini A. Molecular cytogenetic characterization of the DiGeorge syndrome region using fluorescence in situ hybridization. Genomics 1993;17:403–407.

181. Novelli A, Sabani M, Caiola A, Digilio MC, Giannotti A, Mingarelli R, Novelli G, Dallapiccola B. Diagnosis of DiGeorge and Williams syndromes using FISH analysis of peripheral blood smears. Mol Cell Probes 1999; 13:303–307.

182. Keppen LD, Fasules JW, Burks AW, Gollin SM, Sawyer JR, Miller CH. Confirmation of autosomal dominant transmission of the DiGeorge malformation complex. J Pediatr 1988;113:506–507.

183. Lammer EJ, Opitz JM. The DiGeorge anomaly as a developmental field defect. Am J Med Genet Suppl 1986; 2:113–127.

184. Stevens CA, Carey JC, Shigeoka AO. Di George anomaly and velocardiofacial syndrome. Pediatrics 1990;85: 526–530.

185. Hall JG. Editorial: Catch 22. Med Genet 1993;30:801– 802.

186. Scambler PJ. Deletions of human chromosome 22 and associated birth defects. Curr Opin Genet Dev 1993;3: 432–437.

187. Wilson DI, Cross IE, Goodship JA, Coulthard S, Carey AH, Scambler PJ, Bain HH, Hunter AS, Carter PE, Burn J. DiGeorge syndrome with isolated aortic coarctation and isolated ventricular septal defect in three sibs with a 22q11 deletion of maternal origin. Br Heart J 1991; 66:308–312.

188. Wilson, DI, Goodship JA, Burn J, Cross IE, Scambler PJ. Deletions within chromosome 22q11 in familial congenital heart disease. Lancet 1992;340:573–575.

189. Fokstuen S, Arbenz U, Artan S, Dutly F, Bauersfeld U, Brecevic L, Fasnacht M, Rothlisberger B, Schinzel A. 22q11.2 deletions in a series of patients with non-selective congenital heart defects: incidence, type of defects and parental origin. Clin Genet 1998;53:63–69.

190. Vincent MC, Heitz F, Tricoire J, Bourrouillou G, Kuhlein E, Rolland M, Calvas P. 22q deletion in DGS/VCFS monozygotic twins with discordant phenotypes. Genet Couns 1999;10:43–49.

191. Carlson C, Sirotkin H, Pandita R, Goldberg R, McKie J, Wadey R, Patanjali SR, Weissman SM, Anyane-Yeboa K, Warburton D, Scambler P, Shprintzen R, Kucherlapati R, Morrow BE. Molecular definition of 22q11 deletions in 151 velo-cardio-facial syndrome patients. Am J Hum Genet 1997;61:620–629.

192. Ryan AK, Goodship JA, Wilson DI, Philip N, Levy A, Seide, H, Schuffenhauer S, Oechsler H, Belohradsky B, Prieur M, Aurias A, Raymond FL, and 17 others. Spectrum of clinical features associated with interstitial chromosome 22q11 deletions: a European collaborative study. J Med Genet 1997;34:798–804.

193. Karayiorgou M, Morris MA, Morrow B, Shprintzen RJ, Goldberg R, Borrow J, Gos A, Nestadt G, Wolyniec PS, Lasseter VK, Eisen H, Childs B, Kazazian H, Kucher-

lapati R, Antonarakis SE, Pulver AE, Housman DE. Schizophrenia susceptibility associated with interstitial deletions of chromosome 22q11. Proc Natl Acad Sci 1995;92:7612–7616.

194. Goodship J, Cross I, LiLing J, Wren C. A population study of chromosome 22q11 deletions in infancy. Arch Dis Child 1998;79:348–351.

195. Higurashi M, Oda M, Iijima K, Iijima S, Takeshita T, Watanabe N, Yoneyama K. Livebirth prevalece and follow-up of malformation syndromes in 27,472 newborns. Brain Dev 1990;12:770–773.

196. Obregon MG, Mingarelli R, Giannotti A, di Comite A, Spedicato FS, Dallapiccola B. Partial deletion 10p syndrome. Report of two patients. Ann Genet 1992;35:101– 104.

197. Lichtner P, König R, Hasegawa TH, Meitinger T, Schuffenhauer S. An HDR (hypoparathyroidism, deafness, renal dysplasia) syndrome locus maps distal to the DiGeorge syndrome region on 10p13/14. J Med Genet 2000;37:33–37.

198. Greenberg F, Valdes C, Rosenblatt H, Kirkland JL, Ledbetter DH. Hypoparathyroidism and T cell immune defect in a patient with 10p deletion syndrome. J Pediatr 1986;109:489–492.

199. Monaco G, Ciccimarra F, Pignata C, Garofalo S. T cell immunodeficiency in a patient with 10p deletion syndrome (letter). J Pediatr 1989;115:330.

200. Van Esch H, Groenen P, Nesbit MA, Schuffenhauer S, Lichtner P, Vanderlinden G, Harding B, Beetz R, Bilous RW, Holdaway I, Shaw NJ, Fryns JP, Van de Ven W, Thakker RV, Devriendt K. GATA3 haplo-insufficiency causes human HDR syndrome. Nature 2000;406:419– 422.

201. Labastie MC, Bories D, Chabret C, Gregoire JM, Chretien S, Romeo PH. Structure and expression of the human GATA3 gene. Genomics 1994;21:1–6.

202. Bilous RW, Murty G, Parkinson DB, Thakker RV, Coulthard MG, Burn J, Mathias D, Kendall-Taylor P. Autosomal dominant familial hypoparathyroidism, sensineural deafness and renal dysplasia. N Engl J Med 1992; 327:1069–1074.

203. Barakat AY, D'Albora JB, Martin MM, Jose PA. Familial nephrosis, nerve deafness and hypoparathyroidism. J Pediatr 1977;91:61–64.

204. Koenig R, Kessel E, Schoenberger W. Partial monosomy 10p syndrome. Ann Genet 1985;28:173–176.

205. Shaw NJ, Haigh D, Lealmann GT, Karbani G, Brocklebank JT, Dillon MJ. Autosomal recessive hypoparathyroidism with renal insufficiency and development delay. Arch Dis Child 1991;66:1191–1194.

206. Fujimoto S, Yokochi K, Morikawa H, Nakano M, Shibata H, Togari H, Wada Y. Recurrent cerebral infarctions and del(10)(p14p15.1) de novo in HDR (hypoparathyroidism, sensorineural deafness, renal dysplasia) syndrome. Am J Med Genet. 1999;86:427–429.

207. Gencík A, Brönniman V, Tober R, Auf Der Maur P. Partial monosomy of chromosome 10 short arms. J Med Genet 1983;20:107–111.

208. Diaz GA, Gelb BD, Ali F, Sakati N, Sanjad S, Meyer BF, Kambouris M. Sanjad-Sakati and autosomal recessive Kenny-Caffey syndromes are allelic: evidence for an ancestral mutation and locus refinement. Am J Med Genet 1999;85:48–52.

208a. Kelly TE, Blanton S, Saif R, Sanjad SA, Sakati NA. Confirmation of the assignment of the Sanjad-Sakati (congenital hypoparathyroidism) syndrome locus to chromosome 1q42–43. J Med Genet 2000;37:63–64.

209. Parvari RM, Hershkovitz E, Kanis A, Gorodischer R, Shalitin S, Sheffield VC, Carmi R. Homozygosity and linkage-disequilibrium mapping of the syndrome of congenital hypoparathyroidism, growth and mental retardation, and dysmorphism to a 1-cM interval on chromosome 1q42-43. Am J Hum Genet 1998;63:163–169.

210. Sanjad SA, Sakati NA, Abu-Osba YK, Kaddoura R, Milner RD. A new syndrome of congenital hypoparathyroidism, severe growth failure, and dysmorphic features. Arch Dis Child 1991;66:193–196.

210a. Hoffman WH, Kovacs K, Li S, Kulharya AS, Johnson BL, Eidson MS, Cleveland WW. Kenny-Caffey syndrome and microorchidism. Am J Med Genet 1998;80: 107–111.

211. Hershkovitz E, Shalitin S, Levy J, Leiberman E, Weinshtock A, Varsano I, Gorodischer R. The new syndrome of congenital hypoparathyroidism associated with dysmorphism, growth retardation, and developmental delay: a report of six patients. Israel J Med Sci 1995;31:293–297.

212. Richardson RJ, Kirk J. Short stature, mental retardation, and hypoparathyroidism: a new syndrome. Arch Dis Child 1991;65:1113–1117.

213. Richardson RJ, Kirk J. A new syndrome of congenital hypoparathyroidism, severe growth failure, and dysmorphic features (letter). Arch Dis Child 1991;66:1365.

214. Kalam MA, Hafeez W. Congenital hypoparathyroidism, seizure, extreme growth failure with developmental delay and dysmorphic features—another case of this new syndrome. Clin Genet 1992;42:110–113.

215. Khan KTS, Uma R, Usha R, Al Ghanem MM, Al Awadi SA, Farag TI. Kenny-Caffey syndrome in six Bedouin sibships: autosomal recessive inheritance is confirmed. Am J Med Genet 1997;69:26–132.

216. Kenny FM, Linarelli L. Dwarfism and cortical thickening of tubular bones: transient hypocalcemia in a mother and son. Am J Dis Child 1966;111:201–207.

217. Fanconi S, Fischer JA, Weiland P, Atares M, Fanconi A, Giedion A, Prader A. Kenny syndrome: evidence for idiopathic hypoparathyroidism in two patients and for abnormal parathyroid hormone in one. J Pediatr 1986;109: 489–492.

218. Bergada I, Schiffrin A, Abu Srair H, Kaplan P, Dornan J, Goltzman D, Hendy GN. Kenny syndrome: description of additional abnormalities and molecular studies. Human Genet 1988;80:39–42.

219. Abdel-Al YK, Auger LT, ElGharbawy F. Kenny-Caffey syndrome, case report and literature review. Clin Pediatr 1989;28:175–179.

220. Franceschini P, Testa A, Bogetti G, Girardo E, Guala A, Lopez-Bell G, Buzio G, Ferrario E, Piccato E. Kenny-Caffey syndrome in two sibs born to consanguineous parents: evidence for an autosomal recessive variant. Am J Med Genet 1992;42:112–116.

221. Harvey JN, Barnett D. Endocrine dysfunction in Kearns-Sayre syndrome. Clin Endocrinol 1992;37:97–103.

222. Dahlberg PJ, Borer WZ, Newcomer KL, Yutuc WR. Autosomal or X-linked recessive syndrome of congenital lymphedema, hypoparathyroidism, nephropathy, prolapsing mitral valve and brachytelephalangy. Am J Med Genet 1983;16:99–104.

223. Stock JL, Brown RS, Baron J, Coderre JA, Mancilla E, De Luca F, Ray K, Mericq MV. Autosomal dominant hypoparathyroidism associated with short stature and premature osteoarthritis. J Clin Endocrinol Metab 1999; 84:3036–3040.

224. Kuster W, Mahewski F. The Dubowitz syndrome. Eur J Pediatr 1986;144:574–578.

225. Lerman-Sagie T, Merlob P, Shuper A, Kauli R, Kozokaro Z, Grunebaum M, Mimouni M. New findings in patients with Dubowitz syndrome: velopharyngeal insufficiency and hypoparathyroidism. Am J Med Genet 1990;37:241–243.

226. Chandra RK, Jogleker S, Antonio Z. Deficiency of humoral immunity and hypoparathyroidism associated with the Hallerman-Streiff syndrome, clinical note. J Pediatr 1978;93:892–893.

227. Cohen MM Jr. Hallermann-Streiff syndrome: a review. Am J Med Genet 1991;41:488–499.

228. Lipsanen-Nyman M, Perheentupa J. Hypoparathyroidism in an infant with Mulibrey nanism. 1994; unpublished data.

229. Tanner JM, Lejarraga H, Cameron N. The natural history of the Silver-Russel syndrome: a longitudinal study of thirty-nine cases. Pediatr Res 1975;9:611–623.

230. Fanconi A, Prader A. Transient congenital idiopathic hypoparathyroidism. Helv Paediatr Acta 1967;22:342–359.

231. Rosenbloom AL. Transient congenital idiopathic hypoparathyroidism. South Med J 1973;66:666–668.

232. Kooh SW, Binet A. Partial hypoparathyroidism: a variant of transient congenital hypoparathyroidism. Am J Dis Child 1991;145:877–880.

233. Cruz ML, Mimouni F, Tsang RC. "Transient" congenital hypoparathyroidism. J Pediatr 1992;120:332.

234. Cardenas-Rivero N, Chernow B, Stoiko MA, Nussbaum SR, Todres ID. Hypocalcemia in critically ill children. J Pediatr 1989;114:946–951.

235. Zaloga GB. Hypocalcemia in critically ill patients. Crit Care Med 1992;20:251–262.

236. Ryzen E. Magnesium homeostasis in critically ill patients. Magnesium 1989;8:201–212.

237. Gauthier B, Trachtman H, Di Carmine F, Urivetsky M, Tobash J, Chasalow F, Walco G, Schaeffer J. Hypocalcemia and hypercalcitoninemia in critically ill children. Crit Care Med 1990;18:1215–1219.

238. Broner CW, Stidham GL, Westenkirchner DF, Tolley EA. Hypermagnesemia and hypocalcemia as predictors of high mortality in critically ill pediatric patients. Crit Care Med 1990;18:921–928.

239. Klein GL, Langman CB, Herndon DN. Persistent hypoparathyroidism following magnesium repletion in burn-injured children. Pediatr Nephrol 2000;14:301–304.

240. Murphey ED, Chattopadhyay N, Bai M, Kifor O, Harper D, Traber DL, Hawkins HK, Brown EM, Klein GL. Up-regulation of the parathyroid calcium-sensing receptor after burn injury in sheep: a potential contributory factor to postburn hypocalcemia. Crit Care Med 2000;28: 3885–3890.

241. Hanukoglu A, Chalew S, Kowarski A. Late-onset hypocalcemia, rickets, and hypoparathyroidism in an infant of a mother with hyperparathyroidism. J Pediatr 1988; 112:751–754.

242. Bruce J, Strong JA. Maternal hyperparathyroidism and parathyroid deficiency in the child. Q J Med 1955;24: 307–319.

243. Anast CS, Mohns JM, Kaplan SL, et al. Evidence for

parathyroid failure in magnesium deficiency. Science 1972;177:606–608.

244. Anast S. Winnacker JL, Forte LR, Burns TW. Impaired release of parathyroid hormone in magnesium deficiency. J Clin Endocrinol Metab 1976;42:707–717.

245. Suh SM, Tashjian AH, Matsuo N, Parkinson DK, Fraser D. Pathogenesis of hypocalcemia in primary hypomagnesemia: normal end-organ responsiveness to parathyroid hormone, impaired parathyroid gland function. J Clin Invest 1973;52:153–160.

246. Pronicka E, Gruszczynska B. Familial hypomagnesemia with secondary hypocalcemia: autosomal or X-linked inheritance? J Inherit Metab Dis 1991;14:397–399.

247. Woodard CJ, Webster PD, Carr AA. Primary hypomagnesemia with secondary hypocalcemia, diarrhea and insensitivity to parathyroid hormone. Am J Dig Dis 1972;17:612–618.

248. Allgrove J, Adami S, Fraher L, Reuben A, O'Riordan JLH. Hypomagnesaemia: studies of parathyroid hormone secretion and function. Clin Endocrinol 1984;21: 435–449.

249. Wandrup J, Kancir C. Complex biochemical syndrome of hypocalcemia and hypoparathyroidism during cytotoxic treatment of an infant with leukemia. Clin Chem 1986;32:706–708.

250. Freedman DB, Shannon M, Dandona P, Prentice HG, Hoffbrand AV. Hypoparathyroidism and hypocalcemia during treatment for acute leukemia. Br Med J 1982; 284:700–702.

251. Nagant De Deuxchaisnes C, Krane SM. Hypoparathyroidism. In: Alvioli CV, Krane SM, eds. Metabolic Bone Disease, vol II. New York: Academic Press, 1978:218–445.

252. Richards GE, Brewer ED, Conley SB, Saldana LR. Combined hypothyroidism and hypoparathyroidism in an infant after maternal 131I administration. J Pediatr 1981;99:141–143.

253. Gertner JM, Broadus AE, Anast CS, Grey M, Pearson H, Genel M. Impaired parathyroid response to induced hypocalcemia in thalassemia major. J Pediatr 1979;95: 210–213.

254. De Sanctis V, Vullo C, Bagni B, Chiccoli L. Hypoparathyroidism in beta-thalassemia major. Clinical and laboratory observations in 24 patients. Acta Haematol 1992;88:105–108.

255. Carpenter TO, Carnes DL, Anast CS. Hypoparathyroidism in Wilson's disease. N Engl J Med 1983;309:873–877.

256. Bastepe M, Jüppner H. Pseudohypoparathyroidism. New insights into an old disease. Endocrinol Metab Clin North Am 2000;29:569–589.

257. Bell NH, Avery S, Sinha T, Clark LC Jr, Alle, DO, Johnston C Jr. Effects of dibutyryl cyclic adenosine 3′,5′-monophosphate and parathyroid extract on calcium and phosphorus metabolism in hypoparathyroidism and pseudohypoparathyroidism. J Clin Invest 1972;51:816–823.

258. Gilman AG. G proteins: tranducers of receptor-generated signals. Annu Rev Biochem 1987;56:615–649.

259. Barrett D, Breslau NA, Wax MB, Molinoff PB, Downs RW Jr. A new form of pseudohypoparathyroidism with abnormal catalytic adenylate cyclase. Am J Physiol 1989;257:E277–E283.

260. Drezner MK, Neelon FA. Pseudohypoparathyroidism. In: Stanbury JB, Wyngaarden JB, Frederickson DS, et

al, eds. The Metabolic Basis of Inherited Disease. New York: McGraw-Hill, 1983:1508–1527.

261. Poznanski AK, Werder EA, Giedion A. The pattern of shortening of the bones of the hand in PHP and PPHP—a comparison with brachydactyly E, Turner syndrome, and acrodysostosis. Radiology 1977;123:707–718.

262. Izraeli S, Metzker A, Horev G, Karmi D, Merlob P, Farfel Z. Albright hereditary osteodystrophy with hypothyroidism, normocalcemia, and normal Gs protein activity: a family presenting with congenital osteoma cutis. Am J Med Genet 1992;43:764–767.

263. Van Dop C. Pseudohypoparathyroidism: clinical and molecular aspects. Semin Nephrol 1989;9:168–178.

264. Faull CM, Welbury RR, Paul B, Kendall-Taylor P. Pseudohypoparathyroidism: its phenotypic variability and associated disorders in a large family. Q J Med 1991;78: 251–264.

265. Saito T, Akita Y, Fujita H, Furukawa Y, Tsuchiya Y, Yasuda, T, Yamamoto M, Kitagawa T, Nakagawa Y, Takehiro A, Fujita T, Kodama S, Kuzuya T. Stimulatory guanine nucleotide binding protein activity in the erythrocyte membrane of patients with pseudohypoparathyroidism type I and related disorders. Acta Endocrinol (Copenh) 1986;111:507–515.

266. Farfel Z, Friedman E. Mental deficiency in pseudohypoparathyroidism type I is associated with Ns-protein deficiency. Ann Intern Med 1986;105:197–199.

267. Weinstock RS, Wright HN, Spiegel AM, Levine MA. Moses AM. Olfactory dysfunction in humans with deficient guanine nucleotide-binding protein. Nature 1986; 322:635–636.

268. Pace V, Hanski E, Salomen Y, Lanset D. Odorant-sensitive adenylate cyclase may mediate olfactory reception. Nature 1985;316:255–258.

269. Jones DT, Reed RR. Golf: an olfactory neuron-specific G protein involved in odorant signal transduction. Science 1989;244:790–795.

270. Forbes AP. Fingerprints and palmprints (dermatoglyphics) and palmar flexion creases in gonadal dysgenesis, pseudohypoparathyroidism, and Kleinfelter's syndrome. N Engl J Med 1964;270:1268–1277.

271. Werder EA. Pseudohypoparathyroidism. Adv Intern Med Pediatr 1979;42:191–221.

272. Van Dop C, Wang H, Mulakai WJ III, Tolo VT, Rosenbaum AE. Pseudohypoparathyroidism with spinal cord compression. Pediatr Radiol 1988;18:429–431.

273. Brickman AS, Stern N, Sowers JR. Hypertension in pseudohypoparathyroidism type I. Am J Med 1988;85: 785–792.

274. Davies SJ, Hughes HE. Imprinting in Albright's hereditary osteodystrophy. J Med Genet 1993;36:101–103.

275. Wilson LC, Oude Luttikhuis ME, Clayton PT, Fraser WD, Trembath RC. Parental origin of Gs alpha gene mutations in Albright's hereditary osteodystrophy. J Med Genet 1994;31:835–839.

276. Yu S, Yu D, Lee E, Eckhaus M, Lee R, Gorria Z, Accili D, Westphal H, Weinstein LS. Variable and tissue-specific hormone resistance in heterotrimeric Gs protein alpha-subunit (Gsα) knockout mice is due to tissue-specific imprinting of the Gsα gene. Proc Natl Acad Sci USA 1998;95:8715–8720.

277. Lanske B, Karaplis AC, Luz A, Vortkamp A, Pirro A, Karperien M, Defize LHK, Ho C, Mulligan RC, Abou-Samra AB, Juppner H, Segre GV, Kronenberg HM.

PTH/PTHrP receptor in early development and Indian hedgehog-regulated bone growth. Science 1996;273: 663–666.

278. Jüppner H, Schipani E, Bastepe M, Cole DE, Lawson ML, Mannstadt M, Hendy GN, Plotkin H, Koshiyama H, Koh T, Crawford JD, Olsen BR, Vikkula M. The gene reponsible for pseudohypoparathyroidism type Ib is paternally imprinted and maps in four unrelated kindreds to chromosome 20q13.3. Proc Natl Acad Sci USA 1998; 95:11798–11803.

279. Mizunashi K, Furukawa Y, Sohn HE, Miura R, Yumita S, Yoshinaga K. Heterogeneity of pseudohypoparathyroidism type I from the aspect of urinary excretion of calcium and serum levels of parathyroid hormone. Calcif Tissue Int 1990;46:227–232.

280. Breslau NA, Moses AM, Pak CYC. Evidence for bone remodeling but lack of calcium mobilization response to parathyroid hormone in pseudohypoparathyroidism. J Clin Endocrinol Metab 1983;57:638–644.

281. Kolb FO, Steinbach HL. Pseudohypoparathyroidism with secondary hyperparathyroidism and osteitis fibrosa. J Clin Endocrinol Metab 1962;22:59–70.

282. Allen EH, Millard FJC, Nassim JR. Hypo-hyperparathyroidism. Arch Dis Child 1968;43:295–301.

283. Kidd GS, Schaaf M, Adler RA, Lassman MN, Wray HL. Skeletal responsiveness in pseudohypoparathyroidism. A spectrum of clinical disease. Am J Med 1980;68:772–781.

284. Breslau NA. Pseudohypoparathyroidism: current concepts. Am J Med Sci 1989;298:130–140.

285. Stögmann W, Fischer JA. Pseudohypoparathyroidism: disappearance of the resistance to parathyroid extract during treatment with vitamin D. Am J Med 1975;59: 140–144.

286. Drezner MK, Neelon FA, Haussler M, McPherson HT, Lebowitz HE. 1,25-dihydroxycholecalciferol deficiency: the probable cause of hypocalcemia and metabolic bone disease in pseudohypoparathyroidism. J Clin Endocrinol Metab 1976;42:621–628.

287. Werder EA, Kind HP, Egert F, Fischer JA, Prader A. Effective long term treatment of pseudohypoparathyroidism with oral 1α-hydroxy- and 1,25-dihydroxyvitamin D. J Pediatr 1976;89:266–268.

288. Davies M, Hill LF, Taylor CM, Stanbury SW. 1,25-Dihydoxycholecalciferol in hypoparathyroidism. Lancet 1977;1:55–58.

289. Metz SA, Baylink DJ, Hughes MR, Haussler MR, Robertson RP. Selective deficiency of 1,25-hydroxycholecalciferol: a cause of isolated skeletal resistance to parathyroid hormone. N Engl J Med 1977:297:1084–1089.

290. Breslau NA, Notman D, Canterbury JM, Moses AM. Studies on attainment of normocalcemia in patients with pseudohypoparathyroidism. Am J Med 1980;68:856–860.

291. Levine MA, Jap TS, Hung W. Infantile hypothyroidism in two sibs: an unusual presentation of pseudohypoparathyroidism type Ia. J Pediatr 1985;107:919–922.

292. Weisman Y, Golander A, Spirer Z, Farfel Z. Pseudohypoparathyroidism type 1a presenting as congenital hypothyroidism. J Pediatr 1985;107:413–415.

293. Shima M, Nose O, Shimizu K, Seino Y, Yabuuchi H, Saito T. Multiple associated endocrine abnormalities in a patient with pseudohypoparathyroidism type 1a. Eur J Pediatr 1988;147:536–538.

294. Murray TM, Rao LG, Wong MM, Waddel JP, McBroom R, Tam CS, Rosen F, Levine MA. Pseudohypoparathyroidism with osteitis fibrosa cystica: direct demonstration of skeletal responsiveness to parathyroid hormone in cells cultured from bone. J Bone Miner Res 1993;8: 83–91.

295. Prendiville JS, Lucky AW, Malory SB, Mughal Z, Mimouni F, Langman CG. Osteoma cutis as a presenting sign of pseudohypoparathyroidism. Pediatr Dermatol 1992;9: 11–88.

296. Carlson HE, Brickman AS, Burns TW, Langley PE. Normal free fatty acid response to isoproterenol in pseudohypoparathyroidism. J Clin Endocrinol Metab 1985; 61:382–384.

297. Farfel Z, Bourne HR. Pseudohypoparathyroidism: mutation affecting adenylate cyclase. Mineral Electrolyte Metab 1982;8:227–231.

298. Levine MA, Downs RW Jr, Moses AM, Breslau NA, Marx SJ, Lasker RD, Rizzoli RE, Aurbach GD, Spiegel AM. Resistance to multiple hormones in patients with pseudohypoparathyroidism and deficient guanine nucleotide regulatory protein. Am J Med 1983;74:545–556.

299. Farfel Z, Brickman AS, Kaslow, HR, Brothers VM, Bourne HR. Defect of receptor-cyclase coupling protein in pseudohypoparathyroidism. N Engl J Med 1980;303: 237–242.

300. Carlson HE, Brickmann AS, Bottazzo GF. Prolactin deficiency in pseudohypoparathyroidism. N Engl J Med 1977;296:140–144.

301. Kruse K, Gutekunst B, Kracht U, Schwerda K. Deficient prolactin response to parathyroid hormone in hypocalcemic and normocalcemic pseudohypoparathyroidism. J Clin Endocrinol Metab 1981;52:1099–1105.

302. Wägar G, Lehtovuori J, Salven I, Backman R, Sivula A. Pseudohypoparathyroidism associated with hypercalcitoninemia. Acta Endocrinol 1980;93:43–48.

303. Brickman AS, Weitzman RE. Renal resistance to arginine vasopressin in pseudohypoparathyroidism. Clin Res 1977;26:164.

304. Ridderskamp P, Schlaghecke R. Pseudohypoparathyreoidismus und Nebennierenrindeninsuffizienz. Klin Wochenschr 1990;68:927–931.

305. Iiri T, Herzmark P, Nakamoto JM, Van Dop C, Bourne HR. Rapid GDP from $G_s\alpha$ in patients with gain and loss of function. Nature 1994;371:164–168.

306. Fischer JA, Bourne HR, Dambacher MA, Tshopp F, De Meyer F, Devogelaer JP, Werder E, Nagant de Deuxchaisnes C. Pseudohypoparathyroidism: inheritance and expression of deficient receptor-cyclase coupling protein activity. Clin Endocrinol (Oxf) 1983;19:747–754.

307. Levine MA, Tjin-Shing J, Mauseth RS, Downs RW, Spiegel AM. Activity of the stimulatory guanine nucleotide-binding protein is reduced in erythrocytes from patients with pseudohypoparathyroidism and pseudopseudohypoparathyroidism: biochemical, endocrine, and genetic analysis of Albright's hereditary osteodystrophy in six kindreds. J Clin Endocrinol Metab1986;62:497–502.

308. Pickenback A, Lang B, Palitzsch KD, Scholmerich J Straub RH. A 63-year-old patient with worsening general condition, bone demineralization, hypocalcemia and excess parathyroid hormone: late manifestations of pseudohypoparathyroidism. Dtsch Med Wochenschr 1999; 124:551–555.

308a. Farfel Z. Pseudohypohyperparathyroidism-pseudohypoparathyroidism type Ib. J Bone Miner Res 1999;14:1016.

309. Jan de Beur SM, Ding CL, LaBuda MC, Usdin TB, Levine MA. Pseudohypoparathyroidism 1b: exclusion of parathyroid hormone and its receptors as candidate disease genes. J Clin Endocrinol Metab 2000;85:2239–2246.

310. Rodriquez HJ, Villareal H, Klahr S, Slatopolski E. Pseudohypoparathyroidism type II. Restoration of normal renal responsiveness to parathyroid hormone by calcium administration. J Clin Endocrinol Metab 1974;39:693–701.

311. Saito H, Saito M, Saito K, Terauchi A, Kobayashi T, Tominaga T, Hosoi E, Senoo M, Saito K, Saito T. Case report: subclinical pseudohypoparathyroidism type II: evidence for failure of physiologic adjustment in calcium metabolism during pregnancy. Am J Med Sci 1989;297:247–250.

312. Matsuda I, Takekoshi Y, Tanaka M, Matsuura M, Nagai B, Seino Y. Pseudohypoparathyroidism type II and anticonvulsant rickets. Eur J Pediatr 1979;132:303–308.

313. Rao DS, Parfitt AM, Kleerekoper M, Pumo PS, Frame B. Dissociation between effects of endogenous parathyroid hormone on adenosine 3′,5′-monophosphate generation and phosphate reabsorption in hypocalcemia due to vitamin D depletion: an acquired disorder resembling pseudohypoparathyroidism type II. J Clin Endocrinol Metab 1985;61:285–290.

314. Yamada K, Tamura Y, Tomioko H, Kumagai A, Yoshida S. Possible existence of anti-renal tubular plasma membrane autoantibody which blocked parathyroid hormone-induced phosphaturia in a patient with pseudohypoparathyroidism type II and Sjögren's syndrome. J Clin Endocrinol Metab 1984;58:339–343.

315. Kruse K, Kracht U, Wohlfart K, Kruse U. Evaluation of intact serum parathyroid hormone (PTH 1-84) in the diagnosis of disorders of calcium metabolism. Acta Endocrinol Suppl (Copenh) 1988;287:64–65.

316. Allen DB, Friedman AL, Greer FR, Chesney RW. Hypomagnesemia masking the appearance of elevated parathyroid hormone concentrations in familial pseudohypoparathyroidism. Am J Med Genet 1988;31:153–158.

317. Kruse K, Kracht U. A simplified diagnostic test in hypoparathyroidism and pseudohypoparathyroidism type I with synthetic 1-38 fragment of human parathyroid hormone. Eur J Pediatr 1987;146:373–377.

318. Mallette LE. Synthetic human parathyroid hormone 1-34 fragment for diagnostic testing. Ann Intern Med 1988;109:800–804.

319. Miura R, Yumita S, Yoshinaga K, Furukawa Y. Response of plasma 1,25-dihydroxyvitamin D in the human PTH(1-34) infusion test: an improved index for the diagnosis of idiopathic hypoparathyroidism and pseudohypoparathyroidism. Calcif Tissue Int 1990;46:309–313.

320. Cuneo BF, Driscoll DA, Gidding SS, Langman CB. Evolution of latent hypoparathyroidism in familial 22q11 deletion syndrome. Am J Med Genet 1997;69:50–55.

321. Radford DJ, Thong YH. Facial and immunological anomalies associated with tetralogy of Fallot. Int J Cardiol 1989;22:229–239.

322. Winer KK, Yanowski JA, Sarani B, Cutler GB. A randomized, cross-over trial on once-daily versus twice-daily parathyroid hormone 1-34 in treatment of hypoparathyroidism. J Clin Endocrinol Metab 1998;83:3480–3486.

323. Yamamoto M, Furukawa Y, Konagaya Y, Sohn HE, Tomita A, Fujita T, Ogata E. Human PTH (1-34) infusion test in differential diagnosis of various types of hypoparathyroidism: an attempt to establish a standard clinical test. Bone Miner 1989;6:199–212.

324. Levine MA, Downs RW Jr, Moses AMS, Breslau NA, Marx SJ, Lasker RD, Rizzoli RE, Aurbach GD, Spiegel AM. Resistance to multiple hormones in patients with pseudohypoparathyroidism. Association with deficient activity of guanine nucleotide regulatory protein. Am J Med 1983;74:545–556.

324a. Miric A, Vechio JD, Levine MA. Heterogeneous mutations in the gene encoding the α-subunit of the stimulatory G protein of adenylyl cyclase in Albright hereditary osteodystrophy. J Clin Endocrinol Metab 1993;76:1560–1568.

325. Marx SJ. Hypoparathyroidism. In: Krieger DT, Bardin CW, eds. Current Therapy in Endocrinology and Metabolism. Toronto: BC Decker, 1985:329–333.

326. Markowitz ME, Rosen JF, Smith C, DeLuca HF. 1,25-Dihydroxyvitamin D_3-treated hypoparathyroidism: 35 patient years in 10 children. J Clin Endocrinol Metab 1982;55:727–733.

327. Chan JCM, Young RB, Hartenberg MA, Chinchilli VM. Calcium and phosphate metabolism in children with idiopathic hypoparathyroidism or pseudohypoparathyroidism: Effect of 1,25-dihydroxyvitamin D3. J Pediatr 1985;106:421–426.

328. Okano K, Furukawa Y, Morii H, Fujita T. Comparative efficacy of various vitamin D metabolites in the treatment of various types of hypoparathyroidism. J Clin Endocrinol Metab 1982;55:238–243.

329. Mizunashi K, Furukawa Y, Miura R, Yumita S, Sohn HE, Yoshinaga K. Effects of active vitamin D_3 and parathyroid hormone on the serum osteocalcin in idiopathic hypoparathyroidism and pseudohypoparathyroidism. J Clin Invest 1988;82:861–865.

330. Halabe A, Arie R, Mimran D, Samuel R, Liberman UA. Hypoparathyroidism—a long-term follow-up experience with 1α-vitamin D_3 therapy. Clin Endocrinol 1984;40:303–307.

331. Harrison HE, Lifshitz F, Blizzard RM. Comparison between crystalline dihydrotachysterol and calciferol in patients requiring pharmacologic vitamin D therapy. N Engl J Med 1967;276:894–900.

332. Dent CE, Morgans ME, Harper CM, et al. Insensitivity to vitamin D developing during treatment of postoperative tetany. Its specificity as regards the form of vitamin D taken. Lancet 1955;2:687–690.

333. Sutton RAL, Walker, Halabe A, Swenerton K, Coppin CM. Chronic hypomagnesemia caused by cisplatin: effect of calcitriol. J Lab Clin Med 1991;117:40–43.

20
Hyperparathyroidism in Children

Scott A. Rivkees
Yale University School of Medicine, New Haven, Connecticut, U.S.A.

Thomas O. Carpenter
Yale University School of Medicine and Yale–New Haven Hospital, New Haven, Connecticut, U.S.A.

I. INTRODUCTION

Although it makes up less than 1% of total-body calcium stores, extracellular calcium plays a critical role in mammalian physiology. This circulating divalent cation regulates cell membrane electrical potential, neurotransmitter release, renal function, and cardiovascular tone. Thus, maintenance of serum calcium levels in the normal range is a fundamental homeostatic mechanism. The task of maintaining circulating calcium levels in the normal range is the domain of the parathyroid glands. Elevation in calcium levels, as in hyperparathyroidism, impairs renal function and can affect other organ systems. Thus, proper recognition and treatment of hyperparathyroidism are essential.

II. THE PARATHYROID GLANDS

The parathyroid glands are paired structures located behind or within the superior and inferior aspects of the thyroid (1). In 84% of individuals, four parathyroid glands are present (1). The superior pair of glands is generally found 1 cm above the recurrent laryngeal nerve and inferior thyroidal arteries, behind the upper thyroid. The inferior glands are located behind the inferior poles of the thyroid. In 13% of individuals, a fifth gland is present in the region of the thymus (1). Each gland is small, measuring less than 6 × 5 × 2 mm in adulthood (1).

The parathyroid glands are encapsulated by fibrous connective tissue (1). Within the glands, fibrovascular bundles divide the stroma into cordlike structures. Chief cells, of epithelial origin, are typically the only cell type recognized within the glands before puberty. After puberty, fat deposition occurs within the glands, and fat content may reach 10–50% of parathyroid cell mass in adults (2). Oxyphilic cells are rare in children and make up less than 5% of parathyroid tissue in adults (3).

Parathyroid gland embryogenesis occurs during early gestation (4). During gestational week (GW) 6, the dorsum of the third pharyngeal pouch differentiates into the inferior parathyroid glands. The ventral region of this pouch differentiates into the thymus. The thymic and parathyroid primordia are contiguous until GW 10, when the parathyroids separate from the thymus. The fourth pharyngeal pouch gives rise to the superior parathyroid glands. At GW 10, both pairs of glands come to lie on the dorsal surface of the thyroid gland, which completes its migration from the foramen cecum to the pretracheal region by GW 8 (4).

There may be excessive migration of both the superior and inferior parathyroid glands (1). Thus, the final resting location of each gland pair may be inferior to the normal position. The superior glands may migrate to the region of the lower thyroid, and the inferior glands may migrate below the suprasternal notch to within the thymus (1). Parathyroid tissue may also migrate to within thyroid tissue (5).

The factors involved in parathyroid gland formation and migration are unknown. Transgenic animal studies suggest that the homeobox gene *Hox-1.5* may be involved in parathyroid gland development. The selective deletion of *Hox-1.5* in mice results in abnormal differentiation of the third and fourth branchial arches and a phenotype similar to DiGeorge syndrome (parathyroid hypoplasia, cardiac abnormalities, and thymic hypoplasia) (6). In humans, sequences on 22 p11 appear to be essential for parathyroid gland development, since a deletion on this region classically results in the DiGeorge disease phenotype (7).

In X-linked recessive idiopathic hypoparathyroidism, genetic mapping has localized the gene defect region to

Xq 26–Xq 27 (8, 9). However, the specific genes involved have not been identified. Impaired parathyroid gland formation has also been associated with deletions of mitochondrial DNA (10).

Chief cells differentiate during the embryonic period and are functional during fetal life (4). Oxyphil cells do not differentiate until 6 years after birth (3). After birth, parathyroid hormone (PTH)-related peptide levels fall and PTH levels increase (11).

III. PARATHYROID HORMONE AND REGULATION OF ITS SECRETION

A gene on the short arm of chromosome 11 in humans encodes PTH (12, 13). A preprohormone of 115 amino acids is encoded, which is cleaved to an 84 amino acid peptide for secretion (14–16). The hormone is secreted by exocytosis of secretory vesicles. Intravesicular degradation of PTH may occur, and is reduced in the setting of chronic hypocalcemia as to maximize the bioactive intact PTH. PTH secretion is regulated largely by external calcium levels. At low calcium levels PTH secretion is stimulated, whereas PTH release is suppressed at high levels. In vivo and in vitro studies suggest that the ionized calcium concentration required to achieve half-maximal suppression of PTH secretion is 0.99 mmol/l (17, 18). In normal circumstances, circulating levels of intact PTH range between 10 and 65 pg/ml (19). During hypocalcemia, levels may rise fivefold (19). During hypercalcemia, levels are undetectable, or less than 10 pg/ml (19).

The mechanism by which extracellular calcium regulates PTH secretion involves a novel protein found on the parathyroid cell surface that senses ionized extracellular calcium levels. This calcium-sensing receptor (CaSR) has a long extracellular N-terminal moiety where calcium binds in a molecular pocket (17). The receptor is related to the metabotropic glutamate receptors found in the central nervous system (CNS), has seven transmembrane-spanning regions, and an intracellular C-terminal tail that is important for signal transduction via G-proteins. The CaSR is found in the parathyroid glands, kidney, brain, bone, and other sites (20). When activated by binding calcium atoms, the CaSR signals the parathyroid glands to inhibit PTH secretion. As the concentration of ionized calcium declines, CaSR occupancy is reduced, and PTH secretion is restored. Activating mutations in the CaSR result in autosomal dominant hypocalcemia (21, 22). In contrast, inactivating mutations of the CaSR result in familial hypocalciuric hypercalcemia (FHH) in the heterozygous form and severe neonatal hyperparathyroidism in the homozygous state (see below) (21, 22).

Hypomagnesemia may also stimulate PTH secretion, presumably related to the affinity of the CaSR for magnesium (23). However, when magnesium levels drop below 1.5 mg/dl, PTH secretion may be impaired (23). Hyperphosphatemia may also increase PTH secretion. In many clinical situations this is secondary to phosphate-induced suppression of calcium levels (24). However, ambient phosphate levels have been shown to regulate parathyroid secretion when calcium levels are fixed (25). This effect may play a role in the development of secondary hyperparathyroidism in chronic renal failure, when serum calcium levels may not be decreased (25).

The vitamin D metabolite, 1,25-dihydroxy vitamin D, can also directly inhibit PTH secretion, and decrease the abundance of PTH message (26). 24,25 dihydroxy vitamin D has also been shown to inhibit PTH secretion and reduce parathyroid gland mass (27). Thus, these compounds are useful in preventing and treating secondary hyperparathyroidism.

IV. ASSAYS FOR PARATHYROID HORMONE

A variety of assays for PTH are available. Two-site assays detect intact PTH (1–84) utilizing a distinct antibody to the C-terminus to capture the molecule to a solid phase, and then a specific amino-terminus directed antibody coupled to a radioisotope or chemiluminescent moiety, which serves as the detection signal (28, 29). These assays are useful in settings in which clearance of PTH fragments is impaired, such as in renal failure.

In comparison with two-site assays, assays directed to the midmolecule fragment may detect hyperparathyroidism before PTH elevations are evident using the two-site assay (30). We have also used specific radioimmunoassays with antibodies directed toward the N-terminus of the molecule, but have found that the available N-terminal assay is less discriminatory than late midmolecule assays. Thus, measurement of PTH levels using two-site and midmolecule assays may be needed if PTH levels obtained using one assay do not fit with the clinical picture.

Another useful tool for assessing PTH activity is the measurement of nephrogenous camp (31). This assay involves measurement of cAMP and creatinine levels in a 2 h urine collection and measurement of plasma cAMP and creatinine levels at the midpoint of the urine collection (31). The calculated urinary cAMP excretion, corrected for the filtered plasma component, represents the cAMP generated by the kidney and is an excellent index of PTH bioactivity at the kidney.

Evidence of excess PTH activity may also be associated with radiographic evidence of bone resorption, particularly at the tips of phalanges, and at the clavicle (32, 33). However, such changes are apparent after long-standing hyperparathyroidism and provide only a gross estimate of PTH action.

V. PTH/PTHrP RECEPTORS

Parathyroid hormone exerts its many of its biological effects via specific cell surface receptors. The identification of a family of parathyroid hormone receptor has enhanced the understanding of PTH action (34, 35). The first-identified PTH/PTHrP receptor is a monomeric protein of 585 amino acids, with seven transmembrane spanning domains, and has affinity for both PTH and PTHrP. The receptor couples with guanine nucleotide-binding proteins (G proteins). Receptor occupation activates adenylate cyclase, leading to intracellular cAMP accumulation and subsequent activation of protein kinase A. Receptor activation stimulates the protein kinase C pathway as well, activating the membrane phospholipase C, which leads to intracellular accumulation of inositol phosphates and diacylglycerol and increases in intracellular calcium (34, 35).

At least two other members of this family have been subsequently identified, including the PTH-2 receptor, which has much greater affinity for PTH, does not significantly bind PTHrP, and may serve as a receptor for a novel ligand in the hypothalamus (34, 35). A third receptor appears to be a specific receptor for PTHrP, with little affinity for PTH (35).

Activating mutations of the PTH/PTHrP receptor results in Jansen's metaphysical chondrodysplasia demonstrating a critical role for PTH in metaphyseal development (36). In contrast, the absence of functional PTH/PTHrP receptors is seen in Blomstrand chondrodysplasia (37).

VI. MECHANISM OF PARATHYROID HORMONE ACTION

PTH is a major regulator of calcium metabolism and acts on kidney, bone, and the intestine to increase the net flow of calcium into the extracellular fluid space. In the adult, approximately 15 mg/kg calcium is ingested and 12 mg/kg is excreted in the feces, yielding net calcium absorption of 3 mg/kg/day (38). The absorbed calcium is either deposited in the skeleton or excreted in the urine. At calcium intakes above 10 mg/kg/day, net calcium absorption increases only slightly (38).

PTH acts on the kidneys to effect renal tubular reabsorption of calcium (39). The kidneys filter about 8000 mg calcium/m^2 each day (38, 40). The vast amount of filtered calcium is reabsorbed, with only about 5% eliminated in the urine (150–250 mg/m^2/day) (41, 42). During hypercalcemia, urinary calcium excretion may increase more than fourfold, whereas excretion falls during hypocalcemia (41). About 60% of filtered calcium is reabsorbed in the proximal tubule. The remaining calcium is reabsorbed by the loop of Henle or distal tubules, where PTH-stimulated calcium reabsorption acts to maintain serum calcium levels in the normal range.

While promoting calcium reabsorption, PTH induces renal phosphate wasting. Thus, following PTH-induced bone dissolution, calcium returns to the circulation and phosphate is excreted in the urine. The effects of PTH on renal phosphate handling occur primarily at the proximal tubule (43). PTH also influences the tubular reabsorption of bicarbonate, glucose, and amino acids. Bicarbonate,

glucose, and amino acid wasting may attend hyperparathyroidism, resulting in a clinical picture similar to renal tubular acidosis or Fanconi's syndrome (43–45). During hypoparathyroidism, there can be excessive bicarbonate reabsorption, which may result in metabolic alkalosis (43, 45). PTH also stimulates activity of the renal enzyme 25-hydroxyvitamin D-1-alpha-hydroxylase, promoting formation of 1,25-dihydroxyvitamin D (calcitriol) (46) (47). Calcitriol is the most potent vitamin D metabolite with respect to the effect of intestinal transport of calcium (48).

Mechanisms of PTH action on bone are complex (49). Following peripheral injection of PTH, osteoclast proliferation and activity are induced leading to bone dissolution and calcium and phosphate release (50). These effects occur more than 12 h after PTH administration and do not acutely influence calcium levels. These effects are thought to be mediated by a direct effect on osteoblasts, which trigger release of cytokines and other factors that influence bone-resorbing osteoclasts. One recently identified factor that mediates PTH-induced osteoblast stimulation of osteoclast differentiation and action is RANKL, or the osteoprotegerin ligand (50). A pool of rapidly exchangeable bone calcium is thought to mediate the acute effects of PTH on endosteal bone cells. Activation of these cells induces calcium release from bone within a few hours (51).

In contrast to the well-known PTH stimulation of bone resorption, recent data demonstrate an anabolic effect of PTH on bone when administered intermittently (52, 53). These data further indicate that the osteoblast is a primary target of PTH, and emphasized a potential role for PTH as a therapy for osteoporosis.

VII. PATHOGENESIS OF HYPERPARATHYROIDISM

Hyperparathyroidism occurs when PTH is released independently of calcium levels or the so-called set point for calcium-induced suppression of PTH secretion is elevated (18, 54). Hyperparathyroidism is typically a disease of adulthood, presenting between 40 and 60 years of age (55). It is more common in women than in men, and the incidence in the population is between 0.05 and 0.5%. Of individuals with hyperparathyroidism, 85% have parathyroid adenomas (56). The remaining 15% have diffuse parathyroid hyperplasia.

Over the past several years, there have been important advances in our understanding of hyperparathyroidism. Recent data suggest that parathyroid adenomas result from the clonal expansion of individual parathyroid cell lines (57). In some individuals a candidate oncogene (PRDAI: Cylin D1) is abnormally rearranged within the PTH locus (11q13) (58). This gene encodes a 295 amino acid cyclin protein, which may be important in cell cycle regulation (58). It has been postulated that the overexpression of PRAD I plays a role in the development of parathyroid adenomas (58). Abnormalities of the retinoblastoma gene were also recently found in parathyroid adenomas (59). In contrast to PPAD1, mutations in the tumor-suppressor genes RAD51 and RAD54 have not been detected in parathyroid adenomas. Likewise, mutations in the CaSR gene have not been identified in sporadic adenomas. On the other hand, loss of heterozygosity in the MEN1 region on chromosome 11q13 has been found in 30% of sporadic parathyroid tumors (60).

In contrast to adenomas, the pathogenesis of parathyroid hyperplasia may involve different mechanisms. Diffuse hyperplasia of the parathyroid glands may occur following longstanding stimulation of parathyroid activity in response to hypocalcemia. Individuals with chronic hyperphosphatemia from renal failure or exogenous phosphate administration may develop secondary hyperparathyroidism. Over time the calcium concentration needed to suppress PTH secretion gradually increases, leading to a new steady state in which the serum calcium is maintained at a higher level (18, 61). Ionized calcium concentrations of 1.1–1.4 mmol/l may be needed to achieve half-maximal suppression of PTH secretion (normal = 0.99 mmol/l). Eventually, PTH secretion may not be suppressible even by high circulating levels of calcium. Supporting this hypothesis, individuals with tertiary hyperparathyroidism may show a spectrum of evolving parathyroid dysfunction. For example, in one of our patients with multiglandular hyperplasia, the set points for PTH suppression of three distinct glands were 1.1, 1.4, and 1.6 mmol/l, respectively. In the fourth gland, PTH secretion was not suppressible even by high calcium levels (61).

VIII. DIFFERENTIAL DIAGNOSIS

Hyperparathyroidism is rare in children. Thus, other causes should be sought in the hypercalcemic child. The differential diagnosis is extensive, and several specific causes of hypercalcemia are listed here.

In the newborn period, William's syndrome, must be considered (62, 63). These individuals may have hypercalcemia but do not usually have hypophosphatemia. The hypercalcemia usually resolves by the time the child is 1 year of age and is very rarely evident after the fourth year. Affected children may be small for gestational age and have a characteristic facial appearance and supravalvular aortic stenosis. William's syndrome is due to a deletion of the elastin gene locus on chromosome 7 (64). Parathyroid hormone levels are usually suppressed in this disorder, although we have encountered two infants with William's syndrome, proven by FISH analysis of the elastin locus, who have elevated circulating levels of PTH.

It is also important to differentiate FHH from hyperparathyroidism. FHH is characterized by the combination of hypercalcemia and relative hypocalciuria (65, 66). Individuals with FHH do not require parathyroidectomy and almost always have a benign course. FHH is caused by an inactivating mutation of CaSR (21, 67). Thus, PTH levels are usually in the upper range of normal, or are modestly elevated. Serum calcium levels usually range between 10 and 12 mg/dl. Because the CaSR is expressed in the kidney, renal calcium reabsorption is also increased. The generous PTH levels augment renal calcium reabsorption, contributing to hypocalciuria. By examining renal calcium excretion, it may be possible to differentiate FHH from hyperparathyroidism, since more than 99% of filtered calcium is reabsorbed in FHH, whereas renal calcium reabsorption is generally less than that in hyperparathyroidism. However the differentiation between FHH and hyperparathyroidism may not be straightforward. A family history also aids in the diagnosis of FHH. A parent is often found to have the biochemical features of FHH, reflecting the characteristic autosomal dominant mode of inheritance.

Vitamin D intoxication may induce hypercalcemia at dosages more than 100 times the physiological requirement (68). Excessive vitamin D fortification of dairy milk (up to 10,000 u/l; normal 400 u/l) has led to epidemic hypercalcemia (68). Excessive vitamin D supplementation of infant formulas has been described (69). During vitamin D intoxication PTH levels are suppressed and serum phosphate values are normal or modestly elevated.

We have also cared for low-birth-weight infants with hypercalcemia due to unregulated intestinal calcium absorption when placed on breast milk fortifiers. The high calcium load of the supplements plays a large role in this condition. With advancing age intestinal calcium absorption declines, and the tendency for hypercalcemia falls.

Other causes of hypercalcemia include subcutaneous fat necrosis, in which elevated circulating levels of 1,25 dihydoxyvitamin D have been described. Immobilization, vitamin A intoxication, malignancy, granulomatous disease (including cat-scratch fever), and thiazide diuretic therapy should be considered in the differential diagnosis of hypercalcemia in a child.

IX. RECOGNITION AND DIAGNOSIS

Recognition of hyperparathyroidism in its early stages is important because longstanding hypercalcemia may adversely affect several organ systems. The combination of hypercalcemia, hypophosphatemia, and phosphaturia suggests hyperparathyroidism. However, in some individuals calcium elevations may be episodic (70). In individuals with hyperphosphatemia, or those receiving phosphate therapy, hypercalcemia may also be masked (61).

The tubular reabsorption of phosphate (TRP; [1-Up $\times$ SCr/UCr $\times$ SP] 100%) is normally greater than 85%. During parathyroid hormone excess, the TRP may fall to as low as 50%. However, in up to 40% of individuals with hyperparathyroidism, hypophosphatemia may not be present and the TRP is normal (56).

The urinary excretion of calcium is a function of the filtered calcium (which is proportional to the serum calcium level) and the reabsorbed calcium (enhanced by PTH at the distal tubule). Thus, the fractional excretion of calcium is reduced when hyperparathyroidism is present. To assess renal calcium handling, so-called spot urine samples that calcium/creatinine concentration ratios are convenient, eliminating the need for 24 h urine collections, which are often difficult to obtain in young children.

In normal children over 4 years of age, urinary calcium excretion is approximately 2 mg/kg/day, and hypercalciuria is defined as excretion of levels >4 mg/kg/day (38, 40). Over the 24 h day, 10–20 mg/kg creatinine is excreted in the urine. Thus, in children over 4 years of age, the urinary calcium–creatinine ratio is normally less than 0.1 (mg/mg), with a ratio >0.2 defined as hypercalciuria. Urinary calcium excretion is relatively high in infancy. Thus, urinary calcium/creatinine ratios are higher than in older children and range between 0.2 and 0.7 (71, 72).

If suspected, hyperparathyroidism should be confirmed by measurement of circulating PTH levels. If PTH levels are normal when measured using two-site intact PTH assays, measurement of PTH levels by midmolecule should also be performed when the diagnosis remains a possibility.

X. PRIMARY HYPERPARATHYROIDISM

Fewer than 100 cases of isolated primary hyperparathyroidism have been reported in children (73–78). Both parathyroid adenomas and multiglandular hyperplasia have been described. It is postulated that primary hyperparathyroidism in children represents early presentation of the sporadic form of hyperparathyroidism that typically affects adults. No clear pattern of inheritance is generally found; although several kindreds have been reported in whom primary hyperparathyroidism affects several generations (79).

Hypercalcemia is usually not an indication for a parathyroidectomy in FHH, when one mutant copy of the CaSR is present. However, severe neonatal hyperparathyroidism occurs within FHH kindreds in individuals homozygous for mutations of the CaSR (22, 80, 81). In affected individuals, severe hyperparathyroidism presents within the first few days of life, with serum calcium levels as high as 15–30 mg/dl. The serum phosphate level is usually low, and the serum PTH level is elevated. Nephrocalcinosis may be present, reflecting intrauterine hypercalcemia. This is a life-threatening condition that requires emergency extirpation of the parathyroid glands.

Hyperparathyroidism may also be a feature of the inherited multiple endocrine neoplasia syndromes, MEN I and MEN II, which are autosomal dominant disorders (82, 83). Hyperparathyroidism is the most common presenting feature of MEN I (97% of cases), which is also associated with tumors of the pancreas (40%) and pituitary (20%). Hyperparathyroidism may occur in 20% of cases of MEN

IIa (84, 85), which is associated with medullary carcinoma of the thyroid and pheochromocytoma. Hyperparathyroidism typically presents during adulthood, although cases have been reported in children. MEN IIb (MEN III) is not associated with primary hyperparathyroidism, although both MEN IIa and MEN IIb are caused by mutations in different domains of the rearranged during transfection (RET) proto-oncogene (86, 87).

Radiation exposure may be associated with the development of hyperparathyroidism. An increased incidence of hyperparathyroidism has been reported in adult survivors of the Hiroshima atomic blast (88). It has been suggested that the incidence of hyperparathyroidism is greater three decades after head and neck radiotherapy (89, 90). Hyperparathyroidism has also been reported in a few patients treated with radioiodine for Graves' disease (91, 92), however, with no greater frequency than that observed in the normal population (93). Primary hyperparathyroidism has been described in one infant with congenital hypothyroidism (76).

Carcinoma of the parathyroid glands can present with biochemical features similar to those of primary hyperparathyroidism. Although there are very few reports of parathyroid carcinoma in children (94), parathyroid carcinoma has been reported in adolescents with familial hyperparathyroidism (95, 96).

XI. SECONDARY AND TERTIARY HYPERPARATHYROIDISM

Secondary and tertiary hyperparathyroidism are often seen in hypocalcemic and/or hyperphosphatemic states, such as vitamin D deficiency. An appropriate response to hypocalcemia (secondary hyperparathyroidism) may evolve into autonomous PTH secretion (tertiary hyperparathyroidism) following prolonged hypocalcemic stimulation of parathyroid gland activity.

In the newborn period secondary hyperparathyroidism may be seen in children born to hypocalcemic mothers. This typically resolves within several months of birth (97, 98). We have cared for infants with transient hyperparathyroidism whose mothers did not have hypocalcemia; hypercalcemia resolved by 3 months of age.

Secondary hyperparathyroidism is a classic feature of moderate to severe vitamin D-deficient rickets. Diffuse parathyroid hyperplasia has been described in these patients (99) and progression to tertiary hyperparathyroidism may occur in the setting of chronic disease. Efforts should be taken place to prevent this progression since severe parathyroid hyperplasia may not be reversible and surgical extirpation of the parathyroid glands required (61).

Chronic elevation of serum phosphate levels may be the most common cause of secondary hyperparathyroidism in children. The inability of the kidneys to excrete phosphate accounts for this phenomena (100, 101). This scenario is especially troublesome for a skeletal system already at risk for metabolic bone disease. Thus, parathyroid function should be routinely monitored during chronic renal failure, and parathyroidectomy is needed in the setting of irreversible hyperparathyroidism (101–103).

The regulation of parathyroid hormone secretion in X-linked hypophosphatemic rickets (XLH) is complex. Although earlier descriptions of the disorder suggest that circulating levels of PTH are normal prior to the initiation of therapy (104), we have found that many patients with XLH have elevated PTH levels prior to treatment. The recent demonstration that PHEX (the mutated gene in XLH) is expressed in parathyroid glands (105) raises the possibility that disordered regulation of PTH secretion may be part of the XLH phenotype. Phosphate therapy exacerbates the propensity of the parathyroid glands to secrete PTH in patients with XLH, even in the absence of hyperphosphatemia or hypocalcemia. Furthermore, this secondary hyperparathyroidism is a very frequent feature of phosphate-treated patients and may evolve into tertiary hyperparathyroidism. Hyperparathyroidism in XLH is seen more commonly when dosages of phosphate exceed 4 g/day elemental phosphorus (there are about 0.25 g of elemental phosphorus per g of phosphate). Secondary hyperparathyroidism also occurs when lower dosages of phosphorous are used without sufficient calcitriol (61, 106). Thus, phosphate should not be used as solitary treatment of XLH.

Routine measurement of PTH levels in individuals with XLH is an important aspect of disease management, and is critical for making appropriate dosage adjustments in a timely manner. Adjunctive therapy with 24,25 dihydroxyvitamin D also mitigates secondary hyperparathyroidism in XLH and improves skeletal mineralization (27). Thus, improvement in parathyroid status may improve the long-term skeletal outcome of the disease.

XII. COMPLICATIONS OF HYPERPARATHYROIDISM AND HYPERCALCEMIA

The adverse effects of hyperparathyroidism are related to excessive bone resorption and hypercalcemia. Excessive PTH activity leads to loss of skeletal mineral content, microarchitectural defects, and osteopenia (107). In adults with hyperparathyroidism, demineralization may be recognized on standard radiographs (56). Dual-energy x-ray absorptiometry is a much more sensitive means of detecting these changes (108).

Hyperparathyroidism affects the kidneys in several ways. Hypercalcemia can directly reduce the glomerular filtration rate. Longstanding hypercalcemia may lead to deposition of calcium in the tubules, especially during hyperphosphatemia, resulting in nephrocalcinosis (109, 110). Nephrocalcinosis can be detected by ultrasound, which should be performed in individuals with hyperparathyroidism (111). Nephrolithiasis is well described in adults

with hyperparathyroidism (56), yet is unusual in children with hyperparathyroidism. Calcium levels in excess of 15 mg/dl also may result in polyuria secondary to nephrogenic diabetes insipidus.

Hypercalcemia also affects other systems. Hypercalcemia may induce increased cardiovascular tone and hypertension (112). High calcium levels may lead to heart block and shortening of the ST segment (112). The central nervous system is also sensitive to the effects of calcium at high levels (113). Impaired mentation and convulsions may occur at levels above 15 mg/dl (113). Muscle weakness and hyporeflexia may occur (114). Gastric ulcers and constipation may reflect hypercalcemia (115). Anorexia may attend hypercalcemia.

Patients are at increased risk for pancreatitis (116, 117). We have recently cared for a child who presented with recurrent pancreatitis associated with hypercalcemia (11–12 mg/dl) secondary to a parathyroid adenoma.

XIII. TREATMENT OF HYPERPARATHYROIDISM AND HYPERCALCEMIA

Acute therapy of hypercalcemia is indicated for symptomatic individuals or when the total calcium exceeds 13 mg/dl (56, 118, 119). Treatment with intravenous saline (3000 ml/m^2/day; 200–400 ml/kg/day) and furosemide (1 mg/kg every 4–6 h) lowers calcium levels within hours (120). After correction of acute hypercalcemia, a high-sodium diet promotes continued renal calcium excretion. Oral furosemide therapy (1–2 mg/kg/day divided in two or three divided doses) may be of benefit.

Adjunctive therapy with prednisone is usually not effective management of hypercalcemia due to hyperparathyroidism (44). Calcitonin may initially lower serum calcium levels, but patients often become refractory to the medication after several dosages. Bisphosphonates, which inhibit bone resorption, can be used to manage severe hypercalcemia over the short term, but are not recommended as a definitive treatment. Oral or intravenous phosphate therapy can lower circulating calcium levels (56), but leads to precipitation of calcium and phosphate salts in the vascular system and kidneys and is no longer recommended.

Calciomimetic agents that act to inhibit PTH secretion by activating CaSR hold promise as a therapy for parathyroid hyperplasia (121). They are not yet available for widespread clinical use to treat hypercalcemia of any cause. Selective ablation of parathyroid glands by embolization has been shown to be effective only for some ectopic parathyroid glands (122).

Surgery is the definitive cure for hyperparathyroidism. If isolated adenomas are detected, these should be removed. In the setting of multigland parathyroid hyperplasia, our usual approach is to remove three and one-half or four glands. In adults, treatment of the asymptomatic patient with hyperparathyroidism has been the subject of debate (123, 124). Surgery is recommended for asymptomatic individuals with evidence of demineralization, nephrolithiasis, or nephrocalcinosis (118, 119, 123, 124). However, observation may be recommended for individuals without evidence of complications, as long as renal function, bone density, and gastrointestinal status is assessed regularly (118, 119, 123, 125, 126).

Prolonged observation is generally not recommended for children with hyperparathyroidism. Given the longevity of the course in children, progressive skeletal mineral loss, and potential consequences of exposure of the kidneys to long-term hypercalcemia, we choose prompt surgery for patients in this age group.

Preoperative localization of hyperactive parathyroid tissue is a challenging undertaking (118, 119). High-resolution ultrasonography, computed axial tomography, magnetic resonance imaging, and radionuclide scanning have been used to localize parathyroid tissue (127–130). Increasingly we are impressed with the ability of high-resolution Doppler ultrasound to localize parathyroid adenomas. Arteriography and selective venous sampling have been used to localize abnormal parathyroid tissue (131), but successes with this technique are highly variable.

Rapid PTH assays in the intraoperative setting are a new and important means for localizing hyperfunctioning parathyroid tissue (132, 133). The surgeon is able to monitor acutely the effects of gland removal and can be reassured regarding the removal of the abnormal tissue. After removal of the pathological parathyroid gland(s), PTH levels will promptly fall. If PTH levels do not fall after a gland is removed, additional parathyroid tissue must be identified and resected.

XIV. MANAGEMENT AFTER PARATHYROIDECTOMY

After successful resection of hyperactive parathyroid tissue, serum calcium levels may rapidly fall. Intraoperatively, a Chevostek's sign may be elicited by tapping over the facial nerve in the temporal–mandibular region in hypocalcemic patients. Laryngospasm may occur.

Management of postoperative hypocalcemia may require intravenous infusions of calcium if symptoms are present or hypocalcemia is severe. Our usual goal is to maintain serum calcium in the lower range of normal using 30–50 mg/kg/day elemental calcium. When a subtotal parathyroidectomy is performed, the remaining parathyroid tissue that was previously suppressed by hypercalcemia will become functional within 30 h after surgery (134). Thus, calcium levels usually stabilize within 48 h after surgery. If hypocalcemia persists beyond the second postoperative day, oral calcitriol therapy should be started (0.025–0.5 μg twice per day). This potent vitamin D metabolite has a rapid onset of action and increases intestinal

calcium absorption. The dosage may be advanced until serum calcium levels stabilize. When serum calcium levels are stable and intravenous therapy is no longer needed, the calcitriol dosage can be gradually reduced.

Adequate dietary calcium must also be provided for calcitriol to increase calcium levels. Thus, oral calcium supplementation is useful in this setting, since few children and adolescents have adequate dietary calcium intake. We provide up to 1g elemental calcium per day, divided in three doses. Care should also be taken to avoid hypercalcemia during vitamin D therapy, because single episodes of hypercalcemia can induce permanent renal damage in children.

If the serum magnesium concentration is low (<1.5 mg/dl), the function of any residual parathyroid tissue may be compromised. In this event, supplemental magnesium should be given.

Hyperphosphatemia may also occur after parathyroidectomy. This is usually transient and spontaneously corrects with normalization of the serum calcium. If hypocalcemia and hyperphosphatemia persist, lowering serum phosphate levels will allow the serum calcium to rise. This can be accomplished by administering oral calcium or aluminum-based antacids.

If intravenous calcium infusions are needed, they can usually be discontinued shortly after surgery (134). However, individuals with significant skeletal demineralization are at risk for so-called hungry bone syndrome and may require prolonged intravenous infusion of calcium (135). The growing child with hyperparathyroidism and metabolic bone disease is at increased risk for development of hungry bone syndrome.

We have cared for two adolescent girls with XLH who required intravenous calcium infusion for 3 months after total parathyroidectomy to prevent symptomatic hypocalcemia (61). Preoperatively, gross demineralization was noted in radiographs of the hands. To facilitate discharge from the hospital, indwelling central venous catheters were placed, allowing infusions at home. After 45 days, it was possible to administer calcium during the night, allowing schooling during the day. Following the appearance of urinary calcium (calcium/creatinine ratio >0.02), it was possible to stop intravenous therapy within a few weeks.

XV. SUMMARY

Childhood primary hyperparathyroidism is a rare disorder that may present in an extremely severe form in neonates, sporadically in children, or as part of MEN syndromes. Secondary and tertiary hyperparathyroidism may occur in children with chronic hypocalcemia such as in vitamin D deficiency, or in renal disease, accompanied by hyperphosphatemia. Another condition that results in secondary hyperparathyroidism is X-linked hypophosphatemic rickets. The constellation of hypercalcemia, hypophosphatemia, and renal phosphate wasting suggests PTH excess. By measuring PTH levels, hyperparathyroidism can be diagnosed, but requires careful differentiation from FHH. Long-term hyperparathyroidism is likely to lead to skeletal demineralization and renal damage. Thus, surgery is usually indicated for pediatric patients with hyperparathyroidism rather than observation. Children with demineralization and bone disease may be at risk for hungry bone syndrome postoperatively. The child with significant chronic hypocalcemia following parathyroidectomy is best managed with calcitriol and provision of adequate oral calcium.

REFERENCES

1. Wolfe HJ. The anatomy of the parathyroids. In: DeGroot LJ, ed. Endocrinology. Philadelphia: WB Saunders, 1989: 844–847.
2. Dekker A, Dunsford HA, Geyer SJ. The normal parathyroid gland at autopsy: the significance of stromal fat in adult patients. J Pathol 1979; 128:127–132.
3. Christie AC. The parathyroid oxyphil cells. J Clin Pathol 1967; 20:591–602.
4. Moore KL. The Developing Human. Philadelphia: WB Saunders, 1973.
5. Spiegel AM, Marx SJ, Doppman JL, et al. Intrathyroidal parathyroid adenoma or hyperplasia. An occasionally overlooked cause of surgical failure in primary hyperparathyroidism. JAMA 1975; 234:1029–33.
6. Chisaka O, Capecchi MR. Regionally restricted developmental defects resulting from targeted disruption of the mouse homeobox gene hox-1.5. Nature 1991; 350:473–479.
7. Levy-Mozziconacci A, Lacombe D, Leheup B, Wernert F, Rouault F, Philip N. [Microdeletion of the chromosome 22q11 in children: apropos of a series of 49 patients]. Arch Pediatr 1996; 3:761–768.
8. Trump D, Dixon PH, Mumm S, et al. Localisation of X linked recessive idiopathic hypoparathyroidism to a 1.5 Mb region on Xq26-q27. J Med Genet 1998; 35:905–909.
9. Thakker RV, Davies KE, Whyte MP, Wooding C, O'Riordan JL. Mapping the gene causing X-linked recessive idiopathic hypoparathyroidism to Xq26-Xq27 by linkage studies. J Clin Invest 1990; 86:40–45.
10. Tengan CH, Kiyomoto BH, Rocha MS, Tavares VL, Gabbai AA, Moraes CT. Mitochondrial encephalomyopathy and hypoparathyroidism associated with a duplication and a deletion of mitochondrial deoxyribonucleic acid. J Clin Endocrinol Metab 1998; 83:125–129.
11. Burton PB, Moniz C, Quirke P, et al. Parathyroid hormone-related peptide: expression in fetal and neonatal development. J Pathol 1992; 167:291–296.
12. Naylor SL, Sakaguchi AY, Szoka P, et al. Human parathyroid hormone gene (PTH) is on short arm of chromosome 11. Somatic Cell Genet 1983; 9:609–616.
13. Vasicek TJ, McDevitt BE, Freeman MW, et al. Nucleotide sequence of the human parathyroid hormone gene. Proc Natl Acad Sci USA 1983; 80:2127–2131.
14. Naveh-Many T. Post-transcriptional regulation of the parathyroid hormone gene by calcium and phosphate. Curr Opin Nephrol Hypertens 1999; 8:415–419.
15. Silver J, Naveh-Many T. Regulation of parathyroid hor-

16. mone synthesis and secretion. Semin Nephrol 1994; 14: 175–194.
16. Orloff JJ, Reddy D, de Papp AE, Yang KH, Soifer NE, Stewart AF. Parathyroid hormone-related protein as a prohormone: posttranslational processing and receptor interactions. Endocr Rev 1994; 15:40–60.
17. Brown EM, Pollak M, Hebert SC. Sensing of extracellular Ca2+ by parathyroid and kidney cells: cloning and characterization of an extracellular Ca(2+)-sensing receptor. Am J Kidney Dis 1995; 25:506–513.
18. Brown EM, Wilson RE, Thatcher JG, Marynick SP. Abnormal calcium-regulated PTH release in normal parathyroid tissue from patients with adenoma. Am J Med 1981; 71:565–570.
19. Nussbaum SR, Potts JT, Jr. Immunoassays for parathyroid hormone 1–84 in the diagnosis of hyperparathyroidism. J Bone Miner Res 1991; 6 Suppl 2:S43–50; discussion S61.
20. Brown EM, Pollak M, Chou YH, Seidman CE, Seidman JG, Hebert SC. Cloning and functional characterization of extracellular Ca(2+)-sensing receptors from parathyroid and kidney. Bone 1995; 17:7S-11S.
21. Yamaguchi T, Chattopadhyay N, Brown EM. G protein-coupled extracellular Ca2+ (Ca2+o)-sensing receptor (CaR): roles in cell signaling and control of diverse cellular functions. Adv Pharmacol 2000; 47:209–253.
22. Pollak MR, Seidman CE, Brown EM. Three inherited disorders of calcium sensing. Medicine (Baltimore) 1996; 75:115–123.
23. Anast CS, Mohs JM, Kaplan SL, Burns TW. Magnesium, vitamin D, and parathyroid hormone. Lancet 1973; 1: 1389–1390.
24. Sherwood LM, Mayer GP, Ramberg CF Jr, Kronfeld DS, Aurbach GD, Potts JT Jr. Regulation of parathyroid hormone secretion: proportional control by calcium, lack of effect of phosphate. Endocrinology 1968; 83:1043–1051.
25. Rodriguez M, Almaden Y, Hernandez A, Torres A. Effect of phosphate on the parathyroid gland: direct and indirect? Curr Opin Nephrol Hypertens 1996; 5:321–328.
26. Silver J, Yalcindag C, Sela-Brown A, Kilav R, Naveh-Many T. Regulation of the parathyroid hormone gene by vitamin D, calcium and phosphate. Kidney Int Suppl 1999; 73:S2–7.
27. Carpenter TO, Keller M, Schwartz D, et al. 24,25 Dihydroxyvitamin D supplementation corrects hyperparathyroidism and improves skeletal abnormalities in X-linked hypophosphatemic rickets—a clinical research center study. J Clin Endocrinol Metab 1996; 81:2381–2388.
28. Endres DB, Villanueva R, Sharp CF Jr, Singer FR. Measurement of parathyroid hormone. Endocrinol Metab Clin North Am 1989; 18:611–629.
29. Woodhead JS. The measurement of circulating parathyroid hormone. Clin Biochem 1990; 23:17–21.
30. Marcus R. Laboratory diagnosis of primary hyperparathyroidism. Endocrinol Metab Clin North Am 1989; 18:647–658.
31. Thode J. Ionized calcium and cyclic AMP in plasma and urine. Biochemical evaluation in calcium metabolic disease. Scand J Clin Lab Invest Suppl 1990; 197:1–45.
32. Cooper KL. Radiology of metabolic bone disease. Endocrinol Metab Clin North Am 1989; 18:955–976.
33. McAfee JG. Radionuclide imaging in metabolic and systemic skeletal diseases. Semin Nucl Med 1987; 17:334–349.
34. Segre GV, Abou-Samra AB, Juppner H, et al. Character-

ization of cloned PTH/PTHrP receptors. J Endocrinol Invest 1992; 15:11–17.

35. Juppner H. Receptors for parathyroid hormone and parathyroid hormone-related peptide: exploration of their biological importance. Bone 1999; 25:87–90.

36. Schipani E, Langman C, Hunzelman J, et al. A novel parathyroid hormone (PTH)/PTH-related peptide receptor mutation in Jansen's metaphyseal chondrodysplasia. J Clin Endocrinol Metab 1999; 84:3052–3057.

37. Karaplis AC, He B, Nguyen MT, et al. Inactivating mutation in the human parathyroid hormone receptor type 1 gene in Blomstrand chondrodysplasia. Endocrinology 1998; 139:5255–5258.

38. Neer R. Calcium and phosphate homeostasis. In: DeGroot LJ, ed. Endocrinology. Philadelphia: WB Saunders, 1989: 927–953.

39. Aurbach GD, Heath DA. Parathyroid hormone and calcitonin regulation of renal function. Kidney Int 1974; 6: 331–345.

40. Bringhurst FR. Calcium and phosphate distribution, turnover, and metabolic actions. In: DeGroot LJ, ed. Endocrinology. Philadelphia: WB Saunders, 1989:805–843.

41. Peacock M, Nordin BE. Tubular reabsorption of calcium in normal and hypercalciuric subjects. J Clin Pathol 1968; 21:353–358.

42. Nordin BE, Hodgkinson A, Peacock M. The measurement and the meaning of urinary calcium. Clin Orthop 1967; 52:293–322.

43. Nordin BE, Bulusu L. Plasma-phosphate and tubular reabsorption of phosphate. Lancet 1970; 2:212.

44. Coe FL, Canterbury JM, Firpo JJ, Reiss E. Evidence for secondary hyperparathyroidism in idiopathic hypercalciuria. J Clin Invest 1973; 52:134–142.

45. Coe FL, Firpo JJ, Jr. Evidence for mild reversible hyperparathyroidism in distal renal tubular acidosis. Arch Intern Med 1975; 135:1485–1489.

46. Welsh J, Weaver V, Simboli-Campbell M. Regulation of renal 25(OH)D3 1 alpha-hydroxylase: signal transduction pathways. Biochem Cell Biol 1991; 69:768–770.

47. Suda T, Shinki T, Kurokawa K. The mechanisms of regulation of vitamin D metabolism in the kidney. Curr Opin Nephrol Hypertens 1994; 3:59–64.

48. Langman CB. New developments in calcium and vitamin D metabolism. Curr Opin Pediatr 2000; 12:135–139.

49. Norimatsu H, Yamamoto T, Ozawa H, Talmage RV. Changes in calcium phosphate on bone surfaces and in lining cells after the administration of parathyroid hormone or calcitonin. Clin Orthop 1982:271–278.

50. Filvaroff E, Derynck R. Bone remodelling: a signalling system for osteoclast regulation. Curr Biol 1998; 8: R679–682.

51. Norimatsu H, Wiel CJ, Talmage RV. Morphological support of a role for cells lining bone surfaces in maintenance of plasma calcium concentration. Clin Orthop 1979:254–262.

52. Ishii H, Wada M, Furuya Y, Nagano N, Nemeth EF, Fox J. Daily intermittent decreases in serum levels of parathyroid hormone have an anabolic-like action on the bones of uremic rats with low-turnover bone and osteomalacia. Bone 2000; 26:175–182.

53. Brommage R, Hotchkiss CE, Lees CJ, Stancill MW, Hock JM, Jerome CP. Daily treatment with human recombinant parathyroid hormone-(1–34), LY333334, for 1 year increases bone mass in ovariectomized monkeys. J Clin Endocrinol Metab 1999; 84:3757–3763.

54. Mayer GP, Habener JF, Potts JT Jr. Parathyroid hormone secretion in vivo. Demonstration of a calcium-independent nonsuppressible component of secretion. J Clin Invest 1976; 57:678–683.

55. Hellman P, Carling T, Rask L, Akerstrom G. Pathophysiology of primary hyperparathyroidism [in process citation]. Histol Histopathol 2000; 15:619–627.

56. Habener JF, Potts JT. Primary hyperparathyroidism. In: DeGroot LJ, ed. Endocrinology. Philadelphia: WB Saunders, 1989:954–966.

57. Arnold A, Staunton CE, Kim HG, Gaz RD, Kronenberg HM. Monoclonality and abnormal parathyroid hormone genes in parathyroid adenomas. N Engl J Med 1988; 318: 658–662.

58. Mallya SM, Arnold A. Cyclin D1 in parathyroid disease. Front Biosci 2000; 5:D367–371.

59. Cryns VL, Thor A, Xu HJ, et al. Loss of the retinoblastoma tumor-suppressor gene in parathyroid carcinoma. N Engl J Med 1994; 330:757–761.

60. Karges W, Jostarndt K, Maier S, et al. Multiple endocrine neoplasia type 1 (MEN1) gene mutations in a subset of patients with sporadic and familial primary hyperparathyroidism target the coding sequence but spare the promoter region. J Endocrinol 2000; 166:1–9.

61. Rivkees SA, el-Hajj-Fuleihan G, Brown EM, Crawford JD. Tertiary hyperparathyroidism during high phosphate therapy of familial hypophosphatemic rickets. J Clin Endocrinol Metab 1992; 75:1514–1518.

62. Rodd C, Goodyer P. Hypercalcemia of the newborn: etiology, evaluation, and management. Pediatr Nephrol 1999; 13:542–547.

63. Jones KL. Williams syndrome: an historical perspective of its evolution, natural history, and etiology. Am J Med Genet Suppl 1990; 6:89–96.

64. Meng X, Lu X, Morris CA, Keating MT. A novel human gene FKBP6 is deleted in Williams syndrome. Genomics 1998; 52:130–137.

65. Marx SJ, Spiegel AM, Brown EM, et al. Circulating parathyroid hormone activity: familial hypocalciuric hypercalcemia versus typical primary hyperparathyroidism. J Clin Endocrinol Metab 1978; 47:1190–1197.

66. Marx SJ, Stock JL, Attie MF, et al. Familial hypocalciuric hypercalcemia: recognition among patients referred after unsuccessful parathyroid exploration. Ann Intern Med 1980; 92:351–356.

67. Brown EM. Mutations in the calcium-sensing receptor and their clinical implications. Horm Res 1997; 48:199–208.

68. Jacobus CH, Holick MF, Shao Q, et al. Hypervitaminosis D associated with drinking milk. N Engl J Med 1992; 326:1173–1177.

69. Holick MF, Shao Q, Liu WW, Chen TC. The vitamin D content of fortified milk and infant formula. N Engl J Med 1992; 326:1178–1181.

70. Siperstein AE, Shen W, Chan AK, Duh QY, Clark OH. Normocalcemic hyperparathyroidism. Biochemical and symptom profiles before and after surgery. Arch Surg 1992; 127:1157–1166; discussion 1161–1163.

71. Simeckova A, Zamrazil V, Cerovska J. Calciuria, magnesiuria and creatininuria—relation to age. Physiol Res 1998; 47:35–40.

72. Sargent JD, Stukel TA, Kresel J, Klein RZ. Normal values for random urinary calcium to creatinine ratios in infancy. J Pediatr 1993; 123:393–397.

73. Steendijk R. Metabolic bone disease in children. Clin Orthop 1971; 77:247–275.

74. Girard RM, Belanger A, Hazel B. Primary hyperparathyroidism in children. Can J Surg 1982; 25:11–13.

75. Allen DB, Friedman AL, Hendricks SA. Asymptomatic primary hyperparathyroidism in children. Newer methods of preoperative diagnosis. Am J Dis Child 1986; 140: 819–821.

76. Holcomb GWd, Perloff LJ. Primary hyperparathyroidism in a hypothyroid child. Surgery 1990; 108:588–592.

77. Ross AJD. Parathyroid surgery in children. Prog Pediatr Surg 1991; 26:48–59.

78. Damiani D, Aguiar CH, Bueno VS, et al. Primary hyperparathyroidism in children: patient report and review of the literature. J Pediatr Endocrinol Metab 1998; 11:83–86.

79. Marx SJ, Powell D, Shimkin PM, et al. Familial hyperparathyroidism. Mild hypercalcemia in at least nine members of a kindred. Ann Intern Med 1973; 78:371–377.

80. Blair JW, Carachi R. Neonatal primary hyperparathyroidism—a case report and review of the literature. Eur J Pediatr Surg 1991; 1:110–114.

81. Cole DE, Janicic N, Salisbury SR, Hendy GN. Neonatal severe hyperparathyroidism, secondary hyperparathyroidism, and familial hypocalciuric hypercalcemia: multiple different phenotypes associated with an inactivating Alu insertion mutation of the calcium-sensing receptor gene [published erratum appears in Am J Med Genet 1997 Oct 17;72(2):251–252]. Am J Med Genet 1997; 71:202–210.

82. Kraimps JL, Duh QY, Demeure M, Clark OH. Hyperparathyroidism in multiple endocrine neoplasia syndrome. Surgery 1992; 112:1080–6; discussion 1086–1088.

83. Phay JE, Moley JF, Lairmore TC. Multiple endocrine neoplasias. Semin Surg Oncol 2000; 18:324–332.

84. Benson L, Rastad J, Ljunghall S, Rudberg C, Akerstrom G. Parathyroid hormone release in vitro in hyperparathyroidism associated with multiple endocrine neoplasia type 1. Acta Endocrinol (Copenh) 1987; 114:12–17.

85. Benson L, Ljunghall S, Akerstrom G, Oberg K. Hyperparathyroidism presenting as the first lesion in multiple endocrine neoplasia type 1. Am J Med 1987; 82:731–737.

86. Komminoth P. Multiple endocrine neoplasia type 1 and 2: from morphology to molecular pathology 1997. Verh Dtsch Ges Pathol 1997; 81:125–138.

87. Eng C. RET proto-oncogene in the development of human cancer. J Clin Oncol 1999; 17:380–393.

88. Fujiwara S, Sposto R, Ezaki H, et al. Hyperparathyroidism among atomic bomb survivors in Hiroshima. Radiat Res 1992; 130:372–378.

89. Tezelman S, Rodriguez JM, Shen W, Siperstein AE, Duh QY, Clark OH. Primary hyperparathyroidism in patients who have received radiation therapy and in patients who have not received radiation therapy. J Am Coll Surg 1995; 180:81–87.

90. Schneider AB, Gierlowski TC, Shore-Freedman E, Stovall M, Ron E, Lubin J. Dose–response relationships for radiation-induced hyperparathyroidism. J Clin Endocrinol Metab 1995; 80:254–257.

91. Esselstyn CB, Jr., Schumacher OP, Eversman J, Sheeler L, Levy WJ. Hyperparathyroidism after radioactive iodine therapy for Graves disease. Surgery 1982; 92:811–813.

92. Kawamura J, Tobisu K, Sanada S, et al. [Hyperparathyroidism after radioactive iodine therapy for Graves' disease: a case report]. Hinyokika Kiyo 1983; 29:1513–1519.

93. Bondeson AG, Bondeson L, Thompson NW. Hyperparathyroidism after treatment with radioactive iodine: not only a coincidence? Surgery 1989; 106:1025–1027.

94. Wang CA, Gaz RD. Natural history of parathyroid carcinoma. Diagnosis, treatment, and results. Am J Surg 1985; 149:522–527.

95. McHenry CR, Rosen IB, Walfish PG, Cooter N. Parathyroid crisis of unusual features in a child. Cancer 1993; 71:1923–1927.

96. Mallette LE, Bilezikian JP, Ketcham AS, Aurbach GD. Parathyroid carcinoma in familial hyperparathyroidism. Am J Med 1974; 57:642–648.

97. Goldberg E, Winter ST, Better OS, Berger A. Transient neonatal hyperparathyroidism associated with maternal hypoparathyroidism. Isr J Med Sci 1976; 12:199–201.

98. Ghirri P, Bottone U, Coccoli L, et al. Symptomatic hypercalcemia in the first months of life: calcium-regulating hormones and treatment. J Endocrinol Invest 1999; 22: 349–353.

99. Steendijk R. Vitamin D and the pathogenesis of rickets and osteomalacia. Folia Med Neerl 1968; 11:178–186.

100. Pletka PG, Strom TB, Hampers CL, et al. Secondary hyperparathyroidism in human kidney transplant recipients. Nephron 1976; 17:371–381.

101. Hanley DA, Sherwood LM. Secondary hyperparathyroidism in chronic renal failure. Pathophysiology and treatment. Med Clin North Am 1978; 62:1319–1339.

102. Sanchez CP, Salusky IB, Kuizon BD, Abdella P, Juppner H, Goodman WG. Growth of long bones in renal failure: roles of hyperparathyroidism, growth hormone and calcitriol. Kidney Int 1998; 54:1879–1887.

103. Koch Nogueira PC, David L, Cochat P. Evolution of secondary hyperparathyroidism after renal transplantation. Pediatr Nephrol 2000; 14:342–346.

104. Arnaud C, Glorieux F, Scriver C. Serum parathyroid hormone in X-linked hypophosphatemia. Science 1971; 173: 845–847.

105. Rowe PS. The PEX gene: its role in X-linked rickets, osteomalacia, and bone mineral metabolism. Exp Nephrol 1997; 5:355–363.

106. Glorieux FH, Marie PJ, Pettifor JM, Delvin EE. Bone response to phosphate salts, ergocalciferol, and calcitriol in hypophosphatemic vitamin D-resistant rickets. N Engl J Med 1980; 303:1023–1031.

107. Nakaoka D, Sugimoto T, Kobayashi T, Yamaguchi T, Kobayashi A, Chihara K. Prediction of bone mass change after parathyroidectomy in patients with primary hyperparathyroidism. J Clin Endocrinol Metab 2000; 85:1901–1907.

108. Adami S, Braga V, Squaranti R, Rossini M, Gatti D, Zamberlan N. Bone measurements in asymptomatic primary hyperparathyroidism. Bone 1998; 22:565–570.

109. Chan AK, Duh QY, Katz MH, Siperstein AE, Clark OH. Clinical manifestations of primary hyperparathyroidism before and after parathyroidectomy. A case–control study. Ann Surg 1995; 222:402–412; discussion 412–414.

110. Deaconson TF, Wilson SD, Lemann J Jr. The effect of parathyroidectomy on the recurrence of nephrolithiasis. Surgery 1987; 102:910–913.

111. Verge CF, Lam A, Simpson JM, Cowell CT, Howard NJ, Silink M. Effects of therapy in X-linked hypophosphatemic rickets. N Engl J Med 1991; 325:1843–1848.

112. Klein I, Ojamaa K. Clinical review 36: Cardiovascular manifestations of endocrine disease. J Clin Endocrinol Metab 1992; 75:339–342.

113. Petersen P. Psychiatric disorders in primary hyperparathyroidism. J Clin Endocrinol Metab 1968; 28:1491–1495.

114. Patten BM, Bilezikian JP, Mallette LE, Prince A, Engel

WK, Aurbach GD. Neuromuscular disease in primary hyperparathyroidism. Ann Intern Med 1974; 80:182–193.

115. Barreras RF. Calcium and gastric secretion. Gastroenterology 1973; 64:1168–1184.

116. Bess MA, Edis AJ, van Heerden JA. Hyperparathyroidism and pancreatitis. Chance or a causal association? JAMA 1980; 243:246–247.

117. Sitges-Serra A, Alonso M, de Lecea C, Gores PF, Sutherland DE. Pancreatitis and hyperparathyroidism. Br J Surg 1988; 75:158–160.

118. Proceedings of the NIH Consensus Development Conference on diagnosis and management of asymptomatic primary hyperparathyroidism. Bethesda, Maryland, October 29–31, 1990. J Bone Miner Res 1991; 6 Suppl 2:S1–166.

119. NIH conference. Diagnosis and management of asymptomatic primary hyperparathyroidism: consensus development conference statement. Ann Intern Med 1991; 114:593–597.

120. Watson L. Diagnosis and treatment of hypercalcaemia. Br Med J 1972; 2:150–152.

121. Coburn JW, Elangovan L, Goodman WG, Frazao JM. Calcium-sensing receptor and calcimimetic agents. Kidney Int Suppl 1999; 73:S52–58.

122. Doppman JL, Marx SJ, Spiegel AM, et al. Treatment of hyperparathyroidism by percutaneous embolization of a mediastinal adenoma. Radiology 1975; 115:37–42.

123. Potts JT, Jr. Clinical Review 9: Management of asymptomatic hyperparathyroidism. J Clin Endocrinol Metab 1990; 70:1489–1493.

124. Silverberg SJ, Shane E, Jacobs TP, Siris E, Bilezikian JP. A 10-year prospective study of primary hyperparathyroidism with or without parathyroid surgery. N Engl J Med 1999; 341:1249–1255.

125. Silverberg SJ, Bilezikian JP, Bone HG, Talpos GB, Horwitz MJ, Stewart AF. Therapeutic controversies in primary hyperparathyroidism. J Clin Endocrinol Metab 1999; 84:2275–2285.

126. Sosa JA, Powe NR, Levine MA, Udelsman R, Zeiger MA. Profile of a clinical practice: thresholds for surgery and surgical outcomes for patients with primary hyperparathyroidism: a national survey of endocrine surgeons. J Clin Endocrinol Metab 1998; 83:2658–2665.

127. Barraclough BM, Barraclough BH. Ultrasound of the thyroid and parathyroid glands. World J Surg 2000; 24:158–165.

128. Zwas ST, Czerniak A, Boruchowsky S, Avigad I, Wolfstein I. Preoperative parathyroid localization by superimposed iodine-131 toluidine blue and technetium-99m pertechnetate imaging. J Nucl Med 1987; 28:298–307.

129. Gotway MB, Higgins CB. MR imaging of the thyroid and parathyroid glands. Magn Reson Imaging Clin North Am 2000; 8:163–182.

130. Hiromatsu Y, Ishibashi M, Nishida H, Okuda S, Miyake I. Technetium-99m tetrofosmin parathyroid imaging in patients with primary hyperparathyroidism. Intern Med 2000; 39:101–106.

131. Reitz RE, Pollard JJ, Wang CA, et al. Localization of parathyroid adenomas by selective venous catheterization and radioimmunoassay. N Engl J Med 1969; 281:348–351.

132. Wilkinson RH, Jr., Leight GS, Jr., Garner SC, Borges-Neto S. Complementary nature of radiotracer parathyroid imaging and intraoperative parathyroid hormone assays in the surgical management of primary hyperparathyroid disease: case report and review. Clin Nucl Med 2000; 25:173–178.

133. Garner SC, Leight GS Jr. Initial experience with intraoperative PTH determinations in the surgical management of 130 consecutive cases of primary hyperparathyroidism. Surgery 1999; 126:1132–1138.

134. Brasier AR, Wang CA, Nussbaum SR. Recovery of parathyroid hormone secretion after parathyroid adenomectomy. J Clin Endocrinol Metab 1988; 66:495–500.

135. Brasier AR, Nussbaum SR. Hungry bone syndrome: clinical and biochemical predictors of its occurrence after parathyroid surgery. Am J Med 1988; 84:654–660.

21
Neonatal Calcium and Phosphorus Disorders

Winston W. K. Koo

Wayne State University, Detroit, Michigan, U.S.A.

I. INTRODUCTION

The maintenance of calcium (Ca) and phosphorus (P) homeostasis requires a complex interaction of hormonal and nonhormonal factors; adequate functioning of various body systems, in particular, the renal, gastrointestinal, and skeletal systems; and adequate dietary intake. From a clinical perspective, this is reflected in the maintenance of circulating concentrations of Ca and P in the normal range and integrity of the skeleton. In the circulation, the amount of Ca and P constitutes less than 1% of the total body content; however, disturbances in serum concentrations of Ca and P are associated with disturbances of physiological function manifested by numerous clinical symptoms and signs. The skeleton, in contrast, is the major reservoir for Ca (the most abundant mineral in the body) and for P, which together with Ca forms the major inorganic constituent of bone. At all ages, 99% of total body Ca is in the skeleton as is about 89% of the total body P. Thus, the skeleton has the dual function of providing both structural and mechanical support and being a reservoir for mineral homeostasis. Disturbances in Ca and P homeostasis result in osteopenia and rickets in infants and children, and osteomalacia and osteoporosis in adults.

Mechanisms to maintain Ca and P homeostasis in the neonate are the same as for children and adults. However, the newborn infant has a number of unique challenges to maintain Ca and P homeostasis during adaptation to extrauterine life and to continue the rapid rate of growth. These include an abrupt discontinuation of high rate of intrauterine accretion of Ca (>120 mg/kg/day) and P (>70 mg/kg/day) during the third trimester, a smaller skeletal reservoir available for mineral homeostasis, high requirement for Ca and P for the most rapid period of postnatal growth with an average gain in length of >25 cm during the first year, and delay in establishment of adequate nutrient intake for at least a few days after birth. There also

may be diminished end-organ responsiveness to hormonal regulation of Ca and P homeostasis at least during the first days after birth, although the functional capacity of the gut and kidney for Ca and P absorption and retention improves rapidly within days after birth. These issues are exaggerated in infants with heritable disorders of mineral metabolism such as extracellular calcium-sensing receptor mutations, and in infants experiencing adverse prenatal event such as maternal diabetes, intrapartum problems such as perinatal asphyxia, or postpartum complications such as multiple immature organ function with premature birth. In any case, it is important to review the physiology and molecular basis of mineral metabolism to allow a better understanding of the pathophysiology of clinical disorder. This in turn allows a more rational approach in the management of the neonate to minimize iatrogenic causes and the adverse impact of disorders of mineral homeostasis.

II. MAINTENANCE OF CALCIUM AND PHOSPHORUS HOMEOSTASIS

A. Circulating Calcium Concentrations

Serum Ca is found in three forms: approximately 40% is bound predominantly to albumin, approximately 10% is chelated and complexed to small molecules, and approximately 50% is ionized; complexed and ionized Ca are ultrafiltrable. Fetal circulating calcium concentrations as reflected in cord sera are higher than maternal concentrations and are indicative of active placental transfer. Cord serum total calcium concentrations (tCa) increase with increasing gestational age. Serum tCa may be as high as 3 mmol/l (conversion 1 mmol/l = 4 mg/dl) in cord blood from infants born at term, and they are significantly higher than paired material values at delivery (1–4). Serum tCa reaches a nadir during the first 2 days after birth (5–8); thereafter, it increases and stabilizes generally above 2.0

mmol/l (8 mg/dl). In infants exclusively fed human milk, the mean serum tCa increases from 2.3 to 2.7 mmol/l (9.2 to 10.8 mg/dl) over the first 6 months postnatally (9). Serum tCa in infants and children generally remains slightly higher than adult values (9–11). Normally, serum tCa in children and adults remains stable, with a diurnal range of <0.13 mmol/l (0.5 mg/dl) (12). During the third trimester of pregnancy a modest reduction in maternal serum tCa concentration (average 0.1 mmol/l, 0.4 mg/dl) occurs concomitant with a decrease in serum albumin concentration (13).

Serum ionized calcium concentration (iCa) is the best indicator of physiological blood Ca activity (14). Measurement of serum iCa is firmly established in clinical medicine, and the availability of highly reliable iCa analyzers allows simple, rapid, and direct determination of iCa in whole blood, plasma, and serum by ion-selective electrodes. Some differences exist in the reported values for circulating iCa as a result of differences in the design of the reference electrode, formulation of calibrating solutions, and the lack of a reference system for iCa (15,16). Serum iCa also decreases in the presence of high serum albumin (17), magnesium (Mg) (18), phosphorus (P) (19), and bicarbonate levels (20). Clinical situations may affect iCa measurement. For example, the use of heparin may decrease iCa, and iCa is inversely related to blood pH (21). The effect of the latter may be minimized by the immediate analysis of the serum samples for iCa. Freezing serum samples in 5% CO_2-containing tubes may minimize the impact of pH variations if measurement of iCa is delayed for 1 week.

Normal serum iCa range from 1.0 to 1.5 mmol/l (conversion, 1 mmol/l = 4 mg/dl) in the neonate and from 1.18 to 1.32 mmol/l in adults (1,22,23). Cord serum iCa levels increase with gestational age and, similarly serum tCa are higher than paired maternal values (1,2,4,13). In term infants, serum iCa levels average 1.25 mmol/l with 95% confidence limits of 1.1–1.4 mmol/l (4.4–5.6 mg/dl) and there is a decline in serum iCa in the first 48 h of life with a nadir at 24 h (24). Serum tCa and iCa levels are correlated in infants (7,24) and adults (23) but is inadequate to predict one from the other with sufficient accuracy. Serum iCa levels remain generally slightly higher in infants and children than in adults (11). In adults, a circadian rhythm for serum iCa has been reported, with a peak occurring at 10:00 a.m.; the maximal change between peak and trough values is small, averaging 0.08 mmol/l (0.32 mg/dl) (12). Serum iCa levels are stable and normal during pregnancy (2,4,13).

The concentration of iCa is critical to many important biological functions, and there is a finely tuned regulation of extracellular iCa and maintenance of an extremely large iCa concentration gradient across the plasma membrane. In the cell, distribution of Ca is not uniform. The cytosolic compartment contains 50–150 nmol Ca/liter water; a larger intramitochondrial Ca pool contains 500–10,000

nmol Ca/liter cell water. In contrast, extracellular fluid iCa levels are 1 million nM (1 mmol/l). At least two adenosine triphosphate (ATP)-dependent mechanisms are involved in the maintenance of the Ca concentration gradient across the plasma membrane. The Ca messenger system is a nearly universal means by which extracellular messengers regulate cell function (25). Cellular enzyme cascades are activated with a transient increase in intracellular iCa (26,27). The measurement of intracellular Ca is not freely available.

Ca concentration in the extracellular fluid is maintained relatively constant by the effects of interdependent hormonal mechanisms consisting of parathyroid hormone (PTH), 1,25-dihydroxyvitamin D [1,25(OH)2D], and calcitonin (CT) that regulate the influx and efflux of Ca among extracellular fluid, bone, kidney, and gut. Other systemic and local factors also are important in influencing Ca flux, particularly under pathological conditions such as humoral hypercalcemia of malignancy (HHM), and their role in Ca homeostasis under physiological conditions is being studied.

The daily flux of Ca between bone fluid and extracellular fluid across the bone lining cells has been estimated to be as much as 12 mmol (500 mg). It is strongly related to systemic and local factors controlling bone formation and resorption (28–30). In growing infants, there is an extensive exchange of bone Ca with extracellular fluid (31).

The kidney is a major regulator of extracellular fluid Ca concentration, primarily by modulation of Ca excretion. Normally, 98% of the daily renal ultrafiltrate of Ca of about 125 mmol (5000 mg) is reabsorbed. Altered renal regulation of Ca excretion is primarily responsible for the development of some hypercalcemic states, including familial hypocalciuric hypercalcemia; it may also occur during chronic thiazide diuretic therapy. The renal capacity for acute regulation of extracellular fluid Ca concentration, however, may be overwhelmed when net Ca input into the extracellular fluid from the gut or bone exceeds the kidney's capacity for Ca excretion (32,33). The latter situation is exemplified best by hypercalcemia of malignancy. Conversely, in hypocalcemic states, the kidney cannot reduce Ca excretion sufficiently to prevent the occurrence of hypocalcemia.

The gut is important in chronic control of extracellular fluid Ca, primarily through regulation of dietary Ca absorption and the presence of hormonal stimulatory factors, including 1,25(OH)2D (34,35). Gut hyperabsorption of Ca may be associated with hypercalciuria and nephrocalcinosis, but there is no major effect on the development of hypercalcemia (36,37). In the growing skeleton, appropriate dietary Ca intake is of great importance in Ca homeostasis and skeletal mineralization (38).

B. Circulating Phosphorus Concentrations

The total P in serum can be classified into an acid-insoluble fraction, comprising mainly phospholipids, and an acid-soluble fraction, comprising a small amount of organic ester phosphate and all of inorganic phosphate. Normally, more than 90% of the inorganic phosphate is diffusible.

There is also active placental transfer of P. Cord serum P concentrations at term ranges from 1.8 to 2.3 mmol/l (conversion, 1 mmol/l = 3.1 mg/dl). There are large variations in postnatal serum P concentrations. In most newborn infants there is a rise in serum P over the first 48 h after birth (2,4–6), probably unrelated to intestinal absorption of P because dietary P intake is limited at this age. Renal excretion of P is low and contributes to the maintenance of high serum P. Serum P concentrations are high during infancy (1.25–2.60 mmol/l, 3.9–8.0 mg/dl) compared with those in adults (0.9–1.5 mmol/l, 2.8–4.6 mg/dl) (39), and there is a rough correlation between the rate of skeletal growth and serum P concentration. In adults, serum P has a biphasic diurnal rhythm, with peaks in the afternoon and at 3:00 am; maximal change between peak and trough values is <0.4 mmol/l (1.2 mg/dl) (12). Serum P concentrations also fall by about 0.1 mmol/l (0.3 mg/dl) after a meal (40). During pregnancy, maternal serum P concentration remains stable (13).

In the cell, phosphate is the principal intracellular anion and is mostly in the form of organic phosphate. The intracellular inorganic phosphate is normally in equilibrium with both extracellular phosphate and intracellular glyceraldehyde-3-phosphate, an intermediate compound in the regeneration of ATP. The cellular phosphorus/nitrogen ratio is relatively constant. For example, it is 0.07 (by weight) in muscle, and gains or losses of nitrogen by the body are usually accompanied by corresponding gains or losses of extraosseous P (41). The relationship between potassium, the major intracellular cation, and P is more variable.

Maintenance of P concentration in the extracellular fluid requires the effects of interdependent hormonal mechanisms that regulate the influx and efflux of P among extracellular fluid, kidney, gut, and bone. In the growing infant, serum P often varies with the status of calcium homeostasis, in particular, from PTH activity; and to the amount of dietary P intake. The net effect of increased PTH activity is to decrease serum P since its phosphaturic effect is greater than its ability to increase the mobilization of bone P, and to increase gut absorption of P.

Renal function in the neonate is well known to affect serum P concentrations. Renal excretion of P is low in the immediate newborn period and probably contributes to the high serum P. Renal capacity for P excretion can be overwhelm by dietary P ingestion even in otherwise healthy neonates; for example, hyperphosphatemia in those fed cow-milk-based formulas (42). In contrast, hypophosphatemia can occur despite almost total reabsorption of P from the renal ultrafiltrate in infants, especially preterm infants receiving low P intake from human milk (43,44) or parenteral nutrition (45,46). In the growing infant, the gut absorbs dietary P with great efficiency and skeletal turnover involves the release and deposit of P just as it does for Ca. There is a net influx of P from extracellular fluid to bone for mineralization and skeletal growth. Thus dietary P intake has a major role in P homeostasis and maintenance of appropriate skeletal mineralization (47).

III. HORMONAL CONTROL OF CALCIUM AND P HOMEOSTASIS VIA PTH, CT, AND 1,25(OH)2D

PTH and 1,25(OH)2D, and possibly CT, appear to maintain Ca and P homeostasis by intermodulation of their physiological effects on each other and on the classic target organs: kidney, intestine, and bone. PTH serves as the major component of rapid response to hypocalcemia, whereas 1,25(OH)2D, with its major effect on elevating intestinal absorption of Ca, is responsible for a slower but more sustained contribution to the maintenance of normocalcemia. CT, on the other hand, appears to function in the opposite role to PTH but with the capacity to stimulate the production of 1,25(OH)2D, which in theory may serve an additional regulatory role in the maintenance of Ca homeostasis. The direct action of PTH and CT results in a net decrease in serum P, whereas 1,25(OH)2D increases serum P. Maintenance of serum Ca and P in turn are critical to the growing skeleton.

A. Parathyroid Hormone

Parathyroid hormone is synthesized in the chief cells of parathyroid gland. It is stored and secreted mainly as an 84-amino-acid polypeptide. In humans, the PTH gene, along with the genes for insulin, β-globulin, and CT, is located on chromosome 11p15, and restriction site polymorphisms near the PTH gene have been detected (48,49). The initial translational product of the mRNA is a 115-amino-acid prepro-PTH. Prepro-PTH then undergoes proteolytic cleavage in endoplasmic reticulum to remove the amino-terminal signal sequence to form pro-PTH. The prohormone-specific region is cleaved further during subsequent intracellular processing to generate the 84-amino-acid secreted form of the intact hormone. The PTH is stored in secretory granules and colocated and secreted with chromogranin A, a protein that may act in autocrine- or paracrine-regulated release of PTH.

About 50% of the newly generated PTH is also proteolytically degraded intracellularly and some of the inactive fragments also secreted (50). After release into the circulation, the intact PTH molecule has a serum half-life of 5–8 min and undergoes a series of cleavages by endopeptidases in the liver and kidney. The amino-terminal fragments contain the biologically active fractions, with the 1-34 fragment having the most calcemic activity; modifications at the amino terminal, particularly at the first two residuals, can abolish its biological activity. The midregion and carboxyl-terminal fragments are biologically inert, although the latter may have some in vitro biological activity.

Circulating immunoreactive PTH is a complex mixture of intact 1-84 PTH, N-terminal fragments and several inactive C-terminal peptides. The fragments are cleared principally by glomerular filtration and are present in greater concentration than the whole molecule because of their slower clearance rates. PTH molecules reactive in the widely used commercial immunoradiometric assays (IRMA) designed to detect both amino- and carboxy-terminal epitopes of the peptide have been considered as so-called intact IPTH assays. However, there have been reports that large 7–84 fragment of PTH is also detected by these assays. This large fragment is biologically inactive and present in greater concentrations in uremic state or hyperparathyroidism. It increases the PTH concentration by 30–50% using the conventional IPTH technique compared to the latest chemiluminescence or IRMA techniques that measures the so-called whole or bio-intact PTH (51,52). Therefore, the treatment of secondary hyperparathyroidism based on the data from conventional IPTH assays theoretically may lead to oversuppression of biologically active PTH, although the clinical significance of this possibility remains to be defined. In any case, consistency of the PTH assay methodology and serial measurements are critical to the interpretation and management of pathological states.

PTH concentrations in cord blood frequently are low and do not correlate with PTH concentrations in maternal sera (2,4,53). Earlier studies of higher levels of bioactive PTH in cord sera from cytochemical assay (54) may be related to elevated concentrations of parathyroid hormone-related protein (PTHrP) (3,4), since PTH-like bioactivity was tightly correlated with levels of PTHrP in the pig (55) and sheep (56). Small amounts (about 5%) of perfused fragments (34–84, 44–68, and 65–84 amino acids), but probably not the whole PTH molecule, have been reported to cross the human placenta (57). Serum IPTH concentrations increase postnatally coincident with the fall in serum Ca in both term and preterm infants (2,53,58–60). The rise in serum IPTH is greater for preterm infants with hypocalcemia than in term infants (2), reflecting appropriate PTH response. Serum PTH concentrations are similar for children and adults but increased in the elderly (61,62). Serum IPTH showed no change during normal pregnancy (2,4,63). In adults, serum IPTH is present in picomolar concentrations. It has a significant circadian periodicity (64–66), spontaneous episodic pulsatility with distinct peak property (64), and a significant temporal coupling with serum iCa and P (64,66,67) and prolactin secretion (65).

In physiological terms, PTH is the most important regulator of extracellular Ca concentration. PTH acts directly on bone and kidney, and indirectly on intestine. Immediate control of blood Ca is probably due to PTH influence on the mobilization of Ca from bone, probably

synergistically with 1,25(OH)2D; and to increase renal distal tubular reabsorption of Ca. PTH increases acutely within minutes the rate of Ca release from bone into blood. Chronic effects of PTH are to increase the numbers of osteoblasts and osteoclasts and to increase the remodeling of bone. Continuous exposure to elevated levels of PTH leads to increased osteoclastic resorption of bone. Other PTH effects on bone include enhanced collagen synthesis, activities of alkaline phosphatase, ornithine and citrate decarboxylases, and glucose-6-phosphate dehydrogenase; DNA, protein, and phospholipid synthesis; and calcium and phosphate transport. Renal actions of PTH include the stimulation of sodium/calcium exchange and calcium transport channel, decrease reabsorption of sodium, phosphate (decrease in sodium dependent phosphate cotransporter, NPT-2) and bicarbonate, and stimulation of renal 25 OHD-1α-hydroxylase (32,33,67–70). However, in severe phosphate deficiency or hypophosphatemia, there may be paradoxical resistance to PTH action at the renal tubule and clinically manifested as continued calciuria and without phosphaturia (43). Maintenance of steady-state calcium balance is probably from increased intestinal Ca absorption secondary to increased 1,25(OH)2D production. There also may be a direct PTH effect on intestinal Ca absorption (71). In contrast to its classic action on Ca mobilization from bone, the amino terminal fragments of PTH and PTHrP, and small pulses of PTH, have an anabolic effect on bone independent of its resorptive action (72–74). Other tissues such as skin fibroblasts, cardiac cells, and vascular smooth muscle also have PTH-sensitive adenylate cyclase, but the physiological importance of PTH in these nonclassic target tissues is not well defined.

PTH's effects on end-organ systems appear to be mediated through its binding to specific receptors. The type 1 PTH receptor has been identified in bone and kidney. It binds equally to PTH and PTHrP, and belongs to a superfamily of guanine-nucleotide-binding (G) protein-coupled cell membrane receptors (GPCR) including those for CT, growth hormone-releasing hormone, corticotrophin-releasing hormone, glucagon, secretin, vasoactive intestinal polypeptide, and others (75). Another PTH receptor (type 2) responds only to PTH, although its main endogenous ligand appears to be a 39 amino acid peptide, hypothalamic tubular infundibular peptide (TIP-39) (76). It has been found in the brain, pancreas, and intestines but the physiological significance of this receptor remains ill defined. The gene for the PTH/PTHrP receptor is located on chromosome 3p21.1-P24.2. It contains 17 exons and encodes a mature glycoprotein of 593 amino acids (77). The type 1 PTH receptor consists of extended extracellular, ligand-binding amino-terminal, and intracellular G protein-associated carboxyl-terminal domains and seven transmembrane domains. Signal transduction mediated by G proteins results in multiple second messenger pathways to effect both stimulatory and inhibitory end-organ responses. The strongest and best-characterized second messenger signaling pathway is the PTH-stimulated coupling of the type 1 PTH receptor to G_s class protein (composed of three subunits; α, β and γ, and is encoded by *GNAS1* gene localized to 20q13.3), which activates adenyl cyclase, an enzyme that generates cyclic AMP. Coupling of type 1 PTH receptor to the Gq class protein activates phospholipase C that generates inositol phosphate (IP3) and diacylglycerol (DAG). These second messengers in turn lead to stimulation of protein kinases A and C and Ca transport channels and result in a variety of hormone-specific tissue responses.

PTH gene show separate sites for interaction and regulation by Ca and vitamin D. Extracellular Ca is the most potent regulator of PTH secretion and is mediated by the cell-surface Ca-sensing receptor (CaR), which detects minute perturbations in the extracellular iCa concentration and responds with alterations in cellular function that normalize iCa (78). The human CaR gene is located on chromosome 3q13.3-q21 and encodes a cell-surface protein of 1078 amino acids. The CaR gene is developmentally upregulated (79), and CaR transcripts are present in numerous tissues including chief cells of the parathyroid glands, kidneys (in particular the thick ascending limb), brain, and nerve terminals, and also the intestine, lung, and skin (78,80). It is a member of GPCR superfamily and contains at least seven exons of which six encode the large (-600 amino acid) amino-terminal extracellular domain and/or its upstream untranslated regions, while a single exon codes for the remainder of the receptor consisting of a seven-member membrane-spanning domain and a cytoplasmic carboxy-terminal intracellular domain (78).

Low or falling serum Ca levels act within seconds to result in secretion of preformed PTH. There is a sigmoidal type of PTH secretion in response to decreased serum Ca and is most pronounced when serum Ca is in the mildly hypocalcemic range. PTH secretion is 50% of maximal at a serum iCa of 1 mmol/l (4 mg/dl); this is considered as the calcium set point for PTH secretion. Sustained hypocalcemia increases PTH mRNA within hours. Protracted challenge leads within days to cellular replication and increased gland mass. High serum Ca levels suppress PTH secretion via activation of CaR (80,81). It in turn activates phospholipase C and generation of IP3 and DAG, and probably increases the proteolytic destruction of preformed PTH. Hyperphosphatemia stimulates PTH secretion, probably by lowering the serum Ca concentration (67,81). A decrease in serum Mg concentration also can stimulate PTH secretion (82,83), although chronic hypomagnesemia inhibits secretion of PTH possibly from increased target tissue resistance to PTH (84). The latter may be related to inactivity of adenylate cyclase, a Mg-requiring enzyme. Other systemic factors (catecholamines, prostaglandins, growth hormone, CT, estrogen, progesterone, cortisol, and somatostatin) and local factors (interleukin-1) modulate PTH secretion and function (85,86).

However, their role in the regulation of calcium metabolism under physiological conditions is not clear. In chronic renal failure, downregulation in the expression of renal CaR may account for the development of secondary hyperparathyroidism (87) and downregulation of PTH receptors may account for the skeletal resistance to calcemic effect of PTH (88). In the kidney, CaR decreases the basal and PTH-stimulated paracellular reabsorption of Ca, Mg, and sodium via multiple mechanisms. These include inhibition of cAMP accumulation; and stimulation of phospholipase A2 activity, thereby promoting the release of free arachidonic acid that is metabolized via the lipooxygenase pathway to P450 metabolites that inhibit the activities of NaK2Cl cotransporter and the K+ channel. This may affect renal water regulation by inhibition of vasopressin-abated water flow (32,33,68,69,80). Extracellular Ca exerts numerous other actions on parathyroid function, including modulation of the intracellular degradation of PTH, cellular respiration, membrane voltage, the hexose monophosphate shunt, and others (25,26,80). Maintenance of Ca homeostasis through other organs also may be possible with the presence of CaR in the intestinal cells and probable modulation of CT secretion from changes in intracellular calcium (26,89). Vitamin D and its metabolites 25 hydroxyvitamin D (25 OHD) and 1,25(OH)2D, acting through vitamin D receptors decrease the level of PTH mRNA (90).

B. Calcitonin

Calcitonin monomer is a 32-amino-acid peptide secreted primarily from the thyroid C cells and also from many extrathyroidal tissues including brain, putuitary, mammary gland, and other tissues (91–95). CT-containing cells and parathyroid gland cells are thought to derive developmentally from the same tissue source as the neural crest. In the rat, the number of thyroid C cells and secretion of CT increase from fetal life to suckling (93), which are periods of rapid growth. There is probably no placental crossover of CT; the human placental tissue is able to produce CT in response to the presence of Ca in the culture medium (94). In human neonates, the CT content in crude tissue preparations of thyroid is larger than that of the adult thyroid (95).

There are two calcitonin genes, α and β, located on chromosome 11p15.2 near the genes for β-globulin and PTH. Two different RNA molecules are transcribed from the α gene: one is translated into the precursor for CT and the other message is translated into the precursor for CT gene-related peptide (CGRP) (91–97). The initial translational product of the mRNA is prepro-CT, which undergoes proteolytic cleavage to form pro-CT. The larger prohormones include peptides linked to the amino and carboxy terminals of the CT sequence (i.e., flanking peptides). Calcitonin and equimolar amounts of non-CT secretory peptides, corresponding to these flanking peptides, are generated during precursor processing. CGRP is found predominantly in nerve fibers in the central and peripheral nervous system, blood vessels, thyroid and parathyroid glands, liver, spleen, heart, lung, and possibly bone marrow. CGRP, a 37-amino-acid peptide, is also generated from the larger precursor molecule. It is synthesized wherever the CT mRNA is expressed (e.g., in medullary carcinoma of thyroid). The β or CGRP-2 gene is transcribed into the mRNA for CGRP in the central nervous system and does not produce CT. Seventy-five amino-terminal residues of each preprohormone for CT and CGRP are predicted to be identical. Pro-CT is a 116 amino-acid peptide, whereas the pro-CGRP is a 103 amino-acid peptide.

Circulating immunoreactive CT and CGRP are a heterogeneous mixture of different molecular forms and are recognized as long as the antigenic epitopes recognized by the antiserum are expressed. Immunoreactive CT or CGRP concentration is expressed in gravimetric or molar equivalents of synthetic CT or CGRP. Sample preparation with initial extraction, gel chromatography and high-performance liquid chromatography separation, and the use of two-site immunoassay can improve the sensitivity and specificity of CT measurements. Serum CT concentrations during pregnancy are variable (2,98). They are high at birth compared to paired maternal CT concentrations (98). Serum CT further increases during the first few days after birth and may reach levels five- to 10-fold higher than adult CT concentrations (58,59,99,100). Serum CT concentrations decrease progressively during infancy (61,99); however, in preterm infants up to 3 months after birth, the mean serum CT concentrations may remain twice the adult value (99). There is also a small peak of serum CT concentration during late childhood. In human adults, the basal serum CT concentration may be lower in women than in men, but it is not affected by old age. The CT secretory response to Ca infusion is lower in women and with old age (101). In human adults, serum CT and CGRP concentrations are found in the picomolar range. Diurnal variability has been reported for serum CGRP but not for serum CT (102–104). In normal individuals, larger precursor molecules of CT such as procalcitonin is not detected (105).

Classic bioactivity of human calcitonin (hCT) is present in the full 32 amino-acid structure or its smaller fragments, such as hCT 8–32 and hCT 9–32; the ring structure of CT enhances, but is not essential for, hormone action. Basic amino acid substitutions confer a helical structure in this region as found in salmon and other non-mammalian CT, and result in greater potency in lowering serum Ca and probably longer circulating half-life (t1/2) (97). The kidney appears to be the dominant organ in the metabolism of human CT. A small percentage of the metabolic clearance rate of CT in humans may be accounted for by enzymatic degradation in blood. Injected hCT monomer disappears from the blood in vivo with a t1/2 of approximately 10 min; in contrast, the t1/2 of hCT in

plasma incubated in vitro at 37°C may be longer than 20 h (106). Depending on the animal species, other sites such as liver, intestine, and bone may be involved in the metabolism of CT.

In humans, changes in Ca and P metabolism are not seen despite extreme variations in CT production. In the neonate, there is neither an identifiable hypocalcemic response to the postnatal surge in serum CT nor a blunting of CT secretion in the presence of hypocalcemia. In adults, there is no definite effect attributable to CT deficiency, for example, totally thyroidectomized patients receiving only replacement thyroxin; or CT excess, for example, patients with medullary carcinoma of thyroid, except for the chronic suppression of bone remodeling. The clinical significance of CT is related to its use as a tumor marker in the management of medullary carcinoma of the thyroid, and its pharmacological effect to inhibit osteoclast-mediated bone resorption and to increase renal Ca clearance. The pharmacological activities of CT are useful for the suppression of bone resorption in patients with Paget's disease, for limited use in the treatment of osteoporosis, and for early-phase treatment of severe hypercalcemia (92). In addition, CT also increases renal clearance of Mg, P, and sodium and free water clearance (32,33). The net effect of CT is a lowering of serum Ca and P concentrations. Thus, the bioactivity of CT on calcium metabolism frequently is opposite that of PTH; CT probably modulates the effect of PTH on organs.

The clinical role of CT and associated molecules, particularly its non-calcium-related actions, are increasingly being expanded (92,97,105). For example, CT and CT receptors may play an important role in a variety of processes as wide-ranging as embryonic development and sperm function/physiology; and the possible use of serum procalcitonin as a marker of inflammation/sepsis. Its production in neuroendocrine cells in the lung and intestine is increased after exposure to bacterial endotoxin and inflammatory cytokines TNF and IL-6, thus increasing serum procalcitonin.

There are distinct but overlapping effects of CT and CGRP. CGRP primarily affects catecholamine release, vascular tone and blood pressure, and cardiac contractility. Its clinical role probably also lies in its potential pharmacological effect (97,105,107–109). The influence of CGRP on Ca and P homeostasis is minor compared to that of CT. However, amylin, a pancreatic islet-derived or synthetic 37 amino acid peptide, is a member of the CGRP family with a potent hypocalcemic effect despite sharing only 15% of its amino acid sequence with human CT. The hypocalcemic effect of amylin is probably mediated by the CT receptors on osteoclasts, and it is 100-fold more potent than CGRP (110). Both CT and CGRP inhibit gastric acid secretion and food intake.

Calcitonin function is mediated by binding to receptors linked to G proteins, a member of the GPCR superfamily, and activation of adenylate cyclase and phospholipase C. The calcitonin receptor (CTR) gene is located on chromosome 7q21.2-q21.3 and encodes a 490 amino acid, seven-transmembrane G protein-linked receptor. Two isoforms of human calcitonin receptor arise by alternative splicing of an exon of 48 nucleotides that encodes a 16 amino acid insertion within the first intracellular loop. The isoform with the insertion (hCTR-1) activates only adenylate cyclase, whereas the other isoform (hCTR-2) activates both adenylate cyclase and phospholipase C (92,97,111). The role of receptor activity modifying proteins to modify the calcitonin receptor-like receptor (CRLR) posttranslationally is being defined. CGRP functions are also mediated by receptors (109).

Secretion of CT is stimulated by an increase in serum Ca and Mg concentrations and by gastrin, glucagon, and cholecystokinin, along with several other structural analogs of these hormones (e.g., pentagastrin, prostaglandin E2), and by norepinephrine. Secretion of CT is inhibited by hypocalcemia, propranolol, and other adrenergic antagonists, somatostatin, and chromogranin A (92,97). Calcitonin gene transcription is positively regulated by glucocorticoid (112) and negatively regulated by protein kinase C (113), Ca, and vitamin D (114). Calcitonin may activate the 1-hydroxylase system independent of PTH and increase 1,25(OH)2D production (115), whereas 1,25(OH)2D decreases CT gene expression in adult rats but is ineffective in 13-day-old suckling rats (116). The latter observation may be related to fewer 1,25(OH)2D receptors in C cells of immature rats. Calcitonin-induced refractoriness to its own actions is a well known phenomenon in vitro and in vivo, and clinically is manifested as the so-called escape phenomenon during therapy with calcitonin. This probably results from downregulation in the number and functional reduction of receptor mRNA (117).

C. Vitamin D

Vitamin D (Mr 384) can be obtained from diet or synthesized endogenously. It must undergo several metabolic transformations primarily in the liver and kidney to form the physiologically most important metabolite, 1,25(OH)2D, which functions as a hormone in the maintenance of mineral homeostasis. Under in vivo conditions, there are over 30 other vitamin D metabolites, with and without putative functions.

Dietary vitamin D (1 μg = 40 IU) is derived from plants as ergocalciferol (vitamin D2) and from animals as cholecalciferol (vitamin D3). Dietary vitamin D is absorbed into the intestinal lymphatics (118), and about 50% of the vitamin D in chylomicron is transferred to DBP in blood before uptake by the liver (119). In animals, vitamin D3 can be synthesized endogenously in the skin. During exposure to sunlight, the high-energy ultraviolet (UV) photons (290–315 nm) penetrate the epidermis and photolyze 7-dehydrocholesterol (provitamin D3) to previtamin D3. It then undergoes a thermally induced isomerization to vitamin D3 that takes 2–3 days to reach completion. Thus, cutaneous synthesis of vitamin D3 continues for many hours after a single sun exposure. Vitamin D3 is carried in the circulation by DBP to other sites for further metabolism. Vitamin D3 synthesis in the skin is directly dependent on the amount of sunlight exposure and affected by time of day, season and latitude (peak sunlight at midday, in summer and lower latitudes); amount of skin area exposed, and duration of sunlight exposure. Melanin in the skin competes with 7 DHC for ultraviolet photons but the production of vitamin D3 can be compensated for by increasing the duration of sunlight exposure; use of topical sunscreen blocks the ultraviolet photons; and aging, which decreases the capacity for cutaneous synthesis of vitamin D3. Previtamin D3 is photolabile. Continued exposure to sunlight causes the isomerization of previtamin D3 to biologically inert products, principally to lumisterol. No more than 10–20% of the initial provitamin D3 concentrations ultimately end up as previtamin D3, thus preventing the excessive production of previtamin D3 and vitamin D3 (120).

In mammals, vitamins D2 and D3 appear to metabolize along the same pathway, and there is little functional difference between their metabolites. The term vitamin D is frequently used generically to describe vitamins D2 and D3 and, correspondingly, their metabolites.

In the circulation, vitamin D and its metabolites are protein bound, mainly to DBP (about 85%) and to albumin (about 15%) (121). The DBP gene is located on chromosome 4q11-13. It is a member of a gene family that includes serum albumin and α-fetoprotein (122). DBP is a 52 kD globulin in the rat and approximately 58 kD in the human; it is normally <5% saturated with vitamin D metabolite. Its affinity to vitamin D metabolites depends inversely on the distance between the 3β-hydroxy group and other hydroxyl groups on each vitamin D metabolite. Thus, its affinities for 25 OHD, 24,25(OH)2D and 25,26(OH)2D are greater than for vitamin D and 1,25(OH)2D (123). The amount of DBP may influence the concentration of "free" 1,25(OH)2D in plasma, which is important in determining the bioactivity of the hormone.

In the liver, vitamin D is hydroxylated at carbon 25 to 25-hydroxyvitamin D (25-OHD). The vitamin D-25 hydroxylase activity is found predominantly in the cytochrome P450-containing enzyme, CYP-27 protein, on the inner surface of the mitochondrial membrane. This protein also catalyzes 27-hydroxylation of cholesterol derivatives. The CYP-27 gene is located on chromosome 2q33 and encodes a polypeptide of 531 amino acids processed to a mature 56.9 kD protein of 498 amino acids (124). Quantitatively, 25 OHD (1 nmol/L = 0.4 ng/ml) is the most abundant vitamin D metabolite in the circulation and is a useful index of vitamin D reserve.

In the kidney, 25 OHD is hydroxylated further to 1,25(OH)2D with 25-OHD-1α-hydroxylase (CYP 1α), and to 24R,25-dihydroxyvitamin D (24,25(OH)2D) with 25-OHD-24R-hydroxylase (CYP 24). This occurs primarily in the mitochondria of proximal tubules. The genes for these enzymes have been localized to chromosome 12q13-14 and 20q13.3, respectively (125–127). The human gene encoding the CYP 1α is 5 kb in length, located on chromosome 12, and comprises nine exons and eight introns; its exon/intron organization is very similar to other mitochondrial P450 enzymes cloned to date (127). Recent reports that 25 OHD can be metabolized to 1,25(OH)2D in the colon, prostate, and skin have raised the possibility that 1,25(OH)2D may be needed for cellular health of extrarenal tissues in addition to its classic action on mineral metabolism (128).

Regulation of 25-hydroxylase activity is limited and there are few limitations to the production of 25 OHD. At high concentrations of vitamin D, the mitochondrial enzyme will form significant quantities of 25 OHD. This is part explains the serum 25 OHD variations with season and vitamin D intake. The latter can increase serum 25 OHD to more than fivefold of upper normal range. The in vivo administration of 1,25(OH)2D decreases serum 25 OHD (129). Ca deficiency increases the metabolic clearance of 25-OHD (130).

The activity of 1α-hydroxylase, and therefore production of 1,25(OH)2D, are tightly regulated. It is the rate-limiting hormonally regulated step in the bioactivation of vitamin D. PTH increases transcriptional activity of the CYP 1α gene promoter and increases mRNA for 1,25(OH)2D. Decrease in serum or diet Ca or P increase mRNA for (127,130) and serum concentration of 1,25(OH)2D (131). In contrast, hypophosphatemia associated with tumor-induced osteomalacia, autosomal dominant hypophosphatemic rickets (ADHR), and X-linked hypophosphatemia (XLH) do not elicit appropriate phosphate conservation or an increase in 1,25(OH)2D production. They have similar phenotypic manifestations characterized by hypophosphatemia, decreased renal phosphate reabsorption, normal (inappropriately low) or low serum calcitriol concentrations, normal serum Ca and PTH, and defective skeletal mineralization. XLH results from mutations in the PHEX gene, encoding a membrane-bound endopeptidase, whereas ADHR is associated with mutations of the gene encoding FGF-23. The latter is a small heat-sensitive molecule of <25 kD that inhibits sodium-dependent phosphate wasting and probably inhibits CYP 1α. The endopeptidase PHEX degrades native FGF-23, which presumably provides the biochemical link among these clinical syndromes (132).

Other factors that enhance 1,25(OH)2D production include estrogen, prolactin, growth hormone, insulin-like growth factor-I, and PTHrP (133–135). 1,25(OH)2D production is feedback regulated and is inhibited by chronic deficiency or low circulating Mg (82,131,134,136). Mg deficiency also lowers serum 1,25(OH)2D response to low-Ca diet (137) but does not appear to limit 1,25(OH)2D production in animals (138). The effect of Mg on 1,25(OH)2D metabolism is presumably related in part to its role as a cofactor of the 1 α-hydroxylase enzyme (136). In contrast to the rapid increase in PTH secretion and serum PTH concentrations, measurable alteration in serum 1,25(OH)2D concentrations usually occurs only hours after exposure to an appropriate stimulus. Extrarenal production of 1,25(OH)2D in macrophages, particularly in granulomatous disease states, may not be tightly regulated; is stimulated by γ-interferon, but is not responsive to changes in dietary calcium intake (134).

1,25(OH)2D function, like other steroid hormones, is mediated primarily through modulation of the cellular genome by binding to specific nuclear receptors (vitamin D receptor, VDR), a 424-amino-acid phosphoprotein. The VDR gene contains nine exons and is located on chromosome 12q13-14 near the site of the gene for 25 OHD-1α-hydroxylase (125,139). VDR is a member of the nuclear receptor superfamily of steroid–retinoid–thyroid hormone–vitamin D transcription regulatory factors. It has several functional domains including a zinc finger-mediated N-terminal DNA-binding domain, a C-terminal hormone-binding domain, and a hinge region important for nuclear localization. The VDR interacts with the retinoic acid X receptor (RXR) to form a heterodimeric RXR–VDR complex that binds to specific DNA sequences, termed vitamin-D-responsive elements (VDREs) (139). After 1,25(OH)2D binds to the receptor, it induces conformational changes (140) that result in the recruitment of a multitude of transcriptional coactivators that stimulate the transcription of target genes. Vitamin D receptors are upregulated by 1,25(OH)2D at both the mRNA and protein levels. They also are increased during growth, gestation, and lactation but show an age-dependent decrease in mature animals and humans, supporting the notion that vitamin D receptors may be up- or downregulated, depending on Ca needs (126,139,141). All vitamin D target cells that possess VDR can metabolize vitamin D via the 24-hydroxylation pathway (126).

Two basic clinical functions define the major classic action of vitamin D. The first is that vitamin D is required to prevent rickets in children and osteomalacia in adults. The second is the prevention of hypocalcemic tetany. These functions are maintained by 1,25(OH)2D through its effect on a number of target tissues, primarily intestine, kidney, and bone, and modulating effects from other hormones including PTH and CT. However, VDR is present in numerous cell types, and 1,25(OH)2D-VDR action clearly transcends bone and calcium/phosphate homeostasis. Its actions extend into cell growth and differentiation and immune, neural, and endocrine function (126,139).

Intestinal absorption of Ca and P consists of a passive (concentration-dependent) and active component. Classic vitamin D-dependent active Ca absorption in the intestine involves multiple components. At the brush-border membrane, non-genome-mediated action of 1,25(OH)2D occurs within seconds to minutes to transport Ca into the cell, probably mediated through a 1,25(OH)2-D-binding membrane receptor that opens voltage-gated Ca ion channels (71,142). Ca transport through the cytosol is facilitated by binding to Ca-binding proteins (CaBP, or calbindin D). There are at least two CaBPs and their expression depends on the animal species and the organ studied. In mammals, the 7.5–10 kD CaBP (calbindin D 9K) is found mainly in the duodenum, whereas the 28 kD CaBP (calbindin D 28K) is found mainly in the kidney and cerebellum. In avian species, such as the chicken, calbindin D 28K is found in the intestine. 1,25(OH)2D stimulates transcription of the CaBP gene, with resulting accumulation of CaBP mRNA and protein in 1 or more hours after 1,25(OH)2D treatment (143). In the rat, there is an age-dependent increase in intestinal calbindin D 9K extending from the fetal period and reaching adult levels soon after weaning. The level decreases in older rats (144). At the basolateral membrane (BLM), 1,25(OH)2D causes an increase in the concentration of ATP-dependent plasma membrane iCa pump (PMCA) (145) and stimulates the extrusion of Ca (146). Administration of 1,25(OH)2D also induces brush border enzyme activities, such as alkaline phosphatase that facilitates the movement of Ca across cell membranes. The progressive increase in affinity for Ca among the successive components as the Ca is transported from the brush border to the BLM also facilitates Ca transport (143). There are conflicting reports on 1,25(OH)2D-induced changes in membrane fluidity from altered lipid composition of intestinal cell membranes.

Vitamin D metabolites are also needed for the maintenance of P homeostasis by increasing intestinal absorption. Active transport processes of P across the intestine include a saturable, sodium-dependent Na-K-ATPase that involves the endoplasmic reticulum, an unsaturable and sodium-independent component for brush border uptake and basolateral membrane exit processes, and a Ca- and vitamin D-dependent component (147,148). Intestinal P absorption is well established in infants of human and animal species and may be as high as 90% of P intake. In preterm infants, P absorption appears not to be significantly affected by vitamin D intake (149).

The effect of vitamin D and its various metabolites on ion transport is much less marked on the kidney than on the intestine. In humans, conflicting data have been reported on the effect of vitamin D and its metabolites on renal excretion of Ca and P, probably because of the difficulty in controlling the many variables that may influence renal handling of these minerals. The mechanisms of absorption vary significantly from one segment to another, as the extent of hormonal regulation. The active, transcellular component regulated by PTH, 1,25(OH)2D, CT, and Ca-sparing drugs such as thiazide type diuretics, acts primarily at the distal tubule. Both the active (regulated by PTH and CT) and the passive paracellular transport of Ca (32,33,68,142,150) and P (69,151,152) occur at the thick ascending limb. The model for vitamin D-dependent Ca transport across the intestinal epithelial cells also may

be applicable to the active renal Ca transport since VDR, CaBP, and PMCA are found in both cell types and respond similarly to changes in vitamin D, Ca, or P status (143). In the rat kidney, developmental changes in the calbindin D 28K also show an age-dependent change similar to that for the intestinal calbindin D 9K (144). In the human, calbindin D 28K gene is located on chromosome 8. Analogous to rat and chicken, the human calbindin D 28K also contains six EF-hand-like domains, and there are at least four functional binding sites for Ca. Vitamin D depletion is associated with decreased renal P reabsorption that is corrected rapidly by physiological amounts of 1,25(OH)2D, probably from stimulation of sodium-dependent phosphate cotransporter (NPT2) in the brush border membrane of proximal tubules and possibly from changes in the lipid composition of tubular membrane (69,70, 143,151). In any case, renal P retention is extremely effective at low dietary intake in infants (43,45,46) and adults (151,152) with tubular reabsorption of P *approach* 100% in infants with increased P need while receiving low dietary P.

Bone mineralization of skeleton is thought to be predominantly secondary to the action of 1,25(OH)2D in increasing the intestinal absorption of Ca and independently of P; these two actions, thereby, elevate plasma Ca and P concentrations. This is supported by the finding that the skeletal abnormalities present in homozygous VDR knockout mice are completely ablated by normalizing serum Ca and P (153), and that Ca therapy improves bone abnormalities in hereditary hypocalcemic vitamin D-resistant rickets patients (154). Additionally, 1,25(OH)2D acts on receptors of osteoblasts (enhances differentiation and inhibits proliferation) and osteocytes to promote bone formation and the production of osteocalcin, osteopontin, and alkaline phosphatase. Both PTH and 1,25(OH)2D interact with their specific osteoblast surface receptors to induce the production of RANK ligand that interacts with RANK receptors on the immature osteoclast precursor to differentiate into mature osteoclasts (155). This leads to mobilization of bone minerals and contributes to maintenance of Ca and P homeostasis.

Quantification of vitamin D and its metabolites has been achieved by several different methods. The more routine approaches include high-performance liquid chromatography with detection by ultraviolet absorbance or binding assays. Immunoassays based on antibodies raised to vitamin D metabolite conjugates also are available. Values from different laboratories cannot be compared without making direct comparison of their assay procedures. Interlaboratory coefficients of variation for the measurement of 25-OHD, 24,25(OH)2D, and 1,25(OH)2D may range between 35% and 52% (156). Furthermore, differences between vitamins D2 and D3 in their affinity to the vitamin D binding protein and receptors and different chromatographic behavior on various preparative chromatographic systems (157) demand that great care be taken with assay techniques when dealing with patients who have significant vitamin D2 intake. To ensure reliable results, appropriate vitamin D standards must be used for standard curve generation in performing competitive protein binding assays of these compounds.

Maternofetal transfer of vitamin D and its metabolites varies, depending on the species. In humans, the cord serum vitamin D concentration is very low and may be undetectable, probably because of poor maternofetal crossover. The 25 OHD concentration is directly correlated with, but lower than, maternal values, consistent with placental crossover of this metabolite; 1,25(OH)2D concentrations also are lower than maternal values, but there is no agreement on the maternofetal relationship of this and other dihydroxylated vitamin D metabolites (1,158–160). In vitro experiments demonstrate that 25(OH)D and 1,25(OH)2D may cross the perfused human placenta (161). In vivo, some placental crossover may occur after maternal exposure to pharmacological doses of vitamin D (162) or 1,25(OH)2D at 17–36 μg/day (163). In the latter case, consistently elevated (10 times normal) maternal plasma 1,25(OH)2D concentrations (170–500 + pg/ml) resulted in similarly elevated cord serum 1,25(OH)2D concentrations (470 pg/mL) at delivery. However, the placenta, like the kidney, produces 1,25(OH)2D, making it difficult to ascertain just how much fetal 1,25(OH)2D results from placental crossover versus placental synthesis.

Seasonal and racial variations in serum 25 OHD concentrations occur, presumably from variations in endogenous production. Serum 25-OHD is lower in winter and in African-Americans; serum 1,25(OH)2D is higher in African-American mothers. These differences may be reflected in cord serum values (158–160). The vitamin D metabolite 24,25(OH)2D also crosses the placenta and varies with the seasons, being highest in autumn (160). The significance of this finding is unclear as 24,25(OH)2D may be a metabolic product of 25 OHD to prevent vitamin D toxicity. It appears that the human fetus receives the bulk of its vitamin D already metabolized to 25 OHD.

Serum 1,25(OH)2D in the newborn become elevated within 24 h after delivery (1) and appears to vary according to Ca and P intake (45,46). African-Americans have higher 1,25(OH)2D concentrations than whites in infancy and early childhood (164), but not in the older pediatric or adult population. In normal adults, serum 1,25(OH)2D concentrations are relatively constant and maintained within approximately 20% of the overall 24 h mean (165), and show no seasonal variation (166). The latter is consistent with the tightly regulated 1α-hydroxylase activity. Serum 1,25(OH)2D is lowered in the elderly, possibly in part related to a decrease in the responsiveness of 25(OH)D-1α-hydroxylase enzyme activity (167) and, probably low vitamin D production in northern latitudes (168). The circulating t1/2 of 25(OH)D is 2–3 weeks, depending on the vitamin D status of the individual; it is decreased in vitamin D-deficient individuals. 1,25(OH)2D

has a much shorter t1/2 of 3–6 h (169). Metabolites of 25 OHD and 1,25(OH)2D may undergo enterohepatic circulation after exposure to intestinal β-glucuronidase. The physiological role of enterohepatic circulation of vitamin D metabolites has not been precisely quantitated (170, 171).

Human milk vitamin D, but not 25 OHD concentration, correlates with maternal vitamin D intake (169). Infant serum 25 OHD concentration does not correlate with either human milk vitamin D or 25(OH)D concentrations. The major sources of vitamin D for human-milk-fed infants are from endogenous synthesis after sunlight exposure (172–174) or from vitamin D supplementation (172,175,176). It appears that for an infant living in temperate regions, approximately 2 h/week of sunshine exposure while fully clothed but without a hat, or 400 IU vitamin D supplement, is sufficient to maintain normal vitamin D status (173). Neonates, even very-low-birth-weight infants, appear to have adequate capacity to absorb and metabolize vitamin D. In infants receiving standard supplementary vitamin D intake, circulating 25 OHD and 1,25(OH)2D concentrations may be increased to levels comparable to, and sometimes exceeding, adult values (176–178). Circulating 25 OHD and 1,25(OH)2D concentrations in infants also appear to be dependent on Ca and P intake (43,45,46).

The enzyme 25 hydroxyvitamin D-24 hydroxylase (CYP 24) is present in all vitamin D target cells and is strongly induced by 1,25(OH)2D. In kidney and intestine in particular, upregulation of the 24-hydroxylase enzyme in response to 1,25(OH)2D treatment is rapid and occurs within 4 h (179). The 24 hydroxylase catalyzes several steps of 1,25(OH)2D degradation, collectively known as the C24 oxidation pathway, which starts with 24-hydroxylation and culminates in the formation of the biliary excretory form, calcitroic acid. Physiological production of 24R,25(OH)2D is therefore an important means to regulate the circulating concentration of 1,25(OH)2D and catabolism of vitamin D, although it may have a role in bone integrity and fracture healing in the chick model (180). Thus both the synthesis and degradation of 1,25(OH)2D are tightly regulated events, and that the target cells for vitamin D contains the means to regulate its activity at the cellular level. Most of the other vitamin D metabolites are derived primarily from further metabolic alterations to 25 OHD and 1,25(OH)2D through oxidation or side chain cleavage and have poorly defined physiological function. However, many analogs of vitamin D metabolites are been studied for the numerous potential pharmacological actions that involve less calcemic-inducing and greater maturation and differentiation effects (126).

IV. NONCLASSIC CONTROL OF CALCIUM AND P HOMEOSTASIS

Maintenance of mineral homeostasis is intimately related to skeletal health since the skeleton is the major reservoir for Ca and P, and any disturbance in skeletal health can affect Ca and P homeostasis. Skeletal health, particularly in the growing skeleton, requires the integrated actions of classic calciotropic hormones, endocrine modulators of growth, numerous cytokines and growth factors and their receptors, as well as their endogenous modulators. Many factors such as growth hormone, insulin-like growth factor-I, estrogen, progesterone, cortisol, and tumor necrosis factor can affect the secretion or function of one or more of the calciotropic hormones (86,112,133,135,179,181). Many factors such as insulin-like growth factor-I, transforming growth factor-β1, interleukin 1 and 6, and tumor necrosis factor-α in turn can be modulated by calciotropic hormones (85,182,183). The ultimate effect on mineral homeostasis involved bone formation and/or bone resorption and flux of Ca and P between extracellular fluid and bone, with or without direct involvement by calciotropic hormones. Many factors such as cytokines can function in a paracrine (i.e., cell-to-cell) or autocrine (i.e., cell-to-own cell) fashion, particularly under pathological conditions (155,183–188), whereas, some factors such as parathyroid hormone-related protein (PTHrP) may act both systemically and locally (189).

PTHrP and PTH genes appear to be members of the same gene family. PTHrP cDNA encodes a 177 amino acid protein consisting of a 36-amino-acid precursor segment and a 141-amino-acid mature peptide. The mature PTHrP contains several structural or functional domains. The N-terminal 1-13 region has eight of 13 residues similar to PTH. The amino acids 34–111 segment is highly conserved among species while amino acid 118 to the C-terminus is poorly conserved. PTHrP gene expression is found in an extensive variety of normal endocrine and nonendocrine tissues. PTHrP biological activity and immunoreactivity for PTHrP mRNA have been found in many tissues by as early as 7 weeks of gestation, including the fetus, placenta, lactating breasts, and milk in human (190–192) and in various tissues in the pig (55) and sheep (56).

Both PTH and PTHrP appear to bind to the same G-protein-linked receptor. Synthetic and recombinant PTHrPs can mimic the effects of PTH on the classic PTH target organs, involving activation of adenylate cyclase and other second messenger systems (75,77).

Several PTHrP assays with varying sensitivities and specificities have been developed (193) that account for the variability reported between assays. The stability of PTHrP in plasma samples may be enhanced if sample collection is done in the presence of protease inhibitors. Circulating immunoreactive PTHrP concentrations are low or undetectable in normal subjects. Serum PTHrP is increased during pregnancy (3,4) and is similar to (4) or lower than (3) the umbilical cord concentrations. In cord serum, PTHrP concentrations are 10–15-fold higher than that of PTH. Amniotic fluid PTHrP concentrations at midgestation and at term are 13–16-fold greater than the cord

or maternal levels (194), and the concentration of PTHrP in milk is 100-fold higher (192).

PTHrP concentrations in the circulation of individuals with humoral hypercalcemia of malignancy (HHM) are elevated (193). The amino-terminal fragment PTHrP 1-74 appears to be specific for HHM, whereas the carboxy-terminal fragment PTHrP 109-138 is elevated in the serum of patients with HHM or renal failure. The levels of PTHrP in these patients are similar to the concentration of PTH (10^{-12}–10^{-11} mol/l).

In clinical terms, PTHrP, also known as PTH-like peptide, PTH-like protein, or human humoral hypercalcemic factor, is the humoral mediator secreted by tumors that results in the syndrome of HHM. Currently, the measurement of PTHrP is of clinical utility primarily as a tumor marker in HHM. Physiologically, PTHrP is an important paracrine regulator of several tissue-specific functions that may directly or indirectly affect fetal and neonatal mineral homeostasis, probably through its effect on smooth muscle relaxation, placental calcium transport, lactation, fetal bone development, and in the control of cellular growth and differentiation (189,190).

V. HYPOCALCEMIA

Neonatal hypocalcemia may be defined as a serum tCa concentration below 2 mmol/l (1 mmol/l = 4 mg/dl) in term infants and 1.75 mmol/l (7 mg/dl) in preterm infants with iCa below 1.0–1.1 mmol/L (4.0–4.4 mg/dl), depending on the particular ion-selective electrode used. These definitions are made from a clinical viewpoint because serum Ca concentrations are maintained within narrow ranges under normal circumstances and the potential risk for disturbances of physiological function increases as the serum Ca concentration further decreases. Furthermore, improvements in physiological function (e.g., changes in cardiac contractility, blood pressure, and heart rate) are reported in hypocalcemic infants undergoing Ca therapy (195–197), and a higher mortality rate has been reported for children with hypocalcemia in pediatric intensive care setting (198).

Clinically, there are two peaks in the occurrence of neonatal hypocalcemia. An early form typically occurs during the first few days after birth, with the lowest concentrations of serum Ca being reached at 24–48 h of age; late neonatal hypocalcemia occurs toward the end of the first week and generally presents as neonatal tetany. These findings reflect the traditional clinical practice of screening for biochemical abnormalities in small or sick hospitalized infants during the first few days, and in symptomatic infants after hospital discharge. The nadir of the serum Ca concentration may occur at less than 12 h (7,199–201) or not until some weeks after birth (202, 203), and that many neonates, particularly those with genetic defects in Ca metabolism, may be hypocalcemic but remain asymptomatic and undetected during the early neonatal period. This also may contribute to the less frequent diagnosis of late neonatal hypocalcemia compared to early neonatal hypocalcemia. It seems preferable to classify neonatal hypocalcemia based on risk factors (Table 1) rather than the traditional early or late onset.

A. Pathophysiology

The pathophysiological mechanisms of hypocalcemia are varied and frequently interrelated but not fully defined (Table 2). In most cases of neonatal hypocalcemia, there is a decrease in both tCa and iCa. There exists a common basis for its occurrence particularly so-called in early onset hypocalcemia. These include the abrupt discontinuation of placental Ca supply after birth, limited or no dietary calcium, transient limited increase in the serum PTH concentration, possibly end-organ resistance to 1,25(OH)2D, and elevated serum CT concentration. These problems are exaggerated in the preterm infant and accounts for the inverse relationship between the frequency of hypocalcemia with birth weight and gestational age; over 50% of preterm very-low-birth-weight neonates may have hypocalcemia (7,199–201). Small preterm infants often have associated illnesses that preclude early enteral feeding but many clinicians do not use calcium-containing parenteral nutrition for 1 or more days after birth, thus increasing the risk for hypocalcemia. Resistance to pharmacological dosages of 1,25(OH)2D demonstrated in vitro (204) and in vivo (7,200) might contribute to hypocalcemia in small preterm infants. The amount of calcium

Table 1 Risk Factors for Neonatal Hypocalcemia

Maternal
  Insulin-dependent diabetes
  Hyperparathyroidism
  Vitamin D or magnesium deficiency
  Anticonvulsant use (?)
  Narcotic use (?)
Peripartum: Birth asphyxia
Infant
  Intrinsic
    Prematurity
    Malabsorption
    Malignant infantile osteopetrosis
    Parathyroid hormone: impaired synthesis, secretion,
      regulation or responsiveness
  Extrinsic
    Diet
      Inadequate calcium
      Excess phophorus
    Enema: phophate
    Exchange transfusion with citrated blood
    High rate of intravenous lipid infusion
    Phototherapy (?)
    Alkali therapy (?)

retention from milk feeds even in healthy term infants probably is less than 20 mg/kg body weight on the first day, rising to about 45–60 mg or more/kg on the third day; these amounts are significantly lower than the daily in utero Ca accretion of over 100 mg/kg during the third trimester (47). Excessive P load from diet including increased dietary P can be from cow-milk ingestion (6) and even with humanized cow-milk-derived formulas with lower P content (42) or from cereals (205); from accidental overdose of oral phosphate supplement (206) or phosphate-containing enema (207,208) can result in hypocalcemia.

Other clinical situations include any chronic diarrheal condition, especially if associated with steatorrhea, is generally associated with intestinal malabsorption of Ca and possibly impaired enterohepatic circulation of vitamin D and vitamin D metabolites. Specific intestinal malabsorption of Mg (209) may lead to Mg depletion and, secondarily, to hypocalcemia, which can be corrected only when the Mg disturbance is corrected. The most common cause of intestinal malabsorption of Mg is surgical resection of large segments of small bowel, with or without fistula losses of various minerals. The use of high P (106–120 mg/100 kcal) and a fixed Ca (180 mg/100 kcal) content formula can lower the fecal loss of Mg (210) in preterm infants, whereas P depletion may be associated with increased urinary Ca and Mg (32,33,136,211).

Pathophysiology of some situations with hypocalcemia remain ill defined: for example, despite the hypocalcemic effects of CT, the serum CT concentrations continued to increase in neonates of normal and diabetic pregnancies irrespective of the variation in serum calcium (59,201); in neonates with birth asphyxia (201); and in preterm infants (58). The stimulus for the postnatal rise in serum CT, despite falling serum Ca, is unknown. There are conflicting reports on the effect of Ca supplementation to suppress the postnatal surge in CT secretion (58,212). However, serum CT is increased after an intravenous bolus of Ca during exchange blood transfusion (213). Infants with intrauterine growth retardation may have hypocalcemia if they are also preterm (58) or have birth asphyxia (58,201,214); otherwise, there is apparently no increased incidence of hypocalcemia related to growth retardation per se (8,215).

Maternal use of the anticonvulsants phenytoin and phenobarbital may be associated with neonatal hypocalcemia, presumably from increased clearance of vitamin D secondary to the induction of hepatic cytochrome P450 enzyme system (216). However, other maternal factors including seasonal variation in sunlight exposure, increased maternal age and parity, and poor socioeconomic status (217), may contribute to development of neonatal hypocalcemia, presumably in part from varied and probably deficient maternal vitamin D. However, there is no seasonal variation in the rate of early neonatal hypocalcemia (218) despite seasonal variation in maternal and fetal vi-

Table 2 Pathophysiology of Neonatal Hypocalcemia

Physiological basis	Mechanism	Clinical association
Calcium total and ionized	Decreased intake or absorption	Prematurity; malabsorption syndrome
Calcium ionized	Increased Ca complex	Chelating agent (e.g., citrated blood for exchange transfusion, long-chain free fatty acid)
Magnesium	Decreased tissue store or absorption	Infant of insulin-dependent diabetic mother; maternal hypomagnesemia; specific Mg malabsorption (rare)
Phosphorus	Increased	Endogenous and exogenous (e.g., dietary, enema) phosphate loading
pH	Increased	Respiratory or metabolic alkalosis (e.g., shifts Ca from ionized to protein-bound fraction)
Parathyroid hormone	Impair or defective synthesis or secretion	Maternal hypercalcemia; DiGeorge association, hypoparathyroidism, hypomagnesemia; PTH gene mutations
	Impair regulation	Activating mutations of calcium-sensing receptor: autosomal dominant or sporadic hypocalcemia with hypercalciuria
	Impair responsiveness	Chronic hypomagnesemia; inactivating mutation of type 1 PTH receptor (?); pseudohypoparathyroidism
Calcitonin	Increased	Infant of insulin-dependent diabetic mother, birth asphyxia, prematurity
1,25-Dihydroxyvitamin D	Decreased responsiveness	Prematurity
Osteoclast activity	Absent	Malignant infantile osteopetrosis

tamin D status as indicated by maternal and cord 25 OHD concentrations (158,160). Hypomagnesemia may be contributory to hypocalcemia in infants of mothers with insulin-dependent diabetes (219), although it is conceivable that both hypocalcemia and hypomagnesemia may be the result of a common insult from the diabetic pregnancy. Maternal vitamin D or Mg deficiency probably predisposes to but is not the primary cause of hypocalcemia in the neonate. Malignant infantile osteopetrosis may present with neonatal hypocalcemia (220), presumably reflecting continue Ca uptake from unopposed bone formation.

Neonatal hypocalcemia from impaired synthesis or secretion of PTH in the newborn can occur secondary to developmental defects of parathyroid gland, specific mutations of PTH gene, or maternal hypercalcemia. Neonatal hypocalcemia is often the first manifestation that leads to the diagnosis of maternal hyperparathyroidism (202, 203).

Hypocalcemia (in varying degree of severity) from so-called transient congenital hypoparathyroidism (TCHP) may occur in association with DiGeorge and velocardiofacial/Shprintzen syndromes. Both syndromes may represent different degrees of the same disorder with partial or complete absence of derivatives of the third and fourth pharyngeal pouches, and possibly the fifth pouch, and are often associated with defective development of the third, fourth, and sixth aortic arches. Other clinical manifestations may include some combination of congenital heart disease, primarily involving the aortic arch, decreased T-cell number or function, and possibly thyroid C-cell deficiency (221,222). Deletion of 22q.11 has been reported in these patients (223), and DiGeorge association may be

inherited in an autosomal dominant fashion (224). Neonates with TCHP may have prolonged hypocalcemia that requires treatment until late infancy or early childhood, and hypoparathyroidism may recur in later childhood (225–227).

Hypoparathyroidism in the infant is a heterogeneous group of disorders and may occur sporadically or with differing mendelian modes of inheritance (228–232). Synthesis of defective PTH can occur in the autosomal dominant form with a point mutation in the signal peptide-encoding region for the prepro-PTH. The autosomal recessive form is associated with a mutation in the donor splice site leading to transcriptional loss of the second axon and prevention of translation. The X-linked recessive form is associated with embryonic dysgenesis of parathyroid glands. Hypoparathyroidism from fetal parathyroid hypoplasia or dysgenesis usually requires life long treatment to prevent hypocalcemia.

Defects in the regulation of PTH can result in hypocalcemia. A variety of missense, nonsense, deletion, and insertion mutations of CaR gene, some with mendelian modes of inheritance, can result in altered receptor activity and clinical disease. Activating CaR mutations with reduction in EC50 (concentration of extracellular Ca required to elicit half of the maximal increase in intracellular inositol phosphate) manifested as autosomal dominant or sporadic cases of hypocalcemia with hypercalciuria have been reported (233–235). Hypocalcemia is usually mild and asymptomatic, and diagnosis is often delayed beyond the neonatal period, although hypocalcemia was likely to be present during the immediate newborn period.

Neonatal hypocalcemia may result from relative defective or inadequate response to PTH. Inactivating mutation of the type 1 PTH receptor gene as documented in Blomstrand's chondrodystrophy is manifested as the prenatally lethal form of short limb dwarfism (236). Theoretically this defect may result in hypocalcemia but the regulation of serum Ca has not been evaluated in vivo.

Newborn infants increase serum PTH coincident with a fall in serum Ca (53,58–60), presumably reflecting abrupt withdrawal of the placental transfer of Ca, and the increase in PTH may be insufficient to maintain normal serum Ca. This may reflect the relative inadequacy or transient nature of the PTH response. For example, in situations of induced hypocalcemia, such as during an exchange transfusion using citrated blood (213,237) or feeding of the relatively high P content of cow-milk formula (42). The ability of the neonatal parathyroids to respond to hypocalcemic stress increases with age (237). Impaired end-organ response to PTH also occurs with chronic hypomagnesemia and may involve simultaneous impairment in both PTH and 1,25(OH)2D pathways (83,136,137).

End-organ unresponsiveness to PTH associated with genetic defect is classically manifested as pseudohypoparathyroidism type 1a (PHP-1a) or Albright's hereditary osteodystrophy. The biochemical basis of the defect is proximal to cyclic AMP production. It is inherited in an autosomal dominant fashion with heterozygous inactivating mutations in the maternal GNAS1 exons that encode the α-subunit of the stimulating G protein (Gsα). The gene GNAS1 is located on chromosome 20q13.3 and encodes 13 exons that are alternatively spliced to yield four Gsα proteins. Multiple mutations include abnormalities in splice junctions associated with deficient mRNA production and point mutations that result in diminished amount and activity of the G proteins have been reported. The inactivating mutation of the gene impaired the production of adenylate cyclase second messenger system, leading to resistance to multiple hormones (including PTH, vasopressin, and thyrotropin) that activate Gsα. Clinical manifestations include short stature, round face, brachymetacarpals and brachymetatarsals, dental dysplasia, subcutaneous calcifications, abnormalities in taste, smell, hearing, and vision, and developmental delay. Biochemical abnormalities include hypocalcemia, hyperphosphatemia, increased circulating PTH, and insensitivity to the administration of exogenous PTH (unaltered urinary calcium, P, and cAMP) in the absence of compromised renal function. The extent of resistance to other hormones is variable and the complete biochemical picture is usually not evident until 2–3 years after birth (231,238,239).

Parent-specific methylation with parental imprinting of the GNAS1 gene involving selective inactivation of either the maternal or paternal allele is possible and led to different phenotypic expression. In the case of the Gsα gene, it is paternally imprinted (silenced) so that the disease PHP-1a is never inherited from the father carrying the defective allele but only from the mother. However, the defective allele is not imprinted or silenced in all tissues and reflects haplotype insufficiency. For example, PHP type 1b is characterized by isolated resistance to PTH without the accompanied skeletal manifestations. Paternal isodisomy of chromosome 20q in patients that lack the maternal-specific methylation pattern within GNAS1 results in normal Gsα protein and activity in the fibroblast but not in the renal proximal tubules (240). There is a third type, PHP-1c, reported in a few patients that differs from PHP-1a only in having normal erythrocyte levels of Gsα, presumably there is a post-Gsα defect in adenyl cyclase stimulation. All type 1 PHP individuals show a deficient urinary cAMP response to the administration of exogenous PTH. Whereas, individuals with pseudopseudohypoparathyroidism (PPHP) have typical clinical manifestation of PHP-1a but have normal serum Ca and normal response of urinary cAMP to exogenous PTH. The mutated GNAS1 gene is inherited from the father (i.e., paternal imprinting) with suppression of the mutant copy in selected tissues (241) and there is a 50% reduction but not absent Gsα subunit.

Neonatal hypocalcemia with seizure and so-called transient features of pseudohypoparathyroidism has been reported (242). These infants have elevated serum PTH and P with hypocalcemia at diagnosis. Response to exogenous human PTH (1–34) show little phosphaturic effect although there was brisk response in plasma and urine cAMP and alkaline phosphatase. After initial treatment for hypocalcemia, the serum Ca and PTH spontaneously normalized before 6 months of age.

Decreases in serum iCa can occur without decreases in serum tCa. Agents that complex Ca in the blood would be expected to decrease ionized Ca. Such agents include citrate, which is used as an anticoagulant for blood storage. During exchange blood transfusion, iCa can be decreased to 0.5 mmol/l in spite of administration of conventional amounts of Ca (i.e., 0.5–1 ml of 10% Ca gluconate for each 100 ml blood exchanged) during the transfusion (213,237). Increased levels of long-chain free fatty acids from intravenous lipid emulsion can complex Ca and reduce iCa in vitro (243), thus hypocalcemia potentially can occur with excessive rate of intravenous lipid infusion. Alkalosis can result in shifts of Ca from the ionized state to the protein-bound fraction (14,20,21). Because alkalosis per se increases neuromuscular hyperirritability, the combination of decreased serum iCa and alkalosis may precipitate clinical tetany in an infant with borderline serum Ca status. In clinical practice, administration of sodium bicarbonate in the therapy of metabolic acidosis often occurs in situations with high risk of hypocalcemia such as prematurity or perinatal asphyxia, whether it has an independent role in the development of hypocalcemia is not known. Hypocalcemia in neonates receiving phototherapy is thought to result from the stimulation of a complex system of extraretinal photoreception, which results in neuroendocrine sequelae and hypocalcemia (244). For reasons that are unclear, infants born to narcotic-using mothers have been reported to have a lower serum iCa if they manifest withdrawal symptoms (245).

B. Diagnosis

Suspicion of hypocalcemia must be confirmed by measurement of serum tCa and iCa since clinical manifestations are many and varied and may be indistinguishable from other common neonatal diseases. Diagnostic work-ups are listed in Table 3. The less mature the infant, the more subtle and varied are the clinical manifestations and they are frequently asymptomatic. Clinical manifestations may include, irritability, jitteriness, or lethargy; feeding poorly with and without feeding intolerance; abdominal distention; apnea; cyanosis; and seizures and may be confused with manifestations of hypoglycemia, sepsis, meningitis, anoxia, intracranial bleeding, and narcotic withdrawal. Frank convulsions are seen more commonly with so-called late neonatal hypocalcemia. The classic signs of peripheral hyperexcitability of motor nerves: carpopedal spasm (spasm of the wrists and ankles, Trousseau's sign), facial spasm (Chvostek's sign), and laryngospasm (spasm of the vocal cords) are uncommon in newborn infants.

The level of iCa that determines which feature of tetany will be manifested varies among individuals and by other components of the extracellular fluid (e.g., hypo-

magnesemia and alkalosis) lower whereas hypokalemia and acidosis raise the threshold for tetany. At physiological concentrations of hydrogen and potassium ion, tetany may develop in older infants at an iCa less than 0.8 mmol/l (3.2 mg/dl) and will almost always be manifested, with the possible exception of preterm infants, at an iCa less than 0.6 mmol/l (2.4 mg/dl). If serum albumin concentrations are normal, the corresponding serum tCa concentrations usually are less than 1.8 mmol/l (7.2 mg/dl). In the preterm infant, serum iCa may not decrease to the same extent as tCa (7,201,246), presumably in part because of the sparing effect of lower serum albumin and acidosis found frequently in these infants, which tend to increase iCa. This also may partially explain the frequent lack of signs of hypocalcemia in preterm infants. The measurement of electrocardiographic QT intervals, corrected for heart rate (247), and standard nomogram relating serum tCa and total protein to ionized Ca (248), have little value for the prediction of neonatal serum iCa. Serum tCa is correlated with iCa (7,23,24,246) but is also inadequate for the prediction of one from the other. Confirmation of hypocalcemia as the cause of clinical symptoms is its reversibility when serum tCa or iCa has been normalized.

C. Management

Any neonate with seizures should have blood drawn for diagnostic tests before therapy (Table 4). Intravenous administration of Ca salts is the most effective and most rapid means of elevating serum Ca concentrations. Gradual or abrupt decrease in heart rate during the infusion is

Table 3 Diagnostic Work-Up for Neonatal Hypocalcemia

History: Screen for risk factors (see Table 1).
Physical Examination
  General examination with focus on peripheral and central nervous and cardiovascular systems.
  Associated features (e.g., infant of a diabetic mother, prematurity, birth asphyxia, congenital heart disease, pseudohypoparathyroidism etc.).
Investigations[a,b]
  Serum total and ionized calcium (tCa and iCa), magnesium and phosphorus, total protein and albumin, and simultaneous intact or whole parathyroid hormone.
  Acid–base status.
  Complete blood count (lymphocyte count).
  Electrocardiogram (Q-Tc > 0.4 s or Q_o-Tc > 0.2 s).
  Chest x-ray (thymic shadow, aortic arch).
  Urine calcium, phosphorus, magnesium, and creatinine.
  Meconium and urine screen for narcotics.
  Maternal serum total and ionized calcium, magnesium and phosphorus, urine calcium and phosphorus, if suspect maternal or heritable Ca disorder, particularly in persistent neonatal hypocalcemia.
  Additional work-up as indicated: vitamin D metabolites, T-cell number and function, malabsorption studies, response to exogenous PTH, molecular genetic studies (deletion of 22q11, PTH receptor and end-organ responsiveness abnormalities, and calcium-sensing receptor defects, etc.) and family screening.

[a]If serum tCa and iCa levels are normal, diagnostic work-up should focus on non-calcium-related causes of clinical symptoms: serum glucose, sepsis workup, screen for excretion of illicit drugs, neuroimaging studies, and others.
[b]Resolution of clinical symptoms when serum tCa or iCa has been normalized confirms the role of hypocalcemia.

Table 4 Management of Neonatal Hypocalcemia

Acute-phase therapy
    Correction of hypomagnesemia, acid–base problem, or others, if possible.
    Intravenous 10–20 mg elemental Ca/kg as 10% Ca gluconate or 10% Ca chloride (provides 9 mg elemental Ca/ml or 27.2
        mg/ml, respectively) with dextrose water or normal saline infused over 5–10 min under constant electrocardiographic
        (ECG) monitoring; repeat as necessary until resolution of severe symptoms such as seizures.
    In infants that are not fed enterally, this is followed by intravenous continuous infusion at 50–75 mg elemental Ca/kg/day.
        Sometimes parenteral nutrition containing 50 mg elemental Ca/100 ml is preferred and continued until feeding.
    In asymptomatic infants, oral 50–75 mg elemental Ca/kg/day in 4–6 divided doses. Elemental Ca/ml of calcium carbonate
        (40 mg), glubionate (23 mg), gluceptate (18 mg), gluconate (9 mg), lactate (13 mg), or chloride (27 mg). One ml of
        each compound contains 40, 23, 18, 9, 13, and 27 mg elemental Ca, respectively. Should be given appropriate low-
        phosphate milk feeding.
    Once serum tCa normalized, halve the Ca supplement for 2 days, then discontinue.
    Serial serum tCa (+/− iCa) every 12–14 h until clinically stable, every 24 h until normalized, and at 24 h after discontin-
        ued Ca supplement.
Maintenance therapy: treat underlying disorder if possible
    For diet-induced hyperphosphatemia: use very-low-phosphorus formula (PM 60/40, Abbott Laboratories, Columbus, OH)
        until serum Ca and P normalized.
    Higher Ca doses and prolonged therapy, may be needed (e.g., hypoparathyroidism).
Follow-up
    Resolution of acute and residual effects from hypocalcemia and underlying disorder.
    Frequency of clinical and laboratory monitoring depends on underlying disorder.
    Family screening and genetic counseling as appropriate.
Complications
    Treatment-related: minimal with continuous ECG monitoring during Ca infusion, avoid infusion into arterial lines (causes
        arterial spasm and tissue necrosis), check patency of venous lines prior to infusion (extravasation causes tissue necrosis).
        Risk for nephrocalcinosis and nephrolithiasis in patients with absent or nonfunctional parathyroid hormone, since protec-
        tive hypocalciuric effect is absent.
    Short-term: depends on the symptomatic manifestations: seizure, apnea, cyanosis and hypoxia, bradycardia and hypoten-
        sion, and others. Risk of metastatic calcification from aggressive Ca treatment in the presence of hyperphosphatemia.
    Long-term: primarily dependent on underlying cause.
Prevention
    Minimize the predisposing risk factors for hypocalcemia, if possible.
    Early milk feeding and use of calcium-containing parenteral nutrition.

an indication to slow or stop the infusion. There is little information on the comparative efficacy of Ca preparations in the treatment of neonatal hypocalcemia. In neonates, 10% Ca gluconate (0.45 mmol [18 mg] elemental Ca/kg) can effectively increase serum iCa, heart rate, cardiac contractility, and blood pressure (195–197). In children, small equimolar doses (0.07 mmol [2.8 mg] elemental Ca/kg) of 10% Ca chloride compared to 10% Ca gluconate may result in higher mean arterial blood pressure with a slightly greater mean increase (0.06 mmol/l, 0.2 mg/dl) in the measured serum iCa (249). Prolonged use of Ca chloride in high dosages may be associated with acidosis and probably should be avoided. With intravenous Ca therapy, bolus infusion may be associated with a transient slight decrease in blood pH and serum P (250) and with hypercalcemia (237). Continuous infusion probably is more efficacious than intermittent therapy (251) to maintain serum Ca in the normal range.

Arterial infusion of Ca in high concentrations potentially is fraught with many dangers and should be avoided.

Massive sloughing of soft tissue may occur in the distribution of the arterial supply, for example, inadvertent administration into a mesenteric artery theoretically can lead to necrosis of intestinal tissues. if umbilical venous catheter is used, the tip should not be intracardiac as administration of Ca directly into the heart may result in arrhythmia. However, parenteral nutrition solutions containing standard mineral (including calcium) content can be safely infused through appropriately positioned umbilical venous or umbilical arterial catheters. Direct admixture of Ca preparation with bicarbonate or phosphate solution will result in precipitation and must be avoided.

All oral Ca preparations are hypertonic, and there is a theoretical potential for precipitating necrotizing enterocolitis in infants at risk for this condition. Oral Ca preparations generally contains higher Ca concentration than intravenous preparations, and is useful for infants, particularly those requiring fluid restriction. However, syrup-based oral Ca preparations have a high sucrose content that may constitute a significant carbohydrate and osmolar load for small preterm infants and may be associated with an increase in frequency of bowel movements. As an alternative an intravenous preparation can be used orally if the fluid volume is tolerated. Concurrent Mg deficiency, if present, must be treated to obtain maximal response to Ca therapy.

The duration of supplemental Ca therapy is usually 2–3 days for early neonatal hypocalcemia. Vitamin D metabolites, 1,25(OH)2D at 0.05–0.2 μg/kg/day, intravenously or orally (252) and 1α-hydroxyvitamin D at 0.33 μg twice daily orally (253); and exogenous PTH (214) have been used in the treatment of neonatal hypocalcemia. However, there is no practical advantage to the use of these agents in place of Ca for the treatment of acute hypocalcemia.

Vitamin D or one of its analogs is often used in addition to adequate Ca intake for the treatment of severe persistent hypocalcemia. The use of 1,25(OH)2D is preferred because it can raise serum Ca within 1–2 days after initiation of therapy and leaves no residual effects within several days of its discontinuation. Vitamin D has slower onset of action of 2–4 weeks and the residual effect also lasts several weeks after its discontinuation, thus making dosage adjustment more difficult. In situations in which PTH is absent or nonfunctional, its hypocalcuric action cannot occur; therefore raising the serum Ca concentration may cause hypercalciuria, renal stones, nephrocalcinosis, and possible renal damage. These complications have been reported during therapy in patients with activating CaR mutation even while the patients are normocalcemic (234).

Successful management of neonatal hypocalcemia also depends on the resolution, if possible, of the primary cause of hypocalcemia. For example, in phosphate-induced hypocalcemia, high-phosphate formulas and solids should be discontinued, and human milk or a low-phosphate formula should be substituted. Use of aluminum hydroxide gel to bind intestinal phosphate should be avoided because of potential risk for aluminum toxicity (254).

Neonatal hypocalcemia may resolve spontaneously. However, hypocalcemia probably should be corrected, because Ca potentially can alter important cellular functions in which calcium serves either as a first or second messenger in cellular activity. Early milk feeding and the use of calcium-containing parenteral nutrition within hours after birth are the best means to minimize the development and recurrence of hypocalcemia, and may negate the need for use of Ca supplementation. Delaying premature delivery and minimizing perinatal asphyxia, judicious use of bicarbonate therapy and mechanical ventilation, for example, during intentional induction of alkalosis in the treatment of persistent pulmonary hypertension (255) are also useful measures to minimize neonatal hypocalcemia. Maintenance of normal maternal vitamin D status with exogenous vitamin D supplement, if needed, may in theory be helpful in maintaining normal fetal vitamin D

status and may secondarily prevent hypocalcemia in some neonates. Early feeding and provision of Ca to the gut may be important in enhancing the ability of vitamin D metabolites to prevent neonatal hypocalcemia.

Pharmacological prevention of neonatal hypocalcemia has focused primarily on the prophylactic use of Ca salts or vitamin D metabolites. In newborn infants, Ca supplementation results in sustained lowering of serum IPTH concentrations compared to unsupplemented controls (60). Ca supplementation may theoretically decrease the metabolic stress from hypocalcemia and minimize the potential for depletion of tissue Ca stores. Early studies used up to 1.8–2.0 mmol (72–80 mg)/kg/day of oral Ca supplement (256,257) and about half this amount intravenously (258) to prevent hypocalcemia. However, it should be noted that a similar amount of Ca can be provided from an intake of 150–200 ml/kg/day of standard term infant formula or human milk. Standard preterm infant formula can provide almost 5 mmol (200 mg) Ca/kg/day and parenteral nutrition with 1.25–1.5 mmol (50–60 mg) Ca/100 ml can easily provide 1.5 mmol (60 mg) of Ca/kg/day. These amounts of Ca are well tolerated as they have been the standard practice in most neonatal nurseries for over a decade. Early feeding or parenteral nutrition must be considered as the best means to prevent neonatal hypocalcemia particularly for the preterm infant. Vitamin D3 at 30 μg (conversion, 1μg = 40 IU)/day orally (259), 25(OH)D at 10 μg/kg/day orally (260), 1α-hydroxyvitamin D3 at 0.05–0.1 μg/kg/day intravenously (261), and 1,25(OH)2D at 0.5–1 μg/day orally (262) or 0.1–4 μg/kg/day intramuscularly or intravenously (7,200) have been used in attempts to prevent neonatal hypocalcemia with variable degrees of success. In small preterm infants, serum Ca was normalized only at pharmacological dosages of 1,25(OH)2D (7). Regular follow-up clinical and laboratory monitoring such as evaluation of serum Ca and IPTH, are necessary in some situations, because there are no definitive measures to determine whether the infant with so-called transient hypoparathyroidism that may last for several years or is at risk for recurrence of hypoparathyroidism and hypocalcemia as late as adolescence (225–227).

VI. HYPERCALCEMIA

Hypercalcemia in infants is rare. However, it is increasingly being diagnosed because serum Ca is usually part of a panel of chemistry tests, and because of increasing knowledge of its pathogenesis. Hypercalcemia is present when serum tCa levels are more than 2.75 mmol/l (11 mg/dl) or when iCa is more than 1.4 mmol/l (5.6 mg/dl). In pathological hypercalcemia, elevation of serum iCa usually occurs simultaneously with elevation of tCa; however, elevated tCa may occur without elevation of iCa. Elevation of protein available to bind Ca (e.g., prolonged application of tourniquet before venipuncture, transudation of plasma water into tissues, in adult patients with multiple myeloma, and possibly adrenal insufficiency) may result in elevation of serum tCa. A change in serum albumin of 1 g/dl generally results in a parallel change in tCa of about 0.2 mmol/l. Conversely, reduced albumin binding of Ca may result in normal serum tCa in the presence of elevated ionized Ca (263).

A. Pathophysiology

Hypercalcemia in infants, particularly in the neonatal intensive care setting, is often iatrogenic from inadequate provision of dietary phosphate during and after hospitalization (43,44; Table 5). Phosphate deficiency or hypophosphatemia stimulates 1α-hydroxylase and synthesis of 1,25(OH)2D, which enhances intestinal absorption and renal reabsorption of Ca and P. Increased Ca absorbed in the presence of increased 1,25(OH)2D cannot be deposited in bone in the absence of phosphate and contributes to hypercalcemia. Details for the hormonal response to hypophosphatemia are discussed in the previous section. The use of Ca supplementation can result in hypercalcemia if there are periods of absent or inadequate phosphate intake (264) and this is augmented by decreased

Table 5 Pathophysiology of Neonatal Hypercalcemia

Phosphate deficiency
   Low or no phosphate but calcium-containing parenteral
      nutrition
   Very-low-birth-weight infants fed human milk or, less
      commonly, standard formula
Parathyroid-related
   Hereditary primary hyperparathyroidism
      Calcium-sensing receptor inactivating mutations: fa-
         milial hypocalciuric hypercalcemia, neonatal severe
         hyperparathyroidism
      PTH receptor activating mutation
   Secondary hyperparathyroidism
      Maternal: hypocalcemia, renal tubular acidosis
      Neonatal: renal tubular acidosis
Parathyroid hormone-related protein-secreting tumors
Vitamin D
   Excessive intake in
      Mother: increase milk vitamin D
      Neonate: high-dosage vitamin D prophylaxis, overfor-
         tification of milk
   Subcutaneous fat necrosis (increase 1,25 dihydroxyvi-
      tamin D)
Calcitonin response impairment (?) in congenital hypothy-
   roidism
Vitamin A excess
Uncertain pathophysiological mechanism
   Idiopathic infantile hypercalcemia/Williams syndrome
   Extracorporeal membrane oxygenation therapy
   Severe infantile hypophosphatasia
   Blue diaper syndrome

renal Ca excretion in the neonate or from underlying illness.

Neonatal hyperparathyroidism frequently results in marked hypercalcemia. It may be a sporadic congenital occurrence or show a mendelian inheritance, or it may be secondary to maternal hypocalcemia. Hereditary primary hyperparathyroidism manifested in neonates is associated with inactivating mutations of CaR. The severity of hypercalcemia is related to the extent of CaR mutation. Mild hypercalcemia (serum tCa <3.0 mmol/l, 12 mg/dl) associated with heterozygous mutated CaR is manifested clinically in most patients with familial hypocalciuric hypercalcemia (FHH). The normal urinary Ca excretion despite hypercalcemia is an effect of the mutated CaR in the kidneys. Serum PTH is usually within the normal range but is higher than expected for the degree of hypercalcemia. FHH has been reported in patients from 2 h to 82 years of age and is usually diagnosed in infants as part of a screening procedure after diagnosis of a family member with hypercalcemia or familial multiple endocrine neoplasia. It is inherited as an autosomal dominant trait with a high degree of penetrance (265,266). There usually is significant hypophosphatemia and a modest increase in serum Mg concentration, and functional parathyroid glands are needed for full expression (265–268). Neonatal hyperparathyroidism associated with FHH that resolves spontaneously over several months has been reported (269). More severe hypercalcemia with serum tCa of 3 to 3.3 mmol/1 (12–13 mg/dl) has been attributed to coexpression of the normal and mutated CaR, with the latter having a functional equivalent of a so-called dominant negative effect (233,270). The most marked hypercalcemia (serum Ca >4 mmol/l, 16 mg/dl) occurs in neonatal severe hyperparathyroidism with homozygous inactivating germ-line mutations of the Ca-sensing receptor gene; the disorder can be lethal within the first few weeks of life (271,272).

Activating mutations of the PTH/PTHrP receptor gene in Jansen metaphyseal dysplasia presumably have the receptor defects in the kidney, bone, and chondrocytes at the growth plate. The clinical manifestation include postnatal-onset short-limb dwarfism with radiographic rachitic changes, and mild hypercalcemia occurs in about 50% of affected patients (273,274).

Maternal hypocalcemia results in neonatal hyperparathyroidism (275). Neonatal hyperparathyroidism also may occur in the presence of maternal (276) or neonatal (277,278) renal tubular acidosis. In these situations, metabolic acidosis independently increases bone resorption (279), enhances the renal effects of hyperparathyroidism (280), and the hypercalcemic effect is augmented by decreased renal excretory capacity of the neonate.

Elevated serum PTHrP and hypercalcemia are found in an increasing number of infants with a variety of tumors (281–283). There is also associated mortality in some cases although the relative contribution of hypercalcemia and the underlying disease to death is not clear.

Other pathological conditions associated with increased bone turnover or increased intestinal or renal Ca absorption may result in hypercalcemia. Hypercalcemia was reported in 34% of neonates and infants from intermittent high-dosage vitamin D (600,000 IU each 3–5 months) prophylaxis (284). Hypercalcemia also has been reported in infants given human milk with very high vitamin D content (7000 IU/L) from high-dosage vitamin D therapy for maternal hypoparathyroidism (285), milks with excessive vitamin D fortification from errors during processing (286,287), and in preterm infants given chronic vitamin D supplementation in addition to high-Ca and high-P milk formula (288). Neonates with extensive subcutaneous fat necrosis may develop hypercalcemia after a period of low or normal serum Ca concentrations. There is often a history of perinatal asphyxia (289–291) and anecdotal report that body cooling (291) for the treatment of birth asphyxia could augment the development of subcutaneous fat necrosis. Hypercalcemia is reported to occur between 2 and 16 weeks, most commonly at 6–7 weeks. Increased prostaglandin E activity, increased release of Ca from fat and other tissues, and unregulated production of 1,25(OH)2D from macrophages infiltrating fat necrotic lesions have been postulated to be responsible for the hypercalcemia in these conditions (292). Vitamin A toxicity is associated with hypercalcemia presumably secondary to increased bone turnover (293).

Hypercalcemia may develop before and during thyroxine therapy of infants with congenital agoitrous hypothyroidism (294). In theory, deficient CT response to Ca loading or an increased degradation of CT may be responsible for the hypercalcemia.

Neonatal hypercalcemia is reported in other situations in which the pathophysiology remains uncertain. Idiopathic infantile hypercalcemia, often considered as part of Williams syndrome, is associated with varying manifestations including hypercalcemia, mental retardation, elfin facies, and supravalvular aortic stenosis. There also may be prenatal and postnatal growth failure. The presence of hypercalcemia in infants with Williams syndrome is variable, and serum Ca may be normal, but the presence of nephrocalcinosis and soft tissue calcifications in some of these infants suggests that hypercalcemia may have occurred previously. An exaggerated response to pharmacological dosages of vitamin D2 (18,000–100,000 IU) (295) and a blunted CT response to Ca loading and PTH infusion (296) may contribute to the pathogenesis of hypercalcemia of idiopathic infantile hypercalcemia. Several genetic defects in idiopathic infantile hypercalcemia, including hemizygosity at the elastin gene on the long arm of chromosome 7, have been reported (297,298). No mutation of the CT/CGRP gene has been detected (299). However, the cellular mechanism that led to the phenotypic expression remains unknown. Transient hypercalcemia occurs in infants during extracorporeal membrane oxygenation therapy varies from <5% (300,301) to about 30% (302) depending on whether the cutoff point used

was >2.5 or >2.25 mmol (12 mg or 11 mg/dl) respectively. Severe infantile hypophosphatasia is associated with hypercalcemia. It is a rare autosomal recessive disorder associated with decreased synthesis of tissue nonspecific alkaline phosphatase from a deletion or point mutation in its gene located on chromosome 1. These patients have severe bone demineralization, low serum alkaline phosphatase, and elevated urinary pyrophosphate and phosphoethanolamine. The condition may be lethal in utero or shortly after birth because of inadequate bony support of the thorax and skull, although milder phenotypes are compatible with survival to adulthood (303,304). Blue diaper syndrome is a rare familial disorder with defect in intestinal transport of tryptophan. The blue discoloration of the urine results from the hydrolysis and oxidation of urinary indican, an end-product of intestinal degradation of unabsorbed tryptophan and hepatic metabolism of its intermediate metabolites. Hypercalcemia and nephrocalcinosis usually do not manifest until some months after birth (305).

B. Diagnosis

Neonates with hypercalcemia may be asymptomatic despite the onset of hypercalcemia at birth (Table 6). In these cases, there is often delayed for weeks or months before diagnosis is made coincidental to a chemistry panel screening during the course of other illness or because of hypercalcemia in another family member.

Severe hypercalcemia can be fatal (272,281,289,293) although some of the infants have other potentially lethal underlying conditions such as hepatic sarcoma. Symptoms and signs frequently are nonspecific and include lethargy, irritability, poor feeding with or without feeding intolerance, constipation, polyuria, dehydration, and failure to thrive. Hypertension associated with hypercalcemia in adults also may occur in infants, although it may be in part related to relative fluid overload in infants who require extracorporeal membrane oxygen (ECMO) therapy. Ectopic deposition of a solid phase of calcium and phosphate in walls of blood vessels, and in connective tissue about the joints, gastric mucosa, renal parenchyma, and cornea may occur with persistent hypercalcemia, especially when accompanied by normal or elevated levels of serum P. Anatomical anomalies (e.g., elfin facies, evidence of congenital heart disease, subcutaneous fat necrosis) may be present on physical examination.

C. Treatment

Therapy depends on the extent of elevation of serum Ca and whether the infant is symptomatic (Table 7). For mildly elevated serum tCa (<12 mg/dl) in the presence of iatrogenic cause (e.g., phosphate free parenteral nutrition or the use of Ca supplement without any dietary phosphate intake), resolution of the underlying cause should resolve the problem. Dietary P deficiency induced hypercalcemia is becoming less common with the increasing

Table 6 Diagnostic Work-Up for Neonatal Hypercalcemia

History
  Familial or maternal disturbances in calcium (Ca) or
    phosphorus (P) metabolism
  Gestational age, difficult labor, ECMO, and pre-ECMO
    therapy
  Intake of calcium, phosphorus, vitamins D and A:
    mother and infant
Physical Examination
  General examination with focus on growth parameters,
    hydration status, heart rate, blood pressure, cornea
    for band keratopathy (rare)
  Associated features (e.g., subcutaneous fat necrosis, elfin
    facies, congenital heart disease, developmental de-
    lay)
Investigations
  Serum total and ionized Ca, magnesium, P, creatinine
    (Cr), total protein and albumin, alkaline phosphatase
    (total and bone specific), simultaneous so-called in-
    tact or whole parathyroid hormone (PTH), 25 hy-
    droxyvitamin D and 1,25 dihydroxyvitamin D
  Acid–base status
  Urine Ca, P, Cr, amino acids
  X-ray of chest, hands, and long bones
  Ultrasound of kidneys and abdomen, ophthalmological
    examination, eletrocardiogram (shortened QT inter-
    val, bradycardia) for complications
  Other tests if above do not yield diagnosis
    Parental (both parents) serum and urine Ca, P, Cr
    Serum PTH-related protein
    Screen for occult tumor
    Serum vitamin A
    Molecular studies
    Family screening depends on the primary diagnosis

use of commercial fortifier for human-milk-fed preterm infants, and the use of high Ca- and high P-containing infant formula and parenteral nutrition for the preterm infant. In patients with low serum P concentrations, large amounts of phosphate supplement may result in diarrhea and hypocalcemia and the possibility of metastatic calcification (306).

With moderate to severe hypercalcemia, the initial treatment is nonspecific with expansion of extracellular fluid compartment and furosemide-induced diuresis (307). Minimal information is available on the use of hormonal and other drug therapy for neonatal hypercalcemia. Non-mammalian sources of CT (e.g., salmon CT) has a greater hypocalcemic effect and longer duration of action compared with recombinant human CT. However, salmon CT has greater potential for allergic reaction and induction of antibody formation. The hypocalcemic effect decreases after a few days of any CT treatment. Steroid-induced hypertension, hyperglycemia, and gastrointestinal hemor-

rhage are significant problems (308), and thus are not recommended for long-term therapy. Bisphosphonates, oral etidronate (25 mg twice daily), and intravenous pamidronate (0.5 mg/kg) have been used for treatment of hypercalcemia in the mother and neonate (291,309). However, long-term effects on growth plate, bone production, and mineralization remain unknown (310), and its use should be restricted to acute short-term therapy. Dialysis in the neonate is not without technical or metabolic complications. In rare cases, parathyroidectomy may be necessary, although it is not always effective.

Treatment for chronic conditions also includes restriction of dietary intake of vitamin D and Ca and minimizing exposure to sunlight to decrease endogenous vitamin D production. A low-Ca, low-vitamin D3, low-iron infant formula is available for the management of hypercalcemia in infants (Calcilo XD, Abbott Laboratories, Columbus, OH). This formula contains only trace amounts of Ca <10 mg/100 kcal) and no vitamin D. Long-term use of this formula alone will lead to calcium depletion; iatrogenic vitamin D deficiency is also a concern in this situation, and both can result in deleterious consequences.

Neonatal hypercalcemia may not develop until some weeks after the onset of the insult and may resolve spontaneously as in subcutaneous necrosis. Therefore, serum Ca should be monitored at regular intervals in certain situations to determine the onset of hypercalcemia and to determine the need to continue treatment. Family screening for hypercalcemia should be done unless a specific nonfamilial cause for hypercalcemia is established in the index case.

VII. HYPOPHOSPHATEMIA

An infant can be considered to be hypophosphatemic when serum P concentration is <1.3 mmol/l (conversion, 1 mmol/l = 3.1 mg/dl).

A. Pathophysiology

Hypophosphatemia usually has a nutritional basis and occurs most frequently in infants receiving low P intake from parenteral nutrition (45,46) and in preterm infants fed unfortified human milk (43,44,311; Table 8). Hypophosphatemia occurs with administration of glucose, and it may be accentuated during starvation (312,313). The so-called refeeding syndrome from overzealous increase in the delivery of nutrients, particularly calories, can be associated with multiple electrolyte abnormalities, including hypophosphatemia, hypokalemia, hypomagnesemia, and hypocalcemia, and life-threatening complications (313–316). Glucose and P moved from extracellular to intracellular compartments to meet the metabolic needs leads to lowering of serum P. This decreases renal phosphate load and secondarily decreases urinary phosphate excretion. Insulin facilitates these processes (317). Respiratory alkalosis, liver disease, and hypokalemia also

Table 7 Management of Neonatal Hypercalcemia

Acute
  Remove causative factor, if possible (e.g., discontinue vitamin D and Ca supplement).
  Intravenous normal saline (20 ml/kg) and loop diuretic (furosemide 2 mg/kg). Reassess and repeat every 4–6 h as necessary. Monitor fluid balance and serum calcium, magnesium, sodium, potassium, phosphorus, and osmolality every 6–12 h. Prolonged diuresis may require Mg and potassium replacement.
  Use lower Ca content milk or parenteral nutrition if possible to maintain nutrition.
  In neonates with low serum P (<1.3 mmol/l; 4 mg/dl), oral phosphate supplement at 0.5–1 mmol (15–30 mg) elemental P/kg/day in four divided doses may normalize serum P and Ca. In infants not being fed, can use parenteral nutrition containing usual amount of phosphate (1–1.5 mmol (31–46 mg)/100 ml).
  Minimal data on the use of hormone (e.g., subcutaneous or intramuscular recombinant human calcitonin [4–8 IU/kg every 6 h], +/− oral glucocorticoid [prednisone 0.5–1 mg/kg/d]. Other drugs (e.g., bisphonates [pamidronate 0.5 mg/kg intravenously] are experimental.
  Peritoneal or hemodialysis with a low-calcium dialysate may be considered in severely symptomatic patient refractory to medical therapy.
  Parathyroidectomy may be needed when clinically stabilized.
Maintenance
  Depends on underlying cause.
  Additional general therapy may be needed: low-Ca, no-vitamin-D infant formula (Calcilo XD, Abbott Laboratories, Columbus, OH); minimal sunlight exposure to lower endogenous synthesis of vitamin D.
Follow-up
  Resolution of acute and residual effects from hypercalcemia and underlying disorder.
  Frequency of clinical and laboratory monitoring depends on underlying disorder (e.g., in extensive subcutaneous fat necrosis, regular serum calcium is needed to monitor for the later onset and the need to continue treatment).
  Family screening and genetic counseling as appropriate.
Complications
  Acute: fluid electrolyte imbalance.
  Chronic: failure to thrive, nephrocalcinosis, hypocalcemia and bone demineralization from excessive limitation of Ca and vitamin D intake, and those associated with underlying disorders.

may contribute to so-called shift hypophosphatemia. In infants receiving parenteral nutrition, hypophosphatemia is exaggerated if there is an associated rapid increase in delivery of carbohydrates (glucose), probably the result of transcellular shift of P in addition to a relative or absolute deficiency in P intake.

Hypophosphatemia from decreased intestinal P absorption can be an early manifestation of vitamin D deficiency (318,319). In theory, any severe and prolonged malabsorption syndrome may be associated with hypophosphatemia. Excessive nutrient intake, including sodium, glucose, amino acids, particularly if they are delivered intravenously, may exceed the renal reabsorptive capacity or lead to extracellular fluid compartment expansion. Both can result in increased renal loss of water and the infused nutrients including P, since renal excretory mechanisms for most nutrients (including P and water) are interdependent and are generally affected by sodium-dependent cotransport systems. Thus, increase in renal excretion of any of these nutrients potentially can increase the renal P excretion (69).

Nonnutritional causes of neonatal hypophosphatemia are much less frequent than nutritional causes. In the latter situations, the primary mechanism for hypophosphatemia

is probably decreased renal P reabsorption, which may or may not be secondary to elevated PTH.

B. Diagnosis

Serum P is usually normal at birth (Table 9). Hypophosphatemia may occur within days of birth or from the onset of the causative factor such as the use of phosphate-free parenteral nutrition. Acute hypophosphatemia in neonates is usually asymptomatic and may be diagnosed from routine screening because of a family history of disturbances in mineral metabolism. Hypophosphatemia may be an early manifestation of P deficiency. Chronic hypophosphatemia is indicative of P deficiency and may have multiple clinical consequences affecting hematological, immunological, cardiorespiratory, neuromuscular, skeletal, and peripheral and central nervous systems (320). These include impairment of oxygen release from hemoglobin, neutrophil dysfunction, muscle weakness and respiratory failure, and skeletal demineralization and deformity. Clinical signs such as muscle weakness attributed to hypophosphatemia are usually noted when the serum P concentration is <0.7 mmol/l (2.2 mg/dl). However, many of the clinical signs of P deficiency are masked by the un-

Table 8 Pathophysiology of Neonatal Hypophosphatemia

Nutritional
    Low phosphate intake
        Low- or no-phosphate parenteral nutrition
        Human milk or standard milk formula for preterm infants
    Transcellular shift: Refeeding syndrome
    Low phosphorus absorption
        Vitamin D deficiency
        Malabsorption
    Elevated renal phosphorus loss
        Vitamin D deficiency with secondary hyperparathyroidism
        Excessive nutrient intake: sodium, glucose, amino acids
Nonnutritional
    Hyperparathyroidism
    X-linked hypophosphatemic rickets
    Fanconi's syndrome (idiopathic or secondary to inborn errors of metabolism such as cystinosis and tyrosinosis)
    Chronic diuretic therapy

derlying illness or by the therapy administered to the infant; for example, bronchopulmonary dysplasia and hypophosphatemia may occur simultaneously, and it may be difficult to differentiate the relative contribution of each to the respiratory failure in an affected infant. Multiple blood transfusion may mask the effect of decreased oxy-

Table 9 Diagnostic Work-Up for Neonatal Hypophosphatemia

History
    Family history of mineral metabolism disorders
    Gestational age
    Dietary history
    Chronic diuretic therapy
Physical examination
    General examination with focus on growth parameters, muscle tone, and skeletal abnormalities
    Associated features (e.g., inborn errors of metabolism)
Investigations
    Serum phosphorus, total and ionized calcium, magnesium, glucose, creatinine, alkaline phosphatase
    Urine phosphorus, glucose, calcium, creatinine
    Other tests if above do not yield diagnosis
        Serum intact or whole parathyroid hormone, 25 hydroxyvitamin D, 1,25 dihydroxyvitamin D, amino acid
        Urine amino acids
        X-rays of hands and long bones (rachitic and hyperparathyroid changes)

gen delivery associated with hypophosphatemia. More dramatic skeletal manifestations of prolonged and severe hypophosphatemia, such as rickets and osteomalacia, usually are not present until after the neonatal period (38, 47,231,319,321–325). Infants with X-linked hypophosphatemic vitamin-D-resistant rickets (HDDR), a dominantly inherited disorder of renal P wasting, usually do not have hypophosphatemia at birth. However, serial monitoring of infants in these families show hypophosphatemia, decreased percentage renal tubular reabsorption of P (100% × P clearance/creatinine clearance), increased bone turnover as indicated by increased serum alkaline phosphatase and increased urinary hydroxyproline, occur in affected infants as early as 3 weeks after birth (325) and in most affected infants by 3 months (324,325). Onset of growth delay and radiographic rachitic changes depend on the success of therapy and may occur during infancy. In other situations, such as neonatal primary hyperparathyroidism and Fanconi's syndrome, the presenting symptoms and signs may be unrelated to hypophosphatemia.

In most cases of neonatal hypophosphatemia, the diagnosis can be made with a careful review of the history and results of a few laboratory investigations. Severe hypophosphatemia (serum P < 0.7 mmol/l) can result from nutritional causes and is typically associated with hypercalcemia, almost total absence of P in the urine and urine Ca may be elevated (i.e., renal tubules that are resistant to the PTH effects) (43).

C. Treatment

Nutritional hypophosphatemia may be treated with P supplementation at 0.5–1.5 mmol/kg elemental P per day. Calcium supplementation (see Sec. V.C) is useful because it may minimize the fall in serum Ca concentration during P treatment, and it would alleviate Ca deficiency, which also occurs frequently in these infants (47). However, the best means to deliver the appropriate amount of P and Ca is by providing a balanced intake of all nutrients with high-P and high-Ca milk or parenteral nutrition (47). Standard vitamin D supplementation of 400 IU/day is adequate therapy for vitamin-D-deficient rickets in infancy (319). Therapy of nonnutritional hypophosphatemia varies with underlying disorder. For example, early administration of 1,25(OH)2D at 30–40 ng/kg/day and phosphate at 40–50 mg/kg/day in addition to adequate general nutritional intake can improve mineral metabolism and may be useful to obviate severe growth delay and leg deformities (324, 325).

VIII. HYPERPHOSPHATEMIA

An infant can be considered to be hyperphosphatemic when the serum P concentration is >2.6 mmol/l (conversion, 1 mmol/l = 3.1 mg/dl).

A. Pathophysiology

Nutritional causes usually occur with the infusion of excessive P content (45) or alternating delivery of Ca and P in parenteral nutrition solution (264). Ingestion of cows' milk-type formulas (42; Table 10) and early introduction of high-P-containing cereals (205) may lead to neonatal hyperphosphatemia. Accidental overdose of oral phosphate supplement can be fatal (208). Vitamin D (291) and vitamin A (298) toxicity may result in hyperphosphatemia, in addition to hypercalcemia, from increased bone turnover. Nonnutritional causes include an excess phosphate load from the use of P-containing enemas (206,207). Other causes are usually associated with diminished P excretion. Neonates with asphyxia may have increased release of intracellular P to the extracellular compartment in addition to a low renal glomerular filtration. Decreased P excretion and hyperphosphatemia in the neonate can result from intrinsic renal failure, such as congenitally dysplastic kidneys, and from absent or nonfunctional PTH, such as hypoparathyroid and pseudohypoparathyroid states.

B. Diagnosis

History and physical examination consistent with clinical situations (Table 10) are useful for the diagnosis. Clinical features associated with underlying disorder such as Albright's hereditary osteodystrophy may be present. Serum P is usually normal at birth even in neonates with intrinsic renal failure or PTH disorders and increases during the first few days. There is usually concurrent hypocalcemia. Hyperphosphatemia, and hypocalcemia, may occur within hours after a phosphate load (208). Hyperphosphatemia may be asymptomatic, or it may be manifested because of its associated hypocalcemia effects (see Sec. V).

C. Treatment

Removal of excessive P load if possible, for example eliminating or minimizing the P load with the use of so-

Table 10 Pathogenesis of
Neonatal Hyperphosphatemia

Nutritional
  High phosphate load
    Cow-milk-type formula
    Parenteral nutrition
    Cereal
    Accidental overdose
  Hypervitaminosis D and A
Nonnutritional
  High phosphate load from phosphate enema
  Diminished phosphorus excretion
    Perinatal asphyxia
    Renal failure
    Hypoparathyroidism
    Pseudohypoparathyroidism

called humanized formulas with low P content and a high Ca/P ratio of about 2:1, and temporarily discontinuing the use of cereals. A brief period of Ca supplementation is necessary if there is associated hypocalcemia.

Nonspecific lowering of serum P for the acute management of hyperphosphatemia may be achieved with normal saline infusion and forced natriuresis as for hypercalcemia (see Sec. VI). The use of Ca or aluminum salts as chelating agent for intestinal phosphate in the presence of hyperphosphatemia may predispose to metastatic calcification with the former (306) and potential for aluminum toxicity (254) and are not recommended.

For conditions that cause long term hyperphosphatemia, the treatment is aimed at the underlying cause.

IX. SKELETAL MANIFESTATIONS OF DISTURBED MINERAL HOMEOSTASIS

A. Pathophysiology

True fetal or congenital rickets is rare (Table 11). It may result from severe maternal nutritional osteomalacia associated with Ca and vitamin D deficiency (326–328), maternal hypoparathyroidism (203) or hyperparathyroidism (202), or prolonged maternal treatment with Mg sulfate (329) or phosphate-containing enemas (330).

The most frequent cause of skeletal abnormalities in infancy is nutritional deficiency. In the Western world, rickets and osteopenia presenting during infancy occur most frequently in small preterm infants and may occur in more than 30% of extremely low-birth-weight (<1 kg) infants. The rate of occurrence depends on the nutrient intake and is associated most frequently with prolonged

Table 11 Risk Factors for Osteopenia and Rickets
in Infants

Intrauterine
  Severe maternal nutritional osteomalacia (i.e., Ca and vitamin D deficiency)
  Maternal hypoparathyroidism and hyperparathyroidism
  Prolonged maternal magnesium or phosphate treatment
Postnatal
  Nutritional
    Prolonged exclusive human milk feeding
    Macrobiotic diet
    Soy formula or unfortified human milk for small preterm infants
    Prolonged total parenteral nutrition with low Ca and/or low P
    Chronic loop diuretic therapy given to preterm infants
    Aluminum contamination (?)
  Inherited defects
    Renal tubular disorder
    Vitamin D or parathyroid hormone metabolism disorders

Source: From Ref. 347.

intake of soy formula, unfortified human milk, and/or low-Ca and low-P parenteral nutrition (47). In infants born at term, prolonged exclusive human milk feeding with limited exposure to sunshine, macrobiotic diet, and prolonged total parenteral nutrition are factors that contribute to the development of osteopenia and rickets (38, 319,321–323). The common underlying causes in preterm infants appear to be mineral deficiency, particularly Ca and P, whereas in term infants Ca deficiency is also important. Preterm infants fed unfortified human milk or term infants fed standard milk formula often have low serum 25OHD concentrations. The major reason for the low serum 25OHD in these situations is the increased metabolism of 25OHD with mineral deficiency, in particular, Ca deficiency (see Sec. III.C). Ca and P deficiency was demonstrated as the major cause of osteopenia and rickets in preterm infants over 2 decades ago (331). This has been confirmed by many investigators (47) and the use of high-Ca and high-P milk and parenteral intake with a daily supplementation of 400–800 IU vitamin D is sufficient to maintain serum 25OHD in the normal range (177, 331,332). Unfortunately, vitamin D deficiency secondary to inadequate mineral deficiency is still frequently misdiagnosed as the primary cause of osteopenia, fracture, and rickets in preterm infants and treated with more vitamin D supplement without improving the mineral and general nutritional support. Calcium deficiency also is an important cause of rickets in young children living in subtropical regions with adequate vitamin D status (38). Isolated nutritional deficiency of copper and ascorbic acid has been reported in preterm infants with clinical and radiographic manifestations similar to rickets (47). Chronic diuretic therapy, commonly used in infants with bronchopulmonary dysplasia, and contamination of nutrients with toxins such as aluminum are added risk factors (246,323). The extent, however, to which each specific risk factor is responsible for the development of osteopenia, fractures, and rickets is difficult to define in critically ill infants receiving multiple therapies and suboptimal nutritional support.

Acquired and heritable forms of rickets that occur despite adequate availability of vitamin D usually are associated with renal tubular disorders and metabolic defects in vitamin D and PTH metabolism (202,203,231,324, 325). These causes of rickets are rare, and their skeletal manifestations may present during infancy.

B. Diagnosis

History of significant nutritional defect in the mother either from self-selected dietary restriction or cultural habits (e.g., extensive covering of the body with lack of sunlight exposure), or family history of metabolic disorders and disturbed bone mineral metabolism should raise the awareness of the potential for nutritional and skeletal problems in both the mother and infant.

Infants with congenital rickets may be asymptomatic at birth leading to a delay in diagnosis unless investiga-

tions are performed as part of the work-up for disturbances in maternal mineral metabolism. Most postnatal cases of rickets and osteopenia are diagnosed incidentally during the radiographic investigation of skeletal complications such as fractures or nonskeletal problems such as respiratory illness. Radiographic features such as generalized bone demineralization and widening, cupping, and fraying of the distal metaphyses confirm presence of osteopenia and rickets (332–334).

Classic clinical features of rickets such as severe skeletal deformities, including kyphoscoliosis and bowing of the legs, may not be present if the diagnosis is made early in infancy, before significant growth and weight-bearing have occurred. This is particularly true for the preterm infant whose skeletal problem typically is diagnosed between 2 and 6 months postnatally. With the current practice of early discharge of preterm infants from neonatal units, it is possible that some nutritional rickets could be diagnosed after hospital discharge. If there are associated fractures, it may be misdiagnosed as child abuse. Clinical hypotonia is probably due to a decrease in intracellular phosphate pool of skeletal muscle (335).

Serial biochemical changes commonly include persistently low serum inorganic phosphate, elevated serum alkaline phosphatase activity more than five times the normal adult upper limit, and other bone turnover markers in serum and urine also can be elevated. Serum Ca is usually normal except in late severe nutritional rickets. Vitamin D deficiency as indicated by low or undetectable serum 25 OHD is possible; and is usually secondary to mineral deficiency in a small preterm infant. There may be elevated serum 1,25(OH)2D and IPTH with Ca, P, and vitamin D deficiency. The elevated PTH and 1,25(OH)2D still may be relatively insufficient to maintain Ca and P homeostasis if the Ca and P intake remain low. Urine changes may reflect increased serum IPTH with increased urine P excretion and Ca conservation. However, in chronic mineral deficiency, particular of P, urine findings may reflect changes of PTH resistance, in which case urine P would be minimal while there is calcuria. Measurement of specific trace mineral status may be useful if deficiency is suspected (177,336–339). The use of dual energy X-ray absorptiometry (DXA) allows a more accurate quantification of the degree of bone mineralization (340). Additional investigations are needed if inherited renal tubular disorders and for disorders of vitamin D and PTH metabolism are suspected.

C. Prevention and Treatment

Rickets and fractures from nutritional deficiencies respond well to adequate nutrient intake. The best treatment for nutritional osteopenia, fractures and rickets is prevention. For preterm infants, these skeletal problems appear to have become less frequent with increased Ca and P intake through the widespread use of high-Ca and high-P parenteral nutrition until establishment of enteral feeding with human milk containing commercial fortifier or formulas designed specifically for preterm infants (47). Human milk is likely to be low in a number of nutrients including protein, sodium, calcium, P, and possibly other nutrients for the needs of the very small preterm infant (43,47,311,341,342). All very small preterm infants, particularly those with birth weights less than 1500 g should receive commercial fortifier containing multiple nutrients during their hospital stay and probably after hospital discharge.

With established osteopenia with or without fractures or rickets, the use of Ca and P supplementation alone is inappropriate since bone growth requires protein and multiple other nutrients for matrix formation and mineralization. In addition, further large increases in Ca and P intake beyond the current recommended intake is probably not advisable because of the risks of bezoar and even intestinal obstruction with excessive oral intake (47), and hyperphosphatemia with intravenous intake (45). In preterm infants, most fractures show significant callus formation at diagnosis and only require splinting support (343). Short-term analgesia is needed if the fracture is recent and without callus formation. The ingestion of the recommended daily amount of Ca and P should be adequate for otherwise healthy term infants (344,345).

Normal vitamin D status can be maintained in enterally fed healthy term infants without vitamin D supplementation provided adequate sunlight exposure is assured (173–175). In any case, a daily supplementation of 400 IU vitamin D should be adequate (175,176). Enterally fed preterm infants given high Ca- high P- and vitamin-D-fortified preterm infant formula or human milk with similar fortification from commercial human milk fortifiers probably do not require vitamin D supplementation. In any case, a daily supplementation of 400–800 IU vitamin D should be adequate (177,331,332). For infants who require parenteral nutrition as the major source of nutritional support, a maximum total daily intake of 400 IU vitamin D is sufficient to maintain vitamin D status regardless of the gestational age of the infant (45,46). For infants with established nutritional vitamin D deficiency, a daily supplementation of 400 IU vitamin D in addition to adequate overall nutritional support is also adequate (319).

Specific therapies are required for inherited renal tubular disorders and for disorders of vitamin D and PTH metabolism and usually include one or more of the following: calcium, phosphate, and 1,25(OH)2D.

D. Monitoring and Follow-Up

The goal is for affected infants to grow normally without residual defect. Regular clinical assessment and growth measurements are essential. Short-term follow-up of infants with nutritional rickets including preterm infants show no major residual physical deformity (319,343). Skeletal maturation as assessed by ossification centers of the wrists for preterm infants is similar to term infants at 1 year of age (343). However, long-term linear growth in the extremely low-birth-weight infants may remain de-layed (346), indicating that bone mineral status in the smallest preterm infants still may be suboptimal despite the relatively uncommon occurrence of radiographic rickets and fractures on follow-up. Screening for other affected family members and molecular studies may be warranted in heritable conditions.

Biochemical monitoring of nutritional rickets includes maintaining normal serum Ca, P, and alkaline phosphatase levels, while avoiding hypercalciuria (<0.15 mmol, 6 mg Ca/kg/day) every 1–2 weeks until normalized. Measurement of bone turnover markers, IPTH, vitamin D metabolites such as 25OHD and 1,25(OH)2D, and any other abnormal biochemical parameter, every 1–2 months until normalized. Standard skeletal radiographs every 2–4 months to check for healing and remodeling. Serial measurements of bone mineral content by DXA every 2–4 months also may be useful to monitor the progress of bone mineralization during long-term follow-up. Other specific monitoring would depend on the underlying cause.

REFERENCES

1. Steichen JJ, Tsang RC, Gratton TL, Hamstra A, DeLusa HF. Vitamin D homeostasis in the perinatal period: 1,25-dihydroxyvitamin D in maternal, cord and neonatal blood. N Engl J Med 1980; 302:315.
2. Saggese G, Baroncelli GI, Bertelloni S, Cipolloni C. Intact parathyroid hormone levels during pregnancy, in healthy term neonates and in hypocalcemic preterm infants. Acta Pediatr Scand 1991; 80:36.
3. Thiebaud D, Janisch S, Koelbl H, Hanzal E, Jacquet AF, Leodolter S, et al. Direct evidence of a parathyroid related protein gradient between the mother and the newborn in humans. Bone Miner 1993; 23:213.
4. Seki K, Wada S, Nagata N, Nagata I. Parathyroid hormone-related protein during pregnancy and the perinatal period. Gynecol Obstet Invest 1994; 37:83.
5. Tsang RC, Oh W. Neonatal hypocalcemia in low birth weight infants. Pediatrics 1970;45:773.
6. Snodgrass GJ, Stemmler L, Went J, Abrams ME, Will EJ. Interrelations of plasma calcium, inorganic phosphate, magnesium and protein over the first week of life. Arch Dis Child 1973; 48:279.
7. Koo WWK, Tsang RC, Poser JW, Laskarzewski P, Buckley D, Johnson R, et al. Elevated serum calcium and osteocalcin levels from calcitriol in preterm infants. A prospective randomized study. Am J Dis Child 1986; 140:1152.
8. Nelson NA, Finnstrom O, Larsson L. Plasma ionized calcium, phosphate and magnesium in preterm and small for gestational age infants. Acta Paediatr Scand 1989; 78:351.
9. Greer FR, Tsang RC, Levin RS, Searcy JE, Wu R, Steichen JJ. Increasing serum calcium and magnesium concentrations in breast fed infants: longitudinal studies of minerals of human milk and in sera of nursing mothers and their infants. J Pediatr 1982; 100:59.
10. Specker BL, Lichtenstein P, Mimouni F, Gormley C, Tsang RC. Calcium regulating hormones and minerals from birth to 18 months: a cross sectional study. II. Effects of sex, race, age, season and diet on serum minerals, parathyroid hormone, and calcitonin. Pediatrics 1986; 77:891.

11. Soldin S, Hicks JM. Calcium and ionized calcium. Pediatric reference ranges. Washington, DC: American Association for Clinical Chemistry Press, 1995:38.

12. Markowitz M, Rotkin L, Rosen IR. Circadian rhythms of blood minerals in humans. Science 1981; 213:672.

13. Pitkin RM. Calcium metabolism in pregnancy and perinatal period: a review. Am J Obstet Gynecol 1985; 151: 99.

14. Forman D, Lorenzo L. Ionized calcium: its significance and clinical usefulness. Ann Clin Lab Sci 1991; 21:297.

15. Bowers GN, Jr, Brassard C, Sena SF. Measurement of ionized calcium in serum with ion-selective electrodes: a mature technology that can meet the daily service needs. Clin Chem 1986; 32:1437.

16. D'Orazio P, Bowers GN Jr. Design and preliminary performance characteristics of a newly proposed reference cell for ionized calcium in serum. Clin Chem 1992; 38: 1332.

17. Mimouni A, Mimouni F, Mimouni C, Mou S, Ho M. Effects of albumin on ionized calcium in vitro. Pediatr Emerg Care 1991; 7:149.

18. Liu C, Mimouni F, Ho M, Tsang R. In vitro effect of magnesium on ionized calcium concentration in serum. Am J Dis Child 1988; 142:837.

19. Lehmann M, Mimouni F. Serum phosphate concentration. Effect on serum ionized calcium concentration in vitro. Am J Dis Child 1989; 143:1340.

20. Hughes WS, Aurbach GD, Sharp ME, Marx SJ. The effect of the bicarbonate anion on serum ionized calcium concentration in vitro. J Lab Clin Med 1984; 103:93.

21. Fogh-Andersen N, Frederiksen PS, Andersen EA, Thode J. Relation between ionized calcium and pH in infants with acute acid-base disturbances. Clin Chim Acta 1983; 130:357.

22. Wandrup J, Kancir C, Norgaard-Pederson B. The concentration of free calcium ions in capillary blood from neonates on a routine basis using the ICA 1. Scand J Clin Lab Invest 1984; 44:19.

23. Marshall RW, Hodgkinson A. Calculation of plasma ionized calcium from total calcium, protein and pH: comparison with measured values. Clin Chim Acta 1983; 127: 305.

24. Loughead JL, Mimouni F, Tsang RC. Serum ionized calcium concentrations in normal neonates. Am J Dis Child 1988; 142:516.

25. Brown E, Vassilev P, Hebert S. Calcium ions as extracellular messengers. Cell 1995; 83:679.

26. Hurwitz S. Homeostatic control of plasma calcium concentration. Crit Rev Biochem Mol Biol 1996; 31:41.

27. Sorrentino V, Rizzuto R. Molecular genetics of Ca(2+) stores and intracellular Ca(2+) signaling. Trends Pharmacol Sci 2001; 22:459.

28. Parfitt AM. Plasma calcium control at quiescent bone surfaces: a new approach to the homeostatic function of bone lining cells. Bone 1989; 10:87.

29. Canalis E. Systemic and local factors and the maintenance of bone quality. Calcif Tiss Int 1993; 53(Suppl 1): S90.

30. Parfitt AM. The bone remodeling compartment: a circulatory function for bone lining cells. J Bone Miner Res 2001; 16:1583.

31. Abrams SA, Yergey AL, Schanler RJ, Vieira NE, Welch TR. Hypercalciuria in premature infants receiving high mineral-containing diets. J Pediatr Gastroenterol Nutr 1994; 18:20.

32. Seldin DW. Renal handling of calcium. Nephron 1999; 81(Suppl 1):2.

33. Friedman PA. Mechanisms of renal calcium transport. Exp Nephrol 2000; 8:343.

34. Bronner F, Pansu D. Nutritional aspects of calcium absorption. J Nutr 1999; 129:9.

35. Gueguen L, Pointillart A. The bioavailability of dietary calcium. J Am Coll Nutr 2000; 19(Suppl 2):S119.

36. Hess B. Low calcium diet in hypercalciuric calcium nephrolithiasis: first do no harm. Scanning Microsc 1996; 10:547.

37. Audran M, Legrand E. Hypercalcuria. Joint Bone Spine 2000; 67:509.

38. Thacher TD, Fischer PR, Pettifor JM, Lawson JO, Isichei CO, Reading JC, et al. A comparison of calcium, vitamin D, or both for nutritional rickets in Nigerian children. N Engl J Med 1999; 341:563.

39. Soldin S, Hicks JM. Phosphate. Pediatric reference ranges. Washington, DC: American Association for Clinical Chemistry Press 1995:110.

40. Annino JS. Relman AS. The effect of eating on some of the clinically important chemical constituents of blood. Am J Clin Pathol 1959: 31:155.

41. Baldwin D, Robinson PK, Zierler KL, Lilenthal JL Jr. Interrelations of magnesium, potassium, phosphorus, and creatine in skeletal muscle of man. J Clin Invest 1952; 31:850.

42. Specker B, Tsang R, Ho M, Landi T, Gratton T. Low serum calcium and high parathyroid hormone levels in neonates fed humanized cow's milk-based formula. Am J Dis Child 1991; 145:941.

43. Koo WWK, Antony G, Stevens LHS. Continuous nasogastric phosphorus infusion in hypophosphatemic rickets of prematurity. Am J Dis Child 1984; 138:172.

44. Lyon AJ, McIntosh N, Wheeler K, Brooke OG. Hypercalcemia in extremely low birthweight infants. Arch Dis Child 1984; 59:1141.

45. Koo WWK, Tsang RC, Steichen JJ, Succop P, Babcock D, Oestreich AE, et al. Parenteral nutrition for infants: effect of high versus low calcium and phosphorus content. J Pediatr Gastroenterol Nutr 1987; 6:96.

46. Koo WWK, Tsang RC, Succop P, Krug-Wispe SK, Babcock D, Oestreich AE. Minimal vitamin D and high calcium and phosphorus needs of preterm infants receiving parenteral nutrition. J Pediatr Gastroenterol Nutr 1989; 8: 225.

47. Koo WWK, Steichen JJ: Osteopenia and Rickets of Prematurity. In: Polin R, Fox W, eds. Fetal and Neonatal Physiology, 2nd ed. Philadelphia: WB Saunders, 1998; 2335.

48. Kronenberg HM, Igarashi T, Freeman MW, Okazaki T, Brand SI, Wiren KM, et al. Structure and expression of the human parathyroid hormone gene. Rec Prog Horm Res 1986; 42:641.

49. Meyers DA, Beaty TH, Maestri NE, Kittur SD, Antonarakis SE, Kazazian HH Jr. Multipoint mapping studies of six loci on chromosome 11. Hum Hered 1987; 37:94.

50. Cohn DV, Kumarasamy R, Kemp WK. Intracellular processing and secretion of parathyroid gland proteins. Vitam Horm 1986; 43:283.

51. Slatopolsky E, Finch J, Clay P, Martin D, Sicard G, Singer G, et al. A novel mechanism for skeletal resistance in uremia. Kidney Int 2000; 58:753.

52. Gao P, Scheibel S, D'Amour P, John MR, Rao SD, Schmidt-Gayk H, et al. Development of a novel immu-

noradiometric assay exclusively for biologically active whole parathyroid hormone 1-84: implications for improvement of accurate assessment of parathyroid function. J Bone Miner Res 2001; 16:605.

53. Rubin LP, Posillico JT, Anast CS, Brown EM. Circulating levels of biologically active and immunoreactive intact parathyroid hormone in human newborns. Pediatr Res 1991; 29:201.

54. Allgrove J, Adami S, Maning RM, O'Riordan JL. Cytochemical bioassay of parathyroid hormone in maternal and cord blood. Arch Dis Child 1985; 60:110.

55. Abbas SK, Ratcliff WA, Moniz C, Dixit M, Caple IW, Silver M, et al. The role of parathyroid hormone-related protein in calcium homeostasis in the fetal pig. Exp Physiol 1994; 79:527.

56. MacIsaac RJ, Caple JW, Danks JA, Diefenbach-Jagger H, Grill V, Moseley JM, et al. Ontogeny of parathyroid hormone-related protein in the ovine parathyroid gland. Endocrinology 1991; 129:757.

57. Balabanova S, Lang T, Wolfe AS, Henrichs I, Homoki J, Gaedicke G, et al. Placental transfer of parathyroid hormone. J Perinat Med 1986; 14:243.

58. Venkataraman PS, Blick KE, Fry HD, Rao RK. Postnatal changes in calcium-regulating hormones in very-low-birth-weight infants. Effect of early neonatal hypocalcemia and intravenous calcium infusion on serum parathyroid hormone and calcitonin homeostasis. Am J Dis Child 1985; 139:913.

59. Mimouni F, Loughead J, Tsang R, Khoury J. Postnatal surge in serum calcitonin concentrations: no contribution to neonatal hypocalcemia in infants of diabetic mothers. Pediatr Res 1990; 28:493.

60. Dilena BA, White GH. The responses of plasma ionized calcium and intact parathyrin to calcium supplementation in preterm infants. Acta Paediatr Scand 1991; 80:1098.

61. Specker BL, Lichtenstein P, Mimouni F, Gormley C, Tsang RC. Calcium-regulating hormones and minerals from birth to 18 months of age: a cross-sectional study: II. Effects of sex, race, age, season, and diet on serum minerals, parathyroid hormone and calcitonin. Pediatrics 1986; 77:891.

62. Insogna KL, Lewis AM, Lipinski BA, Bryant C, Baran DT. Effect of age on serum immunoreactive parathyroid hormone and its biological effects. J Clin Endocrinol Metab 1984; 53:1072.

63. Davis OK, Hawkins DS, Rubin LP, Posillico JT, Brown EM, Schiff I. Serum parathyroid hormone (PTH) in pregnant women determined by an immunoradiometric assay for intact PTH. J Clin Endocrinol Metab 1988; 67:850.

64. Kitamura N, Shigeno C, Shiomi K, Lee K, Ohta S, Sone T, et al. Episodic fluctuation in serum intact parathyroid hormone concentration in men. J Clin Endocrinol Metab 1990; 70:252.

65. Logue FC, Fraser WD, O'Reilly DS, Cameron DA, Kelly AJ, Beastall GH. The circadian rhythm of intact parathyroid hormone-(1–84): temporal correlation with prolactin secretion in normal men. J Clin Endocrinol Metab 1990; 71:1556.

66. Calvo MS, Eastell R, Offord KP, Bergstralh EJ, Burritt MF. Circadian variation in ionized calcium and intact parathyroid hormone: evidence of sex differences in calcium homeostasis. J Clin Endocrinol Metab 1991; 72:69.

67. Felsenfeld AJ, Rodriguez M. Phosphorus, regulation of plasma calcium, and secondary hyperparathyroidism: a hypothesis to integrate a historical and modern perspective. J Am Soc Nephrol 1999; 10:878.

68. Friedman PA. Codependence of renal calcium and sodium transport. Annu Rev Physiol 1998; 60:179.

69. Tenenhouse HS. Cellular and molecular mechanisms of renal phosphate transport. J Bone Miner Res 1997; 12:159.

70. Taketani Y, Miyamoto K, Tanaka K, Katai K, Chikamori M, Tatsumi S, et al. Gene structure and functional analysis of the human Na+/phosphate co-transporter. Biochem J 1997; 324:927.

71. Nemere I, Norman AW. Parathyroid hormone stimulates calcium transport in perfused duodena of normal chicks: comparison with the rapid effect of 1,25-dihydroxyvitamin D3. Endocrinology 186; 199:1406.

72. Tam CS, Heersche JNM, Murray TM, Parsons JA. Parathyroid hormones stimulates the bone apposition rate independently of its resorptive action: differential effects of intermittent and continuous administration. Endocrinology 1982; 110:506.

73. Whitfield JF, Morley P, Willick G. The parathyroid hormone, its fragments and analogues—potent bone builders for treating osteoporosis. Expert Opin Invest Drugs 2000; 9:1293.

74. Neer RM Arnaud CD, Zanchetta JR, Prince R, Gaich GA, Reginster JY, et al. Effect of parathyroid hormone (1–34) on fractures and bone mineral density in postmenopausal women with osteoporosis. N Engl J Med 2001; 344:1434.

75. Juppner H. Receptors for parathyroid hormone and parathyroid hormone-related peptide: exploration of their biological importance. Bone 1999; 25:87.

76. Usdin TB, Hoare SRJ, Wang T, Mezey E, Kowalak JA. TIP39: a new neuropeptide and PTH2-receptor agonist from hypothalamus. Nat Neurosci 1999; 2:941.

77. Gelbert L, Schipani E, Juppner H, Abou-Samra AB, Segre GV, Naylor S, et al. Chromosomal localization of the parathyroid hormone/parathyroid hormone-related protein receptor gene to human chromosome 3p21.1-p24.2. J Clin Endocrinol Metab 1994; 79:1046.

78. Brown EM, Pollak M, Hebert SC. The extracellular calcium-sensing receptor: its role in health and disease. Annu Rev Med 1998; 49:15.

79. Chattopadhyay N, Baum M, Bai M, Riccardi D, Hebert SC, Harris HW, et al. Ontogeny of the extracellular calcium-sensing receptor in rat kidney. Am J Physiol 1996; 271:F736.

80. Brown EM, Hebert SC. Calcium-receptor-regulated parathyroid and renal function. Bone 1997; 20:303.

81. Moallem E, Kilav R, Silver J, Naveh-Many T. RNA-protein binding and posttranscriptional regulation of parathyroid hormone gene expression by calcium and phosphate. J Biol Chem 1998; 273:5253.

82. Toffaletti J, Cooper DL, Lobaugh B. The response of parathyroid hormone to specific changes in either ionized calcium, ionized magnesium, or protein-bound calcium in humans. Metabolism 1991; 40:814.

83. Fatemi S, Ryzen E, Flores J, Endres DB, Rude RK. Effect of experimental human magnesium depletion on parathyroid hormone secretion and 1,25-dihydroxyvitamin D metabolism. J Clin Endocrinol Metab 1991; 73:1067.

84. MacManus J, Heaton FW, Lucus PW. A decreased response to parathyroid hormone in magnesium deficiency. J Endocrinol 1971; 49:253.

85. Dewhirst FE, Ago JM, Peros WJ, Stashenko P. Synergism between parathyroid hormone and interleukin I in stimulating bone resorption in organ culture. J Bone Miner Res 1987; 2:127.

86. Greenberg C, Kukreja SC, Bowser EN, Hargis GK, Henderson WJ, Williams GA. Parathyroid hormone secretion: effect of estradiol and progesterone. Metabolism 1987; 36:151.

87. Mathias RS, Nguyen HT, Zhang MY, Portale AA. Reduced expression of the renal calcium-sensing receptor in rats with experimental chronic renal insufficiency. J Am Soc Nephrol 1998; 9:2067.

88. Drueke TB. Abnormal skeletal response to parathyroid hormone and the expression of its receptor in chronic uremia. Pediatr Nephrol 1996; 10:348.

89. Eckert RW, Scherubl H, Petzelt C, Raue F, Ziegler R. Rhythmic oscillations of cytosolic calcium in rat C-cells. Mol Cell Endocrinol 1989; 64:267.

90. Demay MB, Kiernan MS, DeLuca HF, Kronenberg HM. Sequences in the human parathyroid hormone gene that binds the 1,25 dihydroxyvitamin D3 receptor and mediate transcriptional repression in response to 1,25 dihydroxyvitamin D3. Proc Nat Acad Sci USA 1992; 89:8097.

91. Bucht E, Telenius-Berg M, Lundell G, Sjoberg HE. Immunoextracted calcitonin in milk and plasma from totally thyroidectomized women. Evidence of monomeric calcitonin in plasma during pregnancy and lactation. Acta Endocrinol 1986; 113:529.

92. Sexton PM, Findlay DM, Martin TJ. Calcitonin. Curr Med Chem 1999; 6:1067.

93. Garel JM, Besnard P, Rebut-Bonneton C. C cell activity during the prenatal and postnatal periods in the rat. Endocrinology 1981; 109:1573.

94. Balabanova S, Kruse B, Wolfe AS. Calcitonin secretion by human placental tissue. Acta Obstet Gynecol Scand 1987; 66:323.

95. Wolfe HJ, DeLellis RA, Volkel EF, Tashjian AH Jr. Distribution of calcitonin-containing cells in the normal neonatal human thyroid gland: a correlation of morphology with peptide content. J Clin Endocrinol Metab 1975; 41: 1076.

96. Lou H, Gagel RF. Alternative RNA processing—its role in regulating expression of calcitonin/calcitonin gene-related peptide. J Endocrinol 1998; 156:401.

97. Pondel M. Calcitonin and calcitonin receptors: bone and beyond. Int J Exp Pathol 2000; 81:405.

98. Samaan NA, Anderson GD, Adam-Mayne ME. Immunoreactive calcitonin in the mother, neonate, child and adult. Am J Obstet Gynecol 1975; 121:622.

99. Hillman LA, Hoff N, Walgate J, Haddad JG. Serum calcitonin concentrations in premature infants during the first 12 weeks of life. Calcif Tissue Int 1982; 34:470.

100. Zamboni G, Avanzini S, Giavarina D, Tato L. Monomeric calcitonin secretion in infants with congenital hypothyroidism. Acta Paediatr Scand 1989; 78:885.

101. Tiegs RD, Body JJ, Barta JM, Health H III. Secretion and metabolism of monomeric human calcitonin: effects of age, sex and thyroid damage. J Bone Miner Res 1986; 1: 339.

102. Robinson MF, Body JJ, Offord KP, Health H III. Variation of plasma immunoreactive parathyroid hormone and calcitonin in normal and hyperparathyroid man during daylight hours. J Clin Endocrinol Metab 1982; 55:538.

103. Trasforini G, Margutti A, Portaluppi F, Menegatti M, Ambrosio MR, Bagni B, et al. Circadian profile of plasma calcitonin gene-related peptide in healthy man. J Clin Endocrinol Metab 1991; 73:945.

104. De Los Santos ET, Mazzaferri EL. Calcitonin gene-related peptide: 24-hour profile and responses to volume contraction and expansion in normal men. J Clin Endocrinol Metab 1991; 72:1031.

105. Maruna P, Nedelnikova K, Gurlich R. Physiology and genetics of procalcitonin. Physiol Res 2000; 49(Suppl 1): S57.

106. Huwyler R, Born W, Ohnhaus EE, Fischer JA. Plasma kinetics and urinary excretion of exogenous human and salmon calcitonin in man. Am J Physiol 1979; 236:EI5.

107. Keith IM. The role of endogenous lung neuropeptides in regulation of the pulmonary circulation. Physiol Res 2000; 49:519.

108. Chovet M. Gastrointestinal functional bowel disorders: new therapies. Curr Opin Chem Biol 2000; 4:428.

109. Juaneda C, Dumont Y, Quirion R. The molecular pharmacology of CGRP and related peptide receptor subtypes. Trends Pharmacol Sci 2000; 21:432.

110. Wimalawansa SJ, Gunasekera RD, Datta HK. Hypocalcemic actions of amylin amide in humans. J Bone Miner Res 1992; 7:1113.

111. Nussenzveig DR, Mathew S, Gershengorn MC. Alternative splicing of a 48-nucleotide exon generates two isoforms of the human calcitonin receptor. Endocrinology 1995; 136:2047.

112. Wada S, Udagawa N, Akatsu T, Nagata N, Martin TJ, Findlay DM. Regulation by calcitonin and glucocorticoids of calcitonin receptor gene expression in mouse osteoclasts. Endocrinology 1997; 138:521.

113. Findlay DM, Michelangeli VP, Robinson PJ. Protein kinase C induced down regulation of calcitonin receptors and calcitonin-activated adenyl cyclase in T47D and BEN cells. Endocrinology 1989; 125:2656.

114. Naveh-Many T, Raue F, Grauer A, Silver J. Regulation of calcitonin gene expression by hypocalcemia, hypercalcemia, and vitamin D in the rat. J Bone Miner Res 1992; 7:1233.

115. Wongsurawat N, Armbrecht HJ. Calcitonin stimulates 1,25-dihydroxyvitamin D production in diabetic rat kidney. Metabolism 1991; 40:22.

116. Besnard P, el M'Selmi A, Jousset U, Collignon H, Garel JM. Effects of 1,25-dihydroxycholecalciferol and calcium on calcitonin mRNA levels in suckling rats. Mol Cell Endocrinol 1991; 79:45.

117. Martin TJ. Calcitonin, an update. Bone 1999; 24:S63.

118. Blomhoff R, Helgerud P, Dveland S, Berg T, Pedersen II. Lymphatic absorption and transport of retinol and vitamin D3 from rat intestine: evidence of different pathways. Biochim Biophys Acta 1984; 772:109.

119. Dueland S, Pedersen JI, Helgerud P, Drevon CA. Transport of vitamin D3 from rat intestine: evidence for transfer of vitamin D3 from chylomicrons to α-globulins. J Biol Chem 1982; 257:146.

120. Holick MF. Photosynthesis of vitamin D in the skin: effect of environmental and life-style variables. Fed Proc 1987; 46:1876.

121. Bikle DD, Siiteri PK, Ryzen E, Haddad JG. Serum protein binding of 1,25-dihydroxyvitamin D: a reevaluation by direct measurement of free metabolite levels. J Clin Endocrinol Metab 1985; 61:969.

122. Cooke NE, David EV. Serum vitamin D binding protein in a third member of the albumin and alpha-fetoprotein gene family. J Clin Invest 1985; 76:2420.

123. Revelle L, Solan V, Londowski J, Bollman S, Kumar R. Synthesis and biologic activity of a C-ring analog of vitamin D3: biologic and protein binding properties of 11 α-hydroxyvitamin D3. Biochemistry 1984; 23:1983.

124. Okuda KI. Liver mitochondrial P450 involved in cholesterol catabolism and vitamin D activation. J Lipid Res 1994; 35:361.
125. Miyamoto KI, Kesterson RA, Yamamoto H, Taketani Y, Nishiwaki E, Tatsumi S, et al. Structural organization of the human vitamin D receptor chromosomal gene and its promoter. Mol Endocrinol 1997; 11:1165.
126. Jones G, Strugnell SA, DeLuca HF. Current understanding of the molecular actions of vitamin D. Physiol Rev 1998; 78:1193.
127. Portale AA, Miller WL. Human 25-hydroxyvitamin D-1alpha-hydroxylase: cloning, mutations, and gene expression. Pediatr Nephrol 2000; 14:620.
128. Holick MF. Calcium and vitamin D. Diagnostics and therapeutics. Clin Lab Med 2000; 20:569.
129. Bell NH, Shaw S, Turner RT. Evidence that 1,25-dihydroxyvitamin D3 inhibits the hepatic production of 25-hydroxyvitamin D in man. J Clin Invest 1984; 74:1540.
130. Clements MR, Johnson L, Fraser DR. A new mechanism for induced vitamin D deficiency in calcium deprivation. Nature 1987; 325:62.
131. Portale AA, Halloran BP, Morris RC Jr. Physiologic regulation of the serum concentration of 1,25-dihydroxyvitamin D by phosphorus in normal man. J Clin Invest 1989; 83:1494.
132. Bowe AE, Finnegan R, Jan de Beur SM, Cho J, Levine MA, Kumar R, et al. FGF-23 inhibits renal tubular phosphate transport and is a PHEX substrate. Biochem Biophys Res Commun 2001; 284:977.
133. Nesbitt T, Drezner MK. Insulin-like growth factor-1 regulation of renal 25-hydroxyvitamin D-1-hydroxylase activity. Endocrinology 1993; 132:133.
134. Bell NH. Renal and nonrenal 25-hydroxyvitamin D-1α-hydroxylases and their clinical significance. J Bone Miner Res 1998; 13:350.
135. Mauras N. Growth hormone, insulin-like growth factor I and sex hormones: effects on protein and calcium metabolism. Acta Paediatr 1999; 88(Suppl 433):81.
136. Saris NE, Mervaala E, Karppanen H, Khawaja JA, Lewenstam A. Magnesium. An update on physiological, clinical and analytical aspects. Clin Chim Acta 2000; 294:1.
137. Saggese G, Federico G, Bertelloni S, Baroncelli GI, Calisti L. Hypomagnesemia and the parathyroid hormone-vitamin D endocrine system in children with insulin-dependent diabetes mellitus: effects of magnesium administration. J Pediatr 1991; 118:220.
138. Weaver VM, Welsh J. 1,25-Dihydroxycholecalciferol and the genesis of hypocalcaemia in magnesium-deficient chicks. Magnes Res 1990; 3:171.
139. Haussler MR, Whitfield GK, Haussler CA, Hsieh JC, Thompson PD, Selznick SH, et al. The nuclear vitamin D receptor: biological and molecular regulatory properties revealed. J Bone Miner Res 1998; 13:325.
140. Yamada S, Yamamoto K, Masuno H, Choi M. Three-dimensional structure–function relationship of vitamin D and vitamin D receptor model. Steroids 2001; 66:177.
141. Ebeling PR, Sandgren ME, DiMagno EP, Lane AW, DeLuca HF, Riggs BL. Evidence of an age related decrease in intestinal responsiveness to vitamin D: relationship between serum 1,25-dihydroxyvitamin D3 and intestinal vitamin D receptor concentrations in normal women. J Clin Endocrinol Metab 1992; 75:176.
142. Norman AW, Nemere I, Zhou LX, Bishop JE, Lowe KE, Maiyar AC, et al. 1,25(OH)2D-vitamin D3: a steroid hormone that produces biologic effects via both genomic and non-genomic pathways. J Steroid Biochem Mol Biol 1992; 41:231.
143. Johnson JA, Kumar R. Renal and intestinal calcium transport: roles of vitamin D and vitamin D-dependent calcium binding proteins. Semin Nephrol 1994; 14:119.
144. Thomasset M, Parkes CO, Cuisinier-Gleizes P. Rat calcium-binding proteins: distribution, development and vitamin D dependence. Am J Physiol 1982; 243:E483.
145. Cai Q, Chandler JS, Wasserman RH, Kumar R. Vitamin D and adaptation to dietary calcium and phosphorus deficiencies increase intestinal plasma membrane calcium pump gene expression. Proc Natl Acad Sci USA 1993; 90:1345.
146. Wasserman RH, Chandler JS, Meyer SA, Smith CA, Brindak ME, Fullmer CS, et al. Intestinal calcium transport and calcium extrusion processes at the basolateral membrane. J Nutr 1992; 122:662.
147. Kurnik BR, Hruska KA. Effects of 1,25-dihydroxycholecalciferol on phosphate transport in vitamin D-deprived rats. Am J Physiol 1984; 247:F177.
148. Ghishan FK, Arab N. Phosphate transport by intestinal endoplasmic reticulum during maturation. Pediatr Res 1988; 23:612.
149. Senterre J, Salle B. Calcium and phosphorus ecomony of the preterm infant and its interaction with vitamin D and its metabolites. Acta Paediatr Scand 1982; 296(Suppl):85.
150. Sooy K, Kohut J, Christokos S. The role of calbindin and 1,25 dihydroxyvitamin D3 in the kidney. Curr Opin Nephrol Hypertens 2000; 9:341.
151. Wesson LG. Homeostasis of phosphate revisited. Nephron 1997; 77:249.
152. Loghman-Adham M. Adaptation to changes in dietary phosphorus intake in health and in renal failure. J Lab Clin Med 1997; 129:176.
153. Amling M, Priemal M, Holzmann T, Chapin K, Rueger JM, Baron R, et al. Rescue of the skeletal phenotype of vitamin D receptor-ablated mice in the setting of normal mineral ion homeostasis: formal histomorphometric and biomechanical analysis. Endocrinology 1999; 140:4982.
154. al-Aqeel A, Ozand P, Sobki S, Sewairi W, Marx S. The combined use of intravenous and oral calcium for the treatment of vitamin D dependent rickets type II (VDDRII). Clin Endocrinol 1993; 39:229.
155. Disthabanchong S, Gonzalez EA. Regulation of bone cell development and function: implications for renal dystrophy. J Invest Med 2001; 49:240.
156. Jongen MJ, Van Ginkel FC, van der Vijgh WJ, Kuiper S, Netelenbos JC, Lips P. An international comparison of vitamin D metabolite measurements. Clin Chem 1984; 30:399.
157. Hollis BW. Comparison of equilibrium and disequilibrium assay conditions for ergocalciferol, cholecalciferol and their major metabolites. J Steroid Biochem 1984; 21:81.
158. Verity CM, Burman D, Beadle PC, Holton JB, Morris A. Seasonal changes in perinatal vitamin D metabolism: maternal and cord blood biochemistry in normal pregnancies. Arch Dis Child 1981; 56:943.
159. Hollis BW, Pittard WB III. Evaluation of the total fetomaternal vitamin D relationship at term: evidence for racial differences. J Clin Endocrinol Metab 1984; 59:652.
160. Nehama H, Weintroub S, Eisenberg Z, Birger A, Milbauer B, Weisman Y. Seasonal variation in paired maternal newborn serum 25 hydroxyvitamin D and 24,25 dihydroxyvitamin D concentrations in Israel. Isr J Med Sci 1987; 23:274.

161. Ron M, Levitz M, Chuba J, Dancis J. Transfer of 25-hydroxyvitamin D3 and 1,25-dihydroxyvitamin D3 across the perfused human placenta. Am J Obstet Gynecol 1984; 148:370.

162. Goodenday LS, Gordon GS. No risk from vitamin D in pregnancy. Ann Intern Med 1971; 75:807.

163. Marx SJ, Swart EG Jr, Hamstra AJ, DeLuca HP. Normal intrauterine development of the fetus of a woman receiving extraordinarily high doses of 1,25-dihydroxyvitamin D3. J Clin Endocrinol Metab 1980; 51:1138.

164. Lichtenstein P, Specker BL, Tsang RC, Mimouni F, Gormley C. Calcium regulating hormones and minerals from birth to 18 months of age: a cross-sectional study. I. Effects of sex, race, age, season and diet on vitamin D status. Pediatrics 1986; 77:883.

165. Halloran BP, Portale AA, Castro M, Morris RC Jr, Goldsmith RS. Serum concentrations of 1,25-dihydroxyvitamin D in the human: diurnal variation. J Clin Endocrinol Metab 1985; 60:1104.

166. Chesney RW, Rosen JF, Hamstra AJ, Smith C, Mahaffey K, DeLuca HF. Absence of seasonal variation in serum concentrations of 1,25-dihydroxyvitamin D despite a rise in 25-hydroxyvitamin D in summer. J Clin Endocrinol Metab 1981; 53:139.

167. Tsai KS, Heath H III, Kumar R, Riggs BL. Impaired vitamin D metabolism with aging in women: possible role in pathogenesis of senile osteoporosis. J Clin Invest 1984; 73:1668.

168. Bouillon RA, Auwerx JH, Lissens WD, Pelemans WK. Vitamin D status in the elderly: seasonal substrate deficiency causes 1,25-dihydroxycholecalciferol deficiency. Am J Clin Nutr 1987; 45:755.

169. Seeman E, Kumar R, Hunder GG, Scott M, Health H III, Riggs BL. Production, degradation and circulating levels of 1,25-dihydroxyvitamin D in health and in chronic glucocorticoid excess. J Clin Invest 1980; 66:664.

170. Kumar R. Hepatic and intestinal osteodystrophy and the hepatobiliary metabolism of vitamin D. Ann Intern Med 1983; 98:662.

171. Clements MR, Chalmers TM, Praser DR. Enterohepatic circulation of vitamin D: a reappraisal of the hypothesis. Lancet 1984; 1:1376.

172. Specker BL, Tsang RC, Hollis BW. Effect of race and diet on human milk vitamin D and 25 hydroxyvitamin D. Am J Dis Child 1985; 139:1134.

173. Specker BL, Valanis B, Hertzberg V, Edwards N, Tsang RC. Sunshine exposure and serum 25 hydroxyvitamin D concentrations in exclusively breast fed infants. J Pediatr 1985; 107:372.

174. Ho ML, Yen HC, Tsang RC, Specker BL, Chen XC, Nichols BL. Randomized study of sunshine exposure and serum 25-OHD in breast-fed infants in Beijing, China. J Pediatr 1985; 107:928.

175. Greer FR, Marshall S. Bone mineral content, serum vitamin D metabolite concentrations, and ultraviolet B light exposure in infants fed human milk with and without vitamin D_2 supplements. J Pediatr 1989; 114:204.

176. Specker BL, Ho ML, Oestreich A, Yin TA, Shui QM, Chen XC, et al. Prospective study of vitamin D supplementation and rickets in China. J Pediatr 1992; 120:733.

177. Koo WWK, Sherman R, Succop P, Ho M, Buckley D, Tsang RC. Serum vitamin D metabolites in very low birth weight infants with and without rickets and fractures. J Pediatr 1989; 114:1017.

178. Salle BL, Delvin EE, Lapillonne A, Bishop NJ, Glorieux FH. Perinatal metabolism of vitamin D. Am J Clin Nutr 2000; 71(Suppl 5):S1317.

179. Shinki T, Jin CH, Nishimura A, Nagai Y, Ohyama Y, Noshiro M, et al. Parathyroid hormone inhibits 25 hydroxyvitamin D3-24-hydroxylase mRNA expression stimulated by 1α,25-dihydroxyvitamin D3 in rat kidney but not in intestine. J Biol Chem 1992; 267:13757.

180. Seo EG, Einhorn TA, Norman AW. 24R,25-dihydroxyvitamin D3: an essential vitamin D3 metabolite for both normal bone integrity and healing of tibial fracture in chicks. Endocrinology 1997; 138:3864.

181. Uy HL, Mundy GR, Boyce BF, Story BM, Dunstan CR, Yin JJ, et al. Tumor necrosis factor enhances parathyroid hormone-related protein-induced hypercalcemia and bone resorption without inhibiting bone formation in vivo. Cancer Res 1997; 57:3194.

182. Pfeilschifter J, Laukhuf F, Muller-Beckmann B, Blum WF, Pfister T, Ziegler R. Parathyroid hormone increases the concentration of insulin-like growth factor-1 and transforming growth factor beta I in rat bone. J Clin Invest 1995; 96:767.

183. Grey A, Mitnick MA, Shapses S, Ellison A, Gundberg C, Insogna K. Circulating levels of interleukin-6 and tumor necrosis factor-alpha are elevated in primary hyperparathyroidism and correlate with markers of bone resorption. J Clin Endocrinol Metab 1996; 81:3450.

184. Ellies LG, Heersche JN, Prusanski W, Vadas P, Aubin JE. The role of phospholipase A2 in interleukin-1 alpha-mediated inhibition of mineralization of the osteoid formed by fetal rat calvaria cells in vitro. J Dent Res 1993; 72:18.

185. Kimble RB, Vannice JL, Bloedow DC, Thompson RC, Hopfer W, Kung VT, et al. Interleukin-1 receptor antagonist decreases bone loss and bone resorption in ovariectomized rats. J Clin Invest 1994; 93:1959.

186. Moe SM, Hack BK, Curnmings SA, Sprague SM. Role of IL-1 beta and prostaglandins in beta 2-microglobulin-induced bone mineral dissolution. Kidney Int 1995; 47:587.

187. Mundy GR, Boyce B, Hughes D, Wright K, Bonewald L, Dallas S, et al. The effects of cytokines and growth factors on osteoblastic cells. Bone 1995; 17:S71.

188. Kimble RB. Alcohol, cytokines, and estrogen in the control of bone modeling. Alcohol Clin Exp Res 1997; 21:385.

189. Martin TJ, Moseley JM, Williams ED. Parathyroid hormone-related protein: hormone and cytokine. J Endocrinol 1997; 154:S23.

190. Moseley JM, Gillespie MT. Parathyroid hormone-related protein. Crit Rev Clin Lab Sci 1995; 32:299.

191. Moseley JM, Hayman JA, Danks JA, Alcorn D, Grill V, Southby J, et al. Immunohistochemical detection of parathyroid hormone-related protein in human fetal epithelia. J Clin Endocrinol Metab 1991; 73:478.

192. Law F, Moate PJ, Leaver DD, Diefenbach-Jagger H, Grill V, Ho PW, et al. Parathyroid hormone-related protein in milk and its correlation with bovine milk calcium. J Endocrinol 1991; 128:21.

193. Bilezikian IP. Clinical utility of assays for parathyroid hormone-related protein. Clin Chem 1992; 38:179.

194. Dvir R, Golander A, Jaccard N, Yedwab G, Otremski I, Spirer Z, et al. Amniotic fluid and plasma levels of parathyroid hormone-related protein and hormonal modulation of its secretion by amniotic fluid cells. Eur J Endocrinol 1995; 133:277.

195. Salsburey DJ, Brown DR. Effect of parenteral calcium treatment on blood pressure and heart rate in neonatal hypocalcemia. Pediatrics 1982;69:605.

196. Mirro R, Brown DR. Parenteral calcium treatment shortens the left ventricular systolic time intervals of hypocalcemic neonates. Pediatr Res 1984; 18:71.

197. Venkataraman PS, Wilson DA, Sheldon RE, Rao R, Parker MK. Effect of hypocalcemia on cardiac function in very low birth weight preterm neonates: studies of blood ionized calcium, echocardiography, and cardiac effect of intravenous calcium therapy. Pediatrics 1985; 76: 543.

198. Broner CW, Stidham GL, Westenkirchner DF, Tolley EA. Hypermagnesemia and hypocalcemia as predictors of high mortality in critically ill pediatric patients. Crit Care Med 1990; 18:921.

199. David L, Salle BL, Putet G, Grafmeyer DC. Serum immunoreactive calcitonin in low birth weight infants. Description of early changes; effect of intravenous calcium infusion; relationship with early changes in serum calcium, phosphorus, magnesium, parathyroid hormone and gastrin levels. Pediatr Res 1981; 15:803.

200. Venkataraman PS, Tsang RC, Steichen II. Early neonatal hypocalcemia in extremely preterm infants: high incidence, early onset, and refractoriness to supraphysiologic dose of calcitrol. Am J Dis Child 1986; 140:1004.

201. Venkataraman PS, Tsang RC, Chen IW, Sperling MA. Pathogenesis of early neonatal hypocalcemia: studies of serum calcitonin, gastrin, and plasma glucagon. J Pediatr 1987; 110:559.

202. Hanukoglu A, Chalew S, Kowardski AA. Late onset hypocalcemia, rickets and hypoparathyroidism in an infant of a mother with hyperparathyroidism. J Pediatr 1988; 112:751.

203. Thomas AK, McVie R, Levine SN. Disorders of maternal calcium metabolism implicated by abnormal calcium metabolism in the neonate. Am J Perinatol 1999; 16:515.

204. Ravid A, Koren R, Rotem C, Amir Y, Reisner S, Novogrodsky A, et al. Mononuclear cells from human neonates are partially resistant to the action of 1,25 dihydroxyvitamin D. J Clin Endocrinol Metab 1988; 67:755.

205. Pierson JD, Crawford JD. Dietary dependent neonatal hypocalcemia. Am J Dis Child 1972; 123:472.

206. Perlman JM. Fatal hyperphosphatemia after oral phosphate overdose in a premature infant. Am J Health-Syst Pharm 1997; 54:2488.

207. Davis RF, Eichner JM, Bleyuer WA, Okamoto G. Hypercalcemia, hyperphosphatemia and dehydration following a single hypertonic phosphate enema. J Pediatr 1977; 90: 484.

208. Walton DM, Thomas DC, Aly HZ, Short BL. Morbid hypocalcemia associated with phosphate enema in a six-week-old infant. Pediatrics 2000; 106(3):E37.

209. Yamamoto T, Kabata H, Yagi R, Takashima M, Itokawa Y. Primary hypomagnesemia with secondary hypocalcemia. Report of a case and review of the world literature. Magnesium 1985; 4:153.

210. Rodder S, Mize C, Forman L, Uauy R. Effects of increased dietary phosphorus on magnesium balance in very low birth weight babies. Magnes Res 1992; 5:273.

211. Quamme GA. Renal magnesium handling: new insights in understanding old problems. Kidney Int 1997; 52:1180.

212. Salle BL, David L, Chopard IP, Grafmeyer DC, Renand H. Prevention of early neonatal hypocalcemia in low birth weight infants with continuous calcium infusion. Effect on serum calcium, phosphorus, magnesium and circulating immunoreactive parathyroid hormone and calcitonin. Pediatr Res 1977; 11:1180.

213. Dincsoy MY, Tsang RC, Laskarzewski P, Ho M, Chen IW, Davis N. Serum calcitonin response to administration of calcium in newborn infants during exchange blood transfusion. J Pediatr 1982; 100:782.

214. Tsang RC, Chen I, Hayes W, Atkinson W, Atherton H, Edwards N. Neonatal hypocalcemia in infants with birth asphyxia. J Pediatr 1974; 84:428.

215. Namgung R, Tsang R, Specker B, Sierra R, Ho M. Reduced serum osteocalcin and 1,25 dihydroxyvitamin D concentrations and low bone mineral content in small for gestational age infants: evidence of decreased bone formation rates. J Pediatr 1993; 122:269.

216. Hahn TI, Hendin BA, Scharp CR, Boisseau VC, Haddad JG. Serum 25-hydroxycholecalciferol levels and bone mass in children on chronic anticonvulsant therapy. N Engl J Med 1975; 292:550.

217. Watney PJM, Chance GW, Scott P, Thompson IM. Maternal factors in neonatal hypocalcemia: a study in three ethnic groups. Br Med J 1971; 2:432.

218. Mimouni F, Mimouni C, Loughead J, Tsang R. A case control study of hypocalcemia in high risk neonates: racial, but no seasonal differences. J Am Coll Nutr 1991; 10:196.

219. Mimouni F, Tsang RC, Hertzberg VS, Miodovnik M. Polycythemia, hypomagnesemia and hypocalcemia in infants of diabetic mothers. Am J Dis Child 1986; 140:798.

220. Srinivasan M, Abinun M, Cant AJ, Tan K, Oakhill A, Steward CG. Malignant infantile osteopetrosis presenting with neonatal hypocalcemia. Arch Dis Child Fetal Neonatal Ed 2000; 83:F21.

221. Conley ME, Beckwith IB, Mancer JF, Tenckoff L. The spectrum of the DiGeorge syndrome. J Pediatr 1979; 94: 883.

222. Burke BA, Johnson D, Gilbert EF, Drut RM, Ludwig J, Wick MR. Thyrocalcitonin-containing cells in the DiGeorge anomaly. Hum Pathol 1987; 18:355.

223. Driscoll D, Salvin J, Sellinger B, Budarf ML, McDonald-McGinn DM, Zackai EH, et al. Prevalence of 22q11 microdeletions in DiGeorge and velocardiofacial syndromes: implications for genetic counselling and prenatal diagnosis. J Med Genet 1993; 30:813.

224. Keppen LD, Fasules JW, Burks AW, Gollin SM, Sawyer JR, Miller CH. Confirmation of autosomal dominant transmission of the DiGeorge malformation complex. J Pediatr 1988; 113:506.

225. Bainbridge R, Mughal Z, Mimouni F, Tsang RC. Transient congenital hypoparathyroidism; how transient is it? J Pediatr 1987; 11:866.

226. Kooh SW, Binet A. Partial hypoparathyroidism. A variant of transient congenital hypoparathyroidism. Am J Dis Child 1991; 145:877.

227. Greig F, Paul E, DiMartino-Nardi J, Saenger P. Transient congenital hypoparathyroidism: resolution and recurrence in chromosome 22q11 deletion. J Pediatr 1996; 128:563.

228. Arnold A, Horst SA, Gardella TJ, Baba H, Levine MA, Kronenberg HM. Mutation of the signal peptide encoding region of the preproparathyroid hormone gene in familial isolated hypoparathyroidism. J Clin Invest 1990; 86:1084.

229. Bilous RW, Murty G, Parkinson DB, Thakker RV, Coulthard MG, Burn J, et al. Autosomal dominant familial hypoparathyroidism, sensorineural deafness, and renal dysplasia. N Engl J Med 1992; 327:1069.

230. Sunthornthepvarakul T, Churesigaew S, Ngowngarmratana S. A novel mutation of the signal peptide of the pre-proparathyroid hormone gene associated with autosomal recessive familial isolated hypoparathyroidism. J Clin Endocrinol Metab 1999; 84:3792.

231. Root AW. Genetic disorders of calcium and phosphorus metabolism. Crit Rev Clin Lab Sci 2000; 37:217.

232. Marx SJ. Hyperparathyroid and hypoparathyroid disorders. N Engl J Med 2000; 343:1863.

233. Bai M, Quinn S, Trivedi S, Kifor O, Pearce SH, Pollak MR, et al. Expression and characterization of inactivating and activating mutations of the human Ca2+-sensing receptor. J Biol Chem 1996; 271:19537.

234. Pearce SH, Williamson C, Kifor O, Bai M, Coulthard MG, Davies M, et al. A familial syndrome of hypocalcemia with hypercalciuria due to mutations in the calcium sensing receptor. N Engl J Med 1996; 335:1115.

235. Baron J, Winer KK, Yanovski JA, Cunningham AW, Laue L, Zimmerman D, et al. Mutations in the Ca(2+)-sensing receptor gene cause autosomal dominant and sporadic hypoparathyroidism. Hum Mol Genet 1996; 5:601.

236. Zhang P, Jobert AS, Couvineau A, Silve C. A homozygous inactivating mutation in the parathyroid hormone/parathyroid hormone-related peptide receptor causing Blomstrand chondrodysplasia. J Clin Endocrinol Metab 1998; 83:3365.

237. Dincsoy MY, Tsang RC, Laskarzewski P, Chen MH, Chen IW, Lo D, et al. The role of postnatal age and magnesium on parathyroid hormone responses during "exchange" blood transfusion in the newborn period. J Pediatr 1982; 100:277.

238. Tsang RC, Venkataraman P, Ho M, Steichen JJ, Witsett J, Greer F. The development of pseudohypoparathyroidism: involvement of progressively increasing serum parathyroid hormone concentrations, increased 1,25-dihydroxyvitamin D concentrations, and "migratory" subcutaneous calcifications. Am J Dis Child 1984; 138:654.

239. Ringel MD, Schwindinger WF, Levine MA. Clinical implications of genetic defects in G proteins: The molecular basis of McCune Albright syndrome and Albright hereditary osteodystrophy. Medicine 1996; 75:171.

240. Bastepe M, Lane AH, Juppner H. Paternal uniparental isodisomy of chromosome 20q and the resulting changes in GNAS1 methylation as a plausible cause of pseudohypoparathyroidism. Am J Hum Genet 2001; 68:1283.

241. Yu S, Yu D, Lee E, Eckhaus M, Lee R, Corria Z, et al. Variable and tissue-specific hormone resistance in heterotrimeric Gs protein alpha subunit (Gsalpha) knockout mice is due to tissue-specific imprinting of the Gsalpha gene. Proc Natl Acad Sci USA 1998; 95:8715.

242. Minagawa M, Yasuda T, Kobayashi Y, Niimi H. Transient pseudohypoparathyroidism of the neonate. Eur J Endocrinol 1995; 133:151.

243. Whitsett J, Tsang RC. In vitro effects of fatty acids on serum ionized calcium. J Pediatr 1977; 91:233.

244. Gutcher GR, Odell GB. Hypocalcemia associated with phototherapy in newborn rats: light source dependence. Photochem Photobiol 1983; 37:177.

245. Oleske JM. Experience with 118 infants born to narcotic-using mothers. Does a lower serum ionized calcium level contribute to the symptoms of withdrawal? Clin Pediatr 1977; 16:418.

246. Scott SM, Ladenson JH, Aguanna JJ, Walgate J, Hillman LS. Effect of calcium therapy in the sick premature infant with early neonatal hypocalcemia. J Pediatr 1984; 104: 747.

247. Colleti RB, Pan MW, Smith EWP, Genel M. Detection of hypocalcemia in susceptible neonates, the QoTc interval. N Engl J Med 1974; 290:931.

248. Zaloga GP, Chernow B, Cook D, Snyder R, Clapper M, O'Brian JT. Assessment of calcium homeostasis in the critically ill surgical patient. The diagnostic pitfalls of the McLean-Hasting normogram. Ann Surg 1985; 202:587.

249. Broner CW, Stidham GL, Westenkirchner DF, Watson DC. A prospective, randomized, double-blind comparison of calcium chloride and calcium gluconate therapies for hypocalcemia in critically ill children. J Pediatr 1990; 117:986.

250. Venkataraman P, Sanchez G, Parker M. Altmiller D. Effect of intravenous calcium infusions on serum chemistries in neonates. J Pediatr Gastroenter Nutr 1991; 13:134.

251. Brown DR, Salsburey DJ. Short term biochemical effects of parenteral calcium treatment of early onset neonatal hypocalcemia. J Pediatr 1982; 100:777.

252. Kooh SW, Fraser D, Toon R, DeLuca HF. Response of protracted neonatal hypocalcemia to 1 alpha,25-hydroxyvitamin D3. Lancet 1976; 2:1105.

253. Barak Y, Milbauer B, Weisman Y, Edelstein S, Spirer Z. Response of neonatal hypocalcemia to 1 alpha-hydroxyvitamin D3. Arch Dis Child 1979; 54:642.

254. Koo WWK, Kaplan LA. Aluminum and bone disorders: with specific reference to aluminum contamination of infant nutrients. J Am Coll Nutr 1988; 7:199.

255. The neonatal inhaled nitric oxide study group. Inhaled nitric oxide in full-term and nearly full-term infants with hypoxic respiratory failure. N Engl J Med 1997; 336:597.

256. Brown DR, Tsang RC, Chen IW. Oral calcium supplementation in premature and asphyxiated neonates. J Pediatr 1976; 89:973.

257. Brown R, Steranko BH, Taylor FH. Treatment of early onset neontal hypocalcemia: effects on serum calcium and ionized calcium. Am J Dis Child 1981; 135:24.

258. Nervez CT, Shott RJ, Bergstrom WH, Williams ML. Prophylaxis against hypocalcemia in low birth weight infants requiring bicarbonate infusion. J Pediatr 1975; 87:439.

259. Salle BL, David L, Glorieux FA, Delvin E, Senterre J, Renaud H. Early oral administration of vitamin D and its metabolites in premature neonates. Effect on mineral homeostasis. Pediatr Res 1982; 16:75.

260. Fleischman AR, Rosen JF, Nathenson G. 25-Hydroxycholecalciferol for early neonatal hypocalcemia. Occurrence in premature newborns. Am J Dis Child 1978; 132: 973.

261. Petersen S, Christensen NC, Fogh-Andersen N. Effect on serum calcium of 1α hydroxyvitamin D3 supplementation in infants of low birth weight with perinatal asphyxia and infants of diabetic mothers. Acta Paediatr Scand 1981; 70: 897.

262. Chan GM, Tsang RC, Chen IW, DeLuca HF, Steichen JJ. The effect of 1,25(OH)2 vitamin D3 supplementation in premature infants. J Pediatr 1978; 93:91.

263. Thode J, Juul-Jorgensen B, Bhatia HM, Kjaerulf-Nielsen M, Bartels PD, Fogh-Andersen N, et al. Comparison of serum total calcium albumin-corrected total calcium, and ionized calcium in 1213 patients with suspected calcium disorders. Scand J Clin Lab Invest 1989; 49:217.

264. Kimura S, Nose O, Seino Y, Harada T, Kanaya S, Yabuuchi H, et al. Effects of alternate and simultaneous administrations of calcium and phosphorous on calcium metabolism in children receiving total parenteral nutrition. J Parenter Enteral Nutr 1986; 10:513.

265. Auwerx J, Brunzell J, Bouillon R, Demedts M. Familial hypocaluria hypercalcemia—familial benign hypercalcemia: a review. Postgrad Med 1987; 63:835.

266. Pearce SH, Trump D, Wooding C, Besser GM, Chew SL, Grant DB, et al. Calcium-sensing receptor mutations in familial benign hypercalcaemia and neonatal hyperparathyroidism. J Clin Invest 1995; 96:2683.

267. Firek AF, Kao PC, Heath H III. Plasma intact parathyroid hormone (PTH) and PTH-related peptide in familial benign hypercalcemia: greater responsiveness to endogenous PTH than in primary hyperparathyroidism. J Clin Endocrinol Metab 1991; 72:541.

268. Firek AF, Carter WB, Heath H III. Cyclic adenosine 3',5'-monophosphate responses to parathyroid hormone, prostaglandin E2, and isoproterenol in dermal fibroblasts from patients with familial benign hypercalcemia. J Clin Endocrinol Metab 1991; 73;203.

269. Wilkinson H, James J. Self limiting neonatal primary hyperparathyroidism associated with familial hypocalciuric hypercalcemia. Arch Dis Child 1993; 69:319.

270. Bai M, Pearce SH, Kifor O, Trivedi S, Stauffer UG, Thakker RV, et al. In vivo and in vitro characterization of neonatal hyperparathyroidism resulting from a de novo, heterozygous mutation in the Ca2+-sensing receptor gene: normal maternal calcium homeostasis as a cause of secondary hyperparathyroidism in familial benign hypocalciuric hypercalcemia. J Clin Invest 1997; 99:88.

271. Pollak M, Chou Y, Marx S, Steimann B, Cole D, Brandi M, et al. Familial hypocalcuric hypercalcemia and neonatal severe hyperparathyroidism. Effects of mutant gene dosage on phenotype. J Clin Invest 1994; 93:1108.

272. Ross AJ, Cooper A, Attie MF, Bishop H. Primary hyperparathyroidism in infancy. J Pediatr Surg 1986; 21:493.

273. Schipani E, Langman C, Parfitt AM, Jensen GS, Kikuchi S, Kooh SW, et al. Constitutively activated receptors for parathyroid hormone and parathyroid hormone-related peptides in Jansen's metaphyseal chondrodysplasia. N Engl J Med 1996; 335:708.

274. Parfitt AM, Schipani E, Rao DS, Kupin W, Han ZH, Juppner H. Hypercalcemia due to constitutive activity of the parathyroid hormone (PTH)/PTH-related peptide receptor: comparison with primary hyperparathyroidism. J Clin Endocrinol Metab 1996; 81:3584.

275. Loughead J, Mughal F, Mimouni F, Tsang R, Oestreich A. The spectrum and natural history of congenital hyperpapathyroidism secondary to maternal hypocalcemia. Am J Perinatol 1990; 7:350.

276. Savani R, Mimouni F, Tsang R. Maternal and neonatal hyperparathyroidism as a consequence of maternal renal tubular acidosis. Pediatrics 1993; 91:661.

277. Igarashi T, Sekine Y, Kawato H, Kamoshita S, Saigusa Y. Transient neonatal distal renal tubular acidosis with secondary hyperparathyroidism. Pediatr Nephrol 1992; 6:267.

278. Rodriguez-Soriano J, Garcia-Fuentes M, Vallo A, Alvarez-Granda JL. Hypercalcemia in neonatal distal renal tubular acidosis. Pediatr Nephrol 2000; 14:354.

279. Chabala JM, Levi-Setti RL, Bushinsky DA. Alteration in surface ion composition of cultured bone during metabolic, but not respiratory acidosis. Am J Physiol 1991; 261:F76.

280. Bichara M, Mercier O, Borensztein P, Paillard M. Acute metabolic acidosis enhances circulating parathyroid hormone, which contributes to the renal response against acidosis in the rat. J Clin Invest 1990; 86:430.

281. Lakhdir F, Lawson D, Schatz D. Fatal parathyroid hormone-related protein-induced humoral hypercalcemia of malignancy in a 3-month old infant. Eur J Pediatr 1994; 153:718.

282. Michigami T, Yamato H, Mushiake S, Nakayama M, Yoneda A, Satomura K, et al. Hypercalcemia associated with infantile fibrosarcoma producing parathyroid hormone-related protein. J Clin Endocrinol Metab 1996; 81:1090.

283. Mahaney C, Cassady C, Weinberger E, Winters W, Benjamin D. Humoral hypercalcemia due to an occult renal adenoma. Pediatr Nephrol 1997; 11:339.

284. Markestad T, Hesse V, Siebenhuner M, Jahreis G, Aksnes L, Plenert W, et al. Intermittent high-dose vitamin D prophylaxis during infancy: effect on vitamin D metabolites, calcium, and phosphorus. Am J Clin Nutr 1987; 46:652.

285. Greer FR, Hollis BW, Napoli JL. High concentrations of vitamin D2 in human milk associated with pharmacologic doses of vitamin D2. J Pediatr 1984; 105:61.

286. Jacobus C, Holick M, Shao Q, Chen T, Holm I, Kolodny J, et al. Hypervitaminosis D associated with drinking milk. N Engl J Med 1992; 326:1173.

287. Holick M, Shao Q, Liu W, Chen T. The vitamin D content of fortified milk and infant formula. N Engl J Med 1992; 326:1178.

288. Nako Y, Fukushima N, Tomomasa T, Nagashima K. Hypervitaminosis D after prolonged feeding with a premature formula. Pediatrics 1993; 92:862.

289. Norwood GA, Lebwohl M, Phelps RG, Raucher H. Subcutaneous fat necrosis of the newborn with hypercalcemia. J Am Acad Dermatol 1987; 16:435.

290. Hicks M, Levy M, Alexander J, Flaitz CM. Subcutaneous fat necrosis of the newborn and hypercalcemia: case report and review of the literature. Pediatr Dermatol 1993; 10:271.

291. Wiadrowski T, Marshman G. Subcutaneous fat necrosis of the newborn following hypothermia and complicated by pain and hypercalcemia. Aust J Dermatol 2001; 42:207.

292. Kruse K, Irle U, Uhlig R. Elevated 1,25 dihydroxyvitamin D serum concentrations in infants with subcutaneous fat necrosis. J Pediatr 1993; 122:460.

293. Bush ME, Dahms BB. Fatal hypervitaminosis A in a neonate. Arch Pathol Lab Med 1984; 108:838.

294. Tau C, Garabedian M, Farriaux JP, Czernichow P, Pomarede R, Balsan S. Hypercalcemia in infants with congenital hypothyroidism and its relation to vitamin D and thyroid hormones. J Pediatr 1986; 109:808.

295. Taylor AB, Stern PH, Bell NH. Abnormal regulation of circulating 25-hydroxyvitamin D in the Williams syndrome. N Engl J Med 1982; 306:972.

296. Culler FL, Jones KL, Deftos LJ. Impaired calcitonin secretion in patients with Williams syndrome. J Pediatr 1985; 107:720.

297. Telvi L, Pinard J, Ion R, Sinet PM, Nicole A, Feingold J, et al. De novo t(X;21) (q28; q11) in a girl with phenotypic features of Williams-Beuren syndrome. J Med Genet 1992; 29:747.

298. Osbourne L, Martindale D, Scherer W, Shi X, Huizenga J, Heng H, et al. Identification of genes from a 500-kb region of 7q11.23 that is commonly deleted in Williams syndrome patients. Genomics 1996; 36:328.

299. Pastores GM, Michels VV, Schaid DJ, Driscoll DJ, Feldt RH, Thibodeau SN. Exclusion of calcitonin/x-CGRP gene defect in a family with autosomal dominant supravalvular aortic stenosis. J Med Genet 1992; 29:56.

300. Zwischenberger JB, Nguyen TT, Upp JR Jr, Bush PE, Cox CS Jr, Delosh T, et al. Complications of neonatal extracorporeal membrane oxygenation. Collective experience from the Extracorporeal Life Support Organizations. J Thorac Cardiovasc Surg 1994; 107:838.

301. Shanley CJ, Hirschl RB, Schumacher RE, Overbeck MC, Delosh TN, Chapman RA, et al. Extracorporeal Life Support for neonatal respiratory failure. A 20 year experience. Ann Surg 1994; 220:269.

302. Fridriksson JH, Helmrath MA Wessel JJ, Warner B. Hypercalcemia associated with extracorporeal life support in neonates. J Pediatr Surg 2001; 36:493.

303. Whyte MP. Hypophosphatasia and the role of alkaline phosphatase in skeletal mineralization. Endocr Rev 1994; 15:439.

304. Barcia J, Strife C, Langman C. Infantile hypophosphatasia: treatment options to control hypercalcemia, hypercalciuria, and chronic bone demineralization. J Pediatr 1997; 130:825.

305. Drummond KN, Michael AF, Ulstrom RA, Good RA. The blue diaper syndrome: familial hypercalcemia with neophrocalcinosis and indicanuria. Am J Med 1964; 37:928.

306. Laflamme GH, Jowsey J. Bone and soft tissue changes with oral phosphate supplements. J Clin Invest 1972; 51: 2834.

307. Bilezikian J. Management of acute hypercalcemia. N Engl J Med 1992; 326:1196.

308. Stark AR, Carlo WA, Tyson JE, Papile LA, Wright LL, Shankaran S, et al. National Institute of Child Health and Human Development Neonatal Research Network. Adverse effects of early dexamethasone in extremely-low-birth-weight infants. National Institute of Child Health and Human Development Neonatal Research Network. New Engl J Med 2001; 344:95.

309. Illidge TM, Hussey M, Godden CW. Malignant hypercalcemia in pregnancy and antenatal administration of intravenous pamidronate. Clin Oncol 1996; 8:257.

310. Shoemaker LR. Expanding role of bisphonate therapy in children. J Pediatr 1999; 134:264.

311. Hall RT, Wheeler RE, Rippetoe LE. Calcium and phosphorus supplementation after initial hospital discharge in breast-fed infants of less than 1800 grams birth weight. J Perinatol 1993; 13:272.

312. Guillou PJ, Morgan DB, Hill GL. Phosphorus: A complication of "innocus dextrose-saline." Lancet 1976; 2: 710.

313. Corredor DO, Sabeb G, Mendelsohn LV, Wassennan RE, Sundennan JH, Danowski TS. Enhanced postglucose hypophosphatemia during starvation therapy of obesity. Metabolism 1969; 18:754.

314. Hill GL, Guinn EJ, Dudrick SJ. Phosphorus distribution in hyperalimentation induced hypophosphatemia. J Surg Res 1976; 20:527.

315. Weinsier RL, Krumdieck CL. Death resulting from overzealous total parenteral nutrition: the refeeding syndrome. Am J Clin Nutr 1980; 34:393.

316. Weisinger JR, Bellorin-Font E. Magnesium and phosphorus. Lancet 1998; 352:391.

317. DeFronzo RA, Cooke CR, Andres R. The effect of insulin on renal handling of sodium, potassium, calcium and phosphate in man. J. Clin Invest 1975; 55:845.

318. Arnaud SB, Stickler OB, Haworth JC. Serum 25-hydroxyvitamin D in infantile rickets. Pediatrics 1976; 57: 221.

319. Venkataraman PS, Tsang RC, Buckely DD, Ho M, Steichen JJ. Elevation of serum 1,25-dihydroxyvitamin D in response to physiologic doses of vitamin D in vitamin D deficient infants. J Pediatr 1983; 103:416.

320. Fouser L. Disorders of calcium, phosphorus, and magnesium. Pediatr Ann 1995; 24:38.

321. Kreiter SR, Schwartz RP, Kirkman HN Jr, Charlton PA, Calikoglu AS, Davenport ML. Nutritional rickets in African American breast-fed infants. J Pediatr 2000; 137:153.

322. Dagnelie PC, Vergote F, van Staveren WA, van den Berg H, Dingjan PG, Hautvast JG. High prevalence of rickets in infants on macrobiotic diets. Am J Clin Nutr 1990; 51: 202.

323. Koo WWK. Parenteral nutrition-related bone disease. J Parenteral Ent Nutr 1992; 16:386.

324. Minamitani K, Minagawa M, Yasuda T, Niimi H. Early detection of infants with hypophosphatemic vitamin D resistant rickets (HDRR). Endocr J 1996; 43:339.

325. Kruse K, Hinkel GK, Griefahn B. Calcium metabolism and growth during early treatment of children with X-linked hypophosphatemic rickets. Eur J Pediatr 1998; 157:894.

326. Russell JGB, Hill LF. True fetal rickets. Br J Radiol 1974; 47:732.

327. Park W, Paust H, Kaufmann HJ, Offermann G. Osteomalacia of the mother—rickets of the newborn. Eur J Pediatr 1987; 146:292.

328. Zhou H. Rickets in China. In: Glorieux FH, ed. Rickets. New York: Raven Press, 1991:253.

329. Lamm CI, Norton KI, Murphy RJ, Wilkins IA, Rabinowitz JG. Congenital rickets associated with magnesium sulfate infusion for tocolysis. J Pediatr 1988; 113:1078.

330. Rimensberger P, Schubiger G, Willi U. Congenital rickets following repeated administration of phosphate enemas in pregnancy: a case report. Eur J Pediatr 1992; 151:54.

331. Steichen JJ, Gratton T, Tsang RC. Osteopenia of prematurity: the cause and possible treatment. J Pediatr 1980; 96:528.

332. Koo WWK, Gupta JM, Nayanar VV, Wilkinson M, Posen S. Skeletal changes in premature infants. Arch Dis Child 1982; 57:447.

333. James JR, Congdon PJ, Truscott J, Horsman A, Arthur R. Osteopenia of prematurity. Arch Dis Child 1986; 61:871.

334. Lyon AJ, McIntosh N, Wheeler K, Williams JE. Radiological rickets in extremely low birthweight infants. Pediatr Radiol 1987; 17:56.

335. Mize CE, Corbett RJT, Uauy R, Nunnally RL, Williamson SB. Hypotonia of rickets: a sequential study by P-31 magnetic resonance spectroscopy. Pediatr Res 1988; 24:713.

336. Koo WWK, Succop P, Hambidge KM. Serum alkaline phosphatase and serum zinc concentrations in preterm infants with rickets and fractures. Am J Dis Child 1989; 143:1342.

337. Koo WWK, Krug-Wispe SK, Succop P, Champlin A, Sherman R, Berry H. Urinary hydroxyproline in infants with and without fractures/rickets. Clin Chem 1990; 36: 642.

338. Koo WWK, Succop P, Hambidge KM. Sequential concentrations of copper and ceruloplasmin in serum from preterm infants with rickets and fractures. Clin Chem 1991; 37:556.

339. Koo WWK. Laboratory assessment of nutritional metabolic bone disease in infants. Clin Biochem 1996; 29:429.

340. Koo WWK, Bush AJ, Walters J, Carlson SE. Postnatal development of bone mineral status during infancy. J Am Coll Nutr 1998; 17:65.

341. Koo WWK, Raju NV, Tan-Laxa MA. Infant nutrition. Hong Kong J Paediatr 1998; 3:103.

342. Koo WWK, McLaughlin K, Saba M. Nutrition support for the preterm infant. In: The ASPEN nutrition support practice manual. Washington DC: American Society for Parenteral and Enteral Nutrition, 1998; 26:1.

343. Koo WWK, Sherman R, Succop P, Krug-Wispe S, Tsang RC, Steichen JJ, et al. Fractures and rickets in very low birth weight infants: Conservative management and outcome. J Pediatr Orthoped 1989; 9:326.

344. Koo WWK, Tsang RC. Building better bones: calcium, magnesium, phosphorus, and vitamin D. In: Tsang RC, Zlotkin SH, Nichols BL, Hansen JW, eds, Nutrition During Infancy: Principles and Practice, 2nd edition. Cincinnati; Digital Educational Publishing Inc., 1997:175.

345. Standing Committee on the Scientific Evaluation of Dietary Reference Intakes, Food and Nutrition Board, Institute of Medicine. Dietary reference intakes for calcium, phosphorus, magnesium, vitamin D, and fluoride. Washington, D.C.: National Academy Press, 1997.

346. Hack M, Taylor HG, Klein N, Eiben R, Schatschneider C, Mercuri-Minich N. School-age outcomes in children with birth weights under 750 g. N Engl J Med 1994; 331:753.

347. Koo WWK, Tsang RC. Calcium and magnesium homeostasis. In Avery GB, Fletcher MA, MacDonald MG (eds), Neonatology—Pathophysiology and Management of the Newborn, 5th edition. Philadelphia: Lippincott-Williams & Wilkins, 1999:715.

22

Metabolic Bone Disease

Joseph M. Gertner

Serono Inc., Rockland, and Children's Hospital, Boston, Massachusetts, U.S.A.

I. INTRODUCTION

Metabolic bone diseases in childhood can be broadly classified into diseases that result from metabolic defects intrinsic to the skeletal system and those that result from an abnormal milieu in which the skeleton is developing. Recent years have seen an explosion of knowledge regarding both types of metabolic bone disease. In the first section I review rickets and rickets-like conditions, which are generally disorders in which bone is affected by an abnormal extraskeletal milieu.

II. RICKETS

The recognition of rickets as a deforming bone disease of childhood is centuries old. Early in the 20th century, Huldschinsky (1) in Vienna made the critical observation that artificial sunlight could cure and prevent rickets, and Mellanby, working in England, showed that a lipid-soluble substance made in the skin or ingested in the diet was necessary to prevent rickets (2). This substance was classified among the essential food factors and called vitamin D, although it differs from true vitamins in that mammals, including humans, can synthesize it in vivo. The last 30 years have seen the recognition that vitamin D needs to be activated, via hepatic and renal hydroxylations, to 1,25 dihydroxyvitamin D (calcitriol) and that the latter is a hormone the production of which is sensitive to hormonal, metabolic, and nutritional regulation. Calcitriol is a sterol derived from cholesterol with considerable structural homology to the adrenal and gonadal steroids. Its principal actions are mediated by the binding of calcitriol to a specific intracellular receptor of the steroid/thyroid/retinoic acid class, followed by interaction of the hormone–receptor complex with the nucleus, where it acts to regulate the transcription of certain specific genes.

In the mid-20th century, Winters in North Carolina and Prader in Zurich described forms of rickets that did not respond to standard replacement therapy with vitamin D. Winter's discovery eventually led to an appreciation of the role of non-vitamin-D-dependent mineral (particularly phosphate) metabolism in skeletal development. The observation by Prader opened a field of inquiry that would eventually link the pathophysiology of vitamin D metabolism and calcitriol–receptor interactions to skeletal disorders in childhood. This section reviews the morphological manifestations of rickets and the associated skeletal histopathology. The specific clinical and biochemical features of rickets as a result of disorders of nutrition, vitamin D metabolism, and calcitriol–receptor interaction are then reviewed. Next, I review the skeletal effects of phosphate depletion, particularly renal phosphate wasting. Finally, rickets and rickets-like conditions caused by renal failure and less common nutritional, metabolic, and genetic disorders are reviewed.

A. Nomenclature

Rickets can be caused by a number of distinct abnormalities of vitamin D intake and metabolism and of mineral homeostasis. As the underlying causes of the varieties of rickets are discovered, more rational names can be applied to individual rachitic syndromes. The terms vitamin-D-resistant rickets and renal rickets are no longer used because they may be applied to a number of conditions that do not resolve with administration of nutritionally adequate dosages of vitamin D or that are attributable to a variety of defects in renal function, respectively. The names of the various kinds of rickets given in this chapter have been selected as the most unambiguous and informative with regard to cause.

B. Definition

Rickets is a bone disease of childhood resulting from the undermineralization of the cartilaginous epiphyseal growth plate. Rickets is confined to children because the growth plate exists only when the skeleton is growing. Widening and flaring of the epiphysis are seen with all forms.

C.   Structural and Clinical Pathology

Softening of the skull (craniotabes) leading to permanent frontal bossing occurs when the onset is in infancy. The ribs (costochondral junctions), ankles, wrists, and knees are other sites commonly affected in growing children. Softening of the long bones is common in severe cases. The nature of the deformity is age dependent. The arms may be affected when used for weight-bearing in babies. The typical lower limb deformity is genu varum when the age of onset is under 3 or 4 years and genu valgum when rickets starts in school-age children. These differences may be caused by the changing relative rates of growth at various epiphyses. (See Fig. 1.)

D.   Extraskeletal Clinical Features

The structural and orthopedic features of the various types of rickets are similar, but this is not true of the extraskeletal manifestations of the conditions that lead to rickets. Hypocalcemia leading to tetany and seizures occurs in vitamin D deficiency and related disorders but not in rickets because of phosphate depletion. Many types of rickets are associated with weakness and myopathy; others are not. Other nonskeletal tissues are also involved in selected forms of rickets, including the hair in calcitriol resistance and the teeth in familial hypophosphatemia. Because of this heterogeneity, nonskeletal manifestations are de-

scribed under the heading of each individual type of rickets.

E.   Nutritional Rickets

Nutritional rickets, once the scourge of poorer children in industrial northern countries, is now largely a disease of developing nations. However, cases occur in the United States and other advanced industrial countries, posing a significant challenge to preventive health services in these countries. Although the term nutritional rickets has generally been reserved for the disease that results from a deficiency of vitamin D, it has been recognized in recent years that calcium deficiency, alone or in combination with vitamin D deficiency (3), can affect large numbers of children in at-risk populations.

F.   Symptoms

Vitamin D deficiency rickets can present at any age during childhood. In severely endemic areas, the deformities and hypocalcemia of rickets may exist at birth (neonatal rickets). When it presents at birth, the softening of the skull (craniotabes) and the neuromuscular consequences of hypocalcemia dominate the clinical picture. More typically, it appears in toddlers aged between 1 and 2 years with a triad of deformity, weakness, and bone pain (Fig. 2). Most frequently, there is enlargement of the epiphyseal growth plates at the ankles and wrists and expansion of the growth plates at the costrochondral junctions (rachitic rosary). The lower limbs may be bowed (genu varum), especially if the child is walking. Because of the proximal muscle weakness of vitamin D deficiency and possibly

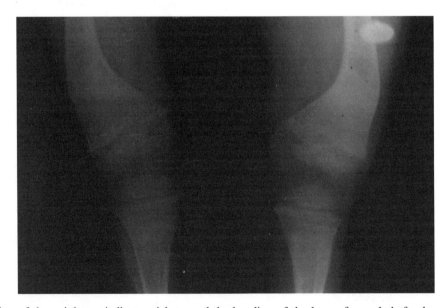

Figure 1   Widening of the epiphyses indicates rickets, and the bending of the lower femoral shafts demonstrates the accompanying osteomalacia in a 5-year-old boy with Fanconi syndrome as a result of cystinosis.

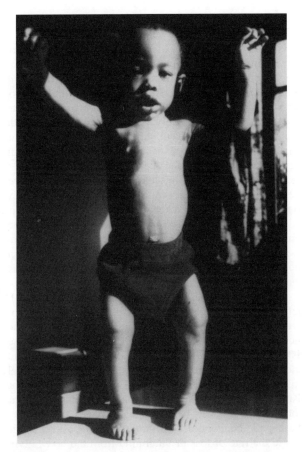

Figure 2 Longstanding nutritional rickets. Note the frontal bossing, rachitic rosary of the costochondral junctions, and deformities of the lower limbs.

G. Radiology

The characteristic radiological changes of rickets are widening cupping, and fraying of the epiphyses (Fig. 3), together with metaphyseal distortion from osteomalacia with malalignment of the long bones resulting from both the epiphyseal and metaphyseal changes. The sites at which these changes are seen vary with the age of the patient and with the cause of the rickets. In infants the wrists and ankles are most likely to show abnormalities, along with the costochondral junctions. In metabolic bone disease of prematurity rickets is often detected at chest x-ray, not only from the costochondral junctions but also because of abnormalities of the proximal humeral and medial clavicular epiphyses. In older children the major epiphyseal changes are more often seen at the knees and hips. The last epiphysis to fuse at adolescence is the iliac crest, which may therefore show rachitic changes in mature teenagers when all other epiphyses are closed. When rickets is treated the widened epiphyses calcify, often to a density higher than seen in the x-rays of healthy children.

because of bone pain, a child who had been walking may become reluctant to walk and revert to crawling or shuffling. There may be tenderness on pressure over the long bones. Growth and weight gain may be impaired either because of a specific deficit in long-bone growth because of vitamin D deficiency or generalized undernutrition of which the vitamin D deficiency is only a part. Associated hypocalcemia may lead to tetany or seizures. In populations in which calcium deficiency appears to be a common cause of rickets the symptoms are quite similar to that seen in vitamin D deficiency (4).

In older children the presentation of nutritional rickets tends to be more subtle, with the gradual appearance of genu varum up to the middle of the first decade and with a knock-kneed or genu valgum deformity occurring in preadolescents. In this age group, as in infants, vitamin D deficiency may also present with hypocalcemia with little or no physical or radiological evidence of skeletal disease. Such children may have a hypocalcemic seizure, or they may complain of distressing paresthesiae or tetany.

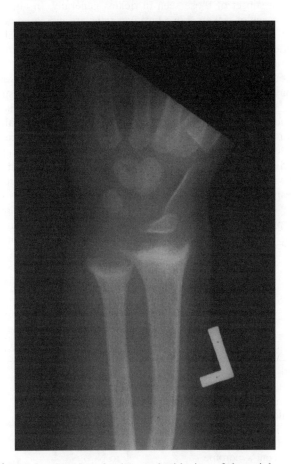

Figure 3 Cupping, fraying, and widening of the epiphyses at the wrist in a young child with nutritional rickets.

In familial hypophosphatemic rickets the upper limbs and costochondral junctions tend to be spared and the major impact is on the lower limbs. The fraying of the upper tibial epiphysis is often much more marked medially than laterally. The osteomalacic bending of long bones (Fig. 1) is not often seen today except in longstanding disease or in those varieties of rickets (such as calcitriol resistance) for which there is no effective treatment.

Malalignment of the lower limbs, on the other hand, is common. Young children tend to show a bow-legged deformity (genu varum), but rickets of onset in an older age group often gives rise to the opposite, knock-kneed (genu valgum) deformity. In contrast to the epiphyseal changes, the changes in alignment do not resolve rapidly with treatment. They may resolve slowly, however, as remodeling and growth proceed over the years following successful treatment of the rickets.

H. Biochemical Changes

Table 1 summarizes the biochemical abnormalities in various types of rickets.

The biochemical abnormalities in nutritional rickets are a subset of those seen in rickets generally. In almost all cases of rickets, bone turnover rates are increased and the attempt to synthesize new osteoid is accompanied by an elevation in serum alkaline phosphatase levels. In nutritional rickets serum calcium levels are usually low, although cases of significant vitamin D deficiency rickets may have normal serum calcium, presumably as a result of parathyroid compensation. The hyperparathyroidism leads to phosphaturia and hypophosphatemia. Eventually parathyroid compensation becomes inadequate and serum calcium falls. Finally, the renal tubule may lose its sensitivity to parathyroid hormone (5), with the result that the renal tubular threshold for phosphate rises with a corresponding increase in serum phosphorus (6).

Vitamin D metabolite levels reflect the nutritional deprivation. The most abundant metabolite in the plasma, the level of which most closely reflects vitamin D nutritional status, is calcidiol (25-hydroxyvitamin D).

I. Epidemiology

In vitamin D deficiency, dietary history may reveal prolonged breastfeeding, a failure to take prescribed vitamin supplements, or, in countries where milk is fortified with vitamin D, an aversion to or intolerance for milk. Disorders of the alimentary tract may also contribute to nutritional rickets, most notably gluten sensitive enteropathy (7), biliary atresia (8), and surgical short gut syndromes (9). Darkly pigmented skin may play a part in reducing the proportion of incident ultraviolet radiation capable of catalyzing the first step in vitamin D formation. However, the nutritional and socioeconomic deprivation conducive to the development of rickets occurs in all human groups.

In contrast to vitamin D deficiency, often associated with prolonged nursing, calcium-deficiency rickets is associated with early discontinuation of breastfeeding and the consumption of diets low in calcium and that may contain inhibitors of calcium absorption (10).

Anticonvulsant rickets is a special case of vitamin-D-deficiency rickets. Patients taking phenobarbital and phenytoin were noted over 30 years ago to have an increased incidence of raised alkaline phosphatase and an increased risk of rickets (11). Subsequent work has shown that phenytoin may be responsible for a variety of relatively mild disturbances of calcium and bone mineral metabolism. These are not necessarily related to vitamin D. Phenobarbital, however, by inducing enzymes that catalyze the hepatic conjugation of vitamin D metabolites, can increase the rate of loss of vitamin D from the body, giving rise to vitamin D deficiency in subjects with marginal states of vitamin D nutrition

III. DISORDERS OF VITAMIN D METABOLISM

As noted, vitamin D is activated by two hydroxylation steps catalyzed by the hepatic microsomal cytochrome P450 enzyme, vitamin D 25-hydroxylase, and the renal mitochondrial cytochrome P450, 25-hydroxyvitamin D 1α-hydroxylase, respectively. Defective activation can oc-

Table 1 Biochemical Abnormalities in Various Types of Rickets

Type of rickets	Serum							Urine Calcium
	Calcium	Phos	AlkPhos	HCO$_3^-$	Calcidiol	Calcitriol	PTH	
Vitamin D deficiency	↓	↓ to ↑	↑	N	↓	↓ to ↑	↑	↓
Calcium deficiency	↓	↑	↑	N	N or ↓	↑	↑	↓
Pseudodeficiency	↓	↓ to ↑	↑	N	N	↓	↑	↓
Calcitriol-resistant	↓	↓ to ↑	↑	N	N	↑	↑	↓
X-linked hypophosphatemia	N	↓	↑	N	N	N	N or ↑	N
Hypercalciuric	N	↓	↑	N	N	↑	↓	↑
Fanconi syndrome	↓ to N	↓	↑	↓	N	↓	N or ↑	N or ↑
Renal failure	↓ to ↑	↑	↑	↓	N or ↓	↓	↑	↓ to ↑

cur if sufficient enzyme-bearing tissue is not available, if enzyme activity is inhibited by the hormonal and ionic milieu, and when genetic disease has reduced or destroyed enzyme activity. In practice, much redundancy exists in the availability of enzyme for the 25-hydroxylation of vitamin D, so that hepatic cirrhosis is not accompanied by a deficiency of calcidiol unless associated biliary obstruction leads to fat malabsorption causing substrate (vitamin D) deficiency. Despite suggestive cases in one family (12), no genetic syndrome caused by a deficiency of vitamin D 25-hydroxylase has been well characterized to date.

The formation of calcitriol in the kidney is tightly regulated and can be pathologically inhibited by a lack of renal tissue or by an excessive extracellular fluid concentration of inorganic phosphate. These conditions prevail in renal failure, which is discussed later. In rare cases, however, the 1α-hydroxylation of calcidiol may be defective in the absence of any other renal dysfunction.

A. Calciferol Deficiency Rickets (Vitamin D Dependency Type 1, or Pseudodeficiency Rickets)

In 1961, Prader and colleagues (13) described an autosomal recessively inherited form of persistent infantile rickets they named pseudodeficiency rickets. The name arises from the close resemblance of the disease to vitamin D deficiency, the major clinical differences lying in the early onset and severity of the rickets and the failure to respond to replacement dosages of vitamin D. A few years later, Fraser, Scriver, and colleagues noted that pseudodeficiency rickets, also called vitamin D dependency rickets, could be treated with low dosages of calcitriol. The condition thus became the first inborn error of vitamin D deficiency to be recognized as such (14). The concept of an abnormality of 1-α hydroxylation was supported when radioreceptor assays for vitamin D metabolites showed patients with pseudodeficiency rickets to have normal levels of calcidiol and very low levels of calcitriol. The assumption that the disease was caused by a mutation of the gene for the 1-α hydroxylase was confirmed after chromosomal mapping of the trait to 12q 1314, cloning of the 1-α hydroxylase gene and sequencing of that gene in affected individuals (15).

Undiagnosed or untreated vitamin D dependency type I can lead to severe deformity, accompanied by hypocalcemia and weakness. However, the disease is readily amenable to treatment with physiological replacement dosages of calcitriol (0.5–2.0 μg/day).

B. Vitamin D Dependency Type II: Calcitriol Resistance (Vitamin-D-Dependent Rickets Type II)

In 1978, two groups independently described patients who appeared to have vitamin D dependency type I but in whom circulating levels of calcitriol were very high. The patients of Marx et al. (16) were siblings with severe hypocalcemic rickets who responded to treatment with high dosages of vitamin D2 or of calcitriol. Three families were described independently 2 years later (from Israel, the United States, and Japan) in which this type of rickets was associated with severe alopecia. The inheritance pattern of the disease and the high frequency of consanguinity in affected kindreds strongly suggest recessive inheritance. The biochemical features resemble those of calcitriol deficiency except that calcitriol levels are high. The patient's condition resists the administration of calcitriol, although some patients respond to dosages as high as 12.5–20 μg/day. The successful use of parenteral and oral calcium to treat this condition (17) is of practical importance because resistance to vitamin D metabolites may be nearly complete in affected patients, offering no other chance for normal bone development. The finding is also of theoretical importance because it implies that the major contribution of calcitriol to skeletal mineralization is the provision of ionized calcium to the extracellular milieu rather than a direct action of calcitriol on bone cells.

The pathogenetic mechanism underlying vitamin D dependency type II is resistance to calcitriol, which has been demonstrated at the subcellular level. The calcitriol receptor may fail to bind hormone because of a mutation at the hormone-binding site (18). Receptor binding may also be normal but hormone action is prevented by impaired interaction of the hormone–receptor complex with the nucleus because of mutations of the DNA-binding so-called zinc fingers (19). In other cases of clear calcitriol resistance, mutations are apparently absent from both the hormone and the DNA-binding regions (20). It is of interest that alopecia accompanies cases of calcitriol resistance of various genetic causes, indicating that normal hair growth may have a direct requirement for functional calcitriol receptors.

IV. DISORDERS OF PHOSPHATE HOMEOSTASIS

Table 2 shows the classification of hypophosphatemic rickets.

A. Physiology

Phosphorus exists in the body largely as phosphate ion bound to organic molecules to form organophosphates. In the serum, about two-thirds of circulating phosphate forms part of such organic molecules bound to protein, but one-third is unbound and is measured after separation from the bound form as so-called inorganic phosphate (Pi). Concentrations of phosphate in the serum are given in molar units or in mass units, which refer to the quantity of elemental phosphorus within molecules of inorganic phosphate.

Table 2 Classification of Hypophosphatemic Rickets

Class of rickets	MIM no.	Inheritance	Comments
Isolated phosphaturia, low urine calcium			
Familial hypophosphatemic rickets	307800	X-linked dominant	Relatively common
Autosomal hypophosphatemic rickets	241520	Autosomal recessive	Very rare, phenotypically identical to 307800
Tumor rickets	—	Not familial	
McCune-Albright syndrome	174800	Not familial	Activation of receptor G proteins
High urine calcium: HHRH	241530	Autosomal recessive	Mild cases may have nephrolithiasis only
Fanconi syndrome: proximal tubular failure			
Cystinosis	219800	Autosomal recessive	Lysosomal cystine storage; progressive uremia
Dent's disease	310468	X-linked	May be a variant of "X-linked nephropathy"

The systems that control phosphate homeostasis tend to regulate total body phosphate content rather than, as in the case of calcium, absolute ionic concentration in the extracellular fluid. This difference accords with the different extracellular roles of calcium and phosphate. Tight control of extracellular Ca^{2+} is essential for the correct function of calcium-dependent cellular activation processes. In contrast, the function of extraskeletal phosphate is mostly as intracellular organophosphates providing intermediaries in energy metabolism, signaling systems, and the genetic code. In accord with these observations is that no well-characterized hormonal system operates primarily to regulate serum phosphate concentration. Instead it is total body phosphate that is sensed and regulated.

The intestinal absorption of dietary phosphate is largely unregulated, about two-thirds of the phosphate content of digested foodstuffs being absorbed. The regulation of phosphate balance lies almost entirely at the level of the proximal renal tubule, which can vary the rate at which filtered Pi is reabsorbed from the tubular fluid. This reabsorption, which normally accounts for 85–95% of filtered Pi, is facilitated by one or more saturable, sodium dependent transporters located on the brush-border membrane. Two genes coding for such transporters in the human have been cloned. Theoretically, the causes of disorders of phosphate homeostasis could be attributable to intrinsic disorders of one or more of these transporter systems or to dysregulation of their function.

1. Dietary Regulation

The renal tubular reabsorption of Pi is extraordinarily sensitive to the dietary intake of phosphorus, specifically to the relationship of the intake of phosphate to that of total calories. In classic studies defining the phosphate-deprived state, Lotz et al. found a sharp reduction in urinary phosphate excretion, increased calciuria, and such symptoms as muscle weakness (21). The reduction in urinary phosphate excretion is rapid, occurring before there is time for serum phosphate to fall significantly, thus leading to the view that there exists a diet-sensitive hormonal system regulating urinary phosphate excretion. The mechanism whereby such a system might influence renal tubular phosphate transport is still unknown but is much closer to elucidation with the recent elaboration of the concept of so-called phosphatonin and the demonstration of the role played by fibroblast growth factor 23 (FGF23) in disorders of phosphate homeostasis (see below).

2. Parathyroid Hormone and PTH-Related Protein

Although primarily functioning as a regulator of Ca^{2+}, parathyroid hormone (PTH) also affects renal phosphate control by inducing phosphaturia. Patients with hyperparathyroidism are hypophosphatemic and, conversely, hypoparathyroidism is associated with hyperphosphatemia. PTH-related protein (PTHrP), circulating in excess in patients with humoral hypercalcemia of malignancy, leads to hypophosphatemia, presumably because of the interaction of PTHrP with renal PTH receptors.

3. Vitamin D Endocrine System

The adequacy of phosphate nutrition and the level of Pi in the serum are major regulators of the renal 1-α hydroxylation of calcidiol to calcitriol. Calcitriol levels are generally high during phosphate deprivation and in the face of hypophosphatemia and are depressed by phosphate excess. Although phosphate regulates the activation of vitamin D, the converse, a vitamin D effect on phosphate homeostasis, appears to play only a minor part in normal physiology.

B. Disordered Control of Serum Phosphate

The control of serum phosphate resides primarily in the proximal renal tubules. Primary disorders of renal tubular phosphate reabsorption, or secondary failure of this process due to lesions outside the tubule, can lead to excessive renal phosphate loss and consequent metabolic bone disease. Phosphate-wasting states are listed in Table 2. Because they lead to hypophosphatemia, their chief manifestations, when chronic, are rickets and osteomalacia, the general features of which have been discussed.

C. X-Linked Hypophosphatemic Rickets

X-linked hypophosphatemic rickets (XLH), a condition dominated by proximal renal tubular phosphate wasting, is by far the most common cause of this type of phosphaturic rickets. Rickets appears in the first year of life. The skeletal changes resemble those of vitamin D deficiency, but the lower limbs are much more severely affected than the upper and the rachitic rosary is not seen. Frontal cranial bossing is common, and rarely there may be a degree of craniosynostosis. There is a striking absence of muscular weakness. Dental deterioration and dental abscess formation are common and may constitute presenting symptoms of the disease. On radiological studies the bones often appear more dense than normal, in contrast to the appearance in nutritional rickets. The lower limbs are more severely affected than the upper, and, characteristically, the lateral portion of the lower femoral epiphysis appears more severely affected than the medial.

Physical growth is impaired. Untreated, the disease results in severe growth retardation and deformity in males, who are hemizygotes. The course is more variable in heterozygous females, some being seriously affected; in others, short stature or the biochemical finding of a reduced renal tubular resorptive capacity for phosphorus may be the only manifestation.

The biochemical findings (Table 1) are dominated by hypophosphatemia with normocalcemia. The renal tubular phosphate threshold (22) is always subnormal in hypophosphatemic rickets. The normal calcitriol concentration is the face of hypophosphatemia (which generally stimulates calcitriol formation) suggests that the underlying defect involves vitamin D metabolism as well as renal tubular phosphate transport. This concept is supported by observation that calcitriol formation stimulated by PTH infusion (23) or by phosphate deprivation (24) is impaired in subjects with FHR relative to normal individuals.

The gene responsible for XLH, originally designated *PEX* and later *PHEX*, has been mapped to the Xp.21 region of the X chromosome and cloned (25). Numerous mutations have been discovered in patients with XLH (26) but there is little evidence of genotype/phenotype associations in this phenotypically rather variable disorder. By homology with genes of known function *PHEX* most probably codes for a membrane metalloprotease and appears to be most strongly expressed in osteoblasts (27). Its precise substrate, and the way in which impaired function lead to phosphate wasting, is still not known but may relate to the role of FGF-23 in the cause of autosomal dominant hypophosphatemia, as discussed in the next section.

D. Autosomal Dominant Hypophosphatemic Rickets

This condition is phenotypically similar to XLH (28). However, its inheritance follows an autosomal dominant pattern. Recent information on the gene responsible for autosomal dominant hypophosphatemic rickets (ADHR) has shown that it codes for FGF-23 (29). This factor appears to be released by the skeleton and to act on the renal tubule as a phosphaturic factor. Work is now (2001) proceeding to determine whether FGF-23 could be a controlling hormone for phosphorus homeostasis (30). This work could radically enhance our understanding of the phosphate homeostatic system.

E. Hereditary Hypophosphatemic Rickets with Hypercalciuria

Low urinary calcium excretion is a biochemical feature common to most types of rickets, including vitamin D deficiency, vitamin D dependency and resistance, and X-linked hypophosphatemia. However, two apparently separate syndromes are known in which hypophosphatemic rickets is accompanied by hypercalciuria.

In 1985, Tieder et al. (31) described an inbred Bedouin family, many members of which had short stature with rickets of infantile onset. Affected subjects had profound hypophosphatemia, parathyroid suppression, elevated calcitriol levels, and marked hypercalciuria, in contrast to FHR patients who suffer from severe muscular weakness. In other described cases, the rickets may be relatively mild, without significant growth impairment.

This form of hypercalciuric rickets, hereditary hypophosphatemic rickets with hypercalciuria (HHRH), is a rare, autosomal recessive inherited condition in which renal phosphate wasting leads to the expected elevation in calcitriol concentrations. Thus, the condition stands in contrast to XLH, in which calcitriol levels are low despite phosphate wasting and hypophosphatemia. As a consequence of elevated calcitriol levels affected subjects may hyperabsorb calcium, which leads to the excessive urinary calcium excretion with resulting nephrolithiasis. Most cases have been described in Middle Eastern and North African populations, but apparently sporadic cases have been seen in North Americans of English and Irish ancestry.

Unlike X-linked familial hypophosphatemic rickets, HHRH has proved relatively easy to control with oral phosphate. Because calcitriol levels are high in the disease and PTH is suppressed, there is no need to supplement with a vitamin D metabolite and no danger of secondary or autonomous hyperparathyroidism. In the author's limited experience and in published reports, the response to therapy has been excellent in terms of increased strength, prevention of deformity, and statural growth.

F. Dent's Disease

Another type of hypercalciuric rickets, now named Dent's disease, was first described by Dent and Friedman (32). Hypophosphatemic hypercalciuric rickets is associated with generalized tubulopathy and eventual renal failure. The disease is inherited as an X-linked recessive trait. Its cause has been identified as a mutation in the gene, CLCN5, coding for a chloride channel and expressed in the proximal renal tubule (33).

G. Tumor (or Oncogenoous) Rickets

Hypophosphatemic rickets is occasionally found in children and adults bearing a small mesenchymal tumor, usually benign (34). The tumor is often classified as a hemangiopericytoma, but benign fibromas, some malignant tumors, and nontumorous conditions such as the linear nevus sebaceus syndrome have been linked to this type of hypophosphatemia. The hypophosphatemia is accompanied by inappropriately low levels of calcitriol, and the degree of osteomalacia or rickets may be severe. Resection of the tumor from affected individuals has resulted in complete and rapid resolution of the hypophosphatemia, leading to the inescapable conclusion that the tumor, often very small, must be secreting an intensely phosphaturic substance that has been called phosphatonin. Since the identification of FGF-23 as the phosphaturic factor in ADHR (see above), this substance has been looked for and found, in tumors associated with hypophosphatemia (30), leading to the strong suspicion that FGF-23 is indeed phosphatonin.

H. McCune-Albright Syndrome

Also called polyostotic fibrous dysplasia, this is a pervasive multisystemic disease of childhood onset that appears to be nonfamilial. Patients show a progressive fibrosis and deformity of bone affecting noncontiguous parts of the skeleton, although completely normal bony architecture is preserved elsewhere. The fibrous dysplasia may lead to pain, weakness, and fractures, with associated disturbances of gait. Children with fibrous dysplasia often manifest hyperactivity of one or more endocrine systems, particularly precocious puberty, thyrotoxicosis, and acromegaly. They also show large, irregularly shaped pigmented skin nevi characteristic of the disease. Many of these children have a phosphaturic state that can lead to rickets and osteomalacia, with worsening of the bone pain and deformity. Following the recognition that most of the manifestations of the disease could be explained by hyperresponsiveness of cyclic AMP-dependent hormone receptors, Weinstein et al. (35) demonstrated that McCune-Albright syndrome is caused by somatic mutations in the gene coding for the α subunit of the G protein gene (GNAS) that controls the regulation of such receptors. The receptors are thus constitutively activated even though the

target organs are not exposed to high levels of the hormonal or other stimulus that would normally be required for activation. In this model the hypophosphatemia would presumably be a result of activation of renal tubular PTH receptors in the absence of excessive PTH concentrations. However, the possibility remains that cells in the abnormal bone are secreting a phosphaturic factor directly reducing tubular phosphate reabsorption.

I. Generalized Tubulopathies (Fanconi Syndrome)

This group of disorders is characterized by excessive urinary losses of all the factors primarily reabsorbed from the proximal tubular fluid. These include glucose, phosphate, bicarbonate, and amino acids. Genetic causes are generally responsible for proximal tubular failure in children.

J. Cystinosis

Severe Fanconi syndrome is seen in cystinosis, an autosomal recessive lysosomal storage disease in which cystine accumulates intracellularly. The onset is in infancy, with failure to thrive and rickets. Affected children are hypophosphatemic and acidotic and go on to develop progressive renal glomerular failure. Treatment with phosphate supplements, calcitriol, and alkalinizing agents, such as the citrates of sodium, potassium, or magnesium, can ameliorate the bone disease. However, until recently only renal transplantation could prevent early death from uremia. The introduction of cysteamine and related sulfur-containing compounds to reverse lysosomal cystine overload and preserve renal cell function has greatly improved the prognosis in this formerly fatal disease (36).

K. Other Causes of Fanconi Syndrome

Genetic conditions in which the impact of the associated Fanconi syndrome is relatively minor include Lowe syndrome (cause of tubular failure unknown), Wilson's disease, and type I glycogen storage disease, which are recessive conditions of copper and carbohydrate metabolism. Another form of Fanconi syndrome that has attracted interest recently is Dent's disease (see above).

L. Nonrenal Disorders: Dietary Phosphate Insufficiency

Dietary phosphate deficiency is very uncommon in adults and older children and is usually seen in association with the abuse of aluminum-containing antacid gels, which bind phosphorus in the gastrointestinal tract. In the premature infant, however, a bone disease that encompasses a spectrum of disturbances resulting in rickets, osteomalacia, and osteoporosis may occur as a result of an oral or parenteral intake insufficient to meet the phosphorus needs of the rapidly growing infant.

V.   RICKETSLIKE CONDITIONS

A.   Hypophosphatasia

This term is used to describe a group of inherited diseases characterized by variable defects in bone mineralization, absent or subnormal serum alkaline phosphatase (ALP) activity, and an excess of natural ALP substrates in the blood or urine. The condition has been classified into five categories according to the age of onset of symptoms and signs: perinatal lethal, infantile, childhood, adult, and odontohypophosphatemia (37). In the last of these dental disease (particularly early shedding of teeth) is the only manifestation. The severity is inversely related to the age of onset. In addition to ricketslike bone deformity, affected individuals may show hypomineralization, fractures, hypercalcemia, and early loss of teeth. Serum ALP levels are low, but vary widely. There appears to be broad correlation of serum tissue-nonspecific alkaline phosphatase (TNSALP) levels with clinical severity (Fig. 4). Increased urinary excretion of phosphoethanolamine and in-

organic pyrophosphate is pathognomonic for the disease. Although the severity, age of onset, and mode of inheritance vary, clinical cases of hypophosphatasia are all attributable to mutations in the same gene, TNSALP mapped to 1p36.1–34. This gene codes for liver and bone alkaline phosphatase but not for placental or intestinal alkaline phosphatase. As shown by Whyte et al. (38), plasma levels of pyridoxal phosphate (a form of vitamin B6) are considerably elevated in patients with hypophosphatasia. This has been attributed to a failure of hydrolysis of pyridoxal phosphate outside the cells and led to the characterization of TNSALP as an ectoenzyme bound to the outside of cell membranes.

B.   Skeletal Manifestations of Trace Metal Disorders

A variety of metallic elements are essential for bone health. Disease can occur both as a result of deficiency and from excess. Table 3 lists the more important ele-

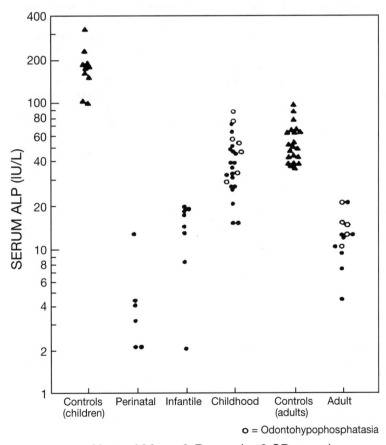

Figure 4   Serum alkaline phosphatase levels in child and adult controls and three categories of hypophosphatasia. (Adapted from Ref. 37.)

Table 3 Effects of Trace Element Nutritional Status on the Skeleton in Childhood

Element	Excess		Deficiency	
	Cause	Manifestation	Cause	Manifestation
Aluminum	Parenteral nutrition, chronic renal dialysis	Rickets, hyperparathyroid bone disease, uremic osteodystrophy		
Copper	Wilson's disease	Osteoporosis	Prematurity, elemental diets	Osteoporosis
Manganese				Osteoporosis (54)
Zinc			Prematurity, elemental diets, absorption defects (e.g., acrodermatitis enteropathica)	Stunting of bone growth

ments concerned, together with the principal causes of imbalance of each element in children, the major skeletal manifestations of excess and deficiency, and references to more detailed information.

VI. METABOLIC AND GENETIC DISORDERS INTRINSIC TO THE SKELETON

A. Introduction

This section reviews the osteoporotic syndromes in childhood followed by some of the skeletal dysplasias. Many of these heritable disorders of the skeleton, with stereotypic deformities, malformations, and growth failure in children can now be explained in terms of genetic disorders of several of the proteinaceous components forming the matrix of bone.

B. Osteoporotic Syndromes in Childhood

1. Definition and Overview

Osteoporosis is the state in which the quantity of material within the bones, both matrix and mineral, is pathologically diminished. It is to be differentiated from osteomalacia in which there is a failure of mineralization on a background of adequate matrix. The term osteopenia is often used to describe an abnormally low density of skeletal material not sufficiently severe to cause symptoms or loss of function. Since osteopenia, thus defined, differs from osteoporosis only in degree the terms are often used interchangeably.

Since osteopenia and osteoporosis are essentially disorders of the proteinaceous matrix of bone they often occur in situations in which protein balance is disturbed by reduced anabolism and/or increased protein catabolism. Another consideration, emphasized by Frost and Schönau (39) comes from the crucial interactivity of bone and muscle at all stages of life and particularly during childhood growth. Given the major trophic role of muscle force on bone development, it is easy to understand why osteo-

porosis should develop alongside neuromuscular diseases such as Duchenne's muscular dystrophy.

Online Inheritance in Man (OMIM) (40) lists 65 inherited disorders involving osteoporosis. Most of these cause symptoms in childhood and most involve disorders of connective tissue matrix. Some of the more important categories of childhood osteoporosis, genetic and acquired, are listed in Table 4.

We generally think of osteoporosis as a disease of later life, particularly common in women and associated in its pathogenesis with the hormonal changes of menopause. This section will touch on developmental topics linking child health to postmenopausal osteoporosis, but its main emphasis will be on osteoporosis occurring in children. Osteopenia and consequent fractures in premature infants are important topics in their own right. The causes, presentation, and treatment of metabolic bone disease of the newborn (41) will, therefore, not be covered here.

2. Clinical Manifestations

Osteoporosis has been called the silent epidemic. Although this alludes to a number of medical and sociologic factors in the elderly population, the description also fits the unobtrusive way in which osteoporosis and its consequences develop. In general, osteoporosis is painless until fractures occur. The prime exception is osteopenia due to malignant infiltration of bone. Osteoporosis in childhood is usually discovered fortuitously by radiological examination or screening in at-risk children, following x-rays done for other purposes, or after a fracture has occurred. Fractures of the peripheral skeleton are more common in the lower limbs and their circumstances may not immediately point to the existence of osteopenia. On the other hand, in the absence of severe trauma, vertebral fractures in children are almost invariably due to osteoporosis, local or generalized. Such fractures cause pain, deformity (kyphosis), and loss of height. The latter may not be as easily appreciated in a growing child as in an adult whose height has been unchanged previously.

Table 4 A Classification of Osteoporosis in Childhood

Category	Diagnosis	Comments
Genetic disorders of connective tissue matrix	Osteogenesis imperfecta Ehlers-Danlos syndrome Osteoporosis-pseudoganglioma syndrome	
Locally mediated bone resorption	Malignancies including leukemia Thalassemia and other causes of myeloid expansion or proliferation	Skeletal pain may be severe May be exacerbated by chelating agents used to treat iron overload
Cytokine-mediated catabolic states affecting connective tissue matrix	Inflammatory bowel disease Inflammatory arthritis	May be worsened by corticosteroid use May be worsened by corticosteroid use
Endocrine and metabolic	Hypercortisolism, iatrogenic or due to pituitary or adrenal disease Thyrotoxicosis Hypogonadism Anorexia nervosa	 Includes failure to convert androgens to estrogens and estrogen receptor defects
Disuse and underuse	Congenital and acquired paraplegia Muscular dystrophy	
Unclassified	Idiopathic juvenile osteoporosis	Usually remits at puberty; heritable disorders of collagen identified in some cases (82)

3. Skeletal Turnover and the Development of Osteoporosis

Once formed, both cortical and trabecular bone are in a state of constant dynamic activity with osteoblasts forming new matrix, calcification of that matrix, and osteoclastic removal of existing bone. Bone cells are able to regulate each others' activity in a paracrine fashion, giving rise to the concept that the processes of bone formation and resorption are coupled (42). During childhood this process leads to a net gain of skeletal material, reaching a plateau in the early 20s and thereafter declining, as

shown in Figure 5. Much of this mineral gain is a consequence of somatic and skeletal growth, but the bones also appear to increase in density (i.e., mass of calcified tissue per unit volume of bone) until early adult life. Adult osteoporosis is due to a preponderance of bone resorption over formation in a skeleton of more or less static proportions. A similar imbalance between formation and resorption may also give rise to osteoporosis in childhood, but a failure to add new bone material as the skeleton grows may lead to a reduction in bone density by a mechanism unique to childhood.

4. Measurement of Bone Density and Normal Ranges

Because the presence or absence of fractures is a crude measure of skeletal integrity, densitometric methods have been devised to diagnose less extreme degrees of osteopenia. In recent years bone densitometric techniques have become sophisticated. The low radiation dosages administered have permitted study of normal children with the publication of normative data from a number of surveys (43). The two methods that can currently provide usable data on bone density in children are dual-energy absorptiometry (DXA) and quantitative computed tomography (qCT). Relatively inexpensive, delivering a low radiation dosage, and with an increasing body of normative data for children, DXA is the most widely used method. The major drawback of DXA bone densitometry in children is that it actually measures the attenuation of an x-ray beam across a projected cross-section of bone. This attenuation

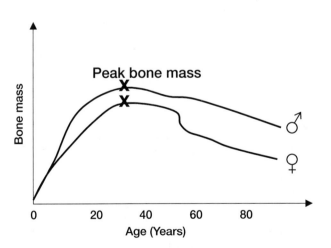

Figure 5 The rapid accumulation and slow loss of bone mineral in males and females.

depends not only on the actual density of skeletal mineral but also on the dimensions of the bone along the axis of the x-ray beam and in the plane perpendicular to that beam. These dimensions and their relation to one another change through childhood, so that corrections based on the child's height and weight have to be applied to the machine's output (44).

Quantitative computed tomography gives a true bone density (mass/unit volume). However, both its cost and radiation dosage preclude the study of large number of child subjects using techniques devised for detailed imaging, so far fewer normative data are available. Low-radiation methods for qCT in children do exist and this method still has potential importance (45).

5. Classification

Following the classification in Table 4, detailed discussion of some of the individual causes follows. The bone matrix consists of collagen and a large number of noncollagenous proteins. Genetic or acquired defects in the structure and/ or assembly of matrix proteins can lead to osteopenia, as exemplified by the defects in collagen synthesis that cause osteogenesis imperfecta.

C. Osteogenesis Imperfecta

The term osteogenesis imperfecta (OI) describes several inherited conditions characterized by an increased incidence of bone fractures on minimal trauma.

1. Causes and Taxonomy

The various types of OI are caused by mutations that affect the nature or synthetic rate of the peptide chains that constitute type I collagen, which is the major collagen of the skeleton. The gene coding for the affected collagen chain is designated by a symbol of the type COLnAm where n is an Arabic numeral denoting type of collagen while the numeral m differentiates between the gene for the A1 chain and A2 chain of the collagen type in question (46). Although some of these affect nonosseous connective tissue, the impact of most falls particularly heavily on the skeleton.

OI is classified into subtypes that are genetically, pathologically, and clinically distinct from one another.

Their taxonomy was clarified by Sillence (Table 5) just as molecular techniques for the analysis of collagen structure and the associated genes were becoming available. The Sillence classification is still useful for clinical purposes and has superseded the formerly used terms OI congenita and OI tarda as well as other descriptive and eponymous terms.

2. Pathophysiology

For a more fundamental understanding of the pathophysiology of the OI syndromes, as well as for genetic counseling and potential prenatal diagnosis, we need a molecular view that is not offered by the Sillence classification. This area remains complicated because of the large size of the collagen molecule and the large number of distinct mutations observed in OI. Although mutations affecting the α-1 chain of collagen are more commonly reported, mutations in both α-1 and α-2 collagen can cause any of the clinical varieties of OI.

3. Inheritance

Both Sillence types II and III were generally considered to be inherited as autosomal recessives. However, some occurrences of multiple cases in siblings born to unaffected parents are now considered to be due to germ-line mutations in which multiple germ cells are heterozygous for a dominant mutation expressed in the offspring.

4. Clinical Features

The clinical features of OI depend on the genetic type of the disorder, the age of onset, and the severity of the skeletal effects. Babies affected at birth have a poor prognosis. Those in Sillence type II are born with multiple fractures that have arisen in utero, some healing with shortening and broadening of the long bones. Stillbirth or early death usually results from respiratory failure or brain damage. In type III the fractures are less widespread, and shortening and deformity of the limbs can be absent at birth. These children often survive for several years with progressive severe deformities of the long bones (Fig. 6). Once again, respiratory failure is often the terminal event. Types I and IV of Sillence are milder conditions in which the mode of inheritance is dominant. The skeletal ten-

Table 5 Sillence Classification of Osteogenesis Imperfecta

Type	Fragility	Sclerae	Teeth	Inheritance	Comments
IA	Present	Blue	Abnormal	Autosomal dominant	Relatively common
IB	Present	Blue	Normal	Autosomal dominant	Variable severity
II	Extreme	Blue[a]	—	? dominant (germ cell)	Perinatal presentation
III	Severe	Normal	Normal	? dominant (germ cell)	Skeletal deformity
IVA	Present	Normal	Abnormal	Autosomal dominant	Uncommon
IVB	Present	Normal	Normal	Autosomal dominant	Variable severity

[a]Sclerae are often blue in normal infants

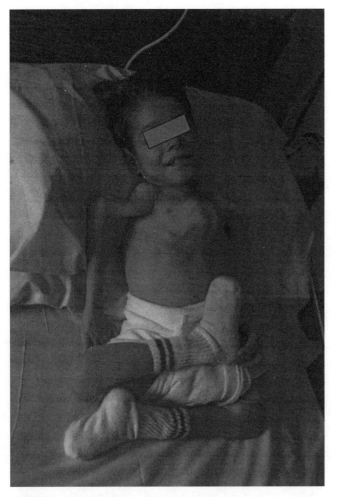

Figure 6 Severe deformity in a young boy with type II osteogenesis imperfecta.

dency to excess fracturing is accompanied by lax-joint-edness, easy bruisability, and conductive deafness. The teeth can be affected by dentinogenesis imperfecta (so-called subtypes Ia and IVa), whereas patients with sub-types Ib and IVb have normal teeth. The identifying characteristic of type I is a persistent blueness of the sclerae (blue sclerae are normal in infancy). Type IV patients present a very similar clinical picture, but the sclerae are a normal white.

D. Homocystinuria

Screening studies of urine from mentally retarded persons revealed some patients with a distinctive appearance, who excreted excess amounts of the sulfur amino acid homocystine. Homocystinuria (MIM #236200) is a recessively inherited disorder caused by the absence or inadequate function of the enzyme cystathionine synthetase. This rare condition has provoked considerable research interest di-

rected toward the high incidence of two very common associated disorders: arterial thromboses and osteoporosis. Tall stature through childhood, and persisting into adult life, is a frequent finding in homocystinuria. The limbs tend to be thin and spindly, with a decreased upper/lower segment ratio. Other skeletal manifestations are severe osteoporosis, beginning in adolescence, and kyphoscoliosis. There is downward dislocation of the lenses, leading to secondary glaucoma, myopia, and retinal detachment. Vascular changes are a frequent source of morbidity in homocystinuria.

E. Hormonal Osteoporosis

1. Hypogonadism
Both androgenic and estrogenic hormones have been considered anabolic for bone and osteoblasts bear receptors for both classes of homones. In both genders there is a sharp increase in bone mineral content during puberty. Osteopenia is seen in adolescents and young adults of either gender in a variety of settings of gonadal hormone deficiency.

2. Turner Syndrome (XO Gonadal Dysgenesis)
Symptomatic osteoporosis used to be common in young women with Turner syndrome before estrogen replacement became routine. There is discussion as to whether osteoporosis is part of the phenotype or entirely secondary to estrogen deficiency manifesting in the early teens. Recent data show that, even with adequate estrogen replacement, osteopenia may persist in patients with Turner syndrome. It is possible that growth hormone, used to promote growth in these short girls, may lead to an increase in bone density acting synergistically with administered estrogens (47).

3. The Exercise–Anorexia–Aamenorrhea Triad
Reduced gonadal hormone output is a hallmark of anorexia nervosa and is also present in many highly trained athletes. Anorexia and athleticism represent different life situations but there are areas of physiological overlap in the anorectic's urge to exercise and the athlete's concern for a trim, muscular, and efficient body. Both in anorexia and in athletic training there are reports that boys as well as girls may suffer from diminished gonadal function, but the diagnosis is made far more commonly in young women and girls and more is known about the skeletal consequences in female subjects. Bone mineral content is reduced in anorexia leading to measurable osteopenia (48) and to concern that these patients will be likely to develop clinically signifcant osteoporosis in middle age. However, it is rare for osteoporotic fractures of the vertebrae or appendicular skeleton to present in young anorectics. It is hard to tell how much of the osteopenia of anorexia is due to hypoestrogenemia and how much to nutritional deficiency, but analogy with more clearly defined varieties

of hypogonadism indicates that hormonal deficiency plays a major causative role.

Exercise, by periodically varying the load imposed on various parts of the skeleton, is anabolic to bone. Nevertheless female athletes (and other trained young women such as ballerinas) lose bone and may become osteoporotic. Undoubtedly the bone loss stems mainly from acquired hypogonadism, the negative effect of which exceeds the benefit from exercise. The major diferences from the anorectic state are that these women are, by and large, well-nourished. In contrast to the situation in anorexia, fractures, particularly cortical microfractures of the lower limbs, are not uncommon. This is related to the great strain imposed upon the limbs by these girls' activities. Bone loss may not be fully reversed with estrogen treatment.

F. Male Hypogonadism

Young men with Kallman syndrome and other causes of hypogonadism are recognized to be osteopenic. Their reduced bone mass is reversible upon administration of androgens. Despite the presence of androgen receptors in bone, doubt has been cast on the role of androgens on bone by the fascinating cases of males who cannot make estrogens (aromatase deficiency) or in whom mutated receptors (49) cause estrogen resistance. In both of these unusual disorders, men developed significant osteopenia despite normal testosterone levels.

G. Glucocorticoid Excess

Cushing's syndrome, endogenous or due to administered glucocorticoids, is a major cause of pathological bone loss in children. It is usually accompanied by severe failure of linear growth. The bone loss can be severe with frequent fractures of the appendicular skeleton as well as vertebral crush fractures. The cellular causes of steroid osteoporosis probably relate more to the catabolic effects of glucocorticoids on matrix protein than to any effect on calcium handling at gut or renal level. No reliable treatment exists for glucocorticoid osteoporosis. Attempts to prevent it have been made by altering the schedule of steroid administration (e.g., alternate-day doses), and by the use of analogs such as deflazacort, designed to have an improved therapeutic ratio. Established disease has been treated with vitamin D, calcium supplements, antiresorptive agents, and anabolic agents such as androgens and growth hormone, all to little avail.

Endogenous and factitious thyrotoxicosis in childhood may cause osteoporosis if untreated for a long period.

Hyperparathyroidism may be associated with bone loss but the sites of skeletal damage are quite specific and different from those seen in patients with true osteoporosis.

H. Nutritional and Metabolic Osteoporosis

1. Liver Disease

The liver is involved in calcium metabolism as the site of the first (25-hydroxylation) step in the activation of vitamin D. In addition, bile production is essential for the normal absorption of both vitamin D and calcium. As a result, severe bone disease, often a combination of rickets and osteoporosis, can affect young children with biliary obstruction (8).

2. Immune and Inflammatory Disease

Cytokines such as those that serve as chemical links between cells of the immune system exert major actions on the relative activities of bone-forming and bone-resorbing cells (42, 50). Conditions as diverse as systemic mastocytosis, inflammatory bowel disease, rheumatoid arthritis, and the hyper IgE syndrome, in which cytokine production is deranged, may be associated with osteoporosis. Juvenile rheumatoid arthritis, in which disuse osteoporosis is combined with steroid effects and, probably, a catabolic effect of immune cytokines, causes a particularly troublesome osteoporosis.

3. Neoplastic Disease

Crush fractures of the vertebrae and pathological fractures through malignant deposits in appendicular bone are not uncommon in patients with childhood malignancy, particularly leukemia and, less commonly, neuroblastoma. The radiological appearances are often patchy, with some areas of the skeleton appearing normal (51). However, diffuse osteopenia is not uncommon. Malignant osteoporosis of childhood is often painful, providing a strong clue to the underlying diagnosis. The rate of bone resorption may be high enough to cause hypercalciuria or even hypercalcemia, but the absence of biochemical abnormalities does not exclude malignancy as a cause for childhood osteoporosis. The evaluation and treatment of the child with leukemias and other malignancies will not be considered further here.

I. Miscellaneous and Unknown

1. Disuse Osteoporosis

Repetitive mechanical stresses are major stimuli to the formation of new bone and the gain of skeletal mass. Conversely, weightlessness, bed rest, and paralysis lead to bone loss. Lower limb fractures are common in nonambulatory children with spina bifida and cerebral palsy. Often nutritional factors contribute to the development of bone disease in these multiply handicapped individuals. A variety of orthopedic approaches may be necessary to handle the fractures but correction of the underlying cause is generally not an option.

Acute paraplegia may cause rapid bone loss, particularly in healthy growing children who have higher bone turnover rates than adults. Although osteoporosis of the paralyzed limbs is the rule in such cases, the major clinical problem is the rapid rise in serum and urinary calcium that may occur in the first few days after injury.

2. Burns

Bone loss after burn injury has been attributed to immobilization. However later work (52) suggested that biochemical markers of bone formation can remain depressed for years after burn injury. The cause of such long-lasting depression of skeletal function after burns remain to be discovered.

3. Idiopathic Juvenile Osteoporosis

Idiopathic juvenile osteoporosis (IJO) describes a severe and rapidly progressive form of osteoporosis seen in the years before puberty (53). The disease affects children of either gender and its cause is unknown. There is now increasing evidence that some cases are due to genetic abnormalities in collagen structure (54).

The most striking feature of IJO is that the bone loss remits with the onset of puberty. At that stage, while residual deformity persists, new growth takes place in the absence of further fractures. IJO is not known to be a familial condition, but the possibility that it is due to an underlying disorder of collagen formation, much like an osteogenesis imperfecta, cannot be ruled out.

The remission of IJO with puberty is a feature shared by many other types of osteoporosis in adolescents, even those whose causes have nothing to do with gonadal hormone status, such as steroid osteoporosis and osteogenesis imperfecta. The natural history of these conditions bears witness to the powerful effect of gonadal hormones on bone.

J. Pediatric Aspects of Adult Osteoporosis

This critically important topic has received much attention. If bone mass increases steadily throughout childhood and the early 20s and is then subject to an inevitble decline, it follows that measures to promote skeletal accretion in youth may prevent the ravages of bone loss later in life. The factors contributing to the gain in bone mass in childhood are complex. They may include calcium nutrition (55), the timing of puberty and other hormonal influences, as well as innate genetic traits. A start in unraveling these genetic factors may have been made by the observation that polymorphisms in the noncoding region of the vitamin D receptor gene are predictors of adult bone mass (56). Doubtless other genetic influences will be discovered since there is certainly a familial component to postmenopausal osteoporosis.

VII. SKELETAL DYSPLASIA

The nomenclature of these conditions seems at first sight to be quite complex. However, in many cases, the con-

nection to the principal clinical and radiological findings is logical and depends on whether the bony dysplasia defects occur in the epiphyses, the metaphyses, or the vertebral bodies (57). An overall classification of the bony dysplasias (Table 6) is provided on the website of the International Nomenclature of Constitutional Disorders of Bone located at Cedars-Sinai Hospital in Los Angeles (58). Names of selected skeletal components together with the names and descriptions of the diseases caused by mutations of these proteins are given in Table 7.

As can be seen from Table 7, the skeletal dysplasias may result not only from abnormalities in structural proteins but also from abnormalities in components of cell-signaling systems active in the skeleton.

Most of these conditions do not disturb the homeostasis of the extracellular biochemical milieu and do not, therefore, show any characteristic biochemical changes in serum. However, there are occasional exceptions to this rule (e.g., Jansen's dysplasia and Albright's hereditary os-

Table 6 A Classification of Skeletal Dysplasias

Achondroplasia group
Spondylodysplastic and other perinatally lethal groups
Metatropic dysplasia group
Short-rib dysplasia (with or without polydactyly) group
Atelosteogenesis-omodysplasia group
Diastrophic dysplasia group
Dyssegmental dysplasia group
Type II collagenopathies
Type XI collagenopathies
Other spondyloepi-(meta)-physeal dysplasias
Multiple epiphyseal dysplasias and pseudoachondroplasia
Chondrodysplasia punctata (stippled epiphyses group)
Metaphyseal dysplasias
Spondylometaphyseal dysplasias
Brachyolmia spondylodysplasias
Mesomelic dysplasias
Acromelic and acromesomelic dysplasias
Dysplasias with prominent membranous bone involvement
Bent-bone dysplasia group
Multiple dislocations with dysplasias
Dysostosis multiplex group
Osteodysplastic slender bone group
Dysplasias with decreased bone density
Dysplasias with defective mineralization
Increased bone density without modification of bone shape
Increased bone density with diaphyseal involvement
Increased bone density with metaphyseal involvement
Neonatal severe osteosclerotic dysplasias
Lethal chondrodysplasias with fragmented bones
Disorganized development of cartilaginous and fibrous
    components of the skeleton
Osteolyses
Patella dysplasias

Source: Ref. 58.

Table 7 Selected Abnormalities of Skeletal Components Giving Rise to Skeletal Dysplasia

Class of disorder	Affected protein	Skeletal dysplasia	MIM code
Matrix collagenopathies	Alpha-1 or alpha-2 chains of type I collagen	Osteogenesis imperfecta types I–IV	166200 166210 166220 166240
	Type II collagen (COL2A1)	Achondrogenesis II Spondyloepiphyseal dysplasia Congenita Spondyloepimetaphyseal dysplasia Strudwick type	200610 183900 184250
	Type X collagen (COL10A1)	Schmidt's metaphyseal dysplasia	156500
Matrix metabolism	Cartilage oligomeric matrix protein	Pseudoachondroplasia	177170
	Solute carrier family 26 (sulfate transporter), member 2	Diastrophic dysplasia	222600
Hormone and growth factor receptors	PTH receptor (PTHR/PTHRPR)	Jansen's metaphyseal dysplasia	156400
	FGFR3	Achondroplasia Thanatophoric dysplasia	100800 187600
	Alphas subunit of G-protein (GNAS1) reduced activity	Albright's hereditary osteodystrophy (pseudohypoparathyroidism)	103580
	Alphas subunit of G-protein (GNAS1) increased activity	McCune-Albright polyostostotic fibrous dysplasia	174800
Control of structural development	Peroxisomal enzymes (Peroxins 1, 2, 5, 6, or 7)	Variants of chondrodyplasia punctata	118650 302950
	Short stature homeobox	Leri-Weill dychondrosteosis	127300
	Cartilage-derived morphogenic protein 1	Several acromelic and acromesomelic dysplasias	177170 132400
Storage diseases	Glycosidases and sulfatases	Several mucopolysaccharidoses	252700 252800 253200 252900 253230 231005 252300

teodystrophy). Although some specific therapies are being explored, the explosion of genetic knowledge about these syndromes has only just begun to generate hypotheses concerning innovative ways to treat some of these distressing disorders.

A selection of these disorders is discussed below. The various syndromes are grouped primarily by cause rather than by morphology.

A. Disorders of Skeletal Structural Protein

1. Type I Collagen

Mutations in the genes coding for this collagen give rise to osteogenesis imperfecta, considered above under the section on osteoporosis.

2. Other Collagenopathies

Mutations in type II collagen (COL 2A1) are responsible for a number of dominantly inherited bony dysplasias including achondrogenesis and hypochondrogenesis and some of the spondyloepiphyseal and the spondyloepimetaphyseal dysplasias.

Some of the defects seen in collagen type II collagenopathies, particularly Stickler-type dysplasia, are mimicked by the effects of mutations in type XI collagen, while other types of multiple ephyseal dysplasias have been traced to mutations in type IX collagen.

Collagen type X is found principally in epiphyseal growth plate cartilage. Mutations can be responsible for Schmid-type epiphyseal dysplasia, which is a dominantly inherited condition that often mimics rickets in its somatic effects and radiological appearances. A major area of differentiation from rickets is that children with Schmid-type epiphyseal dysplasia do not have increased plasma markers of bone turnover, such as alkaline phosphatase, nor any of the other abnomalities of plasma biochemistry that characterize the various forms of rickets.

Cartilage oligomeric matrix protein (COMP) is a matrix protein secreted by chondrocytes that has been found to be mutated in pseudoachondroplasia (PSACH) (59). COMP appears to play a role in the trafficking and organization of other matrix proteins. PSACH is a relatively common disorder usually inherited in an autosomal dominant manner. Patients may not show any abnormality until the second year of life, after which they manifest progressive evidence of limb shortening and disproportion. The face and cranium are not affected in the same way as achondroplasia.

3. Hormone and Growth Factor Receptors

a. Fibroblast Growth Factor Receptor 3: Achondroplasia. A conceptual breakthrough regarding the ways in which the cellular biology of developing bone could affect shape and structure was reached with the discovery that achondroplasia was due to mutations in the gene for the FGFR3. Achondroplasia is a familial autosomal dominant inherited condition characterized by short-limbed growth failure and abnormalities of the cranial and facial bones. The appearances of a large head with frontal bossing and hypoplasia of the midface are easily recognized.

In addition to the morphological abnormalities described, affected individuals may also manifest certain central nervous system disorders including megencephaly, hydrocephalus, and craniocervical instability. In rare cases, the last of these may lead to drastic neurological impairment or to sudden death.

The gene for achondroplasia was mapped to 4 p 16.3 in 1994. Shortly afterwards two groups independently discovered the cause to lie in a specific mutation of FGFR (380 gly_arg) (60). This mutation leads to a gain-of-function for the receptor, which, among other things, leads to premature epiphyseal fusion. Subjects in whom the entire FGFR3 gene is deleted do not have achondroplasia. Hypochondroplasia, a milder form of the disorder, may be caused by the same or other mutations in FGFR3.

Homozygosity for the 380 gly_arg mutation leads to a fatal neonatal skeletal dysplasia called thanatophoric dysplasia.

b. PTH Receptor (Jansen's Metaphyseal Dysplasia). Jansen's metaphyseal dysplasia is much less common than achondroplasia. Its interest lies in the fact that it too is due to an activating mutation of a receptor. However, in this case the receptor is for a systemic hormone system, namely the PTH system. PTH and the PTH-related peptide PTHrP share the same receptor, sometimes referred to as the PTH/PTHRP receptor. Since PTHR

signals the presence of a systemically distributed ligand, it might be expected that constituitive activation of the receptor has systemic consequences, in this case hypercalcemia. It was, in fact this hypercalcemia that provided the first clue as to the molecular cause of the syndrome (61).

c. Alpha Subunit of G-Protein.

Albright's hereditary osteodystrophy. Bony dysplasias may also be related to two separate groups of mutations in the gene coding for the widely distributed alpha subunit of the stimulatory G-protein (GNAS), integrated into a number of membrane bound receptors. AHO is due to loss-of-function mutations in GNAS. When these mutations are inherited from the mother, they lead to reduced function of the PTH receptor with the biochemical features of pseudohypoparathyroidism. However, biochemical abnormality is not the cause of the associated skeletal malformations, which may coexist with a mutant GNAS gene and normal biochemical values.

AHO is characterized by short stature and brachydactyly. Subcutaneous ossifications, which may be extensive, are frequently found and the syndrome is frequently accompanied by cognitive impairment, obesity and hypothyroidism. Where the function of the PTH receptors is affected hypocalcemia, elevated serum PTH level and parathyroid hyperplasia occur.

McCune-Albright syndrome. McCune-Albright syndrome (MAS) is a nonfamilial syndrome due to somatic cell mosaicism conferring constituitive activation of GNAS in various parts of the skeleton and in other organs. Because of the occurrence of hypophosphatemic rickets and osteomalacia in the syndrome, it is discussed above in the section on rickets.

d. Other Abnormalities in the Control of Structural Development: Peroxisomal Enzymes (Peroxins 1, 2, 5, 6, or 7). These enzymes contribute to the turnover of intracellular matrix by controlling the transport of matrix proteins into peroxisomes where they are prepared for catabolism. Dysfunction or absence of the peroxisomes, due to mutations in the peroxins, can lead to a variety of inherited nonskeletal diseases including adrenoleukodystrophy and Zellweger syndrome (62). Skeletal effects include rhizomelic chondrodysplasia punctata (MIM number 215100), an autosomal recessive disorder, and craniofacial dysmorphia and stippled patellas, found in a variant of Zellweger syndrome.

e. SHOX. The short stature homeobox (SHOX) gene, located on the pseudoautomal region of both the X and Y chromosomes, codes for a protein believed to act as a transcription factor. The gene is expressed in osteogenic cells and monosomy of the SHOX gene appears to account for the short stature, and, possibly other skeletal abnormalities (63) seen in Turner syndrome.

Leri-Weil disease is a an apparently dominantly inherited form of skeletal dysplasia with disproportionate short stature and a deformity of the wrist known as Madelung's deformity. The syndrome has been attributed to mutations in SHOX (64). The disorder may be noted at birth and is classified as a dyschondrosteosis because the malformations affect bone derived from cartilaginous growth plates, while growth plate histological examination shows severe disturbance of the arrangement of chondrocytes (65). The reason for the unusual genetics (4:1 female preponderance of cases) was explained when it was understood that the gene involved was located on the X chromosome and the pseudoautosomal region of the Y.

Diastrophic dysplasia is a recessively inherited skeletal dysplasia affecting disparate regions of the skeleton including the vertebrae (scoliosis) and the feet to cause club foot. There is also a characteristic deformity of the position of the thumb designated hitchhiker thumb. The gene responsible has been mapped to 5q32–q33.1 and identified as a sulfate transporter essential for the normal formation of proteoglycans that form the cartilaginous matrix (66).

B.   Storage Diseases

1.   Glycosidases and Sulfatases

A large number of storage diseases affect the skeleton, many of them producing specific skeletal and nonskeletal manifestations. Because the of the extensive effects on the skeleton these disorders are grouped by the International Nomenclature of Constitutional Disorders of Bone as dysostosis multiplex.

The mucopolysaccharidoses are lysosomal storage disorders in which mycopolysachaccharides accumulate due to dysfunction in one of a number of degradative enzymes. Skeletal abnormalities include widening and deformity of the diaphyses of tubular bones and in the spine, kyphosis, vertebral beaking, and other abnormalities in vertebral morphology. Affected patients may also have cognitive impairment, visceromegaly, and involvement of the joints, eyes, and ears.

Other lysosomal storage diseases that can affect the skeleton include the glycoside deficiencies, fucosidosis and the mannosidoses, the GM1 gangliosidoses, the sialidoses, and the mucolipidoses. The reader is referred to the relevant articles in *Online Mendelian Inheritance in Man* for a discussion of the definition, causes, and inheritance patterns of the individual syndromes as well as a tabulation of the relevant original literature (40).

2.   Osteoclast Dysfunction (Osteopetrosis)

Osteopetrosis describes a group of disorders of bone resorption. In its severe form, manifestations are present at birth and prove fatal during infancy or early childhood. The inability to resorb and remodel bone prevents the formation of the intramedullary spaces needed for hematopoiesis and inhibits the development of the cranial nerve foramina in the skull. As a result affected babies are ane-

mic with massive hepatosplenomegaly due to the need for extramedullary hematopoiesis in those organs. Those affected are also often blind and deaf due to maldevelopment of the foramina for the 2nd and 8th cranial nerves.

Children with severe, recessive osteopetrosis are vulnerable to a variety of pyogenic infections including abscesses and osteomyelitis. Neutrophils, monocytes, and lymphocytes from affected children lack the ability to generated superoxide radicals, which are an important component of the process of destruction of phagocytosed micro-organisms (67). Affected infants may show biochemical defects, particularly hypocalcemia due to a failure to mobilize bone from the skeleton and hypophosphatemia due to associated secondary hyperparathyroidism.

One autosomal recessive form that has been well characterized is the form associated with renal tubular acidosis. Acid generation catalyzed by the enzyme carbonic anhydrase is an essential part of successful osteoclastic bone resorption. Absence of enzymic activity results in osteopetrosis and, in the renal tubule, in systemic acidosis. In this form of osteopetrosis the age of onset is higher and severity of the osteopetrosis less than in the so-called malignant infantile form described above. Recently mutations in the CA2 carbonic anhydrase gene have been identified in affected individuals. Other forms of osteopetrosis are much milder and may be noted during adult life following fractures through abnormally sclerotic bone or as an incidental finding on inspection of skeletal x-rays (68).

Infantile osteopetrosis is inherited as an autosomal recessive trait and is, therefore, commonly seen in consanguinous families and within strongly inbred population groups. Within recent years mutations in the osteoclast-specific subunit of the vacuolar proton pump (TCIRG1) have been identified in most, but not all, cases of severe infantile osteopetrosis. A defect in the chloride channel gene, CLCN7, has also been detected in some affected children in whom linkage studies appeared to exclude involvement of TCIRG1.

VIII.   TREATMENT OF SKELETAL DISORDERS

A.   Nutritional Rickets

The treatment of vitamin D deficiency rickets is to provide adequate but not excessive replacement doses of vitamin D. With the recommended daily allowance of vitamin D in childhood at 400 IU (10 μg) we have found that four to five times this dose (i.e., 1600–2000 IU/day) almost always reverses the biochemical and structural changes of vitamin D deficiency. Alkaline phosphatase may rise initially (the so-called flare effect) but after 24 weeks begins to fall toward normal. This approach to treatment constitutes a so-called diagnosis by therapy because unusual and unexpected forms of resistance to standard doses of vitamin D do not respond to replacement doses and then become the focus of more extensive investigations. Treatment may be discontinued when all physical, radiological, and biochemical fractures of rickets have been reversed and the family counseled on dietary and lifestyle changes that can provide the child with the recommended daily allowance (RDA) of vitamin D.

One group of patients who do not respond to vitamin D in doses of four to five times the RDA is that with severe malabsorption syndrome. In such patients, vitamin D should be given intramuscularly, using 100,000–600,000 units. If the malabsorption cannot be reversed by specific therapy, the dose can be repeated after some weeks or months as biochemical indices of osteomalacia begin to worsen again. Intramuscular vitamin D therapy is less often used for children with straightforward nutritional vitamin D deficiency. However, the technique still has its advocates for cases where continued medical supervision and patient adherence to the prescribed regimen are uncertain (69). There is no need to use the hydroxylated metabolites of vitamin D (calcidiol and calcitriol) in the treatment of rickets caused by vitamin D deficiency.

Rickets due to calcium deficiency is being diagnosed increasingly in developing countries in which many children's diets are deficient in this element. In a trial conducted by Thacher et al. (4), 1000 mg/day elemental calcium as an oral supplement, alone or in combination with two intramuscular injections of vitamin D, was clearly superior, over a 3 month interval, to treatment with vitamin D alone.

B. Prevention of Nutritional Rickets

Vitamin D deficiency rickets can be prevented in healthy children by permitting adequate exposure to sunlight and/or by ensuring an adequate dietary intake of the vitamin. Although the majority of the US population is believed to receive most of its vitamin D from solar irradiation (70), this may not apply to impoverished persons living in crowded surroundings or to those immobilized by disability. To target these children and others who may be at risk, the US government has ordered the fortification of milk with vitamin D since the 1930s. In many other advanced countries this policy is not followed, and this difference in public policy may well account for the higher incidence of vitamin D deficiency in the United Kingdom and other European countries than in the United States. Children who do not receive dairy milk may be at increased risk for vitamin D deficiency unless they receive adequate sunshine exposure. This includes infants and lactose-intolerant, vegan, or other milk-averse individuals. Formula-fed infants can be assumed to be receiving adequate nutritional vitamin D. Breastfed babies, however, can receive dietary vitamin D only insofar as the mother is herself adequately nourished. Most of the infantile rickets seen in the United States comes from this breastfed group. Breastfed babies and milk-avoiding growing children should receive vitamin D supplementation according to the RDA, which is 400 IU.

Although US Food and Drug Administration guidelines specify that milk should be fortified with 400 IU per quart (900 ml), reports from Holick and colleagues have shown that many milk samples are inadequately or far too heavily fortified (71). In some cases this has led to vitamin D intoxication and consequent hypercalcemia in heavy drinkers of milk.

The use of calcium fortification to prevent calcium deficiency rickets in children at risk from this deficiency has received considerable recent attention.

C. Pseudodeficiency Rickets

Pseudodeficiency rickets is caused by the inability to hydroxylate calcidiol (25-hydroxivitamin D) at the 1-α position. Since the product of this reaction, the active metabolite of vitamin D, calcitriol, is readily available as a therapeutic agent, simple substitution therapy is possible and has been reported to be fully effective in replacement dosages of 0.5–2.0 ?g/day (72).

D. Calcitriol Receptor Defects

Carefully conducted therapeutic trials have shown that the osteopathy of vitamin D dependency type II can be sharply improved by the intravenous infusion and/or oral administration of calcium (17). The dosages used by Hochberg et al. were high (3.5–9 g elemental calcium/m^2/day) but the treatment was effective in restoring serum calcium levels, reducing deformities, and accelerating linear growth.

E. Familial Hypophosphatemic Rickets

The aims of treatment in familial hypophosphatemic rickets (FHR) are to reduce deformity and optimize statural growth while minimizing the side effects of therapy. The recognition that FHR is primarily a disease of phosphate wasting led Glorieux et al. (73) to propose a regimen of high-dosage phosphate replacement. Such regimens form the mainstay of modern treatment and are always supplemented with a vitamin D preparation, usually calcitriol.

Phosphate is given as a soluble buffered sodium and/or potassium salt. The dosage is calculated in terms of elemental phosphorus and ranges from 0.5 to 1.5 g/day depending on the size of the patient. Emphasis was placed on the need to space doses as widely as possible over 24 h to maximize the period over which phosphate concentrations are enhanced. One of the major untoward effects of this treatment is hyperparathyroidism, which is unusual in untreated XLH (although the author has observed asymptomatic cases) but common during treatment. Rarely this has necessitated parathyroidectomy (74). Evidence that hyperparathyroidism may be exacerbated at night has led to the suggestion that a nocturnal dose of phosphate not be given. Calcitriol is given for two reasons. First, even though calcitriol levels are generally normal in untreated FHR, additional supplementation may promote skeletal mineralization. Second, hyperparathyroidism is minimized by the additional intestinal calcium absorption that follows calcitriol supplementation. There is some evidence that another vitamin D metabolite, 25,25 dihydroxyvitamin D, might be effective in suppressing parathyroid hyperfunction (75) but, this treatment is still experimental.

Treatment is monitored biochemically by measuring serum alkaline phosphatase levels (the most readily accessible marker of bone turnover), urinary calcium excretion, and PTH levels. In affected children, alkaline phosphatase levels should be below the pediatric upper limit, with high levels generally indicating active osteomalacia and requiring higher doses of phosphate. Urinary calcium and PTH measure opposite ends of the spectrum of desirable calcitriol supplementation. This should be increased (and/or the phosphate decreased) if PTH is elevated and decreased if urinary calcium excretion is excessive (above 4 mg/kg/day). Occasionally it is impossible to find a therapeutic combination that achieves all these goals.

Nephrocalcinosis and occasionally nephrolithiasis occur frequently in affected children. These renal changes are probably consequences of excessive urinary calcium excretion during therapy (76); they rarely lead to significant renal glomerular impairment. Thiazide diuretics, which reduce urinary calcium excretion, have been used to reduce the chance of renal damage from hypercalciuria, but they are not widely used in treatment.

The results of treatment of FHR have been surprisingly controversial. Most modern authors are convinced that deformity is reduced and, perhaps less confidently, that treatment leads to improved adult stature. A trial of human growth hormone showed improvement in growth velocity but a worsening in alkaline phosphatase levels, reflecting activity of the rickets. The characterization of the genes and their products responsible for XLH and ADHR may eventually lead to the design of more rational therapy directly targeted at the cellular cause of the phosphaturia.

F. Hypophophatasia

Despite the tremendous progress in understanding the molecular and enzymological pathogenesis of this disease, there are as yet no specific therapies for hypophosphatasia.

G. Childhood Osteoporosis

Childhood osteoporoses are rare and their causes are multifactorial; therefore, a variety of treatment modalities needs to be adopted. As in many rare conditions, it has often proved impractical to prove the efficacy of specific treatments in clinical trials. General approaches include reversal of the cause if known, for example, reducing steroid dosage in steroid osteoporosis and replacing gonadal hormones in osteoporosis due to hypogonadism. As in adult osteoporosis, the administration of calcium supplements is generally held to be helpful.

In recent years there has been strong interest in the use of bisphosphphonates such as palmidronate (77), given intravenously, and alendronate (78) and residronate, given orally. The reader should note that little published literature on the topic relates to controlled clinical trials and that much remains to be learned about the safety, efficacy, and optimal dosing regimens involved in the use of these agents.

H. Osteogenesis Imperfecta

Treatments including fluoride, vitamin D, calcitonin, and zinc have been proposed for OI, but there is no evidence that any are able to lessen the skeletal fragility. Recently it has been shown that bisphosphonates, particularly pamidronate (mean dosage of 6.8 mg/kg intravenously every 4–6 months) can alleviate bone pain and reduce the incidence of fractures in children with osteogenesis imperfecta (79). Conservative treatment and orthopedic correction continue as the mainstays of therapy in OI.

I. Osteopetrosis

The close relationship between the osteoclast line and cellular components of the immune system have led to attempts to treat affected children with compatible bone marrow grafts, where available (80). This method of treatment is still regarded as optimal, but treatment may not be available if a suitable donor cannot be found and still carries a high risk of failure when performed (81). Other forms of treatment include the use of interferon gamma, which can normalize superoxide production in affected osteoclasts, and high dosages of calcitriol.

REFERENCES

1. Huldschinsky K. Heilung von Rachitis durch künstliche Hohensonne. Dtsch Med Wochenschr 1919; 45:712–713
2. Mellanby E. An experimental investigation on rickets. Lancet 1919; 1:407–412.
3. Bhimma R, Pettifor JM, Coovadia HM, Moodley M, Adhikari M. Rickets in black children beyond infancy in Natal. S Afr Med J 1995; 85(7):668–672.
4. Thacher TD, Fischer PR, Pettifor JM, Lawson JO, Isichei CO, Reading JC, et al. A comparison of calcium, vitamin D, or both for nutritional rickets in Nigerian children. N Engl J Med 1999; 341(8):563–568.
5. Kruse K, Bartels H, Kracht U. Parathyroid function in different stages of vitamin D deficiency rickets. Eur J Pediatr 1984; 141:158–162.
6. Robinson D, Flynn D, Dandona P. Hyperphosphataemic rickets in an Asian infant. Br Med J 1985; 290:1318–1319.

7. Stenhammar L. Coeliac disease presenting as vitamin D deficiency rickets in a vegetarian child. Acta Paediatr Scand 1985; 74:972–973.

8. Vanderpas JB, Koopman BJ, Cadranel S, et al. Malabsorption of liposoluble vitamins in a child with bile acid deficiency. J Pediatr Gastroenterol Nutr 1987; 6:33–41.

9. Touloukian RJ, Gertner JM. Vitamin D deficiency rickets as a late complication of the short gut syndrome during infancy. J Pediatr Surg 1981; 16(3):230–235.

10. Pettifor JM, Ross P, Wang J, Moodley G, Couper-Smith J. Rickets in children of rural origin in South Africa: is low dietary calcium a factor? J Pediatr 1978; 92(2):320–324.

11. Lifshitz F, Maclaren NK. Vitamin D-dependent rickets in institutionalized, mentally retarded children receiving long-term anticonvulsant therapy. I. A survey of 288 patients. J Pediatr 1973; 83(4):612–620.

12. Casella SJ, Reiner BJ, Chen TC, Holick MF, Harrison HE. A possible genetic defect in 25-hydroxylation as a cause of rickets. J Pediatr 1994; 124(6):929–932.

13. Prader A, Illig R, Heierli E. Eine besondere Form der primaeren Vitamin-D-resistenten Rachitis mit Hypocalcaemie und autosomal-dominantem Erbgang: die hereditaere Pseudo-Mangelrachitis. Helv Paediatr Acta 1961; 16:452–468.

14. Fraser D, Kooh SW, Kind HP, Holick MF, Tanaka Y, Deluca HF. Pathogenesis of hereditary vitamin-D-dependent rickets. An inborn error of vitamin D metabolism involving defective conversion of 25-hydroxyvitamin D to 1-alpha, 25-dihydroxyvitamin D. N Engl J Med 1973;817–822.

15. Fu GK, Lin D, Zhang MY, Bikle DD, Shackleton CH, Miller WL et al. Cloning of human 25-hydroxyvitamin D-1 alpha-hydroxylase and mutations causing vitamin D-dependent rickets type 1. Mol Endocrinol 1997; 11(13):1961–1970.

16. Marx SJ, Spiegel AM, Brown EM, Gardner DG, Downs RW, Jr., Attie M et al. A familial syndrome of decrease in sensitivity to 1,25-dihydroxyvitamin D. J Clin Endocrinol Metab 1978; 47(6):1303–1310.

17. Hochberg Z, Tiosano D, Even L. Calcium therapy for calcitriol-resistant rickets. J Pediatr 1992; 121:803–808.

18. Kristjansson K, Rut AR, Hewison M, O'Riordan JLH, Hughes MR, Kritz-Silverstein D. Two mutations in the hormone binding domain of the vitamin D receptor cause tissue resistance to 1,25 dihydroxyvitamin D3. Journal of Clinical Investigation 1993; 92:12–16.

19. Hughes MR, Malloy PJ, Kieback DG, Kesterson RA, Pike JW, Feldman D, et al. Point mutations in the human vitamin D receptor gene associated with hypocalcemic rickets. Science 1988; 242:1702–1705.

20. Hewison M, Rut AR, Kristjansson K, et al. Tissue resistance to 1,25-dihydroxyvitamin D without a mutation of the vitamin D receptor gene. Clin Endocrinol 1993; 39:663–670.

21. Lotz M, Zisman E, Bartter FC. Evidence for a phosphorus-depletion syndrome in man. N Engl J Med 1968; 278(8):409–415.

22. Bijvoet OL. Relation of plasma phosphate concentration to renal tubular reabsorption of phosphate. Clin Sci 1969; 37(1):23–36.

23. Lyles KW, Burkes EJ, Ellis GJ, Lucas KJ, Dolan EA, Drezner MC. Genetic transmission of tumoral calcinosis: autosomal dominant with variable clinical expressivity. J Clin Endocrinol Metab 1985; 60:1093–1096.

24. Insogna KL, Broadus AE, Gertner JM. Impaired phosphorus conservation and 1,25 dihydroxyvitamin D generation during phosphorus deprivation in familial hypophosphatemic rickets. J Clin Invest 1983; 71(6):1562–1569.

25. The HYP Consortium. A gene (PEX) with homologies to endopeptidases is mutated in patients with X-linked hypophosphatemic rickets. Nat Genet 1995; 11:130–136.

26. Dixon PH, Christie PT, Wooding C, Trump D, Grieff M, Holm I, et al. Mutational analysis of PHEX gene in X-linked hypophosphatemia. J Clin Endocrinol Metab 1998; 83(10):3615–3623.

27. Guo R, Quarles LD. Cloning and sequencing of human PEX from a bone cDNA library: evidence for its developmental stage-specific regulation in osteoblasts. J Bone Miner Res 1997; 12:1009–1017.

28. Econs MJ, McEnery PT. Autosomal dominant hypophosphatemic rickets/osteomalacia: clinical characterization of a novel renal phosphate-wasting disorder. J Clin Endocrinol Metab 1997; 82:674–681.

29. The ADHR Consortium. Autosomal dominant hypophosphataemic rickets is associated with mutations in FGF23. Nat Genet 2000; 26(3):345–348.

30. White KE, Jonsson KB, Carn G, Hampson G, Spector TD, Mannstadt M, et al. The autosomal dominant hypophosphatemic rickets (ADHR) gene is a secreted polypeptide overexpressed by tumors that cause phosphate wasting. J Clin Endocrinol Metab 2001; 86(2):497–500.

31. Tieder M, Modai D, Samuel R, Arie R, Halabe A, Bab I, et al. Hereditary hypophosphatemic rickets with hypercalciuria. N Engl J Med 1985; 312:611–617.

32. Dent CE, Friedman M. Hypercalciunic rickets associated with renal tubular damage. Arch Dis Child 1964; 39:240–249.

33. Thakker RV. Pathogenesis of Dent's disease and related syndromes of X-linked nephrolithiasis. Kidney Int 2000; 57(3):787–793.

34. Harrison HE. Oncogenous rickets: Possible elaboration by a tumor of a humoral substance inhibiting tubular reabsorption of phosphate. Pediatrics 1975; 52:432–434.

35. Weinstein LS, Shenker A, Gejman PV, Merino MJ, Friedman E, Spiegel AM. Activating mutations of the stimulatory G protein in the McCune-Albright syndrome. N Engl J Med 1991; 325:1688–1695.

36. Markello TC, Bernardini IM, Gahl WA. Improved renal function in children with cystinosis treated with cysteamine. N Engl J Med 1993; 328(16):1157–1162.

37. Whyte MP. Hypophosphatasia and the role of alkaline phosphatase in skeletal mineralization. Endocr Rev 1994; 15(4):439–461.

38. Whyte MP, Mahuren JD, Vrabel LA, Coburn SP. Markedly increased circulating pyridoxal-5′-phosphate levels in hypophosphatasia. Alkaline phosphatase acts in vitamin B6 metabolism. J Clin Invest 1985; 76(2):752–756.

39. Frost HM, Schonau E. The "muscle-bone unit" in children and adolescents: a 2000 overview. J Pediatr Endocrinol Metab 2000; 13(6):571–590.

40. Online Mendelian Inheritance in Man. Baltimore: McKusick-Nathans Institute for Genetic Medicine, Johns Hopkins University; Bethesda, MD: National Center for Biotechnology Information, National Library of Medicine, 2000. World Wide Web URL: http://www.ncbi.nlm.nih.gov/omim/.

41. Gertner JM. Mineral metabolism and skeletal disorders in the newborn. In: Oski FA, ed. Principles and Practice of Pediatrics. Philadelphia: JB Lippincott, 1999: 382–390.

42. Horowitz MC, Xi Y, Wilson K, Kacena MA. Control of osteoclastogenesis and bone resorption by members of the

TNF family of receptors and ligands. Cytokine Growth Factor Rev 2001; 12(1):9–18.

43. Glastre C, Braillon P, David L, Cochat P, Meunier PJ, Delmas PD. Measurement of bone mineral content of the lumbar spine by dual energy x-ray absorptiometry in normal children: correlations with growth parameters. J Clin Endocrinol Metab 1990; 70:1330–1333.

44. Rauch F, Schoenau E. Changes in bone density during childhood and adolescence: an approach based on bone's biological organization. J Bone Miner Res 2001; 16(4):597–604.

45. Gilsanz V. Bone density in children: a review of the available techniques and indications. Eur J Radiol 1998; 26(2):177–182.

46. Prockop DJ. Seminars in medicine of the Beth Israel Hospital, Boston. Mutations in collagen genes as a cause of connective-tissue diseases. N Engl J Med 1992; 326(8):540–546.

47. Rubin K. Turner syndrome and osteoporosis: mechanisms and prognosis. Pediatrics 1998; 102(2 Pt 3):481–485.

48. Sabatini S. The female athlctc triad. Am J Med Sci 2001; 322(4):193–195.

49. Smith EP, Williams TC, Lubahn D, Korach KS, Boyd J, Frank GR, et al. Estrogen resistance caused by a mutation in the estrogen-receptor gene in a man. N Engl J Med 1994; 331:1056–1061.

50. Manolagas SC. The role of IL-6 type cytokines and their receptors in bone. Ann NY Acad Sci 1998; 840:194–204.

51. Gallagher D, Heinrich SD, Craver R, Ward K, Warrier R. Skeletal manifestations of acute leukemia in childhood. Orthopedics 1991; 14(4):485–492.

52. Klein GL, Herndon DN, Langman CB, Rutan TC, Young WE, Pembleton G, et al. Long-term reduction in bone mass after severe burn injury in children. J Pediatr 1995; 126(2):252–256.

53. Dent CE, Friedman M. Idiopathic juvenile osteoperosis. Q J Med 1966; 34:177–210.

54. Dawson PA, Kelly TE, Marini JC. Extension of phenotype associated with structural mutations in type I collagen: siblings with juvenile osteoporosis have an alpha2(I)Gly436 → Arg substitution. J Bone Miner Res 1999; 14(3):449–455.

55. Lloyd T, Andon MB, Rollings N, Martel JK, Landis JR, Demers LM, et al. Calcium supplementation and bone mineral density in adolescent girls. JAMA 1993; 270(7):841–844.

56. Ferrari S, Rizzoli R, Manen D, Slosman D, Bonjour JP. Vitamin D receptor gene start codon polymorphisms (FokI) and bone mineral density: interaction with age, dietary calcium, and 3'-end region polymorphisms. J Bone Miner Res 1998; 13(6):925–930.

57. Taybi H, Lachman RS. Radiology of Syndromes, Metabolic Disorders, and Skeletal Dysplasias. 4th ed. St. Louis: Mosby, 1996.

58. International Nomenclature of Constitutional Disorders of Bone. http://www.csmc.edu/genetics/skeldys/nomenclature.html.

59. Vranka J, Mokashi A, Keene DR, Tufa S, Corson G, Sussman M, et al. Selective intracellular retention of extracellular matrix proteins and chaperones associated with pseudoachondroplasia. Matrix Biol 2001; 20(7):439–450.

60. Bellus GA, Hefferon TW, Ortiz de Luna RI, Hecht JT, Horton WA, Machado M, et al. Achondroplasia is defined by recurrent G380R mutations of FGFR3. Am J Hum Genet 1995; 56:368–373.

61. Schipani E, Kruse K, Juppner H. A constitutively active mutant PTH-PTHrP receptor in Jansen-type metaphyseal chondrodysplasia. Science 1995; 268(5207):98–100.

62. Brul S, Westerveld A, Strijland A, Wanders RJ, Schram AW, Heymans HS, et al. Genetic heterogeneity in the cerebrohepatorenal (Zellweger) syndrome and other inherited disorders with a generalized impairment of peroxisomal functions. A study using complementation analysis. J Clin Invest 1988; 81(6):1710–1715.

63. Clement-Jones M, Schiller S, Rao E, Blaschke RJ, Zuniga A, Zeller R, et al. The short stature homeobox gene SHOX is involved in skeletal abnormalities in Turner syndrome. Hum Mol Genet 2000; 9(5):695–702.

64. Shears DJ, Vassal HJ, Goodman FR, Palmer RW, Reardon W, Superti-Furga A, et al. Mutation and deletion of the pseudoautosomal gene SHOX cause Leri-Weill dyschondrosteosis. Nat Genet 1998; 19(1):70–73.

65. Munns CF, Glass IA, LaBrom R, Hayes M, Flanagan S, Berry M, et al. Histopathological analysis of Leri-Weill dyschondrosteosis: disordered growth plate. Hand Surg 2001; 6(1):13–23.

66. Hastbacka J, de la CA, Mahtani MM, Clines G, Reeve-Daly MP, Daly M, et al. The diastrophic dysplasia gene encodes a novel sulfate transporter: positional cloning by fine-structure linkage disequilibrium mapping. Cell 1994; 78(6):1073–1087.

67. Yang S, Ries WL, Key LL Jr. Superoxide generation in transformed B-lymphocytes from patients with severe, malignant osteopetrosis. Mol Cell Biochem 1999; 199(1-2):15–24.

68. Benichou OD, Laredo JD, de Vernejoul MC. Type II autosomal dominant osteopetrosis (Albers-Schonberg disease): clinical and radiological manifestations in 42 patients. Bone 2000; 26(1):87–93.

69. Shah BR, Finberg L. Single-day therapy for nutritional vitamin D-deficiency rickets: a preferred method. J Pediatr 1994; 125(3):487–490.

70. McKenna MJ. Differences in vitamin D status between countries in young adults and the elderly. Am J Med 1992; 93:69–77.

71. Holick MF, Shao Q, Liu WW, Chen TC. The vitamin D content of fortified milk and infant formula. N Engl J Med 1992; 326:1178–1181.

72. Delvin EE, Glorieux FH, Marie PJ, Pettifor JM. Vitamin D dependency: replacement therapy with calcitriol? J Pediatr 1981; 99(1):26–34.

73. Tayek JA, Brasel JA. Failure of anabolism in malnourished cancer patients receiving growth hormone: a clinical research center study. J Clin Endocrinol Metab 1995.

74. Rivkees SA, El-Hajj-Fuleihan G, Brown EM, Crawford JD. Tertiary hyperparathyroidism during high phosphate therapy of familial hypophosphatemic rickets. J Clin Endocrinol Metab 1992; 75:1514–1518.

75. Carpenter TO, Keller M, Schwartz D, Mitnick M, Smith C, Ellison A, et al. 24,25 Dihydroxyvitamin D supplementation corrects hyperparathyroidism and improves skeletal abnormalities in X-linked hypophosphatemic rickets—a clinical research center study. J Clin Endocrinol Metab 1996; 81:2381–2388.

76. Verge CF, Silink M, Howard NJ, Cowell CT, Simpson JM, Lam A. Effects of therapy in X-linked hypophosphatemic rickets. N Engl J Med 1991; 325:1843–1848.

77. Shaw NJ, Boivin CM, Crabtree NJ. Intravenous pamidronate in juvenile osteoporosis. Arch Dis Child 2000; 83(2):143–145.

78. Bianchi ML, Cimaz R, Bardare M, Zulian F, Lepore L, Boncompagni A, et al. Efficacy and safety of alendronate for the treatment of osteoporosis in diffuse connective tissue diseases in children: a prospective multicenter study. Arthritis Rheum 2000; 43(9):1960–1966.

79. Plotkin H, Rauch F, Bishop NJ, Montpetit K, Ruck-Gibis J, Travers R, et al. Pamidronate treatment of severe osteogenesis imperfecta in children under 3 years of age. J Clin Endocrinol Metab 2000; 85(5):1846–1850.

80. Coccia PF, Krivit W, Cervenka J, Clawson C, Kersey JH, Kim TH, et al. Successful bone-marrow transplantation for infantile malignant osteopetrosis. N Engl J Med 1980; 302(13):701–708.

81. Fasth A, Porras O. Human malignant osteopetrosis: pathophysiology, management and the role of bone marrow transplantation. Pediatr Transplant 1999; 3 Suppl 1:102–107.

82. Saltman PD, Strause LG. The role of trace minerals in osteoporosis. J Am Coll Nutr 1993; 12(4):384–389.

23

Hypoglycemia in the Newborn, Including the Infant of a Diabetic Mother

Hussien M. Farrag
Tufts University School of Medicine and Baystate Medical Center, Springfield, Massachusetts, U.S.A.

Richard M. Cowett
Children's Hospital, Youngstown, and Northeastern Ohio Universities College of Medicine, Rootstown, Ohio, U.S.A.

I. INTRODUCTION

Relative to glucose homeostasis, the neonate is considered to be in a transition between the complete dependence of the fetus and the complete independence of the adult. The neonate must become independent after birth, balancing between glucose deficiency and excess to maintain euglycemia. The dependence of the conceptus on the mother for continuous substrate delivery in utero contrasts with the variable and intermittent exogenous intake orally that is the hallmark of the neonatal period and beyond. The maintenance of euglycemia especially in the sick/or low-birth-weight neonate is difficult. This is especially true in so-called micropremies (birth weight ≤1000 g), who represent a majority of the patient days in the neonatal intensive care nursery (1). Maturation of neonatal homeostasis is influenced by the integrity of the specific pathways of intermediary metabolism important in glucose metabolism. The heterogeneity that is the hallmark of neonatal glucose metabolism is illustrated by the multiplicity of conditions producing or associated with neonatal hypo- and hyperglycemia. This reinforces the concept that the neonate is vulnerable to carbohydrate disequilibrium. This topic has been the subject of a number of recent evaluations (2–7).

II. NEONATAL EUGLYCEMIA AND HYPOGLYCEMIA

A prime example of the heterogeneity that exists in neonatal glucose metabolism is that there are no uniform standards accepted for specific limits for euglycemia. It is well accepted that glucose is the major substrate for carbohydrate metabolism. At birth the maternal supply of glucose to the neonate ceases abruptly. Although the neonatal plasma glucose concentration is usually in the normoglycemic range at delivery, its actual concentration depends on factors such as the last maternal meal, the duration of labor, the route of delivery, and the type of intravenous fluid administered to the mother.

As an example, Figure 1 depicts the mean plasma glucose and insulin concentrations of mothers and their neonates who received either no glucose (Ringer's lactate) ($n = 14$) or glucose (Ringer's lactate + 5% dextrose) ($n = 15$) as a bolus infusion during anesthesia for elective cesarean section (8). Blood samples for plasma glucose and insulin concentrations were taken prior to intravenous fluid administration and at the time of delivery. Corresponding samples were taken from the neonate's umbilical vein and artery at 30 min and hourly after birth for 4 h. As noted in Figure 1, all mothers and infants receiving glucose had hyperglycemia and hyperinsulinemia at delivery. The neonatal plasma glucose concentration declined rapidly during the first 4 h of life. With one exception all neonates evidenced normal plasma glucose concentrations repeatedly and all were clinically asymptomatic. The changes in the neonate following glucose infusion to the mother reflect the differences that can occur in the neonate depending on the type of intravenous infusion administered at delivery.

After normal delivery, the plasma glucose concentration declines to approximately 50 mg/dl by 2 h of age, but equilibrates at approximately 70 mg/dl at 72 h after birth. Cornblath and Reisner have evaluated the blood glucose concentration over time in an old but classic analysis of both term and relatively low birth weight neonates (9).

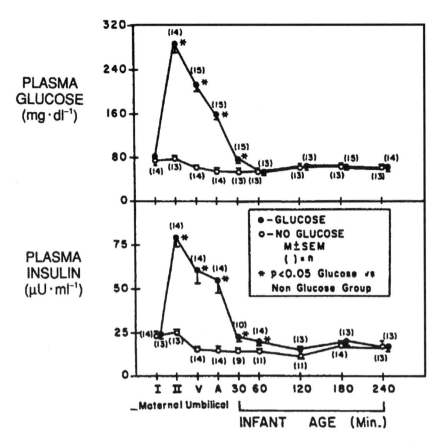

Figure 1 Plasma glucose and insulin concentration for mothers and the neonates. Maternal I and II, samples obtained prior to fluid infusion and at delivery of infants, respectively. V, umbilical venous; A, umbilical arterial samples; (*n*), number of determinations. (From Ref. 8.)

Their data suggested that concentrations below 40 mg/dl or greater than 125 mg/dl are abnormal after 3 days after birth. Critical adjustments are required by the neonate in the first 72 h after birth to maintain glucose homeostasis.

Srinivasan et al. evaluated plasma glucose concentrations in normal full-term neonates who weighed between 2500 and 4000 g and were appropriate for age between 37 and 42 completed weeks of gestation (10). The predicted glucose concentrations during the first week of life are noted in Figure 2. All neonates were fed after 3 h. The data indicated that the nadir in plasma glucose concentration is between 1 and 2 h and that a significant rise occurs during the third hour. The mean glucose concentration in this study ranged from 50 to 80 mg/dl during the first week of life.

No similar evaluation of the limits of euglycemia has been reported for the preterm neonate. This difficult study is clearly necessary because of the general lack of consensus that exists relative to definition of euglycemia. What should be apparent from this discussion is the variation not only in the definition of euglycemia but also in the so-called normal concentration of glucose at any particular time. An obvious example of this latter situation is

noted in Figure 3. In the four types of neonates commonly cared for in a neonatal unit, term appropriate for gestational age (AGA), term small for gestational age (SGA), preterm AGA, and preterm SGA, plasma glucose concentration changed constantly and in an apparent random fashion (11). This chapter will catalog the various causes of hypoglycemia as well as the mechanisms controlling neonatal glucose homeostasis.

A. Definition of Hypoglycemia in the Human Neonate

Although hundreds of papers in the literature focus on the subject of neonatal hypoglycemia, this topic remains controversial. Areas of disagreement involve definition, method/site of sampling, symptoms, significance of asymptomatic status, management, and its effect on neurodevelopmental outcome (12, 13). Koh et al., who surveyed the definition of hypoglycemia in pediatrics textbooks as well as the opinion of over 200 consultant pediatricians in the United Kingdom, considered the controversy relative to the definition (14). They documented substantial variation in the definition of hypoglycemia not

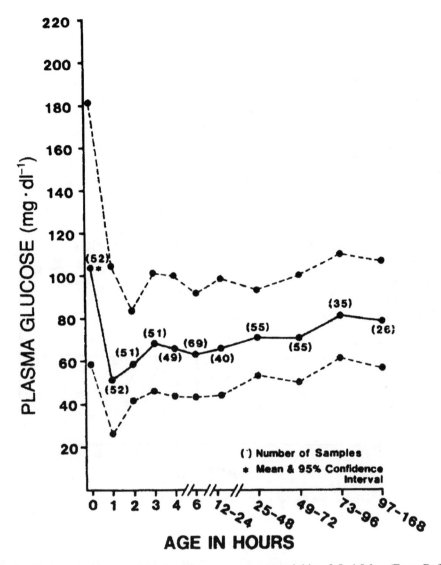

Figure 2 Plasma glucose concentrations in term neonates weighing 2.5–4.0 kg. (From Ref. 10.)

only among the pediatricians surveyed but also among caregivers within the same nursery.

One can postulate four possible approaches to the definition of hypoglycemia in the neonate: statistical, clinical, neurophysiological, and neurodevelopmental.

First, from a statistical standpoint, if a normally distributed curve of glucose concentration exists for the healthy term and preterm neonate, a glucose concentration less than 2 standard deviations of the mean would represent hypoglycemia. In 1965 Cornblath and Reisner reported the data that prevailed in this regard for many years (9). Ninety-five percent of the term neonates in that report had blood glucose concentration >30 mg/dl while 98% of the preterm infants had values >20 mg/dl. Hypoglycemia in the preterm neonate (birth weight [BW] <2.5 kg, in

1965) was defined as blood glucose concentration <20 mg/dl.

Other studies have tried to establish norms for euglycemia in the neonate. Many studies reported concentrations higher than those reported by Cornblath et al. (10, 15). These reports suggested that an average lower limit of 95% CI for neonatal blood glucose concentration is probably ≈45 mg/dl. However, generalization of this knowledge is an inaccurate approach to the problem for multiple reasons. The population studied in these reports varied relative to the following: the source of the blood samples; the methods of assay; whether blood or plasma glucose concentration was measured (i.e., plasma glucose concentration is up to 18% higher than that of the blood) (13); feeding schedules (i.e., early vs. late feeding);

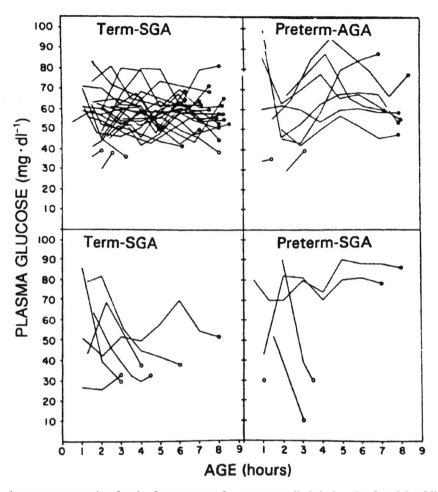

Figure 3 Plasma glucose concentration for the four groups of neonates studied during the first 9 h of life. (From Ref. 11.)

whether the neonate was fed formula or breast milk (i.e., formula induced a higher insulin response than breast milk and may cause lower glucose concentration in formula-fed neonates) (16); cross-sectional vs. longitudinal design; and other metabolic fuels provided at the time of the study, among other issues.

Marconi et al. reported fetal glucose concentration obtained during cordocentesis using venous blood samples (17). We can extrapolate from the data obtained at different gestational ages that venous blood glucose concentrations ranged from 54–108 mg/dl (Fig. 4). That study is probably of greater importance and relevance to the healthy neonate both term and preterm. It is clear that blood glucose concentration was rarely less than 54 mg/dl. This is in agreement with venous cord blood concentrations reported from the neonate by Hawdon et al. that were greater than 47 mg/dl (18).

Second, a clinical approach considers a glycemic concentration to be safe, if clinical symptoms associated with hypoglycemia (Table 1) are not observed, or if these

symptoms have disappeared at that concentration. A classic report, published in 1959 and based on this definition, continues to be influential in clinical practice currently. In that report clinical manifestation of hypoglycemia (i.e., including tremors, irritability, limpness, apnea, seizures, and coma) were observed at a glucose concentration <25 mg/dl and resolved by increasing the blood glucose concentration to >40 mg/dl (19).

There are many concerns with this approach including the observation of extremely low blood concentrations in asymptomatic neonates, especially after glucose screening became a routine clinical practice. If we accept the argument presented in that analysis, we should then consider these extremely low blood glucose concentrations, as observed in the asymptomatic neonates, to be acceptable. The nonspecificity of the symptoms associated with hypoglycemia is another concern, especially when these symptoms are also associated with many other neonatal illnesses. Most of these studies did not evaluate the availability of other energy substrates to the neonate that may

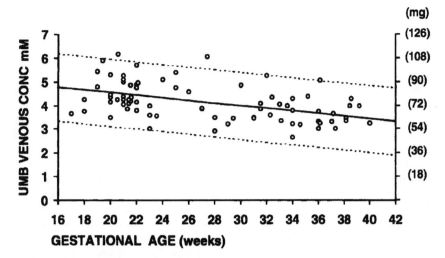

Figure 4 Umbilical venous glucose concentrations (UMB VENOUS CONC) and gestational age for AGA pregnancies (*n* = 77). Dashed lines, mean ± 2 SDs of fetal glucose concentration during pregnancy. Glucose concentrations are noted in mmol/L. Each mmol/L of glucose = 18 mg/dl. (From Ref. 17.)

compensate for the lower glucose concentration. The availability of other substrates may have a protective effect on the brain.

Third, a neurophysiological definition of hypoglycemia has been introduced, based on alteration of neurophysiological functions relative to different glycemic concentrations. Koh et al. evaluated the latency of the auditory evoked response waveform, based on the fact that the inferior colliculus has one of the highest obligatory rates of glucose utilization in the brain (20). They reported that as blood glucose concentration declines (i.e., below 47 mg/dl), the latency between waves 1 and 5 gradually increased until wave 5 disappeared. Restoration of wave 5 was documented when hypoglycemia was corrected; however, it took a few hours in some instances before this restoration was achieved. Among the 17 children they studied, there were only 5 neonates.

Other studies have failed to demonstrate similar effect of hypoglycemia not only on auditory evoked response but also on electroencephalographic (EEG) signals as well as visual evoked potential (21, 22). Future research in the neurophysiological field evaluating electrical signals of different areas of the brain and utilizing other available methodology (e.g., near-infrared spectroscopy or positron emission technology) should be of great value and interest in the future.

Fourth, an approach can be based on neurodevelopmental outcome of the neonate relative to symptomatic or asymptomatic hypoglycemia. The study reported by Lucas et al. provides the most helpful information in this area (23). In their study 661 neonates, all preterm, were evaluated at 18 months of age for neurodevelopmental outcome. Bayley motor and mental developmental scores were blindly assigned to the infants and then these scores

were correlated with their neonatal glycemic concentrations. Data were adjusted for gender, gestational age, birth weight, days of mechanical ventilation, and other social risks. The observed low glucose concentration ranged from 9 to 72 mg/dl.

These investigators demonstrated that two-thirds of the neonates had a blood glucose concentration <47 mg/ dl for a period of time ranging from 3 to 30 days. They found the highest regression coefficient at plasma glucose concentration <47 mg/dl. A more important finding was that if hypoglycemia (level <47 mg/dl) existed for 5 or more consecutive or separate days, the risk of neurodevelopmental deficit (scores <70) significantly increased, regardless of the severity of hypoglycemia during that time. They also suggested that even at lower blood glucose concentration, transient hypoglycemia was tolerated

Table 1 Signs and Symptoms Associated with Hypoglycemia in the Neonate

Apnea
Bradycardia
Cyanosis
Tachypnea
Abnormal cry
Hypothermia
Hypotonia
Lethargy
Apathy
Jitteriness
Seizures

better than prolonged and milder forms of this disequilibrium.

These data reflect the relative inability of the clinician to diagnose hypoglycemia in the neonate. However, there are enough data to support a definition based on the above approaches to the understanding of hypoglycemia in the neonate. A blood glucose concentration of 54–108 mg/dl may represent a more desirable euglycemic range for the term and preterm neonate including the micropremie.

B. Measurement of Neonatal Glucose Concentration

Problems in the definition of euglycemia are accentuated by the lack of attention given to details of measurement of neonatal glucose concentration. Failure to measure the glucose concentration rapidly enough would allow red blood cell oxidation of glucose, resulting in falsely low values. A number of centers previously use the Dextrostix technique, which was thought to be reliable if directions were followed carefully. However, the company cautioned that the reagent strips were not intended for use with neonatal blood. This point is moot since Dextrostix is no longer on the market. However, we suggest that abnormal values, obtained by any strip or meter method either in the hypoglycemic or hyperglycemic range, need to be corroborated with laboratory determination of glucose concentration prior to correction of the suspected disequilibrium, unless the patient is symptomatic (3).

Furthermore, more recent investigations allow one to question if glucose strips should be used at all. Several studies have evaluated various means of assessing blood glucose concentration. Frantz et al. (24) reported that the Dextrostix test strip was able accurately to identify blood glucose concentrations of <50 mg/dl. However, they used fresh heparinized blood from adults to evaluate reliability, which may not be applicable to the neonate. Perelman et al. (25) evaluated rapid glucose determination in the neonate, comparing the Dextrostix Ames Meter, Chemstrip bG test strip, and Stat Tek Meter methods with a glucose analyzer. The investigators concluded that there was modest accuracy in estimating whole blood glucose concentration. They suggested that confirmation by conventional laboratory techniques was necessary before therapeutic intervention. Wilkins and Kaira (26) compared blood glucose test strips for the detection of neonatal hypoglycemia. In 101 blood samples, results of three glucose test strip methods were compared with a laboratory determination of glucose concentration. Two test strips (BM test glycemic 20-800 test strips and the Reflecto-Test hypoglycemia test strips) gave rapid and reliable estimates, but Dextrostix test strips tended to overestimate all blood glucose concentrations.

Conrad et al. (27) suggested that the Glucostix, the Dextrostix, and the Chemstrip bG test strips were relatively unreliable, with r values of 0.73, 0.74, 0.83, respectively, compared with the YSI analyzer in tests of 104 neonatal blood samples obtained by heelstick. They tested one glucose reflectance meter (the Glucometer M), which had an r value of 0.73 when correlated with the YSI analyzer. The investigators suggested that the YSI analyzer should be used preferentially in the determination of blood glucose concentration in the neonatal intensive care unit.

Lin et al. evaluated four glucose reflectance meters in use at the time of their study (28). The manufacturers claimed that these meters could reliably measure whole blood glucose concentrations as low as 20 mg/dl. To determine whether the accuracy of the determination would be affected by the technique of obtaining capillary blood by heelstick, the investigators used cord arterial blood from a separate group of neonates for comparison. All blood was sequentially analyzed five different times on each meter and the YSI analyzer. Evaluation of the data showed that accuracy was limited in heelstick blood whether one evaluated the percentage of difference between the means or the least-squares regression for all the meters tested. The use of cord blood appeared to be associated with greater accuracy than the use of capillary blood obtained by heelstick in the analyses. The reason for the poor correlations with capillary samples and the high variability in the values of blood glucose concentrations remains unclear. There was no relationship between accuracy and reliability of the various glucose reflectance meters. The Diascan S meter, which seemed to have accuracy closest to that of the YSI analyzer, was clearly not the most reliable in comparison with the YSI analyzer. However, the One Touch meter, which had the best reliability among the four glucose reflectance meters tested, was the least accurate. The investigators concluded that, contrary to the manufacturers' claims, glucose reflectance meters should probably not be used for evaluation of capillary blood glucose concentrations in the high-risk neonate.

Holtrop et al. evaluated the sensitivity and specificity of glucose oxidase peroxidase chromogen test strips by comparing values of 272 samples of serum glucose concentration with values obtained by Chemstrip bG (29). The diagnostic sensitivity of a test strip ≤40 mg/dl to predict a serum glucose concentration ≤34 mg/dl was 86% with 78% specificity. The positive predictive value with a 21% prevalence of serum glucose ≤34 mg/dl was 52% with a negative predictive value of 95%. Fifty-eight of the serum glucose concentrations were ≤34 mg/dl and the strips reported values greater than 40 mg/dl in eight. The investigators concluded that more sensitive and specific methods are required for the neonate.

As noted above, it is important to remember that the blood glucose concentration is usually 10–15% lower than the corresponding plasma glucose value. Finally, care must be taken when the test is performed because erroneously high values can be caused by isopropyl alcohol mixing with the blood on the strip that is read by reflectance colorimetry (30).

III. GLUCOSE METABOLISM

A. Methods of Evaluation

Metabolic research in the human neonate is generally limited by several basic ethical constraints, as discussed in a recent review (31). First, the studies must be noninvasive or minimally so. Second, blood samples should be invariably small, particularly those obtained from the very-low-birth-weight neonate. Third, given the limited direct access to most organ systems, the approaches used must allow extrapolation from the sampled data to events occurring in otherwise inaccessible areas. Fourth, the maximal information possible must be obtained from any given study owing to the difficulty of recruiting and the need to study the smallest number of subjects necessary to evaluate the proposed hypotheses adequately.

Many of the above constraints on perinatal metabolic research have been reduced or eliminated by methodological advances in the field. Kinetic studies utilizing stable isotopic tracers in conjunction with mass spectrometric quantification have been the most popular technique in investigating glucose metabolism in the human neonate. This technique is advantageous because both the substrate and the tracer are measured simultaneously with high precision and that minimizes measurement errors. The sample size required for the measurement is small, compared to other analytical methods, which is a major advantage in studies performed in the neonate.

Kinetic studies have been used to evaluate glucose production and utilization (32–34), gluconeogenesis (35), oxidative and nonoxidative disposal of glucose (36–39), insulin sensitivity via the euglycemic hyperinsulinemic clamp (40), as well as other aspects of glucose energy metabolism especially during total parenteral nutrition in the human neonate (41).

B. Evaluation of Hepatic Glucose Production

During kinetic studies utilizing stable isotopic methodology, glucose infusion, glucose absorbed from the gastrointestinal tract, glycogenolysis, and gluconeogenesis may collectively contribute to the rate of glucose appearance in the metabolic pool (i.e., plasma). Only the latter two variables reflect the endogenous rate of glucose production, primarily from the liver.

Measurement of the true rate of glucose production usually gives a good estimate of glucose requirement of the body and the rate of its utilization under basal conditions (42). To measure the true rate of endogenous glucose production, the neonate has to be fasted for at least 3 h prior to the study, resulting in minimal glucose being absorbed from the gastrointestinal tract during the study. No exogenous glucose should be infused during the basal period of the study, except for the tracer isotope that is usually infused at very slow rate. In investigations involve the micropremie (birth weight = 1000 g) the endogenous

glucose production rate under basal conditions cannot be measured for obvious ethical considerations. The rate of glucose infusion, glycemic concentration achieved and the pancreatic β-cell response to the infused glucose during any given study would individually or collectively affect the measured rate of glucose production. The dichotomy that exists in the neonatal literature relative to the endogenous glucose production rate response to plasma-insulin concentration, glycemic concentration and, correspondingly, to the rate of glucose infused, is probably secondary to many of these issues (43).

Our laboratory as well as others has previously demonstrated, in the preterm neonate, that persistent glucose production (glucose production ≥ 1 mg/kg/min) exists during glucose infusion at rates similar to or slightly greater than the basal glucose production rate of the human neonate (i.e., 4 to 7 mg/kg/min) (32, 33, 44). Developmentally this in marked contrast with the adult, in whom glucose production can be suppressed when glucose is infused at a rate equal to or slightly greater than the basal endogenous glucose production rate (i.e., 2–3 mg/kg/min; Fig. 5) (45–48). Other investigators have suggested that plasma glucose concentration of the human neonate, rather than the rate of glucose infusion to the neonate, has an important regulatory effect on the rate of endogenous glucose production (49, 50).

When the results of glucose kinetics studies in three groups of neonates (i.e., the AGA term, the SGA term and the low-birth-weight [LBW] preterm neonate) were combined, Kalhan et al. reported a linear and negative correlation between plasma glucose concentration and endogenous glucose production (33). Complete suppression of glucose production was not achieved in their study.

Zarlengo et al. used the hyperglycemic clamp technique in a group of LBW neonates to evaluate the effect of glycemic concentration on the rate of glucose production (50). They reported complete suppression of glucose production at a plasma glucose concentration of ≥75 mg/dl. An average glucose infusion of 8.7 mg/kg/min was used in that study.

We have previously studied, in a comparable group of neonates, the glucose production response to three different glycemic concentrations (150, 200, and 250 mg/dl) utilizing the hyperglycemic clamp technique (51). A significant reduction in the rate of endogenous glucose production was observed in all groups. Complete suppression of glucose production was not consistent within or among the groups, except in the 250 mg/dl group. To achieve this glycemic level, glucose was infused at an average rate of 16 mg/kg/min.

The dichotomy in results also exists in studies that involve the micropremie. Hertz et al. showed a correlation between glucose production and glycemic concentration in the very LBW (VLBW) neonate (49). They reported a reduction in endogenous glucose production at moderate glucose infusion rate. Complete suppression of glucose

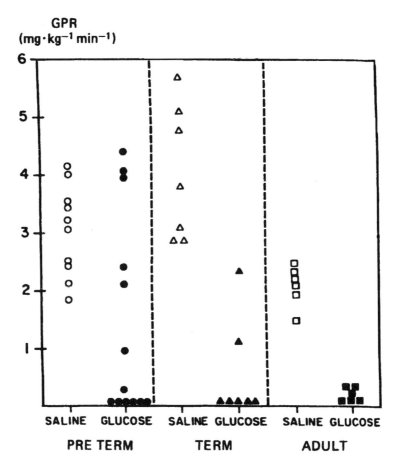

Figure 5 Glucose production rate for each neonate and adult during saline or glucose infusion. (From Ref. 32.)

production was achieved at a relatively high glucose infusion rate and plasma glucose concentration.

Other investigations that evaluated relatively similar groups of VLBW neonates have reported a higher glucose production rate and persistent glucose production during glucose infusion. Sunehag et al. studied 10 neonates born at ≤30 weeks gestation (44). They reported a persistent glucose production during glucose infusion at two consecutive rates of 1.7 and then 6.5 mg/kg/min. Although there was incomplete suppression of glucose production, it is evident that the neonate can partly reduce endogenous glucose production in response to higher rates of glucose infusion. A significant correlation was found between glucose production and plasma insulin concentration but not with glucose concentration. The investigators suggested that insulin plays more important role in the control of endogenous glucose production.

In two groups of smaller AGA neonates (gestational age [GA] 25–27 weeks), Farrag et al. demonstrated persistent glucose production when glucose was infused at both 4 and 8 mg/kg/min (work in progress). There was no significant correlation between endogenous glucose production and either glycemic concentration or plasma

insulin concentration. At the higher glucose infusion rate (8 mg/kg/min) the rate of endogenous glucose production was almost double that reported by Sunehag et al. This is in agreement with the data reported by Keshen et al. and demonstrated a negative correlation between glucose production rate and body weight in the VLBW neonate (35). Table 2 summarizes the results of these three studies.

Although there are differences among the data sets (in weight, gestational age, glycemic concentration, and rate of glucose infused) there is a general agreement that the neonate is able, at least partly, to decrease his or her rate of endogenous glucose production when receiving glucose infusion. However, there is no agreement as to whether glycemic concentration plays a more important role, in the control of hepatic glucose production, than plasma insulin concentration or vice versa.

Relative to the effect of insulin on glucose production, Farrag et al. also reported in the preterm neonate that endogenous glucose production persisted during a wide range of insulin infusion rates (Fig. 6) (40). In that study the investigators applied the euglycemic hyperinsulinemic clamp technique, for the first time, to evaluate insulin sensitivity in the human neonate. When insulin was infused

Table 2 Comparison of Three Studies Evaluating Glucose Production Rate in the Micropremie During Two Different Glucose Infusion Rates for Each Study

Reference	Study weight (g)	Glucose infusion rates (GIR_1 and GIR_2) (mg/kg/min)	Plasma glucose concentration (mg/dl)	Glucose production rate after infusion (mg/kg/min)
49	854 ± 51	GIR_1 = 6.2 ± 0.4	113 ± 12	1.67 ± 0.45
		GIR_2 = 9.5 ± 0.5	136 ± 15	0.32 ± 0.07
44	976 ± 262	GIR_1 = 1.7 ± 0.2	65 ± 20	4.3 ± 1.3
		GIR_2 = 6.5 ± 0.3	110 ± 23	1.4 ± 1.1
Farrag et al., in progress	708 ± 39	GIR_1 = 4.0 ± 0	58 ± 9	3.0 ± 0.8
	677 ± 39	GIR_2 = 8.0 ± 0	83 ± 13	2.5 ± 1.0

at rates that ranged from 0.5 to 4.0 mU/kg/min, that resulted in physiological and pharmacological plasma insulin concentrations (i.e., ranged from 10 to 89 μU/ml), only a reduction of 41–58% of preinsulin glucose production rate was achieved. In a subsequent study this concept was noted to be true for the term, as well as the smaller preterm neonate (28–31 weeks gestation) immediately after birth and in the same preterm neonate when restudied after the conclusion of the neonatal period (≥28 days of age) (52). In that study endogenous glucose production was comparably reduced by 36–60% during insulin infusion at a rate of 2 mU/kg/min. This is again in marked contrast with what is known to be the adult glucose production response to insulin infusion. Our lab-

oratory as well as others has demonstrated complete suppression of glucose production, in the adult, at low plasma insulin concentration and/or minimal insulin infusion rate (32, 45).

Many factors are known to play an important role in glucose homeostasis: glucose infusion rate, glycemic concentration, insulin, and contrainsulin-regulatory hormones. There is no evidence that any of these factors plays a dominant role in the control of hepatic glucose production in the human neonate. Most of the differences between the neonate and the adult in glucose homeostasis are believed to be related to the stress of labor (53, 54). This concept is clearly important in the transition, in the regulation of glucose homeostasis, from the complete de-

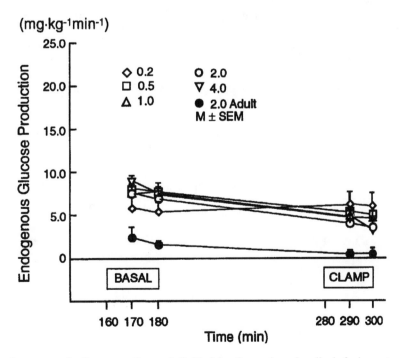

Figure 6 Endogenous glucose production over time subdivided by the various insulin infusion rates (i.e., 0.2, 0.5, 1.0, 2.0, and 4.0 mU/kg/min) administered to the neonate as well as the 2 mU/kg/min rate administered to the adult. (From Ref. 40.)

pendence of the fetus to the complete independence of the neonate in the immediate neonatal period (43). However, there is evidence that these distinctive physiological and metabolic differences between the neonate and the adult continue through the neonatal period and for months afterwards (13, 55). There is also evidence that this pattern of neonatal glucose homeostasis is consistent with the ontogeny of the glucose transporters (i.e., Glut 2) that occurs both at the hepatocyte and at the pancreatic β-cell (56).

Thus the control of glucose production in the neonate is a complex process that is only partially controlled by insulin and glycemic concentrations. This unique response of the liver to insulin and glucose may be of physiological relevance in the human neonate. It is clearly important to ensure adequate glucose delivery to the brain under different metabolic circumstances. This may be of particular importance for the neonate who lacks the autonomy to do so during this critical stage of his or her development. The ontogeny of this process requires further evaluation at both the physiological and molecular levels. The developmental switch to an adultlike response, as has been demonstrated in some of its aspects, most probably requires maturation past the neonatal period (52, 55, 57).

C. Evaluation of Glucose Utilization

It is important to recognize that glucose is utilized by a variety of tissues with different metabolic characteristics (45, 47). First, there are tissues that utilize glucose independent of insulin (e.g., brain). Second are tissues that increase their glucose utilization with increments in plasma glucose concentration independent of increments in insulin concentration (e.g., liver, gut and the red blood cell). Third are tissues dependent on insulin for glucose utilization (e.g., adipose tissues, skeletal and cardiac muscles). It is also important to recognize that these tissues

host different glucose transporters (GLUTS) that are expressed in a tissue-specific pattern (Table 3).

The factors that control the gene expression and function of these transporters probably dictate the metabolic characteristics of the corresponding host tissue (58, 59). The ontogeny of these transporters within any given tissue can explain some of the developmental differences between the neonate and the adult. GLUT-1 is the predominant isoform of the fetus; it is found in virtually all tissues (60–62). It has a very high affinity for glucose and can effectively transport glucose to organs across the blood–tissue barrier. This may be crucial to meet the energy requirement of the fetal tissues during this stage of rapid growth and differentiation. After birth GLUT-1 decreases and other isoforms such as GLUT-2 in the liver, GLUT-3 in the brain, and GLUT-4 in the muscle increase (63–67).

There are two facilitative glucose transporters involved in the brain uptake of glucose. GLUT-1 is primarily responsible for transport of glucose across the blood–brain barrier and GLUT-3 is responsible for the uptake of glucose into the neuron. Evidence from animal studies suggests that GLUT-1 is downregulated by high glucose concentrations while GLUT-3 is not (65, 68). There is otherwise little information available relative to the regulation of GLUT-3. Insulin regulates the expression of GLUT-4 in insulin-sensitive tissues such as adipose tissue and skeletal and cardiac muscle (58). The effect of insulin is rapid and reversible because it primarily translocates intracellular vesicles of glucose transporters to the plasma membrane (69). This step can be rate-limiting for insulin induced glucose uptake under most conditions (70, 71). Except for GLUT-1, which is abundant in fetal life and decreases after birth, some of the other transporters appear to be developmentally regulated. They are found in fetal tissues in smaller amounts that increase after birth and reach adult levels later in life (62, 63, 67, 72).

Table 3 Distribution of Glucose Transporters

Glucose transporter isoform	Primary site of expression	Affinity to glucose
GLUT-1	All fetal tissues, erythrocytes and blood-tissue barriers	High affinity (+++)
GLUT-2	Hepatocyte, pancreatic beta cell and small intestine	Low affinity (+)
GLUT-3	Neurones and testis	Highest affinity (++++)
GLUT-4	Adipose tissue, skeletal muscle and cardiac muscle	Moderate affinity (++)
GLUT-5	Small intestine and sperm	Fructose uptake (+)
GLUT-6	Pseudogene	None
GLUT-7	Liver (endoplasmic reticulum)	Unknown

On the physiological level there is an agreement that neonatal glucose utilization positively correlates to increase of glucose infusion, glycemic concentration, as well as plasma insulin concentration (40, 49, 50). However, it is not clear when this positive correlation would reach plateau in response to each of these factors. In the larger preterm neonate we have demonstrated that endogenous glucose production is sensitive to low insulin concentration, reaches plateau quickly, and then becomes nonresponsive to higher insulin concentrations (Fig. 7) (40). Relative to glucose utilization, although we established a strong positive correlation between insulin concentration and glucose utilization, a plateau was not reached with insulin infusion up to 4.0 mU/kg/min that resulted in a plasma insulin concentration of 89 μU/ml (Fig. 8) (40).

In a comparable group of neonates, we have recently demonstrated that glucose utilization was not significantly different among three groups of neonates evaluated at three glycemic concentrations: 150, 200, and 250 mg/dl

(51). We utilized the hyperglycemic clamp technique in that study. To achieve these glycemic concentrations, glucose was infused at an average rate of 12.8, 14.4, and 16.0 mg/kg/min, respectively. At least in this group of preterm neonates there was no added benefit, in term of glucose utilization (i.e., glucose utilization reached plateau), in increasing glucose infusion from 12.8 to 16.0 mg/kg/min or glycemic concentration from 150 to 250 mg/dl. Similar studies will be important to duplicate in the micropremie to determine the optimal rates of glucose infusion and the appropriate glycemic concentration for these neonates.

D. Oxidative and Nonoxidative Disposal of Glucose

It is important not only to evaluate the overall ability of the neonate to utilize glucose but also to understand how the utilized glucose contributes to his or her energy metabolism. Glucose is generally utilized by either a non-

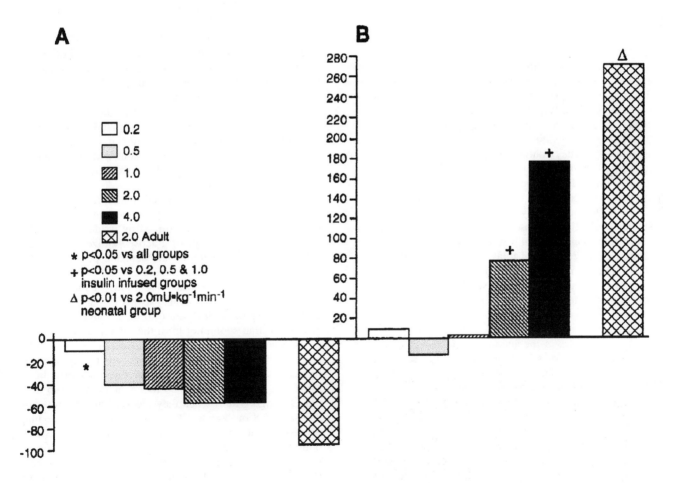

Figure 7 Percentage decrease in endogenous glucose production (A) and percentage increase in glucose utilization (B) subdivided by the various insulin infusion rates (i.e., 0.2, 0.5, 1.0, 2.0, and 4.0 mU/kg/min) administered to the neonate as well as the 2 mU/kg/min insulin rate administered to the adult. (From Ref. 40.)

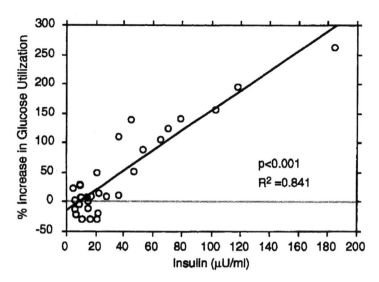

Figure 8 Regression plot correlating the percentage increase in glucose utilization relative to plasma insulin concentration in the neonate. (From Ref. 40.)

oxidative or an oxidative disposal (43, 73). Nonoxidative disposal represents glucose utilized for structural or energy-storage purposes. Only glucose utilized by oxidative disposal will contribute to the energy expenditure of the neonate (73, 74). In the preterm neonate, van Goudoever et al. evaluated the contribution of glucose oxidation to total energy expenditure at glucose infusion rate of 4 mg/kg/min (75). They found that glucose was oxidized at a rate of 2.9 mg/kg/min, which represents 50% of the total glucose utilized by the neonate. They concluded, based on arithmetic calculations, that the contribution of glucose oxidation to total energy expenditure was limited. Other studies evaluating glucose oxidation in the preterm neonate while receiving total parenteral nutrition reported oxidation of up to 65% of total glucose utilized (38, 76). Since glucose represents the main source of energy for the preterm neonate during most of the neonatal period, it is important to determine the extent of glucose oxidation and its contribution to total glucose utilization. It is also important to understand if he or she can adapt to progressive increases in the amount of glucose infused with corresponding increases in the rate of glucose oxidation (77). This knowledge will assist clinically in determination of the optimal rate of glucose infusion, which is the rate appropriate to the neonate's capacity to oxidize glucose.

To answer some of the above questions, we evaluated glucose utilization, both oxidative and nonoxidative, in the preterm neonate (57). We also wanted to determine if hyperglycemia is partly related to diminished glucose oxidation capacity in the preterm neonate. We used stable isotopic infusion of $NaH^{13}CO_3$, followed by $[U-^{13}C]$-glucose, and then analyzed breath and plasma samples to

determine glucose oxidation and total glucose utilization, respectively. This was done over the range of glucose infusion commonly provided clinically in neonatal intensive care units (i.e., 4–8 mg/kg/min). We compared the data obtained within the first 4 days after birth to those obtained from the same neonate at a postnatal age of at least 1 month at the same glucose infusion rates. Thus, we could evaluate the developmental contribution of glucose utilization, both oxidative and nonoxidative, to glucose metabolism in the micropremie.

In that study, we established a significant linear and negative correlation between glycemic concentration and the percentage of glucose utilized by oxidation. We also found that the percentage of glucose oxidized was significantly higher in the immediate neonatal period ($\approx 68\%$) than that oxidized at about 5 weeks of life ($\approx 47\%$) by the same neonate. This was true at both glucose infusion rates with each micropremie serving as his or her own control at the same glucose infusion (4.0 or 8.0 mg/kg/min). We also found that soon after birth the micropremie was able to oxidize significantly higher rates of glucose when glucose was infused at a rate of 8.0 vs. 4.0 mg/kg/min. We found that the preterm neonate was able, soon after birth, to oxidize glucose at rates up to 7.5 mg/kg/min (95% CI 5.5–9.4 mg/kg/min) when they received glucose infusion at a rate of 8 mg/kg/min. The glucose oxidation rate may exceed the rate of glucose infusion, reflecting the contribution of endogenous glucose production to the total pool of glucose available for oxidation. None of these neonates developed hyperglycemia during glucose infusion at 8.0 mg/kg/min and at that rate blood glucose concentration averaged 83 ± 14 mg/dl (mean [M] ± standard error of the mean [SEM]) (57).

These results should encourage the use of glucose infusion at a rate of 8 mg/kg/min in the preterm neonate after the first day of life: the study age ranged from 27 to 96 h. The clinical practice of using as low a glucose infusion rate as possible in the preterm neonate to avoid hyperglycemia limits energy intake not only from glucose but also from fat and protein, since the composition of parenteral alimentation is usually administered proportionally (54). Hyperglycemia did not result from the rates of glucose infusion employed in these studies. However, the addition of fat and/or amino acids can increase the risk of this complication (41, 78). The risk of hyperglycemia should be weighed against the benefit of providing adequate energy, especially when insulin infusion has been shown to improve peripheral glucose utilization and enhance glucose tolerance significantly in the preterm neonate (40, 79).

We found nonoxidative disposal to be significantly higher in the older neonates when they were studied after the conclusion of the neonatal period (the late study) compared to themselves when they were studied in the immediate neonatal period (the early study). It is important to recognize that the metabolic state of the neonate is different during these two periods. Early after birth the caloric intake of the micropremie is insufficient to satisfy his or her energy expenditure, since he or she is in a catabolic state. If the neonate is medically stable after the conclusion of the neonatal period (i.e., similar to our study population) and receiving adequate caloric intake, he or she will be in an anabolic state.

The nonoxidative disposal of glucose represents its utilization by different metabolic pathways (43, 73, 80). In an anabolic state lipogenesis is a major route for nonoxidative disposal (38). Other nonoxidative pathways for glucose may include glycogenesis, cycling in the pentose phosphate pathway, and/or formation of a carbon skeleton for amino acids (73, 74, 76). The extrauterine developmental switch from a catabolic state (the early study) to an anabolic one (the late study) during the course of the current investigation can, at least in part, explain the significant increase in the contribution of the nonoxidative disposal of glucose to total energy metabolism in the late studies. Other factors, such as the change in the substrate available for energy metabolism from primarily glucose to a mixture of fat and carbohydrates, may play an equally important role in that phenomenon.

IV. CLINICAL ASSESSMENT

A. Incidence

It is not surprising that variations in the estimated incidence of hypoglycemia exist in the neonatal literature. Different reports vary relative to populations, definitions, screening methods, clinical status, as well as strategies for nutrition and fluid management. The incidence ranges from 7 to 57% based on these variations (13).

B. General Pathophysiological and Metabolic Considerations

The close relationship between maternal and fetal glucose, the repetitive occurrence of wide swings of neonatal glucose concentration, and the retarded disappearance of an acute glucose load in both term and preterm neonates indicate that the regulation of neonatal carbohydrate metabolism is poorly developed 72 h after birth (81). The birth process brings the necessity of a period of readjustment to allow subsequent control. In the low-birth-weight neonate especially, this adjustment is delicate and may result in abnormal consequences. We have already discussed the difficulties in the definition of hypoglycemia. One of the main clinical difficulties with the definition is the nonspecific symptoms, which include the signs and symptoms listed in Table 1. These difficulties are compounded by the occurrence of symptoms at different concentrations of blood glucose in different neonates and the lack of a universal threshold below or above which symptoms may occur (2, 7).

During steady-state glucose metabolism, glucose production equals glucose utilization and glycemic concentration is maintained within a narrow range. A simplistic approach will attribute hypoglycemia to decreased glucose production and/or increased glucose utilization. As discussed earlier, the neonate, on a per kilogram body weight basis, is able to produce glucose at adequate rates. There is evidence that the enzymatic pathways for glucose production via glycogenolysis as well as gluconeogenesis are intact in the term and preterm neonate (43). It is also recognized that the glycogen stores are limited in the preterm neonate as glycogen accumulation primarily takes place in the third trimester (13, 43, 54). Based on that, gluconeogenesis is the major route of glucose production in these neonates.

The change in metabolic milieu that occurs at birth, including the reduction of plasma insulin concentration as well as the elevation of cortisol concentration, catecholamines, and glucagon, favors the induction of gluconeogenesis. Of course the clamping of the cord and the termination of maternal glucose supplementation initiate and enhance these changes. The time necessary to induce and transcript the involved enzyme's protein of gluconeogenesis, in metabolically functioning amounts (about 2 h), coincides with the clinical observation that the lowest blood glucose concentrations in the neonate were measured between 1–2 h after birth. The absence of stored glycogen in the low-birth-weight neonate makes hypoglycemia almost inevitable in the first few hours after birth if exogenous glucose is not provided.

The brain is the major site of glucose utilization in the neonate and the major site of concern as well. The neonate has the greatest brain to body weight ratio during human development. Some investigations have concluded that up to 90% of the glucose produced is utilized by the brain, via oxidation (82). Other investigations conclude that the entire amount of glucose oxidized, in the term neonate, is insufficient to satisfy brain glucose requirements (83). There is evidence that the neonatal brain utilizes other metabolic substrates soon after birth, including lactate and ketones (73, 84–86). There is evidence from animal and human studies that during hypoglycemia the brain reduces its glucose consumption by more than 50% and increases its utilization of other substrates (e.g., ketones and lactate) by 15-fold or greater (73, 85, 86). There is also evidence that the term neonate can efficiently mobilize similar substrates during fasting (87). Furthermore, free fatty acids, glycerol, and ketone concentrations were negatively correlated with blood glucose concentration in these term neonates (18, 88). This ability to mobilize other energy substrates to adapt to hypoglycemia has a protective effect on the brain.

There is evidence that the preterm neonate lacks this protective ability (89). The lack of energy stores in form of glycogen, as discussed earlier, and adipose tissue is prominent in these neonates. Although fat cannot substitute glucose for brain energy metabolism, its mobilization and oxidation reduce glucose uptake by other tissues and make more glucose available for the brain (13). Levistky et al. demonstrated that nonesterified fatty acids and ketone body concentrations of the preterm infant are significantly lower than those of the term infant (86). Moreover, preterm infants with low blood glucose concentrations did not show increased ketone body concentrations, as did their term counterparts. This discussion emphasizes that, in the micropremie, cerebral defenses against hypoglycemia are limited, and prolonged episodes, even of milder nature, of hypoglycemia may have a more significant effect on the brain of the preterm than that of the term neonate.

There is evidence, as recently reviewed by Simmons, that the immaturity of GLUT-2 function in the hepatocyte as well as in the pancreatic β-cell may play a role in the pathophysiology of neonatal hypoglycemia (58). GLUT-2 is a low-affinity glucose transporter that occurs only in the hepatocyte and pancreatic β-cell. In the mature hepatocyte the low affinity of this transporter allows glucose release into the plasma in response to small reduction in plasma glucose concentration. This process is sensitive even within the normal glucose concentration range, resulting in maintenance of euglycemia.

In the newborn period, studies in multiple species demonstrate that the hepatocyte expresses a relatively high amount of GLUT-1 but relatively low levels of GLUT-2 (56). Decreased GLUT-2 expression may limit the hepatocyte sensitivity and responsiveness to changes in glucose and insulin concentration during hypoglycemia (40). This is in agreement with data from our laboratory demonstrating that the preterm neonatal liver was nonresponsive to progressive increment in insulin rates of infusion and plasma concentrations. We attributed this nonresponsiveness to insulin to intracellular mechanism(s) that probably involve a defect in glucose transporter rather than insulin receptors (40).

In the pancreatic β-cell GLUT-2, in concert with glucokinase, functions as a glucose sensor that allows the β-cell to recognize modest changes in plasma glucose concentration and appropriately secrete insulin (58, 59). Although the β-cell of the neonate responds to changes in the glycemic level, this process is diminished, in part due to decreased expression and/or function of the immature glucose sensor, and in part due to decreased activity of other metabolic linkages in the β-cell. Thus, the immature glucose sensor in the pancreatic β-cell may contribute to its inability to downregulate insulin secretion during hypoglycemia. There is evidence that this phenomenon is developmentally regulated (59). This is in agreement with reports suggesting that the basal insulin/glucose ratio is significantly higher in the preterm than in the term neonate (55).

Pryds et al. reported some evidence of increased cerebral blood flow in preterm infants to support cerebral metabolism during hypoglycemia (<30 mg/dl) (90). They also reported decreased cerebral blood volume during restoration of hypoglycemia in the preterm neonate (91). They concluded from these observations and the rapidity of adjustment of cerebral blood vessels to alteration in glucose concentration that a cerebral glucose sensor exists in the preterm neonate (92). They suggested that this sensor functions by recruiting brain capillaries to maintain adequate glucose transport to the brain during hypoglycemia.

C. Causes of Hypoglycemia

A number of different classifications have been used to categorize the various causes of hypoglycemia seen in the neonatal period. Table 4 lists many mechanisms known to be associated with hypoglycemia in the human neonate. One or a combination of the following three mechanisms generally causes neonatal hypoglycemia: diminished hepatic glucose production; depletion of glycogen stores; increased rate of glucose utilization. Extreme prematurity is a prime example of hypoglycemia due to primary failure to produce and/or store glycogen. Hypoglycemia secondary to depletion of glycogen stores is evident in the prematurely born AGA and/or SGA neonate as well as the neonate with congenital heart disease. Increased rate of glucose utilization, without hyperinsulinism, may explain the hypoglycemia seen in the perinatally stressed and asphyxiated neonate, cold-stressed neonate, as well as the neonate with congestive heart failure [e.g., hemodynamically significant patent ductus anteriosus (PDA)], and/or sepsis. The common thread in all these conditions is poor peripheral circulation and tissue perfusion associated with hypoxemia and lactic acidosis. This will lead to diminished mobilization of substrates as well as energy-inefficient anaerobic glycolysis. Neonatal hyperinsulinemic syndromes, including the infant of diabetic mother, can be associated with significant and/or persistent neonatal hypoglycemia. Neonates may also be hypoglycemic be-

Table 4 Condition Associated with Hypoglycemia in the Neonate

Mechanism and/or origin	Condition, disease, and/or syndrome
Primary failure to produce and/or store glycogen	Extreme prematurity
Depletion of glycogen stores	Prematurity, intrauterine growth restriction/small for gestational age, postmaturity, and congenital heart disease/congestive heart failure
Increased rate of glucose utilization	Perinatal stress/hypoxia, cold stress, and sepsis
Hyperinsulinemia	Infant of diabetic mother, large for gestational age, Rh incompatibility, following exchange transfusion, malposition of umbilical artery catheter, nesidioblastosis, exposure to beta-adrenergic agonists and others
Inherited diseases	Malformation syndromes (e.g., Beckwith-Wiedemann syndrome), autosomal recessive hyperinsulinemia, inborn errors of carbohydrate, protein and lipid metabolism
Endocrine deficiency	Hypopituitarism, growth hormone deficiency, glucagon deficiency, cortisol deficiency/ACTH unresponsiveness
Newly described syndromes	Specific glucose transporter deficiency (neuroglucopenia during euglycemia), neonatal hyperinsulinemia-hypoglycemia and isoimmune thrombocytopenia association

cause of deficits in intermediary metabolic pathways such as glycogen storage disease type I, fructose 1,6 diphosphatase deficiency, or primary glucagon deficiency, reflecting a series of hereditary metabolic and endocrinological disorders in which hypoglycemia may be the initial or most obvious presenting feature.

V. PRETERM APPROPRIATE FOR GESTATIONAL AGE NEONATES

The appropriate for gestational age neonates born before term may develop hypoglycemia. While the first report of this entity concerned small for gestational age neonates, (19) subsequent studies documented hypoglycemia in the low-birth-weight AGA neonate. In 1968, Raivio and Hallman reported a frequency of 1.4% of hypoglycemia in these neonates (93). Fluge reported that as many as 14% of AGA neonates evidenced neonatal hypoglycemia (94).

The diminished oral and parenteral intake in the low-birth-weight neonate in combination with the decreased concentration of substrates may explain the lower plasma glucose seen in these neonates and their propensity to hypoglycemia. Functionally immature gluconeogenic and glycogenolytic enzyme systems present in the neonate potentiate these difficulties. The relatively increased size of the brain (13% of the body mass in the newborn vs. 2% in the adult) may be responsible for the greater proportion of glucose consumption during periods of fasting. This effect is magnified in the low-birth-weight neonate.

VI. SMALL FOR GESTATIONAL AGE INFANTS

Many centers have reported a relatively high frequency of hypoglycemia in SGA neonates ever since Cornblath et

al. in 1959 described its occurrence in eight infants born to mothers with toxemia (19). Lubchenco and Bard (95), deLeeuw and deVries (96), and others have all substantiated the occurrence of hypoglycemia in these neonates. Toxemia has been repeatedly reported to be associated with hypoglycemia, and its incidence has been shown to be highest (61%) in neonates born to mothers with relatively low urinary estriols, compared to a frequency of 19% in neonates born to mothers with normal estriol levels (96, 97). Reduction in energy reserves in the form of decreased glycogen deposition, combined with increased utilization of substrate, may account for the appearance of hypoglycemia.

Kliegman studied the effect of maternal nutritional deprivation on fetal/neonatal metabolism in dogs (98). Besides reduced fetal weight at term (251 ± 7 vs. 277 ± 7 gms), the growth-retarded pups evidenced lower glucose concentrations after 3, 6, and 9 h of fasting, reduced plasma concentrations of free fatty acids at 9 and 24 h, and lower ketone bodies at 24 h compared to controls. Although the systemic rates of palmitate and alanine turnover were not affected, systemic glucose production was reduced for 3–9 h after birth, which resulted in the observed hypoglycemia. The investigator speculated that reduced rates of gluconeogenesis from alanine and reduced oxidation of fuels such as free fatty acids (FFA) contributed to the hypoglycemia. FFA recycling to triglyceride rather than oxidation contributed to the observed hypoglycemia.

Plasma insulin and blood glucose concentrations were measured in umbilical venous samples from 42 SGA and 68 AGA fetuses by cordocentesis at 17–38 weeks of gestation (99). In the AGA fetus plasma insulin and the insulin/glucose ratio increased exponentially with gestation, suggesting maturation of the pancreas. The major determinant of fetal blood glucose concentration was maternal blood glucose concentration. The insulin/glucose ratio in the SGA fetuses was lower than in the AGA fetuses, suggesting that hypoinsulinemia in the former was the result of hypoglycemia and pancreatic dysfunction. The degree of SGA status did not correlate with plasma insulin or the insulin/glucose ratio, which suggested to the authors that insulin is not the primary determinant of fetal size.

Following bilateral maternal uterine artery ligation, Bussey et al. studied the sequential changes in plasma glucose, insulin, and glucagon concentrations, hepatic glycogen, and phosphoenolpyruvate carboxykinase (PEPCK) during the first 4 h in growth-retarded rat pups (100). Hypoglycemia was noted in SGA pups compared to control (AGA pups) as well as reduced hepatic glycogen stores at birth. Plasma glucagon rose, but plasma insulin fell. PEPCK levels did not rise either. The investigators concluded that SGA pups developed hypoglycemia because of limited glycogen stores and retarded gluconeogenesis. They speculated that delayed PEPCK induction in these animals may result from inadequate glycogen release at birth or decrease sensitivity to glucagon.

A number of studies have evaluated the intermediary metabolism of substrate available postnatally. A functional delay in the development of PEPCK, thought to be the rate-limiting enzyme of gluconeogenesis, in SGA neonates was suggested by Haymond et al. (101). This was substantiated by Williams et al., who studied the effect of oral alanine feeding on glucose homeostasis in the SGA neonate compared to AGA neonates (102). Oral alanine feeding enhanced plasma glucagon in both groups but stimulated hepatic glucose output only in the AGA infants.

The effect of intravenously administered glucagon on plasma amino acids has been evaluated in various types of neonates including the SGA neonate. SGA neonates in the first hours of life had significantly lower total amino acids compared to a comparable group of AGA neonates, although the response to glucagon in the SGA neonates mimicked the control (AGA) group. It was speculated that the inability of the SGA neonate to extract specific gluconeogenic amino acids could account for the susceptibility to hypoglycemia in these stressed neonates (103).

Twenty-five SGA neonates received 0.5 mg/day glucagon to treat hypoglycemia (104). Twenty of the 25 responded within 3 h with a rise in blood glucose to greater than 72 mg/dl. Five subsequently required hydrocortisone to maintain euglycemia. Rebound hypoglycemia occurred in nine following discontinuation of the glucagon. The response was poor after maternal beta blockade.

Mestyan et al. also evaluated the role of glucagon by measuring 17 amino acids before and during glucagon infusion in normoglycemic and hypoglycemia SGA neonates (105). In the normoglycemic group most amino acid concentrations declined significantly but this did not occur in the SGA neonates who were hypoglycemic. Although the effect was transient, these results reflect the ability of

glucagon to produce acute changes in hepatic glucose homeostasis. This was demonstrated in neonatal lambs between 1 and 3 days of age with infusions of somatostatin alone or who received insulin and glucagon during a 2 h interval. Plasma glucose concentration fell when both insulin and glucagon were suppressed acutely, suggesting that the latter is of importance in maintaining glucose concentration during short-term fasting. It was suggested that the ratio between the two hormones acutely affected glucose homeostasis (106).

The secretion of glucagon and insulin has been evaluated in SGA neonates. Both SGA and AGA neonates, after being fed oral glucose and protein (1 g/kg each after a 4 h fast), had similar secretion of both pancreatic hormones. The investigators speculated that the instability of glucose metabolism in the SGA neonate resulted from the rapid fall of glucose and probably because of a transient deficiency of hepatic gluconeogenic enzymes, but not from altered secretory patterns of the hormones (107).

The adequacy of the hormonal response was reinforced in a study of glucose-infused SGA neonates who were evaluated by stable isotope kinetic analysis. Under stimulation of glucose infusion, the SGA neonate and his AGA counterpart had similar regulatory responses as well as functional integrity in handling glucose during the second day after birth (108).

Using the newborn piglet model, Flecknell et al. studied the effects of an intravenous glucose infusion on glucose homeostasis in normal and growth-restricted newborn piglets using non-steady-state tracer technique (109). Suppression of hepatic glucose output was noted, but hyperglycemia (plasma glucose >180 mg/dl) developed in the majority of study subjects. The mechanism of the hyperglycemia was thought to be failure to increase glucose utilization in response to the glucose infusion.

The possibility of hormonal excess producing growth retardation has been emphasized by Ogata et al. (110). The investigators adapted methodology to produce maternal hyperinsulinemia in a rat model. This resulted in decreased concentrations of glucose and amino acids in both the mother and fetus, which produced retarded fetal growth, limited hepatic glycogen deposition, and delayed neonatal PEPCK induction.

Sann et al. evaluated the effect of hydrocortisone on intravenous glucose tolerance (1 gm/kg) in eight term SGA neonates compared to seven AGA neonates at mean of 41 h of age (111). The rate of glucose disappearance was decreased in the SGA neonates compared to control neonates. Plasma glucose concentrations were similar in both groups, while plasma insulin concentration did not change in the control group. After hydrocortisone administration, plasma insulin concentration increased. The investigators concluded that hydrocortisone induced a reduced peripheral uptake of glucose independent of insulin secretion.

VII. CONGENITAL HEART DISEASE/ CONGESTIVE HEART FAILURE

An inverse relationship has been noted between the concentration of cardiac glycogen and the level of maturity of the neonate, exemplified by the low levels in the offspring of mammalian species more mature at birth (i.e., human, monkey, sheep, etc.). These reserves are rapidly depleted during anoxia (112). Benzing et al. reported on a series of 27 patients in whom the simultaneous occurrence of hypoglycemia and acute congestive heart failure was noted in association with congenital heart disease (113). Reduced dietary intake in association with diminished hepatic glycogen resulted in hypoglycemia. This has been further substantiated by Amatayakul et al., who noted the association of hypoglycemia with congestive heart failure in neonates without significant heart defects (114). The pathophysiology of hypoglycemia in cyanotic congenital heart disease was studied by Haymond et al. (115). Six subjects were evaluated between 13 and 67 months of age. Glucose and alanine turnover studies utilizing stable isotope labeling in these neonates were compared to controls. A subtle defect in hepatic extraction of gluconeogenic substrates was suspected, possibly secondary to decreased hepatic blood flow. It is apparent that the presence of either hypoglycemia or congestive heart failure should be considered when one or the other appears.

The interrelationship of hypoglycemia and pulmonary edema has been emphasized. Unfortunately, it was unclear whether the pulmonary edema was secondary to the hypoglycemia or due to treatment of the hypoglycemia, since $D_{20}W$ was administered through an umbilical venous catheter into a branch of the left pulmonary vein (116).

Nineteen neonates with symptomatic ventricular septal defect (VSD) were examined by means of an intravenous glucose tolerance test (IVGTT) and compared to 14 neonates who were healthy (117). The VSD neonates were growth-retarded with lower weight for age and length for age. Glucose tolerance was similar in both groups. Plasma insulin concentration was low in the VSD neonates but insulin secretion, as measured by C-peptide concentration, was elevated. The authors speculated that increased insulin extraction occurs in the liver, but the mechanism was unknown.

VIII. PERINATAL STRESS/HYPOXIA

Neonates who utilize glucose at an increased rate may be prone to hypoglycemia. Since the low-birth-weight neonate is subject to hypoxia, the combination of decreased substrate availability and increased rate of utilization may result in hypoglycemia. An increased rate of anaerobic glycolysis in combination with an increased rate of glycogenolysis is probably the underlying biochemical mechanism. Two moles of ATP are generated by the Embden

Meyerhof anaerobic pathway, whereas aerobic oxidation results in 36 moles of ATP; thus, 18 times more glucose is required to generate the same amount of ATP. In addition, increased lactate production may result in an associated acidosis. Beard has emphasized the association between hypoxia and hypoglycemia in the low-birth-weight neonate and noted increased metabolic needs out of proportion to substrate availability (118, 119). The difficulties are all accentuated in neonates who are unable to replace substrate from the usual exogenous (oral) sources because of hypoxia or other clinical problems. Metabolic acidosis and lactic acidemia were noted during the first 24 h of life in 4 term and 11 preterm neonates whose Apgar score had been 5 at 1 min after birth and who were fed oral glucose loads (120). Thus, not only may endogenous stores be depleted but also these neonates may be unable to tolerate an exogenous load.

Another complication of perinatal stress is the presence of hyperinsulinism. In a report by Collins and Leonard, hyperinsulinism was noted unequivocally in three SGA neonates and in three who were asphyxiated (121). The cause of the hyperinsulinism was unclear.

Jansen and co-workers undertook a further evaluation of the metabolic effects of neonatal asphyxia (122). Using a rat preparation, they showed that hypoxia drastically altered both metabolic fuel and glucoregulatory hormone availability. They suggested that persistence of the catecholamine surge and tissue hypoxia and acidosis are responsible for the transient surge in glucose and subsequent delay in decrease of insulin and increase of glucagon in the asphyxiated neonatal rat. That is consistent with the clinical observation that the asphyxiated neonate's initial glucose concentration may be elevated and falsely reassuring. However it is not unusual for the neonate to drop his or her glucose concentration to significantly hypoglycemic levels soon after this initial surge. This emphasizes the importance of careful monitoring of the asphyxiated neonate's blood glucose concentration in the first few hours of life, even if the initial values were reassuring.

IX. COLD INJURY AND SEPSIS

Hypoglycemia has been identified in neonates who experience cold injury. Mann and Elliott described 14 neonates who suffered neonatal cold injury following prolonged exposure to environmental temperatures below 90°F (123). Marked hypoglycemia was documented in three of six neonates in whom it was measured. The hypoglycemia was presumed to be the result of free fatty acid elevation secondary to a cold-induced norepinephrine response (124). Recognition of the potential association of hypoglycemia following cold stress should result in parenteral treatment, if necessary, in conjunction with warming of the neonate. In addition, this relationship needs to be considered in the evaluation of blood glucose levels in neonates with either temperature instability or who are in a suboptimal thermal environment.

Close et al. evaluated the influence of environmental temperature on glucose tolerance and insulin response in the neonatal piglet (125). Temperatures were maintained at 17, 24, and 33°C during which an intravenous infusion of 1 g glucose/kg body weight was administered. Rectal temperatures were maintained in all of the piglets subjected to the two higher temperatures but not the lowest one in which 6 of 18 became hypothermic. A higher glucose disappearance rate was noted—K_G: 2.00 and 2.32%/min was recorded for animals maintaining homeothermic temperatures during 17 and 24°C temperature conditions compared to those kept at thermal neutrality (1.66%/min). The insulin response was comparable. During hypothermia both K_G 0.76 ± 0.12%/min and the insulin response were decreased. Glucose uptake by skeletal muscle was increased in environmentally cold-exposed homeothermic animals, resulting in an increased metabolic rate.

Neonatal sepsis has been identified with increased frequency in association with hypoglycemia. Yeung noted the association in 20 of 56 neonates with signs of sepsis (126). He suggested that inadequate caloric intake in these infected neonates may predispose to hypoglycemia. The possibility of an increased metabolic rate was considered because these neonates were infused with 100 kcalories/kg/day intravenously. A decreased rate of gluconeogenesis has been documented in laboratory animals following Gram-negative bacterial infection (127). The possibility of increased peripheral utilization because of enhanced insulin sensitivity in sepsis has been considered (128). It is likely that one or more of these factors will operate to produce the resultant hypoglycemia.

X. HYPERINSULINISM: THE INFANT OF THE DIABETIC MOTHER

Hypoglycemia following increased plasma insulin concentration has now been associated with several discrete disorders of the islets. It may be found in the infants of diabetic mothers, neonates with hemolytic diseases of the newborn, neonates with pancreatic nesidioblastosis, discrete or multiple islet cell adenomatosis, and neonates undergoing exchange transfusion. The Beckwith-Wiedemann syndrome should be considered along with other causes of hyperinsulinemic hypoglycemia, beta-sympathomimetic treatment to the mother, following high umbilical artery catheter placement, and following maternal ethanol consumption.

The infant of the diabetic mother (IDM) is the premier metabolic example of the morbidity that may exist in the neonate secondary to maternal disease (i.e., diabetes). Although the IDM may have greater morbidity than the neonate of the nondiabetic woman, many infants of insulin-dependent diabetic women experience an uneventful clinical course, and even more infants of women

with gestational diabetes do well (129). In theory the more closely metabolically controlled the diabetic pregnant patient is, the greater the potential for producing a normal neonate. Over the past decade or so, perinatal mortality, except for congenital anomalies, has approached that for the neonate born to a nondiabetic mother (130, 131). Pedersen originally emphasized the relation between maternal glucose concentration and neonatal hypoglycemia (132). His simplified hypothesis recognized that maternal hyperglycemia parallels fetal hyperglycemia, which stimulates the fetal pancreas resulting in islet cell hypertrophy and β-cell hyperplasia with increased insulin content. After separation of the fetus from the mother, the former no longer is supported by placental glucose transfer, which results in neonatal hypoglycemia.

Hyperinsulinemia in utero affects diverse organ systems, including the placenta. Insulin acts as the primary anabolic hormone of fetal growth and development, resulting in visceromegaly, especially of heart and liver, and macrosomia. In the presence of excess substrate such as glucose, increased fat synthesis and deposition occur during the third trimester. Fetal macrosomia is reflected by increased body fat, muscle mass, and organomegaly (insulin-sensitive tissues) but not an increased size of the brain or kidney (insulin-insensitive tissues) (133, 134).

After delivery there is a rapid fall in plasma glucose concentration with persistently low concentrations of plasma FFA, glycerol, and beta-hydroxybutyrate. In response to an intravenous glucose stimulus, plasma insulin-like activity is increased, as is plasma immunoreactive insulin, determined in the absence of maternal insulin antibodies and plasma C-peptide concentration (135). The insulin response to intravenous arginine is also exaggerated in the infant of a gestationally diabetic mother (136). Certainly the pregnancy of the diabetic mother should be considered to be of high risk. Knowledge of the character of the maternal diabetes, prior pregnancy history, and complications occurring during pregnancy allows the physician caring for the neonate to anticipate many of the potential fetal and neonatal complications that are reported in the infant of the diabetic mother (Table 5).

Factors known to influence the degree of hypoglycemia in the IDM include prior maternal glucose homeostasis and maternal glycemia during delivery. An inadequately controlled pregnant diabetic will have stimulated the fetal pancreas to synthesize excessive insulin, which may be readily released. Administration of intravenous dextrose during the intrapartum period, which results in maternal hyperglycemia (>125 mg/dl), will be reflected in the fetus and will exaggerate the normal postdelivery fall in plasma glucose concentration. In addition, hypoglycemia may persist for 48 h or may develop after 24 h.

Fetal hyperinsulinemia is associated with a suppressed concentration of plasma free fatty acids and/or variably diminished hepatic glucose production in the neonate (Fig. 9). Thus, not only is peripheral glucose uti-

Table 5 Neonatal Morbidities Associated with the Infant of the Diabetic Mother

Asphyxia
Birth injury
Caudal regression
Congenital anomalies
Double-outlet right ventricle
Heart failure
Hyperbilirubinemia
Hypocalcemia
Hypoglycemia
Hypomagnesemia
Increased blood volume
Macrosomia
Neurological instability
Organomegaly
Polycythemia and hyperviscosity
Renal vein thrombosis
Respiratory distress
Respiratory distress syndrome
Septal hypertrophy
Small left colon syndrome
Transient hematuria
Transposition of the great vessels
Truncus arteriosus

lization increased due to hyperinsulinemia, but hepatic glucose production is also diminished and other energy substrates are lacking as well.

Other factors that may contribute to the development of hypoglycemia include defective counterregulation by catecholamines and glucagon. The neonate exhibits transitional control of glucose metabolism, which suggests that a multiplicity of factors affect homeostasis. Many of the factors are similar to those that influence homeostasis in the adult. What is different in the neonate are the various stages of maturation that exist. Prior work in conjunction with glucose infusion studies can be summarized to suggest that there is blunted splanchnic (hepatic) responsiveness to insulin in the neonate both in the IDM and the preterm and term neonate of the nondiabetic mother, compared to the adult (32).

What has not been studied, but is of particular interest, are the many contrainsulin hormones that influence metabolism. If insulin is the primary glucoregulatory hormone, then contrainsulin hormones assist in balancing the effect of insulin and other factors. One should probably evaluate all of the contrainsulin hormones, but those of particular interest in the IDM have been those of the sympathoadrenal neural axis. Many studies have evaluated epinephrine and norepinephrine concentrations in the IDM. The results are quite variable. An early study involved 11 infants of diabetic mothers, only two of whom were gestational diabetics. Urinary excretion of catechol-

amines was measured and compared to that in 10 infants of normal mothers. Urinary norepinephrine and epinephrine concentrations did not increase in the IDM who was severely hypoglycemic, but did increase in the neonate whose mother was mildly hyperglycemic (137).

These results parallel investigations of Stern et al. (138), who suggested that hypoglycemia may be secondary to an adrenal medullary exhaustion phenomenon. This would be secondary to longstanding hypoglycemia in the IDM, which would presumably be secondary to poor control of maternal diabetes. In further studies, Keenan et al. (139) noted that when normal plasma glucose concentration increases, plasma insulin concentration declines, and plasma FFA concentration increases in response to exogenous administration of epinephrine. This confirmed the exhaustion theory. In another series, Artel et al. (140) measured plasma epinephrine and norepinephrine concentrations in the IDM. Elevated concentrations of both hormones were reported, although variation was markedly increased in the IDM. The investigators speculated that hypoglycemia after birth may be secondary to adrenal exhaustion, producing temporary depletion later in the neonatal period.

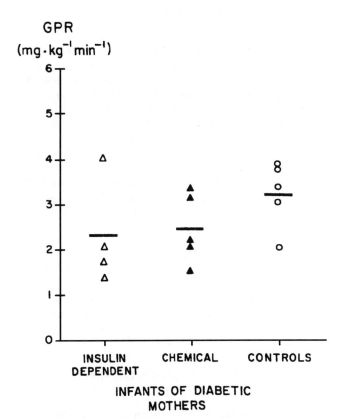

Figure 9 Glucose production rate (GPR) for the infant of the diabetic mother (chemical- and insulin-dependent diabetic mothers) vs. healthy control. The solid bar indicates the mean rate of production within each group. (From Ref. 32.)

Other factors related to sympathoadrenal activity in the neonate may be of importance. In a continuing evaluation of the transitional nature of neonatal glucose metabolism, both of insulin and contrainsulin factors, epinephrine was infused in two dosages (50 mg or 500 mg/kg/min) in a newborn lamb model and glucose kinetics (turnover) were measured with [6-^{3}H]glucose. The newborn lamb showed a blunted response to the lower dosage of epinephrine infused. The investigators speculated that the newborn lamb evidenced blunted responsiveness to this important contrainsulin stimulus (141, 142). This tendency was reaffirmed by recent data from the same laboratory. It is possible that if this occurs in the diabetic state, it would partially account for the presence of hypoglycemia noted clinically.

Thus, the IDM is a prime example of the potential of glucose disequilibrium in the neonate. Because of the transitional nature of glucose homeostasis in the neonatal period in general, accentuation of the disequilibrium may be enhanced in the IDM secondary to metabolic alterations present in the diabetic mother. A great deal of work is necessary to appreciate fully the operative mechanisms.

XI. Rh INCOMPATIBILITY AND HYPOGLYCEMIA

Hyperinsulinism has been implicated as the cause of the hypoglycemia seen in neonates with severe Rh isoimmunization (143, 144–146). These children are invariably severely affected by their disease, with profound anemia and hepatosplenomegaly at birth. The shock and collapse seen on occasion may be caused primarily by the profound hypoglycemia and, under such circumstances, glucose administration in addition to measures taken to correct the anemia may be critical. The IDM and severely Rh-affected neonate share several pathological hallmarks. In addition to the hyperinsulinism and islet cell hyperplasia, both show almost identical edematous placental changes. Both have excessive islands of extramedullary hematopoiesis in both liver and spleen. Although this latter finding may be the result of insulin stimulation, the precise cause of the hyperinsulinism itself in the Rh-affected neonate is uncertain. It has been suggested that an increase in reduced glutathione resulting from massive hemolysis of red blood cells may act as a stimulus to insulin release.

XII. EXCHANGE TRANSFUSION AND UMBILICAL CATHETER

Hypoglycemia, although not often considered, may be a significant problem following exchange transfusion. In this connection, the exchange blood and its preservatives are more critically important in the neonate, in whom a double-volume washout is being undertaken, than in an adult who is receiving 450 ml the blood/preservative mixture to be diluted in a total 5 L or more solvent.

Heparinized blood contains no added glucose. Moreover, the heparin, by raising the free fatty acid levels, contributes to the hypoglycemic potential of the transfusion blood, so that under some circumstances (e.g., severe Rh incompatibility with hyperinsulinism) its use would be contraindicated unless a concomitant IV glucose infusion is administered to prevent and/or treat hypoglycemia (147). With citrated blood, acid citrate dextrose (ACD), or citrate phosphate dextrose (CPD), the added dextrose will yield a blood preservative mixture containing as much as 300 mg % glucose. In this situation, although immediate hypoglycemia is not a problem, the high glucose load may result in a reactive insulin response. This response lags behind the glucose infusion so that when the glucose bolus is suddenly terminated at the end of the exchange procedure, a state of hyperinsulinism ensues. Studies documenting this occurrence have shown a precipitous 2 h postexchange fall in blood glucose to levels below that prior to the exchange procedure (148). Once again, the severely Rh-affected neonate is at greatest risk, but even mildly affected and nonerythroblastotic neonates who undergo an exchange transfusion may respond in such a manner. Recognition of this possibility should lead to its detection and treatment.

Another cause of relative hyperinsulinism was reported secondary to malposition of an umbilical artery catheter. In a neonate requiring supplemental oxygen because of increasing respiratory distress, hypoglycemia was relieved only when a high catheter was repositioned from T 11–12 to L 4. Following repositioning of the catheter, the child became euglycemic (149). Malik and Wilson reported on two neonates who developed hyperinsulinism secondary to malposition of the umbilical arterial catheter. Repositioning resulted in creation of the hyperinsulinemia (150). Puri et al. reported on the association of neonatal hypoglycemia associated with position of an umbilical catheter between the 8th and 9th thoracic vertebrae that is the normal position. In this report, the catheter was moved and neonatal hypoglycemia resolved (151). Three neonates were reported whose catheter were placed between the 8th and 10th thoracic vertebrae. They were noted to have hypoglycemia, which responded to catheter withdrawal to the 3rd–4th lumbar region. The investigators speculated that the cause was a high streaming of glucose to the celiac axis. The mechanism of the hypoglycemia was postulated to be excessive insulin secretion following infusion into the celiac axis (152). This was studied using a neonatal lamb model and the clinical suspicion was confirmed. The mechanism was thought to be decreased production of hepatic glucose secondary to the presumed increased portal insulin following high catheter placement (153).

Jacob and Davis studied differences in serum glucose concentrations from different extremities in neonates with umbilical arterial catheter through which dextrose was being infused. Neonates without catheter had no differences in simultaneous capillary glucose concentrations, obtained from both lower extremities, while neonates with catheters did. Neonates with a high catheter did not. As expected, the highest values were in those extremities into which the catheter was placed. This is another study pointing out the heterogeneity possible in glucose determinations depending on the location from which the blood is taken (154).

XIII. PERSISTENT HYPERINSULINEMIC HYPOGLYCEMIA

Persistent hyperinsulinemic hypoglycemia of infancy (PHHI) consists of persistent neonatal hyperinsulinemia for more than several weeks. Although the infant of the diabetic mother is the premier example of hyperinsulinemia in the newborn, his or her hyperinsulinemia is usually transient and resolves after few or several days. PHHI is a heterogeneous group of disorders and has been given a number of different names in the medical literature (155, 156): leucine-sensitive hypoglycemia, nesidioblastosis (157–159), β-cell hyperplasia, congenital hyperinsulinism, and discrete islet cell adenoma (160, 161), or adenomatosis (162, 163). The term leucine-sensitive hypoglycemia disappeared when leucine was found to function as an insulin secretagogue in patients with PHHI as well as in the healthy infant. Nesidioblastosis (meaning neoformation of islets) refers to the histological finding of newly formed islets budding from pancreatic ductal cells in histopathological specimens from patients who have PHHI. These findings explain the other names used in the literature to describe the syndrome of PHHI as discussed earlier. However, controlled studies have since shown that these histological findings are not unique to PHHI patients. Similar findings do exist in normal controls at different stages of maturation and are quite prominent in the term neonate (164). Hyperinsulinism without other apparent cause and refractory hypoglycemia should point toward this rare but real possibility. Other diagnostic clues include large for gestational age status; nonketotic hypoglycemia associated with low serum levels of FFA and lactate; low levels of insulin-like growth factor (IGF)-binding protein 1 (suppressed by insulin); glucose/insulin ratio less than 3:1 during hypoglycemia; and a glycemic response to glucagon with a rise of more than 30 mg/dl (this rules out depletion of hepatic glycogen store, which is indicative of hyperinsulinism) (165–167).

Solt'esz et al. have reported on 18 children with hyperinsulinemic hypoglycemia born to nondiabetic mothers (168). Thirteen presented within 3 days of birth, three by 20 months, and two aged 9 years. The diagnosis was established by altered insulin/glucose ratio with corresponding low ketone body levels, as well as lactate, alanine, and glycerol concentrations. The subjects required increased rates of glucose administration (between 9 and 25 mg/kg/min) and had an increased glucose disappearance rate of KG 7.6 ± 0.06%. The clinical course was quite variable: four cases had transient hyperinsulinemia; two responded to diazoxide; two required both diazoxide and partial pancreatectomy; two responded to surgical excision of an isolated adenoma; five required total pancreatectomy for nesidioblastosis; and two occurred secondary to drug administration. In this series, heterogeneity existed in the clinical courses of this condition.

Aynsley-Green et al. evaluated plasma proinsulin and C-peptide concentrations in five children with hyperinsulinemic hypoglycemia presenting with severe hypoglycemia (169). Data were compared to those from 13 normal neonates. Three neonates and a 9-year-old child required partial or total pancreatectomy. All evidenced elevated proinsulin concentrations and had elevated C peptide concentrations as well. Given the level of glucose concentration present (normal range for normoglycemia but elevated for hypoglycemia), the investigators concluded that the insulin, proinsulin, and C-peptide concentration profile does not provide a reliable indicator for the underlying pathological mechanism.

Both autosomal recessive and autosomal dominant forms of PHHI have been described (170–172). The autosomal recessive form is common in Saudi Arabia, with an incidence of 1:2675, most probably due to high rates of consanguinity in that country. Genetic mapping linked the disorder to chromosome 11p14–15.1 (170). This finding excluded the involvement of glucokinase gene in chromosome 7 and/or GLUT 2 gene on chromosome 3. Of particular interest was that both the insulin gene and the Beckwith-Wiedemann's gene are located on chromosome 11. In 1995, the sulfonylurea receptor (SUR) was cloned and mapped to chromosome 11p15 (173). Subsequently some cases of PHHI were attributed to mutations in the SUR gene (174). Absence of K_{ATP} activity in the pancreatic β-cell has been documented in patients PHHI (175, 176). The absence of this function was attributed in some cases to SUR mutations, but in other cases mutations other than that of the SUR (e.g., inward rectifier K^+ channel defect) were identified as well (176–178). Of clinical relevance is that patients with PHHI who have these two later mutations usually do not respond well to diazoxide therapy (179).

An autosomal dominant form of hyperinsulinism in infancy has been reported in several families (172). These patients usually have a milder variant of the disease than those with the autosomal recessive form. They often present after the neonatal period and respond well to diazoxide therapy. Treatment has been successfully discontinued after 2–14 years of therapy in many patients. A mutation of the glucokinase gene was reported in one family with an autosomal dominant variant of hyperinsulinism (180). Increased rate of insulin secretion was attributed to greater affinity of glucokinase for glucose, leading to higher rates of glycolysis.

Although rare in the neonatal period, insulin-secreting adenomas have been reported in cases of PHHI. They are usually resistant to diazoxide therapy. Focal adenomatous hyperplasia (FoPHHI) as well as diffuse β-cell hyperplasia (DiPHHI) have been described (181). Differentiating between these two variants of PHHI has important implications for therapy. Of interest in the cases of FoPHHI is that a paternal uniparental disomy was confirmed (182). In these cases both alleles in the chromosome 11p15 region were found to be from a paternal origin with loss of maternal alleles. A similar defect was not found in cases of DiPHHI. It is also fascinating to know that uniparental paternal disomy was reported in some cases of Beckwith-Wiedemann syndrome (183). However, it is not yet known why the maternal allelic loss leads to the observed defect.

Reports have described the potential for hypoglycemia after beta-sympathomimetic tocolytic therapy, which has been used increasingly to inhibit the premature onset of labor. A possible explanation of the relationship involves increased pancreatic secretion of insulin in response to a specific glucose concentration (184, 185). A prospective double-bind study of 35 patients in preterm labor with and without ruptured membranes was conducted. Leake et al. evaluated the neonatal metabolic and cardiovascular effects of Ritodine administration to the mother (186). Patients received intravenous and/or oral ritodrine or a placebo. The shortest time from drug administration to delivery was 6 h. No differences were noted in the Ritodrine vs. the control groups relative to glucose and cardiovascular determinations. The investigators concluded that chronic oral administration did not significantly affect the neonate. In an investigation of the causes of the clinical situation, a neonatal lamb model was used to evaluate the drug (187). Administration of Ritodrine produced both increased insulin secretion from the β-cell and glucose production from the liver. It would follow that the presence of clinical hypoglycemia would depend on the time of administration prior to delivery.

XIV. HYPOGLYCEMIA FOLLOWING MATERNAL ETHANOL CONSUMPTION AND MISCELLANEOUS CAUSES

The association of neonatal hypoglycemia and maternal ethanol ingestion has been reported. Singh et al. evaluated glucose metabolism in neonatal rats exposed to maternal ethanol ingestion (188). Blood glucose concentration, liver glycogen, and plasma insulin concentrations were decreased in ethanol-treated mothers, as was litter size and average fetal body weight. The pups from ethanol-fed mothers evidenced hypoglycemia and hypoinsulinemia. Within 1 h after birth an elevation in blood glucose concentration was followed by a decline to hypoglycemic concentrations. Liver glycogen stores were reduced and they were quickly mobilized. The hypoglycemic tendency

in pups of ethanol-treated mothers disappeared after 4 days.

Witek-Janusek examined the effect of maternal ethanol ingestion on the maternal and neonatal glucose balance in a rat model (189). Controls included an isocaloric liquid pair fed diet or ad libitum rat chow. Blood for glucose concentration and liver was sampled on days 21–22 and pups were studied up to 24 h after birth. Ethanol depressed not only maternal liver glycogen stores but also liver glycogen in the neonatal liver. Ethanol had no effect on plasma insulin concentrations. Postnatal hypoglycemia could be observed following maternal ethanol ingestion. Singh et al. evaluated the combined effect of chronic ethanol ingestion in pregnant rats and three offspring (190). Fetal body weight and liver weight was reduced in fetuses of alcohol-fed mothers. Blood glucose concentrations were also lower, as was liver glycogen.

Isolated instances have been reported that mimic insulin excess and resultant hypoglycemia. Zucker et al. have reported symptomatic neonatal hypoglycemia in association with maternal administration of chlorpropamide (191). This resulted in stimulation of both maternal and fetal β-cells. Because teratogenicity of the drug is a concern, its use is limited, especially since it provides poor control of glucose for the management of diabetes in pregnancy. Benzothiadiazide (thiazide) diuretics have been implicated in producing insulin secretion (192). It has been suggested that these drugs produce elevated maternal blood glucose concentrations and result in stimulation of the fetal islets with subsequent neonatal hypoglycemia. There is a report of a neonate in whom hypoglycemia may have been due to an insulin-releasing substance, possibly from the gut (193).

Hypoglycemia has been noted in individuals who are sensitive to leucine. This amino acid, among others, is known to be associated with increased insulin release and may be seen following ingestion of milk (194). A fourth defect of leucine metabolism, 3-hydroxy-3-methyl glutaryl CoA lyase deficiency, has been reported. Hypoglycemia was noted along with a characteristic excretory pattern of organic acids, but the exact mechanism resulting in the hypoglycemia was not apparent (195).

Neonatal hypoglycemia has followed administration of salicylates, the suggested mechanism being an uncoupling of mitochondrial oxidative phosphorylation (196). The association of congenital adrenal hyperplasia and hypoglycemia has also been recorded (197). Souto et al. studied the effect of equivalent doses of insulin on the adrenal medulla of neonatal and adult rats (198). Glycemia decreased to 33% of the control values in the adult, while an equivalent dose of insulin to the neonate decreased glycemia to about 50%. Morphological evaluation of the adrenal medulla paralleled the metabolic data. The authors speculated that immaturity of the adrenal chromaffin tissue may be present in the neonate and be involved in hypoglycemic catecholamine counterregulation.

Actavia-Loria et al. reported a survey of the frequency of hypoglycemia in 165 children with primary adrenal insufficiency (199). Of these children, 118 had congenital adrenal hyperplasia, 47% had Addison's disease, and 18% had hypoglycemia. One-half of the episodes occurred in the neonatal period. The episodes of hypoglycemia were isolated in 13 children, 4 neonates with congenital adrenal hyperplasia, and in 1 male with 11B-OH deficiency. A significant mechanistic correlation was noted between plasma glucose concentration and cortisol concentration during the episodes of hypoglycemia.

Hypoglycemia has been noted secondary to indomethacin therapy in premature neonates with patent ductus arteriosus. The proposed mechanism of indomethacin-mediated hypoglycemia (i.e., lack of prostaglandin inhibition of insulin release) was not confirmed since there were no significant changes in plasma insulin concentration (200).

XV. BECKWITH-WIEDEMANN SYNDROME

In 1964 Beckwith and associates described a syndrome characterized by omphalocele, muscular macroglossia, and visceromegaly (201). Wiedemann almost simultaneously described a similar clinical picture in three siblings (202). The cause of the syndrome remains unclear. On pathologic examination, islet cell hyperplasia of the pancreas has been demonstrated in these neonates. It was subsequently shown that hypoglycemia may be an associated metabolic component of this syndrome, occurring in approximately 50% of cases reported, with hyperinsulinism responsible for both the hypoglycemia and the somatic and visceral growth abnormalities. The hypoglycemia is ultimately self-limiting but may be protracted and difficult to control. In a patient with resistant hypoglycemia and hyperinsulinism, Schiff and co-workers (203) were ultimately able to achieve adequate control of glucose levels with a combination of Susphrine and diazoxide therapy, which suppressed the release of basal and postprandial insulin. The neonate presented at birth with an umbilical hernia, macroglossia, and hepatosplenomegaly as well as hyperinsulinism and severe, persistent hypoglycemia. Normal glucose control was achieved by 1 month of age. At 6 months, somatic growth was normal, hepatosplenomegaly had receded, but the macroglossia was still present. At 2 years of age growth was normal, and the tongue, although still large, could be kept within the mouth without any evidence of malocclusion. Genetic mapping linked the disorder to a defect in chromosome 11p15, as noted earlier (183).

XVI. DEFECTIVE GLUCONEOGENESIS/ GLYCOGENOLYSIS

Hypoglycemia has been noted in neonates unable to sustain normal gluconeogenesis. Glucagon is influential in

hepatic glucose production since it enhances glycogenolysis and gluconeogenesis. A recent report has documented a neonate with isolated glucagon deficiency and neonatal hypoglycemia (204). The diagnosis was based on a low basal glucagon concentration as well as a diminished response to hypoglycemia and alanine infusion, both of which are potent stimulators of glucagon secretion, in a neonate in whom normal insulin secretion was present. Vidnes has reported three neonates with persistent neonatal hypoglycemia, one of whom evidenced an abnormal subcellular distribution of PEPCK in the extramitochondrial fraction (205, 206).

A specific enzymatic deficiency that may affect gluconeogenesis in the neonate is type I glycogen storage disease (glucose-6-phosphatase deficiency). The deficiency is an autosomal recessive genetic defect, which may occasionally present in the neonatal period with severe hypoglycemia and hepatomegaly. A second enzymatic defect, fructose-1,6-diphosphatase deficiency, has also been associated with hypoglycemia (207–209).

Galactosemia may present in neonates who are septic and/or have hepatocellular jaundice. Later (1 month) galactosemic infants may present with cataract formation. In some neonates, hypoglycemic symptoms have been reported and a positive reducing test in the urine (to copper or iron) noted. The usual biochemical defect is in galactose-1-phosphate uridyl transferase. The diagnosis involves the demonstration of a low true glucose concentration (glucose oxidase) in the presence of normal total hexoses, together with determination of the enzymatic defect, which can be analyzed in both red and white blood cells. Exclusion of milk and mild products (lactose) is the treatment of choice. Because early intervention is preventive, routine neonatal screening has been recommended, since it is inherited as an autosomal recessive condition (210).

Hereditary fructose intolerance may be diagnosed in neonates who are old enough to ingest fruits or juices. The major intolerance is due to fructose-1-phosphate accumulation secondary to fructose-1-phosphate aldolase deficiency. The hypoglycemia is secondary to an inhibition of hepatic glucose release and absence of a hyperglycemic response to glucagon following ingestion or parenteral administration of fructose.

Inborn errors of amino acid metabolism that may present as hypoglycemia in the neonatal period include maple syrup urine disease, propionic acidemia, methylmalonic acidemia, tyrosinemia, and/or 3-hydroxy-3-methylglutaryl CoA lyase deficiency. Disorders of fatty acid metabolism that may present as hypoglycemia in the neonatal period include medium-chain and long-chain acyl CoA dehydrogenase deficiency.

XVII. EVALUATION

Current perinatal clinical practice has significantly reduced hypoglycemia associated with conditions such as the use of glucose infusion during labor, erythroblastosis fetalis, double-volume exchange transfusion, cold stress, and delay of starting enteral feed in the larger neonate or glucose infusion in the low-birth-weight neonate. Many of the clinically observed cases of hypoglycemia occur immediately after birth, as discussed earlier.

As noted with other diagnostic dilemmas in neonatology, a detailed maternal history and thorough physical examination are required to determine the probable cause of neonatal hypoglycemia. Maternal history including family history of diabetes or other glucose intolerance, drug ingestion (chloropropamide, benzothiadiazide diuretics, salicylates, and or ethanol), blood group incompatibility, pre-eclampsia or pregnancy-induced hypertension, and the rate of dextrose administered to the mother during labor should alert the physician to the potential mechanism of the observed hypoglycemia.

A thorough physical examination of the neonate will indicate if the neonate is AGA, SGA, or LGA, as well as the gestational age. The appearance of the infant of the well-controlled diabetic mother of classes A, B, and C can usually be differentiated from that of the infant of classes D, E, F (who may be SGA). The neonate with Beckwith-Wiedemann is usually obvious, with evidence of a protuberant tongue, umbilical hernia, and macrosomia. Prolonged jaundice and cataracts are suggestive of galactosemia, as are reducing substances in the urine, while unexplained hepatomegaly may indicate glycogen storage disease. Abnormalities, which may indicate central defects, include abnormal genitalia indicative of pituitary abnormalities, and cleft lip and palate.

Treating the underlying condition, providing optimal thermal environment, and supporting the cardiocirculatory system, if indicated, are basic concepts in the management of hypoglycemia. Appropriate laboratory evaluation should include evaluation of the following: glucose, insulin, growth hormone, cortisol, and thyroid function. Evaluation of pH, lactate, pyruvate, and ketones is indicated for glycogen storage disease. Studies are usually performed when hypoglycemia is present or at a time following a fast of at least 3–4 h. Tolerance tests are reserved for confirmation of suspected diagnosis, such as a glucagon tolerance test if glycogen storage disease is suspected. A further clinical evaluation of the neonate, infant, and older child has been detailed by Sperling (211).

XVIII. TREATMENT

Treatment of neonatal hypoglycemia begins with identification of its potential in the neonate at risk, documentation of its existence by appropriate laboratory measurement, and determination of appropriate corrective measures.

Oral administration of nutrients generally is advocated, as either 5% dextrose or formula, in the neonate with mild hypoglycemia (glucose concentration 35–45 mg/dl). It should be used only in the neonate who is able quickly to achieve and maintain a glucose concentration in the euglycemic range during oral feedings. It is unreasonable to expect that oral feedings alone will provide for adequate glucose intake in the neonate whose hypoglycemia does not respond quickly to this approach.

In the case of moderate or severe hypoglycemia, we advocate parenteral (intravenous) treatment with a constant-infusion pump to avoid fluctuations in the rate of infusion that would result in irregular rates of endogenous insulin release. Oral feedings should be allowed as tolerated whenever clinically appropriate. Repeated documentation of blood or plasma glucose concentration should be an integral part of the treatment of any neonate. The glucose infusions should be gradually reduced rather than abruptly terminated so that sudden reactive hypoglycemia is avoided. Once oral feedings are initiated, evaluation of the glucose concentration just before a subsequent feeding provides an analysis of the neonate's status.

Parenteral therapy should begin with 6 mg/kg/min followed by graded increases to achieve euglycemia with the minimal concentration of glucose required. A peripheral vein rather than an umbilical vessel is the preferred route of infusion (153). However, other than in an emergency, rates greater than 15 mg/kg/min should be given only when a central venous line is being used. Rates greater than 25 mg/kg/min are probably contraindicated by either route.

There is disagreement about to the beneficial effect of a glucose bolus prior to the administration of continuous glucose infusion. Most authorities appropriately agree that there is no place for a large bolus (i.e., ≥500 mg/kg or 5 ml/kg $D_{10}W$) in the treatment of hypoglycemia in the neonate, because of the high likelihood of pancreatic β-cell stimulation and rebound hypoglycemia (43). Some investigators (Lilien and Hawdon) recommend a so-called minibolus of 2–3 ml/kg $D_{10}W$ (i.e., ≈200–300 mg/kg) given at a rate of 1 ml/kg/min and followed by continuous glucose infusion at a rate of 5–8 mg/kg/min (Fig. 10) (212, 213). The currently popular approach involves infusion of 2 ml/kg 10% dextrose in H_2O (200 mg/kg) given over 1 min, followed by a continuous dextrose infusion of 8 mg/kg/min (213). However, the concept of the minibolus was challenged based on the potential for hyperosmolar cerebral edema at that extremely rapid administration rate, as reported in older children (214). Others also argued that at this high-administration-rate glucose entry far exceeds glucose uptake; the potential for provoking excessive insulin secretion and inhibition of glucagon secretion may, in fact, aggravate the existing hypoglycemia (215).

Based on this discussion, we recommend the use of a minibolus (200 mg/kg, or 2 ml/kg $D_{10}W$, over 5–10 min) only in cases of severe hypoglycemia (i.e., glucose concentration ≤24 mg/dl), followed by continuous glucose infusion at a rate of 6–8 mg/kg/min. For milder or

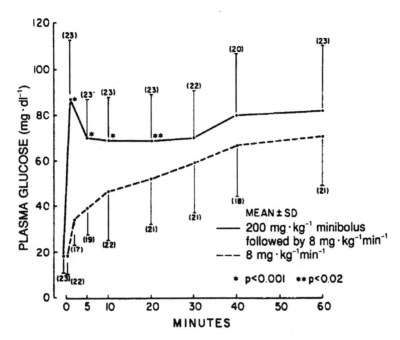

Figure 10 Plasma glucose concentrations in neonates treated with 200 mg/kg minibolus followed by 5–8 mg/kg/min constant glucose infusion compared with plasma glucose concentrations of neonates treated with constant infusion alone. (From Ref. 213.)

improving (i.e., partial correction after an initial bolus) hypoglycemia (i.e., glucose concentration of 25–45 mg/dl), a continuous glucose infusion alone at a rate of 5–8 mg/kg/min is an appropriate approach. In all cases blood glucose concentration should be closely monitored every 30–60 min and glucose infusion rate should be gradually adjusted until hypoglycemia resolves. A number of specific agents (e.g., hydrocortisone and glucagon) are usually recommended when continuous glucose infusion at a rate >15 mg/kg/min is not effective in maintaining euglycemia (43).

Calculation of parenteral glucose therapy must include the actual concentration of glucose present in the administered fluids. A hydrated form of dextrose ($C_6H_{12}O_6 \cdot H_2O$) (molecular weight of 198) is used by most manufacturers to prepare the parenteral fluid so that the actual amount of glucose available is approximately 10% less (216). This is of particular concern when very-low-birth-weight or severely hypoglycemic neonates are being treated.

There are increasing reports of the use of lipid infusion to assist in prevention of hypoglycemia. Sann et al. evaluated the effect of oral lipid supplementation on the prevention of neonatal hypoglycemia in 28 low-birth-weight neonates whose mean gestational age was 36 ± 1 weeks and whose birth weight was 1778 ± 230 g compared to a control group of 23 neonates with comparable demographic data (217). Hypoglycemia ≤31 mg/dl occurred in 8 of 23 neonates in the control group compared

with 2 of 28 in the supplemented group receiving 2.9 g/day of a solution containing 67% medium chain triglycerides. Prospectively this study showed that lipid supplementation can prevent the occurrence of hypoglycemia in the low-birth-weight neonate.

Treatment with a number of specific agents is indicated when parenteral therapy above 15 mg/kg/min is not effective in maintaining euglycemia. Corticosteroids have been shown to be effective in the therapy of hypoglycemia. Although steroids enhance several glucose-producing reactions, the major effect is probably that of gluconeogenesis from noncarbohydrate (protein) sources and decreased peripheral glucose utilization. Hydrocortisone is given at a dosage of 5 mg/kg/day either intravenously or orally every 12 h, or prednisone is used at a dosage of 2 mg/kg/day orally. As with all forms of therapy, gradual diminution of the dosage administered, in concert with decreasing parenteral concentrations of glucose and increasing oral intake of nutrients, should successfully allow for weaning.

The use of glucagon provides a highly effective method of releasing glycogen from the liver and can be a therapeutic means of assessing whether or not the liver contains adequate stores. Its failure in some growth-retarded neonates is considered to be evidence for a lack of hepatic glycogen stores. In the infant of the diabetic mother, there is often a failure to respond to the usual dosages (30 mg/kg), despite the presence of more than adequate hepatic glycogen stores. These neonates will fre-quently respond to higher dosages (300 mg/kg) with a prolonged and sustained hyperglycemia, so that the higher dosage might well be used as initial therapy. Since glu-cagon may stimulate insulin release, its administration in all probability should be accompanied by an intravenous glucose infusion.

Like glucagon, epinephrine is capable of promoting glycogen to glucose conversion, but in far smaller quan-tities. For this effect glucagon is the drug of choice. The hyperglycemic potential of epinephrine in blocking glu-cose uptake by peripheral muscle presupposes an adequate blood level initially and is of little practical benefit in the hypoglycemia state. Epinephrine is a powerful anti-insulin hormone, a fact that explains its success as an effective antihypoglycemic agent in the infant of the diabetic mother as well as in other hyperinsulinemic neonates. The agent most commonly used is a 1:200 epinephrine in aqueous suspension (Sus-Phrine), which can be readily administered subcutaneously (203, 218).

In cases of transient or persistent hyperinsulinism dia-zoxide, octreotide, calcium channel blockers, and/or par-tial pancreatectomy have been used as therapeutic modal-ities (Table 6). It is important to summarize the metabolic signals that lead to insulin gene transcription and then insulin secretion by the pancreatic β-cell, so that the mechanism of action of these therapeutic agents may be understood. Glucose enters the β-cell via the GLUT 2 isoform of glucose transporters. Glycolysis begins with glucokinase, which metabolizes glucose to glucose-6-phosphate. Further glycolysis including interactions in the

tricarboxylic acid (TCA) cycle results in ATP production. Amino acids (AA) and FFA also contribute to ATP pro-duction through metabolism in the TCA cycle. Different intermediate signals from glycolysis lead to insulin gene transcription. Increase of the intracellular ATP/ADP ratio activates the SUR. The K_{ATP} channel then closes, the cell membrane depolarizes, and Ca^{2+} influx through the volt-age-gated calcium channel (VGCC) triggers insulin secre-tion. Figure 11 depicts the metabolic signals involved in insulin production and the sites of action for various drugs used in the treatment of PHHI.

Diazoxide, in a dosage of 10–15 mg/kg/day divided every 8 h is the first drug of choice in the hyperinsu-linemic neonate who cannot be weaned from intravenous glucose. Diazoxide causes hyperglycemia by stabilizing the β-cell K_{ATP} channel in the open state, thereby inhib-iting membrane depolarization and insulin secretion. An intact SUR and inward rectifier K^+ channel are necessary for full action of the drug. Insulin synthesis is uncom-promised by this therapy. A secondary hyperglycemic mechanism is via stimulation of catecholamine; this may reduce insulin secretion and counter its actions peripher-ally as well. A response to diazoxide is usually evident within the first 48 h of therapy. Diazoxide has several important side effects that should be carefully monitored; in some cases the severity of these side effects may ne-cessitate termination of diazoxide therapy. Fluid retention, hypertricosis, and coarse facial changes have been re-ported. Diazoxide therapy can result in hyperglycemia and even diabetic ketoacidosis if the infant is unable to secrete insulin appropriately during time of stress. Uricemia, leu-

Table 6 Therapeutic Modalities for the Treatment of Infants and Children with PHHI

Therapy	Mechanism of action	Dosage	Efficacy and side effect
Diazoxide	Opens K_{ATP} channels	5–20 mg/kg/day orally every 8 h	*Effective in 22–50% of cases* Hypotension, fluid retention, hyperuricemia, hypertrichosis, coarse facial features, leu-kopenia, thrombocytopenia
Octreotide	Activates a G-protein-coupled inward recti-fier K^+ channel	5–40 mg/kg/day subcu-taneously every 4–6 h	*Effective in 25–80% of cases* Abdominal distention, steatorrhea, cholelithi-asis, possible suppression of other hor-mones: growth hormone, thyroid-stimulat-ing hormone, adrenocorticotropic hormone
Calcium channel blockers	Inhibits Ca^{2+} influx via voltage-gated calcium channels	Nifedipine 0.25–0.7 mg/kg/day orally every 8 h	*Case reports suggest efficacy* Potential hypotension, lack of long-term ex-perience
Surgery	Reduction of β-cell mass	Surgical removal of 95% of the pancreas	*Indicated in cases of failure of medical therapy, effective in 75–95% of cases* *Immediate:* injury to the common bile duct and other surgical complications *Long term:* failure to achieve euglycemia; dia-betes mellitus and exocrine pancreatic insuf-ficiency

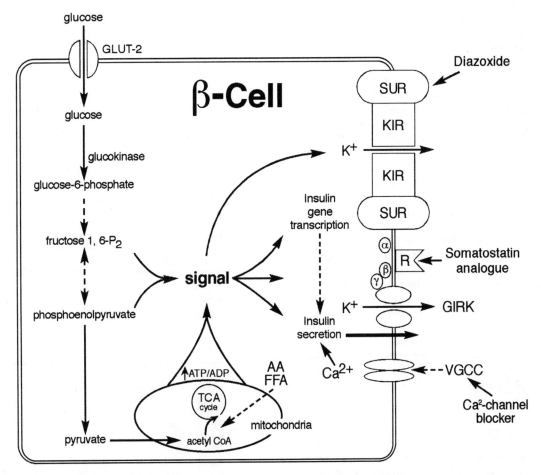

Figure 11 Metabolic signals involved in insulin gene transcription and insulin secretion in the β-cell. Dashed lines represent pathways with intermediate steps, glucose transporter isoform 2 (GLUT2), tricarboxylic acid (TCA) cycle. The right side of the cell membrane represents the sites of action for various drugs used in the treatment of PHHI. Diazoxide binds to the sulfonylurea receptor (SUR) and opens the inward rectifier K$^+$ channel (KIR). Somatostatin analogs bind to the somatostatin receptor (R) and activate a G-protein-coupled inward rectifier K$^+$ channel (GIRK) with its α, β, and γ subunits. These two drugs serve to hyperpolarize the β-cell membrane, which inhibits Ca^{2+} influx and therefore insulin secretion. Ca^{2+} channel blockers inhibit Ca^{2+} influx through voltage-gated calcium channel (VGCC).

kopenia, and thrombocytopenia are rare side effects of this therapy.

Diazoxide is effective in only 22–50% of the patients with PHHI and it is less likely to work in patients presenting in the immediate neonatal period (219–223).

Somatostatin has a very short half-life (1–3 min) prohibits its clinical use. Somatostatin acts via a G-protein-coupled inward rectifier K$^+$ channel. The activation of this channel results in hyperpolarization of the β-cell, which inhibits Ca^{2+} influx, thereby inhibiting insulin release (see Fig. 4). The synthetic analog octreotide, however, has a half-life of 1.5 h, and it has been successfully used at intervals of up to 6–8 h in cases of hyperinsulinemia. A starting dosage of 5–10 μg/kg/day produces favorable initial responses, but because of the development of tolerance, the dosage sometimes has to be increased to as

much as 40 μg/kg/day. Although Thornton et al. advocate octreotide use as an adjunct therapy during the pre and postoperative period of partial pancreatectomy, Glaser et al. demonstrated that aggressive octreotide therapy alone was successful in almost 50% of the cases of PHHI that were resistant to other medical therapy (219, 224). The side effects reported during the course of therapy include vomiting, steatorrhea, and abdominal distention; these were self-limiting within the initial few weeks of therapy (165, 225). Asymptomatic cholelithiasis was reported and concerns relative to the effect of octreotide on other hormonal axis require more careful evaluation.

Because Ca^{2+} influx is required for insulin secretion, calcium channel blockers have been used in the treatment of selective cases of hyperinsulinism. Although there are few encouraging case reports in the literature in which nifedipine was successfully used as adjunct therapy for PHHI, further experience is needed to assess the efficacy of this approach (226).

Surgical intervention is indicated when euglycemia cannot be maintained by medical therapy alone. A 95% pancreatectomy is the surgical procedure of choice. Medical therapy may need to be continued postoperatively, if hypoglycemia persists. If hypoglycemia persists despite added medical therapy, as is the case in 5–25% of the patients, a second surgery would be indicated to remove 99% of the pancreas. Risks associated with surgery other than failure to achieve euglycemia include: injury to the common bile duct, exocrine pancreatic insufficiency, and diabetes mellitus. The later may be transient or persist (219, 227–231).

This review has evaluated the current knowledge of the kinetics of glucose homeostasis in the neonate. Glucose production, glucose utilization, and glucose oxidation have been reviewed in detail. The relationship of the developmental regulation of glucose homeostasis and some of the fundamental differences known to exist in the neonate compared to the adult. The pathophysiological basis and the clinical aspects of neonatal hypoglycemia were discussed. Conditions associated with neonatal hyperinsulinemia, including the infant of the diabetic mother, were also comprehensively reviewed.

ACKNOWLEDGMENT

Some of this work was supported by R01 27287 awarded to Dr. Cowett by the National Institutes of Health.

REFERENCES

1. Cowett RM. Introduction. In: Cowett RM, Hay WW Jr, eds. The micropremie: the next frontier. Report of the ninety-ninth Ross Conference on Pediatric Research. Columbus, OH: Ross Laboratories, 1990:1–3.
2. Farrag HM, Cowett RM. Glucose homeostasis in the micropremie. Clin Perinatol 2000; 27(1):1–22.
3. Cowett RM. Hypo and hyperglycemia in the newborn. In: Polin RA, Fox WW, eds. Neonatal and fetal medicine; physiology and pathophysiology. Philadelphia: WB Saunders, 1998:594–608.
4. Battagliia FC, Thureen PJ. Nutrition of the fetus and premature infant. Nutrition 1997; 13:903–906.
5. Ogata ES. Problems of glucose metabolism in the extremely-low birth weight infant. In: Cowett RM, Hay WW Jr, eds. The micropremie: the next frontier. Report of the ninety-ninth Ross Conference on Pediatric Research. Columbus, OH: Ross Laboratories, 1990:55–63.
6. Cowett RM. Carbohydrate metabolism in the premature and compromised infant. In: Lebenthal E, ed. Textbook of Gastroenterology and Nutrition in Early Childhood, 2nd ed. New York: Raven Press, 1989:311–326.
7. Aynsley-Green A, Hawdon JM. Hypoglycemia in the neonate: current controversies. Acta Paediatr Jpn 1997; 39: S12–S16.
8. Cowett RM, Barcohana Y, Oh W. Human fetal and neonatal insulin response to maternal hyperglycemia at cesarean section (C/S). Pediatr Res 1981; 15:506A.
9. Cornblath M, Reisner SH. Blood glucose in the neonate and its clinical significance. N Engl J Med 1965; 273: 378–381.
10. Srinivasan G, Pildes RS, Cattamanchi G. Plasma glucose values in normal neonates: a new look. J Pediatr 1986; 109:114–117.
11. Stanley CA, Anday EX, Baker L. Metabolic fuel and hormone response to fasting in newborn infants. Pediatrics 1979; 64:613–619.
12. Aynsley-Green A, Hawdon JM. Hypoglycemia in the neonate: current controversies. Acta Paediatr Jpn 1997; 39(1):S12–S16.
13. Williams AF. Hypoglycaemia of the newborn: a review. Bull WHO 1997; 75(3):261–290.
14. Koh T, Eyre JA, Aynsley-Green A. Neonatal hypoglycemia: the controversy regarding definition. Arch Dis Child 1988; 63:1386–1388.
15. Heck LJ, Erenburg A. Serum glucose levels in term neonates during the first 48 hours of life. J Pediatr 1987; 110:119–122.
16. Lucas A. Metabolic and endocrine responses to a milk feed in six-day-old term infants: differences between breast and cow's milk formula feeding. Acta Paediatr Scand 1981; 70:195–200.
17. Marconi AM, Paolini C, Buscaglia M, Zerbe G, Battaglia F, Pardi G. The impact of gestational age and fetal growth on the maternal-fetal glucose concentration difference. Obstet Gynecol 1996; 87:937–942.
18. Hawdon JM, Ward Platt MP, Aynsley-Green A. Patterns of metabolic adaptation for preterm and term infants in the first neonatal week. Arch Dis Child 1992; 67:357–365.
19. Cornblath M, Odell GB, Levin EY. Symptomatic neonatal hypoglycemia associated with toxemia of pregnancy. J Pediatr 1959; 55:545–562.
20. Koh T, Eyre JA, Aynsley-Green A. Neural dysfunction during hypoglycemia. Arch Dis Child 1988; 63:1353–1358.
21. Greisen G, Pryds O. Neonatal hypoglycaemia. Lancet 1989; 1:332–333.
22. Phillips DI, Barker DJ, Fall CH. Elevated plasma cortisol concentrations: a link between low birth weight and the insulin resistance syndrome? J Clin Endocrinol Metabol 1998; 83(3):757–760.
23. Lucas A, Morley R, Cole TJ. Adverse neuro-developmental outcome of moderate neonatal hypoglycemia. Br Med J 1988; 297:1304–1308.
24. Frantz ID III, Medina G, Taeusch HW Jr. Correlation of Dextrostix values with true glucose in the range less than 50 mg/dl. J Pediatr 1975; 87:417–420.
25. Perelman RH, Gutcher GR, Engle MJ. Comparative analysis of four methods for rapid glucose determination in neonates. Am J Dis Child 1982; 136:1051–1053.
26. Wilkins BH, Kaira D. Comparison of blood glucose test strips in the detection of neonatal hypoglycemia. Arch Dis Child 1982; 57:948–960.
27. Conrad PD, Sparks JW, Osberg I. Clinical application of a new glucose analyzer in the neonatal intensive care unit: comparison with other methods. J Pediatr 1989; 114:281–287.
28. Lin HC, Maguire C, Oh W. Accuracy and reliability of glucose reflectance meters in the high risk neonate. J Pediatr 1989; 115:998–1000.

29. Holtrop PC, Madison KA, Kiechle FL. A comparison of chromagen test strip (Chemstrip bG) and serum glucose values in newborns. Am J Dis Childh 1990; 144:183–185.

30. Grazaitis DM, Sexton WR. Erroneously high dextrostix values caused by isopropyl alcohol. Pediatrics 1980; 66:221–223.

31. Bier DM. Methodology for the study of metabolism: kinetic techniques. In: Cowett RM, ed. Principles of Perinatal-Neonatal Metabolism. 2nd ed. New York: Springer-Verlag, 1998:3–15.

32. Cowett RM, Oh W, Schwartz R. Persistent glucose production during glucose infusion in the neonates. J Clin Invest 1983; 71:467–475.

33. Kalhan SC, Oliven A, King KC. Role of glucose in the regulation of endogenous glucose production in the human newborn. Pediatr Res 1986; 20:49–52.

34. Tyrala EE, Chen X, Boden G. Glucose metabolism in the infant weighing less than 1100 grams. J Pediatr 1994; 125:283–287.

35. Keshen T, Miller R, Jahoor F. Glucose production and gluconeogenesis are negatively related to body weight in mechanically ventilated, very low birth weight neonates. Pediatr Res 1997; 41:132–138.

36. Glamour TS, McCullough AJ, Sauer PJJ. Quantification of carbohydrate oxidation by respiratory gas exchange and isotopic tracers. Am J Physiol 1995; 258:E789–E796.

37. Jacot E, Defronzo A, Jequier E. The effect of hyperglycemia, hyperinsulinemia and route of glucose administration on glucose oxidation and glucose storage. Metabolism 1982; 31:922–930.

38. Sauer PJ, Van Aerde JEE, Pencharz PB. Glucose oxidation rates in newborn infants measured with indirect calorimetry and [U-¹³C]glucose. Clin Sci 1986; 70:587–593.

39. Tserng KY, Kalhan SC. Estimation of glucose carbon recycling and glucose turnover with [U-¹³C]glucose. Am J Physiol 1983; 245:E476–E482.

40. Farrag HM, Nawrath LM, Healey JE, Oh W, Cowett RM. Persistent glucose production and greater peripheral sensitivity to insulin in the neonate vs the adult. Am J Physiol 1997; 272:E86–E93.

41. Savich RD, Finley SL, Ogata ES. Intravenous lipid and amino acids briskly increase plasma glucose concentrations in small premature infants. Am J Perinat 1988; 5:201–205.

42. Bier DM, Leake RD, Haymond MW. Measurement of true glucose production rules in infancy and childhood with 6,6 dideutero glucose. Diabetes 1977; 26:1016–1023.

43. Cowett RM, Farrag HM. Neonatal glucose metabolism. In: Cowett RM, ed. Principles of Perinatal-Neonatal Metabolism. 2nd ed. New York: Springer-Verlag, 1998:683–722.

44. Sunehag A, Gustafsson J, Ewald U. Very immature infants (≤30 wk) respond to glucose infusion with incomplete suppression of glucose production. Pediatr Res 1994; 36:550–555.

45. Bergman RN, Hope ID, Yang YJ. Assessment of insulin sensitivity in vivo: A critical review. Diabetes/Metabolism Reviews 1989; 5:411–429.

46. Best JD, Taborsky Jr GJ, Halter JB. Glucose disposal is not proportional to plasma glucose in man. Diabetes 1981; 30:847–850.

47. Vranic M. Banting Lecture: Glucose turnover: A key to

understanding the pathogenesis of diabetes (Indirect effects of insulin). Diabetes 1992; 41:1188–1206.

48. Wolfe R, Allsop JR, Burke JF. Glucose metabolism in man: Responses to intravenous glucose infusion. Metab Clin Exp 1979; 28:210–220.

49. Hertz DE, Karn CA, Liu YM, Denne S. Intravenous glucose suppresses glucose production but not proteolysis in extremely premature newborns. J Clin Invest 1993; 92:1752–1758.

50. Zarlengo KM, Battaglia FC, Fennessey P, Hay W Jr. Relationship between glucose utilization rate and glucose concentration in preterm infants. Biol Neonate 1986; 49:181–189.

51. Farrag HM, Hamill SA, Gelardi NL, Cowett RM. Hyperglycemic clamp studies of pancreatic Beta Cell sensitivity in the human preterm neonate. Pediatr Res Pediatr Res 1999; 45:281A.

52. Farrag HM, Dorcus EJ, Cowett RM. Maturation of the glucose utilization response to insulin occurs before that of glucose production in the preterm neonate. Pediatr Res 1996; 39:308A.

53. Hay WW. Assessing the effect of disease on nutrition of the preterm infant. Clin Biochem 1996; 29(5):399–417.

54. Ogata ES. Carbohydrate metabolism in the fetus and neonate and altered neonatal glucoregulation. Pediatr Clin North Am 1986; 33:25–45.

55. Deshpande S. Persistent immaturity of counter-regulatory ketogenesis in preterm infants (Abstract p. 12). Paper presented at British Paediatric Association Annual Meeting. Warwick, UK, April 12–15, 1994.

56. Lane RH, Simmons RA. Hyperglycemia and other consequences of aggressive intravenous glucose administration. Semin Neonatal Nutr Metab 1997; 4:3–7.

57. Farrag HM, Nawrath LM, Dorcus EJ, Oh W, Cowett RM. Ontogeny of glucose production and glucose oxidation in the micropremie. Pediatr Res 1995; 37:307A.

58. Simmons R. Glucose Transporters: molecular, biochemical, and physiologic aspects. In: Cowett RM, ed. Principles of Perinatal-Neonatal Metabolism. 2nd ed. New York: Springer-Verlag, 1998:121–133.

59. Simmons RA, Flozak AS, Ogata ES. Glucose regulated Glut 1 function and expression in fetal rat lung and muscle in vitro. Endocrinology 1993; 132:2312–2318.

60. Devaskar S, Zahm DS, Holtzclaw L. Developmental regulation of the distribution of rat brain insulin-insensitive (Glut 1) glucose transporter. Endocrine 1991; 129:1530–1540.

61. Santalucia T, Camps M, Castello A. Developmental regulation of Glut 1 (erythroid/Hep2) and Glut 4 glucose transporter expression in rat heart, skeletal muscle, and brown adipose tissue. Endocrinology 1992; 130:837–846.

62. Simmons RA, Flozak AS, Ogata ES. Glut 1 gene expression in growth-retarded juvenile rats. Pediatr Res 1994; 35:382A.

63. Lecturque A, Postic C, Ferre P. Nutritional regulation of glucose transporter and adipose tissue of weaned rats. Am J Physiol 1991; 260:E588–E593.

64. Sadiq F, Holtzclaw L, Chundu K. The ontogeny of the rabbit brain glucose transporter. Endocrinology 1990; 126:2417–2424.

65. Sivitz W, DeSautel S, Walker PS. Regulation of the glucose transporter in developing rat brain. Endocrinology 1989; 124:1875–1880.

66. Studelska DR, Campbell C, Pary S. Developmental expression of insulin-regulatable glucose transporter Glut 4. Am J Physiol 1992; 263:E102–E106.

67. Werner H, Adamo M, Lowe WL. Developmental regulation of rat brain/Hep G2 glucose transporter gene expression. Mol Endocrinol 1989; 3:273–279.

68. Simmons RA, Flozak AS, Ogata ES. Glucose regulated Glut 1 function and expression in fetal rat lung and muscle in vitro. Endocrinology 1993; 132:2312–2318.

69. Slot JW, Gevze HJ, Gigengack S. Immuno-localization of the insulin regulatable glucose transporter in brown adipose tissue of the rat. J Cell Biol 1991; 113:123–135.

70. Eriksson J, Koranyi L, Bourey R. Insulin resistance in type 2 (non-insulin-dependent) diabetic patients and their relatives is not associated with a defect in the expression of the insulin-responsive glucose transporter (Glut-4) gene in human skeletal muscle. Diabetologia 1992; 35:143–147.

71. Koranyi LI, Bouney RE, Vuorinen MH. Levels of skeletal muscle glucose transporter protein correlates with insulin-stimulated whole body glucose disposal in man. Diabetologia 1991; 34:763–765.

72. Hughes SJ. The role of reduced glucose transporter content and glucose metabolism in the immature secretory responses of fetal rat pancreatic islets. Diabetologia 1994; 37:134–140.

73. Vannucci RC. Perinatal brain metabolism. In: Polin RA, Fox WW eds. Fetal and Neonatal Physiology. Philadelphia: WB Saunders, 1992:1510–1519.

74. Altman DI, Perlman JM, Volpe JJ. Cerebral oxygen metabolism in newborns. Pediatrics 1993; 92:99–104.

75. van Goudoever JB, Sulkers EJ, Chapman TE, Sauer P. Glucose kinetics and glucoregulatory hormone levels in ventilated preterm infants on the first day of life. Pediatr Res 1993; 33:583–589.

76. LaFeber HN, Sulkers EJ, Chapman TE, Sauer PJJ. Glucose production and oxidation in preterm infants during total parenteral nutrition. Pediatr Res 1990; 28:153–157.

77. Wolfe RR, O'Donell TF, Stone MD. Investigation of factors determining the optimal glucose infusion rate in total parenteral nutrition. Metabolism 1980; 29:892–900.

78. Yunis KA, Oh W, Kalhan S, Cowett RM. Glucose kinetics following administration of an intravenous fat emulsion to low birth weight neonates. Am J Physiol 1992; 283:E844–E849.

79. Pollak A, Cowett RM, Schwartz R, Oh W. Glucose disposal in low birth weight infants during steady state hyperglycemia: effects of exogenous insulin administration. Pediatrics 1978; 61:546–549.

80. Gleason VA, Hamm C, Jones MD Jr. Cerebral blood flow oxygenation and carbohydrate metabolism in immature fetal sheep in utero. Am J Physiol 1989; 256:R1264–R1268.

81. Shelley HJ, Bassett JM. Control of carbohydrate metabolism in the fetus and newborn. Br Med Bull 1975; 31:37–43.

82. McGowan J. The role of glucose in cerebral function. Semin Neonatal Nutr Metab 1997; 4:2–3.

83. Denne SC, Kalhan SC. Glucose carbon recycling and oxidation in human newborns. Am J Physiol 1986; 251:E71–E77.

84. Fernandes J, Berger R, Smit GPA. Lactate as a cerebral metabolic fuel for glucose-6-phosphatase deficient children. Pediatr Res 1984; 18:335–339.

85. Hernandez MJ, Vannucci RC, Salcedo A, Brennan RW. Cerebral blood flow and metabolism during hypoglycaemia in newborn dogs. J Neurochem 1980; 35:622–628.

86. Levistky LL. Fasting plasma levels of glucose acetoacetate, D-β-hydroxybutyrate, glycerol and lactate in the ba-

boon infant: correlation and cerebral uptake of substrates and oxygen. Pediatr Res 1977; 11:298–302.

87. Bougneres PF. Ketone body transport in the human neonate and infant. J Clin Invest 1986; 77:42–48.

88. Persson B, Gentz J. The pattern of blood lipids, glycerol and ketone bodies during the neonatal period, infancy and childhood. Acta Paediatr Scand 1966; 55:353–362.

89. Cornblath M. Neonatal hypoglycemia 30 years later: does it injure the brain? Historical summary and present challenges. Acta Paediatr Jpn 1997; 39(1):S7–S11.

90. Pryds O, Greisen G, Friis-Hansen B. Compensatory increase of CBF in preterm infants during hypoglycaemia. Acta Paediatr Scand 1988; 77:632–637.

91. Pryds O, Christensen NJ, Friis-Hansen B. Increased cerebral blood flow and plasma epinephrine in hypoglycemic preterm neonates. Pediatrics 1990; 85:172–176.

92. Skov L, Pryds O. Capillary recruitment for preservation of cerebral glucose influx in hypoglycemic preterm newborns: evidence for a glucose sensor? Pediatrics 1992; 90:193–195.

93. Raivio KO, Hallman N. Neonatal hypoglycemia: Occurrence of hypoglycemia in patients with various neonatal disorders. Acta Paediatr Scand 1968; 57:517–521.

94. Fluge G. Clinical aspects of neonatal hypoglycemia. Acta Paediatr Scand 1974; 63:826–832.

95. Lubchenco LO, Bard H. Incidence of hypoglycemia in newborn infants classified by birth weight and gestational age. Pediatrics 1971; 47:831–838.

96. deLeeuw R, deVries IL. Hypoglycemia in small for dates newborn infants. Pediatrics 1976; 58:18–22.

97. Koivisto M, Jouppila P. Neonatal hypoglycemia and maternal toxaemia. Acta Paediatr Scand 1974; 63:743–749.

98. Kliegman R. Alterations of fasting glucose and fat metabolism in intrauterine growth retarded newborn dogs. Am J Physiol 1989; 256:E380–E385.

99. Economides DL, Proudler A, Nicolardes KH. Plasma insulin in appropriate and small for gestational age fetuses. Am J Obstet Gynecol 1989; 160:1091–1094.

100. Bussey ME, Finley S, LaBarbera A. Hypoglycemia in the newborn growth retarded rat delayed phosphoenol pyruvate carboxy kinase induction despite increased glucagon availability. Pediatr Res 1985; 19:363–367.

101. Haymond MW, Karl IE, Pagliara AS. Increased gluconeogenic substrate in the small gestation age infant. N Engl J Med 1974; 291:322–328.

102. Williams PR, Fiser RH Jr, Sperling MA. Effects of oral alanine feeding of blood glucose, plasma glucagon, and insulin concentrations in small for gestational age infants. N Engl J Med 1975; 292:612–614.

103. Reisner SH, Aranda JV, Collc E. The effect of intravenous glucagon on plasma amino acids in the newborn. Pediatr Res 1973; 7:184–191.

104. Carter PE, Lloyd DJ, Duffty P. Glucagon for hypoglycemia in infants small for gestational age. Arch Dis Child 1988; 63:1264–1266.

105. Mestyan MJ, Schultz K, Soltesz G. The metabolic effects of glucagon infusion in normoglycemic and hypoglycemic small for gestational age infants. Changes in plasma amino acids. Acta Paediatr Acad Sci Hung 1976; 17:245–253.

106. Sperling MA, Grajwer L, Leake RD. Effects of somatostatin (SRIF) infusion on glucose homeostasis in newborn lambs: evidence for a significant role of glucagon. Pediatr Res 1977; 11:962–967.

107. Salle BL, Ruiton-Ugliengo A. Effects of oral glucose and protein load on plasma glucagon and insulin concentra-

tions in small for gestational age infants. Pediatr Res 1977; 11:108–112.

108. Cowett RM, Susa JB, Oh W. Glucose kinetics in glucose infused small for gestational age infants. Pediatr Res 1984; 18:74–79.

109. Flecknell PA, Wootton R, Royston JP. Glucose homeostasis in the newborn: effects of an intravenous glucose infusion in normal and intrauterine growth retarded neonatal piglets. Biol Neonate 1987; 52:205–215.

110. Ogata ES, Paul RI, Finley SL. Limited maternal field availability due to hyperinsulinemia retards fetal growth and development in the rat. Pediatr Res 1987; 22:432–437.

111. Sann L, Morel Y, Lasne Y. Effect of hydrocortisone on intravenous glucose tolerance in small for gestational age infants. Helv Paediatr Acta 1983; 38:475–482.

112. Shelley HJ. Glycogen reserves and their changes at birth and in anoxia. Br Med Bull 1972; 17:137–143.

113. Benzing G, Schubert W, Hug G. Simultaneous hypoglycemia and acute congestive heart failure. Circulation 1969; 40:209–216.

114. Amatayakul O, Cumming GR, Haworth JC. Association of hypoglycemia with cardiac enlargement and heart failure in newborn infants. Arch Dis Child 1970; 45:717–720.

115. Haymond MW, Strauss AW, Arnold KJ. Glucose homeostasis in children with severe cyanotic congenital heart disease. J Pediatr 1979; 95:220–227.

116. Kerkering KW, Robertson LW, Kodroff MB. Grand round series: Hypoglycemia and unilateral pulmonary edema in a newborn. Pediatrics 1980; 65:326–330.

117. Lindell KH, Sabel KG, Eriksson BD. Glucose metabolism and insulin secretion in infants with symptomatic ventricular septal defect. Acta Paediatr Scand 1989; 78:620–626.

118. Beard AG, Panos TC, Marasigan BV. Perinatal stress and the premature neonate. Effect of fluid and caloric deprivation on blood glucose. J Pediatr 1966; 68:329–343.

119. Beard AG. Neonatal hypoglycemia. J Perinat Med 1975; 3:219–225.

120. Tejani N, Lipshitz F, Harper RG. The responses to an oral glucose load during convalescence from hypoxia in newborn infants. J Pediatr 1979; 94:792–796.

121. Collins JE, Leonard JV. Hyperinsulinism in asphyxiated and small for dates infants with hypoglycemia. Lancet 1984; 1:311–313.

122. Jansen RD, Hayden MK, Ogata ES. Effects of asphyxia at birth on postnatal glucose regulation in the rat. J Dev Physiol 1984; 6:473–483.

123. Mann TP, Elliott RIK. Neonatal cold injury due to accidental exposure to cold. Lancet 1957; 1:229–234.

124. Schiff D, Stern L, Leduc J. Chemical thermogenesis in newborn infants: Catecholamine excretion and the plasma nonesterified fatty acid response to cold exposure. Pediatrics 1966; 37:577–582.

125. Close WH, LeDividish J, Dulee PH. Influence of environmental temperature on glucose tolerance and insulin response in the newborn piglet. Biol Neonate 1985; 47:84–91.

126. Yeung CY. Hypoglycemia in neonatal sepsis. J Pediatr 1970; 77:812–817.

127. LaNaoue KF, Mason AD Jr, Daniels JP. The impairment of glucogenesis by gram negative infection. Metabolism 1968; 17:606–611.

128. Yeung CY, Lee VMY, Yeung CM. Glucose disappearance rate in neonatal infection. J Pediatr 1973; 83:486–489.

129. Cowett RM. The infant of the diabetic mother. In: Cowett RM, ed. Principles of Perinatal-Neonatal Metabolism, 2nd ed. New York: Springer-Verlag, 1998:1105–1129.

130. Jovanovic L, Druzin M, Peterson CM. Effects of euglycemia on the outcome of pregnancy in insulin-dependent diabetic women as compared with normal control subjects. Am J Med 1980; 68:105–112.

131. Kitzmiller JL, Cloberty IP, Younger MD. Diabetic pregnancy and perinatal morbidity. Am J Obstet Gynecol 1978; 131:560–568.

132. Pedersen J, Molsted-Pedersen L, Andersen B. Assessors of fetal perinatal mortality in diabetic pregnancy. Analyses of 1332 pregnancies in the Copenhagen series 1946–1972. Diabetes 1974; 23:302–305.

133. Naeye RL. Infants of diabetic mothers: a quantitative morphologic study. Pediatric 1964; 35:980–988.

134. Susa JB, McCormick KL, Widness JA. Chronic hyperinsulinemia in the fetal rhesus monkey. Effects on fetal growth and composition. Diabetes 1979; 28:1058–1063.

135. Block MD, Pildes RS, Mossabhou NA. C-peptide immunoreactivity (CRP): a new method for studying infants of insulin-treated diabetic mothers. Pediatrics 1974; 53:923–928.

136. King KC, Adam PAJ, Yamaguchi K. Insulin response to arginine in normal newborn infants and infants of diabetic mothers. Diabetes 1974; 23:816–820.

137. Light IJ, Sutherland JM, Loggie JM. Impaired epinephrine release in hypoglycemic infants of diabetic mothers. N Engl J Med 1967; 277:394–398.

138. Stern L, Ramos A, Leduc J. Urinary catecholamine excretion in infants of diabetic mothers. Pediatrics 1968; 42:598–605.

139. Keenan WJ, Light IJ, Sutherland JM. Effects of exogenous epinephrine on glucose and insulin levels in infants of diabetic mothers. Biol Neonate 1972; 21:44–53.

140. Artel R, Platt LD, Kurnmula RK. Sympatho-adrenal activity in infants of diabetic mothers. Am J Obstet Gynecol 1982; 42:436–439.

141. Cowett RM. Decreased response to catecholamines in the newborn: effect on glucose kinetics in the lamb. Metabolism 1988; 37:736–740.

142. Cowett RM. Alpha adrenergic agonists stimulate neonatal glucose production less than beta adrenergic agonists in the lamb. Metabolism 1988; 37:831–836.

143. Barrett CT, Oliver TK Jr. Hypoglycemia and hyperinsulinism in infants with erythroblastosis fetalis. N Engl J Med. 1968; 278:1260–1263.

144. Molsted-Pedersen L, Trautner H, Jorgensen KR. Plasma insulin and K values during intravenous glucose tolerance test in newborn infants with erythroblastosis foetalis. Acta Paediatr Scand 1973; 62:11–16.

145. Oh W, Yap LL, D'Amodio MD. Hypoglycemia in severely affected Rh erythroblastotic infants. J Pediatr 1969; 74:813 (abstr).

146. Schiff D, Lowy C. Hypoglycemia and excretion of insulin in urine in hemolytic disease of the newborn. Pediatr Res 1970; 4:280–285.

147. Schiff D, Aranda JV, Chan G. Metabolic effects of exchange transfusions. Effect of citrated and of heparinized blood on glucose, non-esterified fatty acids, 2- (4 hydroxybenzeneazo) benzoic acid binding and insulin. J Pediatr 1971; 78:603–609.

148. Schiff D, Aranda JC, Colle E. Metabolic effects of exchange transfusion. Delayed hypoglycemia following exchange transfusion with citrated blood. J Pediatr 1971; 79:589–593.

149. Nagel JW, Sims JS, Aplin CE. Refractory hypoglycemia associated with a malpositoned umbilical artery catheter. Pediatrics 1979; 64:315–317.

150. Malik M, Wilson DP. Umbilical artery catheterization. A potential cause of refractory hypoglycemia. Clin Pediatr 1987; 26:181–182.

151. Puri AR, Alkalay AL, Pomerance JJ. Neonatal hypoglycemia associated with umbilical artery catheter positioned at eighth to ninth thoracic vertebrae. Am J Perinatol 1987; 4:195–197.

152. Carey BE, Zeilinger TC. Hypoglycemia due to high positioning of umbilical artery catheters. J Perinatol 1989; 9:407–410.

153. Cowett RM, Tenenbaum D, Fatoba O. The effects of glucose infusion above the celiac axis in the newborn lamb. Biol Neonate 1985; 47:179–185.

154. Jacob J, Davis RF. Differences in serum glucose determinations in infants with umbilical artery catheters. J Perinatol 1988; 8:40–42.

155. Milner RD. Nesidioblastosis unraveled [comment]. Arch Dis Child 1996; 74:369.

156. Permutt MA, Nestorowicz A, Glaser B. Familial hyperinsulinism: An inherited disorder of spontaneous hypoglycemia in neonates and infants. Diabetes Rev 1996; 4: 347–353.

157. Heitz PU, Kloppel G, Hacki WH. Nesidioblastosis: the pathologic basis of persistent hyperinsulinemic hypoglycemia in infants. Diabetes 1977; 26:637–642.

158. Schwartz SS, Rich BH, Lucky AW. Familial nesidioblastosis: severe neonatal hypoglycemia in two families. Pediatrics 1979; 95:44–53.

159. Woo D, Scopes JW, Polak JM. Idiopathic hypoglycemia in situ with morphological evidence of nesidioblastosis of the pancreas. Arch Dis Child 1976; 51:528–531.

160. Baerentsen H. Case report: neonatal hypoglycemia due to an islet cell adenoma. Acta Paediatr Scand 1973; 62:207–210.

161. Burst NRM, Campbell JR, Castro A. Congenital islet cell adenoma causing hypoglycemia in a newborn. Pediatrics 1971; 47:605–610.

162. Habbick BJ, Cram RW, Miller KR. Neonatal hypoglycemia resulting from islet cell adenomatosis. Am J Dis Child. 1977; 131:210–212.

163. Gruppuso PA, DeLuca F, O'Shea PA. Near total pancreatectomy for hyperinsulinism. Spontaneous remission or resultant diabetes. Acta Paediatr Scand 1985; 74:311–315.

164. Jaffe R, Hashida Y, Yunis EJ. Pancreatic pathology in hyperinsulinemic hypoglycemia of infancy. Lab Invest 1980; 42:356–361.

165. Schwitzgebel VM, Gitelman SE. Neonatal hyperinsulinism. Clin Perinatol 1998; 25(4):1015–1038.

166. Levitt Katz LE, Satin-Smith MS, Collett-Solberg P. Insulin-like growth factor binding protein-1 levels in the diagnosis of hypoglycemia caused by hyperinsulinism. J Pediatr 1997; 131:193–199.

167. Finegold DN, Stanley CA, Baker L. Glycemic response to glucagon during fasting hypoglycemia: an aid in the diagnosis of hyperinsulinism. J Pediatr 1980; 96:257–261.

168. Solt'esz G, Jenkins PA, Aynsley-Green A. Hyperinsulinemic hypoglycemia in infancy and childhood: a practical approach to diagnosis and medical treatment based on experience of 18 cases. Acta Paediatr Hung 1984; 25: 319–332.

169. Aynsley-Green A, Jenkin P, Tronier B. Plasma proinsulin and C peptide concentrations in children with hyperinsulinemic hypoglycemic. Acta Paediatr Scand 1984; 73: 359–363.

170. Glaser B, Chiu KC, Anker R. Familial hyperinsulinism maps to chromosome 11p14-15.1, 30 cM centromeric to the insulin gene. Nat Genet 1994; 7:185–191.

171. Mathew PM, Young JM, Abu-Osba YK. Persistent neonatal hyperinsulinism. Clin Pediatr (Phila) 1988; 27:148–153.

172. Thornton PS, Satin-Smith MS, Herold K. Familial hyperinsulinism with apparent autosomal dominant inheritance: clinical and genetic differences from the autosomal recessive variant. J Pediatr 1998; 132:9–14.

173. Aguilar-Bryan L, Nichols CG, Wechsler SW. Cloning of the β-cell high-affinity sulfonylurea receptor: a regulator of insulin secretion. Science 1995; 268:423–429.

174. Thomas PM, Cote GJ, Wohllk N. Mutations in the sulfonylurea receptor gene in familial persistent hyperinsulinemic hypoglycemia of infancy. Science 1995; 268: 426–431.

175. Kane C, Shepherd RM, Squires PE. Loss of functional K_{ATP} channels in pancreatic β-cells causes persistent hyperinsulinemic hypoglycemia of infancy. Nat Med 1996; 2:1344–1348.

176. Nestorowicz A, Wilson BA, Schoor KP. Mutations in the sulfonylurea receptor gene are associated with familial hyperinsulinism in Ashkenazi Jews. Hum Mol Genet 1996; 5:1813–1818.

177. Dunne MJ, Kane C, Shepherd RM. Familial persistent hyperinsulinemic hypoglycemia of infancy and mutations in the sulfonylurea receptor. N Engl J Med 1997; 336: 703–708.

178. Suzuki M, Fujikura K, Inagaki N. Localization of the ATP-sensitive K^+ channel subunit Kir6.2 in mouse pancreas. Diabetes 1997; 46:1440–1445.

179. Nichols CG, Shyng SL, Nestorowicz A. Adenosine diphosphate as an intracellular regulator of insulin secretion. Science 1996; 272:1785–1790.

180. Glaser B, Kesavan P, Heyman M. Familial hyperinsulinism caused by an activating glucokinase mutation. N Engl J Med 1998; 338:226–231.

181. Dubois J, Brunelle F, Touati G. Hyperinsulinism in children: diagnostic value of pancreatic venous sampling correlated with clinical, pathological and surgical outcome in 25 cases. Pediatr Radiol 1995; 25:512–517.

182. de Lonlay P, Foumet JC, Rahier J. Somatic deletion of the imprinted 11p15 region in sporadic persistent hyperinsulinemic hypoglycemia of infancy is specific of focal adenomatous hyperplasia and endorses partial pancreatectomy. J Clin Invest 1997; 100:802–806.

183. Weksberg R, Shen OR, Fei YL. Disruption of insulin-like growth factor 2 imprinting in Beckwith-Wiedemann syndrome. Nat Genet 1993; 5:143–147.

184. Epstein MF, Nicholls E, Stubblefield PG. Neonatal hypoglycemia after beta-sympathomimetic tocolytic therapy. J Pediatr 1979; 94:449–453.

185. Procianoy RS, Pinheiro CEA. Neonatal hyperinsulinism after short term maternal beta sympathomimetic therapy. J Pediatr 1982; 101:612–614.

186. Leake RD, Hobel CJ, Okada DM. Neonatal metabolic effects of oral retodrine hypochloride administration. Pediatr Pharm 1983; 3:101–106.

187. Tenenbaum D, Cowett RM. The mechanisms of beta sympathomimetic action on neonatal glucose homeostasis in the lamb. J Pediatr 1985; 107:588–592.

188. Singh SP, Sayder AK, Singh SF. Effects of ethanol ingestion on maternal and fetal glucose homeostasis. J Lab Clin Med 1984; 104:176–184.

189. Witer-Janusek L. Maternal ethanol ingestion: effect on maternal and neonatal glucose balance. Am J Physiol 1986; 251:E178–E184.

190. Singh SP, Snyder AK, Pullen GL. Fetal alcohol syndrome: glucose and liver metabolism in term rat fetus and neonate. Alcoholism 1986; 10:54–58.

191. Zucker P, Simon G. Prolonged symptomatic neonatal hypoglycemia associated with maternal chloropropamide therapy. Pediatrics 1968; 42:824–825.

192. Senior B, Slone D, Shapiro S. Benzothiadiazides and neonatal hypoglycemia. Lancet 1976; 2:377–381.

193. Stern C. Idiopathic hypoglycemia. Proc R Soc Med 1973; 66:345–346.

194. Brown RE, Young RB. A possible role for the exocrine pancreas in the pathogenesis of neonatal leucine sensitive hypoglycemia. Am J Dig Dis 1970; 15:65–72.

195. Schutgens RBH, Heymans H, Ketel A. Lethal hypoglycemia in a child with a deficiency of 3-hydroxy-3-methyl glutaryl coenzyme A lyase. J Pediatr 1979; 94:89–91.

196. Pickering D. Neonatal hypoglycemia due to salicylate poisoning. Proc R Soc Med 1968; 61:1256.

197. Gemelli M, DeLuca R, Barberio G. Hypoglycemia and congenital adrenal hyperplasia. Acta Pediatr Scand 1979; 68:285–286.

198. Souto M, Piezzi R, Bianchi R. Effect of insulin on neonatal and adult adrenal medulla in the rat. Acta Anat (Basel) 1985; 122:216–219.

199. Actavia-Loria E, Chaussain JL, Bougneres PF. Frequency of hypoglycemia in children with adrenal insufficiency. Acta Endocrinol Suppl (Copenh) 1986; 279:275–278.

200. Lilien LD, Srinivasan G, Yeh TF. Decreased plasma glucose following indomethacin therapy in premature infants with patent ductus arteriosus. Pediatr Pharm 1985; 5:73–77.

201. Beckwith JB, Wang CI, Donel GN. Hyperplastic fetal visceromegaly with macroglossia, omphalocele, cytomegaly of adrenal fetal cortex, postnatal somatic gigantism, and other abnormalities. Newly recognized syndrome. Proceedings, American Pediatrics Society, Seattle, 1964, June 16–18 (abstr 41).

202. Wiedemann HR. Complexe malformatif familiale avec hernie ombilicale et macroglossie un syndrome nouveau? J Genet Hum 1964; 13:223–225.

203. Schiff D, Colle EC, Wells D. Metabolic aspects of the Beckwith-Wiedemann syndrome. J Pediatr 1973; 82:258–267.

204. Vidnes J, Oyasaeter S. Glucagon deficiency causing severe neonatal hypoglycemia in a patient with normal insulin secretion. Pediatr Res 1977; 11:943–949.

205. Vidnes J, Sovik O. Gluconeogenesis in infancy and childhood. Studies on the glucose production from alanine in three cases of persistent neonatal hypoglycaemia. Acta Paediatr Scand 1976; 65:297–305.

206. Vidnes J, Sovik O. Gluconeogenesis in infancy and childhood. Deficiency of the extramitochondrial form of hepatic phosphoenolpyruvate carboxykinase in a case of persistent neonatal hypoglycemia. Acta Paediatr 1976; 65:307–312.

207. Howell RR, Williams JC. The glycogen storage diseases. In: Stanbury JB, Wyngarden JB, Fredrickson DS, eds. The Metabolic Basis of Inherited Disease. New York: McGraw Hill, 1983:141–152.

208. Pagliara AS, Karl IE, Keating JP. Hepatic fructose-1,6-diphosphatase deficiency: a cause of lactate acidosis and hypoglycemia in infancy. J Clin Invest 1972; 51:2115–2123.

209. Ralleson ML, Mukle AW, Zigrang WD. Hypoglycemia and lactate acidosis associated with fructos-1,6-diphosphatase deficiency. J Pediatr 1979; 94:933–936.

210. Levy HL, Hammersen G. Newborn screening for galactosemia and other galactose metabolic defects. J Pediatr 1978; 92:871–878.

211. Sperling MA. Hypoglycemia in the newborn infant, and child. In: Lifshitz F, ed. Pediatric Endocrinology, a Clinical Guide. 2nd ed. New York: Marcel Dekker, 1990: 803–838.

212. Hawdon JM, Ward Platt M, Aynsley Green A. Prevention and management of neonatal hypoglycaemia. Arch Dis Childh 1994; 70:F60–F65.

213. Lilien LD. Treatment of neonatal hypoglycemia with minibolus and intravenous glucose infusion. J Pediatr 1980; 97:295–298.

214. Settergren G, Lindblad BS, Persson B. Cerebral blood flow and exchange of oxygen, glucose, ketone bodies, lactate, pyruvate and amino acids in infants. Acta Paediatr Scand 1976; 65:343–353.

215. Mehta A. Prevention and management of neonatal hypoglycaemia. Arch Dis Childh 1994; 70:F54–F59.

216. Cowett RM, Susa JB, Schwartz R. Concentration of parenteral glucose solution. Pediatrics 1977; 59:791–794.

217. Sann L, Mousson B, Rousson M. Prevention of neonatal hypoglycemia by oral lipid supplementation in low birth weight infants. Eur J Pediatr 1988; 147:158–161.

218. McCann ML, Likly B. The role of epinephrine prophylactic therapy in infants of diabetic mothers. Proc Soc Pediatr Res 1967; 3:5–11.

219. Glaser B, Hirsch HJ, Landau H. Persistent hyperinsulinemic hypoglycemia of infancy: long-term octreotide treatment without pancreatectomy. J Pediatr 1993; 123:644–651.

220. Grant DB, Dunger DB, Burns EC. Long-term treatment with diazoxide in childhood hyperinsulinism. Acta Endocrinol Suppl (Copenh) 1986; 279:340–344.

221. Labrune P, Bonnefont JP, Nihoul-Fekete C. Evaluation of diagnostic and therapeutic methods in hyperinsulinism in newborn infants and infants. Apropos of a retrospective study of 26 cases. Arch Franc Pediatr 1989; 46:167–173.

222. Thornton PS, Sumner AE, Ruchelli ED. Familial and sporadic hyperinsulinism: Histopathologic findings and segregation analysis support a single autosomal recessive disorder. J Pediatr 1991; 119:721–728.

223. Woolf OA, Leonard IV, Trembath RC. Nesidioblastosis: evidence for autosomal recessive inheritance. Arch Dis Child 1991; 66:529–534.

224. Thornton PS, Alter CA, Katz LE. Short- and long-term use of octreotide in the treatment of congenital hyperinsulinism. J Pediatr 1993; 123:637–642.

225. Stanley CA. Hyperinsulinism in infants and children. Pediatr Clin North Am 1997; 44:363–377.

226. Lindley K, Dunne MJ, Kane C. Ionic control of β-cell function in nesidioblastosis: a possible therapeutic role for calcium channel blockade. Arch Dis Child 1996; 74:373–377.

227. Glaser B, Landau H, Smilovici A, Nesher R: Persistent hyperinsulinemic hypoglycemia of infancy: long-term treatment with the somatostatin analogue Sandostatin. Clin Endocrinol 1989; 31:71–77.

228. Greene SA, Aynsley-Green A, Soltesz G, Baum J. Management of secondary diabetes mellitus after total pancreatectomy in infancy. Arch Dis Child 1984; 59:356–362.

229. Horev Z, Ipp M, Levey P, Daneman D. Familial hyperinsulinism: successful conservative management. J Pediatr 1991; 119:717–724.

230. Landau H, Perlman M, Meyer S. Persistent neonatal hypoglycemia due to hyperinsulinism: medical aspects. Pediatrics 1982; 70:440–445.

231. Leibowitz G, Glaser B, Higazi AA. Hyperinsulinemic hypoglycemia of infancy (nesidioblastosis) in clinical remission: high incidence of diabetes mellitus and persistent β-cell dysfunction at long-term follow-up. J Clin Endocrinol Metab 1995; 80:386–393.

24

Hypoglycemia in Children

Joseph I. Wolfsdorf and David A. Weinstein
Children's Hospital and Harvard Medical School, Boston, Massachusetts, U.S.A.

I. INTRODUCTION

Glucose is normally the predominant fuel for mammalian cells. Because the brain cannot synthesize glucose or store more than a few minutes' supply as glycogen, survival of the brain depends on a continuous supply of glucose (1). Recurrent hypoglycemia during the period of rapid brain growth and differentiation in infancy can result in long-term neurological sequelae, psychomotor retardation, and seizures. Prevention of hypoglycemia and expeditious diagnosis and vigorous treatment are, therefore, essential to prevent the potentially devastating cerebral consequences of hypoglycemia.

Hypoglycemia is most common in the newborn period. During infancy and childhood, it occurs most frequently when nighttime feeding is discontinued and when intercurrent illness interrupts the child's normal feeding pattern, causing periods of relative starvation. Basal energy needs during infancy are high. A full-term newborn baby has a ratio of surface area to body mass more than twice that of an average adult, necessitating a high rate of energy expenditure to maintain body temperature. Also, the infant brain is large relative to body mass and its energy requirement is primarily derived from the oxidation of circulating glucose. To meet the high demand for glucose, the rate of glucose production in infants and young children is two to three times that of older children and mature adults (2). Although the demand for glucose is high, the activity of several liver enzymes involved in energy production is low in the newborn compared to older children and adults. As a consequence, until feeding is well established, maintenance of glucose homeostasis in the newborn period is more precarious than later in childhood.

In the postabsorptive state, the rate of glucose turnover in adults is approximately 2 mg/kg/min (8–10 g/h); whereas the average basal (4–6 h after feeding) rate of glucose turnover is 6 mg/kg/min in newborns, approximately three times the adult rate (2). During prolonged fasting, infants and children cannot sustain the high rate of glucose production. Normal children, 18 months to 9 years of age, fasted for 24 h have a mean whole blood glucose concentration of 52 ± 14 (SD) mg/dl, and 22% have blood glucose concentrations less than 40 mg/dl; blood glucose values conform to a Gaussian pattern of distribution (3). For these reasons, infants and young children are more prone than adolescents and adults to hypoglycemia when normal feeding patterns are disturbed by intercurrent illness.

II. DEFINITION OF HYPOGLYCEMIA

During acute insulin-induced hypoglycemia in normal adults, symptoms appear at an arterialized venous plasma glucose level of approximately 60 mg/dl (3.3 mmol/l) and impairment of brain function occurs at approximately 50 mg/dl (2.8 mmol/l) (4, 5). Comparable levels in venous blood are about 3 mg/dl lower (6). In children, functional changes in the central nervous system (brainstem auditory and somatosensory evoked potentials) occur when the venous plasma glucose concentration falls below 47 mg/dl (2.6 mmol/l) (7). These facts suggest that the physiological threshold is a plasma glucose concentration in the range of 50–60 mg/dl (2.8–3.3 mmol/l). Therefore, for clinical care of children, a venous plasma glucose concentration of 60 mg/dl (3.3 mmol/l) or greater may be regarded as normoglycemia and plasma glucose levels below 50 mg/dl (2.8 mmol/l) as hypoglycemia.

III. OVERVIEW OF FUEL METABOLISM

The physiological mechanisms that normally prevent hypoglycemia ensure that the brain receives a continuous supply of glucose (8). Several tissue-specific glucose transport (GLUT) proteins are responsible for transport of glucose from the extracellular to the intracellular space (Table 1). GLUT-1 and GLUT-3 transporters are found on most cells and are primarily responsible for basal glucose use by the brain and most other body tissues (9). Both GLUT-1 (on glial cells) and GLUT-3 (on neuronal cells) (10) are insulin-independent facilitative glucose transporters. Blood-to-brain glucose transport is a function of the arterial plasma glucose concentration. The supply of glucose to the brain, therefore, is dependent on the precise regulation of systemic glucose balance that maintains the arterial plasma glucose concentration above the critical level that becomes limiting to brain glucose metabolism. None of the glucoregulatory factors, including insulin, modify glucose uptake into the brain. However, chronic exposure to cerebral hypoglycemia results in upregulation of both these transporters (11–13).

Most body tissues, with the exception of the brain, can use free fatty acids (FFA) for oxidative metabolism. Under conditions of fasting, the plasma FFA concentration increases and the uptake and oxidation of glucose decreases. The high rate of tissue oxidation of FFA functionally decreases the use of glucose in accordance with Randle's hypothesis (the glucose–fatty acid cycle) (14). Although FFA are not transported across the blood–brain barrier, β-hydroxybutyrate (BOHB) and acetoacetate (AcAc), the water-soluble products of hepatic β-oxidation of FFA, readily cross the blood–brain barrier (15, 16). In vitro studies in rats have demonstrated that the use of ketones can decrease brain glucose utilization by ~50%. Indirect evidence in humans is consistent with these data (17, 18).

In the interval between meals and during fasting, maintenance of normal plasma glucose concentrations requires adequate endogenous substrate (body fat, hepatic and muscle glycogen, and mobilizable amino acids); intact metabolic and enzymatic pathways; proper hormonal regulation of the mobilization, interconversion, and use of metabolic fuels. An abnormality in any one of these areas may compromise the homeostatic mechanisms that balance the rate of appearance and the rate of disposal of glucose that maintains the plasma glucose concentration in a narrow normal range (19). Glucose is derived from intestinal absorption following digestion of dietary carbohydrate (exogenous glucose delivery) or from endogenous glucose production (glycogenolysis and gluconeogenesis). Gluconeogenesis refers to the formation of glucose from three carbon precursors, including lactate, pyruvate, amino acids (especially alanine and glutamine), and glycerol. The integrated regulatory effects of hormones, neural pathways, and metabolic substrates normally result in the precise matching of glucose utilization

and the sum of exogenous glucose delivery and endogenous glucose production. The key glucoregulatory hormones are insulin, glucagon, and epinephrine. Growth hormone (GH) and cortisol modify the effectiveness of these glucoregulatory hormones.

After feeding, exogenous glucose delivery increases at a rate largely determined by the carbohydrate content of the ingested meal and the rate of gastric emptying. Glucose absorption from the intestine into the portal circulation occurs via a sodium-dependent transport mechanism. The increase in circulating glucose concentration, augmented by incretins (gastric inhibitory polypeptide [GIP] and glucagon-like peptide-1 [GLP-1] secreted by the intestine), stimulates insulin and inhibits glucagon secretion. Increased plasma levels of insulin result in translocation of GLUT-4 transporters from their intracellular location to the cell membrane, thereby enhancing glucose entry into fat and muscle cells (Table 1). More than 80% of ingested glucose enters the systemic circulation; the entire splanchnic bed extracts only 10–20% (20). Over a wide range of carbohydrate consumption in normal individuals, the plasma glucose concentration increases from ~70 mg/dl to ≤150 mg/dl. Endogenous glucose production is suppressed by high postprandial plasma insulin concentrations, which decrease hepatic glycogenolysis and increase glycogen synthesis. Glucose transported into the liver by GLUT-2 transporters replenishes the hepatic glycogen store. Liver and muscle express high levels of glycogen synthase activity and can store appreciable quantities of glucose as glycogen. In the liver, glucose is also converted to fat, which can be stored in the liver or be transported to other tissues in the form of very-low-density lipoproteins. The increase in plasma insulin concentration also decreases rates of proteolysis and lipolysis, thus decreasing the availability of substrates for gluconeogenesis and ketogenesis, respectively.

Increased metabolism of dietary carbohydrate leads to increased cytosolic citrate, which inhibits activity of carnitine palmitoyltransferase-I (CPT-I) and diverts fatty acids away from oxidation in peripheral tissues and away from β-oxidation and ketogenesis in the liver. With decreased hepatic FFA oxidation, activity of pyruvate carboxylase decreases and 3-carbon substrates are directed away from gluconeogenesis and toward formation of acetyl CoA. A reduction in β-oxidation also results in decreased production of reduced nucleotides, which are necessary for gluconeogenesis. With decreased circulating plasma concentrations of FFA and ketone bodies and increased concentrations of glucose and insulin, GLUT-1, GLUT-3, and GLUT-4 transporters efficiently move glucose out of the circulation and into cells.

Despite a substantial increase in glucose influx into the circulation, the increase in plasma glucose concentration is relatively small after a meal, and plasma glucose and insulin concentrations return to basal levels within 2–3 h. As nutrient absorption is completed, flow of glucose

Table 1 Tissue-Specific Glucose Transporters

Glucose transporter	Distribution	Principal function	K_m for glucose (mmol/L)	Gene location	Regulation
GLUT-1	Wide distribution Brain glial cells Erythrocytes Endothelial cells	Constitutive glucose transporter	20	1p35 → 31.3	Minimal
GLUT-2	Liver Pancreatic β cells Small intestine epithelium Kidney	Glucose-sensing in β cells	42	3q26	Zero to minimal
GLUT-3	Wide distribution CNS neurons Fetal muscle Placenta Kidney	High-affinity glucose transporter	10	12p13	None
GLUT-4	Skeletal muscle Cardiac muscle Adipose cells	Insulin-responsive glucose transporter	2–10	17p13	Regulated by insulin
GLUT-5	Liver Small intestine Sperm Adipose cells Brain Muscle	Fructose transporter; very low affinity for glucose	Not defined	1p31	None

from the gut decreases and eventually stops. Plasma glucose concentration frequently decreases to below the pre-meal value. The relative hypoglycemia, together with the decrease in insulin secretion, triggers release of glucagon, which increases hepatic glucose production (21). The transition from endogenous glucose production to exogenous glucose delivery shortly after a meal and the later transition from exogenous glucose delivery back to endogenous glucose production are finely regulated (21). Hypoglycemia normally does not occur in the interval between meals and glucose delivery to the brain continues unabated (Fig. 1A).

Most of the glucose in the body is normally in the extracellular space; the intracellular glucose concentration is low because glucose is rapidly phosphorylated when it enters cells. The extracellular space is ~25% of body weight in children and adolescents. The total glucose present in a person with a plasma glucose concentration of 90 mg/dl is 1.25 mmol/kg body weight or 225 mg/kg. This is equivalent to ~5% of a teaspoon of glucose/kg body weight. Thus, the total pool size of a 10 year old child (30 kg) is approximately 6.75 g glucose (19).

The amount of glycogen stored in the liver is modest: approximately 5% of the wet weight of the liver. For example, the liver of a 10-year-old child who weighs 30 kg contains about 45 g glycogen. This could, theoretically, satisfy the basal requirement for glucose (~9 g/h) for only

5–6 h. Thus, gluconeogenesis soon plays the major part in maintaining normal blood glucose concentrations (Fig. 1B). In children, the precise fraction of glucose derived from glycogenolysis rather than gluconeogenesis at any point in time during feeding and fasting is unknown.

Muscle can store glucose as glycogen, but lacks the enzyme glucose-6-phosphatase, and, therefore, cannot release free glucose. Red cells lack mitochondria; consequently, glycolysis stops with the formation of lactate. In other cells, glucose can be completely oxidized to carbon dioxide and water. During a fast, muscle can oxidize fatty acids to meet its energy needs and substantially reduce its glucose uptake. Proteolysis in muscle provides the liver with amino acids for gluconeogenesis. Whether or not complete oxidation of glucose occurs depends upon the activity of the enzyme pyruvate dehydrogenase, which is inactivated by products of fatty acid oxidation. The availability of other fuels for oxidation (fatty acids or ketones) affects the activity of pyruvate dehydrogenase and determines whether glucose is completely oxidized to carbon dioxide and water, or is conserved via recycling of lactate, pyruvate, and alanine back to glucose in the liver (glucose–lactate–glucose and glucose–alanine–glucose cycles).

In muscle, glucose is metabolized via glycolysis to pyruvate, which can be reduced to lactate, transaminated to form alanine, or undergo oxidation. Lactate and pyru-

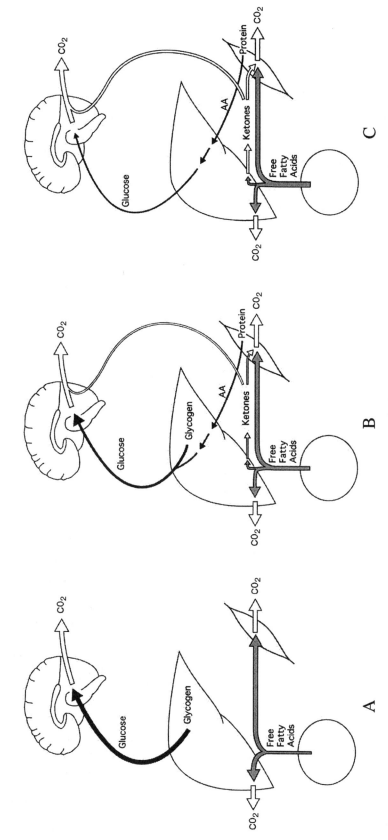

Figure 1 A. Between meals: glucose is from hepatic glycogenolysis; free fatty acids from adipose tissue are an additional source of fuel for muscle. B. Overnight fast: liver glycogen becomes depleted and gluconeogenesis becomes the principal source of glucose. Hepatic ketone production increases and rising plasma ketone body concentrations provide an alternative fuel for brain and muscle. C. Prolonged starvation: Fat-derived fuels are the predominant metabolic substrates. Brain utilization of ketones increases. Glucose is from gluconeogenesis.

vate released from muscle are transported to the liver and serve as gluconeogenic precursors (the Cori or glucose–lactate–glucose cycle). Alanine, glutamine, and other amino acids also flow from muscle to the liver and serve as gluconeogenic precursors. Circulating alanine carbon is largely derived from glucose (glucose–alanine–glucose cycle) (22). Glutamine, the other major amino acid precursor for new glucose formation, is also partially derived from glucose (glucose–glutamine cycle) (23).

Liver and kidney express the critical gluconeogenic enzymes: pyruvate carboxylase, phosphoenolpyruvate carboxykinase (PEPCK), fructose-1,6-bisphosphatase, and glucose-6-phosphatase. Although many tissues have the ability to convert oxaloacetate to glucose-6-phosphate and glycogen, the liver and kidney (owing to the presence of the glucose-6-phosphatase system) are the major organs that produce free glucose that can be released into the circulation. In adults, 40–50% of glucose is derived from gluconeogenesis in the postabsorptive state (after an overnight fast), and this increases to ~90% during a 48–72 h fast (24–26). Thus, in the postabsorptive state, hepatic gluconeogenesis soon plays the major role in maintaining normal blood glucose concentrations. In children and adolescents, the fraction of glucose production from gluconeogenesis is ~50–60% (27) (Fig. 1B).

Over time, the hepatic glycogen store is depleted and all glucose production must be from hepatic and renal gluconeogenesis. Hepatic oxidation of fatty acids produces the energy, reducing equivalents, and metabolic intermediates required to sustain the high rate of hepatic gluconeogenesis that occurs during fasting. FFA are released from adipose tissue stores (lipolysis) and normally are abundant during fasting (28, 29). FFA also provide many tissues (including cardiac and skeletal muscle) with a readily usable energy substrate. A fraction of the FFA undergoes β-oxidation in the liver to form ketone bodies (Fig. 1B,C). High rates of ketone body production are reached during fasting in children. After fasting for 20–22 h, the ketone body turnover rate in young children is comparable to that achieved by adults fasted for several days (30). During fasting, plasma concentrations of ketone bodies increase dramatically as a reflection of increased plasma concentrations of FFA and increased rates of β-oxidation in the liver (28, 31). Within 30 h of fasting, normal children achieve plasma total ketone body concentrations of 5–6 mmol/l, levels that are seen in adult women after fasting for 2.5–3 days and are not achieved in men even after 84 h of fasting (31). Fasting ketonemia provides the brain (which cannot utilize FFA) and other tissues with an alternative source of energy (15, 16, 32). Because the brain can oxidize ketones, it is not solely dependent on glucose as an energy substrate. Normally, the large amounts of ketones generated during fasting results in a decrease in the brain's rate of glucose consumption.

Prolonged fasting ultimately leads to a decrease to about one-half in the basal glucose turnover, resulting in a gradual decrease in the plasma glucose concentration (33). These metabolic responses to fasting (increased gluconeogenesis, lipolysis, and ketogenesis) are finely regulated by changes in the circulating concentrations of hormones including a decrease in insulin secretion and increased plasma concentrations of glucagon, epinephrine, GH, and cortisol, the latter collectively referred to as the counterregulatory hormones.

In summary, the adaptation to fasting involves a major change in the body's fuel economy. As fasting is prolonged, there is decreased dependence on glucose and increased reliance on the products of fat as the primary source of fuel for energy metabolism (Fig. 1C). A failure to oxidize fatty acids or to synthesize or utilize ketones results in greater utilization of glucose, impaired gluconeogenesis, and inability to conserve glucose, which leads to severe hypoglycemia. Examples of these disorders are discussed in detail later in this chapter.

IV. REGULATION OF INSULIN SECRETION

Insulin secretion is regulated by nutritional, hormonal, metabolic, and autonomic nervous system signals. These signals are transduced by a complex system that involves intracellular glucose metabolism, depolarization of the cell membrane, regulation of free intracellular cytosolic calcium concentration, and the movement of insulin-containing secretory granules to fuse with the plasma membrane to release their contents (Fig. 2) (34). ATP-sensitive potassium channels (K_{ATP} channels) in the plasma membrane, which control the polarity of the β-cell membrane, have a pivotal role in regulating insulin secretion. They are formed from two distinct subunit proteins: the high-affinity sulfonylurea receptor (SUR1) and Kir6.2, a weak inward-rectifier (35). The pore of the channel is formed by Kir6.2 in a tetrameric arrangement. At rest, K_{ATP} channels are normally kept open maintaining a membrane potential of about −70 mV. A rise in the blood glucose concentration increases glucose entry into the cell (via GLUT-2 transport) and the rate of glucose metabolism increases in the β-cell. Intracellular glucose is phosphorylated by glucokinase, the rate-limiting step in glucose metabolism (Fig. 2), and is then metabolized resulting in an increased ratio of ATP/ADP, which leads to closure of K_{ATP} channels, depolarization of the β-cell membrane, and opening of voltage-dependent L-type calcium channels with influx of extracellular calcium. The increase in cytosolic free calcium concentration triggers exocytosis of insulin-containing secretory granules (36).

SUR1 encodes for a 39 exon gene with 17 transmembrane domains and produces a 1581 amino acid product; Kir6.2 encodes for a 390 amino acid protein. These genes are located on adjacent regions of chromosome 11p15.1. The SUR protein forms an octameric complex with four SUR1 subunits surrounding four Kir6.2 centrally located channels. ATP acts directly on Kir6.2 resulting in closure

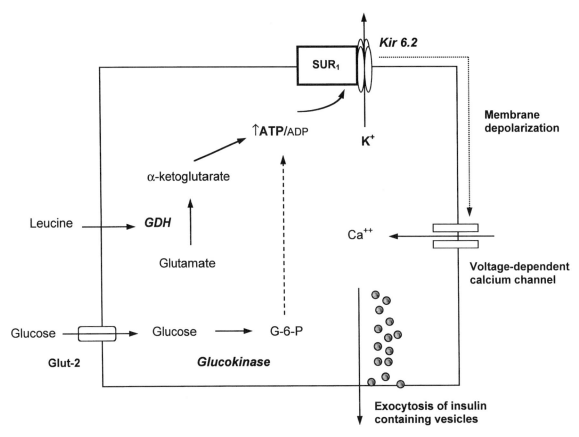

Figure 2 Model of insulin secretion regulation by pancreatic β-cell. Glucose is transported into the β-cell by GLUT-2 and then phosphorylated by glucokinase to glucose-6-phosphate (G-6-P). Glucose metabolism is initiated resulting in an increase in the cytosolic ratio of ATP/ADP, which causes closure of K_{ATP} channels and leads to membrane depolarization and opening of voltage-dependent Ca^{2+} channels. Influx of calcium releases insulin through exocytosis of secretory granules. Leucine stimulates insulin release by allosterically activating glutamate dehydrogenase (GDH), increasing glutamate oxidation, which increases the ATP/ADP ratio and closes K_{ATP} channels.

of the channel, whereas ADP antagonizes the effect via the SUR receptor. Both SUR1 and Kir6.2 are required for the potassium channel to be membrane-bound and functional. Mutations that alter the function of K_{ATP} channels lead to continued membrane depolarization and dysregulation of the voltage-dependent calcium channel, resulting in uncoupling of insulin secretion from glucose metabolism. To date, more than 50 SUR1 mutations have been described; three mutations have been reported in the Kir6.2 component (36, 37).

A constitutive increase in glucokinase activity causes an autosomal dominant form of hyperinsulinism (38). Decreased glucokinase activity causes an unusual form of maturity onset diabetes in youth (MODY-2) characterized by decreased insulin secretion at normal plasma glucose concentrations (39). Other pathways influence the β-cell ATP/ADP ratio and stimulate insulin secretion. For example, leucine stimulates activity of glutamate dehydro-

genase, which converts glutamate to α-ketoglutarate, an intermediary in the Krebs cycle, and results in production of ATP. Glutamate dehydrogenase is constitutively active in patients with the syndrome of hyperinsulinemia and hyperammonemia (40).

V. CLINICAL MANIFESTATIONS OF HYPOGLYCEMIA

The symptoms of hypoglycemia are not specific. Therefore, when a patient's symptoms are suspected to be caused by hypoglycemia, it is essential to measure the blood glucose concentration, confirm that it is low, and demonstrate that administration of glucose promptly relieves the symptoms.

The symptoms of hypoglycemia (Table 2) can be classified into two major categories based on the mecha-

Table 2 Signs and Symptoms of Hypoglycemia

Autonomic	Neuroglycopenic
Sweating	Warmth
Hunger	Fatigue
Paresthesias	Weakness
(tingling, numbness)	Dizziness
Tremors	Headache
Pallor	Inability to concentrate
Anxiety	Drowsiness
Nausea	Blurred vision
Palpitations	Difficulty speaking
	Confusion
	Bizarre behavior
	Loss of coordination
	Difficulty walking
	Coma
	Seizures

nism responsible for their generation: autonomic symptoms result from activation of the autonomic nervous system (both sympathetic and parasympathetic divisions); neuroglycopenic symptoms result from the effects of brain glucose deprivation. The symptoms of hypoglycemia in children are similar to those in adults. In newborn babies and infants hypoglycemia typically manifests as irritability, tremors, feeding difficulty, lethargy, hypotonia, tachypnea, cyanosis, or apnea. Hypoglycemia in this age group is discussed in Chapter 23.

VI. CAUSES OF HYPOGLYCEMIA IN INFANTS AND CHILDREN

The most common cause of hypoglycemia in children is insulin-induced hypoglycemia in individuals with type 1 diabetes mellitus. This is discussed later in this chapter. Almost all cases of hypoglycemia can be classified into one of the five major categories listed in Table 3.

A. Accelerated Starvation (Ketotic Hypoglycemia; Transient Intolerance of Fasting)

So-called ketotic hypoglycemia is the most common noniatrogenic cause of hypoglycemia in children beyond infancy. Hypoglycemia typically first occurs between 18 months and 5 years of age and remits spontaneously by 8 or 9 years of age. Many children with accelerated starvation are small and thin for their age and have decreased muscle mass. Many were born small for gestational age and may have had transient neonatal hypoglycemia. Hypoglycemia typically occurs during periods of intercurrent illness when food intake is limited by anorexia or vomiting, and occurs in the morning before breakfast. Mani-

festations include neurological symptoms ranging from lethargy to seizures and coma. Sometimes, hypoglycemia occurs in the morning after unusually intense physical exertion on the previous day or after the child has eaten poorly or completely omitted an evening meal.

The precise pathophysiological cause of accelerated starvation is unclear. Serum alanine levels are low at the time of hypoglycemia. Hypoglycemia has been attributed to decreased glucose production because of deficient availability of gluconeogenic substrate, especially alanine from muscle (41). The gluconeogenic pathway is intact, and the serum glucose concentration increases appropriately when alanine is infused at the time of hypoglycemia. However, the cause of the hypoalaninemia is the subject of controversy. It may be the result of a specific defect in protein catabolism or reflect decreased muscle mass. An alternative explanation is that hypoalaninemia is a consequence of decreased muscle glucose uptake in response to decreasing plasma glucose concentrations and increasing levels of FFA and ketone bodies, which would affect flux through the glucose–alanine–glucose cycle (22). The plasma epinephrine response to hypoglycemia is reduced in about half the patients with ketotic hypoglycemia (42). It has been suggested that these children may have a deficient catecholamine response to hypoglycemia that results in increased glucose utilization. This conclusion is suspect in light of new knowledge that recent antecedent hypoglycemia elevates the threshold for autonomic, including epinephrine, and symptomatic responses to subsequent hypoglycemia in healthy individuals (43–45).

After 8–16 h, children with accelerated starvation show the same metabolic pattern as normal healthy children fasted for 24–36 h. In many instances, the differentiation between accelerated starvation and the normal response to fasting is indistinct. Because approximately one-fourth of normal children develop hypoglycemia after a fast of 24–36 h duration (3), accelerated starvation may not be a distinct pathological disorder. Rather, it may represent one end of the spectrum of the normal child's response to starvation (46, 47).

B. Diagnosis

Because ketosis (and ketonuria) is a normal response to fasting and a falling plasma glucose concentration, ketotic hypoglycemia should not be regarded as a specific diagnosis (see section on overview of fuel metabolism). The differential diagnosis of the hypoglycemic child with an appropriately suppressed serum insulin concentration and ketosis is shown in Table 4. Accelerated starvation is a diagnosis of exclusion that should only be made when the other causes of so-called ketotic hypoglycemia have been ruled out.

Children with accelerated starvation typically become hypoglycemic in 12–24 h and have a normal metabolic and hormonal response to fasting. At the time of hypoglycemia, blood ketone body concentrations are raised, there is ketonuria, plasma alanine concentration is low,

Table 3 Causes of Hypoglycemia in Children

Accelerated starvation (so-called ketotic hypoglycemia)
Hyperinsulinism
    PHHI
    Insulinoma
    Beckwith-Wiedemann syndrome
    Sulfonylurea ingestion
    Factitious
Hormone deficiency
    ACTH/cortisol
    GH
    Hypopituitarism (ACTH/cortisol and GH)
Metabolic defects
    Disorders of carbohydrate metabolism
        Glycogen synthase deficiency
        Glucose-6-phosphatase deficiency (type I glycogen storage disease)
        Amylo-1,6-glucosidase deficiency (type III glycogen storage disease)
        Phosphorylase deficiency (type VI glycogen storage disease)
        Phosphorylase kinase deficiency (type IX glycogen storage disease)
        Galactose-1-phosphate uridyltransferase deficiency (galactosemia)
        Fructose-1-phosphate aldolase deficiency (fructose intolerance)
        Defects in gluconeogenesis
          • Pyruvate carboxylase deficiency
          • PEPCK deficiency
          • Fructose-1,6-bisphosphatase deficiency
    Disorders of fatty acid oxidation and ketone synthesis
        Carnitine transport and metabolism
        β-oxidation cycle
        Electron transfer
        Hydroxymethylglutaryl CoA synthase deficiency
        Hydroxymethylglutaryl CoA lyase deficiency
    Disorders of protein metabolism
        Maple syrup urine disease (branched-chain ketoacid decarboxylase deficiency)
        Methylmalonic acidemia
        Tyrosinemia
Miscellaneous
    Nonpancreatic tumor hypoglycemia (IGF-II) (250, 251)
    Salicylate intoxication
    Reye syndrome
    Ethanol intoxication
    Malaria
    Diarrhea
    Malnutrition
    Jamaican vomiting sickness (ingestion of unripe ackee)
    Reactive hypoglycemia (dumping syndrome) (252, 253)
    Carbohydrate-deficient glycoprotein syndrome (254)

and blood lactate and pyruvate levels are normal (48). Plasma insulin levels are appropriately suppressed and the concentrations of counterregulatory hormones are increased. The glycemic response to glucagon (0.03 mg/kg intramuscularly (IM) or intravenously (IV); maximum 1 mg) is normal in the fed state, but blunted at the time of hypoglycemia.

C. Treatment

Treatment consists of educating parents to ensure that the child avoids prolonged periods of fasting. A bedtime snack consisting of both carbohydrate and protein prevents further episodes of hypoglycemia. During intercurrent illness, providing carbohydrate-rich drinks at frequent

Table 4 Differential Diagnosis of
Ketotic Hypoglycemia

Liver large
  Glycogen storage diseases (types I, III, VI, IX)
  Disorders of gluconeogenesis (e.g., fructose 1,6-
    bisphosphatase)
Liver normal size
  Accelerated starvation (ketotic hypoglycemia)
  Cortisol/ACTH deficiency
  GH deficiency
  Panhypopituitarism
  Glycogen synthase deficiency
  Short-chain fatty acid oxidation disorders
  Organic acidemias (e.g., maple syrup urine disease,
    methylmalonic acidemia)

intervals during both the day and night can prevent hypoglycemia. Parents are instructed to test urine for ketones during intercurrent illnesses. The appearance of ketonuria precedes the onset of hypoglycemia by several hours. Recently, a new meter (Precision Xtra; Abbott Laboratories, Inc., Bedford, MA, USA) has become available, which accurately measures blood β-hydroxybutyrate concentration on a small drop of blood (49). This may prove quite useful as an alternative method of monitoring the development of ketosis during periods of illness or poor food intake in the child with ketotic hypoglycemia. If the child cannot tolerate oral carbohydrate, intravenous glucose is necessary to avert the development of hypoglycemia.

VII. HYPERINSULINISM

Hyperinsulinism caused by generalized β-cell dysfunction is the most common cause of persistent hypoglycemia in infants and young children. Islet cell adenomas are rare in children less than 1 year of age. Hyperinsulinism that presents in an older child is more likely to be caused by an insulinoma or by exogenous insulin administration (factitious hypoglycemia) (50).

In the past decade, considerable progress has been made toward elucidating the pathophysiology of the heterogeneous disorders that cause hyperinsulinemic hypoglycemia. Several distinct genetic forms of congenital hyperinsulinism have been described (51). The most common variety is an autosomal recessive defect (52) caused by homozygous mutations in either the SUR1 gene (53, 54) or in the Kir6.2 gene (55, 56). Both genes encode components of the K_{ATP} channel involved in glucose-regulated insulin release, and mutations in these genes result in uncoupling of insulin secretion from glucose metabolism.

The principal clinical and biochemical features of hyperinsulinemic hypoglycemia are summarized in Table 5. Patients with autosomal recessive hyperinsulinism due to SUR/Kir6.2 mutations typically present as macrosomic babies with severe intractable hypoglycemia soon after birth. This disorder is discussed in more detail in Chapter 23.

Unlike the autosomal recessive defects of the K_{ATP} channel that result in diffuse β-cell dysfunction, the sporadic form of hyperinsulinemic hypoglycemia (HHI) can result in either focal or diffuse hyperplasia of β-cells. Focal adenomatous hyperplasia occurs in 30–40% of sporadic cases and is caused by a specific somatic loss of the maternal allele imprinted at 11p15 in a patient harboring an SUR1 mutation on the paternal allele (i.e., hemizygous germline mutation together with maternal loss of heterozygosity of 11p15) (57–60). Two hypotheses have been proposed to explain focal hyperplasia. The loss of heterozygosity may unmask a recessively inherited SUR1 or Kir6.2 mutation located on the paternal allele. An alter-

Table 5 Clinical and Biochemical Features of Hyperinsulinemic Hypoglycemia

Usually less than 12 months of age at presentation
Hypoglycemia soon after feeding (0–5.5 h, average ~2 h)
Urinary ketones negative, trace, or small
Serum insulin $\geq$2 μU/ml (15 pmol/l) with plasma glucose <45 mg/dl (2.5 mmol/l)
Increased serum C-peptide concentration
Plasma ketone (β-OH-butyrate and acetoacetate) concentrations inappropriately low
Brisk glycemic response to glucagon >30 mg/dl (1.7 mmol/l)
Parenteral glucose required to maintain normoglycemia is two to four times greater than
  glucose production rate (~6 mg/kg/min)
Decreased plasma branched-chain amino acids (valine, leucine, isoleucine)
Decreased IGF-binding protein-1 (IGFBP-1); all other endocrinologic and metabolic
  abnormalities with fasting hypoglycemia are associated with decreased insulin secretion and
  increased IGFBP-1 levels
Leucine and/or tolbutamide causes an exaggerated hyperinsulinemic response
GH, cortisol concentrations usually normal but may be inappropriately low if hypoglycemia
  occurs gradually or is recurrent (blunted counterregulatory hormone responses)

native hypothesis is that this somatic deletion also results in loss of an associated tumor-suppressor gene, H19. H19 normally inhibits the actions of IGF-2; unopposed IGF-2 action could lead to β-cell proliferation (61). The patient with focal adenomatous hyperplasia cannot be differentiated clinically from the patient with diffuse disease. However, pancreatic venous sampling and intraoperative histopathological examination of the pancreas have been successfully used to differentiate between the two (62, 63). If focal disease can be identified, a more limited pancreatectomy can be performed, thereby curing the patient and obviating the risk of postsurgical diabetes mellitus.

Two distinct forms of autosomal dominant hyperinsulinism have been described, both with milder clinical phenotypes than the autosomal recessive form. Patients are not macrosomic at birth and may not present with hypoglycemia until later in childhood or adulthood; hypoglycemia is usually more easily controlled with either diet alone or with diazoxide (64, 65). It responds well to dietary or pharmacological therapy and is generally associated with an excellent prognosis. One form of autosomal dominant hyperinsulinism is caused by an activating mutation in β-cell glucokinase that results in increased affinity of the enzyme for glucose (38). Glucokinase normally has low affinity for glucose and is the rate-limiting step in β-cell glucose metabolism. In the initial description of this disorder, a single base pair change at codon 455 of the gene was found, resulting in substitution of methionine for valine. This alteration increased the activity of the enzyme (a 65% change in enzyme affinity for glucose; K_m 2.9 mM compared to 8.4 mM in wild type). This causes an abnormally low glucose threshold for insulin secretion, 36–45 mg/dl (2.0–2.5 mM). A defect in glucokinase can be missed if the critical sample is obtained when the plasma glucose concentration is below the threshold for insulin secretion. If this diagnosis is suspected, a fasting study with serial measurements of plasma insulin levels may be required to document inappropriate insulin secretion.

A distinct form of mild hyperinsulinism is associated with persistent mild asymptomatic hyperammonemia (blood ammonia levels are in the range of 100–200 μmol/l or approximately three to six times normal) that is not associated with any abnormality of the amino acids or organic acids characteristic of defects in the urea cycle (40, 66–69). Familial cases with an autosomal dominant pattern of inheritance have been documented; however, the majority of cases have been sporadic. The hypoglycemia may go unrecognized until adulthood. It usually responds well to diet and diazoxide. The syndrome is caused by a gain of function mutation of mitochondrial glutamate dehydrogenase, which causes excessive glutamate oxidation in the β-cell and increased formation of α-ketoglutarate, an intermediary in the Krebs cycle (40). Increased glutamate oxidation increases the ratio of ATP/ADP resulting in unregulated release of insulin. In the

liver, increased glutamate oxidation decreases the glutamate concentration and results in decreased synthesis of N-acetylglutamate, an allosteric activator of carbamoyl phosphate synthetase, which catalyzes the first step in ureagenesis (40).

Despite the extraordinary advances in understanding of the pathophysiology of hyperinsulinism, only 30–50% of patients have a definable genetic abnormality (37, 70). It is likely that other abnormalities will be revealed as the search continues for new defects in the secretory apparatus, including defects in the intracellular control of calcium signaling of exocytosis (70).

A. Diagnosis

Hyperinsulinism should be considered in any infant or child with hypoketotic hypoglycemia (Table 5). Hyperinsulinism is the probable diagnosis in a child with hypoglycemia whose concomitant serum insulin level is >2 μU/ml. Malicious insulin administration should be suspected if severe hypoglycemia is associated with very high serum insulin (>100 μU/ml), and is confirmed by finding concomitantly low or suppressed serum C-peptide levels.

Reliable noninvasive methods are still not available to differentiate among an adenoma, focal adenomatous hyperplasia, and diffuse β-cell dysfunction. Sonographic and computerized axial tomography (CT) are both insensitive imaging modalities. For patients who fail to respond to pharmacological therapy (especially in those without a family history of hyperinsulinism), more extensive evaluation at a specialized center is recommended before undertaking a 95–99% pancreatectomy. The type and location of the pancreatic lesion (diffuse disease vs. focal adenomatous hyperplasia) can be determined by preoperative pancreatic catheterization and intraoperative histopathological studies of the pancreas (evaluation of β-cell nuclear radius and cell density) (62, 71). Armed with this information, the surgeon may be able to choose between a partial pancreatectomy for a focal lesion and a near-total pancreatectomy for a diffuse lesion. It has recently been shown that in neonates with hyperinsulinism about half may have focal islet-cell hyperplasia that can be treated with partial pancreatectomy (63).

B. Treatment

The goal of therapy is to prevent hypoglycemia in order to protect the developing brain from damage. Successful treatment should maintain the plasma glucose concentration above 60 mg/dl (3.3 mmol/l) on a feeding schedule appropriate for the age of the child. For example, for up to 12 h in infants up to 1 year of age, or 16 h or more in older children. Prompt effective treatment is necessary to minimize the risk of long-term adverse neurological sequelae (72).

Oral diazoxide, which opens normal K_{ATP} channels and thereby suppresses insulin secretion, should be given a trial starting at a dosage of 10 mg/kg per day (15–25 mg/kg per day in three doses at 8 h intervals) (70). If no effect is observed at a dosage of 25 mg/kg per day, it is not worthwhile to increase the dose further because this will cause worsening of side effects (edema, hypertrichosis) without improving efficacy. The effect of diazoxide may be potentiated by the addition of a thiazide diuretic (chlorothiazide 7–10 mg/kg per day divided twice daily) which acts synergistically with diazoxide (activates potassium channels by a different mechanism) and decreases edema (70). Diazoxide is ineffective in infants whose hyperinsulinism is caused by mutations resulting in functional inactivation of the K_{ATP} channel.

A long-acting injectable somatostatin analog (Octreotide) may be successful in maintaining normoglycemia in up to 50% of cases of congenital hyperinsulinism. Octreotide inhibits insulin secretion by decreasing intracellular translocation of calcium ions into β cells and through a direct effect on secretory granules. It may also mediate G-protein activity in the potassium channel (73). The starting dosage is 5 μg/kg every 6–8 h. If glucose is not maintained ≥60 mg/dl, the dosage of Octreotide is increased up to a maximum of 40–60 μg/kg daily, divided into three to six doses. Gastrointestinal side effects usually limit the tolerable dosage of Octreotide. Because of the marked variability of response to Octreotide, the therapeutic regimen has to be adapted for each individual patient and its effects closely monitored (74).

More recently, nifedipine (a calcium channel blocker) has been used to treat HHI that is unresponsive to conventional therapy (75–78). Experience with its use is still very limited. However, after failure of diazoxide and/or somatostatin analog to restore euglycemia, nifedipine (0.7–2.5 mg/kg/day) has been used successfully to maintain normoglycemia in at least three patients (76, 77). The clinical response to this drug is highly variable and it is currently not possible to predict which children will respond without a trial.

Continuous subcutaneous (SC) infusions of Octreotide (5–20 μg/kg/day) or glucagon (1–10 μg/kg/hour) IV or SC can be used to stabilize the hypoglycemia in patients prior to surgery. They should be used when the orally administered drugs have been shown not to be effective, particularly if the child remains dependent on a glucose infusion to maintain normoglycemia. When used in high dosages, both hormones cause tachyphylaxis. Many infants fail to respond to medical therapy and require a 95–99% subtotal pancreatectomy to restore normoglycemia (79).

VIII. HORMONE DEFICIENCY

A. ACTH/Cortisol Deficiency

Cortisol limits glucose utilization in several tissues, including skeletal muscle, by directly opposing the action of insulin and, secondarily, by promoting lipolysis. It stimulates protein breakdown and increases release of gluconeogenic precursors from muscle and fat. Cortisol stimulates hepatic gluconeogenesis and glycogen synthesis and exerts permissive effects on the gluconeogenic and glycogenolytic effects of glucagon and epinephrine. As a result of all these effects, cortisol tends to raise the plasma glucose concentration.

Hypoglycemia is an uncommon presentation of primary adrenal failure. Nevertheless, adrenocortical insufficiency should be considered in the differential diagnosis of patients who present with hypoglycemia and ketosis. In infancy and early childhood, adrenocortical insufficiency may be secondary to congenital adrenal hypoplasia or congenital adrenal hyperplasia (rarely). In older children, adrenocortical insufficiency is more likely to be caused by Addison's disease. ACTH deficiency or panhypopituitarism can present with hypoglycemia in infancy or in later childhood. Hypoglycemia caused by isolated deficiency of ACTH is rare (80, 81); it is more common in children with multiple pituitary hormone (including GH and ACTH) deficiencies (82).

B. Diagnosis

A serum cortisol concentration <10 μg/dl at the time of hypoglycemia should suggest the diagnosis. The diagnosis is confirmed by definitive tests that evaluate the hypothalamopituitary–adrenal axis.

Treatment consists of physiological replacement of cortisol and mineralocorticoids (when necessary).

C. Hypopituitarism (Isolated GH Deficiency, Multiple Pituitary Hormone Deficiencies)

GH decreases sensitivity to insulin, stimulates lipolysis, and decreases glucose utilization. Congenital hypopituitarism often presents in the newborn period with hypoglycemia, persistent hyperbilirubinemia, and a microphallus (83). About 20% of children with isolated GH deficiency or multiple anterior pituitary hormone deficiencies present with fasting hypoglycemia and ketosis (84). The occurrence of hypoglycemia in children with GH deficiency is inversely related to age (84, 85). The combination of low serum GH and cortisol concentrations at the time of hypoglycemia suggests hypopituitarism. However, serum GH levels during spontaneous hypoglycemia do not correlate well with GH levels obtained by stimulation tests of pituitary GH secretory reserve. Therefore, a single low serum GH concentration cannot be relied on to make the diagnosis of GH deficiency (86). Patients with insulin-like growth factor 1 (IGF-1) deficiency (Laron syndrome) have high GH levels, but are otherwise indistinguishable from patients with isolated GH deficiency. These patients are prone to symptomatic hypoglycemia in infancy (87); the tendency to develop hypoglycemia ameliorates with advancing age. Pituitary GH secretory reserve should be formally tested if there is any suspicion of GH insufficiency.

Treatment of panhypopituitarism consists of replacing thyroxine, cortisol, and GH.

IX. DISORDERS OF GLYCOGEN SYNTHESIS AND GLYCOGEN DEGRADATION

A. Glycogen Synthase Deficiency

This is a rare autosomal recessive disorder caused by mutations in the human liver glycogen synthase (GYS2) gene (88) on chromosome 12p12.2, resulting in lack of glycogen synthase activity in the liver. Because dietary carbohydrate cannot be stored as glycogen, glucose is preferentially converted to lactate. The disorder causes a unique metabolic disturbance characterized by fasting hypoglycemia and hyperketonemia alternating with daytime hyperglycemia and hyperlacticacidemia after meals. The glycogen content of the liver is markedly decreased (0.5 g/ 100 g wet weight 4–6 h after a meal); the liver is not enlarged. The disorder should be considered in children who have hypoglycemia and ketonuria before the first meal of the day (Table 4) (89).

The goal of treatment is to prevent hypoglycemia and ketosis during the night and hyperglycemia and hyperlacticacidemia during the day. Fasting hypoglycemia is prevented by administration of uncooked cornstarch at bedtime. During the day, patients are fed frequently (e.g., every 4 h). The diet should contain increased amounts of protein to provide substrate for gluconeogenesis (90) and a correspondingly reduced amount of carbohydrate to minimize postprandial hyperglycemia and hyperlacticacidemia (89).

B. Glucose-6-Phosphatase Deficiency (Type I Glycogen Storage Disease)

Type I glycogen storage disease (GSD-I) is an autosomal recessive disease that results from lack of glucose-6-phosphatase activity, the enzyme that catalyzes the final step in the production of glucose from glucose-6-phosphate (91) (Fig. 3). At least 30 different mutations in the gene encoding glucose-6-phosphatase on chromosome 17q21 have been found in patients with GSD-Ia (92). Glucose production both from glycogenolysis and gluconeogenesis is severely impaired, resulting in postprandial hypoglycemia and increased production of lactic acid, uric acid, and triglycerides (Fig. 3). Glycogen and fat accumulate in the liver, resulting in hepatomegaly and a protuberant abdomen. Symptomatic hypoglycemia may be detected soon after birth; however, most infants are asymptomatic as long as they receive frequent feedings containing sufficient glucose to prevent hypoglycemia. Symptoms of hypoglycemia usually appear when the interval between feedings increases and the infant begins to sleep through the night. Characteristic manifestations in untreated patients are a progressive decrease in linear growth, muscle wasting, delayed motor development, and a cushingoid appearance (93). The kidneys are enlarged; renal tubular dysfunction and glomerular hyperfiltration are common in childhood. Increased urinary albumin excretion may be observed in adolescents (94). More severe renal injury (proteinuria, hypertension, decreased creatinine clearance) due to focal segmental glomerulosclerosis and interstitial fibrosis, and hypercalciuria and nephrocalcinosis are common in young adults (95, 96). Inadequate therapy causes severe retardation of physical growth and delayed puberty. Hepatic adenomas usually develop in the second and third decades of life, and may undergo malignant degeneration or hemorrhage (97).

Patients with type Ib glycogen storage disease (deficiency of the glucose-6-phosphate transporter required to move glucose-6-phosphate across the microsomal membrane into the lumen of the endoplasmic reticulum where it is exposed to the hydrolytic function of the glucose-6-phosphatase enzyme system) have similar clinical manifestations (98). In addition, they have either constant or cyclic neutropenia associated with recurrent bacterial infections. Neutropenia of varying severity is a consequence of disturbed myeloid maturation and is accompanied by functional defects of circulating neutrophils and monocytes (99). Some patients develop an inflammatory bowel disease resembling Crohn's disease that is responsive to treatment with granulocyte colony-stimulating factor (GCSF) (100).

C. Diagnosis

In infancy, severe hypoglycemia accompanied by marked hyperlacticacidemia develops 3–4 h after a feed. The serum is often cloudy or milky with very high triglyceride and moderately increased levels of cholesterol. Serum uric acid is increased and serum aspartate aminotransferase (AST) and alanine aminotransferase (ALT) levels are moderately elevated. Glucagon causes either no or only a small increase in blood glucose, whereas the already elevated blood lactate level increases further. Lack of glucose-6-phosphatase activity on a liver biopsy specimen confirms the diagnosis. In many patients mutational analysis can be used to confirm the diagnosis and obviate the need to perform liver biopsy.

Treatment consists of providing a continuous dietary source of glucose at a rate that prevents the blood glucose level from falling below the threshold for glucose counterregulation, approximately 70 mg/dl. When hypoglycemia is prevented by providing an appropriate amount of glucose throughout the day and night, the biochemical abnormalities are ameliorated, liver size decreases, the bleeding tendency is reversed, and growth improves (101). The amount of glucose required varies among patients, but can be approximated, initially, by using the formula for calculating basal glucose production rate as a guide:

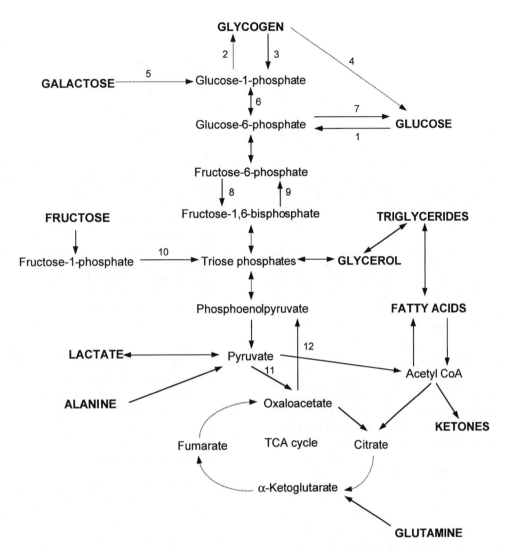

Figure 3 Schematic outline of glucose metabolism shows pathways of glycogen synthesis, glycogen degradation, glycolysis, and gluconeogenesis. Key enzymes are designated by number. 1, hexokinase/glucokinase; 2, glycogen synthase; 3, phosphorylase; 4, Amylo-1,6-glucosidase (glycogen debrancher); 5, galactose-1-phosphate uridyl transferase; 6, phosphoglucomutase; 7, glucose-6-phosphatase; 8, phosphofructokinase; 9, fructose-1,6-bisphosphatase; 10, fructose-1-phosphate aldolase; 11, pyruvate carboxylase; 12, phosphoenolpyruvate carboxykinase.

$$y = 0.0014x^3 - 0.214x^2 + 10.411x - 9.084$$

where y = mg glucose/min, and x = body weight in kg (2). Glucose itself or glucose-containing polymers can be given intermittently during the day and continuously (via a nasogastric tube or gastrostomy) at night. As an alternative, after 6–8 months of age, intermittent feedings of uncooked cornstarch can be used as the source of continuous glucose administration (102). Orally administered uncooked cornstarch appears to act as an intestinal reservoir of glucose that is slowly absorbed into the circulation. It is given in a slurry of water or artificially flavored drink (or in milk or lactose-free formula for infants)

at 3–5 h intervals during the day and 4 or 5 h intervals overnight (103–105).

D. Amylo-1,6-Glucosidase Deficiency (Type III Glycogen Storage Disease; Glycogen Debranching Enzyme Deficiency)

The glycogen debrancher enzyme (GDE) gene is on chromosome 1p21 (106). The disorder is transmitted as an autosomal recessive trait. Absence of GDE activity permits breakdown of glycogen to proceed until the outermost branch points are reached. This leaves a limit dextrin, which consists of the core of the molecule bearing short branches about four glucose units in length. Some 80–85% of patients with GSD III lack GDE activity (deficiency of transferase and glucosidase activities) in both liver and muscle (GDE-IIIa) (91) and show clinical evidence of hepatic dysfunction and myopathy. About 15% of patients have GDE deficiency only in the liver (GSD IIIb) (91). In rare cases, there is selective loss of only one of the two GDE activities (glucosidase [type IIIc] or transferase [type IIId]) (107, 108). GSD types IIIa and IIIb have different prognoses and outcomes. Myopathy and cardiomyopathy are common in GSD IIIa and can lead to early death or debilitation in adult life. Muscle involvement can be inferred from high plasma creatine kinase concentrations.

Several distinct clinical features differentiate type III from type I GSD. Because glucose can be produced from 1,4 segments beyond the outermost branch points and from gluconeogenesis, patients with GDE deficiency are able to tolerate longer periods of fasting and develop less severe hypoglycemia than patients with glucose-6-phosphatase deficiency. Infants who are fed frequently may not have symptoms. Fasting causes hypoglycemia with ketosis (as a result of an accelerated transition to the starving state) (109), mild hypercholesterolemia, and hypertriglyceridemia, without elevation of blood lactate and serum uric acid concentrations. Liver enzyme levels (AST, ALT, alkaline phosphatase, lactic dehydrogenase [LDH]) are consistently elevated in children, but decline at puberty concomitant with a decrease in liver size and may be normal in adults (110). Patients frequently present with growth failure and hepatomegaly, which may be associated with an enlarged spleen at 4–6 years of age in patients who have hepatic fibrosis. The kidneys are not enlarged, nor does renal dysfunction occur. Untreated infants and children have a decreased rate of linear growth and puberty is delayed. The enzyme is lacking in muscle in about 85% of patients; however, weakness is usually minimal and not clinically significant in childhood. A subset of patients primarily manifest myopathic symptoms (usually in their third and fourth decades), and myopathy may be progressive. Abnormal glycogen (limit dextrin) may also accumulate in the heart. Subclinical evidence of cardiac involvement is common and manifests as ventricular hypertrophy on electrocardiography (ECG) and an abnormal echocardiograph (111). Some patients develop a cardiomyopathy similar to hypertrophic obstructive cardiomyopathy (112). Hepatic adenomata occur less frequently in patients with GSD III than in GSD I; and the transformation of an adenoma into a hepatocellular carcinoma is rare. With the exception of myopathy, symptoms and signs characteristically ameliorate with increasing age. The size of the liver tends to decrease to normal during puberty; however, biopsy usually shows hepatic fibrosis and some adult patients develop cirrhosis and its complications (113).

After an overnight fast, the low blood glucose and normal blood lactate concentrations do not increase after administration of glucagon (0.03 mg/kg, maximum dose 1 mg IM or IV). When the test is repeated 2 h after a high-carbohydrate meal, which lengthens the outer branches of glycogen, a glycemic response does occur. Definitive diagnosis and subtyping require a biopsy of both liver and muscle for assay of enzyme activity.

As in type I GSD, continuous provision of an adequate amount of glucose, using uncooked cornstarch, combined with a normal intake of total calories, protein, and other nutrients corrects the clinical and biochemical disorder and restores normal growth. Uncooked cornstarch, 1.75 g/kg at 6 h intervals (e.g. at midnight, 6 a.m., etc.) maintains normoglycemia, increases growth velocity, and decreases serum aminotransferase concentrations (114, 115).

For patients with type III disease who have significant growth retardation and myopathy, continuous nocturnal feeding of a nutrient mixture composed of glucose, glucose oligosaccharides, and amino acids combined with meals that have a high protein content has been shown to improve muscle strength (116). The composition of the diet should be 55–60% carbohydrates, 15–20% protein, and 20–30% fat. Milk products and fruits can be allowed without restriction, as galactose and fructose can be normally converted to glucose.

E. Hepatic Phosphorylase Complex Deficiency

The glycogen storage diseases associated with a reduction in liver phosphorylase activity are a heterogeneous group of disorders that includes autosomal recessive liver glycogen phosphorylase deficiency (type VI or Hers' disease), an autosomal recessive phosphorylase kinase b deficiency (type VIII), and X-linked phosphorylase kinase deficiency (type IX) (93). They are all mild forms of hepatomegalic glycogenosis without hyperlacticacidemia or hyperuricemia.

These disorders present in infancy or early childhood and are characterized by mild to moderate hypoglycemia, ketosis, growth retardation, and prominent hepatomegaly. Blood levels of lactic acid and uric acid are normal. The heart and skeletal muscle are not affected. The clinical course is benign. Symptoms remit and hepatomegaly decreases at puberty. The prognosis is excellent.

F. Phosphorylase Kinase Deficiency

This is the most common disorder in this group, accounting for about 25% of all cases of GSD and occurs with a frequency of approximately 1 in 100,000 births (91, 117). X-linked liver glycogenosis (XLG) is the most common type of phosphorylase kinase (PHK) deficiency and is usually a mild disease. Patients seldom have symptomatic hypoglycemia during infancy unless they fast for a prolonged period of time, in which case they can develop hyperketosis similar to, but usually milder than, that seen in type III GSD. Metabolic acidosis is rare. The disorder is usually discovered in early childhood when an enlarged liver and protuberant abdomen are noted during a physical examination. Physical growth may be retarded, and motor development may be delayed as a consequence of muscular hypotonia in the rare case with reduced enzyme activity in muscle as well as liver. Hypoglycemia is unusual and blood lactate and uric acid levels are normal. Mild hypertriglyceridemia, hypercholesterolemia, and elevated serum AST and ALT levels may be present. Functional tests are not especially useful in evaluating these patients. The administration of glucagon after an overnight fast usually elicits a brisk glycemic response without a rise in the blood lactate level. The glycemic response to glucagon cannot be used to differentiate between phosphorylase kinase deficiency and lack of phosphorylase itself. The enlarged liver regresses when patients reach puberty. With increasing age, clinical and biochemical abnormalities gradually disappear, and most adult patients are asymptomatic despite persistent PHK deficiency.

Liver phosphorylase deficiency can be difficult to diagnose biochemically and difficult to differentiate from deficiency of phosphorylase kinase. Mutation analysis may aid in the laboratory diagnosis of deficiencies of the liver phosphorylase system. Definitive diagnosis of phosphorylase kinase b deficiency requires demonstration of the enzymatic defect in affected tissues.

Most patients do not require treatment; however prolonged fasting should be avoided. For the minority of patients who are prone to fasting hypoglycemia during childhood, a late night snack will usually suffice to prevent morning hypoglycemia. In the unusual patient who experiences overnight hypoglycemia and ketosis, uncooked cornstarch, 2 g/kg at bedtime, prevents hypoglycemia and ketosis (118).

X. DISORDERS OF GLUCONEOGENESIS

Disorders of gluconeogenesis may be caused by deficiency of one of the key gluconeogenic enzymes (pyruvate carboxylase, phosphoenolpyruvate carboxykinase, fructose-1,6-bisphosphatase, and glucose-6-phosphatase) (Fig. 3). In addition to these inborn errors of metabolism, gluconeogenesis is impaired in hereditary fructose intolerance, by ingestion of ethanol, in children with Jamaican vomiting sickness, falciparum malaria, severe diarrhea, and in salicylate intoxication. Hypoglycemia caused by disorders of gluconeogenesis is characteristically accompanied by hyperlacticacidemia and hyperalaninemia.

A. Phosphoenolpyruvate Carboxykinase Deficiency

PEPCK is a unidirectional rate-limiting enzyme of gluconeogenesis that converts oxaloacetate to phosphoenol-

pyruvate (Fig. 3). Hypoglycemia is seen in infancy and may be severe. Fatty infiltration of the liver, kidney, and other organs occurs because there is increased formation of acetyl CoA. Laboratory evaluation reveals high concentrations of lactate and pyruvate, a normal lactate/pyruvate ratio, and ketosis. The definitive diagnosis of PEPCK deficiency depends on the demonstration of impaired enzyme activity on a liver biopsy. Treatment consists of frequent feedings and avoiding fasting.

B. Fructose-1,6-Bisphosphatase Deficiency

The block in gluconeogenesis resulting from failure to convert fructose-1,6-bisphosphate to fructose-6-phosphate causes fasting hypoglycemia and lactic acidosis (Fig. 3). Hypoglycemia occurs during fasting and intercurrent illness and is associated with ketosis, hypertriglyceridemia, and hyperuricemia. In the immediate postprandial period, glucagon elicits a glycemic response (119). The biochemical abnormalities caused by fructose-1,6-bisphosphatase deficiency are similar to glucose-6-phosphatase deficiency. Affected children typically fail to thrive. Hepatomegaly is caused by fatty infiltration of the liver. Diagnosis is based on demonstrating decreased enzyme activity in the liver. Treatment consists of eliminating dietary fructose and sucrose and avoiding prolonged fasts. During intercurrent illness, intravenous glucose must be given to arrest catabolism.

C. Hereditary Fructose Intolerance

This rare disorder is caused by deficiency of fructose-1-phosphate aldolase (Fig. 3). Nursing infants are asymptomatic until fruits and juices are added to their diet. It usually presents following the introduction of a commercial formula containing sucrose, or at the time of weaning when fructose or sucrose are ingested for the first time. Fructose causes vomiting, diarrhea, and hypoglycemia. Chronic exposure to fructose causes hepatomegaly, jaundice, failure to thrive, and renal tubular dysfunction with aminoaciduria. Older children have an aversion to sweets. Fructose-1-phosphate accumulates in the liver and acutely inhibits glycogenolysis via the phosphorylase system and gluconeogenesis at the level of fructose-1,6-bisphosphatase (120). Chronic fructose intoxication can occur after infancy without causing symptoms of acute fructose intoxication and can be expressed as an apparently isolated, reversible retardation of somatic growth. The diagnosis is suggested by fructosuria after meals; a fructose tolerance test results in hypoglycemia. Traditionally, the diagnosis has been made by intravenous fructose challenge or by liver biopsy, both difficult and risky invasive tests. Identification of mutations of the aldolase B gene by analysis of DNA from blood leukocytes is now possible, allowing for the potential of a noninvasive diagnosis (121).

D. Alcohol Intoxication

Ingestion of alcohol by children and adolescents can cause hypoglycemia several hours after its consumption as a result of inhibition of gluconeogenesis (122). Ethanol inhibits gluconeogenesis because its metabolism by alcohol dehydrogenase depletes hepatic nicotinamide adenine dinucleotide, a cofactor critical to the entry of most precursors into the gluconeogenic pathway. It does not inhibit glycogenolysis (123). Ethanol also inhibits cortisol and GH responses to hypoglycemia (122). When hepatic glycogen stores are adequate, ethanol does not cause hypoglycemia. However, severe hypoglycemia occurs when glycogen is depleted as a result of ethanol consumption without food, or after accidental alcohol ingestion after an overnight fast in a young child. Glucagon cannot raise the blood glucose level; treatment of ethanol-induced hypoglycemia should always be with administration of intravenous glucose.

E. Salicylate Poisoning

High dosages of salicylates can lower the plasma glucose concentration (124). Both hyperinsulinemia and reduced gluconeogenesis have been observed following acute ingestion of aspirin (124). However, the precise mechanism causing hypoglycemia is unclear. Salicylates may decrease gluconeogenesis via their ability to uncouple oxidative phosphorylation.

F. Malaria

Hypoglycemia is common in children with severe falciparum malaria in the absence of treatment with quinine (125–128). Impaired gluconeogenesis is suggested by the presence of high blood levels of ketones, lactate, and alanine at the time of hypoglycemia. Gluconeogenesis appears to be limited by an insufficient supply of precursors and is unable to compensate for the decreased availability of glucose from glycogen (129). Hypoglycemia has also been described during treatment with quinine and has been attributed to quinine's hyperinsulinemic effect (124). It has been suggested that the frequency of hypoglycemia in malaria may be no higher than in other serious illnesses associated with severe calorie deprivation (128). Treatment of hypoglycemia associated with malaria is with intravenous glucose.

G. Reye Syndrome

This syndrome typically follows viral infections with varicella and influenza A and B. Aspirin has been implicated in its pathogenesis. It is characterized by recurrent vomiting, an altered level of consciousness, hyperpnea, and hypoglycemia that is mainly the result of altered gluconeogenesis (130). Hypoglycemia occurs most often in children less than 5 years of age. Increased plasma levels of ammonia and free fatty acids suggest impaired urea-

genesis and fatty acid oxidation (131, 132). Recurrent episodes that mimic Reye syndrome should raise suspicion for a fatty acid oxidation defect (see Sec. XIII). Treatment is supportive (133, 134).

H. Diarrhea and Malnutrition

In developing countries, hypoglycemia is a common complication of infectious diarrhea in both well-nourished and poorly nourished children (135–137) and is a major cause of death (138). Children with kwashiorkor frequently suffer from severe hypoglycemia (139–141). Infants with acquired monosaccharide intolerance after an episode of gastroenteritis are also at increased risk for severe and even fatal hypoglycemia when fed a carbohydrate-free diet (142, 143).

Depletion of hepatic glycogen together with hepatic steatosis is observed in children with fatal hypoglycemia and diarrhea (144). Serum insulin levels are appropriately suppressed and glucose counterregulatory hormone concentrations are appropriately elevated in children with diarrhea and hypoglycemia, whereas gluconeogenic substrates are low suggesting that the hypoglycemia may be due to failure of gluconeogenesis (138). Reduced availability of fat-derived fuels (FFA and ketones) may play an important role in the development of hypoglycemia. In children who developed hypoglycemia during acute diarrheal illness, β-hydroxybutyrate concentrations were not significantly higher than in normoglycemic children with diarrhea, suggesting deficient generation of ketones, either because fat stores were diminished as a result of malnutrition or because the oxidation of fat was impaired (138). If fatty acids are less available (as may occur in malnutrition) or when oxidation of fatty acids is defective (e.g., as a result of acquired carnitine deficiency), hypoglycemia is more likely to occur because body tissues and brain (secondary to hypoketonemia) are more dependent on glucose. The failure of gluconeogenesis in diarrheal illness, therefore, may be a consequence of depleted fat stores, defective fatty acid oxidation and ketogenesis, or a defect in the hepatic enzymatic pathways required for gluconeogenesis (145).

Frequent feeding of children during diarrhea may help to prevent hypoglycemia. When patients with diarrhea require parenteral therapy, dextrose-containing electrolyte solutions should be used and the child's blood glucose level must be carefully monitored.

XI. DISORDERS OF AMINO ACID METABOLISM

Several disorders of amino acid metabolism result in hypoglycemia with organic aciduria. These patients typically have a delay in growth and development, recurrent vomiting, and may have hepatomegaly. Laboratory features include hyperammonemia and hyperchloremic metabolic acidosis. Diagnosis depends on identification of specific organic acids in the urine and analysis of liver biopsy specimens or cultured fibroblasts (146).

A. Methylmalonic Acidemia

Methylmalonic acidemia results from a deficiency of methylmalonyl-CoA mutase, a cobalamin-dependent enzyme involved in the carboxylation of propionyl-CoA. Patients typically present in the newborn period with ketoacidosis, hyperammonemia, hypoglycemia, and acute encephalopathy. Hypoglycemia is due to impaired gluconeogenesis (147). Asymptomatic and benign variants are also detected by the analysis of urine organic acids. Plasma amino acid profile shows an increased concentration of glycine.

B. 3-Hydroxy-3-Methyl Glutaric Acidemia

3-Hydroxy-3-methylglutaryl CoA lyase catalyzes the last step of leucine degradation and ketogenesis. Deficiency of this enzyme results in a clinical presentation that includes episodes of hypoketotic hypoglycemia, fatty liver, coma, and mental delay (148).

C. Maple Syrup Urine Disease

Maple syrup urine disease (MSUD) is caused by a deficiency of branched-chain keto acid dehydrogenase, the enzyme that decarboxylates α-keto acids of leucine, isoleucine, and valine (149). The classic clinical presentation consists of failure to thrive, acidosis, hypoglycemia, and neurological symptoms with rapid deterioration when left untreated. The pathogenesis of hypoglycemia is not entirely clear, although it appears to result from defective gluconeogenesis (150). The levels of the branched-chain amino acids (leucine, isoleucine, and valine), particularly leucine, are elevated in plasma and urine. Increased plasma and urine concentrations of leucine, isoleucine, and valine with accumulation of branched-chain keto acids and 2-hydroxy acids are essential for making the diagnosis. Additional metabolites of the branched-chain amino acids may be detected. The enzymatic defect can be detected in leukocytes. Treatment consists of a diet restricted in the precursors to the enzyme defect, avoidance of and aggressive treatment of catabolic states, and supplementation with carnitine and vitamin cofactors. Treatment of acute episodes includes the administration of glucose with or without insulin to increase removal of branched-chain amino acids through enhanced protein synthesis. Long-term treatment requires limiting protein intake.

D. Hereditary Tyrosinemia (Tyrosinemia Type I)

This disorder is caused by deficiency of fumarylacetoacetate hydrolase. Infants present with vomiting, diarrhea, and failure to thrive. Liver disease and hypoglyemia are consistent findings. A large amount of succinylacetone is excreted in the urine. Diagnosis is confirmed by measurement of fumarylacetoacetate hydrolase in the liver. Treatment consists of a diet low in tyrosine and phenylalanine in addition to the administration of 2-(2-nitro-4[trifluoromethyl] benzoyl)-1,3-cyclohexandione. Liver transplant is an effective therapy.

XII. MISCELLANEOUS CAUSES OF HYPOGLYCEMIA

A. Galactosemia

Galactosemia is caused by deficiency of galactose-1-phosphate uridyl transferase (Fig. 3), resulting in an inability to convert galactose-1-phosphate to glucose-1-phosphate (151). A defect in UDP-galactose-4-epimerase may cause a similar presentation (152). Hypoglycemia occurs following milk feedings. Although the precise mechanism causing hypoglycemia is unclear, there is evidence suggesting that the accumulation of galactose-1-phosphate inhibits phosphoglucomutase activity, thereby causing inhibition of glycogenolysis (153). Patients may present with neonatal *Escherichia coli* sepsis, diarrhea, vomiting, failure to thrive, hepatomegaly, jaundice, ascites, cataracts, and mental retardation. The urine contains a reducing substance that is not glucose (urine gives a positive Clinitest reaction but is negative with Clinistix) while the patient is receiving galactose. The increased concentration of galactose-1-phosphate leads to intellectual impairment, cataracts, hepatic dysfunction, renal tubular disease (Fanconi's syndrome), and ovarian failure (154). Diagnosis is confirmed by identifying a marked increase in blood levels of galactose and galactose-1-phosphate and near-absent galactose-1-phosphate uridyl transferase activity in red blood cells (155). Treatment consists of eliminating galactose from the diet.

B. Liver Disease

Fasting hypoglycemia may occur in patients with a variety of diseases and ingestion of various agents that cause extensive damage to the liver parenchyma resulting in fulminant hepatic necrosis and liver failure (156). Hypoglycemia results from impaired glycogenolysis and gluconeogenesis. Treatment is supportive.

C. Jamaican Vomiting Sickness

The unripe ackee fruit of the *Blighia surpida* tree contains a water-soluble toxin, hypoglycin, which produces vomiting, central nervous system depression, acute fatty liver, and severe hypoglycemia. Hypoglycemia is caused by hypoglycin A, which inhibits gluconeogenesis secondary to its interference with oxidation of long chain fatty acids (157). The disease is endemic in Jamaica where ackee is part of the diet of the poor. It has been reported in the United States resulting from the consumption of canned ackee (158).

D. Glucose Transporters

Hypoglycorrhachia despite normal plasma glucose concentrations has been described in infants with a seizure disorder, developmental delay and acquired microcephaly, caused by a defect in the blood–brain GLUT-1. Glucose and lactate concentrations in the cerebrospinal fluid are low. Two distinct classes of mutations cause the functional defect of glucose transport: hemizygosity of GLUT-1 and nonsense mutations resulting in truncation of the GLUT-1 protein (159). Treatment is with a ketogenic diet to provide the brain with an alternative fuel source (160).

XIII. DISORDERS OF CARNITINE METABOLISM, FATTY ACID β-OXIDATION, AND KETONE SYNTHESIS

Disorders of carnitine metabolism and fatty acid β-oxidation are characterized by impaired ability to metabolize free fatty acids to acetyl CoA in various tissues and to synthesize ketones in the liver. During periods of fasting, mitochondrial oxidation of fatty acids becomes the major source of energy. Fatty acids with a chain length of ≤18 carbons undergo a series of reactions that produce acetyl CoA, a Krebs cycle intermediate and a precursor of hepatic ketone body synthesis. Normally, ketones are an alternative source of fuel for a variety of tissues, thereby conserving glucose for oxidation by the brain and heart. The paucity of ketones in fatty acid β-oxidation (FAO) disorders results in continued dependence on and utilization of glucose. FAO disorders result in the inability to maintain fasting plasma glucose concentrations and accumulation of intermediates of β-oxidation, which cause encephalopathy, arrhythmias, cardiac arrest, and sudden death (161, 162).

The oxidation of fatty acids begins with the formation of acyl-coenzyme A, which is transported across the mitochondrial membrane by a carnitine-mediated transport mechanism. Within the mitochondrion, carnitine is removed and four reactions, catalyzed by membrane bound enzymes, result in sequential removal of two carbon moieties (Fig. 4). Although defects in the formation of CoA esters, transport, or β-oxidation all result in impaired energy metabolism, there is a wide spectrum of clinical phenotypes. To date, at least 22 distinct disorders of fatty acid oxidation or transport have been described. Clinical manifestations may appear at any age between birth and adulthood; 69% of patients manifest symptoms before 1 year of age (163). Clinical manifestations usually occur during periods of catabolic stress or reduced caloric consumption (164). Symptoms of an acute metabolic crisis vary in se-

verity and include nausea, vomiting, lethargy, confusion, coma, seizures, or sudden death. Patients may have hypoglycemia (usually, but not always, hypoketotic), liver disease ranging in severity from increased serum transaminase levels to fulminant hepatic failure, skeletal myopathy, or cardiac dysfunction caused by cardiomyopathy (Tables 6, 7).

Approximately one-third of patients with FAO disorders present in the newborn period with lethargy, hypotonia, and neurological depression (163). Dysmorphic features (including facial dysmorphisms, renal dysplasia or cysts, and developmental brain malformations caused by defects in neuronal migration) have been observed in multiple acyl-CoA deficiency (MAD [glutaric acidemia type II]) (165) and in CPT-II deficiency (166). Other disorders that may present in the neonatal period, but are not typically associated with dysmorphology, include translocase deficiency, trifunctional protein deficiency, CPT-I deficiency, and very-long-chain acyl-CoA dehydrogenase (VLCAD) deficiency. Cardiac manifestations, including conduction disturbances and arrhythmias, are common in all of the disorders that present in the newborn period. Although hypoglycemia is a feature of these disorders, severely ill infants usually die within a few days of birth despite treatment of hypoglycemia (167, 168). About 5% of cases of sudden infant death syndrome (SIDS) are believed to be caused by defects in carnitine transport and/ or FAO, including deficiencies of medium-chain acyl-CoA dehydrogenase (MCAD), VLCAD, long-chain hydroxyacyl-CoA dehydrogenase (LCHAD), MAD, and carnitine transport defects (169).

In infancy and childhood, hypoglycemia is the most common presenting abnormality; more than 80% of patients have a low plasma glucose concentration at diagnosis (163). Hypoglycemia is classically associated with hypoketosis; however, enough ketones may be formed in patients with the short-chain fatty acid disorders that patients may appear to have abundant (appropriate) urinary ketones at the time of presentation with hypoglycemia. Moderate hepatomegaly at presentation is caused by fatty infiltration (micro- and macrovesicular steatosis), which may lead to the erroneous impression that the patient has a glycogen storage disease or Reye syndrome. The hepatomegaly rapidly resolves with treatment. In addition to hypoglycemia, most patients show evidence of hepatic dysfunction during episodes of acute metabolic decompensation (161, 164). A clinical picture similar to Reye's syndrome (hepatomegaly, neurological depression, hyperammonemia) is present in about 30% of patients (163). A moderate increase in serum transaminase concentrations (100–800 U/L) is common, and patients with MAD and translocase deficiency may present with frank hepatic failure. The mitochondria may be abnormal in shape and size in both disorders. However, electron microscopy may reveal differences: dense condensation of mitochondria with inclusion bodies in fatty acid oxidation defects compared with mitochondrial swelling in Reye syndrome (170).

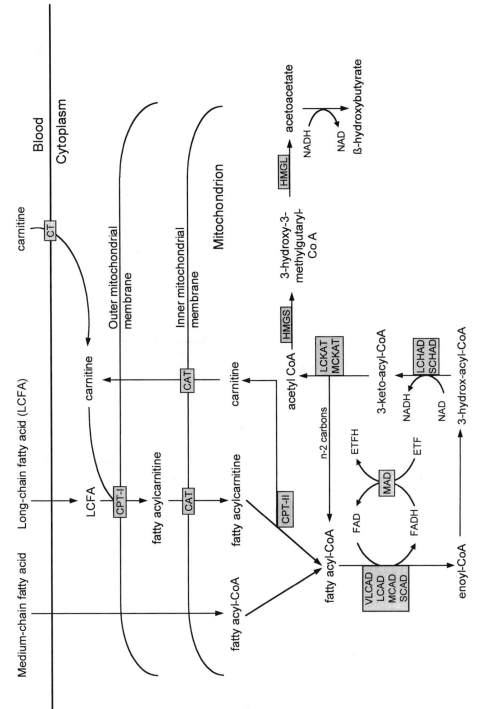

Figure 4 Schema of carnitine metabolism, fatty acid β-oxidation, and ketone synthesis. Reactions associated with known metabolic defects are shown in shaded boxes. CAT, carnitine-acylcarnitine translocase; CT, carnitine transporter; ETF(H), electron transfer flavoprotein (reduced); FAD(H), flavin adenine dinucleotide (reduced); HMGL, 3-hydroxy-3-methylglutaryl-CoA lyase; HMGS, 3-hydroxy-3-methyl-glutaryl-CoA synthetase; LCFA, long-chain fatty acid; LCKAT, long-chain 3-ketoacyl-CoA thiolase; MCKAT, medium-chain 3-ketoacyl-CoA thiolase; NAD(H), nicotinamide adenine dinucleotide (reduced).

Table 6 Disorders of Carnitine Metabolism

Enzyme deficiency	CT	CAT	CPT-I	CPT-II
Clinical				
Fasting intolerance	+	+	+	+
Acute episodes	+	+	+	+
Coma/seizures	+	+	+	+
Muscle weakness/myopathy	+	+	+	+
Muscle pain/myoglobinuria				+
Cardiomyopathy/arrhythmia	+	+		±
Hepatopathy	+	+	+	±
Nephropathy			+	
Congenital anomalies				+
Biochemical				
Hypoglycemia	+	+	+	+
Ketones	Low	Low	Low	Low
Ammonia	+/−High	+/−High	+/−High	+/−High
AST, ALT	Abnormal	Abnormal	Abnormal	Abnormal
Plasma carnitine	Very low	Low/normal	High/normal	Low/normal
Plasma acylcarnitines	Normal	Abnormal	Normal	Abnormal
Dicarboxylic aciduria	No	Yes	No	No
Other abnormal organic acids	No	No	No	No
Urine acylglycines	Normal	Normal	Normal	Normal

CT, carnitine transporter; CAT, carnitine acylcarnitine translocase; CPT-I, carnitine palmitoyltransferase-I; CPT-II, carnitine palmitoyltransfer-ase-II; ±, not common but occasionally reported; +/−high, plasma ammonia level is not invariably high.
Source: From Refs. 161, 162, 164.

Table 7 Disorders of Fatty Acid Oxidation and Ketone Synthesis

Enzyme deficiency	MAD	VLCAD	MCAD	SCAD	LCHAD	SCHAD	KAT	HMGS	HMGL
Clinical									
Fasting intolerance	+	+	+	+	+	+	+	+	+
Acute episodes	+	+	+	+	+	+	+	+	+
Coma/seizures	+	+	+	+	+	+	+	+	+
Myopathy/weakness	+	+		+	+	+	+		+
Myoglobinuria/pain		+			+	+			
Neuropathy		+			+				
Retinopathy					+				
Cardiomyopathy	+	+			+	±	+		
Hepatopathy	+	+	+	+	+	±	+	+	+
Nephropathy		+							
Congenital anomalies	+								
Biochemical									
Hypoglycemia	+	+	+	+	+	+	+	+	+
Ketones	Low	Low	Low	High	Low	High	Low	Low	Low
Ammonia	+/−High	+/−High	+/−High	+/−High	+/−High			N	+/−High
AST, ALT	Abnl	Abnl	Abnl	Abnl	Abnl		Abnl	Abnl	Abnl
Plasma carnitine	Low	Low	Low	Low	Low	Low	Low*	N	N
Plasma acylcarnitines	Abnl	Abnl	Abnl	Abnl	Abnl	N	Abnl	N	N
Dicarboxylic aciduria	Yes	Yes	Yes	Yes	Yes	Yes	Yes	Yes/no	No
Other abnormal OA	Yes	Yes	Yes	Yes	Yes	Yes	Yes	Yes†	Yes
Urine acylglycines	Abnl	N	Abnl	Abnl	N	N	N	N	N

Abnl, abnormal; N, normal; *, may be normal; †, only after MCT loading; OA, organic acids; ±, not common but occasionally reported.
KAT, 3-Ketoacyl-CoA thiolase; HMGS, 3-Hydroxy-3-methylglutaryl-CoA synthase; HMGL, 3-Hydroxy-3-methylglutaryl-CoA lyase.
Source: From Refs. 161, 162, 164, 167, 255, 256.

Patients with defects in carnitine transport and metabolism (other than CPT-I deficiency) or in the oxidation of longer chain fatty acids (long-chain acyl-CoA dehydrogenase [LCAD], VLCAD, LCHAD, MAD deficiency) characteristically have hypertrophic or dilated cardiomyopathy (161, 164, 171). Patients often present with congestive heart failure or cardiac arrest. Arrhythmias have been reported without cardiomyopathy. Conduction disturbances are thought to be due to accumulation of toxic intermediates and can occur before the development of severe hypoglycemia. Cardiac presentations have not been described with CPT-I or MCAD deficiency.

Muscle symptoms are the hallmark of FAO defects that present in adulthood. Progressive muscle weakness, episodic muscle pain, rhabdomyolysis, and myoglobinuria after strenuous physical activity occur in adults with CPT-II, translocase, LCHAD, and VLCAD deficiency (Tables 6, 7). Symptoms may occur after prolonged exercise or exposure to cold, during fasting or an intercurrent infection. Hypoglycemia and alterations in mental status are unusual in the late onset disorders.

The characteristic biochemical features of disorders of carnitine metabolism and FAO are summarized in Tables 6 and 7. Acute metabolic crises are frequently, but not invariably, associated with hypoglycemia and metabolic acidosis. Hypoglycemia results from a combination of failure to decrease utilization of glucose (because of the absence of an alternative energy source) and impaired gluconeogenesis. Metabolic acidosis is accompanied by an increased anion gap. Mild to marked hyperammonemia may occur as a result of secondary inhibition of n-acetylglutamate synthesis in the urea cycle. Hepatic dysfunction generally manifests with increases in serum AST and ALT concentrations. When muscle is affected, serum creatine kinase (CK) increases during symptomatic episodes. The cause of the increased serum uric acid level is unclear.

Urinalysis shows an inappropriately low level of ketonuria relative to the duration of fasting and/or degree of hypoglycemia. Ketones are rarely completely absent from the urine. Note, however, that ketonuria is abundant in patients with defects limited to the oxidation of short chain fatty acids (short-chain acyl-CoA dehydrogenase [SCAD] and short-chain hydroxyacyl-CoA dehydrogenase [SCHAD] deficiency). In these disorders, most of the long-chain fatty acid is oxidized to ketones without difficulty; only the metabolism of the short-chain remnants is impaired.

Quantitative assays of plasma carnitine concentrations measure total carnitine as well as free carnitine and bound (or esterified) carnitine. Normally, the free fraction makes up about 80% of total carnitine. Carnitine transport defects are rare and are characterized by extremely low total and free carnitine levels in blood and urine (generally <10 μmol/l). Carnitine loading (for example, with 100 mg/kg) raises the blood level of carnitine, but produces an inappropriate carnitinuria. Secondary carnitine deficiency is much more common. A low level of total plasma carnitine is usually the result of an inadequate supply of dietary carnitine, and the ratio of the free and esterified fractions to total carnitine generally remains intact. A low free/total carnitine ratio can occur for a number of reasons including physiological ketosis (when acetyl CoA binds free carnitine to form acetylcarnitine), and with certain medications (e.g., valproate binds carnitine forming valproylcarnitine). In disorders of FAO, carnitine binds with intermediate compounds in the pathway (e.g., octanoylcarnitine), resulting in decreased total and free carnitine and increased esterified fractions.

A. Diagnosis

All children with hypoglycemia should be screened for FAO disorders. Failure to make the correct diagnosis in a timely fashion increases the risk of hepatic failure or sudden death. During an episode of hypoglycemia, screening for a FAO defect should routinely include urinalysis for measurement of ketones and an analysis of urinary organic acids. Urinary ketones are usually inappropriately low for the degree of hypoglycemia; complete absence of ketones is unusual. Hypoketosis (unless clearly explained by hyperinsulinism) always warrants an investigation for FAO defects. A moderate or large amount of urinary ketones does not exclude the diagnosis of an FAO disorder.

Analysis of urine organic acids by gas chromatography/mass spectrometry is the most useful method to screen for FAO disorders. The urinary excretion of ketones is reduced (except in SCAD and SCHAD deficiencies). In all defects characterized by impaired ß-oxidation of fatty acids, intermediate compounds accumulate and undergo ω-oxidation, resulting in the production of dicarboxylic acids (adipic, suberic, and sebacic acids, corresponding to the saturated fatty acids hexanoate, octanoate, and decanoate, respectively). The excretion of dicarboxylic acids is not necessarily pathological since this may occur to a limited degree during physiological ketosis. Also, patients receiving medium-chain triglycerides (MCT; e.g., in a formula), have dicarboxylic aciduria. Defects in carnitine transport and metabolism do not directly disrupt ß-oxidation and are not generally associated with dicarboxylic aciduria. In 3-hydroxy-3-methylglutaryl-CoA lyase deficiency, only adipic acid is found in urine during a metabolic crisis. Other metabolites in the organic acid analysis can help to identify the particular site of the metabolic block.

Glycine and carnitine are normal cellular constituents that displace CoA from organic acyl and fatty acyl intermediates, producing acylglycines and acylcarnitines, respectively. The former is analyzed in urine, the latter in plasma or in blood filter paper specimens (172). Certain compounds have a higher affinity for glycine, others for carnitine. The specific pattern of unusual compounds identified by these techniques, in concert with the urine organic acid findings, increases the likelihood of making a specific diagnosis. Quantitative free fatty acid profiles allow direct analysis of all fatty acid intermediates and appears to be the most sensitive test for diagnosing disorders of FAO (162). Because deficiency of carnitine and disorders of carnitine transport do not cause abnormal patterns of fatty acyl-CoA intermediates, measurement of total, free, and esterified carnitine concentrations should be included in the work-up of any patient with a suspected FAO disorder.

The importance of obtaining diagnostic specimens during the acute catabolic phase of illness (or as soon as possible after the patient has been treated) cannot be overstated. Once treatment is begun with oral and/or intravenous glucose, fatty acid flux through the defective pathway decreases so that the characteristic biochemical abnormalities necessary for establishing a diagnosis may no longer be evident. As a consequence, specimens obtained once treatment is well underway may be normal, necessitating a more invasive and potentially dangerous approach to investigating these patients.

Several American states and European regions are using tandem mass spectrometry to screen for FAO disorders and CPT-II deficiency on filter paper blood specimens obtained during the newborn period (173, 174).

There are several options for investigating the asymptomatic patient who has a history suggestive of a defect in carnitine metabolism or FAO. Plasma acylcarnitine and urinary acylgycine should be obtained in the morning after a routine overnight fast of 8–10 h duration when the child is well. Arrangements can be made for diagnostic blood and urine specimens to be obtained when the patient is under catabolic stress (e.g., during a fever or intercurrent illness). The patient can be admitted to the hospital to monitor the response to fasting (29, 175). However, because of the potential hazard of inducing an arrhythmia, hepatic failure, or sudden death, a monitored fast should be performed as a last resort in the child with undiagnosed hypoglycemia in whom all noninvasive methods have failed to yield a diagnosis. A supervised oral fat load is a practical in vivo test to identify defects affecting longer-chain fatty acid metabolism (176). In all cases of potential carnitine transport defects and FAO defects, especially in very young patients or when it is inappropriate for a patient to fast or undergo a provocative study, skin fibroblasts may be obtained for FAO studies and for direct enzyme analysis. In addition, mutational analysis can be performed for diseases with common mutations (e.g., MCAD and LCHAD deficiency).

B. Treatment

The specific treatment of diseases of carnitine metabolism and defects of FAO depends upon the individual defect. The primary recommendation for all disorders of FAO is to avoid prolonged fasting and ensure a regular feeding regimen when patients are at risk for acute decompensation. Provision of a continuous exogenous source of car-

bohydrate obviates dependence on fatty acids and ketones for energy. During intercurrent illnesses, or when calorie intake decreases for any reason, patients should be fed every 4 h around the clock until a normal diet is resumed and symptoms of the illness abate. When vomiting prevents dependable consumption of food or fluids, 10% dextrose solution must be given intravenously at a rate approximately 1.5 times the hepatic glucose production rate to inhibit glucose counterregulation.

Dietary therapy for defects of FAO is controversial. For the young child (above 1 year of age) who is otherwise well, raw cornstarch at night decreases the need for fatty acids as a source of energy. Restriction of fat has been used; however, overzealous fat restriction may lead to deficiencies of essential fatty acids. In defects of long-chain fat oxidation, supplemental dietary medium-chain triglycerides allows ketone synthesis to occur. The availability of fat as a substrate for energy may be of therapeutic benefit even during an acute metabolic crisis.

Carnitine supplementation (usually 100 mg/kg/day) is indicated for carnitine transport defects. Whether carnitine supplementation is beneficial for other defects of FAO is controversial. It is postulated that carnitine displaces coenzyme A bound to toxic intermediates. The liberated CoA is free to participate in other metabolic reactions, allowing excretion of the acylcarnitines.

Patients with later-onset MAD deficiency (i.e., glutaric acidemia type II) may respond to high-dosage (100–200 mg/kg/day) riboflavin supplementation.

Because defects in carnitine metabolism and FAO may be asymptomatic, the siblings of probands should be screened and parents should be counseled regarding the autosomal recessive pattern of inheritance of these diseases. Prenatal diagnosis may be available depending on the specific disorder.

XIV. DETERMINING THE CAUSE OF HYPOGLYCEMIA

The cause of hypoglycemia is often readily apparent; for example, in the child with type 1 diabetes mellitus treated with insulin or when hypoglycemia occurs in a child with fulminant hepatitis or Reye's syndrome. When the cause of hypoglycemia is not obvious, following the diagnostic approach outlined below will usually lead to the specific cause. Determining the cause begins with a detailed history and physical examination. Important features of the history and physical examination are shown in Tables 8 and 9, and a diagnostic algorithm based on key clinical and biochemical features is shown in Figure 5. Infants with hyperinsulinism who do not present in the newborn period usually present within the first 6–12 months of life. Mild forms of congenital hyperinsulinism may present for the first time in childhood or adolescence. When hyperinsulinemic hypoglycemia presents after infancy, one should suspect an islet cell adenoma (often part of mul-

Table 8 History

Birth weight, gestational age, maternal health and
   medications
Symptoms of hypoglycemia at birth or during neonatal
   period
Prolonged neonatal jaundice
Age at onset of symptoms
Family history of hypoglycemia
History of consanguinity
Frequency of hypoglycemia
Temporal relationship to feedings
   <4 h suggests a defect in glycogenolysis or
      hyperinsulinism
   10–12 h suggests a defect in gluconeogenesis or fatty
      acid ß-oxidation
Specific content of feedings and relationship to onset of
   symptoms
Food intolerance or aversion
Unexplained infant deaths or SIDS in family; Reye's
   syndrome, cardiomyopathy, myopathy
Potential drug exposure (oral hypoglycemic agents, insulin)
Hypoglycemia after an adult party: alcohol ingestion
Recurrent "pneumonia": episodes of hyperventilation from
   metabolic acidosis
Unusual odors, especially when sick

tiple endocrine neoplasia type 1 syndrome). Growth hormone and/or cortisol deficiency usually presents in the newborn period or in early childhood. Accelerated starvation usually presents at 18 months to 5 years old. Hepatomegaly, ketosis, and metabolic acidosis suggests an inborn error of metabolism, which may present either in the neonatal period or later in infancy, usually precipitated by cessation of overnight feeding or an infection that interrupts the child's normal feeding pattern and causes catabolic stress.

Glucose meters are widely used in newborn nurseries and in emergency departments to screen for hypoglycemia. These instruments are not consistently reliable at low blood glucose concentrations; therefore, any value below 60 mg/dl (3.3 mmol/l) should be confirmed by a laboratory measurement of the plasma glucose concentration (177). In addition, a simultaneous so-called critical blood sample should be obtained for the measurement of hormones, metabolic substrates, and serum chemistries (see Table 10).

The first urine sample obtained after the episode of hypoglycemia should be tested for the presence of ketones (ketotic vs. nonketotic hypoglycemia), reducing sugars (suggest galactosemia or fructose intolerance), and glucose using a glucose-specific method. An aliquot should be saved and frozen for possible later analysis of amino acids, organic acids, and acylglycines after the initial laboratory investigations have been completed.

The initial laboratory evaluation should include measurement of serum insulin to determine whether the hypoglycemia is associated with a normal (suppressed) or an inappropriately increased serum insulin concentration, and measurement of urinary ketones to determine if the hypoglycemia is associated with ketosis. Absence of urinary ketones or their presence in only trace or small amounts (i.e., nonketotic or hypoketotic hypoglycemia), is characteristic of hyperinsulinism and disorders of carnitine metabolism and FAO and/or ketogenesis. The serum C-peptide concentration is low or undetectable when hyperinsulinism is caused by exogenous insulin administration. If the serum insulin concentration is appropriately suppressed (<2 μU/ml with a highly sensitive insulin assay), the diagnosis is likely to be a disorder of FAO. Encephalopathy is common at the time of acute metabolic decompensation; the liver may be moderately enlarged from acute fatty infiltration (microvesicular steatosis), and liver enzymes (AST, ALT) and plasma ammonia levels are increased during acute episodes of catabolic stress (164). If a disorder of FAO is suspected, plasma total and esterified carnitine, plasma (or filter paper) acylcarnitines (172), and plasma free fatty acids should be measured, and urine analyzed for organic acids and acylglycines (178).

Ketosis with hypoglycemia is a normal physiological response to a falling blood glucose concentration. The differential diagnosis of the hypoglycemic child with an appropriately suppressed serum insulin concentration and ketosis (Table 5) can be further delineated depending on whether or not the liver is large (Fig. 5). Elevated levels of GH and cortisol exclude deficiency of these counterregulatory hormones and obviate the need for further testing. On the other hand, random values that appear to be inappropriately low during a spontaneous episode of hypoglycemia do not constitute definitive evidence of deficient secretion. Specific testing must be performed.

A large liver suggests a glycogen storage disease or disorder of gluconeogenesis (e.g., fructose 1,6-bisphosphatase deficiency). The liver size is normal in patients with accelerated starvation, cortisol deficiency, GH deficiency, glycogen synthase deficiency, maple syrup urine disease, and the other conditions listed in Table 3. Transient enlargement of the liver during an acute metabolic crisis can occur in organic acidemia, FAO defects, and in disorders of carnitine metabolism, and results from acute fatty deposition in the cytosol associated with impaired mitochondrial function.

A specific diagnosis of the cause of the hypoglycemia usually is evident from the analysis of the results of the so-called critical blood sample obtained at the time of hypoglycemia (Table 10) and application of the diagnostic algorithm shown in Figure 5. However, if the laboratory data required to make a diagnosis are not available, it may be necessary to perform a comprehensive evaluation of intermediary metabolism by reproducing the conditions

Table 9 Findings on Physical Examination

Examination	Possible causes
Short stature; growth failure	GH deficiency, hypopituitarism
Microphallus	GH deficiency, hypopituitarism
Midline facial defects	GH deficiency, hypopituitarism
Cleft lip and palate	
Single central incisor	
Optic nerve hypoplasia	
Abnormal skin pigmentation	Addison's disease
Large liver	Glycogen storage disease
	Disorder of gluconeogenesis
	Galactosemia
	Disorder of fatty acid ß-oxidation
	Disorder of carnitine metabolism
	Tyrosinemia type I
Macrosomia	Beckwith-Wiedemann syndrome
Large tongue	
Omphalocele/umbilical hernia	
Visceromegaly	
Horizontal grooves on ear lobes	
Hyperventilation	Metabolic acidosis, hyperammonemia
Odor	Maple syrup urine disease, isovaleric acidemia, 3-methylcrotonyl CoA carboxylase deficiency, multiple acyl CoA dehydrogenase deficiency (glutaric acidemia type II)
Heart	Disorder of fatty acid β-oxidation
Gallop or murmur	Disorder of carnitine transport or metabolism
Cardiomyopathy	

that caused the hypoglycemia. This involves measurement of hormones and metabolic substrates that reflect carbohydrate, fat, and amino acid metabolism during a monitored fast of specified duration depending on the age of the child (175). Fasting may be hazardous and can even be lethal in patients with a disorder of FAO. Before subjecting any child to a monitored fast, one should first attempt to rule out a disorder of FAO by measuring nonfasting plasma acylcarnitines (by tandem mass spectrometry if available) (172) and urinary acylglycines (178).

XV. TREATMENT

Immediately after the critical blood sample has been obtained, 0.3 g/kg glucose is injected intravenously over 10 min to restore the plasma glucose concentration to normal. A continuous infusion of 10% dextrose solution at a rate of ~6–8 mg/kg/min is given to maintain normoglycemia. This rate of glucose infusion is usually sufficient to reverse catabolism. The plasma glucose concentration is monitored and the infusion rate adjusted to maintain a level of ~80 mg/dl (4.5 mmol/l). Valuable diagnostic information can be obtained from the response to treatment. Infants and children with hyperinsulinism characteristi-

cally require considerably higher rates (14.5 ± 1.7 mg/kg/min) of glucose infusion to prevent hypoglycemia (179). In disorders of FAO, administration of glucose at ~1.5 × basal glucose production (10 mg/kg/min) stimulates insulin secretion, inhibits lipolysis, and reverses the acute metabolic disorder and leads to a decrease in liver size to normal over several days.

XVI. HYPOGLYCEMIA AND DIABETES MELLITUS

Hypoglycemia is the most frequent acute complication of the treatment of diabetes mellitus in children and adolescents and is the principal factor that limits attempts to intensify treatment aimed at achieving near-normal glycemic control (180, 181). Patients with type 1 diabetes mellitus are susceptible to hypoglycemia for many reasons, including the nonphysiological nature of insulin replacement therapy, inconsistencies in food intake and exercise, and defective counterregulatory hormone responses to hypoglycemia (Table 11). Because the glucagon response to hypoglycemia is lost early in the course of the disease (182, 183), patients with diabetes mellitus are dependent on sympathoadrenal responses (8) to prevent or

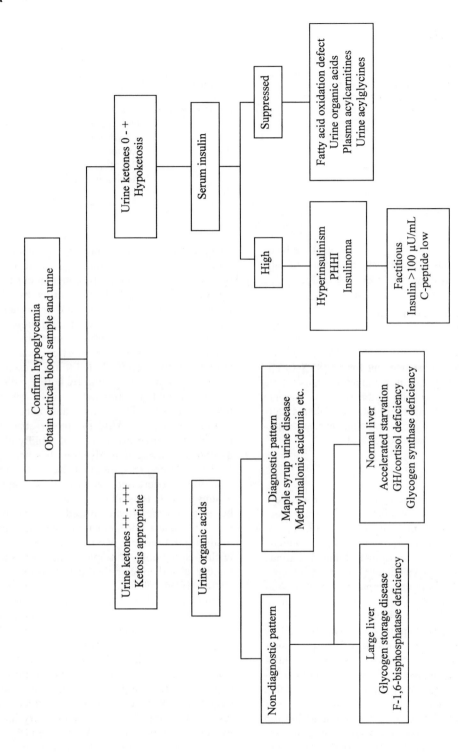

Figure 5 Algorithm for diagnosis of hypoglycemia.

Table 10 Laboratory Investigation of Unexplained Hypoglycemia

	Blood			Urine
Metabolites	Insulin secretion	Counterregulation	Fatty acid oxidation	
Glucose	Insulin	Growth hormone	Free fatty acids	Ketones
Lactate/pyruvate	C-peptide	Cortisol	Fatty acid profile	Reducing sugars
Amino acids (alanine)	Proinsulin	Glucagon	β-hydroxybutyrate	Organic acids
Uric acid		Epinephrine	Acetoacetate	Acylglycines
Serum electrolytes (anion gap)			Carnitine	
pH, bicarbonate			Acylcarnitines	
AST, ALT, CK				

correct hypoglycemia. Mild hypoglycemia itself reduces epinephrine responses and symptomatic awareness of subsequent episodes of hypoglycemia (43, 184, 185).

A. Causes of Hypoglycemia in Diabetes Mellitus

Patient errors relating to insulin dosage, decreased food intake, or unplanned exercise account for 50–85% of episodes of hypoglycemia in children and adolescents (186–191). After years of living with diabetes, some patients and/or their parents conduct their routine diabetes self-care practices without thinking about the intricate interplay among insulin, food, and exercise (192).

B. Symptoms and Signs

Symptoms of hypoglycemia are caused by neuronal deprivation of glucose and are autonomic (adrenergic), neuroglycopenic, or a combination of the two. The most common signs and symptoms of hypoglycemia in diabetic children are pallor, weakness, tremor, hunger, fatigue, drowsiness, sweating, and headache (186, 193). In contrast to adolescents, autonomic symptoms are less common in children younger than 6 years old whose symptoms are more often neuroglycopenic or nonspecific in nature (193). Symptoms of hypoglycemia experienced by adults with diabetes have been categorized into subgroups: autonomic (sweating, palpitations, shaking, hunger), neuroglycopenic (confusion, drowsiness, odd behavior, speech difficulty, incoordination), and nonspecific malaise (hunger and headache) (194).

Manifestations of hypoglycemia in young children with diabetes mellitus tend to differ from those of insulin-treated adults. In young children, behavioral changes are often the primary manifestation of hypoglycemia. This difference has important implications for parent education on hypoglycemia. Also, autonomic and neuroglycopenic symptoms reported by children and their parents tend to cluster. This contrasts with adult patients who are usually able to differentiate between these two types of symptoms. In children, the coalescence of autonomic and neurogly-

copenic symptoms may indicate that both types of symptom are generated at similar glycemic thresholds. Both parents and children report a coherent cluster of symptoms related to behavioral change during hypoglycemia. Behavioral changes, therefore, are important premonitory signs of hypoglycemia in young children (195).

Hypoglycemia is classified in terms of its severity as mild, moderate, or severe; most episodes are mild (193). Parents are most often alerted to the presence of hypoglycemia in a very young child by noting pallor, drowsiness, or unexplained irritability. Cognitive deficits usually do not accompany mild reactions, and older children are able to treat themselves. Mild symptoms abate within 10–15 min after an appropriate dose of rapidly absorbed carbohydrate. Moderate hypoglycemia has neuroglycopenic as well as adrenergic symptoms: headache, mood changes, irritability, decreased attentiveness, and drowsiness. Young patients typically require assistance with treatment because they are often confused and have impaired judgement; weakness and poor coordination may make it difficult to treat oneself. Moderate reactions produce longer-lasting symptoms and may require a second dose of rapidly absorbed carbohydrate. Severe hypoglycemia is characterized by unresponsiveness, unconsciousness, or convulsions and requires emergency treatment with parenteral glucagon administered or intravenous glucose given by an emergency medical technician in the field or in a hospital emergency department. The definition of severe hypoglycemia in the Diabetes Control and Complications Trial (DCCT) was symptoms consistent with hypoglycemia requiring the assistance of another person for treatment, associated with a blood glucose concentration less than 50 mg/dl or prompt recovery after oral carbohydrate, SC glucagon, or IV glucose (181).

Patients with longer duration of diabetes describe a change in their symptomatology over time, characterized by reduced occurrence of autonomic symptoms and increased frequency of neuroglycopenic symptoms (drowsiness, difficulty concentrating, lack of coordination). Patients must learn to recognize the change in symptoms to prevent severe episodes (196). Furthermore, the blood glucose concentration at which symptoms occur varies

Table 11 Causes of Hypoglycemia in Diabetes Mellitus

Insulin errors (inadvertent or deliberate)
  Reversal of morning and evening dose
  Reversal of short- or rapid-acting insulin and
    intermediate-acting insulin
  Improper timing of insulin in relation to food
  Excessive insulin dosage
  Surreptitious insulin administration, suicide gesture, or
    attempt
Erratic or altered absorption
  Inadvertent intramuscular injection
  More rapid absorption from exercising limbs
  Unpredictable absorption from lipohypertrophy at
    injection sites
  More rapid absorption after sauna, hot bath, sunbathing
Diet
  Omission or reduced size of meals or snacks
  Delayed snacks or meals
  Eating disorders
  Gastroparesis
  Malabsorption (e.g., gluten enteropathy)
Exercise
  Unplanned physical activity
  Prolonged duration and/or increased intensity of
    physical activity
  Failure to reduce the dose of intermediate-acting insulin
    to combat the so-called lag effect of exercise
Alcohol and/or drugs
  Impaired gluconeogenesis from excessive consumption
    of ethanol
  Impaired cognition from use of ethanol, marijuana,
    cocaine, other recreational drugs
Hypoglycemia-associated autonomic failure
  Unawareness of hypoglycemia
  Defective glucose counterregulation
Miscellaneous uncommon causes of hypoglycemia
  Adrenocortical insufficiency
  Hypothyroidism
  Growth hormone deficiency
  Renal failure
  Decreased insulin requirement in first trimester of
    pregnancy
  Insulin antibodies

among patients. This threshold may also vary in the same individual in parallel with antecedent glycemic control. For example, children with long-standing hyperglycemia as a result of poor diabetes control experience symptoms of hypoglycemia at higher blood glucose concentrations than children with good glycemic control, similar to adults with diabetes (197).

C. Impact of Hypoglycemia

Occasional, mild symptomatic hypoglycemia may be the price to pay for near-normal glycemic control (198–202).

However, it is important to appreciate that cognitive function deteriorates at low blood glucose levels even in the absence of typical symptoms (203, 204). Moderate and severe hypoglycemia is disabling, affects school performance, and makes driving a car or operating dangerous machinery extremely hazardous (203, 205–207). The utmost effort should be made to avoid such events. Repeated or prolonged severe hypoglycemia can cause permanent central nervous system damage (208), especially in very young children (209). Fortunately, hypoglycemia is an unusual cause of death in children with type 1 diabetes (210). Although diabetes is not typically associated with reduced intelligence in children, subtle neurocognitive impairments may result if onset occurs before 5 years (211) or the child has seizures from hypoglycemia (212, 213). The neurocognitive sequelae of intensive diabetes management in children whose brains are still developing are still largely unknown. Preliminary findings suggest poorer memory skills, presumably the consequence of recurrent and severe hypoglycemia (214).

The confidence of the patient and members of the patient's family is often shaken after an episode of severe hypoglycemia. The fear of hypoglycemia may cause the patient or family to change its diabetes management strategies in an effort to avoid subsequent episodes of hypoglycemia. The fear of hypoglycemia, therefore, can become a barrier to attaining and maintaining optimal glycemic control. Examples of altered patient behaviors that result in worsening metabolic control include chronic overeating or selection of inadequate dosages of insulin to maintain higher blood glucose levels perceived as being safe (215–217). Concern about nocturnal hypoglycemia causes more anxiety for some parents than any other aspect of diabetes, including the fear of long-term complications. Parents may fear that an episode of severe hypoglycemia during the night may not be treated in a timely fashion or that an episode could go entirely undetected and lead to permanent brain damage or death (218).

D. Frequency of Hypoglycemia

The true frequency of mild (self-treated) symptomatic hypoglycemia is almost impossible to ascertain because mild episodes are quickly forgotten and/or are not recorded. In a random sample of 47 children attending a diabetes clinic, the average incidence of symptomatic hypoglycemia was once every 33 days (range, 0–5.2 times per month), and occurred more frequently in children with the lowest glycosylated hemoglobin levels (199). In a 12 month population-based study, Aman et al. found that mild episodes (managed by the child without assistance) occurred in 97% of children and occurred at least once a week in 53% (186). More recently, Tupola et al. (193) prospectively examined the frequency of hypoglycemia (blood glucose <3 mmol/l [54 mg/dl]) in 161 children and adolescents predominantly treated with multiple doses of insulin, who were asked to document hypoglycemia episodes in a 3 month diary. Fifty-two percent of the clinic population experienced episodes of hypoglycemia (0.6 hypoglycemia events per patient per month), most of which (77%) were mild.

The literature is replete with reports of the frequency of severe hypoglycemia in children and adolescents with diabetes (187–191, 198, 200, 201, 219–228). However, various methods of collecting data and different definitions of hypoglycemia and methods of insulin replacement make comparisons among the reports difficult (229). For example, in some studies, severe hypoglycemia is defined as loss of consciousness, whereas others include children who required assistance with treatment. In young children, all episodes of hypoglycemia require the assistance of a third party for treatment regardless of the severity of the symptoms. It is not surprising, therefore, that the reported incidence of moderate or severe hypoglycemia in the pediatric diabetes population varies widely. The incidence of severe hypoglycemia can be assessed with some reliability by defining severe hypoglycemia as requiring the assistance of another person, irrespective of whether it induces loss of consciousness or convulsions. The incidence of severe hypoglycemia varies from 3.1 (227) to 134 episodes per 100 patient-years (202); most studies document a range of 10–40 episodes per 100 patient-years (229, 230). The adolescent cohort of the DCCT had a frequency of severe hypoglycemia of 27.8 and 85.7 episodes per 100 patient-years for the conventional and intensive treatment groups, respectively (201). It is also likely that severe hypoglycemia in pediatric studies has been underreported. This is suggested by the fact that the rate of severe hypoglycemia in conventionally treated adolescents in the year before the DCCT started was 15.7 per 100 patient-years, but increased to 27.8 per 100 patient-years during the course of the study, whereas hemoglobin A1c did not decrease (9.20 ± 1.8% before and 9.76 ± 0.12% during the study) (181, 201).

Many, but not all, studies have found an increased frequency of severe hypoglycemia in younger children (191, 200, 222, 223, 225, 228) and in association with lower hemoglobin A1c concentrations (188, 189, 198, 200, 201, 222, 223, 225, 227). Other factors associated with a higher risk of moderate and severe hypoglycemia are a prior history of severe hypoglycemia (181, 189, 221, 225), relatively higher doses of insulin and low C-peptide secretion (181, 221, 225, 227), longer duration of diabetes (190, 223, 226), and male gender (181, 220).

E. Nocturnal Hypoglycemia

Hypoglycemia, often asymptomatic, frequently occurs during sleep. Moderate and severe (with coma and seizures) hypoglycemia are more common during the night and early morning (before breakfast) than during the daytime (223, 231). In the DCCT, 55% of severe hypoglycemia events occurred during sleep and 43% occurred between midnight and 8 a.m. (181, 231).

Studies of diabetic children and adolescents, in hospital or at home, in which blood glucose concentrations were measured frequently during the night, show a high incidence (14–47%) of asymptomatic hypoglycemia. Such episodes during sleep often exceed 4 h in duration (232–238). Up to half these episodes may be undetected because the subject does not wake from sleep. The incidence of hypoglycemia on any given night may be affected by numerous factors, including the insulin regimen, the timing and content of meals and snacks, and antecedent physical activity. The highest frequency of asymptomatic nocturnal hypoglycemia occurs in children less than 10 years old (234, 236–238). Low blood glucose concentrations in the early morning (before breakfast) are associated with a higher frequency of preceding nocturnal hypoglycemia. Knowledge of this fact is useful in counseling patients to modify the evening insulin regimen and bedtime snack to prevent more severe nocturnal hypoglycemia.

Sleep impairs counterregulatory hormone responses to hypoglycemia in normal subjects and in patients with diabetes mellitus (239). Because a rise in plasma epinephrine levels is normally the main hormonal defense against hypoglycemia, impaired counterregulatory hormone responses to hypoglycemia explain the increased susceptibility to hypoglycemia during sleep. This phenomenon explains the high frequency of nocturnal hypoglycemia. Asymptomatic nocturnal hypoglycemia may itself result in further deficits in counterregulatory hormone responses (240). Thus, impaired defenses against hypoglycemia during sleep may contribute to the vicious cycle of hypoglycemia, impaired counterregulatory responses, and unawareness of hypoglycemia either awake or asleep. Recurrent asymptomatic nocturnal hypoglycemia is an important cause of hypoglycemia unawareness, which, in turn, leads to more frequent and severe hypoglycemia because of failure to experience autonomic warning symptoms before the onset of neuroglycopenia (180).

F. Treatment

Most episodes of symptomatic hypoglycemia are self-treated (except in pre-school-age children) with rapidly absorbed carbohydrate such as glucose tablets, juices, soft drinks, candy, crackers, milk. Glucose tablets raise blood glucose levels more rapidly than do orange juice or milk, and the dosage is easily calibrated (241). Glucose tablets are the treatment of choice for children old enough to chew and swallow large tablets safely. The recommended dosage is 0.3 g glucose/kg body weight. The glycemic response to oral glucose usually lasts less than 2 h (242). Therefore, unless a scheduled meal or snack is due within an hour of the event, following treatment with oral glucose the patient should be given either a mixed snack containing both carbohydrate and protein or a meal.

Severe reactions (unresponsiveness, unconsciousness, or convulsions) require emergency treatment with parenteral glucagon (IM or SC). Buccal and rectal administration of glucose is ineffective (243). Parenteral glucagon is as effective in treating severe hypoglycemia in children (244) as it is in adults (242, 245). Glucagon raises blood glucose levels within 5–15 min and usually relieves symptoms of hypoglycemia (242, 245). Symptoms of experimentally induced hypoglycemia in diabetic children are relieved within 10 min of giving glucagon by either SC or IM injection. Mean blood glucose and plasma glucagon levels are slightly but not significantly higher after IM than SC injection (244). Both 10 μg/kg and 20 μg/kg of glucagon relieve clinical signs and symptoms, but the increment in blood glucose concentration after 10 min is less after the 10 μg/kg dose (1.1 $\pm$ 0.3 vs. 1.7 $\pm$ 0.7 mmol/l). However, after 20 and 30 min the differences in blood glucose concentrations are not significant. Nausea and/or vomiting can be expected to occur after the injection in a minority of children who receive a dose of 20 μg/kg, but usually do not occur after receiving 10 μg/kg. Excessively high plasma glucagon levels are more likely to cause nausea and/or vomiting. The recommended dose, therefore, is 15 μg/kg to a maximum of 1.0 mg. In diabetic children (244) and in healthy adults (245) there appears to be no important difference between the effects of glucagon injected SC or IM. The plasma glucagon levels attained are higher than those in peripheral venous or portal blood of healthy adults during insulin-induced hypoglycemia, and are probably higher than is necessary for maximal effect. The increase in blood glucose concentration after glucagon administration is sustained for at least 30 min; it is therefore not necessary to repeat the dose or force the child to eat or drink for at least 30 min. Intranasal glucagon has a similar effect, but is not available in the United States (246). In an emergency department or hospital, the preferred treatment is intravenous glucose (0.3 g/kg). Because the glycemic response is transient after bolus administration of glucose, the patient should continue to receive intravenous glucose infusion until she or he is able to swallow safely.

If severe hypoglycemia was prolonged and the patient had a seizure, complete recovery of normal mental and neurological function may take many hours despite restoration of a normal blood glucose level (247). Permanent hemiparesis, or other neurological sequelae, is rare (248, 249). The postictal period may be complicated by headache, lethargy, nausea, vomiting, and aching muscles.

REFERENCES

1. Sokoloff L. Circulation and energy metabolism of the brain. In: Siegel G, Agranoff B, Albers R, Molinoff P, eds. Basic Neurochemistry. New York: Raven Press, 1989:565–590.
2. Bier DM, Leake RD, Haymond MW, Arnold KJ, Gruenke LD, Sperling MA, Kipnis DM. Measurement of "true" glucose production rates in infancy and childhood with 6,6-dideuteroglucose. Diabetes 1977; 26: 1016–1023.
3. Chaussain JL. Glycemic response to 24 hour fast in normal children and children with ketotic hypoglycemia. J Pediatr 1973; 82: 438–443.
4. Schwartz NS, Clutter WE, Shah SD, Cryer PE. Glycemic thresholds for activation of glucose counterregulatory systems are higher than the threshold for symptoms. J Clin Invest 1987; 79: 777–781.
5. Mitrakou A, Ryan C, Veneman T, Mokan M, Jenssen T, Kiss I, Durrant J, Cryer P, Gerich J. Hierarchy of glycemic thresholds for counterregulatory hormone secretion, symptoms, and cerebral dysfunction. Am J Physiol 1991; 260: E67–E74.
6. Liu D, Moberg E, Kollind M, Lins PE, Adamson U, Macdonald IA. Arterial, arterialized venous, venous and capillary blood glucose measurements in normal man during hyperinsulinaemic euglycaemia and hypoglycaemia. Diabetologia 1992; 35: 287–290.
7. Koh TH, Aynsley-Green A, Tarbit M, Eyre JA. Neural dysfunction during hypoglycaemia. Arch Dis Child 1988; 63: 1353–1358.
8. Cryer PE. Hypoglycemia: Pathophysiology, Diagnosis, and Treatment. New York: Oxford University Press, 1997.
9. Shepherd PR, Kahn BB. Glucose transporters and insulin action—implications for insulin resistance and diabetes mellitus. N Engl J Med 1999; 341: 248–257.
10. Vannucci SJ, Maher F, Simpson IA. Glucose transporter proteins in brain: delivery of glucose to neurons and glia. Glia 1997; 21: 2–21.
11. Simpson IA, Appel NM, Hokari M, Oki J, Holman GD, Maher F, Koehler-Stec EM, Vannucci SJ, Smith QR. Blood–brain barrier glucose transporter: effects of hypo- and hyperglycemia revisited. J Neurochem 1999; 72: 238–247.
12. Kumagai AK, Kang YS, Boado RJ, Pardridge WM. Up-regulation of blood–brain barrier GLUT1 glucose transporter protein and mRNA in experimental chronic hypoglycemia. Diabetes 1995; 44: 1399–1404.
13. Uehara Y, Nipper V, McCall AL. Chronic insulin hypoglycemia induces GLUT-3 protein in rat brain neurons. Am J Physiol 1997; 272: E716–E719.
14. Randle PJ. Regulatory interactions between lipids and carbohydrates: the glucose fatty acid cycle after 35 years. Diabetes Metab Rev 1998; 14: 263–283.
15. Settergren G, Lindblad BS, Persson B. Cerebral blood flow and exchange of oxygen, glucose, ketone bodies, lactate, pyruvate, and amino acids in infants. Acta Paediatr Scand 1976; 65: 343–353.
16. Hasselbalch SG, Knudsen GM, Jakobsen J, Hageman LP, Holm S, Paulson OB. Blood–brain barrier permeability of glucose and ketone bodies during short-term starvation in humans. Am J Physiol 1995; 268: E1161–E1166.
17. Owen OE, Morgan AP, Kemp HG, Sullivan JM, Herrera MG, Cahill GF Jr. Brain metabolism during fasting. J Clin Invest 1967; 46: 1589–1595.
18. Amiel SA, Archibald HR, Chusney G, Williams AJK, Gale EAM. Ketone infusion lowers hormonal responses to hypoglycaemia: evidence for acute cerebral utilisation of a non-glucose fuel. Clin Sci 1991; 81: 189–194.
19. Haymond MW Sunehag A. Controlling the sugar bowl: regulation of glucose homeostasis in children. Endocrinol Metab Clin North Am 1999; 28: 663–694.
20. Jackson RA, Roshania RD, Hawa MI, Sim BM, DiSilvio L. Impact of glucose ingestion on hepatic and peripheral glucose metabolism in man: an analysis based on simultaneous use of the forearm and double isotope techniques. J Clin Endocrinol Metab 1986; 63: 541–549.

21. Tse TF, Clutter WE, Shah SD, Cryer PE. Mechanisms of postprandial glucose counterregulation in man. Physiologic roles of glucagon and epinephrine vis-a-vis insulin in the prevention of hypoglycemia late after glucose ingestion. J Clin Invest 1983; 72: 278–286.

22. Wolfsdorf JI, Sadeghi-Nejad A, Senior B. Hypoalaninemia and ketotic hypoglycemia: cause or consequence? Eur J Paediatr 1982; 138: 28–31.

23. Perriello G, Jorde R, Nurjhan N, Stumvoll M, Dailey G, Jenssen T, Bier DM, Gerich JE. Estimation of glucose-alanine-lactate-glutamine cycles in postabsorptive humans: role of skeletal muscle. Am J Physiol 1995; 269: E443–E450.

24. Landau BR, Wahren J, Chandramouli V, Schumann WC, Ekberg K, Kalhan SC. Contributions of gluconeogenesis to glucose production in the fasted state. J Clin Invest 1996; 98: 378–385.

25. Hellerstein MK, Neese RA, Linfoot P, Christiansen M, Turner S, Letscher A. Hepatic gluconeogenic fluxes and glycogen turnover during fasting in humans. A stable isotope study. J Clin Invest 1997; 100: 1305–1319.

26. Katz J, Tayek JA. Gluconeogenesis and the Cori cycle in 12-, 20-, and 40-h-fasted humans. Am J Physiol 1998; 275: E537–E542.

27. Sunehag AL, Treuth MS, Toffolo G, Butte NF, Cobelli C, Bier DM, Haymond MW. Glucose production, gluconeogenesis, and insulin sensitivity in children and adolescents: an evaluation of their reproducibility. Pediatr Res 2001; 50: 115–123.

28. Wolfsdorf JI, Sadeghi-Nejad A, Senior B. Fat derived fuels during a 24 hour fast in children. Eur J Pediatr 1982; 138: 141–144.

29. Bonnefont JP, Specola NB, Vassault A, Lombes A, Ogier H, de Klerk JBC, Munnich A, Coude M, Paturneau-Jouas M, Saudubray J-M. The fasting test in paediatrics: application to the diagnosis of pathologogical hypo- and hyperketotic states. Eur J Paediatr 1990; 150: 80–85.

30. Bougneres PF, Ferre P. Study of ketone body kinetics in children by a combined perfusion of 13C and 2H3 tracers. Am J Physiol 1987; 253: E496–E502.

31. Haymond MW, Karl IE, Clarke WL, Pagliara AS, Santiago JV. Differences in circulating gluconeogenic substrates during short-term fasting in men, women, and children. Metabolism 1982; 31: 33–41.

32. Persson B, Settergren G, Dahlquist G. Cerebral arteriovenous difference of acetoacetate and D-β-hydroxybutyrate in children. Acta Paediatr Scand 1972; 61: 273–278.

33. Haymond MW, Campbell C, Ben-Galim E, DeVivo DC. Effects of ketosis on glucose flux in children and adults. Am J Physiol 1983; 245: E373–E378.

34. Matschinsky FM. Banting Lecture 1995. A lesson in metabolic regulation inspired by the glucokinase glucose sensor paradigm. Diabetes 1996; 45: 223–241.

35. Aguilar-Bryan L, Bryan J. Molecular biology of adenosine triphosphate-sensitive potassium channels. Endocr Rev 1999; 20: 101–135.

36. Shepherd RM, Cosgrove KE, O'Brien RE, Barnes PD, Ammala C, Dunne MJ. Hyperinsulinism of infancy: towards an understanding of unregulated insulin release. European Network for Research into Hyperinsulinism in Infancy. Arch Dis Child Fetal Neonatal Ed 2000; 82: F87–F97.

37. Glaser B, Thornton P, Otonkoski T, Junien C. Genetics of neonatal hyperinsulinism. Arch Dis Child Fetal Neonatal Ed 2000; 82: F79–F86.

38. Glaser B, Kesavan P, Heyman M, Davis E, Cuesta A, Buchs A, Stanley CA, Thornton PS, Permutt MA, Matschinsky FM, Herold KC. Familial hyperinsulinism caused by an activating glucokinase mutation. N Engl J Med 1998; 338: 226–230.

39. Froguel P, Zouali H, Vionnet N, Velho G, Vaxillaire M, Sun F, Lesage S, Stoffel M, Takeda J, Passa P, et al. Familial hyperglycemia due to mutations in glucokinase. Definition of a subtype of diabetes mellitus. N Engl J Med 1993; 328: 697–702.

40. Stanley CA, Lieu YK, Hsu BY, Burlina AB, Greenberg CR, Hopwood NJ, Perlman K, Rich BH, Zammarchi E, Poncz M. Hyperinsulinism and hyperammonemia in infants with regulatory mutations of the glutamate dehydrogenase gene. N Engl J Med 1998; 338: 1352–1357.

41. Haymond MW, Karl IE, Pagliara AS. Ketotic hypoglycemia: an amino acid substrate limited disorder. J Clin Endocrinol Metab 1974; 38: 521–530.

42. Hansen IL, Levy MM, Kerr DS. Differential diagnosis of hypoglycemia in children by responses to fasting and 2-deoxyglucose. Metabolism 1983; 32: 960–970.

43. Heller SR, Cryer PE. Reduced neuroendocrine and symptomatic responses to subsequent hypoglycemia after 1 episode of hypoglycemia in nondiabetic humans. Diabetes 1991; 40: 223–226.

44. Widom B Simonson DC. Intermittent hypoglycemia impairs glucose counterregulation. Diabetes 1992; 41: 1597–1602.

45. Davis SN, Shavers C, Mosqueda-Garcia R, Costa F. Effects of differing antecedent hypoglycemia on subsequent counterregulation in normal humans. Diabetes 1997; 46: 1328–1335.

46. Senior B. Ketotic hypoglycemia. J Pediatr 1973; 82: 555–556.

47. Dahlquist G, Gentz J, Hagenfeldt L, Larsson A, Low H, Persson B, Zetterstrom R. Ketotic hypoglycemia of childhood—a clinical trial of several unifying etiological hypotheses. Acta Paediatr Scand 1979; 68: 649–656.

48. Pagliara AS, Karl IE, De Vivo DC, Feigin RD, Kipnis DM. Hypoalaninemia: a concomitant of ketotic hypoglycemia. J Clin Invest 1972; 51: 1440–1449.

49. Byrne HA, Tieszen KL, Hollis S, Dornan TL, New JP. Evaluation of an electrochemical sensor for measuring blood ketones. Diabetes Care 2000; 23: 500–503.

50. Marks V, Teale JD. Hypoglycemia: factitious and felonious. Endocrinol Metab Clin North Am 1999; 28: 579–601.

51. Thomas PM. Genetic mutations as a cause of hyperinsulinemic hypoglycemia in children. Endocrinol Metab Clin North Am 1999; 28: 647–656.

52. Thornton PS, Sumner AE, Ruchelli ED, Spielman RS, Baker L, Stanley CA. Familial and sporadic hyperinsulinism: histopathology and segregation analysis support a single autosomal recessive disorder. J Pediatr 1991; 119: 721–724.

53. Thomas PM, Cote GJ, Wohllk N, Haddad B, Mathew PM, Rabi W, Aguilar-Bryan L, Gagel RF, Bryan J. Mutations in the sulfonylurea receptor gene in familial persistent hyperinsulinemic hypoglycemia of infancy. Science 1995; 268: 426–429.

54. Dunne MJ, Kane C, Shepherd RM, Sanchez JA, James RF, Johnson PR, Aynsley-Green A, Lu S, Clement JP, Lindley KJ, Seino S, Aguilar-Bryan L. Familial persistent hyperinsulinemic hypoglycemia of infancy and mutations in the sulfonylurea receptor. N Engl J Med 1997; 336: 703–706.

55. Thomas P, Ye Y, Lightner E. Mutation of the pancreatic islet inward rectifier Kir6.2 also leads to familial persistent hyperinsulinemic hypoglycemia of infancy. Hum Mol Genet 1996; 5: 1809–1812.

56. Nestorowicz A, Inagaki N, Gonoi T, Schoor KP, Wilson BA, Glaser B, Landau H, Stanley CA, Thornton PS, Seino S, Permutt MA. A nonsense mutation in the inward rectifier potassium channel gene, Kir6.2, is associated with familial hyperinsulinism. Diabetes 1997; 46: 1743–1748.

57. de Lonlay P, Fournet JC, Rahier J, Gross-Morand MS, Poggi-Travert F, Foussier V, Bonnefont JP, Brusset MC, Brunelle F, Robert JJ, Nihoul-Fekete C, Saudubray JM, Junien C. Somatic deletion of the imprinted 11p15 region in sporadic persistent hyperinsulinemic hypoglycemia of infancy is specific of focal adenomatous hyperplasia and endorses partial pancreatectomy. J Clin Invest 1997; 100: 802–807.

58. Verkarre V, Fournet JC, de Lonlay P, Gross-Morand MS, Devillers M, Rahier J, Brunelle F, Robert JJ, Nihoul-Fekete C, Saudubray JM, Junien C. Paternal mutation of the sulfonylurea receptor (SUR1) gene and maternal loss of 11p15 imprinted genes lead to persistent hyperinsulinism in focal adenomatous hyperplasia. J Clin Invest 1998; 102: 1286–1291.

59. Ryan F, Devaney D, Joyce C, Nestorowicz A, Permutt MA, Glaser B, Barton DE, Thornton PS. Hyperinsulinism: molecular aetiology of focal disease. Arch Dis Child 1998; 79: 445–447.

60. Glaser B, Ryan F, Donath M, Landau H, Stanley CA, Baker L, Barton DE, Thornton PS. Hyperinsulinism caused by paternal-specific inheritance of a recessive mutation in the sulfonylurea-receptor gene. Diabetes 1999; 48: 1652–1657.

61. Rahier J, Guiot Y, Sempoux C. Persistent hyperinsulinaemic hypoglycaemia of infancy: a heterogeneous syndrome unrelated to nesidioblastosis. Arch Dis Child Fetal Neonatal Ed 2000; 82: F108–F112.

62. Sempoux C, Guiot Y, Lefevre A, Nihoul-Fekete C, Jaubert F, Saudubray JM, Rahier J. Neonatal hyperinsulinemic hypoglycemia: heterogeneity of the syndrome and keys for differential diagnosis. J Clin Endocrinol Metab 1998; 83: 1455–1461.

63. de Lonlay-Debeney P, Poggi-Travert F, Fournet JC, Sempoux C, Vici CD, Brunelle F, Touati G, Rahier J, Junien C, Nihoul-Fekete C, Robert JJ, Saudubray JM. Clinical features of 52 neonates with hyperinsulinism. N Engl J Med 1999; 340: 1169–1175.

64. Thornton PS, Satin-Smith MS, Herold K, Glaser B, Chiu KC, Nestorowicz A, Permutt MA, Baker L, Stanley CA. Familial hyperinsulinism with apparent autosomal dominant inheritance: clinical and genetic differences from the autosomal recessive variant. J Pediatr 1998; 132: 9–14.

65. Hufnagel M, Eichmann D, Stieh J, Santer R. Further evidence for a dominant form of familial persistent hyperinsulinemic hypoglycemia of infancy: a family with documented hyperinsulinemia in two generations. (letter). J Clin Endocrinol Metab 1998; 83: 2215–2216.

66. Zammarchi E, Filippi L, Novembre E, Donati MA. Biochemical evaluation of a patient with a familial form of leucine-sensitive hypoglycemia and concomitant hyperammonemia. Metabolism 1996; 45: 957–960.

67. Weinzimer SA, Stanley CA, Berry GT, Yudkoff M, Tuchman M, Thornton PS. A syndrome of congenital hyperinsulinism and hyperammonemia. J Pediatr 1997; 130: 661–664.

68. Kitaura J, Miki Y, Kato H, Sakakihara Y, Yanagisawa M. Hyperinsulinaemic hypoglycaemia associated with persistent hyperammonaemia. Eur J Pediatr 1999; 158: 410–413.

69. Miki Y, Taki T, Ohura T, Kato H, Yanagisawa M, Hayashi Y. Novel missense mutations in the glutamate dehydrogenase gene in the congenital hyperinsulinism–hyperammonemia syndrome. J Pediatr 2000; 136: 69–72.

70. Aynsley-Green A, Hussain K, Hall J, Saudubray JM, Nihoul-Fekete C, De Lonlay-Debeney P, Brunelle F, Otonkoski T, Thornton P, Lindley KJ. Practical management of hyperinsulinism in infancy. Arch Dis Child Fetal Neonatal Ed 2000; 82: F98–F107.

71. Rahier J, Sempoux C, Fournet JC, Poggi F, Brunelle F, Nihoul-Fekete C, Saudubray JM, Jaubert F. Partial or near-total pancreatectomy for persistent neonatal hyperinsulinaemic hypoglycaemia: the pathologist's role. Histopathology 1998; 32: 15–19.

72. Aynsley-Green A, Polak JM, Bloom SR, Gough MH, Keeling J, Ashcroft SJ, Turner RC, Baum JD. Nesidioblastosis of the pancreas: definition of the syndrome and the management of severe neonatal hyperinsulinemic hypoglycaemia. Arch Dis Child 1981; 56: 496–508.

73. Kane C, Lindley KJ, Johnson PR, James RF, Milla PJ, Aynsley-Green A, Dunne MJ. Therapy for persistent hyperinsulinemic hypoglycemia of infancy. Understanding the responsiveness of beta cells to diazoxide and somatostatin. J Clin Invest 1997; 100: 1888–1893.

74. Thornton PS, Alter CA, Levitt Katz L, Baker L, Stanley CA. Short- and long-term use of octreotide in the treatment of congenital hyperinsulinisim. J Pediatr 1993; 123: 637–643.

75. Lindley KJ, Dunne MJ, Kane C, Shepherd RM, Squires PE, James RF, Johnson PR, Eckhardt S, Wakeling E, Dattani M, Milla PJ, Aynsley-Green A. Ionic control of β-cell function in nesidioblastosis. A possible therapeutic role for calcium channel blockade. Arch Dis Child 1996; 74: 373–378.

76. Eichmann D, Hufnagel M, Quick P, Santer R. Treatment of hyperinsulinaemic hypoglycaemia with nifedipine. Eur J Pediatr 1999; 158: 204–206.

77. Bas F, Darendeliler F, Demirkol D, Bundak R, Saka N, Gunoz H. Successful therapy with calcium channel blocker (nifedipine) in persistent neonatal hyperinsulinemic hypoglycemia of infancy. J Pediatr Endocrinol Metab 1999; 12: 873–878.

78. Suprasongsin C, Suthutvoravut U, Mahachoklertwattana P, Preeyasombat C. Combined raw cornstarch and nifedipine as an additional treatment in persistent hyperinsulinemic hypoglycemia of infancy. J Med Assoc Thai 1999; 82 Suppl 1: S39–S42.

79. Spitz L, Bhargava RK, Grant DB, Leonard JV. Surgical treatment of hyperinsulinaemic hypoglycaemia in infancy and childhood. Arch Dis Child 1992; 67: 201–205.

80. Aynsley-Green A, Moncrieff MW, Ratter S, Benedict CR, Storrs CN. Isolated ACTH deficiency. Metabolic and endocrine studies in a 7-year-old boy. Arch Dis Child 1978; 53: 499–502.

81. al Jurayyan NA. Isolated adrenocorticotropin deficiency as a rare cause of hypoglycaemia in children. Further studies and report of an additional case. Horm Res 1995; 44: 238–240.

82. Haymond MW, Karl I, Weldon VV, Pagliara AS. The role of growth hormone and cortisone on glucose and gluconeogenic substrate regulation in fasted hypopituitary children. J Clin Endocrinol Metab 1976; 42: 846–856.

83. Lovinger RD, Kaplan SL, Grumbach MM. Congenital hypopituitarism associated with neonatal hypoglycemia and microphallus. J Pediatr 1975; 87: 1171–1181.

84. Hopwood NJ, Forsman PJ, Kenny FM, Drash AL. Hypoglycemia in hypopituitary children. Am J Dis Child 1975; 129: 918–926.

85. Wolfsdorf JI, Sadeghi-Nejad A, Senior B. Hypoketonemia and age-related fasting hypoglycemia in growth hormone deficiency. Metabolism 1983; 32: 457–462.

86. Aynsley-Green A, McGann A, Deshpande S. Control of intermediary metabolism in childhood with special reference to hypoglycaemia and growth hormone. Acta Paediatr Scand Suppl 1991; 377: 43–52.

87. Laron Z. Prismatic cases: Laron syndrome (primary growth hormone resistance) from patient to laboratory to patient. J Clin Endocrinol Metab 1995; 80: 1526–1531.

88. Orho M, Bosshard NU, Buist NRM, Gitzelmann R, Aynsley-Green A, Blümel P, Gannon MC, Nuttall FQ, Groop LC. Mutations in the liver glycogen synthase gene in children with hypoglycemia due to glycogen storage disease type 0. J Clin Invest 1998; 102: 507–515.

89. Gitzelmann R, Spycher MA, Feil G, Muller J, Seilnacht B, Stahl M, Bosshard NU. Liver glycogen synthase deficiency: a rarely diagnosed entity. Eur J Pediatr 1996; 155: 561–567.

90. Aynsley-Green A, Williamson DH, Gitzelmann R. The dietary treatment of hepatic glycogen synthetase deficiency. Helv Paediatr Acta 1977; 32: 71–75.

91. Chen Y-T, Burchell A. Glycogen Storage Diseases. In: Scriver C, Beaudet A, Sly W, Valle D, eds. The Metabolic and Molecular Bases of Inherited Disease. New York: McGraw-Hill, 1995:935–965.

92. Chou JY, Mansfield BC. Molecular genetics of type I glycogen storage diseases. Trends Endocrinol Metab 1999; 10: 104–113.

93. Wolfsdorf JI, Holm IA, Weinstein DA. Glycogen storage diseases. Phenotypic, genetic, and biochemical characteristics, and therapy. Endocrinol Metab Clin North Am 1999; 28: 801–823.

94. Wolfsdorf JI, Laffel LMB, Crigler JF, Jr. Metabolic control and renal dysfunction in type I glycogen storage disease. J Inherit Metab Dis 1997; 20: 559–568.

95. Chen Y-T, Coleman RA, Scheinman JI, Kolbeck PC, Sidbury JB. Renal disease in type I glycogen storage disease. N Engl J Med 1988; 318: 7–11.

96. Lee PJ, Dalton RN, Shah V, Hindmarsh PC, Leonard JV. Glomerular and tubular function in glycogen storage disease. Pediatr Nephrol 1995; 9: 705–710.

97. Labrune P, Trioche P, Duvaltier I, Chevalier P, Odievre M. Hepatocellular adenomas in glycogen storage disease type I and III: a series of 43 patients and review of the literature. J Pediatr Gastroenterol Nutr 1997; 24: 276–279.

98. Hiraiwa H, Pan CJ, Lin B, Moses SW, Chou JY. Inactivation of the glucose 6-phosphate transporter causes glycogen storage disease type 1b. J Biol Chem 1999; 274: 5532–5536.

99. Gitzelmann R Bosshard NU. Defective neutrophil and monocyte functions in glycogen storage disease type Ib: a literature review. Eur J Pediatr 1993; 152: S33–38.

100. Roe TF, Coates TD, Thomas DW, Miller JH, Gilsanz V. Treatment of chronic inflammatory bowel disease in glycogen storage disease type 1b with colony-stimulating factors. N Engl J Med 1992; 326: 1666–1669.

101. Wolfsdorf JI Crigler JF, Jr. Effect of continuous glucose therapy begun in infancy on the long-term clinical course of patients with type I glycogen storage disease. J Pediatr Gastroenterol Nutr 1999; 29: 136–143.

102. Wolfsdorf JI, Keller RJ, Landy H, Crigler JF Jr. Glucose therapy for glycogenosis type 1 in infants: comparison of intermittent uncooked cornstarch and continuous overnight glucose feedings. J Pediatr 1990; 117: 384–391.

103. Chen Y-T, Cornblath M, Sidbury JB. Cornstarch therapy in type 1 glycogen storage disease. N Engl J Med 1984; 310: 171–175.

104. Wolfsdorf JI, Plotkin RA, Laffel LMB, Crigler JF Jr. Continuous glucose for treatment of patients with type 1 glycogen-storage disease: comparison of the effects of dextrose and uncooked cornstarch on biochemical variables. Am J Clin Nutr 1990; 52: 1043–1050.

105. Wolfsdorf JI, Ehrlich S, Landy HS, Crigler JF Jr. Optimal daytime feeding regimen to prevent postprandial hypoglycemia in type 1 glycogen storage disease. Am J Clin Nutr 1992; 56: 587–592.

106. Yang-Feng TL, Zheng K, Yu J, Yang BZ, Chen YT, Kao FT. Assignment of the human glycogen debrancher gene to chromosome 1p21. Genomics 1992; 13: 931–934.

107. Ding JH, de Barsy T, Brown BI, Coleman RA, Chen YT. Immunoblot analyses of glycogen debranching enzyme in different subtypes of glycogen storage disease type III. J Pediatr 1990; 116: 95–100.

108. Van Hoof F, Hers H. The subgroups of type III glycogenosis. Eur J Biochem 1967; 2: 265–270.

109. Fernandes J Pikaar NA. Ketosis in hepatic glycogenosis. Arch Dis Child 1972; 47: 41–46.

110. Coleman RA, Winter HS, Wolf B, Chen YT. Glycogen debranching enzyme deficiency: long-term study of serum enzyme activities and clinical features. J Inherit Metab Dis 1992; 15: 869–881.

111. Moses SW, Wanderman KL, Myroz A, Frydman M. Cardiac involvement in glycogen storage disease type III. Eur J Pediatr 1989; 148: 764–766.

112. Lee PJ, Deanfield JE, Burch M, Baig K, McKenna WJ, Leonard JV. Comparison of the functional significance of left ventricular hypertrophy in hypertrophic cardiomyopathy and glycogenosis type III. Am J Cardiol 1997; 79: 834–838.

113. Markowitz AJ, Chen YT, Muenzer J, Delbuono EA, Lucey MR. A man with type III glycogenosis associated with cirrhosis and portal hypertension. Gastroenterology 1993; 105: 1882–1885.

114. Borowitz SM, Greene HL. Cornstarch therapy in a patient with type III glycogen storage disease. J Pediatr Gastroenterol Nutr 1987; 6: 631–634.

115. Gremse DA, Bucuvalas JC, Balistreri WF. Efficacy of cornstarch therapy in type III glycogen storage disease. Am J Clin Nutr 1990; 52: 671–674.

116. Slonim AE, Weisberg C, Benke P, Evans OB, Burr IM. Reversal of debrancher deficiency myopathy by the use of high-protein nutrition. Ann Neurol 1982; 11: 420–422.

117. Kiliman MW. Glycogen storage disease due to phosphorylase kinase deficiency. In: Swallow DM, Edwards YH, eds. Protein Dysfunction in Human Genetic Disease. Oxford: BIOS Scientific, 1997:57–75.

118. Nakai A, Shigematsu Y, Takano T, Kikawa Y, Sudo M. Uncooked cornstarch treatment for hepatic phosphorylase kinase deficiency. Eur J Pediatr 1994; 153: 581–583.

119. Pagliara AS, Karl IE, Keating JP, Brown BI, Kipnis DM. Hepatic fructose-1,6-diphosphatase deficiency. A cause of lactic acidosis and hypoglycemia in infancy. J Clin Invest 1972; 51: 2115–2123.

120. Gitzelmann R, Steinmann B, Van den Berghe G. Disorders of Fructose Metabolism. In: Scriver C, Beaudet A, Sly W, and Valle D, eds. The Metabolic and Molecular Basis of Inherited Disease. New York: McGraw-Hill, 1995:905–934.

121. Kaiser UB Hegele RA. Case report: heterogeneity of aldolase B in hereditary fructose intolerance. Am J Med Sci 1991; 302: 364–368.

122. Lecavalier L, Bolli G, Cryer P, Gerich J. Contributions of gluconeogenesis and glycogenolysis during glucose counterregulation in normal humans. Am J Physiol 1989; 256: E844–E851.

123. Marks V Teale JD. Drug-induced hypoglycemia. Endocrinol Metab Clin North Am 1999; 28: 555–577.

124. Chan JC, Cockram CS, Critchley JA. Drug-induced disorders of glucose metabolism. Mechanisms and management. Drug Saf 1996; 15: 135–157.

125. White NJ, Warrell DA, Chanthavanich P, Looareesuwan S, Warrell MJ, Krishna S, Williamson DH, Turner RC. Severe hypoglycemia and hyperinsulinemia in falciparum malaria. N Engl J Med 1983; 309: 61–66.

126. White NJ, Miller KD, Marsh K, Berry CD, Turner RC, Williamson DH, Brown J. Hypoglycaemia in African children with severe malaria. Lancet 1987; 1: 708–711.

127. Taylor TE, Molyneux ME, Wirima JJ, Fletcher KA, Morris K. Blood glucose levels in Malawian children before and during the administration of intravenous quinine for severe falciparum malaria. N Engl J Med 1988; 319: 1040–1047.

128. Kawo NG, Msengi AE, Swai AB, Chuwa LM, Alberti KG, McLarty DG. Specificity of hypoglycaemia for cerebral malaria in children. Lancet 1990; 336: 454–457.

129. Dekker E, Hellerstein MK, Romijn JA, Neese RA, Peshu N, Endert E, Marsh K, Sauerwein HP. Glucose homeostasis in children with falciparum malaria: precursor supply limits gluconeogenesis and glucose production. J Clin Endocrinol Metab 1997; 82: 2514–2521.

130. Davis LE, Woodfin BM, Tran TQ, Caskey LS, Wallace JM, Scremin OU, Blisard KS. The influenza B virus mouse model of Reye's syndrome: pathogenesis of the hypoglycaemia. Int J Exp Pathol 1993; 74: 251–258.

131. Corkey BE, Hale DE, Glennon MC, Kelley RI, Coates PM, Kilpatrick L, Stanley CA. Relationship between unusual hepatic acyl coenzyme A profiles and the pathogenesis of Reye syndrome. J Clin Invest 1988; 82: 782–788.

132. Yoshida Y, Singh I, Singh AK, Tecklenberg FW, Brown FR III, Darby CP. Reye syndrome: rate of oxidation of fatty acids in leukocytes and serum levels of lipid peroxides. J Exp Pathol 1989; 4: 133–139.

133. Haymond MW, Karl IE, Keating JP, DeVivo DC. Metabolic response to hypertonic glucose administration in Reye syndrome. Ann Neurol 1978; 3: 207–215.

134. DeVivo DC, Keating JP, Haymond MW. Reye syndrome: results of intensive supportive care. J Pediatr 1975; 87: 875–880.

135. Hirschhorn N, Lindenbaum J, Greenough WB III, Alam SM. Hypoglycemia in children with acute diarrhoea. Lancet 1966; 2: 128–132.

136. Jones R. Hypoglycaemia in children with acute diarrhea. Lancet 1966; 2: 643.

137. Molla AM, Hossain M, Islam R, Bardhan PK, Sarker SA. Hypoglycemia: a complication of diarrhea in childhood. Indian Pediatr 1981; 18: 181–185.

138. Bennish ML, Azad AK, Rahman O, Phillips RE. Hypoglycemia during diarrhea in childhood. Prevalence, pathophysiology, and outcome. N Engl J Med 1990; 322: 1357–1363.

139. Slone D, Taitz L, Gilchrist G. Aspects of carbohydrate metabolism in kwashiorkor: with special reference to spontaneous hypoglycaemia. Br Med J 1961; 1: 32–34.

140. Hadden D. Glucose, free fatty acid, and insulin interrelations in kwashiorkor and marasmus. Lancet 1967; 1: 589–593.

141. Wharton B. Hypoglycaemia in children with kwashiorkor. Lancet 1970; 1: 171–173.

142. Lifshitz F, Coello-Ramirez P, Gutierrez-Topete G. Monosaccharide intolerance and hypoglycemia in infants with diarrhea. I. Clinical course of 23 infants. J Pediatr 1970; 77: 595–603.

143. Lifshitz F, Coello-Ramirez P, Gutierrez-Topete G. Monosaccharide intolerance and hypoglycemia in infants with diarrhea. II. Metabolic studies in 23 infants. J Pediatr 1970; 77: 604–612.

144. Butler T, Arnold M, Islam M. Depletion of hepatic glycogen in the hypoglycaemia of fatal childhood diarrhoeal illnesses. Trans R Soc Trop Med Hyg 1989; 83: 839–843.

145. Haymond MW. Diarrhea, malnutrition, euglycemia, and fuel for thought. N Engl J Med 1990; 322: 1390–1391.

146. Shih VE. Detection of hereditary metabolic disorders involving amino acids and organic acids. Clin Biochem 1991; 24: 301–309.

147. Cheema-Dhadli S, Leznoff CC, Halperin ML. Effect of 2-methylcitrate on citrate metabolism: implications for the management of patients with propionic acidemia and methylmalonic aciduria. Pediatr Res 1975; 9: 905–908.

148. Gibson KM, Breuer J, Nyhan WL. 3-Hydroxy-3-methylglutaryl-coenzyme A lyase deficiency: review of 18 reported patients. Eur J Pediatr 1988; 148: 180–186.

149. Chuang D, Shih V. Disorders of branch chain amino acid and ketoacid metabolism. In: Scriver C, Beaudet A, Sly W, Valle D, eds. The Metabolic and Molecular Bases of Inherited Disease. New York: McGraw-Hill, 1995:1239–1277.

150. Haymond MW, Ben-Galim E, Strobel KE. Glucose and alanine metabolism in children with maple syrup urine disease. J Clin Invest 1978; 62: 398–405.

151. Tyfield L, Reichardt J, Fridovich-Keil J, Croke DT, Elsas LJ II, Strobl W, Kozak L, Coskun T, Novelli G, Okano Y, Zekanowski C, Shin Y, Boleda MD. Classical galactosemia and mutations at the galactose-1-phosphate uridyl transferase (GALT) gene. Hum Mutat 1999; 13: 417–430.

152. Holton JB, Gillett MG, MacFaul R, Young R. Galactosaemia: a new severe variant due to uridine diphosphate galactose-4-epimerase deficiency. Arch Dis Child 1981; 56: 885–887.

153. Segal S, Berry G. Disorders of galactose metabolism. In: Scriver C, Beaudet A, Sly W, and Valle D, eds. The Metabolic and Molecular Basis of Inherited Disease. New York: McGraw-Hill, 1995:967–1000.

154. Holton JB Leonard JV. Clouds still gathering over galactosaemia. Lancet 1994; 344: 1242–1243.

155. Burton BK. Inborn errors of metabolism in infancy: a guide to diagnosis. Pediatrics 1998; 102: E69.

156. Zimmerman HJ, Lewis JH. Chemical- and toxin-induced hepatotoxicity. Gastroenterol Clin North Am 1995; 24: 1027–1045.

157. Tanaka K, Ikeda Y. Hypoglycin and Jamaican vomiting sickness. Prog Clin Biol Res 1990; 321: 167–184.

158. McTague JA, Forney R, Jr. Jamaican vomiting sickness in Toledo, Ohio. Ann Emerg Med 1994; 23: 1116–1118.

159. Seidner G, Alvarez MG, Yeh JI, O'Driscoll KR, Klepper J, Stump TS, Wang D, Spinner NB, Birnbaum MJ, De Vivo DC. GLUT-1 deficiency syndrome caused by haploinsufficiency of the blood–brain barrier hexose carrier. Nat Genet 1998; 18: 188–191.

160. De Vivo DC, Trifiletti RR, Jacobson RI, Ronen GM, Behmand RA, Harik SI. Defective glucose transport across the blood–brain barrier as a cause of persistent hypoglycorrhachia, seizures, and developmental delay. N Engl J Med 1991; 325: 703–709.

161. Roe C, Coates P. Mitochondrial fatty acid oxidation disorders. In: Scriver C, Beaudet A, Sly W, Valle D, eds. The Metabolic and Molecular Bases of Inherited Disease. New York: McGraw-Hill, 1995:1501–1533.

162. Rinaldo P, Raymond K, al-Odaib A, Bennett MJ. Clinical and biochemical features of fatty acid oxidation disorders. Curr Opin Pediatr 1998; 10: 615–621.

163. Saudubray JM, Martin D, de Lonlay P, Touati G, Poggi-Travert F, Bonnet D, Jouvet P, Boutron M, Slama A, Vianey-Saban C, Bonnefont JP, Rabier D, Kamoun P, Brivet M. Recognition and management of fatty acid oxidation defects: a series of 107 patients. J Inherit Metab Dis 1999; 22: 488–502.

164. Hale DE, Bennett MJ. Fatty acid oxidation disorders: a new class of metabolic diseases. J Pediatr 1992; 121: 1–11.

165. Bohm N, Uy J, Kiessling M, Lehnert W. Multiple acyl-CoA dehydrogenation deficiency (glutaric aciduria type II), congenital polycystic kidneys, and symmetric warty dysplasia of the cerebral cortex in two newborn brothers. II. Morphology and pathogenesis. Eur J Pediatr 1982; 139: 60–65.

166. Hug G, Bove KE, Soukup S. Lethal neonatal multiorgan deficiency of carnitine palmitoyltransferase II. N Engl J Med 1991; 325: 1862–1864.

167. Frerman F, Goodman S. Nuclear-encoded defects of the mitochondrial respiratory chain, including glutaric acidemia type II. In: Scriver C, Beaudet A, Sly W, Valle D, eds. The Metabolic and Molecular Bases of Inherited Disease, New York: McGraw-Hill, 1995:1611–1629.

168. North KN, Hoppel CL, De Girolami U, Kozakewich HP, Korson MS. Lethal neonatal deficiency of carnitine palmitoyltransferase II associated with dysgenesis of the brain and kidneys. J Pediatr 1995; 127: 414–420.

169. Boles RG, Buck EA, Blitzer MG, Platt MS, Cowan TM, Martin SK, Yoon H, Madsen JA, Reyes-Mugica M, Rinaldo P. Retrospective biochemical screening of fatty acid oxidation disorders in postmortem livers of 418 cases of sudden death in the first year of life. J Pediatr 1998; 132: 924–933.

170. Treem WR, Witzleben CA, Piccoli DA, Stanley CA, Hale DE, Coates PM, Watkins JB. Medium-chain and long-chain acyl CoA dehydrogenase deficiency: clinical, pathologic and ultrastructural differentiation from Reye's syndrome. Hepatology 1986; 6: 1270–1278.

171. Stanley CA, DeLeeuw S, Coates PM, Vianey L, Divry P, Bonnefont JP, Saudubray JM, Haymond M, Trefz FK, Breningstall GN, Wappner R, Byrd D, Sansaricq C, Tein I, Grover W, Valle D, Rutledge S, Treem W. Chronic cardiomyopathy and weakness or acute coma in children with a defect in carnitine uptake. Ann Neurol 1991; 30: 709–716.

172. Van Hove JLK, Zhang W, Kahler SG, Roe CR, Chen Y-T, Terada N, Chace DH, Iafolla AK, Ding J-H, Millington DS. Medium-chain acyl-CoA dehydrogenase (MCAD) deficiency: diagnosis by acylcarnitine analysis in blood. Am J Hum Genet 1993:958–966.

173. Ziadeh R, Hoffman EP, Finegold DN, Hoop RC, Brackett JC, Strauss AW, Naylor EW. Medium chain acyl-CoA dehydrogenase deficiency in Pennsylvania: neonatal screening shows high incidence and unexpected mutation frequencies. Pediatr Res 1995; 37: 675–678.

174. Seymour CA, Thomason MJ, Chalmers RA, Addison GM, Bain MD, Cockburn F, Littlejohns P, Lord J, Wilcox AH. Newborn screening for inborn errors of metabolism: a systematic review. Health Technol Assess 1997; 1: 1–95.

175. Morris AA, Thekekara A, Wilks Z, Clayton PT, Leonard JV, Aynsley-Green A. Evaluation of fasts for investigating hypoglycaemia or suspected metabolic disease. Arch Dis Child 1996; 75: 115–119.

176. Parini R, Garavaglia B, Saudubray JM, Bardelli P, Melotti D, Zecca G, Di Donato S. Clinical diagnosis of long-chain acyl-coenzyme A-dehydrogenase deficiency: use of stress and fat-loading tests. J Pediatr 1991; 119: 77–80.

177. Holtrop PC, Madison KA, Kiechle FL, Karcher RE, Batton DG. A comparison of chromogen test strip (Chemstrip bG) and serum glucose values in newborns. Am J Dis Child 1990; 144: 183–185.

178. Rinaldo P, O'Shea JJ, Coates PM, Hale DE, Stanley CA, Tanaka K. Medium-chain acyl-CoA dehydrogenase deficiency. Diagnosis by stable isotope dilution measurement of urinary n-hexanoylglycine and 3-phenylpropionylglycine. N Engl J Med 1988; 319: 1308–1313.

179. Antunes JD, Geffner ME, Lippe BM, Landaw EM. Childhood hypoglycemia: differentiating hyperinsulinemic from nonhyperinsulinemic causes. J Pediatr 1990; 116: 105–108.

180. Cryer PE. Banting Lecture. Hypoglycemia: the limiting factor in the management of IDDM. Diabetes 1994; 43: 1378–1389.

181. Diabetes Control and Complications Trial Research Group. Hypoglycemia in the Diabetes Control and Complications Trial. Diabetes 1997; 46: 271–286.

182. Gerich JE, Langlois M, Noacco C, Karam JH, Forsham PH. Lack of glucagon response to hypoglycemia in diabetes: evidence for an intrinsic pancreatic alpha cell defect. Science 1973; 182: 171–173.

183. Bolli G, Calabrese G, De Feo P, Compagnucci P, Zega G, Angeletti G, Cartechini MG, Santeusanio F, Brunetti P. Lack of glucagon response in glucose counter-regulation in type 1 (insulin-dependent) diabetics: absence of recovery after prolonged optimal insulin therapy. Diabetologia 1982; 22: 100–105.

184. Cryer PE. Iatrogenic hypoglycemia as a cause of hypoglycemia-associated autonomic failure in IDDM. A vicious cycle. Diabetes 1992; 41: 255–260.

185. Dagogo-Jack SE, Craft S, Cryer PE. Hypoglycemia-associated autonomic failure in insulin-dependent diabetes mellitus. Recent antecedent hypoglycemia reduces autonomic responses to, symptoms of, and defense against subsequent hypoglycemia. J Clin Invest 1993; 91: 819–828.

186. Aman J, Karlsson I, Wranne L. Symptomatic hypoglycaemia in childhood diabetes: a population-based questionnaire study. Diabet Med 1989; 6: 257–261.

187. Bergada I, Suissa S, Dufresne J, Schiffrin A. Severe hypoglycemia in IDDM children. Diabetes Care 1989; 12: 239–244.

188. Egger M, Gschwend S, Smith GD, Zuppinger K. Increas-

ing incidence of hypoglycemic coma in children with IDDM. Diabetes Care 1991; 14: 1001–1005.

189. Bhatia V, Wolfsdorf JI. Severe hypoglycemia in youth with insulin-dependent diabetes mellitus: frequency and causative factors. Pediatrics 1991; 88: 1187–1193.

190. Limbert C, Schwingshandl J, Haas J, Roth R, Borkenstein M. Severe hypoglycemia in children and adolescents with IDDM: frequency and associated factors. J Diabetes Complications 1993; 7: 216–220.

191. Bognetti F, Brunelli A, Meschi F, Viscardi M, Bonfanti R, Chiumello G. Frequency and correlates of severe hypoglycaemia in children and adolescents with diabetes mellitus. Eur J Pediatr 1997; 156: 589–591.

192. Jacobson AM, Hauser ST, Wolfsdorf JI, Houlihan J, Milley JE, Herskowitz RD, Wertlieb D, Watt E. Psychologic predictors of compliance in children with recent onset of diabetes mellitus. J Pediatr 1987; 110: 805–811.

193. Tupola S, Rajantie J. Documented symptomatic hypoglycaemia in children and adolescents using multiple daily insulin injection therapy. Diabet Med 1998; 15: 492–496.

194. Hepburn DA, Deary IJ, Frier BM, Patrick AW, Quinn JD, Fisher BM. Symptoms of acute insulin-induced hypoglycemia in humans with and without IDDM. Factor-analysis approach. Diabetes Care 1991; 14: 949–957.

195. McCrimmon RJ, Gold AE, Deary IJ, Kelnar CJ, Frier BM. Symptoms of hypoglycemia in children with IDDM. Diabetes Care 1995; 18: 858–861.

196. Dammacco F, Torelli C, Frezza E, Piccinno E, Tansella F. Problems of hypoglycemia arising in children and adolescents with insulin-dependent diabetes mellitus. The Diabetes Study Group of The Italian Society of Pediatric Endocrinology & Diabetes. J Pediatr Endocrinol Metab 1998; 11 Suppl 1: 167–176.

197. Boyle PJ, Schwartz NS, Shah SD, Clutter WE, Cryer PE. Plasma glucose concentrations at the onset of hypoglycemic symptoms in patients with poorly controlled diabetes and in nondiabetics. N Engl J Med 1988; 318: 1487–1492.

198. Goldstein DE, England JD, Hess R, Rawlings SS, Walker B. A prospective study of symptomatic hypoglycemia in young diabetic patients. Diabetes Care 1981; 4: 601–605.

199. Macfarlane PI, Walters M, Stutchfield P, Smith CS. A prospective study of symptomatic hypoglycaemia in childhood diabetes. Diabet Med 1989; 6: 627–630.

200. Daneman D, Frank M, Perlman K, Tamm J, Ehrlich R. Severe hypoglycemia in children with insulin-dependent diabetes mellitus: frequency and predisposing factors. J Pediatr 1989; 115: 681–685.

201. Diabetes Control and Complications Trial Research Group. Effect of intensive diabetes treatment on the development and progression of long-term complications in adolescents with insulin-dependent diabetes mellitus: Diabetes Control and Complications Trial. J Pediatr 1994; 125: 177–188.

202. Boland EA, Grey M, Oesterle A, Fredrickson L, Tamborlane WV. Continuous subcutaneous insulin infusion. A new way to lower risk of severe hypoglycemia, improve metabolic control, and enhance coping in adolescents with type 1 diabetes. Diabetes Care 1999; 22: 1779–1784.

203. Ryan CM, Becker DJ. Hypoglycemia in children with type 1 diabetes mellitus: risk factors, cognitive function, and management. Endocrinol Metab Clin North Am 1999; 28: 883–900.

204. Pramming S, Thorsteinsson B, Theilgaard A, Pinner EM, Binder C. Cognitive function during hypoglycaemia in type I diabetes mellitus. Br Med J (Clin Res Ed) 1986; 292: 647–650.

205. Frier BM, Matthews DM, Steel JM, Duncan LJ. Driving and insulin-dependent diabetes. Lancet 1980; 1: 1232–1234.

206. Songer TJ, LaPorte RE, Dorman JS, Orchard TJ, Cruickshanks KJ, Becker DJ, Drash AL. Motor vehicle accidents and IDDM. Diabetes Care 1988; 11: 701–707.

207. Ratner RE Whitehouse FW. Motor vehicles, hypoglycemia, and diabetic drivers. Diabetes Care 1989; 12: 217–222.

208. Brierley J. Brain damage due to hypoglycaemia. In: Marks V, Rose C, eds. Hypoglycaemia. Oxford: Blackwell Scientific Publications, 1981:488–494.

209. Aynsley-Green A, Soltesz G. Hypoglycaemia in infancy and childhood. In: Aynsley-Green A, Chambers T, eds. Current Reviews in Paediatrics. Vol. 1. Edinburgh: Churchill Livingstone, 1985.

210. Edge JA, Ford-Adams ME, Dunger DB. Causes of death in children with insulin dependent diabetes 1990–96. Arch Dis Child 1999; 81: 318–323.

211. Ryan C, Vega A, Drash A. Cognitive deficits in adolescents who developed diabetes early in life. Pediatrics 1985; 75: 921–927.

212. Rovet JF, Ehrlich RM, Hoppe M. Intellectual deficits associated with early onset of insulin-dependent diabetes mellitus in children. Diabetes Care 1987; 10: 510–515.

213. Rovet JF Ehrlich RM. The effect of hypoglycemic seizures on cognitive function in children with diabetes: a 7-year prospective study. J Pediatr 1999; 134: 503–506.

214. Hershey T, Bhargava N, Sadler M, White NH, Craft S. Conventional versus intensive diabetes therapy in children with type 1 diabetes: effects on memory and motor speed. Diabetes Care 1999; 22: 1318–1324.

215. Cox DJ, Irvine A, Gonder-Frederick L, Nowacek G, Butterfield J. Fear of hypoglycemia: quantification, validation, and utilization. Diabetes Care 1987; 10: 617–621.

216. Gonder-Frederick LA, Clarke WL, Cox DJ. The emotional, social, and behavioral implications of insulin-induced hypoglycemia. Semin Clin Neuropsychiatry 1997; 2: 57–65.

217. Clarke WL, Gonder-Frederick A, Snyder AL, Cox DJ. Maternal fear of hypoglycemia in their children with insulin dependent diabetes mellitus. J Pediatr Endocrinol Metab 1998; 11 Suppl 1: 189–194.

218. Santiago JV. Nocturnal hypoglycemia in children with diabetes: an important problem revisited. J Pediatr 1997; 131: 2–4.

219. Soltesz G, Acsadi G. Association between diabetes, severe hypoglycaemia, and electroencephalographic abnormalities. Arch Dis Child 1989; 64: 992–996.

220. Dumont RH, Jacobson AM, Cole C, Hauser ST, Wolfsdorf JI, Willett JB, Milley JE, Wertlieb D. Psychosocial predictors of acute complications of diabetes in youth. Diabet Med 1995; 12: 612–618.

221. Verrotti A, Chiarelli F, Blasetti A, Bruni E, Morgese G. Severe hypoglycemia in insulin-dependent diabetic children treated by multiple injection insulin regimen. Acta Diabetol 1996; 33: 53–57.

222. Mortensen HB, Hougaard P. Comparison of metabolic control in a cross-sectional study of 2,873 children and adolescents with IDDM from 18 countries. The Hvidore Study Group on Childhood Diabetes. Diabetes Care 1997; 20: 714–720.

223. Davis EA, Keating B, Byrne GC, Russell M, Jones TW. Hypoglycemia: incidence and clinical predictors in a large population-based sample of children and adolescents with IDDM. Diabetes Care 1997; 20: 22–25.
224. Nordfeldt S, Ludvigsson J. Severe hypoglycemia in children with IDDM. A prospective population study, 1992–1994. Diabetes Care 1997; 20: 497–503.
225. Davis EA, Keating B, Byrne GC, Russell M, Jones TW. Impact of improved glycaemic control on rates of hypoglycaemia in insulin dependent diabetes mellitus. Arch Dis Child 1998; 78: 111–115.
226. Rosilio M, Cotton JB, Wieliczko MC, Gendrault B, Carel JC, Couvaras O, Ser N, Bougneres PF, Gillet P, Soskin S, Garandeau P, Stuckens C, Le luyer B, Jos J, Bony-Trifunovic H, Bertrand AM, Leturcq F, Lafuma A. Factors associated with glycemic control. A cross-sectional nationwide study in 2,579 French children with type 1 diabetes. The French Pediatric Diabetes Group. Diabetes Care 1998; 21: 1146–1153.
227. Tupola S, Rajantie J, Maenpaa J. Severe hypoglycaemia in children and adolescents during multiple-dose insulin therapy. Diabet Med 1998; 15: 695–699.
228. Lteif AN, Schwenk WF II. Type 1 diabetes mellitus in early childhood: glycemic control and associated risk of hypoglycemic reactions. Mayo Clin Proc 1999; 74: 211–216.
229. Clarke WL, Gonder-Frederick L, Cox DJ. The frequency of severe hypoglycaemia in children with insulin-dependent diabetes mellitus. Horm Res 1996; 45: 48–52.
230. Aynsley-Green A, Eyre J, Soltesz G. Hypoglycaemia in diabetic children. In: Frier BM, Fisher BM, eds. Hypoglycaemia and Diabetes: Clinical and Physiological Aspects. London: Edward Arnold, 1993:228–240.
231. Diabetes Control and Complications Trial Research Group. Epidemiology of severe hypoglycemia in the diabetes control and complications trial. Am J Med 1991; 90: 450–459.
232. Gale EA, Tattersall RB. Unrecognised nocturnal hypoglycaemia in insulin-treated diabetics. Lancet 1979; 1: 1049–1052.
233. Winter RJ. Profiles of metabolic control in diabetic children-frequency of asymptomatic nocturnal hypoglycaemia. Metabolism 1981; 30: 666–672.
234. Shalwitz RA, Farkas-Hirsch R, White NH, Santiago JV. Prevalence and consequences of nocturnal hypoglycemia among conventionally treated children with diabetes mellitus. J Pediatr 1990; 116: 685–689.
235. Porter PA, Byrne G, Stick S, Jones TW. Nocturnal hypoglycaemia and sleep disturbances in young teenagers with insulin dependent diabetes mellitus. Arch Dis Child 1996; 75: 120–123.
236. Porter PA, Keating B, Byrne G, Jones TW. Incidence and predictive criteria of nocturnal hypoglycemia in young children with insulin-dependent diabetes mellitus. J Pediatr 1997; 130: 366–372.
237. Beregszaszi M, Tubiana-Rufi N, Benali K, Noel M, Bloch J, Czernichow P. Nocturnal hypoglycemia in children and adolescents with insulin-dependent diabetes mellitus: prevalence and risk factors. J Pediatr 1997; 131: 27–33.
238. Lopez MJ, Oyarzabal M, Barrio R, Hermoso F, Lopez JP, Rodriguez M, Blasco L, Gastaldo E. Nocturnal hypoglycaemia in IDDM patients younger than 18 years. Diabet Med 1997; 14: 772–777.
239. Jones TW, Porter P, Sherwin RS, Davis EA, O'Leary P, Frazer F, Byrne G, Stick S, Tamborlane WV. Decreased epinephrine responses to hypoglycemia during sleep. N Engl J Med 1998; 338: 1657–1662.
240. Veneman T, Mitrakou A, Mokan M, Cryer P, Gerich J. Induction of hypoglycemia unawareness by asymptomatic nocturnal hypoglycemia. Diabetes 1993; 42: 1233–1237.
241. Brodows RG, Williams C, Amatruda JM. Treatment of insulin reactions in diabetics. JAMA 1984; 252: 3378–3381.
242. Wiethop BV Cryer PE. Alanine and terbutaline in treatment of hypoglycemia in IDDM. Diabetes Care 1993; 16: 1131–1136.
243. Aman J, Wranne L. Treatment of hypoglycemia in diabetes: failure of absorption of glucose through rectal mucosa. Acta Paediatr Scand 1984; 73: 560–561.
244. Aman J Wranne L. Hypoglycaemia in childhood diabetes. II. Effect of subcutaneous or intramuscular injection of different doses of glucagon. Acta Paediatr Scand 1988; 77: 548–553.
245. Muhlhauser I, Koch J, Berger M. Pharmacokinetics and bioavailability of injected glucagon: differences between intramuscular, subcutaneous, and intravenous administration. Diabetes Care 1985; 8: 39–42.
246. Slama G, Alamowitch C, Desplanque N, Letanoux M, Zirinis P. A new non-invasive method for treating insulin-reaction: intranasal lyophylized glucagon. Diabetologia 1990; 33: 671–674.
247. Lala VR, Vedanarayana VV, Ganesh S, Fray C, Iosub S, Noto R. Hypoglycemic hemiplegia in an adolescent with insulin-dependent diabetes mellitus: a case report and a review of the literature. J Emerg Med 1989; 7: 233–236.
248. Wayne EA, Dean HJ, Booth F, Tenenbein M. Focal neurologic deficits associated with hypoglycemia in children with diabetes. J Pediatr 1990; 117: 575–577.
249. Shehadeh N, Kassem J, Tchaban I, Ravid S, Shahar E, Naveh T, Etzioni A. High incidence of hypoglycemic episodes with neurologic manifestations in children with insulin dependent diabetes mellitus. J Pediatr Endocrinol Metab 1998; 11 Suppl 1: 183–187.
250. Agus MS, Katz LE, Satin-Smith M, Meadows AT, Hintz RL, Cohen P. Non-islet-cell tumor associated with hypoglycemia in a child: successful long-term therapy with growth hormone. J Pediatr 1995; 127: 403–407.
251. Hizuka N, Fukuda I, Takano K, Okubo Y, Asakawa-Yasumoto K, Demura H. Serum insulin-like growth factor II in 44 patients with non-islet cell tumor hypoglycemia. Endocr J 1998; 45 Suppl: S61–S65.
252. Gitzelmann R, Hirsig J. Infant dumping syndrome: reversal of symptoms by feeding uncooked cornstarch. Eur J Pediatr 1986; 145: 504–506.
253. Rivkees SA, Crawford JD. Hypoglycemia pathogenesis in children with dumping syndrome. Pediatrics 1987; 80: 937–942.
254. Babovic-Vuksanovic D, Patterson MC, Schwenk WF, O'Brien JF, Vockley J, Freeze HH, Mehta DP, Michels VV. Severe hypoglycemia as a presenting symptom of carbohydrate-deficient glycoprotein syndrome. J Pediatr 1999; 135: 775–781.
255. Bennett MJ Sherwood WG. 3-Hydroxydicarboxylic and 3-ketodicarboxylic aciduria in three patients: evidence for a new defect in fatty acid oxidation at the level of 3-ketoacyl-CoA thiolase. Clin Chem 1993; 39: 897–901.
256. Kamijo T, Indo Y, Souri M, Aoyama T, Hara T, Yamamoto S, Ushikubo S, Rinaldo P, Matsuda I, Komiyama A, Hashimoto T. Medium chain 3-ketoacyl-coenzyme A thiolase deficiency: a new disorder of mitochondrial fatty acid beta-oxidation. Pediatr Res 1997; 42: 569–576.

25

Diabetes in the Child and Adolescent

Arlan L. Rosenbloom and Janet H. Silverstein
University of Florida College of Medicine, Gainesville, Florida, U.S.A.

I. INTRODUCTION

Until the 1970s, the care and investigation of childhood diabetes were pursued by internists, pediatricians, nephrologists, and general physicians. In 1971 it was estimated that visits for diabetes by those 0–15 years of age were equally divided among internists, general physicians, and general pediatricians (1). At that time there were few pediatric endocrinologists, virtually none in private practice, and most of them did not consider diabetes to be an endocrine disorder. The third (1965) edition of what was then the only textbook of pediatric endocrinology devotes a short paragraph to diabetes mellitus as one of half a dozen causes of hyperglycemia (2). By 1993, pediatric endocrinologists accounted for 35% of all visits of 0–21-year-old diabetes patients and nearly half of these were to private practicing pediatric endocrinologists; the remainder included 37% to internists (most likely the older adolescents and young adults) and 28% to general pediatricians (3). In pediatric endocrinology practice, diabetes now accounts for 50–60% of the workload (3). The movement of diabetology into mainstream pediatric endocrinology has multiple causes beyond the clinical importance and challenge of the problem, including the scientific excitement about diabetes research (and its funding), the extensive endocrine physiology that diabetes affects, and the inclusion of diabetes in the accreditation requirements of training programs and board certification for pediatric endocrinology.

This history deserves consideration and reflection because we are presently engaged in a comparable revolution in what is considered to be within the purview of pediatric endocrinology. The contemporary epidemic of type 2 diabetes in youth has confronted pediatric diabetes specialists with a major responsibility for a condition previously rare in the pediatric age group. Furthermore, pediatric endocrinologists have had to reconsider the associated problem of obesity, which has long been a frequent

reason for referral to the endocrine clinic, but rarely dealt with after ruling out unusual syndromic or medical causes. As they earlier did for diabetes, pediatric diabetologists are becoming involved in creating teams to deal with this difficult and growing clinical challenge of obesity and type 2 diabetes.

II. DIAGNOSIS AND CLASSIFICATION

The diagnosis of diabetes includes a wide variety of diseases characterized by hyperglycemia. Because insulin is the only physiologically significant hypoglycemic hormone, hyperglycemia is the result of either impaired secretion of insulin from the beta cells of the pancreas (type 1 diabetes) or resistance to the effect of insulin in the liver, muscle, and fat cells exceeding a limited capacity of the pancreas to compensate (type 2 diabetes). Criteria for the diagnosis of diabetes have recently been revised and categories of impaired glucose tolerance and impaired fasting glucose added, reflecting the recognition that these preclinical glucose intolerance states are associated with increased cardiovascular morbidity (4). Table 1 lists the current recommendations of the American Diabetes Association (4). There is no reason to apply different criteria with children and adolescents.

In 1997 the American Diabetes Association published revisions of the classification of diabetes, based on etiology, and these were modified in 1999 (4). Early taxonomy had the common forms of diabetes separated by age of onset (juvenile and maturity or adult), which a 1979 report of the U.S. National Diabetes Data Group revised to emphasize treatment, using the terms insulin-dependent (IDDM) and noninsulin-dependent diabetes (NIDDM) for the principal forms (5). Contemporary understanding of the pathogenesis of various forms of diabetes has made this classification based on treatment inappropriate. Table 2 is adapted from the classification published by the ADA expert committee (4).

A. Type 1 Diabetes

Diabetes occurring in childhood remains predominantly immune-mediated type 1 disease associated with histocompatibility locus (HLA) specificities. Type 1 diabetes will be discussed in detail in the next section. Idiopathic type 1 diabetes may be difficult to differentiate from the immune-mediated form. Many, if not most, African-American patients who have type 1 disease without evidence of autoimmunity have what has been termed atypical diabetes mellitus (ADM) or Flatbush diabetes (6, 7). This condition has its onset throughout childhood and rarely past age 40, and is not associated with HLA specificities. Further characteristics are described in Table 3.

B. Type 2 Diabetes

Type 2 diabetes in childhood and adolescence now accounts for 10–50% of new patients with diabetes in this age group, depending on the ethnic/racial mix of the population served (8). Detailed discussion of this form of diabetes is in a subsequent section and the characteristics are listed in Table 3.

C. Maturity-Onset Diabetes of the Young

This is a stable form of youth-onset (under 25 years of age) diabetes inherited in an autosomal dominant fashion and affecting almost exclusively white patients (Table 3). Six molecular causes of MODY have been identified, affecting beta-cell function. Its frequency among patients with diabetes is reported to vary from <0.2 to 5% in various populations (9).

D. Mitochondrial Mutations

Diabetes and deafness may be associated as a result of mutations in mitochondrial DNA (10–12).

Table 1   Criteria for the Diagnosis of Diabetes

Symptoms plus random plasma glucose concentration >200 mg/dl (11 mmol/l), *or*
Fasting plasma glucose >126 mg/dl (7 mmol/l), *or*
2 h plasma glucose >200 mg/dl (11 mmol/l) during oral glucose tolerance test (OGTT). The test should be performed using a glucose load containing the equivalent of 75 g anhydrous glucose dissolved in water for those weighing >43 kg and 1.75 g/kg for those weighing <43 kg.
   In the absence of marked hyperglycemia with decompensation, these criteria should be confirmed by repeat testing on a different day. OGTT is not recommended for routine clinical use.
   Impaired glucose tolerance = 2 h plasma glucose 140–200 mg/dl
   Impaired fasting glucose = 110–125 mg/dl

Table 2   Classification of Causes of Diabetes Mellitus

I. Type 1 diabetes[a] (β-cell destruction), usually leading to absolute insulin deficiency

   A. Immune-mediated
   B. Idiopathic

II. Type 2 diabetes[a]: may range from predominantly insulin resistance with relative insulin deficiency to a predominantly secretory defect with insulin resistance

III. Other specific types

   A. Genetic defects of β-cell function
      1. Maturity-onset diabetes of the young
      2. Mitochondrial defects

   B. Genetic defects in insulin action
      1. Type A insulin resistance
      2. Leprechaunism
      3. Rabson-Mendenhall syndrome
      4. Lipoatrophic diabetes

   C. Diseases of the exocrine pancreas
      1. Pancreatitis
      2. Trauma/pancreatectomy
      3. Neoplasia
      4. Cystic fibrosis
      5. Hemochromatosis
      6. Fibrocalculous pancreatopathy

   D. Endocrinopathies
      1. Acromegaly
      2. Cushing syndrome
      3. Glucagonoma
      4. Pheochromocytoma
      5. Hyperthyroidism
      6. Somatostatinoma
      7. Aldosteronoma

   E. Drug- or chemical-induced
      1. Vacor
      2. Pentamidine
      3. Nicotinic acid
      4. Glucocorticoids
      5. Thyroid hormone
      6. Diazoxide
      7. β-adrenergic agonists
      8. Thiazides
      9. Dilantin
      10. α-Interferon

   F. Infections
      1. Congenital rubella
      2. Cytomegalovirus

   G. Uncommon forms
      1. "Stiff-man" syndrome
      2. Anti-insulin receptor antibodies

Table 2 Continued

   H. Other genetic syndromes sometimes associated with diabetes

      1. Down syndrome
      2. Klinefelter syndrome
      3. Turner syndrome
      4. Wolfram syndrome
      5. Friedreich ataxia
      6. Huntington chorea
      7. Laurence-Moon-Biedl syndrome
      8. Myotonic dystrophy
      9. Porphyria
     10. Prader-Willi syndrome

IV. Gestational diabetes mellitus

[a]Patients with any form of diabetes may require insulin treatment at some stage of their disease. Such use of insulin does not, of itself, classify the patient's disease.

E. Genetic Defects in Insulin Action

Genetically determined abnormalities of insulin action are very rare as a cause of diabetes, ranging from mild hyperinsulinemia with modest hyperglycemia to severe diabetes (13). The structure and function of the insulin receptor are intact in the insulin resistance of lipoatrophic diabetes, indicating that the defect lies in postreceptor transduction (14).

F. Diseases of the Exocrine Pancreas

Diffuse injury to the pancreas needs to be relatively extensive to result in diabetes, because of the small volume occupied by the beta cells, with the exception of carcinoma involving the pancreas, which is a condition not seen in children. With improved survival, increasing numbers of patients with cystic fibrosis are developing diabetes (15).

G. Endocrinopathies

Diabetes has been described in adults with hormone excess syndromes including acromegaly, Cushing syndrome, glucagonoma, and pheochromocytoma (16). There has been recent concern about the use of pharmacological doses of growth hormone in children who do not have growth hormone deficiency, which may be increasing the risk for type 2 diabetes (17, 18).

H. Drug- or Chemical-Induced Diabetes

A large number of drugs used in pediatric care can impair insulin secretion, increase gluconeogenesis, or increase insulin resistance, resulting in hyperglycemia or the precipitation of diabetes in a susceptible individual (19, 20). The rat poison, Vacor, and pentamidine given intravenously can permanently destroy beta cells (21–24). Other drugs can impair insulin action, probably the most common being glucocorticoids (19, 20).

I. Infections

Numerous viruses have been implicated in the induction of diabetes, but the strongest evidence of direct causation comes from the experience with congenital rubella (25) which is, fortunately, now rarely seen.

Table 3 Classification of the Types of Diabetes Seen in Children

	Type 1	ADM	MODY	Type 2
Age at onset	Throughout childhood	Pubertal	Pubertal	Pubertal
Predominant race or ethnic distribution	All (low frequency in Asians)	African American (AA)	White	Nonwhite Hispanic, AA, Native American
Onset	Acute, severe	Acute, severe	Subtle	Subtle to severe
Islet autoimmunity	Present	Absent	Absent	Unusual
Insulin secretion	Very low	Moderately low	Variable	Variable
Insulin sensitivity	Normal (with BG[b] control)	Normal	Normal	Decreased
Ketosis, DKA at onset	Up to 40%	Common	Rare	Up to 33%
Obesity	As in population	As in population	Uncommon	>90%
Proportion of diabetes	~70–80%[a]	<10%	<5%	20–25%[a]
Percentage of probands with affected first-degree relative	5–10%	>75%	100%	~80%
Mode of inheritance	Nonmendelian, generally sporadic	Autosomal dominant	Autosomal dominant	Nonmendelian, strongly familial

[a]The proportion of pediatric diabetes patients having type 2 diabetes will vary with racial/ethnic mix of the population and it is increasing.
[b]BG = blood glucose.
Source: Adapted from Ref. 26.

The distinctions indicated by the typical features in Table 3 are not always as certain as one would like. There are a number of reasons for difficulties in classification. With the increased frequency of obesity in childhood, a substantial number of newly diagnosed type 1 patients and ADM patients will be obese, raising the question of type 2 disease. Because some type 2 patients and almost all ADM have ketoacidosis, this feature is not helpful for differentiating non-type 1 from type 1 diabetes. The specificity of a family history of type 2 disease is low because of the high frequency of this disorder in the general population, particularly in populations of nonwhite heritage. Furthermore, a family history of type 2 diabetes is three times as likely with type 1 diabetes as in the general population; conversely, type 1 diabetes is more frequent in the relatives of patients with type 2 disease. Genetic interaction between type 1 and type 2 diabetes is further suggested by HLA haplotype interaction and the finding of islet autoimmunity markers at onset in some children and adults with typical type 2 disease (27). Insulin or C-peptide measurements at the onset of diabetes may not be helpful because of the recovery phase of autoimmune diabetes indicating reasonable beta cell function and, conversely, glucose toxicity/lipotoxicity in nonautoimmune diabetes, which may impair insulin secretion at the time of testing.

A study of 700 newly diagnosed 5–19-year-old patients from three university centers in Florida over a 5 year period indicated that 3% of those initially classified as having type 1 diabetes (17/605) were later classified as having type 2 disease; 8% of those initially diagnosed as type 2 disease were subsequently reclassified as having type 1 diabetes (6/77) (28). Most of the 17 originally considered to have type 1 disease and later determined to have type 2 diabetes were diagnosed with ketosis or in ketoacidosis. Those six with an initial diagnosis of type 2 diabetes who were subsequently considered to have type 1 disease were, typically, overweight youngsters without diabetes-related antibodies; however, over the next few years they had a clinical course most consistent with type 1 disease. In this relatively sophisticated clinical setting, the proportion of patients in whom classification may be problematic is less than 5% of newly diagnosed children and youth.

Table 4 summarizes clinical characteristics that are helpful in differentiating type 1 and type 2 diabetes in children and adolescents. In those with acute onset who are not obese, and not African-American, type 1 diabetes is highly likely and further testing is not necessary. Non-obese African-American youngsters with acute-onset diabetes who have a three-generation family history of diabetes indicative of autosomal dominant transmission and do not have islet autoimmunity markers are very likely to have ADM. Islet cell autoimmunity testing should be considered in obese patients who have acute onset; if this is not practical or if the patient has acanthosis nigricans, the ability to reduce and stop the acutely required insulin over

the first several months, with weight reduction, exercise, and oral hypoglycemic therapy as necessary, will clarify the diagnosis.

With insidious onset, obese individuals can be considered to have type 2 disease. If the patient is lean, islet autoantibody testing will be helpful and, if results are positive, indicate early detection of type 1 diabetes. Absence of islet cell autoimmunity in the lean individual may indicate MODY, in which case testing of family members will be productive; the pattern of autosomal dominant transmission may not emerge unless apparently unaffected family members are tested. Fasting C-peptide or insulin measurements may be of value, with elevated levels indicative of type 2 diabetes; repeated testing after 1 year or more may be needed for those who have normal results.

III. TYPE 1 DIABETES

A. Epidemiology

The terminology used in discussing the epidemiology of disease includes the following (29):

Incidence: The number of cases diagnosed in a given period of time, within a population or segment thereof, such as males and females, 10–20-year-olds, and so on. For chronic diseases such as diabetes, this is usually expressed as new cases per 100,000 population per year.
Prevalence: The number of cases within a population or a specific segment of the population at any time. This is a cross-section and is usually expressed as number of cases per 1000 individuals.
Frequency: This nonspecific term can denote either prevalence or incidence, or both, depending on how it is used.
Epidemic: A greater number of cases than expected.

The past 20 years have seen a phenomenal increase in knowledge about the epidemiological patterns of type 1 diabetes, which was anticipated to provide insight into the critical environmental contribution to the development of this disease (30). This information has heightened the appreciation of the likely complexity and importance of environmental causation, while casting little light on what those environmental factors might be. The Multi-National Project for Childhood Diabetes (DiaMonde) study was initiated by the World Health Organization in 1990 to investigate and monitor the patterns of incidence of type 1 diabetes (31). This remarkable study encompasses surveillance of 4.5% of the world's population 14 years of age and under, representing probably the largest standardized survey undertaken for any disease (32).

From 1990 to 1994, a total of nearly 20,000 cases of type 1 diabetes in children ≤14 years were diagnosed in the 75 million sample population, and incidence rates calculated per 100,000. There was a >350 fold variation in incidence among the 100 populations studied, from 0.1:100,000 per year in China and Venezuela to 36.8:100,000

Table 4 Differentiating Type 1 from Type 2 Diabetes in Children and Adolescents

Characteristics	Type 1	Type 2	Comment
Demographics			
Family history	3%–5%	74%–100%	Extensive family history suggests T2; T2 affects minorities disproportionately.
Age or pubertal status	Variable	>10 or pubertal[a]	Type 1 can occur at any age; only 10% of type 2 children are younger than 10 or prepubertal.
Gender	F = M	F > M	Some gender difference in T2 may reflect differences in use of medical care.
Presentation			
Asymptomatic	Rare	Common	Type 2 often detected incidentally on routine physical exam.
Symptom duration	Days or weeks	Weeks or months	Predominant symptoms are polyuria, polydipsia, polyphagia, and nocturia.
Weight loss	Common	Common	Type 2 children lose more pounds; type 1 usually lose greater percentage of body weight.
HHS	Very rare	Occurs	Type 2 can develop severe, fatal dehydration, and electrolyte disturbance.
Physical findings			
BMI at diagnosis	≤75 percentile	≤85 percentile	Those with BMI 75–85th percentile often present greatest diagnostic challenge.
Acanthosis	No	Common	Useful marker in hyperglycemic child.
Biochemical findings at diagnosis			
Hyperglycemia	Variable	Variable	Degree of hyperglycemia at diagnosis is not useful in delineating diabetes type.
Ketosis and ketonuria	Common	Common	Not useful for diagnosis of diabetes type.
Acidosis	Common	Moderately common	Not useful for diagnosis of diabetes type.
Other markers			
HbA_1	Elevated	Elevated	Not useful for diagnosis of diabetes type.
Insulin or C-peptide/serum	Low (may be nl early)	Normal-high	Hyperinsulinism reflects insulin resistance. Low levels may be found in type 2 at diagnosis, repeat 3–6 months after diagnosis may be elevated.
Autoimmune markers	Common	Uncommon	Includes anti-islet cell and anti-GAD antibodies; absence does not rule out T1.

[a] Occasionally in 8–10-year-old group and as young as 4 years.
Source: Adapted from Hale DE. Type 2 diabetes: an increasing pediatric problem.

per year in Sardinia and 36.5:100,000 per year in Finland. Very high incidence, considered ≥20:100,000 per year, was also found in Sweden, Norway, Portugal, the United Kingdom, Canada, and New Zealand. When the population was divided into 5 year age groups, incidence increased with age and was highest among those 10–14 years old. Wide variation was seen between neighboring areas in Europe and North America. For example, the rate in Estonia (10.5:100,000) is less than one-third that of Finland. In North America, Alberta and Prince Edward Island have comparable rates of 24 and 24.5:100,000, whereas US rates vary from 11.7:100,000 in Chicago to 17.8:100,000 in Pennsylvania. While the rate in Puerto Rico, 17.4:100,000 is virtually identical to that in Pennsylvania, that in neighboring and ethnically similar Cuba

is only 2.9:100,000 (32). The prevalence of type 1 diabetes is estimated to be 1.7–2.5:1000 in the school-age population younger than 18 years in the United States (33).

Migrant populations provide an interesting perspective on environmental contributions to the development of type 1 diabetes. A number of observations have indicated that susceptibility is affected by environmental change. Japanese living in Hawaii are five times more likely to have type 1 diabetes than those in Japan, a country with a very low incidence of type 1 diabetes. Ethnic French and Italian children in Montreal have twice the incidence of diabetes as those in their native lands (34–36). Israeli children in Canada have a fourfold greater incidence than those in Israel (32). Indian children migrating from South

Africa, where type 1 diabetes in the Indian population is very low, to England had incidence rates comparable to those of English children in the community (33).

There is considerable evidence for an increasing frequency of type 1 diabetes, which is a further profound argument for environmental influences. The temporal trend has been one of steadily increasing incidence in northern European countries (38, 39); Sweden and Norway have reported a 3.3% annual increase while Finland has reported a 2.4% annual rise in incidence (40, 41). Epidemics have been described outside Europe, one striking report being a single year nearly sixfold increase in the Virgin Islands in 1984 (42). There is also evidence that the average age of onset of diabetes is decreasing (43). Consistent with the occasional observation of an epidemic increase in type 1 diabetes, modest seasonality has been documented, with a summertime dip that occurs in both northern and southern parts of the United States (38, 44, 45).

B. Etiology and Prevention

Type 1 diabetes is an autoimmune disease with a long preclinical course. Patients who are genetically predisposed are exposed to an environmental trigger that initiates autoimmune destruction of beta cells. This results in the release of antigens that had previously not been seen by the immune system, resulting in production of antibodies to these antigens. The appearance of insulin autoantibodies, islet cell antibodies, glutamic acid decarboxylase (GAD_{65}) antibodies, and antibodies to tyrosine phosphatase (IA-2 or ICA512) indicates ongoing autoimmune disease. These antibodies may be present in the serum for several years before the development of overt diabetes. As the autoimmune process continues, there is gradual loss of beta-cell mass. The first demonstrable abnormality is loss of first-phase insulin release (FPIR) during intravenous glucose tolerance testing (IVGTT). This is followed by abnormal results of oral glucose tolerance testing and, finally, overt diabetes (46).

The presence of immune markers before the onset of diabetes has allowed for the development of prediction models to determine who is at risk for developing disease. The immunoassays (GAD_{65}, IA-2) are more easily applied for large-scale use than previous assays for islet cell autoimmunity, have a high predictive value for type 1 diabetes, and are more reproducible than islet-cell antibody assays. GAD_{65} antibodies are present in 80% of relatives with newly diagnosed diabetes and IA-2 are present in 50–60% of patients at diabetes onset (46). Multiple autoantibodies to islet antigens confer a cumulative risk of 75–90% over 5–10 years of follow-up in first-degree relatives (47–49). Other risk factors include young age, high-titer antibodies, low first-phase insulin response to IVGTT, and high-risk HLA (DR3/4, DQB0302/DQB0201) (50, 51). The persistent loss of FPIR secretion during IVGTT pre-

dicts progression to overt diabetes over the next 5 years in >85% (52).

Because of this ability to predict diabetes, several trials designed to prevent the disease in high-risk individuals have been initiated. Initial studies were aimed at treatment of newly diagnosed patients with immunosuppressive agents. Cyclosporine appeared promising: there was increased frequency and duration of clinical remission as determined by residual C-peptide secretion, but remission was not long lived and the effect was lost when the cyclosporine was discontinued (53). Furthermore, reports of cyclosporine-induced nephrotoxicity led to concern about the relative risk/benefit ratio of this form of therapy and studies were stopped (54). Azathioprine was also used in patients with newly diagnosed diabetes. Again, the increased C-peptide levels seen in treated patients compared to controls was a short-lived effect despite continued use of the immunosuppressive agent. Predictors of success with these agents were older age, lack of ketoacidosis at diagnosis, early initiation of treatment, and higher C-peptide levels at diabetes onset (55). Treatment with high-dose insulin using the Biostator, a device that measured venous blood glucose every few minutes and provided intravenous insulin to maintain normoglycemia, was as effective in preserving C-peptide as was azathioprine. However, as with the immunosuppressive agents, the results were transient (56). Because of the lack of adequate efficacy to justify the potential toxicities of the immunosuppressive agents used, efforts were made to design trials using safer agents and to initiate treatment at an earlier stage of the disease (i.e., before the appearance of diabetes).

1. North American Diabetes Prevention Trial 1

The North American Diabetes Prevention Trial 1 (DPT-1) was designed to determine if antigen-based therapy could prevent diabetes in at-risk individuals. Insulin was used as the antigen, based on studies showing that low-dose parenteral insulin given to ICA-positive relatives with low FPIR resulted in reduced development of diabetes compared to controls who refused insulin prophylaxis (57). In the DPT-1, patients with ICA were considered high risk if they had low FPIR to IVGTT (>50% risk of developing diabetes over 5 years) and were randomized to receive low-dose subcutaneous insulin or no intervention. Subjects with ICA and normal FPIR were assigned to the intermediate-risk group (25–50% chance of developing diabetes over 5 years) and were randomly assigned to receive oral insulin or placebo. The study revealed no differences in development of diabetes between the high-risk insulin-treated group and controls (58). Enrollment for the oral insulin arm of the study is expected to be complete by 2003. Regardless of the outcome of this large multicenter trial, this undertaking has resulted in the formation of an integrated network with core laboratories providing standardized testing and a centralized data/statistical center, providing a framework for future multicenter intervention trials.

2. Nicotinamide

Nicotinamide is a free radical scavenger that interferes with the autoimmune destruction of beta cells, primarily by acting as an antioxidant. Nicotinamide therapy restores cellular NAD^+ levels, helps to prevent damage from inflammatory macrophages, and promotes increased beta-cell regenerative capacity (59, 60). Animal models have shown nicotinamide to be effective in preventing diabetes. Because nicotinamide is a safe drug, its initial positive results in animal models, as well as in population based studies in New Zealand (below), made it an attractive candidate for diabetes prevention trials.

Nicotinamide decreased the incidence of type 1 diabetes by 41% in a study involving 80,000 5–7-year-old New Zealand school children (61, 62). Among the 20,000 children tested for ICA, 185 were positive and 173 of them accepted treatment with nicotinamide for upwards of 7 years; the incidence of type 1 diabetes in the treated group was ~7:100,000, which was significantly lower than the 16–18:100,000 per year incidence in the background population. These findings led to the initiation of a large European multicenter study, the European Nicotinamide Diabetes Intervention Trial (ENDIT). This trial is a double-blind placebo-controlled study enrolling first-degree relatives who have islet cell antibodies. Enrollment began in 1994 and was completed in 1998. Final results are anticipated in 2003. ENDIT screened 50,000 first-degree relatives of children with type 1 diabetes. Of these, 552 subjects had islet cell antibodies with normal oral glucose testing. The interim analysis demonstrated that none of the criteria for stopping the study had been met: there was neither a higher nor lower incidence of diabetes in the nicotinamide group, using a p value <0.0001 (63).

The Deutsche Nicotinamide Intervention Study (DENIS) was a randomized placebo-controlled trial comparing nicotinamide with placebo in 2415 siblings of children with type 1 diabetes from Germany and Austria. Of those screened, 164 siblings had islet cell antibody titers and, of those, 68 agreed to be randomized to receive nicotinamide or placebo. The study was terminated early (after 2 years) because of failure to demonstrate efficacy of nicotinamide over placebo. Indeed, FPIR during IVGTT was decreased in the nicotinamide group at 2 years compared to the placebo group, in which it remained stable (64).

3. Environmental Triggers

The importance of environmental factors in the initiation of the autoimmune response that ultimately results in diabetes is suggested by the observations that only 30% of identical monozygotic twins are concordant for type 1 diabetes and the incidence of diabetes is rising, with a decrease in mean age of onset, despite a stable genetic pool

(65–67). Several agents have been implicated, but only those figuring in preventive trials will be discussed here. Particularly interesting is the report that vitamin D supplementation of a large group of infants in northern Finland was associated with a relative risk of 0.16 compared to those who did not receive vitamin D (relative risk = 1) (68). Many other factors have been linked to increased risk of diabetes, including perinatal insult, exposure to nitrosamine (69–71), and lack of exposure to early infection (72).

a. Cow's Milk. One of the proposed triggers of diabetes is cow's milk, thought to be due to the structural similarity of a 17 aminoacid fragment (ABBOS) of bovine serum albumin to an islet antigen (ICA 69). This structural similarity invoked the concept of molecular mimicry as the mechanism for autoimmune destruction of beta cells. This hypothesis is controversial, however, with conflicting studies reported. Although Karjalainen et al. found antibodies to bovine serum albumin in children with new-onset diabetes, but not controls (73), the Diabetes Autoimmunity Study of the Young (DAISY) found no association between islet autoimmunity and early cow's milk exposure (74). The Trial to Reduce Type 1 Diabetes in the Genetically at Risk (TRIGR) was designed to test the hypothesis that avoidance of nutritional cow's milk proteins for at least the first 6 months of life would reduce diabetes in the high-risk population. Infants with high-risk HLA genotypes DQB10302 and/or DQB10201 and who were negative for the protective genotypes DQB10602, 0603, or 030 were offered enrollment. Two hundred thirty-four infants have been randomized. Mothers were encouraged to breastfeed. The intervention group received a caseine hydrolysate formula after full breastfeeding, whereas the control group received the cow's-milk-containing formula. The intervention group was advised to avoid beef and cow's milk products in the diet. Fifteen percent of the infants dropped out of the study before 8 months and those infants randomized into the intervention group remained breastfed longer than did those in the control group (8.1 vs 7.2 months). Antibodies to IA-2, insulin, GAD, and islet cell cytoplasm were measured in 173 children at 2 years of age. At least one autoantibody was present in 3.6% of the caseine hydrolysate group and 11.2% of the control group (75). This 10 year prospective trial is not yet complete.

b. Viral Agents/Vaccines. Maternal infection with enterovirus has been reported to increase diabetes risk in the offspring. Studies from Sweden and Finland found increased IgM antibodies to enterovirus in pregnant women whose children subsequently developed diabetes compared to control women (76, 77). Molecular mimicry between the P2-D protein of coxsackievirus and the GAD protein make this an attractive hypothesis. Other viruses implicated have been rubella (acquired in utero), chickenpox, mumps, measles, ECHO, and rotavirus (78, 79). Immunization with diphtheria–pertussis–tetanus and with

Hemophilus influenzae vaccines has also been reportedly associated with increased incidence of type 1 diabetes (80). An expert panel of the National Institutes of Health found no evidence for a relationship between immunizations and diabetes, however.

One approach to diabetes prevention is to shield those who are genetically at risk from potential initiators of pancreatic autoimmunity. The Pediatric Assessment of Newborns for Diabetes Autoimmunity (PANDA) study is a pilot effort in which infants have filter-paper HLA typing done at birth with the rest of the standard neonatal screening (81). Those babies with highest HLA risk haplotypes (DR3 and DR4, DQA0302/501 and DQB0301, 0201) have blood drawn for determination of islet cell antibodies. The families keep records of foods eaten, immunizations, and illnesses and the subjects are tested for islet autoantibodies every 6 months in the initial few years, and then annually. Correlations of the appearance of islet autoimmunity with history of environmental exposure may help to identify the environmental factors that trigger the autoimmune cascade to permit specific preventive intervention.

C. Clinical Picture

Children with type 1 diabetes mellitus are typically diagnosed because of symptoms of polyuria, polydipsia, and weight loss. The classic sign of polyphagia is frequently absent in children, and they are likely to have loss of appetite, presumably because their ketosis results in anorexia. Preschool children often have a shorter duration of symptoms and are more likely to have ketoacidosis with vomiting and lethargy at diabetes diagnosis than are older children. Enuresis in a previously toilet-trained child, or nocturia, may be the first clue to polyuria. Loss of weight despite increased dietary intake is due to tissue catabolism, with gluconeogenesis and urinary glucose loss.

Pyogenic skin infections, candidal diaper rash in babies and toddlers, monilial vaginitis in teenage girls, or dysuria may be present at the time of diagnosis. These findings are rarely isolated features of diabetes in children, and careful history will invariably reveal the coexistence of polyuria and polydipsia. The dehydration associated with polyuria may result in nonspecific symptoms of constipation, headache, and abdominal pain, often interpreted as a viral syndrome, or gastroenteritis if there is vomiting. Ketoacidosis (DKA) is present in 15–40% of newly diagnosed children, depending on the sociodemographic characteristics of the population. Clinical features of DKA are listed in Chapter 27. Vomiting without diarrhea, and continued high urine output despite circumstances associated with dehydration, indicate diabetes.

Children in whom diabetes must be considered may, for practical purposes, be divided into three general categories: those who have typical signs and symptoms of diabetes: polyuria, polydipsia, and weight loss; those who

have glucosuria, without hyperglycemia; and those with transient hyperglycemia.

Renal glucosuria may be an isolated congenital disorder, a feature of Fanconi's syndrome and other renal tubular disorders, due to severe heavy metal intoxication, ingestion of certain drugs (e.g., outdated tetracylcine), or result from inborn errors of metabolism such as cystinosis. When vomiting, diarrhea, or inadequate intake of food occurs in any of these conditions, starvation ketosis may ensue and simulate diabetic ketoacidosis. The absence of hyperglycemia eliminates the possibility of diabetes. Stress of illness, especially in toddlers, may be associated with glucosuria and moderate hyperglycemia. Blood glucose levels usually do not exceed 300–400 mg/dl (17–20 mmol/l), but values up to 800 mg/dl (44 mmol/l) have been reported. This usually occurs in the context of acute exacerbation of asthma or during a hospital admission for infection or other serious illness. The hyperglycemia is usually transient and blood glucose levels normalize with resolution of illness. A similar clinical picture can be seen with glucocorticoid administration (19, 20). The presence of ICA, IA-2, IAA, or GAD antibodies with stress- or glucocorticoid-induced hyperglycemia may indicate limited beta-cell reserve and risk for future development of diabetes (46). Thus, autoantibodies against islet antigens should be measured in all instances of stress hyperglycemia.

D. Complications

Insulin replacement makes it possible for the child with diabetes to attain a level of metabolic control that permits day-to-day functioning in school, play, and at home, with only occasional episodes of mild to moderate hypoglycemia and avoidance of ketoacidosis, despite high average blood sugar concentrations. Awareness that this was the typical situation was limited until the advance of self-monitoring blood glucose and measurement of glycohemoglobin (HbA1c) (82, 83). These advances, and the improvement in insulins and delivery systems, have made it possible to attain a level of glucose control that will reduce the risk of long-term complications, as demonstrated in the Diabetes Control and Complications Trial (84). The contemporary goals of treatment of type 1 diabetes in children, therefore, include the traditional maintenance of a reasonably normal lifestyle and avoidance of the acute complications (see Chapter 26), but with the attainment of near-normal glycemia to reduce the risk of long-term complications involving both microvascular and macrovascular disease. Microvascular disease is responsible for retinopathy, nephropathy, and neuropathy. Macrovascular complications affecting coronary, carotid, and other major vessels are increasingly recognized as beginning during childhood. Of particular interest in children have been skeletal, joint, and skin complications, and the effects of diabetes on growth and development.

1. Skeletal, Joint, and Skin Problems

a. Skeleton. Early studies of bone density, using single-photon absorptiometry, which detects the transmission of radiation from a ^{125}I crystal through the bones of the forearm, described more than 10% loss of bone density in nearly one-half of girls and one-third of boys with type 1 diabetes. This was much more severe in white than in black children, similar to the situation for adult osteopenia in women, and was only seen during the first 5 years of diabetes (85). When spine bone density was examined by computed tomography (CT) scan, a slight but significant decrease was found, which was entirely caused by weight differences between patients and controls (86, 87). More recent study of the lumbar spine in children and adolescents with diabetes, using dual energy x-ray absorptiometry (DEXA), also noted that bone mineral density was highly dependent on stature. There was no abnormality during the first several years of diabetes and no abnormalities in the calcium/phosphorus hormone and metabolic profile (88). Studies of the femoral neck and lumbar spine in 88 younger Spanish adults with young onset type 1 diabetes confirmed no significant osteopenia associated with diabetes (89).

Two recent studies from Venezuela using DEXA examination of the lumbar spine and femoral neck in 26 children with a mean duration of diabetes of 4.3 years are consistent with the initial studies using single-photon absorptiometry of the forearm. Children were compared to controls and restudied after 1 year. There were no significant differences in femoral neck densities or total body densities, but lumbar spine had significantly less bone mineral density in those with diabetes. This did not correlate with duration of diabetes or degree of diabetes control as determined by HbA1c concentration. A variety of measures of bone turnover indicated lower activity in the patients (90). A further study of 23 prepubertal children with an average 6 month diabetes duration also revealed decrease in lumbar spine density and decreased bone formation markers, indicating very early changes (91).

The practical significance of these findings and their consistency remain uncertain. Calcium loss in the urine is characteristic of poorly controlled diabetes (92, 93), but no studies have established a relationship between level of control and bone mineral density. With longstanding diabetes in adults, there is no epidemiological evidence of increased fracture risk (94).

b. Joints. Limited joint mobility (LJM) is the earliest clinically apparent long-term complication of type 1 diabetes in childhood and, following its initial description in 1974, was recognized to be a common feature of both type 1 and type 2 diabetes (95, 96). LJM was described as bilateral, painless, but obvious, contracture of the finger joints and large joints, with thick tight waxy skin and short stature in three older teenagers with longstanding diabetes and early microvascular complications (95).

Milder expression was subsequently recognized as affecting ~30% of youngsters with diabetes, one-third of whom had involvement of more than two fingers or one finger and one large joint bilaterally. Variation in prevalence among various reports is related to the examination technique, criteria, age of the patients, and duration of diabetes. In older adult patients, examination is confounded by the presence of finger contracture related to age, occupation, and non-diabetes-associated problems such as osteoarthritis. It may also be related to other conditions involving the finger joints that are more common in diabetes, such as flexor tenosynovitis, carpal tunnel syndrome, and Dupuytren disease, which are conditions not seen in pediatric patients. It is rare to see bilateral finger contractures in children with diabetes that are not due to LJM, except for the unusual bilateral trauma of the finger or familial camptodactyly of the fifth fingers.

Changes begin in the metacarpophalangeal and proximal interphalangeal joints of the fifth finger and extend radially, with involvement of the distal interphalangeal joints as well. Involvement of larger joints includes particularly the wrist and elbow, but also ankles and the cervical and thoracolumbar spine. The limitation is painless and only mildly disabling when severe. A simple examination method is to have the patient attempt to approximate palmar surfaces of the interphalangeal joints (Fig. 1). Passive examination is essential to confirm that inability to do so is due to LJM. The examiner extends the proximal interphalangeal and distal interphalangeal joints (expected 180 degrees). There may be a sense of resistance to the permitted movement. The metacarpophalangeal joints should extend to >60 degrees and the wrists and elbows to >70 and >180 degrees, respectively. Cervical spine lateral flexion should permit ear to shoulder juxtaposition and thoracolumbar spine lateral flexion should be to at least 35 degrees in young persons. Equivocal or unilateral findings are considered to reflect no limitation (97). There is no associated muscle atrophy or evidence of neuropathy. Involvement of the cervical spine has been found to complicate endotracheal intubation for anesthesia (98).

Diminished pulmonary capacity has also been documented, but it is uncertain whether this is the result of decreased pulmonary compliance or limitation of the thoracic joints (99). Thick, tight, waxy skin, described in the initial patients, was most prominent over the dorsum of the hands and forearms and occurred in one-third of those described later, but only in those who had more than mild changes in the joints (96). Skin biopsy specimens have shown active fibroblasts and extensive collagen polymerization in the rough endoplasmic reticulum. There is a predominance of large fibers that has been found in patients with diabetes whether or not they have had thick skin; this is quite different from the bimodality of collagen fiber sizes seen in scleroderma (100). Radiographic examination of the joints is normal, but there is periarticular thickening that can be quantitated (101).

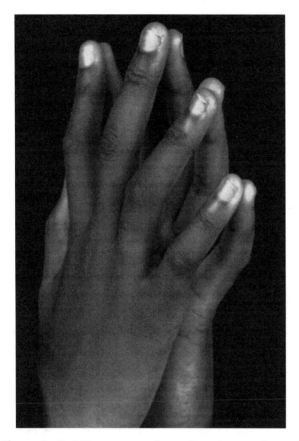

Figure 1 Inability to approximate the palmar surfaces of the fingers in a 14-year-old girl with diabetes for 7 years.

Attained age seems more important than duration of diabetes or age of onset of diabetes in the evolution of LJM. With rare exception, LJM appears after the age of 10 years. The interval between the detection of mild LJM and progression to moderate or severe changes in those who progress beyond mild changes ranges from a few months to 4 years, following which stabilization occurs (102).

The biochemical basis for LJM is likely to be glycation of protein with the formation of advanced glycation end-products (AGE). This results in increased stiffness of the periarticular and skin collagen with decreased range of motion. Increased accumulation of relatively insoluble dermal collagen resistant to enzymatic digestion has long been recognized as a characteristic of connective tissue aging in both type 1 and type 2 diabetes (103). Fluorescence of skin collagen reflects the accumulation of stable end-products of the glycation reaction, with increased cross-linking, dehydration, and condensation of collagen. Such fluorescence increases linearly with age but with abnormal rapidity in patients with type 1 diabetes, correlating with the presence of retinopathy, nephropathy, and LJM (104).

As might be expected, the presence of LJM is associated with increased risk for the development of microvascular (MVC) disease. The initial report of the prevalence of LJM included seven patients with severe changes, of whom five had clinically apparent retinopathy before the age of 18 years (96). In a longitudinal study of 169 patients with diabetes duration >4.5 years, which was the shortest duration at which complications were noted, LJM was associated with an 83% risk for retinopathy, whereas the absence of LJM was associated with a 25% risk after 16 years of diabetes (Fig. 2). The severity of microvascular changes also corresponded with the severity of LJM (97). In a later study of 311 patients aged 6–27 years undergoing fluorescein angiographic examination, 43% of those with LJM and >4 years duration of diabetes had >10 microaneurysms compared to 15% without LJM (105). In another large series, LJM was associated with a 4.3-fold relative risk of clinical neuropathy in those with type 1 diabetes (106). Histopathological changes in renal biopsy specimens from patients without clinically detectable nephropathy also correlate highly with LJM (107).

Although cross-sectional studies had shown no relationship to diabetes control as measured by HbA1c, a longitudinal study of average HbA1c from onset of diabetes revealed a correlation between long-term metabolic control and the development of LJM. For every unit increase in average HbA1c there was an approximately 46% increase in the risk of developing LJM (108).

The impression that LJM had markedly decreased in prevalence and severity since the initial recognition in the 1970s has been confirmed by a recent report comparing subjects examined in 1998 using the same examination methods in the same setting as those examined in 1976–1978. Documented was a >fourfold reduction, from 31% to 7%, in frequency of LJM over this 20 year period, with a marked decrease in the proportion having moderate or severe LJM (9% vs. 35%). This reduction in the prevalence and severity of LJM was considered to be most likely the result of improved glucose control during this era (109). These study results are pertinent to the question of the importance of prepubertal duration and control of diabetes for the development of long-term microvascular complications. Even for the youngest age group studied or those with the shortest duration of diabetes, there was a marked decrease in the prevalence of LJM between the two eras, suggesting that improved control from the first years of childhood diabetes will reduce long-term complication risks.

c. Skin. Necrobiosis lipoidica diabeticorum is a rarely seen pretibial lesion characterized by round or oval indurated plaques, with central atrophy and eventual ulceration. Unless they become infected, the lesions are painless. The relationship to diabetes control is uncertain, but there is an association with smoking, proteinuria, and retinopathy (110). Because these lesions do not heal well, trauma should be avoided and infection vigorously treated.

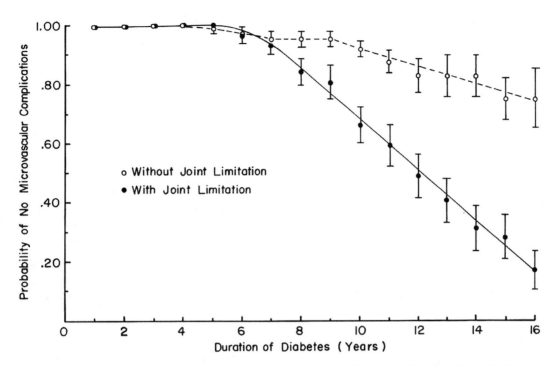

Figure 2   Actuarial analysis of risk for development of microvascular complications with and without limited joint mobility, based on longitudinal study of 169 patients with diabetes duration ≥4.5 years followed from before the development of LJM or microvascular disease. (From Ref. 97.)

Lipoatrophy, seen as indentation or atrophy of the subcutaneous tissue resulting from insulin injection, has become uncommon with the generalized use of recombinant-derived human insulin. It is presumed that the impurities in animal extract insulin or the foreign nature of that insulin led to the problem. It was thought to be immune mediated, frequently following dermatomes and occurring symmetrically, distal from the actual injection sites. The lesions tended to resolve after a few years and were thought to be IgE mediated. Mild atrophy is still seen occasionally with the contemporary insulin, affecting ~3% of patients 1–19 years old in one study (111). Giving insulin injections around the edges of the atrophic area may be helpful.

Lipohypertrophy, which always occurs at the site of injection, is a local reaction to repeated injection trauma, usually from inadequate site rotation, with scarring and decreased sensitivity to pain. The lesion can occur quite early, however, and may not be abolished by site rotation (112). Unlike lipoatrophy, lipohypertrophy continues to be frequent with improved insulin forms, present to some degree in as many as half of patients under 20 years of age (112). Both lipoatrophy and lipohypertrophy are associated with greater insulin antibody concentrations (111). The cosmetic effect is problematic, but most important is the possibility of varying absorption of insulin from areas of hypertrophy, resulting in erratic glycemic control.

2. Cataracts

Cataracts occur rarely during recovery from ketoacidosis, typically in the newly diagnosed patient; they usually disappear rapidly but may persist and require surgical removal (113). In contrast to these sugar cataracts, subcapsular juvenile cataracts, associated with chronic hyperglycemia and caused by sorbitol accumulation, do not regress and always require removal.

3. Growth Failure and Delayed Sexual Maturation

Insulin has important influence on normal growth and development, largely through effects on anabolism and the growth hormone–insulin-like growth factor I (GH–IGF-1) axis. Before the contemporary era of self blood glucose monitoring and more physiological insulin administration, modest growth retardation and delayed puberty were frequently seen in the pediatric diabetes clinic. Nonetheless, despite the generally nonphysiological traditional means of treating diabetes, most children with diabetes did not have serious growth or maturational delay problems. In twin pairs discordant for diabetes, the development of diabetes before the onset of puberty was associated with invariably shorter stature than that of the nonaffected twin (114). More contemporary studies demonstrate normal timing of puberty, with reduced growth and adult height even with modern therapeutic regimens, although these deviations are not substantial (115, 116).

Analyzing the stature of 142 patients with diabetes onset at least 2 years before puberty and with duration longer than 3 years, which provided sufficient time for a growth-inhibiting effect, Rosenbloom et al. in 1982 (117) found that 37% of 68 patients without LJM were below the 25th percentile of NCHS data. The 74 with LJM had four times the proportion with stature below the 25th percentile for age (77%), with no difference between the 31 with mild changes (involving one or two interphalangeal joints, one large joint, or only the metacarpophalangeal joints bilaterally) and those with more severe limitation (*n* = 43). When a similar group of children was examined in 1998, using the same criteria, only 22% of the 157 without LJM were below the contemporary NCHS 25th percentile and only 33% of the 18 with LJM were (118). Thus, contemporary diabetes control methods were resulting in improved growth along with the reduction in frequency of LJM. It will be recalled that the initial patients described with severe LJM had growth failure and delayed puberty (95, 96).

Insulin deficiency is associated with manifold changes in the GH-IGF-I axis. Deficiency of portal insulin delivery to the liver results in reduced circulating GH-binding protein, the extracellular domain of the cell surface receptor for GH, with GH resistance and diminished IGF-I production (119, 120). The deficiency in insulin also results in decreased production of IGF binding protein-3 (IGFBP-3), which is the principal binding protein for circulating IGF-I, and increased production of IGFBP-1 and IGFBP-2 (121). These latter BPs, unlike IGFBP-3, do not deliver their bound IGF-I to tissues. Furthermore, there is increased proteolysis of IGFBP-3, decreasing its viability in the circulation. In addition to the GH resistance, reflected in the lower concentrations of circulating GHBP, there may be postreceptor defects in GH action mediated by the insulin deficiency as well. Diminished circulating total and free IGF-I levels are associated with GH hypersecretion because of the absence of negative feedback from IGF-I. This hypersomatotropism increases glycemia and decreases insulin sensitivity, but is reversible with adequate insulin replacement (122).

Growth failure and maturational delay with hepatomegaly and abdominal distention in insulin-treated children was first described by Mauriac in 1930 (123). The regression of hepatomegaly in 13 such patients, following transfer from regular insulin to protamine zinc insulin, was noted in 1936 (124). Hepatomegaly was apparently a common complication in children in the era when only short-acting insulin was available and aglycosuria was the objective. This was exemplified in a series from the Joslin Clinic in the late 1930s, of 60 youngsters with hepatomegaly, growth failure, delayed sexual maturation, and severe uncontrollable diabetes with frequent hypoglycemia and ketoacidosis (125). Improvement was associated with the change to long-acting protamine zinc insulin.

There appear to be two forms of the Mauriac syndrome. In one form there is associated cushingoid obesity

and documented wide fluctuation between hyper- and hypoglycemia. This is suggestive of a pattern of over- and underinsulinization, which would be expected with treatment using only soluble insulin, with secondary hyperadrenalism. Periods of overinsulinization would appear to be essential for the development of obesity in this form of the syndrome, and for the induction of hyperadrenalism. In addition to the Joslin series, an impressive North American case was reported in 1962 of a 13.5-year-old girl with extremes of blood glucose from 1 to 29 mmol/l, hypertension, edema, hepatomegaly, marked growth failure, sexual immaturity, cushingoid obesity, retarded bone age, hyperlipidemia, and osteoporosis. When her insulin dosage was reduced from 65 units a day (40 NPH/25 soluble) to 20 NPH daily, she had complete clearing of the abnormalities, catch-up growth, and sexual maturation (126). More recent reports are of patients with Mauriac syndrome who are not obese and without a history of alternating hypoglycemia and ketoacidosis; these patients are unmistakably inadequately insulinized continuously (127–129).

Associated autoimmune problems that can result in growth failure include hypothyroidism and celiac disease. Approximately 20% of girls and 15% of boys with type 1 diabetes have evidence of autoimmune thyroid disease, determined by the presence of thyroid autoantibodies (130). Such autoantibodies should be tested for in all youngsters with type 1 diabetes. Those with positive results should have an annual determination of thyroid-stimulating hormone (TSH) level. Celiac disease has been described in 5–8% of children with type 1 diabetes; tissue transglutaminase antibodies should be sought in children with growth failure without obvious cause, even in the absence of diarrhea (131).

Eating disorders are more common in children with diabetes than in the general population and should be considered in the assessment of any child who is not gaining weight or growing normally. Adolescent girls with diabetes are 2.4 times more likely than those without diabetes to have clinical eating disorders and 1.9 times more likely to have a subclinical eating disorder. Mean HbA1c levels were higher in adolescents with diabetes who had an eating disorder than in those who did not (132).

4. Microvascular Complications

a. Pathogenesis. The hallmark of microvascular disease is thickened capillary basement membrane with alterations in membrane permeability and occlusion of small blood vessels. Several theories explain these findings.

Protein glycation. It has been well documented that improved glycemic control is associated with decrease in microvascular disease and its progression (84). This suggests that excess glucose *per se* has deleterious effects on tissues. Some of these effects appear to be through binding to collagen by posttranslational nonenzymatic means.

The amidori glycation products undergo slow (nonenzymatic) chemical rearrangements to form irreversible AGE. These AGE accumulate in the extracellular matrix and vascular intracellular proteins to cause structural tissue alterations with progressive occlusion of blood vessels. This glycation may alter the charge of the proteoglycan component of the basement membrane, resulting in leakage of negatively charged proteins from the plasma. The pores in glomeruli may also undergo alterations in size, resulting in protein leakage. The increased basement membrane thickening found in microvascular disease may be due to this glycation process, with accumulation of proteins that are not degradable. The nonenzymatic glycation of hemoglobin is an example of protein glycation and has been used as an indicator of glycemic control since the late 1970s.

Amidori products may be involved in induction of strand breakage in DNA by interfering with gene transcription. This may explain the hyperglycemic memory observed in the EDIC study 4 years after the conclusion of the Diabetes Control and Complication Trials (DCCT). Although the mean HbA1c levels 4 years after conclusion of the DCCT were similar between the former intensive and former conventional groups (8.38% vs 8.45%), the rate of worsening of retinopathy by three steps or more was lower in the former intensive therapy group than in the former conventional group (84). The prevalence of micro-albuminuria (defined below) was 13.6% for the former conventional treatment group compared to 8.1% in the former intensive treatment group at study closeout; 9.9% of the former conventional group had albuminuria at years 3 and 4 compared to only 1.3% of patients in the former intensive group.

Polyol pathway. Sorbitol (glucose alcohol) is formed enzymatically from glucose by the enzyme aldose reductase. The higher the blood sugar concentration, the more the sorbitol accumulation in a number of tissues, including lens and nerve. This influx of glucose into the polyol pathway is associated with decreased myoinositol uptake and decreased sodium/potassium/ATPase activity. These changes have been related to increased permeability and increased pressure and leakage in blood vessels, which may be related to the increased release of vasoconstrictive prostaglandins and decreased release of nitric oxide that mediates endothelium relaxation. The overall effect of these metabolic abnormalities is decreased vessel wall elasticity and microvascular hypertension (133).

Abnormalities in the coagulation system. Elevated fibrinogen levels and other antithrombotic factors may result in increased platelet stickiness. Increased prostaglandin metabolism increases coagulopathy, resulting in increased red blood cell aggregation and blockage of small capillaries (134).

b. Nephropathy. Micro-albuminuria, defined as urinary albumin excretion rates of 20–200 μg/min or 30–300 mg/24 h, is predictive of renal and cardiovascular

disease (135). Concentration above 300 mg/g is considered overt diabetic nephropathy. HbA1c levels, albumin excretion rate, low-density lipoprotein cholesterol, and body mass index were risk factors for the development of micro-albuminuria in 12.6% of 1134 men and women with type 1 diabetes aged 15–60 years during 7 years of follow-up in the EURO DIAB Prospective Complications Study (136).

The prevalence and progression of micro-albuminuria and of clinical proteinuria were studied in 361 children with type 1 diabetes over the course of 12 years, with the conclusion that micro-albuminuria was rare before adolescence. The incidence of micro-albuminuria, however, increased between the ages of 10 and 18 years with 30.9% of males and 40.4% of females having one or more episodes of micro-albuminuria (137).

A study of 101 normal albuminuric children and adolescents with diabetes found that 11% developed persistent micro-albuminuria during 8 years of follow-up. The odds ratio for the occurrence of micro-albuminuria with elevated vascular endothelial growth factor serum levels was 4.1, indicating that persistently increased serum levels of vascular endothelial growth factor may help to identify patients who are predisposed to persistent albuminuria (138).

In Denmark, high HbA1c and high baseline albumin excretion rates predicted the development of persistent albuminuria over 6 years in 12.8% of 339 children and adolescents with type 1 diabetes (139). These results showed a higher incidence than in a large American cross-sectional survey of 702 children and adolescents with an average diabetes duration of 7.6 years. In this study, albumin excretion rate ≥15 μg/min measured on at least two of three urine collections was defined as micro-albuminuria, which increased from 5.1% to 11.6% after 10 years of diabetes duration and completion of puberty. Maternal hypertension was a significant risk factor, but patients' BP was not, and HbA1c had a borderline effect (140). These findings contrast with other studies in which there is strong association between progression of micro-albuminuria and HbA1c values. A 4 year follow-up of 279 patients with type 1 diabetes found that the rate of progression was 1.3:100 person years in those with HbA1c levels <8%, whereas it was 5.1:100 person years with HbA1c levels between 8 and 9%, 4.2 between 9 and 10%, and 6.7:100 person years if HbA1c was >10%. The risk of progression rose steeply between HbA1c values of 7.5 and 8.5%, emphasizing the importance of improved glycemic control, especially of maintaining HbA1c values below 8.5% (141).

The Pittsburgh Epidemiology of Diabetes Complications (EDC) study is an observational prospective study of 589 patients with onset of type 1 diabetes before the age of 17 years. Baseline low-density lipoprotein (LDL) levels ≥130, triglycerides ≥150, systolic blood pressure ≥130, and diastolic blood pressure ≥85 conferred relative risks of 2.2, 3.2, 2.3, and 2.5, respectively, for developing nephropathy over 10 years (142).

Homocysteine elevation has been considered a risk factor for premature cardiovascular disease. Young patients with type 1 diabetes diagnosed before the age of 12 years and with duration of disease longer than 7 years who had albumin excretion rates >70 μg/min had elevated homocysteine levels, indicating an association of diabetic nephropathy with premature cardiovascular disease (143).

Annual testing of the urine for albumin is recommended for children from puberty and with 3–5 years of diabetes. The most convenient way to assess albuminuria is with the urinary albumin/creatinine ratio obtained on a spot urine sample. Micro-albuminuria in a single specimen may not indicate fixed disease. It is important to repeat the test on at least one other occasion in a random urine sample. A timed 12 h or 24 h urine specimen is preferable. It is also important to differentiate orthostatic proteinuria from that due to diabetic renal disease. With orthostatic proteinuria, a first void morning urine should not contain abnormal concentration of albumin, whereas a late afternoon urine often will.

The DCCT demonstrated that micro-albuminuria and overt nephropathy can be delayed or prevented by intensive diabetes treatment (84). However, the United Kingdom Prospective Diabetes Study (UKPDS) and other studies have shown that blood pressure control is as important as glycemic control in prevention of nephropathy and in decreasing the rate of decline of glomerular filtration rate (GFR) in established disease (144). ACE inhibitors decrease albumin excretion rate in patients with hypertension as well as in nonhypertensive patients (145). Children and adolescents with micro-albuminuria have higher blood pressures than those with normal albuminuria (146–150). Because of this increased risk for development of nephropathy, it is essential to pay close attention to maintaining blood pressure at normal or near normal values.

The treatment of choice for nephropathy has been ACE inhibition, which is effective whether or not the patient has hypertension. In addition to their antihypertensive effects, ACE inhibitors increase afferent vessel dilatation, thereby decreasing elevated intraglomerular pressure, a hallmark of diabetic nephropathy. The role of low-protein diets in treatment of micro-albuminuria has been debated for several years; there are no long-term studies in children. Studies in adults have shown that protein restriction slows the rate of decline of glomerular filtration rate (151). The albumin excretion rate has been decreased in adults with micro-albuminuria with the low protein diet (152). A low-protein diet of 0.8 g/kg body weight may be helpful in decreasing albuminuria and slowing the decline in renal function (153). Thus, high protein intake should be avoided in children with micro-albuminuria. Because of the importance of adequate dietary protein in the growing child, however, protein restriction below 15% of total daily calories is not justified.

Adolescents should be counseled to avoid smoking: nicotine has profound vasoconstrictive effects that have been associated with progression of nephropathy in adults with type 1 diabetes (154).

c. Retinopathy. Retinopathy is the most common microvascular disease in children and adolescents with type 1 diabetes. It is broadly defined to include background retinopathy, with the presence of microaneurysms only or microaneurysms and occasional dot blot hemorrhages, and proliferative retinopathy, with growth of new vessels, glia, and fibrous tissue. Fluorescein angiography is used to document severity of retinopathy by showing areas of retinal ischemia, proliferation of new blood vessels, and permeability of the retinal vessels.

At diabetes diagnosis, there is increased blood flow through the retina. Early on, poor metabolic control may be associated with leakage of injected fluorescein in the vitreous (155, 156), with reversal by improved metabolic control. Anatomical disease begins as background non-proliferative changes within the retina resulting from increased vascular permeability and capillary and arteriolar occlusion. The increased permeability results in edema and the formation of hard exudates, whereas the occlusion results in formation of microaneurysms, hemorrhages, soft exudates, and capillary dropout. The growth of new blood vessels, glia, and fibrous tissue in front of the retina can result in vitreous hemorrhage and retinal detachment from shrinkage of the proliferating tissue.

Although retinopathy has been reported to be present at onset of diabetes (105), it usually is not recognized before 5–10 years' duration. By that time, 20–30% of patients will have background retinopathy, 30–50% after 10–15 years diabetes duration, and 70–80% after 15 years. The progression to blindness is not uniform and varies between 20 and 55% in different series (157). Diabetes accounts for 10–20% of all cases of blindness in adults (158).

The incidence of retinopathy in 764 patients >15 years of age in the EURO DIAB prospective complications study was 56% after 7 years of follow-up. Risk factors for development of retinopathy included albumin excretion rate, cholesterol, triglycerides, and waist-to-hip ratio. In contrast to other studies, there was no association between retinopathy and blood pressure, cardiovascular disease, or smoking in this study (159).

In a cross-sectional study of 725 African–Americans in New Jersey, 3% had macular edema and 20.6% had retinal hard exudates. The severity of retinopathy correlated with the presence of proteinuria, higher LDL cholesterol levels, systolic hypertension, poor glycemic control, and longer duration of disease. Hyperglycemia was strongly associated with retinopathy. Those patients whose HbA1c values were in the highest quartile were three times more likely to have retinopathy than those in the lowest quartile. Patients with renal disease were three times more likely to have retinopathy and 10 times more likely to have proliferative retinopathy than those without renal disease. Patients in the highest quartile of systolic blood pressure were three times more likely to have proliferative retinopathy than patients in the lowest quartile (160, 161).

The Pittsburgh EDC found that systolic BP ≥120 mmHg conferred a relative risk (RR) of 1.6 for the development of proliferative retinopathy and RR was 2.7 if systolic BP ≥130; diastolic BP >79 mmHg conferred RR of 1.8, if ≥85 RR was 2.4, and if ≥90 mmHg, the relative risk of proliferative retinopathy was 4.6 in this population (142). Thus, it is important to maintain blood pressure near normal, because systolic blood pressures above 120 mmHg conferred increased risk of proliferative retinopathy.

Homocysteine concentrations, which, as noted above, are elevated with cardiovascular disease, were higher in adolescents with proliferative retinopathy, further indicating a link between presence of microvascular complications and later onset of macrovascular disease (143).

Because retinopathy is rare before puberty, it is recommended that children begin regular ophthalmological evaluation at the age of 9–10 years and following 3–5 years of diabetes. Once criteria for ophthalmological evaluation have been met, all children with diabetes should be evaluated by an ophthalmologist with serial fundus photographs at annual intervals and photocoagulation performed with the development of proliferative retinopathy. ACE inhibitors have been shown to slow the progression of retinopathy in patients with and without hypertension; thus, the presence of retinopathy is an indication for initiation of such therapy (162, 163).

The use of retinal photocoagulation has markedly improved the prognosis for vision in patients with proliferative retinopathy (164, 165). Although the mechanism of action is uncertain, it is thought that the photocoagulation destroys ischemic retinal tissue, thus removing the stimulus for neovascularization. Laser therapy is also used for macular edema by destroying leaking microaneurysms and dilated capillaries. In cases of proliferative retinopathy, panretinal photocoagulation will destroy retinal tissue outside the macula and optic nerve so that the remaining retina is not ischemic and will, therefore, not produce the growth factors that result in proliferative diabetic retinopathy. The panretinal photocoagulation has the adverse effects of compromising color discrimination, visual fields, and night vision. In the case of vitreous hemorrhage or detached retina, vitrectomy can be used to remove the blood from the vitreous or to reattach a retina in the process of detaching.

d. Neuropathy. Although symptomatic neuropathy is uncommonly seen in children and adolescents with diabetes, findings of sensory and autonomic motor nerve impairment can be demonstrated in young people. Peripheral neuropathy, including motor and sensory disturbances, as well as autonomic neuropathies, including gastrointestinal, cardiovascular, vasomotor instability, and hypoglycemia unawareness, have been described in childhood and adolescence.

The pathogenesis of neuropathy in diabetes is likely multifactorial. The aldose reductase system is present in the lens and peripheral nerves and is responsible for metabolism of glucose to sorbitol. High glucose levels will accelerate the synthesis of sorbitol, which is not freely difusible. The sorbitol thus remains as an osmolar force within the nerve, causing swelling and possible destruction. Myoinositol, a component of neuronal cell membranes, and therefore involved in the control of neural transmission, has been found to be decreased in animals and humans with diabetes. In addition, the basement membrane of the Schwann's cell is thickened and the vasa nervorum has capillary and arteriolar wall thickening by basement membrane accumulation, as part of the generalized microvascular disease of diabetes. Biopsy of affected nerves has shown numerous thrombosed vessels, axonal loss, and a characteristic segmental demyelination.

Peripheral neuropathy. Clinical symptoms of peripheral neuropathy include numbness and paresthesias, especially pain and burning in the lower extremities, which is much worse at night. Usually a decrease in vibratory sense is the first clinical sign of neuropathy, followed by loss of ankle jerks and later by loss of pin prick sensation in a stocking distribution (166). These symptoms are commonly accompanied by anorexia with early satiety and postprandial vomiting due to gastroparesis from autonomic neuropathy. It is possible that undernutrition contributes to the neuropathy (167). The Pittsburgh EDC study found that 3% of 65 children under 18 years of age had neuropathy based on history and physical examination (168). Subclinical neuropathy, assessed by decreased motor nerve conduction velocities and sensory changes, is much more common, however, occurring in as many as 50–72% of adolescents (169). Neuropathy has been correlated with hyperlipidemia and smoking (168) and with LJM (106), but no relationship has been demonstrated between the presence of motor or sensory nerve conduction abnormalities and micro-albuminuria or retinopathy (170, 171). A recent study of 339 patients who were followed for 6 years found that neuropathy, determined by decreased vibration perception threshold, occurred in 62.5% of patients. Risk markers were male gender, age, and increased albumin excretion rate (140).

The Pittsburgh EDC study found the relative risk of developing peripheral neuropathy to be 2.2 if LDL cholesterol was >129 mg/dl and 1.5 if LDL cholesterol was >99 mg/dl. Triglyceride levels >140 mg/dl likewise conferred a 1.5 relative risk. Systolic blood pressure >130 mmHg was associated with a relative risk of 4.0 and diastolic blood pressure >85 mmHg with a 2.0 relative risk. Glycemic control was not evaluated in this report (142).

Improved metabolic control may result in resolution of sensory and motor nerve velocities as well as the sen-

sory and gastrointestinal symptoms. The DCCT showed
that intensive diabetes therapy decreased clinical neuropathy
by 60% (172). Peripheral motor and sensory nerve
conduction velocities were significantly faster after 5
years of intensive therapy than after conventional treatment
in the adolescent cohort (84).

Autonomic neuropathy. Autonomic neuropathy
most commonly results in gastroparesis, cardiovascular reflex
loss, and hypoglycemic unawareness. Diabetic gastroparesis
is associated with decreased gastric motility and
delayed emptying time. Affected patients often complain
of bloating and feelings of satiety following intake of
small amounts of food and they often have anorexia and
weight loss. There are some reports of resolution of gastroparesis
with improved metabolic control (173, 174).
Diagnosis can be made using technetium-coated egg in a
gastric-emptying study. Use of metoclopramide or erythromycin
may result in increased motility with resolution
of symptoms. Diabetic diarrhea is watery, most frequent
at night or following meals, and can result in fecal incontinence
(175).

Autonomic neuropathy of the cardiovascular system
results in persistent tachycardia with a fixed heart rate in
response to standing, Valsalva maneuver, and inspiration.
Because of this, there is an inability to increase cardiac
output resulting in hypotension with standing or exercise,
and hypersensitivity to catecholamines. Patients with this
neuropathy will frequently have a lower blood pressure
when sitting or standing than when supine.

Loss of awareness of hypoglycemia is the loss of the
catecholamine-induced symptoms of sweating, tachycardia,
nausea, sense of fear, and tremulousness that normally
accompany severe drops in the blood glucose level.

5. Macrovascular Disease and Hyperlipidemia

Diabetes mellitus is a strong risk factor for cardiovascular
disease, conferring a two- to fourfold increased risk (176–
178). Risk factors that independently increase cardiovascular
risk in people with diabetes include smoking, hypertension,
dyslipidemia (179), renal dysfunction (179),
and hyperglycemia (180–184). The Pathological Determinants
of Atherosclerosis in Youth (PDAY) study of
more than 3000 people who died between the ages of 15
and 34 evaluated risk factors for coronary heart disease
by correlating pathological findings of fatty streaks and
lipid-laden plaques to blood lipid values, smoking, hypertension,
and tendency towards diabetes. There was a
strong association of extent of disease with smoking, as
measured by serum thiocyanate concentrations. All the
aortas and about half of the right coronary arteries in the
15–19 year age group already had lesions. On average,
7% of the aortas and 12% of the right coronary arteries
had raised lesions or advanced lesions of atherosclerosis
at the young age of 15–19 years. The percentage of intimal
surface involved with lesions in both the aorta and
right coronary artery was positively associated with very-

low-density lipoproteins (VLDL) and LDL cholesterol,
with a 5% increase in surface involvement with each 1
standard deviation increase of LDL and VLDL cholesterol
levels. Conversely, a 1 standard deviation increase in HDL
was associated with a 3% decrease in intimal surface involvement.
HbA1c concentration was associated with
more extensive and more advanced atherosclerosis in the
aorta and right coronary artery, primarily in people between
the ages of 25 and 34 years of age. The prevalence
of raised lesions involving 5% or more of the intimal surface
was twice as great in both the aorta and right coronary
artery of people with hypertension throughout the
entire 15–34 year age span (185).

The Bogalusa heart study reported a study of 43 people
aged 2–39 years who died from accidents or homicide
and in whom premortem data were available. Half of the
children 2–15 years of age had fatty streak lesions in the
coronary arteries and 8% had fibrous plaques in their coronary
arteries. These atherosclerotic lesions correlated
with body mass index (BMI), systolic and diastolic blood
pressure, total and LDL cholesterol, and triglycerides
(186). It is thus important to address each of the risk factors
for cardiovascular disease in order to decrease the risk
of cardiovascular disease early in children with type 1
diabetes because the atherosclerosic process is already
present in childhood. The increased cardiovascular risk in
type 1 diabetes may be due to a number of factors, including
endothelial dysfunction and increased arterial
stiffness (187), and loss of endothelial integrity. Cardiomyopathy,
consisting of interstitial fibrosis, has been described
in adults with type 1 diabetes but is rare in children.
The heart is subject to both microvascular disease,
with microaneurysms and thickened capillary basement
membrane, and macrovascular disease, with accelerated
atherosclerosis.

Recent studies have found higher levels of endothelin-1
(an indicator of endothelial damage) in patients
with diabetes and hyperlipidemia than in controls; those
patients with diabetes who had vascular complications had
significantly higher endothelin-1 levels than did patients
without complications. The patients with diabetes complications
also had significantly higher apolipoprotein B
levels than did healthy controls. Patients without microvascular
or macrovascular disease had levels similar to
those of controls. Thus, it is possible that the susceptibility
to the development of atherosclerosis might be attributed
to the relationship between elevated lipid levels and endothelin-1
(188).

The Heart Outcome Prevention Evaluation (HOPE)
study was a cohort study of 5545 individuals aged 55
years or more with a history of cardiovascular disease or
with diabetes mellitus and at least one cardiovascular risk
factor. Of the 3498 subjects in the latter category, microalbuminuria
increased the relative risk of major cardiovascular
events (relative risk 1.83), all-cause death (relative
risk 2.09), and hospitalization for congestive heart

failure (relative risk 3.23). Any degree of albuminuria was a risk factor for cardiovascular disease, the risk increasing with the albumin/creatinine ratio. The use of the ACE inhibitor ramipril resulted in significant risk reduction of 25% for myocardial infarction, 37% for cardiovascular deaths, 33% for stroke, and 24% for all causes of mortality. ACE inhibition also reduced the risk of overt nephropathy by 22% and dialysis by 15%. Ramipril not only works by decreasing blood pressure but it also has anti-thrombotic effects, reducing collagen-induced platelet aggregation by 18% and ADP-induced platelet aggregation by 39% (189). In addition, ACE inhibitors have effects on endothelium and fibrinolysis that are beneficial in preventing plaque rupture and subsequent thrombosis, which are two key events in the acute formation and progression of atherosclerotic disease (190).

Similar to the findings of the UKPDS in adults with type 2 diabetes, the Pittsburgh EDC found a strong correlation between lipid levels and risk of cardiovascular disease in their 10 year study of patients with diabetes diagnosis in adolescence or earlier. They showed a relative risk of 2.3 for LDL cholesterol levels ≥130 mg/dl, and a relative risk of 1.8 for patients whose LDL levels were ≥100 mg/dl compared to those whose levels are lower. Triglycerides also conferred risk for cardiovascular disease with the relative risk being 2.5 for triglyceride levels ≥90 mg/dl and 3.3 if the levels were ≥150 mg/dl. Systolic blood pressure conferred additional risk with levels of ≥110 mmHg conferring a relative risk of 1.8, 120–129 mmHg, 2.5, and ≥130 mmHg 5.6. Any diastolic blood pressure >80 conferred additional risks but the relative risk was extremely high, 4.2, with diastolic blood pressures ≥90 (142).

The recommended treatment for adults with diabetes is to intervene when LDL cholesterol is >100 mg/dl and triglycerides >140 mg/dl. The data indicating that fatty streaks and atherosclerotic plaques are present during childhood indicate that the process begins early and, therefore, intervention should also begin early. Initial efforts at improving metabolic control with recommendations for diet and exercise should be initiated when lipid levels exceed target. If, after 3 months, fasting lipid profiles are not decreasing, pharmacological therapy should be considered. In our practice we have used HMG Co-A inhibitors (statins) with good success and few adverse reactions.

Triglycerides, too, should be vigorously treated. In some patients optimal blood glucose levels will not be achieved despite intensive attempts to maximize glycemic control, resulting in isolated hypertriglyceridemia. In those instances, agents targeted at lowering triglyceride levels, such as gemfibrizol, should be considered.

6. Hypertension

The UKPDS showed that above a baseline systolic blood pressure of 110 mmHg, the higher the blood pressure, the greater the risk of cardiovascular disease (191). The Hypertension Optimal Therapy (HOT) study compared the outcomes of maintaining diastolic blood pressure to goals of ≤90 mmHg, ≤85 mmHg, or ≤80 mmHg. In the 15,001 patients with diabetes mellitus at baseline, the rate of major cardiovascular events, defined as myocardial infarction, stroke, or death due to any cardiovascular event, revealed that the group randomized to maintain a diastolic blood pressure ≤80 mmHg had half the risk of major cardiovascular events compared to the group randomized to a blood pressure ≤90 mmHg. This differs from the results seen in the group without diabetes, in which the risk reduction was only 10% for the lower compared to the higher blood pressure readings (192), indicating that diabetes conferred an additional risk for cardiovascular disease.

These studies have led to the recommendations that hypertension should be treated to maintain a blood pressure of 130/80 mmHg or less and, as albumin excretion rate is an additional risk factor for cardiovascular disease (>20 mg/min, 30 mg/day, or 30 mg/g creatinine), blood pressure should be treated to a level of 120/75 mmHg or below in those with elevated albumin excretion rates (193).

IV. TYPE 2 DIABETES

A. Epidemiology

The definitions of incidence, prevalence, frequency, and epidemic have been provided in the preceding section on epidemiology of type 1 diabetes. Beginning around 1990, pediatric endocrinologists, who had been aware for decades of a small proportion of their diabetes patients having type 2 disease (194), noticed a sharp increase in the numbers of such patients (195). This was predominantly, but not exclusively, in the African–American and Hispanic–American population, and Native American youth were reported to have a 1% prevalence of type 2 diabetes as early as 1979 (196).

There seems little argument that type 2 diabetes in children and adolescents has become an epidemic. The first recognition of a substantial prevalence was among Pima Indian 15–24-year-olds, 9:1000 (0.9%) having diabetes associated with obesity and long-term complications (196). This was in a population in which 50% of adults have type 2 diabetes. Half of these youngsters had ketoacidosis. By the 1990s, 5% of 15–19-year-olds and 2.2% of 10–14-year-olds (previously 0%) had type 2 diabetes (197). Among First Nations children and youth in Canada, the frequency of type 2 diabetes is comparable to that of type 1 diabetes in the white population (198).

A study in Cincinnati reviewed 1027 consecutive records of children 0–19 years old diagnosed with diabetes and found that the proportion diagnosed as having type 2 increased from 2–4% between 1982 and 1992, to

16% in 1994 (199). It is interesting that this percentage was stable for over 20 years, Knowles having reported that approximately 3.5% of patients in this clinic had type 2 disease in 1971 (194). Thirty-three percent of those in the 10–19 year age group newly diagnosed in 1994 had type 2 disease. The estimated age-specific incidence for the community was 7.2:100,000, which is approximately half the incidence rate for type 1 diabetes in childhood, and a 10-fold increase from 1982 (30). In this study and also in a study from Arkansas, African–Americans accounted for 70–75% of the individuals with type 2 diabetes (200). It is estimated that one-third of Mexican–Americans with diabetes in southern California and over two-thirds of those in south Texas have type 2 disease (201, 202).

In Native North Americans four to six times as many females as males are affected, but among African–American and Mexican–American groups with type 2 diabetes, sex ratio has been far less skewed. It varies from 1.7 females for every male among African–Americans to nearly 1:1 among Mexican–Americans (203).

A study of 682 5–19-year-olds diagnosed between January 1, 1994, and December 31, 1998, at the three University-based diabetes centers in Florida found that 14% of the patients had type 2 disease. While 47% of type 1 patients were female, 63% of type 2 patients were. In contrast to the studies from Arkansas and Cincinnati, African–Americans were only 46% of those with type 2 diabetes while 22% were Hispanic, and the rest non-Hispanic whites. The risk for type 2 diabetes was three times greater for African–American youngsters and 3.5 times greater for Hispanics than for whites. During the initial year of the study, 8.7% of newly diagnosed patients were eventually classified as having type 2 disease, whereas in the last year of the study 19% were thus classified. This indicates a twofold increase in the proportion of new diabetes patients in this age group having type 2 disease over the relatively brief period of 5 years (28).

The recognition of an epidemic of type 2 diabetes is not unique to North America. Libyan Arabs are reported to have an age-specific incidence for the 15–19-year-old group of 6:100,000, increasing to 26:100,000 for the 20–24 year age group. Overall, this represents greater than twice the incidence for type 1 diabetes in males and over four times the incidence of type 1 diabetes in females (204). Among Hong Kong Chinese, type 2 diabetes accounts for >90% of young-onset diabetes and is strongly familial and associated with obesity (205). As with the Chinese, the Japanese have a very low incidence of type 1 diabetes. Annual urine testing for glucose of school-children in the Tokyo area has been carried out since 1975, followed by oral glucose tolerance testing for those with glucosuria. In the 12–15 year age group, there has been a doubling of incidence of type 2 diabetes from 7.2 to 13.9:100,000 paralleling increasing obesity rates (206). Other reports indicate that obese youth who are Bangla-

deshi (207), Australian aborigines (208), New Zealand Maoris (209), or East Indians or Arabs living in the United Kingdom (210) are also being observed with type 2 diabetes. Five obese adolescents aged 13–15 years with type 2 diabetes are the first white youngsters reported from England, and this problem is expected to be more prevalent with the epidemic of childhood obesity in that country (211).

A constant in the emergence of type 2 diabetes in young patients has been the association with obesity and increasing rates of that seminal condition. The U.S. National Health and Nutrition Examination Survey conducted between 1988 and 1994 found that 20% of children 12–17 years of age had BMIs above the 85th percentile for age (the definition of overweight), and that, depending on ethnicity, 8–17% were obese with a BMI >95th percentile. Not only was there a doubling of the frequency of childhood obesity since 1980 but the severity of obesity was also greater (212).

In a 20-year biracial community-based study in Louisiana (the Bogalusa heart study) of 11,564 5–24-year-olds from 1973 to 1994, there was a mean weight increase of 0.2 kg/year along with increased skinfold thickness. Overweight as defined above increased from 15 to 30%, and obesity from 5 to 11% in 5–14-year-olds and increased 5–15% in 15–17-year-olds. The increases in the second 10 years of the study were 50% greater than those in the first 10 years (213). In the National Longitudinal Survey of Youth, a prospective cohort study of 8270 children aged 4–12 years, there was a significant increase in overweight and obesity between 1986 and 1998. The prevalence rates in 1998 for overweight were 38% for African–Americans and Hispanics, and 26% for whites, while 22% of African–Americans and Hispanics and 12% of whites were obese (214).

The epidemic of obesity is also international. Similar trends to those in the United States have been reported for Japan (206) and the United Kingdom (215). In Russia, 6% of ~7000 6–18-year-olds examined in 1992 were obese and 10% were overweight, using US BMI reference data (216). In China, 3.6% of ~3000 6–18-year-olds examined in 1993 were obese and another 3.4% overweight (216). In 1996, in the United Kingdom, 22% of 6-year-olds were overweight, and 10% were obese; by age 15, 31% were overweight and 17% obese. Numerous studies in Europe have indicated that the highest rates of childhood obesity occur in Eastern European countries, particularly Hungary, and in the southern European countries of Italy, Spain, and Greece (217).

B. Etiology

The recent increase in type 2 diabetes prevalence in young patients has been so rapid that it must be explained by changes in the environment, most obviously increasing obesity rates (218, 219). Nonetheless, not all or even a majority of obese youngsters develop type 2 diabetes, emphasizing the importance of genetic factors. The *thrifty genotype* hypothesis, advanced nearly 40 years ago and recently updated (220, 221), explains the insulin resistance and relative beta-cell insufficiency associated with the development of obesity and type 2 diabetes as an adaptation for conserving energy and surviving famine. Until the modern era of continuous feasting, such a genotype would have had great survival advantage.

Numerous studies have demonstrated either insulin resistance preceding the development of type 2 diabetes or that limited pancreatic beta-cell capability to respond to the increased insulin requirements associated with obesity is the basic lesion (222–228).

Insulin resistance can be defined as the impaired ability to respond to physiological effects of insulin on glucose, lipid, and protein metabolism. Normal glycemic control requires the sensing of glucose concentration by the beta cells, the synthesis and release of insulin, binding of insulin to its receptors, and postreceptor insulin activation. This results in increased glucose uptake by muscles, fat, and liver tissue with decreased glucose production by the liver. In type 2 diabetes, there is peripheral insulin resistance in muscle and fat tissue, together with decreased pancreatic insulin secretion, and increased hepatic glucose output (Fig. 3). Note that both insulin resistance and impaired beta-cell function are required for the development of type 2 diabetes in this model (229).

1. Role of Fetal and Childhood Nutrition

The association of lower birth weight, smaller head circumference, and thinness at birth with impaired glucose tolerance or type 2 diabetes and insulin resistance in adults has suggested in utero programming that limited β-cell capacity and induced insulin resistance in peripheral tissues (230, 231). The maternal undernutrition that led to low birth weight was thought to impair development of the endocrine pancreas. The effect of fetal undernutrition on adult glucose tolerance has been confirmed in large

studies in Sweden and the United States (232, 233). Glucose intolerance was also found in adults who were the offspring of mothers who had starved during the last trimester of pregnancy during the Dutch famine of World War II (234).

Low birth weight has also been associated with increased cortisol axis activity in adults. South African non-obese 20-year-olds who had been underweight for gestational age had greater plasma cortisol response to adrenocorticotropin (ACTH), higher blood pressure, and impaired glucose tolerance compared to normal-birth-weight controls (235).

Three studies of young subjects from high-risk populations are consistent with reports of the effect of fetal nutrition on the risk for insulin resistance syndrome (type 2 diabetes, hypertension, hyperlipidemia) in adulthood. Current weight correlated with birth weight among 3061 Pima Indians aged 5–29 years, and 2 h glucose concentrations had a U-shaped relationship with birth weight in those >10 years old, regardless of current weight. Thus, higher blood glucose levels occurred in those with greater than normal and less than normal birth weight, unrelated to their current weight. The 2272 subjects without diabetes had negative correlations between birth weight and insulin concentrations at baseline and at 2 h, and insulin resistance. These findings supported the hypothesis of a survival advantage for insulin resistance in low-birth-weight babies (236).

In a study of 477 8-year-old Indian children, insulin resistance variables and plasma total and LDL cholesterol concentrations were strongly related to current weight. Lower birth weight was associated with elevated systolic BP, fasting plasma insulin and 32–33 split proinsulin concentrations, plasma lipids, glucose and insulin concentrations 30 min after glucose, and calculated insulin resistance. Children who had low birth weight but high fat mass at 8 years had the highest risk of insulin resistance syndrome variables and hyperlipidemia (237). Low-birth-weight white and African–American children (*n* = 139)

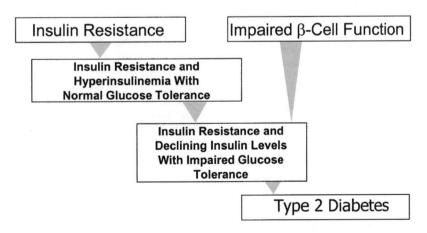

Figure 3   Development of type 2 diabetes. (Adapted from Ref. 229.)

were studied when they were aged 4–14 years. There were significant differences between the two races in the effect of low birth weight on visceral fat mass as measured by DEXA and CT, fasting insulin, acute insulin response and beta cell function, and HDL cholesterol concentrations, indicative of the genetic differences suggested by the thrifty genotype hypothesis (238).

The *thrifty phenotype* hypothesis has emerged from these studies indicating an effect of fetal nutrition on later glucose tolerance and other manifestations of insulin sensitivity. This hypothesis states that poor nutrition in fetal and early infant life would be detrimental to the development and function of the β-cells and insulin-sensitive tissues, primarily muscle, leading to insulin resistance. With obesity in later life, type 2 diabetes would develop. These findings could also be interpreted as a reflection of the *thrifty genotype*: that defective insulin action in utero results in decreased fetal growth and obesity-induced impaired glucose tolerance in later childhood or adulthood (26).

Genetic factors affecting birthweight and glucose metabolism are of interest in this regard. The polymorphism of the variable number of tandem repeats (VNTR) locus of the insulin chain is associated with decreased body length, weight, and head circumference at birth (239). Decreased birthweight has been associated with heterozygosity for a mutation in the glucokinase gene (240). Finally, the glucose transporter 4 (GLUT4) expression is impaired in young adults with insulin resistance who were undernourished in utero (241).

2. Maternal Diabetes

The influence of the diabetic intrauterine environment on the risk of type 2 diabetes in children was first appreciated from studies in the Pima Indian population. The prevalence of diabetes in the offspring of Pima women with diabetes during pregnancy is significantly greater than in nondiabetic mothers or those who develop diabetes after delivery (242). In another population, fetal β-cell function was assessed in 88 pregnancies with pregestational or gestational diabetes by measuring amniotic fluid insulin (AFI) concentration at 32–38 weeks' gestation. The offspring had oral glucose tolerance testing done annually from 18 months of age. Only 1 of 27 adolescents with normal AFI had impaired glucose tolerance, in contrast to one-third of those with elevated AFI (243). These studies suggest a generation-to-generation accumulation of risk for type 2 diabetes that further increases the public health concern about the epidemic of this disease in young persons (244).

3. Role of Puberty

In all reports of type 2 diabetes in childhood, the mean age at diagnosis is ~13.5 years, corresponding to the time of peak adolescent growth and development (198–203). Puberty is associated with relative insulin resistance, re-

flected in a two- to threefold increase in the peak insulin response to oral or intravenous glucose (245). Insulin-mediated glucose disposal is a mean 30% lower in adolescents than in prepubertal children or young adults (246). The physiological insulin resistance of puberty is of no consequence in the presence of adequate beta-cell function. The cause of this physiological resistance is likely to be increased activity of the GH-IGF axis, which is transitory and coincides with the physiological insulin resistance of adolescence (8).

4. Role of Obesity

The insulin resistance associated with obesity is the fundamental problem in type 2 diabetes in children and adolescents, as it is in adults. Total obesity accounts for approximately 55% of the variance in insulin sensitivity (246). That obese children have hyperinsulinism has been known for over 30 years (247, 248). Obese children have ~40% lower insulin-stimulated glucose metabolism than nonobese children (246). African–American 5–10-year-olds, especially girls, have reduced insulin sensitivity in proportion to increases in blood pressure, triglycerides, subcutaneous fat, percentage of total body fat, and stage of sexual maturation (249). The amount of visceral fat in obese adolescents correlates directly with basal and glucose-stimulated insulinemia and inversely with insulin sensitivity (250). Insulin-stimulated glucose metabolism and fasting insulinemia decrease with increasing BMI (246).

Glucose tolerance testing was carried out in 720 Pima Indians aged 10–39 years, including 325 who had been exclusively bottlefed as infants, 144 who were exclusively breastfed, and the rest who had been partially breastfed for the first 2 months of life. Those exclusively breastfed had significantly lower rates of type 2 diabetes than those exclusively bottlefed for each age decade, with an odds ratio for type 2 diabetes in exclusively breastfed individuals of 0.41 (251). Prolonged breastfeeding has been noted in a large study of nearly 10,000 5–6-year-old German children to markedly reduce the risk of overweight; 3.8% of those exclusively breastfed for 2 months were overweight vs. 0.8% of those breastfed for longer than 12 months (252). Lower insulin responses occur in breastfed versus bottlefed infants and breastfed infants have lower energy and protein intake. Association has been made between early high protein intake and later obesity. Breastfeeding results in a more appropriate caloric intake at a critical stage in development, whereas bottlefeeding is more likely to be associated with overfeeding and obesity. The typical overweight of the bottlefed infant may contribute to insulin resistance and obesity in adolescence and young adulthood.

5. Polycystic Ovarian Syndrome and Premature Adrenarche

There is increasing recognition of polycystic ovarian syndrome (PCOS) in the adolescent population (253). Girls with PCOS are reported to have ~40% reduction in insulin-stimulated glucose disposal compared to nonhyperandrogenic control subjects (254, 255). Premature adrenarche, which has been thought to be a benign condition, is now recognized as a risk factor for ovarian hyperandrogenism and PCOS (256). Affected children are also more likely to have been born small for gestational age, indicating another aspect of the association of insulin resistance and intrauterine undernutrition (257, 258).

6. Racial and Familial Influences

A racial difference in the insulin responses to various stimuli parallels the ethnic/racial differential in type 2 diabetes frequency. Greater insulin responses to oral glucose are seen in African–American (AA) children and adolescents than in European–American (EA) children after adjustments are made for weight, age, ponderal (obesity) index, and pubertal stage. This is indicative of compensated insulin resistance in the AA youngsters (259, 260). Both prepubertal and pubertal AA children have higher fasting and stimulated insulin concentrations during glucose clamp studies than do EA youngsters (261). Lipolysis is also significantly less in AA children than in EA children, suggesting an energy conservation phenotype that would have survival value in times of famine but be detrimental with excess nutrition (thrifty genotype) (262).

Prepubertal children who have a family history of type 2 diabetes have lower insulin-stimulated glucose disposal and nonoxidative glucose disposal than do those without such a family history, indicating that family history of type 2 diabetes is a risk factor for insulin resistance in children, as in adults (263).

7. Genetic Considerations

The evidence that type 2 diabetes is a genetic disease includes the family clustering and segregation analyses that indicate that siblings of affected individuals have 3.5 times the general population risk of developing type 2 diabetes; studies of monozygotic twins that indicate a concordance of 80–100%, greater than twice the concordance in dizygotic twins and in monozygotic twins for type 1 diabetes; and the previously noted variations in insulin sensitivity and frequency of type 2 diabetes by ethnic origin (264). With rare exceptions, type 2 diabetes in children and adolescents, as in adults, is polygenic. The rare monogenic (autosomal dominant and mitochondrial) forms, however, provide insights for the study of typical type 2 disease (265).

Autosomal dominant forms include MODY and ADM. Molecular defects in 6 genes have been identified in families with MODY, affecting hepatocyte nuclear factors, glucokinase, and insulin promoter factor-1. Over 200 different mutations have been described. A glucokinase mutation has been identified in 1 of 10 ADM families studied as well (9).

In mitochondrial forms, disease transmission is exclusively from the mother because mitochondria are inherited via the cytoplasm of the ovum. The diabetes is usually indistinguishable from typical type 2 diabetes. In addition to the diabetes, affected individuals may also have sensorineural hearing loss, cardiomyopathy, optic neuropathy, myopathy, encephalopathy, lactic acidosis, strokelike syndrome, or epilepsy (10–12).

The identification of type 2 diabetes susceptibility genes involves choosing between two general approaches: the candidate gene approach and the genome scan approach. In the candidate gene approach, there is a problem identifying or choosing an appropriate candidate, or the candidate may be unknown at the time of the study, as was the case with the MODY genes. In the genome scan approach, the entire genome is examined for linkages within families or associations within populations. In these analyses, microsatellites are particularly useful and microassays of mRNA are able to identify gene patterns that are over- or underexpressed in specific disease states. Figure 4 illustrates possible candidate genes in the beta cell–target cell interaction.

More than 20 loci have been linked to or associated with type 2 diabetes in adults, the most important being *NIDDM1*, described among Mexican–American sibships in Starr County Texas. This county, which is 97% Mexican–American, has the highest disease-specific diabetes mortality in Texas. The gene pool is 31% Native American. Some 474 autosomal markers and 16 X-linked markers were examined in 170 affected sibships involving 300 affected siblings and 78 unaffected siblings. Identified as linked to type 2 diabetes was the *NIDDM1* site on chromosome 2, accounting for ~30% of family clustering. This was equal in importance, therefore, to the linkage with HLA in type 1 diabetes (267). This linkage was not identified in other populations, including non-Hispanic white, Japanese, French, Sardinian, and Finnish (264). The Calpain gene in the *NIDDM1* region of chromosome 2 was subsequently found to be associated with type 2 diabetes in several of these populations, linked to different loci (268).

Calpains are calcium-activated neutral proteases ubiquitously expressed from fetal life through adulthood, which function in signaling, proliferation, differentiation, and insulin-induced downregulation of IRS-1. Multiple polymorphisms of the gene encoding Calpain-10, encoded by the *CAPN10* gene within the *NIDDM1* region, have been found to be associated with type 2 diabetes. The highest-risk combination of polymorphisms give odds ratios of 2.8–3.6 in Mexican–Americans, 2.6 in Finns, and 5.0 in Germans (268). Nondiabetic Pima Indians who are homozygous for a common polymorphism of *CAPN10* have reduced insulin-mediated glucose turnover as the result of decreased glucose oxidation rates (269).

Figure 5 summarizes the factors that have been discussed in the development of type 2 diabetes.

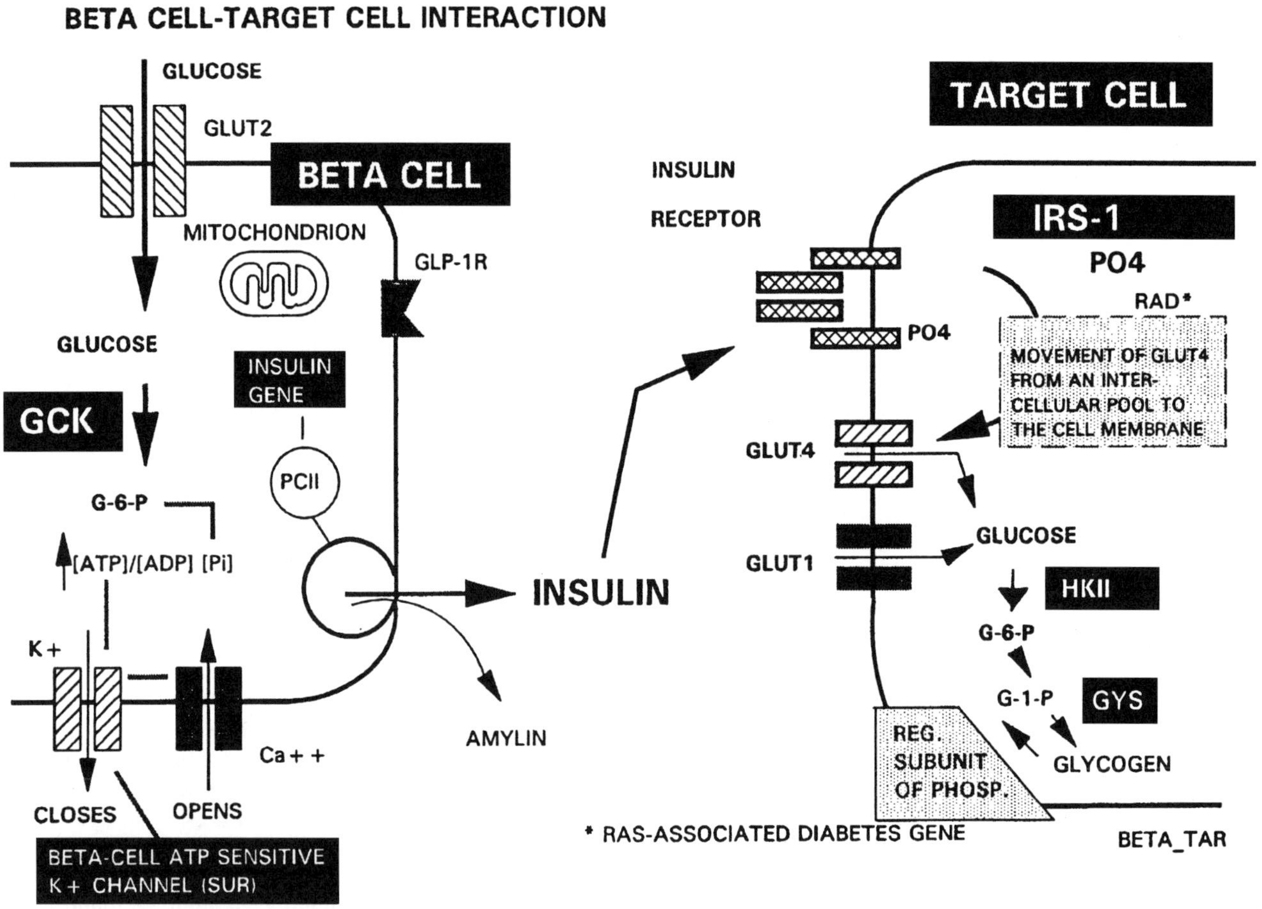

BETA CELL-TARGET CELL INTERACTION

Figure 4 Beta-cell candidate genes in diabetes mellitus include GLUT2 (glucose transporter 2), which is responsible for the facilitative uptake of glucose by beta-cells; glucokinase (GCK), which is the beta-cell glucose sensor; mitochondrial genes that provide power to the beta cell (an increased ratio of ATP to ADP + Pi[(ATP)]/[(ADP) + (Pi)]; the ATP-sensitive potassium (K′) channel (sulfonylurea receptor [SUR]); GLP-1 R (the beta-cell glucagen-like peptide-1 receptor) that responds to GLP from the gastrointestinal tract; insulin; PCII (prohormone convertase II, an example of an insulin-processing protein); and amylin, which is cosecreted with insulin. At the target cell (muscle, fat, or liver), candidate genes include the insulin receptor; intracellular proteins that are phosphorylated (insulin receptor substrate-1 [IRS1]); GLUT1; hexokinase II, which catalyzes the conversion of glucose to glucose-6-phosphate; glycogen synthase (GYS), which regulates glycogen production; and the regulatory subunit of phosphorylase (PHOSP) that regulates glycogen breakdown. GLUT4 is also a candidate gene, but GLUT4 is expressed only in muscle and fat tissues and is not expressed in the liver. (From Ref. 266.)

C. Clinical Features

The most striking difference between type 1 and type 2 diabetes is that in type 2 diabetes hyperglycemia/diabetes is one of many manifestations of the insulin resistance syndrome (diabesity syndrome, syndrome X, or the metabolic syndrome) (see Fig. 6). Common type 1 diabetes is, on the other hand, until the development of long-term complications, a unitary hormone deficiency state (although other autoimmune mediated deficiencies, such as thyroid, may develop).

Insulin resistance is a pathogenic factor in the devel-

opment of a broad spectrum of clinical conditions. These include hypertension, atherosclerosis, dyslipidemia, decreased fibrinolytic activity, impaired glucose tolerance type 2 diabetes, acanthosis nigricans, hyperuricemia, polycystic ovary disease, and obesity, which is the core abnormality (270).

In addition to the metabolic effects related to insulin resistance, obesity has deleterious associations in childhood and adolescence that increase morbidity and contribute to cardiovascular risk. This increased risk has been documented to be the result of the persistence of obesity into adulthood, rather than specific effects during child-

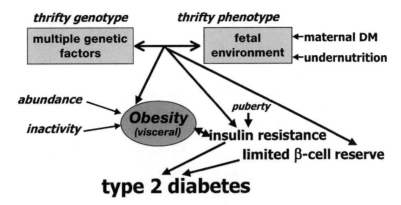

Figure 5 Factors in the development of type 2 diabetes.

hood (271, 272). Childhood obesity has been associated with elevated C-reactive protein and white blood cell counts, which are inflammatory indicators implicated in adult cardiovascular disease (273), proteinuria and focal segmental glomerular sclerosis (274), obstructive sleep apnea and other respiratory problems (275), hepatic steatosis (276), and orthopedic problems (275).

Lipoprotein abnormalities noted in type 2 diabetes include hypertriglyceridemia, elevated VLDL, elevated LDL-cholesterol, elevated lipoprotein (a), decreased high-density lipoprotein (HDL) cholesterol, increased small dense LDL particles, decreased lipoprotein lipase activity, increased lipoprotein glycation, and increased lipoprotein oxidation. The mechanism for this hyperlipidemia pattern is as follows. Fat cells, which are sensitive to insulin, store triglyceride and suppress hormone-sensitive lipase, the enzyme that breaks down triglycerides to release free fatty acids. Insulin also provides glucose to the fat cells for forming glycerol, the triglyceride backbone. With insulin resistance, there is abnormal breakdown of triglyceride and release of free fatty acids and glycerol, the latter contributing to gluconeogenesis. The free fatty acids cause insulin resistance in muscle tissue. In the liver, they are

reconverted to triglyceride, driving the production of LDL, which is the lipoprotein carrier of triglycerides, and the other dyslipidemic changes follow. The hyperinsulinemia of the insulin resistance state further drives the synthesis of fatty acids from glucose in the liver (277).

In adults there is a strong association between the level of hyperglycemia and risk factors for macrovascular disease. Dyslipidemia is one of several factors that accelerate atherosclerosis in type 2 diabetes. Additional factors described include oxidative stress, glycation of numerous vascular proteins, defective endothelium-dependent vasodilatation, and abnormalities of platelet function and coagulation (increased fibrinogen, increased plasminogen activator inhibitor-1, decreased antithrombin III and other anticoagulant and proteins, elevated factors VII and VIII, elevated vascular adhesion molecule 1, increased platelet adhesiveness and aggregation, decreased platelet nitric oxide [NO] production [NO mediates vasodilatation], decreased platelet prostacyclin production, and glycation of platelet proteins) (278).

Hypertension is estimated to account for 35–75% of diabetes complications involving both the microvasculature and macrovasculature (279). Diabetes *or* impaired glucose tolerance doubles the risk of developing hypertension (280). There is emerging evidence of a genetic predisposition to hypertension and type 2 diabetes related to the angiotensin-converting enzyme genotype (281). The hypertension in type 2 diabetes is due to volume expansion and increased vascular resistance, with reduced NO-mediated vasodilatation and increased activity of the renin–angiotensin system (278).

Acanthosis nigricans (AN) is an indicator of insulin resistance, prominent in genetic insulin resistance syndromes not associated with obesity. The frequency of AN in obese adolescents varies greatly by ethnicity: ~90% in Native Americans, ~50% in African–Americans, ~15% in Hispanic–Americans, and <5% in non-Hispanic whites. As an indicator of hyperinsulinism, AN also varies by ethnicity inversely to its frequency of association with

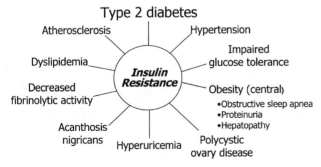

Figure 6 Insulin resistance: associated conditions. (Adapted from Consensus Development Conference of the American Diabetes Association, Diabetes Care, 1997.)

obesity (282). In a study of 139 overweight 6–10-year-olds, AN was present in 50% of African–Americans and 8.2% of whites. Half of those with fasting hyperinsulinemia did not have AN. AN was not considered a reliable marker for hyperinsulinemia in overweight children, despite its presence in a child with diabetes being a diagnostic indicator of type 2 disease (283).

D. Prevention

The concept of prevention of type 2 diabetes arises naturally from the appreciation of its environmental causation. Primary prevention would involve intervention to prevent obesity or to correct obesity before the development of other features of the insulin resistance syndrome. Prevention of obesity is a societal challenge. From the individual physician standpoint, the major question is, "Who should be tested?" (8). The importance of primary prevention of obesity lies in the recognition that preclinical impairment of glucose tolerance as the result of obesity-induced insulin resistance conveys cardiovascular risk; a substantial number of severely obese adolescents have impaired glucose tolerance (284). Considerations of testing for type 2 diabetes in children began with the assumption that this will be done in obese individuals, making the determination of obesity the screening test. The testing for hyperglycemia then becomes a case-finding exercise (285). The justifications for case finding include:

1. That the condition tested for is sufficiently common to provide a reasonable yield
2. That the condition is serious in terms of morbidity and mortality
3. That the condition has a prolonged latency without symptoms during which abnormality can be detected
4. That a test is available that is sensitive (few false-negative results) and accurate with acceptable specificity (a minimum number of false-positive results)
5. That an intervention is available to prevent or delay disease onset or more effectively treat the condition if it is detected in the latency phase

The first three conditions are unquestionably met by type 2 diabetes in children. The fourth criterion is met by plasma glucose measurement, with sensitivity and specificity dependent upon the circumstances of measurement. The last criterion, however, is extremely challenging, as discussed below.

A consensus panel of the American Diabetes Association (8) has recommended criteria for testing children. They should be overweight (BMI >85th percentile for age and sex (Figs. 17 and 27 in Chapter 43), weight for height >85th percentile, or weight >120% of ideal for height). Additionally, they should have two other risk factors, which were considered to be: family history of type 2 diabetes in first or second degree relatives; being of Amer-

ican Indian, African-American, Hispanic, or Asian/Pacific Islander race/ethnicity; and signs of insulin resistance or conditions associated with insulin resistance (acanthosis nigricans, hypertension, dyslipidemia, PCOS). It was recommended that testing begin at age 10 or at the onset of puberty if puberty occurs at a younger age and that repeat testing be done every two years, with fasting plasma glucose as the preferred test.

These criteria were not evidence based, which is why the consensus panel provided the disclaimer that clinical judgment should be used to test for diabetes in high-risk patients who do not meet these criteria. One might also take issue with the suggestion to use fasting plasma glucose. This was considered preferable because of its lower cost and greater convenience: 2 h plasma glucose increases earlier in the course of the development of type 2 diabetes, making it a more sensitive measure. Fasting hyperglycemia is an advanced stage of type 2 diabetes, and therefore highly specific but relatively insensitive as a testing method. Random plasma glucose concentration can be measured in those who have taken food shortly before testing, with a glucose concentration ≥7.8 mmol/L (140 mg/dL) serving as an indication for further testing.

The need for primary prevention efforts in childhood has been the subject of wide publicity for the past several years, with recognition of the epidemic of obesity (286–291). Obesity is associated with diminished school performance due to sleep apnea, torpor associated with physical inactivity, and social stigmatization. Secondary prevention of obesity is rarely successful beyond the short term. Intervention in adult populations indicates the enormous difficulty in altering lifestyle and dietary habits. The challenge for the pediatrician and society is to counter eating and entertainment trends that provide popular social outlets and are highly attractive, heavily promoted, and readily available. Financially stressed school systems often sabotage community efforts by providing fast food concessions and soft drink and snack vending machines in exchange for financial support from the vendors. Food service in middle and high schools typically includes high-fat, high-calorie foods such as pizza and french fries. There are inadequate opportunities for noncompetitive sports permitting participation of all youngsters, such as aerobics and dance, and there has been a sharp reduction in compulsory physical education programs. For some minority youngsters, there is the additional problem of a lack of safe environments in which to be physically active, and lack of funding for afterschool programs. Finally, school curricula have not effectively incorporated healthy lifestyle training.

A number of school-based and community-based programs have been developed targeting high-risk populations (290–295). School-based programs attempt to modify the food provided in school meals, incorporate healthy lifestyle training into classroom education, and create a school environment that promotes physical activity. Preschool and kindergarten through sixth grade programs encourage family involvement; high-school-based programs focus on social networks and peer pressure in an effort to promote behavior change and reduce risk factors. Short-term behavioral change has occurred with these programs, but longer-term studies are needed to determine whether these changes persist and reduce the risk for type 2 diabetes.

Before the contemporary epidemic of type 2 diabetes, we had noted the occasional obese African–American teenager attending our diabetes adventure camp program and rapidly becoming normoglycemic with vigorous exercise, permitting withdrawal of insulin. This phenomenon has been documented in 1 week summer camp programs for North American Indian youth with type 2 diabetes, who are able to achieve normoglycemia after 5 days of increased physical activity. Unfortunately, the behaviors of camp are not maintained, and most of the youngsters return to poor glycemic control at home (292, 296). Programs are in place that emphasize nutrition and exercise in schools, including those on Indian reservations throughout the United States, but their effectiveness has yet to be documented (294, 297).

The health-care system is increasing its appreciation of the magnitude of the obesity/type 2 diabetes problem. All who have contact with at-risk families need to emphasize the importance of intervention. Parent training by pediatricians, WIC and county health-department nurses, and other health personnel should continue to promote prolonged breastfeeding, which, in addition to its other many benefits, reduces the risk of obesity in childhood (251, 252). Parents also need to know that a fat baby is not a more healthy baby: candy, potato chips, and other foods with high caloric density and low nutritional value should not be used as rewards. Because children with normal-weight parents have a much lower risk of overweight (<7% vs. 40% with one overweight parent; and 80% with two overweight parents) obesity prevention is important for the whole family. It will not work for any one member by himself or herself (298). Physical activity must also be a family investment, with habits such as using stairs instead of elevators or escalators, walking or bicycling to school and to shop, and engaging in physically demanding chores such as yardwork. The most effective single thing that can be done to increase children's physical activity is to turn off the television set (299). It is also important that meals be taken on schedule, in one place, with no other activity going on.

Studies in adults have shown improved glucose tolerance or reduction in the rate of development of type 2 diabetes for up to several years as a result of lifestyle interventions, including individualized counseling for weight reduction, reduced total and saturated fat intake, increased fiber intake, and exercise (300–302). Among the most sustained efforts was a 13 year project involving six communities, The Minnesota Heart Health Program.

This included adult education classes for weight control, exercise promotion, and cholesterol reduction; a worksite weight control program; a home correspondence course for weight loss; and a weight gain prevention program. Despite this intensive effort, there was a strong upward trend in weight even when all potentially confounding variables were considered (303). Intervention with children, particularly preadolescents, should be more effective. In one study of family-based intervention involving 113 families, children had greater relative weight loss and better maintenance than the adults with one-third of children remaining nonobese after 10 years (304). In another study involving 24 families, including children 8–12 years old, the intervention was a 10–12 session behavioral modification. Two-thirds of the families completed the treatment program and those children who completed it lost weight. Weight loss was not maintained during 4–13 months of follow-up, however (298). Even modest successes in the reported studies have to be interpreted with caution, because these are selected study populations.

Diabetes prevention programs have to be designed with an understanding of the health beliefs and behaviors of the community. For example, American Indian youth with family members who had diabetes did not relate the complications of retinopathy or amputation to this problem in one study. Over half of the youth thought that diabetes was caused by bad blood, and greater than one-third attributed it to general weakness (305).

No medications are currently approved for the reduction of body weight in children. Medications that have been effective in adults do not result in maintenance of weight loss when the drugs are stopped. The only study of medical intervention for obesity in adolescents has been with metformin. Twenty-nine black and white adolescents aged 12–19 years with BMI >30 kg/m^2, with elevated fasting insulin concentrations (>15 uU/ml), a family history of type 2 diabetes, and normal fasting glucose and HbA1c were randomized to receive metformin 500 mg twice daily or placebo for 6 months. Controls had an increase in BMI of 0.23 SD and metformin-treated subjects a decrease of 0.12 SD, a significant difference. There was also a significant decrease in fasting glucose concentrations and insulin levels in metformin-treated youngsters compared with controls. Transient abdominal discomfort or diarrhea occurred in 40% of those taking metformin (306). In adults, lifestyle intervention was more effective than metformin in preventing progression from impaired glucose tolerance to type 2 diabetes (302).

There are limited data and no guidelines for surgical treatment of obesity in children and adolescents. A report in 1975 indicated a median weight loss of ~25% 3 years after gastric bypass or gastroplasty in 18 morbidly obese adolescents (307). A report 5 years later of 30 patients <20 years of age described average weight loss of 40 kg after 3 years and 26 kg 5 years after gastric bypass or gastroplasty. Major postoperative complications occurred in one-third and there was one postoperative death from anastomosis leakage (308). In 2001, 1 year follow-up of 10 adolescents age 17 years or younger who had undergone gastric bypass surgery by newer techniques was reported. There were no postoperative complications. Morbidities from obesity resolved in seven, including sleep apnea, hypertension, dyspnea, vertebral compression fracture, and refusal to attend school. Nine of the youngsters had >30 kg weight loss. Incisional hernia, gallstones, or small bowel obstruction required surgery in four of the individuals. Medical complications included mild iron deficiency anemia and transient folate deficiency (309).

E. Treatment

1. Challenges

The treatment challenges of type 2 diabetes in children and adolescents differ greatly from those of type 1 diabetes, due largely to the nature of the disease and those most likely affected. While type 1 diabetes is distributed throughout the population, type 2 diabetes disproportionately affects families with fewer resources, paralleling the distribution of obesity in the population. Whereas type 1 diabetes occurs throughout childhood, usually during the time when parental influence predominates, type 2 diabetes affects mostly those in adolescence or beyond, when peer influence is most important. There is also a large difference in family experience, with only ~5% of families with a child with type 1 diabetes having affected family members; 90% or more of youth with type 2 diabetes have family experience. These family members have typically failed to control their weight and glycemia, developing complications and creating an aura of despair and futility. Treatment priorities are also different between type 1 and type 2 diabetes. Extensive lifestyle modification, beyond insulin administration and glucose monitoring, is only required by those patients with type 1 disease who are overweight and inactive. However, the emphasis is on lifestyle modification in all those with type 2 diabetes and secondarily on glucose monitoring and hypoglycemic medication. Finally, technological innovation has revolutionized management of type 1 diabetes with improved insulin purity and delivery, self blood glucose monitoring, and the development of insulin analogs, with an artificial pancreas on the horizon and the likelihood that there will be islet cell replacement.

Technological advances have, however, been the underlying cause of the problem of type 2 diabetes, with advances in home entertainment systems, labor-saving devices, and transportation, and food preparation making calorically dense food increasingly available, desirable, and inexpensive.

2. Treatment Goals

The goals of treatment are to promote weight loss, normalize glycemia and HbA1c, control or prevent hyperten-

sion and hyperlipidemia, reduce acanthosis nigricans, and increase exercise capability.

Treatment is more important than might be indicated by the level of glycemia in some patients, because of the multitude of cardiovascular risk factors associated with insulin resistance. Just as in adults with newly diagnosed type 2 diabetes, young patients may already have evidence of complications, reflecting a prolonged period of impaired glucose tolerance. Among 100 Pima Indian children and adolescents with type 2 diabetes, 7% had high cholesterol ($\geq$200 mg/dl), 18% had hypertension (BP $\geq$140/90, now considered far too high a cut off), and 22% had micro-albuminuria (albumin/creatinine $\geq$30) at the time of diagnosis. Ten years later, while still in their 20s, they had mean HbA1c of 12% indicative of poor control, 60% had micro-albuminuria, and 17% had macro-albuminuria (albumin/creatinine $\geq$300) (310). Japanese investigators have described a high risk of renal failure in those who develop diabetes under 30 years of age (311).

Reduction in the risk of complications may require more stringent glycemic control in the insulin resistance state of type 2 diabetes than is required in type 1 diabetes, with diligent attention to comorbidities. In the UKPDS there was a 25% decrease in the risk of microvascular complications when the average HbA1c decreased from 7.9 to 7.0% (312). Reduction in BP to below 144/82 resulted in a more dramatic decrease of 37% in the risk for microvascular disease, 44% decrease in stroke occurrence, and 36% decrease in heart failure (313).

3. Changing Behavior

The behavioral changes and motivation required are so extensive that the treatment team requires a psychologist or social worker. One of the simplest changes to make is to eliminate the frequent consumption of high-calorie soft drinks, sweetened tea, and juices, substituting water, diet soft drinks, and artificial sweeteners for tea or Kool-Aid (314). Daily exercise should be documented in an attempt to break the vicious cycle of increased weight producing increased torpor, resulting in decreased activity and increased weight. As noted above, the most effective single method for doing this is turning off the television. A relatively small reduction in weight, accomplished by an increase in activity, can restore euglycemia and decrease hyperinsulinemia, as in the camp experience.

The stages of change are outlined in Table 5 (315).

4. Hypoglycemic Agents

Pharmacological therapy can decrease insulin resistance, increase insulin secretion, slow postprandial glucose absorption, or, in the case of insulin injection, supplement inadequate secretion of insulin (Table 6).

a. Biguanides. The biguanides act on insulin receptors in the liver to reduce hepatic glucose production and in muscle and fat tissue to enhance insulin-stimulated glucose uptake. They have an anorexic effect that can pro-

Table 5 Stages of Change

Concept	Definition	Application
1. Precontemplation	Unaware of problem; has no intention of changing in the near future (next 6 months) and may deny need for change. "Everyone in our family is big."	Increase awareness of need for change, personalize information on risks, benefits
2. Contemplation	Thinking about change, in the near future; knows there is an issue but is not ready to change; there may be intent to change in the next 6 months. "I've heard that some overweight kids are getting diabetes. But I don't think I can handle going on a diet."	Motivate, encourage to make specific plans
3. Preparation	Making a plan to change; knows what s/he wants to do; is seeking more information, planning, even starting to change; may tell family and friends; there is an intent to change in the near future. "I found out that if I lose some weight, this smudge on my neck will fade. I've taked to my Mom about it . . ."	Assist in developing concrete action plans, setting gradual goals
4. Action	Implementation of specific action plans; making changes in the environment to support the change. Relapse is normal. This stage may last as long as 6 months. "I'm walking three times a week for half an hour. I've quit drinking sodas . . ."	Assist with feedback, problem solving, social support, reinforcement
5. Maintenance	Continuation of desirable actions; or repeating periodic recommended step(s); may last 6 months to 5 years; some add a sixth stage, termination; "I lost 10 pounds. The smudge on my neck went away. I am going to keep on walking and eating better."	Assist in coping, reminders, finding alternatives, avoiding relapses (as apply)

mote weight loss. As noted above, metformin has also been used for this purpose. It has also been used to reduce acanthosis and ovarian hyperandrogenism. Long-term use is associated with a 1–2% reduction in HbA1c, but a high rate of side effects, including transient abdominal pain, diarrhea, and nausea, limits compliance in adolescents (316). Metformin must not be given to patients with renal impairment or who have hepatic disease, cardiac or respiratory insufficiency, or who are undergoing radiographic contrast studies, because of the risk of lactic acidosis.

Metformin is the only oral hypoglycemic agent for which there are available pediatric data. Eighty previously untreated patients age 8–16 years were randomized to receive metformin or placebo in a multicenter study. Dosage

Table 6 Effects of Drug Action in Diabetes

Drug type	Action	Effect on BG[a]	Risk of low BG[a]	Weight increase	Lipid decrease
Biguanides (metformin)	↓ Hepatic glucose output ↑ Hepatic insulin sensitivity	++	0	0	+
Sulfonylureas	↑ Insulin secretion and sensitivity	++	+	+	0
Metiglinide (repaglinide)	Short-term ↑ insulin secretion	++	+	+	0
Glucosidase inhibitors (acarbose, miglitol)	Slow hydrolysis and absorption of complex CH0	+	0	0	+
Thiazolidinediones (rosi-, pioglitazone)	↑ Insulin sensitivity in muscle and fat tissue ↓ Hepatic glucose output	++	0	+/−	+
Insulin	↓ Hepatic glucose output; overcomes insulin resistance	+++	+	++	+

[a]BG = blood glucose.

began at 500 mg twice daily and increased to 2000 mg/day over 2 weeks. Rescue criteria resulted in few placebo cases remaining by 16 weeks of the study. At 4 months or longer, the mean fasting glucose change from baseline was a decrease of 44 mg/dl with metformin and an increase of 20 mg/dl with placebo. The adjusted mean HbA1c with metformin was 7.5% and with placebo 8.6%. With metformin, there was no weight gain, and modest decrease in some patients, and lipid profiles improved. No serious adverse events were recorded (317).

When metformin is not being effective, it is important to take an in-depth history of medication intake, including refill history from the pharmacy, which may demonstrate that the medication is not being taken. Metformin may normalize ovulatory abnormalities in girls with PCOS or ovarian hyperandrogenism, increasing their pregnancy risk.

b. Sulfonylurea and Metiglinide/Repaglinide. This group of drugs increases insulin secretion and is thus most useful when there is residual beta-cell function. The sulfonylureas bind to specific receptors on the K+/ATP channel complex, while metiglinide and repaglinide bind to a separate site on the complex (Fig. 7). Activating ATP or binding by these drugs causes K+ channels to close, with resultant membrane depolarization, allowing calcium influx and insulin release. ATP-binding sites equilibrate rapidly; sulfonylurea sites do so slowly with prolongation of binding, which explains the sustained effects of traditional sulfonylureas. Metiglinide has an intermediate equilibration and binding duration, explaining its use for more rapid stimulation of insulin secretion and need for premeal dosing (318). The major adverse effects of the sulfonylureas have been hypoglycemia, which, as noted above, can be prolonged, and weight gain, which is particularly troublesome for adolescent patients.

c. Glucosidase Inhibitors. Alpha-glucosidase inhibitors such as acarbose and miglitol reduce the absorption of carbohydrates in the upper small intestine by the inhibition of oligosaccharide breakdown, delaying absorption in the lower small intestine. This results in reduction in postprandial glycemia. Long-term use of glucosidase inhibitors is associated with a reduction in HbA1c of 0.5–1% (319). Flatulence associated with the use of these agents makes them unacceptable to young patients.

d. Thiazolidinediones. These drugs act directly on muscle, adipose tissue, and liver to increase insulin sensitivity, and are, therefore, considered specific agents for the manifold problems of the insulin sensitivity syndrome. They bind to nuclear proteins, activating peroxisome proliferator activator receptors (PPAR), which are orphan steroid receptors particularly abundant in adipocytes, thus increasing formation of proteins involved in the nuclear-based actions of insulin. These include cell growth, adipose cell differentiation, regulation of insulin receptor activity, and glucose transport into cells. Long-term treatment with thiazolidinediones has been associated with a

reduction in HbA1c of 0.5–1.3% (320). Side effects have included edema, weight gain, and anemia. The original member of this group of drugs, troglitazone, was associated with liver enzyme elevations in ~1% of those taking the drug, with mortality in some who had existing liver problems. For these reasons it was withdrawn from the market. The newer thiazolidinediones, rosiglitazone and pioglitazone, have not been shown to have significant hepatotoxicity.

The binding of thiazolidinediones to PPARγ receptors is ubiquitous and includes arterial walls that contain muscle, affecting the growth of muscle cells and their migration in response to growth factors (321). These drugs also improve lipid profiles, decreasing LDL-cholesterol and triglycerides, while increasing HDL-cholesterol. These effects on vascular muscle and lipids could be important for the reduction of macrovascular disease associated with type 2 diabetes (322).

Although studies are in progress, there is no published data yet on the use of rosiglitazone and pioglitazone in children.

e. Insulin. The development of type 2 diabetes is an indicator of limited beta-cell function, estimated to be ~50% by the time of diagnosis in adults, most of whom will be insulin-requiring by 6 or 7 years later (323). Despite the insulin resistance, relatively low dosages of supplemental insulin (a few units) may be sufficient to maintain euglycemia. The newly available long-acting insulin analog without peak effects, insulin glargine, may be especially useful for type 2 diabetes in combination with premeal megilitinide, particularly in individuals unwilling to take metformin. Hypoglycemia has not been a common side effect of insulin in type 2 diabetes, but weight gain is an important adverse effect. All patients with type 2 diabetes eventually require treatment with insulin because of continuing loss of beta-cell function.

f. Treatment Recommendations. Treatment decisions are based on symptoms, severity of hyperglycemia, the presence or absence of ketosis/ketoacidosis (DKA), or dehydration. Dehydration signs may be less obvious in the obese. Symptomatic youngsters with type 2 diabetes, in addition to frequently having ketoacidosis at onset, are at particular risk for the hyperglycemic hyperosmolar state (HHS) which carries a high mortality (324). Acute management of DKA is discussed in Chapter 27. A treatment decision tree for outpatient management is given in Figure 8 (328).

Metformin should be the first oral agent used, because it is associated with HbA1c reductions similar to those resulting from use of sulfonylureas, without the risk of hypoglycemia and without weight gain. Furthermore, there may be greater effect on reducing LDL cholesterol and triglyceride levels. If there is failure of monotherapy using metformin over 3–6 months, sulfonylurea, metiglinide, or insulin can be added. Thiazolidinediones may

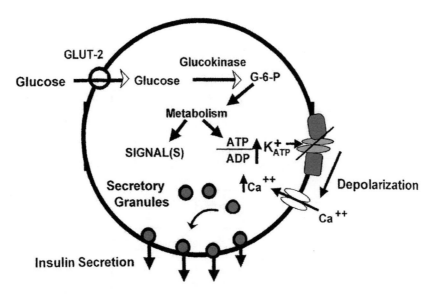

Figure 7   Insulin secretory control mechanism affected by sulfonylurea and metiglinide.

be used in older adolescents. Combination formulations may result in better compliance.

It is important to counsel adolescents with type 2 diabetes about sexuality and pregnancy, and provide contraceptive advice, as necessary. Metformin and thiazolidinediones may restore normal periods (326), and none of these oral agents should be used during pregnancy.

Although routine self-monitoring of blood glucose may not be needed as frequently as with type 1 diabetes, frequent monitoring is needed during periods of acute illness, during dosage adjustment, or with symptoms that indicate hyper- or hypoglycemia. It is also necessary to monitor for asymptomatic hypoglycemia in individuals who are taking insulin or sulfonylureas. The frequency of routine self-monitoring of blood glucose needs to be individualized, but should include a combination of fasting and postprandial measurements.

Assessments of HbA1c concentration should be done at least twice a year and, if metabolic control is unsatisfactory and requires treatment adjustment, every 3 months. The involvement of a dietitian with skill in the management of nutritional problems in children with diabetes is essential. Dietary recommendations need to be culturally appropriate, sensitive to family style and resources, and understood by all caregivers.

g. Treating Comorbidities.   Hypertension is an independent risk factor for the development of albuminuria, retinopathy, and cardiovascular disease in type 2 diabetes in adults. Its importance is emphasized by the experience of the UKPDS, in which hypertension control was more important than blood glucose control in reducing the risk of cardiovascular disease (313). Blood pressure should be measured at diagnosis and at least quarterly and compared to standards appropriate for age and height percentiles, as

noted in the tables in Chapter 38 (327). Elevations must be treated aggressively if there is persistent elevation above the usual percentile for the child or above the 90th percentile for either systolic or diastolic pressure. Angiotensin-converting enzyme inhibitors (ACEI) are the initial drug of choice. As with type 1 diabetes, many physicians use ACEI prophylactically.

Lipid levels and urine albumin excretion should be measured shortly after diagnosis and annually, or more often if there is abnormality and if treatment effects need monitoring. Exercise, weight loss, and glycemic control may be sufficient to correct hyperlipidemia. Dietary recommendations should be for the reduced-fat diet consistent with step 1 American Heart Association guidelines. Lipid-lowering medications should be added if lipid levels do not normalize after 2–3 months of dietary and diabetes control efforts. HMG CoA reductase inhibitors (statins) are the most commonly used lipid-lowering agents in children; they are contraindicated in pregnancy or if there is risk of pregnancy (328).

Unlike the recommendations for type 1 diabetes, in which is recommended that regular monitoring for complications not begin until adolescence and several years of diabetes, monitoring lipids and urinary albumin excretion, and examining the retina in those with type 2 diabetes, should begin at the time of diagnosis (8).

V.   OTHER TYPES OF DIABETES

A.   Cystic-Fibrosis-Related Diabetes

Cystic-fibrosis-related diabetes (CFRD) occurs in a substantial percentage of patients with CF and impaired glucose tolerance can be seen in most adolescents, which is

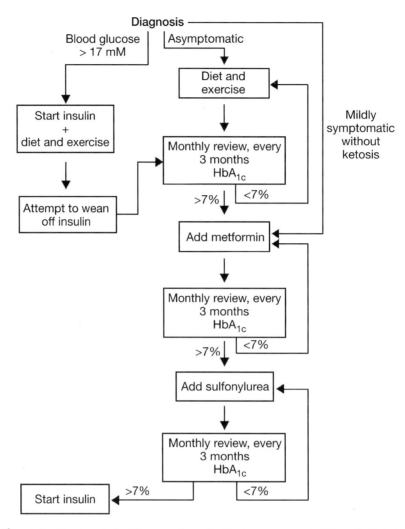

Figure 8 Treatment decision tree for outpatient management of type 2 diabetes.

the result of progressive pancreatic damage (329). Earlier reports suggested a prevalence of 2.5–7.6% in North America (330–332), but more recent reports indicate prevalences of 10–15% for overt diabetes (333–337). These rates continue to increase with the increase in longevity of patients with CF.

Pancreatic involvement beginning in utero progresses throughout life (338, 339). It eventually results in impaired insulin secretion in the vast majority of CF patients who have pancreatic exocrine deficiency, even in the presence of normal glucose tolerance (332, 340–343). The development of CFRD is considered an indicator of deterioration in the clinical state (330, 344, 345). Decrease in pulmonary function has been noted 2–4 years before the onset of CFRD, with improvement with insulin therapy (346). The course of CFRD is complicated by the need for high caloric intake to counter malabsorption and catabolism, the intermittent use of glucocorticoids, and re-

current infection. The diabetes has features of type 1 and type 2 disease, with insulin dependency and resistance (15, 335, 347, 348).

A recent report noted impaired glucose tolerance in 20% of 18 children with cystic fibrosis aged 9.5–15 years who were studied for the relationship of insulin secretion, IGF axis, and growth. However, impaired insulin secretion was present in 65% and was related to poor linear growth. It was considered that the increased demands for insulin during the pubertal growth period could indicate the need for treatment of growing children before the appearance of overt diabetes (349).

B. Infantile Diabetes

1. Transient Diabetes of the Newborn

This rare condition occurs from the first few hours to 6 weeks of life in small for gestational age infants who appear hyperalert with marked subcutaneous wasting (350). Onset is sudden, with severe dehydration in the absence of vomiting or diarrhea. Histological appearance of the pancreas has been reported as normal (351, 352), showing decrease in islet cells (353, 354) or increased numbers of islets (355). Approximately one-third of reported patients have a family history of type 1 diabetes (350) and have siblings who have been reported with transient diabetes of the newborn (356–358). Insulin may be required for a few days to a few months. Some infants may have permanent diabetes and a number have been reported to develop diabetes 8–20 years later (359–363).

2. Pancreatic Dysgenesis/Agenesis

Infants with transient diabetes who subsequently develop permanent diabetes (358–363) are thought to have dysgenesis of the pancreas. In one of these patients, no evidence of islet cell or other organ-specific autoimmunity was detected (361).

Only a few patients with severe pancreatic dysgenesis or agenesis have been reported, with permanent neonatal diabetes. Some have not survived, particularly those with associated anomalies such as gallbladder achalasia, diaphragmatic hernia, and cardiac defects (364, 365). Several infants without associated anomalies have survived, including siblings from our clinic, both with onset at 4 months of age, who are now in their mid-30s and have long-term complications (366–368). Such patients have exocrine and endocrine deficiency.

REFERENCES

1. Rosenbloom AL, Ongley JP. Who provides what services to children in private medical practice? Am J Dis Child 1974; 127:357–361.
2. Wilkins L. The Diagnosis and Treatment of Endocrine Disorders in Childhood and Adolescence, 3rd edition. Springfield IL: Charles C. Thomas, 1965:542.
3. Rosenbloom AL, Deeb LC, Allen L, Pollock BH. Characteristics of pediatric endocrinology practice: a workforce study. Endocrinologist 1998; 8:213–218.
4. The Expert Committee on the Diagnosis and Classification of Diabetes Mellitus. Report of the Expert Committee on the Diagnosis and Classification of Diabetes Mellitus. Diabetes Care 2001; 24:S5–20.
5. National Diabetes Data Group. Classification and diagnosis of diabetes mellitus and other categories of glucose intolerance. Diabetes 1979; 28:1039–1057.
6. Winter WE, Maclaren NK, Riley WJ, et al. Maturity-onset diabetes of youth in black Americans. N Engl J Med 1987; 316:285–291.
7. Banerji MA, Chaiken RL, Juey H, Tuomi T, Norin AJ, Mackay IR, Rowley MJ, Zimmet PZ, Lebovitz HE. GAD antibody negative NIDDM in adult with black subjects with diabetic ketoacidosis and increased frequency of human leukocyte antigen DR3 and DR4: Flatbush diabetes. Diabetes 1994; 43:741–745.
8. American Diabetes Association. Type 2 diabetes in children and adolescents: consensus conference report. Diabetes Care 2000; 23:381–389.
9. Winter WE. Molecular and biochemical analysis of the MODY syndromes. Pediatr Diabetes 2000; 1:88–117.
10. Reardon W, Ross RJM, Sweeney MG, Luxon LM, Pembrey ME, Harding AE, Trembath RC. Diabetes mellitus associated with a pathogenic point mutation in mitochondrial DNA. Lancet 1992; 340:1376–1379.
11. van den Ouwenland JMW, Lemkes HHPJ, Ruitenbeek W, Sandkuijl LA, de Vijlder MF, Struyvenberg PAA, van de Kamp JJ, Maassen JA. Mutation in mitochondrial tRNA (Leu(URR) gene in a large pedigree with maternally transmitted type II diabetes mellitus and deafness. Nature Genet 1992; 1:368–371.
12. Kadowaki T, Kadowaki H, Mori Y, Tobe K, Sakuta R, Suzuki Y, Tanabe Y, Sakura H, Awata T, Goto Y, et al. A subtype of diabetes mellitus associated with a mutation of mitochondrial DNA. N Engl J Med 1994; 330:962–968.
13. Taylor SI. Lilly Lecture: molecular mechanisms of insulin resistance: lessons from patients with mutations in the insulin-receptor gene. Diabetes 1992; 41:1473–1490.
14. Rosenbloom AL, Goldstein S, Yip CC. Normal insulin binding to cultured fibroblasts from patients with lipoatrophic diabetes. J Clin Endocrinol Metab 1977; 44:803–806.
15. Moran A, Doherty L, Wang X, Thomas W. Abnormal glucose metabolism in cystic fibrosis J Pediatr 1998; 133:10–17.
16. Berelowitz M, Eugene HG. Non-insulin-dependent diabetes mellitus secondary to other endocrine disorders. In: LeRoith D, Taylor SI, Olefsky JM, eds. Diabetes Mellitus. New York: Lippincott-Raven, 1996:496–502.
17. Cutfield WS, Wilton P, Bennmarker H, Albertsson-Wikland K, Chatelain P, Ranke MB, Price DA. Incidence of diabetes mellitus and impaired glucose tolerance in children and adolescents receiving growth hormone treatment. Lancet 2000; 355:610–613.
18. Rosenbloom AL. Hot topic. Fetal growth, adrenocortical function, and the risk for type 2 diabetes. Pediatr Diabetes 2000; 1:150–154.
19. Pandit MK, Burke J, Gustafson AB, Minocha A, Peiris AN. Drug-induced disorders of glucose tolerance. Ann Intern Med 1993; 118:529–540.
20. O'Byrne S, Feely J. Effects of drugs on glucose tolerance in non-insulin-dependent diabetes (parts I and II). Drugs 1990; 40:203–219.
21. Bouchard P, Sai P, Reach G, Caubarrere I, Ganeval D, Assan R. Diabetes mellitus following pentamidine-induced hypoglycemia in humans. Diabetes 1982; 31:40–45.
22. Assan R, Perronne C, Assan D, Chotard L, Mayaud C, Matheron S, Zucman D. Pentamidine-induced derangements of glucose homeostasis. Diabetes Care 1995; 18:47–55.
23. Gallanosa AG, Spyker DA, Curnow RT. Diabetes mellitus associated with autonomic and peripheral neuropathy after Vacor poisoning: a review. Clin Toxicol 1981; 18:441–449.
24. Esposti MD, Ngo A, Myers MA. Inhibition of mitochondrial complex I may account for IDDM induced by intoxication with rodenticide Vacor. Diabetes 1996; 45:1531–1534.
25. Forrest, JA, Menser MA, Burgess JA. High frequency of diabetes mellitus in young patients with congenital rubella. Lancet 1971; 2:332–334.
26. Rosenbloom AL. Type 2 diabetes in children. American

Association for Clinical Chemistry. Diagn Endocrinol Immunol Metabol 2000; 18:143–153.

27. Hathout EH, Thomas W, El-Shahawy, Nabab F, Mace JW. Diabetic autoimmune markers in children and adolescents with type 2 diabetes. Pediatrics 2001 http://www. pediatrics.org/cgi/content/full/107/6/e102.

28. Macaluso CJ, Bauer UE, Deeb LC, Malone JI, Chaudhari M, Silverstein J, Eidson M, Arbelaez AM, Goldberg RB, Gaughan-Bailey B, Brooks RG, Rosenbloom AL. Type 2 diabetes mellitus among Florida children, 1994 through 1998. Public Health Rep (in press).

29. Fletcher RH, Fletcher SW, Wagner EH. Clinical Epidemiology, The Essentials. 2nd ed. Baltimore: Williams & Wilkins, 1988.

30. Sekikawa A, LaPorte RE. Epidemiology of insulin-dependent diabetes mellitus. In Alberti KGMM, Zimmet P, DeFronzo RA, eds. International Textbook of Diabetes Mellitus. 2nd ed, vol 1. West Sussex, UK: John Wiley & Sons, 1997:89–96.

31. LaPorte RE, Tuomilehto J, King H. WHO Multinational Project for Childhood Diabetes. Diabetes Care 1990; 13: 1062–1068.

32. Karvonen M, Viik-Kajander M, Moltchanova E, Libman I, LaPorte R, Tuomilehto J, for the Diabetes Mondiale (DiaMond) Project Group. Incidence of childhood type 1 diabetes worldwide. Diabetes Care 2000; 23:1516–1526.

33. LaPorte RE, Matsushima M, Chang Y-F. Prevalence and incidence of insulin-dependent diabetes. In National Diabetes Data Group, eds. Diabetes in America, 2nd ed. Washington, DC: National Institutes of Health, National Institute of Diabetes and Digestive and Kidney Diseases, NIH Publication No. 95-1468, 1995:37–46.

34. Mimura G. Present status and future view of the genetics of diabetes in Japan. In Mimura G, Baba S, Goto W, Kobberling J, eds. Clinical Genetics of Diabetes Mellitus, International Congress Series 597. Amsterdam: Excerpta Medica, 1982:13–18.

35. Kitagawa T, Fujita H, Hibi I, et al. A comparative study of the epidemiology of IDDM between Japan, Norway, Israel and the United States. Acta Paediatr Jpn 1984; 26: 275–281.

36. Siemaitycki J, Colle E, Campbell S, Dewar R, Aubert D, Bellmonte, M. Incidence of IDDM in Montreal by ethnic group and by social class and comparisons with ethnic groups living elsewhere. Diabetes 1988; 37:1096–1112.

37. Burden AC, Burden ML, Williams ER, et al. Evidence of frequent epidemics of childhood diabetes. Diabetes 1991; 40:373A.

38. Karvonen M, Tuomilehto J, Libman I, LaPorte R for the World Health Organization DiaMond Project Group. A review of the recent epidemiological data on the worldwide incidence of type 1 (insulin-dependent) diabetes mellitus. Diabetologia 1993; 36:83–892.

39. Diabetes Epidemiology Research International Group. Secular trends in incidence of childhood IDDM in 10 countries. Diabetes 1990; 39:858–864.

40. Dahlquist G, Blom L, Holmgren G, Hagglof B, Larson Y, Sterky G, Wall S. The epidemiology of diabetes in Swedish children 0–14 years—a six-year prospective study. Diabetologia 1985; 28:802–808.

41. Joner G, Sovik O. Incidence, age at onset and seasonal variation of diabetes mellitus in Norwegian children. Acta Paediatr Scand 1981; 70:329–325.

42. Tull ES, Roseman JM, Christian CLE. Epidemiology of childhood IDDM in U.S. Virgin Islands from 1979 to 1998. Diabetes Care 1991; 14:558–564.

43. Zhao HX, Stenhouse E, Soper C, Hughes P, Sanderson E, Baumer JH, Demaine AG, Millward BA. Incidence of childhood-onset type 1 diabetes mellitus in Devon and Cornwall, England, 1975–1996. Diabet Med 1999; 16: 1030–1035.

44. Fleegler FM, Rogers KD, Drash A, Rosenbloom AL, Travis LM, Court JM. Age, sex, and season of onset of childhood diabetes in different geographic areas. Pediatrics 1979; 63:374–379.

45. Karvonen M, Tuomilehto J, Virtala E, Pitkaniemi J, Feunanen A, Tuomilehto-Wolf E, Akerblom KA for the Childhood Diabetes in Finland (DiMe) Study Group. Seasonality in the clinical onset of insulin-dependent diabetes mellitus in Finnish children. Am J Epidemiol 1996; 143: 167–176.

46. Atkinson MA, Maclaren NK. The pathogenesis of insulin-dependent diabetes. N Engl J Med 1994; 331:1428–1436.

47. Maclaren NK, Lan M, Coutant R, et al. Only multiple autoantibodies to islet cells (ICA), insulin, GAD65, IA-2 and IA-2β predict immune mediated (type 1) diabetes in relatives. J Autoimmun 1999; 12:279–287.

48. Bingley PJ, Christie MR, Bonifacio E, et al. Combined analysis of autoantibodies improves prediction of IDDM in islet sell antibody-positive relatives. Diabetes 1994; 43: 1304–1310.

49. Kulmala P, Savola K, Peterson JS, and the Childhood Diabetes in Finland (DiMe) Study Group. Prediction of insulin-dependent diabetes mellitus in siblings of children with diabetes. J Clin Invest 1998; 101:327–336.

50. Krischer JP, Schatz D, Riley WJ, Spillar RP, Silverstein JH, Schwartz S, Malone J, Shah S, Vadheim CM, Rotter JI, Quatrin T, Maclaren NK. Insulin and islet cell autoantibodies as time dependent co-variates in the development of insulin dependent diabetes: a prospective study in relatives. J Clin Endocrinol Metab 1993; 77:743–749.

51. Riley WJ, Maclaren NK, Krischer JP, Spillar RP, Silverstein JH, Schatz D, Shah S, Vadheim CM, Rotter JI. A prospective study of the development of diabetes in relatives of patients with insulin dependent diabetes. N Engl J Med 1990; 323:1167–1172.

52. DPT-1 Study Group. The Diabetes Prevention Trial Type 1 Diabetes (DPT-1). Diabetes 1994; 43(Suppl)159A.

53. Bougneres PF, Carel JC, Castano L, et al. Factors associated with early remission of type 1 diabetes in children treated with cyclosporine. N Engl J Med 1988; 318:663–670.

54. Lipton R, LaPorte RE, Becker DJ, et al. Cyclosporin therapy for prevention and cure of IDDM. Epidemiologic perspective of benefits and risks. Diabetes Care 1990; 13: 776–74.

55. Silverstein J, Maclaren N, Riley W, Spillar R, Radjenovic D, Johnson S. Immunosuppression with azathioprine and prednisone in recent-onset insulin-dependent diabetes mellitus. N Engl J Med 1988; 319:599–604.

56. Shah SC, Malone JI, Simpson NE. A randomized trial of intensive insulin therapy in newly diagnosed insulin-dependent diabetes mellitus. N Engl J Med 1989; 320:550–554.

57. Keller RJ, Eisenbarth GS, Jackson RA. Insulin prophylaxis in individuals at high risk of type 1 diabetes. Lancet 1993; 341:927–928.

58. Diabetes Prevention Trial—Type 1 Diabetes Study Group. Effects of insulin in relatives of patients with type 1 diabetes mellitus. N Engl J Med 2002; 346:1685–1691.

59. Pozzilli P, Andreani D. The potential role of Nicotinamide in the secondary prevention of IDDM. Diabetes Metab Rev 1993; 9:219–230.

60. Kolb H, Burkert V. Nicotinamide in type 1 diabetes. DiabetesCare 1999; 22:B16–B20.

61. Elliott RB, Chase HP. Prevention or delay to type 1 (insulin-dependent) diabetes mellitus in children using nicotinamide. Diabetologia 1991; 34:362–365.

62. Elliott R, Pilcher C, Fergusson D, Stewart A. A population based strategy to prevent insulin-dependent diabetes using nicotinamide. J Pediatr Endocrinol Metab 1996; 9: 501–509.

63. Rosenbloom AL, Schatz DA, Krischer JP, et al. Therapeutic controversy. Prevention and treatment of diabetes in children. J. Clin Endocrinol Metab 2000; 85:494–508.

64. Lampeter EF, Klinghammer A, Scherbaum WA, et al. The Deutsche Nicotinamide Intervention Study: an attempt to prevent type 1 diabetes. DENIS group. Diabetes 1998; 47:980–994.

65. Green A, Patterson CC, EURO DIAB TIGER Study Group. Trends in the incidence of childhood-onset diabetes in Europe 1989–98 Diabetologia 2001; 44(Suppl 3): B3–B8.

66. Karvonen M, Pitkaniemi J, Tuomilehto J. The onset age of type 1 diabetes in Finnish children has become younger. Diabetes Care 1999; 22:1066–1070.

67. Gardner SG, Bingley PJ, Sawtell PA, Weeks S, Gale EAM. Rising incidence of insulin dependent diabetes in children aged under 5 years in the Oxford region. Br Med J 1997; 315:713–717.

68. Hyppönen E, Läärä E, Reunanen A, Järvelin M-R, Virtanen S. Intake of vitamin D and risk of type 1 diabetes: a birth-cohort study. Lancet 2001; 358:1500–1503.

69. Schein PS, Alberti KG, Williamson DH. Effects of streptozotocin on carbohydrate and lipid metabolism in the rat. Endocrinology 1971; 89:827–834.

70. Banerjee S. Effect of certain substances of the prevention of diabetogenic action of alloxan. Science 1947;128–130.

71. Pont A, Rubino JM, Bishop D. Diabetes mellitus and neuropathy following Vacor ingestion in man. Arch Intern Med 1979; 139:185–187.

72. McKinney PA, Okasha M, Parslow RC, Law GR, Gurney KA, Williams R, Bodansky HJ. Early social mixing and childhood type 1 diabetes mellitus: a case–control study in Yorkshire, UK. Diabet Med 2000; 17:236–242.

73. Karjalainen J, Martin JM, Knip M, et al. A bovine serum albumin peptide as a possible trigger of insulin-dependent diabetes mellitus. N Engl J Med 1992; 327:302–307.

74. Norris JM, Beaty B, Klingensmith G, Hoffman MN, Yu L, Chase HP, Erlich HA, Hamman RF, Eisenbarth GS, Rewers M. Lack of association between early exposure to cow's milk protein and beta-cell autoimmunity: Diabetes Autoimmunity Study in the Young. JAMA 1996; 276:609–614.

75. Papaccio G, Ammendola E, Pisanti FA. Nicotinamide decreases MHC class II but not MHC class I expression and increases intercellular adhesion molecule-1 structures in non-obese diabetic mouse pancreas. J Endocrinol 1999; 160:389–400.

76. Hyoty H, Hiltunen M, Knip M, Laakkonen M, Vahasalo P, Karjalainen J, Koskela P, Roivainen M, Leinikki P, Hovi T, Akerblom HK. A prospective study of the role of coxsackie B and other enteroviral infections in the pathogenesis of IDDM. Diabetes 1995; 44:652–657.

77. Dahlquist GG, Ivarsson S, Lindberg B, Forsgren M. Maternal enteroviral infection during pregnancy as a risk factor for childhood IDDM. Diabetes 1995; 44:408–413.

78. Uriarte A, Cabrera E, Ventura R, Vargas J. Islet cell antibodies and ECHO-4 virus infection. Diabetologia 1987; 30:590A.

79. Honeyman MC, Coulson BS, Stone NL, Gellert SA, Goldwater PN, Steele CE, Couper JJ, Tait BD, Colman PG, Harrison LC. Association between rotavirus infection and pancreatic islet autoimmunity in children at risk of developing type 1 diabetes. Diabetes 2000; 49:1219–1324.

80. Helmke K, Otten A, Willems WR, Brockhaus R, Mueller-Eckhardt G, Stief T, Bertrams J, Wolf H, Federlin K. Islet cell antibodies and the development of diabetes mellitus in relation to mumps infection and mumps vaccination. Diabetologia 1986; 29:30–33.

81. Silverstein JH, Rosenbloom AL. New developments in type 1 (insulin-dependent) diabetes. Clin Pediatr 2000; 39:257–266.

82. Malone JI, Hellrung JM, Malphus EW, Rosenbloom AL, Grgic A, Weber FT. Good diabetic control—a study in mass delusion. J Pediatr 1976; 88:943–947.

83. Rosenbloom AL, Silverstein JH, Riley WJ, Malone JI, Lezotte DC, McCallum M, Maclaren NK, Neufeld M. Total glycosylated hemoglobin estimation in the management of children and youth with diabetes. Bull Int Study Group Diabetes Child Adolesc 1980; 4:24–25.

84. Diabetes Control and Complications Trial (DCCT)/Epidemiology of Diabetes Intervention and Complications (EDIC) Research Group. Beneficial effects of intensive therapy of diabetes during adolescence: outcomes after the conclusion of the Diabetes Control and Complications Trial (DCCT). J Pediatr 2001; 139:804–812.

85. Rosenbloom AL, Lezotte DC, Weber FT, Gudat J, Heller DR, Weber ML, Klein S, Kennedy BB. Diminution of bone mass in childhood diabetes. Diabetes 1977; 26: 1052–1055.

86. Ponder SW, McCormick DP, Fawcett HD, Tran AD, Oglesby GW, Brouhard BH, Travis LB. Bone mineral density of the lumbar vertebrae in children and adolescents with insulin-dependent diabetes mellitus. J Pediatr 1992; 120:541–545.

87. Roe TF, Mora S, Costin G, Kaufman F, Carlson ME, Gilsanz V. Vertebral bone density in insulin-dependent diabetic children. Metabolism 1991; 40:967–971.

88. De Schepper J, Smitz J, Rosseneu S, Bollen P, Louis O. Lumbar spine bone mineral density in diabetic children with recent onset. Horm Res 1998; 50:193–196.

89. Rozadilla A, Nolla JM, Montana E, Fiter J, Gomez-Vaquero C, Sorler J, Roig-Escofet D. Bone mineral density in patients with type 1 diabetes mellitus. Joint Bone Spine 2000; 67:215–218.

90. Gunczler P, Lanes R, Paz-Martinez V, Martins R, Esaa S, Colmenares V, Weisinger JR. Decreased lumbar spine bone mass and global turnover in children and adolescents with insulin-dependent diabetes mellitus followed longitudinally. J Pediatr Endocrinol Metab 1998; 11:413–419.

91. Gunczler P, Lanes R, Paoli M, Martinis R, Villaroel O, Weisinger JR. Decreased bone mineral density and bone formation markers shortly after diagnosis of clinical type 1 diabetes mellitus. J Pediatr Endocrinol Metab 2001; 14: 525–528.

92. Malone JI, Lowitt S, Duncan JA, Shah S, Vargas A, Root A. Hypercalciuria, hyperphosphaturia, and growth retar-

dation in children with diabetes mellitus. Pediatrics 1986; 78:298–304.

93. Thalassinor NC, Hadjiyauni P, Tzanela M, Akvizaki C, Philokiprou D. Calcium metabolism and diabetes mellitus: effect of improved blood glucose control. Diabet Med 1993; 10:341–344.

94. Heath H, Melton LJ, Chic GP. Diabetes mellitus and risk of skeletal fracture. N Engl J Med 1980; 303:567–570.

95. Rosenbloom AL, Frias JL. Diabetes mellitus, short stature and joint stiffness—a new syndrome. Clin Res 1974; 22: 92A.

96. Grgic A, Rosenbloom AL, Weber FT, Giordano B, Malone JI, Shuster JJ. Joint contracture—common manifestation of childhood diabetes mellitus. J Pediatr 1976; 88: 584–588.

97. Rosenbloom AL, Silverstein JH, Lezotte DC, Richardson K, McCallum M. Limited joint mobility in childhood diabetes mellitus indicates increased risk for microvascular disease. N Engl J Med 1981; 305:191–194.

98. Salzarulo HH, Taylor LA. Diabetic "stiff joint syndrome" as a cause of difficult endotracheal intubation. Anesthesiology 1986; 64:366–368.

99. Schnapf BM, Banks R, Silverstein JH, Rosenbloom AL, Chesrown S, Loughlin G. Pulmonary function in insulin dependent diabetes mellitus with limited joint mobility. Am Rev Respir Dis 1984; 130:930–932.

100. Hanna W, Friesen D, Bombardier C, Gladman D, Hanna A. Pathological features of diabetic thick skin. J Am Acad Dermatol 1987; 16:546–553.

101. Rosenbloom AL, Williams J, Linda SB. Quantitative assessment of limited joint mobility (LJM) in diabetes from radiographs. J Pediatr Endocrinol 1991; 4:243–247.

102. Rosenbloom AL, Silverstein JH, Lezotte DC, Riley WJ, Maclaren NK. Limited joint mobility in diabetes mellitus of childhood: natural history and relationship to growth impairment. J Pediatr 1982; 101:874–878.

103. Kohn RR, Schnider SL. Glucosylation of a of human collagen. Diabetes 1982; 31(suppl 3):47–51.

104. Monnier VM, Vishwanath V, Frank KE, Elmets CA, Dauchot P, Kohn RR. The relation between complications of type 1 diabetes mellitus and collagen-linked fluorescence. N Engl J Med 1986; 314:403–408.

105. Rosenbloom AL, Malone JI, Yucha J, Van Cader TC. Limited joint mobility and diabetic retinopathy demonstrated by fluorescein angiography. Eur J Pediatr 1984; 141:163–164.

106. Starkman HS, Gleason RE, Rand LI, Miller DE, Soeldner J. Limited joint mobility (LJM) of the hand in patients with diabetes mellitus: relation to chronic complications. Ann Rheum Dis 1986; 45:130–135.

107. Silverstein JH, Fennell R, Donnelly W, Banks R, Stratton R, Spillar R, Rosenbloom AL. Correlates of biopsy-studied nephropathy in young patients with insulin-dependent diabetes mellitus. J Pediatr 1985; 106:196–201.

108. Silverstein JH, Gordon G, Pollock BH, Rosenbloom AL. Long term glycemic control influences the development of limited joint mobility in type 1 diabetes. J Pediatr 1998; 132:944–947.

109. Infante J, Rosenbloom AL, Silverstein JH, Garzarella L, Pollack BH. Changes in frequency and severity of limited joint mobility in children with type 1 diabetes mellitus between 1976–78 and 1998. J Pediatr 2001; 138:33–37.

110. Kelly WF, Nicholas J, Adams J, Mahmood R. Necrobiosis lipoidica diabeticorum: association with background retinopathy, smoking, and proteinuria. A case control study. Diabet Med 1993; 10:725–728.

111. Raile K, Noelle V, Landgraf R, Schwarz HP. Insulin antibodies are associated with lipoatrophy but also with lipohypertrophy in children and adolescents with type I diabetes. Exp Clin Endocrinol Diabetes 2001; 109:393–396.

112. Roper NA, Bilous RW. Resolution of lipohypertrophy following change of short-acting insulin to insulin lispro (Humalog). Diabet Med 1998; 15:1063–1064.

113. Muritano ML, La Roche GR, Stevens JL, Gloor BRD, Schoenle EJ. Acute cataracts in newly diagnosed IDDM in five children and adolescents. Diabetes Care 1995; 18: 1395–1396.

114. Tattersall RB, Pyke DA. Growth in diabetic children: studies in identical twins. Lancet 1973; 2:1105–1109.

115. Holl RW, Heinze E, Seifert M, Grabert M, Teller WM. Longitudinal analysis of somatic development in pediatric patients with IDDM: genetic influences on weight. Diabetologia 1994; 37:925–929.

116. Salerno M, Argenziano A, Di Maio S, Gasparini N, Formicola S, De Filippo G, Tenore A. Pubertal growth, sexual maturation, and final height in children with IDDM. Diabetes Care 1997; 20:721–724.

117. Rosenbloom AL, Silverstein JH, Lezotte DC, Riley WJ, Maclaren NK. Limited joint mobility in diabetes mellitus of childhood: natural history and relationship to growth impairment. J Pediatr 1982; 101:874–878.

118. Infante JR, Rosenbloom AL, Silverstein JH, Garzarella L, Pollack BH. Limited joint mobility (LJM) and stature in childhood type 1 diabetes (DM1): improved methods of control are making a difference. Proceedings, Endocrinology Society 81st Annual Meeting. San Diego, CA, 1999.

119. Menon RK, Arslanian S, May B, Cutfield WS, Sperling MA. Diminished growth hormone binding protein in children with insulin-dependent diabetes mellitus. J Clin Endocrinol Metab 1992; 74:934–938.

120. Massa G, Dooms L, Bouillon R, Vanderschueren-Lodeweyckz. Serum levels of growth hormone binding protein and insulin like growth factor I in children and adolescents with type 1 (insulin-dependent) diabetes mellitus. Diabetologia 1993; 36:239–243.

121. Munoz MT, Barrior, Pozo J, Argente J. Insulin like growth factor I, its binding proteins 1 and 3, and growth hormone binding protein in children and adolescents with insulin-dependent diabetes mellitus: clinical implications. Pediatr Res 1996; 39:992–998.

122. Bereket A, Lang CH, Wilson TA. Alterations in the growth hormone insulin like growth factor axis in insulin-dependent diabetes mellitus. Horm Metab Res 1999; 31: 172–181.

123. Mauriac P. Gros ventre, hépatomégalie, troubles de croissance chez les enfants diabétiques traités depuis plusiers année par l'insuline. Gaz Hebd Med Bordeaux 1930; 26:402–410.

124. Rosenbloom AL, Clarke DW. Excessive insulin treatment and the Somogyi effect. In Pickup J, ed. Difficult Diabetes. Oxford: Blackwell, 1985: 103–131.

125. Marble A, White P, Bogan I, Smith R. Enlargement of the liver in diabetic children: I. Its incidence etiology and nature. Arch Intern Med 1938; 62:740–750.

126. Lasalle R, Chicoine L. Le syndrome de Mauriac: une observation clinique. Union Med Can 1962; 91:963–968.

127. Lee RG, Bode HH. Stunted growth and hepatomegaly in diabetes mellitus. J Pediatr 1977; 91:82–84.

128. Dorchy H, van Vliet G, Toussaint D, Ketelbant-Balasse

P, Loeb H. Mauriac syndrome: three cases with retinal angiofluorescein study. Diabete Metab 1979; 5:195–200.

129. Winter R, Phillips L, Green O, Traisman H. Somatomedin activity in the Mauriac syndrome. J Pediatr 1980; 97: 589–600.

130. Riley WJ, Maclaren NK, Lezotte DC, Spillar RP, Rosenbloom AL. Thyroid autoimmunity in insulin-dependent diabetes mellitus. The case for routine screening. J Pediatr 1981; 98:350–354.

131. Aktay AN, Lee PC, Kumar V, Parton E, Wyatt DT, Werlin SL. The prevalence and clinical characteristics of celiac disease in juvenile diabetes in Wisconsin. J Pediatr Gastroenterol Nutr 2001; 33:462–465.

132. Affenito SG, Adams CH. Are eating disorders more prevalent in females with type 1 diabetes mellitus when the impact of insulin omission is considered? Nutr Rev 2001; 59:179–182.

133. Greene DA, Lattimer SA, Simon AAF. Sorbitol, inositides and sodium potassium-ATPase in the pathogenesis of diabetic complications. N Engl J Med 1987; 316:599–606.

134. Lee P, Jenkins P, Bourke C, et al. Prothrombotic and antithrombotic factors are elevated in patients with type 1 diabetes complicated by microalbuminuria. Diabet Med 1993; 10:122–128.

135. Viberti GC, Hill RD, Jarret TRJ, et al. Microalbuminuria as a predictor of clinical nephropathy in insulin-dependent diabetes mellitus. Lancet 1982; 1:1430–1432.

136. Chaturvedi N, Bandinelli S, Mangill R, Penno G, Rottiers RE, Fuller JH. Microalbuminuria in type 1 diabetes: rates, risk factors and glycemic threshold. Kidney Int 2001; 60: 219–227.

137. Twyman S, Rowe D, Mansell P, Schapira D, Betts P, Leatherdale B. Longitudinal study of urinary albumin excretion in young diabetic patients—Wessex Diabetic Nephropathy Project. Diabet Med 2001; 18:402–408.

138. Santilli F, Spagnoli A, Mohn A, Tumini S, Verrotti A, Cipollone F, Mezzetti A, Chiarelli F. Increased vascular endothelial growth factor serum concentrations may help to identify patients with onset of type 1 diabetes during childhood at risk for developing persistent microalbuminuria. J Clin Endocrinol Metab 2001; 86:3871–3876.

139. Olsen BS, Sjolie A, Hougaard P, Johannesen J, Borch-Johnsen K, Marinelli K, Thorsteinsson B, Pramming S, Mortensen HB. A 6-year nationwide cohort study of glycaemic control in young people with type 1 diabetes. Risk markers for the development of retinopathy, nephropathy and neuropathy. Danish Study Group of Diabetes in Childhood. J Diabetes Complications 2000; 14:295–300.

140. Levy-Marchal C, Sahler C, Cahane M, Czernichow P. Risk factors for microalbuminuria in children and adolescents with type 1 diabetes. J Pediatr Endocrinol Metab 2000; 13:613–620.

141. Warram JH, Scott LJ, Hanna LS, et al. Progression of microalbuminuria to proteinuria in type 1 diabetes: nonlinear relationship with hyperglycemia. Diabetes 2000; 49:94–100.

142. Orchard TJ, Forrest KYZ, Kuller LH, Becker DJ. Lipid and blood pressure treatment goals for type 1 diabetes: 10-year incidence data from the Pittsburgh Epidemiology of Diabetes Complications Study. Diabetes Care 2001; 24:1053–1059.

143. Chiarelli F, Pomilio M, Mohn A, et al. Homocysteine levels during fasting and after methionine loading in ad-

olescents with diabetic retinopathy and nephropathy. J Pediatr 2000; 137:386–392.

144. UKPDS Group. Tight blood pressure control and risk of macrovascular and microvascular complications in type 2 diabetes: UKPDS 38. Br Med J 1998; 317:703–713.

145. Mathiesen ER, Hommel E, Giese J, Parving HH. Efficacy of captopril in postponing nephropathy in normotensive insulin dependent diabetic patients with microalbuminuria. Br Med J 1991; 303:81–87.

146. Dahlquist G, Rudberg S. The prevalence of microalbuminuria in diabetic children and adolescents and its relation to puberty. Acta Pediatr Scand 1987; 76:795–800.

147. Joner G, Brinchmann-Hansen O, Torres CG, Hanssen KF. A nationwide cross-sectional study of retinopathy and microalbuminuria in young Norwegian type 1 (insulin dependent) diabetic patients. Diabetologia 1992; 35:1049–1054.

148. Mortensen HB, Marinelli K, Norgaard K, et al. A nationwide cross-sectional study of urinary albumin excretion rate, arterial blood pressure and blood glucose control in Danish children with type 1 diabetes mellitus. Diabet Med 1990; 7:887–897.

149. Davies AG, Price DA, Poslethwaite RJ, Addison GM, Burn JL, Fielding BA. Renal function in diabetes mellitus. Arch Dis Child 1985; 60:299–304.

150. Mathiesen ER, Ronn B, Jensen T, Storm B, Deckert T. Relationship between blood pressure and urinary albumin excretion in development of microalbuminuria. Diabetes 1990; 39:245–249.

151. Walker C, Dodds RA, Murrells TJ, et al. Restriction of dietary protein in progression of renal failure in diabetic nephropathy. Lancet 1989; 2:1411–1444.

152. Dullart RP, Beusekump BJ, Meijer S, et al. Long term effects of protein restricted diet on albuminuria and renal function in IDDM patients without clinical nephropathy and hypertension. Diabetes Care 1993; 16:483–492.

153. Morgensen CE. The kidney and diabetes: how to control renal and related cardiovascular complications. Am J Kidney Dis 2001; 37(Suppl 2):S2–S6.

154. Sawicki PT, Didjurgeit U, Muhlhäuser I, et al. Smoking is associated with progression of diabetic nephropathy. Diabetes Care 1994; 17:126–131.

155. Kohner E, et al. The retinal blood flow in diabetes. Diabetologia 1975; 2:27–33.

156. Cunha-Vaz JG, et al. Early breakdown of the blood–retinal barrier in diabetes. Br J Ophthalmol 1975; 59:649–656.

157. Keen H. Chronic complications of diabetes mellitus In: Galloway JP, Patvin JH, Shuman CR, eds. Diabetes Mellitus. Indianapolis: Eli Lilly, 1988:178–305.

158. Will JC, Geiss LSM, Wetterhall SF. Diabetic retinopathy. N Engl J Med 1990; 323:613.

159. Chaturvedi N, Sjoelie AK, Porta M, Aldington SJ, Fuller JH, Songini M, Kohner EM. Markers of insulin resistance are strong risk factors for retinopathy incidence in type 1 diabetes. Diabetes Care 2001; 24:284–289.

160. Roy MS. Diabetic retinopathy in African American with type 1 diabetes: New Jersey 725: II. Risk factors. Arch Ophthalmol 2000; 118:105–115.

161. Roy MS, Klein R. Macular edema and retinal hard exudates in African Americans with type 1 diabetes: the New Jersey 725. Arch Ophthalmol 2001; 119:251–259.

162. Chaturvedi N, Sjolie AK, Stephenson JM. Effect of lisinopril on progression of retinopathy in normotensive people with type 1 diabetes. The EUCLID study group

EURO DIAB controlled trial of lisinopril in insulin dependent diabetes mellitus. Lancet 1998; 351:28–31.
163. Neely KA, Quillen DA, Schachatap, et al. Diabetic retinopathy. Med Clin North Am 1998; 82:847–87637.
164. The Diabetic Retinopathy Study Research Group. Photocoagulation of proliferative diabetic retinopathy. Trans Am Acad Ophthalmol Ontolaryngol 1978; 85:82–106.
165. Elfervig LS, Elfervig JL. Proliferative diabetic retinopathy. Insight 2001; 26:88–91.
166. Bell DHS, Ward J. Peripheral and cranial neuropathies in diabetes. In Davidson JD, ed. Clinical diabetes mellitus. 3rd ed. New York: Thieme, 2000:621–635.
167. White NH, et al. Reversal of neuropathic and gastrointestinal complications relate to diabetes mellitus in adolescents with improved metabolic control. J Pediatr 1981; 99:41–45.
168. Maser RE, Steenkiste R, Dorman JS, et al. Epidemiological correlates of diabetic neuropathy: report from Pittsburgh Epidemiology of Diabetes Complications Study. Diabetes 1989; 38:1456–1461.
169. Käär ML, Saukkonen AL, Pitkänen, Akerblom HK. Peripheral neuropathy in diabetic children and adolescents. A cross-sectional study. Acta Paediatr Scand 1983; 73: 373–378.
170. Dorchy H, Noel P, Kruger M, et al. Peroneal motor nerve conduction velocity in diabetic children and adolescents. Relationship to metabolic control, HLA-DR antigens, retinopathy and EEG. Eur J Pediatr 1985; 44:310–315.
171. Becker DJ, Greene DA, Aono SA, et al. Assessment of subclinical autonomic and peripheral neuropathy in childhood insulin-dependent diabetes mellitus. Pediatr Adolesc Endocrinol 1988; 17:173–178.
172. Diabetes Control and Complications Trial Research Group. The effect of intensive treatment of diabetes on the development and progression of long-term complications in insulin dependent diabetes mellitus. N Engl J Med 1993; 329:977–986.
173. Reid B, DiLorenzo C, Trains L, et al. Diabetic gastroparesis due to postprandial antral hypomobility in childhood. Pediatrics 1992; 90:43–46.
174. White N, Waltman S, Krupi T, et al. Reversal of neuropathic and gastrointestinal complications related to diabetes mellitus in adolescents with improved metabolic control. J Pediatr 1981; 99:41–45.
175. Reid B, DiLorenzo C, Trains L, et al. Diabetic gastroparesis due to postprandial antral hypomobility in childhood. Pediatrics 1992; 90:43–46.
176. Kannel WB, McGee DL. Diabetes and cardiovascular disease: the Framingham study. JAMA 1979; 241:2035–2038.
177. Stamler J, Vaccaro O, Neaton JD, Wentworth D. Diabetes, other risk factors, and 12-year cardiovascular mortality for men screened in the Multiple Risk Factor Intervention Trial. Diabetes Care 1993; 16:434–444.
178. Goldbourt U, Yaari S, Medalie JH. Factors predictive of long-term coronary heart disease mortality among 10059 male Israeli civil servants and municipal employees. Cardiology 1993; 82:100–121.
179. Mudrikova T, Gmitrov J, Tkac I, Gonsorcik J, Szakacs M. Cardiovascular risk factors as predictors of mortality in type II diabetic patients. Wien Klin Wochenschr 1999; 111:66–69.
180. Turner RC, Millns H, Neil HAW, et al. Risk factors for coronary artery disease in non-insulin dependent diabetes mellitus: United Kingdom Prospective Diabetes Study (UKPDS: 23). Br Med J 1998; 16:823–828.
181. Wei M, Gaskill SP, Haffner SM, Stern NP. Effects of diabetes and level of glycemia on all-cause and cardiovascular mortality: the San Antonio Heart Study. Diabetes Care 1998; 21:1167–1172.
182. Moss DR Klein BEK, Meuer SM. The association of glycemia and cause-specific mortality in a diabetic population. Arch Intern Med 1994; 154:2473–2479.
183. Anderson DKG, Svardsudd K. Long-term glycemic control relates to mortality in type II diabetes. Diabetes Care 1995; 18:1534–1543.
184. Kuusisto J, Mykkanen L, Pyorala K, Lasko M. NIDDM and its metabolic control predic coronary heart disease in elderly subjects. Diabetes 1994; 43:960–967.
185. Malcom GT, Oalmann MC, Strong JP. Risk factors for atherosclerosis in young subjects: The PDAY Study—Pathobiological Determinants of Atherosclerosis in Youth. Ann NY Acad Sci 1997; 817:179–188.
186. Berenson GS, Srinivasan SR, Bao W, Newman WP, Tracy RE, Wattigney WA. The Bogalusa Heart Study association between multiple cardiovascular risk factors and atherosclerosis in children and young adults. N Engl J Med 1998; 338:1650–1656.
187. Wilkinson IB, MacCallum H, Rooijmans DF, Murray GD, Cockcroft JR, McKnight JA, Webb DJ. Increased augmentation index and systolic stress in type 1 diabetes mellitus. Q J Med 2000; 93:441–448.
188. Sarman B, Farkas K, Toth M, Somogyi A, Tulassay Z. Circulating plasma endothelin-1, plasma lipids and complications in Type 1 diabetes mellitus. Diabetes Nutr Metab 2000; 13:142–148.
189. Gerstein HC, Mann JF, Yi Z, Zinman B, Dinneen SF, Hoogwef B, Halle JP, Young J, Rashkow A, Joyce C, Nawaz S, Yusuf S. Albuminuria and risk of cardiovascular events, death, and heart failure in diabetic and nondiabetic individuals. JAMA 2001; 286:421–426.
190. Skowasch D, Lentini S, Andrie R, Jabs A, Bauriedel G. Verminderte Plattchenaggregation bei ACE-Hemmertherapie. Ergebnisse einer Pilotstudie. [Decreased platelet aggregation during angiotensin-converting enzyme inhibitor therapy. Results of a pilot study.] Dtsch Med Wochenschr 2001; 126:707–711.
191. Adler AI, Stratton IM, Neil HA, et al. Association of systolic blood pressure with microvascular and microvascular complications of type 2 diabetes (UKPDS 36): prospective observational study. Br Med J 2000; 321:394–395.
192. Hansson L, Zanchetti A, Carruthers SG, Dahlöf B, Elmfeldt D, Julius S, Ménard J, Rahn KH, Wedel H, Westerling S for the HOT Study Group: effects of intensive blood-pressure lowering and low-dose aspirin in patients with hypertension: principal results of the Hypertension Optimal Treatment (HOT) randomized trial. Lancet 1998; 351:1755–1762.
193. The Sixth Report of the Joint National Committee on Prevention, Detection, Evaluation and Treatment of High Blood Pressure. Arch Intern Med 1997; 157:2413–2446.
194. Knowles HC. Diabetes mellitus in childhood and adolescence. Med Clin North Am 1971; 55:975–987.
195. Rosenbloom AL, Joe JR, Young RS, Winter WE. The emerging epidemic of type 2 diabetes mellitus in youth. Diabetes Care 1999; 22:345–354.
196. Savage PJ, Bennett PH, Senter RG, Miller M. High prevalence of diabetes in young Pima Indians. Diabetes 1979; 28:937–942.
197. Dabelea D, Hanson RL, Bennett PH, Roumain J, Knowler WC, Pettitt DJ. Increasing prevalence of type 2 diabetes

in American Indian children. Diabetologia 1998; 41:904–910.

198. Dean HJ. NIDDM-Y in First Nation children in Canada. Clin Pediatr 1998; 39:89–96.

199. Pinhas-Hamiel O, Dolan LM, Daniels SR, et al. Increased incidence of non-insulin-dependent diabetes mellitus among adolescents. J Pediatr 1996; 128:608–615.

200. Pihoker C, Scott CR, Lensing SY, et al. Non-insulin dependent diabetes mellitus in African-American youths of Arkansas. Clin Pediatr 1998; 37:97–102.

201. Glaser NS, Jones KL. Non-insulin-dependent diabetes mellitus in Mexican-American children. West J Med 1998; 168:11–16.

202. Neufeld ND, Raffal LF, Landon C, Chen Y-DI, Vadheim CM. Early presentation of type 2 diabetes in Mexican-American youth. Diabetes Care 1998; 21:80–86.

203. Fagot-Campagna A, Pettitt DJ, Engelgau MM, Burrows MT, Geiss LS, Valdez R, Beckles GLA, Saaddine J, Gregg EW, Villiamson DF, Narayan KMV. Type 2 diabetes among North American children and adolescents: an epidemiological review and a public health perspective. J Pediatr 2000; 136:664–72.

204. Kadiki OA, Reddy MR, Marzouk AA. Incidence of insulin-dependent diabetes (IDDM) and non-insulin-dependent diabetes (NIDDM) (0–34 years at onset) in Benghazi, Libya. Diabetes Res Clin Pract 1996; 32:165–173.

205. Chan JCN, Cheung CK, Swaminathan R, et al. Obesity, albuminuria, and hypertension among Hong Kong Chinese with non-insulin-dependent diabetes mellitus (NIDDM). Postgrad Med J 1993; 69:204–210.

206. Kitagawa T, Owada M, Urakami T, Yamauchi K. Increased incidence of non-insulin dependent diabetes mellitus among Japanese schoolchildren correlates with an increased intake of animal protein and fat. Clin Pediatr 1998; 37:111–115.

207. Sayeed MA, Hussain MZ, Banu A, Rumi MAK, Azad Khan AK. Prevalence of diabetes in a suburban population of Bangladesh. Diabetes Res Clin Pract 1997; 34:149–155.

208. Braun B, Zimmerman MB, Kretchmer N, Spargo RM, Smith RM, Gracey M. Risk factors for diabetes and cardiovascular disease in young Australian aborigines. A 5-year follow-up study. Diabetes Care 1996; 19:472–479.

209. McGrath NM, Parker GN, Dawson P. Early presentation of type 2 diabetes mellitus in young New Zealand Maori. Diabetes Res Clin Pract 1999; 43:205–209.

210. Ehtisham S, Barrett TG, Shawl NJ. Type 2 diabetes mellitus in UK children—an emerging problem. Diabetic Med 2000; 17:867–871.

211. Drake AJ, Smith A, Betts PR, Crowne EC, Shield JP. Type 2 diabetes in obese white children. Arch Dis Child 2002; 86:207–208.

212. Troiano RP, Flegal KM. Overweight children and adolescents: description, epidemiology, and demographics. Pediatrics 1998; 101(suppl):497–504.

213. Freedman DS, Srinivasan SR, Valdez RA, Williamson DF, Berenson GS. Secular increases in relative weight and obesity among children over two decades: the Bogalusa Heart Study. Pediatrics 1997; 99:420–426.

214. Strauss RS, Pollack HA. Epidemic increase in childhood overweight, 1986–1998. JAMA 2001; 286:2845–2848.

215. Reilly JJ, Dorosty AR. Epidemic of obesity in UK children. Lancet 1999; 354:1874–1875.

216. Wang Y. Cross-national comparison of childhood obesity: the epidemic and the relationship between obesity and socioeconomic status. Int J Epidemiol 2001; 30:1129–1136.

217. Livingstone B. Epidemiology of childhood obesity in Europe. Eur J Pediatr 2000; 159(suppl 1):S14–S34.

218. Yanovski SZ, Yanovski JA. Obesity. N Engl J Med 2002; 346:591–602.

219. Blair SN, Nichaman MZ. The public health problem of increasing prevalence rates of obesity and what should be done about it. Mayo Clin Proc 2002; 77:109–113.

220. Neel JV. Diabetes mellitus: a "thrifty" genotype rendered detrimental by "progress"? Am J Hum Genet 1962; 14:353–362.

221. Lev-Ran A. Thrifty genotype: how applicable is it to obesity and type 2 diabetes? Diabetes Rev 1999; 7:1–22.

222. Lillioja S, Mott DM, Spraul M, et al. Insulin resistance and insulin secretory dysfunction as precursors of non-insulin-dependent diabetes mellitus: prospective studies of Pima Indians. N Engl J Med 1993; 329:1988–1992.

223. Haffner SM, Stern MP, Dunn J, et al. Diminished insulin sensitivity and increased insulin response in non-obese, non-diabetic Mexican Americans. Metabolism 1990; 39:842–847.

224. Haffner SM, Miettinen H, Stern MP. Insulin secretion and resistance in non-diabetic Mexican Americans and non-Hispanic whites with a parental history of diabetes. J Clin Endocrinol Metab 1996; 81:1846–1851.

225. Groop L, Forsblom C, Lehtovirta M, Tuomi T, Karanko S, Nissén M, Ehrnström B-O, Forsén B, Isomaa B, Snickers B, Taskinen N-R. Metabolic consequences of a family history of NIDDM (the Botnia Study): evidence for sex specific parental effects. Diabetes 1996; 45:1585–1593.

226. Martin BC, Warram JH, Krolewski AS, Bergman RN, Soeldner JS, Kahn CR. Role of glucose and insulin resistance in development of type 2 diabetes mellitus: results of a 25 year follow-up study. Lancet 1992; 340:925–929.

227. Pigon J, Giacca A, Ostenson C-G, Lam L, Vranic M, Efendi S. Normal hepatic insulin sensitivity in lean, mild non-insulin-dependent diabetic patients. J Clin Endocrinol Metab 1996; 81:3702–3708.

228. O'Rahilly S, Turner RC, Matthew D. Impaired pulsatile secretion of insulin in relatives of patients with non-insulin-dependent diabetes. N Engl J Med 1988; 318:1225–30.

229. AR Saltiel, Olefsky JM. Thiazolidinediones in the treatment of insulin resistance and type II diabetes. Diabetes 1994; 45:1661–1669.

230. Philipps K, Barker DJP. Fetal growth and impaired glucose tolerance in men and women. Diabetologia 1993; 36:225–228.

231. Philips DIW, Barker DJP, Hales CN, et al. Thinness at birth and insulin resistance in adult life. Diabetologia 1994; 37:150–154.

232. Lithell HO, McKeigue PM, Gerglund L, et al. Relation at birth to non-insulin-dependent diabetes and insulin concentrations in men aged 50–60 years. Br Med J 1996; 312:406–410.

233. Curhan GC, Willett WC, Rimm EB, et al. Birth weight and adult hypertension, diabetes mellitus, and obesity in US men. Circulation 1996; 94:3246–3250.

234. Ravelli AC, van der Meulen JH, Michels RP, et al. Glucose tolerance in adults after prenatal exposure to famine. Lancet 1998; 351:173–177.

235. Levitt NS, Lambert EV, Woods D, et al. Impaired glucose tolerance and elevated blood pressure in low birth weight,

nonobese, young South African adults:early programming of cortisol axis. J Clin Endocrinol Metab 2000; 85:4611–4618.

236. Dabelea D, Pettitt DJ, Hanson RL, et al. Birthweight, type 2 diabetes, and insulin resistance in Pima Indian children and young adults. Diabetes Care 1999; 22:944–950.

237. Bavdekar A, Yajnik CS, Fall CHD, et al. Insulin resistance syndrome in 8-year old Indian children. Small at birth, big at 8 years, or both? Diabetes 1999; 48:2422–2429.

238. Li C, Johnson MS, Goran MI. Effects of low birth weight on insulin resistance syndrome in Caucasian and African-American children. Diabetes Care 2001; 24:2035–2042.

239. Dunger DB, Ong KK, Huxtable SJ, Sherriff A, Woods KA, Ahmed ML, Golding J, Pembrey ME, Ring S, Bennett ST, Todd JA. Association of the INS VNTR with size at birth. ALSPAC study team. Avon longitudinal study of pregnancy and childhood. Nat Genet 1998; 19:98–100.

240. Hattersley AT, Beards F, Ballantyne E, Appleton M, Harvey R, Ellard S. Mutations in the glucokinase gene of the fetus result in reduced birthweight. Nat Genet 1998; 268–270.

241. Jaquet D, Vidal H, Hankard R, Czernichow P, Levy-Marchal C. Impaired regulation of glucose transporter 4 gene expression in insulin resistance associated with in utero undernutrition. J Clin Endocrinol Metab 2001; 86:3266–3271.

242. Pettitt DJ, Aleck KA, Baird HR, et al. Congenital susceptibility to NIDDM: role of intrauterine environment. Diabetes 1988; 37:622–628.

243. Silverman BL, Metzger BE, Cho NH, Loeb CA. Impaired glucose tolerance in adolescent offspring of diabetic mothers. Relationship to fetal hyperinsulinism. Diabetes Care 1995; 18:611–617.

244. Dabelea D, Knowler WC, Pettitt DJ. Effect of diabetes in pregnancy on offspring: follow-up research in the Pima Indians. J Matern Fetal Med 2000; 9:83–88.

245. Rosenbloom AL, Wheeler L, Bianchi R, et al. Age adjusted analysis of insulin responses during normal and abnormal oral glucose tolerance tests in children and adolescents. Diabetes 1975; 24:820–828.

246. Caprio S, Tamborlane WV. Metabolic impact of obesity in childhood. Endocrinol Metab Clin North Am 1999; 28:731–747.

247. Drash AM. Relationship between diabetes mellitus and obesity in the child. Metabolism 1973; 22:337–344.

248. Martin MM, Martin AL. Obesity, hyperinsulinism, and diabetes mellitus in childhood. J Pediatr 1973; 192–201.

249. Young-Hyman D, Schlundt DG, Herman L, DeLuca F, Counts D. Evaluation of the insulin resistance syndrome and 5- to 10-year old overweight/obesity African-American children. Diabetes Care 2001; 24:1359–1364.

250. Caprio S. Relationship between abdominal visceral fat and metabolic risk factors in obese adolescents. Am J Hum Biol 1999; 11:259–266.

251. Pettitt DJ, Forman MR, Hanson RL, Knowler WC, Bennett PH. Breastfeeding and incidence of non-insulin-dependent diabetes mellitus in Pima Indians. Lancet 1997; 350:166–168.

252. Von Kries R, Koletzko R, Sauerwald T, et al. Breast feeding and obesity: cross-sectional study. Br Med J 1999; 319:147–150.

253. Legro RS, Kunselman AR, Dodson WC, Dunaif A. Prevalence and predictors of risk for type 2 diabetes mellitus and impaired glucose tolerance in polycystic ovary syn-

drome: a prospective, controlled study in 254 affected women. J Clin Endocrinol Metab 1999; 84:165–169.

254. Lewy V, Danadian K, Arslanian SA. Early metabolic abnormalities in adolescents with polycystic ovarian syndrome (PCOS). Pediatr Res 1999; 45:93A.

255. Lewy V, Danadian K, Arslanian SA. Roles of insulin resistance and B-cell dysfunction in the pathogenesis of glucose intolerance in adolescents with polycystic ovary syndrome. Diabetes 1999; 48:A292.

256. Banerjee S, Raghavan S, Wasserman EJ, et al. Hormonal findings in African-American and Caribbean Hispanic girls with premature adrenarche: implications for polycystic ovarian syndrome. Pediatrics 1998; 102:E36.

257. Vuguin P, Linder B, Rosenfeld RG, et al. The roles of insulin sensitivity, insulin-like growth factor I (IGF-I), and IGF-binding protein-1 and -3 in the hyperandrogenism of African American and Caribbean Hispanic girls with premature adrenarche. J Clin Endocrinol Metab 1999; 84:2037–2042.

258. Ibañez L, Potau N, Marcos MV, deZegher F. Exaggerated adrenarche and hyperinsulinism in adolescent girls born small for gestational age. J Clin Endocrinol Metab 1999; 84:4739–4741.

259. Svec F, Nastasi K, Hilton C, et al. Black-white contrasts and insulin levels during pubertal development: the Bogalusa Heart Study. Diabetes 1992; 41:313–317.

260. Jiang X, Srinivasan SR, Radhakrishnamurthy B, et al. Racial (black–white) differences in insulin secretion and clearance in adolescents: the Bogalusa heart study. Pediatrics 1996; 97:357–360.

261. Arslanian S. Insulin secretion and sensitivity in healthy African-American vs. American-white children. Clin Pediatr 1998; 37:81–88.

262. Danadian K, Lewy V, Janosky JJ, Arslanian S. Lipolysis in African–American children: is it a metabolic risk factor predisposing to obesity? J Clin Endocrinol Metab 2001; 86:3022–3026.

263. Danadian K, Balasekaran G, Lewy V, et al. Insulin sensitivity in African-American children with and without a family history of type 2 diabetes. Diabetes Care 1999; 22:1325–1329.

264. Lindgren CM, Hirschhorn JN. The genetics of type 2 diabetes. Endocrinologist 2001; 11:178–187.

265. Rosenbloom AL, Joe JR, Young RS, Winter WE. The emerging epidemic of type 2 diabetes mellitus in youth. Diabetes Care 1999; 22:345–354.

266. Rosenbloom AL, House DV, Winter WE. Non-insulin dependent diabetes mellitus (NIDDM) in minority youth: research priorities and needs. Clin Pediatr 1998; 37:143–152.

267. Hanis CL, Boerwinkle E, Chakraborty R, et al. A genome-wide search for human non-insulin-dependent (type 2) diabetes genes reveals a major susceptibility locus on chromosome 2. Nat Genet 1996; 13:161–6.

268. Horikawa Y, Oda N, Cox NJ, et al. Genetic variation in the gene encoding calpain-IO is associated with type 2 diabetes mellitus. Nat Genet 2000; 26:163–75.

269. Baier LJ, Permana PA, Yang X, et al. A calpain 10 gene polymorphism is associated with reduced muscle mRNA levels and insulin resistance. J Clin Invest 2000; 106:R69–R73.

270. American Diabetes Association Consensus Development Conference On Insulin Resistance. Diabetes Care 1998; 21:310–314.

271. Steinberger J, Moran A, Hong C-P, Jacobs DR, Sinaiko AR. Adiposity in childhood predicts obesity and insulin

resistance in young adulthood. J Pediatr 2001; 138:469–473.

272. Freedman DS, Khan LK, Dietz WH, Srinivasan SR, Berenson GS. Relationship of childhood obesity to coronary heart disease risk factors in adulthood: the Bogalusa heart study. Pediatrics 2001; 108:712–718.

273. Visser M, Bouter LM, McQuillan GM, Wener MH, Harris TB. Low-grade systemic inflammation in overweight children. Pediatrics 2001; 107:e13.

274. Adelman RD, Restaino IG, Alon US, Blowey DL. Proteinuria and focal segmental glomerulosclerosis in severely obese adolescents. J Pediatr 2001; 138:481–485.

275. Smith JC, Field C, Braden DS, Gaymes CH, Kastner J. Coexisting health problems in obese children and adolescents that might require special treatment considerations. Clin Pediatr 1999; 38:305–307.

276. Strauss RS, Barlow SE, Dietz WH. Prevalence of abnormal serum amrinotransferase values in overweight and obese adolescents. J Pediatr 2000; 136:727–733.

277. Goldberg IJ. Diabetic dyslipidemia: causes and consequences. J Clin Endocrinol Metab 2001; 86:965–971.

278. Kirpichnikov D, Sowers JR. Diabetes mellitus and diabetes-associated vascular disease. Trends Endocrinol Metab 2001; 12:225–230.

279. Gress TW, Nieto FJ, Shahar E, Wofford MR, Brancati FL. Hypertension and antihypertensive therapy has risk factors for type 2 diabetes mellitus. Atherosclerosis Risk in Community Study. N Engl J Med 2000; 342:905–912.

280. Salomaa VV, Strandberg TE, Vanhanen H, Naukkarinen V, Sarna S, Miettinen TA. Glucose tolerance and blood pressure: long-term follow-up in middle-age men. Br Med J 1991; 302:493–496.

281. Wierzbicki AS, Nimmo L, Feher MD, Cox A, Foxton J, Lant AF. Association of angiotensin-converting enzyme DD genotype with hypertension in diabetes. J Hum Hypertens 1995; 9:671–673.

282. Stuart CA, Gilkison CR, Smith MM, Bosma AM, Keenan BS, Nagamani M. Acanthosis nigricans as a risk factor for non-insulin dependent diabetes mellitus. Clin Pediatr 1998; 37:73–79.

283. Nguyen TT, Keil MF, Russell DL, et al. Relation of acanthosis nigricans to hyperinsulinemia and insulin sensitivity in overweight African-American and white children. J Pediatr 2001; 138:474–480.

284. Sinha R, Fisch G, Teague B, et al. Prevalence of impaired glucose tolerance among children and adolescents with marked obesity. N Engl J Med 2002; 346:802–810.

285. Sackett DL, Holland WW. Controversy in detection of disease. Lancet 1965; 2:357–359.

286. Sokol RJ. The chronic disease of childhood obesity: the sleeping giant has awakened. J Pediatr 2000; 136:711–713.

287. Tersbakovec AM, Watson MH, Wenner WJ, Marx AL. Insurance reimbursement for treatment of obesity in children. J Pediatr 1999; 134:573–578.

288. Zwiaur KFM. Prevention and treatment of overweight and obesity in children and adolescents. Eur J Pediatr 2000; 159(suppl 1):S56–S68.

289. Segel DG, Sanchez JC. Childhood obesity in the year 2001. Endocrinologist 2001; 11:296–306.

290. Trevino RP, Pugh JA, Hernadez AE, Menchaca VD, Ramirez RR, Mendoza M. Bienestar: a diabetes risk factor prevention program. J School Health 1998; 68:62–66.

291. Epstein LH, Myers MD, Raynor HA, Saelens BE. Treatment of pediatric obesity. Pediatrics 1998; 101:554–570.

292. Cook VV, Hurley JS. Prevention of type 2 diabetes in childhood. Clin Pediatr 1998; 37:123–129.

293. Teufel NI, Ritenbaugh CK. Development of a primary prevention program: insight gained in the Zuni Diabetes Prevention Program. Clin Pediatr 1998; 37:131–141.

294. Gortmaker SL, Cheung LWY, Peterson KE, Chomitz G, Cradle JH, Dart H, Fox MK, Bullock RB, Sobol AM, Colditz G, Field AE, Laird N. Impact of a school-based interdisciplinary intervention on diet and physical activity among urban primary school children. Arch Pediatr Adolesc Med 1999; 153:975–983.

295. Macaulay AC, Paradis G, Potvin L, et al. The Kahnawake Schools Diabetes Prevention Project: intervention, evaluation and baseline results of a diabetes primary prevention program with a native community in Canada. Prev Med 1997; 26:779–790.

296. Dean HJ. NIDDM-Y in the first nation children in Canada. Clin Pediatr 1998; 39:89–96.

297. Perry CL, Stone EJ, Parcel GS, et al. School-based cardiovascular health promotion: the child and adolescents trial for cardiovascular health (CATCH). J School Health 1998; 68:406–413.

298. Levine MD, Ringham RM, Kalarchian MA, Wisniewski L, Marcus MD. Is family based behavioral weight control appropriate for severe pediatric obesity? Int J Eat Disord 2001; 30:318–328.

299. Robinson TM. Reducing children's television viewing to prevent obesity. A randomized controlled trial. JAMA 1999; 282:1561–1567.

300. Swinburn BA, Metcalf PA, Ley SJ. Long-term (five-year) effects of a reduced fat diet intervention in individuals with glucose intolerance. Diabetes Care 2001; 24:619–624.

301. Tuomilehto J, Lindstrom J, Eriksson JG, et al. Prevention of type 2 diabetes mellitus by changes in lifestyle among subjects with impaired glucose tolerance. N Engl J Med 2001; 344:1343–1350.

302. Diabetes Prevention Program Research Group. Reduction in the incidence of type 2 diabetes with lifestyle intervention or metformin. N Engl J Med 2002; 346:393–403.

303. Jeffrey RW. Community programs for obesity prevention: the Minnesota Heart Health Program. Obesity Res 1995; 3(suppl 2):283S–288S.

304. Epstein LH, Valoski AM, Kalarchian MA, McCurley J. Do children lose and maintain weight easier than adults: a comparison of child and parent weight changes from six months to ten years. Obesity Res 1995; 3:411–417.

305. Joe JR. Perceptions of diabetes by Indian adolescents. In: Joe JR, Young RS, eds. Diabetes as a Disease of Civilization: the Impact of Culture Change on Indigenous Peoples. Berlin: Mouton de Gruyter, 1994:329–356.

306. Freemark M, Bursey D. The effects of metformin on body mass index and glucose tolerance in obese adolescents with fasting hyperinsulinemia and a family history of type 2 diabetes. Pediatrics 2001;107. http://www.pediatrics.org/cgi/content/full/107/4/e55.

307. Soper RT, Mason EE, Printen KJ, Ellweger H. Gastric bypass for morbid obesity in children and adolescents. J Pediatr Surg 1976; 10:51–58.

308. Anderson AE, Soper RT, Scott DH. Gastric bypass for morbid obesity in children and adolescents. J Pediatr Surg 1980; 15:876–881.

309. Strauss RS, Bradley LJ, Brolin RE. Gastric bypass surgery and adolescents with morbid obesity. J Pediatr 2001; 138:499–504.

310. Fagot-Compagna A, Knowler WC, Pettitt DJ. Type 2 diabetes in Pima Indian Children: Cardiovascular risk factors at diagnosis and 10 years later. Diabetes 1998; (suppl 1):A155.

311. Yokoyama H, Okudaira M, Otani T, et al. High incidence of diabetic nephropathy in early-onset Japanese NIDDM patients. Risk analysis. Diabetes Care 1998; 21:1080–1085.

312. UKPDS Group: Intensive blood glucose control with sulphonylureas or insulin compared with conventional treatment and risk of complications in patients with type 2 diabetes (UKPDS 33). Lancet 1998; 352:837–853.

313. UKPDS Group. Tight blood pressure control and risk of macrovascular and microvascular complications in type 2 diabetes: UKPDS 38. Br Med J 1998; 317:703–713.

314. Ludwig DS, Peterson KE, Gortmaker SL. Relation between consumption of sugar sweetened drinks and childhood obesity: a prospective observational analysis. Lancet 2001; 357:505–508.

315. Kids, teens, and type 2 diabetes: what you need to know. An essential reference for school nurses. University of Texas Health Science Center at San Antonio: Department of Pediatrics; and The Children's Center At the Texas Diabetes Institute, 2000.

316. DeFronzo RA, Goodman AM. Efficacy of metformin in patients with non-insulin dependent diabetes mellitus. The multicenter metformin study group. N Engl J Med 1995; 333:541–549.

317. Jones KL, Arslanian S, Peterokova VA, Park JS, Tomlinson MJ. Effect of metformin in pediatric patients with type 2 diabetes: a randomized controlled trial. Diabetes Care 2002; 25:89–94.

318. Lebovitz HE. Insulin secretagogues, old and new. Diabetes Rev 1999; 7:139–152.

319. Chiasson J, Josse R, Hunt J, Palmason C, Rodger NW, Ross SA, Ryan EA, Tan MH, Wolever TM. The efficacy of acarbose in the treatment of patients with non-insulin-dependent diabetes mellitus. A multicenter controlled clinical trial. Ann Intern Med 1994; 121:928–935.

320. Schwartz S, Raskin P, Fonseca V, Graveline JF. Effect of troglitazone a in insulin treated patients with type 2 diabetes. N Engl J Med 1998; 338:861–866.

321. Law RE, Goetze S, Xi X-P, et al. Expression and function of PPARγ rat and human vascular smooth muscle cells. Circulation 2000; 101:1311–1318.

322. Olefsky JM, Saltiel AR. PPARγ and the treatment of insulin resistance. Trends Endocrinol Metab 2000; 11:362–367 .

323. UKPDS Group. Intensive blood glucose control with sulphonylureas or insulin compared with conventional treatment and risk of complications in patients with type 2 diabetes (UKPDS 33). Lancet 1998; 352:837–853.

324. Morales A, Rosenbloom AL. Death at the onset of type 2 diabetes (T2DM) in African-American youth. Pediatr Res 2002; 51:124A.

325. Silverstein JH, Rosenbloom AL. Treatment of type 2 diabetes in children and adolescents. J Pediatr Endocrinol Metab 2000; 13(suppl 6):1403–1409.

326. Azziz R, Ehrmann RS, Legro RS, et al. Troglitazone improves a ovulation and hirsutism in the polycystic ovary syndrome: a multicenter, double-blind, placebo-controlled trial. J. Clin Endocrinol Metab 2001; 86:1626–1632.

327. National Heart, Long, and Blood Institute. Report of the second task force on blood pressure control in children —1987. J Pediatr 1987; 79:1–25.

328. Haffner SM, Alexander CM, Cook TJ, Boccuzzi SJ, Musliner TA, Pederson TR, Kjekshus J, Pyarola K, for the Scandinavian Simvastatin Survival Study Group. Reduced coronary events in Simvastatin treated patients with coronary heart disease and diabetes or impaired fasting glucose levels. Arch Intern Med 1999; 59:2661–2667.

329. Handwerger S, Roth J, Gorden P, Di SantAgnese P, Carpenter D, Peter G. Glucose intolerance in cystic fibrosis. N Engl J Med 1969; 56:451–461.

330. Finkelstein SM, Wielinski CL, Elliott GR, Warwick WJ, Barbosa J, Wu SC, Klein DJ. Diabetes mellitus associated with cystic fibrosis. J Pediatr 1998; 56:373–377.

331. FitzSimmons SC. The changing epidemiology of cystic fibrosis. J Pediatr 1993; 122:1–9.

332. Rodman HM, Doershuk CJ, Roland JM. The interaction of 2 diseases: diabetes mellitus and cystic fibrosis. Medicine (Baltimore) 1986; 65:389–397.

333. Lanng S, Thorsteinsson B, Nerup J, Koch C. Diabetes mellitus in cystic fibrosis: effect of insulin therapy on lung function and infections. Acta Paediatrica 1994; 56: 849–853.

334. Hayes F, OBrien A, Fitzgerald MX, McKenna MJ. Diabetes mellitus in an adult cystic fibrosis population. Irish Med J 1995; 56:102–104.

335. Yung B, Kemp M, Hooper J, Hodson ME. Diagnosis of cystic fibrosis related diabetes: a selective approach in performing the oral glucose tolerance test based on a combination of clinical and biochemical criteria. Thorax 1999; 56:40–43.

336. Cotellessa M, Minicucci L, Diana MC, et al. Phenotype/genotype correlation and cystic fibrosis related diabetes mellitus (Italian Multicenter Study). J Pediatr Endocrinol Metabol 2000; 56:1087–1093.

337. Milla CE, Warwick WJ, Moran A. Trends in pulmonary function in patients with cystic fibrosis correlate with the degree of glucose intolerance at baseline. Am J Respir Crit Care Med 2000; 56:891–895.

338. Kopito L, Shwachman H, Vawter G, Edlow J. The pancreas in cystic fibrosis: chemical composition and comparative morphology. Pediatr Res 1976; 56:742–749.

339. Ornoy A, Arnon J, Katznelson D, Granat M, Caspi B, Chemke J. Pathological confirmation of cystic fibrosis in the fetus following prenatal diagnosis. Am J Med Genet 1987; 56:935–947.

340. Lippe B, Sperling M, Dooley R. Pancreatic alpha and beta cell functions in cystic fibrosis. J Pediatr 1977; 56:751–755.

341. Moran A, Diem P, Klein D, Levitt M, Robertson RP. Pancreatic endocrine function in cystic fibrosis. J Pediatr 1991; 56:715–723.

342. Arrigo T, Cucinotta D, Conti Nibali S, Di Cesare E, Di Benedetto A, Magazzu G, De Luca F. Longitudinal evaluation of glucose tolerance and insulin secretion in non-diabetic children and adolescents with cystic fibrosis: results of a two-year follow-up. Acta Paediatr 1993; 56: 249–253.

343. Cucinotta D, De Luca F, Gigante A, Arrigo A, Di Benedetto A, Tedeschi A, Lombardo F, Romano G, Sferlazzas C. No changes of insulin sensitivity in cystic fibrosis patients with different degrees of glucose tolerance: an epidemiological and longitudinal study. Eur J Endocrinol 1994; 56:253–258.

344. Lanng S, Thorsteinsson B, Nerup J, Koch C. Influence of the development of diabetes mellitus on clinical status in patients with cystic fibrosis. Eur J Pediatr 1992; 56:684–687.

345. Hardin DS, Stratton R, Kramer JC, Reyes de la Rocha S, Govaerts K, Wilson DP. Growth hormone improves weight velocity and height velocity in prepubertal children with cystic fibrosis. Horm Metab Res 1998; 56:636–641.

346. Lanng S, Thorsteinsson B, Lund Andersen C, Nerup J, Schiotz PO, Koch C. Diabetes mellitus in Danish cystic fibrosis patients: prevalence and late diabetic complications. Acta Paediatr 1994; 56:72–77.

347. Austin A, Kalhan SC, Orenstein D, Nixon P, Arslanian S. Roles of insulin resistance and beta cell dysfunction in the pathogenesis of glucose intolerance in cystic fibrosis. J Clin Endocrinol Metab 1994; 56:80–85.

348. Hardin DS, Sy JP. Effects of growth hormone treatment in children with cystic fibrosis: the National Cooperative Growth Study experience. J Pediatr 1997; 56:S65–S69.

349. Ripa P, Robertson I, Cowley D, Harris M, Masters IB, Cotterill AM. The relationship between insulin secretion, the insulin like growth factor access and growth in children with cystic fibrosis. Clin Endocrinol 2002; 56:383–389.

350. Gentz JCH, Cornblath M. Transient diabetes of the newborn. Adv Pediatr 1969; 16:345.

351. Hickish G. Neonatal diabetes. Br Med J 1956; 1:95–96.

352. Dourov M, Buyl-Strouvens ML. Agénésie du pancréas. Observation anatomoctinique d'un cas de diabète sucré, avec stéatorrhée et hypotrophie, chez un nouveau-né. Arch Franc Pédiatr 1969; 26:641–650.

353. Lewis E, Eisenberg H. Diabetes mellitus neonatorum. Am J Dis Child 1935; 49:408–410.

354. Tidd JT, Stanage WF. Congenital diabetes mellitus. S D J Med 1965; 18:15–19.

355. Osboume GR. Congenital diabetes. Arch Dis Child 1965; 40:332.

356. Ferguson AW, Milner RDG, Naidu SH. Transient neonatal diabetes rnellitus in three successive male siblings. Arch Dis Child 1971; 46:724–729.

357. McGill JJ, Roberton DM. A new type of transient diabetes mellitus of infancy? Arch Dis Child 1986; 61:334–336.

358. Coffey JD, Killelea DE. Transient neonatal diabetes mellitus in half-sisters: a sequel. Am J Dis Child 1982; 136:66–727.

359. Campbell IW, Fraser DM, Duncan LJP, Keay AJ. Permanent insulin-dependent diabetes rnellitus after congenital temporary diabetes mellitus. Br Med J 1978; 2:174.

360. Geffner ME, Clare-Salzler M, Kaufman DL, et al. Permanent diabetes developing after transient neonatal diabetes. Lancet 1993; 341:1095.

361. Gottschalk ME, Schatz DA, Clare-Salzler M, et al. Permanent diabetes without serologic evidence of autoimmunity after transient neonatal diabetes. Diabetes Care 1992; 15:1273–1276.

362. Weimerskirch D, Klein DJ. Recurrence of insulin-dependent diabetes mellitus after transient neonatal diabetes: a report of two cases. J Pediatr 1993; 122:598–600.

363. Edidin DV. Permanent diabetes developing after transient neonatal diabetes. Lancet 1993; 341:1095.

364. Töpke B, Menzel K. Die Pankreasagenesie des Neugeborenen; ein seltenes, klinisch aber charakteristisches Krankheitsbild. Acta Paediatr Acad Sci Hung 1976; 17:147–51.

365. Wöckel W, Scheibner K. Aplasie des Pankreas mit Diabetes mellitus, intrahepatische Gallengangsaplasie und weitere Missbildungen bei einem hypotrophen Neugeborenen. Zentralbl Pathot Anat 1977; 121:186–194.

366. Howard CP, Go VLW, Infante AJ, et al. Long-term survival in a case of functional pancreatic agenesis. J Pediatr 1980; 97:786–789.

367. Winter WE, Maclaren NK, Riley WR, Toskes PP, Andres J, Rosenbloom A. Congenital pancreatic hypoplasia: a syndrome of exocrine and endocrine insufficiency. J Pediatr 1986; 109:465–468.

368. Wright NM, Metzger DL, Clarke WL. Permanent neonatal diabetes mellitus and pancreatic exocrine insufficiency resulting from pancreatic agenesis. Am J Dis Child 1993; 147:607–608.

26
Management of the Child with Diabetes

Oscar Escobar, Dorothy J. Becker, and Allan L. Drash

*University of Pittsburgh School of Medicine and Children's Hospital of Pittsburgh,
Pittsburgh, Pennsylvania, U.S.A.*

I. INTRODUCTION

Three distinct aspects of diabetes management have occupied the minds of physicians and researchers for decades: the *control* of the disease, its *prevention*, and its *cure*. Simultaneous with significant advancements in the control of the metabolic disturbances of diabetes and its complications, immense efforts have recently been carried out through large-scale clinical trials to find a strategy to prevent the disease in susceptible individuals, and, through arduous bench, animal, and clinical research, to find a definitive cure. These latter two objectives have been elusive, but as more people and resources are committed to this endeavor their attainment looks closer.

Since the first recognition of diabetes as a clinical entity, utmost attention has been paid to its control. Initial efforts were directed toward amelioration of the symptoms of polyuria and polydipsia, which would lead to severe cachectic states and eventually to death within weeks or months. Severe dietary restriction, especially in the intake of sugars and other carbohydrates, high-fat diets, and even complete starvation were the only available strategies to achieve that goal before the discovery of insulin. This therapeutic approach did not prevent death as an almost immediate outcome of the disease and, surely enough, contributed to the progression through the final stages of the disease.

The discovery of insulin by Banting and Best in 1922 divided the history of diabetes in two. When injections of pancreas extracts started to be used as management for this disease, the expectations of the outcome changed drastically. Survival beyond the first months after diagnosis was now possible, starvation was not necessary, and patients could recover from their initial cachexia. Progressive refinement by the pharmaceutical industry

lead to improved purification techniques, which helped to circumvent initial problems with nonpurified pancreas extracts such as local and generalized reactions and immune-mediated inactivation of insulin through antibody production. Years of research and sophistication of molecular engineering have lead to the production of human insulin through recombinant DNA technology and the design of insulin analogs with particular pharmacokinetic profiles that allow extrarapid or retarded insulin action of injected insulin.

II. METABOLIC DISTURBANCES AS A CONSEQUENCE OF INSULIN DEFICIENCY

The hormone insulin has pervasive effects on overall energy homeostasis. Although diabetes mellitus is usually considered a disease of carbohydrate metabolism, in fact, equally serious alterations are present in the area of lipid and protein metabolism. The actions of insulin referable to carbohydrate metabolism are multifold. Insulin promotes the translocation of glucose from the intravascular space to the intracellular space by activation of insulin receptors that promote glucose transport. Intracellularly, insulin promotes the utilization of glucose as a direct energy source, or storage of glucose as glycogen (primarily in the liver, muscle and kidney), or converted into lipids with accumulation within the cell via the lipid synthesis pathway. Insulin also inhibits the release of glucose from the liver, promoting hepatic glucose storage. The actions of insulin on lipid metabolism include the transfer of so-called excess dietary carbohydrate calories into the lipid synthesis and storage pool and the inhibition of lipid mobilization from adipose tissue stores. Insulin has both direct and indirect effects on protein metabolism. The insulin molecule, apparently through specialized cell membrane receptors, works in a coordinated fashion with pituitary growth hormone to stimulate amino acid uptake into cells and promote cell growth and multiplication. Insulin promotes glycolysis and inhibits gluconeogenesis indirectly.

Insulin release is stimulated by dietary intake (glucose, amino acids and, to a much lesser extent, fats and ketones). The body energy metabolism is under the direct control of insulin during the prandial and immediate postprandial periods, whereas it is probably under the control of glucagon and epinephrine in the distal postprandial periods, growth hormone and cortisol being added during intervals of fasting. The overall effect in the normal healthy individual is very narrow variations in the concentration of all nutrients throughout the course of each day, despite feasting and fasting cycles. These well-regulated nutrient concentrations include glucose, amino acids, triglyceride, cholesterol, ketone bodies, and a number of energy intermediates such as lactate, pyruvate, and glycerol. The extremes of both hyper- and hypoglycemia are avoided, as are significant variations in lipid and protein concentration.

The deficiency of insulin results in a reversal of all these normal patterns. Hyperglycemia results as a consequence of impaired peripheral glucose uptake and increased hepatic glucose production, from an increased rate of both glycogenolysis and gluconeogenesis.

Hyperlipidemia results from a marked increase in the mobilization of preformed fat in adipose tissues, and ketonuria results if this process continues unabated, without intervention of insulin therapy. The concentration of several counterregulatory hormones is increased, including growth hormone, adrenocorticotropic hormone (corticotropin), cortisol, glucagon, and, in extreme stress, the catecholamines. Insulin deficiency and counterregulatory hormone excess combine to complicate the metabolic picture further, exacerbating hyperglycemia, hyperlipidemia, and ketogenesis. This leads to an increased rate of proteolysis and gluconeogenesis, placing the individual in negative nitrogen balance (1, 2). Acidosis, which is an additional complicating factor, ensues as the result of direct and indirect effect of insulin deficiency. Increased serum ketone concentration is the main cause of acidosis in insulin deficiency. Two additional sources of acidosis in the individual with moderate to severe fluid deficit are build-up of excretable organic acids resulting from decreased renal clearance and accumulation of lactic acid resulting from anaerobic metabolism of peripheral tissues.

III. MANAGEMENT

We are currently in the midst of changes in the strategies, techniques and objectives of diabetes management. There are continual improvements in techniques used for short- and intermediate-term assessment of metabolic control using capillary blood glucose monitoring and measurements of glycosylated proteins, particularly glycosylated hemoglobin, as well as attempts to standardize their laboratory measurements. The widespread utilization of these monitoring techniques has provided the patient and the therapeutic team with quantitative means of assessing metabolic status over time. There have been also advancements in other areas, since the improvement in the purification of pork insulin and the introduction of human insulin produced by DNA technology. More recently, beef insulin has been taken off the US market and there is widespread use of insulin analogs. The latter may allow much more precise tailoring of an individual patient's insulin therapeutic needs based on the individual's lifestyle (3, 4). An improvement of insulin infusion devices, both external and implanted, also provides the potential for more physiological insulin delivery (5). Ultrasound-enhanced transdermal delivery of insulin and oral insulin therapy is appearing as a possible way to treat diabetic patients. Trials of inhaled insulin are currently underway (6–10).

With these methodological advances has come an increasing interest in attempting to normalize energy metabolism, with the anticipation that this will eliminate or reduce the serious vascular complications of diabetes. This increasingly popular therapeutic movement has been improperly referred to as intensive insulin therapy rather than the more appropriate intensive diabetes therapy (11). Unfortunately, many, both physicians and patients have concluded that the way to improve diabetes management is simply to give insulin more often. This is a serious misconception. Intensive diabetes therapy also includes the need for intensive blood glucose monitoring and close attention to the patient's dietary regimen. Successful therapeutic management of the child and adolescent with diabetes mellitus requires a highly integrated four-pronged approach: insulin administration, dietary management, physical activity, and education and emotional support (12–15).

IV. INSULIN THERAPY

A. Insulin Requirements

Initial insulin requirements are approximately 1.0 unit/kg/day. A partial remission, referred to as the honeymoon period, is identified as a decline in insulin requirement below 0.5 units/kg/day associated with very good metabolic control as measured by near-normal glycosylated hemoglobin levels. This occurs in more than 65% of all newly diagnosed patients during the first several weeks after diagnosis, with the nadir in insulin requirement reached on average between 12 and 16 weeks after diagnosis. During this period, insulin doses must be carefully adjusted downward to prevent hypoglycemia. In some cases the evening dose can be entirely eliminated.

This is particularly true in children under 6 years of age. We believe that the duration of this remission period is usually longer than experienced in the past and in some cases may last longer than 2 years before increasing insulin needs are again expressed. The maintenance of some residual C-peptide secretion by intensive therapy must be a goal of treatment in view of the beneficial effects on the prevention of microvascular complications seen in the Diabetes Control and Complications Trial (DCCT) (16). Eventually, in all patients, insulin requirements begin to climb after the nadir of remission and generally plateau at about 0.8 units/kg/day in the preadolescent and somewhat above 1.0 units/kg/day in the adolescent. Pubertal development is associated with increased insulin requirements secondary to insulin resistance induced by changes in the hormonal millieu. It is not infrequent to find adolescent patients who require 1.5–1.8 units/kg/day to maintain target hemoglobin A1c (HbA1c) levels (17).

B. Available Insulin Preparations and Insulin Management Strategies

The last 20 years have witnessed major changes in all aspects of insulin treatment. Improvement in manufacturing techniques has resulted in a remarkably increased purity of commercially available insulin preparations. Mixed beef and pork insulin, formerly the standard of therapy, has been removed from the marketplace for the most part. Highly purified pork insulin is currently available in some but not all countries. Human insulins produced by recombinant DNA technologies are the most frequently available choices. New synthetic insulin analogs have been engineered to provide either extra-rapid action or prolonged, peakless pharmacokinetics.

Human insulin has been thought to have both theoretical and practical advantages and has been the insulin of choice. Two issues have raised concern about this apparently reasonable conclusion. Several investigators, particularly Europeans, have reported that severe hypoglycemia, usually without typical hypoglycemic symptoms, is far more common in patients treated with human insulin preparations. This suggests that there is something uniquely different about the body's response to human insulin that increases the likelihood of hypoglycemia. The controversy remains unresolved, with most studies not supportive of a uniquely dangerous hypoglycemic potential for human insulin (18, 19). The second issue has to do with the time course of human insulin. It relates to our own experience and decision to prefer pork insulin, especially in children under 10 years of age. All the human insulin preparations appear to have a quicker onset time and a shorter duration of effect than the comparable pork insulin preparations (20). Diabetes in very young children can be controlled using a split-dose regimen of NPH insulin plus lispro or regular insulin given before breakfast and before the evening meal using pork NPH. When using this schedule with human insulin, the shorter time course

of human NPH, particularly overnight, did not provide adequate glucose control. Raising the dosage increased the likelihood of nocturnal hypoglycemia. If a two injection/day regimen is used, we recommend highly purified pork NPH insulin, which provides better and more prolonged coverage especially through the night. Insulin antibody formation is the same whether pure pork or human insulins are used. Although we still support the use of pork insulin, we have recently faced the problem of decreased availability of these preparations. For this reason and where flexibility of schedule is needed, we recommend using alternative insulin injection regimens that circumvent the problem of poor overnight coverage. One such regimen involves the administration of human NPH insulin before breakfast and before the bedtime snack. We have found human ultralente insulin useful only in the context of a four shot/day regimen when it can provide basal coverage, but with significant variation in its effect.

The use in the near future of long-acting insulin analogs may provide another strategy to avoid this problem, as discussed below. A fast-acting insulin analog is also given before breakfast and before dinner and, if necessary, with a bedtime snack. Regular insulin was, until not too long ago, the only fast-acting insulin available. The introduction of insulin lispro, an extra-rapid acting insulin analog, in the last decade has broadened the repertoire of therapeutic options. Insulin lispro is synthetically produced by recombinant DNA technology, introducing a reversal of the natural occurring sequence of proline and lysine in positions B-28 and B-29, respectively to LysB28, ProB29. It is highly homologous with human insulin, yet it does not self-associate into dimers as does human insulin. The stabilized hexamer complexes of insulin lispro immediately dissociate into monomeric subunits upon injection into the subcutaneous tissue. This characteristic confers on insulin lispro at least three differences compared to human regular insulin: the action starts earlier (10–15 min), the peak insulin concentration in plasma is higher (more than double), and the duration of action is shorter (less than 4 h). A similar pharmacokinetic profile is found in insulin aspart, another analog also produced by recombinant DNA technology substituting proline in position B28 with Aspartate (21–23).

These rapid analogs provide a more precise action profile at mealtimes. Our current practice in the treatment of the great majority of school-age patients involves three insulin shots: human or pork NPH plus insulin lispro before breakfast, insulin lispro before supper, and human or pork NPH insulin before bedtime snack. Variations in this basic regimen are designed depending on the need. They include, but are not limited to, substitution of regular insulin for insulin lispro; the use of an insulin injection (either regular or lispro) before lunch or lispro before an afternoon snack; and the use of fast-acting insulin in conjunction with the bedtime dose of NPH insulin, depending on the blood glucose and the size of the snack. Advantages of these short-acting analogs include lower post-prandial blood glucose levels, less hypoglycemia, and thus better hypoglycemia awareness and counterregulation in response to low blood sugar levels. An additional advantage in pediatric patients, especially infants, is that medication can be given after eating due to these agents' rapid initiation of action. This allows dosing adjustments depending on the food intake, which in infants is very frequently unpredictable. More recently, long-acting insulin analogs have been synthesized with the idea of providing peakless basal insulin concentrations. Also produced by recombinant DNA technology, these analogs are designed to have a longer period of action by changing their isoelectric point (i.e., insulin glargine) or by promoting their binding to serum proteins such as albumin (fatty acid acylated insulins) (21).

Insulin glargine has already been approved by the Food and Drug Administration (FDA) and became available a few months before completion of this chapter. Two arginine molecules are added at the C-terminus of the B-chain. With these two extra positive charges, the isoelectric point changes and creates a molecule that is soluble at a more acidic pH and less soluble at the physiological pH of subcutaneous tissue. Another modification of the molecule, a substitution of Asparagine in position 21 of the A-chain by Glycine, is intended to protect it from deamidation and dimerization that would otherwise occur in the acidic solution in which it is formulated. The acidity of its formulation (pH 4.0) allows insulin glargine to remain soluble. Once injected in the subcutaneous tissue, the solution is neutralized and forms microprecipitates from which insulin glargine is slowly released, providing virtually no peak concentrations and duration of action for at least 24 h (24). Disadvantages of this type of insulin include the fact that it cannot be mixed with any other type of insulin. Therefore, two separate injections must be given when the action of a rapid action insulin is needed at the same time. The acidic pH of the preparation seems to be responsible for a burning sensation at the injection site for some patients. Large multicenter trials of the effectiveness of these newer analogs in the pediatric population are soon to be initiated in the United States.

It should be possible in the near future to tailor the individual patient's insulin management carefully to his or her lifestyle and changing requirements. The availability of this new family of synthetic insulins will make the demise of animal insulin less painful for all of us. Premixed insulins, such as 70/30 or 75/25 H are used only in patients with compliance problems because of the inablity to adjust doses according to planned food intake, meal plans, or ambient blood sugar levels.

C. Insulin Dosage Adjustments

By applying glucose goals derived from self-monitoring of blood glucose, insulin adjustments are made as necessary to attempt continually to bring the patient's glucose variation into the target range. Diet and exercise alterations are also considered and applied as necessary. We use a 10% rule for insulin changes: By summing the total insulin dose and dividing by 10, one obtains the number of units of insulin that is generally safe to increase or decrease in a patient who requires change. However, a maximum increase is 6 units (total insulin dose of 60 units). If the patient's blood glucose levels are generally high throughout, then the distribution of the increase follows the current distribution: usually two-thirds added to the morning and one-third to the evening dosage. On the other hand, if the patient is persistently out of range at a particular time, for example before dinner, then the dose modification applies only to the morning or lunch-time insulin and the amount is determined by calculating 10% of the morning dose. The distribution between NPH insulin and regular insulin or insulin lispro depends upon both the pre- and postprandial blood glucose levels. In the asymptomatic patient, we prefer to make insulin adjustments relatively slowly, after 3–5 days on a particular dose. On the other hand, if the patient is symptomatic and/or ketonuric, one must be more aggressive in moving toward a more acceptable blood glucose excursion. Most patients are provided with insulin scales for their short-acting insulin doses that can be used in anticipation of planned activity, food intake, and to correct current hyperglycemia.

V. INTENSIVE DIABETES THERAPY

There has been a gradual movement toward intensification of diabetes management, climaxed by the results of the DCCT. The term "intensive insulin therapy" has unfortunately become embedded in our terminology and to the uninitiated may be interpreted to mean that overall diabetes management can be improved simply by increasing the frequency of insulin administration. The proper message, of course, is that improved results are accomplished in the great majority of patients only with intensification of all aspects of management. The therapeutic set of the diabetes team, with full cooperation of the patient and family, is directed toward achieving either optimal management utilizing whatever resources are available or something less. The concept of conventional vs. intensive management must be set aside. We must undertake to do the very best we can with each patient, understanding that there are major differences in resources and abilities as well as many barriers to the achievement of metabolic near-normality (25–28). Intensive diabetes therapy almost always includes frequent insulin injections or continuous insulin infusion.

A. Continuous Subcutaneous Insulin Therapy

In the early days of insulin pumps in the 1980s, we developed extensive pump experience with our adolescent patients. Their initial metabolic response was gratifying in terms of decreasing glycosylated hemoglobin and blood glucoses. As we evaluated these patients over time, however, the enthusiasm for living with a pump declined and their compliance with the intensive therapeutic regimen diminished. Thus, the early successes were lost. At that time we concluded that the rigors of insulin pump therapy with the available pumps were such that few children or adolescents would adapt successfully to it. We essentially discontinued pump use in our general clinic population (29). More recently, however, advances in delivery systems have made pump therapy much easier for the patient, with more reliable insulin delivery and less complications. The potential for success with pump therapy has been demonstrated in carefully selected patients who are either very mature and have made a clear commitment to improved health or have very dedicated families.

Determining patient eligibility for continuous subcutaneous insulin infusion (CSII) therapy has been a subject of controversy. Among the factors involved are the age of the patient, the degree of prior glycemic control and multiple psychological, familial, cultural, and socioeconomic issues. The American Diabetes Association suggests four basic conditions that should be met by the patient to increase the chances of obtaining benefit from CSII: motivation, willingness to work in conjunction with the health care team, demonstrated understanding of the technical aspects of correct use of the pump, and ability to obtain and interpret data to make decisions regarding pump programming (30, 31). Patient's age and the degree of prior glycemic control are major factors accounting for the heterogeneity of eligibility criteria for CSII in different centers. Some centers have been more liberal with the use of insulin pumps in younger patients including young children and even infants, while others prefer to reserve this mode of therapy for older children, adolescents, and young adults capable of independent decision-making. The involvement of parents or caregivers is a *sine qua non* in the former group. The parental share of responsibility approaches 100% in the youngest patients, and should decrease in the older ones, although at least a certain degree of supervision continues to be highly recommended in the latter. Improvement of glycemic control achieved by adolescent patients with the participation of their parents or responsible adults decreases significantly when these patients are left on their own (32). This most probably reflects a decrease in the frequency of blood glucose monitoring and/or failure to give premeal insulin boluses. Poor judgment at the time of deciding on pump programming and bolus calculation according to the blood sugar level, the food to be eaten, and the amount of exercise predicted for the next minutes or hours would be additional concerns in some adolescents managed through CSII without parental involvement.

Our most recent experience with CSII (33) showed that metabolic control improved in patients switched from multiple daily insulin injections (MDI) to CSII as manifested by a decrease of 0.5% of HbA1c at 3 and 6 months after initiation. HbA1c levels at 9 and 12 months after initiation of CSII were not significantly different from baseline. A similar difference in Hb1Ac levels was observed between patients managed with MDI and those receiving CSII during the same observation period, with lower HbA1c levels in the latter. The patients who had worsening of their diabetic control when switched to CSII were older than the patients whose condition improved. They also had higher baseline levels of HbA1c. We found that the patients more likely to experience improved metabolic control are those with better control to begin with than patients in poorer control who are older adolescents and whose condition tends to worsen.

A beneficial effect of CSII found by us and others is the reduction in the frequency of severe hypoglycemia. We have not seen an increase in body weight in patients managed with CSII, as would be expected according to the results of DCCT. Despite the lack of improvement in metabolic control in older adolescents with poorer control, reduction in the frequency of DKA has been reported (34).

Approximately one-third of DCCT's intensively managed patients were using an insulin infusion device. The general experience did not clearly document a benefit of either pump or MDI therapy. Since then, uncontrolled studies have suggested improved glycemic control and less hypoglycemia in children and adolescents in CSII (35), although similar results are not universally reported (36). Our own experience suggests that CSII does not improve glycemic control in those with high HbA1cs but can improve quality of life. The biggest risk is exaggerated expectations of pump therapy.

VI. SOMOGYI EFFECT AND DAWN PHENOMENON

A very common management problem is illustrated by the child whose fasting blood glucose levels are consistently elevated. The usual strategy is to increase the evening NPH insulin until these levels are satisfactory. The common complication of this technique is that nocturnal hypoglycemia may be induced, leading to the Somogyi reaction and rebound hyperglycemia the next morning. This is particularly true with human insulin because of its shorter duration time. This hypoglycemia is masked by counterregulation or waning of insulin action. If fasting glucose levels are high, with NPH given at bedtime the addition of lispro at this time may be beneficial. In essentially all patients, excluding some toddlers, a minimum program of three injections per day program is needed. This is due to the need to continue covering the postprandial glucose rise after dinner with regular insulin or insulin lispro and administration of lispro as late as possible. This change has been frequently successful and surprisingly well accepted by most patients and parents (37, 38).

Elevated plasma glucose concentrations in the morning (after 5 am), without preceding hypoglycemia characterize the so-called dawn phenomenon. This occurs as a result of increased insulin requirements in the early morning, which could be related to either increased insulin clearance or decreased insulin action. An early-morning surge of growth hormone, one of the insulin-counterregulatory hormones, has been hypothesized as a causal factor. Whether long-acting insulin analogs are able to avoid this morning rise in blood glucose levels as a result of the dawn phenomenon in children and adolescents remains to be demonstrated in larger-scale pediatric trials. The once-popular concept of the Somogyi effect is unlikely to explain early-morning hyperglycemia, although counterregulation can account for past hypoglycemic euglycemia. Rebound hyperglycemia probably only occurs after active food therapy of low blood sugar (although this is not well reported in children).

VII. DIETARY MANAGEMENT

As stated above, the nutritional component is one of the cornerstones of diabetes management. Recommendations on nutritional intervention in diabetes have changed over the years. Before the discovery of insulin, the concept of dietary management relied on severe restriction of caloric intake leading to starvation diets. This was followed by low-carbohydrate–high-fat diets and, most recently, higher-carbohydrate–lower-fat diets (see Table 1). Our own recommendations since the early 1970s have been 50–55% carbohydrate, 15–20% protein, and 30% fat with limitation of saturated fat and cholesterol to <10%.

The design of nutritional strategies for the management of diabetes must be based on the procurement of basic goals, including the maintenance of near-normal glucose and lipid levels; the delivery of adequate amount of calories to achieve normal growth and development in children, and to avoid weight loss or excessive weight gain in all patients; and the prevention of nutrition-related complications such as hypoglycemia, renal disease, cardiovascular disease, hypertension, and autonomic neuropathy. Therefore, diabetic patients should have individually designed meal plans based on their needs and goals, taking into consideration cultural, ethnic, and financial issues. This clearly opposes the obsolete concept of a unique diabetic or American Diabetes Association diet. Furthermore, the term *diet* should be avoided, given its connotation of imposed and punitive restriction.

The food plan for a diabetic child, as well as that of any healthy child, should be balanced. It should contain adequate amounts of carbohydrates, protein, fat, minerals, vitamins, fiber, and water. Current recommendations suggest that carbohydrates should provide 55–60% of the total caloric intake; no more than 30% of the calories should come from fat; and 10–20% should derive from protein. It is evident from Table 1 that carbohydrate intake has become less restricted according to recent recommendations. Carbohydrates are mainly of two kinds: complex carbohydrates, or starches; and simple sugars. Great emphasis has been given in the past to the avoidance of simple sugar intake in diabetic individuals. Although this continues to be true, the restriction need not be as severe as originally proposed. Simple sugars naturally occurring in fruits (fructose) and milk (galactose), for instance, should be allowed in the meal plan. Fructose induces a smaller rise in blood sugar than isocaloric amounts of sucrose or other carbohydrates; however, it may induce an undesirable increase in serum cholesterol and low-density lipoprotein (LDL) cholesterol. Therefore, its intake in diabetic individuals should be moderate and its use as a sweetener should be considered as not advantageous. Sucrose may also be part of the meal plan, as long as it is not abused and is part of a meal rather than eaten alone. Glycemic excursions after ingestion of sucrose have been found to be of similar magnitude to those occurring after intake of white bread, refined rice, and cooked potatoes. Therefore, more attention has been paid to the total amount of carbohydrate and not the source of carbohydrate. Less attention has been paid to patient factors that affect absorption of the carbohydrate, such as the rapid absorption in the liquid state or delay when eaten with fat or fiber.

Within the 30% of calories coming from fat, it is accepted that less than 10% could come from saturated fat, another 10% from polyunsaturated fat, and yet another 10% or more from monounsaturated fat. Because LDL cholesterol is a major risk factor for both micro- and macrovascular disease in patients with type 1 diabetes (39, 40), we advise that more attention be paid to the fat content of the diet. This is in addition to the importance of the role of fat in influencing glycemic excursions after a meal.

Limitations of protein content in the meals prior to albuminuria have been recommended because of the detrimental effect of protein excesses in animals. Although

Table 1 Historical Perspective on Nutrition Recommendations

	Distribution of calories		
Year	% Carbohydrate	% Protein	% Fat
Before 1921	Starvation diets		
1921	20	10	70
1950	40	20	40
1971	45	20	35
1986	Up to 60	12–20	<30
1994	a	10–20	a,b

[a]Based on nutritional assessment and treatment goals.
[b]Less than 10% from saturated fats.
Source: Ref. 38a.

this effect has not yet been proven in children and adolescents, preventing protein overload to the kidneys appears to be prevalent.

Food exchange lists have been created to deal with the heterogeneity of nutrient composition of different foods, so as to provide some standardization when designing a meal plan. These lists group certain foods together based on similarities in their composition. The carbohydrate group includes several lists: starch, fruit, milk (skim, reduced fat, whole), other carbohydrates, and vegetables. The meat and meat substitute group also includes several lists: very lean, lean, medium fat, and high fat. The fat group includes lists of monounsaturated fats, polyunsaturated fats, and saturated fats. These lists are not a dietary formulation *per se*. The meal plan should be individually tailored by a skilled dietician for each patient. This can be made on the basis of the exchange lists to help the patient understand better the rationale for the prescription, and to make it easier when making decisions about food choices and alternatives.

A balanced diet must provide adequate amounts and proportions of all macronutrients and micronutrients. The food exchange list system is a tool to help accomplish this goal; however, tailoring insulin needs according to food exchanges and vice versa is not a straightforward task. Because more than 90% of the calories from carbohydrates end up as glucose (compared to far fewer of the calories from protein and fat), carbohydrate is considered the main dietary driver for blood glucose concentration. Carbohydrate counting has been suggested as a means to assist diabetic patients in designing their meal plan, especially when their glycemic control has proven inadequate through other ways of meal planning or no meal planning at all. Such counting offers the possibility of calculating, by a simple mathematical operation that involves initial training and attainment of skills, the amount of insulin that should be given to cover the predicted blood glucose rise after a certain food is eaten. This approach has proven particularly useful to calculate insulin boluses to cover meals in patients receiving insulin through an infusion pump. However, it should not be limited to this mode of insulin delivery. In addition, when teaching carbohydrate counting, the importance of stabilizing the other meal constituents should not be forgotten.

VIII. EXERCISE AS A THERAPEUTIC MODALITY

An increasing body of scientific data suggests, but does not definitively prove, that physical fitness is beneficial and highly desirable for the patient with diabetes mellitus (41–45).

We have taken on faith that this is true and, consequently, recommend to our patients that they incorporate a regular exercise program into their daily lives. Exercise increases glucose utilization, and highly fit muscles have an increased sensitivity to insulin and, consequently, glucose uptake. Our clinical observations include the following. Highly fit children and adolescents with diabetes usually require less insulin per level of metabolic control. These individuals are generally in better metabolic control than their relatively unfit diabetic peers. The physically fit individual, particularly the competitive athlete, usually has a better self-image and a better appreciation of the importance of good diabetes management. Episodic exercise, as opposed to regular exercise that leads to an improved level of physical fitness, may be dangerous in terms of both hypoglycemia or the induction of diabetic ketoacidosis in very poorly controlled patients. Our long-term diabetes complication studies indicate that persons who participate in competitive athletics during high school and college had a significant reduction in both diabetes-related morbidity and mortality when evaluated 10–30 years later.

Our recommendation to our patients is that they undertake a daily exercise regimen (7 days per week) that involves a fairly vigorous level of exercise for approximately 1 h each day. This is usually most easily achieved by participating in competitive programs at school. If this is neither possible nor desirable, other entirely satisfactory exercise activities can be substituted: vigorous walking, jogging, swimming, aerobic dancing, tennis, and golf. The patients must understand the effects of exercise on blood glucose and be ready to make necessary adjustment in his or her insulin dosage or diet. In general, we prefer to increase caloric intake before exercise rather than reduce insulin in the normal-weight child, although either or both may be satisfactory solutions to problems of hypoglycemia associated with exercise. The very poorly controlled patient who desires to embark on an exercise program should be encouraged to improve overall metabolic control by increasing insulin dosage beforehand.

IX. EDUCATION AND EMOTIONAL SUPPORT

The importance of education as part of the integral management of diabetes cannot be overemphasized. Education should start at the very moment when the diagnosis of diabetes is made. However, the initial phase of shock experienced by parents in response to the new diagnosis in their child may interfere with their understanding of basic principles. For this reason a well-balanced combination of emotional support and objective teaching is essential for the success of the initial education process. Previous misconceptions about diabetes that patients and their families may have when they are first faced with this diagnosis should be clearly addressed. When the child presents in severe diabetic ketoacidosis, starting the education process should be deferred until the parents see signs of recovery and the child is able to participate in a teaching conversation depending on his or her age. However, the diabetes management team should be readily available to answer questions from family members during this critical period, to soothe their fears and to start building a nurturing relationship. That opportunity can be used to explain in very basic language the pathophysiology of DKA and the reason for the clinical manifestations during the days prior to the diagnosis and at presentation. This will help the family to recognize later the signs of decompensation that need to be avoided.

The education process may start immediately when the newly diagnosed child does not present in DKA or comes with a very mild DKA. Doing this initial education when the child is an inpatient or an outpatient depends on several considerations: resources available to the diabetes management team, third-party reimbursement issues, and patient-related issues. Several investigators have addressed the question of differences in the outcome when comparing inpatient and outpatient education in the newly diagnosed patient. Initial retrospective studies by Lee, Chase, and Swift suggested that the patients who received outpatient education at the time of diagnosis had lower rate of hospital readmission for diabetes-related problems than those who received inpatient education (46–48).

In a prospective study comparing the outpatient education programs at Texas Children's Hospital (Houston, TX) and Denver Children's Hospital (Denver, CO), with the inpatient education program at Children's Hospital of Pittsburgh (Pittsburgh, PA), no significant differences were found in the outcome of multiple variables among the two approaches. The outcome measures considered in this study included rates of hospital readmissions and/or emergency room visits, knowledge test scores, sharing of responsibilities, adherence to the diabetes regimen, family functioning scores, coping skills, and perceptions of quality of life. Because very sick patients are always hospitalized initially, the problems with these studies are that they may be comparing outcomes in milder and more severe onset (49–51).

In our service we usually provide this initial education to the patient and the family in the hospital on an inpatient basis. Attempts to move to an outpatient setting have encountered obstacles, especially in terms of reimbursement by third-party payers.

Both inpatient and outpatient approaches have advantages and disadvantages, as listed in Table 2.

X. THE THERAPEUTIC TEAM

Medical care of the child with diabetes is different from that of patients with most other diseases handled by the pediatrician. The primary focus is on education. A major responsibility for the physician is to ensure that the patient and family members are well educated about the diversity of problems associated with diabetes. This cannot be a one-time experience: it must be a constantly renewed and continuing activity. However, attainment of the knowl-

Table 2 Advantages and Disadvantages of Inpatient and Outpatient Diabetes Education

Inpatient setting
  Advantages
    Interaction between patient and family with the team in one place and during a few days.
    Supervised environment, rapid response to possible complications. Patients/family may feel safer.
    Fewer trips for patient/family for medical facility.
    Fewer difficulties in team member reimbursement.
    Less reticence in early initiation of tight metabolic control.
  Disadvantages
    Hospital stay increases general cost.
    Less comfort for patient and family.
    Removal of child from home environment.
Outpatient setting
  Advantages
    Change is reduced because hospital stay is avoided.
    Family starts building self-confidence early in the process.
  Disadvantages
    Needs well-mounted and coordinated infrastructure of outpatient resources, including sufficient well-trained personnel on 24 h call.
    If families cannot commute from home, housing at no cost to family must be available.

edge is only half of the battle. The knowledge gained about insulin administration, the utilization of monitoring information, dietary principles, and the incorporation of exercise into daily life must be accepted by the patient, with adherence to the therapeutic regimen as a personal commitment for improved health. Each patient and family has their own unique barriers to full acceptance and incorporation of the recommended therapeutic regimen. Although most of these barriers are in the psychological sphere, other factors, such as peer group pressures, financial problems, or unavailability of parents at appropriate times, may make the recommended therapeutic regimen difficult, if not impossible, to follow.

The physician diabetologist must serve as captain of the therapeutic team. It is his or her responsibility to assess the unique characteristics of each patient and family and to determine the general therapeutic strategies to be used in an attempt to help the child achieve and maintain good health. Several other team members are essential for the creation of an effective diabetes therapeutic program. The diabetes nurse educator plays a pivotal role. Although the experienced physician must always be involved in reinforcing the educational components of therapy, it is unlikely that he or she has sufficient time to carry the primary educational activities. The nurse educator must become involved with the family as early as possible, usually at the initial diagnosis. It is clear from a number of studies that this is not an optimal time for teaching because of the family's shock at the diagnosis of diabetes. However, we believe it important to begin this process and ensure that the family has at least rudimentary survival skills when the child is discharged from the hospital 3–5 days later. The educational process continues at each clinic visit and, if necessary, special educational sessions are set up with the diabetes educator outside the normal clinic schedule.

The dietitian assesses the family's knowledge of food and nutrition at the initial visit and begins constructing a diet appropriate to the particular child. At least an annual review of the patient's nutritional status by the dietitian is desirable. Specific issues about the appropriateness of particular food substances and insulin coverage can usually be handled by telephone consultation or at clinic visits.

The psychiatric social worker plays a special role in the diabetes therapeutic team. It is the social worker's responsibility to assess the strengths and weaknesses of the family as they relate to emotional issues, economic and community support, educational activities, and other issues. Usually the social worker's assessment and recommendations determine whether other professionals, such as clinical psychologists and psychiatrists, become promptly involved with the family. The appearance of psychiatric problems over time as a consequence of stresses of the disorder also calls for the social worker's reinvolvement. The social worker can be particularly useful in families with limited financial resources, helping them to obtain support for diabetes medications and supplies, and transportation to clinic appointments.

The core diabetes therapeutic team includes the physician diabetologist, diabetes nurse educator, dietitian, and psychiatric social worker. However, the central member of the team is the patient. The patient, when old enough to be involved in a meaningful way in decisions, or the parents of the younger child, must be incorporated from the beginning in planning therapeutic strategies and all other major decisions. It is not therapeutically meaningful to insist on an insulin therapy of three to four injections daily or using an insulin pump and a monitoring program of four glucose determinations daily when the patient frequently misses some injections of insulin and/or refuses any monitoring. Although one continues to try to educate the patient and the family about the importance of a more comprehensive approach at the same time, it is essential to deal with reality. Most patients understand and appreciate the responsibility being placed upon them as part of the therapeutic team and respond maturely and appropriately to it.

The need for the diabetes therapeutic team cannot be minimized. Creative new ways must be found to make these resources available to all children and adolescents with diabetes mellitus. University diabetes centers must provide the leadership and direction for the development of networks of diabetes therapeutic programs across ge-

ographic areas, involving small communities with apparently limited diabetes-related resources. The local family physician or pediatrician must be incorporated into the therapeutic team and given encouragement for periodic re-education to function locally as the diabetes leader. In every community, it should be possible to identify nurses and dietitians who are willing to accept increased responsibility with appropriate, specifically pediatric diabetes training to become the local diabetes educator or special diabetes dietitian. The university-based diabetes center or speciality clinic must be able to provide outreach to the local community diabetes program by providing periodic visiting specialists, local patient and professional teaching conferences, and referral services for especially difficult management problems.

Opportunities for educational renewal by local team members must be available on a periodic basis. Such a networking program should provide the benefits of diabetes team management to the great majority of children and adolescents with type 1 diabetes. Although the initial costs of such a program will clearly be greater than for current management activities, the long-term reduction in vascular complications will greatly reduce the health care costs associated with visual loss, end-stage renal disease, peripheral vascular disease, heart attacks, and strokes.

XI. THERAPEUTIC OBJECTIVES AND MONITORING REQUIREMENTS

It is the therapeutic goal of all of us to put our patients right. We would like to be able to provide such comprehensive management to our patients with diabetes mellitus that they are metabolically normal, physically and emotionally healthy, and free of diabetes-related complications, both acute and chronic, as they go through life. Unfortunately, even with the advances of the DCCT, this is not now possible. We regularly find ourselves making therapeutic compromises between what we and the patients would like to achieve and what is reasonable within their personal situations. Table 3 lists the principles of diabetes therapy as they have evolved over the last several years in the diabetes clinic at Children's Hospital of Pittsburgh.

Certainly a primary therapeutic objective is to eliminate the obvious symptoms of poorly controlled diabetes, including polyuria, polydipsia, and polyphagia. Conversely, both serious and frequent mild hypoglycemia should be avoided. Careful attention to physical growth and sexual maturation is important. Inadequate insulin therapy results in slow growth and delayed maturation. Unfortunately, the achievement of these important therapeutic goals is not enough. Many patients deny symptoms of either hyper- or hypoglycemia and are able to maintain normal growth and maturation while maintaining blood glucose and glycosylated hemoglobin levels that are persistently too high.

Table 3 Principles of Diabetic Therapy

Elimination of the clinical features of inadequately
  controlled diabetes, including polyuria, polydipsia, and
  polyphagia.
Prevention of diabetic ketoacidosis.
Avoidance of hypoglycemia.
Maintenance of normal growth and sexual maturation.
Prevention of obesity.
Early detection of associated diseases. A number of
  autoimmune diseases (such as Hashimoto's thyroiditis)
  and celiac disease occur with increased frequency in
  patients with IDDM. Routine surveillance is important to
  detect these conditions in the early stages.
Prevention of hyperlipidemia.
Prevention of emotional disorders. The chronic and
  unrelenting demands of the disease and the therapeutic
  regimentation necessary to achieve reasonable control
  result in behavioral disability in a large number of
  families. The therapeutic program should be designed to
  prevent such problems or provide prompt and effective
  therapy as required.
Prevention of chronic vascular complications of diabetes.

Specific therapeutic objectives are presented in Table
4. Based on the DCCT results, primary therapeutic emphasis should be placed on achieving a near-normal metabolic status while avoiding the known complications of
this approach, including hypoglycemia and excessive
weight gain. The primary biochemical guides to management include glycosylated hemoglobin measurements obtained every 3 months and self-monitoring for blood glucose carried out at least four times daily. A number of
commercial techniques are available for determination of
glycosylated hemoglobin. It is imperative that the physician be well acquainted with his or her own laboratory
assay, its normal range, and any special peculiarities of
the assay. The currently used assays measure either gly-
cated Hb or HbA1c. The DCCT used a highly standardized method for measuring HbA1c that had a higher limit
of normal of 6.05% to which all other assays should be
standardized. This was the therapeutic goal of the intensively managed patients, a goal achieved in only about
5%. At the close of the study, the mean HbA1c in the
intensively managed adults was 7.1% , compared with 9%
in the conventionally treated cohort. In those individuals
who entered the study as adolescents, mean values were
approximately 1% higher with the intensively treated adolescents, with a mean of 8.1% and the conventional at
9.8%. Because the effectiveness of the management appears to be comparable in both adults and adolescents, in
terms of minimizing rates of progression of vascular
change, it seems reasonable to use the HbA1c value of
8.0% as a maximum therapeutic goal for adolescents participating in an optimized management program. Different

assays have different normal ranges and may not read parallel to each other despite excellent statistical correlations.

There were no patients younger than 13 years of age
at entry in to the DCCT, and at the conclusion of the
study, there were no individuals under 20 years of age.
One must therefore translate the conclusions of the DCCT
to younger children with extreme caution. It is our view
that although the general principle of moving all patients
toward physiological homeostasis should be embraced,

Table 4 Specific Monitoring and Objectives

1. Glycosylated hemoglobin (total HbA1 or HbA1c) should
   be obtained at least every 3 months; the goal in patients
   participating in an optimized management program
   should be an HbA1c of 8% (the average of adolescents
   in the DCCT) or lower in older patients.
2. Self-monitoring for blood glucose should be carried out
   daily before each meal and at bedtime, and at 3:00 a.m.
   three or four times per month; the blood glucose goals
   in optimized patients should be in the range of 80–120
   mg/dl in the fasting state and 80–140 mg/dl at other
   times. (See text for goals for younger patients.)
3. Urine testing: daily dipstick testing for glucose and
   ketones of the first voided urine in the morning unless
   blood sugar is measured more often at night; presence
   of ketonuria should lead to prompt consultation with the
   therapeutic team; minimal or no glycosuria or ketonuria
   is the goal.
4. Urine testing for albuminum: dipstick screening testing
   for albuminuria should be performed on a single voided
   specimen at each clinic visit; presence of albuminuria
   should promptly lead to assessment of an overnight or
   24 h urine collection; in the absence of postural
   proteinuria, overt proteinuria should result in a detailed
   renal evaluation and appropriate therapeutic intervention;
   microalbumin methods are now becoming available and
   are recommended for routine assessment; a timed
   overnight specimen is more convenient as it decreases
   the chances of detection of postural proteinuria. Spot
   urine albumin/creatinine ratios are more costly and
   introduce two variables.
5. Blood lipids: Blood should be obtained annually for
   determination of total cholesterol, HDL, LDL, very-low-
   density lipoproteins, and triglycerides; the lipid fractions
   should be between the normal range for nondiabetic
   children and adolescents. If the LDL level is greater
   than 100–110 mg/dl, a fasting level should be measured.
   Increases may reflect inadequate diabetes management
   or genetic lipid alterations.
6. Thyroid function should be assessed annually by
   determination of TSH; thyroid antibodies should be
   obtained in the presence of a goiter.
7. Poor growth, erratic glycemic control, or abdominal
   symptoms may be indicative of celiac disease and
   transglutaminase antibodies should be measured. The
   need for routine screening remains controversial.

glycemic goals may have to be higher in the preadolescent, particularly the preschooler. It is important to focus on blood glucose variation in these two younger groups, with a significant emphasis on avoiding hypoglycemia in preschoolers (52).

Because of the impossibility of monitoring amino acid and lipid fluctuations on a day-to-day basis, blood glucose measurements have traditionally been the sole modality to assess and manipulate insulin and food therapies. It is important to recognize that although monitoring is "glucocentric," our therapy should be global in terms of insulin action. Routine frequent self-monitoring for blood glucose is an essential component of good diabetes management. We recommend that, at a minimum, the patient measure blood glucose before each meal and at bedtime. In addition, periodical blood glucose determination at 2–3 a.m. should be obtained to document whether hypoglycemia is occurring during sleep. It is obvious that postprandial blood glucose determinations should be obtained under certain circumstances. It is also important to document symptomatic hypoglycemia by promptly performing a blood glucose test. During illness, blood glucose monitoring should be more frequent, as well as ketone checks. Although there is a general correlation between the frequency of blood glucose determinations and control, this is true only if the individual uses this information to make informed decisions regarding alteration in insulin dosage or other aspects of management. Recording of the blood glucose levels on a log sheet or computer can be useful in this regard. A single determination of blood glucose at any one time gives valuable information that may lead to immediate therapeutic decisions. However, the other half of the information lies in the analysis of patterns appearing day to day when multiple measurements are reviewed as a whole. For instance, finding a significantly low blood sugar level in the midmorning might prompt immediate management of hypoglycemia with the use of a fast-acting carbohydrate such as glucose tablets or orange juice. However, the recognition of a pattern of low blood sugar levels in the midmorning over several consecutive days would call for its prevention by a decrease in the prebreakfast fast-acting insulin dosage, an adjustment in the content of breakfast, or both, to avoid this hypoglycemia on a continuous basis.

Although it is difficult for US patients to measure blood glucose values at school before lunch, we insist that prelunch values be obtained routinely to assess properly the need for regular insulin in the morning injection. Schools should make this as easy as possible for the patient. There are major advantages to the use of meters with extensive memory capacity, primarily to cross-check the patient's accuracy in the recording of blood glucose results. However, the meter memory should not be used as an excuse for not recording the daily results in a format available for review by the parent as well as the team, at and between outpatient visits.

The DCCT blood glucose goals should be adopted for adolescent patients who have made a commitment to optimize management. The blood glucose goals are to achieve a normal fasting blood glucose level in the range of 80–120 mg/dl (or 80–140 with meters calibrated to serum). Any other daytime determination should fall in the range of 80–140 mg/dl, with 3 a.m. values in excess of 70 mg/dl. The DCCT results, based on seven-point glucose profiles performed once monthly, gave a mean daily blood glucose level of 153 mg/dl in the intensively management cohort compared with 230 mg/dl in the conventionally treated group. The results, although documenting the improved status of the intensively managed patients, further illustrates the difficulty in achieving blood glucose goals close to the normal range. We are pleased if our patients met the agreed goals about 80% of the time.

Pediatric diabetologists are currently attempting to come to grips with issues surrounding the general implementation of DCCT guidelines in the younger child. In the preadolescent (6–13 years of age) preprandial fasting levels should be moved as close as possible to adolescent blood glucose goals: 80–140 mg/dl. This should be done as soon as patients can reliably detect and respond to hypoglycemic symptoms. Some preadolescent patients are stable and have predictable enough blood glucose excursions that careful management adjustments can be made to bring them into line with adolescent recommendations. For the preschool child we strongly recommend that higher blood glucose goals be implemented to minimize the danger of hypoglycemia. Our specific recommendations are for fasting blood glucose levels in the 100–180 mg/dl range and postprandial values in the 100–200 mg/dl range in toddlers, and 80–180 mg/dl for 3–6 years. Allowable glycosylated hemoglobin results may be 1–1.5% higher than those of the adolescent if frequent hypoglycemia cannot be avoided.

With the widespread acceptance of routine self-monitoring of blood glucose, urine glucose testing has largely been relegated to an assay of historical interest only. We think that this is a mistake. The value of assessing night time control is significant and can be achieved by routine daily testing for urine glucose and ketones in the first voided morning urine. A dipstick method is used to measure both glucose and ketones. The presence of ketonuria is always of importance. Ketonuria associated with negative or minimal glucose spill is suggestive of nighttime hypoglycemia. The combination of high urinary glucose and ketones must be considered a strong indication of impending serious metabolic deterioration that requires careful follow-up. Under these circumstances, each successive voiding should be checked until ketonuria is clear. Communication with the therapeutic team is necessary to alter management as needed to prevent progression to DKA.

Urine protein determination is an essential component of routine management. A freshly voided specimen should be checked at each visit using one of the microalbumin screening methods. More sensitive methods for albumin determination to detect microalbuminuria can detect that protein levels of 30–300 mg/24 h may be indicative of impending, progressive renal disease. If positive, overt proteinuria should be assessed using a protein dipstick method that becomes positive with a urine albumin concentration of about 300 mg/l or total protein level of 500. Proteinuria at this level or higher, if related to diabetes renal damage, is indicative of significant and serious pathology once infection is excluded. A carefully obtained 24 h urine specimen or a timed overnight urine specimen obtained the morning before the clinic or office visit is possibly easier and more helpful in excluding orthostatic proteinuria. A spot urine albumin/creatinine ratio is the most convenient, but also the most costly and erratic assessment of microalbuminuria; it does not exclude orthostatic proteinuria.

Patients with poorly controlled diabetes mellitus frequently have elevations in several of the blood lipid fractions. As a component of assessment of control, we recommend that nonfasting lipids be screened annually for the determination of total cholesterol, LDL, high-density lipoproteins (HDL), and triglycerides. Total cholesterol values should be below 160 mg/dl, LDL below 100–110 mg/dl, and triglycerides below 140 mg/dl. If any levels are elevated, this should be confirmed on a fasting specimen. Elevated lipid values may be a result of either inadequate diabetes management or one of the forms of genetic hyperlipidemia. If the patient's diabetes control is unsatisfactory, the first objective should be to improve overall diabetes management and determine whether the elevated lipid fractions return toward the normal range. If persistent hyperlipidemia is identified in individuals with satisfactory diabetes control, then an evaluation for genetic hyperlipidemia should follow. Strict diet or pharmacological therapy with lipid-lowering agents may be necessary.

Thyroid disease is commonly seen in association with IDDM. Hashimoto's thyroiditis, an autoimmune destructive process, appears to share many similarities with the mechanism of β-cell destruction leading to IDDM. In our experience, approximately 40% of our patients, particularly during the adolescent years, have evidence of Hashimoto's thyroiditis, including goiter and/or elevations in thyroid antibodies. Approximately 10% of these patients develop hypothyroidism; a significantly smaller number develop hyperthyroidism. Timely diagnosis and appropriate management of these conditions are obviously important to the patent's well-being. Careful examination of the patient's neck should be a part of each clinic visit, and assessment of thyroid function should occur as specifically indicated or on an annual basis. We recommend annual screening with measurement of thyroid-stimulating hormone (TSH). In the patient whose TSH level is abnormally elevated or in whom a goiter or signs or symp-

toms of hypothyroidism are present, measurement of free thyroxine (free T4) and thyroid antibodies are also indicated; thyroglobulin antibodies (TG-Ab) and thyroid peroxidase antibodies (TPO-Ab). Measurement of thyrotropin receptor antibodies (TR-Ab) is indicated when a hyperthyroid state is suspected as a work-up to rule out Graves' disease. Unexplained persistent hypoglycemia may be a subtle manifestation of hypothyroidism; conversely, unexplained persistent hyperglycemia may be a subtle manifestation of a hyperthyroid state.

Another relatively common association has been documented between type 1 diabetes mellitus and celiac disease. The prevalence of celiac disease using screening tests among type 1 diabetics has been calculated by different authors in Europe, Australia, and the United States showing rates between 1.0 and 7.8% (53–55). Based on this, it has been suggested that all patients with type 1 diabetes be screened for celiac disease. However, this recommendation remains controversial. The measurement of tissue transglutaminase antibodies is currently accepted as the most sensitive test to screen for celiac disease. The diagnosis, when suspected, is confirmed only with biopsy. We do not routinely perform "universal" screening for celiac disease in all our diabetic patients, but we certainly request measurement of transglutaminase antibodies in those patients who display poor linear growth, weight loss, or poor weight gain not clearly explainable by their degree of metabolic control, and obviously in patients showing signs or symptoms of the disease. A similar genetic background, especially the high frequency of HLA-DR3 genotypes, has been postulated as the explanation for the simultaneous occurrence of type 1 diabetes mellitus and celiac disease (56) Gluten, the protein responsible for celiac disease, has also been suggested as a possible determinant for islet autoimmunity (57).

XII. CONSULTATIONS AND REFERRALS

For the child and adolescent with diabetes mellitus, there may be several occasions on which the advice of physicians outside the therapeutic team is especially valuable. According to current guidelines, children with type 1 diabetes of at least 5 years' duration, as well as all patients during their adolescent years, undergo a thorough retinal exam through dilated pupils performed by an ophthalmologist or a trained optometrist on an annual basis. Many advocate waiting until 8 years of diabetes duration in the prepubertal child in good control, but doing the exam after 2 years in patients with poorly controlled disease. Ideally the eye specialist should have experience in detecting early diabetic retinal changes. Fundus photography, either stereo color photography or fluorescein angiography, may be appropriate as a more sensitive assessment during the adolescent years. The detection of vascular changes in the eye by either the family physician or diabetologist should promptly result in referral to an ophthalmologist. Although in most cases the ophthalmologist provides no therapeutic intervention at that time, the visit may provide an opportunity for the therapeutic team to re-emphasize the importance of good diabetes management. Adolescent girls should be referred to a gynecologist or adolescent medicine clinic when they become sexually active.

The stress of diabetes and its management requirements exact a heavy toll in terms of behavioral problems and disabilities. In prospective studies carried out in our institution, nearly 50% of our patients experience significant psychopathology during adolescence (58). In most cases, this was pathological depression, requiring professional intervention. Other problems include antisocial acting-out behaviors, eating disorders, and adjustment problems. It is essential for all therapeutic team members to be sensitive to behavioral issues and be prepared for referral to colleagues in psychiatry or psychology if necessary. There is a natural reticence on the part of most patients and families to accept psychiatric referrals. By including the behavioral scientist as an integral member of the therapeutic team from the beginning, and emphasizing the importance of psychological well-being as part of the management of the patient with diabetes, the likelihood of family cooperation, if active intervention therapy is needed, is increased.

Annual evaluation of possible renal involvement is also advised. Measurement of microalbuminuria is recommended on an annual basis in patients who have had diabetes for at least 5 years or those who are reaching puberty, and after 2 years if the disease is poorly controlled. Albumin excretion rate above 21 μg/min should be confirmed by repetition of the test within the following few weeks or months. A persistent overt proteinuria should ideally prompt the referral of the patient to a nephrologist. If the patient has not had poor glycemic control, causes other than diabetes should be excluded.

Eventually the patient evaluated by the pediatric diabetes specialist must be referred for adult care based on age. It is our preference to continue to work with these patients through adolescence; high school or college graduation is a natural time to terminate this therapeutic relationship and hand the patient's case over to an adult diabetologist. All too often the young adult diabetic, following high school graduation and either entry into the work force or departure from home for university, is lost from the healthcare system and may not return for several years. Unfortunately the return is frequently precipitated by an acute event, such as retinal hemorrhage or other diabetic complications. It is not enough simply to refer the patient to the family doctor and assume that proper future management will be arranged locally. These patients deserve the opportunity to continue in a therapeutic environment characterized by the diabetes therapeutic team and led by a skilled internist or diabetologist. Assuring that this connection is made will go a long way toward minimizing serious complications during patients' young adult years.

XIII. CLINICAL ASSESSMENT AND THERAPEUTIC DECISION-MAKING

Children and adolescents with insulin-dependent diabetes mellitus require regular physical, biochemical, and emotional assessment and modification in all aspects of management to meet their changing needs and individual lifestyle requirements. Because of the complexity of this problem, we are convinced that this process should be carried out in a setting in which the talents of several diabetes therapeutic team members can be brought to bear on the situation of the patient and family.

We recommend that routine care involve a full clinic visit at a minimum of 3 month intervals, with interim visits with the nurse educator or dietitian as required. The physician's routine evaluation should include a careful review of general health and diabetes management issues in the interval since the last examination. Frequency, severity and management of hypoglycemia should be specifically investigated. Symptoms of hyperglycemia, such as nocturia or urinary frequency, should be documented. Dietary management should be reviewed by the physician, and specific dietary problems should be referred to the dietitian. An evaluation of physical activity should be obtained and the patient encouraged to participate in daily exercise to achieve superior physical fitness and assistance with dose adjustment made. Psychological issues should be reviewed, including how the patient is handling the personal problems of diabetes and its management, school performance, and interpersonal relationships at school and at home. Issues of sexuality and drug and alcohol abuse should be approached directly in a nonjudgmental fashion. Sexually active girls should be referred to a gynecologist for additional counseling.

Physical examination should be complete. Height and weight measurements should be transferred to a standard percentile growth grid in which assessment of growth parameters over time can be followed accurately. A declining growth rate or inadequate weight gain should result in careful review to determine whether this is a reflection of inadequate diabetes management or another problem. In the adolescent patient, the physical examination should include determination of Tanner staging and information about menses in girls. Blood pressure should be carefully obtained with the patient in a relaxed state. Even moderate elevations above the appropriate blood pressure range for the age should lead to additional determinations during the visit and, if necessary, periodically by the school nurse or even with use of an ambulatory monitor. Persistent hypertension is a serious problem in the diabetic patient and must be aggressively evaluated and treated. The diabetologist should be comfortable and confident in carrying out a routine ophthalmological examination looking for early changes indicative of background retinopathy. Insulin injection sites should be carefully examined. Lipohypertrophy may result in impairment of insulin absorption and contribute to inadequate management.

A major portion of the routine visit is review of the patient-generated blood glucose records by the diabetologist. This is an opportunity to teach about diabetes therapeutics and encourage the patient's and parents' participation in therapeutic decision-making. The individual's blood glucose goals in the fasting and postprandial state are reviewed, and an assessment of the interim performance provided . The focus is on insulin adjustments, but the integration of diet and physical activity must also be emphasized in these discussions. Any therapeutic changes must be followed by a telephone conversation between the patient and the therapeutic team, which may include faxing the most recent blood glucose results to a member of the therapeutic team. The results of the biochemical assessment are shared with the family and referring physician by letter within days of the clinic visit. Elevations in glycosylated hemoglobin levels, for example, may dictate more vigorous therapeutic changes than the initial review of the patient's blood glucose record would suggest. When biochemical therapeutic goals are met, congratulations are due to the patient and family, with encouragement to keep up the good work. Lack of achievement of goals should not be presented in a negative or punitive fashion but rather as encouragement to the patient and family to try even harder in the future with the assistance of the therapeutic team.

REFERENCES

1. Feldman JM. Pathophysiology of diabetes mellitus. In Galloway JA, Potvin JH, Shuman CR, eds. Diabetes Mellitus. 9th ed. Indianapolis: Eli Lilly, 1988:28–44.
2. Gerich JA. Hormonal control of homeostasis. In Galloway JA, Potvin JH, Shuman CR, eds. Diabetes Mellitus. 9th ed. Indianapolis: Eli Lilly, 1988:45–64.
3. Galloway JA. New directions in drug development: mixtures, analogs, modeling. Diabetes Care 1993; 16(3):16–23.
4. Chance RE, Frank BH. Research, development, production and safety of biosynthetic human insulin. Diabetes Care 1993; 16(3):133–142.
5. Saudek CD. Future developments in insulin delivery systems. Diabetes Care 1993; 16(3):122–132.
6. Laube BL. Treating diabetes with aerosolized insulin. Chest 2001; 120(3 Suppl):99S–106S.
7. Tamborlane WV, Bonfig W, Boland E. Recent advances in treatment of youth with Type 1 diabetes: better care through technology. Diabet Med 2001; 18(11):864–870.
8. Steiner S, Pfutzner A, Wilson BR, Harzer O, Heinemann L, Rave K. Technosphere™/Insulin—proof of concept study with a new insulin formulation for pulmonary delivery. Exp Clin Endocrinol Diabetes 2002; 110(1):17–21.
9. Gerber RA, Cappelleri JC, Kourides IA, Gelfand RA. Treatment satisfaction with inhaled insulin in patients with type 1 diabetes: a randomized controlled trial. Diabetes Care 2001; 24(9):1556–1559.
10. Skyler JS, Cefalu WT, Kourides IA, Landschulz WH, Balagtas CC, Cheng SL, Gelfand RA. Efficacy of inhaled human insulin in type 1 diabetes mellitus: a randomised proof-of-concept study. Lancet 2001; 357(9253):331–335.
11. Schade DS, Santiago JV, Skyler JS, Rizza RA. Intensive Insulin Therapy. Amsterdam: Excerpta Medica, 1983.
12. Drash AL. Clinical care of the diabetic child. Chicago: Year Book Medical Publishers, 1987.
13. Santiago JV. Insulin therapy in the last decade: a pediatric perspective. Diabetes Care 1993; 16(3):143–154.
14. Becker DJ. Management of insulin-dependent diabetes mellitus in children and adolescents. Curr Opin Pediatr 1991; 3:710–723.
15. Rother KT, Levitsky LL. Diabetes mellitus during adolescence. Adolescent endocrinology. Endocrinol Metab Clin North Am 1993; 22:553–572.
16. The Diabetes Control and Complications Trial Research Group. Effect of intensive therapy on residual beta-cell function in patients with type 1 diabetes in the diabetes control and complications trial. A randomized, controlled trial. Ann Intern Med 1998; 128(7):517–523.
17. Becker D. Individualized insulin therapy in children and adolescents with type 1 diabetes. Acta Pediatr Suppl 1998;425:20–24.
18. Cryer P. Human insulin and hypoglycemia unawareness. Diabetes Care 1990; 13:536–538.
19. Orchard TJ, Maser RE, Becker DJ, Doman JN, Drash AL. Human insulin use and hypoglycemia: insights from the Pittsburgh Epidemiology of Diabetes Study. Diabetic Med 1991; 8:469–474.
20. Heineman L, Richter B. Clinical pharmacology of human insulin. Diabetes Care 1993; 16(3):90–100.
21. Bolli GB, Di Marchi RD, Park GD, Pramming S, Koivisto VA. Insulin analogs and their potential in the management of diabetes mellitus. Diabetologia 1999; 42:1151–1167.
22. Brange J. The new era of biotech insulin analogues. Diabetologia 1997; 40:S48–S53.
23. Berger M, Heinemann L. Are presently available insulin analogues clinically beneficial? Diabetologia 1997; 40: S91–S96.
24. Ratner RE, Hirsch IB, Neifing JL, Garg SK, Mecca TE, Wilson CA. Less hypoglycemia with insulin glargine in intensive therapy for type 1 diabetes. Diabetes Care 2000; 23(5):639–643.
25. Rovet JF, Ehrlich RM. The effect of hypoglycemic seizures on cognitive function in children with diabetes: a 7-year prospective study. J Pediatr 1999; 134:503–506.
26. Becker D. Intensive diabetes therapy in childhood: is it achievable? Is it desirable? Is it safe? J Pediatr 1999; 134: 392–394.
27. Ludvigsson J, Bolli GB. Intensive insulin treatment in diabetic children. Diabetes Nutr Metab 2001; 14(5):292–304.
28. White NH, Cleary PA, Dahms W, Goldstein D, Malone J, Tamborlane WV. Beneficial effects of intensive therapy of diabetes during adolescence: outcomes after the conclusion of the Diabetes Control and Complications Trial (DCCT). J Pediatr 2001; 139(6):804–812.
29. Becker DJ, Kerensky KM, Transue D, et al. Current status of pump therapy in childhood. Acta Pediatr Jpn 1984; 6: 347–358.
30. American Diabetes Association Clinical Education Series. Insulin infusion pump therapy. In: Intensive Diabetes

Management. 2nd ed. Alexandria, VA: American Diabetes Association, 1998:99–120.

31. Kaufman FR, Halvorson M, Fisher L, Pitukcheewanont P. Insulin pump therapy in type 1 patients. J Pediatr Endocrinol Metab 1999; 12(3):759–764.

32. Anderson B, Ho J, Brackett J, Finkelstein D, Laffel L. Parental involvement in diabetes management tasks: relationship to blood glucose monitoring adherence and metabolic control in young adolescents with insulin dependent diabetes mellitus. J Pediatr 1997; 130:257–265.

33. Kandemir N, Becker DJ. Subcutaneous insulin infusion therapy in children and adolescents with type 1 diabetes mellitus: identification of factors contributing to outcome. In preparation, 2001.

34. Steindel BS, Roe TR, Costin G, Carlson M, Kaufman FR. Continuous subcutaneous insulin infusion (CSII) in children and adolescents with chronic poorly controlled type 1 diabetes mellitus. Diabetes Res Clin Pract 1995; 27(3): 199–204.

35. Boland EA, Grey M, Oesterle A, Fredrickson L, Tamborlane WV. Continuous subcutaneous insulin infusion. A new way to lower risk of severe hypoglycemia, improve metabolic control, and enhance coping in adolescents with type 1 diabetes. Diabetes Care 1999; 22(11):1779–1784.

36. Maniatis AK, Klingensmith GJ, Slover RH, Mowry CJ, Chase HP. Continuous subcutaneous insulin infusion therapy for children and adolescents: an option for routine diabetes care. Pediatrics 2001; 107(2):351–356.

37. Zinman B. Insulin regimens and strategies for IDDM. Diabetes Care 1993; 16(3):24–28.

38. Bolli GB, Peniello G, Carmine G, Famelli P, DeFeo P. Nocturnal blood glucose control in type 1 diabetes mellitus. Diabetes Care 1993; 16(3):71–89.

38a. Nutrition recommendations and principles for people with diabetes mellitus. Diabetes Care 1994; 17(5):519–522.

39. Orchard TJ, Forrest KY, Kuller LH, Becker DJ. Lipid and blood pressure treatment goals for type 1 diabetes: 10-year incidence data from the Pittsburgh Epidemiology of Diabetes Complications Study. Diabetes Care 2001; 24(6):1053–1059.

40. Fried LF, Forrest KY, Ellis D, Chang Y, Silvers N, Orchard TJ. Lipid modulation in insulin-dependent diabetes mellitus: effect on microvascular outcomes. J Diabetes Complications 2001; 15(3):113–119.

41. LaPorte R, Dorman JS, Tajima N, Cruickshanks KJ, Orchard TJ, Cavender DE, Becker DJ, Drash AL. Pittsburgh insulin-dependent diabetes mellitus morbidity and mortality study: physical activity and diabetic complications. Pediatrics 1986; 78:1027–1033.

42. Moy CS, Songer TJ, LaPorte RE, Dorman JS, Kriska AM, Orchard TJ, Becker DJ, Drash AL. Physical activity, insulin dependent diabetes mellitus and death. Am J Epidemiol 1993; 137(1):74–81.

43. Zinman B. Exercise in the patient with diabetes mellitus. In: Galloway JA, Potvin JH, Schuman CR, eds. Diabetes Mellitus. 9th ed. Indianapolis: Eli Lilly, 1988:215–224.

44. Arslanian S, Nixon PA, Becker D, Drash AL. Impact of physical fitness and glycemic control on in vivo insulin action in adolescents with IDDM. Diabetes Care 1990; 13:9–15.

45. Rigla M, Sanchez-Quesada JL, Ordonez-Llanos J, Prat T, Caixas A, Jorba O, Serra JR, de Leiva A, Perez A. Effect of physical exercise on lipoprotein(a) and low-density lipoprotein modifications in type 1 and type 2 diabetic patients. Metabolism 2000; 49(5):640–647.

46. Chase P, Crews K, Garg S, Crews M, Cruickshanks K, Klingensmith G, Gay E, Hamman R. Outpatient management vs. min-hospital management of children with new-onset diabetes. Clin Pediatr 1992; 31(8):450–456.

47. Swift P, Hearnshaw J, Botha J, Wright G, Raymond N, Jamieson K. A decade of diabetes: keeping children out of hospital. Br J Med 1993; 307:96–98.

48. Lee P. An outpatient-focused program for childhood diabetes: design, implementation, and effectiveness. J Tex Med 1992; 88(7):64–68.

49. Siminerio LM. Comparing outpatient to inpatient diabetes education for newly diagnosed pediatric patients: an exploratory study. A thesis in health education. The Pennsylvania State University, Graduate School Department of Health Education, 1998.

50. Siminerio LM, Charron-Prochownik D, Banion C, Schreiner B. Comparing outpatient and inpatient diabetes education for newly diagnosed pediatric patients. Diabetes Educ 1999; 25(6):895–906.

51. Charron-Prochownik D, Maihle T, Siminerio L, Songer T. Outpatient versus inpatient care of children newly diagnosed with IDDM. Diabetes Care 1997; 20(4):657–660.

52. Ryan CM, Becker DJ. Hypoglycemia in children with type 1 diabetes mellitus. Risk factors, cognitive function, and management. Endocrinol Metab Clin North Am 1999; 28(4):883–900.

53. Cronin CC, Shanahan F. Insulin-dependent diabetes mellitus and coeliac disease. Lancet 1997; 349:1096–1097.

54. Hummel M, Ziegler AG, Bonifacio E. Type 1 diabetes mellitus, celiac disease and their association—lessons from antibodies. J Pediatr Endocrinol Metab 2001; 14 Suppl 1:607–610.

55. Schuppan D, Hahn EG. Celiac disease and its link to type 1 diabetes mellitus. J Pediatr Endocrinol Metab 2001; 14 Suppl 1:597–605.

56. Shanahan F, Mckenna R, McCarthy CF, Drury MI. Coeliac disease and diabetes mellitus: a study of 24 patients with HLA typing. QJM 1982; 51:329–335.

57. Bonifacio E, Ziegler AG, Hummel M, Dittler J, Lampasona V, Pastore MR, Bosi E. Gluten: is it also a determinant of islet autoimmunity? Diabetes Metab Rev 1998; 14(3):258–259.

58. Drash AL, Becker DJ. Behavioral issues in patients with diabetes mellitus, with special emphasis on the child and adolescent. In: Rifkin H, Porte D, eds. Ellenberg and Rifkin's Diabetes Mellitus Theory and Practice. 4th ed. New York: Elsevier, 1990:992–934.

27

Diabetic Ketoacidosis

Dorothy J. Becker, Allan L. Drash, and Oscar Escobar
University of Pittsburgh School of Medicine and Children's Hospital of Pittsburgh, Pittsburgh, Pennsylvania, U.S.A.

I. INTRODUCTION

Diabetic ketoacidosis (DKA) is a potential complication in every patient with type 1 or insulin-dependent diabetes mellitus (IDDM). It is an inevitable consequence of untreated or inadequately controlled IDDM, and may be part of the initial presentation. Ketoacidosis is the most common cause of rehospitalization in the child with known type 1 diabetes or atypical or type 1½ diabetes.

DKA is a serious, life-threatening acute metabolic complication of IDDM. The frequency of DKA in our center and others in the United States is declining, both as the presenting feature of IDDM and as a later-recurring problem. There appears to be considerable variation in the frequency of DKA in children and adults in different geographic areas of the world. Although these data are poorly documented and scanty, physicians from Israel and parts of Europe report that DKA is uncommon in their countries. However, DKA remains a major frequent problem in diabetic children in many parts of the world including the United States. From our experience at Children's Hospital of Pittsburgh, DKA (defined as a serum bicarbonate level less than 18 mEq/l and/or pH equal to or less than 7.3), as the new presenting feature of newly diagnosed patients has declined from 80% of cases in the 1950s to 55% of cases in the early 1980s and to 40% among whites in the late 1990s. However, there was no change in the frequency of DKA among black patients. DKA is more frequent and more severe in children <6 years of age (64%), with one-third of these presenting with impaired levels of consciousness in the youngest children, in contrast to 9% in the older age groups (1).

The severity of DKA in these children also appears to have lessened. Severe acidosis with dehydration has been more common in our newly diagnosed girls than boys, and is associated with higher mean glycosylated hemoglobin and serum cholesterol levels. They also had a greater frequency of evidence of infection or pre-existing infection. The reason for gender differences in DKA is not apparent (2).

Despite improvement in therapy, DKA remains a major cause of death in IDDM around the world and, until the 1980s, was the most common cause of death in the diabetic patient under 20 years of age (3). Although there was some decline during that period, within our own institution deaths have become extremely rare and have occurred only in patients transferred from other hospitals in a moribund state. This suggests that with improved therapy and more rapid diagnosis, death from DKA may be preventable. There is little new data regarding DKA mortality in the United States (3). The overall mortality rate due to DKA was approximately 7% in the United States and the United Kingdom, with reports ranging from 1 to 19% before 1980 (4). Approximately 65% of all DKA admissions reported in this study occurred in children and adolescents. However, the mortality was far higher in adults, with death mostly resulting from complications of myocardial infarction and cerebral vascular accident.

It is hoped that with increasing understanding of the pathogenesis of this disorder and careful therapy, together with education of the physician and patient population, the overall morbidity and mortality rates of this acute complication can be appreciably lessened in the future.

II. PRESENTATION AND CLINICAL FEATURES

Insulin deficiency results in a series of understandable and predictable metabolic events, which have associated clinical concomitants. The pathogenesis of these events is described later. In patients with new-onset diabetes, presumably there is a gradual drop in the release of insulin from the β cells with an associated impairment in the metabolism of energy intermediates, including carbohydrates, fat, and protein. The first recognizable symptoms are associated with postprandial hyperglycemia and glycosuria, because the concomitant hyperlipidemia and alterations in protein metabolism are not yet clinically evident (5). Thus, the classic initial features of IDDM include polyuria, polydipsia, polyphagia, and visual disturbances, all associated with hyperglycemia. This condition progresses to a catabolic state with fatigue and weight loss due to muscle proteolysis and lipolysis. The abnormal fat metabolism results in hypercholesterolemia and ketosis. If the diagnosis of IDDM or of poor control of IDDM is not made at this phase, the symptoms progress to vomiting, abdominal pain, anorexia, dehydration, so-called sighing respiration, and, later, impairment of the central nervous system (CNS) or coma. In our experience, most patients have a clinical course of approximately 4–8 weeks before development of DKA. In some cases, the symptoms have been identified for only a few days and, in previously diagnosed patients, often for only few hours prior to their presentation with severe metabolic derangement.

Very severe DKA is seen most commonly in the infant and toddler. It declines in frequency with the presentation of IDDM in the older child (1). Hyperosmolar diabetic coma (severe hyperglycemia with no ketosis) also occurs more often in the younger child (6). The degree of metabolic derangement in DKA can vary widely from severe uncompensated metabolic acidosis to diabetic ketosis in which there is hyperglycemia and ketonemia with ketonuria and normal acid–base balance. Diabetic ketosis occurs in approximately 50% of our patients. Although the clinical presentation of patients usually parallels the severity of the biochemical changes, one frequently sees patients who are in surprisingly good clinical condition relative to the severity of their metabolic derangement. One also sees patients who are in poor clinical condition with marked dehydration relative to the mildness of metabolic acidosis.

The biochemical alterations of DKA are hyperglycemia, dehydration, ketosis, acidosis, and electrolyte disturbance. Often a linear relationship exists between the concentration of blood glucose and the severity of the metabolic acidosis. Exceptions at either extreme occur frequently. Thus, patients may have severe hyperglycemia and hypernatremia with resultant hyperosmolarity and minimal or no ketosis. Hyperosmolar diabetic coma, which is a rare complication of diabetes in childhood, is at one extreme of this biochemical derangement with marked hyperglycemia but no ketosis and little acidosis. Conversely, a number of children have severe metabolic acidosis and only mild to moderate hyperglycemia with blood glucose levels in the range of 200–300 mg/dl. These patients usually have an acute onset with severe vomiting and frequently have previously diagnosed diabetes. We consider any patient to have DKA whose serum bicarbonate level is less than 18 mEq/l, irrespective of serum pH (i.e., whether or not the acidosis is compensated). We define a serum pH of less than 7.2 in a diabetic

patient as severe ketoacidosis. Hyperlipidemia is almost invariably present in patients with DKA with elevations in both serum cholesterol and triglyceride concentrations. Increases or decreases in the serum levels of electrolytes, blood urea nitrogen (BUN), and creatinine also occur, depending upon the degree of dehydration, acidosis, and vomiting. The hemoglobin value, hematocrit, and white blood cell count may likewise be high.

Although the serum sodium concentration is usually high when associated with severe dehydration, it may be mildly or moderately depressed. The depressed sodium level results from both excessive urinary losses and movement of sodium from the extracellular space into the intracellular space, secondary to the hyperosmolarity associated with hyperglycemia. Serum sodium may also be spuriously low in association with the concomitant hyperlipidemia with increased fat displacing plasma water (7). Most clinical laboratories today displace these circulating lipids by ultracentrifugation, and it is important to determine whether or not hyperlipidemia has been allowed for in each laboratory (8). Serum potassium levels are usually initially normal or even elevated, depending upon the degree of acidosis and dehydration. This occurs despite severe total body potassium deficit with markedly diminished intracellular concentrations of potassium. During therapy, even with adequate replacement of potassium, there is usually a decline in the serum concentrations of potassium (9). Like potassium concentration, the concentration of phosphorus in the blood is variable at presentation but usually drops markedly during therapy because of excessive urinary losses with an associated total body phosphorus deficit (9). Reduction of the intracellular phosphate content is associated with a loss of 2,3-diphosphoglycerate (2,3-DPG), which is most important in the red blood cells. Thus, 2,3-DPG, which controls the oxygen affinity of hemoglobin, may be important in oxygen transfer at the tissue level (10). However, this subject is highly controversial. Although severe hypophosphatemia frequently occurs during therapy in DKA, identifiable associated complications have not been reported in this condition. The clinical effect of hypophosphatemia is therefore not yet clear in DKA (11).

Routine urinary test findings in DKA indicate glucosuria and ketonuria. Proteinuria and hyaline casts are frequently found at presentation. Both findings depend on the degree of dehydration. The glycosylated hemoglobin concentrations in DKA are variable and probably depend on both the prior duration and severity of hyperglycemia.

III. PATHOGENESIS

A. Insulin Deficiency

The pathophysiology and presenting features of DKA are the subject of a number of reviews (12–14). Ketoacidosis in the newly diagnosed diabetic patient may have a fairly extensive prodrome consisting of the classic symptoms of polydipsia, polyuria, and polyphagia, or it may develop within a few hours in an insulin-treated diabetic child who had otherwise previously been in good health. The first case appears associated with relative insulin deficiency due to failure of insulin secretion by the pancreatic β cells, although circulating levels may be detectable in the low-normal or, in the face of obesity, even the normal range at the time of presentation. Circulating insulin levels are lower than the body's requirement at that time (5,15). In the insulin-treated diabetic child, the cause is usually absolute insulin deficiency with frequently very low circulating free insulin levels when measured on presentation (despite a history of not missing insulin injections). However, insulin deficiency may also be relative to increased insulin requirements (12).

Reasons for the apparently greater requirement for insulin may be infection, dehydration, physical or emotional stress with overproduction of counterregulatory hormones, insulin antagonism by elevation of free fatty acid levels, and diminished number of insulin receptors associated with acidosis. Circulating insulin antibodies are usually of low affinity and are an unlikely cause of an acute reduction of insulin action.

The absolute or relative insulin deficiency produces a situation of acute intracellular starvation in most of the cells of the body. The accompanying metabolic changes in diabetic ketoacidosis are thus very similar to those found in prolonged starvation. The major effects are those of insulin deficiency, which is accompanied by an acute elevation of the counterregulatory hormones, presumably stimulated by the insulin deficit and its metabolic consequences (16). The metabolic consequences of the insulin deficit are enhanced glycogenolysis and gluconeogenesis resulting in greater hepatic glucose output, increased lipolysis, and reduction of peripheral glucose utilization, lipogenesis, and protein synthesis.

B. Counterregulatory Hormones

As suggested previously, absolute insulin deficiency, per se, does not account for the development of ketoacidosis in the majority of patients. Even when insulin therapy is omitted, ketoacidosis is not precipitated without the concomitant increment of some, if not all, the counterregulatory hormones (12). These hormones—glucagon, catecholamines, cortisol, and growth hormone—which are also known as the stress hormones, antagonize the action of insulin on carbohydrate, protein, and fat metabolism. In DKA of both adults and children there is almost invariably an elevation of at least three, if not all, of the counterregulatory hormones. The most important for the development of ketogenesis appear to be glucagon and catecholamines because of the rapid onset of their metabolic effect (12,17). The actions of glucagon include the following: glycogenolysis; elevated gluconeogenesis; enhanced ketogenesis, by suppression of malonyl CoA,

which regulates the carnitine acyl transferase enzymes; and proteolysis (18,19). Catecholamine actions are as follows: lipolysis by stimulation of lipase, gluconeogenesis, possible ketogenesis, and reduction of peripheral glucose utilization (18).

Cortisol and growth hormone excesses, both of which occur in DKA, have much slower actions but play an important role in the pathogenesis of DKA after a number of hours (12,18). The actions of increased circulating cortisol are catabolism of protein, reduction of peripheral utilization of glucose, augmentation of both gluconeogenesis and ketogenesis, along with some lipolysis. The effects of growth hormone elevation are lipolysis, gluconeogenesis (by an undefined mechanism), augmentation of ketogenesis, and reduction of peripheral glucose utilization.

C. Mechanism of Hyperglycemia

The degree of hyperglycemia in DKA varies and does not necessarily correlate with the severity of acidosis. The major source of blood glucose elevation is the continued hepatic glucose output due initially to glycogenolysis. Later it is due to continued gluconeogenesis stimulated by the combination of insulin deficiency and glucagon and catecholamine excess, augmented by the action of cortisol and growth hormone (20,21). Superimposed on the elevated glucose output is the reduction of peripheral glucose utilization caused by the absolute or relative insulin deficiency as well as the catecholamine action on muscle and adipose tissue (22).

Most of the glucose formed is excreted in the urine, resulting in a major caloric loss. As long as there is normal renal function, the circulating blood glucose does not increase much above 300–400 mg/100 ml. However, once severe dehydration ensues owing to osmotic diuresis, the diminished glomerular filtration rate prevents further excretion of glucose and the serum glucose level increases markedly. The more dehydrated the patient, the higher the serum glucose level (23). However, some patients exhibit initially very high serum glucose levels without concomitant dehydration. This occurs when thirst is quenched with sugar-containing fluids, resulting in extremely large glucose loads that can be partially excreted by the kidney without insulin therapy.

D. Mechanism of Hyperlipidemia

DKA is associated almost invariably with hypertriglyceridemia and elevated circulating nonesterified fatty acids (NEFA). The major source of these lipids is lipolysis of the adipose tissue due to stimulation of lipase caused by a combination of insulin deficiency and catecholamine, cortisol, and growth hormone excess (24). Another major source of serum triglycerides and NEFA may be the hepatocytes (25). As a result of extensive lipolysis, the serum in DKA may be extremely turbid, with increased viscosity and the danger of sludging in small blood vessels. A major complicating factor caused by severe hyperlipidemia is the spuriously low measurement of plasma electrolytes due to displacement of plasma water by the lipids. Thus, severe hyponatremia may be an artifact of hyperlipidemia unless the lipid is extracted prior to analysis (7,8).

E. Aminoacidemia

Because DKA is a catabolic condition, with reduced protein synthesis and continued proteolysis associated with both insulin deficiency and cortisol and glucagon excess, it causes increased concentrations of circulating branch-chain aminoacids (i.e., leucine, isoleucine, and valine). By contrast, the gluconeogenic aminoacid concentrations, particularly those of alanine and glutamine, are diminished because of greater hepatic uptake (26,27).

F. Mechanism of Ketogenesis

The liver is the sole source of ketone-body production. Acetoacetate and β-hydroxybutyrate are metabolized from the increased circulating NEFA delivered from the adipose cells. The liver is set in the ketogenic mode by a combination of insulin deficiency and glucagon excess. The higher ketone body production is controlled by the rate of lipolysis and thus by the substrate availability, and to a minor extent by the supply of ketogenic aminoacids, which are leucine and isoleucine. Continued gluconeogenesis, stimulated by glucagon with possibly an additive action of catecholamines and cortisol, produces sufficient NAD for ketone production. The long-chain fatty acids are transported into the mitochondria after combining with carnitine by the action of two carnitine acyl transferase enzymes. Sequential β-oxidation results in the formation of acetoacetate that is in equilibrium with β-hydroxybutyrate. Acetone may be formed by spontaneous decarboxylation of acetoacetate and excreted through the lungs or kidneys. Under the condition of severe acidosis, particularly that associated with hypoxia or lactic acidosis, most of the ketone bodies exist as β-hydroxybutyrate. This finding is important because β-hydroxybutyrate does not react with nitroprusside when the serum and urine are tested for ketones. Only acetoacetate will give the classic purple color. As the acidosis resolves, β-hydroxybutyrate is converted to acetoacetate and may give the impression of an increased production of ketones if one is not aware of this so-called factitious increased ketosis. The production of acetoacetate occurs at a time when there is an actual reduction in the total plasma ketone body concentration (28). New meters appearing on the market measure serum β-hydroxybutyrate and thus circumvent this problem.

Two studies have shown that the hepatic overproduction of ketone bodies alone cannot account for the huge increase in the circulating ketone concentration in DKA (29,30). It is suggested that a reduction in ketone body clearance and utilization is also necessary to explain the severe ketoacidosis. Insulin deficiency and catecholamine excess have been shown to lessen peripheral ketone body utilization, particularly by muscle. Excretion of ketone bodies through the lungs and kidneys is not sufficient to compensate for the greater hepatic production and lesser muscle utilization, particularly when glomerular filtration is diminished due to dehydration.

G. Mechanism of the Metabolic Acidosis

In children with DKA, the major cause of acidosis is the accumulation of ketone bodies. β-Hydroxybutyrate and acetoacetate both are strong acids and contribute to the classic anion gap found in DKA (31). When severe dehydration is found with peripheral vascular shutdown and anoxia, an accumulation of lactic acid with lactic acidosis contributes to the general metabolic acidosis (32). Patients with DKA usually have a normochloremic acidosis with an elevated anion gap. However, during therapy, despite continued excretion of the ketone bodies, acidosis frequently persists with the appearance of hyperchloremia and disappearance of the anion gap. Excretion of ketone bodies is not associated with a rise in serum bicarbonate concentration, suggesting the loss of a great deal of alkali together with the ketones in the urine. However, it is likely that the apparent loss of bicarbonate may also occur on a dilutional basis or may be associated with alterations in anion distribution. It is thought that the administration of chlorides during rehydration can only partially account for the hyperchloremia, and that there is increased renal tubular chloride reabsorption. The associated lack of adequate amounts of alkali causes the persistent metabolic acidosis. Serum electrolyte balance is maintained by elevated chloride concentration (33).

H. Effects of Renal Function

1. Water Loss
A major effect of uncontrolled diabetes is osmotic diuresis associated with glucosuria. This water loss results in severe dehydration and, eventually, reduced glomerular filtration. If the decrease in plasma volume is severe, diminished peripheral circulation, shock, and, occasionally, renal tubular necrosis can result.

2. Electrolyte Loss
The glycosuria of DKA classically is accompanied by a loss of sodium, potassium, calcium, phosphate, and magnesium in the urine. The loss of sodium, calcium, and phosphate is apparently related to both insulin deficiency and glucagon excess, which have a direct effect on the renal tubules. The contraction of the intravascular circulating volume together with the sodium loss stimulates

both aldosterone and ADH secretion. Aldosterone's action on the tubules may account for some of the potassium loss. However, most of the potassium and phosphate loss is due to movement of these cations from the intracellular space into the intravascular space and into the urine due to insulin deficiency. Glucagon excess may induce resistance to the sodium-retaining actions of mineralocorticoids so that circulating aldosterone does not exert its sodium-retaining action (34,35). High levels of ADH add to the Na excretion in the urine, contributing to the total body sodium deficit. As mentioned previously, the alkali loss through the kidney associated with the excretion of ketone bodies can result in a total body bicarbonate deficit that must be replenished. As mentioned previously, sodium moves from the intravascular to extravascular space in the face of severe hyperglycemia. An approximate formula to calculate this effect is a decrease of sodium in the serum of 1.6 mE/l for every 100 mg increase in serum glucose above normal.

I. Effects on the Brain

Changes in the level of consciousness are a hallmark of severe DKA. These changes can vary from lethargy to stupor and coma. Even when there is not clinical change in the level of consciousness. DKA, particularly when associated with severe hyperosmolarity, is associated with major electroencephalographic (EEG) abnormalities that are usually reversible (36). Alterations in the level of consciousness appear to be more closely associated with hyperosmolarity due to hyperglycemia, with or without hypernatremia. If there is severe ketoacidosis and dehydration, there may be relative cerebral anoxia, which can also contribute to changes in the level of consciousness. Severe phosphate loss will result in deficiency of 2,3-DPG. This loss results in increased oxygen affinity of hemoglobin and relatively decreased delivery of oxygen to the tissues (i.e., a shift of the Bohr curve to the left) (10). When a patient is severely acidotic the Bohr curve is effectively shifted to the right. Thus acidosis and 2,3-DPG reduction counterbalance each other. Severe phosphate depletion without severe acidosis shifts the Bohr curve to the left and, theoretically, is associated with tissue anoxia. However, measurements of oxygen partial pressure in peripheral tissues were not abnormal in a series of studies, but the effect in the brain has not been well studied.

J. Hyperosmolar Nonketotic Coma

In pediatric practice, hyperosmolar nonketotic coma is an unusual condition that occurs mainly in very young or mentally retarded children (6). It is assumed that these patients are unable to obtain access to sufficient water to prevent severe dehydration. This condition occurs in the presence of a relative insulin deficiency, resulting in excessive glucose production and an osmotic diuresis. How-

ever, there appears to be enough insulin to suppress lipolysis and thus prevent an excess production of ketone bodies. There is assumed to be an unexplained limitation to the output of glucagon that would usually occur in a stress situation and stimulate ketogenesis. Coma in these patients is associated with severe hyperosmolarity, metabolic acidosis, and high incidence of death associated with cerebral edema. It should be remembered that an equal degree of hyperosmolarity could occur in the presence of ketoacidosis with similar detrimental effects.

IV. CAUSES OF DIABETIC KETOACIDOSIS

In both newly diagnosed patients and insulin-treated patients with diabetes, DKA is usually associated with a precipitating factor, making the relative insulin deficiency functionally absolute. In the known diabetic, the most common precipitating cause is disruption of insulin delivery by omitting injections, malfunction of an insulin pump, or inappropriate decreases of doses during illness. In contrast, in newly diagnosed patients DKA is often precipitated by an acute infection that carries with it an increase in the insulin requirement. Relatively routine pediatric illnesses such as flu, otitis media, and gastroenteritis may rapidly induce ketosis and subsequent acidosis in a previously apparently healthy child. Acute infection is a less common precipitant in known diabetic children. It occurs only in the face of inadequate insulin delivery. The progression to DKA usually suggests that prompt intervention at home was not accomplished, often because of failure to recognize the early deterioration. The mild insulin deficiency results in acute DKA only if it is accompanied by an increase in the counterregulatory hormones, particularly glucagon. Less common precipitating causes of DKA after diagnosis are physical and mental stress. In most diabetic children the occurrence of DKA after diagnosis is not common. A small group of patients has recurrent DKA in response to emotional stress. It has long been held that this response seems related to an acute rise in catecholamine secretion, with an accompanying rise in free fatty acid (FFA) production due to lipolysis and subsequent ketogenesis. This response can occur within hours in a previously apparently healthy person.

Our recent experience suggests that this phenomenon is rare in the majority of children with recurrent DKA. These children appear to have an excessive biochemical response to stress or a defect in the clearance rates of related hormones or substrates. Such patients are referred to as psychogenic diabetics and are often adolescents from disorganized homes. Like the rapid onset of DKA in these children, the response to medical therapy is unusually prompt. Our institution of measurements of free insulin levels has revealed that a more common mechanism of this recurrent DKA is failure to receive insulin, even sometimes when a parent claims to have administered the injection. The problem will recur unless underlying behavioral problems are identified and resolved. Exercise can also precipitate acute ketoacidosis in a patient who is already partially decompensated due to underinsulinization. Again, this is presumed to be related to an elevation of catecholamines and glucagon levels in excess of available insulin.

V. DIFFERENTIAL DIAGNOSIS

If the patient has known history of diabetes, the differential diagnosis of alterations in consciousness is between DKA and hypoglycemia. Measurement of blood glucose levels by a blood glucose monitor and serum or urine ketones should give the accurate diagnosis (remembering that hypoglycemia can induce ketosis).

Because patients with ketoacidosis often have abdominal pain with vomiting, an acute abdomen must enter the differential diagnosis. A patient with diabetes may have an acute abdomen most commonly from appendicitis, and this can coexist with DKA.

Severe gastroenteritis with hypernatremia and acidosis is occasionally associated with ketoacidosis due to inhibition of insulin secretion, with accompanying hyperglycemia and ketosis. Such patients have temporary diabetes and sometimes may require a few doses of very small amounts of insulin. Some drugs induce nondiabetic ketoacidosis, the most common being salicylate intoxication in children. In addition, high dosages of diazoxide or salbutamol have been reported to induce nondiabetic ketoacidosis. Chronic alcoholism associated with reduced food intake can cause severe hyperketonemia with acidosis. However, alcoholism is usually associated with hypoglycemia.

VI. CLINICAL ASSESSMENT

Most of the diagnostic signs and symptoms of DKA are sequelae of the metabolic disorder with clear pathogenesis. The only feature that is not fully explained is the devastating effect of DKA on the CNS. Patients will almost always present with polyuria and polydipsia of variable duration. These symptoms eventually result in dehydration with consequent hypovolemia, tachycardia, and shock. Ketosis is usually accompanied by abdominal pain, nausea, and vomiting, the mechanism of which is totally unclear. DKA typically causes hyperventilation (Kussmaul breathing), which is deep sighing ventilation with a long air column. If the patient is extremely acidotic (pH < 7.0), CNS depression often occurs and the respiratory rate may fall in association with carbon dioxide retention. When acidosis is severe, the serum potassium level may be high. However, because of insulin deficiency, there is a great deal of intracellular potassium loss due mainly to potassium diuresis, which accounts for gastric stasis, ileus,

muscle weakness and cramps, and the risk for cardiac arrhythmia. The loss of intracellular magnesium and phosphate may add to these symptoms (37).

The presenting abdominal symptoms and signs may be similar to those of an acute abdomen. Because of the frequent increase in serum amylase levels in DKA, a number of workers have suggested an association of DKA with acute pancreatitis in some of these patients. However, serum amylase levels increase in approximately 70% of patients with DKA, most of whom have no clinical evidence of pancreatitis. The raised serum amylase levels are usually associated with severe hyperglycemia, and the origin of the enzyme is likely to be the salivary glands (38). Because DKA is often precipitated by infection, accompanying signs and symptoms should be sought. It is important to note that even in the absence of infection, pyrexia is rare in association with DKA, and leukocytosis frequently occurs despite the absence of infection.

Reports indicate that approximately 10% of patients with DKA are comatose and coma is associated with a greater mortality risk. We have noted that the incidence of coma is diminishing at our center because of earlier recognition of decompensating diabetes. Disturbances in the level of consciousness are more common, varying from lethargy to disorientation and agitation. Cerebral edema at presentation is unusual but may occur, and the mechanism of CNS abnormalities appears to be related mainly to the degree of hyperosmolarity.

Initial clinical assessment of the patient should be made rapidly and should include state of hydration; blood pressure and cardiac output; renal function (polyuria or anuria); cerebral function, including a very careful evaluation of the optic discs for papilledema; and complicating and precipitating factors.

Immediately after the clinical assessment, baseline biochemical evaluation of the patient should be made prior to initiation of insulin therapy. This evaluation should include:

1. Urinalysis for glucose and ketones, recognizing that interfering substances such as salicylates, antibiotics, and degraded strips may possibly give false-negative or false-positive results for acetonuria (39).
2. Serum glucose level using a sensitive laboratory technique after screening with one of the available bedside blood glucose monitors.
3. Serum electrolyte levels.
4. Values of arterial or venous gases. In our experience, we have not found measurement of arterial gases necessary for monitoring patients, and we have used venous blood unless there is peripheral vascular collapse. The measurement of blood gases should include pH, PCO_2, and bicarbonate.
5. Plasma osmolarity should be measured or calculated using the formula:

$$Osm\ (serum) = 2 \times Na\ (mEq/l)$$
$$+ \frac{Glucose\ (mg/dl)}{18} + \frac{BUN\ (mg/dl)}{2.8}$$

6. Serum or plasma ketone levels should be measured using an Acetest tablet or a meter.
7. BUN and creatinine levels.
8. Calcium and phosphorus values.
9. Serum amylase level (if indicated).
10. Hemoglobin value, hematocrit, and white blood cell count.
11. Microscopic examination of the urine.

VII. THERAPY

The development of DKA is usually relatively slow and should be corrected relatively slowly. The only indication for very rapid correction is impending or actual shock. This maxim is probably even more important in treatment of children than of adults.

A. Rehydration

Because a major feature of DKA is water loss associated with loss of electrolytes, rehydration is the cornerstone of therapy. It is probably more important in the early stages of therapy than insulin delivery. An initial 1 h bolus of 10–20 cc/kg 0.9% normal saline should be given prior to the administration of insulin while awaiting report of laboratory results and assessing fluid losses. The most common fluid used is normal saline without the addition of potassium until urine excretion has been confirmed and serum potassium levels have been measured. Ringers' lactate, while effective, is less than optimal because of possible delay in lactate metabolism by the liver. The advantage of this initial hour or even 2 h of rehydration is that it allows one to assess the degree of dehydration and rate of blood glucose decrement associated with volume expansion rather than insulin action. Rehydration is very useful in the child in whom the degree of dehydration is not apparent based on clinical assessment. Some of the plasma glucose reduction during this period is probably caused by improved insulin action in previously treated patients, or elimination of a large oral glucose load by improved renal function in the face of enhanced glomerular filtration rate. The fluid deficit is calculated according to the body weight, and the deficit is corrected over 24 h with one-half the correction over the first 8 h. It is extremely important to assess water balance continually in the patient with an actual measurement of the total fluid infused or taken orally and the total urine volume lost.

The initial fluid rate required should be between 10 and 20 ml/kg/h depending on the patient's hydration and hemodynamic status. Excessive infusion should be avoided unless it is needed for correction of hypotension

and shock. Excessively rapid rehydration with volumes above this is thought by some (40,41) but not all (42,43) to be related to the development of cerebral edema. Unless severe hyperosmolarity or hyponatremia persists after the first hour, the rehydration fluid is changed to half-normal saline in order to supply maintenance fluid, correct the deficit, and replace continual losses. Fluid status must be reassessed on a regular basis; fluid requirements should not be calculated based on the initial status without reevaluation.

Maintenance and replacement fluid volumes can be calculated on a weight or surface area basis, with allowances made for age (Fig. 1). Most of the rehydration treatment should be administered intravenously and oral fluids should be avoided in the very ill patient, particularly if there has been prior vomiting. Even when oral fluids are tolerated, gastric stasis and ileus may prevent rapid absorption of fluids and make it difficult to calculate actual delivery to the intravascular space. Composition of the rehydration fluids depends on the patient's serum sodium and potassium levels and the serum osmolarity. In general, one should attempt to rehydrate, at least initially, with iso-osmolar solutions. As the serum osmolarity diminishes, some free water should be administered. There is almost never an indication for administration of intravenous fluids that do not contain sodium. In contrast, hyponatremia, which may occur during therapy, may require continuation or reinstitution of 0.9% normal saline therapy. The aim should be to reduce the serum osmolarity slowly by constant administration of solutions containing sodium (unless the serum sodium levels rise), and later to add glucose (see following section). The concentration of K^+ usually should not exceed 40 mEq/l but in rare circumstances up to 80 mEq/l may be required. Maintenance and replacement fluid volumes can be calculated according to body weight in kilograms (Fig. 1).

There are some differences of opinion as to whether the rehydration period should be 24, 36, or 48 h in duration. In our experience, a period longer than 24 h with very slow correction of hydration results in persistent acidosis. However, if there is severe hyperosmolarity, a 36–48 h rehydration period should be calculated.

B. Insulin

For many years, the conventional mode of insulin therapy in DKA was intermittent subcutaneous injections of crystalline insulin. Fairly high doses (100–200 units) were recommended, particularly in adults (44). In children, the tendency was to use slightly lower doses, although these would still be considered high compared with the low doses currently shown to be effective. Since the mid-1970s, a number of studies in both adults and children have shown that low-dose intravenous or intramuscular insulin delivery corrects the hyperglycemia and ketoacidosis in DKA as rapidly and effectively as the previously used high doses. With lower insulin doses, more physio-

	Maintenance Fluid	Deficit (10% dehydration)
Fluid	100 ml/kg	100 ml/kg
	50 ml/kg	
	20 ml/kg	
Na	3 mEq/kg	6 mEq/kg
K	2 mEq/kg	5 mEq/kg

Thus, a 30-kg patient with 10% dehydration would need:

	Maintenance	Deficit	Total
Fluids	1700 ml	3000 ml	4700 ml
Na	90 mEq	180 mEq	270 mEq
K	60 mEq	150 mEq	210 mEq

Fluids could be given according to the following procedure:

Hour	ml/kg/hr	Fluid composition	
1st	15	Normal saline	
2nd	10	Half-normal saline plus 40 mEq KCl/L	Add 5% glucose when necessary
3rd-8th	8	Half-normal saline plus 30 mEq KCl/L	
9th-24th	5	Quarter-normal saline plus 20-30 mEq KCl/L	

Figure 1   Calculation of maintenance fluid levels.

logical circulating insulin levels are achieved, and hypoglycemia, hypokalemia, and hypophosphatemia have been shown to occur less frequently in comparative studies (45,46). Thus, low-dose insulin therapy compared to that used in adults is the treatment of choice in children with DKA because this level of insulin delivery achieves its goal in the majority of cases (47,48). Occasionally, a patient appears to have a greater than usual degree of insulin resistance, requiring slightly higher doses for reversal of the ketoacidotic state.

The choice of insulin delivery route should depend on the condition of the patient and the facilities available. If DKA is very mild with minimal acidosis and dehydration, the subcutaneous route is convenient and effective, especially if the patient does not require intravenous rehydration. The dosage regimen is approximately 0.25 units/kg regular insulin given every 4–6 h prior to meals. Regular insulin given subcutaneously delivers therapeutic doses for approximately 4 h, with the duration of action being 6 h at most. Therefore, patients must receive insulin at least every 4–6 h, even during the night, and if they are not eating, in order to prevent recurrent ketosis. The dose given during the night can be decreased slightly if ketosis is nearly cleared and should always be accompanied by a small meal.

If the patient is significantly dehydrated, subcutaneous insulin is poorly and irregularly absorbed. Under these circumstances, the intravenous route is preferred for insulin delivery by means of a continuous infusion of 0.1 units/kg/h after an initial loading bolus of 0.1 units/kg.

Although some investigators believe that a loading dose is not necessary (49), it seems logical to achieve physiological insulin levels immediately, particularly in the patient who has not had prior insulin therapy. The insulin is delivered in a fairly concentrated solution (approximately 1 unit/ml in normal saline) with the infusion controlled by a syringe pump through a line, which is connected piggyback to the rehydration intravenous infusion set using as short tubing as possible. A change of the syringe or infusion bag every 12 or 24 h and the use of concentrated solution of insulin minimize the problems of insulin adherence to the plastic of the infusion system. Thus, the use of albumin has not been necessary (50). Mixing insulin in the rehydration fluid directly is dangerous because the delivery rate will depend on the rate of rehydration rather than on insulin need. In addition, these dilute solutions of insulin have a greater propensity for loss of insulin onto the surface of the infusion apparatus.

The advantage of the intravenous delivery of insulin is the smooth pattern of circulating insulin levels achieved. The physician is able to increase or decrease the amount of insulin delivered with immediate effect, since intravenous insulin has a half life of 3–8 min. Contrary to popular belief, the patient does not require greater vigilance from a biochemical standpoint when insulin is infused intravenously. The same care is needed irrespective of the route of insulin delivery. However, greater care is required to ensure that the intravenous delivery system and the pump are working effectively. A number of clinicians believe that constant intravenous infusion of insulin should not be used in community hospitals that do not have adequate facilities, particularly the use of some type of pump system. The use of intravenous insulin boluses should be discouraged, as it results in supraphysiological levels with a rapid decline, possibly stimulating an enhanced secretion of counterregulatory hormones (47,51).

Intramuscular insulin delivery with a loading dose of 0.25 units/kg followed by 0.1 units/kg/h has been used with the same success as the continuous intravenous routes (52). The disadvantage of this mode of therapy is the repeated pain of an intramuscular injection, which is avoided with the use of intravenous routes.

The amount of insulin given initially should be tailored so that the drop in blood glucose level is approximately, but no more than, 100 mg/dl/h. If the blood glucose level drops more rapidly than this rate after the first 2 h of rehydration, the insulin dose should be reduced. If it drops to less than 75 mg/dl/h, the insulin dose rarely may have to be increased. In general, as long as there is ketosis, it is preferable to add 5% dextrose water to the hydration solution to prevent excessive glucose decrements once the serum glucose is below 500 mg/dl, but this is rarely needed.

Continuous intravenous insulin is administered until the acidosis is corrected, the hyperglycemia under control, and ketonemia virtually absent. Ketonuria will persist for some time after correction of metabolic acidosis. If a patient is able to eat meals prior to achievement of these goals, a small increment of insulin should be given to cover the anticipated hyperglycemia. A dose of subcutaneous insulin (0.1–0.25 units/kg, depending on the ambient blood glucose level, ketosis, and appetite) should be given approximately 30 min prior to the discontinuation of intravenous insulin. The patient should then be given subcutaneous insulin, 0.2–0.25 units/kg every 4–6 h. The next 24 h should be used to evaluate the patient's total dose requirements. Thereafter, a regimen of intermediate-acting plus short-acting insulin can be started, with the total long-acting dose requirement approximately close to the previous day's total crystalline insulin dose. Short-acting insulin is given as needed, starting with approximately the same dose of short-acting insulin as had been used in a single injection on the prior day.

C. Potassium

Potassium should be started when the initial insulin dose is given, unless severe hyperkalemia ($K^+ > 6$ mEq/l) is present. Potassium is given prophylactically to prevent dangerous hypokalemia from occurring with the movement of serum potassium back into the cells or into the urine. Electrocardiographic (ECG) monitoring is very useful in indicating hyperkalemia and hypokalemia, by demonstrating peaked T waves in the former and U waves in the latter. Intracellular potassium deficiency, even when it occurs without accompanying hypokalemia, can result in

gastric stasis, ileus, and arrhythmia. Failure to replace potassium was a frequent cause of death in DKA in the past and is required even when low-dose insulin therapy is used. If bicarbonate is administered, a greater amount of potassium may be needed. In all dehydrated patients, potassium should be started at a rate of 20–40 mEq/l with the intravenous rehydration fluid. If, despite this therapy, the plasma potassium levels drop into the hypokalemic range ($K^+ < 3.5$ mEq/l), a higher concentration even up to 60 and rarely 80 mEq/l may be necessary. Hourly serum potassium monitoring is required until the patient is stable (usually 6–8 h) and thereafter the frequency can be decreased. Under most circumstances, it is safe to give the potassium in the form of potassium chloride: it is unlikely that the additional chloride administration will significantly contribute to the degree of hyperchloremia that is sometimes seen. If necessary, half the potassium can be given as potassium chloride and the other one-half as potassium phosphate (see discussion below). It should be remembered that 80% of the administered potassium can be lost in the urine during the first 24 h, and continued oral potassium supplementation in the diet is recommended after an episode of ketoacidosis. Most normal diets contain enough potassium to replenish the body's stores.

D. Phosphate

Phosphate is lost from the intracellular space by the same mechanism as that causing potassium depletion. The institution of insulin therapy causes a drop in serum phosphate in the majority of patients, resulting occasionally in severe hypophosphatemia. The inclusion of phosphate in the rehydration solution is a subject of continued controversy. The administration of phosphate supplements in the treatment of DKA can prevent early but not late hypophosphatemia and has been reported to maintain normal 2,3 DPG levels, although this has not been shown to be associated with improved peripheral oxygen delivery (10). Although there is one report of phosphate therapy improving the level of consciousness in patients with DKA (53), such is not the case in our experience (11). High-dosage phosphorus supplementation, in children particularly, which is a risk in dehydrated patient requiring large fluid volumes, is associated with the development of severe hypocalcemia and tetany (54). By contrast, low-dosage phosphate therapy in our studies does not prevent late hypophosphatemia because most of the supplement is lost in the urine, particularly in patients with severe initial acidosis who require bicarbonate therapy (11). Total serum calcium, but not ionized serum calcium, is diminished in many ill patients with DKA even without the use of phosphate supplements (11). Because the severe complications of hypophosphatemia are rarely, if ever, described in children with DKA, and because the benefits of phosphate therapy are not demonstrated conclusively, many pediatricians believe that there is at present no indication for routine phosphate therapy because of the concomitant risk of hypocalcemia. However, others hold that severe hypophosphatemia per se may be dangerous and that careful supplementation with phosphate with continuous monitoring of serum calcium and phosphorus levels and clinical signs of hypocalcemia is a logical form of therapy. In the severely ill patient with DKA, a rational approach is administration of half the potassium as potassium chloride and the other half as potassium phosphate once the serum phosphorus level starts falling below 3 mg/dl. Phosphate should preferably be given independent of potassium needs as a sodium phosphate solution in a dosage of approximately 4 mM/kg over 12 h. Dietary phosphate supplements may need to be continued after intravenous rehydration has stopped, in order to correct the total body phosphate deficit and maintain normal intracellular levels of 2,3 DPG.

E. Magnesium

Although magnesium loss in the urine with intracellular depletion has been documented in DKA, its clinical effects are not clear (37). Thus the replacement of magnesium in the rehydration fluid is not commonly carried out. However, severe magnesium depletion can be associated with transient hypoparathyroidosm and hypocalcemia. Improvement in resistant hypocalcemia and carpopedal spasm has been reported in one child with DKA after magnesium supplementation (54).

F. Bicarbonate

Bicarbonate administration is, perhaps, one of the most controversial areas in the therapy of DKA (55). It is agreed that severe acidosis, particularly in very young children, should be treated with bicarbonate because the risk of arrhythmia, reduced cardiac contractility, and possible contribution to circulatory collapse and insulin resistance. The most important danger is impaired ventilatory capacity. There is a debate about the definition of severe acidosis. The reason for avoiding the use of bicarbonate is its potential effect on cerebrospinal fluid pH (56), the production of severe hypokalemia (55), the possibility of hypophosphatemia (11), and the excessively rapid shift of the oxygen dissociation curve to the left. This would result in reduced tissue oxygenation, particularly in the presence of diminished 2,3 DPG (55), and the possibility of persistent ketosis as shown in a small-human and animal study (57). Because the paradoxical drop in CNS pH occurs in patients given bicarbonate and in those not given bicarbonate (58), this danger has been de-emphasized recently. However, the effect of bicarbonate administration on CNS oxygen tension, and its possible role in the production of cerebral edema in dogs, have made a number of physicians very cautious about its use (59). This concern has been emphasized by the identification of treatment of DKA with bicarbonate in very dehydrated

children being a major risk factor for cerebral edema (60,61).

Our current recommendation is to add bicarbonate to the rehydration fluid if the serum pH is less than 7.2. The amount to be replaced is calculated to correct the serum bicarbonate to a level of 12 mEq/l, and it is given over 4–6 h without any bolus administration. Bicarbonate therapy is discontinued as soon as the venous bicarbonate level has reached 12 mEq/l, even when the calculated amount has not yet been delivered. To calculate the amount of bicarbonate needed, one subtracts the actual serum bicarbonate level from 12, and multiplies that value by the weight in kilograms and a correction factor of 0.6. The calculated amount of bicarbonate to be given is added to the intravenous fluids as sodium bicarbonate, taking into consideration that the concentration of sodium chloride has to be decreased proportionally to reach an adequate concentration of sodium in the fluid. This bicarbonate is to be delivered to the patient in a slow infusion over 4–8 h and never as a rapid (IV push) bolus.

G. Glucose

As the patient's serum glucose level approaches 250–300 mg/dl, or possibly when the serum glucose level falls at a rate greater than 100 mg/dl/h, glucose is added to the intravenous fluid, usually as 5% dextrose water and half-normal saline. If the serum glucose level continues to fall rapidly, 10% dextrose water is given to provide calories to the patient who has had a major caloric loss over the preceding few weeks. Preventing the drop in blood glucose level below 250 mg/dl is based on studies by Arieff and Kleeman showing that cerebral edema can be induced in rabbits if the blood glucose level drops rapidly below this level from hyperglycemic levels (62). Thus glucose is added to prevent both a blood glucose decrement of more than 100 mg/dl/h from high levels and to allow the development of normoglycemia from 250 mg/dl slowly. Avoidance in a rapid drop of osmolarity is probably more important than the actual serum glucose level, but this has not been studied formally.

H. Other Therapeutic Considerations

If the patient is extremely acidotic and in shock, the administration of oxygen for a short time may improve peripheral oxygen delivery. Catheterization of the bladder is rarely necessary and carries with it the risk of infection. If the patient is unconscious, nasogastric suction is necessary to prevent the aspiration of vomitus. Under all circumstances, the event precipitating the episode of DKA should be sought and treated accordingly. During therapy, continuous clinical and biochemical monitoring is mandatory. Initially, hourly measurements should be made of plasma glucose, electrolyte levels, osmolarity, and blood gas values. Serum calcium and phosphorus concentrations should be measured intermittently. The frequency of electrolyte measurements can be decreased as the patient's condition improves, although blood glucose levels should be obtained every hour. Accurate measurements of fluid intake and output should be made with appropriate changes in the therapeutic regimen. If possible, the patient should be treated in a metabolic ward or intensive care unit, where the staff is fully conversant with the therapy of DKA. Careful watch for the complications of DKA should be maintained throughout the first 12–24 h of therapy.

VIII. COMPLICATIONS OF DKA

A. Persistent Acidosis

Persistent acidosis may or may not be accompanied by continued hyperglycemia and may be related to insulin resistance, requiring a higher insulin dose regimen. However, the usual cause is unrecognized or untreated infection or inadequate fluid replacement.

B. Overhydration

Overhydration results from overestimation of the initial fluid deficit or failure to monitor the patient's fluid balance during the course of therapy. Overhydration may result in peripheral edema or even cardiac failure in the very young child. Peripheral edema (known as insulin edema) may also be caused by hypoalbuminemia, which is frequently seen during the correction of DKA because of shifts of albumin from the intra- to the extravascular space (11).

C. Hypoglycemia

Often hypoglycemia occurs 8–12 h after the initiation of therapy if serum glucose levels are not monitored regularly. This complication is less likely to occur with the use of low-dosage insulin regimens (63). Hypoglycemia is a possible cause of lethargy, disorientation, and recurrence of coma or seizures. It is easily preventable by increasing glucose delivery or reducing the insulin dose as soon as low serum glucose levels are seen during hourly monitoring.

D. Hypokalemia

Low serum potassium levels reflect even lower intracellular concentrations. These intracellular potassium deficits account for some of the symptoms accompanying DKA, such as gastric stasis and ileus. If sufficient potassium supplements are not given, classic ECG changes of hypokalemia are observed. Hypokalemia is potentially lethal, causing cardiac arrhythmia. Serum potassium levels should be monitored carefully even if insulin is given subcutaneously and oral hydration is possible.

E. Cerebral Edema

Cerebral edema is the most feared complication of DKA, occurring in 0.2–1% of children with DKA and more frequently in children than in adults. It has very high mortality and morbidity rates. It most commonly occurs after 3–12 h of therapy, even in patients who did not have significant hyperosmolarity. After initial improvement in clinical, biochemical, and CNS signs, patients experience greater irritability, CNS depression, and, later, seizures and coma. These conditions may occur even without obvious papilledema. The pathogenesis remains an enigma. A number of theories attempt to explain cerebral edema, none of which is entirely satisfactory or proven (43,64). These theories include the following:

1. A rapid drop in the blood glucose levels below 250 mg/dl. However, of the 17 patients reported in the medical literature, only nine had glucose levels that reached this range (43).

2. A rapid drop in serum osmolarity or severe hyponatremia. It is difficult to assess accurate sodium levels because of the associated hyperlipidemia in some of these patients. Despite this difficulty, the serum sodium levels were not lower than 130 mEq/l in seven of the reported cases. Also, rapid changes in serum osmolarity could not be documented (43,65). However, another study reports that progressive hyponatremia was a distinctive factor in children who developed cerebral edema (66). This supports our experience.

3. Overhydration or rapid fluid administration. Again, the theory is difficult to prove because many patients who receive the same amount of intravenous fluids as those who develop cerebral edema do not have any adverse effects. In the patients reported, the amounts and rates of fluid administration were variable. In addition, two patients had received only oral fluids prior to the development of cerebral edema (43).

4. Increased polyol activity in the brain. It is postulated that the accumulation of osmotically active sorbitol in the brain can account for the elevated CNS pressure documented in the majority of patients with DKA who were studied. However, it seems that the osmotic contribution of sorbitol is not sufficient to cause cerebral edema (67,68).

5. Cerebral anoxia associated with decreased 2,3 DPG levels. Rapid bicarbonate infusion or change in pH could precipitate such an event (59). This treatment was not unusual in the patients reported in the medical literature. However, cause and effect have not been proven.

6. An increase in the insulin induced Na+/H+ antiporter pump activity, which increases the accumulation of intracellular fluid by increasing sodium movement into the brain cells. An exchange with ketone bodies may also be involved (69).

A number of other mechanisms have also been postulated, but none has been proven (64). However, the fact that the frequency of cerebral edema appears to be decreasing suggests that slow, careful therapy with insulin fluid and electrolytes may be important in its prevention.

A patient who shows any signs of cerebral edema should be immediately treated with mannitol with appropriate cerebrospinal fluid pressure monitoring in an intensive care unit. Confirmation with a CT scan is not always possible and may be difficult without a baseline image. However, magnetic resonance imaging (MRI) may be useful to exclude infarction as a cause of the cerebral pathology seen in the pediatric DKA population in our center and elsewhere (64).

IX. PREVENTIVE THERAPY

The development of DKA in the child or adolescent with previously diagnosed diabetes mellitus is caused by a failure of therapy, the responsibility of which must be borne by the patient, the family, the physician, and the entire therapeutic team. DKA certainly should be preventable in the patient with previously diagnosed diabetes. Proper daily blood or urine monitoring, or both, by the patient or family should identify metabolic alterations that may lead to DKA and thus allow initiation of therapeutic intervention, which should prevent the progression of the metabolic problem. Frequent daily monitoring of blood glucose and the initial morning urine specimen for ketones should allow appropriate preventive therapy. The presence of ketones necessitates that each voiding thereafter be checked. The persistence of small amounts of ketones for more than 3 h or the presence of large concentrations is an indication to contact the physician for specific directions.

General principles for preventive management include an increase in oral fluid intake and the administration of additional regular insulin at a dosage of 0.1–0.25 units/kg every 3–4 h or ultra-short-acting insulin every 2–3 h in the presence of persistent ketonuria. The development of nausea and continuous vomiting requires examination by a physician and, frequently, hospitalization. Temperature elevation should also be reason for direct observation by the physician. The usual childhood illnesses, such as flu, laryngitis, tonsillitis, and otitis media, which may be tolerated by the average child with little or no major disability, may rapidly lead to major metabolic disorder in the child with diabetes. The parents must understand that early contact with their physician is essential to prevent DKA. The availability of a 24 h hotline is most important in ensuring that the families of diabetic children receive prompt and accurate direction for the management of impending illnesses.

A particular problem has arisen since the widespread acceptance of home blood glucose monitoring. It is the position of most patients and many physicians that the utilization of blood glucose level observations makes ketone testing superfluous. This is not true. Observation of blood glucose concentration provides no information on the presence or absence of ketonuria or ketonemia. Although it is true that DKA rarely occurs in the presence of normal or modestly elevated blood glucose values, it is also true that many children and adolescents do not perform accurate measurements of blood glucose concentrations. The child who is performing only one or two blood glucose determinations daily may not record persistent or episodic hyperglycemia. Those patients with previously diagnosed diabetes admitted for treatment of ketoacidosis who were supposedly monitoring blood glucose concentrations carefully almost certainly would have been alerted earlier about a change in metabolic status if ketones had been checked.

Despite the best intentions and careful observation and intervention by the family, a small number of cases of DKA in individuals with known diabetes will almost inevitably continue to occur. Most of these cases will be the result of emotional stress in children and family without a rapid response and early intervention. The use of very-short-acting insulin in insulin pumps is another more recent common factor. The interruption of its delivery can cause rapid ketoacidosis because there is no insulin reservoir. The other major group of patients who may develop acute-onset DKA are those with acute infections, usually viral and associated with gastroenteritis. A preventive approach to DKA is essential if the cost and the mortality associated with IDDM in children are to be reduced. Education about diabetes and its complications is the cornerstone upon which this approach must be constructed. The utilization of a therapeutic team, including physician, diabetes nurse–educator, dietician, and social worker–behaviorist, will enhance the likelihood that adequate education will be delivered and continuing needs met. Prompt attention to recurrent illnesses, even minor ones, is essential. DKA in the child can and should be prevented.

REFERENCES

1. Nitadori Y, Fukushima K, Libman I, Nishimura R, Becker D. Changes in onset features of children with type I diabetes. Submitted for publication.
2. Eberhardt MS, Wagener DK, Orchard TJ, LaPorte RE, Cavender DE, Rabin BS, Atchison RW, Kuller LH, Drash AL, Becker DJ. HLA heterogeneity of insulin-dependent diabetes mellitus at onset: The Pittsburgh IDDM Study. Diabetes 1985;34:1247–1252.
3. Dorman J, Laporte R, Kuller LH, et al. The Pittsburgh Insulin Dependent Diabetes Registries: the mortality experience. Diabetes 1984;33:271.
4. Schade DS, Eaton RP, Alberti KGMM, Johnston DG. The importance of diabetic coma. In Diabetic Coma. Albuquerque, NM: University of New Mexico Press, 1981: 3–9.
5. Children's Hospital of Pittsburgh Diabetes Registry. Unpublished observations.
6. Rubin HM, Kramer R, Drash A. Hyperosmolarity complicating diabetes mellitus in childhood. J Pediatr 1969;74: 177–186.

7. Frier BM, Steer CR, Baird JD, Bloomfield S. Misleading plasma electrolytes in diabetic children with severe hyperlipidemia. Arch Dis Child 1980;55:771–775.

8. Steffes MW, Freier EF. A simple and precise method of determining true sodium, potassium and chloride concentrations in hyperlipemia. J Lab Clin Med 1976;88:683–688.

9. Bradley RF. Diabetic ketoacidosis and coma. In: Marble A, White P, Bradley RF, eds. Joslin Diabetes Mellitus. Philadelphia: Lea & Febiger, 1971:361–416.

10. Gibby OM, Veale KE, Hayes TM, Jones JG, Wardrop CA. Oxygen availability from the blood an effect of the phosphate replacement of erythrocyte 2,3-diphosphoglycerate and hemoglobin oxygen affinity in diabetic ketoacidosis. Diabetologia 1978;15:381–385.

11. Becker DJ, Brown DR, Steranka BH, Drash AL. Comparison of the effects of potassium phosphate and potassium chloride on calcium and phosphorus homeostasis during the treatment of diabetic ketoacidosis. Am J Dis Child 1983; 137:241–246.

12. Schade DS, Eaton RP. Pathogenesis of diabetic ketoacidosis: a reappraisal. Diabetes Care 1979;2:269–306.

13. Alberti KGMM, Hockaday TDR. Diabetic coma: a reappraisal after 5 years. Clin Endocrinol Metab 1977; 6:421–455.

14. McGillivray MH, Brock E, Voorhess ML. Acute diabetic ketoacidosis in children: role of the stress hormones. Pediatr Res 1981;15:99–106.

15. Parker ML, Pildes RS, Chao KL, Cornblath M, Kipnis DM. Juvenile diabetes mellitus: a deficiency of insulin. Diabetes 1968;17:27–32.

16. Levine R, Goldstein MS. On the mechanism of action of insulin. Recent Prog Horm Res 1955;11:343–380.

17. Gerich JE, Lorenzi M, Bier DM et al. Effects of physiological levels of glucagon and growth hormone on human carbohydrate and lipid metabolism. J Clin Invest 1976;57:875–884.

18. Schade DS, Eaton RP, Alberti KGMM, Johnston DG. Regulation of intermediary metabolism in normal man. In: Diabetic Coma. Albuquerque, NM: University of New Mexico Press, 1981:10–19.

19. Unger RH. Glucagon physiology and pathophysiology. N Engl J Med 1971;285:443–448.

20. Bearn AG, Billing BH, Sherlock S. The response of the liver to insulin in normal subjects and in diabetes mellitus. Hepatic vein catheterization studies. Clin Sci 1952;11:151–165.

21. Owen OE, Block BSP, Patel M, Boden G, McDonough M, Kreulen T, Shuman CR, Richard GA Jr. Human splanchnic metabolism during diabetic ketoacidosis. Metabolism 1977; 26:381–398.

22. Forbath N, Hetenyi G Jr. Glucose dynamics in normal subjects and diabetic patients before and after a glucose load. Diabetes 1966;15:778–789.

23. Clements RS Jr, Vourganti B. Fatal diabetic ketoacidosis: major causes and approaches to their prevention. Diabetes Care 1978;1:314–325.

24. McGarry JD, Foster DW. Hormonal control in ketogenesis. Arch Intern Med 1977;137:495–501.

25. McGarry JD, Foster DW. Regulation of hepatic fatty acid oxidation and ketone body production. Annu Rev Biochem 1980;49:395–420.

26. Felig P, Marliss E, Ohman JL, Cahill GE. Plasma aminoacid levels in diabetic ketoacidosis. Diabetes 1970;19:727–729.

27. Blackshear PJ, Alberti KGMM. Sequential aminoacid measurements during experimental diabetic ketoacidosis. Am J Physiol 1975;228:205–211.

28. Stephens JM, Sulway MJ, Watkins PJ. Relationship of blood acetoacetate and 3-hydroxybutyrate in diabetes. Diabetes 1971;20:485–489.

29. Balasse EO, Havel RJ. Evidence for an effect of insulin on the peripheral utilization of ketone bodies in dogs. J Clin Invest 1971;40:801–803.

30. Miles JM, Rizza RA, Haymond MW, Gerich JE. Effects of acute insulin deficiency on glucose and ketone body turnover in man: evidence for the primacy of overproduction of glucose and ketone bodies in the genesis of diabetic ketoacidosis. Diabetes 1980;29:926–930.

31. Adrogue HJ, Wilson H, Boyd AE III, Suki WN, Eknoyan G. Plasma acid–base patterns in diabetic ketoacidosis. N Engl J Med 1982;307:1603–1610.

32. Hockaday TDR, Albert KGMM. Diabetic coma. Clin Endocrinol Metab 1972;1:751–788.

33. Oh MS, Banerji MA, Carrol HJ. The mechanism of hyperchloremic acidosis during the recovery phase of diabetic ketoacidosis. Diabetes 1981;30:310–313.

34. DeFronzo R, Cooke CR, Andres R, Faloona GR, Davis PJ. The effect of insulin on the renal handling of sodium, potassium, calcium, and phosphate in man. J Clin Invest 1975;55:845–855.

35. Saudek CD, Boulier PR, Arky RA. The natriuretic effect of glucagon and its role in starvation. J Clin Endocrinol Metab 1975;36:761–765.

36. Tsalikian E, Becker DJ, Crumrine PK, et al. Electroencephalographic changes in diabetic ketoacidosis in children. J Pediatr 1981;99:355–359.

37. Escobar O, Lifshitz F, Mimouni F. Dynamics of ionized magnesium and ionized calcium during recovery from diabetic ketoacidosis managed with conventional treatment. Magnes Res 1998;11(2)111–115.

38. Knight AH, Williams DN, Ellis G, Goldberg DM. Significance of hyperamylasemia and abdominal pain in diabetic ketoacidosis. Br J Med 1973;3:128–131.

39. Rosenbloom AL, Malone J. Recognition of impending ketoacidosis by ketone reagent strip failure. JAMA 1978;240:2462–2464.

40. Duck SC, Wyatt DT. Factors associated with brain herniation in the treatment of diabetic ketoacidosis. J Pediatr 1988;113(1 Pt 1):10–14.

41. Duck SC, Kohler E. Cerebral edema in diabetic ketoacidosis. J Pediatr 1981;98(4):674–676.

42. Rosenbloom AL. Intracerebral crises during treatment of diabetic ketoacidosis. Diabetes Care 1990;13(1):22–33.

43. Rosenbloom AL, Riley WJ, Weber FT, Malone JI, Donnelly WH. Cerebral edema complicating diabetic ketoacidosis in childhood. J Pediatr 1980;96(3 Pt 1):357–361.

44. Arky RA, Hurwitz D. Management of emergencies: VII. The therapy of diabetic ketoaciodosis. N Engl J Med 1966; 274:1135–1137.

45. Alberti KGMM, Nattrass M. Severe diabetic ketoacidosis. Med Clin North Am 1978;62:799–814.

46. Drop SLS, Duval-Arnaud BJM, Gober AE, et al. Low-dose intravenous insulin infusion versus subcutaneous insulin injection: a controlled comparative study of diabetic ketoacidosis. Pediatrics 1977;59:733–738.

47. Schade DS, Eaton RP, Alberti KGMM, Johnston DG. Insulin dosage. In: Diabetic Coma. Albuquerque, NM: University of New Mexico Press, 1981:144–160.

48. Drash AL. The treatment of diabetic ketoacidosis. J Pediatr 1977;91:858–860.

49. Fort P, Waters SM, Lifshitz F. Low-dose insulin infusion in the treatment of diabetic ketoacidosis: bolus versus nonbolus. J Pediatr 1980;96:36–40.

50. Page M, Alberti KGMM, Greenwood R. Treatment of diabetic coma with continuous low-dose infusion of insulin. Br Med J 1974;2:687–690.

51. Clumeck N, DeTroyer A, Naeije R. Treatment of diabetic coma with small intravenous boluses. Br Med J 1976;11:394–396.

52. Moseley J. Diabetic crises in children treated with small doses of intramuscular insulin. Br Med J 1975;1:59–61.

53. Martin HE, Smith K, Wilson MI. The fluid and electrolyte therapy of severe diabetic acidosis and ketosis. Am J Med 1958;24:376–389.

54. Zipf WB, Bacon GF, Spencer ML, et al. Hypocalcemia, hypomagnesemia, and transient hypoparathyroidism during therapy with potassium phosphate in diabetic ketoacidosis. Diabetes Care 1979;2:265–268.

55. Schade DS, Eaton RP, Alberti KGMM, Johnston DG. Bicarbonate administration. In: Diabetic Coma. Albuquerque, NM: University of New Mexico Press, 1981:171–183.

56. Posner JB, Plum F. Spinal fluid pH and neurologic symptoms in systemic acidosis. N Engl J Med 1967;277:605–613.

57. Okuda Y, Adrogue HJ, Field JB, Nohara H, Yamashita K. Counterproductive effects of sodium bicarbonate in diabetic ketoacidosis. J Clin Endocrinol Metab 1996;81:314–320.

58. Assal JP, Aoko TT, Manzano FM, Kozak GP. Metabolic effects of sodium bicarbonate in the management of diabetic ketoacidosis. Diabetes 1974;23:405–411.

59. Bureau MA, Begin R, Berthiaume Y, et al. Cerebral anoxia from bicarbonate infusion in diabetic acidosis. J Pediatr 1980;96:968–973.

60. Glaser N, Barnett P, McCaslin I, Nelson D, Trainor J, Louie J, Kaufman F, Quayle K, Roback M, Malley R, Kuppermann N. The Pediatric Emergency Medicine Collaborative Research Committee of the American Academy of Pediatrics. N Engl J Med 344:264–69, 2001.

61. Edge JA, Hawkins MM, Winter DL, Dunger DB. The risk and outcome of cerebral oedema developing during diabetic ketoacidosis. Arch Dis Child 2001;85(1):16–22.

62. Arieff AL, Kleeman CR. Cerebral edema in diabetic comas. 2. Effects of hyperosmolality, hyperglycemia and insulin in diabetic rabbits. Clin Endocrinol Metab 1974;38:1057–1067.

63. Kitabchi AE. Treatment of diabetic ketoacidosis with low-dose insulin. Adv Intern Med 1978;23:115–135.

64. Rosenbloom AJ, Schatz DA, Krischer JP, Skyler JS, Becker DJ, Laporte RE, Libman I, Pietropaolo M, Dosch HM, Finberg L, Muir A, Tamborlane WV, Grey M, Silverstein JH, Malone JI. Therapeutic controversy: prevention and treatment of diabetes in children. J Clin Endocrinol Metab 2000;85(2):494–522.

65. Duck SC, Weldon VV, Pagliara AS, Haymond MW. Cerebral edema complicating therapy for diabetic ketoacidosis. Diabetes 1976;25:111–115.

66. Hale PM, Rezvani I, Braunstein AW, Lipman TH, Martinez N, Garibaldi L. Factors predicting cerebral edema in young children with diabetic ketoacidosis and new onset type 1 diabetes. Acta Paediatr 1997;86:626–31.

67. Clements RR, Blumenthal SA, Morrison AD, Winegrad AI. Increased cerebrospinal fluid pressure during treatment of diabetic ketosis. Lancet 1971;2:671–678.

68. Arieff AL, Kleeman CR. Studies on mechanisms of cerebral edema in diabetic comas: effects of hyperglycemia and rapid lowering of plasma glucose in normal rabbits. J Clin Invest 1973;52:571–583.

69. Van der Meuten JA, Klip A, Grinstein S. Possible mechanism for cerebral edema in diabetic ketoacidosis. Lancet 1987;2:306–308.

28
Autoimmune Endocrinopathies

William E. Winter
University of Florida College of Medicine, Gainesville, Florida, U.S.A.

I. AUTOIMMUNITY AND AUTOIMMUNE DISEASES

A. Role of the Immune System

Cells of the immune system, including macrophages, T lymphocytes (e.g., T cells), and B lymphocytes (e.g., B cells), must recognize one another as well as somatic cells of the body to achieve proper intercellular communication (1) (Fig. 1). This recognition is afforded by polymorphic cell surface molecules encoded by genes within the major histocompatibility complex (MHC), as well as by various adhesion and other cell-cell recognition molecules (2). The human MHC, which is termed the human leukocyte antigen (HLA) complex, is located on the short arm of chromosome 6. By differentiating self from nonself (a process sustained by thymic T-lymphocyte education, B-lymphocyte education, and peripheral T-cell tolerance), the immune system is able to recognize and react to foreign antigens, providing protection from microbiological invasion and certain cancers that express "new" antigens.

The immune system must survey or monitor two major spaces of the body: the cytoplasmic space and the extracellular/intravesicular space. Class I MHC molecules (HLA-A, B, and C in humans) monitor the cytoplasm of nucleated cells whereas the extracellular/intravesicular space is surveyed by class II MHC molecules (HLA-DR, DQ, and DP in humans). The intravesicular space is the space that exists within cellular vesicles formed during pinocytosis and phagocytosis of extracellular materials.

B. Communication Between Cells via MHC Molecules: Class I MHC Molecules

Class I MHC heavy chains are each encoded by single loci within the HLA complex. At the cell surface, each HLA-encoded chain is coexpressed with beta-2-micro-

globulin as the class I MHC molecule. The molecules present cytoplasmic peptides, both self and nonself, to CD8 T cells (e.g., lymphocytes). Class I MHC molecules are found on the surfaces of all nucleated cells. If an activated CD8 T cell recognizes a peptide, usually viral in origin, presented by a class I MHC molecule, that CD8 T cell will function as a cytolytic-T lymphocyte (CTL or Tk [killer] cell) and will induce apoptosis in the cell presenting the peptide that was recognized (Fig. 2). Differences in MHC molecules between donor and recipient play a major role in foreign tissue rejection serving as the classically described transplantation antigens.

Apoptosis is programed cell death. In apoptosis, the apoptotic cell essentially involutes, breaks into fragments contained within plasma membrane, and undergoes an "intracellular" necrosis where intracellular materials are not released to the extracellular space until the cell has fully autodigested. In response to viral infection, apoptosis does not release viable virions: as the cell autodigests, the intracellular virus is also digested, protecting adjacent cells from exposure to potentially infectious virus. Cytolytic-T lymphocytes (e.g., T killer cells) represent the "effector" stage of activated CD8 positive T lymphocytes. T cells, both CD4 and CD8, predominantly use alpha/beta T-cell receptors to recognize MHC-presented peptides (3). Gamma/delta-bearing T cells represent about 5% of circulating T cells and are in high concentration along mucosal surfaces such as in the Peyer's patches in the gut. The role of such gamma/delta T cells is still poorly understood.

Upon recognizing a "target" cell, the CD8-positive Tk cell juxtaposes its cell membrane against the target cell and inflicts cell membrane damage by the release of perforin, a C9-like protein that forms pores in the target cell membrane. In the target cell, plasma membrane holes are produced by perforin, and granzymes enter the target cell cytoplasm through these holes to induce apoptosis. Apoptosis can also be induced in the target cell via membrane

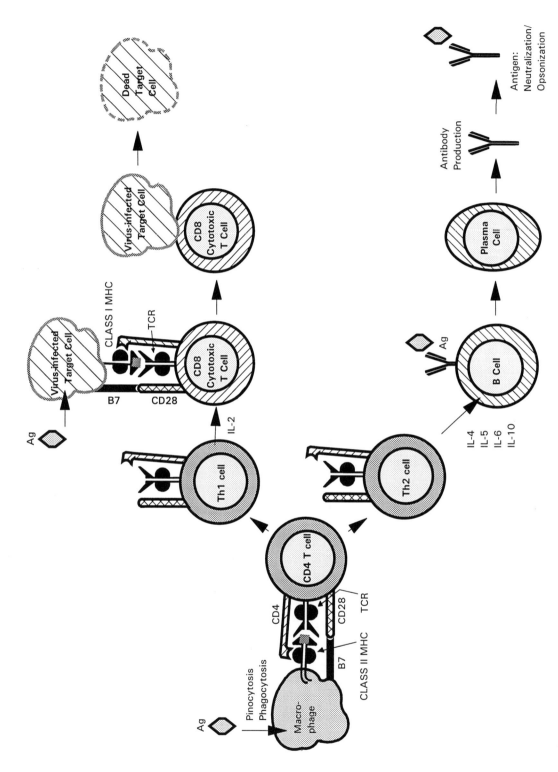

Figure 1 Initial contact of CD4 T cells with antigen peptide plus microenvironmental influences stimulation and differentiation of the Th0 CD4 T cell into a Th1 cell or a Th2 cell CD4 T cell (e.g., IFN-γ from natural killer cells and IL-12 from dendritic cells push CD4 T cells towards a Th1 phenotype, IL-4 from CD4 T NK1.1+ cells pushes CD4 T cells towards a Th2 phenotype).

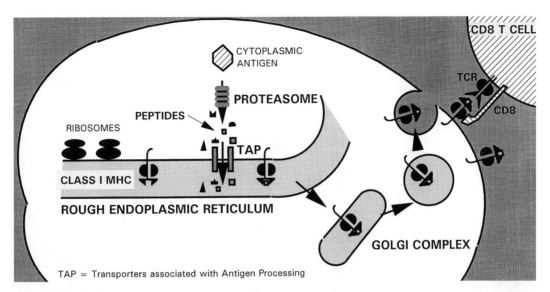

TAP = Transporters associated with Antigen Processing

Figure 2 Cytoplasmic antigens, either endogenous or exogenous (e.g., viral infection), are processed by proteasomes to peptides. These peptides are transported into the lumen of the rough endoplasmic reticulum (RER) by transporters associated with antigen processing (TAP). Once the class I MHC molecule is loaded with peptide, a transport vesicle buds from the RER. This vesicle passes through the Golgi complex to fuse eventually with the plasma membrane, where the class I MHC molecules and peptides are oriented to the outside of the cell. In this way, class I MHC molecules display cytoplasmic contents (e.g., peptides) to CD8 T cells. MHC, major histocompatibility complex; TCR, T-cell receptor.

contact between the CD8-Tk-cell-expressed cell-surface molecule FAS ligand and FAS on the target cell surface.

C. Communication Between Cells via MHC Molecules: Class II MHC Molecules

Class II MHC molecules present extracellular peptides to CD4-positive T-helper cells to initiate immune responses that culminate in humoral and/or cell-mediated responses designed to remove the invader from the body (Fig. 3). These heterodimeric molecules (HLA-DR, DP, and DQ in humans) are restricted in their distributions to specialized antigen-presenting cells (APCs): monocyte-derived cells, B lymphocytes, and dendritic cells found in lymph nodes. Monocyte derived-cells include tissue macrophages, Kupffer's cells that line the liver sinusoids, alveolar macrophages, central nervous system microglia, and glomerular mesangial cells. Via class II MHC molecules, such APCs present (e.g., display) extracellular-derived peptides to the alpha/beta T-cell receptors of CD4 T cells. Almost all infectious agents in some stage of their life cycle pass through the extracellular space of the cell and thus these agents (or their toxic products) can be presented to CD4 T cells.

Initial MHC typing (e.g., allele identification and classification) in animals was discovered and accomplished by tissue transplantation. This lead to the naming of these molecules as histocompatibility antigens. Serological typing of class I and class II MHC molecules followed. In the 1990s DNA-sequence-based allele typing

became a reality using a variety of molecular techniques including allele-specific polymerase chain reactions (PCR), allele-specific oligonucleotide probes, and direct sequencing of PCR-amplified gene segments. Based on classic cellular immunology, the in vitro mixed lymphocyte reaction results primarily from differences in class II MHC molecules.

As a population, humans express a large number of different class I and class II MHC alleles. This ensures that the population as a whole should be able to present peptides from any potential pathogen to T cells and thus react to that pathogen in a protective manner. In a single individual, up to six different class I MHC molecules can be expressed when the individual is heterozygous at each of the HLA-A, HLA-B, and HLA-C loci. Because some class II MHC alpha and beta DP and DQ chains from the maternal and paternal chromosomes can pair (e.g., transcomplementation), theoretically a single individual can express up to 12 different class II MHC molecules. Molecular cloning of the HLA genes and sequence analysis has revealed a tremendous degree of MHC genomic polymorphism in the human population. A recent count of the various MHC alleles is presented in Table 1.

D. Coordination of the Acquired Immune Response: CD4 Th1 and Th2 Cells

The CD4 T cells orchestrate (e.g., direct) the immune response. CD4 T-cell function can be described in two polarized functional modes: Th1 cells and Th2 cells. The

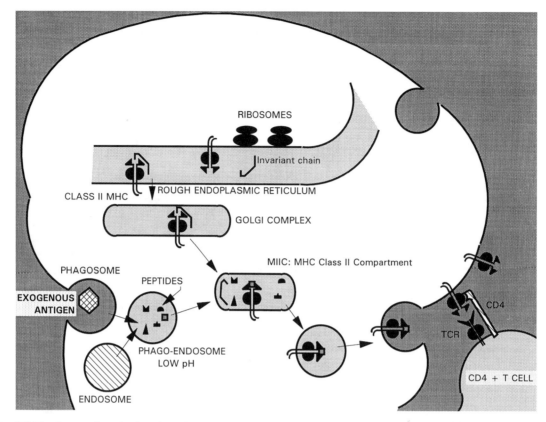

Figure 3 Within the rough endoplasmic reticulum (RER), class II MHC molecules bind the invariant chain that protects the class II MHC molecule from inadvertent loading by cytoplasmic peptides. A transport vesicle containing the class II MHC-invariant chain complex buds from the RER and passes through the Golgi complex. Extracellular antigens are taken up by specific antigen-presenting cells via phagocytosis or pinocytosis. The resulting phagosome then fuses with an endosome. Within the phagoendosome, antigen is degraded and peptides result. Fusion of the phagoendosome with the class II MHC transport vesicle forms the MHC class II compartment (MIIC). The low pH of the phagoendosome degrades the invariant chain, allowing peptide loading into the class II MHC molecule. Fusion of the MIIC with the plasma membrane allows the class II MHC molecules to be placed on the plasma membrane displaying peptides to CD4 T cells.

Table 1 Number of MHC Alleles per locus

MHC Alleles	No.
Class I MHC molecules	
HLA-A	95
HLA-B	20
HLA-C	50
Class II MHC chains	
DPβ	80
DPα	12
DQβ	35
DQα	20
DRβ	239
DRα	1

Th1 cells are responsible for stimulating cell-mediated immunity including activation of CD8 T cells, macrophages, and natural killer (NK) cells (4). Th1 and Th2 cells can both play a role in activating B cells, thereby stimulating humoral (antibody-mediated) immunity. Extracellular invaders such as bacteria and viruses are opsonized by antibody and complement and are then phagocytosed by granulocytes or macrophages to clear these pathogens. Fungi are phagocytosed and destroyed by Th1-activated macrophages. If the pathogen has reached the cell's cytoplasm, the CD8 T cell will activate apoptosis in that host cell to destroy the pathogen and its site of reproduction.

The primary difference between Th1 and Th2 cells is in the cytokines that they secrete: Th1 cells release interleukin-2 (IL-2, T-cell growth factor), gamma interferon (IFN-γ) and IL-12, whereas Th2 cells release IL-4, IL-5, IL-6, and IL-10. Each subset secretes cytokines that also regulate the other subset: IFN-γ from Th1 cells suppresses

Th2 cells and IL-10 and transforming growth factor beta (TGF-β) (5) from Th2 cells suppress Th1 cells. A third subset of CD4 T cells has also been described that is present in mucosa activated by mucosal antigen presentation. These so-called Th3 cells secrete the immunosuppressive cytokine TGF-β as do Th2 cells.

E. Autoimmunity and Central Tolerance: T Cells

Autoimmunity is a disorder of self–nonself recognition whereby self is recognized aberrantly as nonself and an autoreactive process occurs. If sufficient damage is incurred in the target tissues, circulating proteins, or cells, a clinically recognizable autoimmune disease results. Pathological autoreactivity could result in pathogenic autoantibodies and/or an antiself cell-mediated immune responses that would serve as the effectors of the autoimmune process. Autoreactivity to self-antigens that could induce autoimmune diseases is normally restricted by the phenomenon of immunological tolerance.

Tolerance is the active process by which the immune system does not normally develop an effector response to self-antigens (6). T-cell tolerance is acquired by the time of birth and is necessary to ensure that the body does not mount an immune response to self. Central T-cell tolerance results from self–nonself discrimination that occurs in the thymus during T-cell development (7). In the thymus, T cells must express CD4, CD8, and a TCR during T-cell thymic ontogeny. Developing T cells, called thymocytes, must be able to recognize self-MHC to avoid apoptosis; however, excessive adherence to self-MHC (which might trigger autoimmunity) also leads to apoptosis. This destruction of antiself T cells in the thymus results in so-called clonal deletion.

In the process of clonal deletion, T cells that have been rescued by their initial interaction with self-MHC will be induced to undergo apoptosis at the thymic corticomedullary junction if their TCR interaction with MHC is excessively strong. Ultimately in the thymus, CD8 T cells survive because of their modest ability to perceive class I MHC molecules; CD4 T cells survive because of their modest ability to perceive class II MHC molecules.

Normally T-cell thymic ontogeny results in T cells exiting the thymus that recognize self-MHC molecules and, presumably, foreign peptides. However, these T cells do not strongly recognize self-peptides. The ability of T cells to recognize MHC is critical to the antigen–peptide-presenting role of MHC molecules. There would be no purpose for TCRs to interact, for example, with self-surface molecules that do not present peptides. The ability of TCRs to perceive peptides presented by one's own MHC molecules is termed MHC restriction. The TCR recognizes the presented peptide plus a portion of the MHC molecule.

F. Autoimmunity and Central Tolerance: B Cells

Tolerance towards self antigens is primarily a function of T cells. However developing B cells can undergo tolerization: IgM-positive, IgD-negative immature, naive B cells upon exposure to antigen will either be anergized or induced to undergo apoptosis. When a B cell is tolerized but does not die, the B cell is said to be anergized. If the tolerized B cell is induced to undergo programed cell death, the B cell undergoes apoptosis. Anergy results when few antigenic epitopes interact with the B-cell receptors. On the other hand, apoptosis is triggered when multiple antigenic epitopes interact with the B-cell receptors, providing a more powerful tolerization signal. B-cell tolerance is a continuing process because B cells are produced by the bone marrow throughout an individual's life.

G. Autoimmunity and Peripheral Tolerance: T Cells

Peripheral tolerance (or anergy) has evolved, presumably, because not all antigens necessarily enter the thymus during T-cell ontogeny (8) (Fig. 4). Initial T-cell activation, regardless of whether the cell is a CD4 or CD8 T cell, requires two signals. One signal is antigen–peptide-specific via MHC-TCR whereas the second signal is antigen-nonspecific (e.g., CD28 of the T cell interacting with B7 on the cell expressing the MHC molecule). Peripheral tolerance results when the antigen-specific signal is present (e.g., self-MHC do present self-peptides) but the second activation signal is absent. In fact, once exposed to antigen peptide in the absence of the second signal, the T cell can not respond in the future and is thus essentially permanently anergized. This aspect of peripheral tolerance produces so-called clonal anergy. Defects in T-cell signaling are hypothesized to play a role in loss of tolerance in type 1 diabetes (9).

H. Autoimmunity and Peripheral Tolerance: B Cells

Peripheral tolerance in terms of B cells occurs via T-cell tolerance. Like T cells, B cells require two sets of signals to become activated. One set of signals comes from the interaction of the B-cell receptor (surface antibody) and the antigen, and the second set of signals comes from helper CD4 T cells of either the Th1 or Th2 subclasses. If the antigen is bound by B-cell surface antibody but there is no T-cell help, the B cell will not be activated, will not proliferate, will not class switch, and will not undergo affinity maturation. Therefore naive mature B cells without T-cell help (because the T cells are tolerant) should not produce large amounts of high-affinity IgG autoantibodies.

THYMUS   PERIPHERY

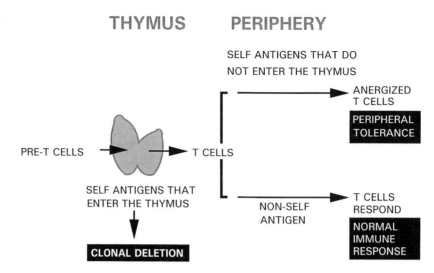

Figure 4 In the thymus, exposure of developing T cells to antigen peptides produces clonal deletion of such potentially autoreactive T cells. This process can be described as central thymic tolerance. T cells that leave the thymus and subsequently encounter novel self-antigen not previously seen in the thymus can be anergized producing peripheral tolerance. The remaining T cells are then available to respond to nonself antigens, elaborating a protective immune response.

I. Autoimmunity and Loss of Tolerance

When a breakdown in tolerance occurs, the immune system recognizes self as foreign and mounts a humoral and/or cell-mediated immune response that can result in an autoimmune disease (10). Only one autoimmune disease has been shown to be monogenic (autoimmune polyglandular syndrome type 1) (11), while all other autoimmune diseases are polygenic (12). Loss of tolerance can occur by many theoretical routes. However, loss of peripheral tolerance is thought to be the most reasonable explanation based upon the highly selective nature of organ-specific autoimmune responses and diseases. As an alternative, tolerance may have never been initially developed (13). Loss of peripheral tolerance most likely results from molecular mimicry (14). Molecular mimicry occurs, theoretically, when an immune response to a foreign antigen cross reacts with a self antigen leading to clinical disease. Molecular mimicry is likely in the prototypic autoimmune disease rheumatic fever. Examples of molecular mimicry include similarities in the antigenic structure of group A, β-hemolytic *Streptococcus*, and antigens found in the heart (producing carditis), joints (resulting in arthritis), and basal ganglia (eliciting chorea). For example, cardiac myosin shares certain antigenic epitopes with streptococcal M protein. Similarities between HLA antigens and bacterial antigens have been described in reactive arthritides associated with intestinal infection (e.g, *Proteus*). For example *Klebsiella* nitrogenase and HLA-B2 are cross-reactive and implicated in the pathogenesis of ankylosing spondylitis and Reiter's syndrome (arthritis, conjunctivitis, and urethritis). Further cross-reactivities are described among collagen antigens and mycobacteria.

Mycobacterial proteoglycan wall component and cartilage protein cross-reactivity has been described in rheumatoid arthritis. Other theories of how tolerance fails or is broken include failure of thymic clonal deletion (15), failure of peripheral tolerance, sequestered antigen theory, altered self-antigen (16), aberrant class II MHC expression, superantigen theory of autoimmunity, and polyclonal B-cell stimulation.

The factors that lead to a disruption in self-tolerance, resulting in autoimmunities, have not been fully identified (17). To a large degree, this phenomenon is genetically programmed, since autoimmune diseases are frequently associated with specific immune response gene alleles (e.g., specific HLA types). For example, ankylosing spondylitis is increased in frequency in men who especially carry the HLA-B27 allele. Systemic lupus erythematosus (SLE) is more common in HLA-DR2 positive individuals. Environmental influences, including viral infections and diet, are also often implicated in the triggering of autoimmune processes. As noted previously, molecular mimicry between an environmental antigen and an endogenous antigen could lead to autoimmunity. Amino acid sequence homologies have been described between Coxsackievirus and the beta-cell autoantigen, glutamic acid decarboxylase (GAD). Whereas eradication of virally infected cells by T-cell lysis provides an important defense against viral illnesses, this mechanism may expand beyond its immunological defense function and lead to an autoimmune disorder. Th1 cells may play a crucial role in the process (18).

With refinements in laboratory technique, intracellular antigens (i.e., thyroglobulin) can now be found in the circulation of normal subjects. This discovery discredits much of the so-called sequestered antigen theory of autoimmune disease for at least several endocrinopathies. It is of great interest that many autoantigens are enzymes whose distribution is often limited to specific tissues (19,20). During the aging process, there is a progressive breakdown in self-tolerance and an increased appearance of autoimmune phenomena with self-reactive autoantibodies. However, clinically apparent autoimmune disease may not be obvious in older persons because of the decreased efficiency of the immune system with advancing age, and the limited duration of an autoimmune process that begins in an elderly person. Thus with aging a higher prevalence of various autoantibodies will be recorded; however, fewer of those individuals harboring such autoantibodies will actually express disease. In contrast in younger individuals, autoantibodies will be of lower prevalence yet more of the individuals expressing those autoantibodies will be affected with clinically apparent disease.

II. CLASSIFICATION AND RECOGNITION OF AUTOIMMUNE DISEASES

Autoimmune diseases can be classified as organ-specific (e.g., autoimmune endocrinopathies) (21–23; Table 2) or non-organ-specific or systemic (e.g., collagen vascular diseases) (Table 3). Autoimmune diseases in which an antibody is made to a circulating hormone (e.g., insulin autoantibodies: autoimmune hypoglycemia), thyroid hormone autoantibodies (24), thyroid-stimulating hormone (TSH) autoantibodies (25), adrenocorticotropin (ACTH) autoantibodies (26), and testosterone autoantibodies (27) form a subgroup of the organ-specific autoimmunities.

Four types of findings support an autoimmune cause for a disease: Evidence of humoral (antibody/B cell) and/or cell-mediated (T-cell) autoreactivity; ability to transfer disease with either serum or lymphocytes (this is usually performed in animal models of autoimmune disease); disease recurrence in transplanted tissue in the absence of

Table 2 Organ-Specific Autoimmune Disorders

Antireceptor diseases
  Atopic diseases involving B$_2$-adrenergic receptors
  Atrophic thyroiditis
  Graves' disease
  Insulin-resistant diabetes/acanthosis nigricans syndrome
  Hypoglycemia–insulinomimetic autoantibodies
  Myasthenia gravis
Autoimmune endocrinopathies
  Addison's disease
  Autoimmune diabetes insipidus
  Autoimmune hypoparathyroidism
  Autoimmune polyglandular syndrome type 1
  Autoimmune polyglandular syndrome type 2
  Autoimmune primary gonadal failure
  Hashimoto's thyroiditis
  Hypophysitis
  Pancreatic alpha-cell autoimmunity
  Pancreatic delta-cell autoimmunity
  Type 1 diabetes mellitus
Anti-circulating-protein disorders
  Anti-ACTH autoantibodies
  Anti-TSH autoantibodies
  Insulin autoantibodies–hypoglycemia
  Thyroid hormone autoantibodies
Autoimmune cytopenias
  Immune hemolytic anemia
  Immune leukopenia
  Immune thrombocytopenic purpura
Gastrointestinal autoimmunities
  Celiac disease
  Chronic lymphocytic gastritis/pernicious anemia
  Crohn disease
  Ulcerative colitis

Hepatobiliary autoimmunities
  Chronic active hepatitis
  Cryptogenic cirrhosis
  Primary biliary cirrhosis
  Sclerosing cholangitis
Dermatological autoimmunity
  Autoimmune alopecia totalis or areata
  Autoimmune vitiligo
  Bullus pemphigoid (bullus, gestationis, and cicatricial)
  Chronic bullous disease of childhood
  Dermatitis herpetiformis
  Epidermolysis bullosa acquisita
  Erythema nodosa
  Linear IgA disease
  Pemphigus (vulgaris, foliaceous, and paraneoplastic)
Neuromuscular
  Acute disseminated encephalomyelitis
  Chronic inflammatory demyelinating polyradiculoneuropathy
  Chronic neuropathy with monoclonal gammopathy
  Eaton-Lambert syndrome
  Guillain-Barré syndrome
  Multifocal motor neuropathy with conduction block
  Multiple sclerosis
  Myasthenia gravis
  Polymyositis
  Stiff-man syndrome
Paraneoplastic syndrome
  Cerebellar degeneration
  Encephalomyelitis
  Opsoclonus–myoclonus syndrome
  Retinopathy
Basement-membrane autoimmunity
  Goodpasture syndrome

Table 3 Non-Organ-Specific Autoimmune Disorders

Connective tissue diseases
    Ankylosing spondylitis
    Behçet syndrome
    Dermatomyositis
    Mixed connective tissue disease
    Progressive systemic sclerosis (scleroderma)
    Psoriasis
    Reactive arthritides
    Reiter syndrome
    Rheumatic fever
    Rheumatoid arthritis
    Sjögren (sicca) syndrome
    Systemic lupus erythematous
Vasculopathies
    Hypersensitivity vasculitis
    Kawasaki disease
    Polyarteritis nodosa
    Takayasu arteritis
    Temporal arteritis
    Thromboangiitis obliterans
    Wegener's granulomatosis
Sarcoidosis
Graft-vs.-host disease

Table 4 Identification of Autoantibodies

Methods
Cytoplasmic autoantibodies
    Indirect immunofluorescence, Ig and complement-fixing Ig, using unfixed human tissue sections as substrates.
    Immunohistochemical methods.
    Immunoprecipitation: sera or Ig against cell extracts.
    Hemagglutination of tissue antigen-coated red blood cells.
    Other methods: radioimmunoassay, complement-fixation assays, ELISA.
Cell-surface autoantibody determinations
    (using isolated xenogeneic or allogeneic target cells) by indirect immunofluorescence; binding of [^{125}I] protein A, antigen precipitation by serum from an affected individual; or as measured by flow cytometry with a fluorescein-labeled second antibody.
Determination of autoantibody effects
Cell metabolism/products
    Measurement of changes in cell metabolism (i.e., cAMP production) or cell products (hormones) after exposure to sera, or purified or partially purified Ig serum fractions. Target cells are isolated from tissue, tissue culture, or tissue slices.
Cytolysis
    Measurement of cytolysis by ^{51}Cr release or supravital staining after the addition of sera, or purified or partially purified Ig serum fractions.
Transplacental passage
    Study of the clinical effects of autoantibodies transplacentally passed from mother to fetus or neonate.
Passage to animals
    Purification of Ig (Protein A or NH$_4$ [SO$_4$]$_2$) and passage to animals.

immunosuppression; and ability to prevent or cure disease with immunotherapy through either immunosuppression or induction of tolerance (28).

Autoantibodies, which are the hallmark of B-cell autoimmunity, can be identified by several methods (Table 4). Their participation in an autoimmune disorder can be assessed by complement fixation and lysis of target cells in tissue culture or by promoting cytolysis of target cells by NK cells or macrophages in the process of antibody-dependent cell cytolysis. In other diseases, autoantibodies may bind to membrane receptors stimulating target cells, as in Graves' disease or insulinomimetic hypoglycemia; or interfere with receptor functions, as occurs in myasthenia gravis or Eaton-Lambert syndrome. In myasthenia gravis the target autoantigen is the acetylcholine receptor. On the other hand, in Eaton-Lambert syndrome the autoantigen is the presynaptic voltage-gated calcium channel. Autoantibodies to ganglionic acetylcholine receptors in autoimmune autonomic neuropathies have been described (29).

The finding of lymphocytic infiltration of a target organ or tissue is histopathological evidence of cell-mediated autoimmunity. Cell-mediated autoreactivity can also be shown in vivo by positive delayed-type hypersensitivity reactions during skin testing with specific syngeneic, allogenic, or xenogeneic self antigens. Cell-mediated autoimmunity can be assessed in vitro by the production of cytokines such as IL-1, IL-2, tumor necrosis factor, or interferon production, or by proliferation of T cells mea-

sured by [^{3}H]thymidine incorporation. T-cell cytolysis of target cells in tissue culture can be measured by ^{51}Cr release or supravital staining of damaged cells. Healthy cells retain ^{51}Cr once labeled for a specific length of time and exclude supravital stains.

Cytokines and reactive oxygen intermediates (O$_2^-$) are also incriminated as mediators or final effectors of autoimmune cell damage (30). IL-1 is often implicated along with IFN-γ and tumor necrosis factor in damaging beta cells. In the case of type 1 diabetes mellitus, in tissue culture IL-1 is toxic to isolated islets. At low dosages, IL-1 inhibits glucose-stimulated insulin release, while at higher dosages IL-1 is directly toxic and leads to islet cell death. Certain lymphokines (i.e. IFN-γ) may induce high levels of class I MHC expression as well as low levels of class II MHC expression that may propagate autoimmune responses once initiated.

Several other lines of evidence can support an autoimmune cause for a particular disease: clinical association with known autoimmune diseases; disease association with particular HLA alleles; the ability to induce a similar disease in animals after injection of self antigens (often in Freund's adjuvant to exaggerate the response); increased disease frequency in females compared with males; and increased disease frequency with advancing age. A wide variety of autoimmune mechanisms have been proposed as outlined in Table 5.

This chapter will discuss endocrinopathies believed to have an autoimmune cause with particular reference to genetics and HLA relationships; classify endocrinopathies into autoimmune polyglandular syndromes and describe their relationship to other nonendocrine autoimmune diseases; discuss available diagnostic tests (31); and elaborate a clinical approach to the endocrinopathies.

III. AUTOIMMUNITY TO THE PANCREATIC ISLETS, INSULIN RECEPTORS, AND INSULIN

A. Type 1 Diabetes Mellitus

1. Classification

In 1997, the American Diabetes Association (ADA) (32) reclassified diabetes mellitus according to cause. Thus the term type 1 diabetes mellitus replaced the term insulin-dependent diabetes mellitus. Type 1 diabetes is insulinopenic diabetes that results from autoimmune beta-cell destruction (type 1A diabetes) or whose cause is unknown (type 1B diabetes). Likewise noninsulin-dependent dia-

Table 5 Suggested Pathogenic Mechanisms of Autoimmune Endocrinopathies

Autoantibody hormone-receptor binding
  Blocking of receptor-hormone activation (e.g., atrophic thyroiditis)
  Stimulation by autoantibodies with receptor activation (e.g., Graves' disease)
Autoantibody-induced target cell destruction/dysfunction
  Formation of local immune complexes with subsequent local inflammation
  Complement-dependent cytolysis
  Antibody-dependent cell cytolysis by macrophages, natural killer cells, possible role for subsequent IL-1, TNF mediated cytolysis
Autoantibody binding to a circulating protein with inappropriate levels of circulating free hormone producing excessive or deficient hormone effects (e.g., autoimmune hypoglycemia)
Immune complex formation with distal localization and destruction (e.g., immune complex nephritis secondary to autoimmune thyroid disease)
Cell-mediated (classic CD8+ killing or delayed-type hypersensitivity) target cell destruction by T cells without participation of autoantibodies
Cytokine and/or free radical destruction of target organ
Combinations of the above

betes mellitus (NIDDM) was reclassified as type 2 diabetes that results from insulin resistance in combination with relative insulinopenic beta-cell failure.

Nonautoimmune forms of insulinopenic diabetes for which a cause has been identified are classified as other specific types of diabetes in the 1997 ADA scheme. These disorders include diabetes secondary to transcription factor mutations (hepatocyte nuclear factor [HNF] 4β, HNF-1β, insulin promoter factor-1, and HNF-1α), glucokinase mutations (33), certain types of mitochondrial mutations (34), drugs and poisons (e.g., the rodenticide Vacor [35], drug toxicity [36]), and viral infections (e.g., Coxsackie B4 [37]; rubella [38]).

2. Clinical Impact of Type 1 Diabetes

Type 1 diabetes is a major clinical problem in both children and adults, and approximately 1 in 500 children are affected (39). It can be argued that diabetes is the most significant endocrine disorder affecting developed populations. Before the introduction of rigorous glycemic control as the standard of care as dictated by the Diabetes Control and Complications Trial results (40), expected life span from the time of diagnosis was reduced by one-third. For example, if the normal life expectancy of a 10 year child was to age 70 with 60 more years of life expected, in type 1 diabetes the expected life span would be reduced to age 50. Microvascular complications (retinopathy and nephropathy) are major causes of morbidity and mortality in type 1 diabetes. Premature macrovascular disease (coronary artery, carotid artery, and peripheral vascular disease) and neuropathy are also major contributors to morbidity and mortality (see Chapter 25). The leading causes of premature death in type 1 diabetes are coronary artery disease and renal failure. With better diabetes management, there is hope that these grim statistics can be avoided and revised.

3. Causes

The majority of cases of type 1 diabetes result from a cell-mediated autoimmune process (41) that selectively destroys the pancreatic beta cells. Both CD8 T cells and macrophages are believed to be responsible for beta-cell necrosis. Islet-cell autoimmunity can develop very early in life (42); it has been reported to develop prenatally (43) and is transferable by bone marrow transplantation (44). Roles for Th1 and Th2 cells have been implicated (45).

Multiple lines of evidence support an autoimmune basis for type 1 diabetes. In patients dying within 6 months of diagnosis of type 1 diabetes, 60–~90% have pancreatic insulitis (46). Insulitis is the histological description of lymphocytic infiltration of the pancreatic islets with destruction of the beta cells and a depletion in insulin content. With increasing duration of the disease, there is progressive disappearance of pancreatic beta cells. Non-beta cells (alpha, gamma, and pancreatic polypeptide cells) are not subject to autoimmune targeting or permanent damage. Thus, the beta cell most likely carries antigens unique to insulin-producing cells. Of the major antigens so far discovered that are targeted in type 1 diabetes (e.g., glutamic acid decarboxylase, insulinoma-associated antigen 2, and islet sialoglycoconjugate), only insulin appears to be absolutely beta-cell-specific (47).

4. Natural History of Type 1 Diabetes

The natural history of type 1 diabetes can be addressed in five stages. Stage 1 is defined as genetic susceptibility; stage 2: evidence of humoral and/or cell-mediated autoimmunity without detectable metabolic perturbations; stage 3: declining first-phase insulin response to intravenously administered glucose; stage 4: oral glucose intolerance; stage 5: frank clinical type 1 diabetes (48). Issues of genetic susceptibility will be addressed in the next section. Following a discussion of the genetics, environmental triggers will be examined. Next, islet autoantibodies and immune abnormalities in type 1 diabetes will be analyzed. Finally metabolic progression to type 1 diabetes will be reviewed under the heading of prediction and prevention.

5. Genetics of Type 1 Diabetes

Susceptibility to type 1 diabetes can be inherited, although most cases (~85%) of type 1 diabetes are sporadic. Whereas the general population frequency of type 1 diabetes in the United States is ~1:500 (0.2% of the population affected), siblings of type 1 diabetes patients experience a 25-fold higher risk of type 1 diabetes (e.g., 1: 20 or 5% affected). Likewise offspring of a type 1 diabetes father or mother are also at increased risk: 1:14 (7%; 35-fold increased risk) and 1:50 (2%; 10-fold increased risk), respectively. Ethnic origin greatly influences risk for type 1 diabetes. Finns experience the highest risk in the world (1:100) while Chinese and Japanese have the lowest risk for type 1 diabetes worldwide (1:10,000) (49). Risks for type 1 diabetes in white North Americans and southern Europeans, and African–Americans are intermediate: 1:500 and 1:1000, respectively. Nevertheless, inheritance of susceptibility to type 1 diabetes is not mendelian but instead is multifactorial and polygenic. Clearly no single gene allele is always associated with type 1 diabetes nor are unique DNA sequences observed in subjects with type 1 diabetes (50). The association of specific HLA-loci and type 1 diabetes was first recognized in the 1970s for HLA-B alleles and then, more powerfully, associated with DR alleles in the late 1970s and early 1980s. In the mid to late 1980s the predominant role of HLA-DQB1 and A1 alleles was discovered in providing proclivity to type 1 diabetes.

In studies from the University of Florida involving more than 1000 individuals with type 1 diabetes, ~95% express at least one HLA-DR3 and/or DR4 allele. Compared with a general population frequency of ~3%, ~40% of type 1 diabetes patients are heterozygous for HLA-DR3 and DR4. After DR3/DR4 heterozygotes, DR4 homozygosity is the next highest risk genotype followed by DR3 homozygotes and DR4/DRx heterozygotes (X = nonDR3/DR4 allele). Only 5% of type 1 diabetes patients lack both HLA-DR3 and DR4. In individuals with HLA-DR3 or DR4, the second antigen excluding DR3 and DR4 is most commonly DR1. DR2 and DR5 are usually protective of type 1 diabetes (51).

In contrast to the data in whites, in African–Americans with type 1 diabetes only 70% have a HLA-DR3 and/or DR4 allele, suggesting a greater heterogeneity of causes of youth-onset diabetes in African–Americans than in whites (52). In African–Americans, while HLA-DR4 is associated with type 1 diabetes DR3 is not. Thirty percent of African–Americans with youth-onset diabetes lack both DR3 or DR4 alleles. Islet-cell autoantibody (ICA) frequencies at diabetes onset in African–Americans are also considerably lower than in whites (40% vs. ~75%), thus providing further evidence of etiological heterogeneity.

Using recombinant DNA methodologies, the serological DQw3 antigen associated with DR4 has been divided by analysis of DR4-related DQβ genes (DQw3) into type 1 diabetes-susceptible (DQB1*0302) and type 1 diabetes-resistant or neutral (DQB1*0301 and DQB1*0303) type 1 diabetes-risk subtypes (53). The susceptibility to type 1 diabetes is inherited, at least in part, by way of inheritance of DQA1*0501-DQB1*0201 (associated with DR3) and DQA1*0301-DQB1*0302 (associated with DR4) or closely linked alleles (54). Individuals heterozygous for DQA1*0501-DQB1*0201/DQA1*0301-DQB1*0302 can have a 32-fold increased risk for type 1 diabetes. This would be an absolute risk of ~6.4% risk based on a general population frequency of type 1 diabetes of 1:500. HLA-DQB1*0602 is highly protective of type 1 diabetes, with only 1:15,000 persons carrying this allele developing type 1 diabetes (55). HLA-DQB1*0602 is also protective of type 1 diabetes in subjects with autoimmune polyglandular syndrome type 1 (56). The DR4 molecular split DR*0403 is also highly protective of the development of type 1 diabetes.

For the DQB1 alleles associated with type 1 diabetes, at position 57 of the β1 exon, there are non-aspartic-acid residues (e.g., serine, valine, and alanine) as opposed to type 1 diabetes-resistance alleles where aspartic acid is present (57). This amino acid difference alters the class II MHC antigen-binding cleft and thus influences which antigen peptides are presented (58). Many studies have associated nonaspartic acid alleles with type 1 diabetes susceptibility (59). Arginine at position 52 in the DQα chain has also been related to type 1 diabetes susceptibility (60). A combination of these DQA1 and DQB1 alleles (particularly in the *trans* configuration) further increases risk for type 1 diabetes (61). The DR2 and DR5 associated DQA1-DQB1 haplotypes are, respectively, DQA1*0102-DQB1*0602 and DQA1*0501-DQB1*0301. As opposed to whites and DQB1, in Japanese DQA1 alleles are the major MHC susceptibility factors (62). However Korean and white type 1 diabetes subjects display similar HLA susceptibility patterns (63). Dorman et al. have proposed that variations in population frequencies of DQB1 non-aspartic-acid alleles correlate with the population frequency of type 1 diabetes (64). She et al. have recently presented a excellent overview of the genetics of type 1 diabetes with reference to the MHC (65). The influence of various DQ loci is summarized in Table 6.

Studies of multiplex families show that the inheritance of type 1 diabetes is associated with particular parental haplotypes. In sibling pairs with type 1 diabetes, instead of the expected random haplotype distribution (25% HLA identical, 50% haploidentical, 25% nonidentical) a predominance of like haplotypes is found (60% HLA identical, 25% haploidentical, less than 5% nonidentical). There is an apparent transmission bias for type 1 diabetes: ~7% of children fathered by type 1 diabetes men develop type 1 diabetes as opposed to 2% of the offspring of type 1 diabetes mothers (66). This is due to the preferential inheritance of a DR4-bearing haplotype from the affected type 1 diabetes father (70% transmission to offspring vs. expected 50% transmission) (67). In both type 1 diabetes fathers and mothers, there is transmission bias of DR3 (60% transmission to offspring vs. expected 50% transmission).

Polygenic inheritance of susceptibility to type 1 diabetes is certain (68). Polymorphisms in at least 14 different genetic loci have been associated with type 1 diabetes in humans (69–73). The loci have been identified by population studies and sib-pair analysis. The loci can be classified according to the certainty with which the data support a genetic association with type 1 diabetes (Table 7). Despite this surfeit of loci, the MHC remains the most important susceptibility factor (Table 8) and provides 40–50% of genetic susceptibility to type 1 diabetes. The next most influential gene may be the insulin gene and its hypervariable region (74).

6. Environmental Triggers in the Pathogenesis of Type 1 Diabetes

Because concordance for type 1 diabetes in identical twins is only 33–50%, environmental factors are thought to play a role in triggering type 1 diabetes (75). Environmental triggers of beta-cell autoimmunity under investigation include diet/breastfeeding (76), toxins, drugs, immunizations (77), viral infections (78–80), and stress. Suspected toxins include alloxan-like or streptozotocin-like agents that induce oxidant beta-cell damage, and smoked or cured mutton. Viral infections hypothesized to trigger type 1 diabetes include coxsackie A, coxsackie B (81), cytomegalovirus, ECHO virus (82), Epstein–Barr virus, rubella, mumps, and retroviruses. There is no unequivocal evidence to suggest that children should avoid cows' milk products to prevent type 1 diabetes (83), although cow's

Table 6 Relative Influence of HLA-DQ Alleles on Susceptibility to Type 1 Diabetes

DQ alleles DQB1	DQA1	Associated HLA-DR	Type 1 DM influence	Relative influence
0602	0102	DR15[a]	Protective	++++
0301	0501	DR5	Protective	+++
0302	0301	DR4	Susceptible	++
0201	0501	DR3	Susceptible	+

[a]DR15, split of DR2.

Table 7 Susceptibility Loci in Type 1 Diabetes

Loci	Location	Gene
Confirmed		
IDDM1	6p21	HLA-DR and DQ
IDDM2	11p15	Insulin
IDDM4	11q13	Unknown
IDDM5	6q25	Unknown
IDDM8	6q2	Unknown
IDDM12	2q33	CTLA-4
Unconfirmed		
IDDM3	15q26	
IDDM6	18q	
IDDM7	2q33	
IDDM9	3q	
IDDM10	10p13-q11	
IDDM11	14q24-q31	
IDDM13	2q33	
IDDM15	6q21	

Table 8 Risk Effect of Specific HLA Alleles for the Development of Type 1 Diabetes

HLA-DRB1	Absolute risk	Relative risk
Within families		
Random sibling risk	1:20	25
Sibling HLA identical to affected sib	1:7	70
Sib shares DR3/DR4 with affected sib	1:4	125
Genetically identical to affected sib (identical twin)	1:3–1:2	167–250
General population		
Random risk	1:500	1
DR3 (+)	1:400	1.25
DR4 (+)	1:400	1.25
DR3/DR4 (+)	1:40	12.5

milk (vs. breastfeeding), bovine serum albumin, and beta-lactoglobulin exposure have been found in various studies to act as diabetogenic influences (84).

Because of the inherent plasticity of the genome, especially with respect to T-cell receptor and immunoglobulin gene rearrangements, the supposition that monozygotic twins are immunogenetically identical can be questioned (85). In persons who develop type 1 diabetes, the relative contributions of genetic and interacting environmental factors appear to be highly variable. Genetic factors may predominate early in life whereas environmental exposures may become more important with advancing age. It is assumed that once a person is predisposed to type 1 diabetes by the possession of particular immune response genes (HLA-associated and those outside the MHC) and nonimmune response genes, the proper environmental exposure may trigger or foster the initiation of the autoimmune process. It is unfortunate that the triggers to the development of type 1 diabetes remain largely unknown (86–91).

7. Islet Autoantibodies

Although many types of autoantibodies have been described in the sera of persons with type 1 diabetes (Table 9) (92), investigators have focused their studies on four types of islet autoantibodies: ICA (107), insulin autoantibodies (IAA) (108), glutamic acid decarboxylase autoantibodies (GADA) (109), and insulinoma-associated-2 autoantibodies (IA-2A) (110).

The ICA and ICSA autoantibodies (111,112) have been described in the sera of patients with type 1 diabetes since the mid-1970s. At the time of diagnosis, 70–80% of caucasian children with type 1 diabetes have ICA; how-

Table 9 Autoantigens to Which Autoantibodies Have Been Detected in Type 1 Diabetes

Carboxypeptidase H (93)
Aromatic-L-amino-acid decarboxylase (94)
30 kD pancreatic autoantigen related to chymotrypsinogen (95)
DNA topoisomerase II (96)
Islet cell 69 kD (ICA69)[a] (97,98)
M_r 38,000 (38 Ka) insulin-secretory granule protein (99)
Rubella-related M_r 52,000 (52 Ka) islet autoantigen (100)
Proinsulin (101)
Insulin receptor autoantibodies (102)
Glima 38 autoantibodies (103)
GLUT2 autoantibodies (104)
Heat shock protein[a] (105)
Islet cell surface autoantibodies
SOX13 (106)

[a]Controversial.

ever, the frequency falls thereafter (113). By 5 years' duration of type 1 diabetes, ICA frequency has declined to approximately 25%, and after 10 years ICA persists in sera in less than 5%. First-degree relatives of type 1 diabetes patients have a frequency of type 1 diabetes similar to their ICA frequency: 3–5%. In Pasco County, Florida, in a study of ~10,000 normal school children, ICA were detected in 1:~250 children (114).

In patients with clinically apparent type 2 diabetes, some 5–15% are ICA positive (115–117), and, with time, these patients tend to progress to insulin dependence. These individuals also express higher frequencies of the type 1 diabetes-associated HLA-DR alleles DR3 and DR4. Autoantibodies to GAD have also been described in such patients with apparent type 2 diabetes. Such islet-autoantibody-positive individuals with type 2 diabetes, according to the 1997 ADA scheme, are now classified as having autoimmune diabetes and in reality have type 1 diabetes. Because of the attenuated pace of beta-cell destruction and older-onset of disease, the term latent autoimmune diabetes of adulthood (LADA) has been applied to such clinical circumstances (118–121).

Since ICA react with intracellular antigens of all cells of the pancreatic islets, ICA are not involved in the pathogenesis of type 1 diabetes. However sera containing ICSA have been shown in vitro to be cytotoxic to rodent islet cells (122) and can inhibit glucose-stimulated insulin release by islets (123). ICSA may also react preferentially with beta cells, unlike other islet autoantibodies that react with all cells of the islet (e.g., ICA and GADA).

ICA usually predate the clinical presentation of type 1 diabetes by months or years (124). ICA-positive nondiabetic patients evaluated serially by glucose tolerance testing often show insulinopenia to intravenous glucose injection; later, rises in fasting and stimulated glucose concentrations occur after oral glucose challenges (125). Work by Schatz et al. has shown that ICA are polyclonal including both kappa and lambda light chains and all four IgG subclasses (126). Higher-titer ICA appear to predict an increased risk for the development of type 1 diabetes in nondiabetic individuals. Furthermore, newly diagnosed individuals with type 1 diabetes who have higher ICA titers are at higher risk to lose endogenous C-peptide secretion more rapidly (127). A similar claim has been made for higher-titer GADA (128).

Standardization of ICA testing has been accomplished by workshops held under the aegis of the Juvenile Diabetes Foundation. This lead to the establishment of ICA titers being reported as JDF units. To calculate JDF units, the next to last positive titer is multiplied by 10. Thus if a serum level were last positive at a dilution of 1:64 (e.g., negative at 1:128), the next to last positive dilution is 1:32. Multiplying 32 by 10 gives a JDF titer of 320 JDF units.

With greater than 90% beta-cell destruction, significant insulinopenia results with consequent hyperglycemia, unrestricted ketogenesis, and clinical insulin-dependent diabetes. Data from the Pasco County, Florida, study (114) indicate that ICA in the general population predicts type 1 diabetes as well as ICA in nondiabetic first-degree relatives of patients with type 1 diabetes. The ability to predict type 1 diabetes in the general population is most important because ~85% of type 1 diabetes patients do not have a first-degree relative with type 1 diabetes.

Another type of autoantibody found in ~40% of newly-diagnosed patients with type 1 diabetes is the IAA (129). The enzyme-linked immunosorbent assay (ELISA) method for the detection of IAA does not correlate with the development of type 1 diabetes (130,131). However, IAA detected by a serum-binding assay when present with ICA is highly predictive of insulinopenia and the eventual development of type 1 diabetes.

In 1990, the M_r 64,000 (64 Ka) islet immunoprecipitable autoantigen was shown to be GAD (109). ICA react with GAD as well as a sialoglycoconjugate target antigen (132) and recombinant IA-2 (133). Non-GAD ICA have been noted by Richter et al. (134). GAD normally converts glutamate to γ-aminobutyric acid (GABA). GAD is expressed predominantly in the central and peripheral nervous systems but also in testes, ovary, adrenal, pituitary, thyroid, islets, and kidney (135). GAD comes in two molecular weights coded for by separate genes (GAD65 on chromosome 2 and GAD 6 on chromosome 10). GAD65 and GAD67 exhibit ~70% amino acid homology. GADA are most commonly directed against GAD65 (136–138). Radiobinding immunoprecipitation assays for GADA require that labeled GAD be kept in solution (as opposed to an ELISA format) because GADA recognize conformational determinants. Epitope reactivity for GADA among nondiabetic and diabetic individuals may explain why not all GADA in nondiabetic individuals predicts type 1 diabetes (139).

A primary sequence homology between portions of GAD and the P2-C protein expressed by Coxsackie virus has been described (140). GAD cellular autoimmunity has been shown (141). In addition to GAD, cell-mediated immune responses to other islet antigens have been described such as insulin secretory granule proteins and beta-cell membrane antigens (142). One group of investigators proposed that cellular and humoral GAD reactivity are inversely associated with type 1 diabetes risk (145). Using the older immunoprecipitation assay, Atkinson et al. (146) showed that 64 kDa autoantibodies were highly predictive of type 1 diabetes. Since this initial report, many studies have confirmed that GADA in nondiabetic individuals predicts the later development of type 1 diabetes. GADA in patients with clinical so-called type 2 diabetes correlates with insulin deficiency similar to ICA.

The most recently identified autoantigen of great importance is a member of the plasma membrane protein tyrosine phosphatase family: insulinoma-associated antigen-2 (IA-2) (147–149). Located on lymphocytes, CD45 is another example of a protein tyrosine phosphatase. Recent work has identified a second transmembrane protein tyrosine phosphatase: IA-2β (150). IA-2 and IA-2β share several common epitopes while other epitopes are unique to each molecule.

In the prediction of type 1 diabetes in nondiabetic individuals using islet autoantibody testing, it is now clear that the presence of a single autoantibody is not as powerful a predictor of the later development of type 1 diabetes as positive findings of multiple islet autoantibodies. When multiple islet autoantibodies are present, the risk for developing type 1 diabetes rises substantially (151–154). Furthermore in children when multiple autoantibody positivity islet autoimmunity is coupled with depressed first-phase insulin response to intravenously administered glucose, risk for type 1 diabetes can exceed 50% over 5 years follow-up and approaches 100% over 10 years. Although the biochemical autoantibodies GADA and IA-2A provide many methodological advantages over ICA testing, ICA testing should not abandoned because of its higher specificity than GAD or IA-2A and its ability to detect autoimmunity to several islet autoantigens not detected by the single GADA or IA-2A assays (155).

8.   Immune Abnormalities in Type 1 Diabetes

Besides insulitis and islet autoantibodies (e.g., ICA, IAA, GADA, and IA-2A), a number of other immunological abnormalities have been described in type 1 diabetes: elevated levels of Ia (class II MHC) and TAC- (transferrin receptor) positive T cells (activated T cells), increased K-cell levels, perturbed numbers or ratios of T-helper/inducer (CD4) and T-cytotoxic/suppressor (CD8) cells, lymphocytotoxic autoantibodies, circulating immune complexes, possible decreased IL-2 production by lymphocytes from type 1 diabetes patients, impaired CD4-positive T-lymphocyte function, and potentially decreased class I MHC expression. In vitro, lymphocytes from type 1 diabetes patients have been shown to produce migration inhibition factor when exposed to xenogeneic islets or islet homogenates. Lymphocytes in vitro have produced islet adherence and cytolysis and have inhibited insulin release. Recently Clare-Salzler and colleagues have described variations in antigen-presenting cell function in type 1 diabetes and prostaglandin synthase 2 expression (156).

Further evidence of an autoimmune cause for type 1 diabetes is found in the association of type 1 diabetes with other recognized autoimmune diseases (particularly chronic lymphocytic thyroiditis [157] and atrophic gastritis), and with disturbed frequencies of particular HLA-DR and DQ types (158). In contrast to many other autoimmune disorders, type 1 diabetes is slightly more common in males than females and more commonly presents in childhood than in adult life.

9. Prediction, Immunotherapy, and Prevention of Type 1 Diabetes

In the natural history of type 1 diabetes, autoantibody-positive individuals progress through varying stages of glucose intolerance to clinical diabetes (159). The earliest clinical abnormality is a decline in first-phase insulin response to intravenously administered glucose at time 1 plus 3 min (160,161). Later, intolerance to oral glucose challenges appears. After 1–2 years of glucose intolerance upon oral testing, a typical history of polyuria and polydipsia is found as the patient presents with frank clinical diabetes. Weight loss and diabetic ketoacidosis may occur if the diagnosis of diabetes is delayed.

In studies undertaken largely in the 1980s, immunosuppression of newly diagnosed type 1 diabetes patients with cyclosporin or azathioprine and glucocorticoids produced short-lived remissions (162–164). Because of the limited success of these trials and the intrinsic toxicities of such immunosuppressive agents, researchers have recently attempted to induce immunological tolerance to beta-cell antigens as a method of preventing type 1 diabetes (165). The first beta-cell antigen to be used in such trials is insulin by subcutaneous injection for high-risk individuals and oral insulin in lower-risk individuals (166). This is the basis for the Diabetes Prevention Trial 1 study that started in 1993 (167). However, oral insulin administration begun at disease onset is ineffective in changing the disease course over the first 12 months following diagnosis (168).

Nasal insulin administration is being attempted in Finland in the Diabetes Prediction and Prevention (DIPP) trial (169). In New Zealand (170) and Canada, Texas, and Europe (European Nicotinamide Intervention Trial [ENDIT]) (171), nicotinamide is being studied as a beta-cell-selective antioxidant. However, several papers have disputed the claim that nicotinamide is of any benefit in preventing or treating type 1 diabetes (172,173). Islet beta-cell (174) and stem-cell (175) transplantation is a promising field in beta-cell reconstitution.

Success in such trials may lead to the routine treatment of prediabetic individuals, enabling one to forestall or actually prevent type 1 diabetes (176). Such trials are to be considered strictly experimental at this time (177).

B. Type B Insulin-Resistant Diabetes and Acanthosis Nigricans

In this rare syndrome, insulin resistance occurs as a result of autoantibodies directed towards the insulin receptor that interfere with insulin binding (type B insulin resistance and acanthosis nigricans) (178). Acanthosis nigricans of the skin is recognized as raised, waxy plaques that occur in skin folds especially around the neck and upper trunk, under the arms, breasts, and in the groin where skin abrasion occurs. In severe cases, the elbows, knees, and periumbilical skin can become exceptionally rough.

Type B disease, which has been described in a few adolescents, is more common in females and is associated with other autoimmune disorders. Type B patients may display antinuclear antibodies, anti-DNA antibodies, episodic hypocomplementemia, hypergammaglobulinemia, and leukopenia. A number of type B patients have been reported with systemic lupus erythematosus, scleroderma, Sjögren's syndrome, and ataxia–telangiectasia (179). In one patient, a dramatic remission was induced with steroid therapy (180). Insulin receptor autoantibodies and a type-B-like syndrome have been described in an adult with pheochromocytoma (181). The diagnosis of type B insulin-resistant diabetes should be pursued in patients with type 2 diabetes and acanthosis nigricans who require high dosages of insulin (>100–1000 units/day) for treatment of hyperglycemia. The presence of non-organ-specific autoantibodies or non-organ-specific autoimmune diseases increases the likelihood of type B disease.

In contrast to the type B syndrome, another nonimmunological form of severe insulin resistance and acanthosis nigricans (type A) is associated with hypogonadism and/or the Stein-Leventhal polycystic ovary syndrome phenotype. In this disorder, there is a decrease in receptor number with normal receptor affinity and no antireceptor autoantibodies.

C. Hypoglycemia Secondary to Insulinomimetic Autoantibodies

Antireceptor autoantibodies usually block insulin action. Patients have been described with antireceptor autoantibodies that displayed insulin-like action producing hypoglycemia (182). This disorder has been reported in children (183). Hypoglycemia secondary to insulinomimetic autoantibodies has been identified in adults with Hodgkin's disease (184) and lupus erythematosus (185,186). Insulinomimetic autoantibodies, which are a rare cause of hypoglycemia, can be considered when the biochemical determinations suggest hyperinsulinism (e.g., nonketotic hypoglycemia) yet insulin concentrations are depressed. Tests for insulin receptor autoantibodies are available generally only from research laboratories.

D. Autoimmune Hypoglycemia

In this disorder, an autoantibody is produced against circulating insulin (187,188). Whereas insulin antibodies are common in patients who have received exogenous insulin (including human insulin), patients with autoimmune hypoglycemia spontaneously develop such antibodies (189). Pediatric cases have been identified (190). This condition is most often recognized in Japan (191), but it has been reported in Norway and the Netherlands (192). Some subjects have developed this syndrome following exposure to antithyroid medications used to treat Graves' disease (193). Nevertheless, a recent report noted a decline in insulin autoantibodies despite continuation of methimazole therapy in a patient with Graves' disease and autoimmune hypoglycemia (194).

The circulating autoantibody–insulin complexes can release insulin inappropriate to metabolic needs, increasing the free insulin concentration (195). At these times, hypoglycemia results from relative hyperinsulinism. The amount of circulating insulin complexed to autoantibodies may also lead to glucose intolerance or a mild diabetic state as well as hyperglycemia during fasting.

Similar to insulin antibodies resulting from exogenous insulin administration, autoimmune hypoglycemia is associated with HLA-DR4 (196). IAA described above in prediabetic individuals do not appear to be associated with hypoglycemia. In so-called prediabetes, IAA serve as markers of beta-cell autoimmunity.

E. Pancreatic Alpha-Cell and Delta-Cell Autoimmunity

Bottazzo and Lendrum in 1976 first described autoantibodies that reacted solely with the cytoplasm of the pancreatic glucagon-producing alpha cells and with the somatostatin-secreting delta cells (197). The Pasco County, Florida, ICA study found that the frequency of alpha-cell autoantibodies (ACA) was similar in controls and relatives of type 1 diabetes patients (0.5% vs. 0.6%, respectively). ACA are apparently very rare in type 1 diabetes patients because they were not found in any of 62 ICA-negative type 1 diabetes patients studied. Eleven ACA-positive patients were also studied using arginine infusion and did not display glucagon deficiency (198). Del Prete et al. had previously shown normal glucagon responses to arginine infusion in two patients with ACA (199). Asymptomatic autoantibodies to the glucagon molecule have been reported (200). ACA is a very interesting autoantibody because as yet there are no disease associations with it. Subjects with ACA do not display disturbed HLA-DR frequencies, in contrast to nondiabetic individuals with ICA who exhibit increased frequencies of HLA-DR3 and DR4.

IV. AUTOIMMUNE THYROID DISEASE

Autoimmune thyroid disease (AITD) can present clinically as goiter and/or thyroid dysfunction: either hyper- or hypothyroidism. AITD includes a spectrum of disorders bridging chronic thyroiditis (201) and Graves' disease (202). Graves' disease is the most common form of primary hyperthyroidism in which thyrotoxicosis results from agonistic TSH receptor autoantibodies. AITD is commonly seen in both children and adults and rarely develops prenatally (203).

Thyroid inflammation (so-called thyroiditis) can be classified as acute (suppurative) resulting from bacterial thyroid gland infection, subacute (deQuervain) resulting from viral thyroid gland infection, or chronic resulting

from an autoimmune lymphocytic infiltration of the gland. There are two clinical forms of chronic thyroiditis: goitrous and atrophic thyroiditis. Hashimoto originally described the association of chronic lymphocytic thyroiditis and goiter in 1912 and it is this form of thyroiditis that bears his name (Hashimoto's thyroiditis). Taken together, all forms of AITD represent the most common causes of autoimmune endocrinopathies in humans. Among all forms of AITD there is a striking female predominance (see Chapter 17).

A. Chronic Lymphocytic Thyroiditis

1. Thyroiditis

Chronic lymphocytic thyroiditis (CLT) is the most common cause of goiter and acquired hypothyroidism in childhood (204). Patients presenting with a goiter may progress to frank hypothyroidism because of continued gland destruction, while other patients may pass through a transient state of hyperthyroidism (hashitoxicosis) with release of thyroid hormone from a period of accelerated thyroid gland destruction, with later development of hypothyroidism. In atrophic thyroiditis, an autoantibody to the TSH receptor may be present that blocks TSH action (e.g., an antagonistic TSH receptor autoantibody) (205,206). About 20–25% of individuals with atrophic thyroiditis exhibit antagonistic TSH receptor autoantibodies compared with 10% of individuals with goitrous thyroiditis. Goiter is not present in the patients with atrophic thyroiditis, unlike patients with CLT. With disappearance of antagonistic TSH receptor autoantibodies, hypothyroidism can spontaneously remit (207).

Atrophic thyroiditis, goitrous thyroiditis, and Graves' disease often coexist in single pedigrees. About 50% of first-degree relatives will be affected with AITD, suggestive of autosomal dominant inheritance. Higher levels of dietary iodine are associated with higher population frequencies of CLT.

Histological examination of the thyroid of patients with CLT reveals lymphocytic infiltration with germinal center formation. In the late stages of disease, fibrosis and atrophy are present. The intrathyroidal plasma cells are a major source of thyroid autoantibody production. T-cell lines derived from the thyroid glands of subjects with AITD demonstrate a predominance of CD4 expression (208) and Th1 cytokine patterns (209). These data are consistent with the destruction of thyroid follicular cells effected through a Th1-cell-mediated autoimmune response. In contrast, Graves' disease may represent a predominantly Th2 disease with pathogenic autoantibody production.

An interesting phenomenon is the finding of class II MHC (e.g., HLA-DR) expression on thyroid follicular cells in both patients with Hashimoto's thyroiditis (~100% of cases) and Graves' disease (~70% of cases). Two competing hypotheses explain the role of such aberrant class II MHC expression. A proautoimmune hypothesis states that T-cell secretion of IFN-γ elicits HLA-DR expression and that the follicular cells then present autoantigens to CD4 T cells to foster the autoimmune response (210). Stimulation of naive CD4 T cells could not occur, however, because thyroid follicular cells fail to express the costimulatory molecule B7. An alternative hypothesis is that aberrant class II MHC expression actually downregulates autoimmunity by inducing anergy in naive T cells, because of the absence of B7 co-expression with class II MHC. Both hypotheses could be true: naive cells could be anergized, yet activated cells that do not require B7 activation could be stimulated. Cytokine secretion such as IL-1, TNF, and IFN-γ can all depress thyroid cell function in vitro (211,212). IL-1β induces Fas expression on normal thyroid follicular cells in vitro (213). Once Fas is expressed, such thyroid follicular cells could trigger so-called bystander apoptosis by interacting with Fas ligand on adjacent cells. Increased apoptosis has been recognized in glands of patients with Hashimoto's thyroiditis (214).

Autoantibodies to the thyroid microsomes (thyroid microsomal autoantibodies, TMA), to thyroglobulin (thyroglobulin autoantibodies, TGA), and to nonthyroglobulin colloid antigen (CA2) can be found very frequently in affected patients (215). The major microsomal autoantigen is thyroperoxidase (TPO) whose autoantibodies are termed TPOAb (216). A thyroid-growth-promoting autoantibody that does not interact with the TSH receptor has been suggested (217). In clinical practice, the finding of TMA, TPOAb, and/or TGA in the presence of euthyroid goiter or goitrous hypothyroidism is consistent with Hashimoto's thyroiditis. When these autoantibodies are present in cases of nongoitrous hypothyroidism, atrophic thyroiditis is diagnosed.

The TMA autoantigen has been shown to be TPO as noted above (218). Existing in two molecular forms (105 and 110 kDa), thyroperoxidase is a glycosylated hemoprotein located on the apical plasma membrane of thyroid follicular cells. Located on chromosome 2, the thyroperoxidase genes covers >150 kb and contains 17 exons. TPO functions to oxidize iodide and to organify iodine covalently bound to thyroglobulin tyrosine residues, forming monoiodothyronine (MIT) and diiodothyronine (DIT). TPO is next responsible for the coupling reaction forming triiodothyronine and tetraiodothyronine. The catalytic domain of TPO is oriented toward the colloid space where organification of iodide and iodination of thyroglobulin occur. On the immediate extracellular N-terminal portion of TPO, an epidermal growth factor precursor-like domain and complement protein C4b-like domain are recognized. TPO demonstrates extensive homology with myeloperoxidase, an autoantigen in some forms of systemic vasculitis (219).

The TMA autoantibody reacts with TPO in its native conformation (220). Antibodies to TPO (e.g., TPOAb) are more sensitive for the detection of AITD; however, because such TPOAbs are more common in the general population than TMA, TPOAb may be less specific than TMA. This may lead to improvements in the TMA assay but this is still somewhat controversial (221).

Autoantibodies to thyroglobulin (e.g., TGA) are not as common as TMA/TPOAb in all forms of AITD and CLT. Thyroglobulin is a 2748 amino acid, 330 kD homodimeric glycosylated iodoprotein that can represent 75% of the total protein content of the thyroid gland. There are multiple regions of repeated structure within the protein. The coding portion of the thyroglobulin gene covers >250 kb of DNA and 42 exons. The gene is located on chromosome 8q24. Synthesized by thyroid follicular cells, thyroglobulin is secreted into the lumen of the thyroid follicle forming the colloid, where it becomes the substrate for thyroid hormone synthesis.

Two new autoantigens have been recognized in AITD: megalin (GP330) and the thyroid Na$^+$/I$^-$ symporter. Megalin is a multiligand receptor found on the apical surface of selected epithelial cells including the thyroid gland. Antibodies to megalin were found in 50% of subjects with autoimmune thyroiditis and 10% of Graves' disease subjects (222). Megalin is also referred to as a polyspecific receptor protein. Na$^+$/I$^-$ symporter is not believed to be a major thyroid autoantigen because autoantibodies to the symporter are found in only 10% of subjects with Hashimoto's thyroiditis and 20% of Graves' disease subjects (223).

In children, TMA correlates best with the presence of CLT; virtually 100% of children with CLT will have TMA, albeit some also have TGA (224,225). About 2% of the general childhood population have at least one antithyroid autoantibody. Thyroid autoimmunity is also highly associated with gastric parietal cell autoimmunity: approximately 25% of TMA-positive patients also have gastric parietal cell autoantibodies (PCA). About 25% of PCA-positive patients likewise also have TMA, indicating an underlying genetic predisposition to both thyroid and gastric (thyrogastric) autoimmunities in such patients (226). The histological correlate of PCA is chronic lymphocytic gastritis that can cause achlorhydria, iron deficiency, and intrinsic factor deficiency. Long-term deficiency of intrinsic factor can cause cobalamine deficiency and pernicious anemia. A major target autoantigen in atrophic gastritis is the H+/K+ ATPase pump. Both the 95 kDa alpha subunit and 60–90 kDa beta subunits of the gastric H+/K+ ATPase pump (proton pump) are targeted (227,228).

Thyrogastric autoimmunities appear to be frequently inherited as an autosomal dominant trait with increased expression in female patients. Unlike type 1 diabetes, CLT and thyrogastric autoimmunities are not inherited in association with particular parental HLA haplotypes (229). HLA does appear to modulate (230) the clinical expression of the disease: DR4 and/or DR5 are associated with CLT and pernicious anemia in population studies and DR3 is associated with Graves' disease. A model can be created in which a non-HLA gene provides the predominant susceptibility to AITD that, in the presence of DR4 or DR5, stimulates a Th1-mediated antithyroid attack presenting as autoimmune thyroiditis, whereas the presence of DR3 stimulates a Th2-mediated antithyroid attack presenting as Graves' disease.

Genetics does play a major role in the pathogenesis of CLT in studies of adults. No data in children have been reported. In a study of 2945 female Danish twin pairs, concordance for autoimmune hypothyroidism was 55% in monozygotic twins and 0% in dizygotic twins (231). Concordance in TPOAb and/or TGA positive results was 80% in monozygotic twins and 40% in dizygotic twins. Besides the genetic influence of HLA, association studies strongly suggest that the cytotoxic T-lymphocyte-associated serine esterase-4 (CTLA-4) gene located on chromosome 2q33, or genes closely linked to CTLA-4, influence the development of AITD including Graves' disease and Hashimoto's thyroiditis (232). CTLA-4 is expressed on the surface of activated T cells. Interaction of CTLA-4 with B7 from antigen-presenting cells provides a suppressive influence to downregulate activated T cells. Therefore failure to turn off activated T cells could theoretically lead to autoimmunity. Kotsa et al. showed that microsatellite-defined CTLA-4 allele 106 was increased in autoimmune hypothyroidism (233). Donner et al. from Germany demonstrated that the alanine CTLA-4 leader sequence polymorphism (threonine/alanine) at amino acid 17 was more frequent in Hashimoto's thyroiditis (22%) than controls (15%) (234). One year later these investigators described that a −318 cytosine/thymine promoter variant associated with AITD (both Graves' and Hashimoto's thyroiditis) was linked to an exon 1 polymorphism (235). However, by itself, Hashimoto's thyroiditis was not significantly associated with a promoter polymorphism. Thymine in the promoter was linked to adenine in exon 1 of the CTLA-4 gene. In contrast to these German data, researchers from the United Kingdom did not find evidence for genetic association of the −318 polymorphism with Graves' disease, autoimmune hypothyroidism, or systemic lupus erythematosus (236). It is controversial whether CTLA-4 plays a role in the association of AITD and type 1 diabetes. Djilali-Saia et al. (237) found no influence for CTLA-4 on the association of type 1 diabetes and AITD. While the CTLA-4 codon 17 A/G polymorphism was associated with autoimmune hypothyroidism, the polymorphism was no more strongly associated with type 1 diabetes plus AITD than Graves' disease or Hashimoto's thyroiditis alone. On the other hand in Japanese type 1 diabetes subjects under age 30 years (238), the G-variant of the Thr17Ala CTLA-4 exon polymorphism was more common in type 1 diabetes subjects than controls (39% vs. 28%) and was more common in type 1 diabetes subjects with AITD (54%) than either of the other groups. The authors point out that while there are no data to suggest that the Thr17Ala polymorphism influences the func-

tion of CTLA-4, this polymorphism may be linked to an AT microsatellite polymorphism that could affect mRNA stability.

A new locus on chromosome 13 termed Hashimoto's thyroiditis locus-1 (HD-1) was detected in linkage studies in 1999 (239). This locus was uniquely linked to Hashimoto's thyroiditis and did not show linkage to Graves' disease. In a subset of the families studied, a locus on chromosome 12 was linked to Hashimoto's thyroiditis. One locus on chromosome 6 (AITD locus-1 [AITD-1]) was linked to both Hashimoto's thyroiditis and Graves' disease. This locus was close to, but distinct from, the HLA complex.

As opposed to the above population association studies, using family-based linkage studies many candidate gene loci have been excluded as affecting AITD including CTLA-4, the T-cell receptor Vα and Vβ complexes, the Ig heavy chain locus (240), the estrogen receptor alpha gene, and the aromatase gene (241). The Graves' disease-1 locus (GD-1) on chromosome 14 is also not linked to Hashimoto's thyroiditis (242) nor is the TSH receptor gene associated with AITD (243).

Thus the current state of the genetics of CLT can be summarized as follows. In families, AITD including CLT, atrophic thyroiditis, or Graves' disease appears to be inherited as a dominant trait. HLA DR4 and/or DR5 are associated with an increased risk for CLT. Loci on chromosomes 2 (CTLA-4) and 13 also influence the development of CLT. Non-MHC regions on chromosome 6 and chromosome 12 deserve further study.

2. Effects of AITD on the Fetus and Newborn: Congenital Hypothyroidism and Transient Hyperthyrotropinemia

Women with CLT do not have a significantly increased risk of bearing a infant with congenital hypothyroidism because TMA, TPOAb, and TGA that do cross the placenta are not pathogenic. This has been known for over 20 years (244). However, if the mother has antagonistic TSH receptor autoantibodies, transient congenital hypothyroidism or transient hyperthyrotropinemia can result (245). In one study, 15 of 34 women giving birth to children with congenital hypothyroidism had evidence of TSH receptor antagonist autoantibodies (246). Variable neonatal thyroid function can be observed in babies born to mothers with AITD, ranging from hypothyroidism to hyperthyroidism depending upon the mix and titer of agonist vs. antagonist TSH receptor autoantibodies (247). A report of familial nongoitrous congenital hypothyroidism due to maternal AITD was reported as early as 1960 (248). In a North American study, TSH receptor-blocking autoantibodies accounted for 2% of infants with congenital hypothyroidism identified in a T4 screening program and overall affected 1:180,000 newborns (249).

Thyrotropin-binding inhibitory immunoglobulins have been identified in infant and maternal sera (250).

Finding thyroid-binding inhibitory immunoglobulins in mothers of infants with congenital hypothyroidism suggests that the hypothyroidism will be transient. However, thyroid replacement therapy in such infants should be continued until age 3 or 4 years when a trial without hormone replacement can be carried out to confirm or deny that the hypothyroidism is persistent (251).

3. Postpartum Thyroiditis

With an increasing frequency of adolescent girls becoming mothers (intended or unintended teenage pregnancy), pediatricians and pediatric endocrinologists must be aware of postpartum thyroiditis that occurs in 5–10% of women following delivery (252). Postpartum thyroiditis is a variant of autoimmune thyroiditis: following delivery, mothers can express any one of several possible clinical courses including hypothyroidism (3–6 months following delivery; ~40% of cases of postpartum thyroiditis), hyperthyroidism (~35% of cases), or hyperthyroidism followed by hypothyroidism (~25% of cases) (253,254). In many cases, euthyroidism supervenes by 12 months postpartum yet there is an high risk of hypothyroidism in the long term (255). After 3–5 years, up to 25% of such women can develop hypothyroidism. About one-third of women with postpartum hyperthyroidism appear to have Graves' disease (256). Postpartum thyroiditis recurs very commonly in subsequent pregnancies. An increased rate of miscarriage in women with thyroid autoantibodies has been suggested (257).

Postpartum thyroiditis may represent a rebound of thyroid autoimmunity following delivery with release of the general immunosuppressive state imposed on the immune system by pregnancy (258). Effervescence of autoimmune disease following parturition is also seen in women with other autoimmune diseases such as Graves' disease and systemic lupus erythematosus. Women who are positive for thyroid autoantibodies in the first trimester have a 33–50% risk of experiencing postpartum thyroiditis. Women with type 1 diabetes are at threefold higher risk for postpartum thyroiditis than women in the general population (259).

During episodes of hypothyroidism, thyroid hormone replacement in postpartum thyroiditis is appropriate to restore the euthyroid state. Thyroid hormone can be discontinued at ~9 months to observe whether the euthyroid state has recurred. During a phase of hyperthyroidism, if symptoms are mild, no therapy is indicated because thyrotoxicosis rarely lasts more than 1–2 months. Similar to hashitoxicosis, postpartum thyrotoxicosis is usually the consequence of thyroid gland destruction and release of thyroid hormone; thus antithyroid drugs such as propylthiouracil or methimazole are not indicated. Radioactive iodine uptake in a hyperthyroid stage of postpartum thyroiditis is not elevated unless true Graves' disease is present. If therapy is required for thyrotoxicosis, a beta-blocker such as propranolol can be used but the drug's

dosage should be tapered once the destructive phase of postpartum thyroiditis remits.

B. Graves' Disease

Graves' disease is the result of thyroid-stimulating autoantibodies (TSAb) that mimic the action of TSH by binding to and activating the TSH receptor (260). These immunoglobulins, upon binding to TSH receptors on the surface of thyroid epithelial follicular cells, stimulate cyclic AMP production, and thus lead to excessive thyroid hormone production and clinical hyperthyroidism (261). Some TSAbs may also activate phospholipase A_2 and these autoantibodies may be particularly goitrogenic. The TSH receptor is the major thyroid autoantigen in Graves' disease. As opposed to CLT, in which thyroid gland destruction is mediated by a CD4 Th1-mediated cell-mediated response, Graves' disease results from a CD4 Th2 response against the TSH receptor (262).

Covering 60 kb, the 10 exon TSH receptor gene is located on chromosome 14q31 (263). Smaller mRNA transcripts can be observed, but the major mRNA is 4.3 kb. Prior to glycosylation, the TSH receptor apoprotein core weighs 84.5 kDa and ~100 kDa after glycosylation. The first nine exons encode the N-terminal extracellular domain of 398 amino acids. Six N-glycosylation sites are identified in the extracellular domain. TSH binds to this region of the TSHR. Encoded by a single large exon (exon 10), the 346 amino acid carboxyl half of the receptor contains the seven hydrophobic transmembrane segments that are connected by three extra- and three intracellular loops and the cytoplasmic tail of the TSHR. This portion of the TSHR demonstrates homology with other G protein-coupled receptors and activates the G_s protein complex upon TSH binding to the extracellular domain. The TSH receptor is a member of the superfamily of G-protein-coupled receptors. Other members of this receptor superfamily include the ACTH receptor, α-adrenergic and β-adrenergic catecholamine receptors, luteinizing hormone (LH) receptor, follicle-stimulating hormone (FSH) receptor, human chorionic gonadotropin (hCG) receptor, glucagon receptor, parathyroid hormone (PTH) receptor, and somatostatin receptor. TSH receptor autoantibodies bind to the extracellular domain of the receptor as expected (264).

TSAbs were first described in the McKenzie mouse assay system as long-acting thyroid stimulator (LATS) (265). LATS was observed as delayed, but prolonged, thyroid gland stimulation after the injection of human immunoglobulin into mice. In some patients with low levels of LATS a substance that blocked LATS absorption by thyroid cells was termed LATS protector (LATS-P) (266). LATS-P corresponds more closely to human-specific LATS. In commercial radioimmunoassays to measure TRAbs, either thyrotrophin-binding inhibitory immunoglobulins (TBII) or thyroid-stimulating immunoglobulins (TSI) can be determined (267). TBII detect autoantibodies that can bind to the TSH receptor by the ability of human serum to compete with radioactively labeled TSH for binding to the TSH receptor. TBII titers are higher when more [^{125}I]TSH binding is inhibited. The TBII assay does not differentiate agonistic autoantibodies as seen in Graves' disease from antagonistic autoantibodies as observed in many cases of atrophic thyroiditis and some cases of Hashimoto's thyroiditis. On the other hand, the TSI assay detects antibodies with stimulatory effects on the TSH receptor as seen in Graves' disease. The TSI assay is typically negative in cases of autoimmune thyroiditis. The action of TSIs can be measured as the production and release of cAMP or thyroid hormone from slices of thyroid glands or cultured thyroid cells such as the FRTL-5 thyrocyte line. The titer of TSIs does not correlate with the severity of Graves' disease.

Being IgG autoantibodies, TRAbs can cross the placenta. In about 1% of pregnancies in which the mother presently has Graves' disease or had Graves' disease in the past, TRAbs with agonistic activity against the TSH receptor produce fetal and neonatal hyperthyroidism. In cases of maternal Graves' disease, some experts have suggested that testing for TRAbs should be undertaken in the third trimester of pregnancy to assess the risk of neonatal Graves' disease. If the TRAb titer is high, there is an increased risk of fetal and neonatal hyperthyroidism. Cord blood testing for TRAbs is another approach if maternal testing has not been pursued previously. TRAbs may be persistent even if the mother has had a thyroidectomy for treatment of Graves' disease or is spontaneously euthyroid.

The clinical appearance of neonatal hyperthyroidism may be delayed for 3–10 days if the mother was treated with the antithyroid drugs propylthiouracil or methimazole. Because TRAbs can represent a mixture of agonistic (e.g., TSIs) and antagonistic TSH receptor autoantibodies, the clinical course in the neonate born to a woman with Graves' disease can be variable. If there is sustained fetal tachycardia, treatment of fetal hyperthyroidism with maternal administration of propylthiouracil and concurrent T4 can be considered because of the increased risk of poor fetal outcome (268).

TMA/TPOAb and/or TGA are found in the sera of a large percentage of patients with Graves' disease. These autoantibodies, therefore, do not differentiate CLT from Graves' disease. In patients with sustained hyperthyroidism, and exophthalmos and/or pretibial myxedema, who are positive for TMA/TPOAb and/or TGA, the diagnosis of Graves' disease is appropriate. However with positive TMA/TPOAb and/or TGA, if the patient is predominantly clinically euthyroid with goiter or hypothyroid and an episode of hyperthyroidism lasted only 2 months or less, the appropriate diagnosis is CLT with temporary hashitoxicosis from transient accelerated thyroid gland destruction. The radioactive iodine uptake in Graves' disease is elevated; the radioactive iodine uptake in hashitoxicosis is not elevated.

In terms of genetic susceptibility to Graves' disease, it has already been mentioned that AITD, including Graves' disease, is often inherited in an apparent autosomal dominant mode within affected families (269). First-degree family members of individuals with Graves' disease display a high frequency of thyroid autoantibodies and AITD as well as GPCA, pernicious anemia, islet autoantibodies, and type 1 diabetes (270). Graves' disease is associated with HLA-DR3 (271), but, within families, inheritance of AITD is not linked to the inheritance of specific HLA haplotypes (272). In the HLA-DQ region, Graves' disease is associated with DQA1*0501 (273). Recently the HLA DRB3*020/DQA1*0501 haplotype has been associated with Graves' disease in African–Americans (274).

In the mid-1990s, CTLA-4 polymorphisms on chromosome 2q33 were implicated in influencing genetic susceptibility to Graves' disease (275). Researchers studied a CTLA-4 gene (AT)n microsatellite polymorphism within the 3′ untranslated region of exon 3. The relative risk for Graves' disease with the 106-base pair allele was 2.82. Two years later the CTLA-4 exon 1, 49 A/G polymorphism interchanging alanine for threonine was associated with Graves' disease (276). Graves' disease patients show more alanine alleles than controls (73% vs. 58%). The CTLA-4 A/G polymorphism was substantiated in a new data set from the United Kingdom in 1999 (277). These investigators also found preferential transmission of the A allele to offspring with Graves' disease. Researchers from the University of Newcastle-upon-Tyne calculated that 50% of inherited susceptibility to Graves' disease was provided by the CTLA-4 and MHC regions (278).

Loci on chromosomes 14q31 (termed GD-1 [242, 279]), 12q (IFN-γ [280]), 6 (TAP1 and TAP2 [281]), 20q11.2 (termed GD-2 [282,283]) and the X chromosome (termed GD-3 [279]), IL-4 promoter (chromosome 5q31.1 [284]), vitamin D receptor (285) and chromosome 18q21 (286) have subsequently been linked to or associated with Graves' disease. Loci shown not be associated with Graves include the TSH receptor (287,288),TNF receptor 2 (chromosome 1p36.3-p36.2 [289]), IL-1α, IL-1β, IL-1 receptor antagonist, IL-1 receptor, IL-4 receptor, IL-6, IL-10, and TGF-β (284,290). Although the MHC and CTLA-4 loci appear to have the greatest influence on the development of Graves' disease, many other loci are under investigation on multiple chromosomes (291).

Exophthalmos in Graves' disease and other thyroid disorders is also believed to be immunologically mediated (292). The spectrum of such associations is termed thyroid-associated ophthalmopathy (TAO). Clinically euthyroid patients presenting with exophthalmos often have TMA, TGA, and LATS-P (293). Even without frank exophthalmos, 68% of patients with Graves' disease have abnormally increased intraocular pressure on upward gaze (294).

Since part of the thyroid's lymphatic drainage traverses the retro-orbital space, it has been postulated that thyroid antigens such as thyroglobulin might attach to the eye muscles and cause tissue damage as immune complexes are formed between thyroglobulin and anti-thyroglobulin autoantibodies. An exophthalmos-stimulating autoantibody has been described. Antibody to a soluble eye-muscle antigen has also been demonstrated. A older hypothesis that is again gaining favor proposes that growth of retro-orbital tissues in autoimmune exophthalmos is due to TSH receptors on fat cells and muscle cells that are affected by thyroid-stimulating immunoglobulins. The nature of the orbital antigens is unresolved and controversial, revolving around discussions of the TSH receptor, a 64 kD autoantigen (295), a 72 kD heat shock protein (296), and the G2s gene product (297). Regarding the causes of ophthalmopathy associated with Graves' disease, there is evidence for both CD4 Th1 and CD4 Th2 subset involvement (298). Various therapies for extreme exophthalmos that threaten vision include prednisone, orbital irradiation, surgical decompression, and newer uses of immunomodulatory agents such as nicotinamide (299).

V. AUTOIMMUNE ADDISON'S DISEASE

Addison's disease is manifested as glucocorticoid and mineralocorticoid deficiency. Second only to iatrogenic adrenal cortical suppression from exogenous glucocorticoid administration, autoimmune adrenalitis with lymphocytic infiltration of the adrenal cortex is the most common cause of Addison's disease. In the era before antibiotics were available, tuberculosis was the most common cause of adrenal failure.

Complement-fixation testing using saline extracts of adrenal tissue was the first methodology employed to detect adrenal autoantibodies (300). Shortly thereafter, indirect immunofluorescence using cryocut sections of unfixed human adrenal cortical tissue became the method of choice for the detection of adrenal autoantibodies. Cytoplasmic fluorescence of the adrenal cortical cells demonstrates that adrenal cytoplasmic autoantibodies are present in the serum being tested (301). All layers of the adrenal cortex often fluoresce, whereas the medulla rarely fluoresces (302). The adrenal cortical cytoplasmic autoantigens were localized to the microsomes of the adrenal cortical cells by examination of ultracentrifuged adrenal fractions (303). A peroxidase-labeled protein A technique has been also been developed to detect adrenal autoantibodies (304). However, the results of such autoantibody testing were not identical to those using indirect immunofluorescence. Adrenal cytoplasmic autoantibodies are detected in up to 75–80% of new-onset subjects with Addison's disease (305).

Autoantibodies to the surface of human or murine adrenocortical cells can be detected in some patients by indirect immunofluorescence. In one study, 24 of 28 individuals (86%) with Addison's disease displayed auto-antibodies to the adrenal cell surface (306). Cytoplasmic and surface autoantibodies are strongly correlated. Because of the difficulty and expense of obtaining isolated viable adrenal cortical cells, such tests for surface autoantibodies are relegated to research laboratories and have been replaced by the enzyme autoantibody immunoassays discussed below.

In the 1990s, with the molecular cloning of the adrenal steroidogenic enzymes, various immunoassays were developed to detect autoantibodies directed against these enzymes. The adrenal enzymes 17-alpha-hydroxylase (307), 21-hydroxylase (308,309), and the side chain cleavage enzyme P450$_{scc}$ have been shown to be autoantigens targeted in individuals with adrenalitis. The P450$_{scc}$ enzyme autoantibody is identified in sera from patients with autoimmune polyglandular syndrome type 1 but not in patients with isolated autoimmune Addison's disease (310). The 21-hydroxylase autoantibodies are believed to be most clearly associated with Addison's disease and adrenal cytoplasmic autoantibodies (311). Germane to 21-hydroxylase as a major autoantigen in Addison's disease is that in-vitro-demonstrated suppression of in-vivo 21-hydroxylase activity does not advance progression to adrenal failure (312). This illustrates that while adrenal autoantibodies are plentiful in autoimmune Addison's disease, these autoantibodies are not pathogenic.

Similarly to the natural history of type 1 diabetes, the development of Addison's disease passes through various sequential, cumulative stages: elevated renin and normal to low aldosterone, deficient cortisol response to ACTH injection, elevated basal ACTH concentrations, and deficient basal aldosterone and cortisol secretion (313). Similarly to the predictive function of islet autoantibodies for the development of type 1 diabetes, autoantibodies directed against the adrenal cortical cytoplasm or steroidogenic enzymes precede the first appearance of the clinical manifestations of Addison's disease (314).

Adrenal cytoplasmic autoantibodies are predictive of the development of Addison's disease in children and, to a lesser degree, in adults (315). Complement-fixing adrenal cytoplasmic autoantibodies may be more strongly associated with progression to adrenal failure than those that do not fix complement (316). This likely reflects the fact that complement-fixing autoantibodies are higher-titer autoantibodies. This certainly appears to the case for "non-complement-fixing" ICA vs. "complement-fixing" ICA: higher-titer ICA more strongly predict the development of type 1 diabetes in nondiabetic individuals.

Addison's disease occurs in less than 3 years in up to 50% of initially asymptomatic adrenal cytoplasmic autoantibody-positive individuals. In adrenal cytoplasmic autoantibody-positive children, 9 of 10 developed Addison's disease during follow-up of up to 10 years. The nonaddisonian child, nevertheless, still had laboratory evidence of adrenal insufficiency (317).

The relationship between increased titers of adrenal autoantibodies (both cytoplasmic and 21-hydroxylase autoantibodies) and more severe degrees of impaired adrenocortical function and increased risk of progression to Addison's disease has been recognized (318). In the natural history of the development of Addison's disease, adrenal autoantibody concentrations were reported to rise until the development of clinical disease, when autoantibody reactivity waned.

Excluding autoimmune polyglandular syndrome 1, isolated autoimmune Addison's disease and autoimmune Addison's disease associated with autoimmune polyglandular syndrome 2 has been associated with HLA-B8 and HLA-DR3. These associations are no stronger than the HLA associations discussed for AITD and are considerably weaker than the HLA associations described for type 1 diabetes. Adrenalitis commonly occurs with other autoimmune diseases (autoimmune polyglandular syndrome types 1 and 2 [319]) and Addison's disease by itself or as part of autoimmune polyglandular syndrome 2 has also been associated with HLA-DR4 in addition to HLA-DR3. Therefore, the genetic basis for type 1 diabetes and Addison's disease is, in part, similarly linked to an HLA-associated gene or genes.

Polymorphisms of the CTLA-4 gene at the 49 A/G site were associated with Addison's disease in subjects with the HLA-DQA1*0501 allele (320). In studies of the (AT)n microsatellite within exon 3, the 106 base pair allele was more common in English patients with Addison's disease than controls but no difference was observed in Norwegians, Finns, or Estonians (321). In 2000, a study from the United Kingdom demonstrated an association between the G allele of the CTLA-4 A/G polymorphism in isolated Addison's disease as well as Addison's disease that was part of autoimmune polyglandular syndrome type 2 (322).

VI. ACQUIRED PRIMARY GONADAL FAILURE

In patients with hypergonadotropic hypogonadism, the presence of serum steroidal cell autoantibodies (SCA) detected by indirect immunofluorescence supports the diagnosis of an autoimmune cause for primary gonadal failure (323). SCA were described using indirect immunofluorescence as early as 1968 (324). In patients of either gender, such autoantibodies react with steroid hormone-producing cells in the theca interna/granulosa layer of graafian follicles, cells of the corpus luteum, the placental syncytiotrophoblast, Leydig's cells of the testes, and cells of the normal adrenal cortex. If SCA are present, an independent determination about the presence of adrenal cytoplasmic autoantibodies cannot be made.

Premature menopause, male climacteric, or infertility are clinical manifestations of gonaditis (325). Gonaditis is seen more often in female patients and is usually recognized in association with autoimmune polyglandular syndrome type 1 but can occur in autoimmune polyglandular

syndrome type 2. Approximately 1:4 women with autoimmune Addison's disease will exhibit amenorrhea and 10% will develop premature ovarian failure (326). In the absence of associated autoimmune disorders, SCA specifically against the ovary can be rare (327). On the other hand, Fenichel et al. (328) observed gonadal autoantibodies in ~60% of cases of idiopathic premature ovarian failure. SCA frequently predict later ovarian failure. Over 12 years of follow-up, ovarian failure occurred in 100% of SCA-positive women with autoimmune polyglandular syndrome type 1 (329).

Autoantibodies directed against steroidogenic enzymes in cases of gonaditis should not be surprising given the embryological commonality of the adrenal cortex and gonads. However, in the absence of associated adrenal autoimmunity, autoantibodies to P450scc 17-hydroxylase and 21-hydroxylase are uncommon (330,331), while autoantibodies to 3β-hydroxysteroid dehydrogenase have been reported in at least one study (332). Autoantibodies to 3β-hydroxysteroid dehydrogenase in women with premature ovarian failure have been associated with DQB1 alleles with aspartic acid at position 57 (333). This might be somewhat surprising since non-aspartic-acid residue 57 DQB1 alleles increase risk for type 1 diabetes.

VII. IDIOPATHIC HYPOPARATHYROIDISM

Idiopathic (presumed autoimmune) hypoparathyroidism in children is often seen in association with mucocutaneous candidiasis or autoimmune Addison's disease as part of autoimmune polyglandular syndrome type 1 (334). Lymphocytic infiltration of the parathyroid glands is observed in cases of idiopathic hypoparathyroidism, especially if associated with autoimmune polyglandular syndrome type 1. This attests to the autoimmune nature of so-called idiopathic hypoparathyroidism in at least some patients.

There is continued controversy about whether parathyroid autoantibodies can be detected by indirect immunofluorescence (335,336). Parathyroid autoantibodies detected by indirect immunofluorescence can be preabsorbed with human mitochondria, indicating that such parathyroid autoantibodies are not tissue-specific (337). Using Western blotting, autoantibodies to the extracellular domain of the calcium receptor in patients with hypoparathyroidism have been reported (338). However this finding has yet to be substantiated by other research laboratories. Autoantibodies cytotoxic for cultured bovine parathyroid cells in subjects with hypoparathyroidism have been described (339). Finally autoantibodies to circulating parathyroid hormone (340,341) and the renal tubular parathyroid hormone receptor (342) have been observed in adults but have not so far been described in children.

In the absence of recognized causes of hypoparathyroidism (eg., postparathyroidectomy or DiGeorge syndrome), and in the absence of candidiasis and Addison's disease (or adrenal autoantibodies), it is presently not possible to confirm the diagnosis of idiopathic hypoparathyroidism as autoimmune in etiology because of the lack of confirmed autoantibodies to the parathyroid gland that can be easily measured (see Chapter 19).

VIII. HYPOPHYSITIS AND AUTOIMMUNE DISEASE OF THE PITUITARY

In rare cases of hypopituitarism in which mass lesions of the pituitary were suspected, histological examination of surgical specimens has revealed hypophysitis (343). Such idiopathic lymphocytic hypophysitis is believed to be autoimmune in etiology. In some patients with type 1 diabetes, as well as their immediate relatives, autoantibodies reactive with prolactin and growth-hormone-secreting cells have been visualized by indirect immunofluorescence (344). No associations between such autoantibodies and clinical disease were recognized in these individuals. By Western blotting, pituitary autoantigens of 40 kDa and 49 kDa have been identified, although expression of these proteins was not restricted to the pituitary (345). For the 49 kDA autoantibody, positive sera were most common in subjects with lymphocytic hypophysitis (70%) with lower frequencies in subjects with Addison's disease (42%), thyroid autoimmunity (15%), rheumatoid arthritis (13%), and normal subjects (10%). In a group of Swedish patients with hypopituitarism, 28% had 49 kDa autoantibodies (346). Cases of lymphocytic hypophysitis continue to be reported (347) and definitely occur in children (348). However idiopathic hypopituitarism in children is believed generally to be rarely caused by autoimmunity (349).

IX. AUTOIMMUNE DIABETES INSIPIDUS

In some patients with idiopathic diabetes insipidus (DI), autoantibodies to the antidiuretic-hormone-producing cells of the hypothalamus have been recognized (350). Problematic is the need for fresh human hypothalamus as substrate for indirect immunofluorescence. DI-associated hypothalamic (vasopressin-cell) autoantibodies are not removed by preabsorption with vasopressin, oxytocin, neurophysin I, or neurophysin II (351). Up to one-third of children with otherwise idiopathic DI may have an autoimmune process responsible for their condition. An adult has been reported with scleroderma and DI (352). Suspected autoimmune DI has also been observed in cases of autoimmune polyglandular syndrome type 1 (353) and other autoimmune conditions (354–356). Adolescents with autoimmune DI and hypophysitis have been reported (357,358). Most cases of hypophysitis do not involve the posterior pituitary. DI-associated hypothalamic (vasopressin-cell) autoantibodies can precede the development of DI and appear to be predictive of the development of DI in initially unaffected subjects (359,360).

X. ASSOCIATED NONENDOCRINE AUTOIMMUNE DISEASES

A. Chronic Lymphocytic Gastritis Producing Atrophic Change

Gastritis has been classified as type A gastritis with sparing of the antrum, evidence of autoimmunity to the gastric parietal cells, destruction of the parietal cells and hypergastrinemia; or as type B gastritis due to *Helicobacter pylori* infection with involvement of the antrum and hypogastrinemia (361). Autoimmune atrophic gastritis (type A gastritis) due to chronic lymphocytic infiltration of the gastric fundus, as noted previously, is commonly associated with thyroiditis and type 1 diabetes (362–364). In this process the gastric parietal cells in the fundus and body of the stomach are destroyed along with their ability to secrete hydrochloric acid and intrinsic factor. Achlorhydria can be frequently found; however, intrinsic factor secretion is usually preserved except in cases of long-standing gastric autoimmunity. With prolonged deficiency of intrinsic factor, pernicious anemia manifested as a megaloblastic anemia and neuropathy may occur during mid to late life.

Autoantibodies to the cytoplasm of the gastric parietal cell (PCA) and autoantibodies that block vitamin B12 binding to intrinsic factor (IF-blocking autoantibodies), or block the absorption of the IF–vitamin B12 complex, are markers for chronic lymphocytic gastritis. PCA are assayed by indirect immunofluorescence using stomach fundus as substrate. As noted previously, the target autoantigen in chronic lymphocytic gastritis is the H^+/K^+ ATPase pump. An ELISA methodology for the detection of H^+/K^+ ATPase pump autoantibodies has been described (365).

Gastric parietal cell autoantibodies often appear early in the course of the disease, are associated with achlorhydria, and are absent in about half the patients by the time pernicious anemia is clinically apparent. Intrinsic factor autoantibodies can appear late in the course of disease, often close to the onset of pernicious anemia and thereafter.

B. Chronic Hepatitis

In the absence of a previous hepatitis B or hepatitis C infection, chronic hepatitis may result from an autoimmune process. Chronic autoimmune hepatitis is observed frequently in autoimmune polyglandular syndrome type 1. The presence of autoantibodies to smooth muscle (SMA; ~50% prevalence), mitochondria (antimitochondrial antibodies [AMA]; ~15% prevalence) and liver–kidney–mitochondrion-1 [LKM1]) can serve as markers for autoimmune hepatitis (366). Although nonspecific, antinuclear antibodies (ANA) can also be observed in ~80% of cases of autoimmune hepatitis.

Nine different mitochondrial antigens have been described termed M1 through M9. The E2 subunit of the pyruvate dehydrogenase complex (the M2 AMA antigen), the asialoglycoprotein receptor (367), cytochrome P450, UDP-glucuronosyl-transferases (368), and F-actin (the SMA autoantigen) are autoantigens described in chronic hepatitis.

C. Celiac Disease

Celiac disease (also known as celiac sprue or gluten-induced enteropathy) is characterized by gluten intolerance, abnormal small bowel histological changes, and malabsorption. IgA autoantibodies against gliadin, reticulin, and endomysium have been described in subjects with celiac disease, but the major autoantigen appears to be the enzyme transglutaminase (369). Individuals with transglutaminase autoantibodies (370) should undergo periodic small bowel biopsy. If the histological findings of celiac disease are identified, wheat and wheat products should be eliminated from the diet. Transglutaminase autoantibodies have been detected in ~10% of subjects with type 1 diabetes.

XI. AUTOIMMUNE DISEASE ASSOCIATIONS

The concurrence of multiple autoimmune endocrinopathies (with or without other nonendocrine autoimmune diseases) is common. Two consistent associations have been classified into the autoimmune polyglandular syndromes (APS) (371,372) (Table 10). Almost every disease combination (Table 11) has been noted clinically.

A. APS-1

In APS-1, the primary diseases usually present clinically in the order listed in Table 10. If a component disease is skipped, it usually does not present later. Malabsorption, early-onset pernicious anemia, alopecia, vitiligo, primary

Table 10 Autoimmune Polyglandular Syndromes

Type	Diagnostic criteria
1	At least two of the following: Mucocutaneous candidiasis Hypoparathyroidism Addison's disease or adrenal autoantibodies
2	Addison's disease (or adrenal autoantibodies) plus Autoimmune thyroid disease (Schmidt syndrome) Insulin dependent diabetes, or Autoimmune thyroid disease and insulin-dependent diabetes (Carpenter syndrome)

Table 11 Autoimmune Polyglandular Syndromes

	Diabetes	
	Type 1	Type 2
Adrenalitis/Addison's disease	+++	+++
Hypoparathyroidism	+++	−
Mucocutaneous candidiasis	+++	−
Dental enamel hypoplasia/nail dystrophy	++	−
AITD	+	+++
Type 1 diabetes	+	+++
Gonaditis	++	+
Hypophysitis	−	+
Autoimmune hepatitis	++	+
Vitiligo/alopecia	+	+
Dermatitis herpetiformis	−	+
Fat malabsorption	+	−
IgA deficiency	+	+
Celiac disease	−	+
Autoimmune pernicious anemia	+	+
Pure red cell aplasia	+	−
Immune thrombocytopenic purpura	−	+
Progressive myopathy	+	−
Myasthenia gravis	−	+
Stiff man syndrome	−	+
Parkinson's disease	−	+

−, unobserved or rare; +, observed; ++, common; +++, pathognomonic.

hypogonadism, and chronic active hepatitis may frequently accompany APS-1. AITD and/or type 1 diabetes are infrequently encountered. Another term used for APS-1 is autoimmune polyendocrinopathy–candidiasis–ectodermal dystrophy (APECED), emphasizing that selective immunoendocrinopathies are associated with candidiasis and ectodermal problems.

APS-1 can be identified in siblings although most cases are sporadic. The greatest recent development in the genetics of autoimmune endocrine disease was the identification of a single gene locus termed the autoimmune regular (AIRE) that is responsible for APS-1 (373) [located on chromosome 21 (374)]. Homozygosity or compound heterozygosity for AIRE mutations produces APS-1 in an autosomal recessive pattern of inheritance (375). The predicted protein sequence of AIRE suggests that AIRE functions as a transcription factor (376).

B. APS-2

APS-2 was first described by Schmidt (Schmidt syndrome: Addison's disease plus chronic lymphocytic thyroiditis) and later as Carpenter syndrome (Schmidt syndrome plus type 1 diabetes). Unlike APS-1, which presents in childhood, APS-2 can occur at any age, but occurs more commonly in midlife and shows a female

Table 12 Autoimmune Endocrinopathy Associations

A. Type 1 diabetes	Autoimmune thyroid disease
	Chronic lymphocytic thyroiditis
	Graves' disease
	Pernicious anemia
	Addison's disease
B. Genetic syndromes (Down, Turner, Klinefelter)	Type 1 diabetes
	Autoimmune thyroid disease
	Chronic lymphocytic thyroiditis
	Graves' disease
	Pernicious anemia
C. Congenital infections (rubella)	Type 1 diabetes
	Chronic lymphocytic thyroiditis

C. Other Autoimmune Endocrinopathy Associations

The association of type 1 diabetes with thyrogastric autoimmunity is of great clinical importance (378) (Table 12). Approximately 20% of patients with type 1 diabetes have TMA, and 9% have PCA. These autoantibodies are usually present at the time of diagnosis of type 1 diabetes. Of type 1 diabetes patients with TMA, almost one-half will eventually manifest thyroid dysfunction. Of these, 80% develop primary hypothyroidism, while the remaining 20% will manifest Graves' disease. Hyperthyroidism may precede the clinical onset of type 1 diabetes.

In childhood, frank pernicious anemia is unusual in type 1 diabetes patients with PCA; however, achlorhydria is commonly associated with the PCA autoantibody. Adrenal cytoplasmic autoantibodies are present in 2% of type 1 diabetes patients and are most commonly associated with TMA and PCA (APS-2). Six percent of children and young adults with type 1 diabetes and TMA have adrenal cytoplasmic autoantibodies. Approximately one-half of patients with adrenal cytoplasmic autoantibodies will show evidence of chemical hypoadrenocorticalism (i.e., raised basal renin/ACTH levels) while 20% will have more overt features of adrenocortical insufficiency when

predominance (2:1) in contrast to APS-1 in which the gender ratio is unbiased. APS-2 is strongly associated with HLA-DR3 and DR4 and may share certain common genetic origins with type 1 diabetes (377). However, when subjects with type 1 diabetes are excluded from the APS-2–HLA analysis, the strong HLA association disappears.

Table 13 Clinically Useful Tests for the Diagnosis of Autoimmune Endocrinopathies and Related Diseases

Disease	Autoantibody	Technique
Type 1 diabetes	**ICA:** Islet cell cytoplasmic autoantibody	IFL (unfixed blood group O pancreas)
	IAA: Insulin autoantibody	RBA
	GADA: GAD autoantibody	RBA
	IA-2A: IA-2 autoantibody	RBA
Chronic lymphocytic thyroiditis	**TMA:** Thyroid microsomal autoantibody	HA, IFL, RIA, CF, latex agglutination
	TPOAb: thyroperoxidase autoantibody	RIA or immunochemiluminometric assay
	TGA: Thyroglobulin autoantibody	HA, IFL, RIA, CF, latex agglutination
Graves' disease	**TMA, TPOAb, TGA**	See above
	TBII: Thyrotropin-binding inhibitory immunoglobulin	Radioreceptor assay
	TSI: Thyroid-stimulating immunoglobulin	In vitro bioassay, RIA
Addison's disease	**ACA:** Adrenal cytoplasmic autoantibody	IFL
	21-hydroxylase autoantibody	RBA
Primary gonadal failure	**SCA:** Steroidal cell autoantibody	IFL
	3β-hydroxysteroid dehydrogenase autoantibody	RBA
Associated nonendocrine diseases		
Chronic lymphocytic gastritis/ pernicious anemia	**PCA:** Gastric parietal cell autoantibody	IFL
	IFAb: Intrinsic factor blocking autoantibody	RIA
Chronic active hepatitis	**SMA:** Smooth muscle autoantibody	IFL
	Mitochondrial autoantibody	IFL
Celiac disease	**Transglutaminase** autoantibody	ELISA
Vitiligo	Melanocyte or tyrosinase autoantibody	IFL
		WB

CF, complement fixation; ELISA, enzyme-linked immunosorbent assay; HA, hemagglutination; IFL, indirect immunofluorescence; RBA, radiobinding assay; RIA, radioimmunoassay; WB, Western blot.

studied (379). At least 1:6 such patients will ultimately develop clinical Addison disease, giving an overall prevalence of Addison disease in type 1 diabetes patients of 0.33% (1:300).

In many genetic syndromes, especially those with chromosomal abnormalities (i.e., Down, Turner, and Klinefelter syndromes), increased frequencies of autoimmune endocrinopathies (especially thyrogastric autoimmunity and type 1 diabetes) are recognized. In patients with congenital infections such as rubella, the frequencies of AITD and type 1 diabetes are increased. Undoubtedly new autoimmune polyendocrinopathies will continue to be described in the future such as the triple H syndrome (dysfunction of the hippocampus [impaired anterograde memory], hair follicle [alopecia areata], and hypothalamic–pituitary–adrenal axis from isolated ACTH deficiency) (380).

Table 13 outlines a variety of tests available for autoantibody detection. Those in bold are often of greatest potential value to the clinician. A positive autoantibody result in an unaffected individual can predict the later development of autoimmune disease. In an affected individual, a positive autoantibody result can demonstrate that the disease in question has an autoimmune cause. A clinical approach to the testing of clinically unaffected yet autoantibody-positive individuals is presented in Table 14 (see below). Again, prediction and prevention studies concerning type 1 diabetes should only be carried out in a research setting.

XII. CLINICAL APPROACH TO THE AUTOIMMUNE ENDOCRINOPATHIES AND RELATED DISEASES

In general, whenever one autoimmune disease is suspected or diagnosed, a search for other autoimmune diseases should be launched guided by knowledge of the common associations noted previously (381,382).

Any patient with TMA/TPOAb should be studied for PCA and vice versa. Any patient with TMA/TPOAb and/or PCA should be evaluated for adrenocortical cytoplasmic or 21-hydroxylase autoantibodies, especially if type 1 diabetes is present. Because of the high frequency of CLT and atrophic gastritis in patients with type 1 diabetes, all type 1 diabetes patients should be screened

Table 14 Clinical Evaluation of Individuals Positive for Various Autoantibodies

Condition/autoantibody(s)	Yearly clinical evaluation/measurement
ICA, GADA, IA-2A and/or IAA[a]	Frequently sampled intravenous glucose tolerance test: if first-phase insulin response is repeatedly <1% percentile, enter into research trial to prevent type 1 diabetes*; in established type 1 diabetes: measure TMA/TPOAb and/or TGA, and PCA; islet autoantibody positivity usually confirms autoimmune diabetes from beta-cell attack.
TMA, TPOAb, and/or TGA	TSH measurement; if abnormal: measure FT4; treat either hypo- or hyperthyroidism; measure PCA (because of thyrogastric autoimmunity association)
Adrenal cytoplasmic autoantibody (or) 21-hydroxylase autoantibody	Cortrosyn stimulation test; supine renin; treat glucocorticoid and/or mineralocorticoid deficiency (Addison's disease)
Steroidal cell autoantibody (or) 3β-hydroxysteroid dehydrogenase autoantibody	Estradiol in women or testosterone in men, LH and FSH; treat hypogonadism; also: evaluate adrenal function as per adrenal cytoplasmic autoantibody or 21-hydroxylase autoantibody positive
Gastric parietal cell autoantibody	Vitamin B12 (if >100 and <300 pg/ml: measure plasma or urine methylmalonic acid); ferritin; treat vitamin B12 and/or iron deficiency; measure TMA/TPOAb and TGA (because of thyrogastric autoimmunity association)
Smooth muscle autoantibody (or) mitochondrial autoantibody	Alanine amino transferase; if abnormal: total protein, albumin, total and direct bilirubin, alkaline phosphatase; liver biopsy; if hepatitis is detected, treat autoimmune hepatitis (e.g., glucocorticoid therapy)
Transglutaminase autoantibodies	Small bowel biopsy
Autoimmune polyglandular syndrome type 1 without apparent hypoparathyroidism	Calcium and phosphate; if hypocalcemia and/or hyperphosphatemia detected: measure intact PTH; treat hypoparathyroidism
Autoimmune polyglandular syndrome type 1 without apparent hypoadrenalism	Adrenal cytoplasmic autoantibody (or) 21-hydroxylase autoantibody [and] cortrosyn stimulation test and supine renin; manage as above per adrenal cytoplasmic or 21-hydroxylase autoantibody-positive
Mucocutaneous candidiasis and/or isolated hypoparathyroidism	Test for adrenal cytoplasmic or 21-hydroxylase autoantibodies; if positive, follow up as per adrenal cytoplasmic autoantibody or 21-hydroxylase autoantibody-positive

[a]For research purposes only.

at the time of diagnosis of type 1 diabetes for TMA/TPOAb and PCA (383). Patients with serological evidence of thyroid autoimmunity should have thyroid-stimulating hormone (TSH) measured yearly to detect incipient hypo- or hyperthyroidism in their earliest stages (384). PCA-positive patients should have yearly measurements of serum vitamin B12 and ferritin levels, and be given replacement treatment accordingly.

At present, screening for ICA, IAA, GADA, and IA-2A in the general population and first-degree relatives of type 1 diabetes patients is not recommended outside of the research setting because definitive, safe, and totally efficacious immunotherapy is not currently available. Likewise HLA typing to assess risk for type 1 diabetes is not recommended. On the other hand, individuals with a family history of CLT or atrophic gastritis should be screened for TMA/TPOAb and PCA.

Patients with mucocutaneous candidiasis and/or hypoparathyroidism should be tested for adrenal cytoplasmic or 21-hydroxylase autoantibodies. Patients with such autoantibodies should then undergo yearly assessment of adrenal function consisting of a cortrosyn stimulation test and/or morning cortisol and ACTH measurements and peripheral plasma renin activity after the patient has been supine for at least 30 min. Patients with APS-1 should be tested for steroidal cell autoantibodies and the development of gonadal failure near the time of puberty. This can be accomplished by measuring levels of sex steroids and gonadotropins. Such patients should also be screened for mitochondrial and smooth-muscle autoantibodies as indicators of chronic active hepatitis. At that time, serial studies of liver function (e.g., ALT) would be indicated.

XIII. SUMMARY

Numerically, the majority of endocrine disorders seen in childhood are the result of autoimmune processes. Recognition of the interrelationships among the autoimmune endocrinopathies provides the rationale for autoantibody screening. Identification of autoantibody-positive individuals followed by appropriate endocrine testing allows the clinician to anticipate and treat disease states before their frank clinical presentation. This can lower the morbidity and mortality of autoimmune endocrine disorders in childhood. In the long run, this should lower the costs of caring for patients with these highly prevalent conditions.

REFERENCES

1. Janeway CA. How the immune system recognized invaders. Sci Am 1993; September:73–79.
2. Unanue ER. The concept of antigen processing and presentation. JAMA 1995;274:1071–1073. Strominger JL, Wiley DC: The class I and class II proteins of the human major histocompatibility complex. JAMA 1995; 274: 1074–1076.
3. Delves PJ, Roitt IM. The immune system. First of two parts. N Engl J Med. 2000 343(1):37–49. Delves PJ, Roitt IM. The immune system. Second of two parts. N Engl J Med 2000; 343(2):108–117.
4. Abbas AK, Murphy KM, Sher A. Functional diversity of helper T lymphocytes. Nature 1996; 383:787–793.
5. Blobe GC, Schiemann WP, Lodish HF. Role of transforming growth factor beta in human disease. N Engl J Med 2000; 342(18):1350–1358.
6. Kroemer G, Martinez-A C. Immunol Today 1992; 13(10): 401–404.
7. Nossal GJV. Life, death and the immune system. Sci Am 1993; September 53–62; Ramsdell F, Fowlkes BJ. Clonal deletion versus clonal anergy: the role of the thymus in inducing self tolerance. Science 1990; 248:1342–1348.
8. Marrack P, Kappler JW. How the immune system recognizes the body. Sci Am 1993; September:81–89.
9. Buchs AE, Rapoport MJ. T cell signaling and autoimmune diabetes. J Pediatr Endocrinol Metab 2000; 13(9): 1549–1554.
10. Sinha AA, Lopez MT, McDevitt HO. Autoimmune diseases: the failure of self tolerance. Science 1990; 248: 1380–1388.
11. Bjorses P, Aaltonen J, Horelli-Kuitunen N, Yaspo ML, Peltonen L. Gene defect behind APECED: a new clue to autoimmunity. Hum Mol Genet 1998; 7(10):1547–1553.
12. Theofilopoulos AN. The basis of autoimmunity: part II. Genetic predisposition. Immunol Today 1995; 16(3):150–159.
13. Theofilopoulos AN. The basis of autoimmunity: part I. Mechanisms of aberrant self-recognition. Immunol Today 1995; 16(2):90–98.
14. Albert LJ, Inman RD. Molecular mimicry and autoimmunity. N Engl J Med. 1999; 30:341(2):2068–2074.
15. Ridgway WM, Fathman CG. The association of MHC with autoimmune diseases: understanding the pathogenesis of autoimmune diabetes. Clin Immunol Immunopathol 1998; 86(1):3–10.
16. Bodansky HJ, Dean BM, Grant PJ, et al. Does exposure to rubella virus generate endocrine autoimmunity? Diabet Med 1990; 7(7):611–614; Röcken M, Urban JF, Shevach EM. Infection breaks T-cell tolerance. Nature 1992; 359(6390):79–82.
17. Bellgrau D, Eisenbarth GS. Immunobiology of autoimmunity. In: Eisenbarth GS, ed. Endocrine and Organ-Specific Autoimmunity. RG Landes Co. 1999:1–11.
18. Liblau RS, Singer SM, McDevitt HO. Th1 and Th2 CD4+ T cells in the pathogenesis of organ-specific autoimmune diseases. Immunol Today 1995; 16(1):34–38.
19. Riley WJ. Enzymes as antigens in autoimmune endocrinopathies. Clin Chem 1995; 41(3):33–39.
20. Song YH, Li Y, Maclaren NK. The nature of autoantigens targeted in autoimmune endocrine diseases. Immunol Today 1996; 17(5):232–238.
21. Winter WE. The immunoendocrinopathies. Part 1: Overview and insulin-dependent diabetes mellitus. AACC Diagnostic Endocrinology and Metabolism In-Service Training and Continuing Education 1996; 14(1):13–21.
22. Winter WE. The immunoendocrinopathies. Part 2: Autoimmune thyroid disease, autoimmune Addison disease, and related disorders. AACC Diagnostic Endocrinology and Metabolism In-Service Training and Continuing Education 1996; 14(2):45–52.
23. Wilkin TJ. Receptor autoimmunity in endocrine disorders. N Engl J Med 1990; 323:1318–1324.

24. Volpe R. Autoimmunity causing thyroid dysfunction. Endocrinol Metab Clin North Am 1991; 20:565–587.

25. Raines K B, Baker JR, Lukes YG, Wartofsky L, Burman KD. Antithyrotropin antibodies in the sera of Graves' disease patients. J Clin Endocrinol Metab 1985; 61:217–222.

26. Carstensen H, Krabbe S, Wulffraat NM, Nielsen MD, Ralfkiaer E, Drexhage HA. Autoimmune involvement in Cushing syndrome due to primary adrenocortical nodular dysplasia. Eur J Pediatr 1989; 149:84–87.

27. Kuwahara A, Kamada M, Irahara M, Naka O, Yamashita T, Aono T. Autoantibody against testosterone in a woman with hypergonadotropic hypogonadism. J Clin Endocrinol Metab 1998;83(1):14–16.

28. Rose NR, Bona C. Defining criteria for autoimmune diseases. Immunol Today 1993; 14(9):426–430.

29. Vernino S, Low PA, Fealey RD, Stewart JD, Farrugia G, Lennon VA. Autoantibodies to ganglionic acetylcholine receptors in autoimmune autonomic neuropathies. N Engl J Med 2000; 343(12):847–855.

30. Rabinovitch A. An update on cytokines in the pathogenisis of insulin-dependent diabetes mellitus. Diabetes/Metabol Rev 1998; 14:129–151.

31. Nakamura RM. Human autoimmune diseases: progess in clinical laboratory tests. Med Lab Observ 2000; 32(10): 32–34.

32. American Diabetes Association. Clinical Practice Recommendations 2000: Report of the Expert Committee on the Diagnosis and Classification of Diabetes Mellitus. Diabetes Care 2000; 23(Suppl.1):S4–S19.

33. Taylor SI, Arioglu E. Genetically defined forms of diabetes in children. J Clin Endocrinol Metab 1999; 84: 4390–96; Winter WE, Nakamura M, House DV. Monogenic diabetes mellitus in youth: the MODY syndromes. Endocrinol Metab Clin North Am 1999; 28(4):765–785.

34. van den Ouweland JM, Lemkes HH, Trembath RC, et al. Maternally inherited diabetes and deafness is a distinct subtype of diabetes and associates with a single point mutation in the mitochondrial tRNA(Leu(UUR)) gene. Diabetes 1994; 43(6):746–751.

35. Karam JH, Lewitt PA, Young CW. Insulinopenic diabetes after rodenticide (Vacor) ingestion: a unique model of acquired diabetes in man. Diabetes 1980; 29:971–978.

36. Hauser L, Sheehan P, Simpkins H. Pancreatic pathology in pentamidine-induced diabetes in acquired immunodeficiency syndrome patients. Hum Pathol 1991; 229:926–929.

37. Yoon JW, Austin M, Onodera T, Notkins AL. Virus-induced diabetes mellitus. N Engl J Med 1979; 300:1173–1179.

38. Forrest JM, Menser MA, Burgess JA. High frequency of diabetes mellitus in young adults with congenital rubella. Lancet 1971; 2:332–334.

39. Winter WE. Diabetes mellitus: pathophysiology, etiologies, complications, management, and laboratory evaluation. Washington D.C.: American Association for Clinical Chemistry, Inc. (monograph), 1999:1–99.

40. The Diabetes Control and Complications Trial Research Group. The effect of intensive treatment of diabetes on the development and progression of long-term complications in insulin-dependent diabetes mellitus. N Engl J Med 1993; 329:977–986.

41. Kukreja A, Maclaren NK. Autoimmunity and diabetes. J Clin Endocrinol Metab 1999; 84(12):4371–8; Kawasaki E, Gill RG, Eisenbarth GS. Type 1 diabetes mellitus. In Eisenbarth GS, ed. Endocrine and Organ Specific Autoimmunity. Austin, TX: RG Landes Company, 1999:149–182.

42. Ziegler AG, Hummel M, Schenker M, Bonifacio E. Autoantibody appearance and risk for development of childhood diabetes in offspring of parents with type 1 diabetes: the 2-year analysis of the German BABYDIAB Study. Diabetes 1999; 48(3):460–468.

43. Cilio CM, Bosco A, Moretti C, Farilla L, Savignoni F, Colarizi P, Multari G, Di Mario U, Bucci G, Dotta F. Congenital autoimmune diabetes mellitus. N Engl J Med 2000; 342(20):1529–1531.

44. Lampeter EF, Homberg M, Quabeck K, Schaefer UW, Wernet P, Bertrams J, Grosse-Wilde H, Gries FA, Kolb H. Transfer of insulin-dependent diabetes between HLA-identical siblings by bone marrow transplantation. Lancet 1993; 341(8855):1243–1244.

45. Almawi WY, Tamim H, Azar ST. Clinical review 103: T helper type 1 and 2 cytokines mediate the onset and progression of type I (insulin-dependent) diabetes. J Clin Endocrinol Metab 1999; 84(5):1497–1450.

46. Gepts W, Lecompte PM. The pancreatic islets in diabetes. Am J Med 1981; 70:105–115.

47. House DV, Nakamura M, Winter WE. Autoimmune markers of type I diabetes mellitus. In Nakamura RM, Burek CL, Cook L, Folds JD, eds. Clinical Diagnostic Immunology: Protocols In Quality Assurance and Standardization. Cambridge, MA: Blackwell Science, 1998:234–249.

48. Gottlieb PA, Eisenbarth GS. Diagnosis and treatment of pre-insulin dependent diabetes. Annu Rev Med 1998; 49: 391–405.

49. Karvonen M, Viik-Kajander M, Moltchanova E, Libman I, LaPorte R, Tuomilehto J. Incidence of childhood type 1 diabetes worldwide. Diabetes Mondiale (DiaMond) Project Group. Diabetes Care 2000; 23(10):1516–1526.

50. Becker KG. Comparative gentics of type 1 diabetes and autoimmune disease, common loci, common pathways? Diabetes 1999; 48:1353–1358.

51. Maclaren N, Riley W, Skordis N, Atkinson M, Spillar R, Silverstein J, Klein R, Vadheim C, Rotter J. Inherited susceptibility to insulin-dependent diabetes is associated with HLA-DR1, while DR5 is protective. Autoimmunity 1988; 1:197–205.

52. Winter WE, Maclaren NK, Riley WJ, Clarke DW, Kappy MS, Spillar RP. Maturity-onset diabetes of youth in Black Americans. N Engl J Med 1987; 316:285–291.

53. Khalil I, Deschamps I, Lepage V, al-Daccak R, Degos L, Hors J. Dose effect of cis- and trans-encoded HLA-DQ alpha beta heterodimers in IDDM susceptibility. Diabetes 1992; 41:378–384.

54. Ronningen KS. Genetics in the prediction of insulin-dependent diabetes mellitus: from theory to practice. Ann Med 1997; 29:387–392.

55. Greenbaum CJ, Schatz DA, Cuthbertson D, Zeidler A, Eisenbarth GS, Krischer JP. Islet cell antibody-positive relatives with human leukocyte antigen DQA1*0102, DQB1*0602: identification by the Diabetes Prevention Trial-type 1. J Clin Endocrinol Metab 2000; 85(3):1255–1260.

56. Gylling M, Tuomi T, Bjorses P, Kontiainen S, Partanen J, Christie MR, Knip M, Perheentupa J, Miettinen A. B-cell autoantibodies, human leukocyte antigen II alleles, and type 1 diabetes in autoimmune polyendocrinopathy–candidiasis–ectodermal dystrophy. J Clin Endocrinol Metab 2000; 85(12):4434–4440.

57. Todd JA, Bell JI, McDevitt HO. HLA-DQβ gene contributes to susceptibility and resistance to insulin-dependent diabetes mellitus. Nature 1987; 329:599–604.

58. Todd JA, Acha-Orbea H, Bell JI, Chao N, Fronek Z, Jacob CO, McDermott M, Sinha AA, Timmerman L, Steinman L, McDevitt HO. A molecular basis for MHC class II-associated autoimmunity. Science 1990; 240:1003–1008.

59. Baisch JM, Weeks T, Giles R, Hoover M, Stastny P, Capra JD. Analysis of HLA-DQ genotypes and susceptibility in insulin-dependent diabetes mellitus. N Engl J Med 1990; 322:1836–1841.

60. Owerbach D, Gunn S, Ty G, Wible L, Gabby KH. Oligonucleutide probes for HLA-DQA and DQB genes define susceptibility to type 1 (insulin-dependent) diabetes mellitus. Diabetologia 1988; 31:751–757.

61. Gutierrez-Lopez MD, Bertera S, Chantres MT, Vavassori C, Dorman JS, Trucco M, Serrano-Rios M. Susceptibility to type 1 (insulin-dependent) diabetes mellitus in Spanish patients correlates quantitatively with expression of HLA-DQ alpha Arg 52 and HLA-DQ beta non-Asp 57 alleles. Diabetologia 1992; 35:583–588.

62. Ikegami H, Tahara Y, Topyon C, Yamato E, Ogihara T, Noma Y, Shima K. Aspartic acid at position 57 of the HLA-DQβ chain is not protective against insulin-dependent diabetes mellitus in Japanese people. J Autoimmun 1990; 3:167–174.

63. Park Y, She JX, Wang CY, Lee H, Babu S, Erlich HA, Noble JA, Eisenbarth GS. Common susceptibility and transmission pattern of human leukocyte antigen DRB1-DQB1 haplotypes to Korean and Caucasian patients with type 1 diabetes. J Clin Endocrinol Metab 2000; 85(12):4538–4542.

64. Dorman JS, LaPorte RE, Stone RA, Trucco M. Worldwide differences in the incidence of type I diabetes are associated with amino acid variation at position 57 of the HLA-DQ β chain. Proc Natl Acad Sci USA 1990; 87:7370–737.

65. She JX. Susceptibility to type I diabetes: HLA-DQ and DR revisited. Immunol Today 1996l; 17(7):323–329.

66. Warram JH, Krolewski AS, Gottlieb MS, Kahn CR. Differences in risk of insulin-dependent diabetes in offspring of diabetic mothers and diabetic fathers. N Engl J Med 1984; 311:149–152.

67. Vadheim CM, Rotter JI, Maclaren NK, Riley WJ, Anderson CE. Preferential transmission of diabetic alleles within the HLA gene complex. N Engl J Med 1986; 315:1314–1318.

68. She JX, Marron MP. Genetic susceptibility factors in type 1 diabetes: linkagc, discquilibrium and functional analyses. Curr Opin Immunol 1998; 10(6):682–689.

69. Davies JL, Kawaguchi Y, Bennett ST, Copeman JB, Cordell HJ, Pritchard LE, Reed PW, Gough SC, Jenkins SC, Palmer SM, et al. A genome-wide search for human type 1 diabetes susceptibility genes. Nature 1994; 371(6493):130–136.

70. Buzzetti R, Quattrocchi CC, Nistico L. Dissecting the genetics of type 1 diabetes: relevance for familial clustering and differences in incidence. Diabetes Metab Rev 1998; 14(2):111–128.

71. Luo DF, Buzzetti R, Rotter JI, Maclaren NK, Raffel LJ, Nistico L, Giovannini C, Pozzilli P, Thomson G, She JX. Confirmation of three susceptibility genes to insulin-dependent diabetes mellitus: IDDM4, IDDM5 and IDDM8. Hum Mol Genet 1996; 5(5):693–698.

72. Pugliese A: Unraveling the genetics of insulin-dependent type 1A diabetes: the search must go on. Diabetes Rev 1999; 7:39–54.

73. Marron MP, Zeidler A, Raffel LJ, Eckenrode SE, Yang JJ, Hopkins DI, Garchon HJ, Jacob CO, Serrano-Rios M, Martinez Larrad MT, Park Y, Bach JF, Rotter JI, Yang MC, She JX. Genetic and physical mapping of a type 1 diabetes susceptibility gene (IDDM12) to a 100-kb phagemid artificial chromosome clone containing D2S72-CTLA4-D2S105 on chromosome 2q33. Diabetes 2000; 49(3):492–499.

74. She JX, Bui MM, Tian XH, Muir A, Wakeland EK, Zorovich B, Zhang LP, Liu MC, Thomson G, Maclaren NK. Additive susceptibility to insulin-dependent diabetes conferred by HLA-DQB1 and insulin genes. Autoimmunity 1994; 18(3):195–203.

75. Akerblom HK, Knip M. Putative environmental factors in type 1 diabetes. Diabetes/Metabol Rev 1998; 14:31–67.

76. Couper JJ, Steele C, Beresford S, Powell T, McCaul K, Pollard A, Gellert S, Tait B, Harrison LC, Colman PG. Lack of association between duration of breast-feeding or introduction of cow's milk and development of islet autoimmunity. Diabetes 1999; 48(11):2145–2149.

77. Graves PM, Barriga KJ, Norris JM, Hoffman MR, Yu L, Eisenbarth GS, Rewers M. Lack of association between early childhood immunizations and beta-cell autoimmunity. Diabetes Care 1999; 22(10):1694–1697.

78. Maclaren NK, Atkinson MA. Insulin-dependent diabetes mellitus: the hypothesis of molecular mimicry between islet cell antigens and microorganisms. Mol Med Today 1997; 76–83.

79. Law GR, McKinney PA, Staines A, Williams R, Kelly M, Alexander F, Gilman E, Bodansky HJ. Clustering of childhood IDDM. Links with age and place of residence. Diabetes Care. 1997; 20(5):753–756.

80. Honeyman MC, Coulson BS, Stone NL, Gellert SA, Goldwater PN, Steele CE, Couper JJ, Tait BD, Colman PG, Harrison LC. Association between rotavirus infection and pancreatic islet autoimmunity in children at risk of developing type 1 diabetes. Diabetes 2000; 49(8):1319–1324.

81. Hyoty H, Hiltunen M, Knip M, Laakkonen M, Vahasalo P, Karjalainen J, Koskela P, Roivainen M, Leinikki P, Hovi T, et al. A prospective study of the role of coxsackie B and other enterovirus infections in the pathogenesis of IDDM. Childhood Diabetes in Finland (DiMe) Study Group. Diabetes 1995; 44(6):652–657.

82. Vreugdenhil GR, Schloot NC, Hoorens A, Rongen C, Pipeleers DG, Melchers WJ, Roep BO, Galama JM. Acute onset of type I diabetes mellitus after severe echovirus 9 infection: putative pathogenic pathways. Clin Infect Dis 2000; 31(4):1025–1031.

83. Maclaren NK, Atkinson MA. Is insulin-dependent diabetes mellitus environmentally induced? N Engl J Med 1992; 327:347–349.

84. Karjalainen J, Martin J, Knip M. A bovine albumin peptide as a possible trigger of insulin-dependent diabetes mellitus. N Engl J Med 1992; 327:302–307.

85. Verge CF, Gianani R, Yu L, Pietropaolo M, Smith T, Jackson RA, Soeldner JS, Eisenbarth GS. Late progression to diabetes and evidence for chronic beta-cell autoimmunity in identical twins of patients with type I diabetes. Diabetes 1995; 44(10):1176–119.

86. Krokowski M, Caillat-Zucman S, Timsit J, Larger E, Pehuet-Figoni M, Bach JF, Boitard C. Anti-bovine serum

albumin antibodies: genetic heterogeneity and clinical relevance in adult-onset IDDM. Diabetes Care 1995; 18(2): 170–173.

87. Hummel M, Fuchtenbusch M, Schenker M, Ziegler AG. No major association of breast-feeding, vaccinations, and childhood viral diseases with early islet autoimmunity in the German BABYDIAB Study. Diabetes Care 2000; 23(7):969–974.

88. Cainelli F, Manzaroli D, Renzini C, Casali F, Concia E, Vento S. Coxsackie B virus-induced autoimmunity to GAD does not lead to type 1 diabetes. Diabetes Care 2000l; 23(7):1021–1022.

89. Casu A, Carlini M, Contu A, Bottazzo GF, Songini M. Type 1 diabetes in sardinia is not linked to nitrate levels in drinking water. Diabetes Care 2000; 23(7):1043–1044.

90. Lonnrot M, Korpela K, Knip M, Ilonen J, Simell O, Korhonen S, Savola K, Muona P, Simell T, Koskela P, Hyoty H. Enterovirus infection as a risk factor for beta-cell autoimmunity in a prospectively observed birth cohort: the Finnish Diabetes Prediction and Prevention Study. Diabetes 2000; 49(8):1314–1318.

91. Juhela S, Hyoty H, Roivainen M, Harkonen T, Putto-Laurila A, Simell O, Ilonen J. T-cell responses to enterovirus antigens in children with type 1 diabetes. Diabetes 2000; 49(8):1308–1313.

92. Winter WE. The use of islet autoantibody markers in the prediction of autoimmune type 1 diabetes. Clin Immunol Newslett 1999; 19(3):25–39.

93. Castano L, Russo E, Zhou L, Lipes MA, Eisenbarth GS. Identification and cloning of a granule autoantigen (carboxypeptidase-H) associated with type I diabetes. J Clin Endocrinol Metab 1991; 3:119–1201.

94. Rorsman F, Husebye ES, Winqvist O, Bjork E, Karlsson FA, Kampe O. Aromatic-L-amino-acid decarboxylase, a pyridoxal phosphate-dependent enzyme, is a beta-cell autoantigen. Proc Natl Acad Sci USA 1995; 92(19):8626–8629.

95. Kim YJ, Zhou Z, Hurtado J, Wood DL, Choi AS, Pescovitz MD, Warfel KA, Vandagriff J, Davis JK, Kwon BS. IDDM patients' sera recognize a novel 30-kD pancreatic autoantigen related to chymotrypsinogen. Immunol Invest 1993; 22(3):219–2.

96. Chang YH, Hwang J, Shang HF, Tsai ST. Characterization of human DNA topoisomerase II as an autoantigen recognized by patients with IDDM. Diabetes 1996; 45(4):408–414.

97. Pietropaolo M, Castaño L, Babu S, Buelow R, Kuo Y-LS, Martin S, Martin A, Powers AC, Prochazka M, Naggert J, Leiter EH, Eisenbarth GS. Islet cell autoantigen 69 kD (ICA69): molecular cloning and characterization of a novel diabetes-associated autoantigen. J Clin Invest 1993; 92:359–371.

98. Lampasona V, Ferrari M, Bosi E, Pastore MR, Bingley PJ, Bonifacio E. Sera from patients with IDDM and healthy individuals have antibodies to ICA69 on western blots but do not immunoprecipitate liquid phase antigen. J Autoimmun 1994; (5):665–664.

99. Pak CY, Cha CY, Rajotte RV, McArthur RG, Yoon JW. Human pancreatic islet cell specific 38 kilodalton autoantigen identified by cytomegalovirus-induced monoclonal islet cell autoantibody. Diabetologia 1990; 33(9):569–572.

100. Karounos DG, Thomas JW. Recognition of common islet antigen by autoantibodies from NOD mice and humans with IDDM. Diabetes 1990; 39(9):1085–1090.

101. Bohmer K, Keilacker H, Kuglin B, Hubinger A, Bertrams J, Gries FA, Kolb H. Proinsulin autoantibodies are more closely associated with type 1 (insulin-dependent) diabetes mellitus than insulin autoantibodies. Diabetologia 1991; 34(11):830–834.

102. Maron R, Elias D, DeJongh BM, Bruining GF, VanRood JJ, Shechter Y, Cohen IR. Autoantibodies to the insulin receptor in juvenile onset insulin-dependent diabetes. Nature 1983; 303:81–88.

103. Aanstoot HJ, Kang SM, Kim J, Lindsay LA, Roll U, Knip M, Atkinson M, Mose Larsen P, Fey S, Ludvigsson J, Landin M, Bruining J, Maclaren N, Akerblom HK, Baekkeskov S. Identification and characterization of glima 38, a glycosylated islet cell membrane antigen, which together with GAD65 and IA2 marks the early phases of autoimmune response in type 1 diabetes. J Clin Invest 1996; 97(12):2772–2783.

104. Johnson JH, Crider BP, McCorkle K, Alford M, Unger RH. Inhibition of glucose transport into rat islet cells by immunoglobulins from patients with new-onset insulin-dependent diabetes mellitus. N Engl J Med 1990; 332:653–659.

105. Atkinson MA, Holmes LA, Scharp DW, Lacy PE, Maclaren NK. No evidence for serological autoimmunity to islet cell heat shock proteins in insulin dependent diabetes. J Clin Invest 1991; 8:21–24.

106. Kasimiotis H, Myers MA, Argentaro A, Mertin S, Fida S, Ferraro T, Olsson J, Rowley MJ, Harley VR. Sex-determining region Y-related protein SOX13 is a diabetes autoantigen expressed in pancreatic islets. Diabetes 2000; 49(4):555–561.

107. Bottazzo GF, Florin-Christensen A, Doniach D. Islet-cell autoantibodies in diabetes mellitus with autoimmune polyendocrine deficiencies. Lancet 1994; 2:1279–1283.

108. Palmer JP, Asplin CM, Clemons P, Lyen K, Tatpati O, Raghu PK, Paquette TL. Insulin antibodies in insulin-dependent diabetics before insulin treatment. Science 1983; 222(4630):133–139.

109. Baekkeskov S, Aanstoot HJ, Christgau S, Reetz A, Solimena M, Cascalho M, Folli F, Richter-Olesen H, DeCamilli P, Camilli PD. Identification of the 64K autoantigen in insulin-dependent diabetes as the GABA-synthesizing enzyme glutamic acid decarboxylase. Nature 1990; 34:151–156.

110. Rabin DU, Pleasic SM, Shapiro JA, Yoo-Warren H, Oles J, Hicks JM, Goldstein DE, Rae PM. Islet cell antigen 512 is a diabetes-specific islet autoantigen related to protein tyrosine phosphatases. J Immunol 1994; 152(6):3183–3188.

111. Lernmark A, Freedman ZR, Hofmann C, Rubenstein AH, Steiner DF, Jackson RL, Winter RJ, Traisman HS. Islet-cell-surface antibodies in juvenile diabetes mellitus. N Engl J Med 198; 299:375–380.

112. Maclaren NK, Huang S-W. Antibody to cultured human insulinoma cells in insulin-dependent diabetes. Lancet 195; 1:997–999.

113. Neufeld M, Maclaren NK, Riley WJ, Lezotte D, McLaughlin JV, Silverstein J, Rosenbloom AL. Islet cell and other organ-specific antibodies in U.S. Caucasians and Blacks with insulin-dependent diabetes mellitus. Diabetes 19080; 29:589–592.

114. Schatz D, Krischer J, Horne G, Riley W, Spillar R, Silverstein J, Winter W, Muir A, Derovanesian D, ShahS, MaloneJ, Maclaren N. Islet cell antibodies predic insulin-dependent diabetes in United States school age children

as powerfully as in unaffected relatives. J Clin Invest 1994; 93:2403–2407.

115. Irvine WJ, McCallum CJ, Gray RS, Duncan LJP. Clinical and pathogenic significance of pancreatic islet-cell antibodies in diabetics treated with oral hypoglycemic agents. Lancet 1977; 1:1025–1027.

116. Di Mario U, Irvine WJ, Borsey DQ, Kyner JL, Weston J, and Galfo C. Immune abnormalities in diabetic patients not requiring insulin at diagnosis. Diabetologia 1983; 25: 392–395.

117. Niskanen L, Karjalaienen J, Sarlund H, Siitonen O, Uusitupa M. Five year follow-up of islet-cell antibodies in (non-insulin dependent) diabetes mellitus. Diabetologia 1991; 34:402–408.

118. Tuomi T, Groop LC, Zimmet PZ, Rowley MJ, Knowles W, Mackay IR. Antibodies to glutamic acid decarboxylase reveal latent autoimmune diabetes mellitus in adults with a non-insulin-dependent onset of disease. Diabetes 1993; 42:359–362.

119. Seissler J, de Sonnaville JJ, Morgenthaler NG, Steinbrenner H, Glawe D, Khoo Morgenthaler UY, Lan MS, Notkins AL, Heine RJ, Scherbaum WA. Immunological heterogeneity in type I diabetes: presence of distinct autoantibody patterns in patients with acute onset and slowly progressive disease. Diabetologia 1998; 41(8): 891–897.

120. Carlsson A, Sundkvist G, Groop L, Tuomi T. Insulin and glucagon secretion in patients with slowly progressing autoimmune diabetes (LADA). J Clin Endocrinol Metab 2000; 85(1):76–80.

121. Pietropaolo M, Barinas-Mitchell E, Pietropaolo SL, Kuller LH, Trucco M. Evidence of islet cell autoimmunity in elderly patients with type 2 diabetes. Diabetes 2000; 49(1):32–38.

122. Dobersen MJ, Scharff JE, Ginsberg-Fellner F, Notkins AL. Cytotoxic autoantibodies to beta cells in the serum of patients with insulin-dependent diabetes mellitus. N Engl J Med 1980; 303:1493–1498.

123. Kanatsuna T, Lernmark A. Rubinstein AH, Steiner DF. Block in insulin release from column-perfused pancreatic beta cells induced by islet cell surface antibodies and complement. Diabetes 1981; 30:231–234.

124. Riley WJ, Maclaren NK, Krischer J, Spillar RP, Silverstein JH, Schatz DA, Schwartz S, Malone J, Shah S, Vadheim C. A prospective study of the development of diabetes in relatives of patients with insulin-dependent diabetes. N Engl J Med 1990; 323:1167–1172.

125. Palmer JP. Predicting IDDM: use of humoral immune markers. Diabetes Rev 1993; 1:104–115.

126. Schatz DA, Barrett DJ, Maclaren NK, Riley WJ. Polyclonal nature of islet cell antibodies in insulin-dependent diabetes. Autoimmunity 1988; 1:45–50.

127. Decochez K, Keymeulen B, Somers G, Dorchy H, De Leeuw IH, Mathieu C, Rottiers R, Winnock F, ver Elst K, Weets I, Kaufman L, Pipeleers DG, Rottiers R. Use of an islet cell antibody assay to identify type 1 diabetic patients with rapid decrease in C-peptide levels after clinical onset. Belgian Diabetes Registry. Diabetes Care 2000; 23(8):1072–1078.

128. Torn C, Landin-Olsson M, Lernmark A, Palmer JP, Arnqvist HJ, Blohme G, Lithner F, Littorin B, Nystrom L, Schersten B, Sundkvist G, Wibell L, Ostman J. Prognostic factors for the course of B cell function in autoimmune diabetes. J Clin Endocrinol Metab 2000; 85(12): 4619–4623.

129. Atkinson MA, Maclaren NK, Riley WJ, Winter WE, Fisk DD, Spillar RP. Are insulin autoantibodies markers for insulin-dependent diabetes mellitus? Diabetes 1986; 35: 894–898.

130. Greenbaum CJ, Palmer JP, Kuglin B, Kolb H: Insulin autoantibodies measured by radioimmunoassay methodology are more related to insulin-dependent diabetes mellitus than those measured by enzyme-linked immunosorbent assay: results of the Fourth International Workshop on the Standardization of Insulin Autoantibody Measurement. J Clin Endocrinol Metab 1992; 74(5):1040–1044.

131. Levy-Marchal C, Bridel MP, Sodoyez-Goffaux F, Koch M, Tichet J, Czernichow P, Sodoyez JC Superiority of radiobinding assay over ELISA for detection of IAAs in newly diagnosed type I diabetic children. Diabetes Care 1991; 14(1):61–63.

132. Nayak RC, Omar MAK, Rabizadeh A, Srikanta S, Eisenbarth GS. "Cytoplasmic" islet cell antibodies. Evidence that the target antigen is a sialoglycoconjugate. Diabetes 1985; 34:617–619.

133. Lan MS, Wasserfall C, Maclaren NK, Notkins AL. IA-2, a transmembrane protein of the protein tyrosine phosphatase family, is a major autoantigen in insulin-dependent diabetes mellitus. Proc Natl Acad Sci USA 1996; 93(13): 636–640.

134. Richter W, Seissler J, Northemann W, Wolfahrt S, Meinch H-M, Scherbaum WA. Cytoplasmic islet cell antibodies recognize distinct islet antigens in IDDM but not in stiff man syndrome. Diabetes 1993; 42:1642–1648.

135. Vives Pi M, Somoza N, Vargas F, Armengol P, Sarri Y, Wu JY, Pujol-Borrell R. Expression of glutamic acid decarboxylase (GAD) in the alpha, beta and delta cells of normal and diabetic pancreas: implications for the pathogenesis of type I diabetes. Clin Exp Immunol 1993; 92(3):391–396.

136. Kaufman DL, Erlander MG, Clare-Salzler M, Atkinson MA, Maclaren NK, Tobin AJ. Autoimmunity to two forms of glutamate decarboxylase in insulin-dependent diabetes mellitus. J Clin Invest 1992; 89:283–292.

137. Hagopian WA, Michelsen B, Karlsen AE, et al. Autoantibodies in IDDM primarily recognize the 65,000-M(r) rather than the 6,000-M(r) isoform of glutamic acid decarboxylase. Diabetes 1993; 42(4):631–636.

138. Luhder F, Schlosser M, Mauch L, Haubruck H, Rjasanowski I, Michaelis D, Kohnert KD, Ziegler M. Autoantibodies against GAD65 rather than GAD6 precede the onset of type 1 diabetes. Autoimmunity 1994; 19(2):1–80.

139. Hampe CS, Hammerle LP, Bekris L, Ortqvist E, Kockum I, Rolandsson O, Landin-Olsson M, Torn C, Persson B, Lernmark A. Recognition of glutamic acid decarboxylase (GAD) by autoantibodies from different gad antibody-positive phenotypes. J Clin Endocrinol Metab 2000; 85(12):4671–4679.

140. Kaufman DL, Erlander MG, Clare-Salzler M, Atkinson MA, Maclaren NK, Tobin AJ. Autoimmunity to two forms of glutamate decarboxylase in insulin-dependent diabetes mellitus. J Clin Invest 1992; 89:283–292.

141. Atkinson MA, Kaufman DL, Campbell L. Response of peripheral blood mononuclear cells to glutamate decarboxylase in insulin-dependent diabetes. Lancet 1992; 339: 458–459.

142. oep BO, Arden SD, de Vries RRP, et al. T-cell clones from a type-1 diabetes patient respond to insulin secretory granule proteins. Nature 1990; 345:632–634.

143. Roep BO, Kallan AA, Duinkerken G, et al. T-cell reactivity to beta-cell membrane antigens associated with beta-cell destruction in IDDM. Diabetes 1995; 44:278–283.

144. Hummel M, Durinovic-Bello I, Ziegler A-G. Relation between cellular and humoral immunity to islet cell antigens in type I diabetes. J Autoimmun 1996; 9:427–430.

145. Harrison LC, Honeyman MC, DeAizpurua HJ, Schmidli RS, Colman PG, Tait BD, Cram DS. Inverse relation between humoral and cellular immunity to glutamic acid decarboxylase in subjects at risk of insulin-dependent diabetes. Lancet 1993; 341:1365–1369.

146. Atkinson MA, Maclaren NK, Scharp DW, Lacy PE, Riley WJ. 64 000 M_r autoantibodies as predictors of insulin-dependent diabetes. Lancet 1990; 335:1357–1360.

147. Rabin DU, Pleasic SM, Shapiro JA, Yoo-Warren H, Oles J, Hicks JM, Goldstein DE, Rae PM. Islet cell antigen 512 is a diabetes-specific islet autoantigen related to protein tyrosine phosphatases. J Immunol 1994; 152(6): 3183–3188.

148. Payton MA, Hawkes CJ, Christie MR. Relationship of the 37,000- and 40,000-M(r) tryptic fragments of islet antigens in insulin-dependent diabetes to the protein tyrosine phosphatase-like molecule IA-2 (ICA512). J Clin Invest 1995; 96(3):1506–1511.

149. Bonifacio E, Lampasona V, Genovese S, Ferrari M, Bosi E. Identification of protein tyrosine phosphatase-like IA2 (islet cell antigen 512) as the insulin-dependent diabetes-related 37/40K autoantigen and a target of islet-cell antibodies. J Immunol 1995; 155(11):5419–5426.

150. Lu J, Li Q, Xie H, Chen ZJ, Borovitskaya AE, Maclaren NK, Notkins AL, Lan MS. Identification of a second transmembrane protein tyrosine phosphatase, IA-2beta, as an autoantigen in insulin-dependent diabetes mellitus: precursor of the 3-kDa tryptic fragment. Proc Natl Acad Sci USA 1996; 93(6):2307–2311.

151. Bonifacio E, Genovese S, Braghi S, Bazzigaluppi E, Lampasona V, Bingley PJ, Rogge L, Pastore MR, Bognetti E, Bottazzo GF, et-al. Islet autoantibody markers in IDDM: risk assessment strategies yielding high sensitivity. Diabetologia 1995; 38(7):816–822.

152. Verge CF, Gianani R, Kawasaki E, Yu L, Pietropaolo M, Jackson RA, Chase HP, Eisenbarth GS. Prediction of type I diabetes in first-degree relatives using a combination of insulin, GAD, and ICA512bdc/IA-2 autoantibodies. Diabetes 1996; 45(7):926–933.

153. Maclaren N, Lan M, Coutant R, Schatz D, Silverstein J, Muir A, Clare-Salzer M, She JX, Malone J, Crockett S, Schwartz S, Quattrin T, DeSilva M, Vander Vegt P, Notkins A, Krischer J. Only multiple autoantibodies to islet cells (ICA), insulin, GAD65, IA-2 and IA-2beta predict immune-mediated (type 1) diabetes in relatives. J Autoimmun 1999; 12(4):279–278.

154. Gardner SG, Gale EA, Williams AJ, Gillespie KM, Lawrence KE, Bottazzo GF, Bingley PJ. Progression to diabetes in relatives with islet autoantibodies. Is it inevitable? Diabetes Care 1999; 22(12):2049–2054.

155. Dupre J, Mahon JL. Diabetes-related autoantibodies and the selection of subjects for trials of therapies to preserve pancreatic beta-cell function in recent-onset type 1 diabetes. Diabetes Care 2000; 23(8):1057–1058.

156. Litherland SA, Xie XT, Hutson AD, Wasserfall C, Whittaker DS, She JX, Hofig A, Dennis MA, Fuller K, Cook R, Schatz D, Moldawer LL, Clare-Salzler MJ. Aberrant prostaglandin synthase 2 expression defines an antigen-presenting cell defect for insulin-dependent diabetes mellitus. J Clin Invest 1999; 104(4):515–523.

157. McCanlies E, O'Leary LA, Foley TP, Kramer MK, Burke JP, Libman A, Swan JS, Steenkiste AR, Mccarthy BJ, Trucco M, Dorman JS. Hashimoto's thyroiditis and insulin-dependent diabetes mellitus: differences among individuals with and without abnormal thyroid function. J Clin Endocrinol Metab 1998; 83(5):1548–1551.

158. Nepom GT, Kwok WW. Molecular basis for HLA-DQ associations with IDDM. Diabetes 1998; 47(8):1177–1184.

159. Thai A-C, Eisenbarth GS. Natural history of IDDM. Diabetes Rev 1990; 1:1–14.

160. Srikanta S, Ganda OP, Jackson RA, Brink SJ, Fleischnick E, Yunis E, Alpen C, Soeldner JS, Eisenbarth GS. Pre-type 1 (insulin-dependent) diabetes: common endocrinological course despite immunological and immunogenetic heterogeneity. Diabetologia 1984; 27:146–148.

161. Srikanta S, Ganda OP, Gleason RE, Jackson RA, Soeldner JS, Eisenbarth GS. Pre-type 1 diabetes, linear loss of beta cell response to intravenous glucose. Diabetes 1984; 33: 717–720.

162. Harrison LC, Colman PG, Dean B, Baxter R, Martin FI. Increase in remission rate in newly diagnosed type I diabetic subjects treated with azathioprine. Diabetes 1985; 34:1306–1308.

163. Silverstein J, Maclaren N, Riley W, Spillar R, Radjenovic D, Johnson S. Immunosuppression with azathioprine and prednisone in recent-onset insulin-dependent diabetes mellitus. N Engl J Med 1988; 319:599–604.

164. Martin S, Schernthaner G, Nerup J, Gries FA, Koivisto VA, Dupre J, Standl E, Hamet P, McArthur R, Tan MH, et-al. Follow-up of cyclosporin A treatment in type 1 (insulin-dependent) diabetes mellitus: lack of long-term effects. Diabetologia 1991; 34(6):429–434.

165. Silverstein JH, Rosenbloom AL. New developments in type 1 (insulin-dependent) diabetes. Clin Pediatr 2000, 39:257–266.

166. Fuchtenbusch M, Rabl W, Grassl B, Bachmann W, Standl E, Ziegler AG. Delay of type I diabetes in high risk, first degree relatives by parenteral antigen administration: the Schwabing Insulin Prophylaxis Pilot Trial. Diabetologia 1998; 41(5):536–541.

167. Rabinovitch A, Skyler JS. Prevention of type 1 diabetes. Med Clin North Am 1998; 82(4):739–755.

168. Pozzilli P, Pitocco D, Visalli N, Cavallo MG, Buzzetti R, Crino A, Spera S, Suraci C, Multari G, Cervoni M, Manca Bitti ML, Matteoli MC, Marietti G, Ferrazzoli F, Cassone Faldetta MR, Giordano C, Sbriglia M, Sarugeri E, Ghirlanda G. No effect of oral insulin on residual beta-cell function in recent-onset type I diabetes (the IMDIAB VII). IMDIAB Group. Diabetologia 2000; 43(8):1000–1004.

169. Hahl J, Simell T, Ilonen J, Knip M, Simell O. Costs of predicting IDDM. Diabetologia 1998; 41(1):79–85.

170. Elliott RB, Chase HP. Prevention or delay of type 1 (insulin-dependent) diabetes mellitus in children using nicotinamide. Diabetologia 1991; 34(5):362–365.

171. Manna R, Migliore A, Martin LS, Ferrara E, Ponte E, Marietti G, Scuderi F, Cristiano G, Ghirlanda G, Gambassi G. Nicotinamide treatment in subjects at high risk of developing IDDM improves insulin secretion. Br J Clin Pract 1992; 46(3):1–9.

172. Herskowitz RD, Jackson RA, Soeldner JS, Eisenbarth GS. Pilot trial to prevent type I diabetes: progression to

overt IDDM despite oral nicotinamide. J Autoimmun 1989; 2(5):733–737.

173. Vidal J, Fernandez-Balsells M, Sesmilo G, Aguilera E, Casamitjana R, Gomis R, Conget I. Effects of nicotinamide and intravenous insulin therapy in newly diagnosed type 1 diabetes. Diabetes Care 2000; 23(3):360–364.

174. Shapiro AM, Lakey JR, Ryan EA, Korbutt GS, Toth E, Warnock GL, Kneteman NM, Rajotte RV. Islet transplantation in seven patients with type 1 diabetes mellitus using a glucocorticoid-free immunosuppressive regimen. N Engl J Med 2000; 343(4):230–238.

175. Ramiya VK, Maraist M, Arfors KE, Schatz DA, Peck AB, Cornelius JG. Reversal of insulin-dependent diabetes using islets generated in vitro from pancreatic stem cells. Nat Med 2000; 6(3):278–282.

176. Pozzilli P. Prevention of insulin-dependent diabetes mellitus 1998. Diabetes Metab Rev 1998; 14(1):69–84.

177. Rosenbloom AL, Schatz DA, Krischer JP, Skyler JS, Becker DJ, Laporte RE, Libman I, Pietropaolo M, Dosch HM, Finberg L, Muir A, Tamborlane WV, Grey M, Silverstein JH, Malone JI. Therapeutic controversy: prevention and treatment of diabetes in children. J Clin Endocrinol Metab 2000; 85(2):494–522.

178. Taylor SI. Insulin action and inaction. Clin Res 1987; 35(5):459–72.

179. Bloise W, Wajchenberg BL, Moncada VY, et al. Atypical antiinsulin receptor antibodies in a patient with type B insulin resistance and scleroderma. J Clin Endocrinol Metab 1989; 68:227–231.

180. Duncan JA, Shah SC, Shulman DI, Siegel RL, Kappy MS, Malone JI. Type b insulin resistance in a 15-year-old white youth. J Pediatr 1983; 103(3):421–424.

181. Matsuoka LY, Goldman J, Wortsman J, Kleinsmith D, Kupchella CE. Antibodies against the insulin receptor in paraneoplastic acanthosis nigricans. Am J Med 1987; 82(6):1253–1256.

182. Flier JS, Kahn CR, Roth J. Receptors, antireceptor antibodies, and mechanisms of insulin resistence. N Engl J Med 1979; 300:413–419.

183. Elias D, Cohen IR, Schechter Y, Spirer Z, Golander A. Antibodies to insulin receptor followed by anti-idiotype antibodies to insulin in child with hypoglycemia. Diabetes 1987; 36:348–354.

184. Braund WJ, Naylor BA, Williamson DH, Buley ID, et al. Autoimmunity to insulin receptor and hypoglycaemia in patient with Hodgkin's disease. Lancet 1987; 1:237–240.

185. Moller DE, Ratner RE, Borenstein DG, Taylor SI. Autoantibodies to the insulin receptor as a cause of autoimmune hypoglycemia in systemic lupus erythematosus. Am J Med 1988; 84:334–338.

186. Varga J, Lopatin M, Boden G. Hypoglycemia due to antiinsulin receptor antibodies in systemic lupus erythematosus. J Rheumatol 1990; 17:1226–1229.

187. Virally ML, Timsit J, Chanson P, Warnet A, Guillausseau PJ. Insulin autoimmune syndrome: a rare cause of hypoglycaemia not to be overlooked. Diabetes Metab 1999; 25(5):429–431.

188. Uchigata Y, Hirata Y. Insulin autoimmune syndrome (IAS, Hirata disease). Ann Med Intern (Paris) 1999; 150(3):245–253.

189. Burch HB, Clement S, Sokol MS, et al. Reactive hypoglycemic coma due to insulin autoimmune syndrome: case report and literature review. Am J Med 1992; 92:681–685.

190. Meschi F, Dozio N, Bognetti E, Carra M, Cofano D, Chiumello G. An unusual case of recurrent hypoglycae-

mia: 10-year follow up of a child with insulin auto-immunity. Eur J Pediatr 1992; 151:32–34.

191. Takayama S, Eguchi Y, Sato A, et al. Insulin autoimmune syndrome is the third leading cause of spontaneous hypoglycemic attacks in Japan. Diabetes Res Clin Pract 1990; 10:211–214.

192. Schlemper RJ, Uchigata Y, Frolich M, Vingerhoeds AC, Meinders AE. Recurrent hypoglycaemia caused by the insulin autoimmune syndrome: the first Dutch case. Neth J Med 1996; 48:188–192.

193. Hirata, Y. Methamizole and insulin autoimmune syndrome with hypoglycemia. Lancet 1983; 2:1037–1038.

194. Okabe R, Inaba M, Hosoi M, Ishimura E, Kumeda Y, Nishizawa Y, Morii H. Remission of insulin autoimmune syndrome in a patient with Grave's disease by treatment with methimazole. Intern Med 1999; 38(6):482–485.

195. Dozio N, Scavini M, Beretta A, Sarugeri E, Sartori S, Belloni C, Dosio F, Savi A, Fazio F, Sodoyez JC, Pozza G. Imaging of the buffering effect of insulin antibodies in the autoimmune hypoglycemic syndrome. J Clin Endocrinol Metab 1998; 83(2):643–648.

196. Uchigata Y, Kuwata S, Tokunaga K, Eguchi Y, Takayama Hasumi S, Miyamoto M, Omori Y, Juji T, Hirata Y. Strong association of insulin autoimmune syndrome with HLA-DR4. Lancet 1992; 339:393–394.

197. Bottazzo GF, Lendrum R. Separate autoantibodies to human pancreatic glucagon and somatostatin cells. Lancet 1976; 2:873–876.

198. Winter WE, Maclaren NK, Riley WJ, Unger, RH, Ozand P, Neufeld M. Pancreatic alpha cell autoantibodies and glucagon response to arginine. Diabetes 1984; 33:435–437.

199. Del Prete GF, Tiengo A, Nosadini R, Bottazzo GF, Betterle C, Bersani G. Glucagon secretion in two patients with autoantibodies to glucagon producing cells. Horm Metab Res 1978; 10:260–261.

200. Baba S, Morita S, Mizuno N, Okada K. Autoimmunity to glucagon in a diabetic not on insulin. Lancet 1976; 12: 585; Sanke T, Kondo M, Moriyama J, Nanjo K, Iwo K, Miyamura K. Glucagon binding autoantibodies in a patient with hyperthyroidism treated with methimazole. J Clin Endocrinol Metab 1983; 57:1140–1144.

201. Dayan CM, Daniels GH. Chronic autoimmune thyroiditis. N Engl J Med 1996; 335(2):99–107.

202. Weetman AP. Medical progress: Graves' disease. N Engl J Med 2000; 343(17):1236–1248.

203. Foley TP Jr, Abbassi V, Copeland KC, Draznin MB. Brief report: hypothyroidism caused by chronic autoimmune thyroiditis in very young infants. N Engl J Med 1994; 330(7):466–468.

204. Hunter I, Greene SA, MacDonald TM, Morris AD. Prevalence and aetiology of hypothyroidism in the young. Arch Dis Child 2000; 83(3):207–210.

205. Strakosch CR, Wenzel BE, Row VV, Volpe R. Immunology of autoimmune thyroid diseases. N Engl J Med 1982; 307:1499–1507.

206. Akamizu T, Kohn LD, Hiratani H, Saijo M, Tahara K, Nakao K. Hashimoto's thyroiditis with heterogeneous antithyrotropin receptor antibodies: unique epitopes may contribute to the regulation of thyroid function by the antibodies. J Clin Endocrinol Metab 2000; 85(6):2116–2121.

207. Takasu N, Yamada T, Takasu M, Komiya I, Nagasawa Y, Asawa T, Shinoda T, Aizawa T, Koizumi Y. Disappearance of thyrotropin-blocking antibodies and spontaneous

recovery from hypothyroidism in autoimmune thyroiditis. N Engl J Med 1992; 326(8):513–518.

208. Massart C, Caroff G, Maugendre D, Genetet N, Gibassier J. Peripheral blood and intrathyroidal T cell clones from patients with thyroid autoimmune diseases. Autoimmunity 1999; 31(3):163–174.

209. Drugarin D, Negru S, Koreck A, Zosin I, Cristea C. The pattern of a T(H)1 cytokine in autoimmune thyroiditis. Immunol Lett 2000; 71(2):73–77.

210. Zantut-Wittmann DE, Boechat LH, Pinto GA, da Silva Trevisan MA, Vassallo J. Autoimmune and non-autoimmune thyroid diseases have different patterns of cellular HLA class II expression. Sao Paulo Med J 1999; 117(4): 161–164.

211. Rasmussen AK. Cytokine actions on the thyroid gland. Dan Med Bull 2000; 47(2):94–114.

212. Paolieri F, Salmaso C, Battifora M, Montagna P, Pesce G, Bagnasco M, Richiusa P, Galluzzo A, Giordano C. Possible pathogenetic relevance of interleukin-1 beta in "destructive" organ-specific autoimmune disease (Hashimoto's thyroiditis). Ann NY Acad Sci 1999; 876:221–228.

213. Giordano C, Stassi G, De Maria R, Todaro M, Richiusa P, Papoff G, Ruberti G, Bagnasco M, Testi R, Galluzzo A. Potential involvement of Fas and its ligand in the pathogenesis of Hashimoto's thyroiditis. Science 1997; 275(5302):960–963.

214. Hammond LJ, Lowdell MW, Cerrano PG, Goode AW, Bottazzo GF, Mirakian R. Analysis of apoptosis in relation to tissue destruction associated with Hashimoto's autoimmune thyroiditis. J Pathol 1997; 182(2):138–144.

215. Doniach D, Bottazzo GR, Russell RCG. Goitrous autoimmune thyroiditis. Clin Endocrinol Metab 1979; 8:63–80.

216. Vakeva A, Kontiainen S, Miettinen A, Schlenzka A, Maenpaa J. Thyroid peroxidase antibodies in children with autoimmune thyroiditis. J Clin Pathol 1992; 45:106–109.

217. Valenti WA, Vitti P, Rotella CM, Vaughn MM, Aloj SM, Grollam EF, Ambesi-Impiombato FS, Kohn LD. Antibodies that promote thyroid growth, a distinct population of thyroid-stimulating autoantibodies. N Engl J Med 1983; 309:1028–1034.

218. Mariotti S, Caturegli P, Piccolo P, Barbesino G, Pinchera A. Antithyroid peroxidase autoantibodies in thyroid diseases. J Clin Endocrinol Metab 1990; 71:661–669; Banga JP, Barnett PS, McGregor AM. Immunological and molecular characteristics of the thyroid peroxidase autoantigen. Autoimmunity 1991; 8:335–343.

219. Falk RJ, Jennette JC. Anti-neutrophil cytoplasmic autoantibodies with specificity for myeloperoxidase in patients with systemic vasculitis and idiopathic necrotizing and crescentic glomerulonephritis. N Engl J Med 1988; 318(25):1651–1657.

220. Berthold H, Steffens U, Northemann W. Human thyroid peroxidase: autoantibody recognition depends on the natural conformation. J Clin Lab Anal 1993; 7:401–404.

221. Vakeva A, Kontiainen S, Miettinen A, Schlenzka A, Maenpaa J. Thyroid peroxidase antibodies in children with autoimmune thyroiditis. J Clin Pathol 1992; 45:106–109.

222. Marino M, Chiovato L, Friedlander JA, Latrofa F, Pinchera A, McCluskey RT. Serum antibodies against megalin (GP330) in patients with autoimmune thyroiditis. J Clin Endocrinol Metab 1999; 84(7):2468–2474.

223. Seissler J, Wagner S, Schott M, Lettmann M, Feldkamp J, Scherbaum WA, Morgenthaler NG. Low frequency of autoantibodies to the human Na(+)/I(-) symporter in patients with autoimmune thyroid disease. J Clin Endocrinol Metab 2000; 85(12):4630–4634.

224. Mariotti S, Caturegli P, Piccolo P, Barbesino G, Pinchera A. Antithyroid peroxidase autoantibodies in thyroid diseases. J Clin Endocrinol Metab 1990; 71:661–669.

225. Banga JP, Barnett PS, McGregor AM. Immunological and molecular characteristics of the thyroid peroxidase autoantigen. Autoimmunity 1991; 8:335–343.

226. Irvine WJ. The association of atrophic gastritis with autoimmune thyroid disease. Clin Endocrinol Metab 1975; 4:351–377.

227. Toh BH, van Driel IR, Gleeson PA. Autoimmune gastritis: tolerance and autoimmunity to the gastric H+/K+ ATPase (proton pump). Autoimmunity 1992; 13(2):165–72.

228. Callaghan JM, Khan MA, Alderuccio F, van Driel IR, Gleeson PA, Toh BH. Alpha and beta subunits of the gastric H+/K(+)-ATPase are concordantly targeted by parietal cell autoantibodies associated with autoimmune gastritis. Autoimmunity 1993; 16(4):289–295.

229. Roman SH, Greenberg D, Rubinstein P, Wallenstein S, Davies TF. Genetics of autoimmune thyroid disease: lack of evidence for linkage to HLA within families. J Clin Endocrinol Metab 1992; 74:496–503.

230. Wick G. Concept of a multigenic basis for the pathogenesis of spontaneous autoimmune thyroiditis. Acta Endocrinol Suppl Copenh 1987; 281:63–69.

231. Brix TH, Kyvik KO, Hegedus L. A population-based study of chronic autoimmune hypothyroidism in Danish twins. J Clin Endocrinol Metab 2000; 85(2):536–539.

232. Barbesino G, Chiovato L. The genetics of Hashimoto's disease. Endocrinol Metab Clin North Am 2000; 29(2): 357–74.

233. Kotsa K, Watson PF, Weetman AP. A CTLA-4 gene polymorphism is associated with both Graves disease and autoimmune hypothyroidism. Clin Endocrinol (Oxf) 1997; 46(5):551–554.

234. Donner H, Braun J, Seidl C, Rau H, Finke R, Ventz M, Walfish PG, Usadel KH, Badenhoop K. Codon 17 polymorphism of the cytotoxic T lymphocyte antigen 4 gene in Hashimoto's thyroiditis and Addison's disease. J Clin Endocrinol Metab 1997; 82(12):4130–4132.

235. Braun J, Donner H, Siegmund T, Walfish PG, Usadel KH, Badenhoop K. CTLA-4 promoter variants in patients with Graves' disease and Hashimoto's thyroiditis. Tissue Antigens 1998; 51(5):563–566.

236. Heward JM, Allahabadia A, Carr-Smith J, Daykin J, Cockram CS, Gordon C, Barnett AH, Franklyn JA, Gough SC. No evidence for allelic association of a human CTLA-4 promoter polymorphism with autoimmune thyroid disease in either population-based case-control or family-based studies. Clin Endocrinol (Oxf) 1998; 49(3): 331–334.

237. Djilali-Saiah I, Larger E, Harfouch-Hammoud E, Timsit J, Clerc J, Bertin E, Assan R, Boitard C, Bach JF, Caillat-Zucman S. No major role for the CTLA-4 gene in the association of autoimmune thyroid disease with IDDM. Diabetes 1998; 47(1):125–127.

238. Takara M, Komiya I, Kinjo Y, Tomoyose T, Yamashiro S, Akamine H, Masuda M, Takasu N. Association of CTLA-4 gene A/G polymorphism in Japanese type 1 diabetic patients with younger age of onset and autoimmune thyroid disease. Diabetes Care 2000; 23(7):975–978.

239. Tomer Y, Barbesino G, Greenberg DA, Concepcion E, Davies TF. Mapping the major susceptibility loci for familial Graves' and Hashimoto's diseases: evidence for genetic heterogeneity and gene interactions. J Clin Endocrinol Metab 1999; 84(12):4656–4664.

240. Barbesino G, Tomer Y, Concepcion E, Davies TF, Greenberg DA. Linkage analysis of candidate genes in autoimmune thyroid disease: 1. Selected immunoregulatory genes. International Consortium for the Genetics of Autoimmune Thyroid Disease. J Clin Endocrinol Metab 1998; 83(5):1580–1584.

241. Barbesino G, Tomer Y, Concepcion ES, Davies TF, Greenberg DA. Linkage analysis of candidate genes in autoimmune thyroid disease. II. Selected gender-related genes and the X-chromosome. International Consortium for the Genetics of Autoimmune Thyroid Disease. J Clin Endocrinol Metab 1998; 83(9):3290–3295.

242. Tomer Y, Barbesino G, Greenberg DA, Concepcion E, Davies TF. Linkage analysis of candidate genes in autoimmune thyroid disease. III. Detailed analysis of chromosome 14 localizes Graves' disease-1 (GD-1) close to multinodular goiter-1 (MNG-1). International Consortium for the Genetics of Autoimmune Thyroid Disease. J Clin Endocrinol Metab 1998; 83(12):4321–4327.

243. Sunthornthepvarakul T, Kitvitayasak S, Ngowngarmaratana S, Konthong P, Deerochanawong C, Sarinnapakorn V, Phongviratchai S. Lack of association between a polymorphism of human thyrotropin receptor gene and autoimmune thyroid disease. J Med Assoc Thai 1999; 82(12): 1214–1219.

244. Dussault JH, Letarte J, Guyda H, Laberge C. Lack of influence of thyroid antibodies on thyroid function in the newborn infant and on a mass screening program for congenital hypothyroidism. J Pediatr 1980; 96(3 Pt 1):385–389.

245. Matsuura N, Yamada Y, Nohara Y, Konishi J, Kasagi K, Endo K, Kojima H, Wataya K. Familial neonatal transient hypothyroidism due to maternal TSH-binding inhibitor immunoglobulins. N Engl J Med 1980; 303(13):738–741.

246. van der Gaag RD, Drexhage HA, Dussault JH. Role of maternal immunoglobulins blocking TSH-induced thyroid growth in sporadic forms of congenital hypothyroidism. Lancet 1985; 1(8423):246–250.

247. Fort P, Lifshitz F, Pugliese M, Klein I. Neonatal thyroid disease: differential expression in three successive offspring. J Clin Endocrinol Metab 1988; 66(3):645–647.

248. Sutherland JM, Esselborn VM, Burket RL, Skillman TB, Benson JT. Familial nongoitrous cretism apparently due to maternal antithyroid antibody. N Engl J Med 1960; 263:336–341.

249. Brown RS, Bellisario RL, Botero D, Fournier L, Abrams CA, Cowger ML, David R, Fort P, Richman RA. Incidence of transient congenital hypothyroidism due to maternal thyrotropin receptor-blocking antibodies in over one million babies. J Clin Endocrinol Metab 1996; 81(3): 1147–1151.

250. Iseki M, Shimizu M, Oikawa T, Hojo H, Arikawa K, Ichikawa Y, Momotani N, Ito K. Sequential serum measurements of thyrotropin binding inhibitor immunoglobulin G in transient familial neonatal hypothyroidism. J Clin Endocrinol Metab 1983; 57(2):384–387; Connors MH, Styne DM. Transient neonatal 'athyreosis' resulting from thyrotropin-binding inhibitory immunoglobulins. Pediatrics 1986; 78(2):287–290.

251. Francis G, Riley W. Congenital familial transient hypothyroidism secondary to transplacental thyrotropin-block-ing autoantibodies. Am J Dis Child 1987; 141(10):1081–1083.

252. Roti E, Emerson C. Clinical review 29. Postpartum thyroiditis. J Clin Endocrinol Metab 1992; 74:3–5.

253. Stagnaro-Green A. Recognizing, understanding, and treating postpartum thyroiditis. Endocrinol Metab Clin North Am 2000; 29(2):417–430.

254. Premawardhana LD, Parkes AB, Ammari F, John R, Darke C, Adams H, Lazarus JH. Postpartum thyroiditis and long-term thyroid status: prognostic influence of thyroid peroxidase antibodies and ultrasound echogenicity. J Clin Endocrinol Metab 2000; 85(1):71–75.

255. Smallridge RC. Postpartum thyroid dysfunction: a frequently undiagnosed endocrine disorder. Endocrinologist 1996, 6:44–50.

256. Smallridge RC. Postpartum thyroid disease: a paradigm of immune dysfunction. Advance/Laboratory 1999:69–71.

257. Stagnaro-Green A, Roman SH, Cobin RH, el-Harazy E, Alvarez-Marfany M, Davies TF. Detection of at-risk pregnancy by means of highly sensitive assays for thyroid autoantibodies. JAMA 1990; 264(11):1422–1425.

258. Stagnaro-Green A, Roman SH, Cobin RH, el-Harazy E, Wallenstein S, Davies TF. A prospective study of lymphocyte-initiated immunosuppression in normal pregnancy: evidence of a T-cell etiology for postpartum thyroid dysfunction. J Clin Endocrinol Metab 1992; 74(3): 645–653.

259. Weetman AP. Editorial: insulin-dependent diabetes mellitus and postpartum thyroiditis: an important association. J Clin Endocrin Metabol 1994; 79:7–9.

260. Weetman AP. Medical progress: Graves' disease. N Engl J Med 2000; 343(17):1236–1248.

261. Orgiazzi J. Anti-TSH receptor antibodies in clinical practice. Endocrinol Metab Clin North Am 2000; 29(2):339–335.

262. Itoh M, Uchimura K, Makino M, Kobayashi T, Hayashi R, Nagata M, Kakizawa H, Fujiwara K, Nagasaka A. Production of IL-10 and IL-12 in CD40 and interleukin 4-activated mononuclear cells from patients with Graves' disease. Cytokine 2000; 12(6):688–693.

263. Duprez L, Parma J, Van Sande J, Rodien P, Sabine C, Abramowicz M, Dumont JE, Vassart G. Pathology of the TSH receptor. J Pediatr Endocrinol Metab 1999; 12 Suppl 1:295–302.

264. Seetharamaiah GS, Zhuang J, Huang J, Patibandla SA, Kaithamana S, Tahara K, Kohn LD, Prabhakar BS. Selective binding of thyrotropin receptor autoantibodies to recombinant extracellular domain of thyrotropin/lutropin-chorionic gonadotropin receptor chimeric proteins. Thyroid 1999; 9(9):879–886.

265. McKenzie JM. Humoral factors in the pathogenesis of Graves' disease. Physiol Rev 1968; 48:252–310.

266. Adams DD, Kennedy TH. Evidence to suggest that LATS-protector stimulates human thyroid gland. J Clin Endocrinol Metab 1971; 33:47–51.

267. Fisher DA, Pandian MR, Carlton E. Autoimmune thyroid disease: an expanding spectrum. Pediatr Clin North Am 1987; 34:907–918.

268. Burrow GN. The management of thyrotoxicosis in pregnancy. N Engl J Med 1985; 313(9):562–565.

269. Phillips D, McLachlan S, Stephenson A, Roberts D, Moffitt S, McDonald D, Ad'Hiah A, Stratton A, Young E, Clark F. Autosomal dominant transmission of autoantibodies to thyroglobulin and thyroid peroxidase. J Clin Endocrinol Metab 1990; 70:742–746.

270. Riley WJ, Maclaren NK, Lezotte DC, Spillar RP, Rosenbloom AL. Thyroid autoimmunity in insulin-dependent diabetes mellitus: the case for routine screening. J Pediatr 1981; 98:350–354.

271. Farid NR, Stone E, Johnson G. Graves' disease and HLA: clinical and epidemiologic associations. Clin Endocrinol (Oxf) 1980; 13(6):535–544.

272. Roman SH, Greenberg D, Rubinstein P, Wallenstein S, Davies TF. Genetics of autoimmune thyroid disease: lack of evidence for linkage to HLA within families. J Clin Endocrinol Metab 1992; 74:496–503.

273. Yanagawa T, Mangklabruks A, Chang YB, Okamoto Y, Fisfalen ME, Curran PG, DeGroot LJ. Human histocompatibility leukocyte antigen-DQA1*0501 allele associated with genetic susceptibility to Graves' disease in a Caucasian population. J Clin Endocrinol Metab 1993; 76(6): 1569–1574.

274. Chen QY, Nadell D, Zhang XY, Kukreja A, Huang YJ, Wise J, Svec F, Richards R, Friday KE, Vargas A, Gomez R, Chalew S, Lan MS, Tomer Y, Maclaren NK. The human leukocyte antigen HLA DRB3*020/DQA1*0501 haplotype is associated with Graves' disease in African Americans. J Clin Endocrinol Metab 2000; 85(4):1545–1549.

275. Yanagawa T, Hidaka Y, Guimaraes V, Soliman M, DeGroot LJ. CTLA-4 gene polymorphism associated with Graves' disease in a Caucasian population. J Clin Endocrinol Metab 1995; 80(1):41–45.

276. Donner H, Rau H, Walfish PG, Braun J, Siegmund T, Finke R, Herwig J, Usadel KH, Badenhoop K. CTLA4 alanine-17 confers genetic susceptibility to Graves' disease and to type 1 diabetes mellitus. J Clin Endocrinol Metab 1997; 82(1):143–146.

277. Heward JM, Allahabadia A, Armitage M, Hattersley A, Dodson PM, Macleod K, Carr-Smith J, Daykin J, Daly A, Sheppard MC, Holder RL, Barnett AH, Franklyn JA, Gough SC. The development of Graves' disease and the CTLA-4 gene on chromosome 2q33. J Clin Endocrinol Metab 1999; 84(7):2398–2401.

278. Vaidya B, Imrie H, Perros P, Young ET, Kelly WF, Carr D, Large DM, Toft AD, McCarthy MI, Kendall-Taylor P, Pearce SH. The cytotoxic T lymphocyte antigen-4 is a major Graves' disease locus. Hum Mol Genet 1999; 8(7): 1195–1199.

279. Tomer Y, Barbesino G, Keddache M, Greenberg DA, Davies TF. Mapping of a major susceptibility locus for Graves' disease (GD-1) to chromosome 14q31. J Clin Endocrinol Metab 1997; 82(5):1645–1648.

280. Siegmund T, Usadel KH, Donner H, Braun J, Walfish PG, Badenhoop K. Interferon-gamma gene microsatellite polymorphisms in patients with Graves' disease. Thyroid 1998; 8(11):1013–1017.

281. Rau H, Nicolay A, Usadel KH, Finke R, Donner H, Walfish PG, Badenhoop K. Polymorphisms of TAP1 and TAP2 genes in Graves' disease. Tissue Antigens 1997; 49(1):16–22.

282. Tomer Y, Barbesino G, Greenberg DA, Concepcion E, Davies TF. A new Graves disease-susceptibility locus maps to chromosome 20q11.2. International Consortium for the Genetics of Autoimmune Thyroid Disease. Am J Hum Genet 1998; 63(6):1749–1755.

283. Pearce SH, Vaidya B, Imrie H, Perros P, Kelly WF, Toft AD, McCarthy MI, Young ET, Kendall-Taylor P. Further evidence for a susceptibility locus on chromosome 20q13.11 in families with dominant transmission of Graves disease. Am J Hum Genet 1999; 65(5):1462–1465.

284. Hunt PJ, Marshall SE, Weetman AP, Bell JI, Wass JA, Welsh KI. Cytokine gene polymorphisms in autoimmune thyroid disease. J Clin Endocrinol Metab 2000; 85(5): 1984–1988.

285. Ban Y, Taniyama M, Ban Y. Vitamin D receptor gene polymorphism is associated with Graves' disease in the Japanese population. J Clin Endocrinol Metab 2000; 85(12):4639–4643.

286. Vaidya B, Imrie H, Perros P, Young ET, Kelly WF, Carr D, Large DM, Toft AD, Kendall-Taylor P, Pearce SH. Evidence for a new Graves disease susceptibility locus at chromosome 18q21. Am J Hum Genet 2000; 66(5):1710–1714.

287. Watson PF, French A, Pickerill AP, McIntosh RS, Weetman AP. Lack of association between a polymorphism in the coding region of the thyrotropin receptor gene and Graves' disease. J Clin Endocrinol Metab 1995; 80(3): 1032–1035.

288. de Roux N, Shields DC, Misrahi M, Ratanachaiyavong S, McGregor AM, Milgrom E. Analysis of the thyrotropin receptor as a candidate gene in familial Graves' disease. J Clin Endocrinol Metab 1996; 81(10):3483–3486.

289. Rau H, Donner H, Usadel KH, Badenhoop K. Polymorphisms of tumor necrosis factor receptor 2 are not associated with insulin-dependent diabetes mellitus or Graves' disease. Tissue Antigens 1997; 49(5):535–536.

290. Chistyakov DA, Savost'anov KV, Turakulov RI, Petunina NA, Trukhina LV, Kudinova AV, Balabolkin MI, Nosikov VV. Complex association analysis of graves disease using a set of polymorphic markers. Mol Genet Metab 2000; 70(3):214–218.

291. Gough SC. The genetics of Graves' disease. Endocrinol Metab Clin North Am 2000; 29(2):255–266.

292. Bahn RS. Understanding the immunology of Graves' ophthalmopathy. Is it an autoimmune disease? Endocrinol Metab Clin North Am 2000; 29(2):287–296.

293. Solomon DH, Chopra IJ, Chopra U, Smith FJ. Identification of subgroups of euthyroid Graves' ophthalmopathy. N Engl J Med 1997; 296:181–186.

294. Gamblin GT, Harper DG, Galentine P, Buck DR, Chernow B, Eil C. Prevalence of increased intraocular pressure in Graves' disease—evidence of frequent subclinical opthalmopathy. N Engl J Med 1983; 308:420–424.

295. Kubota S, Gunji K, Ackrell BA, Cochran B, Stolarski C, Wengrowicz S, Kennerdell JS, Hiromatsu Y, Wall J. The 64-kilodalton eye muscle protein is the flavoprotein subunit of mitochondrial succinate dehydrogenase: the corresponding serum antibodies are good markers of an immune-mediated damage to the eye muscle in patients with Graves' hyperthyroidism. J Clin Endocrinol Metab 1998; 83(2):443–447.

296. Heufelder AE, Wenzel BE, Bahn RS. Cell surface localization of a 72 kilodalton heat shock protein in retroocular fibroblasts from patients with Graves' ophthalmopathy. J Clin Endocrinol Metab 1992; 74(4):732–736.

297. Gunji K, De Bellis A, Li AW, Yamada M, Kubota S, Ackrell B, Wengrowicz S, Bellastella A, Bizzarro A, Sinisi A, Wall JR. Cloning and characterization of the novel thyroid and eye muscle shared protein G2s: autoantibodies against G2s are closely associated with ophthalmopathy in patients with Graves' hyperthyroidism. J Clin Endocrinol Metab 2000; 85(4):1641–1647.

298. Aniszewski JP, Valyasevi RW, Bahn RS. Relationship between disease duration and predominant orbital T cell

subset in Graves' ophthalmopathy. J Clin Endocrinol Metab 2000; 85(2):776–780; Wakelkamp IM, Gerding MN, Van Der Meer JW, Prummel MF, Wiersinga WM. Both Th1- and Th2-derived cytokines in serum are elevated in Graves' ophthalmopathy. Clin Exp Immunol 2000; 121(3):453–457.

299. Hiromatsu Y, Yang D, Miyake I, Koga M, Kameo J, Sato M, Inone Y, Nonaka K. Nicotinamide decreases cytokine-induced activation of orbital fibroblasts from patients with thyroid-associated ophthalmopathy. J Clin Endorinol Metabol 1998; 83:121–124.

300. Maclaren NK, Blizzard RM. Adrenal autoimmunity and autoimmune polyglandular syndromes. In: Rose NR, MacKay IR, eds. The Autoimmune Diseases. Academic Press, 1985:201–225.

301. Riley WJ, Maclaren NK, Neufeld M. Adrenal autoantibodies and Addison's disease in insulin-dependent diabetes mellitus. J. Pediatr 1980; 97:191–195.

302. Drexhage HA. Autoimmune adrenocortical failure. In: Volpe R, ed. Contemporary Endocrinology: Autoimmune Endocrinopathies. Totowa, NJ: Humana Press, 1999:309–336.

303. Bright GM, Singh I. Adrenal autoantibodies bind to adrenal subcellular fractions enriched in cytochrome-c reductase and 5'-nucleotidase. J Clin Endocrinol Metab 1990; 70(1):95–99.

304. Silva RC, Faical S, Laureti S, Falorni A, Dib SA, Kater CE. Detection of adrenocortical autoantibodies in Addison's disease with a peroxidase-labelled protein A technique. Braz J Med Biol Res 1998; 31(9):1141–1148.

305. Muir AM, Maclaren NK. Autoimmune diseases of the adrenal glands, parathyroid glands, gonads, and hypothalamic-pituitary axis. Endocrinol Metabol Clin North Am 1991; 20(3):619–644.

306. Khoury EL, Hammond L, Bottazzo GF, Doniach D. Surface-reactive antibodies to human adrenal cells in Addison's disease. Clin Exp Immunol 1981; 45(1):48–55.

307. Krohn K, Uibo R, Aavik E, Peterson P, Savilahti K. Identification by molecular cloning of an autoantigen associated with Addison's disease as steroid 17 alpha-hydroxylase. Lancet 1992; 339:770–773.

308. Baumann-Antczak A, Wedlock N, Bednarek J, Kiso Y, Krishnan H, Fowler S, Smith BR, Furmaniak J. Autoimmune Addison's disease and 21-hydroxylase. Lancet 1992; 340:429–430.

309. Bednarek J, Furmaniak J, Wedlock N, Kiso Y, Baumann-Antczak A, Fowler S, Krishnan H, Craft JA, Rees Smith B. Steroid 21-hydroxylase is a major autoantigen involved in adult onset autoimmune Addison's disease. FEBS Lett 1992; 309(1):51–55.

310. Winqvist O, Gustafsson J, Rorsman F, Karlsson FA, Kämpe O. Two different cytochrome P450 enzymes are the adrenal antigens in autoimmune polyendocrine syndrome type I and Addison's disease. J Clin Invest 1993; 92:2377–2385.

311. Peterson P, Salmi H, Hyoty H, Miettinen A, Ilonen J, Reijonen H, Knip M, Akerblom HK, Krohn K. Steroid 21-hydroxylase autoantibodies in insulin-dependent diabetes mellitus.Childhood Diabetes in Finland (DiMe) Study Group. Clin Immunol Immunopathol 1997; 82(1): 37–42.

312. Boscaro M, Betterle C, Volpato M, Fallo F, Furmaniak J, Rees Smith B, Sonino N. Hormonal responses during various phases of autoimmune adrenal failure: no evidence for 21-hydroxylase enzyme activity inhibition in vivo. J Clin Endocrinol Metab 1996; 81(8):2801–2804.

313. Betterle C, Scalici C, Presotto F, Pedini B, Moro L, Rigon F, Mantero F. The natural history of adrenal function in autoimmune patients with autoantibodies. J Endocrinol 1988; 117(3):467–475.

314. Betterle C, Scalici C, Pedini B, Mantero F. Addison's disease: principal clinical associations and description of natural history of the disease. Ann Ital Med Int 1989; 4: 195–206.

315. Betterle C, Volpato M, Rees Smith B, Furmaniak J, Chen S, Greggio NA, Sanzari M, Tedesco F, Pedini B, Boscaro M, Presotto F. I. Adrenal cortex and steroid 21-hydroxylase autoantibodies in adult patients with organ-specific autoimmune diseases: markers of low progression to clinical Addison's disease. J Clin Endocrinol Metab 1997; 82(3):932–938.

316. Betterle C, Zanette F, Zanchetta R, Pedini B, Trevisan A, Mantero F, Rigon R. Complement fixing adrenal autoantibodies: a marker for predicting the onset of idiopathic Addison's disease. Lancet 1983; 1:1238–1240.

317. Betterle C, Volpato M, Rees Smith B, Furmaniak J, Chen S, Zanchetta R, Greggio NA, Pedini B, Boscaro M, Presotto F. II. Adrenal cortex and steroid 21-hydroxylase autoantibodies in children with organ-specific autoimmune diseases: markers of high progression to clinical Addison's disease. J Clin Endocrinol Metab 1997; 82(3):939–942.

318. Laureti S, De Bellis A, Muccitelli VI, Calcinaro F, Bizzarro A, Rossi R, Bellastella A, Santeusanio F, Falorni A. Levels of adrenocortical autoantibodies correlate with the degree of adrenal dysfunction in subjects with preclinical Addison's disease. J Clin Endocrinol Metab 1998; 83(10): 3507–3511.

319. Neufeld M, Maclaren NK, Blizzard RM. Two types of autoimmune Addison's disease associated with different polyglandular autoimmune (PGA) syndromes. Medicine 1981; 60:355–362; Papadopoulos KI, Hallengren B. Polyglandular autoimmune syndrome type II in patients with idiopathic Addison's disease. Acta Endocrinol Copenh 1990; 122:472–478.

320. Donner H, Braun J, Seidl C, Rau H, Finke R, Ventz M, Walfish PG, Usadel KH, Badenhoop K. Codon 17 polymorphism of the cytotoxic T lymphocyte antigen 4 gene in Hashimoto's thyroiditis and Addison's disease. J Clin Endocrinol Metab 1997; 82(12):4130–4132.

321. Kemp EH, Ajjan RA, Husebye ES, Peterson P, Uibo R, Imrie H, Pearce SH, Watson PF, Weetman AP. A cytotoxic T lymphocyte antigen-4 (CTLA-4) gene polymorphism is associated with autoimmune Addison's disease in English patients. Clin Endocrinol (Oxf) 1998; 49(5):609–613.

322. Vaidya B, Imrie H, Geatch DR, Perros P, Ball SG, Baylis PH, Carr D, Hurel SJ, James RA, Kelly WF, Kemp EH, Young ET, Weetman AP, Kendall-Taylor P, Pearce SH. Association analysis of the cytotoxic T lymphocyte antigen-4 (CTLA-4) and autoimmune regulator-1 (AIRE-1) genes in sporadic autoimmune Addison's disease. J Clin Endocrinol Metab 2000; 85(2):688–691.

323. Elder M, Maclaren N, Riley W. Gonadal autoantibodies in patients with hypogonadism and/or Addison's disease. J Clin Endocrinol Metab 1981; 52:1137–1142.

324. Irvine WJ, Chan MM, Scarth L, Kolb FO, Hartog M, Bayliss RI, Drury MI. Immunological aspects of premature ovarian failure associated with idiopathic Addison's disease. Lancet 1968; 2(7574):883–887.

325. Moncayo R, Moncayo HE. Autoimmunity and the ovary. Immunol Today 1992; 13(7):255–258.

326. Gargiulo AR, Hill JA. Autoimmune endocrinopathies in female reproductive dysfunction. In Volpe R, ed. Contemporary Endocrinology: Autoimmune Endocrinopathies. Totowa, NJ: Humana Press, 1999:365–383.

327. Kirsop R, Brock CR, Robinson BG, Baber RJ, Wells JV, Saunders DM. Detection of anti-ovarian antibodies by indirect immunofluorescence in patients with premature ovarian failure. Reprod Fertil Dev 1991; 3(5):537–541.

328. Fenichel P, Sosset C, Barbarino-Monnier P, Gobert B, Hieronimus S, Bene MC, Harter M. Prevalence, specificity and significance of ovarian antibodies during spontaneouspremature ovarian failure. Hum Reprod 1997; 12(12):2623–2628.

329. Ahonen P, Miettinen A, Perheentupa J. Adrenal and steroidal cell antibodies in patients with autoimmune polyglandular disease type I and risk of adrenocortical and ovarian failure. J Clin Endocrinol Metab 1987; 64(3):494–500.

330. Chen S, Sawicka J, Betterle C, Powell M, Prentice L, Volpato M, Rees Smith B, Furmaniak J. Autoantibodies to steroidogenic enzymes in autoimmune polyglandular syndrome, Addison's disease, and premature ovarian failure. J Clin Endocrinol Metab 1996; 81(5):1871–1876.

331. Reimand K, Peterson P, Hyoty H, Uibo R, Cooke I, Weetman AP, Krohn KJ. 3beta-hydroxysteroid dehydrogenase autoantibodies are rare in premature ovarian failure. J Clin Endocrinol Metab 2000; 85(6):2324–2326.

332. Arif S, Vallian S, Farzaneh F, Zanone MM, James SL, Pietropaolo M, Hettiarachchi S, Vergani D, Conway GS, Peakman M. Identification of 3 beta-hydroxysteroid dehydrogenase as a novel target of steroid cell autoantibodies: association of autoantibodies with endocrine autoimmune disease. J Clin Endocrinol Metab 1996; 81(12):4439–4445.

333. Arif S, Underhill JA, Donaldson P, Conway GS, Peakman M. Human leukocyte antigen-DQB1* genotypes encoding aspartate at position 57 are associated with 3beta-hydroxysteroid dehydrogenase autoimmunity in premature ovarian failure. J Clin Endocrinol Metab 1999; 84(3):1056–1060.

334. Irvine WJ, Barnes EW. Addison's disease, ovarian failure and hypoparathyroidism. Clin Endocrinol Metab 1975; 4:379–434.

335. Blizzard RM, Chee P, David W. The incidence of parathyroid and other autoantibodies in the sera of patients with idiopathic hypoparathyroidism. Clin Exp Immunol 1966; 1:119–128.

336. Chapman CK, Bradwell AR, Dykks PW. Do parathyroid and adrenal autoantibodies coexist? J Clin Pathol 1986; 39(7):813–814.

337. Betterle C, Caretto A, Zeviani M, Pedini B, Salviati. Demonstration and characterization of anti-human mitochondria autoantibodies in idiopathic hypoparathyroidism and in other conditions. Clin Exp Immunol 1985; 62(2):353–360.

338. Li Y, Song YH, Rais N, Connor E, Schatz D, Muir A, Maclaren N. Autoantibodies to the extracellular domain of the calcium sensing receptor in patients with acquired hypoparathyroidism. J Clin Invest 1996; 97(4):910–914.

339. Brandi ML, Aurbach GD, Fattorossi A, Quarto R, Marx SJ, Fitzpatrick LA. Antibodies cytotoxic to bovine parathyroid cells in autoimmune hypoparathyroidism. Proc Natl Acad Sci USA 1986; 83(21):8366–8369.

340. Juppner H, Atkinson MJ, Baethke R, Hesch RD. Autoantibodies against parathyroid hormone in a patient with terminal renal insufficiency. Lancet 1(8391):1379–1381.

341. Cavaco B, Leite V, Loureiro MM, Ferreira MF, Pereira MC, Santos MA, Sobrinho LG J. Spontaneously occurring anti-PTH autoantibodies must be considered in the differential diagnosis of patients with elevated serum PTH levels. Endocrinol Invest 1999; 22(11):829–834.

342. Yamada K, Tamura Y, Tomioka H, Kumagai A, Yoshida S. Possible existence of anti-renal tubular plasmamembrane autoantibody which blocked parathyroid hormone-induced phosphaturia in a patient with pseudohypoparathyroidism type II and Sjogren's syndrome. J Clin Endocrinol Metab 1984; 58(2):339–343.

343. Supler M, Mickle JP. Lymphocytic hypophysitis: report of a case in a man with cavernous sinus involvement. Surg Neurol 1992; 37:472–476.

344. Mirakian R, Bottazzo GF, Cudworth AG, Richardson CA, Doniach D. Autoimmunity to anterior pituitary cells and the pathogenesis of insulin-dependent diabetes mellitus. Lancet 1982; 1:775–759.

345. Crock PA. Cytosolic autoantigens in lymphocytic hypophysitis. J Clin Endocrinol Metab 1998; 83(2):609–618.

346. Stromberg S, Crock P, Lernmark A, Hulting AL. Pituitary autoantibodies in patients with hypopituitarism and their relatives. J Endocrinol 1998 Jun;157(3):475–80.

347. Ruelle A, Bernasconi D, Tunesi G, Andrioli G. Lymphocytic hypophysitis. Case report. J Neurosurg Sci 1999; 43(3):205–208.

348. Heinze HJ, Bercu BB. Acquired hypophysitis in adolescence. J Pediatr Endocrinol Metab 1997; 10(3):315–321.

349. Maghnie M, Lorini R, Vitali L, Mastricci N, Carra AM, Severi F. Organ- and non-organ-specific auto-antibodies in children with hypopituitarism on growth hormone therapy. Eur J Pediatr 1995; 154(6):450–453.

350. Scherbaum WA, Czernichow P, Bottazzo GF, Doniach D. Diabetes insipidus in children. IV. A possible autoimmune type with vasopressin cell antibodies. J Pediatr 1985; 107:922–925.

351. Scherbaum WA, Bottazzo GF. Autoantibodies to vasopressin cells in idiopathic diabetes insipidus: evidence for an autoimmune variant. Lancet 1983; 1(8330):897–901.

352. Harada M, Yoshida H, Mimura Y, Ohtsubo K, Kawaguchi T, Murashima S, Sasatomi K, Komai A, Miyazato M, Iwao T, Sata M, Tanikawa K. Systemic sclerosis associated with diabetes insipidus. Intern Med 1997; 36(1):73–76.

353. Maghnie M, Cosi G, Genovese E, Manca-Bitti ML, Cohen A, Zecca S, Tinelli C, Gallucci M, Bernasconi S, Boscherini B, Severi F, Arico M. Central diabetes insipidus in children and young adults. N Engl J Med 2000; 343(14):998–1007.

354. Scherbaum WA, Wass JA, Besser GM, Bottazzo GF, Doniach D. Autoimmune cranial diabetes insipidus: its association with other endocrine diseases and with histiocytosis X. Clin Endocrinol (Oxf) 1986; 25(4):411–420.

355. De Bellis A, Bizzarro A, Di Martino S, Savastano S, Sinisi AA, Lombardi G, Bellastella A. Association of arginine vasopressin-secreting cell, steroid-secreting cell, adrenal and islet cell antibodies in a patient presenting with central diabetes insipidus, empty sella, subclinical adrenocortical failure and impaired glucose tolerance. Horm Res 1995; 44(3):142–146.

356. Paja M, Estrada J, Ojeda A, Ramon y Cajal S, Garcia-Uria J, Lucas T. Lymphocytic hypophysitis causing hypopituitarism and diabetes insipidus, and associated with autoimmune thyroiditis, in a non-pregnant woman. Postgrad Med J 1994; 70(821):220–224.

357. Weimann E, Molenkamp G, Bohles HJ. Diabetes insipidus due to hypophysitis. Horm Res 1997; 47(2):81–84.

358. Cemeroglu AP, Blaivas M, Muraszko KM, Robertson PL, Vazquez DM. Lymphocytic hypophysitis presenting with diabetes insipidus in a 14-year-old girl: case report and review of the literature. Eur J Pediatr 1997; 156(9):684–688.

359. De Bellis A, Bizzarro A, Amoresano Paglionico V, Di Martino S, Criscuolo T, Sinisi AA, Lombardi G, Bellastella A. Detection of vasopressin cell antibodies in some patients with autoimmune endocrine diseases without overt diabetes insipidus. Clin Endocrinol (Oxf) 1994; 40(2):173–177.

360. De Bellis A, Colao A, Di Salle F, Muccitelli VI, Iorio S, Perrino S, Pivonello R, Coronella C, Bizzarro A, Lombardi G, Bellastella A. A longitudinal study of vasopressin cell antibodies, posterior pituitary function, and magnetic resonance imaging evaluations in subclinical autoimmune central diabetes insipidus. J Clin Endocrinol Metab 1999; 84(9):3047–3051.

361. Toh BH, van Driel IR, Gleeson PA. Pernicious anemia. N Engl J Med 1997; 337(20):1441–1448.

362. Irvine WJ. The association of atrophic gastritis with autoimmune thyroid disease. Clin Endocrinol Metab 1975; 4:351–377.

363. Riley WJ, Toskes PP, Maclaren NK, Silverstein JH. Predictive value of gastric parietal cell autoantibodies as a marker for gastric and hematologic abnormalities associated with insulin-dependent diabetes. Diabetes 1982; 31:1051–1055.

364. De Block CE, De Leeuw IH, Van Gaal LF. High prevalence of manifestations of gastric autoimmunity in parietal cell antibody-positive type 1 (insulin-dependent) diabetic patients. The Belgian Diabetes Registry. J Clin Endocrinol Metab 1999; 84(11):4062–4067.

365. Chuang JS, Callaghan JM, Gleeson PA, Toh BH. Diagnostic ELISA for parietal cell autoantibody using tomato lectin-purified gastric H+/K(+)-ATPase (proton pump). Autoimmunity 1992; 12(1):1–7.

366. Meek F, Khoury EL, Doniach D, Baum H. Mitochondrial antibodies in chronic liver diseases and connective tissue disorders: Further characterization of the autoantigens. Clin Exp Immunol 1980; 41:43–54.

367. Czaja AJ. Autoantibodies. Baillieres Clin Gastroenterol 1995; 9(4):723–744.

368. Obermayer-Straub P, Manns MP. Cytochromes P450 and UDP-glucuronosyl-transferases as hepatocellular autoantigens. Baillieres Clin Gastroenterol 1996; 10(3):501–532.

369. Korponay-Szabo IR, Sulkanen S, Halttunen T, Maurano F, Rossi M, Mazzarella G, Laurila K, Troncone R, Maki M. Tissue transglutaminase is the target in both rodent and primate tissues for celiac disease-specific autoantibodies. J Pediatr Gastroenterol Nutr 2000; 31(5):520–527.

370. Kawasaki E, Eisenbarth GS. High-throughput radioassays for autoantibodies to recombinant autoantigens. Front Biosci 2000; 5:E181–E190.

371. Obermayer-Straub P, Manns MP. Autoimmune polyglandular syndromes. Baillieres Clin Gastroenterol 1998; 12(2):293–315.

372. Muir A, She JX. Advances in the genetics and immunology of autoimmune polyglandular syndrome II/III and their clinical applications. Ann Med Intern (Paris) 1999; 150(4):301–312.

373. Nagamine K, Peterson P, Scott HS, Kudoh J, Minoshima S, Heino M, Krohn KJ, Lalioti MD, Mullis PE, Antonarakis SE, Kawasaki K, Asakawa S, Ito F, Shimizu N. Positional cloning of the APECED gene. Nat Genet 1997; 17(4):393–398.

374. Chen Q-Y, Lan Michael, She J-X, Maclaren. The gene responsible for autoimmune polyglandular syndrome type 1 maps to chromsome 221q22.3 in US patients. J Autoimmunity 1998; 11:177–183.

375. An autoimmune disease, APECED, caused by mutations in a novel gene featuring two PHD-type zinc-finger domains. The Finnish-German APECED Consortium. Autoimmune Polyendocrinopathy-Candidiasis-Ectodermal Dystrophy. Nat Genet 1997; 17(4):399–403.

376. Bjorses P, Aaltonen J, Horelli-Kuitunen N, Yaspo ML, Peltonen L. Gene defect behind APECED: a new clue to autoimmunity. Hum Mol Genet 1998; 7(10):1547–1553.

377. Maclaren NK, Riley WJ. Inherited susceptibility to autoimmune Addison's disease is linked to hukman leukocyte antigens-DR3 and/or DR4, except when associated with type I autoimmune polyglandular syndrome. J Clin Endocrinol Metab 1986; 62(3):455–459.

378. Riley WJ, Winer A, Goldstein D. Coincident presence of thyrogastric autoimmunity at onset of type I diabetes. Diabetologia 1983; 24:418–421.

379. Ketchum C, Riley WJ, Maclaren NK. Adrenal dysfunction in asymptomatic patients with adrenocortical autoantibodies. J Clin Endocrinol Metab 1984; 58:1166–1170.

380. Farooqi IS, Jones MK, Evans M, O'Rahilly S, Hodges JR. Triple H syndrome: a novel autoimmune endocrinopathy characterized by dysfunction of the hippocampus, hair follicle, and hypothalamic-pituitary adrenal axis. J Clin Endocrinol Metab 2000; 85(8):2644–2648.

381. Neufeld M, Maclaren N, Blizzard R. Autoimmune polyglandular syndromes. Pediatr Ann 1980; 9:43–53.

382. Winter WE, Maclaren NK. To what extent is "polyendocrine" serology related to the clinical expression of disease. In: Doniach D, Bottazzo GF, eds. Clinical Immunology and Allergy. Bailliere Tindall, 1987:1:109–123.

383. Riley W, Maclaren N, Rosenbloom A. Thyroid disease in young diabetics. Lancet 1982; 2:489–490.

384. Maclaren NK, Riley WJ. Thyroid, gastric, and adrenal autimmunities associated with insulin-dependent diabetes mellitus. Diabetes Care 1985; 8 (Suppl 1):34–38.

29

Multiple Endocrine Neoplasia Syndromes

Giulia Costi and Noel K. Maclaren

Weill Medical College of Cornell University, New York Presbyterian Hospital, New York, New York, U.S.A.

I. INTRODUCTION

The multiple endocrine neoplasia (MEN) syndromes are inherited diseases characterized by the occurrence of tumors in two or more endocrine glands in a single patient and/or the family member of the patient. Although they are relatively rare, their importance is due to their risk of malignancies, which can be reduced by early diagnosis and treatment, especially among family members. There are two types of MEN syndromes, types 1 and 2, with distinct patterns of tissue involvement (Table 1).

II. MEN-1

Multiple endocrine neoplasia type 1 (Wermer syndrome) is an autosomal dominant disorder defined by a collective predisposition to tumors of the endocrine glands of the parathyroids, anterior pituitary, and pancreatic islets. More rarely, foregut carcinoid tumors may arise, while nonendocrine tumor expressions such as lipomas, facial angiofibromas, and skin collagenomas are relatively frequent. The prevalence of MEN-1 as estimated by autopsy studies approximates 2.5:1000 (1). However 1–18% of patients with primary hyperparathyroidism have been reported to have underlying MEN-1 (the prevalence is age dependent) while among patients with a gastrinoma the prevalence has been reported from 16 to 38%, and to near 3% among patients with pituitary tumors (2). All age groups may be affected, but in 80% of patients, the clinical manifestations will have appeared by the fifth decade of life (3). PTH secreting tumors are very rare in children, but they are increasingly common through late mid-life.

A. Genetics and Pathogenesis

In 1997 the gene responsible for MEN-1 syndrome was identified on chromosome 11q13 (4), consisting of 10 exons with an 1830 base-pair coding region that encodes a novel protein, named *menin* that is 610 amino acids long. Many different mutations in the MEN1 gene have been discovered, and most (75%) are functionally inactivating, consistent with MEN1 being a tumor-suppressor gene (5). In 5–10% of the cases where the mutations are not in the coding region of the MEN1 gene, they may occur in the promoter or enhancer regions that affect MEN1 transcription rates (6). No correlations have been reported between genotype and phenotype (7). The menin protein has a nuclear location, with two nuclear-binding domains located in the C-terminus (8). All the truncated MEN1 proteins seen in MEN-1 lack at least one of these nuclear localization signals resulting from nonsense and frame-shift mutations. *Menin* binds to junD, a jun/fos transcription factor, and it inhibits tumor-suppressor transcriptions stimulated by junD (9).

B. Clinical Features

The most common clinical problem in this syndrome results from the hypersecretion of the hormones by the glands affected.

1. Primary Hyperparathyroidism

Primary hyperparathyroidism is the most common expression of MEN1, occurring in 95% of patients (10). The disease presents usually as a long preclinical asymptomatic stage characterized by hypercalcemia followed by the onset of polyuria, polidipsia, muscular weakness, constipation, nephrolithiasis, and back pain from demineralized bone/osteitis fibrosa cystica. Older patients may develop characteristic subperiosteal absorptions of the second phalanges and so-called salt and pepper changes resulting from alternating hypo- and hyperdensities in the skull x-rays. Older patients are prone to changes in affect and mental problems that can have them erroneously diagnosed as senility or psychiatric disorders. A hypercalcemic storm or crisis is rare, as is the development of

Table 1 Genetics and Clinical Features of MEN Syndromes

	Locus	Gene	Mutation distribution	Mutation effect	Encoded protein	Inheritance	Age of onset (years)	Clinical features	Age to perform gene analysis in family members (years)
MEN-1	11q13	*MEN1*	Spread over nine coding exons	Gene inactivation	Nuclear protein, binding junD	Autosomal dominant	15–25	Primary hyperparathyroidism Pituitary tumors Pancreatic tumors	15
MEN-2									
MEN-2a			Exons 10, 11				30–40	Medullary thyroid carcinoma Pheochromocytoma Primary hyperparathyroidism	5
MEN-2b	10q11.2	*Rat*	Exon 16	Gene activation	Transmembrane glycoprotein, tyrosine kinase	Autosomal dominant	1–18	Medullary thyroid carcinoma Pheochromocytoma	Neonatal
FMTC			Exons 10, 11, 13, 14				30–40	Medullary thyroid carcinoma	5

parathyroid cancer. Laboratory findings document total (serum) calcium and ionized calcium (plasma) levels plus low serum phosphate levels in the face of elevated and nonsuppressed concentrations of plasma parathyroid hormone (PTH). Measurement of PTH by immunoassays often detects fragments, which have no biological activity. Measurements of more intact molecules or those determining the midportion of the molecule have lower margins of error. Replicate elevations of serum calcium over 10.2 mg/dl are consistent with the diagnosis; levels over 13 mg/dl can be life-threatening and require urgent treatment. Patients have hypercalcinuria exceeding 200–300 mg/day on normal diets. In such cases, or with acute symptoms, hydration with saline infusions and diuretics to force natriuresis is helpful in the emergency situation. Oral phosphate can be given with more chronic effects, however, the dosages given should be initially low (1–2 gm daily) to avoid precipitation of calcium phosphate in cardiac tissues. Later, higher dosages (2–4 g daily) can be given. Mithramycin is a cytotoxic antibiotic that can inhibit bone resorption, but is toxic and best reserved for cancer-related hypercalcemias. Bisphosphonate compounds will be increasingly used to control both acute and chronic hypercalcemias.

MEN1 can be differentiated from sporadic parathyroid adenoma by the earlier age of onset of the hypercalcemia (typically 15–25 vs. 50–60 years), and the lack of female bias (the male/female ratio of MEN-1 is 1:1), the autosomal dominant pattern of inheritance in pedigrees, and the presence of pituitary or pancreatic manifestations. MEN-1 should also be differentiated from familial hypocalciuric hypercalcemia that has its onset from birth and is characterized by low levels (<100 mg in adults) of calcium in the urine and normal level of PTH in the serum (11).

Surgical removal of the hyperfunctioning tumors is the treatment of choice, which is best accomplished by a good preoperative work-up involving ultrasound or magnetic resonance imaging (MRI) studies, and sometimes preoperative venous sampling for PTH since 20% of all parathyroid tumors are located in the upper mediastinum. Management of the hyperparathyroidism is controversial; surgery may be put off if the patient has only mildly elevated serum calcium level, no renal or bone problems, no previous hypercalcemic crisis, and is prepared to be closely monitored. Surgical intervention is, however, indicated when the calcium level increases more than 11.0 mg/dl, and/or renal stones or bone density decreases occur.

2. Pituitary Tumors

Pituitary tumors occur in 15–20% of patients with MEN-1 (12). Some 60% of these tumors are prolactinomas, fewer than 25% are growth-hormone-secreting, and about 5% secrete adenocorticotropic hormone (ACTH). Nonfunctioning tumors can also be observed clinically. The clinical characteristics of these tumors are similar to those found in sporadic neoplasias and they depend on the hormone(s) secreted and the size of the tumor. Patients can present with amenorrhea, infertility, and galactorrhea in women; impotence in men; and acromegaly or Cushing disease. Pituitary tumors can also compress the optic chiasm, causing bilateral peripheral hemianopsia. The diagnostic and therapeutic approach to pituitary tumors in the context of MEN-1 is not different from that in sporadic cases and consists of medical therapy (bromocryptine or the long-acting somatostatin analog Octreotide) or selective hypophysectomy and radiotherapy for residual unresectable tumor.

3. Pancreatic Tumors

The occurrence of *pancreatic tumors* in MEN-1 syndromes is important because of their malignant potential. The incidence of pancreatic islet cell or gastrointestinal tumors in MEN-1 is age dependent but varies from 30 to 80% (13). The most common cause of symptomatic disease is the Zollinger-Ellison syndrome leading to persistent peptic ulcerations and hyperacidity due to the hypersecretion of gastrin, often from a pancreatic islet cell. The hypercalcemia from parathyroid adenoma can exacerbate the symptoms and further elevate serum gastrin concentration. Patients with Zollinger-Ellison syndrome may also present with diarrhea or steatorrhea. The diagnosis is made by demonstrating a raised fasting serum gastrin concentration in association with an increased basal gastric acid secretion. Whereas H_2 receptor histamine antagonists cimetidine or Tagamet, ranitidine (Zantac), or famotidine (Pepcid) usually reduce gastric acidity, they often fail in this condition. However, reduction of basal acid output may be achieved by the substituted benzimidazoles (e.g. Omeprazole), which are potent inhibitors of parietal cell H^+/K^+-ATPase (14).

Because of the multifocal nature of the tumors in MEN-1 syndrome, surgical therapy is controversial and often not successful. Only 16% of patients so treated become free from symptoms after surgical intervention (15). In some islet tumors, watery diarrhea hypokalemia and hypochloremia can be seen in the absence of increased gastrin levels, due to vasoactive intestinal peptide (vipoma) and prostaglandins, while hypersecretion of glucagons can induce weight loss, hyperglycemia, venous thromboses, and a characteristic necrotizing migratory erythema.

Insulinoma is the second most common pancreatic islet cell tumor in patients with MEN-1 and occurs more often in patients under 40 years of age (3). The tumors are typically multicentric and may become malignant. Patients present with hypoglycemia especially after fasting. Biochemical investigations reveal inappropriately raised plasma insulin concentrations in association with hypoglycemia. Elevated plasma C-peptide and proinsulin levels are useful to confirm the diagnosis, since proinsulin levels may be disproportionately high. Surgery is the optimal treatment and is usually curative when a discrete tumor is found (16).

Besides alpha and beta islet cell tumors, others may secrete pancreatic polypeptide or, more rarely ACTH, serotonin, or somatostatin. However, surgical removal of the tumor may be difficult when metastases have already occurred by the time of diagnosis. In some patients the administration of Octreotide may be helpful.

Thymic carcinoid tumors develop in about 5% of the patients, especially in men who are heavy smokers. The tumors are usually nonfunctioning and aggressive (17). Other tumors seen on occasion in MEN-1 include adrenal adenomas (sometimes ACTH secreting) and carcinomas, and cell thyroid tumors that are never of the medullary type.

C. Screening of Family Members

Family members of patients with MEN-1 are at risk for carrying the defective gene; and the closer the relationship, the higher the risk. Screening for the MEN-1 gene is of great importance because early diagnosis and treatment of these tumors can reduce morbidity and mortality. Recently DNA testing for the inherited MEN-1 mutation has become available (18), but the proper role of this test still needs to be defined. Individuals found to be carriers of a mutant gene should nevertheless undergo biochemical screening (serum concentration of calcium, gastrointestinal hormones especially gastrin and prolactin) at least once a year. Every 5 years, pituitary and abdominal imaging should be performed from the age of 5 years on.

III. MEN-2

MEN-2 (Sipple syndrome) is a genetic disease, inherited by an autosomal dominant pattern as is MEN-1, and with high grade of penetrance. It is classified into three different forms. MEN-2a is characterized by C-cell (calcitonin-secreting) tumors of the thyroid (medullary thyroid carcinoma) in virtually every patient, with pheochromocytoma, and/or primary parathyroid hyperplasia. Recently, lichen amyloidosis has been recognized to be part of the syndrome (19). In MEN-2b, patients present with medullary thyroid carcinoma and pheochromocytoma, but do not develop hyperparathyroidism. The thyroid carcinoma is more aggressive than in MEN-2a, and occurs at an earlier age. Patients can also present with mucosal neuromas, intestinal ganglioneuromas, and a marfanoid habitus. Familial medullary thyroid cancer is a variant of MEN-2a, in which the tendency to develop thyroid carcinoma is not associated with other clinical manifestations. There are no accurate population studies for the incidence of the MEN-2 syndromes; however, it is generally assumed that 20–25% of medullary thyroid cancers are heritable.

A. Genetics and Pathogenesis

The gene responsible for MEN-2 has been identified as the *ret* gene located on the chromosome 10q11.2 (20,21). The coding sequence of *ret* consists of 21 exons over a total length of 55 kb. It is a proto-oncogene and the gene product is a cell-surface glycoprotein. The protein is a member of the receptor tyrosine–kinase family, which transduces growth and proliferation signals in tissues derived from the neuronal crest, from which all of the tissues involved in the MEN-2 (thyroid C cells, adrenal medulla and autonomic ganglia) are derived (22). Three ligands have been identified: glial cell-line-derived neurotrophic factor (GDNF) (23), neuturin, and persephin (24). They are expressed in the nervous system and promote the survival of neurons during development. A glycosyl-phosphatidylinositol protein (GFR α1, GFR α2) binding of the ligand is also necessary for the activation of *ret* (25). MEN-2a and the MEN-2b are caused by different mutations of the *ret* gene. In the MEN-2a and in familial medullary thyroid carcinoma, most of the mutations occur in the cysteine-rich region of the extra-cellular domain encoded by exon 10. These mutations cause the substitution of cysteine by another amino acid. A few mutations have been found in exons 13, 14, and 15 (26). By contrast, 95% of MEN-2b cases are caused by a mutation in exon 16 with the substitution of methionine with threonine, which alters the substrate-recognition pocket in the tyrosine kinase protein (27). All the mutations both in the MEN-2a and MEN-2b lead to activation of the protein. This is different from almost all other inherited predispositions to neoplasia, which are due to mutations that inactivate tumor suppressor protein (Table 1).

B. Clinical Features

1. Medullary Thyroid Carcinoma

Medullary thyroid carcinoma (MTC) is usually preceded by multicentric hyperplasia of the parafollicular C cells. The clinical manifestation of this tumor is no different from that in the sporadic case, in which it presents as a thyroid nodule or cervical lymphadenopathy. Sometimes MTC can cause Cushing syndrome because of ectopic production of ACTH. Serum levels of calcitonin are usually high, especially if the tumor is palpable. In patients with C-cell hyperplasia or small C-cell tumors, the resting serum levels of calcitonin can be normal but will rise after calcium infusion (28). The necessary treatment of MTC in any MEN-2 syndrome is total thyroidectomy. This should be performed as early as possible, especially in MEN-2b syndrome, in which the MTC tends to be more aggressive and undergo malignant transformation. Metastatic disease has been reported as early as in 1-year-old children (29). Radiation therapy can be useful to reduce the tumor dimension and prevent local recurrence.

2. Pheochromocytoma

Some 40% of patients with MEN-2a and MEN-2b develop pheochromocytomas, usually 10 years or so later than MTC (30). Generally the tumors are nonmalignant at least until they are of large size. Symptoms can include anxiety, headache, diaphoresis, and palpitations. Laboratory evaluations reveal raised excretions of epinephrine and norepinephrine or metanephrines (31). In patients with MEN-2a there is an increased risk of bilateral tu-

mors; imaging studies should be performed to detect possible bilateral disease before surgery is undertaken. Unilateral adrenalectomy is the treatment of choice in cases of unilateral tumor. Bilateral adrenalectomy should be limited to patients with bilateral tumors or, more specifically, in those with a family history of aggressive bilateral adrenal medullary disease.

3. Primary Hyperparathyroidism

Involvement of the parathyroid glands in this syndrome is always benign. It has been reported in 10–25% of patients (32). Hyperplasias or benign adenomas can occur and are often clinically silent. Otherwise symptoms of hypercalcemia or renal stones have been reported. The diagnosis can be achieved finding high or normal level of PTH in the presence of hypercalcemia, as discussed above under MEN-1. The indications for surgery are similar to those in patients with sporadic primary hyperparathyroidism.

C. Screening in Family Members

The early detection of affected family members is essential so that thyroidectomy can be performed as soon as possible. Before DNA testing was available, biochemical screening was performed using intravenous pentagastrin or calcium infusion to stimulate the secretion of calcitonin from malignant or hyperplastic C cells. False-positive responses could, however, occur (33). In family members, such tests, if found to be negative, should be performed yearly. Recently DNA analysis became the optimal test in the MEN-2 syndrome. In a MEN-2 family the affected patient should be analyzed to determine the specific mutation responsible for the disease. The number of possible mutations in the *ret* gene are small and a single mutation can be detected in 90% of cases. Once the mutation in the proband has been found, all other family members should be tested before the age of 4–5 years in case of MEN-2a and familial medullary thyroid carcinomas, and in the neonatal period in the case of MEN-2b (Table 1).

IV. ADRENAL ADENOMA

Benign adenomas are the most common cause of an adrenal mass. The majority of cases are clinically silent, being usually found incidentally during a computed tomographic (CT) scan of the abdomen performed for an unrelated reason. The prevalence of so-called incidentalomas gradually increases from 3 years of age, to be as high as 7% in adults over the age of 50 years (34).

A. Genetics

The molecular mechanisms of the adrenal tumorigenesis have been studied extensively. Evidence has accumulated to show that tumorigenesis in the adrenal gland is different from that in other endocrine tissues. Cyclic AMP is a second messenger involved in the proliferation and hypersecretion of many endocrine tissues. The activation of G-protein-coupled receptors and GTP-binding proteins, and the regulatory proteins of cAMP, have been involved in the pathogenesis of acromegaly and toxic thyroid adenomas. However, the activation of cAMP/protein kinase A pathway seems not to be important in the development of neoplasia in the adrenal gland (35). Cytogenetic studies have shown that adrenal tumorogenesis is characterized by the amplification of chromosomes not commonly affected in other tumors, suggesting the possible presence of adrenal-specific oncogenes. Adrenal adenoma or carcinoma can occur in several hereditary tumor syndromes such as Li-Fraumeni syndrome, Beckwith-Wiedemann syndrome, MEN-1, Carney complex, and familial adenomatosis polyposis. The discovery of the genetic defects underlying these disorders increases the potential understanding of adrenal tumorigenesis.

Li-Fraumeni syndrome is a rare family tumor syndrome characterized by breast cancer, leukemias, soft tissue sarcomas, gliomas, and adrenocortical carcinomas. The genetic defect has been identified as germ-line point mutations in the p53 tumor-suppressor gene. The other nonaffected p53 allele is inactivated in tumor tissue by deletion of the short arm of chromosome 17, thus eliminating all wild-type p53 activity (36).

In Beckwith-Wiedemann syndrome (BWS), a rare disease characterized by macroglossia, gigantism, earlobe pits, and increased risk of Wilms' tumor of the kidney, rhabdomyosarcoma, hepatoblastoma, and adrenal carcinoma are caused by the allelic loss of a tumor suppressor gene mapped to chromosome 11p15 (37).

The Carney complex is a disorder characterized by myxomas of the heart, tumors involving the peripheral nervous system, spotty pigmentation of the skin, and endocrine neoplasia (e.g., adrenocortical tumors). The molecular defect has been identified in mutations of the protein kinase A type 1-α regulatory subunit on chromosome 2p16 (38).

In familial adenomatous polyposis, an autosomal dominant disorder in which patients develop more than 100 adenomatous polyps in the large intestine with a strong tendency to undergo malignant degeneration, adrenocortical neoplasms also occur with an abnormally high prevalence (39). The disease is caused by a mutation in the adenomatous polyposis coli (APC) gene located at 5q21.

The discovery of the genetic defects underlying the familial syndrome and the fact that most of the benign and malign neoplasia of adrenal are monoclonal suggest that genetic changes at a specific locus are necessary for the development of such tumors. Several candidate genes have been investigated. For aldosterone-producing tumors, the aldosterone synthase receptor (the CYP11B2 gene), the corticotropin-regulated promoter (the CYP11B1), and the angiotensin II type-1 receptor (ATR-1) have been studied but they seem not to be associated with sporadic adrenal adenoma (40). In cortisol-producing tumors, the loss of heterozygosity of the corticotropin receptor (MC2R) has been discovered to occur frequently in adrenocortical carcinomas but not in adenomas (41). Because there is the loss of heterozygosity on chromosome 11q13 in 20% of sporadic adenomas, some authors studied the expression of the MEN1 gene, located on 11q13, in sporadic adenomas and found mutations in less than 10% of the tumors. This suggests that another tumor suppressor gene is important for the predisposition to adrenal tumors encoded by the 11q13 region (42).

B. Clinical Features

Adenomas that can develop in the adrenal gland can be subclassified in glucocorticoid secreting, adrenocorticoid secreting, and nonfunctioning adenomas.

1. Aldosterone-Producing Adenomas

The clinical manifestations of *aldosterone-producing adenoma* derive from the hypernatremia and hypokalemias and metabolic alkalosis. Patients can present with hypertension, urinary frequency, muscular weakness, paraesthesias, cramps, and tetany. Determination of plasma aldosterone (high), plasma renin activity (low), and 24 h urinary aldosterone excretion (high) should be performed in newly diagnosed hypertensive patients with hypokalemia or young age of onset. A ratio of plasma aldosterone to plasma renin activity of 20 or more indicates the presence of a primary hyperaldosteronism. The relationship is best demonstrated by obtaining a renin level with the patient standing up, in which position the release of renin is normally greatly stimulated.

Once primary hyperaldosteronism is diagnosed, the differential diagnosis lies among aldosterone-producing adrenal tumor, idiopathic adrenal hyperplasia, and glucocorticoid-suppressible hyperaldosteronism in which aldosterone biosynthesis is regulated by ACTH rather than by renin. A postural test can differentiate between adenoma and idiopathic hyperaldosteronism (42). If plasma aldosterone and renin activity are measured in the morning after overnight recumbency and 2 h of ambulation, aldosterone levels increase in patients with adenoma, because of the diurnal fall of the ACTH, which is a minor stimulus to aldosterone production. In the case of idiopathic hyperaldosteronism, the level of plasma aldosterone will rise during the test under the stimulus of angiotensin II that increases in the upright position. Moreover, the level of 18-hydroxycorticosterone is elevated in patients with aldosterone-producing adenomas but is lower in patients with idiopathic hyperaldosteronism. The diagnosis of glucocorticoid-suppressible hyperaldosteronism can be obtained by measuring the plasma level of 18-hydroxycortisol and 18-oxocortisol, which are products of the methyloxidation of cortisol by the aldosterone synthase that is typically elevated in this condition. The enzyme is the product of a chimeric gene that arose from an unequal crossover. The hybrid gene can catalyze the reaction but is regulated by ACTH instead of the renin–angiotensin system. The administration of dexamethasone for 4 days inhibits the secretion of ACTH and suppresses the production of aldosterone. Recently, DNA analysis for the identification of the hybrid gene mutation responsible for the glucocorticoid-suppressible hyperaldosteronism has become available (43).

Computer tomography is the best imaging technique to identify adrenal mass. It can identify masses of 10 mm, and gives information about size, homogeneity, presence of calcifications or areas of necrosis, and eventual local infiltration.

2. Glucocorticoid-Producing Adenomas

Glucocorticoid-producing adenomas are one cause of Cushing's syndrome that is ACTH-independent. Hyperproduction of cortisol determines the severity of symptoms such as hypertension, obesity, and hirsutism in females. To detect hypersecretion by the adrenal gland, the best test is the 24 h urinary free cortisol level, which, in a patient with adrenal adenoma and subclinical Cushing disease, will be more than 551.8 nmol/day. A dexamethasone suppression test can also be performed.

C. Treatment

If the tumor is hormone-secreting, or is clinically silent but larger than 5 cm, the patient should undergo surgery. The treatment of choice for benign adrenal adenoma is laparoscopic adrenalectomy when the retroperitoneal approach is preferred. If the tumor is suspected to be malignant, classic transperitoneal surgery should be performed (44). Patients with aldosterone-producing adenomas must have their blood pressure carefully controlled and their potassium level monitored before surgery. Hypertension can still be present after the intervention, however, because of long-term vascular damage resulting from prolonged hyperaldosteronism (45). In case of aldosteronomas, moreover, the patient can have a period of hyponatremia and hyperkalemia after the surgery due to continued suppression of the renin–angiotensin–aldosterone system. A high-salt diet and mineralocorticoid therapy may have to be given temporally. Patients with corticoid-secreting adenomas may likewise need hormonal replacement therapy because of atrophy of the hypothalamic corticotropin-releasing hormone-secreting cells.

V. THYROID ADENOMAS

Thyroid adenomas represent 90% of the nodular lesions of the thyroid. Single nodules are more common in women than in men, but the incidence of thyroid nodules increases throughout life in patients of both genders. The typical thyroid adenoma is a solitary encapsulated lesion demarcated from the surrounding parenchyma. Adenomas derive from follicular epithelia and, microscopically, the cells form uniform follicles that contain colloid. On histological examination the adenomas can be classified into subtypes based on the degree of follicle formation and their colloid content. These are classified as macrofollicular, microfollicular, Hürthle's cell adenoma, atypical adenoma, and adenoma with papillae.

A. Genetics

Most thyroid tumors are sporadic and nonfamilial, suggesting that the underlying genetic abnormality is likely to be a somatic, acquired mutation. Pituitary thyroid-stimulating hormone (TSH) is the main stimulator of growth and function of normal follicular thyroid cells. When TSH binds to its membrane receptor, it actives guanine–nucleotide-binding protein Gs and stimulates the adenylate cyclase cAMP pathway (46). Increases in the intracellular levels of cAMP activate protein kinase, which in turn stimulates thyroid hormone production and induces the proliferation of thyroid epithelial cells. Adenylate cyclase activity decreases when the GTP is hydrolyzed by the intrinsic GTPase activity of Gs-α. Many thyroid adenomas are caused by activating somatic mutations in genes that encode for the TSH receptor, or the α subunit of the guanyl-nucleotide stimulatory protein (Gs) that results in constitutive activation of thyroid epithelial cells in the absence of TSH (47, 48).

Most of the mutations causing adenomas have been found in the third cytoplasmic loop on the sixth transmembrane segment of the TSH receptor, and in the C-terminus of Gs-α that is critical to the receptor interaction (so-called hot spot sequence) (49,50). These mutations do not explain all the tumors, or toxic adenomas that are not secondary to TSH-R mutations. Other genes encoding for proteins involved in the TSH-R pathway could be activated and responsible for the tumorigenesis. Mutations of the Ras oncogenes have been found in both benign and malignant thyroid tumors. There are three ras proteins: K-ras, N-ras, and H-ras. All of them are membrane-anchored and they mediate signaling through many tyrosine kinases, including those of hormone receptors. The hydrolysis of the GTP to GDP that is bound to the ras protein determines the inactivation of the signal. Mutations in the GTP-binding domain (codons 12,13) or the GTP-ase domain (codon 61) cause activation of the ras oncogenes (51). In thyroid tumors, point mutations or amplifications of all three ras oncogenes can occur (52). There is a general agreement on the role of the ras oncogenes in the early phases of the tumorigenesis, but the real prevalence of these mutations still needs to be determined. The angiogenic and the soluble factors that stimulate them have been recently studied in their pathogenesis. Vascular endothelial growth factor (VEGF), the principal cytokine that mediates angiogenesis, has been associated with tumorigenic potential of thyroid cancer cell lines (53). Other authors found overexpression of VEGF in follicular adenomas, Hürthle's cell neoplasia, and papillary carcinomas; in follicular carcinoma and anaplastic carcinomas, VEGF was suppressed, suggesting an important role for the cytokine in the early stages of the thyroid carcinogenesis (54).

B. Clinical Features

Thyroid adenomas often present as a mass without any other clinical sign or symptoms, discovered during an examination or radiological procedure. In a minority of cases, adenomas can be hyperfunctional and cause clinical features of hyperthyroidism. Neoplasia must be strongly considered when nodules are "cold" and do not take up ^{131}I on scanning.

VI. PITUITARY ADENOMAS

Pituitary adenomas are common neoplasia derived from adenohypophyseal cells. They can be small, nonfunctioning lesions that are discovered casually, similiarly to radiological incidentalomas or during autopsy. In some cases they produce hormones that can cause severe clinical syndromes such as acromegaly or Cushing disease. They are typically benign lesions with a very small possibility (0.1%) of becoming malignant. However, they can present from the effects of aggressive local growth invading the brain parenchyma, the cavernous and paranasal sinuses, the bony clivius, and cause symptoms of intracranial mass, hypopituitarism, and/or peripheral visual field disturbances from pressure effects on the optic chiasm (55).

Although the true incidence of pituitary adenomas is not known, recent data suggest that pituitary adenomas occur in as many as 20% of the general population (56). At autopsy, careful histological assessment identifies pituitary adenoma in 22.5–27% of patients, with no gender-based differences in incidence (57). The incidence increases with aging: more than 30% of people 60 years of age have clinically silent tumors. Pituitary adenomas are, however, rare in children, with only 3.5–8.5% of these tumors diagnosed during childhood. At such time they manifest clinically especially in girls, and it has been reported that they are less aggressive and invasive than tumors of adults (58). Pituitary adenomas represent approximately 15% of all intracranial tumors (59). Prolactinomas are the most common type of adenoma; GH- and ACTH-producing adenomas each represent 10–15% (often they are mixed), while TSH-secreting tumors are rare (60).

A. Genetics and Pathogenesis

For many years there has been controversy regarding the molecular basis of pituitary tumorigeneisis. Several animal studies have suggested a fundamental role for hypothalamic hormones in the development of pituitary tumors. Recently the question was resolved when it became clear that all the pituitary tumors arise from a single cell. This monoclonality implies that intrinsic genetic alterations account for the initiating event. Furthermore, the tissue surrounding the pituitary adenoma is usually normal, suggesting that independent cellular events do not necessarily precede adenoma formation. It is likely that the majority of pituitary adenomas develop from transformed cells that are dependent on hormonal stimulation for tumor progression (61). The dysregulation of cell proliferation and differentiation may occur by the activation of oncogenes or inactivation of tumor-suppressor genes. Oncogene activation may occur as a result of an activating single-point mutation. Because the gain of function is a dominant event, a single altered allele may be sufficient to produce the phenotypic change. By contrast, the tumor-suppressor genes (TSG) are recessive oncogenes that require the inactivation of both alleles (by deletion, rearrangement, or silencing through methylation) to cause proliferation of the cell in a clonal neoplastic fashion. Heterozygous activating somatic point mutations in the α-subunit of the stimulatory Gs proteins (Gs) were the earliest dominant activating mutations described in endocrine tumors (62). Activation results when a missense mutation replaces residue 201 or 227. The resulting oncogene encodes for mutated G protein called *gsps*, which were first described in a subset of somatotroph adenomas, nonfunctioning adenomas, and other functional pituitary neoplasms. The mutation result in a ligand-independent, constitutively elevated cAMP and hormone hypersecretion.

Recently Melmed and colleagues isolated a novel pituitary tumor-transforming gene (PTTG) (63). They showed increased levels of PTTG mRNA in GH-, prolactin-secreting, and nonfunctional pituitary tumors. In vitro and in vivo experiments showed the strong transforming potential of PTTG. Because of its widespread and abundant expression in pituitary tumors, PTTG most likely has a key role in the early induction of pituitary cell transformation. It potently induces the expression of fibroblast growth factor, a known mediator of cell growth and angiogenesis. Another oncogene involved in pituitary tumorigenesis seems to be the cyclin D1 gene (*CCND1*) located on 11q13. Gene amplification leads to overexpression of cyclin D. Habbers et al. found an allelic imbalance of the *CCND1* gene in the pituitary tumors. They studied the expression of cyclin D1 by an immunohistochemical assay and found that 25% of the tumor cells showed expression of cyclin D1. Both nuclear and cytoplasmic staining was found more frequently in nonfunctional tumors than in somatotropinomas (64). The loss of tumor-suppressor gene function has also been implicated. *MEN1* gene, the TSG located on the long arm of the chromososme 11 (11q13) responsible for the MEN-1 syndrome, has been studied, but menin expression is not downregulated in the majority of the sporadic pituitary tumors (65). However, these tumors present loss of heterozygosity at the same locus 11q13 in 20% of cases, suggesting that an additional TSG at this locus is involved in the pathogenesis of pituitary adenomas.

The retinoblastoma gene (*RB1*) is another TSG implicated in several neoplasms. Adenocarcinomas of intermediate lobe corticotroph differentiation have been found in RB1 transgenic knockout mice (66) induced in order to study this gene in the humans, but no mutations have been found in the pituitary adenoma (67). However, preliminary data show loss of heterozygosity at sites telomeric and centromeric to the RB locus in some aggressive pituitary adenomas. These data suggest the presence of another TSG located at 13q that is closely linked to RB1 (68). The frequent loss of heterozygosity of 9p21 also has been found in pituitary adenomas (69). The *CDKN2A* gene maps to this locus and its protein product p16 is a cell cycle regulator that is often disrupted in human neoplasias. It prevents the phosphorylation of RB and is responsible for inhibiting progress through the G1/S cell cycle checkpoint. Loss of p16 results in RB remaining in its hyperphosphorylated form, negating its ability to inhibit the progression of the cell cycle.

Several growth factors have been implicated in the pathway of the tumorogenesis. They are polypeptides that can regulate cell replication and differentiation, altering the expression of specific genes. The pituitary is a site of synthesis and action of growth factors including insulin-like growth factor-I and II (IGF-I, IGF-II), nerve growth factor (NGF) (70), transforming growth factor-α and β, and basic fibroblast growth factor (bFGF). Some studies suggest that peptides derived from human pituitary tumor cells can stimulate rat adenohypophysial cells replication in vitro (71). The role of these growth factors in pituitary tumorogenesis remains to be established. The understanding of the exact mechanism involved in pituitary adenoma will have relevance in clinical practice. The identification of specific molecular markers of tumor invasiveness and recurrence will permit the selection of appropriate follow-up protocols and earlier subcellular therapies.

B. Clinical Features

1. Prolactinoma

Prolactin-secreting adenoma (prolactinoma) is the most common hormonally active pituitary adenoma. When the tumor is less than 1 cm in diameter, it is defined as a microadenoma. If it is 1 cm or larger, then it is classified as a macroadenoma.

In women the first clinical manifestations usually are galactorrhea and ovulatory disorders probably due to inhibition of luteinizing hormone (LH) and perhaps follicle-stimulating hormone (FSH) secretion, because of inhibition of the release of gonadotropin-releasing hormone (GnRH). In men, hyperprolactinemia results in decreased libido, infertility, and impotence. Women usually present with symptoms at a younger age and tend to have mi-

croadenoma. Men tend to present at older ages with larger adenoma that cause visual field abnormalities and hypopituitarism owing to pituitary tissue destruction (72). They only rarely develop galactorrhea. Some patients with a lactrotoph adenoma are noted to have subtle acromegalic features. Even if the hypersecretion of GH cannot be documented, the tumors contain prolactin and GH. This kind of tumor is known as acidophil stem cell adenoma, which can be differentiated from the usual lactotroph adenomas because of aggressivity and tendency to recur (73).

In children, prolactinomas are rare, but their clinical presentations have been reported in small numbers of studies. However the frequency of such tumors is likely underestimated since symptoms tend to occur later in life. As reported in adults, prolactinomas in children occur mostly in girls, causing menstrual disturbances (74). Delayed puberty can also be associated with prolactinomas because of the effect of hyperprolactinemia on the hypothalamic-gonadotropic activity. The symptoms of hyperprolactinemia correlate with its severity. Serum prolactin concentrations greater than 20 ng/ml are abnormal. The measurement can be performed at any time, since usual daily activities have little effect on prolactin secretion. However, physical stress and high-protein meals can increase the prolactin concentrations; therefore, a slightly high value should be confirmed. In case of persistent slightly elevated serum prolactin values or when levels are clearly pathological, an MRI to search for a mass lesion in the hypothalamic–pituitary region is required.

A dopamine agonist is the first-line treatment for patients with micro- or macro-adenomas because it decreases the size and secretion of the tumors. Bromocriptine is an ergot derivate that has been used for decades for treatment of hyperprolactenemia. Other dopamine agonists such as Pergolide or Carbegoline can be used if the patient does not respond. Bromocriptine must be given twice a day and the principal side effects are nausea, postural hypotension, and mental dulling (75). If the patient cannot tolerate the dopamine agonists, or if the adenoma does not respond to agonist therapy, transphenoidal surgery should be performed. If a significant amount of hormonally secreting tissue remains after surgery, radiation therapy should follow.

2. GH-Secreting Adenoma

GH-secreting adenoma is the most common cause of acromegaly or gigantism. These adenomas account for about one third of all hormone-secreting pituitary adenomas. The hyperproduction of GH by the tumor stimulates the hepatic secretion of IGF-I, which in turn causes most of the clinical features. In adults the typical sign is acromegaly, which is insidious in onset and progresses slowly. The characteristic findings are enlarged jaw and enlarged swollen soft tissues of the hands and feet. The facial features became coarse, with enlargement of the nose and frontal bones (76). Bone density can be increased and cardiovascular disease including hypertension, left ventricular hypertrophy, and cardiomyopathy can occur (77). In children GH excess results in rapid and excessive growth and attainment of adult height beyond the genetic potential. Typical manifestations of acromegaly can also appear. The diagnosis of acromegaly can be confirmed by measurement of both serum GH concentrations that do not suppress after a glucose load and GH-dependent circulating molecules, such as IGF-I and IGFBP-3. IGF-I concentrations during the day are not influenced by food intake, exercise, or sleep. The result must be interpreted, however, with the age, because IGF-I concentrations are highest during puberty and decline gradually thereafter. In contrast, GH concentrations reflect their pulsatile secretion and are stimulated by a variety of factors including short-term fasting, exercise, stress, and sleep. To obviate this problem, it is best not to obtain random measurements of serum GH.

The most specific dynamic test for establishing the diagnosis of acromegaly is an oral glucose tolerance test in which postglucose values remain greater than 2 ng/ml in 85% of patients with GH hypersecretion (78). Additional hyperprolactinemia occurs in 30% of the patients because the cosecretion of prolactin and GH by a somammotroph adenoma. Once GH hypersecretion has been confirmed, the next step is an MRI study of the pituitary. Pituitary tumors as small as 2 mm in diameter can be detected by this technique and the dimension and the exact extension of the tumor can be identified.

Selective transsphenoidal surgical resection is the treatment of choice for patients with somatotroph adenoma that are small enough to be removed surgically (79). Medical therapy is indicated in patients with adenomas that are too large to be completely removed, or when resection has failed. Somatostatin analogs such like Octreotide inhibit GH secretion by binding to specific receptors for somatostatin (80). The long-acting form of Octreotide, which is administrated intramuscularly every 2 or 4 weeks, is now available in the United States.

Somatostatin analogs are usually well tolerated but about one-third of patients may experience nausea, fat malabsorption, and decreased gallbladder postprandial contractility (81). Dopamine agonists such as bromocryptine, Pergolide and Cabergoline inhibit GH secretion in patients with sommamotroph adenoma. They have a limited efficacy but combined therapy with Octreotide and a dopamine may be successful when either alone is not. If GH hypersecretion cannot be controlled by surgery or medical therapy, external radiation can be used.

3. TSH-Secreting Adenoma

This kind of adenoma accounts for less than 1% of all hormone-secreting pituitary adenomas and less than 1% of all cases of hyperthyroidism. Adenomas secreting TSH are equally common in men and women, whereas tumors secreting both TSH and prolactin are about five times more common in women. Most patients have the typical symptoms and signs of hyperthyroidism, but a few patients have mild or even no symptoms (82). Other clinical features in addition to hyperthyroidism are visual field defect, menstrual disturbances, and galactorrhea. In childhood, these tumors are very rare. Patients have an enlarged gland and clinical symptoms and signs of thyrotoxicosis but without exophthalmos.

The characteristic biochemical abnormalities in patients with TSH-secreting adenoma are normal or high serum TSH concentrations and high serum total and free thyroxine (T4) and triiodothyronine (T3) concentrations. The autonomous TSH secretion usually does not increase in response to thyrotropin-releasing hormone (TRH) and does not decrease in response to exogenous thyroid hormone administration. Any patients with hyperthyroidism and elevated serum TSH should undergo a CT or MRI study of the pituitary. MRI is the most sensitive test for the detection of pituitary tumors.

The treatment of choice is transsphenoidal resection of the tumor, even if the surgery will result in no change in one-third of patients. Therefore, many patients also require medical therapy. Dopamine agonists (Bromocryptine, Carbegoline) have proven to be effective but the somatostatine analog Octreotide is effective in almost all patients.

4. Gonadotropin-Secreting Adenoma

Gonadotroph adenomas are the most common clinically nonfunctioning pituitary macroadenoma. They usually inefficiently secrete or secrete noneffective hormones. Thus they are often identified only when they are large enough to produce neurological symptoms. The most common symptom is impaired vision due to compression of the optic chiasm (83). The patient will complain of diminished vision in the temporal field. Headache and diplopia due to the compression of the oculomotor nerves can occur. Sometimes gonadotroph adenomas became clinically manifest because of excess hormone secretion. The hypersecretion of follicle-stimulating hormone (FSH) determines ovarian hyperstimulation in premenopausal women. In men the hypersecretion of LH can cause elevated testosterone concentrations, which in children will lead to premature puberty (84).

5. ACTH-Secreting Adenoma

Pituitary-dependent hypercortisolism is responsible for approximately two-thirds of cases of Cushing syndrome. The majority of these cases are attributable to basophilic microadenomas. In children and adolescents the clinical manifestation are somewhat different from those seen in adults. Younger patients usually present with weight gain that tends to be generalized, growth failure as direct effect of hypercortisolemia, compulsive behavior, and overachievement in school in contrast with the typical adult emotional lability and depression (85). Menstrual irregularity or amenorrhea is a common symptom in adolescent girls.

Confirmation of Cushing disease can be obtained from results of the 24 h urine free cortisol measurement. In children the value should be corrected by reference to the body surface. To establish that Cushing syndrome is due to a pituitary adenoma, stimulation of ACTH and cortisol following injection of CRH and suppression of cortisol by administration of dexamethasone should be shown. All patients should undergo MRI with the administration of gadolinium. If the MRI is negative, CRH-stimulated bilateral inferior petrosal sinus sampling can be used to confirm that the excessive ACTH comes from the pituitary. Surgical excision by transphenoidal adenomectomy is the treatment of choice. The remission rate after surgery is 85–95% in both children and adults (86).

VII. PANCREATIC ADENOMAS

The pancreatic islet contains alpha cells (glucagon), beta cells (insulin), and delta cells (somatostatin), as well as enterochromaffin cells (serotonin). These cells are all part of the APUD system, and tumors so derived secrete a wide variety of polypeptides. Gastrinoma and insulinoma are the most common form. According to a Mayo Clinic Study, the incidence of insulinoma is 0.4:100,000 person-years, and the average age of patients at presentation of insulinoma is in the mid-40s with very low incidence during childhood or adolescence (87). The adenomas are usually small and solitary; the lesion is generally well-encapsulated and highly vascular. Malignant insulinomas occur only in the 5% of cases of adenomas, tend to be larger, and metastasize to the liver and regional lymph nodes.

A. Genetics and Pathogenesis

The molecular mechanism leading to pancreatic tumor is still unclear but several tumor-suppressor genes have been implicated. The tumor-suppressor gene Smad/DPC4 has been found mutated in nonfunctional pancreatic tumors (88). Loss of heterozygosity in on chromosomes 1, 3q, 3p, 11p, 16p, 17p, and 22q has been noted in several studies (89). Guo and colleagues found overexpression of p27^{Kip1} in sporadic pancreatic endocrine tumors without differences between benign and malignant tumors (90). p27^{Kip1} is a universal cyclin-dependent kinase inhibitor, which acts as a tumor suppressor and a negative regulator of cell cycle. In various types of human cancers, the suppression of p27^{Kip1} expression is linked to aggressive behavior. However, the overexpression of p27^{Kip1} in the pancreatic endocrine tumor can be secondary to the other primary molecular disregulations or be a unique molecular pathway leading to endocrine tumorigenesis. Another molecule involved in pancreatic tumorigenesis is the paired-homeodomain transcription factor PAX4. The PAX gene family encodes highly conserved paired-box-containing transcription factors that control the tissue-specific expression of genes during embryogenesis. Because of this important role in the differentiation and development of pancreatic beta-cells, Miyamoto et al. studied PAX4 expression in the insulinomas. They found an overexpression of PAX4 mRNA in the tumors, but little or none in the normal islets, suggesting a fundamental role in the development of insulinoma (91).

B. Clinical Features

A patient with insulinoma will characteristically present with fasting hypoglycemia with neurological symptoms such as confusion, personality change, or seizures (92). The release of catecholamine due to the hypoglycemia will result in anxiety, palpitations, weakness, tremor, and sweating. Weight gain has been described.

Diagnosis is based on demonstrating Whipple's triad: hypoglycemic symptoms, blood glucose level less than 50 mg/dl, and relief of symptoms after glucose ingestion. Unfortunately, these symptoms are not specific for insulinoma. Because a single overnight fasting blood sugar level combined with a simultaneous plasma insulin level fails to establish the presence of fasting organic hypoglycemia in more than 35% of patients, a 72 h fast is usually done with blood glucose and insulin levels determined at 2–4 h intervals. Recently a study based on 127 patients with insulinoma demonstrated that a 48 h test is as effective as the 72 h one (93).

Measurement of C-peptide at the end of the fast can help to differentiate endogenous from exogenous (factitious) hyperinsulinemia. C-peptide will be proportionally elevated with insulin in patients with insulinoma, and low or normal in patients who abuse insulin or hypoglycemic agents. Nesidioblastosis and familial hyperinsulinemic hypoglycemia simulate the insulinoma's biochemical findings.

The treatment of choice is surgery, but preoperative localization of the tumor is necessary because of the small tumor size. The imaging techniques available are spiral CT, arteriography, and transabdominal and endoscopic ultrasonography. Patients with metastatic insulinoma or those who are not candidates for or refuse surgery, require medical therapy. Diazoxide, verapamil, phenytoin, and Octreotide have all been used to prevent symptomatic hypoglycemia. Diazoxide, which diminishes insulin secretion, is the most effective and should be given in divided doses of up to 1200 mg/day. However, it causes unwanted hair growth and edema.

REFERENCES

1. Teh BT, McArdle J, Parameswaran V, David R, Larsson C, Shepherd J. Sporadic primary hyperparathyroidism in the setting of multiple endocrine neoplasia type 1. Arch Surg 1996; 131:1230–1232.

2. Brandi ML, Marx SJ, Aurbach GD, Fitzpatrick LA. Familial multiple endocrine neoplasia type 1: a new look at pathophysiology. Endocrine Rev 1987; 8:391–405.
3. Trump D, Farren B, Wooding C, Pang JT, Besser GM, Buchanan KD, Edwards CR, Heath DA, Jackson CE, Jansen S, Lips K, Monson JP, O'Halloran D, Sampson J, Shalet SM, Wheeler MH, Zink A, Thakker RV. Clinical studies of multiple endocrine neoplasia type 1 (MEN-1) in 220 patients. Q J Med 1996; 89:653–669.
4. Chandrasekharappa SC, Guru SC, Manickam P, Olufemi SE, Collins FS, Emmert-Buck MR, Debelenko LV, Zhuang Z, Lubensky IA, Liotta LA, Crabtree JS, Wang Y, Roe BA, Weisemann J, Boguski MS, Agarwal SK, Kester MB, Kim YS, Heppner C, Dong Q, Spiegel AM, Burns AL, Marx SJ. Positional cloning of the gene for multiple endocrine neoplasia type 1. Science 1997; 276:404–407.
5. Pannett AA, Thakker RV. Multiple endocrine neoplasia type 1 (MEN1). Endocr Rel Ca 1999; 6:449–473.
6. Teh BT, Kytola S, Farnebo F, Bergman L, Wong FK, Weber G, Hayward N, Larsson C, Skogseid B, Beckers A, Phelan C, Edwards M, Epstein M, Alford F, Hurley D, Grimmond S, Silins G, Walters M, Stewart C, Cardinal J, Khodaei S, Parente F, Tranebjaerg L, Jorde R. Mutation analysis of the MEN 1 gene in multiple endocrine neoplasia type 1, familial acromegaly and familial isolated hyperparathyroidism. J Clin Endocrinol Metab 1998; 83:2621–2626.
7. Bassett JH, Forbes SA, Pannett AA, Lloyd SE, Christie PT, Wooding C, Harding B, Besser GM, Edwards CR, Monson JP, Sampson J, Wass JA, Wheeler MH, Thakker RV. Characterisation of mutations in patients with multiple endocrine neoplasia type 1 (MEN1). Am J Hum Genet 1998; 62:232–244.
8. Guru SC, Goldsmith PK, Burns AL, Marx SJ, Spiegel AM, Collins FS, Chandrasekharappa SC. Menin, the product of the MEN1 gene, is a nuclear protein. Proc Natl Acad Sci USA 1998; 95:1630–1634.
9. Agarwal SK, Guru SC, Heppner C, Erdos MR, Collins RM, Park SY, Saggar S, Chandrasekharappa SC, Collins FS, Spiegel AM, Marx SJ, Burns AL. Menin interacts with the AP1 transcription factor JunD and represses JunD-activated transcription. Cell 1999; 96:143–152.
10. Benson L, Ljunghall S, Akerstrom G, Oberg K. Hyperparathyroidism presenting as the first lesion in multiple endocrine neoplasia type 1. Am J Med 1987; 82:731–737.
11. Law WM Jr, Health H. Familial benign hypercalcemia (hypocalciuric hypercalcemia): clinical and pathogenetic studies in 21 families. Ann Intern Med 1985; 102:511–519.
12. Burgess JR, Shepherd JJ, Parameswaran V, Hoffman L, Greenaway TM. Spectrum of pituitary disease in multiple endocrine neoplasia type 1 (MEN 1): clinical, biochemical, and radiological features of pituitary disease in a large MEN 1 kindred. J Clin Endocrinol Metab 1996; 81:2642–2646.
13. Skogseid B, Oberg K. Prospective screening in multiple endocrine neoplasia type 1. Henry Ford Hosp Med J 1992; 40:167–170.
14. Jensen RT. Managment of the Zollinger-Ellison syndrome in patients with multiple endocrine neoplasia type 1. J Intern Med 1998; 243:477–488.
15. Norton JA, Fraker DL, Alexander HR, Venzon DJ, Doppman JL, Serrano J, Goebel SU, Peghini PL, Roy PK, Gibril F, Jensen RT. Surgery to cure the Zollinger-Ellison syndrome. N Engl J Med 1999; 341:635–644.
16. Thompson NW. Managment of pancreatic endocrine tu-

mors in patients with multiple endocrine neoplasia type 1. Surg Oncol Clin North Am 1998; 1998:881–891.
17. Teh BT, McArdle J, Chan SP, Menon J, Hartley L, Pullan P, Ho J, Khir A, Wilkinson S, Larsson C, Cameron D, Shepherd J. Clinicopathologic studies of thymic carcinoids in multiple endocrine neoplasia type 1. Medicine 1997; 76:21–29.
18. Larsson C, Shepherd J, Nakamura Y, Blomberg C, Weber G, Werelius B, Hayward N, Teh B, Tokino T, Seizinger B. Predictive testing for multiple endocrine neoplasia type 1 using DNA polymorphisms. J Clin Invest 1992; 89:1344–1349.
19. Donovan DT, Levy ML, Furst EJ, Alford BR, Wheeler T, Tschen JA, Gagel RF. Familial cutaneous lichen amyloidosis in association with multiple endocrine neoplasia type 2A: a new variant. Henry Ford Hosp J 1989; 37:147–150.
20. Mulligan LM, Eng C, Healey CS, Clayton D, Kwok JB, Gardner E, Ponder MA, Frilling A, Jackson CE, Lehnert H, et al. Specific mutations of the RET proto-oncogene are related to disease phenotype in MEN-2A and FMTC. Nat Genet 1994; 6:70–74.
21. Hofstra RM, Landsvater RM, Ceccherini I, Stulp RP, Stelwagen T, Luo I, Pasini B. A mutation in the RET proto-oncogene associated with multiple endocrine neoplasia type 2B and sporadic medullary thyroid carcinoma. Nature 1994; 367:375–380.
22. Mulligan LM, Ponder BA. Genetic basis of endocrine disease: Multiple endocrine neopplasia type 2. J Clin Endocrinol Metab 1995; 80:1989–1995.
23. Durbec P, Marcos-Gutierrez CV, Kilkenny C, Grigoriou M, Wartiowaara K, Suvanto P, Smith D, Ponder B, Costantini F, Saarma M, et al. GDNF signaling through the Ret receptor tyrosine kinase. Nature 1996; 381:789–793.
24. Kotzbauer PT, Lampe PA, Heuckeroth RO, Golden JP, Creedon DJ, Johnson EM Jr, Milbrandt J. Neurturin, a relative of glial-cell-line-derived neurotrophic factor. Nature 1996; 384:467–470.
25. Treanor JJ, Goodman L, de Sauvage F, Stone DM, Poulsen KT, Beck CD, Gray C, Armanini MP, Pollock RA, Hefti F, Phillips HS, Goddard A, Moore MW, Buj-Bello A, Davies AM, Asai N, Takahashi M, Vandlen R, Henderson CE, Rosenthal A. Characterization of a multicomponent receptor for GDNF. Nature 1996; 382:80–83.
26. Eng C, Clayton D, Schuffenecker I, Lenoir G, Cote G, Gagel RF, van Amstel HK, Lips CJ, Nishisho I, Takai SI, Marsh DJ, Robinson BG, Frank-Raue K, Raue F, Xue F, Noll WW, Romei C, Pacini F, Fink M, Niederle B, Zedenius J, Nordenskjold M, Komminoth P, Hendy GN, et al. The relationship between specific RET proto-oncogene mutations and disease phenotype in multiple endocrine neoplasia type 2. International Consortium analysis. JAMA 1996; 276:1575–1579.
27. Gimm O, Marsh DJ, Andrew SD, Frilling A, Dahia PL, Mulligan LM, Zajac JD, Robinson BG, Eng C. Germline dinucleotide mutation in codon 883 of the RET proto-oncogene in multiple endocrine neoplasia type 2B without codon 918 mutation. J Clin Endocrinol Metab 1997; 82:3902–3904.
28. Parthemore JG, Bronzert D, Roberts G, Deftos LJ. A short calcium infusion in the diagnosis of medullary thyroid carcinoma. J Clin Endocrinol Metab 1974; 39:108–111.
29. Duh QY, Sancho JJ, Greenspan FS, Hunt TK, Galante M, deLorimier AA, Conte FA, Clark OH. Medullary thyroid carcinoma: the need for early diagnosis and total thyroidectomy. Arch Surg 1989; 124:1206–1210.

30. Raue F, Frank-Raue K, Grauer A. Multiple endocrine neoplasia type 2: clinical features and screening. Endocrinol Metab Clin North Am 1994; 23:137.

31. Gagel RF, Tashjian AH Jr, Cummings T, Papathanasopoulos N, Kaplan MM, DeLellis RA, Wolfe HJ, Reichlin S. The clinical outcome of prospective screening for multiple endocrine neoplasia type 2a. An 18-years experience. N Engl J Med 1988; 318:478–484.

32. Schuffenecker I, Virally-Monod M, Brohet R, Goldgar D, Conte-Devolx B, Leclerc L, Chabre O, Boneu A, Caron J, Houdent C, Modigliani E, Rohmer V, Schlumberger M, Eng C, Guillausseau PJ, Lenoir GM. Risk and penetrance of primary hyperparathyroidism in multiple endocrine neoplasia type 2A families with mutations at codon 634 of the RET proto-oncogene. J Clin Endocrinol Metab 1998; 83: 487–491.

33. Marsh DJ, McDowall D, Hyland VJ, Andrew SD, Schnitzler M, Gaskin EL, Nevell DF, Diamond T, Delbridge L, Clifton-Bligh P, Robinson BG. The identification of false positive responses to the pentagastrin stimulation test in RET mutation negative members of MEN 2A families. Clin Endocrinol 1996; 44:213–220.

34. Latronico AC, Chrousos GP. Extensive personal experience: adrenocortical tumors. J Clin Endocrinol Metab 1997; 82:1317–1324.

35. Reincke M, Beuschlein F, Slawik M, Borm K. Molecular adrenocortical tumourigenesis. Eur J Clin Invest 2000; 30: 63–68.

36. Srivastava S, Zou Z, Pirollo K, Blattner W, Chang EH. Germ-line transmission of a mutated p53 gene in a cancer-prone family with Li-Fraumeni syndrome. Nature 1990; 348:747–749.

37. Henry I, Bonaiti-Pellie C, Chehensse V, Beldjord C, Schwartz C, Utermann G. Uniparental paternal disomy in a genetic cancer-predisposing syndrome. Nature 1991; 351: 667–670.

38. Stratakis CA, Carney JA, Lin JP, Papanicolaou DA, Karl M, Kastner DL, Pras E, Chrousos GP. Carney complex: a familial multiple neoplasia and lentiginosis syndrome: analysis of 11 kindred and linkage to the short arm of chromosome 2. J Clin Invest 1996; 97:699–705.

39. Marchesa P, Fazio VW, Church JM, McGannon E. Adrenal masses in patients with familial adenomatous polyposis. Dis Colon Rectum 1997; 40:1023–1028.

40. Torpy D, Stratakis CA, Chrousos GP. Hyper- and hypo-aldosteronism. Vitam Horm 1999; 46:177–216.

41. Reincke M, Mora P, Beuschlein F, Arlt W, Chrousos GP, Allolio B. Deletion of the adrenocorticotropin receptor gene in human adrenocortical tumors: implications for tumorigenesis. J Clin Endocrinol Metab 1997; 82:3054–3058.

42. Schulte KM, Heinze M, Mengel M, Simon D, Scheuring S, Kohrer K, Roher HD. MEN I gene mutations in sporadic adrenal adenomas. Hum Genet 1999; 105:603–610.

43. Jonnsson JR, Klemm SA, Tunny TJ, Stowasser M, Gordon RD. A new genetic test for familial hyperaldosteronism type 1 aids in the detection of curable hypertension. Biochem Biophys Res Commun 1995; 207:565–571.

44. Chee C, Ravinthiran T, Cheng C. laparoscopic adrenalectomy: experience with transabdominal and retroperitoneal approches. Urology 1998; 51:29–32.

45. Costantine A, Stratakis MD, Chrousos GP. Adrenocortical tumors: recent advances in basic concepts and clinical managment. Ann Intern Med 1999; 130:759–771.

46. Dumont JE, Lamy F, Roger P, Maenhaut C. Physiological and pathological regulation of thyroid cell proliferation and differentiation by thyrotropin and other factors. Physiol Rev 1992; 72:667–697.

47. Procellini A, Ruggiano G, Pannain S, Ciullo I, Amabile G, Fenzi G, Avvedimento EV. Mutations of thyrotropin receptor isolated from thyroid autonomous functioning adenomas confer TSH-independent growth to thyroid cells. Oncogene 1997; 15:781–789.

48. Suarez HG, du Villard JA, Caillou B, Schlumberger M, Parmentier C, Monier R. Gsp mutations in human thyroid tumors. Oncogene 1991; 6:677–679.

49. Dhanasekaran N, Heasley L, Johnson GL. G protein-coupled receptor system invoved in cell growth and oncogenesis. Endocrinol Rev 1995; 16:259–270.

50. Kosugi S, Okajima F, Ban T, Hidaka A, Shenker A, Kohn LD. Substitutions of different regions of the third cytoplasmic loop of the thyrotropin (TSH) receptor have selective effects on constitutive, TSH, and TSH receptor autoantibody-stimulated phosphoinositide and 3′,5′-cyclic adenosine monophosphate signal generation. Mol Endo 1993; 7:1009–1018.

51. Fagin JA. Molecular genetics of human thyroid neoplasm. Annu Rev Med 1994; 45:45–52.

52. Namba H, Gutman RA, Matsuo K. H-ras proto-oncogene mutations in human thyroid neoplasms. J Clin Endocrinol Metab 1990; 71:223–229.

53. Viglietto G, Maglione D, Rambaldi M, Cerutti J, Romano A, Trapasso F, Fedele M, Ippolito P, Chiappetta G, Botti G. Upregulation of vascular endothelial growth factor (PIGF) associated with malignancy in human thyroid tumors and cell lines. Oncogene 1995; 11:1569–1579.

54. Huang SM, Lee JC, Wu TJ, Chow NH. Clinical relevance of vascular endothelial growth factor for thyroid neoplasm. World J Surg 2001; 25:302–303.

55. Sautner D, Saeger W. Invasiveness of pituitary adenomas. Pathol Res Pract 1991; 187:632–636.

56. AD Elster. Modern imaging of the pituitary. Radiology 1993; 187:1–14.

57. Burrow GN Wortzman G, Rewcastle NB. Microadenomas of the pituitary and abnormal sellar tomograms in an unselected autopsy series. N Engl J Med 1981; 304:156–158.

58. Kane LA, Leinung MC, Scheithauer BW, Bergstralh EJ, Laws ER Jr, Groover RV, Kovacs K, Horvath E, Zimmerman D. Pituitary adenomas in childhood and adolescence. J Clin Endocrinol Metab 1994; 79:1135–1140.

59. Ogishima T, Shibata H, Shimada H. Aldosterone synthase cytochrome P-450 expressed in the adrenal of patients with primary aldosteronism. J Biol Chem 1991; 266:10731–10734.

60. Mindermann T, Wilon CB. Age-related and gender-related occurence of pituitary adenomas. Clin Endocrinol (Oxf) 1994; 41:359–364.

61. Asa SL, Ezzet S. The cytogenesis and pathogenesis of pituitary adenomas. Endocrinol Rev 1998; 19:798–827.

62. Landis CA, Masters SB, Spada A, Pace AM, Bourne HR, L Vallar. GTPase inhibiting mutations activate the alpha chain of Gs and stimulate adenyl cyclase in human pituitary tumors. Nature 1989; 340:692–696.

63. Pei L, Melmed S. Isolation and characterization of pituitary tumor-transforming gene (PTTG). Mol Endocrinol 1997; 11:433–441.

64. Hibberts NA, Simpson DJ, Bicknell JE, Broome JC, Hoban PR, Clayton RN, Farrel WE. Analysis of cyclic D1 (CCND1) allelic imbalance and overexpression in sporadic pituitary tumors. Clin Cancer Res 1999; 5:2133–2139.

65. Asa SL, Somers K, Ezzat S. The MEN-1 gene is rarely

down-regulated in pituitary adenoma. J Clin Endocrinol Metab 1998; 83:3210–3212.

66. Hu N, Gutsmann A, Herbert DC, Bradley A, Lee W-H, Lee EY. Heterozygous Rb-1delta/+ mice are predisposed to tumors of the pituitary gland with a nearly complete penetrance. Oncogene 1994; 9:1021–1027.

67. Cryns VL, Alexander JM, Klibanski A, Arnold A. The retinoblastoma gene in human pituitary tumors. J Clin Endocrinol Metab 1993; 77:644–646.

68. Pei L, Melmed S, Scheithauser B, Kovacs K, Benedict WF, Prager D. Frequent loss of heterozygosity at the retinoblastoma susceptibility gene (RB) locus in aggressive pituitary tumors: evidence for a chromosome 13 tumor suppressor gene other then RB. Cancer Res 1995; 55:1613–1616.

69. Simpson DJ, Bicknell JE, McNicol AM, Clayton RN, Farrell WE. Hypermethylation of the p16/CDKN2A/MTS1 gene and loss of protein expression is associated with nonfunctional pituitary adenomas but not somatotropinomas. Genes Chrom Cancer 1999; 24:328–336.

70. Patterson J, Childs GV. Nerve growth factor in the anterior pituitary: regulation of secretion. Endocrinology 1994; 135:1697–1704.

71. Webster J, Ham J, Bevan JS, ten Horn CD, Scalon MF. Preliminary characterization of growth factors secreted by human pituitary tumors. J Clin Endocrinol Metab 1991; 72:687–692.

72. Vance ML, Thorner MO. Prolactinomas. Endocrinol Metab Clin North Am 1987; 16:731–753.

73. Horvath E, Kovacs K, Killinger DV et al. Acidophil stem cell adenoma of the human pituitary: clinicopathologic analysis of 15 cases. Cancer 1981; 47:761–771.

74. Colao AM, Loche S, Cappa M, Di Sarna A, Landi ML, Sarnacchiaro F, Facciolli G, Lombardi G. Prolactinomas in children and adolescents. Clinical presentation and long-term follow-up. J Clin Endocrinol Metab 1998; 83:2777–2780.

75. Vance ML, Evans WS, Thorner MO. Drugs five years later. Bromocriptine. Ann Intern Med 1984; 100:78–91.

76. Molitch ME. Clinical manifestation of acromegaly. Endocrinol Metab Clin North Am 1992; 21:597–614.

77. Lopez-Velasco R, Escobar-Morreale HF, Vega B, Villa E, Sancho JM, Moya-Mur JL, Garcia-Robles R. Cardiac involvement in acromegaly: specific myocardiopathy or consequence of systemic hypertension? J Clin Endocrinol Metab 1997; 82:1047–1053.

78. Hartman ML, Veldhuis JD, Vance ML, Faria AC, Furlanetto RW, Thorner MO. Somatotropin pulse frequency and basal concentration are increased in acromegaly and reduced by successful therapy. J Clin Endocrinol Metab 1990; 70:1375–1384.

79. Fahlbusch R, Honegger J, Buchfelder M. Surgical managment of acromegaly. Endocrinol Metab Clin North Am 1992; 21:669–692.

80. Shimon I, Taylor JE, Dong JZ, Bitonte RA, Kim S, Morgan B, Coy DH, Culler MD, Melmed S. Somatostatin receptor subtype specificity in human fetal pituitary cultures. Differential role of SSTR2 and SSTR5 for growth hormone, thyroid-stimulating hormone, and prolactin regulation. J Clin Invest 1997; 99:789–798.

81. Lamberts SW, van der Lely AJ, de Herder WW, Hofland LJ. Octrotide. N Engl J Med 1996; 334:246–254.

82. Brucker-Davis F, Oldfield EH, Skarulis MC, Doppman JL, Weintraub BD. Thyrotropin-secreting pituitary tumors: diagnostic criteria, thyroid hormone sensitivity, and treatment outcome in 25 patients followed at the National Institutes of Health. J Clin Endocrinol Metab 1999; 84:476–486.

83. Snyder PJ. Gonadotroph cell adenomas of the pituitary. Endocrinol Rev 1985; 6:552–563.

84. Ambrosi B, Bassetti M, Ferrario R, Medri G, Giannattasio G, Faglia G. Precocious puberty in a boy with a PRL-LH and FSH-secreting pituitary tumor: hormonal and immunocytochemical studies. Acta Endocrinol (Copenh) 1990; 122:569–576.

85. Kunwar S, Wilson CB. Pediatric pituitary adenomas. J Clin Endocrinol Metab 1999; 84:4385–4389.

86. Lafferty AR, Chousos GP. Pituitary tumors in children and adolescents. J Clin Endocrinol Metab 1999; 12:4317–4323.

87. Service FJ, McMahon MM, O'Brien PC, Ballard DJ. Functioning insulinoma—incidence, recurrence and long-term survival of patients: a 60-year study. Mayo Clin Proc 1991; 66:711–719.

88. Bartsch D, Hahn SA, Danichevski KD, Ramaswamy A, Bastian D, Galehdari H, Barth P, Schmiegel W, Simon B, Rothmund M. Mutations of the DPC4/Smad4 gene in neuroendocrine pancreatic tumors. Oncogene 1999; 18:2367–2371.

89. Ebrahimi S, Wang EH, Wu A, Schreck RR, Passaro E Jr, Sawicki MP. Deletion of chromosome 1 predicts prognosis in pancreatic endocrine tumors. Cancer Res 1999; 59:311–315.

90. Guo S, Xinyi W, Shimoide AT, Wong J, Sawicki MP. Anomalous overexpression of p27kip1 in sporadic pancreatic endocrine tumors. J Surg Res 2001; 96:284–288.

91. Miyamoto T, Kakizawa T, Ichikawa K, Nishio S, Kajikawa S, Hashizume K. Expression of dominant negative form of PAX4 in human insulinoma. Biochem Biophys Res Commun 2001; 282:34–40.

92. Dizon AM, Kowalyk S, Hoogwerf BJ. Neuroglycopenic and other symptoms in patients with insulinomas. Am J Med 1999; 106:307–310.

93. Hirshberg B, Livi A, Bartlett L, Libutti SK, Alexander HR, Doppman JL, Skarulis MC, Gorden P. Forty-eight hours fast: the diagnostic test for insulinoma. J Clin Endocrinol Metab 2000; 85:3222–3226.

30

Endocrine Tumors in Children

Muhammad A. Jabbar

Hurley Medical Center, Michigan State University School of Medicine, Flint, Michigan, U.S.A.

I. INTRODUCTION

Endocrine tumors in children pose a number of fundamental questions: is the tumor a nonfunctioning, functioning, or hyperfunctioning entity? Is it a malignant or a benign process or a hyperplasia responsive to physiological regulations? Apart from clinical presentation, the answers to these questions often depend on specific hormonal–biochemical, radiological, and histopathologic findings. Consequently, the optimal assessment and management of these patients remains a challenging task and must include the efforts of endocrinologists, oncologists, surgeons, and other support personnel.

This chapter reviews the clinical approach to children with adrenal, gonadal, and pancreatic tumors. Pituitary, thyroid and parathyroid tumors are covered in Chapters 2 and 20, respectively.

II. ADRENAL TUMORS

The incidence of adrenal tumors in children is not known (see Chapter 6 for adrenal cortex and Chapter 8 for adrenal medulla). Of 58 patients reported by Bertagna (1), 11 (19%) were between 0.8 and 15 years of age. Adrenal carcinoma represented about 10% of the carcinomas in childhood, according to a registry-based data from England (2). The age of appearance is usually during the first decade of life (3). Girls are more frequently affected than boys, with ratio of 2.5:1 (4). While familial cases are reported (5), occurrence of adrenal carcinoma in patients with Li-Fraumeni syndrome (6), Beckwith syndrome (7) hemihypertrophy (8), and congenital malformations of the genitourinary tract are well known.

Incidence of nonmalignant tumors increases with age. Malignant tumors show a bimodal distribution with the first peak below age 5 years and the second peak in the fourth to fifth decade (9). Industrial pollutants may play a causative role, as reported from Brazil (10).

On a pathological basis, corticotropin-independent cortisol overproduction represents a spectrum ranging from benign nodular hyperplasia to malignant adrenal tumors. In the 1960s, Meador et al. (11) described primary adrenocortical nodular dysplasia, characterized by non-malignant, autonomously secreting lesions. In another recent review (12), a similar condition predominantly affecting children and young adults has been described with bilateral nodular disease, internodular cortical atrophy, and varying degrees of pigmentation. This condition has also been described in association with the Carney complex, which includes myxomas, pigmented skin lesions, peripheral nerve tumors, and various endocrine tumors (13).

The cause of the nodule formation or dysplasia remains to be established. An adrenal-stimulating immunoglobulin has been implicated in the pathogenesis (14). In McCune-Albright syndrome, nodular hyperplasia of the adrenal glands has been reported as the cause of hypercortisolism (Chapter 9) (15). In these patients, somatic mutation of the alpha subunit of the G-protein occurs during fetal development, creating a mosaicism of normal and mutant-bearing cells. In the latter, G-protein activation of adenylate cyclase increases cyclic AMP with formation of multiple nodules and overproduction of cortisol. Inverted diurnal rhythm, subnormal morning cortisol concentration, and low corticotropin in association with gastric inhibitory peptide (GIP) recently were described. Although the causative role of GIP in cortisol overproduction remains undetermined, data support the hypothesis of abnormal expression of receptors in the adrenal (16,17).

A. Clinical Features

Adrenal tumors in children are usually functional, giving rise to a constellation of symptoms or signs (Chapter 6). Depending on the duration of the disease and the action of the metabolic, androgenic, and salt-retaining hormones, the clinical spectrum may include Cushing syndrome and virilization to hypertension. A majority of the tumors secrete cortisol, while androgen and aldosterone secretion follow in decreasing frequency. Occasionally there is alteration of the clinical course with evidence of initial glucocorticoid predominance being overlapped by the androgenic effects or vice versa, as the disease progresses. An incidental adrenal tumor without any clinical manifestation is a distinct entity in adults; this represents only about 5% of all adrenal tumors in children.

Weight gain, truncal obesity, moon face, and buffalo hump are observed in 40–60% of children with functional adrenal tumors (Table 1). Obesity and short stature are common presenting features (18–20), although the latter may be the only manifestation of hypercortisolemia in children (21).

Normal or accelerated linear growth may be encountered in children with androgen-producing adrenal tumors. In such cases, the presence of acne, hirsutism, hypertrichosis of the face and trunk, deepening of the voice, and clitoromegaly in females, are the distinguishable physical signs. In prepubertal children, excess androgen will lead to virilization with excess body hair, adrenarche, acne, clitoromegaly or abnormal phallic growth, rapid skeletal growth, along with excess weight gain (22,23). The disorder tends to be more severe and the clinical findings more flagrant in infants than when the onset occurs in

older children (24,25). Premature adrenarche, a common problem in clinical practice, may be the initial presentation, although the severity of the signs and symptoms will help to differentiate the adrenal tumor from benign adrenarche. In postmenarcheal girls, rapid weight gain and menstrual irregularity often results from increased androgens (Chapter 12). Estrogen-secreting tumors of the adrenals are rare in childhood. In prepubertal boys, these may lead to gynecomastia along with enhancement of growth and skeletal maturation; in girls, sexual precocity characterized by premature thelarche and advanced growth may occur (26). If there is evidence of virilization or elevation of blood pressure, concomitant secretion of androgens or mineralocorticoids should be suspected.

Hypertension, plethora, and fluid retention are also common in children with adrenal tumor, being present in up to 70% (Chapter 38). In aldosterone-producing tumors, elevated blood pressure is one of the most common manifestations. Both systolic and diastolic blood pressure is abnormally elevated. Muscle weakness, cramping, paresthesia, polydipsia, and polyuria may occur. Despite fluid retention and increase in the intravascular volume, there is no clinical evidence of edema in these patients. Sodium retention is only mild to moderate. Hypokalemia is the most reliable laboratory abnormality, with electrocardiographic signs of prolonged ST segment and inverted T-wave. Alkalosis is also a frequent finding, causing tetany and Trousseau's sign in untreated patients.

A small percentage of patients are known to have psychiatric symptoms, ranging from acute psychosis and depression to manic-depressive behavior. Asymptomatic hypercortisolemia with normal blood pressure has been reported in children. Diffuse osteoporosis, more noticeable in the vertebral column, is also common in these patients. Impaired glucose tolerance is more frequent than overt diabetes, and the incidence of renal stones is higher than in the general population.

Preoperative differentiation of an adenoma from carcinoma is difficult. Although Cushing syndrome is frequently caused by adenoma, while virilization is associated with carcinoma, benign and malignant tumors may be functionally identical and, thus, clinically inseparable. A normal or exaggerated response to exogenous ACTH stimulation is more often encountered in adenoma than carcinoma but lack of dexamethasone suppression is observed in both (1). Size of the tumor has been noted to be a predictor, with tumor size greater than 75 g being more likely to be malignant (19). Histopathological criteria such as mitoses, necrosis, and capsular and vascular invasion were not reliable predictors of a malignant tumor, as demonstrated by the presence of these findings in patients with benign adenomas (27,28).

Table 1 Clinical Features of Hypercortisolemia in Children and Adults

Symptoms/signs	Children (CS)	Children (CS)	Adult (CD)
General			
Obesity (moon facies)	25	100	85
Growth failure	0	85	NR
Hypertension	13	77	75
Cutaneous			
Plethora	13	77	80
Striae	0	54	50
Acne	88	85	35
Hirsutism	75	85	75
Bruising	0	38	35
Hyperpigmentation	0	38	5
Musculoskeletal			
Osteoporosis	NR	54	80
Weakness	0	46	50
Metabolic			
Glucose intolerance	NR	38	75
Renal stones	NR	15	15
Neuropsychiatric symptoms			
Fatigue, weakness	50	46	85

CS, Cushing syndrome; CD, Cushing's disease; NR, not reported.
Source: Data adapted from Pediatr Clin North Am 1990; 37:1313–1329.

B. Diagnosis

Because of the anatomical location deep in the abdomen as well as nonfunctioning nature of the tumors, adrenal adenoma or carcinoma often remains undiagnosed for a considerable period of time. The size attained by these tumors is therefore enormous in many instances. During evaluation of nonspecific complaints or routine physical examination, abdominal mass may be detected in such patients.

Hormonal studies are of vital importance in the diagnosis of adrenal tumors. Levels of urinary free cortisol, 17-KS, and 17-OHCS are significantly elevated in patients with a functioning adrenal tumor (29). Plasma cortisol is elevated, along with loss of diurnal rhythm. Complete androgen profile including DHEA, androstenedione, and testosterone levels should be studied in patients with clinical evidence of virilization (Chapter 17). Differentiation from congenital adrenal hyperplasia is an important but difficult task. In the hypercortisolemic state, lack of suppression of plasma cortisol following administration of dexamethasone is characteristic of adrenal tumors. Therefore, performance of a low-dose or high-dose dexamethasone test should be a priority in these patients (Chapter 41).

Differentiation of pituitary disease from adrenal disease is challenging. Apart from providing further understanding about the functional relations between the pituitary and the adrenal, the metyrapone test may be useful in differentiating adrenal adenomas from carcinomas. In about 50% of cases, adrenal adenoma are responsive to metyrapone while carcinomas are usually nonresponsive. Because the tumors do not respond and the normal adrenal cortices are atrophic, ACTH stimulation test has very limited use in the diagnosis of adrenal tumors. Differentiation of central precocious puberty from estrogen-secreting adrenal tumors in girls may be necessary. Urinary estrogens and 17-KS and plasma DHEA, DHEAS, and estrogens are elevated along with absent gonadotropin response following GnRH stimulation in adrenal tumors. Measurement of serum and 24 h urinary aldosterone levels as well as plasma renin activity is useful for initial evaluation of suspected aldosterone-producing tumors. To differentiate secondary hyperaldosteronism and avoid false-positive results, all medications, particularly diuretics, should be discontinued prior to laboratory studies. In patients with elevated serum aldosterone levels, complete suppression of aldosterone secretion by administration of dexamethasone differentiates dexamethasone-suppressible hyperaldosteronism from primary hyperaldosteronism. Elevated aldosterone levels, low renin activity, and high urinary aldosterone with lack of dexamethasone suppression establishes a diagnosis of hyperaldosteronism (Chapter 6). Further diagnostic studies, including the imaging studies, should be performed in these patients (Chapter 38).

Radiological studies are an important component in the diagnosis of adrenal tumors. CT scan and MRI aim to localize the tumor and define the extent of the disease. Intravenous pyelography is useful to delineate the relationship of the kidney to the tumor mass. Ultrasonography shows an adrenal mass in the majority of cases. CT scan is, however, the ideal method since it allows visualization of other abdominal organs. Angiography is often required to provide the surgeon with a map of the tumor's blood supply.

C. Treatment

Complete surgical excision with replacement steroid therapy provides the best choice for treatment of these patients (30). Preoperative, operative, and postoperative management are of critical importance. For primary pigmented nodular adrenocortical disease, bilateral adrenalectomy with steroid replacement is preferred (27). For adrenal adenoma, unilateral adrenalectomy or resection of the tumor followed by replacement steroid therapy is the treatment of choice. Replacement therapy with glucocorticoid is necessary until normal function in the contralateral gland is restored. This is usually for 6–12 months, although suppression from the tumor can persist for up to 2 years.

For adrenal carcinoma, surgical therapy aims to excise the tumor and local metastasis completely to enhance the chance of cure. For inoperable or partially resectable carcinoma, combination chemotherapy may offer an alternative management approach (31,32). However, experience with pediatric patients is largely anecdotal. Mitotane therapy has been successful in patients with intrauterine adrenal carcinoma and metastasis (34). In addition, medical therapy with metyrapone and aminoglutethimide in combination is useful for control of symptoms. Ketoconazole, an inhibitor of steroid biosynthesis, is the preferred drug to decrease cortisol secretion in selected cases. RU 486, a glucocorticoid antagonist, has also been employed to control the symptoms secondary to hypercortisolism.

D. Prognosis and Follow-Up

Early diagnosis and surgery offer the best hope for long-term survival, with adenoma exhibiting an extremely good outcome. Adrenal carcinoma in children, on the other hand, is an extremely progressive disease. Final adult stature is stunted in most of these patients. Replacement therapy with glucocorticoid is required for an indefinite period of time. Careful follow-up at a 3–6 month interval is mandatory. Clinical assessment and serum levels of cortisol, DHEA, androstenedione, testosterone, and plasma rennin activity are necessary to detect recurrent or metastic disease. The 24 h urinary 17-KS, 17-OHCS, and free cortisol, along with the other hormones that were initially abnormal, should be measured. A repeat dexamethasome stimulation test should be done to assess the suppressibility of cortisol production.

III. GONADAL TUMORS

A. Testicular Tumors

1. Causes and Presentation

Constituting about 1% of all cancers in men, testicular tumors occur most commonly during the third and fourth decades of life. Germ cell tumors, accounting for about 90% of all testicular tumors in the pediatric age group, include embryonal carcinoma, endodermal sinus tumor, and teratoma, representing a spectrum of progressive histological differentiation. In young adults, however, the spectrum includes seminoma, which represent 30–50% of all germ cell tumors (35,36).

The best-documented risk factor for the development of germ cell tumors is cryptorchidism, which is associated with about 10% of germ cell tumors (Chapter 13) (37–39). The degree of lack of descent of the testes correlates with the likelihood of tumor formation, with abdominal tests more at risk than those in the inguinal area. Orchidopexy performed before the age of 6, however, reduces this risk significantly. The pathogenesis of these tumors is not clear. Incidence of tumor in the contralateral normally descended testis is higher than that of controls. Although several factors including higher temperature, higher gonadotropin levels, and congenitally abnormal germ cells have been proposed, none has provided compelling evidence to attain wide acceptance.

Dysgenetic gonads associated with androgen insensitivity, persistent mullerian syndrome, true hermaphroditism and Klinefelter syndrome have a higher incidence of germ cell tumors (38–40). Down syndrome and cutaneous icthyosis (40–42) with steroid sulfatase deficiency also has been reported to be associated with occurrence of testicular tumors. One of the strongest risk factors for the development of a germ cell tumor is having a history of prior contralateral tumor (43–45), although a specific causative factor remains undetermined. Familial occurrence of tumor has been reported, with sixfold increase for a son whose father had a germ cell tumor (46).

Inadequately treated congenital adrenal hyperplasia has been observed to be associated with testicular tumors (47,48). It is presumed that the development and progression of these tumors is enhanced by the chronic stimulatory effect of elevated corticotropin.

Painless mass is the common mode of presentation; however, pain and tenderness are found in half the cases. Symptoms or signs due to metastasis to the retroperitoneal lymph nodes or lungs are the initial findings in a small proportion of patients. Tumors of Leydig cell origin may secrete testosterone, producing signs of sexual development. Unilateral or bilateral gynecomastia may occur as a result of secretion of estrogen or of chorionic gonadotropin by the stromal or germ cell tumors (49).

2. Diagnosis

Careful examination is crucial to the diagnosis testicular tumors. An area of hardness, nodularity, or altered consistency should be determined. Localization of the tumor and differentiation of simple hydrocele from reactive hydrocele with testicular tumor can be reliably performed by sonographic study. Patients suspected of having germ cell tumor should undergo radiographic or imaging studies of the chest, abdomen, and skeletal system to detect metastatic disease. The functional and histological behavior of various testicular tumors is detailed in Table 2.

Malignant behavior of Sertoli cell tumors correlates directly with large size (50). Preoperatively as well as during the follow-up, measurement of biomarkers such as serum human chorionic gonadotropin (hCG) and alphafetoprotein (AFP) x-fetoprotein (51) are useful, particularly for monitoring these patients.

3. Treatment

Following diagnosis of testicular tumor, immediate surgery is indicated. For teratoma, surgery alone is usually sufficient while localized germ cell tumor requires radical surgery (involving excision of the spermatic cord structures and the testicle). Periodic evaluation of the chest and abdomen and measurement of serum AFP level allows identification of tumor recurrence. For malignant tumors with metastatic or recurrent disease, radical surgery and chemotherapy (cisplatin, vinblastine, bleomycin) offer the best outcome. However, controversy remains about the

Table 2 Classification, Median Age, Frequency, Secretory, and Histological Characteristics of Childhood Testicular Tumors

Classification	Median age (years)	Frequency (%)	Secretory activity	Tumor characteristics
Germ cell tumors				
Endodermal sinus tumor	2	26	AFP	Malignant
Teratoma	3	24	None	Usually benign
Embryonal carcinoma	Late teens	20	AFP, hCG	Both
Teratocarcinoma	Late teens	13	None	Both
Gonadoblastoma	5–10	<1	None	Both
Non-germ-cell tumors				
Leydig cell tumor	5	6	Androgen	Benign
Sertoli cell tumor	1	4	Androgen, estrogen	Benign

AFP, Alpha-fetoprotein; hCG, human chorionic gonadotropin.
Source: Data adapted from Ref. 51.

need for retroperitoneal lymph node resection in pediatric patients.

B. Ovarian Tumors

Ovarian tumors, which represent approximately 1% of childhood malignancies (52), are classified into two categories on the basis of their cells of origin: germ cell tumor and non-germ-cell tumor. Germ cell tumors, which are more common than non-germ-cell tumors in all age groups, account for 90% of ovarian tumors in premenarcheal girls (53). The majority of these germ cell tumors are teratoma, having a histologically benign and functionally inactive nature. Non-germ-cell tumors such as granulosa, theca, Sertoli and Leydig cell tumors represent a small proportion of the ovarian tumors; however, these are of additional clinical significance because of their secretory activity. The granulosa and theca cell tumors predominantly produce estrogens while Sertoli's and Leydig's cell tumors secrete androgens.

Classification, median age, distribution, secretory and histological characteristics, and the common presentation of ovarian tumors are provided in Table 3. Dysgerminoma, the most common germ cell tumor of the ovary, presents with painless abdominal mass. Endodermal sinus tumor, the most aggressive type of the germ cell tumors, presents as a painful mass with rapid metastasis to distant sites. Teratomas, the most common and benign tumor of germ cell origin, usually remain hormonally inactive. In contrast, embryonal carcinomas, which are typically found as an admixture of dysgerminoma, endodermal sinus tumor, or teratoma, may undergo differentiation, become

hormonally active, and manifest with effect of hormone production. Gonadoblastomas are uncommon tumors, yet an important ovarian tumor in girls for two reasons. First, these tumors occur more in phenotypic females with abnormal karyotype containing components of Y chromosomes (46,XY; 45,X/46,XY; 45,X/46,X fra). A recent report has shown the occurrence of gonadoblastoma in 7–10% of Y-chromosome-positive Turner's syndrome patients (54). Second, these tumors, which occur in dysgenetic gonads where differentiation into tesis or ovary has been absent or incomplete, usually contain both germ cell and stromal cell components and frequently exhibit a tendency to recur. Since all the gonadal tissue is potentially involved and carcinoma in situ is always a possibility, removal of the gonads is recommended at early stage (55).

About 5% of granulosa cell tumors develop in prepubertal girls. In these girls, with a median age of 8 years, presenting symptoms are attributed to the hormones produced by the tumors. Precocious sexual development characterized by premature breast development, pubic and axillary hair, white vaginal discharge, or irregular uterine bleeding may be the mode of presentation (55). Excessive weight gain with or without acceleration of linear growth may also occur with advancement in the skeletal age (Chapter 9). On rare occasions, androgen production may lead to virilization with hirsutism, clitoromegaly, along with acceleration of growth. In postmenarcheal girls, unregulated estrogen production may lead to irregular bleeding or amenorrhea. Although hormonally inactive tumors may remain asymptomatic, acute abdominal symptoms may be the presentation in a small proportion of these patients. This is largely the result of torsion or rupture of

Table 3 Classification, Median Age, Frequency, Secretory, and Histological Characteristics and Presentation of Ovarian Tumors in Childhood

Classification	Median age (Years)	Frequency (%)	Secretory activity	Tumor and presentation
Germ cell tumors				
Dysgerminoma	16	17	HCG	M[a]/mass
EST	18	11	AFP	H/mass, pain
Embryonal carcinoma	14	4	AFP, HCG	M/Sexual precocity
Choriocarcinoma	—	rare	HCG	M/Sexual precocity
Teratoma	10–15	29	None	B/mass
Gonadoblastoma	8–10	rare	A, HCG	M/Virilization
Carcinoid	—	rare	Serotonin	Nonspecific
Struma ovarii	—	rare	Thyroxine	Hyperthyroidism
Non-germ-cell tumors				
Granulosa-theca cell	8	13	E, P	L/Sexual precocity
Sertoli-Leydig cell	8	17	A, P	L/Virilization

EST, endodermal sinus tumor; A, androgens; E, estrogens; P, progesterone; AFP, alpha-fetoprotein; HCG, human chorionic gonadotropin.
[a]Indicates degree of malignant behavior: L, low-grade malignancy; M, moderately malignant; H, highly malignant.
Source: Data adapted from Refs. 61 and 62.

the tumor. Adequate clinical evaluation of these girls should include pelvic examination, to be performed under sedation or anesthesia, since palpable mass is almost always diagnostic of tumor.

To complete the endocrine evaluation, the pituitary–ovarian axis and estrogen profile should be studied. Estradiol level is usually elevated while luteinizing hormone (LH) and follicle-stimulating hormone (FSH) levels are suppressed, thereby excluding the differential diagnosis of central precocious puberty. Vaginal cytology reveals maturation of squamous cells, reflecting the effect of estrogen. Sonographic study helps in localizing the mass in the ovary, although it is not a useful method to exclude adrenal disease. Laparoscopy and biopsy are often necessary. Surgical resection of the lesion (i.e., unilateral salpingo-oophorectomy), usually yields good outcome. Recurrence of the disease is unusual. Compared to adult granulosa cell tumors, juvenile granulosa cell tumors have distinct histological features characterized by luteinized cells, irregular follicles, and fibroblast-like cells and the absence of Call-Exner bodies. The tumors may be cystic, solid or both. Theca cell tumors are often hormonally active and manifest by premature breast development, which is similar to that of granulosa cell tumors. They are usually slow-growing and lack the acuteness often encountered in patients with granucosa cell tumor. Diagnostic studies and management approach are, however, identical in both of these conditions.

Classic virilizing ovarian neoplasms often called arrhenoblastoma, Sertoli-Leydig cell tumors occur most commonly during the teenage or early adult years (56). Due to the effect of androgens, the early symptoms and signs consist of weight gain, amenorrhea, hirsutism, acne, deepening of the voice, and clitoromegaly. Abdominal mass and nonspecific gastrointestinal and urinary symptoms may be present concurrently. Although symptoms and signs are more intense and the progression of the course is more rapid compared to congenital adrenal hyperplasia, androgen-producing adrenal tumor, and polycystic ovarian disease, clinical differentiation may be difficult. ACTH-stimulated adrenal study, GnRH-stimulated gonadotropin profile, and estrogen levels are essential to confirm or exclude these differential diagnoses. Sonographic study of the ovary often provides adequate information to detect cystic lesions. However, computed tomographic (CT) scan is often required to assess the adrenal disease in noncystic ovarian lesions. Histologically, these tumors show an intermediate to poor degree of differentiation (57).

Identification of the cellular origin of such tumors is possible; the presence of mRNA for P450c11 and P450c21 and ACTH receptor will indicate adrenal tissue (58). Prediction of prognosis based on the cells of origin is a possibility.

Because of patients' relatively young age, conservative surgical management with preservation of the uterus

and contralateral ovary is the goal of therapy. In advanced or recurrent disease, chemotherapy and irradiation remain the alternative (59,60), although the benefits of such therapy are not proven.

IV. TUMORS OF ENDOCRINE PANCREAS

A. Nesidioblastosis

This is defined, from the pathologist's point of view, as the diffuse proliferation of islet cells budding off from the pancreatic duct, leading to the formation of numerous small clusters of the B-cells (63–65).

Males and females are equally affected and familial occurrence has been reported. Clinically, the condition is encountered in neonates and infants with persistent symptomatic hypoglycemia (Chapters 23 and 24). Almost exclusively, neonatal hypoglycemia is attributed to impaired hepatic glucose output due to hyperinsulinemia. Severe persistent hypoglycemia determines the clinical picture (66–68). Seizures, apnea, respiratory distress, listlessness, and cyanosis are the common manifestations (69). Neonates are usually macrosomic, and infants frequently weigh above than the 97th percentile. Physical examinations are otherwise unremarkable in these patients. Demonstration of hyperinsulinemia in the face of hypoglycemia, normal liver function, as well as other glucoregulatory hormones confirms diagnosis.

While diagnostic imaging studies are performed and the patient awaits surgical treatment, medical therapy should be instituted. This includes diazoxide, corticosteroids, and epinephrine (69–72). However, partial pancreatectomy is recommended in these patients. Surgery should be performed at the earliest opportunity to minimize episodes of hypoglycemia and the risk of consequent neurologic impairment (69).

Such terms as nesidioblastoma, multifocal ductuloinsular proliferation, microadenomatosis, nesidiodysplasia, and islet-cell dysmaturation syndrome have been used to describe the morphological variants of nesidioblastosis (64,73). Clinical and biochemical means are not helpful to characterize the morphological patterns in these patients (Table 4). At the functional level, further controversy exists about the relationship between hypoglycemia and

Table 4 Distribution (%) of Morphological Patterns in Nesidioblastosis

Lesions	Reference 68	Reference 76
Hyperplasia	33	29
Nesidioblastosis	17	34
Discrete adenomas	16	29
Normal pancreas	30	8

*Report was not available in 4% of the patients.

nesidioblastosis: pathological characteristics similar to nesidioblastosis are known to exist in patients with normoglycemia, while normal pancreatic morphology has been described in patients with hypoglycemia (74–76).

B. Insulinoma

Functioning beta-cell tumors have been found in patients from birth to old age, with approximately 10% of all cases occurring in individuals below 20 years of age (78,79). There is slight preponderance to females, with adequate reasons for this observation being unclear (80).

Although insulinomas may belong to a spectrum that includes islet cell tumors, nesidioblastosis, and multiple endocrine neoplasia (MEN) type 1 (81,82), it is important to differentiate this entity from the rest because of therapeutic implications (Chapter 28). If it is part of MEN type 1, long-term follow-up has to focus on the detection of other tumors. Nesidioblastosis requires more radical surgical resection than what is necessary for a discrete tumor.

1. Clinical Features

In patients with insulinoma, the hypoglycemia due to hyperinsulinemia determines the clinical pictures. Combinations of adrenergic and neuroglycopenic symptoms, as shown in Table 5, are present in vast majority of patients (83,84), although the latter tends to predominate in individuals with organic hyperinsulinism. The time of the day that symptoms occur and the relationship of these symptoms to meals are important. If the symptoms are present in the morning during fasting state, hyperinsulinemic hypoglycemia remains a strong possibility; if symptoms are reported during the postmeal period, excessive insulin response due to leucine sensitivity becomes a possibility. Presence or absence of other diseases, such as pituitary, adrenal, hepatic, renal, or autoimmune diseases, should likewise be ascertained. Family history of MEN-type I, possible access to hypoglycemic agents, history of ethanol

ingestion, and the nutritional status of the patient should be specifically determined.

Apart from the symptoms being nonspecific, physical examinations are also noncontributory. Thus, clinical diagnosis of insulin producing tumor is an almost impossible task. As shown in Table 6, initial diagnosis in patients with proven insulinoma is extremely variable, with 50% of patients being diagnosed inappropriately. The duration of symptoms in patients with islet-cell tumor is also variable and may be as short as 2 weeks or as long as 20 years. Because they learn to avoid symptoms by eating frequently throughout the day and night, some patients with longstanding disease may present with obesity and increased linear growth, which may also be the direct consequence of the anabolic and growth-promoting effect of insulin.

2. Laboratory Tests

Although normoglycemia and normal serum insulin levels have been documented in a small percentage of patients with insulinoma (85), this condition is usually suspected in nondiabetic individuals with hyperinsulinemic hypoglycemia during the fasting state. Indeed, absolute values of blood glucose and serum insulin as well as their ratio, normally up to 0.3, at the fasting state requires documentation in these patients before one undertakes more definitive and expensive tests (86). Lack of ketonemia, ketonuria, and acidosis in the presence of fasting hypoglycemia is also strongly supportive of a diagnosis of hyperinsulinemic hypoglycemia.

An amended insulin glucose ratio, calculated by multiplying the insulin level by 100 and then dividing by the blood glucose minus 30, is considered a better discriminator between normal and abnormal insulin secretion. This ratio of normally 50 or less measures the degree of suppression of the pancreatic insulin secretion and reduces false-negative results.

Table 5 Symptoms of Hypoglycemia

Adrenergic	Neuroglycopenic
Anxiety	Headache
Nervousness	Blurred vision
Tremulousness	Paresthesias
Sweating	Weakness
Hunger	Tiredness
Palpitation	Confusion
Irritability	Dizziness
Pallor	Amnesia
Nausea	Incoordination
Flushing	Behavioral change
Angina	Seizures, coma

Source: Ref. 81.

Table 6 Initial Diagnosis in 46 of 91 Patients with Proven Insulinoma

Diagnosis	Number of patients
Epilepsy	14
Nervous exhaustion	6
Psychoses	6
Stroke	4
Hysteria	4
Menopause	3
Tetany	2
Brain tumor	2
Diabetes	2
Inebriation	2
Heart attack	1

Source: Ref. 88.

Measurement of plasma C-peptide and proinsulin levels are also useful in differentiating factitious hypoglycemia from islet-cell tumor (87). Normally, the pancreatic insulin secretion parallels the plasma level of peptides. In children with suspected hypoglycemia due to insulinoma, a limited fast of variable duration (6–72 h) is often necessary (88). This is especially the case when hypoglycemia is observed in the absence of inappropriate elevation of insulin levels.

Duration of the fast should be determined on the basis of age, concurrent conditions, and severity of symptoms. Infants and young children should fast 4–12 h under close observation in the hospital. In adults, prolonged fast of 72 h has been used. However, with the availability of insulin, proinsulin, and C-peptide assays, the 72 h fast is not necessary (89).

For detection of symptoms of hypoglycemia and measurements of blood glucose, insulin, and urine ketones at the time of the symptoms, hospitalization is necessary. In patients with insulinoma, the time of symptom development during the fast has been variable, ranging from 7 to 60 h. Spontaneous increase in blood glucose levels has also been reported in such patients.

Provocative tests for assessment of insulin secretion are sometimes necessary (90). This is particularly advantageous when the clinical evidence is compelling, yet time limitations do not allow hospitalization for prolonged fasting. Glucagon, leucine, and tolbutamide are beta-cell-stimulatory agents used for this purpose (90–92). Intravenous calcium infusion is also used as a stimulus to insulin secretion (93,94). However, the tolbutamide test should not be used because it may be dangerous.

Depressed glucosylated hemoglobin and fructosamine levels may be present in patients with insulinoma, supporting the presence of hypoglycemia during the preceding 6–8 weeks.

3. Differential Diagnosis

Hypoglycemia due to various systemic diseases is frequently encountered in clinical practice. Hyperinsulinemia is the primary differentiating feature between these patients and those with insulinoma. The most difficult differential diagnosis is nesidioblastosis.

4. Localization of the Lesion

Once clinical and biochemical evidence of hyperinsulinism is established, anatomical localization of the insulin-secreting lesion is indicated. This is accomplished by ultrasonography, CT scan, highly selective arteriography, or percutaneous transhepatic pancreatic venous sampling.

Of all the methods of study, preoperative ultrasonography is the most inexpensive and least invasive technique to localize pancreatic tumors. However, the accuracy is low, with detection of 25% of pancreatic lesions (95). On the other hand, this will avoid the false-negative results of laparotomy that can occur in patients with nesidioblas-tosis where no identifiable tumor is present. Preoperative endoscopic ultrasonography increases the accuracy of diagnosis and has been the choice for many surgeons (96).

Using intraoperative ultrasonography by applying the probe on the surface of the pancreas, lesions too small to be palpable have been detected. CT scan performed with contrast enhancement can improve the sensitivity of detection up to 40% (97). Detection of the lesion also depends on its size and location: lesions measuring less than 2 cm or located on the head or tail of the pancreas are most likely to be missed. Although ultrasonography and CT scan have low accuracy, these are reasonable first choices for tumor staging and detection of metastasis. Selective arteriography is useful to demonstrate insulinomas, with a success rate ranging from 30 to 90% (98); lesions as small as 0.5 cm in diameter have been detected. Preoperative angiography is utilized to determine the number, size, and location of the tumors. Tumors located in the head or tail of the pancreas are the most likely to be missed.

Transhepatic venous sampling with simultaneous arterial blood sampling has been useful in detecting small tumors that were missed during preoperative imaging studies (99). Apart from obtaining blood samples from different points in the portal, splenic, and mesenteric venous system, it is important to draw simultaneous peripheral blood samples to allow for changing during the course of the procedure. During this study, venous insulin concentration at least 50% higher than the arterial level is considered to be diagnostic of insulinoma. There is a considerable degree of risk of complication, such as peritonitis, hemorrhage, or perforation of the gallbladder. As a consequence, this procedure should be considered if insulinoma is likely based on the hypoglycemia and hyperinsulinemia and yet ultrasound, CT scan, and arteriography have all been negative. Biochemical markers using alpha-hCG, beta-hCG, or immunostaining technique have been found to be helpful in some patients. Differentiation of malignant lesions from benign by the histological criteria has been unreliable, because the morphological characteristics fail to correlate with the metastatic disease (100).

5. Treatment and Prognosis

To avoid irreversible neurological sequelae of persistent profound hypoglycemia, intense preoperative management is mandatory. Dietary management should be judicious, particularly ensuring a snack before the bedtime. However, treatment is particularly difficult in infants and children due to the uncertainty in ensuring food intake at a timely manner and the variability of the pathology. Diffuse islet cell involvement is more frequent than solitary adenomas, thus making complete surgical removal of the tumor difficult for the surgeons.

For preoperative patients as well as those with inoperable or undetectable tumor, pharmacological agents are indicated. Diazoxide, a benzothiadiazine derivative, reduces insulin secretion and increases the epinephrine release. When administered at a dosage of 100–800 mg daily this maintains normoglycemia. Although side effects such as fluid retention and hypertrichosis are unacceptable, it is tolerated by most patients. Corticosteroid, used in conjunction with other agents, enhances the effectiveness of maintaining normoglycemia. A long-acting somatostatin analog, SMS 201-995, has shown promise in correcting hypoglycemia (101). Surgical removal of the tumor is the mode of therapy in patients with insulinoma (102) and should be performed at the earliest possible time. Almost 90% of the tumors are benign, and carry a favorable diagnosis.

C. Glucagonoma

Clinical and diagnostic features of glucagonoma, in comparison with vipoma and somatostatinoma, are presented in Table 7. Apart from insulin, endocrine tumors of the pancreas can produce glucagon, pancreatic polypeptide, and somatostatin along with peptides that are not normally present therein, such as VIP, peptide histidine methionine, growth hormone-releasing factors, gastrin, and calcitonin. Due to cosecretion of these hormones by various tumors, clinical syndromes may overlap and appear to be nonspecific. It consequently becomes impractical to pursue the diagnosis in all patients who present with these symptoms. However, glucagonoma, vipoma, and somatostatinoma, despite being rare in children, are interesting because of the cause and effect relationship between the increased hormone levels and the distinct clinical syndromes (glucagon and hyperglycemia, vasoactive intestinal peptide and diarrhea, somatostatin and reduced motility of the gastrointestinal–biliary tract). For a practicing physician, the importance of being familiar with these syndromes is, therefore, obvious: distinct clinical expression caused by altered biochemical environment, increased availability of precise diagnostic tools, and, most of all, specific therapeutic implications.

The true incidence of glucagonoma is not really known. Postmortem studies in adult patients with neither clinical symptoms nor diabetes have disclosed the presence of glucagonoma (103). However, there are no such data available in children. Glucagon, a 29-aminoacid polypeptide, is secreted mostly by the alpha cells of the pancreatic islets. It stimulates the glycogenolytic process, resulting in elevation of blood glucose.

1. Clinical Features

A characteristic skin rash is the major manifestation in patients with glucagon-secreting islet cell tumor (103–105). Commonly starting in the groin area as erythematous blotches, the lesions migrate to the buttocks, thighs, perineum, and distal extremeties. The lesions are necrolytic, with raised and vesiculopustular appearance and gradually become confluent. During the acute stage, these lesions are intensely painful and pruritic. After scaling, the lesions heal and become indurated and hyperpigmented. However, remission and relapse are typical of these lesions, which are due to the glycogenolytic action of glucagon. Glossitis, angular stomatitis, venous thrombosis, and occasional blackout spells occur in association with these lesions. The most common gastrointestinal symptoms are diarrhea and constipation, which is attributed to the altered motility of the intestine. Other findings include anemia and weight loss, which is primarily due to the anorexic and catabolic effect of glucagon. Specific biochemical findings include hypoproteinemia, hypoaminoacidemia, and hypocholesterolemia. Mild hyperglycemia, due to the glycogenolytic effect of glucagon, is also observed in some patients (106).

2. Diagnosis and Management

In the presence of suggestive clinical findings, the diagnosis is readily confirmed by the finding of elevated serum

Table 7 Characteristic Features of Glucagonoma, Vipoma, and Somatostatinoma

Character	Glucagonoma	Vipoma	Somatostatinoma
Amino acid	29	28	14
Normal source	a-cells of pancreatic islet	Intestinal mucosa, central and peripheral nervous system	D cells of pancreatic islet, hypothalamus-pituitary, intestinal mucosa
Physiological action	Raise blood glucose	Neurotransmitter; Enhances intestinal secretion	Reduces intestinal secretion and motility
Characteristics Clinical features	Rash, glossitis, stomatitis	Persistent and profuse diarrhea mimics cholera	Diabetes, cholestasis, steatorrhea; may have hypoglycemia
Malignancy (%)	75	60	60
Incidence in children	Not known, cases reported	Not known	Not known
Diagnosis	Elevated plasma level glucagons, insulin; CT scan	Elevated plasma level of VIP or PHM; hypokalemia; CT scan; laparotomy	Elevated serum level of somatostatin; CT scan to detect tumor mass

glucagon concentrations. Plasma insulin levels are also elevated, which explains the mildness of diabetes. A paradoxic rise of plasma glucagon during an oral glucose tolerance test or intravenous tolbutamide test provides additional support to the diagnosis of glucagonoma. However, these tests are superfluous in most cases. Preoperatively, CT scan is necessary to localize the primary and metastatic disease. However, the most valuable technique for tumor localization is selective arteriography: glucagonomas are highly vascular and produce prominent tumor blush.

Treatment involves surgical resection, which leads to dramatic improvement of the rash (106,107). Chemotherapy with dacarbazine (108) and stretpzotocin (109) have been useful in case of nonresectable tumors. Somatostatin use alleviates the symptoms, because of the reduction of glucagon (110,111). Although zinc levels in the blood do not correlate with the presence or absence of the rash, oral zinc administration has been shown to improve the skin lesions (112). Adequate nutritional support and reversal of negative nitrogen balance stand at the center of the medical and surgical management of these patients. Parenteral infusions of specific amino acids to correct the catabolic hypoaminoacidemia has led to disappearance of the skin lesions (113).

D. Vipoma

Since the first description of this condition in 1957 by Priest and Alexander (114), various investigators have reported its manifold clinical features (115–119). Various synonyms such as Verner-Morrison syndrome, watery diarrhea hypokalemia–achlorhydria (WDHA) syndrome, and pancreatic cholera syndrome have described the same condition (118). In 1973, Bloom and colleagues renamed this condition vipoma syndrome (116).

VIP is a 28-amino-acid peptide, distributed diffusely in the gastrointestinal submucosa as well as the central nervous system (120). It stimulates water and electrolyte secretion, leading to profuse water loss in the small intestine and colon. Sodium and potassium secretion into the lumen of the bowel also features prominently due to VIP's action. Relaxation of the smooth muscles of gastrointestinal and vascular system, reduction of the gastric acid output, and decrease in the motility of the gall bladder are also caused by the vipoma.

1. Clinical Features

Vipoma is an uncommon disorder in children. Mekhjian reported 6 patients (119), out of 29 diagnosed cases of this syndrome, who were below 5 years of age. Mean age of presentation is 47 years (121), and the incidence has been estimated at 1:10 million per year. There is a female preponderance.

Diarrhea, the major manifestation of the vipoma syndrome, is characterized as persistent, secretory, and large in volume, exceeding 700 ml/day. Stool is isotonic with plasma and mimics the description of cholera. Apart from the massive water loss, large amounts of potassium and bicarbonate are lost in the stool. Thus, dehydration, hypokalemia, and acidosis lead to significant morbidity and mortality.

Due to the inhibitory effect of VIP on pentagastrin-mediated acid secretion, gastric acid secretion is frequently decreased in these patients. Differentiation from Zollinger-Ellison syndrome is therefore based on diminished basal acid output. Although the serum phosphorus level is normal, hypercalcemia and hypomagnesemia occur in patients with vipoma syndrome. Hypercalcemia is explained on the basis of excessive bone resorption mediated by the VIP. Hyperglycemia, due to the glucagonlike effect of the VIP, is also reported.

2. Diagnosis and Management

Correction of volume deficit, electrolyte abnormalities, hypercalcemia, and hypomagnesemia should be the priority before establishing the diagnosis of vipoma and localizing the tumor.

In the presence of characteristic clinical syndrome, the elevated plasma VIP concentration is diagnostic (122). However, normal plasma VIP levels with increased level of peptide histidine-methionine (PHM), another intestinal secretagogue similar in effect to the VIP, have been described in patients with this syndrome. An intestinal perfusion study is useful to document intestinal secretion and confirm the diagnosis of vipoma syndrome. Anatomical localization of the tumor and its metastasis is obtained by ultrasound and CT scan study. However, false-negative studies are reported, making exploratory laparotomy the most definitive diagnostic modality.

Surgical resection offers the best chance of cure and provides relief of symptoms. In patients with nonresectable or metastatic disease, chemotherapy with streptozotocin may produce remission of symptoms and normalize the plasma VIP levels. Other drugs such as corticosteroids and lithium carbonates have been reported to control the symptoms of diarrhea. Treatment with octreotide, a somatostatin analogue, represents a newer method of nonsurgical management of these patients.

E. Somatostatinoma

1. Clinical Features

This is also an unusual disorder in children. Most of the reported cases in literature involve adult patients. Somatostatin, a 14-amino-acid cyclic peptide, is present in the anterior pituitary, hypothalamus, thyroid follicle, D-cells of the pancreatic islet, and intestinal mucosa (123–126). As indicated by its name, it inhibits the pituitary, pancreatic, gastric, and biliary secretion. Thus, in patients with somatostatinoma and consequent increased serum somatostatin concentration, provocative GH and TSH response is inhibited, insulin and glucagon levels are diminished, and gastrointestinal and biliary secretion is decreased. Motility of the gastrointestinal and biliary tract is also reduced. Clinically, pancreatic somatostatinoma produces a triad of diabetes, cholelithiasis, and steatorrhea (127,128). Diabetes is usually mild, cholelithiasis is associated with gallbladder stasis, and steatorrhea is due to insufficient exocrine function of the pancreas. However, cosecretion of the hormones can alter the picture, contributing to various nonspecific symptoms. For instance, diarrhea may be the prominent feature in case of calcitonin oversecretion. Due to the altered insulin/glucagon balance, hypoglycemia has been reported in some patients with somatostatinoma (129). Extrapancreatic somatostatinoma, usually located in the duodenal mucosa, is more likely to present with biliary obstruction than the above-mentioned constellation of the syndrome. Weight loss and anemia are also present in patients with longstanding disease.

2. Diagnosis and Management

In presence of clinical syndrome, the serum somatostatin level is usually elevated in patients with somatostatinoma. Provocative endocrine studies using tolbutamide, arginine, or the glucose tolerance test may be required in doubtful cases to document lack of change in the insulin and glucagon (129,130). Detection of tumor mass and metastasis requires radiological imaging study, usually with CT scan. Although total surgical resection offers the most favorable outcome, advanced or recurrent disease may require chemotherapy with streptozotocin and 5-fluorouracil (129, 131). Prognosis for treatment depends on the extent of the disease at the time of diagnosis.

REFERENCES

1. Bertagna C, Orth DN. Clinical and laboratory findings and results of therapy in 58 patients with adrenocortical tumors admitted to a single medical center (1951 to 1978). Am J Med 1981; 71:855–875.
2. McWhirter WR, Stiller CA, Lennox EL. Carcinoma in childhood. A registry-based study of incidence and survival. Cancer 1989; 63:2242–2246.
3. Kaplan SA. Disorders of the adrenal cortex I. Pediatr Clin North Am 1979; 26:65–76.
4. Luton J, Cedras S, Billard L, et al. Clinical features of adrenocortical carcinoma, prognostic factors and the effect of mitotane therapy. N Engl J Med 1990; 325:1195–1201.
5. Donaldson MDC, Grant DB, O'Hare MJ, Schackleton CHL. Familial congenital Cushing syndrome due to bilateral nodular adrenal hyperplasia. Clin Endocrinol 1981; 14:519–525.
6. Reincke M, Karl M, Travis WH, et al. Mutations in human adrenocortical neoplasms; immunohistochemical and molecular studies. J Clin Endocrinol Metab 1994; 78: 790–794.
7. Sotelo-Avila C, Gonzales-Crussi F, Fowler JW. Complete and incomplete forms of Beckwith-Weidemann syndrome: their oncogenic potential. J Pediatr 1980; 96:47–50.
8. Fraumeni JF Jr, Miller RW. Adrenocortical neoplasms with hemihypertrophy, brain tumors, and other disorders. J Pediatr 1967; 70:129–138.
9. Latronico AC, Chrousos GP. Adrenocortical tumors. J Clin Endocrinol Metab 1997; 82:1317–1324.
10. Sandrini R, Ribeiroo RC, Delacerda L. Childhood adrenocortical tumors. J Clin Endocrinol Metab 1997; 92: 2027–2031.
11. Meador CK, Bowdoin B, Owen WC, Farmer TA. Primary adrenocortical nodular dysplasia: a rare cause of Cushing's syndrome. J Clin Endocrinol Metab 1967; 27:125–163.
12. Larsen JL, Cathey WJ, Odell WD. Primary adrenocortical nodular dysplasia, a distinct subtype of Cushing's syndrome. Case report and review of the literature. Am J Med 1986; 80:976–984.
13. Carney JA, Hruska LS, Beauchamp GD, et al. Dominant inheritance of the complex of myxomas, spotty pigmentation, and endocrine overactivity. Mayo Clin Proc 1986; 61:165–172.
14. Wulffraat NM, Drexhage HA, Wiersinga RD, et al. Immunoglobulins of patients with Cushing's syndrome due to pigmented adrenocortical micronodular dysplasia stimulate in vitro steroidogenesis. J Clin Endocrinol Metab 1988; 66:301.
15. Weinstein LS, Shenker A, Gejman PV, Merino MJ, Friedman E, Spiegel AM. Activating mutations of the stimulatory G-protein in the McCune-Albright Syndrome. N Engl J Med 1991; 325:1688–1695.
16. Lacroix A, Bolte E, Tremblay J, et al. Gastric inhibitory polypeptide-dependent cortisol hypersecretion: a new cause of Cushing's Syndrome. N Engl J Med 1992; 327: 974–980.
17. Reznik Y, Allili-Zerah V, Chayvialle, et al. Food-dependent Cushing's syndrome mediated by aberrant adrenal sensitivity to gastric inhibitory polypeptide. N Engl J Med 1992; 327:981–986.
18. McArthur RG, Cloutier MD, Hayles AB, et al. Cushing's disease in children. Mayo Clin Proc 1972; 47:318–326.
19. Thomas CG Jr, Smith AT, Griffith JM, et al. Hyperadrenalism in childhood and adolescence. Ann Surg 1984; 199:538–548.
20. Tyrell JB. Cushing's disease. N Engl J Med 1978; 298: 753–758.
21. Lee PA, Weldon VV, Migeon CJ. Short stature as the only clinical sign of Cushing syndrome. J Pediatr 1975; 86: 89–91.
22. Lee PDK, Winter RJ, Green OC. Virilising adrenocortical tumors in childhood. Eight cases and review of literature. Pediatrics 1985; 76:437–444.
23. Lanes R. Adrenocortical carcinoma in a 4 year old. Clin Pediatr 1982; 21:164–166.
24. Giombetti R, Hagstrom JW, Landey S, Young MC, New MI. Cushing's syndrome in infancy: a case complicated by monilia endocarditis. Am J Dis Child 1971; 122:264–266.
25. Dahms WT, Gray G, Vrana M, New MI. Adrenocortical adenoma and a ganglineuroblastoma in a child: a case presenting as Cushing's syndrome with virilization. Am J Dis Child 1973; 125:608–611.
26. Comite F, Schiebinger RJ, Albertson BD, et al. Isosexual precocious pseudopuberty secondary to a feminizing adrenal tumor. J Clin Endocrinol Metab 1984; 58:435–440.
27. Cagle PT, Hough AJ, Pysher TJ, et al. Comparison of adrenal cortical tumors in children and adults. Cancer 1986; 57:2235–2237.

28. Moore L, Barker AP, Byard RW, Bourne AJ, Ford WDA. Adrenocortical tumors in childhood—clinicopathological features of six cases. Pathology 1991; 23:94–97.

29. Mendonca BB, Lucon AM, Menezes CAV, et al. Clinical, hormonal and pathological findings in a comparative study of adrenortical neoplasms in childhood and adulthood. J Urol 1995; 154:2004–2009.

30. Zeiger MA, Nieman LK, Cutler GB, et al. Primary bilateral adrenocortical causes of Cushing's syndrome. Surgery 1990; 110:1106–1115.

31. Arico M, Bossi G, Livieri C, Raiteri E, Severi F. Partial response after intensive chemotherapy for adrenocortical carcinoma in a child. Med Pediatr Oncol 1992; 20:246–248.

32. Crock PA, Clark ACL. Combination chemotherapy for adrenal carcinoma: response in a 5 and half year old male. 1989; 17:62–65.

33. Schlumberger M, Brugieres L, Gicquel C, Travagli J, Groz J, Parmentier C. 5-Fluorouracil, doxorubicin, and cisplatin as treatment for adrenal carcinoma. Cancer 1991; 67:2997–3000.

34. Godil MA, Atlas MP, Parker RI, et al. Metastic congenital adrenocortical carcinoma: a case report with tumor remission at $3\frac{1}{2}$ years. J Clin Endocrinol Metab 2000; 85:3964–3967.

35. Ulbright TM, Roth LM. Recent developments in the pathology of germ cell tumors. Semin Diagn Pathol 1987; 4:304–319.

36. Jacobson GK, Barlebo H, Olsen J, et al. Testicular germ cell tumors in Denmark 1976–1980: Pathology of 1058 consecutive cases. Acta Radiol Oncol 1984; 23:239–247.

37. Batata MA, Whitmore WFJ, Chu FCH. Cryptorchidism and testicular cancer. J Urol 1980; 124:382–387.

38. Martin DC. Germinal cell tumors of the testis after orchiopexy. J Urol 1979; 121:422–424.

39. Benson RJ, Beard CM, Kelalis PP, et al. Malignant potential of the cryptorchid testis. Mayo Clin Proc 1991; 66:372–378.

40. Cassio A, Cacciari E, D'Errico A, et al. Incidence of intratubular germ cell neoplasia in androgen insensitivity syndrome. Acta Endocrinol (Copenh) 1990; 123:416–422.

41. Dexeus FH, Logothetis CJ, Chong C, et al. Genetic abnormalities in men with germ cell tumors. J Urol 1988; 140:80–84.

42. Lykkesfeldt G, Bennet P, Lykkesfeldt AE, et al. Testis cancer. Icthyosis constitutes a significant risk factor. Cancer 1991; 67:730–734.

43. Aristizabal S, Davis JR, Miller RC, Moore MJ, Boone LM. Bilateral primary germ cell testicular tumors. Report of four cases and review of literature. Cancer 1978; 42:591–597.

44. Thompson J, Williams CJ, Whitehouse JM, Mead GM. Bilateral testicular germ cell tumors: an increasing incidence and prevention by chemotherapy. Br J Urol 1988; 62:374–376.

45. Patel SR, Richardson RL, Kuols L. Synchronous and metachronous bilateral testicular tumors. Mayo Clinic experience. Cancer 1990; 65:1–4.

46. Tollerud DJ, Blattner WA, Fraser MC. Familial testicular cancer and urogenital developmental anomalies. Cancer 1985; 55:1849–1854.

47. Radfar N, Bartler FC, Easley R, et al. Evidence for endogenous LH suppression in a man with bilateral testicular tumors and congenital adrenal hyperplasia. J Clin Endocrinol Metab 1977; 45:1194–1203.

48. Srikanth MS, West BR, Ishitani M, et al. Benign testicular tumors in children with congenital adrenal hyperplasia. J Pediatr Surg 1992; 27:639–641.

49. Morrish DW, Venner PM, Siy O, et al. Mechanisms of endocrine dysfunction in patients with testicular cancer. J Natl Cancer Inst 1990; 82:412–418.

50. Borer JG, Tan PE, Diamond DA. The spectrum of Sertoli cell tumors in children. Urol Clin North Am 2000; 27:529–541.

51. Castleberry RP, Kelly DR, Joseph DB, Cain WS. Gonadal and extragonadal germ cell tumors. In: Fernbach DJ, Vietti TJ, eds. Clinical Pediatric Oncology, 4th ed. Chicago: Mosby Year Book, 1991:577–594.

52. Young JL, et al. Cancer, incidence, survival and mortality for children younger than age 15 years. Cancer 1986; 58:598–602.

53. Abell MR, Johnson VJ, Holtz F. Ovarian neoplasms in childhood and adolescence. Am J Obstet Gynecol 1965; 92:1059–1081.

54. Gravholt CH, Fedder J, Naeraa RW, Muller J. Occurrence of gonadoblastoma in female with Turner syndrome and Y chromosome material: a population study. J Clin Endocrinol Metab 2000; 85:3199–3202.

55. Young RH, Dickerson RG, Scully RE. Juvenile granulosa cell tumor of the ovary. A clinicopathological analysis of 125 cases. Am J Surg Path 1984; 8:575–596.

56. Young RH, Scully RE. Ovarian Sertoli-Leydig cell tumors. A clinicopathologic analysis of 207 cases. Am J Surg Pathol 1985; 9:534–569.

57. Roth LM, Anderson MC, Govan ADT, Langley FA, Gowing NFC, Woodcock AS. Sertoli-Leydig cell tumors: a clinicopathological study of 34 cases. Cancer 1981; 48:187–197.

58. Lin CJ, Jorge AAL. Latronico Acietal. Origin of an ovarian steroid cell tumor causing isosexual psuedoprecocious puberty demonstrated by the expression of adrenal steroidogenic enzymes and adrenocorticotrophin receptor. J Clin Endocrinol Metab 2000; 85:1211–1214.

59. Zaloudek C, Norris HJ. Sertoli-Leydig tumors of the ovary. A clinicopathologic study of 64 intermediate and poorly differentiated neoplasm. Am J Surg Pathol 1984; 8:405–418.

60. Schwartz PE, Smith JP. Treatment of ovarian stromal tumors. Am J Obstet Gynecol 1976; 125:402–411.

61. Carr BR. Disorders of the ovary and female reproductive tract. In: Wilson JD, Foster DW, eds. Williams Textbook of Endocrinology, 8th ed. Philadelphia: WB Saunders, 1992:779.

62. Castleberry RP, Kelly DR, Joseph DB, Cain WS. Gonadal and extragonadal germ cell tumors. In: Fernbach DJ, Vietti T, eds. Clinical Pediatric Oncology, 4th ed. Chicago: Mosby Year Book, 1991:577–594.

63. Laidlaw G. Nesidioblastoma, the islet tumor of the pancreas. Am J Pathol 1938; 14:12–34.

64. Heitz PV, Kloppel G, Haiki WH, et al. Nesidioblastosis. The pathologic basis of persistent hyperinsulinemic hypoglycemia in infants: morphologic and quantitative analysis of seven cases based on specific immunostaining and electron microscopy. Diabetes 1971; 26:632–642.

65. Nathan DM, Axelrod L, Proppe KH, et al. Nesidioblastosis associated with insulin-mediated hypoglycemia in an adult. Diabetes Care 1981; 4:383–388.

66. Vance JE, Stoll RW, Kitabchi AE, et al. Nesidioblastosis in familial endocrine adenomatosis. JAMA 1969; 207:1679–1682.

67. Schwartz SS, Rich BM, Lucky AW, et al. Familial nesidioblastosis: severe neonatal hypoglycemia in two families. J Pediatr 1979; 95:44–53.

68. Woo D, Scopes JW, Polak JM. Idiopathic hypoglycemia in sibs with morphological evidence of nesidioblastosis of the pancreas. Arch Dis Child 1976; 51:528–531.

69. Thomas CG Jr, Underwood LE, Carney CN, et al. Neonatal and infantile hypoglycemia due to insulin excess: new aspects and diagnosis in surgical management. Ann Surg 1977; 185:505–517.

70. Fajans SS, Floyd JC Jr. Diagnosis and medical management of insulinomas. Annu Rev Med 1979; 30:313–329.

71. Fajans SS, Floyd JC Jr, Thiffault CA, et al. Further studies on diazoxide suppression of insulin release from abnormal and normal islet tissue in man. Ann NY Acad Sci 1968; 150:261–280.

72. Field JB, Remer A, Drapanas T. Clinical and physiologic studies using diazoxide in the treatment of hypoglycemia. Ann NY Acad Sci 1968; 150:415–428.

73. Carlson T, Eikhauser ML, DeBoz B, et al. Nesidioblastosis in an adult: an illustrative case and collective review. Am J Gastroenterol 1987; 82:566–571.

74. Rahier J. Relevance of endocrine pancrease nesidioblastosis to hyperinsulinemic hypoglycemia. Diabetes Care 1989; 12:164–166.

75. Karnauchow PN. Nesidioblastosis in adults without insular hyperfunction. Am J Clin Pathol 1982; 78:511–513.

76. Fong T, Warner NE, Kumar D. Pancreatic nesidioblastosis in adults. Diabetes Care 1989; 12:108–114.

77. Field JB. Insulinoma. In: Mazzaferi EL, Samaan NA, eds. Endocrine Tumors, 1st ed. Oxford: Blackwell Scientific Publications, 1993:517–518.

78. Crain EL, Thorn GW. Functioning pancreatic islet cell adenomas: a review of the literature and presentation of two new differential tests. Medicine 1949; 28:427–447.

79. Stefanini P, Carboni M, Pitrassi N, Bosali A. Beta-islet cell tumors of the pancreas. Results of a study on 1067 cases. Surgery 1989; 75:597–609.

80. Brunelle F, Negre V, Barth MD. Pancreatic venous sampling in infants and children with primary hyperinsulinism. Pediatr Radiol 1989; 19:100–103.

81. Field JB. Hypoglycemia. Definition, clinical presentations, classification, and laboratory tests. Endocrinol Metab Clin North Am 1989; 18:27–43.

82. Jensen RT. Pancreatic endocrine tumors: recent advances. Ann Oncol 1999; 10:5710–5176.

83. Turner RC, Oakley NW, Naborro JDN. Control of basal insulin secretion with special reference to the diagnosis of insulinoma. Br Med J 1971; 2:132–135.

84. Johnson RG, Bauman WA, Warshaw A, et al. Factitious hypoglycemia due to administration of human synthetic insulin: new diagnostic challenge. Diabetes Care 1987; 10:253–255.

85. Carlett JA, Mako ME, Rubinstein AH, et al. Factitious hypoglycemia: diagnosis by measurement of serum C-peptide immunoreactivity and insulin-binding antibodies. N Engl J Med 1977; 297:1029–1032.

86. Turner RC, Heding LG. Plasma proinsulin, C-peptide and insulin in diagnostic suppression tests for insulinomas. Diabetologia 1977; 13:571–577.

87. Fajans SS, Vinick AI. Insulin-producing islet cell tumors. Endocrinol Metab Clin North Am 1989; 18:45–74.

88. Breidahl HD, Priestly JT, Rynearson EH. Hyperinsulinemia: surgical aspects and results. Ann Surg 1955; 142:698–708.

89. Hirshberg B, Livi A, Bartlet DL, et al. Forty-eight hour fast: the diagnostic test for insulinoma. J Clin Endocrinol Metab 2000; 85:3222–3226.

90. Service FJ, Dale AJ, Elveback R, Jiang NS. Insulinomas: clinical and diagnostic features of 60 consecutive cases. Mayo Clin Proc 1976; 51:417–431.

91. Pun KK, Young RTT, Wang C, et al. The use of glucagon challenge tests in the diagnostic evaluation of hypoglycemia due to hepatoma and insulinoma. J Clin Endocrinol Metab 1988; 67:546–550.

92. Kaplan EL, Arganine M, Kong SJ. Diagnosis and treatment of hypoglycemic disorder. Surg Clin North Am 1987; 67:395–410.

93. Kaplan EL, Rubinstein AH, Evans R, et al. Calcium infusion—a new provocative test for insulinoma. Ann Surg 1979; 190:501–507.

94. Roy BK, Abuid J, Wendorff H, et al. Insulin release in response to calcium in the diagnosis of insulinoma. Metabolism 1979; 28:246–252.

95. Gorman B, Charboneau JW, James EM, et al. Benign pancreatic insulinoma. Preoperative and intraoperative sonographic localisation. Am J Roengenol 1986; 147:929–934.

96. Chun J, Doherty GM. Pancreatic endocrine tumors. Curr Opin Oncol 2001; 13:52–56.

97. Dagget PR, Goodburn EA, Kurtz AB, et al. Is preoperative localization of insulinomas necessary? Lancet 1981; 1:483–486.

98. Galiher AR, Reading CC, Charbonneau JW, et al. Localization of pancreatic insulinoma: comparison of pre- and intoperative US with CT and arteriography. Radiology 1988; 166:405–408.

99. Cho KJ, Vinik AI, Thompson NW, et al. Localization of the source of hyperinsulinism: percutaneous transhepatic portal and pancreatic vein catheterization with hormone assay. Am J Roengenol 1982; 139:237–245.

100. Kenny BD, Sloan JM, Hamilton PW, et al. The role of morphometry in predicting prognosis in pancreatic islet cell tumors. Cancer 1989; 64:460–465.

101. Osei K, O'Dorisio TM. Malignant insulinoma: effects of somatostatin analog (compound 201-995) on serum glucose, growth and gastroenteropancreatic hormones. Ann Intern Med 1985; 103:223–225.

102. Koivunen DG, Harrison TS. The hypoglycemic syndrome: endogenous hyperinsulinism. In: Friesen SR, Thompson NW, eds. Surgical Endocrinology: Clinical Syndromes, 2nd ed. Philadelphia; JB Lippincott, 1990: 221–225.

103. Mallinson CN, Bloom SR, Warin AP, et al. A glucagonoma syndrome. Lancet 1974; 2:1–3.

104. Printz RA, Dorsch TR, Lawrence AM. Clinical aspects of glucagon producing islet cell tumors. Am J Gastroenterol 1981; 76:125–131.

105. Stacpole PW. The glucagonoma syndrome: clinical features, diagnosis and treatment. Endocr Rev 1981; 2:347–361.

106. Higgins GA, Recant L, Fischman AB. The glucagonoma syndrome: surgically curable diabetes. Am J Surg 1979; 137:142–148.

107. Boden G, Owen OE, Rezvani I, et al. An islet cell carcinoma containing glucagon and insulin. Chronic glucagon excess and glucose homeostasis. Diabetes 1977; 26:128–137.

108. Strauss GM, Weitzman SA, Aoki TT. Dimethyltriazionoimidazole carboxamide therapy of malignant glucagonoma. Ann Intern Med 1979; 80:57–58.

109. Danforth DN Jr, Triche T, Doppman JL, Beazley RM, Perrino PV, Recant L. Elevated plasma glucagon-like component with -secreting tumor: effect of streptozotocin. N Engl J Med 1976; 295:242–245.

110. Kahn CR, Bhathena SJ, Recant L, et al. Use of somatostatin and somatostatin analogs in a patient with a glucagonoma. J Clin Endocrinol Metab 1981; 53:543–549.

111. Sohier H, Jeanmougin M, Lombrail P. Rapid improvement of skin lesions in glucagonoma with intravenous somatostatin infusion (letter). Lancet 1980; 1:40.

112. Mallinson C, Bloom SR. The hyperglycemic, cutaneous syndrome: pancreatic glucagonoma. In: Friesen SR, ed. Surgical Endocrinology: Clinical Syndromes. Philadelphia: JB Lippincott, 1978:171–202.

113. Norton JA, Kahn CR, Scheibinger R, Gorscboth C, Brennan MF. Amino acid deficiency and the skin rash associated with glucagonoma. Ann Intern Med 1979; 91:213–215.

114. Priest WM, Alexander MK. Islet-cell tumor of the pancreas with peptic ulceration, diarrhea and hypokalemia. Lancet 1957; 2:1145–1147.

115. Verner JV, Morrison AB. Islet cell-tumor and a syndrome of refractory watery diarrhea and hypokalemia. Am J Med 1958; 25:374–380.

116. Bloom SR, Polak JM, Pearse AGE. Vasoactive intestinal peptide and watery diahhrea syndrome. Lancet 1973; 2:14–16.

117. Murray JS, Paton RR, Pope CE. Pancreatic tumor associated with flushing and diarrhea. Report of a case. N Engl J Med 1961; 264:436–439.

118. Matsumoto KK, Peter JB, Schultze RG, et al. Watery diarrhea and hypokalemia associated with pancreatic islet cell adenoma. Gastroenterology 1966; 50:231–242.

119. Mekhjian HS, O'Dorisio TM. Vipoma syndrome. Semin Oncol 1987; 14:282–291.

120. Pearse AGE. Peptides in brain and intestine. Nature 1976; 262:92–94.

121. Verner JV, Morrison AB. Non-beta islet cell tumors and the syndrome of watery diarrhea, hypokalemia and hypochlorhydria. Clin Gastroenterol 1974; 3:595–608.

122. Gardner JD. Plasma VIP in patients with watery diarrhea syndrome. Am J Dig Dis 1978; 23:370–373.

123. Brazeau P, Vale W, Burgus R, et al. Hypothalamic polypeptide that inhibits the secretion of immunoreactive pituitary growth hormone. Science 1973; 179:77–79.

124. Yamada Y, Ito S, Matsubara Y. Immunohistochemical demonstration of somatostatin-containing cells in the human, dog and rat thyroids. Tohoku J Exp Med 1977; 122:87–92.

125. Sundler F, Alumets J, Hokanson R, et al. Somatostatin immunoreactive cells in medullary carcinoma of thyroid. Am J Pathol 1977; 88:381–386.

126. Reichlin S. Somatostatin, part I. N Engl J Med 1983; 309:1495–1501.

127. Gunther KJ, Orci L, Conlon JM, et al. Somatostatinoma syndrome. Biochemical, morphologic and clinical features. N Engl J Med 1979; 285:285–292.

128. Friesen SR. Tumors of the endocrine pancreas. N Engl J Med 1982; 306:580–590.

129. Pipeleers D, Coutourier E, Gepts W, Reynders J, Somers G. Five cases of somatostatinoma: clinical heterogeneity and diagnostic usefulness of basal and tolbutamide-induced hypersomatostatinoma. J Clin Endocrinol Metab 1983; 56:1236–1242.

130. Boyce EL, Guenter KJ. The inhibitory syndrome: somatostatinoma. In: Friesen FR, Thompson TW, eds. Surgical Endocrinology, 2nd ed. Philadelphia: JB Lippincott, 1990:249–266.

131. Ganda OP, Weir GC, Soeldner S, et al. Somatostatinoma: a somatostatin-containing tumor of the endocrine pancreas. N Engl J Med 1977; 296:963–967.

31

Nontraditional Inheritance of Endocrine Disorders

Judith G. Hall

University of British Columbia and British Columbia Children's Hospital, Vancouver, British Columbia, Canada

I. INTRODUCTION

Over the last few years many new developments in the area of molecular genetics have uncovered alternative genetic mechanisms leading to human genetic disorders and disease.

Disorders that were previously thought to have a straightforward mendelian inheritance are now being recognized as involving nontraditional forms of inheritance, such as uniparental disomy, mosaicism, cytoplasmic elements, unstable DNA, and genomic imprinting. With the complete analyses of the human genome, many additional mechanisms of disease are likely to be defined. These newly recognized nontraditional forms of inheritance and their importance in endocrine disorders are reviewed in this chapter.

II. UNIPARENTAL DISOMY

Chromosomes are inherited in pairs. Humans usually have 23 chromosome pairs. The usual normal chromosome pair consists of one chromosome contributed from the father and one from the mother. Occasionally, however, both chromosomes of a particular pair come from only one of the parents. This is called uniparental disomy (1), from uni meaning one; parental and disomy meaning normal number of normal paired chromosomes.

Uniparental disomy (UPD) has now been described with many different human chromosomes. Patients with UPD who have been described so far are usually sporadic, but can be expected to be seen rarely in families with translocations. Three types of problems occur with UPD: genomic imprinting is uncovered, autosomal recessive disorders are produced, and vestigial aneuploidy can be seen.

A. Genomic Imprinting

Uniparental disomy may be associated with abnormalities of growth and behavior, placental abnormalities, and in-

trauterine death. This seems to be related to genomic imprinting (see below).

The classic examples of genomic imprinting being uncovered in UPD involve Prader-Willi syndrome (PWS) (2–4) and Angelman syndrome (AS) (5,6). Prader-Willi syndrome is a disorder that may be present to the endocrinologist. Affected individuals have a round face, obesity, mental retardation, and hypogonadism. In the newborn period, they are usually markedly hypotonic. PWS is associated with an absence of the paternal contribution of chromosome 15 because of a deletion or due to maternal UPD for chromosome 15. Angelman syndrome, on the other hand, presents with a very long face, mental retardation, uncontrolled bouts of laughter, and seizures, and is associated with an absence of the maternal contribution of chromosome 15 because of a deletion or due to paternal UPD for chromosome 15.

Maternal UPD for chromosome 7 is associated with intrauterine and postbirth growth retardation (7–10). These individuals present as or in a similar manner to those with Russell–Silver syndrome. It has been estimated that 10% of Russell Silver syndrome patients have maternal UPD 7 as the cause of their growth deficiency.

Paternal UPD of chromosome 6 is associated with transient neonatal diabetes (11). Although it is not seen in all cases of transient neonatal diabetes, it should be screened for since the natural history may be different from non-UPD cases.

B. Autosomal Recessives

Uniparental disomy, as mentioned, occurs when the two chromosomes in a pair have been inherited from only one parent (1). UPD may be uniparental *isodisomy*, in which the two homologs originate from the same parental chromosome and are identical; or uniparental *heterodisomy*, in which the two chromosomes originate from the two different parental chromosomes and are not identical. When two copies of exactly the same chromosome are inherited from one parent, an abnormal gene may be present, and thereby both copies of the gene are abnormal. This may lead to an autosomal recessive disease. This is a very unusual situation for an autosomal recessive disease because only one parent is a carrier. A long list of autosomal recessive disorders associated with UPD is accumulating (12) (see Table 1). UPD should also be considered whenever a patient has two autosomal recessively inherited disorders.

C. Vestigial Aneuploidy

UPD is likely to arise from trisomy rescue (14). Most trisomies are embryonic or fetal lethal conditions. The only way such a conception is likely to survive is if a so-called normal diploid cell line develops by the loss of one of the trisomy chromosomes. When that happens, one-third of the time UPD will occur. Such a conception may harbor some trisomic cells in some tissues, which can lead to malfunction, cancer, or anomalies. Thus individuals with UPD must be viewed with concern.

UPD for many other chromosomes has not been associated with an abnormal phenotype (14). Several reports have shown that UPD for other chromosomes, for example chromosome 9 (15) and chromosome 1 (16) has no phenotypic abnormalities. The UPDs of concern seem to be maternal 7, 14, 15, 16, and paternal 6, 11, 15.

In summary, it is important to keep in mind that UPD for certain chromosomes or chromosome regions must be considered a possible mechanism producing disease, particularly related to disorders of growth, many different autosomal disorders (particularly the associations of two recessive disorders), and/or patches of chromosomally abnormal tissue.

III. MOSAICISM

Mosaicism describes an individual who has two different cell lines derived from a single zygote. Studies of placental tissues from chorionic villus sampling have shown that at least 2% of all conceptions are mosaic for chromosomal anomalies at or before 10 weeks of pregnancy (13). This suggests that mosaicism may be quite frequent in humans. Among early abortuses, 50% have a chromosomal anomaly, the most common being trisomy and triploidy. Complete trisomies are usually nonviable, and in most cases are aborted. However, the development of a normal cell line may rescue or allow a trisomic conception to come to term and be viable. In trisomies 13 and 18, Kalousek (17) has shown that all pregnancies that survive to birth have some normal cells in the placenta.

Depending upon the point at which the new cell line arises during early embryogenesis, a patient may have a variety of clinical presentations. In some situations, the trisomic cell line may be lost or overgrown. Mosaicism

Table 1 Uniparental Isodisomy and Recessive Disorders

Chromosome	Transmission	Recessive Disorders
1	Maternal	Epidermolysis bullosa
	Paternal	Pyknodysostosis
5	Paternal	Spinal muscular atrophy
6	Paternal	Complement deficiency
	Paternal	Methylmalonic acidemia
	Maternal	Congenital adrenal hyperplasia
7	Maternal	Cystic fibrosis
	Maternal	Osteogenesis imperfecta
	Paternal	Situs inversus and immotile cilia
	Paternal	Congenital chloride diarrhea
8	Paternal	Lipoprotein lipase deficiency
9	Maternal	Cartilage hair hypoplasia
10	Paternal	Multiple endocrine neoplasia
11	Maternal	Beta thalassemia
13	Paternal	Retinoblastoma
14	Maternal	Rod monochromacy
15	Maternal	Bloom syndrome
16	Paternal	Alpha thalassemia
	Maternal	Familial Mediterranean fever
X	Paternal	Hemophilia transmitted from father to son
	Maternal	Duchenne muscular dystrophy in a female
	Maternal	Androgen insensitivity

Source: Ref. 12.

may be present in some tissues, but not in others. Mosaicism may lead to patchy or asymmetrical distribution for abnormal tissue. There are many conditions that are asymmetrical or patchy (such as Ollier syndrome, multiple exostosis, and McCune-Albright syndrome) that are best explained on the basis of mosaicism.

McCune-Albright is a sporadic disorder characterized by polyostotic fibrous dysplasia, café-au-lait pigmentation, sexual precocity, and hyperfunction of multiple endocrine glands (Chap. 9). Because MAS is usually sporadic and has a characteristic lateralized pattern of cutaneous hyperpigmentation, it has been thought for some time to be likely caused by a somatic mutation occurring early in development, with some cells affected but others not affected. The occurrence and severity of the disease in bone, skin, and endocrine abnormalities in a patient depend on the number of cells carrying the mutated gene in the specific tissue.

MAS has been shown to result from a specific mutation in the alpha subunit of the G_s protein of adenyl cyclase (18,19). This type of mutation leads to constitutive activation of the G_s protein, inducing proliferation and hyperfunction of cells' responsiveness to hormones. The mutation is not the same in all patients, and different patients have different specific mutations and different distributions of tissue involvement. However the mutation is always consistent within an affected individual. It would be a lethal mutation if there were not normal cells present in some tissues. Many other patchy disorders are being found to represent somatic mutations, or so-called second hits to the normal allele leaving no normal gene. This obviously occurs in cancer, but is also seen in patchy disorders.

IV. GERMLINE MOSAICISM

Germline mosaicism refers to mosaicism of the germ cells (eggs and sperm), and occurs when some germ cells are normal and others carry a genetic abnormality, such as a mutation or differences in chromosome number. Because this situation may be exclusive to the germ cells, it does not become apparent until a couple has children (20). In this type of situation, parents can have two or more children with the same new dominant mutation, but the parents appear to be and test as normal. Germline and somatic mosaicism have been documented on a bichemical and DNA level in some cases of osteogenesis imperfecta (21) and pseudoachondroplasia.

V. GENOMIC IMPRINTING

Genomic imprinting refers to the differences in the phenotype of a disorder depending on the parent from whom it is inherited (22–24). Much of the information on imprinting comes from studies done in mice (25) but, more

recently, several specific clinical disorders have been defined in humans.

One of the first indications that male and female genetic contributions were different came from pronuclear transplantation experiments. Pronuclear transplantation allows the pronuclei of the oocyte and the sperm to be manipulated before fertilization. This technique was used in mice to produce zygotes that have two female pronuclei (gynogenetic) or two male (androgenetic) pronuclei. These studies showed that the zygote with two maternal contributions developed embryos, but the embryos were very small. However, when two paternal contributions were present, a placenta developed but no embryo did. These studies clearly showed that both maternal and paternal genetic contributions are different, complementary, and necessary (26,27).

Mouse and human chromosomes have homologous regions. This has prompted the suggestion that several genes known to be imprinted in mice may also be imprinted in homologous chromosomal regions in humans. Several genes known to be imprinted in mice have been associated with disorders of growth in humans (Table 2) (26–28).

Insulin-like growth factor type II and the H19 genes, for example, are located in the mouse chromosome 7 (29). In humans these genes map to 11p15, which is the area associated with Beckwith-Wiedemann syndrome (30–32), a fetal overgrowth disorder characterized by a predisposition to tumors and hyperinsulinism (Chap. 5).

Because disorders that are imprinted in humans show a difference in the phenotype depending on the parent transmitting the gene, endocrine and other disorders

Table 2 Endocrine Disorders at Risk to Be Imprinted

Chromosome	Endocrine Disorder
6	Insulin-dependent diabetes
	H-Y antigen
	Prolactin
	21-OH
	Paget's disease of bone
	Estrogen receptor
	MEN I
11	Hypoparathyroidism
	Adrenocortical cancer
	MODY
19	Insulin receptor
	Infertility (LH)
	Chorionic gonadotrophic cluster
20	Diabetes insipidus
	Albright hereditary osteodystrophy
	Growth hormone releasing factor
22	Thyroid-stimulating hormone
	MEN II

MEN, multiple endocrine neoplasia; LH, luteinizing hormone.

should be suspected to be imprinted if varying phenotypes are seen in a pedigree (Figs. 1 and 2) depending on the transmitting parent. Two disorders suspected of being imprinted on the basis of varying phenotype in the pedigrees are Albright's hereditary osteodystrophy and paragangliomas.

Albright's hereditary osteodystrophy (AHO), also known as pseudopseudohypoparathyroidism, is characterized by short stature, mental retardation, round face, obesity, brachydactyly, and subcutaneous calcifications in the presence of hypocalcemia and parathyroid hormone resistance.

A review of reported cases of AHO showed that there is a marked difference in the phenotype of AHO depending on the parent transmitting the disorder. Davies and Hughes (33) collected data on 36 AHO-transmitting parents. They found that in 92% of the affected cases the allele was inherited from the mother, and the phenotype was fully expressed (AHO + hormone resistance + pseudohypoparathyroidism). The remaining 8% were paternally inherited, and the phenotype was only partially expressed (AHO alone).

Subsequently, mutations of the G_s protein have been observed in patients with AHO, but in contrast to MAS patients these mutations cause deficient expression of the various alternatively spliced isoforms of the G_s protein (34). The gene for G_s protein, which has been isolated on 20q13.11, shows alternative splicing. Several of the isotypes are imprinted.

VI. CYTOPLASMIC INHERITANCE

It is well known that mitochondria (and consequently mitochondrial-associated diseases) are maternally inherited. Some of these mitochondrial mutations lead to endocrine disorders such as Pearson syndrome. However, other cytoplasmic structures, such as the cell wall, nuclear membrane, and endoplasmic reticulum, receive their template for protein folding from the oocyte. Thus, there are likely

PATERNAL

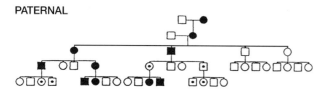

Figure 1 Pedigree suggestive of paternal imprinting. Phenotypic effects occur only when the gene is transmitted from the mother but not when transmitted from the father. An equal number of males or females are affected or unaffected phenotypically in each generation. A nonmanifesting transmitter gives a clue to the gender of the parent who passes the expressed genetic information; in other words, in paternal imprinting there are "skipped" male nonmanifesting individuals.

MATERNAL

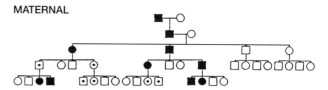

Figure 2 In pedigrees suggestive of maternal imprinting, phenotypic effects occur only when the gene is transmitted from the father, but not when transmitted from the mother. Equal numbers of males or females are affected or unaffected phenotypically in each generation. A nonmanifesting transmitter gives a clue to the gender of the parent who passes the expressed genetic information; in other words, in paternal imprinting there are "skipped" female nonmanifesting individuals.

to be a variety of other diseases that will be influenced by maternal factors.

VII. SUMMARY

It is clear that nontraditional mechanisms of inheritance may be playing a major role in a number of endocrine disorders, and it is important to look for parent of origin effects in all disorders. This will allow better understanding of some of the genetic mechanisms causing disease, which could lead to better diagnosis, therapy, and counseling of patients and their families.

ACKNOWLEDGMENT

The author acknowledges the input of Elena Lopez-Rangel.

REFERENCES

1. Engel E, Delozier-Blanchet D. Uniparental disomy, isodisomy and imprinting: probable effects in man and strategies for their detection. Am J Hum Genet 1991; 40:432–439.
2. Lee S, Wevrick R. Identification of novel imprinted transcripts in the Prader-Willi syndrome and Angelman syndrome deletion region: further evidence for regional imprinting control. Am J Hum Genet 2000; 66:848–858.
3. Boccaccio I, Glatt-Deeley H, Watrin F, Roeckel N, Lalande M, Muscatelli F. The human MAGEL2 gene and its mouse homologue are paternally expressed and mapped to the Prader-Willi region. Hum Mol Genet 1999; 8:2497–2505.
4. Nicholls RD, Saitoh S, Horsthemke B. Imprinting in Prader-Willi and Angelman syndromes. Trends Genet 1998; 14:194–200.
5. Jiang Y-H, Lev-Lehman E, Bressler J, Tsai T-F, Beaudet AL. Neurogenetics '99: genetics of Angelman syndrome. Am J Hum Genet 1999; 65:1–6.
6. Moncla A, Malzac P, Voelckel M-A, Auquier P, Girardot L, Mattei M-G, Philip N, Mattei J-F, Lalande M, Livet M-O. Phenotype-genotype correlation in 20 deletion and

20 non-deletion Angelman syndrome patients. Eur J Hum Genet 1999; 7:131–139.

7. Price SM, Stanhope R, Garrett C, Preece MA, Trembath RC. The spectrum of Silver-Russell syndrome: a clinical and molecular genetic study and new diagnostic criteria. J Med Genet 1999; 36:837–842.

8. Bernard LE, Penaherrera MS, Van Allen MI, Wang MS, Yong S-L, Gareis F, Langlois S, Robinson WP. Clinical and molecular findings in two patients with Russell-Silver syndrome and UPD7: comparison with non-UPD7 cases. Am J Med Genet 1999; 87:230–236.

9. Blagitko N, Schultz U, Schinzel AA, Ropers H-H, Kalscheuer, VM. y2-COP, a novel imprinted gene on chromosome 7q32, defines a new imprinting cluster in the human genome. Hum Mol Genet 1999; 8:2387–2396.

10. Kosaki K, Kosaki R, Craigen WJ, Matsuo N. Isoform-specific imprinting of the human PEG1/MEST Gene. Am J Hum Genet 2000; 66:309–312.

11. Marquis E, Robert JJ, Benezech C, Junien C, Diatloff-Zito C. Variable features of transient neonatal diabetes mellitus with paternal isodisomy of chromosome 6. Eur J Hum Genet 2000; 8:137–140.

12. Hall JG. Human diseases and genomic imprinting. In: Ohlsson R, ed. Genomic imprinting: an interdisciplinary approach. Berlin/Heidelberg/New York: Springer-Verlag, 1999:119–132.

13. Genuardi M, Tozzi C, Grazia Pomponi M, Letizia Stagni M, Della Monica M, Scarano G, Calvieri F, Torrisi L, Neri G. Mosaic trisomy 17 in amniocytes: phenotypic outcome, tissue distribution, and uniparental disomy studies. Eur J Hum Genet 1999; 7:421–426.

14. Kotzot D. Abnormal phenotypes in uniparental disomy (UPD): fundamental aspects and a critical review with bibliography of UPD other than 15. Am J Med Genet 1999; 82:265–274.

15. Bjorck EJ, Anderlid B-M, Blennow E. (1999). Maternal isodisomy of chromosome 9 with no impact on the phenotype in a woman with two isochromosomes: i(9p) and i(9q). Am J Med Genet 1999; 87:49–52.

16. Leigh Field L, Tobias R, Robinson WP, Paisey R, Bain S. Maternal uniparental disomy of chromosome 1 with no apparent phenotypic effects. Am J Hum Genet 1998; 63:1216–1220.

17. Kalousek DK. The role of confined placental mosaicism in placental function and human development. GGH 1988; 4:1–3.

18. Weinstein LE, Shenker A, Gejman P, Merino MJ, Friedman E, Spiegel AM. Activating mutation of the stimulatory G protein in the McCune-Albright syndrome. N Engl J Med 1991; 325:1688–1695.

19. Schuwindinger WF, Francomano CA, Levine ME. Identification of a mutation in the gene encoding the alpha subunit of the stimulatory G protein of adenylyl cyclase in McCune-Albright syndrome. Proc Natl Acad Sci USA 1992; 89:5152–5156.

20. Cohn DH, Starman BJ, Blumberg B, Byers PH. Recurrence of lethal osteogenesis imperfecta due to parental mosaicism for a dominant mutation in a human type I collagen gene (COL1A1). Am J Hum Genet 1990; 46:591–601.

21. Wallis GA, Starman BJ, Zinn AB, Byers PH. Variable expression of osteogenesis imperfecta in a nuclear family is explained by somatic mosaicism for a lethal point mutation in the alpha 1 (I) gene (COL1A1) of type I collagen in a parent. Am J Hum Genet 1990; 46:1034–1040.

22. Ohlsson R. Genomic imprinting: an interdisciplinary approach. Berlin/Heidelberg/New York: Springer-Verlag, 1999.

23. Ohlsson R, Hall K, Ritzen M. Genomic Imprinting: Causes and Consequences 1995. Cambridge: Cambridge University Press.

24. Trends Genet (Special Epigenetics Issue) 1997; 13:293–341.

25. Cattanach BM, Kirk M. Differential activity of maternally and paternally derived chromosome regions in mice. Nature 1989; 315:496–498.

26. Solter D. Differential imprinting and expression of maternal and paternal genomes. Annu Rev Genet 1988; 22:127–226.

27. Surani MA, Reik W, Allen ND. Transgenes as molecular probes for genomic imprinting. Trends Genet 1988; 4:59–62.

28. Surani MA, Kothary R, Allen ND, et al. Genome imprinting and development in the mouse. Development 1990; 108:203–211.

29. Ekstrand J, Ehrenborg E, Sten I, Stellan B, Zech L, Luthman H. The gene for insulin-like growth factor-binding protein is localized to human chromosome region 7p14-p12. Genomics 1990; 6:413–418.

30. Li M, Squire JA, Weksberg R. Molecular genetics of Wiedemann-Beckwith syndrome. Am J Med Genet 1998; 79:253–259.

31. Lee MP, Hu R-J, Johnson LA, Feinberg AP. Human KVLQT1 gene shows tissue-specific imprinting and encompasses Beckwith-Wiedemann syndrome chromosomal rearrangements. Nat Genet 1997; 15:181–185.

32. Moore ES, Ward RE, Escobar LF, Carlin ME. Heterogeneity in Wiedemann-Beckwith syndrome: anthropometric evidence. Am J Med Genet 2000; 90:283–290.

33. Davies SJ, Hughes HE. Imprinting in Albright's hereditary osteodystrophy. J Med Genet 1992; 30:101–103.

34. Hayward BE, Moran V, Strain L, Bonthron DT. Bidirectional imprinting of a single gene: GNAS1 encodes maternally, paternally, and biallelically derived proteins. Proc Natl Acad Sci 1998; 95:15475–15480.

32

Disorders of Water Homeostasis

Joseph A. Majzoub

Children's Hospital and Harvard Medical School, Boston, Massachusetts, U.S.A.

Louis J. Muglia

St. Louis Children's Hospital and Washington University School of Medicine,
St. Louis, Missouri, U.S.A.

I. INTRODUCTION

Maintenance of the tonicity of extracellular fluids within a very narrow range is crucial for proper cell function (1, 2). Extracellular osmolality regulates cell shape, as well as intracellular concentrations of ions and other osmolytes. Furthermore, proper extracellular ionic concentrations are necessary for the correct function of ion channels, action potentials, and other modes of intercellular communication. Extracellular fluid tonicity is regulated almost exclusively by the amount of water intake and excretion, whereas extracellular volume is regulated by the level of sodium chloride intake and excretion. In children and adults, normal blood tonicity is maintained over a 10-fold variation in water intake by a coordinated interaction among the thirst, vasopressin, and renal systems. Dysfunction in any of these systems can result in abnormal regulation of blood osmolality, which, if not properly recognized and treated, may cause life-threatening dysfunction in neuronal and other cellular activities.

The posterior pituitary, or neurohypophysis, secretes the nonapeptide hormone vasopressin, which controls water homeostasis by its interaction with the renal V2 vasopressin receptor. This receptor regulates the activity of the water channel, aquaporin-2, in the distal nephron, which controls the reabsorption of water from the urine. Disorders of vasopressin secretion and its action in the kidney lead to clinically important derangements in water metabolism.

II. REGULATION OF THIRST AND FLUID BALANCE

A. Osmotic Sensor and Effector Pathways

1. Vasopressin and Oxytocin Biochemistry

The sequence and synthesis of biologically active 9-amino-acid-long vasopressin peptide was performed by du Vigneaud and colleagues during the mid 1950s (3). Vasopressin was found to be closely related to oxytocin, differing by only two amino acids. By replacement of L-arginine with D-arginine at position 8 of the vasopressin molecule, and amino-terminal deamidation, an analog with enhanced, prolonged antidiuretic to pressor activity ratio was found (desamino-D-arginine vasopressin [d-DAVP]) (4). dDAVP is now routinely used in clinical practice.

Vasopressin is initially synthesized as part of a larger precursor protein that also contains neurophysin. After biosynthesis, vasopressin and neurophysin are cleaved, but remain associated within the cell prior to their secretion into the bloodstream. The function of neurophysin is not clear, but may include stabilization of vasopressin against degradation during intracellular storage, and its more efficient packaging of posttranslational processing by the proenzyme convertases within secretory granules.

In all mammalian species thus far analyzed the oxytocin and vasopressin genes are adjacent in chromosomal location [chromosome 20 in the human (5)] and linked tail to tail, in opposite transcriptional orientation. In the human, they are separated by 12 kilobases (5). This likely explains their origin from the ancient duplication of a common ancestral gene (6). Whether this adjacent linkage is of regulatory significance is under investigation.

Expression of the vasopressin and oxytocin genes occurs in the hypothalamic, paraventricular, and supraoptic nuclei (7, 8). The magnocellular components of each of these nuclei are the primary neuronal populations involved in water balance, with vasopressin synthesized in these areas carried via axonal transport to the posterior pituitary, its primary site of storage and release into the systemic circulation. The bilaterally paired hypothalamic paraventricular and supraoptic nuclei are separated from each other by relatively large distances (approximately 1 cm). Their axons course caudally, converge at the infundibulum, and terminate at different levels within the pituitary stalk and posterior pituitary gland. Vasopressin is also synthesized in the parvocellular neurons of the paraventricular nucleus, where it has a role in modulation of hypothalamic–pituitary–adrenal axis activity. In this site, vasopressin is colocalized in cells that synthesize corticotropin-releasing hormone (9, 10), which are both secreted at the median eminence and carried via the portal–hypophyseal capillary system to the anterior pituitary, where together they act as the major regulators of adrenocorticotropin synthesis and release (11). Vasopressin is also present in the hypothalamic suprachiasmatic nucleus, the circadian pacemaker of the body, where its function is unknown.

2. Regulation of Vasopressin Secretion and Thirst

a. Osmotic Regulation. The rate of secretion of vasopressin from the paraventricular and supraoptic nuclei is influenced by several physiological variables, including plasma osmolality and intravascular volume, as well as nausea and a number of pharmacological agents. The major osmotically active constituents of blood are sodium, chloride, and glucose (with insulin deficiency). Normal blood osmolality ranges between 280 and 290 mOsm/kg H_2O.

The work of Verney (12) first demonstrated the relationship of increased vasopressin release in response to increasing plasma osmolality, as altered by infusion of sodium chloride or sucrose. At that time, it was postulated that intracranial sensors are sensitive to changes in plasma osmolality. Multiple researchers have subsequently confirmed that plasma vasopressin concentration rises in response to increasing plasma tonicity, although the exact nature of the osmosensor had not been defined (13, 14). Neurons of the supraoptic nucleus can respond directly to hypertonic stimuli with depolarization and vasopressin secretion (15), but the majority of evidence indicates that osmosensor and vasopressin-secreting neurons are anatomically distinct (16, 17). The osmosensor is likely to reside outside the blood–brain barrier as implicated by

differential vasopressin secretory response to similar changes in plasma osmolality, depending upon whether the change was induced by salt, sucrose, or urea (12, 18). The organ vasculosum of the lamina terminalis (OVLT) and the subfornical organ (SFO), areas of the preoptic hypothalamus outside the blood–brain barrier, are likely sites of osmosensing because lesions of the OVLT result in impaired AVP secretion and hypernatremia (16, 17). Also, the site of action of angiotensin II infused intracerebrally or peripherally to produce vasopressin secretion and antidiuresis resides within the OVLT (19–21).

The pattern of secretion of vasopressin into blood has been characterized extensively in normal individuals and those with abnormalities in water homeostasis. Normally, at a serum osmolality of less than 280 mOsm/kg, plasma vasopressin concentration is at or below 1 pg/ml, which is the lower limit of detection of most radioimmunoassays (13, 14). Above 283 mOsm/kg, the normal threshold for vasopressin release, plasma vasopressin concentration rises in proportion to plasma osmolality, up to a maximum concentration of about 20 pg/ml at a blood osmolality of approximately 320 mOsm/kg (Fig. 1). The osmosensor

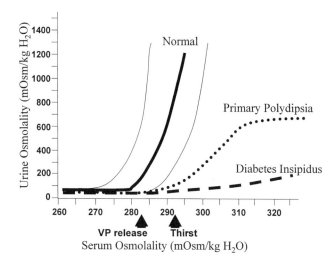

Figure 1 Relationship between serum and urine osmolalities during a water deprivation test. With water deprivation, serum osmolality rises above the threshold for vasopressin secretion, causing antidiuresis and concentration of the urine. In normal persons, when serum osmolality exceeds 300 mOsm/kg H_2O, urine osmolality exceeds 600 mOsm/kg H_2O (solid thick and thin lines, mean and 95% confidence intervals for normal children). In patients with diabetes insipidus (dashed line), urine osmolality does not exceed 200–300 mOsm/kg H_2O, even with marked serum hyperosmolality. In patients with primary polydipsia (dotted line), urine osmolality may not exceed 600 mOsm/kg H_2O, due to partial nephrogenic diabetes insipidus caused by dilution of the osmotic gradient in the renal interstitium (see text). Solid arrowheads denote the thresholds for vasopressin (VP) release and thirst sensation.

can detect as little as a 1% change in blood osmolality. Plasma concentrations in excess of 5 pg/ml are also found with nausea, hypotension, hypovolemia, and insulin-induced hypoglycemia, but further increments in urine concentration do not occur since peak antidiuretic effect is achieved at 5 pg/ml. The rate of rise of plasma vasopressin concentration, and thus the sensitivity of the osmosensor, exhibits substantial (as much as 10-fold) interindividual variation as plasma osmolality increases (22). The set point for vasopressin secretion varies in a single individual in relation to changes in volume status and hormonal environment [e.g., pregnancy (23) or glucocorticoid status (24, 25)]. After the seventh week of gestation, osmotic thresholds for both vasopressin release and thirst are reduced by approximately 10 mOsm/kg, such that normal blood osmolality during pregnancy is approximately 273 mOsm/kg (serum sodium 135 mEq/L) (23, 26).

The sensation of thirst, a more integrated cortical activity, is determined by other anatomically distinct hypothalamic neurons, with afferents involving the ventromedial nucleus (27). The activation of the thirst mechanism is also probably mediated by angiotensin II (28). Whether the osmosensor for thirst and vasopressin release is the same is not certain, although this is suggested by lesions in the anteroventral region of the third ventricle that abolish both thirst sensation and vasopressin release (29). It makes physiological sense that the threshold for thirst (~293 mOsm/kg) is approximately 10 mOsm/kg higher than that for vasopressin release (Fig. 1). Otherwise, during the development of hyperosmolality, the initial activation of thirst and water ingestion would result in polyuria without activation of vasopressin release, causing a persistent diuretic state. Immediately following water ingestion, prior to a change in blood osmolality or volume, vasopressin concentration falls and thirst ceases (30). The degree of suppression is directly related to the coldness (31) and volume (32) of the ingested fluid. This effect is probably mediated by chemoreceptors present in the oropharynx, which guard against the rapid overdrinking of fluids after intense thirst during the time before the lowering of blood osmolality.

As noted above, water balance is regulated in two ways: vasopressin secretion stimulates water reabsorption by the kidney, thereby reducing future water loss; and thirst stimulates water ingestion, thereby restoring previous water loss. Ideally, these two systems work in parallel to regulate extracellular fluid tonicity efficiently (Fig. 2). However, each system by itself can maintain plasma osmolality in the near-normal range. For example, in the absence of vasopressin secretion but with free access to water, thirst drives water ingestion up to the 5–10 l/m² urine output seen with vasopressin deficiency. Conversely, an intact vasopressin secretory system can compensate for some degree of disordered thirst regulation. However, when both vasopressin secretion and thirst are compromised, either by disease or iatrogenic means, there is great

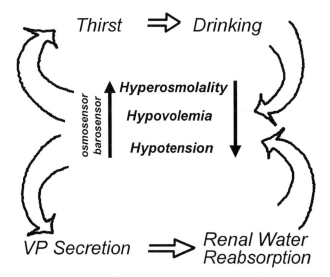

Figure 2 Regulation of vasopressin secretion and serum osmolality. Hyperosmolality, hypovolemia, or hypotension is sensed by osmosensors, volume sensors, or barosensors, respectively. These stimulate both vasopressin (VP) secretion as well as thirst. Vasopressin, acting on the kidney, causes increased reabsorption of water (antidiuresis). Thirst causes increased water ingestion. The results of these dual negative feedback loops cause a reduction in hyperosmolality or hypotension/hypovolemia. (From Muglia L, Majzoub J. Disorders of the posterior pituitary. In: Sperling M, ed. Pediatric Endocrinology, 2d ed. Philadelphia: Saunders, 2002:289–322.)

risk for the occurrence of life-threatening abnormalities in plasma osmolality.

b. Nonosmotic Regulation. Separate from osmotic regulation, vasopressin has been shown to be secreted in response to alterations in intravascular volume. Afferent baroreceptor pathways arising from the right and left atria, and the aortic arch (carotid sinus) are stimulated by increasing intravascular volume and stretch of vessel walls, and they send signals via the vagus and glossopharyngeal nerves, respectively, to the brainstem nucleus tractus solitarius (33, 34). Nonadrenergic fibers from the nucleus tractus solitarius synapse upon the hypothalamic paraventricular nucleus and supraoptic nucleus and, on stimulation, inhibit vasopressin secretion (35, 36). Experimental verification of this pathway has included demonstration of increased vasopressin concentration following interruption of baroreceptor output to the brainstem, and decreased plasma vasopressin concentration following mechanical stimulation of baroreceptors, an effect that is diminished by vagotomy (37, 38).

The pattern of vasopressin secretion in response to volume as opposed to osmotic stimuli is markedly different (Fig. 3). Although minor changes in plasma osmolality above 280 mOsm/kg evoke linear increases in plasma va-

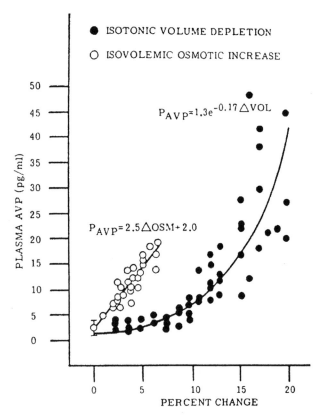

Figure 3 Relationships between osmotic and nonosmotic stimuli for vasopressin release. Reaction of plasma vasopressin (AVP) concentration to the percentage increase in blood osmolality (open circles) or decrease in blood volume (closed circles). (Reproduced with permission from Dunn FL, Brennan TJ, Nelson AE, et al. The role of blood osmolality and volume regulating vasopressin secretion in the rat. J Clin Invest 1973; 52:3212.

sopressin, substantial alteration in intravascular volume is required for alteration in vasopressin output (39–41). No change in vasopressin secretion is seen until blood volume decreases by approximately 8%. With intravascular volume deficits exceeding 8%, vasopressin concentration rises exponentially. Furthermore, osmotic and hemodynamic stimuli can interact in a mutually synergistic fashion, so that the response to either stimulus may be enhanced by the concomitant presence of the other. When blood volume [or blood pressure (42–44)] decreases by approximately 25%, vasopressin concentrations 20–30-fold above normal and vastly exceeding those required for maximal antidiuresis are evident. It is surprising that the use of vasopressin antagonists has suggested that the high concentration of vasopressin observed with hypotension does not contribute to the maintenance of blood pressure in humans (45).

Nausea, as evoked by apomorphine (46), motion sickness (47), and vasovagal reactions, is a very potent stim-

ulus for vasopressin secretion. This effect is likely mediated by afferents from the area postrema of the brainstem, and may result in vasopressin concentrations two to three orders of magnitude above basal levels. Nicotine is also a strong stimulus for vasopressin release (48). These pathways probably do not involve osmotic or hemodynamic sensor systems, since blockade of the emetic stimulus with dopamine or opioid antagonists does not alter the vasopressin response to hypernatremia or hypovolemia.

Vasopressin secretion is inhibited by glucocorticoids; because of this, the loss of negative regulation of vasopressin secretion occurs in the setting of primary or secondary glucocorticoid insufficiency (49, 50). The effects of cortisol loss both enhancing hypothalamic vasopressin production and directly impairing free water excretion (51) are important considerations in the evaluation of the patient with hyponatremia, as is subsequently discussed.

3. Vasopressin Metabolism

Once in the circulation, vasopressin has a half-life of only 5–10 min, due to its rapid degradation by a cysteine amino terminal peptidase, called vasopressinase. A synthetic analog of vasopressin, dDAVP (desmopressin), is insensitive to amino terminal degradation, and thus has a much longer half-life: 8–24 h. During pregnancy, the placenta secretes increased amounts of this vasopressinase (52), resulting in a fourfold increase in the metabolic clearance rate of vasopressin (53). Normal women compensate with an increase in vasopressin secretion, but women with pre-existing deficits in vasopressin secretion or action (54), or those with increased concentrations of placental vasopressinase associated with liver dysfunction (55) or multiple gestations (56), may develop diabetes insipidus in the last trimester, which resolves in the immediate postpartum period (57). As expected, this form of diabetes insipidus responds to treatment with dDAVP but not with vasopressin (58, 59).

4. Sites of Vasopressin Action

a. Vasopressin Receptors. Vasopressin released from the posterior pituitary and median eminence affects the function of several tissue types by binding to members of a family of G protein-coupled cell surface receptors, which subsequently transduce ligand binding into alterations of intracellular second-messenger pathways (60). Biochemical and cell biological studies have defined at least three receptor types, designated V1, V2, and V3 (or V1b). The major sites of V1 receptor expression are on vascular smooth muscle (61) and hepatocytes (62–65), where receptor activation results in vasoconstriction (66, 67) and glycogenolysis (68), respectively. The latter activity may be augmented by stimulation of glucagon secretion from the pancreas (68). The V1 receptor on platelets also stimulates platelet aggregation (69). V1 receptor activation mobilizes intracellular calcium stores through phosphatidylinositol hydrolysis (66, 70). Despite its initial characterization as a powerful pressor agent, the concentration of vasopressin needed to increase blood pressure significantly is several times higher than that required for maximal antidiuresis (71), although substantial vasoconstriction in renal and splanchnic vasculature can occur at physiological concentrations (72). The recent cloning of the V1 receptor (61–63) has greatly elucidated the relationship of the vasopressin [and oxytocin (73, 74)] receptors and, through sensitive in situ hybridization analysis, has further localized V1 expression to the liver and vasculature of the renal medulla, as well as to many sites within the brain, including the hippocampus, amygdala, hypothalamus, and brainstem (64, 65). The V3 (or V1b) receptor is present on corticotrophs in the anterior pituitary (75), and acts through the phosphatidylinositol pathway (76) to increase ACTH secretion. Its binding profile for vasopressin analogs resembles more closely that of the V1 than the V2 receptor. The structure of this receptor has recently been determined in human via cloning of its complementary DNA (76, 77). Its structure is similar to that of the V1 and oxytocin receptors and is expressed in the kidney as well as in the pituitary.

Modulation of water balance occurs through the action of vasopressin upon V2 receptors located primarily in the renal collecting tubule, along with other sites in the kidney including the thick ascending limb of Henle's loop and periglomerular tubules (64, 65, 78). It is also present on vascular endothelial cells in some systemic vascular beds, where vasopressin stimulates vasodilation (79), possibly via activation of nitric oxide synthase (80). Vasopressin also stimulates von Willebrand's factor, factor VIIIa, and tissue plasminogen activator via V2-mediated actions. Because of this, dDAVP is used to improve the prolonged bleeding times characteristic of uremia, type I von Willebrand's disease, and hemophilia (81). The V2 receptor consists of 370 amino acids encoding seven transmembrane domains characteristic of the G protein-coupled receptors (78, 82). These transmembrane domains share approximately 60% sequence identity with the V1 receptor, but substantially less with other members of this family. Unlike the V1 and V3 receptors, the V2 receptor acts through adenylate cyclase to increase intracellular cAMP concentration. The human V2 receptor gene is located on the long arm of the X chromosome (Xq28) (83, 84), at the locus associated with congenital, X-linked vasopressin-resistant diabetes insipidus.

b. Renal Cascade of Vasopressin Function. Vasopressin-induced increases in intracellular cAMP as mediated by the V2 receptor trigger a complex pathway of events, resulting in increased permeability of the collecting duct to water and efficient water transit across an otherwise minimally permeable epithelium (85) (Fig. 4). Activation of a cAMP-dependent protein kinase imparts remodeling of cytoskeletal microtubules and microfilaments that culminate in the insertion of aggregates of water channels into the apical membrane (86). Insertion of

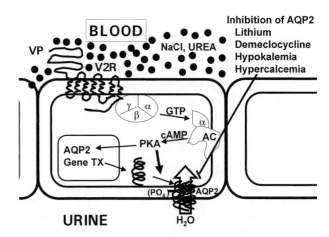

Figure 4 Action of vasopressin in the collecting duct cell. Vasopressin (AVP) binds to the V2 receptor (V2R), causing the binding of GTP to the stimulatory alpha G protein subunit (α). This activates adenylate cyclase (AC), resulting in an increase in cAMP and activation of protein kinase A (PKA). The catalytic subunit of PKA, via phosphorylation of serine 256 of the water channel, aquaporin-2 (AQP2), causes aggregation of AQP2 homotetramers in membrane vesicles and their fusion with the collecting duct luminal membrane, resulting in an increase in water flow from the urine into the renal medullary interstitium. Demeclocycline, lithium, high calcium, and low potassium interfere with these processes, possibly at the level of cAMP generation and AQP2 synthesis or action. (From Majzoub, J. Primary disturbances of water homeostasis. In: Rudolf CD et al., ed. Rudolf's Pediatrics, 21st ed. New York: McGraw-Hill, 2002:2025–2028.)

the water channels causes an up to 100-fold increase in water permeability of the apical membrane, allowing water movement along its osmotic gradient into the hypertonic inner medullary interstitium from the tubule lumen and excretion of a concentrated urine (Fig. 4). Molecular analysis of water channels has revealed a family of related proteins, designated aquaporins, which differ in their sites of expression and pattern of regulation (87). Each protein consists of a single polypeptide chain with six membrane-spanning domains. Although functional as monomers, they are believed to form homotetramers in the plasma membrane (85). Aquaporin-2 is expressed mostly within the kidney (88), primarily within the collecting duct (89). It is also expressed in the vas deferens, at least in the rat, although it is not regulated by vasopressin in this location (90). Studies with immunoelectron microscopy have demonstrated large amounts of aquaporin-2 in the apical plasma membrane and subapical vesicles of the collecting duct, consistent with the so-called membrane-shuttling model of water channel aggregate insertion into the apical membrane after vasopressin stimulation (91). In response to water restriction or dDAVP infusion in humans, the content of urinary aquaporin-2 in both soluble and membrane-bound forms has been found to increase (92). In addition to aquaporin-2, different aquaporins appear to be involved in other aspects of renal water handling. In contrast to the apical localization of aquaporin-2, aquaporins 3 and 4 are expressed on the basolateral membrane of the collecting duct epithelium. They appear to be involved in the flow of water and urea from the inside of the collecting duct cell into the extracellular renal medullary space.

B. Volume Sensor and Effector Pathways

1. Renin–Angiotensin–Aldosterone System

In contrast to the vasopressin system, the classic, or peripheral, renin–angiotensin system primarily affects maintenance of intravascular volume as opposed to plasma tonicity. In addition to the well-established endocrine regulatory system, several local renin–angiotensin systems have emerged, with both autocrine and paracrine effects in their tissue of synthesis, whose regulation is independent of the classic system. Finally, brain and pituitary angiotensin systems involved in blood pressure, autonomic function, and fluid balance have recently been characterized with extensive interaction with the vasopressin system.

a. Endocrine Anatomy and Biochemistry. Renin, which is synthesized by the renal juxtaglomerular apparatus, is a proteolytic enzyme that catalyzes the cleavage of angiotensinogen, synthesized by hepatocytes, into the decapeptide angiotensin (93, 94). Angiotensin I possesses no intrinsic vasoreactive or mineralocorticoid secretagogue activity, but is efficiently cleaved by angiotensin-converting enzyme in the lungs, as well as other peripheral sites, to generate the octapeptide angiotensin II. Angiotensin II is further metabolized to the heptapeptide angiotensin III by removal of one amino-terminal amino acid. Angiotensin II possesses greater vasopressor activity, and is present in approximately fourfold greater amount than angiotensin III. Angiotensins II and III possess equivalent mineralocorticoid secretory activity on the adrenal glomerulosa cells.

Aldosterone, which is the primary and most potent endogenous mineralocorticoid released by the zona glomerulosa, acts on target tissues expressing the nuclear mineralocorticoid (or type I glucocorticoid) receptor to promote sodium absorption and potassium excretion. For control of intravascular volume, the primary target of action of aldosterone is the distal nephron. Here, aldosterone increases synthesis of apical membrane sodium channels, mitochondrial enzymes involved in ATP production, and components of the Na^+-K^+ ATPase to cause increased sodium reabsorption and potassium excretion (95).

b. Regulation of Secretion. Decreased intravascular volume as sensed by the renal juxtaglomerular apparatus results in release of renin (93, 96). Increased plasma renin activity then allows increased conversion of angiotensinogen to angiotensin I, which in turn is converted peripherally to angiotensins II and III. Increased angiotensin II activity causes vasoconstriction and blood pressure elevation, whereas both angiotensins II and III stimulate aldosterone release from the zona glomerulosa and subsequent salt and water retention and potassium, excretion by the distal tubule of the kidney. Expanded intravascular volume, on the other hand, causes decreased renin output and less sodium and water resorption in the kidney, serving to decrease intravascular volume and restore homeostasis.

Changes in vascular volume are not the only regulators of the renin–angiotensin–aldosterone system. Serum potassium concentration directly modulates aldosterone release by the adrenal glomerulosa by its effects on plasma membrane potential and activation of voltage-gated calcium channels (94, 97). By membrane depolarization, increased serum potassium leads to increased aldosterone synthesis, which promotes renal potassium excretion, whereas low serum potassium reduces aldosterone synthesis and decreases urinary potassium losses. Pituitary adrenocorticotropin hormone and vasopressin act via their respective receptors on the glomerulosa cells to increase acute aldosterone secretion. These effects are of short duration because long-term chronic infusions do not chronically elevate aldosterone concentrations. Direct inhibitors of aldosterone secretion, and thus promoters of natriuresis, include atrial natriuretic peptide (98, 99), somatostatin (100–102), and dopamine (103, 104).

2. The Natriuretic Peptide System

In addition to the classic vasopressin and renin–angiotensin–aldosterone systems, the recently defined natriuretic peptide families of ligands and their receptors add further potential for modulation of salt and water balance. The interaction of the natriuretic peptide system occurs both in the central nervous system via effects on vasopressin secretion and peripherally, through its ability both to promote natriuresis directly in the kidney, and inhibit adrenal aldosterone production indirectly.

a. Anatomy and Biochemistry. Atrial natriuretic peptide (ANP) was initially discovered as a component of cardiac atrial muscle that was able to induce natriuresis, a decrease in blood pressure, and rise in hematocrit when injected into rats (105, 106).

The biologically active form of ANP consists of a 28 amino acid peptide that includes a 17 amino acid ring structure (107). The primary sequence of the peptide has been conserved among mammalian species, and in addition to synthesis in cardiac atrial tissue (108) it has been detected in brain, spinal cord, pituitary, and adrenal gland (109–112).

Subsequent investigation defined a second peptide from porcine brain with structural homology to ANP (113). This peptide, designated brain natriuretic peptide (BNP), was later found to be secreted by the heart as well, in this case from both ventricular and atrial tissue (114–116).

A third member of this family, C-type natriuretic peptide (CNP), was also isolated from porcine brain (117). Little CNP can be detected in plasma, and in marked contrast to ANP and BNP, CNP does not increase in plasma in the setting of cardiac failure (118, 119).

b. Regulation of Secretion and Action. Secretion of ANP by cardiac tissue occurs in response to increasing atrial transmural pressure, from both left and right atria (118, 120). Also, increased heart rate, especially increased atrial contractile frequency, results in increased ANP secretion. Ventricular production of ANP has also been demonstrated; it is increased in states of left sided overload associated with ventricular hypertrophy (116).

The physiological ramifications of increased ANP production are several. Infusion of ANP in the setting of normovolemia causes natriuresis, diuresis, and a small increase in divalent cation excretion (118, 119, 121). ANP, through the NPR-A receptor, primarily inhibits sodium reabsorption within the renal inner medullary collecting duct, but also opposes the salt-retaining effects of angiotensin II at the level of the proximal tubule (121). ANP similarly inhibits the actions of vasopressin and aldosterone in the renal tubules (122–124).

ANP modulates mineralocorticoid production in a manner that results in the reduction of intravascular volume of pressure. Although direct reduction in plasma renin activity has been described with ANP infusion (125, 126), the most dramatic response to ANP occurs at the level of the adrenal glomerulosa cell. ANP inhibits aldosterone production by inhibiting action of most aldosterone secretagogues, with the most pronounced reduction being angiotensin II activity (119–121).

BNP synthesis and secretion from cardiac ventricular tissue are augmented in congestive heart failure, and, as for ANP, with hypertension, chronic renal, and chronic liver failure (115, 118).

III. CENTRAL DIABETES INSIPIDUS

A. Causes

Central (hypothalamic, neurogenic, or vasopressin-sensitive) diabetes insipidus can be caused by disorders of vasopressin gene structure; accidental or surgical trauma to vasopressin neurons; congenital anatomical hypothalamic or pituitary defects; neoplasms; infiltrative, autoimmune, and infectious diseases affecting vasopressin neurons or fiber tracts; and increased metabolism of vasopressin. In approximately 10% of children with central diabetes insipidus, the cause is not apparent (127, 128).

1. Genetics

Familial autosomal dominant central diabetes insipidus is manifest within the first half of the first decade of life (129). Vasopressin secretion, initially normal, gradually declines until diabetes insipidus of variable severity en-

sues. Patients respond well to vasopressin replacement therapy. The disease has a high degree of penetrance, but may be of variable severity within a family (130) and may spontaneously improve in middle age (130, 131). Vasopressin-containing neurons are absent from the magnocellular paraventricular neurons (132) but are present in parvocellular regions (133). Several different oligonucleotide mutations in the vasopressin structural gene have been found to cause the disease (www.medcon.mcgill.ca/nephros/avp_npii.html). To date, there have been mutations detected in 22 amino acids of the vasopressin gene, including 15 missense, 5 nonsense, 1 deletion, and 1 frameshift mutations. Vasopressin deficiency is also found in the syndrome consisting of diabetes insipidus, diabetes mellitus, optic atrophy, and deafness (DIDMOAD) (134, 135). One (136), but not another (137), study has suggested that a mitochondrial defect is responsible for the disease. The gene for this syndrome complex, also known as Wolfram syndrome, was localized to human chromosome 4p16 by polymorphic linkage analysis (138), and has recently been isolated (139).

2. Trauma

The axons of vasopressin-containing magnocellular neurons extend uninterrupted to the posterior pituitary over a distance of approximately 10 mm. Trauma to the base of the brain can cause swelling around or severance of these axons, resulting in either transient or permanent diabetes insipidus (140). Permanent diabetes insipidus can occur after seemingly minor trauma. Approximately one-half of patients with fractures of the sella turcica will develop permanent diabetes insipidus (141), which may be delayed as long as 1 month following the trauma, during which time neurons of severed axons may undergo retrograde degeneration (142).

Septic shock (143) and postpartum hemorrhage associated with pituitary infarction (Sheehan syndrome) (144, 145) may involve the posterior pituitary with varying degrees of diabetes insipidus. Diabetes insipidus is never associated with cranial irradiation of the hypothalamic–pituitary region, although this treatment can cause deficits in all of the hypothalamic releasing hormones carried by the portal–hypophyseal system to the anterior pituitary (see Chapter 36). Because vasopressin is carried directly to the posterior pituitary via magnocellular axonal transport, radiation may affect hypothalamic releasing hormone function by interruption of the portal–hypophyseal circulation.

3. Neurosurgical Intervention

One of the most common causes of central diabetes insipidus is the neurosurgical destruction of vasopressin neurons following pituitary–hypothalamic surgery. It is important to differentiate polyuria associated with the onset of acute postsurgical central diabetes insipidus from polyuria due to the normal diuresis of fluids given during surgery. In both cases, the urine may be very dilute and of high volume, exceeding 200 ml/m²/h. In the former case, serum osmolality will be high; in the latter case it will be normal. A careful examination of the intraoperative record should also help to differentiate between these two possibilities. Vasopressin axons traveling from the hypothalamus to the posterior pituitary terminate at various levels within the stalk and gland (Fig. 5). Since surgical interruption of these axons can result in retrograde degeneration of hypothalamic neurons, lesions closer to the hypothalamus will affect more neurons and cause greater permanent loss of hormone secretion. Of special interest is the triphasic pattern of vasopressin secretion, often, but not always, seen following neurosurgical procedures interfering with the supraoptic–hypophyseal tract (146). Following surgery, an initial phase of transient diabetes insipidus is observed lasting $\frac{1}{2}$–2 days, and possibly due to edema in the area interfering with normal vasopressin secretion (Fig. 5). If significant vasopressin cell destruction has occurred, this is often followed by a second phase of SIADH, which may last up to 10 days, secondary to release of prestored vasopressin from damaged neurons. A third phase of permanent neurogenic diabetes insipidus may follow if more than 90% of vasopressin cells are destroyed. Usually a marked degree of SIADH in the second phase portends significant permanent diabetes insipidus in the final phase of this response. In patients with coexisting vasopressin and cortisol deficits (e.g., in combined anterior and posterior hypopituitarism following neurosurgical treatment of craniopharyngioma), symptoms of diabetes insipidus may be masked because cortisol deficiency impairs renal free water clearance, as discussed below. In such cases, institution of glucocorticoid therapy alone may precipitate polyuria, leading to the diagnosis of diabetes insipidus.

4. Congenital Anatomical Defects

Midline brain anatomical abnormalities such as septo-optic dysplasia with agenesis of the corpus callosum (147), the Kabuki syndrome (148), holoprosencephaly (149), and familial pituitary hypoplasia with absent stalk (150) may be associated with central diabetes insipidus. These patients need not have external evidence of craniofacial abnormalities (149). Central diabetes insipidus due to midline brain abnormalities is often accompanied by defects in thirst perception (147), suggesting that a common osmosensor may control both vasopressin release and thirst perception. Some patients with suspected defects in osmosensor function but with intact vasopressin neurons may have recumbent diabetes insipidus, with baroreceptor-mediated release of vasopressin while upright and vasopressin-deficient polyuria while supine (151).

5. Neoplasms

Several important clinical implications follow from knowledge of the anatomy of the vasopressin system. Because hypothalamic vasopressin neurons are distributed over a large area within the hypothalamus, tumors that cause diabetes insipidus must be very large, or infiltrative, or be strategically located at the point of convergence of the hypothalamoneurohypophyseal axonal tract in the infundibulum. Germinomas and pinealomas typically arise near the base of the hypothalamus where vasopressin axons converge before their entry into the posterior pituitary. For this reason they are among the most common primary brain tumors associated with diabetes insipidus. Germinomas causing the disease can be very small (152, 153) and undetectable by magnetic resonance imaging (MRI) for several years following the onset of polyuria (154). For this reason, quantitative measurement of the β subunit of human chorionic gonadotropin, often secreted by germinomas and pinealomas, and regularly repeated MRI scans should be performed in children with idiopathic or unexplained diabetes insipidus. Empty sella syndrome, possibly due to unrecognized pituitary infarction, can be associated with diabetes insipidus in children (155). Craniopharyngiomas and optic gliomas can also cause central diabetes insipidus when very large, although this is more often a postoperative complication of the treatment for these tumors. Hematological malignancies can cause diabetes insipidus. In some cases, such as with acute myelocytic leukemia, the cause if infiltration of the pituitary stalk and sell (156–158). However, more than 30 patients with monosomy or deletion of chromosome 7 associated with acute blast transformation of myelodysplastic syndrome presented with central diabetes insipidus (159–162), without evidence of infiltration of the posterior pituitary by neoplastic cells, leaving the cause of the diabetes insipidus unresolved.

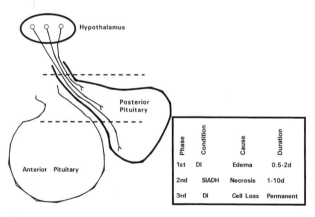

Figure 5 Diabetes insipidus following neurosurgery. Vasopressin neurons terminate at different levels of the posterior pituitary. Depending on the level of neurosurgical damage (dashed lines), different numbers of vasopressin neurons will be permanently damaged. The three phases of the triple phase response to neural damage, along with their causes and duration, are noted in the box.

6. Infiltrative, Autoimmune, and Infectious Diseases

Langerhans cell histiocytosis and lymphocytic hypophysitis are the most common types of infiltrative disorders causing central diabetes insipidus. Approximately 10% of patients with histiocytosis will have diabetes insipidus. These patients tend to have more serious, multisystem disease for longer periods of time than those without diabetes insipidus (163, 164), and anterior pituitary deficits often accompany posterior pituitary deficiency (165). MRI characteristically shows thickening of the pituitary stalk (166). One report suggests that in patients with Langerhans cell histiocytosis, radiation treatment to the pituitary region within 14 days of onset of symptoms of diabetes insipidus may result in return of vasopressin function in more than one-third of affected patients (167).

Lymphocytic infundibuloneurohypophysitis may account for over one-half of patients with so-called idiopathic central diabetes insipidus (168). This entity may be associated with other autoimmune diseases (169). Image analysis discloses an enlarged pituitary and thickened stalk (168, 170), and biopsy of the posterior pituitary reveals lymphocytic infiltration of the gland, stalk, and magnocellular hypothalamic nuclei (171). A necrotizing form of this entity has been described that also causes anterior pituitary failure and responds to steroid treatment (172). Diabetes insipidus can also be associated with pulmonary granulomatous diseases (173) including sarcoidosis (174). Whether antibody-mediated destruction of vasopressin cells occurs is controversial. Over one-half of patients with central diabetes insipidus of a nontraumatic cause have antibodies directed against vasopressin-containing cells (175), and patients with other autoimmune diseases have such antibodies without evidence of diabetes insipidus (176). Many patients with central diabetes insipidus also have antivasopressin peptide antibodies, although their appearance usually follows institution of vasopressin treatment (177). It is very possible that antibodies directed against vasopressin-containing cells or vasopressin are not pathogenetic, but instead are markers of prior neuronal cell destruction.

Infections involving the base of the brain, such as meningococcal (178), cryptococcal, *Listeria* (179), and toxoplasmosis (180) meningitis, congenital cytomegalovirus infection (181), and nonspecific inflammatory disease of the brain (182), can cause central diabetes insipidus. The disease is often transient, suggesting that it is due to inflammation rather than destruction of vasopressin-containing neurons.

7. Brain Death

Central diabetes insipidus can appear in the setting of hypoxic brain death (183). Although its presence has been suggested as a marker for brain death in children (184), in some studies only a minority of patients with brain death manifest the disorder (185), and up to 15% of patients with cerebral insults and diabetes insipidus ultimately recover brain function (186). Polyuria in the setting of brain death can be accompanied by high concentrations of plasma vasopressin (187), suggesting that some cases mistaken for diabetes insipidus are actually due to other causes, such as cerebral salt wasting with polyuria, as discussed subsequently.

8. Increased Metabolism of Vasopressin

The metabolic clearance rate of vasopressin increases fourfold during pregnancy due to the elaboration of a vasopressinase by the placenta (53). If the mother cannot respond with a concomitant increase in vasopressin action because of pre-existing subclinical central or nephrogenic diabetes insipidus (54), overt, transient disease will appear, usually early in the third trimester and resolve within 1 week of delivery (57, 188). Even without prior defects in vasopressin function, an extreme elevation in vasopressinase concentrations in primigravidas with pre-eclampsia, liver dysfunction, or multiple gestation (55, 56, 189–191) may result in development of the syndrome.

9. Drugs

The most common agent associated with inhibition of vasopressin release and impaired urine concentrating ability is ethanol (192). Since inhibition of vasopressin release by ethanol can be overcome in the setting of concurrent hypovolemia, clinically important diabetes insipidus due to ethanol ingestion is uncommon (193). Phenytoin, opiate antagonists, halothane, and α-adrenergic agents have also been associated with impaired vasopressin release (194, 195).

B. Diagnostic Approach and Differential Diagnosis

The salient features of neurogenic diabetes insipidus are polyuria and polydipsia. In children, it must first be determined whether pathological polyuria or polydipsia (exceeding 2 l/m²/day) is present, by asking the following questions: Is there a psychosocial reason for either polyuria or polydipsia? Can either be quantitated? Has either polyuria or polydipsia interfered with normal activities? Is nocturia or enuresis present? If so, does the patient also drink following nocturnal awakening? Does the history (including longitudinal growth data) or physical examination suggest other deficient or excessive endocrine secretion or an intracranial neoplasm? If pathological polyuria or polydipsia is present, the following should be obtained in the outpatient setting: serum osmolality; serum concentrations of sodium, potassium, glucose, calcium, and blood urea nitrogen (BUN); and urinalysis, including measurement of urine osmolality, specific gravity, and glucose concentration. A serum osmolality greater than 300 mOsm/kg, with urine osmolality less than 300 mOsm/kg, establishes the diagnosis of diabetes insipidus.

If serum osmolality is less than 270 mOsm/kg, or urine osmolality is greater than 600 mOsm/kg, the diagnosis of diabetes insipidus is unlikely. If, on initial screening, the patient has a serum osmolality less than 300 mOsm/kg, but the intake/output record at home suggests significant polyuria and polydipsia that cannot be attributed to primary polydipsia (i.e., the serum osmolality is greater than 270 mOsm/kg), the patient should undergo a water deprivation test to establish a diagnosis of diabetes insipidus and to differentiate central from nephrogenic causes.

After a maximally tolerated overnight fast (based on the outpatient history), the child is admitted to the outpatient testing center in the early morning of a day when an 8–10 h test can be carried out and is deprived of water (196, 197). The physical signs and biochemical parameters shown in Figure 6 are measured. If, at any time during the test, the urine osmolality exceeds 1000 mOsm/kg, or 600 mOsm/kg and is stable over 1 h, the patient does not have diabetes insipidus. If, at any time, the serum osmolality exceeds 300 mOsm/kg and the urine osmolality is less than 600 mOsm/kg, the patient has diabetes insipidus. If the serum osmolality is less than 300 mOsm/kg and the urine osmolality is less than 600 mOsm/kg, the test should be continued unless vital signs disclose hypovolemia. A common error is to stop a test too soon, based on the amount of body weight lost, before either urine osmolality has plateaued above 600 mOsm/kg or a serum osmolality above 300 mOsm/kg has been achieved. Unless the serum osmolality rises above the threshold for vasopressin release, a lack of vasopressin action (as inferred by a nonconcentrated urine) cannot be deemed pathological. If the diagnosis of diabetes insipidus is made, aqueous vasopressin (Pitressin, 1 U/m^2), should be given subcutaneously. If the patient has central diabetes insipidus, urine volume should fall and osmolality should at least double during the next hour, compared with the value prior to vasopressin therapy. If there is less than a twofold rise in urine osmolality following vasopressin administration, the patient probably has nephrogenic diabetes insipidus. dDAVP should not be used for this test, since it has been associated with water intoxication in small children in this setting (198). Patients with longstanding primary polydipsia may have mild nephrogenic diabetes insipidus because of dilution of their renal medullary interstitium. This should not be confused with primary nephrogenic diabetes insipidus, since patients with primary polydipsia should have a tendency towards hyponatremia, rather than hypernatremia, in the basal state. Patients with a family history of X-linked nephrogenic diabetes insipidus can be evaluated for the disorder in the prenatal or perinatal period by DNA sequence analysis, as will be discussed, allowing therapy to be initiated without delay (199).

The water deprivation test should be sufficient in most patients to establish the diagnosis of diabetes insipidus, and to differentiate central from nephrogenic causes. Plasma vasopressin concentration may be obtained during the procedure (Fig. 6), although it is rarely needed for diagnostic purposes in children (200). It is particularly helpful in differentiating between partial central and nephrogenic diabetes insipidus, in that it is low in the former and high in the latter situation (201). If urine osmolality concentrates normally, but only after serum osmolality is well above 300 mOsm/kg, the patient may have an altered threshold for vasopressin release, also termed a reset osmostat. This may occur following head trauma, neurosurgery, or with brain tumors (202). Magnetic resonance imaging is not very helpful in differentiating central from nephrogenic diabetes insipidus (203). Normally, the posterior pituitary is seen as an area of enhanced brightness in T1-weighted images following administration of gadolinium (204). The posterior pituitary bright spot is diminished or absent in both forms of diabetes insipidus, presumably because of decreased vasopressin synthesis in central, and increased vasopressin release in nephrogenic, disease (204–206). In primary polydipsia, the bright spot is normal, probably because vasopressin accumulates in the posterior pituitary during chronic water ingestion (204), whereas it is decreased in the syndrome of inappropriate antidiuretic hormone (SIADH), presumably because of increased vasopressin secretion (203). Dynamic, fast-frame, magnetic resonance image analysis has recently allowed estimation of blood flow to the posterior pituitary (207). With this technique, both central and nephrogenic diabetes insipidus are associated with delayed enhancement in the area of the neurohypophysis (208).

In the inpatient, postneurosurgical setting, central diabetes insipidus is likely if hyperosmolality (serum osmolality >300 mOsm/kg) is associated with urine osmolality less than serum osmolality. One must beware of intraoperative fluid expansion with subsequent hypo-osmolar polyuria masquerading as diabetes insipidus.

C. Treatment

1. Fluid Therapy

Patients with otherwise untreated diabetes insipidus crave cold fluids, especially water. With complete central diabetes insipidus, maximum urine concentrating ability is approximately 100 mOsm/kg. Since 5 l urine would be required to excrete an average daily solute load of 500 mOsm/m^2, fluid intake must match this to maintain normal plasma tonicity. With an intact thirst mechanism and free access to oral fluids, a person with complete diabetes insipidus can maintain plasma osmolality and sodium in the high normal range, although at great inconvenience. Furthermore, longstanding intake of these volumes of fluid in children can lead to hydroureter (209) and even hyperfluorosis in communities that provide fluoridated water (210).

There are two situations in which central diabetes insipidus is sometimes best treated solely with high levels

Water Deprivation Test

ENDOCRINE FUNCTION TEST	MR
DIAGNOSIS: Rule out Diabetes Insipidus	
TEST: Water Deprivation	

Present Health ____ Good ____ Fair ____ Poor

Diet for previous two days (attach diet history): ____ Good ____ Fair ____ Poor

Period of Fast ____ Hours Recent Medications ____

Body Weight ____ Kg

No	Hour	Interval Minutes	BS mg/dL	Serum Na	Serum OSM	Serum BUN	Serum VP*	Body weight	Vital signs	Urine Na	Urine OSM	Urine S.G.	Urine vol/hr
		-30	Place IV hep lock										
		0		X	X	X	X	X	X	X	X	X	X
		60		X	X			X	X	X	X	X	X
		120		X	X			X	X	X	X	X	X
		180		X	X			X	X	X	X	X	X
		240		X	X		X	X	X	X	X	X	X
		300		X	X			X	X	X	X	X	X
		360		X	X			X	X	X	X	X	X
		420		X	X			X	X	X	X	X	X
		480		X	X		X	X	X	X	X	X	X

*If patient has DI, last VP sample at last time point before VP administration (see below)

AT ANY TIME DURING TEST:

If serum osm <300 (Na<145), urine osm <600, continue test unless vital signs disclose hypovolemia

If urine osm >1000, or >600 and stable (<30 mosm change for 2 time points), stop test = NORMAL

If serum osm >300 and urine osm<600=DIABETES INSIPIDUS. Give Pitressin, 1U/m^2 SQ and measure:

TIME AFTER PITRESSIN ADMINISTRATION:

No	Hour	Interval Minutes	BS mg/dL	Serum Na	Serum OSM	Serum BUN	Serum VP*	Body weight	Vital signs	Urine Na	Urine OSM	Urine S.G.	Urine vol/hr
		0									X	X	X
		30									X	X	X
		60									X	X	X

COMMENTS: *VP = vasopressin (ADH)

Figure 6 Protocol for evaluation of diabetes insipidus using water deprivation. IV, intravenous; OSM, osmolality; S.G., urinary specific gravity; SQ, subcutaneous. (From Muglia L, Majzoub J. Disorders of the posterior pituitary. In: Sperling, ed. Pediatric Endocrinology, 2d ed. Philadelphia: Saunders, 2002:289–322.)

of fluid intake, without vasopressin. Vasopressin therapy coupled with excessive fluid intake (usually greater than 1 l/m^2/day as discussed subsequently) can result in unwanted hyponatremia. Because neonates and young infants receive all of their nutrition in liquid form, the obligatory high oral fluid requirements for this age (3 l/m^2/day) combined with vasopressin treatment are likely to lead to this dangerous complication (211). Such neonates are better managed with fluid therapy alone. Although children managed with such a regimen may be chronically thirsty, parents may have difficulty keeping up with the voluminous fluid intake and urine output, and poor growth may occur if adequate calories are not provided along with water (212). These problems are more easily addressed than is life-threatening hyponatremia. In difficult cases, thiazide and/or amiloride diuretics may be added to facilitate renal proximal tubular sodium and water reabsorption (213) and thereby decrease oral fluid requirements. In older children, the use of short-acting agents such as arginine vasopressin (Pitressin) or lysine vasopressin (Diapid) will decrease fluid needs while minimizing the possible occurrence of hyponatremia (see section below on vasopressin and vasopressin analogs).

In the acute postoperative management of central diabetes insipidus occurring after neurosurgery in young children, vasopressin therapy may be successfully employed (214, 215), but extreme caution must be exerted with its use. While under the full antidiuretic effect of vasopressin, a patient will have a urine osmolality of approximately 1000 mOsm/kg and become hyponatremic if she or he receives an excessive amount of fluids, depending on the solute load and nonrenal water losses. With a solute excretion of 500 mOsm/m^2/day, normal renal function, and nonrenal fluid losses of 500 ml/m^2/day, fluid intake greater than 1 l/m^2/day will result in hyponatremia. In addition, vasopressin therapy will mask the emergence of the SIADH phase of the triple-phase neurohypophyseal response to neurosurgical injury (as discussed above). For these reasons, it is often best to manage acute postoperative diabetes insipidus in young children with fluids alone, avoiding the use of vasopressin (216). This method consists of matching input and output hourly using between 1 and 3 l/m^2/day (40–120 ml/m^2/h). If intravenous therapy is used, a basal 40 ml/m^2/h should be given as 5% dextrose (D5) in one-fourth normal saline (normal saline = 0.9% sodium chloride) and the remainder, depending on the urine output, as 5% dextrose in water. Potassium chloride (40 mEq/l) may be added if oral intake is to be delayed for several days. No additional fluid should be administered for hourly urine volumes under 40 ml/m^2/h. For hourly urine volumes above 40 ml/m^2/h, the additional volume should be replaced with 5% dextrose up to a total maximum of 120 ml/m^2/h. For example, in a child with a surface area of 1 m^2 (approximately 30 kg), the basal infusion rate would be 40 ml/h of 5% dextrose in one-fourth normal saline. For an hourly urine output of

60 ml, an additional 20 ml/h 5% dextrose would be given, for a total infusion rate of 60 ml/h. For urine outputs above 120 ml/h, the total infusion rate would be 120 ml/h. In the presence of diabetes insipidus, this will result in a serum sodium level in the 150 mEq/l range and a mildly volume contracted state, which will allow one to assess both thirst sensation and the return of normal vasopressin function or the emergence of SIADH. Patients may become mildly hyperglycemic with this regimen, particularly if they are also receiving postoperative glucocorticoids. However, because it does not use vasopressin this fluid management protocol prevents any chance of hyponatremia.

2. Vasopressin and Vasopressin Analogs

Intravenous therapy with synthetic aqueous vasopressin (Pitressin) is useful in the management of central diabetes insipidus of acute onset (214, 215). If continuous vasopressin is administered, fluid intake must be limited to 1 l/m^2/day (assuming normal solute intake and nonrenal water losses as described). The potency of synthetic vasopressin is still measured using a bioassay and is expressed in bioactive units, with 1 milliunit (mU) equivalent to approximately 2.5 ng vasopressin. For intravenous vasopressin therapy, 1.5 mU/kg/h results in a blood vasopressin concentration of approximately 10 pg/ml (217), twice that needed for full antidiuretic activity (218). Vasopressin's effect is maximal within 2 h of the start of infusion (218), and one must beware of it sticking to intravenous bottles and tubing. Occasionally following hypothalamic (but not transsphenoidal) surgery, higher initial concentrations of vasopressin are required to treat acute diabetes insipidus, which may be attributable to the release of a substance related to vasopressin from the damaged hypothalamoneurohypophyseal system, which acts as an antagonist to normal vasopressin activity (219).

Much higher rates of vasopressin infusion, resulting in plasma concentrations above 100 pg/ml, should be avoided, as they may cause cutaneous necrosis (220), rhabdomyolysis (220, 221), and cardiac rhythm disturbances (222). Patients treated with vasopressin for postneurosurgical diabetes insipidus should be switched from intravenous to oral fluid intake at the earliest opportunity, because thirst sensation, if intact, will help regulate blood osmolality, as discussed. Intravenous dDAVP should not be used in the acute management of postoperative central diabetes insipidus, because it offers no advantage over vasopressin, and its long half-life (8–12 h) compared with that of vasopressin (5–10 min) is a distinct disadvantage, because it may increase the chance of causing water intoxication (198). In fact, the use of intravenous dDAVP (0.3 μg/kg) to shorten the bleeding time in a variety of bleeding disorders (as has been discussed) has been associated with water intoxication (223), particularly in young children who have high obligate oral fluid needs.

A special problem arises when a patient with established central diabetes insipidus must receive a high volume of fluid for therapeutic reasons (e.g., accompanying cancer chemotherapy). Such patients can be managed either by discontinuing antidiuretic therapy and increasing fluid intake to 3–5 l/m²/day (rendering the patient moderately hypernatremic), or by using a low dosage of intravenous vasopressin (0.1 mU/kg/h, approximately one-eighth the full antidiuretic dosage). The partial antidiuretic effect allows the administration of higher amounts of fluid without causing hyponatremia (224).

In the outpatient setting, treatment of central diabetes insipidus in older children should begin with oral dDAVP in dosages of 25–300 µg every 8–12 h. Oral dDAVP tablets have recently come into widespread use. Although when given orally dDAVP is at least 20-fold less potent than when given via the intranasal route, it is reported to be highly effective and safe in children (225–227). Intranasal dDAVP (10 µg/0.1 ml), 0.025 ml (2.5 µg) is given by rhinal tube at bedtime and the dosage is increased to the lowest amount that gives an antidiuretic effect. If the dosage is effective, but has too short a duration, it should be increased further or a second, morning dose should be added. Patients should escape from the antidiuretic effect for at least 1 h before the next dose, to ensure that any excessive water will be excreted. Otherwise, water intoxication may occur. dDAVP is also available as a nasal spray in the same concentration, with each spray delivering 10 µg (0.1 ml). This is the standard preparation used for treatment of primary enuresis. Lysine vasopressin (Diapid) nasal spray (50 units/ml) may be used if a duration less than that of dDAVP is desired. One spray delivers 2 units (0.04 ml), with a duration of action between 2 and 8 h.

In addition to polyuria and polydypsia, decreased bone mineral density has been reported in patients with central diabetes insipidus (228). The decreased bone density was not corrected by vasopressin analog treatment alone, suggesting that institution of bisphosphonate or other therapies designed to prevent bone loss may be of long-term benefit in the treatment of diabetes insipidus.

3. Children with Primary Enuresis

Although normal children have a nocturnal rise in plasma vasopressin associated with an increase in urine osmolality and a decrease in urine volume, those with primary enuresis have a blunted or absent rise in vasopressin, and excrete a higher urine volume of lower tonicity (229, 230). This has suggested that enuretic children have a primary deficiency in vasopressin secretion, although the same outcome could be caused solely by excessive water intake in these children. The use of the V2 agonist dDAVP is highly effective in abolishing bed-wetting episodes, although relapse is high once therapy is stopped (231–233). Fluid intake must be limited while a child is exposed to

the antidiuretic action of dDAVP to guard against water intoxication.

IV. NEPHROGENIC DIABETES INSIPIDUS

A. Causes

Nephrogenic (vasopressin-resistant) diabetes insipidus can be due to genetic or acquired causes. Genetic causes are less common but more severe than acquired forms of the disease, although genetic causes are more common in children than in adults.

1. Genetic Causes

a. Congenital X-Linked Diabetes Insipidus: V2 Receptor Mutations. Congenital X-linked nephrogenic diabetes insipidus is caused by inactivating mutations of the vasopressin V2 receptor. Due to its mode of transmission, it is a disease of males, although rarely females may be affected, presumably due to extreme Lyonization during X-chromosome inactivation (234). In keeping with a germline, as opposed to somatic, mutation in the V2 receptor, these patients are deficient in all systemic V2 receptor-mediated actions (235, 236) and have intact V1-receptor-mediated responses (237, 238). As expected, the V2 receptor defect is proximal to the activation of renal adenylate cyclase (239, 240). Unlike the function of other G protein-coupled seven transmembrane receptors such as the parathyroid hormone (PTH) and thyroid-stimulating hormone (TSH) receptors, that of the V2 receptor is unaffected in patients with pseudohypoparathyroidism, who have inactivating mutations in the alpha subunit of G_s (241).

Because of vasopressin resistance in congenital nephrogenic diabetes insipidus, the kidney elaborates large volumes of hypotonic urine with osmolality ranging between 50 and 100 mOsm/kg. Manifestations of the disease are usually present within the first several weeks of life (242), but may only become apparent after weaning from the breast. The predominant symptoms are polyuria and polydipsia. Thirst may be more difficult to satisfy than in central diabetes insipidus. Many infants initially present with fever, vomiting, and dehydration, often leading to an evaluation for infection. Growth failure in the untreated child may be secondary to the ingestion of large amounts of water, which the child may prefer over milk and other higher-caloric substances (243). Mental retardation of variable severity as a result of repeated episodes of dehydration was described frequently in early reports (244). However, the majority of patients reported in recent studies have a normal intelligence, very likely due to an early diagnosis and appropriate treatment (245).

Intracerebral calcification of the frontal lobes and basal ganglia is not uncommon in children with X-linked nephrogenic diabetes insipidus (246–249). Because this appears early and is not seen in children with central diabetes insipidus of equivalent severity, cerebral calcification is probably unrelated to the level of dehydration or therapeutic intervention. It is possible that elevated vasopressin concentrations, acting via intact V1 or V3 receptors, contribute to some of the unique manifestations of X-linked nephrogenic diabetes insipidus, such as cerebral calcification, intense thirst, vomiting, and growth failure. Older children may present with enuresis or nocturia. They may learn to reduce food intake (and therefore solute load) to decrease polyuria, which may contribute to growth failure. After longstanding ingestion and excretion of large volumes of water, patients may develop non-obstructive hydronephrosis, hydroureter, and megabladder (209).

Although one founder (arriving in North America from Scotland in 1761 on the ship *Hopewell*) was initially postulated to be the ancestor of most North American subjects with congenital, X-linked nephrogenic diabetes insipidus (250), more than 180 mutations in the V2 receptor have been found, with some appearing to have arisen independently more than once (251–264). These are mostly single base mutations that result in amino acid substitutions, translational frame shifts, or termination of peptide synthesis, and are distributed fairly evenly throughout the receptor protein (www.medcon.mcgill.ca/nephros/avpr2. html). Mutations may affect vasopressin binding, cyclic AMP generation, or possibly transcriptional regulation (265–269). Patients with different mutations will likely be found to exhibit phenotypic heterogeneity, including severity of disease and response to treatment. Genetic heterogeneity may underlie the variable response of patients with X-linked diabetes insipidus to dDAVP treatment. In a family with a known mutation, prenatal or early postnatal DNA screening can unambiguously identify affected males, allowing the institution of appropriate therapy (199).

b. Congenital, Autosomal, Nephrogenic Diabetes Insipidus: Aquaporin-2 Mutations. After the initial description of X-linked nephrogenic diabetes insipidus (270), several patients were reported with similar clinical findings except for autosomal recessive transmission of the disease (271) or normal V2 receptor function outside of the kidney (272). With cloning of the complementary DNA for the renal water channel, aquaporin-2, many patients with autosomal recessive nephrogenic diabetes insipidus have been reported who have a total of 21 mutations different in this gene (Oksche, 1998 #3453) (*www. medcon.mcgill.ca/nephros/aqp2.html*). Most are missense mutations, although four are nonsense or frameshift mutations. They are scattered throughout the molecule, including within four of the five transmembrane domains, two of three extracellular domains, and two of four intracellular domains. Recently, an autosomal dominant mode of inheritance for nephrogenic diabetes insipidus has been described, associated with mutations in aquaporin-2. One of these dominant mutations results in mixed tetramers of the wild type and mutant alleles being retained in the

Golgi apparatus (273). Aquaporin-2 mutations impair the ability of the luminal membrane to undergo an increase in water permeability following signaling through the V2 receptor. They could include patients previously described who had a normal rise in urinary cyclic AMP in response to vasopressin, without a concomitant increase in urine osmolality (239). Aquaporin-2 protein has recently been shown to be excreted in the urine in both soluble and membrane-bound forms. Aquaporin-2 excretion is low in untreated central and nephrogenic diabetes insipidus, but following dDAVP administration increases markedly in the former, but not latter, disease (92). For this reason, its measurement in urine has been suggested as an aid in the differential diagnosis of diabetes insipidus (92).

2. Acquired Causes

Acquired causes of nephrogenic diabetes insipidus are more common and less severe than genetic causes. Nephrogenic diabetes insipidus may be caused by drugs such as lithium and demeclocycline, both of which are thought to interfere with vasopressin-stimulated cyclic AMP generation or action. Approximately 50% of patients receiving lithium have impaired urinary concentrating ability, although only 10–20% of them develop symptomatic nephrogenic diabetes insipidus, which is almost always accompanied by a reduction in the glomerular filtration rate (274, 275). The risk increases with duration of therapy. Lithium impairs the ability of vasopressin to stimulate adenylate cyclase (276), resulting in a 90% fall in aquaporin-2 messenger RNA expression in renal collecting ducts (277) and may be the basis for its causing nephrogenic diabetes insipidus.

Demeclocycline treatment causes nephrogenic diabetes insipidus by inhibiting transepithelial water transport (278). For this reason, it is useful in the treatment of dilutional hyponatremia associated with inappropriate secretion of vasopressin, as will be discussed. Other agents that cause nephrogenic diabetes insipidus include hypercalcemia, hypokalemia, and therapy with foscarnet (used in treatment of cytomegalovirus infection in immunosuppressed patients) (279, 280), clozapine (280), amphotericin (281), methicillin (282), or rifampin (283). Whether any of these agents causes nephrogenic diabetes insipidus by interfering with the expression or insertion into apical collecting duct membranes of aquaporin-2 water channels is not yet known. Ureteral obstruction (284), chronic renal failure, polycystic kidney disease, medullary cystic disease, Sjögren syndrome (285), and sickle cell disease can also impair renal-concentrating ability. Osmotic diuresis due to glycosuria in diabetes mellitus, or to sodium excretion with diuretic therapy, will interfere with renal water conservation. Primary polydipsia can result in secondary nephrogenic diabetes insipidus because the chronic excretion of a dilute urine lowers the osmolality of the hypertonic renal interstitium, thus decreasing renal-concentrating ability. Finally, decreased protein or sodium uptake also can lead to diminished tonicity of the renal medullary interstitium and nephrogenic diabetes insipidus.

B. Treatment of Nephrogenic Diabetes Insipidus

The treatment of acquired nephrogenic diabetes insipidus focuses on elimination, if possible, of the underlying disorder, such as offending drugs, hypercalcemia, hypokalemia, or ureteral obstruction. Congenital nephrogenic diabetes insipidus is often difficult to treat. The main goals should be to ensure the intake of adequate calories for growth and to avoid severe dehydration. Foods with the highest ratio of caloric content to osmotic load should be ingested, to maximize growth and minimize the urine volume required to excrete urine solute. However, even with the early institution of therapy, growth and mental retardation are not uncommon (286).

Thiazide diuretics in combination with amiloride or indomethocin are the most useful pharmacological agents in the treatment of nephrogenic diabetes insipidus. Thiazides promote sodium excretion by interfering with sodium reabsorption in the distal tubule of the nephron and altering inner medullary osmolality; the former promotes increased proximal tubule reabsorption of sodium and the latter leads to increased free water reabsorption from the collecting duct (213, 287). Indomethacin, 2 mg/kg/day, further enhances proximal tubular sodium and water reabsorption (213, 288, 289), although this effect is not mediated by inhibition of cyclo-oxygenase (290). The combination of thiazide and amiloride diuretics is the most commonly used regimen for the treatment of congenital, X-linked nephrogenic diabetes insipidus, because amiloride counteracts thiazide-induced hypokalemia (242), avoids the nephrotoxicity associated with indomethacin therapy, and is well tolerated, even in infants (291). In addition, amiloride decreases the uptake of lithium by renal epithelial cells, and for this additional reason has been proposed in combination with thiazide as treatment for lithium-induced nephrogenic diabetes insipidus (292). High-dosage dDAVP therapy, in combination with indomethacin, has been reported to be helpful in treating some subjects with nephrogenic diabetes insipidus (293). This treatment may prove to be useful in patients with genetic defects in the V2 receptor that reduce the binding affinity for vasopressin.

V. HYPONATREMIA AND THE SYNDROME OF INAPPROPRIATE SECRETION OF VASOPRESSIN

The evaluation of hyponatremia requires the exclusion of states of hyperproteinemia, hyperlipidemia, and hyperglycemia that may falsely lower the measurement of serum sodium by flame-emission spectrophotometry.

Hyponatremia (serum sodium <130 mEq/l) in children is usually associated with severe systemic disorders. It is most often due to intravascular volume depletion or excessive salt loss, as will be discussed, and is also encountered with hypotonic fluid overload, especially in infants. Inappropriate excess secretion of vasopressin is one of the least common causes of hyponatremia in children, except following vasopressin administration for treatment of diabetes insipidus.

In evaluating the cause of hyponatremia, one should first determine whether the patient is dehydrated and hypovolemic. This is usually evident from the physical examination (decreased weight, skin turgor, central venous pressure) and laboratory data (high blood urea nitrogen, renin, aldosterone, uric acid). With a decrease in the glomerular filtration rate, proximal tubular reabsorption of sodium and water will be high, leading to a urinary sodium less than 10 mEq/l. Patients with decreased effective intravascular volume due to congestive heart failure, cirrhosis, nephrotic syndrome, or lung disease will present with similar laboratory data, but will also have obvious signs of their underlying disease, which often includes peripheral edema. Patients with primary salt loss will also appear volume depleted. If the salt loss is from the kidney (e.g., diuretic therapy or polycystic kidney disease), urinary sodium will be elevated, as may be urine volume. Salt loss from other regions (e.g., the gut in gastroenteritis or the skin in cystic fibrosis) will cause urine sodium to be low, as in other forms of systemic dehydration. Cerebral salt washing is encountered with central nervous system insults, and results in high serum atrial natriuretic peptide concentrations, leading to high urine sodium and urine excretion.

The syndrome of inappropriate antidiuretic hormone (vasopressin) secretion (SIADH) exists when a primary elevation in vasopressin secretion is the cause of hyponatremia. It is characterized by hyponatremia, an inappropriately increased urinary osmolality (>100 mOsm/kg), normal or slightly elevated plasma volume, and a normal to high urine sodium level (because of volume-induced suppression of aldosterone and elevation of atrial natriuretic peptide). Serum uric acid is low in patients with SIADH, whereas it is high in those with hyponatremia due to systemic dehydration or other causes of decreased intravascular volume (294). Measurement of plasma vasopressin is not very useful because it is elevated in all causes of hyponatremia except for primary hypersecretion of atrial natiuretic peptide (295). Because cortisol and thyroid deficiency cause hyponatremia by several mechanisms discussed subsequently, they should be considered in all hyponatremic patients. Drug-induced hyponatremia should be considered in patients taking potentially contributory medications, as discussed below. In children with SIADH who do not have an obvious cause, a careful search for a tumor (thymoma, glioma, bronchial carcinoid) causing the disease should be considered. Patients present clinically with nonspecific symptoms of hyponatremia: anorexia, lethargy, weakness, and in severe cases obtundity and convulsions. Signs of diminished intravascular volume, edema, hypothyroidism, adrenal insufficiency, and renal disease are absent by definition.

A. Hyponatremia with Normal Regulation of Vasopressin

1. Hyponatremia with Appropriate Decreased Secretion of Vasopressin

a. Increased Water Ingestion (Primary Polydipsia). In a hypo-osmolar state with vasopressin secretion normally suppressed, the kidney can excrete urine with an osmolality as low as 50 mOsm/kg. Under these conditions, a daily solute load of 500 mOsm/m^2 could be excreted in 10 l/m^2 urine/day. Neonates cannot dilute their urine to this degree, and are prone to develop water intoxication at levels of water ingestion above 4 l/m^2/day (approximately 60 ml/h in a newborn). This may happen when concentrated infant formula is diluted with excess water, either by accident or in a misguided attempt to make it last longer (296). A primary increase in thirst, without apparent cause, leading to hyponatremia has been reported in infants as young as 5 weeks of age (212). In older children, with a normal kidney and the ability to suppress vasopressin secretion, hyponatremia does not occur unless water intake exceeds 10 l/m^2/day, a feat that is almost impossible to accomplish. Longstanding ingestion of large volumes of water will decrease the hypertonicity within the renal medullary interstitium, which will impair water reabsorption and guard against water intoxication (297). However, hyponatremia will occur at lower rates of water ingestion when renal water clearance is impaired, either because of inappropriately elevated vasopressin secretion (as has been discussed) or for other reasons (see below).

The rare patient in whom the osmotic thresholds for thirst and vasopressin release are reversed illustrates the importance of the normal relationship between these two responses to osmotic stimulation (298). If thirst is activated below the threshold for vasopressin release, water intake and hypo-osmolality will occur and suppress vasopressin secretion, leading to persistent polydipsia and polyuria. As long as daily fluid intake is less than 10 l/m^2, hyponatremia will not occur. Despite the presence of polyuria and polydipsia, this entity should not be confused with diabetes insipidus because of the presence of hypernatremia. However, dDAVP treatment of such a patient may lower serum osmolality below the threshold for thirst, suppressing water ingestion and the consequent polyuria.

b. Decreased Renal Free Water Clearance. Adrenal insufficiency, either primary or secondary, has long been known to result in compromised free water excretion (25, 51). The mechanisms by which glucocorti-

coids and mineralocorticoids modulate water diuresis have been the subject of substantial investigation. Some studies have demonstrated increased plasma vasopressin activity in the context of glucocorticoid insufficiency (299, 300), consistent with more recent molecular biological evidence that glucocorticoids inhibit transcription of the vasopressin gene (301). However, other investigators have failed to detect vasopressin in plasma of patients with adrenal insufficiency and abnormal water clearance (302). Consistent with vasopressin-independent actions of adrenal steroids on water metabolism, Brattleboro rats with hypothalamic diabetes insipidus manifest impaired excretion of a water load after adrenalectomy (51). In adrenalectomized Brattleboro rats, glucocorticoid administration restored urine flow rate but did not restore maximal urinary diluting capacity. In converse fashion, mineralocorticoid administration restored maximal urinary diluting capacity but not flow rate. Thus, both mineralocorticoids and glucocorticoids are required for normal free water clearance.

In part, these vasopressin-independent actions of mineralocorticoids and glucocorticoids have been attributed to the increased glomerular filtration rate arising from reexpansion of extracellular fluid volume (reduced due to salt-wasting) and improved cardiovascular tone, respectively (24, 303, 304). By restoring the glomerular filtration rate, more free water is delivered to the distal tubule for excretion. In addition, volume repletion reduces the nonosmotic stimuli for vasopressin release of volume depletion and hypotension. Nitric oxide has recently been found to stimulate cyclic GMP-dependent membrane insertion of aquaporin 2 into renal epithelial cells (305). Since glucocorticoid has been shown to inhibit endothelial nitric oxide, it is possible that under conditions (306) of glucocorticoid deficiency, high levels of nitric oxide synthase result in elevated levels of endothelial nitric oxide in the renal vasculature, which in the distal renal tubule stimulate increased, vasopressin-independent aquaporin 2 activity and decreased free water clearance.

Direct effects of glucocorticoid or mineralocorticoid insufficiency on aquaporin expression and function have not been reported. In addition to impairing maximal renal diluting capacity, adrenal insufficiency compromises maximal urine-concentrating capacity (307). This effect has been shown to result from reduced tubular response to vasopressin.

Thyroid hormone is also required for normal free water clearance, and its deficiency likewise results in decreased renal water clearance and hyponatremia. Some studies suggest that vasopressin mediates the hyponatremia of hypothyroidism because ethanol increases free water excretion in hypothyroid patients, but this effect has not been found in other reports (308). In severe hypothyroidism, hypovolemia is not present, and hyponatremia is accompanied by appropriate suppression of vasopressin (309). Similar to the consequences of isolated glucocorticoid deficiency described above, hypothyroidism impairs free water clearance more than maximal urine-diluting capacity (310). This decrease in free water clearance may result from diminished glomerular filtration rate (GFR) and delivery of free water to the diluting segment of distal nephron, as suggested by both animal (311) and human studies (312).

Given the often subtle clinical findings associated with adrenal and thyroid deficiency, all patients with hyponatremia should be suspected of these disease states and undergo appropriate diagnostic tests if indicated. Moreover, patients with coexisting adrenal failure and diabetes insipidus may have no symptoms of the latter until glucocorticoid therapy unmasks the need for vasopressin replacement (313, 314). Resolution of diabetes insipidus in chronically polyuric and polydipsic patients may likewise suggest inadequate glucocorticoid supplementation or noncompliance with glucocorticoid replacement.

Some drugs may cause hyponatremia by inhibiting renal water excretion without stimulating secretion of vasopressin (Table 1), an action that could be called *nephrogenic SIADH*. In addition to augmenting vasopressin release, both carbamazepine (315, 316) and chloropropamide (317, 318) increase the cellular response to vasopressin. Acetaminophen also increases the response of the kidney to vasopressin (317); however, this has not been found to cause hyponatremia. High-dosage cyclophosphamide treatment (15–20 mg/kg intravenous bolus) is often associated with hyponatremia, particularly when it is followed by a forced water diuresis to prevent hemorrhagic cystitis (319–321). Plasma vasopressin concentrations are normal, suggesting a direct effect of the drug on increasing water resorption (322). Vinblastine, inde-

pendent of augmentation of plasma vasopressin concentration or vasopressin action (323), and cis-platinum (324, 325) likewise cause hyponatremia. These drugs may damage the collecting duct tubular cells, which are normally highly impermeable to water, or may enhance aquaporin-2 water channel activity and thereby increase water reabsorption down its osmotic gradient into the hypertonic renal interstitium.

B. Treatment

Hyponatremia due to cortisol or thyroid hormone deficiency reverses promptly following institution of hormone replacement. Because the hyponatremia is often chronic, too rapid a rise in serum sodium should be avoided if possible. When drugs that impair free water excretion must be used, water intake should be limited, as if the patient has SIADH to 1 l/m^2/24 h, using the regimen proposed.

1. Hyponatremia with Appropriate Increased Secretion of Vasopressin

Increased vasopressin secretion causing hyponatremia may either be an appropriate response or an inappropriate response to a pathological state. Inappropriate secretion of vasopressin, also called SIADH, is the much less common of the two entities (326, 327). Whatever the cause, hyponatremia is a worrisome sign often associated with increased morbidity and mortality (328).

a. Systemic Dehydration. Systemic dehydration (water in excess of salt depletion) initially results in hypernatremia, hyperosmolality, and activation of vasopres-

Table 1 Drugs Impairing Free Water Clearance

Class	Drug	Increases vasopressin secretion
Angiotensin-converting enzyme inhibitors	Lisinopril	
Anticonvulsants	Carbamazepine/oxabarbazepine	Yes
	Valproic acid	
Antineoplastics	Cis-platinum	
	Cyclophosphamide	No
	Vinblastine	Yes
	Vincristine	Yes
Antiparkinsonian	Amantadine	Yes
	Trihexyphenidyl	
Antipsychotics	Haloperidol, thioridazine	
Antipyretics	Acetaminophen	
Hypolipidemics	Clofibrate	Yes
Oral hypoglycemics	Chlorpropamide	Yes
	Tolbutamide	
Selective serotonin uptake inhibitors	Fluoxetine, sertraline, others	Likely
Tricyclic antidepressants	Imipramine, amitriptyline	Yes

Source: Adapted from Refs. 316–318, 323, 385–391.

sin secretion as reviewed above. In addition, the associated fall in the renal glomerular filtration rate results in an increase in proximal tubular sodium and water reabsorption, with a concomitant decrease in distal tubular water excretion. This limits the ability to form a dilute urine and, along with the associated stimulation of the renin–angiotensin–aldosterone system and suppression of atrial natriuretic peptide secretion, results in the excretion of urine that is very low in sodium. As dehydration progresses hypovolemia and/or hypotension become major stimuli for vasopressin release that are much more potent than hyperosmolality (see above). This effect, by attempting to preserve volume, decreases free water clearance further and may lead to water retention and hyponatremia, especially if water replacement in excess of salt is given. In many cases, hyponatremia due to intravascular volume depletion is evident from physical and laboratory signs such as decreased skin turgor, low central venous pressure, hemoconcentration, and elevated blood urea nitrogen. However, the diagnosis may be subtle. For example, patients with meningitis may present with hyponatremia, for which water restriction has been advocated in the belief that it is due to SIADH. However, several studies have found that volume depletion, rather than SIADH, is often the cause of the hyponatremia (329, 330), and that it resolves more readily when supplemental, rather than restricted, fluid and solute are administered (331). In patients with hyponatremia following head trauma, volume depletion rather than SIADH is the cause in approximately one-half (332).

b. Primary Loss of Sodium Chloride. Salt can be lost from the kidney, such as in patients with congenital polycystic kidney disease, acute interstitial nephritis, and chronic renal failure. Mineralocorticoid deficiency, pseudohypoaldosteronism (sometimes seen in children with urinary tract obstruction or infection), diuretic use, and gastrointestinal disease (usually gastroenteritis with diarrhea and/or vomiting) can also result in excess loss of sodium chloride. Hyponatremia can also result from salt loss in sweat in cystic fibrosis, although obstructive lung disease with elevation of plasma vasopressin probably plays a more prominent role, as reviewed above. With the onset of salt loss, any tendency toward hyponatremia will initially be countered by suppression of vasopressin and increased water excretion. However, with continuing salt loss, hypovolemia and/or hypotension ensue causing nonosmotic stimulation of vasopressin. This plus increased thirst, which leads to ingestion of hypotonic fluids with low solute content, result in hyponatremia. Weight loss is usually evident, as is the source of sodium wasting. If it is the kidney, it is accompanied by a rate of urine output and a urine sodium content greater than those associated with most other causes of hyponatremia except a primary increase in atrial natriuretic peptide secretion.

c. Decreased Effective Plasma Volume. Congestive heart failure, cirrhosis, nephrotic syndrome, positive

pressure mechanical ventilation (333), severe burns (334), and lung disease (bronchopulmonary dysplasia (335–337) [in neonates], cystic fibrosis with obstruction (338, 339), and severe asthma (340, 341)) are all characterized by a decrease in so-called effective intravascular volume (308, 342). This occurs because of impaired cardiac output, an inability to keep fluid within the vascular space, or impaired blood flow into the heart, respectively. As with systemic dehydration, in an attempt to preserve intravascular volume, water and salt excretion by the kidney are reduced, and decreased barosensor stimulation results in a compensatory, appropriate increase in vasopressin secretion, leading to an antidiuretic state and hyponatremia (343). Because of the associated stimulation of the renin–angiotensin–aldosterone system, these patients also have an increase in the total body content of sodium chloride and may have peripheral edema, which differentiates them from those with systemic dehydration. In patients with impaired cardiac output and elevated atrial volume (e.g., congestive heart failure or lung disease), atrial natriuretic peptide concentrations are elevated, which contributes to hyponatremia by promoting natriuresis (see below).

d. Treatment. Patients with systemic dehydration and hypovolemia should be rehydrated with salt-containing fluids such as normal saline or lactated Ringer's solution. Because of activation of the renin–angiotensin–aldosterone system, the administered sodium will be avidly conserved, and a water diuresis will quickly ensue as volume is restored and vasopressin concentrations fall (344). Under these conditions, caution must be taken to prevent too rapid a correction of hyponatremia, which may itself result in brain damage (see below).

Hyponatremia due to a decrease in effective plasma volume caused by cardiac, hepatic, renal, or pulmonary dysfunction is more difficult to reverse. The most effective therapy is the least easily achieved: treatment of the underlying systemic disorder. Patients weaned from positive pressure ventilation undergo a prompt water diuresis and resolution of hyponatremia as cardiac output is restored and vasopressin concentrations fall. The only other effective route is to limit water intake to that required for the renal excretion of the obligate daily solute load of approximately 500 mOsm/m^2 and to replenish insensible losses. In a partial antidiuretic state with a urine osmolality of 750 mOsm/kg and insensible losses of 500 ml/m^2, oral intake would have to be limited to approximately 1200 ml/m^2/day.

Because of concomitant hyperaldosteronism, the dietary restriction of sodium chloride needed to control peripheral edema in patients with heart failure may reduce the daily solute load and further limit the amount of water that can be ingested without exacerbating hyponatremia. However, hyponatremia in these settings is often slow to develop, rarely causes symptoms, and usually does not need treatment. If the serum sodium levels fall below 125 mEq/l, water restriction to 1 l/m^2/day is usually effective in preventing a further decline. Since water retention in patients with these disorders is a compensatory response to decreased intravascular volume, an attempt to reverse it with drugs such as demeclocycline or specific V2-receptor antagonists (which induce nephrogenic diabetes insipidus, as discussed above) could result in worsening hypovolemia, with potentially dire consequences (345).

In general, patients with hyponatremia due to salt loss (including those with cerebral salt-wasting syndrome) require continued supplementation with sodium chloride and fluids. Initially, intravenous replacement of urine volume with fluid containing sodium chloride, 150–450 mEq/l depending on the degree of salt loss, may be necessary; oral salt supplementation may be required subsequently (295). This treatment contrasts with that of SIADH, for which water restriction without sodium supplementation is the mainstay.

e. Precautions in Emergency Treatment. Severe hyponatremia requires rapid treatment but not rapid correction. Most children with hyponatremia develop the disorder gradually, are asymptomatic, and should be treated with water restriction alone. However, the development of acute hyponatremia, or a serum sodium concentration below 120 mEq/l, may be associated with lethargy, psychosis, coma, or generalized seizures, especially in younger children. Acute hyponatremia causes cell swelling due to the entry of water into cells which can lead to neuronal dysfunction from alterations in the ionic environment, or to cerebral herniation because of the encasement of the brain in the cranium. If present for more than 24 h, cell swelling triggers a compensatory decrease in intracellular organic osmolytes, resulting in the partial restoration of normal cell volume in chronic hyponatremia (346).

The proper emergency treatment of cerebral dysfunction depends on whether the hyponatremia is acute or chronic (1, 347). In all cases, water restriction should be instituted. If hyponatremia is acute, and therefore probably not associated with a decrease in intracellular organic osmolyte concentration, rapid correction with hypertonic 3% sodium chloride administered intravenously may be indicated. As a general guide, this solution, given in the amount of 12 ml/kg body weight, will result in a rise in serum sodium of approximately 10 mEq/l. If hyponatremia is chronic, hypertonic saline treatment must be undertaken with caution, because it may result in both cell shrinkage (Fig. 7) and the associated syndrome of central pontine myelinolysis (348). This syndrome, affecting the central portion of the basal pons as well as other brain regions, is characterized by axonal demyelination, with sparing of neurons. It becomes evident within 24–48 h following too rapid correction of hyponatremia, has a characteristic appearance by computed tomographic and MRI, and often causes irreversible brain damage (348–350). If hypertonic saline treatment is undertaken, the serum sodium level should be raised only high enough to cause an improvement in mental status, and in no case

faster than 0.5 mEq/l/h or 12 mEq/l/day (347–350). In the case of systemic dehydration, the rise in serum sodium levels may occur very rapidly using this regimen. The associated hyperaldosteronism will cause avid retention of the administered sodium, leading to rapid restoration of volume and suppression of vasopressin secretion, and resulting in a brisk water diuresis and a rise in serum sodium (344).

Acute treatment of hyponatremia is more difficult in patients with decreased effective plasma volume. This is both because the underlying disorder makes it difficult to maintain the administered fluid within the intravascular space, and because an associated increase in atrial natriuretic peptide promotes natriuresis and loss of the administered salt. Furthermore, patients with cardiac disease who are given hypertonic saline may require concomitant treatment with a diuretic such as furosemide to prevent worsening of heart failure, which will also increase natriuresis.

C. Hyponatremia with Abnormal Regulation of Vasopressin

1. Hyponatremia with Inappropriate Increased Secretion of Vasopressin (SIADH)

a. Causes. SIADH is uncommon in children (326, 327, 351). It can occur with encephalitis, brain tumor (352), head trauma (332, 353), or psychiatric disease (354), after generalized seizures (355), after prolonged nausea (356, 357), pneumonia (358, 359), or acquired immunodeficiency syndrome (AIDS) (360). Many drugs have been associated with impaired free water clearance as indicated in Table 1. Impaired free water clearance can result from alteration in vasopressin release, increased vasopressin effect at the same plasma vasopressin concentration, or vasopressin-independent changes in distal collecting tubule water permeability. Common drugs shown to increase ADH secretion and result in hyponatremia include carbamazepine (316), chlorpropamide (361), vinblastine (323), vincristine (362), and tricyclic antidepressants (363, 364). Newer sulfonylurea agents, including glyburide, are not associated with SIADH (365). Although it has been believed to be the cause of hyponatremia associated with viral meningitis, volume depletion is more commonly the cause (329, 331).

In contrast, the majority of children with tuberculous meningitis have hyponatremia and SIADH, which predict more severe disease and poor outcome (366–368). SIADH is the cause of the hyponatremic second phase of a triple-phase response seen after hypothalamic–pituitary surgery, as reviewed previously. Hyponatremia with elevated vasopressin secretion is found in up to 35% of patients 1 week after transsphenoidal pituitary surgery (369, 370). The mechanism is most likely retrograde neuronal degeneration with cell death and vasopressin release. Secondary adrenal insufficiency causing stimulation of va-

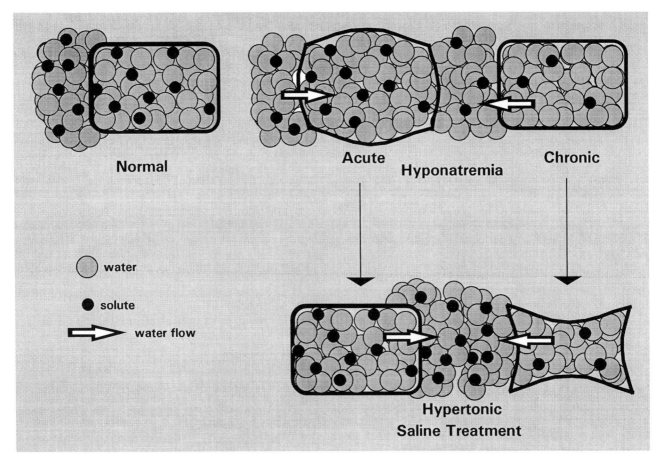

Figure 7 Changes in organic osmolytes with hyponatremia and after its correction. Under normal conditions, osmotic balance exists between extracellular and intracellular compartments. With acute hyponatremia, water enters cells, causing cell swelling. After approximately 24 h continued hyponatremia, intracellular organic osmolytes decrease, restoring cell volume towards normal. Hypertonic saline treatment of acute hyponatremia results in restoration of normal cell volume, whereas the same treatment of chronic hyponatremia results in cell shrinkage. Large circle, water; closed smaller circle, solute; arrow, direction of water flow. (From Muglia L, Majzoub J. Disorders of the posterior pituitary. In: Sperling M, ed. Pediatric Endocrinology, 2d ed. Philadelphia: Saunders, 2002:289–322.)

sopressin release (49) may also play a role, since hyponatremia most commonly follows the removal of adrenocorticotropin hormone-secreting corticotroph adenomas (370). In the vast majority of children with SIADH, the cause is the excessive administration of vasopressin, whether to treat central diabetes insipidus (198, 211) or, less commonly, bleeding disorders (223) (see above), or, most uncommonly, following dDAVP therapy for enuresis.

b. Treatment. Chronic SIADH is best treated by chronic oral fluid restriction. Under full vasopressin antidiuretic effect (urine osmolality of 1000 mOsm/kg), a normal daily obligate renal solute load of 500 mOsm/m^2 would be excreted in 500 ml/m^2 water. This, plus a daily nonrenal water loss of 500 ml/m^2, would require that oral fluid intake be limited to 1000 ml/m^2/day to avoid hypo-

natremia. In young children, this degree of fluid restriction may not provide adequate calories for growth. In this situation, the creation of nephrogenic diabetes insipidus using demeclocycline therapy may be indicated to allow sufficient fluid intake for normal growth (371). Demeclocycline is superior to lithium for this purpose (372). However, its use is not recommended in children under 8 years of age and pregnant women, since tetracyclines are extensively incorporated into bones and tooth enamel. Specific V2 receptor antagonists are also being developed for this purpose (373). Acute treatment of hyponatremia due to SIADH is only indicated if cerebral dysfunction is present. In that case, treatment is dictated by the duration of hyponatremia and the extent of cerebral dysfunction, as has been discussed. Because patients with SIADH have volume expansion, salt administration is not very effective in raising the serum sodium level: it is rapidly excreted in the urine due to suppressed aldosterone and elevated atrial natriuretic peptide concentrations.

2. Hyponatremia with Inappropriate Decreased Secretion of Vasopressin, Due to Increased Secretion of Atrial Natriuretic Peptide (Cerebral Salt-Wasting Syndrome)

Although atrial natriuretic peptide does not usually play a primary role in the pathogenesis of disorders of water metabolism, it may have an important secondary role (335, 374–376). Patients with SIADH have elevated atrial natriuretic peptide concentrations, probably due to hypervolemia, which may contribute to the elevated natriuresis of SIADH and which decrease as water intake is restricted (374). Likewise, the suppressed atrial natriuretic peptide concentrations found in patients with central diabetes insipidus, probably due to the associated hypovolemia, rise after dDAVP therapy (374). However, hyponatremia in some patients, primarily those with central nervous system disorders including brain tumor, head trauma, hydrocephalus, neurosurgery, cerebral vascular accidents, and brain death, may be due to the primary hypersecretion of atrial natriuretic peptide (295, 377–379). This syndrome, called cerebral salt-wasting, is defined by hyponatremia accompanied by elevated urinary sodium excretion (often more than 150 mEq/l), excessive urine output, hypovolemia, suppressed vasopressin, and elevated atrial natriuretic peptide concentrations (>20 pmol/L). Thus, it is differentiated from SIADH, in which normal or decreased urine output, euvolemia, only modestly elevated urine sodium concentration, and elevated vasopressin concentration occur. Direct measurement of intravascular volume status with a central venous line is often helpful. The distinction is important because the therapies of the two disorders are markedly different. Treatment of patients with cerebral salt wasting consists of restoring intravascular volume with sodium chloride and water, as with the treatment of other causes of systemic dehydration. The underlying cause of the disorder, which is usually due to acute brain injury, should also be treated if possible.

D. Other Causes of True and Factitious Hyponatremia

True hyponatremia is associated with hyperglycemia, which causes the influx of water into the intravascular space. Serum sodium will decrease by 1.6 mEq/l for every 100 mg/dl increment in blood glucose above 100 mg/dl. Glucose is not ordinarily an osmotically active agent, and does not stimulate vasopressin release, probably because it is able to equilibrate freely across plasma membranes. However, in the presence of insulin deficiency and hyperglycemia, glucose acts as an osmotic agent presumably because its normal intracellular access to osmosensor sites is prevented (380). Under these circumstances, an osmotic

gradient exists, and this stimulates vasopressin release. In diabetic ketoacidosis, this, together with the hypovolemia caused by the osmotic diuresis secondary to glycosuria, results in marked stimulation of vasopressin secretion (381–384). Rapid correction of hyponatremia may follow soon after the institution of fluid and insulin therapy. Whether this contributes to the pathogenesis of cerebral edema occasionally seen following treatment of diabetic ketoacidosis is not known. Elevated concentrations of triglycerides may cause factitious hyponatremia, as can obtaining a blood sample downstream from an intravenous infusion of hypotonic fluid.

VI. CONCLUDING REMARKS

Precise regulation of water balance is necessary for the proper function of multiple cellular pathways. Vasopressin released from the posterior pituitary, stimulated by both hyperosmolar and nonosmotic factors, acts via the kidney V2 vasopressin receptor to stimulate both an increase in aquaporin-2 expression and its insertion into collecting duct luminal membrane, thereby enhancing renal water reabsorption to minimize subsequent water loss. Thirst controls the second major physiological response to hyperosmolality and results in increased water intake to make up for past water loss. The renin–angiotensin–aldosterone and atrial natriuretic peptide systems also make important contributions to water and volume regulation by modulating sodium intake and output.

The proper diagnosis of disorders caused by deficient and excessive action of vasopressin requires a thorough understanding of the physiological regulation of this hormone. Recent advances in molecular medicine have revealed mutations in the vasopressin gene, and the V2 receptor or aquaporin-2 genes, responsible for familial central and nephrogenic diabetes insipidus, respectively. Molecular methods allow the diagnosis of these disorders in the prenatal or early postnatal periods. Nevertheless, the most frequent cause of central diabetes insipidus remains a destructive lesion of the central nervous system caused by tumor or neurosurgical insult, and pharmacological toxicity remains the most common cause of nephrogenic diabetes insipidus.

Hyponatremia is a common occurrence in childhood, but is rarely due to a primary increase in vasopressin secretion (SIADH). It is more commonly caused by hypovolemia (either primary or secondary to decreased effective vascular volume), salt loss, excessive ingestion of hypotonic fluids, or cortisol deficiency. Hyponatremia due to increased vasopressin action is most commonly caused by excessive vasopressin administration during the treatment of central diabetes insipidus or coagulopathies.

Central diabetes insipidus is best treated in infants with fluid therapy, which avoids the administration of vasopressin or its V2 receptor analog, dDAVP. In older children, dDAVP is the drug of choice. Nephrogenic diabetes insipidus remains a therapeutic challenge. Hyponatremia due to SIADH is best managed by restricting water intake, whereas salt and water replacement are indicated when hyponatremia is due to hypovolemia or excessive secretion of atrial natriuretic peptide, as occurs in cerebral salt wasting. Hyponatremia causing central nervous system dysfunction is a medical emergency. Blood sodium must be raised promptly, but at a rate not greater than 0.5 mEq/l to avoid the occurrence of central pontine myelinolysis.

REFERENCES

1. Strange K. Regulation of solute and water balance and cell volume in the central nervous system (editorial). (Review). J Am Soc Nephrol 1992; 3:12–27.
2. Vokes TJ, Robertson GL. Disorders of antidiuretic hormone. (Review). Endocrinol Metab Clin North Am 1988; 17:281–299.
3. Du Vigneaud V, Gish DT, Katsoyannis PG. A synthetic preparation possessing biological properties associated with arginine-vasopressin. J Am Chem Soc 1954; 76:4751–4752.
4. Vavra I, et al. Effect of a synthetic analogue of vasopressin in animals and in patients with diabetes insipidus. Lancet 1968; 1:948–952.
5. Summar ML, et al. Linkage relationships of human arginine vasopressin–neurophysin-II and oxytocin-neurophysin-I to prodynorphin and other loci on chromosome 20. Mol Endocrinol 1990; 4:947–950.
6. Ruppert SD, Schere G, Schutz G. Recent gene conversion involving bovine vasopressin and oxytocin precursor genes suggested by nucleotide sequence. Nature 1984; 308:554–557.
7. Brownstein MJ, Russell JT, Gainer H. Synthesis, transport, and release of posterior pituitary hormones. Science 1980; 207:373–378.
8. Vandesande F, Dierickx K. Identification of the vasopressin producing and of the oxytocin producing neurons in the hypothalamic magnocellular neurosecretory system of the rat. Cell Tissue Res 1975; 164:153–162.
9. Whitnall MH, Mezey E, Gainer H. Co-localization of corticotropin-releasing factor and vasopressin in median eminence neurosecretory vesicles. Nature 1985; 317:248–252.
10. Sawchenko PE, Swanson LW, Vale WW. Co-expression of corticotropin-releasing factor and vasopressin immunoreactivity in parvocellular neurosecretory neurons of the adrenalectomized rat. Proc Natl Acad Sci USA 1984; 81:1883–1887.
11. Holm IA, Majzoub JA. Adrenocorticotrophin. In Melmed S, ed. The Pituitary. Cambridge: Blackwell Scientific, 1994.
12. Verney EB. The antidiuretic hormone and the factors which determine its release. Proc R Soc 1947; 135:25–105.
13. Robertson GL, Shelton RL, Athar S. The osmoregulation of vasopressin. Kidney Int 1976; 10:25–37.
14. Hammer M, Ladefoged J, Olgaard K. Relationships between plasma osmolality and plasma vasopressin in human subjects. Am J Physiol 1980; 238:E313–E317.
15. Leng G. Rat supraoptic neurones: the effects of locally applied hypertonic saline. J Physiol (Lond) 1980; 304:405–414.
16. Bealer SL, Crofton JT, Share L. Hypothalamic knife cuts alter fluid regulation, vasopressin secretion and natriuresis during water deprivation. Neuroendocrinology 1983; 36:364–370.
17. Thrasher TN, Keil LC, Ramsay DJ. Lesions of the organum vasculosum of the lamin terminalis (OVLT) attenuate osmotically-induced drinking and vasopressin secretion in the dog. Endocrinology 1982; 110:1837–1839.
18. McKinley MJ, Denton DA, Weisinger RS. Sensors for antidiuresis and thirst-osmoreceptors or CSF sodium detectors? Brain Res 1978; 141:89–103.
19. Phillips MI. Functions of angiotensin in the central nervous system. Annu Rev Physiol 1987; 49:413–435.
20. Simpson JB. The circumventricular organs and the central action of angiotensin. Neuroendocrinology 1981; 32:248–256.
21. Yamaguchi K, Koike M, Hama H. Plasma vasopressin response to peripheral administration of angiotensin in conscious rats. Am J Physiol 1985; 248:R249–R256.
22. Robertson GL. The regulation of vasopressin function in health and disease. Rec Progr Horm Res 1977; 33:333–385.
23. Davison JM, et al. Altered osmotic thresholds for vasopressin secretion and thirst in human pregnancy. Am J Physiol 1984; 246:F105–F109.
24. Linas SL, et al. Role of vasopressin in the impaired water excretion of glucocorticoid deficiency. Kidney Int 1980; 18:58–67.
25. Boykin J, et al. Role of plasma vasopressin in impaired water excretion of glucocorticoid deficiency. J Clin Invest 1978; 62:738–744.
26. Lindheimer MD, Barron WM, Davison JM. Osmoregulation of thirst and vasopressin release in pregnancy (published erratum appears in Am J Physiol 1989; 257(4 Pt 2):preceding F503). (Review). Am J Physiol 1989; 257:F159–F169.
27. Kucharczyk J, Morgenson GJ. Separate lateral hypothalamic pathways for extracellular and intracellular thirst. Am J Physiol 1975; 228:295–301.
28. Phillips PA, et al. Angiotensin II-induced thirst and vasopressin release in man. Clin Sci 1985; 68:669–674.
29. Gruber KA, Wilkin LD, Johnson AK. Neurohypophyseal hormone release and biosynthesis in rats with lesions of the anteroventral third ventricle (AV3V) region. Brain Res 1986; 378:115–119.
30. Thompson CJ, Burd JM, Baylis PH. Acute suppression of plasma vasopressin and thirst after drinking in hypernatremic humans. Am J Physiol 1987; 252:R1138–R1142.
31. Salata RA, Verbalis JG, Robinson AG. Cold water stimulation of oropharyngeal receptors in man inhibits release of vasopressin. J Clin Endocrinol Metab 1987; 65:561–567.
32. Williams TD, Seckl JR, Lightman SL. Dependent effect of drinking volume on vasopressin but not atrial peptide in humans. Am J Physiol 1989; 257:R762–R764.
33. Gauer OH, Henry JP. Circulatory basis of fluid volume control. Physiol Rev 1963; 43:423–481.
34. Thrasher TN. Baroreceptor regulation of vasopressin and renin secretion: low-pressure versus high-pressure receptors. (Review). Front Neuroendocrinol 1994; 15:157–196.
35. Cunningham ET Jr, Sawchenko PE. Reflex control of

magnocellular vasopressin and oxytocin secretion. (Review). Trends Neurosci 1991; 14:406–411.

36. Sawchenko PE, Swanson LW. Central noradrenergic pathways for the integration of hypothalamic neuroendocrine and autonomic responses. Science 1981; 214:685.

37. Blessing WW, Sved AF, Reis DJ. Destruction of noradrenergic neurons in rabbit brainstem. Science 1983; 217:661.

38. Schrier RW, Berl T, Harbottle JA. Mechanisms of the antidiuretic effect associated with interruption of parasympathetic pathways. J Clin Invest 1972; 51:2613.

39. Robertson GL. The regulation of vasopressin function in health and disease. (Review). Rec Progr Horm Res 1976; 33:333–385.

40. Robertson GL, Athar S. The interaction of blood osmolality and blood volume in regulating plasma vasopressin in man. J Clin Endocrinol Metab 1976; 42:613–620.

41. Goetz KL, Bond GC, Smith WE. Effect of moderate hemorrhage in humans on plasma ADH and renin. Proc Soc Exp Biol Med 1974; 145:277–280.

42. Arnauld E, et al. The effects of hypotension and hypovolaemia on the liberation of vasopressin during haemorrhage in the unanaesthetized monkey (Macaca mulatta). Pflugers Arch Eur J Physiol 1977; 371:193–200.

43. Wiggins RC, et al. Vasovagal hypotension and vasopressin release. Clin Endocrinol 1977; 6:387–393.

44. Murase T, Yoshida S. Effect of hypotension on levels of antidiuretic hormone in plasma in dogs. Endocrinol Japon 1971; 18:215–219.

45. Hirsch AT, et al. Contribution of vasopressin to blood pressure regulation during hypovolemic hypotension in humans. J Appl Physiol 1993; 75:1984–1988.

46. Feldman M, Samson WK, O'Dorisio TM. Apomorphine-induced nausea in humans: release of vasopressin and pancreatic polypeptide. Gastroenterology 1988; 95:721–726.

47. Koch KL, et al. Vasopressin and oxytocin responses to illusory self-motion and nausea in man. J Clin Endocrinol Metab 1990; 71:1269–1275.

48. Seckl JR, et al. Endogenous opioids inhibit oxytocin release during nicotine-stimulated secretion of vasopressin in man. Clin Endocrinol 1988; 28:509–514.

49. Oelkers W. Hyponatremia and inappropriate secretion of vasopressin (antidiuretic hormone) in patients with hypopituitarism (see comments). N Engl J Med 1989; 321:492–496.

50. Ishikawa S, et al. Role of antidiuretic hormone in hyponatremia in patients with isolated adrenocorticotropic hormone deficiency. Endocrinol Japon 1991; 38:325–330.

51. Green HH, Harrington AR, Valtin H. On the role of antidiuretic hormone in the inhibition of acute water diuresis in adrenal insufficiency and the effects of gluco- and mineralocorticoids in reversing the inhibition. J Clin Invest 1970; 49:1724–1736.

52. Viinamaki O, Erkkola R, Kanto J. Plasma vasopressin concentrations and serum vasopressinase activity in pregnant and nonpregnant women. Biol Res Pregnancy Perinatol 1986; 7:17–19.

53. Davison JM, et al. Changes in the metabolic clearance of vasopressin and in plasma vasopressinase throughout human pregnancy. J Clin Invest 1989; 83:1313–1318.

54. Iwasaki Y, et al. Aggravation of subclinical diabetes insipidus during pregnancy (see comments). N Engl J Med 1991; 324:522–526.

55. Kennedy S, et al. Transient diabetes insipidus and acute fatty liver of pregnancy. Br J Obstet Gynaecol 1994; 101:387–391.

56. Katz VL, Bowes WA Jr. Transient diabetes insipidus and preeclampsia. South Med J 1987; 80:524–525.

57. Durr JA, et al. Diabetes insipidus in pregnancy associated with abnormally high circulating vasopressinase activity. N Engl J Med 1987; 316:1070–1074.

58. Krege J, Katz VL, Bowes WA Jr. Transient diabetes insipidus of pregnancy. (Review). Obstet Gynecol Surv 1989; 44:789–795.

59. Davison JM, et al. Metabolic clearance of vasopressin and an analogue resistant to vasopressinase in human pregnancy. Am J Physiol 1993; 264:F348–F353.

60. Jard S. Vasopressin isoreceptors in mammals: relation to cyclic-AMP dependent and cyclic-AMP-independent transducer mechanisms. Curr Top Membr Transp 1983; 18:225–285.

61. Hirasawa A, et al. Cloning, functional expression and tissue distribution of human cDNA for the vascular-type vasopressin receptor. Biochem Biophys Res Commun 1994; 203:72–79.

62. Thibonnier M, et al. Molecular cloning, sequencing, and functional expression of a cDNA encoding the human V1a vasopressin receptor. J Biol Chem 1994; 269:3304–3310.

63. Morel A, et al. Molecular cloning and expression of a rat V1a arginine vasopressin receptor. Nature 1992; 356:523–526.

64. Ostrowski NL, et al. Expression of vasopressin V1a and V2 receptor messenger ribonucleic acid in the liver and kidney of embryonic, developing, and adult rats. Endocrinology 1993; 133:1849–1859.

65. Ostrowski NL, et al. Distribution of V1a and V2 vasopressin receptor messenger ribonucleic acids in rat liver, kidney, pituitary and brain. Endocrinology 1992; 131:533–535.

66. Takeuchi K, et al. Phosphoinositide hydrolysis and calcium mobilization induced by vasopressin and angiotensin II in cultured vascular smooth muscle cells. Tohoku J Exp Med 1992; 166:107–122.

67. Johnson EM, et al. Characterization of oscillations in cytosolic free Ca2+ concentration and measurement of cytosolic Na+ concentration changes evoked by angiotensin II and vasopressin in individual rat aortic smooth muscle cells. Use of microfluorometry and digital imaging. J Biol Chem 1991; 266:12618–12626.

68. Spruce BA, et al. The effect of vasopressin infusion on glucose metabolism in man. Clin Endocrinol 1985; 22:463–468.

69. Inaba K, et al. Characterization of human platelet vasopressin receptor and the relation between vasopressin-induced platelet aggregation and vasopressin binding to platelets. Clin Endocrinol 1988; 29:377–386.

70. Briley EM, et al. The cloned vasopressin V1a receptor stimulates phospholipase A2, phospholipase C, and phospholipase D through activation of receptor-operated calcium channels. Neuropeptides 1994; 27:63–74.

71. Montani JP, et al. Hemodynamic effects of exogenous and endogenous vasopressin at low plasma concentrations in conscious dogs. Circ Res 1980; 47:346–355.

72. Altura BM, Altura BT. Actions of vasopressin, oxytocin, and synthetic analogs on vascular smooth muscle. Fed Proc 1984; 43:80–86.

73. Rozen F, et al. Structure, characterization, and expression of the rat oxytocin receptor gene. Proc Natl Acad Sci USA 1995; 92:200–204.

74. Kimura T, et al. Structure and expression of a human oxytocin receptor. Nature 1992; 356:526–529.

75. Baertschi AJ, Friedli M. A novel type of vasopressin receptor on anterior pituitary corticotrophs. Endocrinology 1985; 116:499–502.

76. de Keyzer Y, et al. Cloning and characterization of the human V3 pituitary vasopressin receptor. FEBS Lett 1994; 356:215–220.

77. Sugimoto T, et al. Molecular cloning and functional expression of a cDNA encoding the human V1b vasopressin receptor. J Biol Chem 1994; 269:27088–27092.

78. Lolait SJ, et al. Cloning and characterization of a vasopressin V2 receptor and possible link to nephrogenic diabetes insipidus. Nature 1992; 357:336–339.

79. Hirsch AT, et al. Vasopressin-mediated forearm vasodilation in normal humans. Evidence for a vascular vasopressin V2 receptor. J Clin Invest 1989; 84:418–426.

80. Tagawa T, et al. Vasodilatory effect of arginine vasopressin is mediated by nitric oxide in human forearm vessels. J Clin Invest 1993; 92:1483–1490.

81. Kobrinsky NL, et al. Shortening of bleeding time by 1-deamino-8-D-arginine vasopressin in various bleeding disorders. Lancet 1984; 1:1145–1148.

82. Birnbaumer M, et al. Molecular cloning of the receptor for human antidiuretic hormone. Nature 1992; 357:333–335.

83. Seibold A, et al. Structure and chromosomal localization of the human antidiuretic hormone receptor gene. Am J Hum Genet 1992; 51:1078–1083.

84. Frattini A, et al. Type 2 vasopressin receptor gene, the gene responsible nephrogenic diabetes insipidus, maps to Xq28 close to the LICAM gene. Biochem Biophys Res Commun 1993; 193:864–871.

85. Harris HW, Paredes A, Zeidel ML. The molecular structure of the antidiuretic hormone elicited water channel. (Review). Pediatr Nephrol 1993; 7:680–684.

86. Harris HW, Strange K, Zeidel ML. Current understanding of the cellular biology and molecular structure of the antidiuretic hormone-stimulated water transport pathway. J Clin Invest 1991; 88:1–8.

87. Knepper MA. The aquaporin family of molecular water channels. Proc Natl Acad Sci USA 1994; 91:6255–6258.

88. Sasaki S, et al. Cloning, characterization, and chromosomal mapping of human aquaporin of collecting duct. J Clin Invest 1994; 93:1250–1256.

89. Deen PM, et al. Requirement of human renal water channel aquaporin-2 for vasopressin-dependent concentration of urine. Science 1994; 264:92–95.

90. Stevens AL, et al. Aquaporin 2 is a vasopressin-independent, constitutive apical membrane protein in rat vas deferens. Am J Physiol 2000; 278(4):C791–C802.

91. Nielsen S, et al. Cellular and subcellular immunolocalization of vasopressin-regulated water channel in rat kidney. Proc Natl Acad Sci USA 1993; 90:11663–11667.

92. Kanno K, et al. Urinary excretion of aquaporin-2 in patients with diabetes insipidus (see comments). N Engl J Med 1995; 332:1540–1545.

93. Gibbons GH, et al. Interaction of signals influencing renin release. (Review). Annu Rev Physiol 1984; 46:291–308.

94. Quinn SJ, Williams GH. Regulation of aldosterone secretion. Annu Rev Physiol 1988; 50:409–426.

95. Morris DJ. The metabolism and mechanism of action of aldosterone. (Review). Endocr Rev 1981; 2:234–247.

96. Dzau VJ. Molecular and physiological aspects of tissue renin-angiotensin system: emphasis on cardiovascular control. (Review). J Hypertens Suppl 1988; 6:S7–S12.

97. Chartier L, Schiffrin EL. Role of calcium in effects of atrial natriuretic peptide on aldosterone production in adrenal glomerulosa cells. Am J Physiol 1987; 252:E485–E491.

98. Chartier L, Schiffrin EL. Atrial natriuretic peptide inhibits the effect of endogenous angiotensin II on plasma aldosterone in conscious sodium-depleted rats. Clin Sci 1987; 72:31–35.

99. Chartier L, et al. Atrial natriuretic factor inhibits the stimulation of aldosterone secretion by angiotensin II, ACTH and potassium in vitro and angiotensin II-induced steroidogenesis in vivo. Endocrinology 1984; 115:2026–2028.

100. Hausdorff WP, Aguilera G, Catt KJ. Inhibitory actions of somatostatin on cyclic AMP and aldosterone production in agonist-stimulated adrenal glomerulosa cells. Cellular Signalling 1989; 1:377–386.

101. Rebuffat P, et al. Further studies on the involvement of dopamine and somatostatin in the inhibitory control of the growth and steroidogenic capacity of rat adrenal zona glomerulosa. Exp Clin Endocrinol 1989; 93:73–81.

102. Robba C, Mazzocchi G, Nussdorfer GG. Further studies on the inhibitory effects of somatostatin on the growth and steroidogenic capacity of rat adrenal zona glomerulosa. Exp Pathol 1986; 29:77–82.

103. Gallo-Payet N, et al. Dual effects of dopamine in rat adrenal glomerulosa cells. Biochem Biophys Res Commun 1990; 172:1100–1108.

104. Missale C, et al. Dopaminergic regulation of aldosterone secretion. Biochemical mechanisms and pharmacology. (Review). Am J Hypertens 1990; 3:93S–95S.

105. de Bold AJ. Tissue fractionation studies on the relationship between an atrial natriuretic factor and specific atrial granules. Can J Physiol Pharmacol 1982; 60:324–330.

106. de Bold AJ, et al. A rapid and potent natriuretic response to intravenous injection of atrial myocardial extract in rats. Life Sci 1981; 28:89–94.

107. Yandle TG. Biochemistry of natriuretic peptides. (Review). J Intern Med 1994; 235:561–576.

108. Hamid Q, et al. Localization of atrial natriuretic peptide mRNA and immunoreactivity in the rat heart and human atrial appendage. Proc Natl Acad Sci USA 1987; 84:6760–6764.

109. Inagaki S, et al. Atrial natriuretic peptide-like immunoreactivity in the rat pituitary: light and electron microscopic studies. Regul Peptides 1986; 14:101–111.

110. Ritter D, et al. Localization, synthetic regulation, and biology of renal atriopeptin-like prohormone. Am J Physiol 1992; 263:F503–F509.

111. Inagaki S, et al. Immunoreactive atrial natriuretic polypeptide in the adrenal medulla and sympathetic ganglia. Regul Peptides 1986; 15:249–260.

112. Imura H, Nakao K, Itoh H. The natriuretic peptide system in the brain: implications in the central control of cardiovascular and neuroendocrine functions. Front Neuroendocrinol 1992; 13:217–249.

113. Sudoh T, et al. A new natriuretic peptide in porcine brain. Nature 1988; 332:78–81.

114. Hasegawa K, et al. Ventricular expression of brain natriuretic peptide in hypertrophic cardiomyopathy. Circulation 1993; 88:372–380.

115. Yoshimura M, et al. Different secretion patterns of atrial natriuretic peptide and brain natriuretic peptide in patients with congestive heart failure. Circulation 1993; 87:464–469.

116. Hasegawa K, et al. Ventricular expression of atrial and brain natriuretic peptides in dilated cardiomyopathy. An immunohistocytochemical study of the endomyocardial biopsy specimens using specific monoclonal antibodies. Am J Pathol 1993; 142:107–116.

117. Sudoh T, et al. C-type natriuretic peptide (CNP): a new member of natriuretic peptide family identified in porcine brain. Biochem Biophys Res Commun 1990; 168:863–870.

118. Espiner EA. Physiology of natriuretic peptides. (Review). J Intern Med 1994; 235:527–541.

119. Cuneo RC, et al. Renal, hemodynamic, and hormonal responses to atrial natriuretic peptide infusions in normal man, and effect of sodium intake. J Clin Endocrinol Metab 1986; 63:946–953.

120. Espiner EA, et al. Studies on the secretion, metabolism and action of atrial natriuretic peptide in man. J Hypertens Suppl 1986; 4:S85–S91.

121. Cuneo RC, et al. Effect of physiological levels of atrial natriuretic peptide on hormone secretion: inhibition of angiotensin-induced aldosterone secretion and renin release in normal man. J Clin Endocrinol Metab 1987; 65:765–772.

122. Kimura T, et al. Effects of human atrial natriuretic peptide on renal function and vasopressin release. Am J Physiol 1986; 250:R789–R794.

123. Williams TD, et al. Atrial natriuretic peptide inhibits postural release of renin and vasopressin in humans. Am J Physiol 1988; 255:R368–R372.

124. Thrasher TN, Ramsay DJ. Interactions between vasopressin and atrial natriuretic peptides. (Review). Ann NY Acad Sci 1993; 689:426–437.

125. Wittert GA, et al. Atrial natriuretic factor reduces vasopressin and angiotensin II but not the ACTH response to acute hypoglycaemic stress in normal men. Clin Endocrinol 1993; 38:183–189.

126. Florkowski CM, et al. Renal, endocrine, and hemodynamic interactions of atrial and brain natriuretic peptides in normal men. Am J Physiol 1994; 266:R1244–R1250.

127. Greger NG, et al. Central diabetes insipidus. 22 years' experience. Am J Dis Child 1986; 140:551–554.

128. Wang LC, Cohen ME, Duffner PK. Etiologies of central diabetes insipidus in children. Pediatr Neurol 1994; 11:273–277.

129. Pedersen EB, et al. Familial cranial diabetes insipidus: a report of five families. Genetic, diagnostic and therapeutic aspects. Q J Med 1985; 57:883–896.

130. Os I, Aakesson I, Enger E. Plasma vasopressin in hereditary cranial diabetes insipidus. Acta Med Scand 1985; 217:429–434.

131. Toth EL, Bowen PA, Crockford PM. Hereditary central diabetes insipidus: plasma levels of antidiuretic hormone in a family with a possible osmoreceptor defect. Can Med Assoc J 1984; 131:1237–1241.

132. Nagai I, et al. Two cases of hereditary diabetes insipidus, with an autopsy finding in one. Acta Endocrinol 1984; 105:318–323.

133. Bergeron C, et al. Hereditary diabetes insipidus: an immunohistochemical study of the hypothalamus and pituitary gland. Acta Neuropathol 1991; 81:345–348.

134. Thompson CJ, et al. Vasopressin secretion in the DIDMOAD (Wolfram) syndrome. Q J Med 1989; 71:333–345.

135. Grosse Aldenhovel HB, Gallenkamp U, Suleman CA. Juvenile onset diabetes mellitus, central diabetes insipidus and optic atrophy (Wolfram syndrome)—neurological findings and prognostic implications. Neuropediatrics 1991; 22:103–106.

136. Rotig A, et al. Deletion of mitochondrial DNA in a case of early-onset diabetes mellitus, optic atrophy, and deafness (Wolfram syndrome, MIM 222300). J Clin Invest 1993; 91:1095–1098.

137. Jackson MJ, et al. Biochemical and molecular studies of mitochondrial function in diabetes insipidus, diabetes mellitus, optic atrophy, and deafness. Diabetes Care 1994; 17:728–733.

138. Polymeropoulos MH, Swift RG, Swift M. Linkage of the gene for Wolfram syndrome to markers on the short arm of chromosome 4. Nat Genet 1994; 8:95–97.

139. Inoue H, et al. A gene encoding a transmembrane protein is mutated in patients with diabetes mellitus and optic atrophy (Wolfram syndrome). Nat Genet 1998; 20:143–148.

140. Labib M, McPhate G, Marks V. Post-traumatic diabetes insipidus combined with primary polydipsia. Postgrad Med J 1987; 63:33–35.

141. Defoer F, et al. Posttraumatic diabetes insipidus. Acta Anaesth Belg 1987; 38:397–399.

142. Hadani M, et al. Unusual delayed onset of diabetes insipidus following closed head trauma. Case report. J Neurosurg 1985; 63:456–458.

143. Jenkins HR, Hughes IA, Gray OP. Cranial diabetes insipidus in early infancy. Arch Dis Childh 1988; 63:434–435.

144. Piech JJ, et al. [Twin pregnancy with acute hepatic steatosis followed by antehypophyseal insufficiency and diabetes insipidus]. (French). Presse Med 1985; 14:1421–1423.

145. Iwasaki Y, et al. Neurohypophyseal function in postpartum hypopituitarism: impaired plasma vasopressin response to osmotic stimuli. J Clin Endocrinol Metab 1989; 68:560–565.

146. Seckl JR, Dunger DB, Lightman SL. Neurohypophyseal peptide function during early postoperative diabetes insipidus. Brain 1987; 110:737–746.

147. Masera N, et al. Diabetes insipidus with impaired osmotic regulation in septo-optic dysplasia and agenesis of the corpus callosum. Arch Dis Childh 1994; 70:51–53.

148. Tawa R, et al. A case of Kabuki make-up syndrome with central diabetes insipidus and growth hormone neurosecretory dysfunction. Acta Paediatr Jpn 1994; 36:412–415.

149. Van Gool S, et al. Alobar holoprosencephaly, diabetes insipidus and coloboma without craniofacial abnormalities: a case report. Eur J Pediatr 1990; 149:621–622.

150. Yagi H, et al. Familial congenital hypopituitarism with central diabetes insipidus. J Clin Endocrinol Metab 1994; 78:884–889.

151. Villadsen AB, Pedersen EB. Recumbent cranial diabetes insipidus. Studies in a patient with adipsia, hypernatremia, poikilothermia and polyphagia. Acta Paediatr Scand 1987; 76:179–183.

152. Ono N, et al. Suprasellar germinomas; relationship between tumour size and diabetes insipidus. Acta Neurochir 1992; 114:26–32.

153. Tarng DC, Huang TP. Diabetes insipidus as an early sign of pineal tumor. Am J Nephrol 1995; 15:161–164.

154. Appignani B, Landy H, Barnes P. MR in idiopathic central diabetes insipidus of childhood. Am J Neuroradiol 1993; 14:American Jo–American 10.

155. Hung W, Fitz CR. The primary empty-sella syndrome and diabetes insipidus in a child. Acta Paediatr 1992; 81:459–461.

156. Eichhorn P, et al. [Diabetes insipidus in chronic myeloid leukemia. Remission of hypophyseal infiltration during busulfan treatment]. (German). Schweiz Med Wochenschr 1988; 118:275–279.

157. Puolakka K, Korhonen T, Lahtinen R. Diabetes insipidus in preleukaemic phase of acute myeloid leukaemia in 2 patients with empty sella turcica. A report of 2 cases. Scand J Haematol 1984; 32:364–366.

158. Foresti V, et al. Central diabetes insipidus due to acute monocytic leukemia: case report and review of the literature. (Review). J Endocrinol Invest 1992; 15:127–130.

159. de la Chapelle A, Lahtinen R. Monosomy 7 predisposes to diabetes insipidus in leukaemia and myelodysplastic syndrome. (Review). Eur J Haematol 1987; 39:404–411.

160. Kanabar DJ, et al. Monosomy 7, diabetes insipidus and acute myeloid leukemia in childhood. Pediatr Hematol Oncol 1994; 11:111–114.

161. La Starza R, et al. 3q aberration and monosomy 7 in ANLL presenting with high platelet count and diabetes insipidus. Haematologica 1994; 79:356–359.

162. Ra'anani P, et al. Acute leukemia relapse presenting as central diabetes insipidus. (Review). Cancer 1994; 73:2312–2316.

163. Dunger DB, et al. The frequency and natural history of diabetes insipidus in children with Langerhans-cell histiocytosis. N Engl J Med 1989; 321:1157–1162.

164. Grois N, et al. Diabetes insipidus in Langerhans cell histiocytosis: results from the DAL-HX 83 study. Med Pediatr Oncol 1995; 24:248–256.

165. Broadbent V, et al. Anterior pituitary function and computed tomography/magnetic resonance imaging in patients with Langerhans cell histiocytosis and diabetes insipidus. Med Pediatr Oncol 1993; 21:649–654.

166. Tien RD, et al. Thickened pituitary stalk on MR images in patients with diabetes insipidus and Langerhans cell histiocytosis. Am J Neuroradiol 1990; 11: American Jo–American J8.

167. Minehan KJ, et al. Radiation therapy for diabetes insipidus caused by Langerhans cell histiocytosis (see comments). Int J Radiat Oncol Biol Phys 1992; 23:519–524.

168. Imura H, et al. Lymphocytic infundibuloneurohypophysitis as a cause of central diabetes insipidus. N Engl J Med 1993; 329:683–689.

169. Paja M, et al. Lymphocytic hypophysitis causing hypopituitarism and diabetes insipidus, and associated with autoimmune thyroiditis, in a non-pregnant woman. Postgrad Med J 1994; 70:220–224.

170. Koshiyama H, et al. Lymphocytic hypophysitis presenting with diabetes insipidus: case report and literature review. (Review). Endocr J 1994; 41:93–97.

171. Kojima H, et al. Diabetes insipidus caused by lymphocytic infundibuloneurohypophysitis. Arch Pathol Lab Med 1989; 113:1399–1401.

172. Ahmed SR, et al. Necrotizing infundibulo-hypophysitis: a unique syndrome of diabetes insipidus and hypopituitarism. J Clin Endocrinol Metab 1993; 76:1499–1504.

173. Rossi GP, et al. Bronchocentric granulomatosis and central diabetes insipidus successfully treated with corticosteroids. Eur Respir J 1994; 7:1893–1898.

174. Lewis R, Wilson J, Smith FW. Diabetes insipidus secondary to intracranial sarcoidosis confirmed by low-field magnetic resonance imaging. Magnet Reson Med 1987; 5:466–470.

175. Scherbaum WA, et al. Autoimmune cranial diabetes insipidus: its association with other endocrine diseases and with histiocytosis X. Clin Endocrinol 1986; 25:411–420.

176. De Bellis A, et al. Detection of vasopressin cell antibodies in some patients with autoimmune endocrine diseases without overt diabetes insipidus. Clin Endocrinol 1994; 40:173–177.

177. Vokes TJ, Gaskill MB, Robertson GL. Antibodies to vasopressin in patients with diabetes insipidus. Implications for diagnosis and therapy. Ann Intern Med 1988; 108:190–195.

178. Christensen C, Bank A. Meningococcal meningitis and diabetes insipidus. Scand J Infect Dis 1988; 20:341–343.

179. Sloane AE. Transient diabetes insipidus following listeria meningitis. Irish Med J 1989; 82:132–134.

180. Brandle M, et al. [Cerebral toxoplasmosis with central diabetes insipidus and panhypopituitarism in a patient with AIDS]. (German). Schweiz Med Wochenschr 1995; 125:684–687.

181. Mena W, et al. Diabetes insipidus associated with symptomatic congenital cytomegalovirus infection. J Pediatr 1993; 122:911–913.

182. Watanabe A, et al. Central diabetes insipidus caused by nonspecific chronic inflammation of the hypothalamus: case report. Surgic Neurol 1994; 42:70–73.

183. Arisaka O, et al. Central diabetes insipidus in hypoxic brain damage. Childs Nerv Syst 1992; 8:81–82.

184. Outwater KM, Rockoff MA. Diabetes insipidus accompanying brain death in children. Neurology 1984; 34:1243–1246.

185. Fiser DH, et al. Diabetes insipidus in children with brain death. Crit Care Med 1987; 15:551–553.

186. Barzilay Z, Somekh E. Diabetes insipidus in severely brain damaged children. J Med 1988; 19:47–64.

187. Hohenegger M, et al. Serum vasopressin (AVP) levels in polyuric brain-dead organ donors. Eur Arch Psychiatry Neurol Sci 1990; 239:267–269.

188. Durr JA. Diabetes insipidus in pregnancy. (Review). Am J Kidney Dis 1987; 9:276–283.

189. Hadi HA, Mashini IS, Devoe LD. Diabetes insipidus during pregnancy complicated by preeclampsia. A care report. J Reprod Med 1985; 30:206–208.

190. Harper M, et al. Vasopressin-resistant diabetes insipidus, liver dysfunction, hyperuricemia and decreased renal function. A case report. J Reprod Med 1987; 32:862–865.

191. Frenzer A, et al. [Triplet pregnancy with HELLP syndrome and transient diabetes insipidus]. (German). Schweiz Med Wochenschr 1994; 124:687–691.

192. Kleeman CR, et al. Studies on alcohol diuresis. II. The evaluation of ethyl alcohol as an inhibitor of the neurohypophysis. J Clin Invest 1955; 34:448–455.

193. Tata PS, Buzalkov R. Vasopressin studies in the rat. III. Inability of ethanol anesthesia to prevent ADH secretion due to pain and hemorrhage. Pfluegers Arch 1966; 290:294–297.

194. Miller M, Moses AM. Clinical states due to alteration of ADH release and action. In Moses AM, Share L, eds. Neurohypophysis. Basel: Karger, 1977:153–166.

195. Sklar AH, Schrier RW. Central nervous system mediators of vasopressin release. Physiol Rev 1983; 63:1243–1280.

196. Frasier SD, et al. A water deprivation test for the diagnosis of diabetes insipidus in children. Am J Dis Child 1967; 114:157–160.

197. Richman RA, et al. Simplifying the diagnosis of diabetes insipidus in children. Am J Dis Child 1981; 135:839–841.

198. Koskimies O, Pylkkanen J. Water intoxication in infants caused by the urine concentration test with the vasopressin analogue (DDAVP). Acta Paediatr Scand 1984; 73: 131–132.

199. Bichet DG. Molecular and cellular biology of vasopressin and oxytocin receptors and action in the kidney. (Review). Curr Opin Nephrol Hypertens 1994; 3:46–53.

200. Milles JJ, Spruce B, Baylis PH. A comparison of diagnostic methods to differentiate diabetes insipidus from primary polyuria: a review of 21 patients. Acta Endocrinol 1983; 104:410–416.

201. Zerbe RL, Robertson GL. A comparison of plasma vasopressin measurements with a standard indirect test in the differential diagnosis of polyuria. N Engl J Med 1981; 305:1539–1546.

202. Andersson B, Leksell LG, Rundgren M. Regulation of water intake. (Review). Annu Rev Nutr 1982; 2:73–89.

203. Papapostolou C, et al. Imaging of the sella in the syndrome of inappropriate secretion of antidiurectic hormone. J Intern Med 1995; 237:181–185.

204. Moses AM, Clayton B, Hochhauser L. Use of T1-weighted MR imaging to differentiate between primary polydipsia and central diabetes insipidus (comment) (see comments). Am J Neuroradiol 1992; 13:J7.

205. Maghnie M, et al. Correlation between magnetic resonance imaging of posterior pituitary and neurohypophyseal function in children with diabetes insipidus. J Clin Endocrinol Metab 1992; 74:795–800.

206. Halimi P, et al. Post-traumatic diabetes insipidus: MR demonstration of pituitary stalk rupture. J Comput Assist Tomogr 1988; 12:135–137.

207. Maghnie M, et al. Evolving pituitary hormone deficiency is associated with pituitary vasculopathy: dynamic MR study in children with hypopituitarism, diabetes insipidus, and Langerhans cell histiocytosis. Radiology 1994; 193: 493–499.

208. Sato N, et al. Posterior lobe of the pituitary in diabetes insipidus: dynamic MR imaging. Radiology 1993; 186: 357–360.

209. Uribarri J, Kaskas M. Hereditary nephrogenic diabetes insipidus and bilateral nonobstructive hydronephrosis. (Review). Nephron 1993; 65:346–349.

210. Seow WK, Thomsett MJ. Dental fluorosis as a complication of hereditary diabetes insipidus: studies of six affected patients (see comments). Pediatr Dent 1994; 16: 128–132.

211. Crigler JF Jr. Commentary: on the use of pitressin in infants with neurogenic diabetes insipidus. J Pediatr 1976; 88:295–296.

212. Davidson S, Frand M, Rotem Y. Primary polydipsia in infancy: a benign disorder simulating diabetes insipidus. Clin Pediatr 1978; 17:419–420.

213. Jakobsson B, Berg U. Effect of hydrochlorothiazide and indomethacin treatment on renal function in nephrogenic diabetes insipidus. Acta Paediatr 1994; 83:522–525.

214. McDonald JA, et al. Treatment of the young child with postoperative central diabetes insipidus. Am J Dis Child 1989; 143:201–204.

215. Ralston C, Butt W. Continuous vasopressin replacement in diabetes insipidus. Arch Dis Childh 1990; 65:896–897.

216. Muglia LJ, Majzoub JA. Diabetes insipidus. In Burg F, Inglefinger J, Wald E, eds. Gellis and Kagan's Current Pediatric Therapy 14. Philadelphia: WB Saunders, 1993: 318–319.

217. Aylward PE, et al. Effects of vasopressin on the circula-

tion and its baroreflex control in healthy men. Circulation 1986; 73:1145–1154.

218. Andersen LJ, et al. Antidiuretic effect of subnormal levels of arginine vasopressin in normal humans. Am J Physiol 1990; 259:R53–R60.

219. Seckl JR, et al. Vasopressin antagonist in early postoperative diabetes insipidus. Lancet 1990; 335:1353–1356.

220. Moreno-Sanchez D, et al. Rhabdomyolysis and cutaneous necrosis following intravenous vasopressin infusion. (Review). Gastroenterology 1991; 101:529–532.

221. Pierce ST, Nickl N. Rhabdomyolysis associated with the use of intravenous vasopressin. Am J Gastroenerol 1993; 88:424–427.

222. Mauro VF, et al. Torsade de pointes in a patient receiving intravenous vasopressin. Crit Care Med 1988; 16:200–201.

223. Smith TJ, et al. Hyponatremia and seizures in young children given DDAVP. Am J Hematol 1989; 31:199–202.

224. Bryant WP, et al. Aqueous vasopressin infusion during chemotherapy in patients with diabetes insipidus. Cancer 1994; 74:2589–2592.

225. Williams TD, et al. Antidiuretic effect and pharmacokinetics of oral 1-desamino-8-D-arginine vasopressin. 1. Studies in adults and children. J Clin Endocrinol Metab 1986; 63:129–132.

226. Cunnah D, Ross G, Besser GM. Management of cranial diabetes insipidus with oral desmopressin (DDAVP). Clin Endocrinol 1986; 24:253–257.

227. Stick SM, Betts PR. Oral desmopressin in neonatal diabetes insipidus. Arch Dis Childh 1987; 62:1177–1178.

228. Pivonello R, et al. Impairment of bone status in patients with central diabetes insipidus. J Clin Endocrinol Metab 1998; 83:2275–2280.

229. Rittig S, et al. Abnormal diurnal rhythm of plasma vasopressin and urinary output in patients with enuresis. Am J Physiol 1989; 256:F664–F671.

230. Wille S, et al. Plasma and urinary levels of vasopressin in enuretic and nonenuretic children. Scand J Urol Nephrol 1994; 28:119–122.

231. Terho P, Kekomaki M. Management of nocturnal enuresis with a vasopressin analogue. J Urol 1984; 131:925–927.

232. Evans JH, Meadow SR. Desmopressin for bed wetting: length of treatment, vasopressin secretion, and response (see comments). Arch Dis Childh 1992; 67:184–188.

233. Steffens J, et al. Vasopressin deficiency in primary nocturnal enuresis. Results of a controlled prospective study. Eur Urol 1993; 24:366–370.

234. Moses AM, Sangani G, Miller JL. Proposed cause of marked vasopressin resistance in a female with an X-linked recessive V2 receptor abnormality. J Clin Endocrinol Metab 1995; 80:1184–1186.

235. Kobrinsky NL, et al. Absent factor VIII response to synthetic vasopressin analogue (DDAVP) in nephrogenic diabetes insipidus. Lancet 1985; 1:1293–1294.

236. Bichet DG, et al. Hemodynamic and coagulation responses to 1-desamino[8-D-arginine] vasopressin in patients with congenital nephrogenic diabetes insipidus. N Engl J Med 1988; 318:881–887.

237. Knoers VV, et al. Evidence for intact V1-vasopressin receptors in congenital nephrogenic diabetes insipidus. Eur J Pediatr 1992; 151:381–383.

238. Brink HS, et al. 1-Desamino-8-D-arginine vasopressin (DDAVP) in patients with congenital nephrogenic diabetes insipidus. Neth J Med 1993; 43:5–12.

239. Ohzeki T. Urinary adenosine 3′,5′-monophosphate (cAMP) response to antidiuretic hormone in diabetes in-

sipidus (DI): comparison between congenital nephrogenic DI type 1 and 2, and vasopressin sensitive DI. Acta Endocrinol 1985; 108:485–490.

240. Bichet DG, et al. Epinephrine and dDAVP administration in patients with congenital nephrogenic diabetes insipidus. Evidence for a pre-cyclic AMP V2 receptor defective mechanism. Kidney Int 1989; 36:859–866.

241. Moses AM, et al. Evidence for normal antidiuretic responses to endogenous and exogenous arginine vasopressin in patients with guanine nucleotide-binding stimulatory protein-deficient pseudohypoparathyroidism. J Clin Endocrinol Metab 1986; 62:221–224.

242. Knoers N, Monnens LA. Nephrogenic diabetes insipidus: clinical symptoms, pathogenesis, genetics and treatment. (Review). Pediatr Nephrol 1992; 6:476–482.

243. Vest M, Talbot NB, Crawford JD. Hypocaloric dwarfism and hydronephrosis in diabetes insipidus. Am J Dis Child 1963; 105:175–181.

244. Macaulay D, Watson M. Hypernatremia in infants as a cause of brain damage. Arch Dis Childh 1967; 42:485–491.

245. Van Lieburg AF, Knoers NV, Monnens LA. Clinical presentation and follow-up of 30 patients with congenital nephrogenic diabetes insipidus. J Am Soc Nephrol 1999; 10:1958–1964.

246. Freycon MT, Lavocat MP, Freycon F. [Familial nephrogenic diabetes insipidus with chronic hypernatremia and cerebral calcifications]. (Review). (French). Pediatrie 1988; 43:409–413.

247. Nozue T, et al. Intracranial calcifications associated with nephrogenic diabetes insipidus (see comments). Pediatr Nephrol 1993; 7:74–76.

248. Schofer O, et al. Nephrogenic diabetes insipidus and intracerebral calcification. Arch Dis Childh 1990; 65:885–887.

249. Tohyama J, et al. Intracranial calcification in siblings with nephrogenic diabetes insipidus: CT and MRI. Neuroradiology 1993; 35:553–555.

250. Bode HH, Crawford JD. Nephrogenic diabetes insipidus in North America. The Hopewell hypothesis. N Engl J Med 1969; 280:750–754.

251. Rosenthal W, et al. Molecular identification of the gene responsible for congenital nephrogenic diabetes insipidus. Nature 1992; 359:233–235.

252. Bichet DG, et al. Nature and recurrence of AVPR2 mutations in X-linked nephrogenic diabetes insipidus. Am J Hum Genet 1994; 55:278–286.

253. Bichet DG, et al. X-linked nephrogenic diabetes insipidus: from the ship Hopewell to RFLP studies. Am J Hum Genet 1992; 51:1089–1102.

254. Birnbaumer M, Gilbert S, Rosenthal W. An extracellular congenital nephrogenic diabetes insipidus mutation of the vasopressin receptor reduces cell surface expression, affinity for ligand, and coupling to the Gs/adenylyl cyclase system. Mol Endocrinol 1994; 8:886–894.

255. Holtzman EJ, et al. Mutations in the vasopressin V2 receptor gene in two families with nephrogenic diabetes insipidus. J Am Soc Nephrol 1994; 5:169–176.

256. Holtzman EJ, et al. A Null mutation in the vasopressin V2 receptor gene (AVPR2) associated with nephrogenic diabetes insipidus in the Hopewell kindred. Human Mol Genet 1933; 2:1201–1204.

257. Knoers NV, et al. Inheritance of mutations in the V2 receptor gene in thirteen families with nephrogenic diabetes insipidus. Kidney Int 1994; 46:170–176.

258. Yuasa H, et al. Novel mutations in the V2 vasopressin receptor gene in two pedigrees with congenital nephrogenic diabetes insipidus. J Clin Endocrinol Metab 1994; 79:361–365.

259. Oksche A, et al. Two novel mutations in the vasopressin V2 receptor gene in patients with congenital nephrogenic diabetes insipidus [published erratum appears in Biochem Biophys Res Commun 1995 Feb 27; 207(3):1059]. Biochem Biophys Res Commun 1994; 205:552–557.

260. Pan Y, et al. Mutations in the V2 vasopressin receptor gene are associated with X-linked nephrogenic diabetes insipidus. Nature Genet 1992; 2:103–106.

261. Tsukaguchi H, et al. Two novel mutations in the vasopressin V2 receptor gene in unrelated Japanese kindreds with nephrogenic diabetes insipidus. Biochem Biophys Res Commun 1993; 197:1000–1010.

262. van de Ouweland AM, et al. Mutations in the vasopressin type 2 receptor gene (AVPR2) associated with nephrogenic diabetes insipidus. Nat Genet 1992; 2:99–102.

263. Wenkert D, et al. Novel mutations in the V2 vasopressin receptor gene of patients with X-linked nephrogenic diabetes insipidus. Human Mol Genet 1994; 3:1429–1430.

264. Wildin RS, et al. Heterogeneous AVPR2 gene mutations in congenital nephrogenic diabetes insipidus. Am J Human Genet 1994; 55:266–277.

265. Pan Y, Wilson P, Gitschier J. The effect of eight V2 vasopressin receptor mutations on stimulation of adenylyl cyclase and binding to vasopressin. J Biol Chem 1994; 269:31933–31937.

266. Rosenthal W, et al. Nephrogenic diabetes insipidus. A V2 vasopressin receptor unable to stimulate adenylyl cyclase. J Biol Chem 1993; 268:13030–13033.

267. Rosenthal W, et al. Mutations in the vasopressin V2 receptor gene in families with nephrogenic diabetes insipidus and functional expression of the Q-2 mutant. Cell Mol Biol 1994; 40:429–436.

268. Friedman E, et al. Nephrogenic diabetes insipidus: an X chromosome-linked dominant inheritance pattern with a vasopressin type 2 receptor gene that is structurally normal. Proc Nat Acad Sci USA 1994; 91:8457–8461.

269. Oksche A, Rosenthal W. The molecular basis of nephrogenic diabetes insipidus. J Mol Med 1998; 76(5):326–337.

270. Waring AJ, Kajdi L, Tappan V. A congenital defect of water metabolism. Am J Dis Child 1945; 69:323.

271. Langley JM, et al. Autosomal recessive inheritance of vasopressin-resistant diabetes insipidus. Am J Med Genet 1991; 38:90–94.

272. Knoers N, Monnens LA. A variant of nephrogenic diabetes insipidus: V2 receptor abnormality restricted to the kidney. Eur J Pediatr 1991; 150:370–373.

273. Mulders SM, et al. An aquaporin-2 water channel mutant which causes autosomal dominant nephrogenic diabetes insipidus is retained in the Golgi complex. J Clin Invest 1998; 102:57–66.

274. Boton R, Gaviria M, Batlle DC. Prevalence, pathogenesis, and treatment of renal dysfunction associated with chronic lithium therapy. (Review). Am J Kidney Dis 1987; 10:329–345.

275. Bendz H, et al. Kidney damage in long-term lithium patients: a cross-sectional study of patients with 15 years or more on lithium. Nephrol Dialysis Transplant 1994; 9:1250–1254.

276. Yamaki M, et al. Cellular mechanism of lithium-induced nephrogenic diabetes insipidus in rats. Am J Physiol 1991; 261:F505–F511.

277. Marples D, et al. Lithium-induced downregulation of aquaporin-2 water channel expression in rat kidney medulla. J Clin Invest 1995; 95:1838–1845.

278. Hirji MR, Mucklow JC. Transepithelial water movement in response to carbamazepine, chlorpropamide and demeclocycline in toad urinary bladder. Br J Pharmacol 1991; 104:550–553.

279. Navarro JF, et al. Nephrogenic diabetes insipidus and renal tubular acidosis secondary to foscarnet therapy. Am J Kidney Dis 1996; 27:431–434.

280. Bendz H, Aurell M. Drug-induced diabetes insipidus: incidence, prevention and management. Drug Safety 1999; 21:449–456.

281. Hohler T, et al. Indomethacin treatment in amphotericin B induced nephrogenic diabetes insipidus. Clin Invest 1994; 72:769–771.

282. Vigeral P, et al. Nephrogenic diabetes insipidus and distal tubular acidosis in methicillin-induced interstitial nephritis. Adv Exp Med Biol 1987; 212:129–134.

283. Quinn BP, Wall BM. Nephrogenic diabetes insipidus and tubulointerstitial nephritis during continuous therapy with rifampin. Am J Kidney Dis 1989; 14:217–220.

284. Kato A, et al. Nephrogenic diabetes insipidus associated with bilateral ureteral obstruction. Intern Med 1994; 33:231–233.

285. Nagayama Y, et al. Acquired nephrogenic diabetes insipidus secondary to distal renal tubular acidosis and nephrocalcinosis associated with Sjogren's syndrome. J Endocrinol Invest 1994; 17:659–663.

286. Hartenberg MA, Cory M, Chan JC. Nephrogenic diabetes insipidus. Radiological and clinical features. Int J Pediatr Nephrol 1985; 6:281–286.

287. Alon U, Chan JC. Hydrochlorothiazide-amiloride in the treatment of congenital nephrogenic diabetes insipidus. Am J Nephrol 1985; 5:9–13.

288. Libber S, Harrison H, Spector D. Treatment of nephrogenic diabetes insipidus with prostaglandin synthesis inhibitors. J Pediatr 1986; 108:305–311.

289. Rascher W, et al. Congenital nephrogenic diabetes insipidus-vasopressin and prostaglandins in response to treatment with hydrochlorothiazide and indomethacin. Pediatr Nephrol 1987; 1:485–490.

290. Vierhapper H, et al. Comparative therapeutic benefit of indomethacin, hydrochlorothiazide, and acetyl-salicylic acid in a patient with nephrogenic diabetes insipidus. Acta Endocrinol 1984; 106:311–316.

291. Uyeki TM, et al. Successful treatment with hydrochlorothiazide and amiloride in an infant with congenital nephrogenic diabetes insipidus. Pediatr Nephrol 1993; 7:554–556.

292. Batlle DC, et al. Amelioration of polyuria by amiloride in patients receiving long-term lithium therapy. N Engl J Med 1985; 312:408–414.

293. Weinstock, RS, Moses AM. Desmopressin and indomethacin therapy for nephrogenic diabetes insipidus in patients receiving lithium carbonate. South Med J 1990; 83:1475–1477.

294. Assadi FK, John EG. Hypouricemia in neonates with syndrome of inappropriate secretion of antidiuretic hormone. Pediatr Res 1985; 19:424–427.

295. Ganong CA, Kappy MS. Cerebral salt wasting in children. The need for recognition and treatment [published erratum appears in AM J Dis Child 1993 Apr; 147(4):369]. Am J Dis Child 1993; 147:167–169.

296. Medani CR. Seizures and hypothermia due to dietary water intoxication in infants. South Med J 1987; 80:421–425.

297. Kovacs L, et al. Renal response to arginine vasopressin in premature infants with late hyponatraemia. Arch Dis Childh 1986; 61:1030–1032.

298. Robertson GL. Dipsogenic diabetes insipidus: a newly recognized syndrome caused by a selective defect in the osmoregulation of thirst. Trans Assoc Am Physicians 1987; 100:241–249.

299. Dingman JF, Despointes RH. Adrenal steroid inhibition of vasopressin release from the neurohypophysis of normal subjects and patients with Addison's disease. J Clin Invest 1960; 39:1851–1863.

300. Ahmed AB, et al. Increased plasma arginine vasopressin in clinical adrenocortical insufficiency and its inhibition by glucosteroids. J Clin Invest 1967; 46:111–123.

301. Iwasaki Y, et al. Positive and negative regulation of the rat vasopressin gene promoter. Endocrinology 1997; 138:5266–5274.

302. Kleeman CR, Czaczkes JW, Cutler R. Mechanisms of impaired water excretion in adrenal and pituitary insufficiency. IV. Antidiuretic hormone in primary and secondary adrenal insufficiency. J Clin Invest 1964; 43:1641–1648.

303. Kamoi K, et al. Hyponatremia and osmoregulation of thirst and vasopressin secretion in patients with adrenal insufficiency. J Clin Endocrinol Metab 1993; 77:1584–1588.

304. Laczi F, et al. Osmoregulation of arginine-8-vasopressin secretion in primary hypothyroidism and in Addison's disease. Acta Endocrinol 1987; 114:389–395.

305. Bouley R, et al. Nitric oxide and atrial natriuretic factor stimulate cGMP-dependent membrane insertion of aquaporin 2 in renal epithelial cells. J Clin Invest 2000; 106(9):1115–1126.

306. Wallerath T, et al. Down-regulation of the expression of endothelial NO synthase is likely to contribute to glucocorticoid-mediated hypertension. Proc Natl Acad Sci USA 1999; 96(23):13357–13362.

307. Schwartz MJ, Kokko JP. Urinary concentrating defect of adrenal insufficiency. Permissive role of adrenal steroids on the hydroosmotic response across the rabbit cortical collecting tubule. J Clin Invest 1980; 66:234–242.

308. Schrier RW, Berl T. Nonosmolar factors affecting renal water excretion (first of two parts). (Review). N Engl J Med 1975; 292:81–88.

309. Iwasaki Y, et al. Osmoregulation of plasma vasopressin in myxedema. J Clin Endocrinol Metab 1990; 70:534–539.

310. Discala VA, Kinney MJ. Effects of myxedema in the renal diluting and concentrating mechanism. Am J Med 1971; 50:325–335.

311. Michael UF, et al. Renal handling of sodium and water in the hypothyroid rat. Clearance and micropuncture studies. J Clin Invest 1972; 51:1405–1412.

312. Yount E, Little JM. Renal clearance in patients with myxedema. J Clin Endocrinol Metab 1955; 15:343–346.

313. Iwasaki Y, et al. Osmoregulation of plasma vasopressin in three cases with adrenal insufficiency of diverse etiologies. Horm Res 1997; 47:38–44.

314. Yamada K, Tamura Y, Yoshida S. Effect of administration of corticotropin-releasing hormone and glucocorticoid on arginine vasopressin response to osmotic stimulus in normal subjects and patients with hypocorticotropinism without overt diabetes insipidus. J Clin Endocrinol Metab 1989; 69:396–401.

315. Kamiyama T, et al. Carbamazepine-induced hyponatremia in a patient with partial central diabetes insipidus. Nephron 1993; 64:142–145.

316. Van Amelsvoort T, et al. Hyponatremia associated with carbamazepine and oxcarbazepine therapy: a review. (Review). Epilepsia 1994; 35:181–188.

317. Lozada ES, et al. Studies of the mode of action of the sulfonylureas and phenylacetamides in enhancing the effect of vasopressin. J Clin Endocrinol Metab 1972; 34: 704–712.

318. Moses AM, Numann AM, Miller M. Mechanism of chlorpropamide-induced antidiuresis in man: evidence for release of ADH and enhancement of peripheral action. Metabolism 1973; 22:59–66.

319. Bressler RB, Huston DP. Water intoxication following moderate-dose intravenous cyclophosphamide. Arch Intern Med 1985; 145:548–459.

320. Harlow PJ, et al. A fatal case of inappropriate ADH secretion induced by cyclophosphamide therapy. Cancer 1979; 44:896–898.

321. Larose P, Ong H, du Souich P. The effect of cyclophosphamide on arginine vasopressin and the atrial natriuretic factor. Biochem Biophys Res Commun 1987; 143:140–144.

322. Bode U, Seif SM, Levin AS. Studies on the antidiuretic effect of cyclophosphamide: vasopressin release and sodium excretion. Med Pediatr Oncol 1980; 8:295–303.

323. Zavagli G, et al. Life-threatening hyponatremia caused by vinblastine. Med Oncol Tumor Pharmacother 1988; 5:67–69.

324. Ritch PS. Cis-dichlorodiammineplatinum II-induced syndrome of inappropriate secretion of antidiuretic hormone. Cancer 1988; 61:448–450.

325. Hutchison FN, et al. Renal salt wasting in patients treated with cisplatin. Ann Intern Med 1988; 108:21–25.

326. Judd BA, et al. Hyponatraemia in premature babies and following surgery in older children. Acta Paediatr Scand 1987; 76:385–393.

327. Gerigk M, et al. Clinical settings and vasopressin function in hyponatraemic children. Eur J Pediatr 1993; 152:301–305.

328. Anderson RJ, et al. Hyponatremia: a prospective analysis of its epidemiology and the pathogenetic role of vasopressin. Ann Intern Med 1985; 102:164–168.

329. Kanakriyeh M, Carvajal HF, Vallone AM. Initial fluid therapy for children with meningitis with consideration of the syndrome of inappropriate anti-diuretic hormone. Clin Pediatr 1987; 26:126–130.

330. Padilla G, et al. Vasopressin levels in infants during the course of aseptic and bacterial meningitis (see comments). Am J Dis Child 1991; 145:991–993.

331. Powell KR, et al. Normalization of plasma arginine vasopressin concentrations when children with meningitis are given maintenance plus replacement fluid therapy (see comments). J Pediatr 1990; 117:515–522.

332. Vingerhoets F, de Tribolet N. Hyponatremia hypo-osmolarity in neurosurgical patients. "Appropriate secretion of ADH" and "cerebral salt wasting syndrome." Acta Neurochir 1988; 91:50–54.

333. Zanardo V, et al. Plasma arginine vasopressin, diuresis, and neonatal respiratory distress syndrome. Padiatr Padol 1989; 24:297–302.

334. Potts FL, May RB. Early syndrome of inappropriate secretion of antidiuretic hormone in a child with burn injury. Ann Emerg Med 1986; 15:834–835.

335. Kojima T, et al. Changes in vasopressin, atrial natriuretic factor, and water homeostasis in the early stage of bronchopulmonary dysplasia. Pediatr Res 1990; 27:260–263.

336. Rao M, et al. Antidiuretic hormone response in children with bronchopulmonary dysplasia during episodes of acute respiratory distress. Am J Dis Child 1986; 140:825–828.

337. Sulyok E, et al. Late hyponatremia in premature infants: role of aldosterone and arginine vasopressin. J Pediatr 1985; 106:990–994.

338. Stegner H, et al. Urinary arginine-vasopressin (AVP) excretion in cystic fibrosis (CF). Acta Endocrinol Suppl 1986; 279:448–451.

339. Cohen LF, et al. The syndrome of inappropriate antidiuretic hormone secretion as a cause of hyponatremia in cystic fibrosis. J Pediatr 1977; 90:574–578.

340. Iikura Y, et al. Antidiuretic hormone in acute asthma in children: effects of medication on serum levels and clinical course. Allergy Proc 1989; 10:197–201.

341. Arisaka O, et al. Water intoxication in asthma assessed by urinary arginine vasopressin. Eur J Pediatr 1988; 148: 167–169.

342. Schrier RW, Berl T. Nonosmolar factors affecting renal water excretion (second of two parts). (Review). N Engl J Med 1975; 292:141–145.

343. O'Rahilly S. Secretion of antidiuretic hormone in hyponatraemia: not always "inappropriate." Br Med J Clin Res Ed 1985; 290:1803–1804.

344. Kamel KS, Bear RA. Treatment of hyponatremia: a quantitative analysis. (Review). Am J Kidney Dis 1993; 21: 439–443.

345. Schrier RW. Treatment of hyponatremia (editorial). N Engl J Med 1985; 312:1121–1123.

346. Videen JS, et al. Human cerebral osmolytes during chronic hyponatremia. A proton magnetic resonance spectroscopy study. J Clin Invest 1995; 95:788–793.

347. Ayus JC, Arieff AI. Pathogenesis and prevention of hyponatremic encephalopathy. (Review). Endocrinol Metab Clin North Am 1993; 22:425–446.

348. Sterns RH, Riggs JE, Schochet SS Jr. Osmotic demyelination syndrome following correction of hyponatremia. N Engl J Med 1986; 314:1535–1542.

349. Ayus JC, Krothapalli RK, Arieff AI. Treatment of symptomatic hyponatremia and its relation to brain damage. A prospective study. (Review). N Engl J Med 1987; 317: 1190–1195.

350. Ayus JC, Krothapalli RK, Arieff AI. Changing concepts in treatment of severe symptomatic hyponatremia. Rapid correction and possible relation to central pontine myelinolysis. Am J Med 1985; 78:897–902.

351. Sklar C, Fertig A, David R. Chronic syndrome of inappropriate secretion of antidiuretic hormone in childhood. Am J Dis Child 1985; 139:733–735.

352. Tang TT, et al. Optic chiasm glioma associated with inappropriate secretion of antidiuretic hormone, cerebral ischemia, nonobstructive hydrocephalus and chronic ascites following ventriculoperitoneal shunting. Childs Nerv Syst 1991; 7:458–461.

353. Padilla G, et al. Vasopressin levels and pediatric head trauma. Pediatrics 1989; 83:700–705.

354. Goldman MB, Luchins DJ, Robertson GL. Mechanisms of altered water metabolism in psychotic patients with polydipsia and hyponatremia. N Engl J Med 1988; 318: 397–403.

355. Meierkord H, Shorvon S, Lightman SL. Plasma concentrations of prolactin, noradrenaline, vasopressin and oxy-

tocin during and after a prolonged epileptic seizure. Acta Neurol Scand 1994; 90:73–77.

356. Edwards CM, et al. Arginine vasopressin—a mediator of chemotherapy induced emesis? Br J Cancer 1989; 59: 467–470.

357. Coslovsky R, Bruck R, Estrov Z. Hypo-osmolal syndrome due to prolonged nausea. Arch Intern Med 1984; 144:191–192.

358. Dhawan A, Narang A, Singhi S. Hyponatraemia and the inappropriate ADH syndrome in pneumonia. Ann Trop Paediatr 1992; 12:455–462.

359. van Steensel-Moll HA, et al. Excessive secretion of antidiuretic hormone in infections with respiratory syncytial virus. Arch Dis Childh 1990; 65:1237–1239.

360. Tang WW, et al. Hyponatremia in hospitalized patients with the acquired immunodeficiency syndrome (AIDS) and the AIDS-related complex. Am J Med 1993; 94:169–174.

361. Weissman PN, Shenkman L, Gregerman RI. Chlorpropamide hyponatremia: drug-induced inappropriate antidiuretic-hormone activity. N Engl J Med 1971; 284:65–71.

362. Escuro RS, Adelstein DJ, Carter SG. Syndrome of inappropriate secretion of antidiuretic hormone after infusional vincristine. Clevel Clin J Med 1992; 59:643–644.

363. Liskin B, et al. Imipramine-induced inappropriate ADH secretion. J Clin Psychopharmacol 1984; 4:146–147.

364. Parker WA. Imipramine-induced syndrome of inappropriate antidiuretic hormone secretion. Drug Intell Clin Pharmacy 1984; 18:890–894.

365. Moses AM, Howanitz J, Miller M. Diuretic action of three sulfonylurea drugs. Ann Intern Med 1973; 78:541–544.

366. Cotton MF, et al. Plasma arginine vasopressin and the syndrome of inappropriate antidiuretic hormone secretion in tuberculous meningitis (see comments). Pediatr Infect Dis J 1991; 10:837–842.

367. Cotton MF, et al. Raised intracranial pressure, the syndrome of inappropriate antidiuretic hormone secretion, and arginine vasopressin in tuberculous meningitis. Childs Nerv Syst 1993; 9:10–15.

368. Hill AR, et al. Altered water metabolism in tuberculosis: role of vasopressin (see comments). Am J Med 1990; 88: 357–364.

369. Olson BR, et al. Isolated hyponatremia after transsphenoidal pituitary surgery. J Clin Endocrinol Metab 1995; 80:85–91.

370. Sane T, et al. Hyponatremia after transsphenoidal surgery for pituitary tumors. J Clin Endocrinol Metab 1994; 79: 1395–1398.

371. Anmuth CJ, et al. Chronic syndrome of inappropriate secretion of antidiuretic hormone in a pediatric patient after traumatic brain injury. Arch Phys Med Rehab 1993; 74: 1219–1221.

372. Forrest JN Jr, et al. Superiority of demeclocycline over lithium in the treatment of chronic syndrome of inappropriate secretion of antidiuretic hormone. N Engl J Med 1978; 298:173–177.

373. Ohnishi A, et al. Potent aquaretic agent. A novel nonpeptide selective vasopressin 2 antagonist (OPC-31260) in men. J Clin Invest 1993; 92:2653–2659.

374. Kamoi K, et al. Atrial natriuretic peptide in patients with the syndrome of inappropriate antidiuretic hormone secretion and with diabetes insipidus. J Clin Endocrinol Metab 1990; 70:1385–1390.

375. Manoogian C, et al. Plasma atrial natriuretic hormone levels in patients with the syndrome of inappropriate antidiuretic hormone secretion. J Clin Endocrinol Metab 1988; 67:571–575.

376. Kojima T, et al. Role of atrial natriuretic peptide in the diuresis of a newborn infant with the syndrome of inappropriate antidiuretic hormone secretion. Acta Paediatr Scand 1989; 78:793–796.

377. Wijdicks EF, et al. Atrial natriuretic factor and salt wasting after aneurysmal subarachnoid hemorrhage. Stroke 1991; 22:1519–1524.

378. Isotani E, et al. Alterations in plasma concentrations of natriuretic peptides and antidiuretic hormone after subarachnoid hemorrhage. Stroke 1994; 25:2198–2203.

379. Diringer M, et al. Sodium and water regulation in a patient with cerebral salt wasting. Arch Neurol 1989; 46: 928–930.

380. Vokes TP, Aycinena PR, Robertson GL. Effect of insulin on osmoregulation of vasopressin. Am J Physiol 1987; 252:E538–E548.

381. Zerbe RL, Vinicor F, Robertson GL. Plasma vasopressin in uncontrolled diabetes mellitus. Diabetes 1979; 28:503–508.

382. Ishikawa S, et al. Prompt recovery of plasma arginine vasopressin in diabetic coma after intravenous infusion of a small dose of insulin and a large amount of fluid. Acta Endocrinol 1990; 122:455–461.

383. Tulassay T, et al. Atrial natriuretic peptide and other vasoactive hormones during treatment of severe diabetic ketoacidosis in children. J Pediatr 1987; 111:329–334.

384. Zerbe RL, Vinicor F, Robertson GL. Regulation of plasma vasopressin in insulin–dependent diabetes mellitus. Am J Physiol 1985; 249:E317–E325.

33
Emergencies of Inborn Metabolic Diseases

Jose E. Abdenur

Foundation for the Study of Neurometabolic Diseases and University of Buenos Aires School of Dentistry, Buenos Aires, Argentina

I. INTRODUCTION

Baby JO was born full term, after an uneventful pregnancy and delivery. He had a normal physical examination and was discharged home at 36 h of age. Twelve hours later, the mother noted poor sucking and a weak cry. He was brought to the hospital and found to be lethargic. A sepsis work-up was performed and, as a blood gas revealed respiratory alkalosis, an ammonium level was obtained. The value was 1600 μM (normal up to 80). Blood was sent for analysis of plasma amino acids and he was treated with sodium benzoate, sodium phenylacetate, arginine, and a high glucose infusion rate (GIR). Citrulline levels were 2300 μM and the arginine dosage was adjusted for the treatment of argininosuccinic acid synthetase deficiency. The patient improved and was discharged after 2 weeks on a special diet. His family history revealed that a brother had died at 5 days of age. He had also presented with poor suck and lethargy early in life, was admitted to a hospital, had seizures and lapsed into coma. The diagnosis was sepsis.

This story shows two dramatically different outcomes for two siblings who, undoubtedly, had the same disease. Inborn metabolic diseases (IMD) are a group of genetic disorders in which there is a block in a metabolic pathway. They are usually the product of a single gene defect that affects the activity of an enzyme either directly or through abnormalities in its cofactors or activating proteins. IMD comprise a variety of disorders affecting the metabolism of small (i.e., aminoacids) or large molecules (i.e., sphingolipids). Many patients present with a catastrophic collapse in the neonatal period. However, the age and clinical presentation of patients with IMD are highly variable. Therefore a disease-free period of months or years, or a subacute presentation does not rule out the possibility of an IMD (1). A variable phenotype can be seen in patients with the same enzyme deficiency and clinical heteroge-

neity has even been observed between siblings carrying the same mutations. Nevertheless, when possible, the molecular defect of the patient should be identified. This information is useful for prenatal diagnosis and, in some cases, may allow one to predict the clinical course of the disease (genotype–phenotype correlation), helping one to find the best therapeutic option for each individual.

A complete description of the different IMD can be found in excellent textbooks (2–4). In this chapter, we will describe the most common IMD that can present with acute, life-threatening illness, focusing on the diagnosis and treatment of these emergencies.

II. UREA CYCLE DEFECTS

A. Pathophysiology: The Urea Cycle

High ammonium levels can be found in a variety of diseases, but the most severe causes of hyperammonemia are the urea cycle defects (UCD) (Table 1). The urea cycle prevents the toxic accumulation of ammonium and other nitrogen compounds by incorporating nitrogen not used for protein synthesis into urea. Each molecule of urea contains two atoms of waste nitrogen: one derived from ammonia and the other from aspartate (5,6) (Fig. 1). The urea cycle is also responsible for the biosynthesis of arginine. Abnormalities in the urea cycle produce hyperammonemia and elevation of glutamine. The former may have a deleterious effect on the central nervous system (CNS) through different mechanisms, including alteration in trafficking of amino acids and monoamines between neurons and astrocytes, as well as deficit in cerebral energy metabolism due to inhibition of 2-ketoglutarate-dehydrogenase (5,7). High levels of glutamine produce an intracellular osmotic effect with secondary swelling of astrocytes and increased intracranial pressure, which is clinically expressed by acute encephalopathy (5,7,8,9).

Table 1   Causes of Hyperammonemia

Inborn errors of metabolism

Urea cycle defects
  N-acetylglutamate synthetase deficiency
  Carbamylphosphate synthetase deficiency
  Ornithine transcarbamylase deficiency
  Argininosuccinic acid synthetase deficiency
  Argininosuccinic acid lyase deficiency
  Arginase deficiency
Organic acidemias: Propionic acidemia, methylmalonic
    acidemia, isovaleric acidemia, and others
Fatty acid oxidation defects
  Medium-chain acyl-CoA-dehydrogenase deficiency, long-
    chain 3-hydroxyacyl-CoA-dehydrogenase, and others
Transport defects of urea cycle intermediates
  Lysinuric protein intolerance
  Hyperammoniemia–hyperornithinemia–homocitrullinuria
    syndrome
Glutamato dehydrogenase deficiency (hyperammonemia and
    hyperinsulinism)
Mitochondrial diseases: Mitochondrial DNA depletion, and
    others
Pyruvate carboxylase deficiency (neonatal form)

Acquired causes

Transient hyperammonemia of the newborn
Muscular hyperactivity (seizures, respiratory distress syn-
    drome)
Infections with urease positive bacteria (skin, intestine, uri-
    nary tract)
Asparaginase treatment
Deficient arginine supply in diet
Treatment with valproate and other anticonvulsants
Hepatocellular carcinoma
Liver insufficiency: Reye syndrome, infections, intoxication,
    and others
Portocava shunt (liver bypass): Vascular malformations, cir-
    rhosis

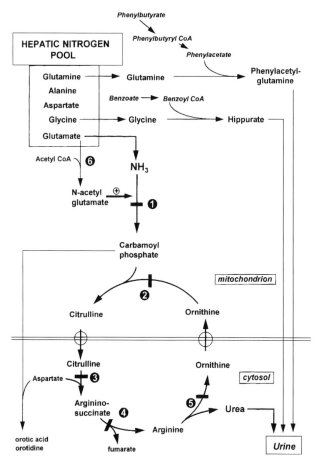

Figure 1   The urea cycle and alternative pathways of nitrogen excretion. Enzymes: 1, carbamyl phosphate synthetase;
2, ornithine transcarbamylase; 3, argininosuccinate synthetase; 4, argininosuccinate lyase; 5, arginase; 6, N-acetylglutamate synthetase. Enzyme defects are shown by solid bars
across the arrows. (From Ref. 6.)

There are five enzymes involved in the urea cycle
(Fig. 1): carbamylphosphate synthetase (CPS), ornithine
transcarbamylase (OTC), argininosuccinic acid synthetase
(AS), argininosuccinic acid lyase (AL), and arginase. Because N-acetylglutamate (NAG) is required for the activity of CPS, the enzyme responsible for NAG biosynthesis
(NAG synthetase) is also considered to be a part of the
pathway (5,6). Defects for each of these enzymes have
been described. Except for OTC deficiency, which is X-
linked, inheritance in all UCD is autosomal recessive.

B. Clinical Presentation

1. Neonatal Form

Patients with UCD can present with symptoms from birth
to adulthood. Neonatal presentation is the most common
and is due to a complete deficiency of CPS, OTC, AS, or

AL, all of which have almost identical clinical expression
(5,6). These patients are usually born at full term and have
a normal physical exam at birth. Between the first 24 and
72 h, depending on protein intake, the neonate presents
with poor suck, vomiting, and hypotonia followed by lethargy, seizures, vasomotor instability, hypothermia, and
coma. Slight liver enlargement and hyperventilation are
also constant findings. AS-deficient patients may present
with hypertonicity and trismus; pulmonary hemorrhage
has been described as a complication of OTC deficiency
(6). If hyperammonemia is not detected, the patient might
die with a suspected diagnosis of sepsis, respiratory distress, and/or intracranial bleeding (5,6).

Although infrequent, NAG synthetase deficiency can
also have a similar severe neonatal course, but its clinical
presentation appears to be variable (5,10).

2. Late-Onset Form

Beyond the neonatal period, the clinical expression of UCD is highly variable, depending on the degree of the enzyme defect, nitrogen intake, and endogenous catabolism. Common presentations are intermittent episodes of vomiting associated with headaches, irritability, agitation, ataxia, and/or lethargy, sometimes progressing to coma. Recovery from these episodes may be complete, or with different degrees of neurological sequelae. These episodes can be triggered by an exogenous protein load or increased endogenous catabolism (i.e., fever, fasting, steroid treatment, surgery, etc.). Strokelike episodes and central pontine myelinolysis have been reported in patients with OTC deficiency (11,12). Hepatomegaly is common in AS deficiency and severe liver involvement, mimicking a Reye's syndrome has been described in several urea cycle defects (1,5,6). Brittle hair (trichorrhexis nodosa) is characteristic of AS- and AL-deficient patients.

A history of anorexia, poor weight gain and a self-imposed protein restriction is frequently overlooked in these patients.

Female carriers for OTC deficiency can have a similar variability in clinical presentation, ranging from completely asymptomatic to severe neonatal hyperammonemia, due to the different degree of Lyonization in the hepatocytes (5,13). Some of these women have presented with severe hyperammonemia in the postpartum period (14).

Common misdiagnoses of the late presentation of UCD include migraine, cyclic vomiting, esophageal reflux, food allergies, behavioral problems, or hepatitis (5,6).

Clinical presentation of arginase deficiency differs from the other urea cycle defects. The disease is characterized by chronic encephalopathy progressing to spastic tetraplegia, seizures, and microcephaly. Episodic vomiting and hyperammonemia are less common (5,15).

C. Diagnosis

In the severe neonatal presentation, or during the acute decompensation in the late-onset forms, the most important biochemical finding in patients with NAGS, CPS, OTC, AS, or AL deficiency is severe hyperammonemia (usually greater than 300 μM), with low blood urea nitrogen (BUN) and slight or moderate elevation in liver transaminase levels. It is important to note that in common diseases of the neonatal period such as sepsis, seizures, or asphyxia, ammonia levels rarely exceed the 200 μM level. Also ammonia levels can be falsely elevated if specimens are not collected and processed properly. Respiratory alkalosis, due to the toxic effect of the ammonia to the respiratory center, is another key to the diagnosis (5), but this sign is frequently overlooked. More rarely, patients with UCD can present with metabolic acidosis, probably secondary to dehydration. When severe hyperammonemia in a sick neonate is found, quantitative measurements of plasma and urine amino acids (AA), acylcarnitines (AC), urine organic acids analysis (UOA) and orotic acid should be performed as soon as possible. Diagnosis of the specific block in the urea cycle is determined by the AA and orotic acid results. Low or undetected citrulline levels are present in NAGS, CPS, and OTC deficiencies (5,6) (Fig. 1). In OTC deficiency, the accumulated carbamyl phosphate will be diverted to the pyrimidine synthetic pathway, producing an increased excretion of orotic acid (and orotidine), which is the basis for the differential diagnosis between OTC and NAGS or CPS deficiencies (5,6,16). Orotic acid can also be increased in AS, AL, and arginase deficiencies but in lesser amounts. Uracil, another pyrimidine, may be found in the UOA of these enzyme deficiencies. Differentiation between NAGS and CPS requires assessment of CPS enzyme activity in hepatocytes and/or an oral load with N-carbamyl glutamate, an analog of N-acetyl glutamate (6).

Patients with AS deficiency have markedly increased citrulline levels (usually more than 1000 μM) and patients with AL deficiency have milder elevations of citrulline (100–300 μM) and increased levels of argininosuccinic acid (5). The latter is detected more easily in urine than in serum amino acids. Other abnormalities in the amino acid profile, common to all of the above-mentioned enzyme deficiencies, are increased glutamine and alanine, due to nonspecific nitrogen accumulation; and decreased arginine and ornithine, due to the impaired arginine biosynthesis (5,6).

In arginase deficiency, in contrast, hyperammonemia is uncommon and the characteristic serum AA profile shows a marked elevation of arginine. Urine amino acids also show a marked elevation of arginine with milder increase in lysine, cystine, and ornithine (15). A liver biopsy, for measurement of enzyme activity, is seldom necessary for diagnostic purposes, except for the differential diagnosis between NAGS and CPS as mentioned above. The most common differential diagnoses of UCD are transient hyperammonemia of the newborn (THAN), organic acidemias (OA), and fatty acid oxidation (FAO) defects. Patients with THAN are usually preterm babies who present in the first 24 h of life with respiratory distress and severe hyperammonemia (even higher than in UCD) (17). Neonates with OA (mainly propionic and methylmalonic) classically present with metabolic acidosis with high anion gap, ketonuria and hyperammonemia. The latter can be as severe as in the UCD. In exceptional cases, metabolic acidosis and ketonuria may be absent but AC and/or UOA are diagnostic (see review organic acidemias, below).

Children with FAO defects can present as neonates but, in general, hyperammonemia is not severe and hypoketotic hypoglycemia and severe liver or cardiac involvement are common in these patients. Acylcarnitines are the main tool for their diagnosis (see review of fatty acid oxidation defects, below).

Other causes of hyperammonemia are outlined in Table 1 (5,6,18,18a).

Diagnosis of UCD in patients out of crisis is more difficult, specially for the female heterozygous for OTC deficiency. Amino acid levels in these female patients are slightly different from normal controls (14,19), but might still fall within the normal range, even during a mild crisis Enzyme activity measured in liver biopsy samples is unreliable (5). The allopurinol test is useful for diagnosis and carrier detection, but it might not be completely specific (5,19,20). When possible, mutation analysis of the OTC gene should be done. Even though the majority of mutations are private, recent information allows for the establishment of some degree of genotype to phenotype correlations (21,22). This information is also essential for prenatal diagnosis.

D. Treatment: The Acute Episode

For teaching purposes we classify treatment of this emergency into three areas: supportive therapy, anabolism, and detoxification.

1. Supportive Therapy

A hyperammonemic episode is a life-threatening condition with risk for severe brain damage. Nitrogen intake should be discontinued. A central venous line should be placed for intravenous (IV) infusion and an arterial line should be available for blood drawing and blood pressure monitoring. The hemodialysis team should be alerted. Blood samples for measurement of ammonia, blood gas, electrolytes, BUN, glucose, and calcium should be obtained prior to the beginning of the treatment and every 4–6 h thereafter. If intracranial pressure is elevated, therapy with mannitol can be started. Corticosteroids should be avoided, as they will produce a negative nitrogen balance (5). Many patients are dehydrated due to the previous history of vomiting and poor feeding. However, IV fluids should be given cautiously, since cerebral edema is frequently present in severely ill patients. Infections should be searched for and treated accordingly.

2. Anabolism

In order to decrease endogenous protein catabolism, calories to cover at least the basal energy expenditure should be provided (60 Cal/kg/day in newborns) (23) but, when possible, a higher caloric intake (100–120 Cal/kg/day) is desirable. This requires the use of a high glucose infusion rate (GIR), for which a central line is required. The different GIR and calories delivered using different concentrations of dextrose are listed in Tables 2 and 3. In less severely ill patients who can tolerate oral or nastogastric feedings, IV calories can be supplemented by using glucose polymers (10% solution) or one of the protein-free powders available: Pro-Phree (Ross Laboratories, Columbus, OH), Mead-Johnson 80056 (Mead Johnson Labora-

Table 2 GIR Calculated from Different Glucose Concentrations (D%) and Fluid Infusion Rates (ml/kg)[a]

cc/kg	D5%	D7.5%	D10%	D12.5%	D15%	D20%
40	1.4	2.1	2.8	3.5	4.2	5.6
50	1.7	2.6	3.5	4.3	5.2	6.9
60	2.1	3.1	4.2	5.2	6.2	8.3
67	2.3	3.5	4.6	5.8	7.0	9.3
75	2.6	3.9	5.2	6.5	7.8	10.4
100	3.5	5.2	6.9	8.7	10.4	13.9
120	4.2	6.2	8.3	10.4	12.5	16.7
150	5.2	7.8	10.4	13.0	15.6	20.8
180	6.2	9.4	12.5	15.6	18.8	25.0

[a]Concentrations of dextrose greater than 12.5% should not be used through a peripheral vein.

tories, Evansville, IN). If the gastrointestinal (GI) tract cannot be used, IV lipids (0.5–2 g/kg/day) can be given as long as sepsis is not present and liver enzyme and triglyceride levels are within normal limits.

3. Detoxification

Hemodialysis is the treatment of choice for severe hyperammonemia and can usually normalize ammonium levels in less than 24 h (5,24). If that is not possible, continuous hemodiafiltration, hemofiltration, peritoneal dialysis, or exchange transfusion, in that order, are the alternatives (25,26). Pharmacological treatment with sodium benzoate and sodium phenylacetate should be carried on until dialysis procedures are available. These drugs activate alternative pathways for nitrogen excretion. After being

Table 3 Calories/kg/day Provided at Different GIR[a]

mg/kg/min	Cal/kg/day
4.0	19.6
5.0	24.5
6.0	29.4
7.0	34.3
8.0	39.2
9.0	44.0
10.0	49.0
11.0	53.9
12.0	58.8
13.0	63.6
14.0	68.5
15.0	73.4
16.0	78.3
17.0	83.2
18.0	88.1

[a]The 3.4 Cal provided by 1 g intravenous glucose was used for the calculations.

esterified to their CoA-esters, sodium benzoate and phe-nylacetate will produce hippurate and phenylacetylglu-tamine, respectively. The latter two compounds are ex-creted through the urine, diverting nitrogen from the urea cycle (5,27) (Fig. 1). Intravenous preparations are rec-ommended for the acutely ill patient by giving a priming infusion of 250 mg/kg in 25–35 ml/kg of 10% dextrose solution over 90 min, followed by a sustaining infusion of 250 mg/kg given over 24 h in maintenance fluids (5). Lower dosages (5.5 g/m^2 in 400–600 ml/m^2) are used in older patients. When D10% is used to prepare the priming infusion, the resulting GIR infusion is very high (28–39 mg/kg/min), and we have observed hypoglycemia with hyperinsulinism as a result of the sudden change in IV glucose infusion when the priming dose finishes. To avoid this problem we dilute the drugs in D5%.

Repeat priming doses are not recommended due to the potential toxic effect of these drugs. It is also impor-tant that dosages of the IV medications be carefully cal-culated as cases of overdose with toxic effects have been reported (28). Because drug levels in blood are not rou-tinely measured, we have evaluated levels of benzoylcar-nitine by tandem mass spectrometry as a rapid and simple means of estimating the benzoate levels.

Sodium benzoate and sodium phenylacetate provide 6.9 and 6.4 mEq sodium/g, respectively. Therefore, the amount of sodium given to the patient with both drugs in 24 h will be approximately 6.7 mEq/kg. The use of these salts can produce potassium loss (5), which, in association with the increased potassium uptake secondary to the high GIR, may result in hypokalemia. Therefore, serum elec-trolyte levels must be followed closely, and IV fluids ad-justed accordingly. Nausea and vomiting are frequent side effects of the treatment and could be avoided by using antiemetics (5). As an alternative to the IV medications, sodium benzoate or sodium phenylbutyrate can be given via NG tube. Sodium phenylbutyrate is converted into phenylacetate in the body and is twice as effective as so-dium benzoate on a molar basis. Recommended dosages are up to 500 mg/kg/day for sodium benzoate and up to 600 mg/kg/day for sodium phenylbutyrate (5,6,27).

Arginine, which becomes an essential amino acid in UCD, should also be provided. The recommended dosage is 210 mg/kg/day for CPS, OTC, and AS deficiencies and 660 mg/kg day for AL deficiency (4.0 and 12.0 g/m^2 re-spectively, for older patients). It is also recommended to give a priming infusion over 90 min followed by a sus-taining infusion, of a similar dosage, given over 24 h (5). An IV preparation of arginine HCl (10% solution) is avail-able. As an alternative, oral arginine can be given diluted in water via NG tube. A side effect of the treatment with arginine HCl is the development of hyperchloremic met-abolic acidosis, which may require treatment with sodium bicarbonate (5). The use of potassium acetate, rather than KCl, is useful to decrease the hyperchloremia resulting from the arginine administration.

E. Long-Term Management

When ammonia levels are close to normal, protein can be added to the parenteral nutrition at an initial dosage of 0.5 g/kg/day. Nasogastric (NG) or oral (PO) feeds can be started as soon as the clinical condition is stable. Pro-tein can be then provided by administration of an infant formula, increasing the intake gradually according to am-monium levels. In general 1.5–2 g/kg/day can be given to newborns and young infants, but protein tolerance de-creases after 6 months of age. The use of special for-mulas with essential amino acids mixtures, to provide about 50% of the total protein intake, is recommended for OTC and CPS and could also be used in AS and AL deficiencies. This approach is used to meet the require-ments for essential amino acids and to reutilize waste nitrogen for the synthesis of the nonessential ones (6). To achieve the desired caloric intake (120–140 Cal/kg for a newborn), the formula should be supplemented with one of the protein-free powders available (see above). As an alternative, glucose polymers and oil can be added to the infant formula as a source of calories. Minerals, vitamin, and trace element requirements should be met and enough water must be added to meet the patient's needs and maintain the caloric density at 20–24 Cal/oz. Hyperosmolar preparations may cause di-arrhea. The diet should be adjusted frequently to ensure weight gain and growth. Protein and calorie requirements per kg body weight will decrease with age and vary from patient to patient according to the disease, growth rate, and residual enzyme activity. Fasting plasma ammonium, branched-chain AA, arginine, and serum plasma protein levels should be maintained within normal limits; plasma glutamine should be below 1000 μM (5).

Because carnitine deficiency may develop in patients with UCD (27), carnitine should be given to these pa-tients (50–100 mg/kg/day, divided in three doses). The dosage should be adjusted according to free carnitine levels.

When PO intake is satisfactory, the appropriate med-icines for long-term treatment (sodium phenylbutyrate, ar-ginine, and/or citrulline) can be given orally, mixed with the formula. Recommended dosages of sodium phenyl-butyrate are 0.45–0.60 g/kg/day for newborns and young children, and 9.9–13.0 g/m^2/day for older patients. When phenylbutyrate is not available, sodium benzoate 0.25–0.5 g/kg/day can be prescribed as alternative. These de-toxifying agents might not be needed in patients with AL deficiency (5,6).

Arginine (free base) is given at a dosagee of 0.40–0.70 g/kg/day for young children and 0.8–15.4 g/m^2/day for older patients. The dosage can be adjusted to maintain normal arginine levels for age. Patients with AS and AL deficiencies require the higher dosages. In patients with severe CPS or OTC deficiencies, arginine can be substi-tuted by citrulline, 0.17 g/kg/day or 3.8 g/m^2/day, accord-ing to age. Citrate has been also used to provide a substrate for Krebs-cycle intermediates and might be useful in the treatment of AL deficiency (6).

NAGS deficiency might only require treatment with oral N-carbamyl glutamate (100–300 mg/kg/day. (6).

If anticonvulsant agents are needed, valproic acid should be avoided (29).

The outcome for patients with UCD remains very guarded. In general it depends on the disease, age at diagnosis, residual enzyme activity, and compliance with treatment (5,6,30,31). Neurological damage may be directly related to the duration and degree of the initial hyperammonemic episode; therefore, neurological impairment is common in almost all forms with neonatal presentation. Patients with AS deficiency seem to have a better prognosis than OTC- or CPS-deficient patients (5). It is surprising that AL patients appear to have poor outcome in spite of infrequent decompensations (31). Prospective treatment of children with confirmed prenatal diagnosis or at risk of having UCD has been more effective in patients with AS and AL than in OTC and CPS deficiencies (32). Liver transplantation has been performed in several patients. Correction of the hyperammonemia can be obtained but neurological outcome is mainly related to the condition prior to transplantation (31,33). Further studies are still needed to confirm long-term benefits of this therapeutic approach. Efforts to develop gene therapy for UCD are underway (34,35).

III. ORGANIC ACIDEMIAS

A. Pathophysiology

Organic acidemias (OA) are a group of IMDs characterized by an abnormal accumulation of one or more organic acids in body fluids. The majority of the OA are due to defects in the catabolic pathways of AA. However, because the site of the enzymatic block is far from the step where the amino group is lost, AA do not accumulate. The fatty acid oxidation defects and the primary lactic acidemias, which also produce abnormal amounts of organic acids, are described in other sections of this chapter.

For teaching purposes we can classify the OA into three groups (Table 4). The first one includes defects in the metabolism of branched-chain aminoacids. In general, they present with acute "intoxication-like" episodes dominated by metabolic acidosis and increased anion gap (1, 36,37).

In the second group, the clinical picture is characterized by a progressive neurological deterioration (38,39, 40). These patients appear to be normal in infancy or early childhood. Thereafter, mental retardation, movement disorders, ataxia, and/or seizures become apparent. Some of these OA have characteristic neuroradiological findings (38,41,42,43). The most common of these conditions, and one of the most common organic acidemias, is glutaric aciduria type 1 (glutaryl-CoA dehydrogenase deficiency)

(38,41,44). Clinical presentation of these OA highlights the importance of requesting organic acid analysis in every patient with mental retardation, movement disorder, dystonia, and/or macrocephaly of unknown origin, even if episodes of acute metabolic decompensation are absent (45).

In the third group we have listed miscellaneous disorders that are usually diagnosed based on the UOA but have a clinical presentation that differs from the other two groups. In the same group we have included OA with a still unknown enzymatic defect.

For the purpose of this chapter we will focus on the organic acidemias due to defects in branched-chain AA metabolism. They are inherited as autosomal recessive conditions and have a variable phenotype (Fig. 2; Table 4). The most common are isovaleric acidemia (IVA), propionic acidemia (PA), and methylmalonic acidemia (MMA).

Isovaleric acidemia, a defect of leucine metabolism, results from a deficiency of isovaleryl-CoA dehydrogenase. Patients with IVA accumulate isovaleric acid and isovaleryl-CoA. The former is a volatile compound and is responsible for the characteristic sweaty feet odor found in the urine and skin of affected patients (36,37,46).

PA results from a defect in propionyl-CoA carboxylase, a biotin-dependent enzyme (37,60); and MMA from a deficiency of methylmalonyl-CoA mutase. Activity of the latter could be impaired due to defects in the mutase itself (mut$^+$ or mut$^-$) or due to defects in the synthesis of its cofactor, adenosylcobalamin (37,61–65). Both PA and MMA accumulate propionyl-CoA, which derives from the catabolism of valine, isoleucine, threonine, methionine, odd-chain fatty acids, and cholesterol side-chain and is also produced by the anaerobic gut flora (87, 88). In general, patients with OA accumulate acyl-CoA esters and organic acids in the mitochondria. These abnormal metabolites inhibit several mitochondrial enzymes, leading to a series of secondary biochemical abnormalities (61). Inhibition of N-acetyl-glutamate-synthetase and carbamyl phosphate synthetase are responsible for the hyperammonemia, which usually correlates with the level of organic acid accumulation (89,90). Impairment of pyruvate carboxylase and the shunt of malate explain the hypoglycemia and ketosis found in these patients, and inhibition of the glycine cleavage system may be responsible for the hyperglycinemia (61). Decreased ATP synthesis and hyperlactacidemia may result from inhibition of citrate synthase and pyruvic dehydrogenase (37).

B. Clinical and Common Laboratory Manifestations

The clinical presentation of patients with OA can be organized schematically into a severe neonatal form with metabolic distress, a chronic intermittent late-onset form, and a chronic progressive form (37). Asymptomatic patients have been found as a result of screening programs and studies performed in relatives of affected individuals (36,37).

1. Neonatal Form

This is the most common and severe. The usual presentation is a neonate with a history of normal pregnancy, delivery, and a short disease-free period, who presents with poor sucking, vomiting, respiratory distress, hypotonia or dystonia, lethargy, and coma. These symptoms are usually attributed to sepsis or, in less severe cases, pyloric stenosis (1,37). Mild dehydration is frequent in MMA and PA (due to vomiting and osmotic diuresis) and a strong sweaty feet odor in urine and skin is present in patients with IVA. Seizures and a Reye's-like syndrome can be present in severely ill patients (1,37). Neutropenia, thrombocytopenia, or pancytopenia is frequent and acute pancreatitis has been diagnosed in decompensated patients with OA (91–93). Other complications include infections, generalized staphyloccocal epidermolysis, and alopecia (37,94–96). Acute basal ganglion dysfunction should be suspected in any patient with sudden onset of dystonia and/or movement disorder. The globus pallidum is more frequently affected in MMA and PA (37,97–99), while abnormalities in the caudate and putamen are the most frequent basal ganglia involved in patients with glutaric aciduria type I (38,41,44,67).

The most characteristic biochemical abnormalities are metabolic acidosis, with elevated anion gap and ketosis. Mild hyperammonemia (200–500 μM) is usually present but levels could be as high as those in patients with urea cycle defect (>1000 μM) (89,90). Mild hyperlactacidemia and hypocalcemia, probably due to parathyroid hormone (PTH) resistance, are common (37,96). Amylase and lipase are increased if pancreatitis is present (91–93). Blood glucose levels are usually low, but in some patients they may be high, even before IV fluids have been started (100,101). This is particularly frequent in patients with ketolysis defects (i.e., 2-methyl-acetoacetyl-CoA thiolase, succinyl-acetoacetate-CoA-transferase deficiencies), who can present with hyperglycemia and ketosis resembling an episode of diabetic ketoacidosis (52). In contrast, patients with 3-OH 3-methyl glutaryl-CoA lyase deficiency, a defect affecting leucine catabolism and ketone bodies synthesis, present with metabolic acidosis (characteristic of OA) and hypoketotic hypoglycemia (characteristic of fatty acid oxidation defects) (51–52).

2. Late-Onset Form

In the intermittent, late-onset form, patients present with recurrent attacks of coma or lethargy with ataxia or dystonia. Acute hemiplegia, hemianopsia, and cerebellar hemorrhage have also been described (36–37). Increased protein intake or endogenous catabolism, due to an intercurrent illness, may trigger these crisis. The first attack may present at several months or years of age, or even in adolescence or adulthood, and has frequently been preceded by episodes of dehydration, anorexia, vomiting, failure to thrive, hypotonia, developmental delay, and/or other symptoms (37,102,103). Between attacks, clinical and laboratory evaluations may appear normal. However, the laboratory profile obtained during the attacks is similar to that described for the severe neonatal form, with the exception of hyperammonemia, which is less frequent (37).

3. Chronic Form

The chronic progressive form is characterized by persistent anorexia, failure to thrive, and vomiting. These symptoms are frequently attributed to gastrointestinal problems. Renal Fanconi syndrome or osteoporosis may develop. Hypotonia and muscle weakness can be present, mimicking congenital or metabolic myopathies. Developmental delay, progressive mental retardation, self-mutilation, and seizures sometimes accompany the above-mentioned symptoms (1,36,37,104).

C. Diagnosis

The most important test is the analysis of UOA performed by gas chromatography and mass spectrometry (GC/MS). Diagnostic possibilities of this test greatly increase if the urine is collected during the acute episode, when the characteristic profile for each OA is most likely to be found (45,105). In an acutely sick patient, the laboratory performing the test must be alerted so that the result can be available as soon as possible. Typical UOA profiles show elevated excretion of 3-OH-isovaleric acid and isovalerylglycine in IVA; and 3-OH-propionic acid, 3-hydroxyvaleric acid, methylcitrate, tiglylglycine and propionylglycine in PA. In MMA, there is a large increase of methylmalonic acid, with or without mild elevation of some of the propionate metabolites (37,45). Ketone bodies (3-OH-butyrate and acetoacetate) may be increased in decompensated patients with any of the above-mentioned OA. Another reliable and fast methodology for the diagnosis of several OA is the analysis of AC by tandem mass spectrometry (TMS). This methodology is highly sensitive and can be performed in blood spots on filter paper (Guthrie card), plasma, urine, or cerebrospinal fluid (CSF) (106–107). AC analysis allows the diagnosis of more than 20 different diseases (OA, fatty acid oxidation defects, and aminoacidopathies) and is being used not only for the diagnosis of symptomatic patients but also for mass newborn screening (108–110). Abnormal profiles can even be obtained from cord blood in asymptomatic newborns (111–112).

A typical AC profile shows a large increase of isovalerylcarnitine in IVA. However, other AC species, such as pivaloylcarnitine and 2-methylbutyrylcarnitine, have the same molecular weight and should be considered when the profile is being interpreted (53,113). In PA and MMA there is a large increase of propionylcarnitine. A slight increase of methylmalonylcarnitine is also usually

Table 4 Organic Acidemias

Common name	Enzyme deficiency	Pathway involved	Comments	References
Organic acidemias due to defects in branched-chain aminoacids				
Isovaleric aciduria	Isovaleryl-CoA dehydrogenase	Leu		36,37,46
3-Methyl crotonylglycinuria	3-Methyl crotonyl-CoA carboxylase	Leu	a	36,37,47–49
3-Methyl glutaconic aciduria type I	3-Methyl glutaconyl CoA hydratase	Leu		36,37,50
3-OH 3-methyl glutaric aciduria	3-OH 3-methyl glutaryl-CoA lyase	Leu, ketone bodies synthesis		51,52
2-Methyl butyrylglycinuria	2-methylbutyryl-CoA-dehydrogenase/short-branched-chain acyl-CoA dehydrogenase	Ileu	b	53,54
2-methyl-3-hydroxybutyric aciduria	2-methyl-3-hydroxybutyryl-CoA dehydrogenase	Ileu, 2-methyl fatty acids.		55
2-Methyl acetoacetic aciduria	2-methyl acetoacetyl-CoA thiolase (B-keto-thiolase)	Ketolysis, Ileu		52
—	Succynyl-CoA: 3-ketoacid CoA transferase	Ketolysis, Leu		52
3-OH-isobutyric aciduria	Isobutyryl-CoA dehydrogenase	Val		56
3-OH-isobutyric aciduria	3-OH isobutyryl-CoA deacilase	Val		36,37,57,58
3-OH-isobutyric aciduria	3-OH isobutyric-acid dehydrogenase (?)	Val		36,37,57
3-OH-isobutyric aciduria	Methylmalonate semialdehyde dehydrogenase	Val. (B-ala, L-alloisoleucine)		36,37,57,59
Propionic aciduria	Propionyl-CoA carboxylase	Val, Ileu, Met, Treo, OCFA, Ch.	a	37,48,49,60
Methylmalonic aciduria	Methylmalonyl-CoA mutase (mut+/mut−)	Val, Ileu, Met, Treo, OCFA, Ch.		37,61,62
Methylmalonic aciduria	Cobalamin defect B: adenosyltransferase deficiency	AdoCbl. synthesis defect. Val, Ileu, Met, Treo, OCFA, Ch.	Methylmalonic aciduria without homocystinuria	62–64
Methylmalonic aciduria	Cobalamin defect A: Reductase deficiency	AdoCbl. Synthesis. Val, Ileu, Met, Treo, OCFA, Ch.	Methylmalonic aciduria without homocystinuria	62–64
Methylmalonic aciduria	Cobalamin defects C, D and F	AdoCbl and MetCbl synthesis. Val, Ileu, Met, Treo, OCFA, Ch.	Homocystinuria and methylmalonic aciduria	63–65
—	Acetyl CoA carboxylase	Leu, Ileu		37
Malonic aciduria	Malonyl-CoA decarboxylase	Leu, Ileu	Secondary FAO inhibition. Combined malonic/methylmalonic aciduria	36,37,66
Organic acidemias with primary CNS involvement				
Glutaric aciduria type I	Glutaryl-CoA dehydrogenase	Lys, Try		38,41,44,67
L-2-Hydroxyglutaric aciduria	?	Lys, Try		38,42,68,69

Disease	Enzyme/defect	Metabolite	Comments	Ref.
D-2-Hydroxyglutaric aciduria	Dehydrogenase (?)	Unknown		43,70
2-Ketoadipic aciduria	2-Ketoadipic dehydrogenase	Lys,Try		71
4-OH butyric aciduria	Succinic semialdehyde dehydrogenase	Glu, GABA	Neurotransmitter defect	39
N-acetylaspartic aciduria	Aspartoacylase deficiency	N-acetyl-aspartic acid		40,72
Miscellaneous organic acidemias				
Hyperoxaluria type I	Alanine/glyoxylate aminotransferase	Oxalate	Peroxisomal defect	73
Hyperoxaluria type II	D-Glyceric dehydrogenase	Oxalate	Peroxisomal defect	73
Glyceroluria	Glycerol kinase (isolated or as a contiguous gene defect)	Glycerol	X-linked.	74
Alkaptonuria	Homogentisic acid oxidase	Tyrosine, homogentisic acid		75
Pyroglutamic aciduria	Glutathione synthetase	Gamma glutamyl cycle		76
Mevalonic aciduria/hyper-IgD and periodic fever syndrome	Mevalonate kinase	Cholesterol and non sterol isoprenes		77–80
Encephalopathy, petechiae, and ethylmalonic aciduria syndrome	Unknown	Unknown	Differential diagnosis with SCAD and mild MAD	81–83
3-Methyl glutaconic aciduria type II Barth syndrome: X-linked cardiomyopathy and neutropenia	Acyltransferase deficiency (?) Normal 3-methyl glutaconyl CoA hydratase activity.	Synthesis of phospholipids (?)		50,84
3-Methyl glutaconic aciduria, type III and IV	Unknown Normal 3-methyl glutaconyl CoA hydratase activity	Unknown	Found in Costeff syndrome, Pearson syndrome, ATPase syntase deficiency, and others	37,50
Malonic aciduria	Normal malonyl-CoA decarboxylase activity	Unknown		37,85

Val, valine; Ileu, isoleucine; Met, methionine; Treo, treonine; Lys, lysine; Try, tryptophan; Glu, glutamic acid; GABA, 4-aminobutyric acid; FA, fatty acids; OCFA, odd-chain fatty acids; Ch, cholesterol (side-chain); AdoCbl, adenosylcobalamin; MetCbl, methylcobalamin; FAO, fatty acid oxidation; SCAD, short-chain acyl-CoA dehydrogenase deficiency; MAD, multiple acyl-CoA dehydrogenase deficiency.

[a]3-Methyl crotonyl-CoA carboxylase, propionyl-CoA carboxylase and pyruvate carboxylase (see prymary lactic acidemias) are impared in holocarboxylase syntethase and biotinidase deficiency (48,49,86).

[b]Impaired protein and fatty acid metabolism.

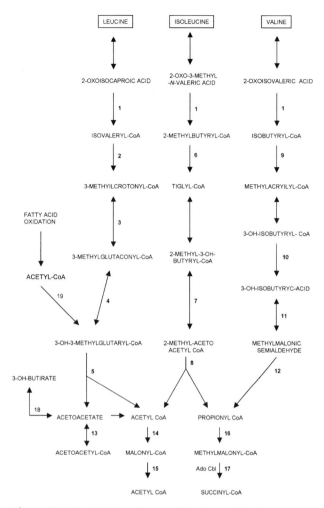

present in the latter. It is important to consider that the increase in diagnostic AC species is limited in patients with severe carnitine deficiencies.

Acylglycines by GC/MS stable isotope dilution or TMS may also be used for diagnosis (53,105,113a).

Quantitative AA usually show a nonspecific elevation of glycine. Glutamine is also elevated, reflecting the hyperammonemia usually seen in these patients, with the exception of PA (113b,113c). Total and free carnitine levels are low, with elevation of the acylcarnitine/free carnitine ratio (37).

D. Treatment: The Acute Episode

Rapid recognition and treatment of the acute metabolic decompensation in patients with OA can be life-saving. Treatment should provide supportive therapy, promote anabolism, and remove the offending toxins and should be carried out in specialized centers (37,114).

1. Supportive Therapy

The treatment will depend on the patient's clinical condition. A central line to ensure IV access and an arterial line for blood pressure monitoring and frequent blood drawing should be placed. Assisted ventilation, inotropics, albumin, and/or blood products are frequently needed.

Acutely ill patients with OA are usually dehydrated due to poor intake, vomiting, hyperventilation, and increased urinary losses. After fluid resuscitation is provided, IV hydration should be aimed at correcting dehydration over a period of 48 h. Rapid rehydration should be avoided due to the risk of cerebral edema. If pH is less than 7.20, metabolic acidosis should be only partially corrected with sodium bicarbonate at an initial dosage of 1–3 mEq/kg, repeated as needed. Overcorrection of the metabolic acidosis should be avoided, since this can increase cerebral edema. In severely acidotic patients sodium overload can be prevented by giving 30–50% of the sodium requirements as sodium bicarbonate instead of sodium chloride.

Blood gases, electrolytes, BUN, glucose, calcium, ammonium, and urine ketones should be monitored every 2–4 h. Initial potassium levels are usually normal or high in acutely ill patients, but these levels might be artificially increased due to the acidosis. In fact, potassium requirements are elevated due to the usual history of vomiting that precedes the admission and to the treatment with a high GIR and insulin (see below). Liver function tests, creatinine, amylase, and lipase levels should be checked initially and repeated as needed. Acute pancreatitis should be treated when present (91–93). Cultures should be obtained and antibiotics started. Staphylococcal and *Candida* infections should be considered in the differential diagnosis, and complete blood count (CBC) and platelet count should be evaluated daily.

Figure 2 Metabolic pathway of the branched-chain amino acid catabolism and related compounds. Numbers denote sites of the known enzymatic blocks. 1, Branched-chain-oxo-acid dehydrogenase; 2, Isovaleryl-CoA dehydrogenase; 3, 3-Methylcrotonyl-CoA-carboxylase; 4, 3-Methylglutaconyl-CoA-hydratase; 5, 3-OH 3-methyl glutaryl-CoA lyase; 6, 2-methylbutyryl-CoA-dehydrogenase; 7, 2-methyl-3-hydroxy-butyryl-CoA dehydrogenase; 8, 2-methyl acetoacetyl-CoA thiolase (B-keto-thiolase); 9, Isobutyryl-CoA-dehydrogenase; 10, 3-OH isobutyryl-CoA deacilase; 11, 3-OH isobutyric-acid dehydrogenase; 12, Methylmalonate semialdehyde dehydrogenase; 13, Succynyl-CoA: 3-ketoacid CoA transferase; 14, Acetyl CoA carboxylase (cytosolic); 15, Malonyl-CoA decarboxylase; 16, Propionyl-CoA carboxylase; 17, Methylmalonyl-CoA mutase, cobalamin defects A, B, C, D, and F; 18, 3-OH-butyric-acid dehydrogenase; 19, 3-OH 3-methyl glutaryl-CoA synthase. (Adapted from Ref. 37.)

2. Anabolism

It has been shown that endogenous production is an important source of abnormal metabolites in nonacutely ill patients with OA. This production is probably due to protein turnover (115,116) and is increased by fatty acid breakdown and intestinal production of propionate in patients with PA and MMA (87,88). These endogenous sources of toxic metabolites become even more important in severely ill patients and treatment should be aggressive to decrease their production (37). Oral intake is usually not possible and IV nutrition should be used to promote anabolism. Initially, this goal can be partially achieved by giving a high GIR to provide at least 8–10 mg/kg/min (Table 2). It is important to note that even with such a GIR, caloric intake is not sufficient to cover the patient's needs (Table 3), which are increased during the decompensation (117). Patients with OA can develop hyperglycemia and glycosuria, even with low GIR. We have documented an inadequate insulin response to hyperglycemia during the acute decompensation (118), which may or not be associated with pancreatitis (91). If hyperglycemia develops, insulin should be used (37,119). The requirements vary depending on the severity of the patient's condition and the GIR. In our experience, in a severely ill patient receiving a GIR of 8–10 mg/kg/min, a dosage of 0.10–0.15 U/kg/h is enough to control hyperglycemia, but it is advisable to start with a lower dosage (0.05 U/Kg/h) and to adjust it according to blood sugar levels. Insulin requirements decrease when acidosis improves.

Plasma ammonia levels decrease in parallel with those of the organic acids (90). Once acidosis has been corrected and ammonia and transaminase levels are close to normal, fats can be added to the treatment. If amylase and lipase levels are high or oral intake is not possible, IV lipids (Intralipid) should be used, starting at 0.5 g/kg/day and increasing gradually to 2 g/kg/day. When the oral route can not be used for more than 48 h, total parenteral nutrition (TPN) should be considered. TPN has been successfully used in chronic and acutely ill patients with OA and allows an effective anabolism that cannot be achieved with glucose and lipids alone (119,120). An ideal IV amino acid mixture should contain lower concentration of those AAs that are precursors of the increased organic acid (i.e., leucine in IVA). Such preparations are not available in the majority of the medical centers. As an alternative, any available amino acid solution can be used cautiously. We start with an amount that provides 30–50% of the recommended intake of the AA involved in the metabolic block. This amount can be increased gradually depending on the results of blood gases, ammonium, and serum AA. Levels of the abnormal metabolites in urine (UOA) or blood (acylcarnitines) should also be evaluated to monitor the response to treatment. With a high caloric supply from carbohydrates and fat, an IV amino acid dosage of 1–1.5 g/kg/day can be achieved, but special mixtures, deprived of the offending amino acids, might be required to supply more protein. As patient improves, the oral/NG tube route can be restarted (see section on long-term treatment).

3. Detoxification

In IVA and MMA, the organic acids are effectively excreted through the urine. Therefore, detoxification procedures should be indicated only in those severely ill patients who do not respond rapidly to treatment in spite of maintaining a good urinary output (37,114). In contrast, urinary excretion of propionic acid is poor, therefore detoxifying procedures should be considered early in the treatment in patients with PA (37,121). The most effective detoxification method is hemodialysis, which allows a high clearance of organic acids, amino acids and ammonium. Hemofiltration, peritoneal dialysis, or blood exchange transfusions can be used when the former is not available. Continuous venovenous hemofiltration is well tolerated by newborns or infants and allows rapid toxin removal (114). Peritoneal dialysis is available in most centers and is more effective in newborns than children. The dialysate should be warmed and buffered with bicarbonate. Hypertonic solutions can be used when overhydration is present. In those circumstances, hyperglycemia can develop and insulin might be needed.

To treat the hyperammonemia, sodium benzoate (250 mg/kg/day) can be used alone, or in conjunction with any of the above-mentioned detoxification procedures (37,122). The amount of sodium provided through this source should be accounted for when the daily sodium requirements are calculated (see section on treatment of urea cycle defects). Intravenous carnitine is another resource for toxin removal. This therapy will correct the decreased levels of free carnitine, provide enough substrate for the synthesis of nontoxic acylcarnitine compounds (i.e., isovalerylcarnitine, propionylcarnitine, etc.) that are excreted through the urine, and restore the intramitochondrial levels of CoA (36,37). After obtaining a sample for basal levels, a dosage of 100–400 mg/kg/day (divided every 4–6 h) should be given. The highest dosage should be used in newly diagnosed patients who may have severe carnitine depletion.

In patients with IVA, treatment with L-glycine increases the conversion of isovaleryl-CoA to the nontoxic compound isovalerylglycine, which is excreted through the urine (36,123). Oral or nasogastric-tube supplementation of L-glycine (250–600 mg/kg/day, divided in four to eight doses) prepared in a 100 mg/ml water solution should be given during the acute episode (36,37). Another potential resource for toxin removal is the administration of cofactors: biotin (10–20 mg/day) in PA and hydroxycobalamin (1–2 mg/day IM) in MMA (37). However, patients with severe neonatal presentation rarely respond to vitamin treatment. Clinical improvement correlates with correction of the metabolic acidosis, hyperammonemia, and ketonuria. Patients with MMA may develop persistent lactic acidemia due to chronic glutathione deficiency, which can be corrected with high dosages of vitamin C (2 g/day) (124). Lactic acidosis secondary to thiamine deficiency has been described in PA patients (125).

E. Long-Term Management

When the patient's condition allows for it, PO or NG feedings can be started. Natural protein is restricted to meet the recommended amounts of the AAs involved in the metabolic block, and can be initially provided with an infant formula. Total protein requirements for age and gender are achieved by adding special formulas devoid of the offending amino acids (36,37).

Recent studies suggest that energy requirements might be normal or even low in OA patients out of crisis (126). However, energy intake should be adequate to meet the patient's needs for normal growth, to maintain anabolism when poor appetite is present, and also should cover the increased requirements during intercurrent illnesses (37). Caloric requirements can be met with the use of protein-free powders (i.e., Prophree, Ross Laboratories; 80056, Mead Johnson; Duocal, SHS). As an alternative, carbohydrate supplements or oil (except for olive oil in PA and MMA patients) can be added to the formula when these products are not available. Osmolarity of the final preparation should be considered to prevent diarrhea.

Long fasting periods should be avoided (115) and dietary treatment should meet all the requirements for micronutrients and minerals. Iron and calcium supplements are frequently needed. Oral carnitine (in IVA, PA, and MMA) and/or glycine (for IVA) supplementation should be maintained, and vitamin therapy should only continue if a positive response has been documented. Metronidazole has been shown to be effective in decreasing the production of propionate by the gut flora (37,88,127). Recommended dosage is 10–20 mg/kg/day. Due to the possible side effects of metronidazole (leukopenia, peripheral neuropathy, and pseudomembranous colitis), it has been recommended to restrict its use to 10 consecutive days every month (37). We have not seen adverse effects after using the drug at 10 mg/kg/day daily for prolonged periods of time.

The long-term prognosis varies depending upon the particular OA, age at onset, response to vitamin therapy, and residual enzyme activity. Several mutations have been found (128–130), and clear genotype/phenotype has been described for a particular group of MMA patients (131).

Family compliance, psychological adjustment, and education are important for successful treatment. Nasogastric or gastrostomy feedings are usually needed and frequent hospitalizations are common in the most severe cases. Guidelines should be given to parents and primary physicians for special situations such as intercurrent illnesses, immunizations, anesthesia, or surgery (37,132, 133).

Reported long-term outcome has varied from a normal development to different degrees of neurological involvement, including mental retardation and movement disorders (134–140). Other long-term complications, including poor growth, malnutrition, cutaneous lesions (141), deficiency of trace elements (142), and osteoporosis can be prevented if good metabolic control and proper nutritional treatment can be achieved. Cardiomyopathy has been reported in some patients with OA (37,56,143). Tubular dysfunction and progressive renal insufficiency are common in MMA patients (37,144–148). It is not clear if these long-term manifestations can be prevented with optimum metabolic control. Kidney transplantation or combined kidney and liver transplantation have been performed in several patients with MMA. In general, better metabolic control and higher protein tolerance were obtained, but decompensations, mental deterioration, or acute basal ganglia lesions could not be prevented with these treatments (149,151). Similar experience has been reported for PA patients undergoing liver transplant (140,152).

Early diagnosis and intensive treatment are key factors in improving long-term prognosis (36,37). Therefore, the availability of newborn screening with tandem mass spectrometry opens a new chapter for the outcome of these diseases (108–111).

IV. FATTY ACID OXIDATION DEFECTS

A. Pathophysiology: Mitochondrial Fatty Acid Oxidation

Mitochondrial fatty acid oxidation (FAO) disorders are a relatively new group of IMD of increasing relevance. Understanding the FAO process is essential to interpret the pathophysiology of these diseases and to develop adequate strategies for treatment. FAO is the major source of energy for skeletal muscle and the heart, while liver oxidizes fatty acids (FA) primarily during fasting (153,154). The FAO process begins when triglycerides, stored in adipose tissue, are broken down to glycerol and fatty acids, mainly long-chain. The latter are transported in blood bound to albumin and enter liver cells through a specific transport system (155). Carnitine, an important metabolite in fatty acid oxidation, is transported into the tissues by a plasma membrane carnitine transporter (CT) specific for kidney, muscle, and heart (153,154). Once inside the cell, FFA of carbon length 18 or shorter are oxidized in the mitochondria, while longer-chain fats are metabolized in the peroxisomes (156). Fatty acids are activated to their corresponding acyl-CoA by specific acyl-CoA synthetases. The resulting acyl-CoAs enter the mitochondria in different ways, depending on their chain length. Short- (4–6 carbons) and medium-chain (6–10 carbons) acyl-CoAs directly enter the mitochondrial matrix. In contrast, long-chain acyl-CoAs (12–18 carbons) enter the mitochondria through a complex active transport system (Fig. 3). Initially, long chain acyl-CoAs are conjugated to carnitine by carnitine palmitoyl transferase I (CPT-I), located in the outer mitochondrial membrane. There are two tissue-specific isoforms of CPT-I, hepatic and muscular, but only patients with the hepatic form have been described so far (154). Long-chain acylcarnitines are carried through the intermembranous space by a carnitine–acylcarnitine translocase (translocase). Finally, another enzyme, carnitine palmitoyl-transferase II (CPT II), bound to the inner mitochondrial membrane, releases carnitine and long-chain acyl-CoAs into the mitochondrial matrix (153,154). Carnitine is recycled and acyl-CoAs of all chain lengths undergo a series of cyclic enzymatic reactions (Fig. 3).

The first step in the mitochondrial FAO of saturated straight-chain fats is a dehydrogenation of the acyl-CoA to enoyl-CoA. This reaction is catalyzed by four related enzymes, the acyl-CoA dehydrogenases (ACDs): very long-, long-, medium-, and short-chain acyl-CoA dehydrogenases (VLCAD, LCAD, MCAD, and SCAD, respectively), which differ in their chain-length specificity (153,156). Nevertheless, there is some degree of overlap in their activity. Recent data suggest that the main enzyme involved with long straight-chain fatty acid metabolism is VLCAD and that LCAD may play a role in the metabolism of branched-chain fatty acids (157). All dehydrogenases have flavin adenine dinucleotide (FAD) bound at the active site. Electrons released during these reactions are channeled by the electron transfer flavoprotein (ETF), a mitochondrial matrix enzyme with α- and β-subunits, and the ETF-ubiquinone oxidoreductase (ETF-QO), a component of the inner mitochondrial membrane that feeds the electrons into the respiratory chain via ubiquinone (156,158). ETF and ETF-QO defects impair not only

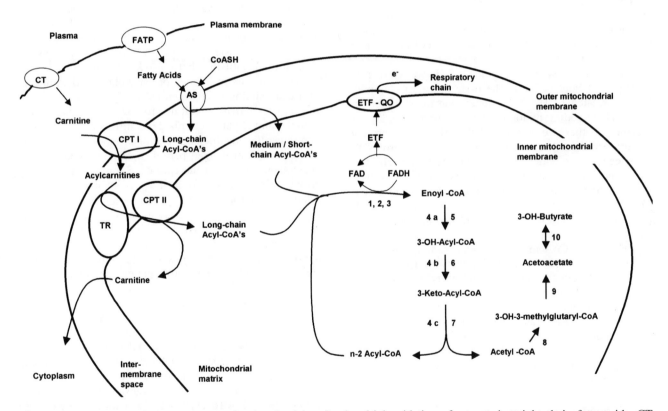

Figure 3 Enzymes and transporter proteins involved in mitochondrial oxidation of saturated straight-chain fatty acids. CT, carnitine transporter; FATP, fatty acid transport proteins; AS, acyl-CoA synthetase(s); CPT I, carnitine palmitoyltransferase I; TR, carnitine-acylcarnitine translocase; CPT II, carnitine palmitoyltransferase II; ETF, electron transfer flavoprotein; ETF-QO, ETF-ubiquinone-oxidoreductase; 1, very long-chain acyl-CoA-dehydrogenase; 2, medium-chain acyl-CoA-dehydrogenase; 3, short-chain acyl-CoA-dehydrogenase; 4, mitochondrial trifunctional protein (MTP): 4a, long-chain-enoyl-CoA-hydratase; 4b, long-chain 3-hydroxy-acyl-CoA-dehydrogenase; 4c, long-chain-ketoacyl-CoA thiolase; 5, short-chain-enoyl-CoA-hydratase (crotonase); 6, short-chain 3-hydroxy-acyl-CoA-dehydrogenase; 7, medium-chain 3-ketoacyl-CoA thiolase; 8, hydroxymethylglutaril-CoA-sinthetase; 9, hydroxymethylglutaril-CoA-lyase (enzyme involved in ketogenesis and leucine metabolism);10, 3-OH-butyric-acid dehydrogenase. CoA, Coenzyme A; CoASH, free CoA; FAD, flavin adenine dinucleotide; FADH, reduced form of FAD.

the dehydrogenases involved in fatty acid oxidation but also those involved in the metabolism of branched-chain aminoacids (valine, isoleucine, and leucine), lysine, hydroxylysine, tryptophan, and sarcosine.

In the second step of FAO, the enoyl-CoAs produced by the ACDs are hydrated to hydroxyacyl-CoAs by an enoyl-CoA-hydratase. Then, the hydroxyacyl-CoAs undergo dehydrogenation to ketoacyl-CoAs by a hydroxyacyl-CoA dehydrogenase and finally there is a cleavage of the thioester bond by an acyl-CoA ketothiolase (Fig. 3). This process completes one turn of the FAO cycle and results in the release of acetyl-CoA and a new acyl-CoA molecule that is two carbons shorter (153,156). The exact mechanism of the last three steps varies for substrates of different chain length. For long-chain acyl-CoA substrates the reactions are carried by a mitochondrial trifunctional protein (MTP) with enoyl-CoA-hydratase, hydroxyacyl-CoA dehydrogenase, and ketoacyl-CoA thiolase activities (159,160). This protein is an octamer composed of four α- and four β-subunits. The α-subunits contain the long-chain 3-enoyl-CoaA hydratase activity and the long-chain 3-hydroxy-acyl-CoA dehydrogenase (LCHAD) activities; the β subunit has the long-chain 3-ketoacyl-CoA thiolase activity (161).

Biochemical studies have identified two groups of LCHAD-deficient patients. The first, and most common, has an isolated LCHAD deficiency due to mutations in the LCHAD coding region of the α-subunit gene. Activities of the other two enzymes of the trifunctional protein are preserved in these patients. In the second group all three enzyme activities are deficient (162). For shorter-chain fatty acids, individual enzymes, each one with a single activity, have been identified: short-chain-enoyl-CoA-hydratase (crotonase), short-chain 3-hydroxyacyl-CoA dehydrogenase (SCHAD), and medium-chain 3-ketoacyl-CoA thiolase (153,156).

The acetyl-CoA moieties produced during the FAO are used as a source of energy through the tricarboxylic acid cycle. Under fasting conditions, acetyl-CoA moieties produced in the liver become the substrate for the synthesis of ketone bodies that are used as fuel by several tissues, including the brain. Two enzymes are involved in ketone bodies synthesis: hydroxymethylglutaryl-CoA-synthase and hydroxymethylglutaryl-CoA lyase (Fig. 3) (52,163). The latter is also the final enzyme of leucine catabolic pathway.

B. Clinical Presentation

Several enzymatic defects in FAO and ketogenesis have been found in humans, all inherited as autosomal recessive diseases. These defects have become one of the most important group of IMD, due to the number of patients and the severe outcome. In a series of 107 patients, Saudubray et al. found that 50 patients and 47 siblings died, 30% within the first week and 60% before age 1 year (164).

1. Main Clinical Features

The most common diseases are MCAD, LCHAD, and MAD deficiencies, but it is possible that many patients with long-chain fatty acid oxidation defects still die without recognition of their underlying disease. Table 5 summarizes the known defects in saturated straight-chain fatty acid metabolism found in humans and their most distinctive features. Clinical presentation in patients with FAO defects ranges from completely asymptomatic to severe malformations or unexplained sudden death in infancy or adulthood. As expected by the important role of FAO in liver, heart, and muscle the main clinical presentation of FAO defects is dominated by symptoms related to these organs. Neurological symptoms are also common during the acute crisis and they might be in part related to hypoglycemia and impaired ketogenesis.

Neonatal presentations, including malformations, lethargy, hypotonia, heart-beat abnormalities, liver involvement, or sudden death, were thought to be limited to CPT-II, translocase, and MAD deficiencies (158, 164,182) but neonatal cases of MCAD, LCHAD, and VLCAD deficiencies have also been reported (164, 183,184). In classic cases, patients with FAO defects appear normal until the first episode of metabolic decompensation occurs in infancy or early childhood. A history of a dead sibling is common (164). The metabolic crisis is characterized by vomiting, followed by lethargy, hypotonia, and slight liver enlargement. Respiratory distress due to cardiac insufficiency and/or metabolic acidosis can be present. A prolonged period of fasting, and/or hypercatabolism can trigger the episode. Symptoms are usually erroneously attributed to an intercurrent illness or cyclic vomiting syndrome (153,164). Patients can recover from the initial crisis, and repeat another episode, remaining asymptomatic in between. Liver insufficiency can be severe, leading to a Reye-like syndrome, complicated by hypothermia and gastrointestinal bleeding (185). Cholestasis has also been reported in patients with LCHAD deficiency (164,175,186).

Cardiac involvement is characterized by hypertrophic or, less commonly, dilated cardiomyopathy. Severe arrhythmia (ventricular and supraventricular tachycardia, ventricular fibrillation), conduction defects (bundle branch block, atrioventricular (AV) block, sinus node dysfunction), and cardiac insufficiency can be found in neonates, especially in those with CPT-II, translocase, and LCHAD deficiencies (154,164,170,182), which are diseases in which there is an accumulation of long-chain-acyl-CoAs and long-chain acylcarnitines. Heart-beat disorders have not been observed in CT, CPT-I, or MCAD deficiencies. Pericardial effusion and endocardial fibroelastosis have been described (187).

Symptoms of skeletal muscle involvement have been described for the majority of the FAO defects, and they are especially common in patients with CPT II-adult type-, LCHAD and mild MAD deficiencies. Usual mani-

Table 5 Defects in Mitochondrial Oxidation of Saturated Straight-Chain Fatty Acids

Known enzyme deficiencies in humans	Main organ involved			Distinctive features
	Liver	Muscle	Heart	
Defects in plasmatic membrane transport				
Carnitine transporter (CT)	Yes	Yes	Yes	Very low plasma carnitine levels (165).
Fatty acid transport protein (FATP)	Yes	No	No	Severe episodic liver failure. Two patients reported (155).
Defects in mitochondrial transport				
Carnitine palmitoyltransferase I (CPT-I)	Yes	No	No	Plasma carnitine elevated or normal. Renal tubular acidosis reported (166).
Carnitine-acylcarnitine translocase (translocase)	Yes	Yes	Yes	Neonatal presentation. Heart beat abnormalities. Hyperammonemia (167).
Carnitine palmitoyltransferase II (CPT-II)				
Neonatal	Yes	Yes	Yes	Severe neonatal presentation. Renal and brain abnormalities reported (168,169).
Infantile	Yes	No	Yes	Less frequent (169,170).
Late onset (most frequent)	No	Yes	No	Most common cause of rhabdomyolysis and myoglobinuria (169).
Mitochondrial beta oxidation				
Very long-chain acyl-CoA-dehydrogenase (VLCAD)	Yes	Yes	Yes	Neonatal and infantile presentation. Arrhythmias (171).
Medium-chain acyl-CoA-dehydrogenase (MCAD)	Yes	No	No	Most frequent FAO defect. Reye-like episodes. Sudden death (172).
Short-chain acyl-CoA-dehydrogenase (SCAD)	Yes	Yes	No	Variable phenotype. Ophthalmoplegia, myopathy, metabolic acidosis (173,174).
Long-chain 3-hydroxy-acyl-CoA-dehydrogenase (LCHAD)	Yes	Yes	Yes	Retinitis pigmentosa, peripheral neuropathy (175,176).
Mitochondrial trifunctional protein (MTP)	Yes	Yes	Yes	Few cases reported. More severe than LCHAD deficiency (177).
Short-chain 3-hydroxy-acyl-CoA-dehydrogenase (SCHAD)	Yes	Yes	Yes	Few cases reported. Variable phenotype. Ketonuria, muscle and liver isoforms (?) (178).
Medium-chain 3-ketoacyl-CoA thiolase deficiency (MCKAT)	Yes	Yes	Yes	Few patients known. Typical organic acid profile (179,180).
Electron transfer				
Multiple acyl-CoA-dehydrogenase (MAD)	Yes	Yes	Yes	Great phenotypic variation from severe neonatal form with malformations
Electron transfer flavoprotein (ETF)	Yes	Yes	Yes	to progressive muscle weaknes with lipidic myopathy (158).
ETF-ubiquinone-oxidoreductase (ETF-QO)				
Ketone body synthesis				
Hydroxymethylglutaril-CoA-synthetase (HMG-S)	Yes	No	No	Few patients reported (163,181).
Hydroxymethylglutaril-CoA-lyase[a] (HMG-L)	Yes	No	No	Hypoketotic hypoglycemia and severe metabolic acidosis. (51,52,163).

Abnormalities related to liver, muscle, and heart involvement are described in the text.
[a]Enzyme involved in ketogenesis and leucine catabolism.

festations are hypotonia and/or progressive proximal weakness. Acute episodes of muscle pain or cramps, fatigue, and/or exercise intolerance with rhabdomyolysis can appear in response to stress, prolonged exercise, or cold, and can produce acute renal failure. Muscle involvement has not been associated to CPT-I deficiency (154,164,188). Malformations are mainly associated with MAD deficiency, but have also been described in CPT-II deficiency. Most common dysmorphic features are a high forehead, wide-spaced eyes, and low-set ears, resembling a Zellweger syndrome. Renal dysplasia (polycystic kidneys) and brain malformations have also been reported (153,158,164).

Retinitis pigmentosa and peripheral neuropathy have been found in patients with LCHAD deficiency. The former seems to be related to deficiency of docosahexaenoic acid (DHA). Endogenous synthesis of DHA may be impaired in LCHAD-deficient patients and a preliminary study treating these children with oral DHA has shown promising results (189). Mental retardation and/or other neurological sequelae are observed mostly in patients who had severe encephalopathy associated to Reye's-like syndrome (164,185).

Other manifestations, specific for a given defect, are outlined in Table 1.

2. Maternal Complications During Pregnancy of Affected Fetuses

The association between LCHAD deficiency in the fetus and maternal pre-eclampsia, the syndrome of hemolysis, elevated liver enzymes, and low platelets (HELLP syndrome) or acute fatty liver of pregnancy (AFLP) has been well documented (162,190–192). These complications have been reported in up to 79% of pregnancies with fetuses affected with LCHAD, while there were no complications if the fetus was heterozygous or normal. Ibdah et al. reported that the complications were related to the presence of the prevalent E474Q mutation on one or both alleles (homozygous or compound heterozygous) of the LCHAD-affected fetus (162,191). However, a recent report describes three families with trifunctional enzyme deficiency and maternal hepatic dysfunction in pregnancy not associated with the common E474Q mutation (193).

Affected LCHAD patients show a higher incidence of prematurity, asphyxia, intrauterine growth retardation, and intrauterine death than their unaffected siblings (190). These findings highlight the importance of obtaining molecular diagnoses for patients and parents, and to provide adequate genetic counseling and molecular prenatal diagnosis when indicated (194). More recently, AFLP has also been reported in pregnancies with fetal CPT-1, MCAD, and SCAD deficiencies, raising the possibility of a common mechanism producing liver disease in mothers carrying fetuses affected with FAO defects (195–197).

3. Sudden Infant Death

Many FAO defects have been associated with episodes of sudden, unexpected, infant death. Different studies analyzing postmortem specimens of liver, bile, cultured fibroblasts, or blood spots in filter paper have estimated that 2–5% of sudden infant death syndrome (SIDS) can be attributed to FAO defects (198–200). They include deficiencies of the carnitine transporter, translocase, VLCAD, LCHAD, MCAD, SCHAD, and MAD (171,198–204). The mechanism of sudden death in these patients is not clear, but acute arrhythmia may account for the unexpected deaths in children with abnormalities in long-chain fatty acid metabolism (182). Acylcarnitine analysis by tandem mass spectrometry in postmortem bile or in the newborn screening samples (Guthrie card) stored by state programs have significantly expanded the retrospective diagnosis of fatty acid oxidation disorders (200,204,205). With the availability of newborn screening by tandem mass spectrometry and early treatment, it is reasonable to expect that the number of patients who experience sudden death due to FAO defects will decrease significantly.

Other metabolic diseases, not involving fatty acid metabolism, have also been found in children who experience sudden or unexpected death in infancy. Among others they include glutaric aciduria type I, myophosphorilase deficiency, lysinuric protein intolerance, and defects of the respiratory chain (1,200,206–209).

C. Laboratory Abnormalities

The most common laboratory abnormality found during an acute episode is hypoglycemia. Ketone bodies can be detected in urine, but in smaller amounts than expected for the degree of hypoglycemia (hypoketotic hypoglycemia). Total nonesterified fatty acids (NEFA) are increased, and the NEFA to ketone body ratio is abnormally high (>3) when the sample is obtained before IV glucose is started (210). As an exception to the rule, patients with SCHAD deficiency may present with large amounts of ketones in urine (178).

Elevated liver enzymes, mild hyperammonemia, and slight metabolic acidosis are common. Abnormal clotting factors are seldom observed. Very high levels of CK (several thousands) and aldolase reveal muscle involvement. Hyperuricemia appears to be a common finding in MCAD deficiency and mild elevation of lactic acid is present in LCHAD deficiency (175,211). Myoglobinuria can be present in any FAO defect affecting skeletal muscle, and is a common presentation in the adult form of CPT II deficiency (153,154,164).

During the acute episode, a liver biopsy under light microscopy shows micro- and macrovesicular steatosis. These abnormalities usually lead to the diagnosis of Reye syndrome. However, the electron microscopy will lack the characteristic mitochondrial changes of Reye syndrome (188,212). Fibrosis and cirrhosis has been described in liver biopsies of VLCAD and LCHAD deficiencies. Pathology of skeletal and cardiac muscle shows fatty infiltration (lipidic myopathy) (153,158,188).

D. Diagnosis

Once the diagnosis of a FAO defect is suspected, samples should be immediately obtained for specialized metabolic studies. They must include blood spots in filter paper (Guthrie card), serum, and urine. Analysis of acylcarnitines (AC) by TMS in plasma or blood spots in filter paper have become the most important tool for diagnosis of FAO defects. This methodology is highly sensitive and abnormal profiles can be obtained even when samples are collected out of crisis. In rare cases an AC profile can be misread as normal when free carnitine levels are very low or when the sample is obtained out of crisis in nonfasting conditions. Typical AC profiles can be identified for CPT-II/translocase, LCAD/VLCAD, MCAD, SCAD, LCHAD, and MAD as well as for HMG-CoA-lyase deficiencies (106,107,213–215). In the transport defects of long-chain fatty acids and the carnitine uptake deficiency AC are uninformative; in CPT-I deficiency, low levels of all AC species (including acetylcarnitine), combined with high levels of free carnitine, are suggestive of the defect (216). AC have been reported as normal in children with SCHAD (203) and HMG-CoA-synthase deficiencies (217). AC analysis performed in the newborn screening card have allowed retrospective diagnosis in patients who died of MCAD, CPT II, VLCAD, translocase, and MAD deficiencies (111,169,185,202,204,218). Tandem mass spectrometry is also being employed by many screening programs around the world for the neonatal detection of FAO defects as well as other IMD (109–111,219,220). It is likely that early diagnosis and treatment will change the natural history of the disease for many patients (221).

Urine OA profile is the second choice for the diagnosis of FAO defects. It is important that analysis and interpretation be performed in an experienced center. Several defects can be diagnosed if samples are obtained during the acute episode; they include HMG-CoA-lyase, MCAD, LCHAD, SCAD, MCKAT, SCHAD, and MAD. However, frequently the results may be suggestive of, but nonspecific for, an FAO defect or give a false-negative result when samples are collected after the patient has been started on supportive therapy (105,188,222). Therefore, patients with FAO defects can be misdiagnosed if only standard OA analysis is performed.

Quantitative analysis of acylglycines by GC/MS stable isotope dilution or tandem mass spectrometry is an alternative method for diagnosis when acylcarnitines are not available and/or when UOA analysis gives a negative result (105,223).

Carnitine levels are informative. Total and free carnitine levels are normal or high in CPT-I deficiency and extremely low in the CT defect. In all other FAO diseases, total and free carnitine are usually decreased, and the percentage of acylcarnitines is increased (164,188). Another method for the diagnosis of FAO defects is to measure the levels of individual free fatty acids in plasma by GC/MS (224). This method is sensitive but time consuming. We have shown that in MCAD and MAD deficiencies, levels of individual fatty acids correlate well with those of the acylcarnitine of the same carbon length (221,225). However, short-chain-3-hydroxy fatty acids are not esterified with carnitine and therefore their measurement might be important for the diagnosis of SCHAD, when the acylcarnitine profile is noncontributory (226).

In vitro flux studies with labeled fatty acids in lymphocytes of fibroblasts are another useful tool for diagnosis (227,228). Fasting or loading tests are less frequently needed and should only be performed in experienced centers if the above-mentioned specialized tests are not informative (164). Enzyme activity can be measured in the majority of these conditions in cultured fibroblasts, liver, and/or muscle. Tissue specificity is known for CT, and CPT-I, and has also been postulated for SCHAD, while HMG-CoA-synthase is only expressed in liver.

Molecular studies are available for most of the FAO defects (229). Common mutations have been described in MCAD and LCHAD deficiencies. Several studies have shown that a missense mutation 985 A>G, accounts for the majority of the mutant alleles in MCAD deficiency, being more prevalent in northern Europeans (219,229–231). In LCHAD deficiency, a common 1528 G>C mutation has been identified (175,229).

E. Treatment: The Acute Episode

Acutely ill patients with suspected FAO defect should be treated in an experienced pediatric intensive care unit. Delay in proper treatment may result in death or permanent brain damage (164,188).

1. Supportive Therapy

Intravenous hydration should be given cautiously because patients with hyperammonemia may have cerebral edema and patients with heart involvement may develop cardiac insufficiency. Intracranial pressure monitoring should be considered if brain swelling is suspected and mannitol can be used if needed. Clotting factors may be required in patients with severe liver dysfunction and H2 blockers should be given to prevent gastrointestinal bleeding.

Salicylates and valproic acid are contraindicated due to their potential mitochondrial toxicity and should be investigated as a potential cause of the metabolic crisis (232). Epinephrine and glucagon have a lipolytic effect and therefore should be avoided.

2. Anabolism

In order to suppress lipolysis, intravenous fluids should provide a glucose infusion rate of 10 mg/kg/min or more, regardless of the blood sugar levels found on admission (164,188). If patients develop hyperglycemia, IV insulin can be given. Due to the required high glucose concentration in the IV fluids, a central line is needed. As an alternative, glucose (10% glucose polymers solution) can be provided via NG tube. In patients known to have long-chain fatty acid defects, medium-chain triglycerides (1–3 grams/kg/day) can be added via NG tube as soon as the GI tract allows for it.

3. Detoxification

Treatment with intravenous carnitine (100–200 mg/kg/day) is life saving for the carnitine transport defect (CTD). There is general agreement to the use of carnitine (50–100 mg/kg/day) in patients with short- and medium-chain defects (153,156,164). However, use of carnitine for defects involving long-chain fatty acids is still controversial, due to the possible role of long-chain acylcarnitines in the development of heart beat abnormalities (164). A recent study also shows that medium- and long-chain acylcarnitines suppress mitochondrial fatty acid transport through inhibition of translocase (233). A conservative approach is to start treatment with 50% of the usual dosage and adjust it to maintain free carnitine levels within normal limits.

Riboflavin (100–200 mg/day) should be tried in patients with MAD and SCAD deficiencies, even though only a few patients with mild variants have been reported to respond to it (188).

F. Long-Term Management

Carnitine is the only treatment needed for the CT deficiency. For all other FAO defects, the key to chronic treatment is to avoid prolonged fasting and to use a fat-restricted diet. Guidelines for treatment of the different conditions are outlined in Table 6. The formula to be used depends on the enzymatic defect. There is a rationale for the use of medium-chain triglycerides (MCT) in patients with impaired metabolism of long-chain fatty acids (FATP,

CPT-I, translocase, CPT-II, VLCAD, LCHAD, MTP). In contrast, the use of MCT is contraindicated for patients with short- or medium-chain FAO defects as well as for MAD and defects in ketogenesis. Enough essential fatty acids (linoleic and α-linolenic) acids should be provided to avoid deficiencies. Dietary supplementation with DHA appears to be beneficial in LCHAD-deficient patients to prevent retinal damage (189). In addition to the low-fat diet, patients with MAD should also have a mild protein restriction. Patients HMG-CoA-lyase may likewise benefit from leucine restriction.

Blood glucose, liver enzymes, uric acid, ammonia, and CK are late markers of a metabolic crisis (188) and cannot be used to monitor fasting tolerance or response to dietary changes. In contrast, acylcarnitines have been shown to be a sensitive marker. AC levels tend to increase rapidly during short fasting periods and reflect the accumulation of toxic metabolites (221,225). Treatment of infants and young children with severe enzyme deficiencies needs to be aggressive and may require frequent feedings during the day and overnight NG or G-tube feedings (164). In children over 2 years of age, the diet can be supplemented with uncooked cornstarch. In children with poor appetite who have severe enzyme deficiencies, cornstarch can be given at regular intervals throughout the 24 h, as used for patients with glycogen storage diseases. In less severely affected patients uncooked cornstarch (1–2 g/kg) can be used at bedtime only. We have documented the beneficial effect of uncooked cornstarch in decreasing abnormal metabolites in children with MCAD, MAD (221,225), and LCHAD deficiencies. As an alternative for young children whose amylase activity is deficient, we have successfully used cornstarch with exogenous amylase (221).

Education and family compliance are essential to avoid life-threatening decompensations, which can occur very rapidly in young patients. Long-term prognosis varies according to the disease, residual enzyme activity, age at diagnosis, and long-term treatment. The mortality rate has been estimated at 25% for MCAD deficiency; the ma-

Table 6 Guidelines for the Nutritional Treatment of Fatty Acid Oxidation Defects

	Metabolic abnormality		
	Long-chain FAO	Medium- and short-chain FAO, HMG-CoA-synthase	Electron transfer (MAD), HMG-CoA-lyase
Calories	>20% RDA	>20% RDA	>20% RDA
Protein	RDA	RDA	7%
Fat	25–30%	15–25%	15–20%
MCT	15–20% (1–3 g/kg/d)	Contraindicated	Contraindicated
LCFA	±10%	—	—
EFA	4%	4%	4%
CHO	60–65%	60–75%	73–78%

MCT, medium-chain triglycerides; LCFA, long-chain fatty acids; EFA, essential fatty acids; CHO, carbohydrates. Fat and CHO are expressed as % or total calories.

jority of these patients die in the initial episode (185,234). Long-term complications in MCAD deficiency include developmental delay, muscle weakness, failure to thrive, and cerebral palsy (172,185,234). To prevent the mortality and severe morbidity of MCAD, it would be mandatory to implement newborn screening programs (108,172,185, 219).

Limited information is still available for the long-term prognosis of patients with other FAO defects, but it is likely that, as shown for MCAD deficiency, newborn screening may change the natural history of these diseases (221).

V. PRIMARY LACTIC ACIDEMIAS

The primary lactic acidemias (PLA) are a group of IMD with variable clinical presentation, including life-threatening episodes of metabolic acidosis, and complex biochemical, enzymatic, and molecular diagnosis. They represent abnormalities in pyruvate metabolism that are recognized biochemically by its primary consequence, hyperlactacidemia, and clinically by symptoms reflecting energy deficiency (1,235). Pyruvic acid produced by the glycolytic pathway can follow different metabolic fates. To produce energy, pyruvate enters the mitochondria and undergoes aerobic catabolism via acetyl-CoA, the tricarboxylic acid cycle (TCA) and the respiratory chain (Fig. 4). During fasting periods, pyruvic acid can also be an intermediary substrate for gluconeogenesis, via oxaloacetic acid. A block in any of the many enzymatic steps involved in those pathways can increase pyruvic acid levels, with simultaneous elevation of lactic acid and alanine, and limit the production of energy or glucose synthesis. In general, the PLA can be classified into four groups:

Defects in pyruvate dehydrogenase complex
Defects in the TCA cycle
Defects in gluconeogenesis
Defects in oxidative phosphorylation (respiratory chain)

A. Pathophysiology and Clinical Presentation

Correlation between symptoms and enzymatic block is difficult: one enzymatic defect can present with different phenotypes and different enzyme deficiencies can give a similar clinical presentation. A detailed description of each enzymatic defect is beyond the scope of this chapter, so we will mainly address those conditions that can present with severe hyperlactacidemia, requiring emergency treatment.

1. Pyruvate Dehydrogenase Complex

Deficiency of pyruvate dehydrogenase complex (PDHC) is one of the most frequent causes of PLA. This thiamine-dependent enzymatic complex is responsible for the decarboxylation of pyruvate to acetyl-CoA (Fig. 4) and is

made of four different components: E_1-α, E_1-β, E_2, and E_3. Two regulatory components at the E_1 level are known: pyruvate dehydrogenase kinase and pyruvate dehydrogenase phosphatase, which inactivate and activate, respectively, the enzyme activity. An E_3-binding protein (formerly called X-lipoate protein) is also part of the complex (235,236). Deficiencies in different components of the PDHC have been reported, but the most common is the deficiency of the E_1-α subunit.

Three different clinical presentations have been outlined. The most severe is neonatal, characterized by overwhelming lactic acidosis at birth. These children present soon after birth with poor feeding, hypotonia, lethargy, and respiratory distress. Mild dysmorphism (frontal bossing, low nasal bridge, upturned nose, long philtrum) has been described, and death occurs within the first weeks of life (236,237). A less severe picture appears in infants and young children with hypotonia, developmental delay, and seizures. The third form presents with acute, intermittent episodes of ataxia, which can be triggered by a high-carbohydrate intake (235–237). The E_1-α subunit is encoded by an X-linked gene. However, due to the important role of the PDHC in energy metabolism, males as well as females can be affected. Most defects of E_1-α gene are de novo, with point mutations being more common in males and deletions or insertions in females (236,238). This information is extremely important for genetic counseling.

Defects in the E_2 component, the E_3-binding protein, and the pyruvate dehydrogenase phosphatase, while rare, have been reported (236,239,240). Described phenotypes have ranged from severe mental retardation to Leigh syndrome and refractory lactic acidosis.

The E_3 component (dihydrolipoamide dehydrogenase) is common to three other enzymatic complexes: the α-ketoglutarate dehydrogenase (α-KGD) (involved in TCA cycle), the branched-chain 2-ketoacid dehydrogenase (BCKD), which is the enzyme deficient in maple syrup urine disease (MSUD), and the glycine cleavage system (involved in glycine catabolism). Few patients with deficiency of the E_3 component (lipoamide dehydrogenase) are known. Their clinical and biochemical presentation is variable, with a combination of the different manifestations of the PDHC, α-KGD, and BCKD deficiencies. Recurrent episodes of liver failure, cardiomyopathy and myoglobinuria have also been reported (235,236, 241–243).

Progressive involvement of the basal ganglia and brainstem is frequent in PDHC-deficient patients, and can lead to nystagmus, dystonia, apnea, or sudden, unexpected death. Magnetic resonance imaging (MRI) findings in these patients are suggestive of subacute necrotizing encephalopathy (Leigh syndrome). However, it is important to note that Leigh syndrome has also been described in patients with pyruvate carboxylase, the TCA cycle, and respiratory chain deficiencies (see below) as well as in other inborn metabolic diseases (IMD) (1,244,245). Other

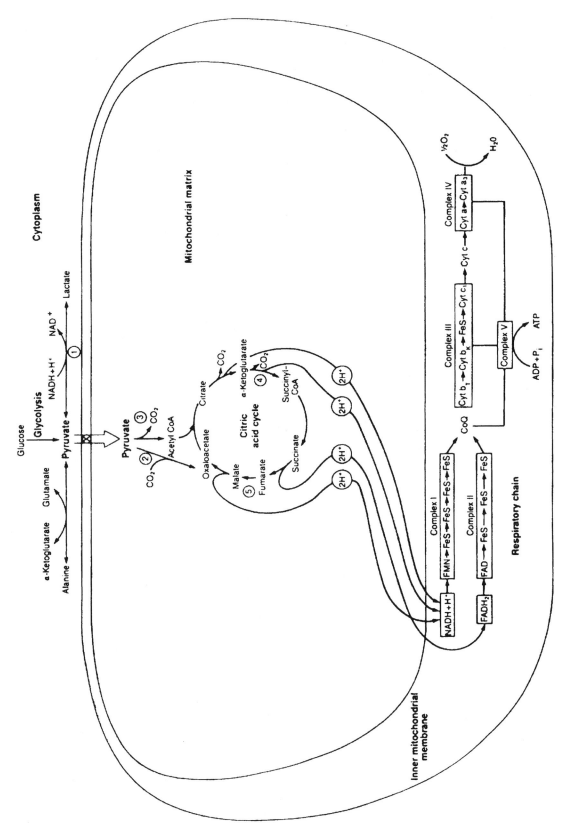

Figure 4 Pyruvate metabolism, the TCA cycle, and the respiratory chain. See explanation in the text. Enzymes: 1, lactate dehydrogenase; 2, pyruvate carboxylase; 3, pyruvate dehydrogenase complex; 4, α-ketoglutarate dehydrogenase; 5, fumarase. (From: D.C. De Vivo and S. Di Mauro. Disorders of pyruvate metabolism, the citric acid cycle and the respiratory chain. In: Inborn Metabolic Diseases. Diagnosis and management. J. Fernandes, JM Saudubray and Tada. Eds. Springer Verlag-1st Ed., 1990, pp. 127–160.)

frequent abnormalities of the CNS in PDHC deficiency are congenital malformations of the brain, including agenesis or hypoplasia of the corpus callosum (235–237).

2. Defects in the TCA Cycle

The TCA cycle is responsible for the oxidative decarboxylation of citrate to oxaloacetate (Fig. 4). Several enzymes are involved, and defects in α-ketoglutarate dehydrogenase (α-KGD), fumarase, and succinate dehydrogenase (SDH) have been characterized. Structure of α-KGD is similar to the PDHC and the BCKD, sharing with them the E_3 component. Therefore the three enzymes can be affected in E_3 deficiency (see section on PDHC deficiency above). A few patients with isolated α-KGD have also been reported. They present in infancy or early childhood with severe neurological involvement, including developmental delay, hypo- or hypertonia, and ataxia (235,246–248). Structural brain abnormalities can be present.

Fumarase deficiency appears to be more common. Clinical presentation ranges from severe neurological involvement, seizures, and death in childhood to mild mental retardation and survival into adulthood (235,248–250). Dysmorphic facial features and neonatal polycythemia have been recently reported (251). Structural brain malformations such as diffuse polymicrogyria, hypomyelination, agenesis of the corpus callosum, Leigh syndrome, decreased white matter, and cortical atrophy are common (250,251). A few patients with SDH are known. This TCA cycle enzyme is also part of complex II of the respiratory chain (succinate–ubiquinone oxidoreductase) and these patients' clinical presentation resembles more a respiratory chain defect (see below) (235). A combined deficiency of SDH, aconitase, complex I and III has been reported (252). This defect is apparently caused by abnormalities in the iron–sulfur clusters common to these enzymes.

3. Defects in Gluconeogenesis

Gluconeogenic defects involve deficiencies in the four regulatory enzymes of this pathway: pyruvate carboxylase, phosphoenolpyruvate carboxykinase, fructose-1,6-diphosphatase, and glucose-6-phosphatase. Deficiency of the latter affects gluconeogenesis as well as glycogen degradation and is responsible for the glycogen storage disease type 1. In general, patients with gluconeogenic defects present not only lactic acidosis but also hypoglycemia and hepatomegaly. Pyruvate carboxylase (PC), a biotin-dependent enzyme responsible for the carboxylation of pyruvate to oxaloacetate (Fig. 4), plays an important role in gluconeogenesis, lipogenesis, and energy production. Decreased availability of oxaloacetate also impairs the synthesis of aspartate and glutamate with secondary abnormalities in the urea cycle and the synthesis of glutamine-derived neurotransmitters. Deficiency of the PC can be isolated or as a part of the biotinidase or ho-

locarboxylase synthetase deficiencies (see organic acidemias). Isolated PC deficiency has been described in about 40 patients. Three clinical presentations are differentiated. The most severe form presents in neonates with lactic acidosis, hypotonia, and seizures, progressing to coma and death in the first few months of life (235,236). A less severe phenotype, mainly described in North American Indians, presents in infancy with developmental delay, failure to thrive, and seizures, progressing to severe mental retardation. Mild hepatomegaly is present in both clinical presentations. Macrocephaly and brain abnormalities, including decreased myelination, ischemia-like lesions, cyst, periventricular leukomalacia, Leigh syndrome, subdural hematomas, and brain atrophy have been described (235,236,253,254). These abnormalities are thought to be related to the important role of PC in astrocyte metabolism. The third, less common, phenotype is characterized by episodic attacks of lactic acidosis with slight neurological involvement (235,236).

Phosphoenolpyruvate carboxykinase (PEPCK) deficiency is very rare. Symptoms appear in the newborn period or early infancy and include failure to thrive, hypotonia, lethargy, and hepatomegaly. Renal tubular acidosis as well as skeletal and cardiac muscular involvement have been reported (235).

Fructose-1,6-diphosphatase (FDP) deficient patients present in the newborn period with symptoms of hypoglycemia, hypotonia, and liver enlargement. Neurological involvement in these patients is only related to the hypoglycemic episodes (255).

4. Defects in Oxidative Phosphorylation

The oxidative phosphorylation (OXPHOS) is a complex system that carries electrons through a series of reactions to generate ATP. Our understanding of this system has greatly increased in the last few years with significant advances in molecular genetics. The OXPHOS is composed of five different complexes (I, II, III, IV, and V), located in the inner mitochondrial membrane. Each complex has several protein components, some of them encoded by nuclear DNA (nDNA) and others by mitochondrial DNA (mtDNA) (256,257). The only exception is complex II, which has only nDNA-encoded proteins. Differentiation between abnormalities in the OXPHOS caused by defects in nDNA or mtDNA is important for prenatal diagnosis and genetic counseling: nDNA defects follow a mendelian inheritance, while mtDNA is maternally transmitted.

The nuclear DNA is responsible for the synthesis of about 70 OXPHOS subunits, their transport into the mitochondria, and their proper processing and assembly (256). A great number of the nuclear genes, the majority of them still unidentified, are responsible for these processes.

The mtDNA is a small circular molecule (16.5 kb) that encodes for 13 OXPHOS subunits together with ribosomal RNAs and the 22 mitochondrial transfer RNAs necessary for mRNA expression (256,257). Each cell contains hundreds of mitochondria and thousands of mtDNA. In patients with mtDNA abnormalities, normal and abnormal mtDNA coexist in the same cells (heteroplasmy). During cell division, mitochondria are randomly distributed to the new cells (replicative segregation) and, as the cells divide, the relative proportions of normal and abnormal mtDNA change (256). These characteristics of the mtDNA have clinical implications. In the same patient some tissues/organs may or may not be affected depending on their proportion of normal and abnormal mtDNA. Furthermore, tissues that are not affected at one point may become affected when the number of abnormal mitochondria reaches a threshold for phenotypic expression. These facts explain why the same molecular defect can present with different phenotypes, which can also change over time (256–258).

Clinical presentation of patients with OXPHOS diseases is extremely variable. Neonatal decompensation, with severe metabolic acidosis, is not frequent but has been described in fatal and benign infantile myopathy due to complex IV (COX deficiency) as well as in deficiencies of other complexes (257–260). These children present in the neonatal period with severe hypotonia, abnormal movements, poor sucking, lethargy, respiratory distress, and severe lactic acidosis. Ketosis is usually present. A picture resembling neonatal-onset diabetes mellitus, with hyperglycemia, ketosis, and hyperlactacidemia has been reported in patients with OXPHOS defects (261). Another severe neonatal presentation is seen in one of the variants of the mitochondrial DNA depletion syndrome (see below). These children develop severe liver failure, with hypoglycemia, lactic acidosis, and elevated liver enzymes within the first day of life. Liver histopathological examination reveals micronodular cirrhosis, cholestasis, microvesicular steatosis, and accumulation of iron. Electron microscopy shows abnormal proliferation of mitochondria. Less severe infantile forms of this syndrome have been reported in children with failure to thrive, vomiting, ypotonia, hypoglycemia, and progressive liver dysfunction (258,262–264).

Because OXPHOS is present in all cells, patients with a subacute or chronic course can have different combinations of symptoms and signs. In general, an OXPHOS defect must be considered when there is an unexplained association of symptoms, with early onset and a rapidly progressive course involving seemingly unrelated organs (257,258). A list of the most frequent signs and symptoms is presented in Table 7. Patients with OXPHOS diseases are prone to multiorgan involvement; therefore abnormalities in tissues with high energy needs including muscle, liver, kidney, pancreas, bone marrow, heart, brain, retina, auditory nerve, and endocrine system should be searched for. In patients with CNS involvement MRI of the brain will provide useful information (Table 7) (265). Different combinations of symptoms and signs are possible, and classification of OXPHOS diseases has been difficult.

Table 7 Most Frequent Findings Associated with OXPHOS Diseases

Hypotonia
Developmental delay
Progressive encephalopathy, regression
Seizures, myoclonus
Strokelike episodes
Recurrent ataxia
Cortical blindness
Brain abnormalities
    Absence of corpus callosum
    Porencephalic cysts
    Abnormal signaling of the basal ganglia
    Leukodystrophy
    Cortical atrophy/poliodystrophy
    Leigh's disease
Sudden infant death
Muscle weakness, myopathy
Myalgia, exercise intolerance, myoglobinuria
Palpebral ptosis, progressive external ophthalmoplegia
Cataracts, corneal opacities
Retinitis pigmentosa
Sensorineural hearing loss
Cardiomyopathy (mainly hyperthrophic)
Heart block (A-V, and others)
Failure to thrive, intrauterine growth retardation
Renal Fanconi's syndrome
Tubulointerstitial nephritis, renal failure
Episodic vomiting
Chronic diarrhea, villous atrophy
Exocrine pancreatic dysfunction
Liver failure
Anemia (sideroblastic), myelodysplasia
Diabetes mellitus
Growth hormone deficiency
Hypothyroidism, hypoparathyroidism
Recurrent hypoglycemia
Craniofacial dysmorphic features
Hair abnormalities (dry, thick, brittle hair)
Skin abnormalities (mottled pigmentation in exposed areas)

Source: Refs. 256–258.

They have been categorized based on their molecular defect in mtDNA or nDNA. Known mtDNA abnormalities include point mutations, deletions, and duplications. In general, point mutations follow a pattern of maternal inheritance while deletions tend to be sporadic. Many of them correlate with well-defined syndromes, but significant overlapping and variation exist (Table 8).

In the last few years, an increasing number of mutations in nuclear OXPHOS genes are being recognized. The most frequent inheritance in this group is autosomal recessive, but any mendelian pattern is possible. Some clinical entities are defined but their genes are still unidentified. They include, among others, the mtDNA depletion syndrome, hereditary spastic paraplegia, and the

Table 8 Most Common Clinical Syndromes Associated with mtDNA Defects

Mainly associated with mtDNA mutations

Mitochondrial encephalomyopathy, lactic acidosis, and stroke-like episodes (MELAS) (266)
Myoclonic epilepsy and ragged-red fibers (HERRF) (267)
Neuropathy, ataxia, and retinitis pigmentosa (NARP) (268)
Leber's hereditary optic neuropathy (LHON) (269)
Diabetes mellitus and deafness (270)

Mainly associated with mtDNA deletions/duplications

Pearson syndrome: Anemia (sideroblastic)/pancytopenia, exocrine pancreatic insufficiency, failure to thrive, liver dysfunction, myopathy, lactic acidosis (271,272)

Kearns Sayre syndrome: Age before 20 years, progressive external ophthalmoplegia, retinitis pigmentosa, cerebellar ataxia, increased CSF protein, complete heart block, diabetes mellitus (273)

Wolfram syndrome: Diabetes insipidus, diabetes mellitus, optic atrophy, and deafness (274)

Progressive external ophthalmoplegia (275)

Source: Refs. 256–258.

myoneurogastrointestinal encephalopathy (MNGIE) (256, 258,264). Nuclear genes responsible for specific deficiencies of subunits in complex I (producing Leigh disease) and complex IV (citochrome oxidase deficiency) have been identified (256,259). More important, nuclear genes affecting the OXPHOS have been found to be the cause of Friedreich's ataxia (276) and the Barth syndrome (277). It is likely that in the next few years more chronic diseases associated with nDNA defects affecting OXPHOS will be described.

B. Diagnosis

Initial laboratory work-up for a patient with suspected PLA with an acute or chronic presentation is similar. In patients with intermittent symptoms, diagnostic possibilities increase when samples are obtained during the acute decompensation. Fasting blood levels for lactate (L), pyruvate (P), ammonia, and AAs and urine for organic acids should be obtained.

Additional information can be obtained by measuring blood levels of 3-OH-butyrate (3OHB), acetoacetate (AcAc), total and free carnitine, and urine amino acids. Accurate measurement of L and P requires rapid and proper handling of the specimens. Arterial samples are preferred, and the use of a tourniquet should be avoided if venous samples are to be obtained.

In patients with acute decompensations, laboratory tests disclose severe metabolic acidosis, high anion gap, and markedly elevated lactic acid. The lactic/pyruvate (L/P) molar ratio should be calculated (normally 10–20). A low to normal value suggests PDHC deficiency. By contrast, PC and respiratory chain defects (complex I, III, and IV) show elevated L/P ratios (278). Reduced 3OHB/AcAc ratio is seen in PC deficiency (235,278). Lactic acidosis due to poor perfusion, hypoxia, liver insufficiency, sepsis, or sedation with propofol (2,6-di-isopropylphenol) (Diprivan, Zeneca Pharma, Mississauga, ON, Canada) should be ruled-out (278,279). In general they do not present with ketosis.

In patients with chronic disease, even slight elevations of lactate provide a clue for diagnosis. More severe biochemical abnormalities might only be present during attacks, which are usually triggered by intercurrent illnesses. In some patients increased lactic acid levels are only detected when they are measured 1–2 h after a regular or a high-carbohydrate meal. Elevated fasting levels of lactic acid that decrease after a high-CHO meal, with simultaneous increase in ketone bodies, are suggestive of PC deficiency (235). In patients with CNS involvement and normal lactic acid in blood, L and P levels have to be measured in cerebral spinal fluid.

Hypoglycemia is associated with lactic acidemia during fasting in patients with gluconeogenic defects, while hyperglycemia can be found in OXPHOS and PDHC deficiencies (261,278). Mild hyperammonemia is present in neonates with PC and fumarase deficiencies and increased uric acid and hypophosphatemia are found in those with FDP deficiency. In the latter, provocative tests with fructose and glycerol, performed under close supervision, are useful for diagnosis. Glucose tolerance tests should be avoided because they can trigger an acute decompensation in PDHC-deficient patients.

Urine organic acids analysis provides useful information in PLA patients, but, with the exception of the TCA cycle defects, cannot determine the site of the metabolic block. Usual findings are elevated lactic, pyruvic, and 2-hydroxybutyric acids. Elevation of TCA cycle intermediates (succinic, fumaric, malic, and α-ketoglutaric acids) might be present in patients with OXPHOS defects. Ketonuria suggests PC deficiency. However, increased ketones can also be found in patients with other PLA defects. Glycerol and glycerol-3-phosphate can be found in the urine of patients with FDP deficiency. A recent report suggests that glycerol intolerance syndrome might be indeed a partial FDP defect (280). α-Ketoglutaric and lactic acids are increased in α-keto glutarate dehydrogenase. However, abnormal excretion of the former could be intermittent (247). Increased α-ketoglutaric is also found in patients with glycogen storage disease type I. In patients with lipoamide dehydrogenase (E$_3$ deficiency), the increased levels of lactic and α-keto glutaric acids are accompanied by metabolites of 2-hydroxy- and 2-ketoacids. Fumarase deficiency is characterized by increased fumaric acid with different degrees of lactic, succinic, and α-ketoglutaric acids (235). Methylglutaconic acid has been reported in several patients with OXPHOS defects, as well as in other diseases (see section on organic acidemias) (278).

Isolated elevations of lactic acid in urine can be found in patients with urinary infections due to *E. cloacae* (281) and in patients with short gut or blind loop syndrome, who excrete high amounts of D-lactic acid, which is undistinguishable from the L-isomer (282). Quantitative plasma AAs have similar limitations to UOA. A common finding for all PLA is an elevation of alanine, while elevated glutamate and glutamine may be present in patients with PDHC, α-KGD, and OXPHOS deficiencies (235, 278). Serum amino acids are characteristic in the neonatal form of PC deficiency, with increased elevation of alanine, proline, citrulline, and lysine and decreased levels of aspartate and glutamine (235,236,253,254). In the E3 subunit deficiency, mild elevations of branched-chain AAs and alanine are characteristic.

A muscle biopsy is another important tool for the diagnosis of PLA, especially for OXPHOS diseases. Specimens should be obtained for light and electron microscopy and tissue should be immediately frozen for enzymatic studies. The specimens should be referred to an experienced laboratory. The presence of ragged red fibers (modified Gomori trichrome stain) are suggestive of an OXPHOS defect. Important information is also obtained from succinate dehydrogenase and cytochrome oxidase reactions, immunohistochemistry, mtDNA quantification, and electron microscopy (245,258,283).

Enzymatic diagnosis for defects in pyruvate oxidation, the TCA cycle, and gluconeogenesis can be done in blood, fibroblasts, or other tissues (235,236). The reference laboratory should be contacted for the best specimen to be obtained for each particular enzyme. Enzyme activity for the respiratory chain is best measured in muscle. However, the assessment is complicated due to several factors, including different percentages of abnormal mtDNA and different isoforms of the same enzyme in different tissues (245,257,258). Point mutations in a tRNA of the mtDNA, or mtDNA depletion can affect the enzyme activity of several respiratory chain complexes. Secondary deficiencies of the respiratory chain due to defects in mitochondrial β-oxidation and other enzyme deficiencies are possible (257). In patients who die unexpectedly, enzymatic studies can be done on frozen samples (skeletal muscle, heart, liver, and brain) if they are obtained no more than 4 h postmortem.

Molecular diagnosis for the majority of the enzymes described is available. Regarding the OXPHOS defects, the mutations or deletions should be searched for, according to the clinical presentation (245,256,258).

C. Treatment: The Acute Episode

Treatment of acute neonatal lactic acidemia requires an intensive care unit. Sodium bicarbonate in large amounts is usually required to control the metabolic acidosis. If hypernatremic metabolic acidosis develops, it should be treated with peritoneal or hemodialysis. Special solutions with sodium bicarbonate (instead of sodium chloride) and devoid of acetate or lactate should be used in those procedures. A high GIR can severely worsen the lactic acidemia in patients with PDHC deficiency. Therefore, initial intravenous fluids should provide a low GIR that can be increased according to clinical and biochemical response. A high GIR is indicated in patients with PC deficiency.

After the appropriate samples for diagnosis have been obtained, treatment with one or several drugs can be started in patients with life-threatening lactic acidemia (Table 9). A wide range of dosages have been used. Assessment of the response to vitamin therapy is difficult and well-documented data are rare. The most commonly used are biotin, thiamine, riboflavin, and coenzyme-Q_{10}. These compounds are cofactors involved in the different metabolic pathways. Vitamins C and K have been used as artificial electron acceptors (235,256,284). Dichloroacetate (DCA) stimulates the activity of the PDHC and is used, in dosages of 15–200 mg/kg/day in the treatment of PLA of unknown origin as well as in PDHC and complex I deficiencies (235,256,284). In patients with low carnitine levels, carnitine supplementation (50–100 mg/kg/day) should be used to maintain normal free carnitine levels. A recent report documents a marked improvement of a cardiomyopathy following treatment with idebenone, a synthetic analog of coenzyme Q_{10} (285). Treatment with succinate, nicotinamide, corticosteroids, chloranphenicol, vitamin-E, methylene blue, and acetylcarnitine have been advocated for some conditions (256,284). When final diagnosis becomes available, an attempt to withdraw those vitamins not involved in the metabolic block should be done, one at a time, with careful monitoring of the clinical and biochemical response.

Table 9 Pharmacological Treatment for PLA

Agent	Dosage (range)	Deficiency
Thiamine	500–2000 mg/day	PDHC
	200–300 mg/day	OXPHOS
Lipoic acid	10–50 mg/kg/day	PDHC
Dichloroacetate	15–200 mg/kg/day	PDHC, OXPHOS
Biotin	10–50 mg/day	PC
Riboflavin	50–300 mg/day	OXPHOS
Coenzyme-Q_{10}	60–360 mg/day	OXPHOS
Idebenone	30–90 mg/day	OXPHOS
Vitamin C	500–4000 mg/day	OXPHOS
Vitamin K_3, menadione or K_1, phylloquinone	50–100 mg/day	OXPHOS

D. Long-Term Management

In patients with chronic disease it is advisable to add one drug or vitamin at a time, according to the suspected diagnosis, and maintain careful monitoring of the patient's response. However well-documented long-term studies are difficult and, in general, prognosis is poor. In patients with PDHC deficiencies, thiamine (500–2000 mg/day), lipoic acid (which is bound to the E_2 component), carnitine, and DCA have been tried with variable results (235,242). A high-fat (75–80%), low-CHO (5%) diet has been useful in some patients. The rationale is to provide alternative sources of Acetyl-CoA, not derived from pyruvate (235,284). However, a detailed study showed mild improvement in development but not change in long-term survival of these patients (286). In PDHC deficiency due to abnormalities in the E_3 component, dietary treatment is more difficult because the affected enzymes impair protein, carbohydrate, and fat metabolism. Restriction of branched-chain amino acids (as in MSUD) is helpful to reduce blood levels of branched-chain AAs and their metabolites in urine (235).

In patients with PC deficiency, treatment with biotin (10–50 mg/day) is indicated. Citrate and aspartate have also been tried in the treatment of this condition, with improvement in blood chemistry but poor long-term neurological outcome (254). A low-fat–high-CHO diet with frequent feeds is also indicated in patients with PC deficiency as well as in all the other gluconeogenic defects (235,284). Restriction of protein intake to reduce production of gluconeogenic substrates has also been proposed in PC deficiency.

In patients with FDP deficiency, mild restriction of sucrose and fructose is indicated. Controlled exercise has been helpful in some patient with OXPHOS defects to enhance the aerobic capacity and decrease lactic acid levels (256). Liver transplantation has been performed in patients with hepatic respiratory chain disorders, but extrahepatic manifestations may appear later despite successful transplantation (287). Treatment with valproic acid and phenobarbital should be avoided because they inhibit the respiratory chain (257). Supportive treatment for the different manifestations of OXPHOS diseases (exocrine pancreatic deficiency, anemia, diabetes, renal Fanconi's syndrome, etc.), as well as psychological support for patients and family should be provided.

VI. MAPLE SYRUP URINE DISEASE

A. Pathophysiology

Maple syrup urine disease (MSUD) is an autosomal recessive disease affecting the metabolism of the branched-chain amino acids (BCAA) leucine, isoleucine, and valine. BCAA play an important role in intermediate metabolism. They are substrates for gluconeogenesis and ketogenesis, and their end-catabolic product, acetyl-CoA, is a precursor for fatty acid and cholesterol synthesis. The defect in MSUD is located in the branched-chain 2-ketoacid dehydrogenase complex (BCKD), which is made of four different components: E_1-α, E_1-β, E_2, and E_3 (288). The E_1 component is thiamine dependent. BCKD deficiency results in the elevation of BCAA and their corresponding branched-chain 2-ketoacids (BCKA) 2-ketoisocaproic, 2-keto-3-methylvaleric, and 2-ketoisovaleric. Accumulation of these compounds is responsible for the characteristic odor as well as the clinical course of the disease.

B. Clinical and Laboratory Manifestations

Five phenotypes have been described, based on the clinical presentation and response to thiamine therapy: classic, intermediate, intermittent, thiamine-responsive, and E_3-(dihydrolipoamide dehydrogenase) deficient (288). The classic form is the most common. Children appear normal at birth, but between the first and the second week of life present with poor feedings, lethargy, dystonic posturing, seizures, and apneas. The characteristic maple syrup odor can easily be detected in urine. This intoxication-like encephalopathy resembles that of the organic acidemias. Biochemical abnormalities include ketoacidosis and hypoglycemia; hyperammonemia may be mild or absent (37,288). Diagnosis can be made by measurement of either plasma AAs or UOA. Typical findings in the former are elevated levels of BCAA, mainly leucine (1000–5000 μM/l), and the presence of L-alloisoleucine, which is a transamination product of the 2-keto-3-methylvaleric acid (105). Routine UOA analysis shows an elevation of branched-chain 2-OH-acids and BCKA. The latter are better detected when the sample is previously oximated. Ketone bodies are also usually present.

The intermediate form of MSUD presents in infancy to young adulthood with neurological impairment, seizures, failure to thrive, and ataxia. Ketoacidosis is less severe and acute crisis may be absent. In these patients BCAA are always abnormal, with leucine levels ranging between 400 and 2000 μM/l (289).

The intermittent form presents in children or adults with episodes of acute decompensation (ataxia, seizures, coma, and ketoacidosis) triggered by infections or high protein ingestion. Plasma leucine values are mildly elevated during the crisis, but they can be normal while compensated (288).

The thiamine-responsive patients are a heterogeneous group. Their clinical presentation resembles that of patients with the intermediate form of the disease. Treatment with thiamine tends to normalize the BCAA levels, and some patients can be completely off diet. Thiamine dosages have ranged from 10 to 1000 mg/day and response was achieved days or weeks after starting the treatment (37,288,290).

The E_3 component of the BCKD is common to other three enzymatic complexes: pyruvate dehydrogenase complex (PDHC), α-ketoglutarate dehydrogenase (α-KGD), and the glycine cleavage system (involved in glycine catabolism). Clinical presentation in these patients is variable, combining features of BCKD and primary lactic acidemias (see section on PDHC deficiency above).

MSUD is transmitted as an autosomal recessive condition and has been diagnosed in all ethnic groups. The general incidence of the disease is estimated at 1:185,000, but the incidence is much higher for some inbred communities, such as the Mennonites (288). Mutations in the genes encoding for the different components of the BCKD have been identified. Different genotypes correlate with the severity of clinical presentation (288,289).

C. Treatment: The Acute Episode

Acute management of MSUD patients follows the same principles outlined for the treatment of organic acidemias (see section on organic acidemias above). Patients with MSUD usually require less bicarbonate than OA to correct the metabolic acidosis. High-energy nutrition alone is not sufficient to lower leucine levels rapidly (37). Therefore dialysis should be considered early in the treatment, especially in patients with acute and severe encephalopathy and/or with leucine levels above 1500 μMol. Hemodialysis, hemofiltration, and continuous blood exchange transfusion, in this order, are the preferred methods for toxin removal (24,114,291). As in OA, pancreatitis and brain edema have been reported in acutely ill MSUD patients (37,292–294). The latter has been documented in CT and MR studies, which also showed dysmyelination of several areas of the brain in patients under poor metabolic control (295). Unlike in OA, secondary carnitine deficiency is not common in MSUD patients.

D. Long-Term Management

Long-term treatment of UCD patients is also based on the same principles as the organic acidemias (see section on organic acidemias above). Because leucine is considered the most toxic of the BCAA, leucine requirements are followed to prescribe the diet. Occasionally, small amounts of valine and isoleucine need to be added to the diet because the tolerance for leucine is lower than of the other two BCAA. Administration of thiamine is indicated for thiamine-responsive patients. Prognosis of MSUD patients has dramatically improved due to the early diagnosis achieved through newborn screening programs (NBS), intensive treatment, and availability of special formulas. NBS programs are being performed using the traditional bacterial inhibition assay or new techniques such as TMS. The later is being used in many centers to detect not only MSUD but also many other IEM (109,110,296). We have detected abnormal levels of leucine + isoleucine and valine before 24 h of age in a patient with MSUD whose sibling had a classic form of the disease (111). These results suggest that TMS will lower the impact of early discharge on newborn screening.

For children treated in specialized centers, survival is 100% (37,288). However, some degree of psychomotor impairment seems to be present, even in patients with early diagnosis and strict dietary treatment (294,297,298). Successful pregnancies have been reported in patients with intermediate MSUD who were evaluated with close monitoring (288).

ACKNOWLEDGMENTS

Thanks to CVA, NA, and MA for their support.

REFERENCES

1. Saudubray JM, Ogier de Baulny H, Charpentier C. Clinical approach to inherited metabolic disorders. In: Fernandes J, Saudubray JM, van den Berghe G, eds. Inborn Metabolic Diseases. 2nd eds. Berlin: Springer-Verlag, 2000:3–42.
2. Scriver CR, Beaudet AL, Sly WS, Valle D. ed. The Metabolic and Molecular Bases of Inherited Disease. 8th ed. New York: McGraw-Hill, 2001.
3. Fernandes J, Saudubray JM, van den Berghe G. ed. Inborn Metabolic Diseases. 2nd ed. Berlin: Springer-Verlag, 2000.
4. Nyhan WL, Ozand PT, eds. Atlas of Metabolic Diseases. 1st ed. London: Chapman & Hall Medical, 1998.
5. Brusilow SW, Horwich AL. Urea cycle enzymes. In: Scriver CR, Beaudet AL, Sly WS, Valle D, eds. The Metabolic and Molecular Bases of Inherited Disease. 8th ed. New York: McGraw-Hill, 2001: 1909–1963.
6. Leonard JV. Disorders of the urea cycle. In: Fernandes J, Saudubray JM, van den Berghe G, eds. Inborn Metabolic Diseases. 2nd ed. Berlin: Springer-Verlag, 2000: 214–222.
7. Butterworth RF. Effects of hyperammonemia on brain function. J Inherit Metab Dis 1998; 21 (Suppl 1) 1998: 6–20.
8. Voorhies TM, Ehrlich ME, Duffy TE, Petito CK, Plum F. Acute hyperammonemia in the young primate: physiologic and neurophathologic correlates. Pediatr Res 1983; 17:971–975.
9. Connelly A, Cross JH, Gadian DG, et al. Magnetic resonance spectroscopy shows increased brain glutamine in ornithine carbamoyl transferase deficiency. Pediatr Res 1993; 33:77–81.
10. Schubiger G, Bachmann C, Barben P, et al. N-acetylglutamate synthetase deficiency: diagnosis, management and follow-up of a rare disorder of ammonia detoxification. Eur J Pediatr 1991; 150:353–356.
11. Christodolou J, Qureshi IA, McInnes RR, et al. Ornithine transcarbamylase deficiency presenting with stroke-like episodes. J Pediatr 1993; 122:423–427.
12. Mattson LR, Lindor NM, Goldman DH, et al. Central pontine myelinolysis as a complication of partial ornithine carbamoyl transferase deficiency. Am J Med Genet 1995; 60:210–213.
13. Rowe PC, Newman SL, Brusilow SW. Natural history of symptomatic partial ornithine transcarbamylase deficiency. N Engl J Med 1986; 314:541–47.
14. Arn PH, Hauser ER, Thomas GH, et al. Hyperammonemia in women with a mutation at the ornithine trans-

carbamylase locus. N Engl J Med 1990:322: 1652–1655.

15. Nyhan WL, Ozand PT, ed. Argininemia. In: Atlas of Metabolic Diseases. 1st ed. London: Chapman & Hall Medical, 1998: 194–198.

16. Webster DR, Simmonds HA, Barry DMJ, Becroft DMO. Pyrimidine and purine metabolites in ornithine carbamoyl transferase deficiency. J Inherit Metab Dis 1981; 4:27–31.

17. Hudak ML, Jones D, Brusilow S. Differentiation of transient hyperammonemia of the newborn and urea cycle enzyme defects by clinical presentation. J Pediatr 1985: 107:712–719.

18. Stanley CA, Lieu YK, Hsu BY, et al. Hyperinsulinism and hyperammonemia in infants with regulatory mutations of the glutamate dehydrogenase gene. N Engl J Med 1998;338:1352–1357.

18a. Tuchman, Lichtenstein GR, Rajagopal BS, et al. Hepatic glutamine synthetase deficiency in fatal hyperammonemia after lung transplantation. Ann Intern Med 1997; 127:446–449.

19. Maestri NE, Lord CR Glynn M, et al. The phenotype of ostensibly healthy women who are carriers for ornithine transcarbamylase deficiency. Medicine 1998; 77:389–397.

20. Bonham JR, Guthrie P, Downing M, et al. The allopurinol load test lacks specificity for primary urea cycle defects but may indicate unrecognized mitochondrial disease. J Inherit Metab Dis 1999; 22:174–184.

21. Tuchman M, Morizono H, Rajagopal BS, et al. The biochemical and molecular spectrum of ornithine transcarbamylase deficiency. J Inherit Metab Dis 1998; 21(Suppl. 1):40–58.

22. McCullogh BA, Yudkoff M, Batshaw ML, et al. Genotype spectrum of ornithine transcarbamylase deficiency: correlation with the clinical and biochemical phenotype. Am J Med Genet 2000; 93:313–319.

23. Hendricks KM. Estimation of energy needs. In: Hendricks KM, Walker WA, ed. Manual of Pediatric Nutrition. 2nd ed. Philadelphia: B.C. Decker, 1990:59–71.

24. Rutledge SL, Havens PL, Haymond MW, et al. Neonatal hemodialysis: effective therapy for the encephalopathy of inborn errors of metabolism. J Pediatr 1990; 116:125–128.

25. Chen CY, Chen YC, Fang JT, Huang CC. Continuous arteriovenous hemodiafiltration in the acute treatment of hyperammonaemia due to ornithine transcarbamylase deficiency. Ren Fail 2000; 22:823–836.

26. Donn SM, Schwartz RD, Thoene JG. Comparison of exchange transfusion, peritoneal dialysis and hemodialysis for the treatment of hyperammonemia in an anuric newborn infant. 1979; J Pediatr 95:67–70.

27. Feillet F, Leonard JV. Alternative pathway therapy for urea cycle disorders. J Inherit Metab Dis 1998; 21(Suppl 1):101–111.

28. Praphanphoj V, Boyadjiev SA, Waber LJ, et al. Three cases of intravenous sodium benzoate and sodium phenylacetate toxicity occurring in the treatment of severe hyperammonaemia. J Inherit Metab Dis 2000; 23:129–136.

29. Oechsner M, Steen C, Sturenburg HJ, Kohlschutter A. Hiperammonaemic encephalopathy after initiation of valproate therapy in unrecognised ornithine transcarbamylase deficiency. J Neurol Neurosurg Psychiatry 1998; 64:680–682.

30. Uchino T, Endo F, Matsuda I. Neurodevelopmental outcome of long-term therapy of urea cycle dissorders in Japan. J Inherit Metab Dis 1998; 21(Suppl. 1):151–159.

31. Saudubray JM, Touati G, Delonay P, et al. Liver transplantation in urea cycle disorders. Eur J Pediatr 1999; 158(Suppl. 2):S55–S59.

32. Maestri NE, Hauser ER, Bartholomew D, Brusilow SW. Prospective treatment of urea cycle disorders. J Pediatr 1991; 119:923–928.

33. Whitington PF, Alonso EM, Boyle JT, et al. Liver transplantation for the treatment of urea cycle disorders. J Inherit Metab Dis 1998; 21(Suppl. 1):112–118.

34. Raper SE, Wilson JM, Yudkoff M, et al. Developing adenoviral-mediated in vitro gene therapy for ornithine transcarbamylase deficiency. J Inherit Metab Dis 1998; 21(Suppl 1):119–137.

35. Lee B, Dennis JA, Healy PJ, et al. Hepatocyte gene therapy in a large animal: a neonatal bovine model of citrullinemia. Proc Natl Acad Sci USA 1999; 96:3981–3986.

36. Sweetman L, Williams JC. Branched chain organic acidurias. In: Scriver CR, Beaudet AL, Sly WS, Valle D, ed. The Metabolic and Molecular Bases of Inherited Disease. 8th ed. New York: McGraw-Hill, 2001:2125–2164.

37. Ogier de Baulny H, Saudubray JM. Branched-chain organic acidurias. In: Fernandes J, Saudubray JM, van den Berghe G, eds. Inborn Metabolic Diseases. 2nd ed. Berlin: Springer-Verlag, 2000:195–212.

38. Hoffmann GF. Disorders of Lysine catabolism and related cerebral organic-acid disorders. In: Fernandes J, Saudubray JM, van den Berghe G, eds. Inborn Metabolic Diseases. 2nd ed. Berlin: Springer-Verlag, 2000:241–254.

39. Gibson KM, Hoffmann GF, Hodson AK, Bottiglieri T, Jacobs C. 4-Hydroxybutyric acid and the clinical phenotype of succinic semialdehyde dehydrogenase deficiency, an inborn error of GABA metabolism. Neuropediatrics 1998; 29:14–22.

40. Traeger EC, Rapin I. The clinical course of Canavan disease. Pediatr Neurol 1998; 18:207–212.

41. Goodman SI, Frerman FE. Organic acidemias due to defects in Lysine oxidation: 2-ketoadipic acidemia and glutaric acidemia. In: Scriver CR, Beaudet AL, Sly WS, Valle D, eds. The Metabolic and Molecular Bases of Inherited Disease. 8th ed. New York: McGraw-Hill, 2001:2195–2205.

42. Barth PG, Hoffmann GF, Jaeken J, et al. L-2-hydroxyglutaric acidaemia: Clinical and biochemical findings in 12 patients and preliminary report on L-2-hydroxyacid dehydrogenase. J Inherit Metab Dis 1993;16:753–761.

43. van der Knaap MS, Jacobs C, Hoffmann GF, et al. D-2-hydroxyglutaric aciduria. Biochemical marker or clinical disease entity? Ann Neurol 1999; 45:111–119.

44. Superti-Furga A, Hoffmann GF. Glutaric aciduria type 1 (glutaryl-CoA-dehydrogenase deficiency): advances and unanswered questions. Eur J Pediatr 1997; 156: 821–828.

45. Hoffmann GF. Organic acid analysis. In: Blau N, Duran M, Blaskovics ME, eds. Physician's Guide to the Laboratory Diagnosis of Metabolic Diseases. 1st ed. London: Chapman & Hall Medical, 1996:32–49.

46. Nyhan WL, Ozand PT, eds. Isovaleric acidemia. In: Atlas of Metabolic Diseases. 1st ed. London: Chapman & Hall Medical, 1998:41–45.

47. Nyhan WL, Ozand PT, eds. 3-methylcrotonyl-CoA-carboxylase deficiency/3-methylcrotonylglycinuria. In: At-

las of metabolic diseases. 1st ed. London: Chapman & Hall Medical, 1998:53–56.

48. Nyhan WL, Ozand PT, eds. Multiple carboxylase deficiency/holocarboxylase synthetase deficiency. In: Atlas of Metabolic Diseases. 1st ed. London: Chapman & Hall Medical, 1998:27–32.

49. Nyhan WL, Ozand PT, eds. Multiple carboxylase deficiency/biotinidase deficiency. In: Atlas of Metabolic Diseases. 1st ed. London: Chapman & Hall Medical, 1998: 33–40.

50. Nyhan WL, Ozand PT, eds. 3-methylglutaconic aciduria. In: Atlas of Metabolic Diseases. 1st ed. London: Chapman & Hall Medical, 1998:57–63.

51. Nyhan WL, Ozand PT, ed. 3-hydroxy-3-methyl-glutaryl-CoA-lyase deficiency. In: Atlas of Metabolic Diseases. 1st ed. London: Chapman & Hall Medical, 1998:253–258.

52. Morris AA. Disorders of ketogenesis and ketolysis. In: Fernandes J, Saudubray JM, van den Berghe G, eds. Inborn Metabolic Diseases. 2nd ed. Berlin: Springer-Verlag, 2000:151–156.

53. Gibson KM, Burlingame TG, Hogema B, et al. 2-methylbutyryl-CoA-dehydrogenase deficiency: a new inborn error of L-Isoleucine metabolism. Pediatr Res 2000; 47: 830–833.

54. Andresen BS, Christensen E, Corydon TJ, et al. Isolated 2-methylbutyrylglycinuria caused by short/branched-chain acyl CoA dehydrogenase deficiency: identification of a new enzyme defect, resolution of its molecular basis, and evidence for distinct acyl-CoA dehydrogenases in isoleucine and valine metabolism. Am J Hum Genet 2000; 67: 1095–1103.

55. Zschocke J, Ijlst L, Brand J, et al. 2-methyl-3-hydroxybutyryl-CoA-dehydrogenase deficiency: a novel neurodegenerative disorder. J Inherit Metab Dis 2000; 23: Suppl 1:109(A).

56. Roe CR, Cederbaum SD, Roe DS, et al. Isolated isobutyryl-CoA-dehydrogenase deficiency: an unrecognized defect in human valine metabolism. Mol Gene Metab 1998; 65:264–271.

57. Nyhan WL, Ozand PT, eds. 3-Hydroxyisobutyric aciduria. In: Atlas of Metabolic Diseases. 1st ed. London: Chapman & Hall Medical, 1998:64–68.

58. Brown GK, Hunt SM, Scholem R, et al. B-hydroxyisobutyril-CoA-deacylase deficiency: a defect in valine metabolism associated with physical malformations. Pediatrics 1982; 70:532.

59. Chambliss KL, Gray RG, Rylance G, Pollit RJ, Gibson KM. Molecular characterization of methylmalonate semialdehyde dehydrogenase deficiency. J Inherit Metab Dis 2000; 23:497–504.

60. Nyhan WL, Ozand PT, eds. Propionic acidemia. In: Atlas of Metabolic Diseases. 1st ed. London: Chapman & Hall Medical, 1998:4–12.

61. Fenton WA, Gravel RA, Rosenblatt DA. Disorders of propionate and methylmalonate metabolism. In: Scriver CR, Beaudet AL, Sly WS, Valle D, eds. The Metabolic and Molecular Bases of Inherited Disease. 8th ed. New York: McGraw-Hill, 2001:2165–2194.

62. Nyhan WL, Ozand PT, ed. Methylmalonic acidemia. In: Atlas of Metabolic Diseases. 1st ed. London: Chapman & Hall Medical, 1998:13–23.

63. Rosenblatt DS. Disorders of Cobalamin and folate transport and metabolism. In: Fernandes J, Saudubray JM, van den Berghe G, eds. Inborn Metabolic Diseases. 2nd ed. Berlin: Springer-Verlag, 2000:283–300.

64. Andersson HC, Shapira E. Biochemical and clinical response to hydroxycobalamin versus cyanocobalamin in patients with methylmalonic acidemia and homocystinuria (cblC). J Pediatr 1998; 132:121–124.

65. Nyhan WL, Ozand PT, eds. Methylmalonic aciduria and homocystinuria/Cobalamin C and D disease. In: Atlas of Metabolic Diseases. 1st ed. London: Chapman & Hall Medical, 1998: 24–26.

66. Bennet MJ, Harthcock PA, Boriack RL, Cohen JC. Impaired fatty acid oxidation (FAO) in malonyl-CoA decarboxylase (MCD) deficiency. J Inherit Metab Dis 2000; 23:Suppl 1:99(A).

67. Nyhan WL, Ozand PT, eds. Glutaric aciduria (type I). In: Atlas of Metabolic Diseases. 1st ed. London: Chapman & Hall Medical, 1998:46–52.

68. Nyhan WL, Ozand PT, eds. L-2-hydroxyglutaric aciduria. In: Atlas of Metabolic Diseases. 1st ed. London: Chapman & Hall Medical, 1998:76–78.

69. Topcu M, Coskun T, Saatci I, et al. L-2-hydroxyglutaric aciduria: report of 18 turkish patients. J Inherit Metab Dis 2000; 23:Suppl 1:104(A).

70. Nyhan WL, Ozand PT, eds. D-2-hydroxyglutaric aciduria. In: Atlas of Metabolic Diseases. 1st ed. London: Chapman & Hall Medical, 1998:73–75.

71. Nyhan WL, Ozand PT, eds. 2-Oxoadipic aciduria. In: Atlas of Metabolic Diseases. 1st ed. London: Chapman & Hall Medical, 1998:79–81.

72. Nyhan WL, Ozand PT, eds. Canavan disease/aspartoacylase deficiency. In: Atlas of Metabolic Diseases. 1st ed. London: Chapman & Hall Medical, 1998:637–642.

73. Danpure C. Primary hyperoxaluria. In: Scriver CR, Beaudet AL, Sly WS, Valle D, ed. The Metabolic and Molecular Bases of Inherited Disease. 8th ed. New York: McGraw-Hill, 2001:3323–3370.

74. McCabe E. Disorders of glycerol metabolism. In: Scriver CR, Beaudet AL, Sly WS, Valle D, ed. The Metabolic and Molecular Bases of Inherited Disease. 8th ed. New York: McGraw-Hill, 2001:3323–3370.

75. Nyhan WL, Ozand PT, eds. Alkaptonuria. In: Atlas of Metabolic Diseases. 1st ed. London: Chapman & Hall Medical, 1998:104–108.

76. Glutathione synthetase deficiency and other disorders of the γ-glutamyl cycle. In: Scriver CR, Beaudet AL, Sly WS, Valle D, eds. The Metabolic and Molecular Bases of Inherited Disease. 8th ed. New York: McGraw-Hill, 2001:3323–3370.

77. Nyhan WL, Ozand PT, eds. Mevalonic aciduria. In: Atlas of Metabolic Diseases. 1st ed. London: Chapman & Hall Medical, 1998:510–514.

78. Houten SM, Wanders RJ, Waterham HR. Biochemical and genetic aspects of mevalonate kinase and its deficiency. Biochem Biophys Acta 2000; 1529:19–32.

79. Houten SM, Frenkel J, Kuis L, et al. Molecular basis of classical mevalonic aciduria and the hyperimmunoglobulinaemia D and periodic fever syndrome: high frequency of 3 mutations in the mevalonate kinase gene. J Inherit Metab Dis 2000; 24: 367–370.

80. Di Rocco N, Caruso U, Waterham HR, et al. Mevalonate kinase deficiency in a child with periodic fever without hyperimmunoglobulin D. J Inherit Metab Dis 2000; 23: Suppl 1:109(A).

81. Burlina AB, Dionici-Vici C, Bennett MJ, et al. A new syndrome with ethylmalonic aciduria and normal fatty acid oxidation in fibroblasts. J Pediatr 1994; 124:79–86.

82. Garcia Silva MT, Ribes A, Campos Y, et al. Syndrome

of encephalopathy, petechiae and ethylmalonic aciduria. Pediatr Neurol 1997; 17:165–170.

83. Nyhan WL, Ozand PT, eds. Ethylmalonic aciduria. In: Atlas of Metabolic Diseases. 1st ed. London: Chapman & Hall Medical, 1998:646–650.

84. Vreken P, Valianpour F, Grivell LA, Nijtmans, LG, Wanders RJA, Barth PG. Abnormal cardiolipin and phosphatidylglycerol remodeling in Barth syndrome. J Inher Metab Dis 2000; 23:Suppl.1: 150(A).

85. Nyhan WL, Ozand PT, eds. Malonic aciduria with normal malonil-CoA-decarboxylase. In: Atlas of Metabolic Diseases. 1st ed. London: Chapman & Hall Medical, 1998:69–72.

86. Wolf B. Disorders of biotin metabolism. In: Scriver CR, Beaudet AL, Sly WS, Valle D, ed. The Metabolic and Molecular Bases of Inherited Disease. 8th ed. New York: McGraw-Hill, 2001:3935–3964.

87. Thompson GN, Walter JH, Bresson JL, et al. Sources of propionate in inborn errors of metabolism. Metabolism 1990; 11:1133–1137.

88. Leonard JV. Stable isotope studies in propionic and methylmalonic acidaemia. Eur J Pediatr 1996; 156[suppl 1]: S67–S69.

89. Coude FX, Sweetman L, Nyhan WL. Inhibition by propionyl-coenzyme A of N-Acetyglutamate synthtase in rat liver mitochondria. J Clin Invest 1979:1544–1551.

90. Coude FX, Ogier H, Grimber G, Parvy P, Dinh DP, Charpentier C, Saudubray JM. Correlation between blood ammonia concentration and organic acid accumulation in isovaleric and propionic acidemia. Pediatrics 1982; 69:115–117.

91. Khaler SG, Sherwood WG, Woolf D, et al. Pancreatitis in patients with organic acidemias. J Pediatr 1994; 124: 239–243.

92. Fiumara A, Barone R, Nigro F, Ribes A, Pavone L. Pancreatitis in organic acidemias. J Pediatr 1995; 126:852.

93. Burlina AB, Dionisi-Vici C, Piovan S, et al. Acute pancreatitis in propionic acidemia. J Inher Metab Dis 1995; 18: 169–172.

94. Al essa M, Rahbeeni Z, Jumaah S, et al. Infectious complications of propionic acidemia in Saudi Arabia. Clin Genet 1998; 54:90–94.

95. Koopman RJJ, Happle R. Cutaneous manifestations of methylmalonic acidemia. Arch Dermatol Res 1990; 282: 272–273.

96. Griffin TA, Hostoffer RW, Tserng KY, et al. Parathyroid resistance and B cell lymphopenia in propionic acidemia. Acta Paediatr 1996; 85:875–878.

97. Heidenreich R, Natowicz M, Hainline B, Berman P, Kelley R, Hillman R, Berry GT. Acute extrapyramidal syndrome in methylmalonic acidemia: "metabolic stroke" involving the globus pallidus. J Pediatr 1988; 113:1022–1027.

98. Haas RH, Marsden DL, Capistrano-Estrada S, et al. Acute basal ganglia infarction in propionic acidemia. J Child Neurol 1995; 10:18–22.

99. Bergman AJ, Van der Knaap MS, Smeitink JA, et al. Magnetic resonance imaging and spectroscopy of the brain in propionic acidemia: clinical and biochemical considerations. J Pediatr 1996; 129:758–760.

100. Boeckx RL, Hicks JM. Methylmalonic acidemia with the unusual complication of severe hyperglycemia. Clin Chem 1982; 28:1801–1803.

101. Attia N, Sakati N, al Ashawal A, et al. Isovaleric acidemia appearing as diabetic ketoacidosis. J Inherit Metab Dis 1996; 19:85–86.

102. Shapira SK, Ledley FD, Rosenblatt DS, Levy HL. Ketoacidotic crisis as a presentation of mild methylmalonic acidemia. J Pediatr 1991; 119:80–84.

103. Sethi KD, Ray R, Roesel RA, Carter AL, Gallagher BB, Loring DW, Hommes FA. Adult onset chorea and dementia with propionic acidemia. Neurology 1989; 39: 1343–1345.

104. Nyhan WL, Bay C, Beyer EW, Mazi M. Neurologic nonmetabolic presentation of propionic acidemia. Arch Neurol 1999; 56:1143–1147.

105. Rinaldo P. Laboratory diagnosis of inborn errors of metabolism. In: Suchy FJ, ed. Liver disease in children. 1st ed. St. Louis: Mosby, 1994:295–308.

106. Rashed MS, Bucknall MP, Little D, et al. Screening blood spots for inborn errors of metabolism by electrospray tandem mass spectrometry with a microplate batch process and a computer algorithm for automated flagging of abnormal profiles. Clin Chem 1997; 43:1129–1141.

107. Vreken P, van Lint AEM, Bootsma AH, et al. Quantitative plasma acylcarnitine analysis using electrospray tandem mass spectrometry for the diagnosis of organic acidemias and fatty acid oxidation defects. J Inherit Metab Dis 1999; 22:302–306.

108. Levy HL. Newborn screening by tandem mass spectrometry: a new era. Clin Chem 1998; 44: 2401–2402.

109. Naylor EW, Chace DH. Automated tandem mass spectrometry for mass newborn screening for disorders in fatty acid, organic acid, and aminoacid metabolism. J Child Neurol 1999; 14(Suppl 1):S4–S8.

110. Rashed MS, Rahbeeni Z, Ozand P. Application of electrospray tandem mass spectrometry to neonatal screening. Semin Perinatol 1999; 23:183–193.

111. Abdenur JE, Chamoles NA, Schenone AB, et al. Supplemental newborn screening of aminoacids (AA) and acylcarnitines by electrospray tandem mass spectrometry: experience in Argentina (abstr.). J Inherit Metab Dis 2000; 23:Suppl. 1:13.

112. Patterson AL, Pourfarzam M, Henderson MJ. The utility of cord blood analysis in the diagnosis of organic acidemias (abstr.). J Inherit Metab Dis 2000; 23:Suppl. 1:84.

113. Abdenur JE, Chamoles NA, Schenone AB, et al. Diagnosis of isovaleric acidemia by tandem mass spectrometry: false positive result due to pivaloylcarnitine in a newborn screening programme. J Inherit Metab Dis 1998; 21:624–630.

113a. Bonafe L, Troxler H, Kuster T, et al. Evaluation of urinary acylglycines by electrospray tandem mass spectrometry in mitochondrial energy metabolism defects and organic acidurias. Mol Genet Metab 2000; 69:302–311.

113b. Tuchman M, Yudkoff M. Blood levels of ammonia and nitorgen scavenging aminoacids in patients with inherited hyperammonemia. Mol Genet Metab 1999; 66:10–15.

113c. Ierardi-Curto L, Kaplan S, Saitta S, et al. The glutamine paradox in a neonate with propionic acidemia and severe hyperammonaemia. J Inherit Metab Dis 2000; 23:85–86.

114. Ogier de Baulny H, Saudubray JM. Emergency treatments. In: Fernandes J, Saudubray JM, van den Berghe G, eds. Inborn Metabolic Diseases. 2nd ed. Berlin: Springer-Verlag, 2000:53–61.

115. Thompson GN, Chalmers RA. Increased urinary metabolite excretion during fasting in disorders of propionate metabolism. Pediatr Res 1990; 27:413–416.

116. Millington DS, Roe ChR, Maltby DA, Inoue F. Endogenous catabolism is the major source of toxic metabolites in isovaleric acidemia. J Pediatr 1987; 110:56–60.

117. Bodamer OAF, Hoffman GF, Visser GH, et al. Assessment of energy expenditure in metabolic disorders. Eur J Pediatr 1997; 156(Suppl 1):S24–S28.

118. Abdenur J, Greene C. Unpublished observation, 1992.

119. Kalloghlian A, Gleispach H, Ozand PT. A patient with propionic acidemia managed with continuous insulin infusion and total parenteral nutrition. J Child Neurol 1992; 7(Suppl):S88–S91.

120. Khaler SG, Millington DS, Cederbaum SD, et al. Parenteral nutrition in propionic and methylmalonic acidemia. J Pediatr 1989; 115:235–241.

121. Roth B, Younossi A, Skopnik H, Leonard JV, Lehnert W. Haemodialysis for metabolic decompensation in propionic acidemia. J Inherit Metab Dis 1987; 10:147–151.

122. Praphanphoj V, Brusilow S, Hamosh A, Geraghty MT. The use of intravenous sodium benzoate and sodium phenylacetate in propionic acidemia with hyperammonemia. J Inherit Metab Dis 2000; 23:Suppl. 1:91(A).

123. Fries MH, Rinaldo P, Schmidt-Sommerfeld E, et al. Isovaleric acidemia: response to a leucine load after three weeks of supplementation with glycine, L-carnitine, and combined glycine-carnitine therapy. J Pediatr 1996; 129:449–452.

124. Tracy E, Arbour L, Chessex P, et al. Glutathione deficiency as a complication of methylmalonic acidemia: response to high doses of ascorbate. J Pediatr 1996; 129:445–448.

125. Matern D, Seydewitz HH, Lehnert W, et al. Primary treatment of propionic acidemia complicated by thiamine deficiency. J Pediatr 1996; 129:758–760.

126. Feillet F, Bodamer OA, Dixon M, et al. Resting energy expenditure in disorders of propionate metabolism. J Pediatr 2000; 136:659–663.

127. Thompson GN, Chalmers RA, Walter JH, et al. The use of metronidazole in management of methylmalonic and propionic acidemias. Eur J Pediatr 1990; 149:792–796.

128. Vockley J, Rogan PK, Anderson BD, et al. Exon skipping in IVD RNA processing in isovaleric acidemia caused by point mutations in the coding region of the IVD gene. Am J Hum Genet 2000; 66:356–367.

129. Ugarte M, Perez Cerda C, Rodriguez Pombo P, et al. Overview of mutations in the PCCA and PCCB genes causing propionic acidemia. Hum Mutat 1999; 14: 275–282.

130. Fuchshuber A, Mucha B, Baumgartner ER, et al. Mut0 methylmalonic acidemia: eleven novel mutations of the methylmalonyl CoA mutase including a deletion-insertion. Hum Mutat 2000; 16:179.

131. Crane AM, Martin LS, Valle D, Ledley FD. Phenotype of disease in three patients with identical mutations in methylmalonyl CoA mutase. Hum Genet 1992; 89:259–264.

132. Weinberg GL, Laurito CE, Geldner P, et al. Malignant ventricular disrythmias in a patient with isovaleric acidemia receiving general and local anesthesia for suction lipectomy. J Clin Anesth 1997; 9:668–670.

133. Harker HE, Emhardt JD, Hainline BE. Propionic acidemia in a four-month-old male: a case study and anesthetic implications. Anesth Analg 2000; 91:309–311.

134. North KN, Korson MS, Gopal YR, et al. Neonatal onset propionic acidemia: neurologic and developmental profiles and implications for management. J Pediatr 1995; 126:916–922.

135. van der Meer SB, Poggi F, Spada M, et al. Clinical outcome and long term management of 17 patients with propionic acidemia. J Pediatr 1996; 155:205–210.

136. van der Meer SB, Poggi F, Spada M, et al. Clinical outcome of long term management of patients with vitamin B-12 unresponsive methylmalonic acidemia. J Pediatr 1994; 125:903–908.

137. Varvogli L, Repetto GM, Waisbren SE, Levy HL. High cognitive outcome in an adolescent with mut- methylmalonic acidemia. Am J Med Genet 2000; 96:192–195.

138. Anderson HC, Marble M, Shapira E. Long-term outcome in treated combined methylmalonic acidemia and homocystinemia. Genet Med 1999; 1:146–150.

139. Nicolaides P, Leonard JV, Surtees R. Neurological outcome of methylmalonic acidemia. Arch Dis Child 1998; 78:508–512.

140. Saudubray JM, Touati P, Delonlay P, et al. Liver transplantation in propionic acidaemia. Eur J Pediatr 1999; 158[suppl 2]:S65–S69.

141. De Raeve L, Meirleir L, Ramet J, Vandenplas Y, Gerlo E. Acrodermatitis enteropathica-like cutaneous lesions in organic aciduria. J Pediatr 1994; 124:416–420.

142. Yannicelli S, Hambidge KM, Picciano MF. Decreased selenium intake and low plasma selenium concentrations leading to clinical symptoms in a child with propionic acidemia. J Inher Metab Dis 1992; 15:261–268.

143. Massoud AF, Leonard JV. Cardiomyopathy in propionic acidaemia. Eur J Pediatr 1993; 152:441–445.

144. D'angio CT, Dilon MJ, Leonard JV. Renal tubular dysfunction in methylmalonic acidemia. Eur J Pediatr 1991; 150:259–263.

145. Dudley J, Allen J, Tizard J, McGraw M. Benign methylmalonic acidemia in a sibship with distal renal tubular acidosis. Pediatr Nephrol 1998; 12:564–566.

146. Rutledge SL, Geraghty M, Mroczek E, et al. Tubulointerstitial nephritis in methylmalonic acidemia. Pediatr Nephrol 1993; 7:81–82.

147. Baumgartner ER, Viardot, et al. Long term follow-up of 77 patients with isolated methylmalonic acidemia. J Inher Metab Dis 1995:138–142.

148. Dechaux M, Touati G, Vargas Poussou R, et al. Renal function in children with methylmalonic acidaemia. J Inher Metab Dis 2000; 23:Suppl. 1:97(A).

149. van't Hoff WG, Dixon M, Taylor J, et al. Combined liver–kidney transplantation for methylmalonic acidemia. 1998; J Pediatr 132:1043–1044.

150. van't Hoff WG, McKiernan PJ, Surtees RAH, Leonard JV. Liver transplantation for methylmalonic acidemia. 1999; Eur J Pediatr 1999; 158[suppl 2]:S70–S74.

151. Packman S, Rosenthal P, Weisiger K, et al. Liver transplantation in Cbl B methylmalonic acidemia. J Inherit Metab Dis 2000; 23:Suppl. 1:95(A).

152. Yorifuji T, Muroi J, Uematsu A, et al. Living-related liver transplantation for neonatal-onset propionic acidemia. J Pediatr 2000; 137:572–574.

153. Roe CR, Ding J. Mitochondrial fatty acid oxidation disorders. In: Scriver CR, Beaudet AL, Sly WS, Valle D, eds. The Metabolic and Molecular Bases of Inherited Disease. 8th ed. New York: McGraw-Hill, 2001:2297–3327.

154. Brivet M, Boutron A, Slama A, et al. Defects in activation and transport of fatty acids. J Inher Metab Dis 1999; 22:428–441.

155. Al Odaib A, Shneider AL, Bennet M, et al. A defect in the transport of long-chin fatty acids associated with acute liver failure. N Engl J Med 1998; 339:1752–1757.

156. Wanders RJA, Vreken P, den Boer MEJ, et al. Disorders of mitochondrial fatty acyl-CoA B-oxidation. J Inher Metab Dis 1999; 2:442–487.

157. Wanders RJ, Denis S, Ruiter JP, Ijlst L, Dacremont G. 2,6-Dimethylheptanoyl-CoA is a specific substrate for long-chain acyl-CoA dehydrogenase (LCAD): evidence for a major role of LCAD in branched-chain fatty acid oxidation. Biochem Biophys Acta 1998; 1393:35–40.

158. Frerman FE, Goodman SI. Defects of electron transfer flavoprotein and electron transfer flavoprotein-ubiquinone oxidoreductase: Glutaric acidemia type II. In: Scriver CR, Beaudet AL, Sly WS, Valle D, eds. The Metabolic and Molecular Bases of Inherited Disease. 8th ed. New York: McGraw-Hill, 2001:2357–2366.

159. Uchida Y, Izai K, Orii T, Hashimoto T. Novel fatty acid B-oxidation enzymes in rat liver mitochondria. II. Purification and properties of enoyl-CoA hydratase/3-hydroxyacyl-CoA dehydrogenase/3-keto-acyl-CoA thiolase trifunctional protein. J Biol Chem 1992;267:1034–1041.

160. Carpenter K, Pollit RJ, Middleton B. Human liver long-chain 3-hydroxyacyl-coenzyme A dehydrogenase is a multifunctional membrane bound beta oxidation enzyme of mitochondria. Biochem Biophys Res Commun 1992; 183:443–448.

161. Ushikubo S, Ayoama T, Kamijo T, et al. Molecular characterization of mitochondrial trifunctional protein deficiency: formation of the enzyme complex is important for stabilization of both α- and β-subunits. Am J Hum Genet 1996; 58:979–988.

162. Ibdah JA, Yang Z, Bennet M. Liver disease in pregnancy and fetal fatty acid oxidation defects. Mol Genet Metab 2000; 71:182–189.

163. Mitchell GA, Fukao T. Inborn errors of ketone body metabolism. In: Scriver CR, Beaudet AL, Sly WS, Valle D, eds. The Metabolic and Molecular Bases of Inherited Disease. 8th ed. New York: McGraw-Hill, 2001:2327–2356.

164. Saudubray JM, Martin D, de Lonlay P, et al. Recognition and management of fatty acid oxidation defects: a series of 107 patients. J Inherit Metab Dis 1999; 22:488–502.

165. Stanley CA, De Leeuw S, Coates P, et al. Chronic cardiomyopathy and weakness or acute coma in children with a defect in carnitine uptake. Ann Neurol 1991; 30:709–716.

166. Olpin SE, Allen J, Bonham JR, et al. Features of palmitoyltransferase type I deficiency. J Inherit Metab Dis 2001; 24:3542.

167. Lopriore E, Gemke RJ, Verhoeven NM, et al. Carnitine-acylcarnitine translocase deficiency: phenotype, residual enzyme activity and outcome. Eur J Pediatr 2001; 160:101–104.

168. North K, Hoppel CL, De Girolami U, et al. Lethal neonatal deficiency of carnitine palmitoyl transferase II associated with dysgenesis of the brain and kidneys. J Pediatr 1995; 127:414–420.

169. Bonnefont JP, Demaugre F, Prip-Buus C, et al. Carnitine palmitoyltransferase deficiencies. Mol Genet Metab 1999; 68:424–440.

170. Vianney-Saban C, Stremler N, Paul O, et al. Infantile form of carnitine palmitoyltransferase type II deficiency in a girl with rapid fatal onset. J Inher Metab Dis 1995; 18:362–363.

171. Mathur A, Sims HF, Gopalakrishnan D, et al. Molecular heterogeneity in very-long-chain Acyl-CoA dehydrogenase deficiency causing pediatric cardiomyopathy and sudden death. Circulation 1999; 99:1337–1343.

172. Wilson CJ, Champion MP, Collins JE, et al. Outcome of medium chain acyl-CoA dehydrogenase deficiency after diagnosis. Arch Dis Child 1999; 80:459–462.

173. Bhala A, Willi S, Rinaldo P, et al. Clinical and biochemical characterization of short-chain acyl-CoA dehydrogenase deficiency. J Pediatr 1995; 126:910–915.

174. Tein I, Haslam RH, Rhead W, et al. Short chain acyl-CoA-dehydrogenase deficiency. A cause of ophthalmoplegia and multicore myopathy. Neurology 1999; 52:366–372.

175. Tyni T, Palotie A, Viinikka L, et al. Long-chain 3-hydroxyacyl-CoA dehydrogenase deficiency with the G1528 mutation: clinical presentation of thirteen patients. J Pediatr 1997; 130:67–76.

176. Gillingham M, Van Calcar S, Ney D, et al. Dietary management of long-chain 3-hydroxyacyl-CoA dehydrogenase deficiency (LCHADD). A case report and survey. J Inherit Metab Dis 1999; 22:123–131.

177. Ibdah JA, Tein I, Dionisi-Vici C, et al. Mild trifunctional protein deficiency is associated with progressive neuropathy and myopathy and suggest a novel genotype-phenotype correlation. J Clin Invest 1998; 102:1193–1199.

178. Bennett MJ, Spotswood SD, Ross KF, et al. Fatal short-chain L-3-hydroxyacyl-coenzyme A dehydrogenase deficiency: clinical, biochemical and pathological studies on three subjects with this recently identified disorder of mitochondrila beta oxidation. Pediatr Dev Pathol 1999; 2:337–345.

179. Kamijo T, Indo Y, Souri M, et al. Medium chain 3-ketoacyl-coenzyme A thiolase deficiency: a new disorder of mitochondrial fatty acid B-oxidation. Pediatr Res 1997; 42:569–576.

180. Rinaldo P, Raymond K, Al-odaib A, et al. Clinical and biochemical features of fatty acid oxidation disorders. Curr Opin Pediatr 1998; 10:615–621.

181. Mitchell G, Bouchard L, Robert MF, et al. Mitochondrial 3-hydroxy-3-methyl-glutaryl-CoA synthase deficiency. Clinical course and description of causal mutations in the two known patients. J Inherit Metab Dis 2000; 23[Suppl. 1]:108(A).

182. Bonnet D, Martin D, Lonlay P, et al. Arrhytmias and conduction defects as presenting symptoms of fatty acid oxidation disorders in children. Circulation 1999; 100:2248–2255.

183. Christodolou J, Hoarse J, Hammond J, et al. Neonatal onset of medium-chain-acyl-Coenzyme A dehydrogenase deficiency with confusing biochemical features. J Pediatr 1995; 126:65–68.

184. Thiel C, Baudach S, Schnackenberg U, Vreken P, Wanders R. Long-chain 3-hydroxyacyl-CoA dehydrogenase deficiency: neonatal manifestation at the first day of life presenting with tachipnoea. J Inherit Metab Dis 1999; 22:839–840.

185. Iafolla AK, Thompson RJ, Roe CR. Medium-chain acyl-coenzyme A dehydrogenase deficiency: clinical course in 120 affected children. J Pediatr 1994; 124:409–415.

186. Ibdah JA, Dasouki MJ, Strauss AW. Long-chain 3-hydroxyacyl-CoA dehydrogenase deficiency: variable expressivity of maternal illness during pregnancy and unusual presentation with infantile cholestasis and hypocalcemia. J Inherit Metab Dis 1999; 22:811–814.

187. Tripp M, Katcher M, Peters HA, et al. Systemic carnitine deficiency presenting as familial endocardial fibroelastosis. N Engl J Med 305:385–390.

188. Stanley CA. Disorders of fatty acid oxidation. In: Fernandes J, Saudubray JM, van den Berghe G, eds. Inborn

Metabolic Diseases. 2nd ed. Berlin: Springer-Verlag, 2000:140–149.

189. Harding CO, Gillingham MB, van Calcar SC, et al. Docosahexaenoic acid and retinal function in children with long-chain 3-hydroxyacyl-CoA dehydrogenase deficiency. J Inherit Metab Dis 1999; 2:276–280.

190. Tyni T, Ekholm E, Pihko H. Pregnancy complications are frequent in long-chain-3hydroxyacyl-coenzyme A dehydrogenase deficiency. Am J Obstet Gynaecol 1998; 178:603–608.

191. Ibdah JA, Bennett MJ, Rinaldo, et al. A fetal fatty-acid oxidation disorder as a cause of liver disease in pregnant women. N Engl J Med 1999; 340:1723–1731.

192. Treem WR. Pregnancy and liver disease. Beta oxidation defects. Clin Liver Dis 1999; 3:50–67.

193. Chakrapani A, Olpin S, Cleary M, et al. Trifunctional protein deficiency: three families with significant maternal hepatic dysfunction in pregnancy not associated with E474Q mutation. J Inher Metab Dis 2000; 23:826–834.

194. Ibdah JA, Zhao Y, Viola J, et al. Molecular prenatal diagnosis in families with fetal mitochondrial trifunctional protein mutations. J Pediatr 2001; 138:396–399.

195. Innes AM, Seargeant LE, Balachandra K, et al. Hepatic carnitine palmitoyltransferase I deficiency presenting as maternal illness in pregnancy. Pediatr Res 2000; 47:43–45.

196. Nelson J, Lewis B, Walters B. The HELLP syndrome associated with fetal medium-chain acyl-CoA dehydrogenase deficiency. J Inherit Metab Dis 2000; 23:518–519.

197. Matern D, Hart P, Murtha AP, et al. Acute fatty liver of pregnancy associated with short-chain acyl-coenzyme A dehydrogenase deficiency. J Pediatr 2001; 138:585–588.

198. Boles RG, Buck EA, Blitzer MG, et al. Retrospective biochemical screening of fatty acid oxidation disorders in post mortem liver of 418 cases of sudden death in the firs year of life. J Pediatr 1998; 132:924–933.

199. Lundemose JB, Kolvraa S, Gregersen N, et al. Fatty acid oxidation disorders as primary cause of sudden and unexpected death in infants and young children: an investigation performed on cultured fibroblasts from 79 children who died aged between 0–4 years. Mol Pathol 1997; 50:212–217.

200. Rashed MS, Ozand PT, Bennet MJ, et al. Inborn errors of metabolism diagnosed in sudden death cases by acylcarnitine analysis of postmortem bile. Clin Chem 1995; 41:1109–1114.

201. Rinaldo P, Stanley CA, Hsu BY, et al. Sudden neonatal death in carnitine transporter deficiency. J Pediatr 1997; 131:304–305.

202. Nuoffer JM, de Lonlay P, Costa C, et al. Familial neonatal SIDS revealing carnitine-acylcarnitine translocase deficiency. Eur J Pediatr 2000; 159:82–85.

203. Treacy E, Lambert D, Barnes R, et al. Short-chain hydroxyacyl-CoA dehydrogenase deficiency presenting as unexpected infant death: a family study. J Pediatr 2000; 137:257–259.

204. Poplawski NK, Ranieri E, Harrison JR, Fletcher JM. Multiple acyl-CoA-dehydrogenase deficiency: diagnosis by acylcarnitine analysis of a 12 year old newborn screening card. J Pediatr 1999, 134:764–766.

205. Rinaldo P, Yoon HR, Yu C, et al. Sudden and unexpected neonatal death: a protocol for the postmortem diagnosis of fatty acid oxidation disorders. Semin Perinatol 1999; 23:204–210.

206. El-schahawi M, Bruno C, Tsujino S, et al. Sudden infant death syndrome (SIDS) in a family with myophosphorilase deficiency. Neuromusc Disord 1997 7:81–3.

207. de Klerk JB, Duran M, Huijmans JG, Mancini GM. Sudden infant death and lysinuric protein intolerance. Eur J Pediatr 1996; 155:256–257.

208. Pastores GM, Santorelli FM, Shanske S, et al. Leigh syndrome and hypertrophic cardiomyopathy in an infant with a mitochondrial DNA point mutation (T8993G). Am J Med Genet 1994; 50:265–71.

209. Dionisi-Vici C, Seneca S, Zeviani M, et al. Fulminant Leigh syndrome and sudden unexpected death in a family with the T9176C mutation of the mitochondrial ATPase 6 gene. J Inher Metab Dis 1998: 21:2–8.

210. Treem WR. Inborn defects in mitochondrial fatty acid oxidation. In: Suchy FJ, ed. Liver disease in children. 1st ed. St. Louis: Mosby, 1994:852–887.

211. Davidson-Mundt A, Luder A, Greene C. Hyperuricemia in medium-chain-acyl-coenzyme-A dehydrogenase deficiency. J Pediatr 1992; 120:444–446.

212. Treem WR, Witzleben CA, Picoli DA, et al. Medium-chain and long-chain acyl CoA dehydrogenase deficiency: clinical, pathologic and ultrastructural differentiation from Reye's syndrome. Hepatology 1986; 6: 1270–1278.

213. Millington DS, Terada, Chase DH, et al. The role of tandem masss spectrometry in the diagnosis of fatty acid oxidation disorders. In Coates PM, Tanaka K, eds. New Developments in Fatty Acid Oxidation. Progress in Clinical and Biochemical Research. New York: Wiley-Liss, 1992:339–354.

214. van Hove JLK, Zhang W, Kahler SG, et al. Medium-chain acyl-CoA-dehydrogenase deficiency: diagnosis by acylcarntine analysis in blood. Am J Hum Genet 1993; 52:958–966.

215. van Hove, Kahler SG, Feezor, et al. Acylcarnitines in plasma and blood spots of patients with long-chain 3-hydroxyacyl-CoA dehydrogenase deficiency. J Inherit Metab Dis 2000; 23:571–582.

216. Sim KG, Wiley V, Wilken B. Carnitine palmitoyltransferase I deficiency in neonates identified by dried blood spot free carnitine and acylcarnitine profile. J Inherit Metab Dis 2001; 24:51–59.

217. Zschocke J, Hegardt FG, Casals N, et al. Clinical biochemical and molecular characterization of 3-hydroxy-3-methylglutaryl-CoA synthase deficiency. J Inherit Metab Dis 2000; 23:Suppl. 1:107(A).

218. Brivet M, Slama A, Millington DS, et al. Retrospective diagnosis of carnitine acylcarnitine translocase deficiency in the proband Guthrie card and enzymatic studies in parents. J Inherit Metab Dis 1996; 19:181–184.

219. Ziadeh R, Hoffman EP, Finegold DN, et al. Medium-chain Acyl-CoA dehydrogenase deficiency in Pennsylvania: neonatal screening shows high incidence and unexpected mutation frequencies. Pediatr Res 1995; 37: 675–678.

220. Wilcken B, Wiley V, Carpenter K. Two years of routine newborn screening by tandem mass spectrometry in New South Wales, Australia (abstr.). J Inherit Metab Dis 2000; 23:Suppl. 1:4.

221. Abdenur JA, Chamoles NA, Schenone AB, et al. Multiple acyl-CoA-dehydrogenase deficiency: use of acylcarnitines and fatty acids to monitor the response to dietary treatment. Pediatr Res 2001; 50:61–66.

222. Bennet MJ, Weinberger MJ, Sherwood WG, Burlina AB. Secondary 3-hydroxydicarboxylic aciduria mimicking

long-chain 3-hdroxyacyl-CoA dehydrogenase deficiency. J Inherit Metab Dis 1994; 17:283–286.

223. Bonafe L, Troxler H, Kuster T, et al. Evaluation of urinary acylglycines by electrospray tandem mass spectrometry in mitochondrial energy metabolism defects and organic acidurias. Mol Genet Metab 2000; 69:302–311.

224. Costa CG, Dorland L, Holwerda U, et al. Simultaneous analysis of plasma free fatty acids and their 3-hydroxy analogs in fatty acid β-oxidation disorders. Clin Chem 1998; 44:463–471.

225. Abdenur JA, Chamoles NA, Specola N, Schenone AB, et al. MCAD deficiency: Acylcarnitines by tandem mass spectrometry (MS-MS) are useful to monitor dietary treatment. Adv Exp Med Biol 1999; 46:353–363.

226. Jones PM, Burlina AB, Bennet MJ. Quantitative measurement of total and free 3-hydroxy fatty acids in serum or plasma samples: short-chain 3-hydroxy fatty acids are not esterified. J Inherit Metab Dis 2000; 23:745–750.

227. Brivet M, Slama A, Saudubray JM, et al. Rapid diagnosis of long chain and medium chain fatty acid oxidation disorders using lymphocytes. Ann Clin Biochem 1995; 32:154–159.

228. Shen JJ, Matern D, Millington D, et al. Acylcarnitines in fibroblasts of patients with long-chain 3-hydroxyacyl-CoA dehydrogenase deficiency and other fatty acid oxidation disorders. J Inherit Metab Dis 2000; 23:27–44.

229. Gregersen N, Andresen BS, Bross P. Prevalent mutations in fatty acid oxidation disorders: diagnostic considerations. Eur J Pediatr 2000; 159[Supp. 3]:S213–218.

230. Matsubara Y, Narisawa K, Tada K, et al. Prevalence of K329E mutation in medium chain acylCoA dehydrogenase gene determined from Guthrie cards. Lancet 1991; 338:552–553.

231. Andresen BS, Bross P, Szabolcs U, et al. The molecular basis of medium-chain-acyl-CoA dehydrogenase (MCAD) deficiency in compound heterozygous patients: is there a correlation between genotype and phenotype? Hum Mol Genet 1997; 6:695–707.

232. Njolstad PR, Skjeldal OH, Agsteribbe A, et al. Medium chain acyl-CoA dehydrogenase deficiency and fatal valproate toxicity. Pediatr Neurol 1997; 16:160–162.

233. Baillet L, Mullur RS, Esser V, McGarry JD. Elucidation of the mechanism by which (+)-acylcarnitines inhibit mitochondrial fatty acid transport. J Biol Chem 2000; 275:36766–36768.

234. Pollit, Leonard JV. Prospective surveillance study of medium chain acyl-CoA dehydrogenase deficiency in the UK. Arch Dis Child 1998; 79:116–119.

235. Kerr DS, Wexler I, Zinn AB. Disorders of pyruvate metabolism and the tricarboxylic acid cycle. In: Fernandes J, Saudubray JM, van den Berghe G, eds. Inborn Metabolic Diseases. 2nd ed. Berlin: Springer-Verlag, 2000: 126–138.

236. Robinson BH. Lactic acidemia: Disorders of pyruvate carboxylase and pyruvate dehydrogenase. In: Scriver CR, Beaudet AL, Sly WS, Valle D, eds. The Metabolic and Molecular Bases of Inherited Disease. 8th ed. New York: McGraw-Hill, 2001:2275–2295.

237. Nyhan WL, Ozand PT, eds. Deficiency of pyruvate dehydrogenase complex. In: Atlas of Metabolic Diseases. 1st ed. London: Chapman & Hall Medical, 1998:278–284.

238. Lissens W, De Meirleir L, Seneca S, et al. Mutations in the X-linked pyruvate dehydrogenase (E1) subunit gene (PDHA1) in patients with a pyruvate dehydrogenase complex deficiency. Hum Mutat 2000; 15:209–219.

239. Robinson BH, Mac Kay N, Petrova-Benedict R, et al. Defects in the E2 lipoyltransacetylase and the X-lipoyl containing component of the pyruvate dehydrogenase complex in patients with lactic acidemia. J Clin Invest 1990; 85:1821–1824.

240. Ito M, Kobashi H, Naito E, et al. Decrease of pyruvate dehydrogenase phosphatase activity in patients with congenital lactic acidemia. Clin Chim Acta 1992; 209:1–7.

241. Yoshida I, Sweetman L, Kulovich S, Nyhan WL, Robinson B. Effect of lipoic acid in a patient with defective activity of pyruvate dehydrogenase, 2-oxoglutarate dehydrogenase and branched-chain keto acid dehydrogenase. Pediatr Res 1990; 27:75–79.

242. Elpeleg ON, Ruitenbeek W, Jakobs C, et al. Congenital lactic acidemia caused by lipoamide dehydrogenase deficiency with favorable outcome. J Pediatr 1995; 126: 72–74.

243. Saada A, Aptowitzer I, Link E, Elpeleg ON. ATP synthesis in lipoamide dehydrogenase deficiency. Biochem Biophys Res Commun 2000; 16:382–386.

244. Makino M, Horai S, Goto Y, Nonaka I. Mitochondrial DNA mutations in Leigh syndrome and their phylogenetic implications. J Hum Genet 2000; 45:69–75.

245. DiMauro S, Bonilla E, De Vivo D. Does the patient have a mitochondrial encephalomyopathy? J Child Neurol 1999; 14(Suppl 1):S23–S35.

246. Kohlschutter A, Behbehani A, Langenbeck U, et al. A familial progressive neurodegenerative disease with 2-oxo-glutaric aciduria. Eur J Pediatr 1982; 138:32–37.

247. Dunckelmann RJ, Ebinger F, Schulze A, et al. 2-ketoglutarate dehydrogenase deficiency with intermittent 2-ketoglutaric aciduria. Neuropediatrics 2000; 31:35–38.

248. Rustin P, Bourgeron T, Parfait B, et al. Inborn errors of the Krebs cycle: a group of unusual mitochondrial diseases in human. Biochim Biophys Acta 1997; 1361: 185–197.

249. Bourgeron T, Chretien D, Poggi-bach J, et al. Mutation of the fumarase gene in two siblings with progressive encephalopathy and fumarase deficiency. J Clin Invest 1994:2514–2518.

250. Coughlin EM, Christensen E, Kunz P, et al. Molecular analysis and prenatal diagnosis of human fumarase deficiency. Mol Genet Metab 1998; 63:254–262.

251. Kerrigan JF, Aleck KA, Tarby TJ, et al. Fumaric aciduria: clinical and imaging features. Ann Neurol 2000; 47:583–588.

252. Hall RE, Henriksson KG, Lewis SF, et al. Mitochondrial myopathy with succinate dehydrogenase and aconitase deficiency. Abnormalities of several iron sulfur proteins. J Clin Invest 1993; 92:2660–2666.

253. Brun N, Robitaille Y, Grignon A, et al. Pyruvate carboxylase deficiency: prenatal onset of ischemia-like brain lesions in two sibs with acute neonatal form. Am J Med Genet 1999; 84:94–101.

254. Ahmad A, Khaler S, Kishnani PS, et al. Treatment of pyruvate carboxylase deficiency with high doses of citrate and aspartate. Am J Med Genet 1999; 87:331–338.

255. Nyhan WL, Ozand PT, eds. Fructose 1,6-diphosphatase deficiency. In: Atlas of Metabolic Diseases. 1st ed. London: Chapman & Hall Medical, 1998:273–277.

256. Shoffner JM. Oxidative phosphorylation diseases. In: Scriver CR, Beaudet AL, Sly WS, Valle D, eds. The Metabolic and Molecular Bases of Inherited Disease. 8th ed. New York: McGraw-Hill, 2001:2367–2423.

257. Munnich A. Defects of the respiratory chain. In: Fernandes J, Saudubray JM, van den Berghe G, eds. Inborn Metabolic Diseases. 2nd ed. Berlin: Springer-Verlag, 2000:158–168.

258. Munnich A, Rotig A, Cormier-Daire V, Rustin P. Clinical presentation of respiratory chain deficiency. In: Scriver CR, Beaudet AL, Sly WS, Valle D, eds. The Metabolic and Molecular Bases of Inherited Disease. 8th ed. New York: McGraw-Hill, 2001:2261–2274.

259. Robinson BH. Human citochrome oxidase deficiency. Pediatr Res 2000; 48:581–585.

260. Pastores GM, Santorelli FM, Shanske S, et al. Leigh syndrome and hypertrophic cardiomyopathy in a patient with a mitochondrial DNA point mutation (T8993G). Am J Med Genet 1994; 50:265–71.

261. Munnich A, Rotig A, Chretien D, et al. Clinical presentation of mitochondrial disorders in childhood. J Inherit Metab Dis 1996; 19:521–527.

262. Naviaux R. The mitochondrial DNA depletion syndromes. In: Nyhan WL, Ozand PT, eds. Atlas of Metabolic Diseases. 1st ed. London: Chapman & Hall Medical, 1998: 314–320.

263. Mazziota MRM, Ricci E, Bertini E, et al. Fatal infantile liver failure associated with mitochondrial DNA depletion. J Pediatr 1992; 121:896–901.

264. Vu TH, Sciacco M, Tanji K, et al. Clinical manifestations of mitochondrial DNA depletion. Neurology 1998; 50:1783–1790.

265. van der Knaap MS, Jakobs C, Valk J. Magnetic resonance imaging in lactic acidosis. J Inher Metab Dis 1996; 19:535–547.

266. Nyhan WL, Ozand PT, eds. Mitochondrial encephalomyopathy, lactic acidosis and stroke-like episodes (MELAS) In: Atlas of Metabolic Diseases. 1st ed. London: Chapman & Hall Medical, 1998:297–304.

267. Nyhan WL, Ozand PT, eds. Myoclonic epilepsy and ragged red fibers (MERRF). In: Atlas of Metabolic Diseases. 1st ed. London: Chapman & Hall Medical, 1998: 292–297.

268. Nyhan WL, Ozand PT, eds. Neurodegeneration, ataxia and retinitis pigmentosa (NARP). In: Atlas of Metabolic Diseases. 1st ed. London: Chapman & Hall Medical, 1998:304–309.

269. Wallace DC, Lott MT, Brown MD, Kerstann K. Mitochondria and neuro-ophthalmological diseases. In: Scriver CR, Beaudet AL, Sly WS, Valle D, eds. The Metabolic and Molecular Bases of Inherited Disease. 8th ed. New York: McGraw-Hill, 2001:2425–2512.

270. Kadowaki T, Kadowaki H, Mori Y, et al. A subtype of diabetes mellitus associated with a mutation of mitochondrial DNA. N Engl J Med 1994; 330:962–966.

271. Rotig A, Bourgeron T, Chretien D, et al. Spectrum of mitochondrial DNA rearrangements in the Pearson marrow–pancreas syndrome. Hum Mol Genet 1995; 4: 1327–1331.

272. Nyhan WL, Ozand PT, eds. Pearson syndrome. In: Atlas of Metabolic Diseases. 1st ed. London: Chapman & Hall Medical, 1998:309–313.

273. Moraes CT, DiMauro S, Zeviani M, Lombes A, et al. Mitochondrial DNA deletions in progressive external ophthalmoplegia and Kearns-Sayre syndrome. N Engl J Med 1989; 320:1293.

274. Rotig A, Cormier V, Chatelain P, et al. Deletion of the mitochondrial genome in a case of early onset diabetes mellitus, optic atrophy and deafness (Wolfram syndrome). J Clin Invest 1993; 91:1095–1102.

275. Zeviani M, Servidei S, Gellera C, et al. An autosomal dominant disorder with multiple deletions of mitochondrial DNA starting at the D-loop region. Nature 1989; 339:309–313.

276. Rotig A, De Lonlay P, Chretien D, et al. Frataxin expansion causes aconitase and mitochondrial iron-sulfur protein deficiency in Friedreich ataxia. Nat Genet 1997; 17:215.

277. Bionne S, D'Adamo P, Maestrini E, et al. A novel X-linked gene, G4.5 is responsible for Barth syndrome. Nat Genet 1996; 12:385.

278. Poggi-Travert F, Martin D, Billette de Villemeur T, et al. Metabolic intermediates in lactic acidosis: compounds samples and interpretation. J Inherit Metab Dis 1996; 19: 478–488.

279. Cray SH, Robinson B, Cox PN. Lactic acidemia and bradyarrhythmia in a child sedated with profolol. Crit Care Med 1998; 26:2087–2092.

280. Beatty ME, Zhang YH, Mc Cabe ER, Steiner RD. Fructose-1-6-diphosphatase deficiency and glyceroluria: one possible etiology for GIS. Mol Genet Metab 2000; 69: 338–340.

281. Rogers JG, Wilkinson RG, Skelton I, Danks DM. Tertiary lactic acidosis. J Pediatr 1981; 99: 272–273.

282. Bongaerts G, Bakkeren J, Severijen R, et al. Lactobacilli and acidosis in children with short small bowel. J Pediatr Gastroenterol Nutr 2000; 30:288–293.

283. Romero NB, Lombes A, Touati G, et al. Morphological studies of skeletal muscle in lactic acidosis. J Inher Metab Dis 1996; 19:528–534.

284. Morris AAM, Leonard JV. The treatment of congenital lactic acidoses. J Inherit Metab Dis 1996; 19:573–580.

285. Lerman-Sagie T, Rustin P, Lev D, et al. Dramatic improvement in mitochondrial cardiomyopathy following treatment with idebenone. J Inher Metab Dis 2001; 24: 28–34.

286. Wexler ID, Hemalatha SG, McConnell J, et al. Outcome of pyruvate dehydrogenase deficiency treated with ketogenic diets. Studies in patients with identical mutations. Neurology 1997; 49:1655–1661.

287. Sokal EM, Sokol R, Cormier V, et al. Liver transplantation in mitochondrial respiratory chain disorders. Eur J Pediatr 1999; 158(Suppl 2):S81–S84.

288. Chuang DT, Shih V. Maple syrup urine disease (branched-chain ketoaciduria. In: Scriver CR, Beaudet AL, Sly WS, Valle D, eds. The Metabolic and Molecular Bases of Inherited Disease. 8th ed. New York: McGraw-Hill, 2001:1971–2005.

289. Peinemann, Danner DJ. Maple syrup urine disease 1954 to 1993. J Inherit Metab Dis 1994; 17:3–15.

290. Fernhoff P, Lubitz D, Danner DJ, et al. Thiamine responsive maple syrup urine disease. Pediatr Res 1985; 19:1011–1016.

291. Jouvet P, Poggi F, Rabier D, et al. Continuous venovenous haemofiltration in the acute phase of neonatal maple syrup urine disease. J Inher Metab Dis 1997; 20: 463–472.

292. Friedrich CA, Marble A, Maher J, et al. Successful control of branched-chain aminoacids in maple syrup urine disease using elemental aminoacids in total parenteral nutrition during acute pancreatitis. Am J Hum Genet 1992; 51:A350.

293. Riviello JJ, Rezvani I, Digeorge AM, et al. Cerebral edema causing death in children with maple syrup urine disease. J Pediatr 1991; 119:42–47.

294. Treacy E, Clow CL, Reade TR, et al. Maple syrup urine disease: interrelations between branched-chain amino-oxo- and hydroxyacids; implications for treatment: associations with CNS dysmyelination. J Inherit Metab Dis 1992;15:121–135.

295. Brismar J, Aqeel A, Brismar G, et al. Maple syrup urine disease: findings on CT and MRI scans of the brain in 10 infants. Am J Neuroradiol 1990; 11:1219.

296. Chase DH, Hillman SL, Millington DS, et al. Rapid diagnosis of MSUD in blood spots from newborns by tandem mass spectrometry. Clin Chem 1995; 41:62–68.

297. Nord A, van Doorninck WJ, Greene C. Developmental profile of patients with maple syrup urine disease. J Inherit Metab Dis 1991; 14:881–89.

298. Hilliges C, Awiszus D, Wendel U. Intellectual performance of children with maple syrup urine disease. Eur J Pediatr 1993; 152:144–147.

34

Obesity in Children

Ramin Alemzadeh
Medical College of Wisconsin, Milwaukee, Wisconsin, U.S.A.

Russell Rising and Maribel Cedillo
EMTAC, Inc., Miami, Florida, U.S.A.

Fima Lifshitz
Miami Children's Hospital and University of Miami School of Medicine, Miami, Florida; State University of New York Health Science Center at Brooklyn, Brooklyn, New York; Pediatric Sunshine Academics; and Sansum Medical Research Institute, Santa Barbara, California, U.S.A.

I. PREVALENCE

Childhood obesity is one of the most complex and poorly understood clinical syndromes in pediatrics. Obesity is a common nutritional disorder among children and adolescents in the United States, with an estimated prevalence of 20% as compared to 30% in the adult population. A study in Europe found that 15 and 22% of adult men and women, respectively, were obese (1). Furthermore, 60 and 75% of men and women, respectively, in urban Samoa were obese (2). It is estimated that obesity affects 7% of the world's adult population. The percentage of overweight children and adolescents has increased by almost 50% in the past two decades (3). This disturbing trend in childhood and adolescent obesity parallels a concurrent increase in prevalence of this disorder (4). It is estimated that 10–20% of obese infants will remain overweight (5). It has also been observed that about 40% of overweight children will continue to have increased weight during adolescence and 75–80% of obese adolescents become obese adults (6). Moreover, more than one-third of overweight children will eventually become obese adults (7). Obesity in children is expected to continue to increase into the 21st century.

Obesity is present in every continent. This includes the established market economies including the economies of Europe, Latin America, the Caribbean, and the Middle East. More worrisome is the fact that the body mass index (BMI) in adults is expected to almost double in most of the major market economies of the world by the year 2030 (8). France, the Netherlands, United Kingdom, and the United States also report increasing prevalence of obesity in children and adolescents. Data from 79 developing countries and a number of industrialized nations suggests that 22 million children under 5 years of age are overweight (>+2 standard deviations above National Child Health Survey (NCHS) reference median weight for height) (9). These increases in obesity may be partly due to the greater social economic status of the market economies (10). In the future, the prevalence of childhood obesity may be as much as the current rise in adult obesity, but the consequences may be more severe as the duration of obesity will be longer. It may therefore have a greater deleterious impact on health and the rate of morbidity and mortality than obesity starting in adulthood.

Many children are at high risk of becoming overweight between the ages of 3 and 10 years. This is the time they begin school and socialization with other children. Furthermore, the risk of becoming an obese adult was 3–10 times greater if the child's weight was greater than the 95th percentile for their age. Obese parents impose even a greater risk that their children will be overweight. There is a 75% chance that children aged 3–10 will be overweight if both parents were obese. This drops to a 25–50% chance with just one obese parent. These statistics suggest that behavior modification or treatment intervention at an early age may be important for preventing future adolescent and adulthood obesity (11).

II. MORBIDITY

Obesity in childhood is a major public health problem and is strongly linked to persistence into adulthood. This increases the obese individual's risks for hypertension (12), hyperlipidemia (13), respiratory diseases (14), diabetes (15), orthopedic conditions (16, 17), psychosocial disorders (18), and social and economic consequences (19).

The altered nutritional state in obesity results in many endocrine changes that disappear with weight loss. These include excess insulin secretion, insulin resistance, and alterations at the level of the hypothalamic pituitary gonadal and adrenal axis. Hyperinsulinemia of obesity is strongly linked with cardiovascular diseases, including type 2 diabetes mellitus, hyperlipidemia, and hypertension (20). Obesity is associated with hypertension in 10–30% of children (12) regardless of age, gender, and duration. Obese children and adolescents tend to have elevated levels of total serum cholesterol, triglycerides, and low-density lipoprotein, and decreased levels of high-density lipoproteins (12). They are also at increased risk for coronary heart disease as they grow into obese adults (21, 22). With few exceptions, the clinical features of cardiovascular heart disease are not apparent until the third or fourth decade of life. However, there is substantial evidence that the atherosclerotic process is initiated during childhood (23, 24).

In a study by Must et al., long-term morbidity and mortality of overweight adolescents were examined (25). They demonstrated that obesity in adolescent subjects were associated with an increased risk of mortality from all causes and disease-specific mortality among men, but not among women. On the other hand, the risk of morbidity from coronary heart disease and atherosclerosis was increased in both men and women who had been obese in adolescence. This suggests that body weight reduction among the young may decrease the risks for many of the obesity-related health disorders.

Increased cholesterol turnover and its concentration in the bile of obese individuals predispose them to a high incidence of steatohepatitis (26) and gallbladder disease (27). Indeed, gallstones (cholelithiasis) have been reported to be three times more common in morbidly obese people than in normal subjects. Gallstones may also result while the obese person is on a hypocaloric diet. This may be due to mobilization of adipose tissue cholesterol during weight loss (28). Furthermore, the risk of colorectal cancer and gout was increased among women who had been obese in adolescence. Finally, obesity in adolescence was a more significant predictor of these risks than being overweight in adulthood (29).

Syndrome X is a clinical quartet of hyperinsulinemia, hyperlipidemia, hypertension, and subsequent cardiovascular disease (30). It is believed that obesity is a component of this metabolic syndrome and has been described in obese children (31) and adolescents (32). In a more recent study, Chen et al. suggested that syndrome X is characterized by the linking of a metabolic entity (hyperinsulinemia/insulin resistance, hyperlipidemia, and obesity) to a hemodynamic factor (hypertension) through a shared correlation with hyperinsulinemia/insulin resistance. Clustering features of syndrome X are independent of gender and age in both black and white populations (33).

Nonautoimmune forms of youth-onset diabetes are becoming increasingly prevalent as rates of obesity in children and adolescents accelerate (15). Many health professionals have recognized an emerging epidemic of type 2 diabetes mainly affecting minorities (34–36). Epidemiological data obtained from various centers suggest an almost fourfold increase in the prevalence of type 2 diabetes among minority groups such as Native, African, and Hispanic Americans aged 10–19 years over the past 10 years (15, 37). Increasing prevalence of type 2 diabetes in the youth is not limited to North America. For instance, among Japanese junior high school students, the incidence of type 2 diabetes is almost seven times that for type 1 diabetes (38). It is believed that the increasing incidence of type I diabetes is associated with changing food patterns and rising obesity rates among Japanese school children (39). Children have hyperinsulinism as a result of obesity, as do adults, and childhood obesity is commonly associated with impaired glucose tolerance (40). The stress of obesity and the increased demand for insulin during adolescence explain the predominantly pubertal and postpubertal onset of type 2 diabetes in obese children (41).

Orthopedic complications of obesity are believed to be largely of mechanical nature. During childhood, slipped capital femoral epiphysis, Legg-Calve-Perthes disease, and genu valgum tend to be more common in obese subjects. Orthopedic disorders such as Blount's disease (tibia vara) and slipped capital femoral epiphysis are frequently seen in obese adolescents (16, 17).

Rapid weight gain or obesity during infancy and childhood tends to be a risk factor for frequent respiratory infections (14). The work of breathing is increased in obese individuals and larger body mass places increased demands for oxygen consumption and carbon dioxide elimination. Many obese subjects suffer from chronic hypoxemia secondary to ventilation–perfusion mismatch. This is characterized by increased ventilation of upper lobes and increased perfusion of the lower lobes. Insufficient elimination of carbon dioxide, in some obese subjects, leads to hypoventilation (pickwickian) syndrome (42), which is characterized by chronic hypoxemia and hypercapnia. These subjects have blunted respiratory drive to both hypoxemia and hypercapnia.

Sleep apnea is also seen in severe obesity and is characterized by cessation of air flow for 10 s or longer on 30 occasions during 7 h of sleep. Parents of obese children and adolescents usually report that their children snore loudly and sometimes appear to stop breathing. Sleep apnea is a major problem found to be associated with increased risk of traffic accidents (43). The apnea may be obstructive, central, or combined. In most patients, no anatomical abnormalities of the upper airway can contribute to the development of obstructive sleep apnea (OSA). It has been shown that the occurrence of OSA in obese subjects is related to the size of the region enclosed by the mandible (44, 45) and sites and sizes of fat deposits around the pharynx, as well as subjects' weight. In patients with OSA, alveolar hypoventilation results from increased oxygen demand during the apneic episode. Coexistent cardipulmonary or neuromuscular disease in subjects with OSA can play a role in the development of alveolar hypoventilation. During the apneic episodes, the systemic blood pressure increases whereas the heart rate and cardiac output decrease. Apnea-associated cardiac arrhythmias have been frequently observed in patients with OSA and increases their risk for cardiovascular mortality (46). Relief of respiratory obstruction alleviates OSA. This may be accomplished by weight loss and continuous positive airway pressure (CPAP) during sleep.

Obesity is also accompanied by advanced skeletal maturity (bone age) and early menarche (29). Amenorrhea, oligomenorrhea, and/or dysfunctional uterine bleeding are common among obese adolescent females. Some of these patients will also develop polycystic ovarian syndrome (47–49).

A. Psychosocial Impact of Obesity

In addition to the medical complications associated with obesity, the juvenile-onset obese subject is also at risk for psychological morbidity (18). It has also been shown that obesity tends to confer disability greater than that associated with other forms of chronic illness (19). This disability seems to be linked to the public nature of obesity. Peer group discrimination is the factor that prompts parents to seek treatment in their obese child. Even young school-aged children have been observed to view their overweight classmates as less desirable playmates (50). Overweight children are frequently teased on the playground and usually excluded from games. Obese children are under considerable psychological stress and are generally viewed by society as clumsy, unattractive, and overindulgent.

Overweight children as young as 5 years of age have been found to associate their obesity with lower body esteem and lower perceived cognitive ability. A parent's concern about obesity and restriction of food were associated with negative self-evaluations among girls (51). In one study a mothers' own dietary restraint and concern about their daughter's obesity predicted child feeding practices. This suggests that a mother's control over her daughter's feeding practices and concern about the child's obesity may be an important, nonshared, environmental influence on the daughter's eating habits and relative weight (52). Moreover, obese elementary school-aged girls were more likely to be dieting and express concern about their overweight than similarly aged boys (53). All of these results suggest that childhood obesity can occur early in a child's life and has to be addressed by the whole family.

Lowered self-image, heightened self-consciousness, and impaired social functioning have been noted in some individuals who either become or remain obese during adolescence (54). Studies of obese adolescents have demonstrated obsession with being overweight, passivity, and withdrawal from social contact (18). Some investigators have found similarities between the behavior of obese subjects and racial minorities expressing prejudice (55). In fact, it has been shown that the obese persons were less likely to get admitted to a college than their lean counterparts, although there were no significant differences in their application rates, academic standing, or economic background (56). Moreover, obese individuals are 20% less likely to marry and are of lower income status than normal-weight individuals with other chronic medical conditions.

B. Economic Impact of Obesity

The increasing prevalence of obesity in adults is associated with rising health care costs. The cost of treating obesity-related illnesses to the economy of United States business sector has escalated in recent years. In one study employees of United States businesses between 25 and 64 years old were classified as nonobese (BMI < 25 kg), mildly obese (BMI 25–29), or moderately to severely obese (BMI > 29). The cost of obesity to the medical insurers of these businesses in 1994 was $12.7 billion, including $2.6 billion as a result of mild and $10.1 billion due to more severe obesity. Health insurance expenditures for treating obesity-related illnesses such as hypertension, type 2 diabetes, and coronary artery disease amounted to 43% of the total amount. The rest was the result of increased sick leave, and life and disability insurance payments. Overall, obesity was responsible for 5% of all health-related expenditures in the United States in 1994 (57).

Other countries have seen similar obesity-related increases in health care costs in adults. For example, total obesity-related health care costs for Canada in 1997 was $1.8 billion or 2.4% of total health care expenditures. The major contributors were hypertension ($656.6 million), type 2 diabetes ($423.2 million), and coronary artery disease ($346.0 million). This represents a considerable amount of available health care dollars for treating obesity-related comorbidities in Canada (58).

Health care cost can be tracked according to increases or decreases in a standard measure of obesity, such as the BMI. For example, health care costs for 5689 adults more than 40 years old, who were enrolled in a Minnesota health plan, were evaluated. Data were adjusted for age, race, gender, and chronic disease status. Physical activity was associated with 4.7% lower health care charges per active day per week while BMI was associated with 1.9% higher charges per BMI unit. Never-smokers with a BMI of 25 and who participated in physical activity 3 days per week had mean annual health care charges that were approximately 49% lower than physically inactive smokers with a BMI of 27.5. These data suggest that adverse health risks translate into significantly higher health care costs (59).

The recent advent of specialized programs for treating childhood obesity limits the amount of data available to track specific costs. This is due to many of these programs either being supported by outside funding or to their operating costs being incorporated into adult obesity program budgets. However, managed care organizations are now beginning to offer benefits for the treatment of childhood obesity through better access to established community childhood obesity programs (60).

III. SOCIAL OBESITY

People want to be thin. They like to be slim and trim and they fear being even a little bit overweight. This fear is present among all individuals, even those who are not overweight, but who want to be thinner (61, 62). The likes and dislikes of the population have changed. In the past, excess body fat was a symbol of wealth, power, and status. Now people do not like this type of appearance. Even children, by the time they reach the first grade, prefer other disabilities to obesity (63). The desire to be thin constitutes a problem that must be considered as a form of social obesity. This phenomenon often translates as a fear of obesity (61).

The fear of obesity may lead people to both health-promoting and health-compromising eating behaviors. Health promoting activities include exercising; eating fruits, vegetables, and reduced-fat food; limiting the amount of food eaten; and avoiding sweets and junk food. Health-compromising activities involve the use of diet pills, laxatives, or water pills; self-induced vomiting; skipping meals; dieting and fasting (64).

A. Children

Currently, a large portion of the population, including children, is attempting to lose weight. While children should be learning to enjoy food, it appears that they are dieting without supervision. Dieting in childhood is becoming a common habit. Very young children are reporting frequent dieting. A recent national survey found that 31% of fifth grade girls have dieted (64). Abramovitz and

Birch explored 5-year-old girls' ideas, concepts, and beliefs about dieting. They found that 34–64% of the girls had ideas about dieting and weight loss and understood the link between eating and body shape. Girls' knowledge about how people diet is inappropriate. These included descriptions of modified eating behaviors, such as drinking diet shakes and sodas, eating more fruits and vegetables, and use of special diet foods and restrictive eating behaviors. Mothers seem to be modeling both health-promoting and health-compromising eating behaviors to their daughters. Girls whose mothers reported current or recent food restriction were more than twice as likely to have ideas about dieting (65). Another factor found to influence girls' ideas, concepts, and beliefs about dieting is family history of overweight. The media was also mentioned by 55% of the children as a source of dieting ideas (66).

Children not only diet, they also worry about their body appearance. More and more children are concerned about and dissatisfied with their body image. Studies have shown that 55% of girls and 35% of boys in grades 3–6 want to be thinner (66). The Children's Version of the Eating Attitudes Test showed a negative correlation with children's BMI (66). It was found that 4.8% of them had scores suggestive of anorexia nervosa. Stice et al. found that eating disturbances that emerged during childhood led to inhibited and secretive eating, overeating, and vomiting. Maternal body dissatisfaction, internalization of the thin ideal, dieting, bulimic symptoms, and maternal and paternal body mass prospectively predicted the emergence of childhood eating disturbances. Infant feeding behavior and body mass during the first month of life also predicted the emergence of eating disturbances (67).

Parents who worry about their children becoming overweight may set the stage for a vicious cycle. Johnson and Birch found those parents who control what and how much their children eat may impede energy self-regulation and put these children at higher risk for overweight (68). These findings suggest that the optimal environment for children's development of self-control of energy intake is that in which parents provide healthy food choices but allow children to assume control of how much they consume (68). The Framingham Children's Study showed that children whose parents had high degrees of dietary control had greater increases in body fatness than did children whose parents had the lowest levels of dietary restraint and disinhibition (69).

B. Adolescents

There is a high prevalence of extreme measures taken by high school students throughout the country to avoid obesity (70–72). They often diet and have inappropriate eating habits and purging behaviors. Young persons, even when they are not overweight, diet to avoid obesity at a time when they are still growing and developing (73, 74). This can adversely affect their growth, resulting in nutritional dwarfing (75).

Neumark recently published results from a national survey examining weight-related behaviors among 6728 American adolescents in grades 5–12 (64). Almost half of the female population (45%) and 20% of male adolescents reported dieting. Older adolescent girls were significantly more likely to diet than younger ones. Dieting was reported by 31% of fifth graders and increased consistently to 62% among the 12th graders. The largest increase was among adolescent girls between the eighth (40%) and ninth (53%) grades. Thirteen percent of the girls and 7% of the boys reported disordered eating behaviors (64).

In another study, Neumark studied 3832 adults and 459 adolescents from four regions of the United States for weight-control behaviors. Based on gender, weight-control behaviors were found in 56.7% of adult women, 50.3% of adult men, 44.0% of adolescent girls, and 36.8% of adolescent boys (76).

Moses et al. showed that high school adolescents in an affluent suburban location were dieting at a very high rate. Forty-one percent of the adolescents were dieting on the day of the survey. Sixty-seven percent of all the adolescents had made on their own important dietary efforts during the past 4–8 weeks. Dieting occurred in normal-weight and underweight students. About 30% of dieters were among the underweight and those of normal weight for height. However, the proportion of the overweight students who were dieting was relatively low: 50–60% (62).

A distorted perception of ideal body weight (below appropriate body weight for height) is very prevalent among high school students. Adolescents often know what their ideal weight should be, but some prefer to be 10% less than their ideal weight for their height (62). Health-compromising behaviors and the fear of obesity may have detrimental consequences in children. Inappropriate nutrient intake may lead to nutritional dwarfing, failure to thrive, and various other nutritional problems, as described in another chapter of this book and elsewhere (76).

C. Dieting/Body Image Problem

It is important to pay close attention to the new classification scheme related to behavioral and mental health concerns for children and adolescents published in 1996 by the American Academy of Pediatrics. The *Diagnostic and Statistical Manual for Primary Care* (DSM-PC) is now paying attention to dieting/body image behaviors that were, in the past, not considered to be eating disorders. Older children and younger adolescents may exhibit behaviors that do not meet full DSM-IV criteria, yet still deserve attention. The two specific complexes in the DSM-PC related to eating disorders are: dieting/body image behaviors and purging/binge-eating behaviors (77). There are two levels of pathology for both of these behavior patterns that are not healthy, but do not fulfill DSM-IV criteria for an eating disorder. In DSM-PC, *var-*

iations constitute minor deviations from normal that still might be of concern for a parent or clinician (77).

An adolescent with a dieting/body image problem will be one who exhibits voluntary food limitation in a pursuit of thinness. He or she experiences a systematic fear of gaining weight that extends beyond a simple dieting/body image variation. However, the intensity of the problem does not meet criteria for anorexia. An obese adolescent who exhibits dieting/body image behaviors and or purging/binge-eating behaviors has a more complicated problem which adds to the difficulties in treatment and long-term health.

IV. GROWTH ASSESSMENT

The measurement of body weight, the parameter commonly used to assess adiposity, is not an optimal method to differentiate between being overweight and being obese. Indeed, individuals with larger than average body frames or excess muscle mass (athletes) may be mistakenly considered obese since they have excess body weight. Since they do not have excess body fat, they are not obese but their relative weight for height may be above 120%, which is a commonly used criterion of obesity in children.

Age-specific growth charts (73) allow a more precise assessment of a child's nutritional status. These charts help the clinician to evaluate a child's weight and its relationship to height. They also provide a view of the previous growth patterns and thus establish the presence of obesity more accurately. However, weight and height nomograms also fail to take into account the frame size and body composition of the patient. The importance of growth charts in the evaluation of childhood obesity is illustrated in the example shown in Figure 1. Julie is a 5-year-old girl with a pattern of morbid obesity. Review of her growth records revealed that Julie's rate of weight gain became excessive after 3 months of age and progressed at an accelerated pace after 1 year of age. This coincided with acceleration of linear growth. The final point on Julie's growth chart (weight: 50 kg; height: 116.5 cm) represents 249% of her ideal body weight for height. In contrast, in Figure 2 the growth chart of Michael with a pattern of constitutional overweight is shown. In this patient, body weight progression was constant throughout, being two major percentiles above that of height with an excess weight for height of 38% throughout his life span. These two types of growth patterns provide clear evidence of two distinct clinical patterns necessitating different approaches. In Julie's case, all efforts need to be made to stop the disproportionate body weight accretion; in Michael's case, caution must be exercised not to interfere with the balance and adjustment already achieved by the patient in maintaining body weight. In a survey of high school children, Moses et al. showed that constitutional patterns of overweight are encountered in about 25% of

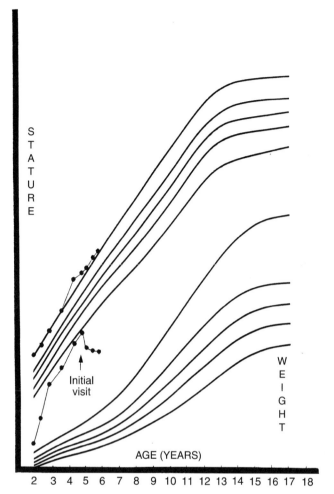

Figure 1 Growth pattern of a patient with severe obesity before and after treatment was initiated. Note that the patient was gaining excess weight for height that started after 3 months of age. Her BMI was 36.8 at the time of his first visit.

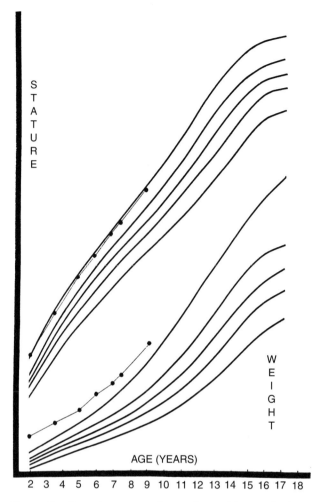

Figure 2 Growth pattern of a patient with constitutional overweight. Note that the patient's weight was in excess for height but remained proportional throughout his life. His BMI at 10 years old was 24.

the students with excess body weight for height, remaining proportional throughout their school years (62). The morbid obesity pattern of growth is rare, observed in 0.8% of students. Therefore, the clinical assessment of an obese child must include measurements of height and weight progression for the proper assessment and recommendations for treatment.

A. BMI

Body mass index (BMI) is a widely used method to define the relationship between weight and height (78). The BMI is calculated as weight (kg)/height(m^2) and provides a practical clinical tool for classification of individuals with normal and those with various degrees of obesity (grades I–III): grade I, BMI 25–29; grade II, BMI 30–40; and

grade III, >40 BMI. The BMI system of classification of obesity is important because it has been found that the risk for medical complications of obese patients increases at BMI levels above 25 (79). According to the National Center for Health Statistics' Health and Nutrition Examination Survey (80), individuals with a BMI above 27 have a markedly increased risk for hypertension, hypercholesterolemia, and diabetes mellitus. In contrast, when the BMI index is less than 25, there are no apparent physical effects of obesity on the individual, although there may be social problems and psychological concerns with body appearance. However, the use of BMI has limited applications in the assessment of overweight children since its calculation is based primarily on a stable height, which is not applicable to growing children. Also, the BMI can underestimate the percentage of lean body mass since it does not account for variations in musculature; this could lead to classification of normal children as being overweight.

Charts of BMI relative to age are used in many countries to determine childhood obesity. They are easy to use, nonintrusive, and have been validated against measures of body fat. Many countries, including the United States, use the 85th percentile for BMI to define children who are overweight and then above the 95th percentile for obesity in children. Furthermore, no differences in the relationship between BMI and age exist among boys and girls up to age 20 from the United States, United Kingdom, Japan, and Singapore (81).

The stage of maturity may cause additional errors when BMI is used to determine obesity in children and adolescents from different ethnic groups (82). In spite of these ethnic differences, BMI correlates (>0.8) with body fat as determined by both skinfold thickness measurements and by densitometry (83). This suggests that BMI is a reasonable criterion for determining obesity in children and adolescents.

There are several potential errors associated with BMI as an indicator of obesity in children. The increasing height in children from birth until adulthood may cause a difference in the weight-for-height relationship assumed in current BMI-for-age charts. Gender and age also affect body weight and height. Furthermore, puberty may introduce another change in the weight-for-height relationship. Ethnic origin and social class may also affect both body weight and height. However, in adults, these relations are simpler because adult height is assumed to be fixed. Therefore, body weight is adjusted for height only. Usually this adjustment takes the form of body weight/height^2. However, this is not always the best adjustment depending on the age of the child. One study found that the power used to adjust height (Benn index) changed from 2.0 to 3.5 over the first 20 years of life in order to maintain the best relationship with skinfold thickness. The strongest relationships with skin-fold thickness were obtained in children between 9 and 10 years old. Using only a Benn index of 2.0 may introduce subtle errors in BMI when used in younger children. Taller children will tend to have greater BMIs than shorter children. However, trying to define which Benn index to use at certain ages will lead to more errors than if just one standard Benn index is used, such as the current Benn index of 2.0 (84).

B. Key Indicators

In the United States, percentiles are the most commonly used method for clinical monitoring of individual growth. In 2000 the National Center for Health Statistics (NCHS) growth charts were revised. The revised growth charts will include growth curves for BMI and utilize newer mathematical methods for curve smoothing. New data from the third cycle of the National Health and Nutrition Examination Survey (NHANES III) showed increased prev-

alence of overweight in children. Currently being debated is whether it is appropriate to exclude the heavier NHANES III children in the revised growth reference data. For height and weight, percentiles increase monotonically with age. This should be preserved in any curve-smoothing process while still maintaining some variability. Methodologies for smoothing curves include cubic splines, kernel regression, locally weighted regression, and running medians. Locally weighted regression is currently being applied to the NCHS chart revisions. Revised NCHS growth charts for BMI may eliminate subtle errors in some of the percentiles currently used to define childhood obesity.

C. Skinfolds

Skinfold thickness from several separate sites, including both trunk and extremities, provide a reliable estimate of obesity and regional fat distribution. The correlation of multiple skinfold measurements with total body adiposity is in the range of 0.7–0.8. One problem with skinfold measurements is that the equations used must be changed for age, gender, and ethnic background. Body fat increases with age, even through the sum of the skinfolds remains constant. This means that the fat deposition with age occurs in large part at sites other than subcutaneous ones (85). Also, triceps skinfold (TSF), which is typically the site of measurement, is often difficult to grasp and measurement reliability can be poor. It has been observed that there is a strong correlation between BMI and TSF among age- and gender-matched groups, suggesting that these measures are interchangeable for use in classification of individuals and in the evaluation of secular trends of obesity and super obesity (86).

D. Body Fat

Several methods are available for the estimation of body fat content. These include methods that measure body density derived from its specific gravity, that is, the weight of body in and out of the water. This process makes it possible to fractionate the body into its fat and lean components, assuming a density for fat of 0.91 g/cm^2. The technique remains basically a research method; however, bioelectrical impedance analysis (BIA) has been commonly used as a noninvasive and inexpensive method for estimation of body fat and lean mass (87). Bioelectrical impedance relies on the association between conductivity and tissue fluid and electrolyte content. It has proved to be fairly reliable in assessing total body water, but is less reliable in the estimation of body fat, especially in obese children (88, 89). Other noninvasive methods, such as the use of ultrasound waves applied to the skin, can provide a measure of fat depth. In a group of children, Czinner et al. demonstrated a significant correlation (r = 0.969) between the body adiposity (skin fold thickness) measured with ultrasound and calipers (90). However the data derived from ultrasound method were 15–25% lower than fat obtained by calipers. The authors concluded that the ultrasound-derived body fat estimates represented only the subcutaneous body fat and not the whole body adiposity (i.e., visceral fat). On the other hand, other studies have shown that sonography is a reliable tool in measuring small variations in quantities of intra-abdominal (visceral) fat and is superior to waist to hip ratio (WHR) in evaluating regional fat distribution and visceral adiposity (91).

Dual energy x-ray absorptiometry (DEXA) has been used as a reliable method for estimating fat-free mass and body fat. It has a unique ability to provide precise measures of regional fat mass, lean mass, and bone mineral content (92, 93). The DEXA technique can also be utilized for the evaluation of fat distribution and its role in insulin resistance syndrome and cardiovascular risk factors (94). Computerized axial tomography (CT) scan and magnetic resonance imaging (MRI) can also be used to quantitate lean and fat tissue. They provide accurate anatomical details and can reliably measure total and regional body adiposity. Numerous studies have shown the feasibility of using CT scans to measure human adiposity (95). In a recent study, Ross et al. (96) demonstrated that MRI can provide a reliable measure of subcutaneous and visceral adipose tissue in obese subjects. A principal benefit of measuring adipose tissue by MRI or CT is the development of mathematical equations from external anthropometry that can predict MRI adipose tissue.

E. Total Body Electrical Conductivity

Validation for the use of total body electrical conductivity (TOBEC) for body composition measurements in infants has allowed accurate determinations of fat-free mass and fat mass without the assumptions associated with other methods. This method is appealing due to its ease of use, lack of radiation exposure, and the fact that little subject cooperation is required. The entire procedure takes only 5 min and does not require that infants or young children be sedated. This method involves passing an individual through a large solenoidal coil driven by a 2.5 MHz oscillating radiofrequency that generates a magnetic field. Upon passage through the instrument, all electrolytes, with fat-free mass containing the majority, contribute to disruption of the magnetic field. The instrument registers the magnitude of the magnetic field disruption and provides a value referred to as the TOBEC number. The TOBEC number depends on the conductivity, the length and cross-sectional area of the conductor, as well as electrical and coil parameters. The TOBEC number equals the instrument constants multiplied by the length and volume of the conductor. The square root of the TOBEC number (SQRT TOBEC # × length) has been found to be directly correlated with fat-free mass and fat mass in Hanford piglets (97).

F. Air Displacement Plethysmography

Until recently, there was no easy-to-use and accurate method to determine body composition in adults. The recent availability of the BodPod Body Composition System has allowed accurate determinations of body composition without the associated problems with hydrostatic weighting (98). The principle of the method is similar to hydrostatic weighting except that body volume is now obtained by air displacement. Subjects sit for 2 min in a 450 l chamber and a moving diaphragm determines the difference in air pressure between where the subject is sitting in the front chamber and a rear reference chamber. The pressure difference, along with the subject's body weight, are used to calculate body volume. From these results, body density is calculated and any of the standard equations for calculating fat-free mass and fat mass can be used. The procedure is entirely safe and requires no special cooperation on the part of the subject. In a validation study with 68 subjects, no differences were found in fat-free mass and percentage body fat when determined by both the BodPod Body Composition System and hydrostatic weighting (99). Furthermore, the BodPod Body Composition System can accommodate adults up to 160 kg (350 lb).

In children the BodPod Body Composition System may underestimate body fat. In one study body density was determined in 54 boys and girls from 10 to 18 years of age by both the BodPod Body Composition System and hydrostatic weighing. Body fat values calculated from both of these densities were compared to those determined by DEXA. Body fat calculated from both the Bodpod and DEXA were correlated; however, body fat estimates from the Bodpod were 2.9% lower than those derived from DEXA. This may be due to the significantly higher body density obtained from the Bodpod Body Composition System. These results suggest that body fat percentages in children derived from the Bodpod Body Composition System may not be as accurate (100).

G. Fat Distribution

In recent years, several studies have revealed major morphological and metabolic features that differentiate upper from lower body obesity (101–103). In adults, body fat distribution is more important than percentage body fat in predicting morbidity. Adults with a preponderance of abdominal fat ("android") have a higher frequency of hypertension, hyperinsulinernia, diabetes, and hyperlipidernia than equally obese individuals with predominantly pelvic ("gynecoid") fat distribution. The distribution of body fat is assessed using WHR. Increasing WHR in excess of 0.8 has been accompanied by abnormalities in glucose, insulin, and lipoprotein homeostasis (104, 105). Thus, the evaluation of body fat distribution is an essential element in the assessment of obesity. However, it has been observed that WHR cannot predict visceral adiposity in obese individuals (90, 93). On the other hand, using CT scan, MRI, or visceral-to-subcutaneous fat tissue ratio (VSR) has been shown to be a better index of regional fat distribution than WHR (106, 107). Furthermore, VSR correlates more closely with metabolic variables such as levels of serum lipids, insulin, and glucose than WHR. A WHR greater than 0.8 has been associated with hyperinsulinernia, insulin resistance, and future development of noninsulin-dependent diabetes mellitus (NIDDM) in adults. In Julie's case (Fig. 1), the WHR was 0.96 with significant upper body adiposity, whereas Michael's WHR was 0.76 with modest subcutaneous adiposity. The presence of upper body obesity in markedly obese children may be associated with development of acanthosis nigricans (brownish discoloration of skin) along the skin creases of posterior cervical, axillary, and other flexural areas.

V. WHO IS AT RISK?

A. Infants and Children

It has been shown that parental fatness is related to future obesity in their children. When both parents are overweight, about 80% of their children will be obese. When one parent is obese, this incidence decreases to 40%; and when both parents are lean, obesity prevalence drops to approximately 14% (107). However, the reasons for these associations are not clear since most of the studies fail to separate the genetic and environmental influences in a critical way.

The susceptibility to obesity may begin at birth as a consequence of metabolic variations in energy expenditure. Roberts et al. (108) demonstrated that excessive weight gain among a group of infants born to obese mothers was accompanied by reduced level of physical energy expenditure (108). This was probably the result of infants mimicking the activity patterns of their moderately inactive parents or siblings. Furthermore, Ravussin et al. observed decreased levels of energy expenditure in obese compared to nonobese families (109). These findings are similar to another study in which energy intake at 6 months predicted body fatness by 1 year of age (110). In contrast, several studies have found that energy intake in infants less than 3 months old is not a determinant of body fatness by 2–3 years of age (111, 112). Later studies have verified that parental fatness is related to the incidence of their children becoming obese.

Previous metabolic studies in infants cited above (109–112), which tried to identify alterations in metabolic rate that may contribute to future obesity, were inconclusive. Recent improvements in indirect calorimetry technology have enabled more accurate measurements of infant energy expenditure. The new Enhanced Metabolic Testing Activity Chamber (EMTAC) has been validated for accurate measurements of the components of energy

expenditure, such as resting and sleeping metabolic rates, along with physical activity, in infants from birth to 6 months old (113). Furthermore, during metabolic measurements in the EMTAC, parents have unrestricted access to their infants in a comfortable environment that is as close to normal as possible. This eliminates potential errors in energy expenditure due to stress caused by forced separation between parents and infants for long periods of time. With this new technology future metabolic studies in infants will be able to determine if changes in just one or more of the components of energy expenditure contribute to future childhood obesity.

Some of the physiological components of obesity found in adults may apply to infants from the time of birth. For example, a change in the utilization of nutrients as determined by the RQ (114), a lower than average body temperature (115), and sleeping body core temperature (116) may contribute to additional positive energy balance, thus leading to body weight gain in infants. A recent study using microneurographic recordings of sympathetic nervous system activity found that lower sympathetic nervous system activity occurs in obese adults (117). However, no current studies have addressed any of these potential causes of childhood obesity.

Weight gain and adiposity in infancy and early childhood are also influenced by several environmental factors (118). For instance, birth weight, duration of feeding, male gender, and age at the introduction of solid foods seem to affect significantly the rate of weight gain during the first year of life. Maternal weight only becomes a significant determinant for adiposity during the second year of life. The latter probably reflects the maternal environmental influences that may contribute significantly to the development of obesity since they determine child's energy intake and expenditure (119).

Vigorous feeding of infants and children may set the ground for the development of obesity (120, 121). Overweight children have been observed to eat more rapidly and chew their food less than those of normal weight (121). The influence of many environmental factors on the rate of weight gain, with or without a genetic susceptibility, has been evaluated by some investigators (122). Body adiposity and growth of newborns are influenced significantly by maternal weight and rate of weight gain during the prenatal period (123). It has long been observed that infants of diabetic mothers have increased body adiposity at birth and at 1 year of age (124). It has also been shown that macrosomic infants of mothers with gestational diabetes mellitus (GDM) have evidence of increasing body size and adiposity with increasing age and that maternal GDM and maternal prepregnant adiposity are significant predictors of their unique growth patterns (125).

In a subsequent study, differences of up to 500 calories per day in energy expended as a result of spontaneous physical activity (i.e., fidgeting) were observed among obese children compared to normal-weight children (126). Differences in basal metabolic rate (BMR) and physical activity were found in 3–5-year-old offspring of obese parents. Basal metabolic rate of children with at least one obese parent was 10% lower than that of children with lean parents (127). Children of lean parents had about twice the energy expenditure for physical activities of children with at least one obese parent, suggesting that children of obese parents are less physically active.

B. Teens

Obesity in teenagers is fast becoming a national concern. The latest results from NHANES III (1988–1994) found a high prevalence of adolescent obesity. Of 2850 children ages 12–18 years, 16% were overweight (85th percentile < BMI < 95th percentile), and 10% were obese (BMI > 95th percentile). However, a South Carolina Health Maintenance Organization (HMO) determined BMI in 30,445 children during the years 1995–1997 to determine the prevalence of childhood obesity in their members' population (128). The criteria for overweight and obesity were similar to those mentioned for NHANES III. In this subject sample 35 and 34% of the boys and girls, respectively, aged 12–17 years, were overweight. This means that 1:3 children in this HMO was above normal weight. Furthermore, 19% of the boys and 18% of the girls in this population were obese. The prevalence of obesity in this adolescent population was greater than that obtained from NHANES III (128). These surveys suggest that more programs specific for treating obesity in teenagers may be necessary.

VI. GENETICS

It has long been known that obesity runs in families. Obese parents impose even a greater risk that their children will be overweight. There is a 75% chance that children aged 3–10 will be overweight if both parents were obese. This drops to a 25–50% chance with just one obese parent. These statistics suggest that behavior modification or treatment intervention at an early age may be important for preventing future adolescent and adulthood obesity (11).

A. Twin Studies

The role of genetic factors in obesity was evaluated by Stunkard et al., who demonstrated no relationship between the body fat indices of adoptive parents and their adoptive children (129). They showed that BMI of biological parents was more closely correlated with the weight status of their offspring although they did not live together. The importance of the genetic component was also confirmed by a more recent study involving monozygotic twins (130). The BMIs of identical twins reared apart compared with those reared together were essentially the same. Also,

the use of skinfolds as genetic markers in twins has been reported (131). With the use of correlation coefficients to estimate the heritability of skinfold thickness, it has been shown that there was a significant environmental component among children less than 10 years, whereas heritability estimated in twins more than 10 years of age was very high. In a recent study involving Swedish adult twins, Heitmann et al. (132) recently suggested that although food choices seemed to play a role in the frequency of consumption of various foods, genetics also influenced the preference for several foods. However, there was no evidence that the consumption frequency of any of the foods was differentially associated with expression of genes responsible for weight gain.

B. Leptin

A major advance in understanding the pathogenesis of obesity is the discovery of the hormone leptin. It is produced by adipose tissue and has been found to modify feeding behavior in rodents by suppressing food intake and stimulating energy expenditure (133, 134). Leptin exerts its actions centrally on appetite and thermogenic control centers located in the hypothalamus. It is believed that obesity in humans is due to a desensitization of leptin reception within the hypothalamus, resulting in hyperphagia (133–135). Obese individuals have marked elevation of their plasma levels of leptin directly proportional to body fat mass (136). Sustained elevated levels of plasma leptin are proposed to uncouple leptin actions on its receptors in the hypothalamus, thereby attenuating signal transduction pathways that exert the effects of the hormone on satiety and energy expenditure (133, 137). Furthermore, leptin acts directly on receptors in pancreatic beta-cells to suppress insulin secretion in rodents (138–140). Thus, some have proposed the existence of an adipoinsular axis in which insulin stimulates adipogenesis and leptin production, and leptin inhibits insulin secretion through its effect on beta-cell ATP-sensitive potassium channels (141). Seufert et al. recently proposed that in obese individuals leptin reception by beta cells is desensitized, similar to what is proposed to occur at the level of the hypothalamus (142). This desensitization of suppression of insulin secretion of beta cells contributes to the hyperinsulinemia of obesity. Hyperinsulinemia, in turn, leads to increased adipogenesis and insulin resistance, culminating in some individuals in the development of diabetes.

The recent discovery of the obese (*Lep*) gene (143) has provided new insights into the regulation of energy metabolism in the body (Fig. 3). The *Lep* gene is specifically expressed in adipocytes (143, 144) and encodes a 167 amino-acid-secreted protein called leptin. The physiological importance of quantitative changes in leptin concentration indicates that regulation of the *Lep* gene is a critical control point (145–147). Leptin receptors have been found in several hypothalamic nuclei, including the

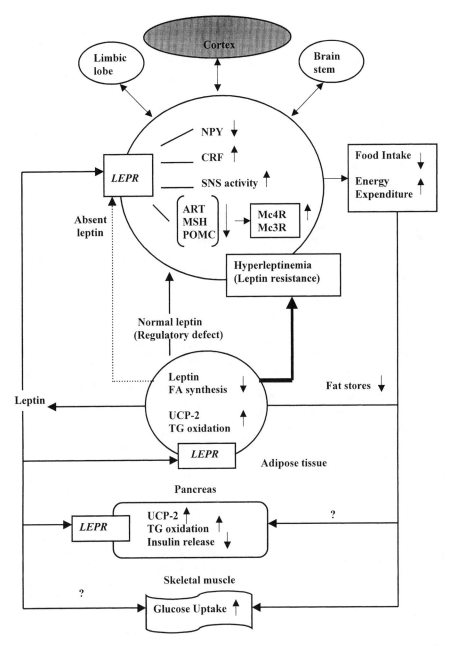

Figure 3 Schematic of the current view of the roles of leptin in energy homeostatsis.

arcuate nucleus, ventromedial, lateral, dorsomedial, and paraventricular hypothalamic nuclei (148). These hypothalamic nuclei express one or more neuropeptides and neurotransmitters that regulate food intake and/or body weight. Genetic data indicate that neuropeptide Y (NPY) and one or more of its receptors act in response to absent (and possibly low) leptin, whereas melanocyte-stimulating hormone (MSH), its receptor, the melanocortin-4 receptor, and possibly the agouti-related transcript (ART) are re-

quired for the response to an increased plasma leptin concentration (149). Neuropeptide Y is the most potent orexigenic agent known when administered intrathecally. Neuropeptide Y mRNA is increased in *ob/ob* mice and decreases after leptin treatment (150). Leptin also increases corticotropin-releasing hormone (CRH) gene expression and synthesis (151), which, in turn, inhibits food intake and increases energy expenditure (152). Conversely, food intake has effects on both the plasma leptin concentration and *Lep* gene expression. Fasting decreases and refeeding increases *Lep* gene expression (153, 154) and the plasma leptin concentration (155).

It is believed that decreased leptin expression per adipocyte could lead to obesity with normal (but inappropriately low) plasma leptin concentrations. This hypothesis is supported by the observation that *ob/ob* mice carrying a poorly expressed leptin transgene are obese, despite having relatively normal leptin levels (147). Similarly, 5–10% of obese human subjects have relatively low levels of leptin, indicative of a reduced rate of leptin production in this subgroup (156). Low leptin levels also predispose preobese Pima Indians to weight gain (157). In almost all cases, obese subjects express at least some leptin, indicating that human *Lep* gene mutations are likely to be rare. Except for a few reported cases of *Lep* mutations in massively obese subjects (158, 159), researchers have not been able to demonstrate *Lep* mutations in most obese subjects (160). Although the *Lep* gene has been linked to severe obesity in some family studies, mutations in the leptin-coding sequence were not identified (161, 162). The molecular basis for this association is unknown but could be related to differences in the amount of expression of leptin mRNA. Loci on human chromosome 2 may be linked to leptin levels and, to a lesser extent, to BMI (163). These loci are near the gene for human proopiomelanocortin (POMC), which is a precursor of MSH. It has been shown that abnormal melanocortin signaling in yellow agouti (A^y) or melanocortin-4-knockout mice leads to obesity and leptin resistance (164). A subset of neurons expresses both *Lep* receptor and POMC, and leptin modulates POMC gene expression (165). Krude et al. (166) recently described two red-haired subjects with severe obesity and adrenal insufficiency. It has also been shown that agonists of beta MSH and MSH decrease food intake and pretreatment of animals with a beta-MSH antagonist blunts the anorectic effect of injected leptin (167). Therefore, association of mutations in leptin and its receptor with massive obesity confirms its importance in regulating human body weight (168). However, these syndromes are rare.

Changes in *Lep* gene expression have been shown to be associated with parallel changes in plasma insulin concentration (169). Since insulin itself has a stimulatory effect on *Lep* gene expression and leptin secretion (170), it is likely that feeding-induced changes in leptin concentrations are dependent on insulin. Furthermore, insulinemia has been shown to regulate plasma leptin and to be a determinant of its plasma concentration in normal-weight and obese human subjects (171). In fact, plasma leptin level in obese children and adults correlates not only with the degree of insulinemia but also with percentage of body fat (171), suggesting that human obesity is generally associated with an insensitivity to leptin. However, investigators have recently reported that inadequate insulin-induced leptin production in obese insulin-resistant subjects may contribute to the development of obesity (172).

Lahlou et al. recently suggested that increased circulating leptin concentrations during the dynamic phase of childhood obesity are indicative of leptin resistance (173). They observed that leptin did not act as an appetite regulator in the obese children without a significant impact on basal energy expenditure. These investigators also showed that obese girls had higher leptin levels than boys. A comparable gender-related difference was found in non-obese children. This sexual dimorphism of circulating leptin levels could reflect a physiological role in the regulation of reproduction in humans. In mice, while the *ob/ob* males are normally fertile, administration of leptin to infertile female *ob/ob* mice is needed to restore fertility (174). It is therefore possible that leptin plays a role in the female gonadostat as a signaling hormone reflecting the amount of fat stores at the hypothalamic–pituitary level or directly at the ovarian level (175). It is likely that quantitative and possible functional changes in adipose tissue of girls entering puberty may physiologically increase leptin to levels that allow the hypothalamic–pituitary–gonadal axis to complete sexual maturation and prepare for pregnancy. The sexual dimorphism for circulating leptin levels observed in lean girls and boys is consistent with these metabolic considerations. Thus, the lack of premature puberty despite hyperleptinemia in massively obese girls could be taken as an additional index of central leptin resistance.

Finally, leptin increases energy expenditure by direct effects on CNS and the peripheral tissues. Leptin infusion into the CNS increases sympathetic activity to brown adipose tissue, kidney, and adrenal gland (176). However, it is not yet known whether blockage of beta-adrenergic receptors attenuates leptin-induced weight loss. Thus the role of the sympathetic nervous system in mediating the weight-reducing effect of leptin is not yet established. Leptin also prevents reduced energy expenditure normally associated with decreased food intake (145). Administration of leptin also decreases blood glucose and insulin concentrations in *ob/ob* mice (177). Leptin induces depletion of triglyceride in adipose tissue and pancreas by increasing intracellular fatty acid oxidation and gene expression of the enzymes involved in fatty acid oxidation (178, 179). Leptin also increases the expression of uncoupling protein-2 (UCP-2) in adipose tissue and pancreas (179). Uncoupling proteins disrupt the mitochondrial proton gradient in brown fat (and possibly other tissues), resulting in the generation of heat rather than ATP. However, it has been suggested that leptin treatment does not cause a net increase in 24 h energy expenditure but instead blunts the decreased energy expenditure that generally accompanies food restriction (145). It is thus uncertain whether leptin increases energy expenditure or activates uncoupling protein. In summary, a complex physiological system has evolved to regulate fuel stores and energy balance at an optimum level. Leptin and its receptors are integral components of this system. Although the entire pathogenesis of human obesity is unknown, it is assumed to be, in part, the result of differences in leptin secretion and/or leptin sensitivity and its interaction with underlying genetic and environmental factors.

C. Ghrelin

Ghrelin is an acylated peptide hormone recently purified from rat stomach. The hormone consists of 28 amino acids in which the serine-3 residue is n-octanolylated. It is primarily synthesized in the stomach but its principal site of action is growth hormone secretagogue receptors located on hypothalamic neurons and in the brainstem. Only two amino acids are not conserved between rat and human ghrelin. The main function of ghrelin is the regulation of pituitary growth hormone secretion independent of growth-hormone-releasing hormone and somatostatin. It has been suggested that ghrelin is an endocrine link between the stomach, hypothalamus, and pituitary. This may be important for the regulation of energy balance (180–182).

There may be different effects between rodents and humans in regard to the action of ghrelin. For example, peripheral daily administration of ghrelin to both rats and mice caused body weight gain by reducing fat utilization. Furthermore, intracerebroventricular administration of ghrelin in increasing amounts generated a dose-dependent increase in food intake and body weight gain. Through the measurement of 24 h energy expenditure in a rodent calorimeter, ghrelin was found to exhibit its effect by increasing carbohydrate and reducing fat utilization without any changes in food intake. This was determined from the RQ derived from the ratio of carbon dioxide production and oxygen consumption. This change in nutrient utilization resulted in an increased amount of body fat without any corresponding changes in fat-free mass or bone mineral content. Furthermore, no changes occurred in energy expenditure or physical activity (182). It was theorized that the concentration of serum ghrelin will be increased in obese humans. Furthermore, predominantly obese ethnic groups, such as the Pima Indians of Southern Arizona, would have the greatest plasma concentrations of ghrelin. In one study, 15 lean and obese white subjects and 15 lean and obese Pima Indian adults had plasma ghrelin, insulin, and leptin determined. In contrast to the hypothesis, both obese groups had significantly lower plasma ghrelin concentrations than the respective lean groups. Furthermore, plasma insulin and leptin concentrations were increased. Moreover, plasma ghrelin concentrations were negatively correlated with body weight, percentage body fat, as well as plasma leptin and insulin. These data suggest that plasma ghrelin is downregulated in obesity. This may result from increased concentrations of both leptin and insulin. These investigators further suggest that reduced plasma ghrelin concentrations may represent adaptation to a positive energy balance associated with obesity (183).

D. Adipose Tissue Endocrine Functions

Adipose tissue is comprised of lipid-filled cells surrounded by a matrix of collagen fibers, vessels, fibroblasts, and immune cells. Its main function is the storage of triglycerides for times of energy deprivation. However, adipose tissue may be involved in other aspects of metabolism that may affect the onset of obesity. Adipose tissue metabolizes sex steroids and glucocorticoids. For example, 17 beta-hydroxysteroid oxidoreductase converts androstenedione to testosterone and estrone to estradiol. This may be important for fat distribution. Estrogens stimulate fat accumulation in the breast and subcutaneous tissue, while androgens promote central obesity. Alteration of these interconversions may predispose individuals to reproductive disorders and certain cancers (184, 185).

Adipose tissue also produces and secretes certain inflammatory cytokines, for example tumor necrosis factor alpha (TNF-alpha) and interleukin-6 (IL-6). It has been suggested that both of these cytokines prevent obesity through inhibition of lipogenesis, increased lipolysis, and promotion of adipocyte death via apotosis. However, TNF-alpha has been found to be a mediator of insulin resistance in obesity (186, 187). C-reactive protein, stimulated by elevated IL-6, has been found to be correlated with obesity, insulin resistance, elevated THF-alpha, and endothelial dysfunction (188).

Alteration of coagulation and complement factors may contribute to the obesity associated cardiovascular disease. Fibrinogen and plasma activator inhibitor type-1 (PAI-1) are altered in obesity and may be involved in cardiovascular disease. For example, high levels of PAI-1 have been detected after myocardial infarction. Much of the PAI-1 is synthesized by adipose tissue and is increased in proportion to visceral adiposity. This may serve as a link between abdominal/central obesity and cardiovascular disease (189).

E. Adiponectin

Plasma concentrations of adiponectin, a novel adipose-specific protein with putative antiathrogenic and anti-inflammatory effects, were recently found to be decreased in Japanese individuals with obesity, type 2 diabetes, and cardiovascular diseases conditions commonly associated with insulin resistance and hyperinsulinemia (190). It has also been shown that the degree of hypoadiponectinemia is more closely related to the degree of insulin resistance and hyperinsulinemia than the degree of adiposity and glucose intolerance.

F. Mutations

In monogenetic or dysmorphic forms of obesity, transmitted by both recessive and dominant modes of inheritance, there are also alterations in energy balance that result in obesity. Patients with Prader-Willi syndrome are characterized by hyperphagia, hypotonia, developmental delay, hypogonadism, and short stature (191). In these children, obesity may start during the first year of life and becomes prominent by the second year, which in the presence of hyperphagia can result in morbid obesity. It was previously suggested that a low metabolic rate caused the obesity in these children (192). However, it has been demonstrated that a lower energy requirement of these children is due to less fat-free mass and not to an unusually low metabolic rate (193).

Translocation or deletion of chromosome 15 has been reported in about 50% of these patients (194). In contrast, Lawrence-Moon-Biedl syndrome is another dysmorphic form of obesity characterized by retinitis pigmentosa, hypogonadism, mental retardation, and polydactyly. It is inherited by an autosomal recessive gene (195). It is believed that excessive weight gain in these children is caused by disturbance of hypothalamic appetite center(s), which leads to increased food intake. Pseudohypoparathyroidism is also associated with obesity and short stature and is characterized by short fourth metacarpal, short thick neck, rounded facies, mental retardation, and hypocalcemia (196). It is commonly inherited as a sex-linked dominant trait and may be accompanied by hypothyroidism and gonadal failure. Other genetic syndromes that include obesity are Alstrom's, Carpenters, and Cohen's. The mechanisms of excess weight in these patients have not been elucidated as yet.

VII. ENERGY BALANCE

Obesity is a heterogenous group of disorders that can result from an energy imbalance over an extended period of time in which energy intake exceeds expenditure. It is superficially apparent that obese subjects ingest more food relative to their needs. However, caloric intakes have been reported to be comparable among overweight and normal weight adults (197), suggesting that obese subjects have "increased metabolic efficiency."

It has been shown that low total and resting energy expenditure are risk factors for long-term weight gain in infants (198) and adults (199), respectively. However, Dwyer et al. (200) showed that obese children might not eat more than their normal-weight peers and they may expend relatively fewer calories to maintain their body weight. This phenomenon has been referred as adaptation and results after frequent dieting efforts have taken place. This results in lower energy requirements due to loss of lean body mass (201). Repeated weight reduction attempts result in alterations in body composition and decreased fat-free mass. This leads to decreased metabolic demands and thus fewer calories needed to maintain weight (202).

Reduced meal frequency, or gorging (i.e., one to two meals daily), has been associated with an increased risk of obesity (203, 204). This is also associated with high fasting serum lipid and insulin levels. Insulin stimulates hepatic synthesis of cholesterol and tissue lipogenesis (205, 206). Increasing meal frequency, or nibbling has been shown to significantly lower serum cholesterol and insulin levels (207). This is thought to have a beneficial effect in decreasing triglyceride synthesis in adipose tissue through a reduction in postprandial glucose and insulin levels. However, this effect may be significantly minimized by a parallel reduction in the postprandial thermogenesis stimulated by insulin and glucose (208).

The main determinant of BMR is fat-free mass (FFM) and the main determinant of energy expenditure is physical activity. It is believed that minor alterations in any of these could result in positive energy balance and lead to obesity over prolonged periods of time. For example, obligatory energy expenditure, reflected by a decreased resting metabolic rate, could be the consequence of an increased metabolic efficiency in obese persons. On the other hand, a reduced level of activity could also lead to an increased energy balance and weight gain. The resting energy expenditure and the baseline activity levels are thought to be genetically determined. In fact, studies among obese Pima Indians have demonstrated low BMR values and, therefore, enhanced metabolic efficiency of energy consumption among some families with obesity (209, 210). However, other studies demonstrated that BMR values, corrected for FFM, among obese subjects were relatively higher than those in nonobese subjects (211), suggesting that attainment of energy balance and weight maintenance in obese individuals requires a larger energy intake than in nonobese individuals.

VIII. PHYSICAL ACTIVITY

It is not clear whether inactivity is a cause or consequence of obesity. However, it is believed that a sedentary lifestyle increases the risk for obesity. Furthermore, low cardiorespiratory fitness is an independent predictor of cardiovascular heart disease in obese adult men. This is comparable to diabetes mellitus, high blood pressure, and smoking (212). Physical activity in children has declined over recent decades implying an increasingly sedentary lifestyle in Western industrialized countries. Reports have indicated that physical activity declines almost 50% during adolescence, with girls becoming increasingly more sedentary than boys (213). A recent observation is that this pattern is due to a gender dimorphism in the developmental changes in energy expenditure before adolescence, independent of body composition, with a conservation of energy use in girls achieved through an appreciable reduction in physical activity (214). Social and environmental influences are also believed to have major roles in the gender and developmental variation in physical activity (215).

The role of physical energy expenditure in the development of obesity is not very clear. Obese individuals have often been described as sluggish or lazy. A study of children and adolescents by Bullen et al. (216) indicated that obese youngsters were less active than their peers. However, an earlier study, which measured caloric expenditure by measuring oxygen consumption, found that obese individuals actually expended more calories through activity than did normal-weight individuals (217). Maffeis et al. (218) recently demonstrated that walking and running are energetically more expensive for obese children than for nonobese children.

The estimates of energy requirements for children were derived in a time when more physical exertion was needed for daily living; therefore, energy requirements for children may be overestimated for today's sedentary lifestyle. Prentice et al. (219) measured energy expenditure in children aged 0–3 years by the doubly labeled water method and found that energy needs were overestimated by 15% as originally recommended by the World Health Organization (WHO) (220). Goran et al. (221) likewise showed that energy requirements were 25% overestimated for 4–6-year-old children. Fontvieille et al. (222) found that energy requirements for 5–6-year-old children were overestimated by 24% in comparison to that calculated according to the WHO. The sedentary lifestyles of today's children may easily account for consistent overestimates of childhood energy requirements. Indeed, children living a sedentary lifestyle with unlimited access to food are prone to consuming more energy than they expend, and therefore are at increased risk of obesity.

Child obesity experts have suggested that the relationship between television and obesity may be the consequence of enhanced food consumption during viewing. This may be due to the influence of food advertisements (223, 224). Experimental studies have demonstrated that a causal relationship exists between specific televised messages and children's eating behavior (225) and between television viewing and participation in sports (226). Earlier studies among children and adolescents found an association between hours of television viewing and the development of obesity (227). Indeed, this association was further supported by a recent observation that the levels of physical activity and hours of television viewing tend to have a strong relationship with body weight and degree of obesity among children (228). It is also possible that the way a child watches television and the content of the television programs may be more important than the number of viewing hours. However, it has been recently shown that television viewing has a fairly profound lowering effect on metabolic rate in both lean and obese individuals. This may be an important factor in susceptible children who are at risk for weight gain and potentially lead to obesity (224).

IX. HYPERINSULINISM

Syndrome X is a clinical quartet of hyperinsulinemia, hyperlipidemia, hypertension, and subsequent cardiovascular disease (30). It is believed that obesity is a component of this metabolic syndrome and has been described in obese children (31) and adolescents (32). In a more recent study Chen et al. suggested that syndrome X is characterized by the linking of a metabolic entity (hyperinsulinemia/insulin resistance, hyperlipidemia, and obesity) to a hemodynamic factor (hypertension) through a shared correlation with hyperinsulinemia/insulin resistance. Clustering features of syndrome X are independent of gender and age in both black and white populations (33).

Hyperinsulinism and insulin resistance are characteristic features of obesity (229). It has been demonstrated that insulin secretion increases as the severity of obesity increases (210), and this increase in insulin secretion is accompanied by varying degrees of resistance to insulin-mediated glucose uptake (230). Indeed, the observed abnormalities in glucose tolerance in some obese adolescents are consistent with the presence of hyperinsulinemia and insulin resistance. Occasionally, young patients with a strong positive family history of type 2 diabetes develop the disease. Also, insulin resistance may result in the development of acanthosis nigricans, a hyperpigmentation of skin, which is commonly seen in the back of the neck, axillae, and other flexural areas (71). Hyperinsulinemia is usually accompanied by hyperandrogenism, which leads to hirsutism.

The presence of hyperinsulinemia favors the maintenance of the obese state by stimulating lipogenesis via activation of lipoprotein lipase and by inhibiting lipolysis. The hyperinsulinemia and insulin resistance are believed to cause preferential shunting of substrates to adipose tissue, with conversion of periadipocytes to adipocytes; this is associated with hyperplasia and hypertrophy of fat cells, inducing an unabated lipogenic state and obesity (231). It has also been shown that the lipogenic action of insulin occurs at a lower insulin concentration than its glycoregulatory action (232). Additionally, Le Stunff et al. (233) demonstrated that hyperinsulinemic obese children oxidized more fat and less glucose than their lean counterparts. This impairment of glucose metabolism may, in part, by caused by an excessive utilization of fatty substrate (234). This finding supports the concept of decreased glucose utilization and its shunting to fatty acid and triglycerides synthesis.

The hyperinsulinemia of obesity is apparently due to a combination of increased pancreatic secretion and a reduction of in heptatic extraction (235). The extent of the changes in insulin level is correlated with increasing fat cell size and degree of obesity and is more prominent in individuals with central obesity (235, 236). The mechanisms for the enhanced insulin secretion are not well understood, but one explanation is that it is an adaptive response to the diminished insulin-binding sites (237). However, dysregulation of beta-cell function has been described in obese children in the absence of insulin resistance (233). Odeleye et al. (238) found high fasting insulin levels in lean prepubertal Pima Indian children are predicative of the development of adolescent obesity (238).

The observed metabolic alterations in the insulin-resistant state are predominant with regard to glucose metabolism, especially with respect to cellular glucose uptake and hepatic glucose production, whereas effects on amino acid metabolism and fat metabolism are less significant. These metabolic changes lead to blood glucose elevation (239) and enhanced fatty acid storage in adipose tissue. Kida et al. (240) demonstrated diminished insulin receptor binding in monocytes of obese children that inversely correlated with their degree of obesity. Both receptor and postreceptor binding defects appear to play a role in insulin resistance of obesity. However, it is not clear whether hyperinsulinemia-induced downregulation of insulin receptors and/or decreased receptor-induced hyperinsulinernia are the mechanisms for the observed alterations. These abnormalities correct towards normal range with weight loss.

Other investigators have evaluated the rate of body fat distribution and altered fatty acid metabolism in insulin resistance and hyperinsulinemia of obesity. For instance, obese subjects with an abdominal fat distribution have reduced hepatic insulin binding (241, 242). A possible cellular mechanism may be the result of high physiological free fatty acid (FFA) concentrations. It has been suggested that the inhibitory effect of FFA is energy dependent and does not change the total cellular number of insulin receptors or their binding characteristics, indicating that the receptor internalization or recycling is influenced (243). Svedberg et al. (244) demonstrated that obesity with high ambient FFA levels influences internalization/recycling of hepatic insulin receptors, leading to reduced cell surface binding (244). An increased supply of FFAs to muscle has been suggested to restrain glucose transport and disposal through the inhibitory action of the products of FFA oxidation (citrate, acetyl-CoA, adenosine 5-triphospate, etc.). This is due to the FFA oxidation products' influence on key enzymes of glucose metabolism (pyruvate dehydrogenase, phosphofructokinase, and hexokinase) (234). The observed substrate competition is suggested to impede insulin action on glucose metabolism through derangement in lipid metabolism (245, 246). In children, progressive augmentation of fat stores and lipid oxidation during the first years of obesity could therefore induce a progressive reduction in glucose oxidation and decreased insulin action (233). This suggests that the increase in lipid oxidation precedes the changes in glucose oxidation and insulin levels associated with long-duration obesity.

Finally, elevated circulating levels of insulin due to insulin-producing tumor (insulinoma) or to excessive administration of insulin to an insulin-dependent diabetic patient can lead to obesity. These patients develop obesity, short stature, and hepatomegaly (Mauriac syndrome) (247).

X. HORMONAL ALTERATIONS

A. Adrenals

Adrenal glucocorticoid production is enhanced in obese children (248). Obese children tend to maintain normal serum cortisol levels due to its increased urinary clearance and in direct proportion to an increase in lean body mass. Increased clearance of cortisol has a stimulatory effect on pituitary adrenocorticotrophic hormone (ACTH) release. Adrenocorticotrophic hormone stimulates increased production of adrenal sex steroids such as dehydroepiandrosterone and testosterone. Increased production of adrenal sex steroids leads to early adrenarche (pubarche) in obese children (248).

The release of cortisol is maintained under a normal circadian rhythm. Furthermore, it is believed that elevated plasma cortisol in some obese individuals is related to the hyperinsulinernia of obesity and contributes to the characteristic body fat distribution and altered body composition (249). In obese children, serum levels of epinephrine and norepinephrine remain normal. Adrenal hypercorticolism has long been recognized in the differential diagnosis of pediatric obesity. Although some patients have a fat distribution suggestive of Cushing syndrome, the use of corticosteroid therapy for a variety of inflammatory and allergic conditions is also associated with the development of obesity. In this type of obesity the problem is transient and resolves once use of the drug is stopped. Cushing syndrome is a rare cause of obesity and these patients can be differentiated from those with exogenous obesity by the cessation of growth that accompanies excess cortisol.

B. Growth

Obese children are commonly tall for their age. This is associated with advanced skeletal maturity and early onset of puberty as well as premature pubarche (248). The lean body mass is often increased in these children (250). Reduced serum concentrations of growth hormone (GH) are characteristically seen in obese individuals and have been attributed to diminished GH secretion as well as accelerated GH clearance (251). The concentrations of insulin-like growth factor (IGF)-1 tend to vary because, unlike insulin, it circulates bound to specific proteins such as IGF-binding proteins (IGFBPs) with variable affinities (252–254). Six IGFBPs have been structurally identified, but only IGFBP-1, -2, and -3 have been well characterized in humans (251). In contrast to the lack of diurnal variation of IGFBP-2 and IGFBP-3, circulating levels of IGFBP-1 vary widely throughout the day in an inverse relationship with changes in plasma insulin (255, 256). Acute and chronic elevations in plasma insulin lower IGFBP-1 by suppressing its production by the liver, which, in turn, increases the bioavailability of free IGF-1 (257, 258). The blunted growth hormone response in obese subjects could be secondary to negative feedback inhibition by IGF-1 (259). However, other investigators have suggested that IGF-1 levels are maintained or even enhanced by the hyperinsulinemia of obesity (260). The metabolic syndrome induced by increased adiposity appears to have profound effects on the complex interplay among GH, IGF-1, and IGFBPs during puberty. However, the effect is an increase in the ratio of free to total IGF-1 in obese subjects, which may help to explain the lack of alteration of the pubertal growth spurt in obese adolescents even in the presence of lower GH levels. On the other hand, GH deficiency or pituitary dwarfism is reported to result in a mild degree of obesity compared to other causes of weight gain. It is believed that weight gain in a growth-deficient child is caused by diminished energy expenditure. Indeed, it has been observed that GH stimulates the growth of muscle tissue and breakdown of fat tissue, therefore affecting body composition (261).

There is a potential for reduced growth performance during obesity treatment. This may be due to the inherent reduction in nutrient intake associated with various obesity treatment programs. For example, a reduction in height velocity was found in children undergoing an energy-restrictive 6 month obesity treatment protocol. However, children undergoing a 12 month, less energy restrictive obesity treatment showed no reductions in height velocity. Furthermore, both groups had similar heights from baseline until 12 months, suggesting that the children undergoing the more restrictive 6 month protocol showed catch-up growth following treatment (262). The situation was not similar in regard to increases in fat-free mass. The more restrictive group had smaller increases in fat-free mass after 12 months than the 12 month treatment groups (263). A recent review of 10 year follow-up data in children found no significant changes in final height in regard to the amount of energy restriction during obesity treatment. Furthermore, multiple regression analysis found that childhood percentage of overweight did not contribute to predicting height change. However, a reduction in the percentile for height did occur in children from baseline to 10 years after treatment. The mean height of the children was over the 70th percentile for height prior to, and it decreased to just over the 50th percentile 10 years after, obesity treatment. These studies suggest that children participating in comprehensive obesity treatment programs, which include energy restriction, may attain an appropriate adult height and this will be similar to their parents (263). Children who diet without appropriate supervision do have growth failure (61).

C. Prolactin

Basal prolactin levels are normal or slightly elevated in obese children. However, the prolactin response to provocative stimuli is often diminished (264). Donders et al. suggested that decreased serotonin in the brain was a potential mechanism for the blunted prolactin response. Oth-

ers have hypothesized that this may be due to a hypothalamic defect that contributes to the abnormal prolactin response and aberrant appetite regulation, especially when prolactin response does not return to normal with weight loss in the same obese patients.

D. Thyroid

No evidence links thyroid dysfunction to exogenous obesity. Serum levels of thyroxine, free thyroxine, and thyroid-stimulating hormone (TSH) are normal in obese individuals. Hypothyroidism is not a common cause of obesity. Excessive weight gain, secondary to an underactive thyroid gland, is due to a combination of decreased metabolic rate and enhanced fluid retention (265). In children, hypothyroidism is associated with poor linear growth. Therefore, a normally growing but overweight child is not likely to be hypothyroid.

E. Reproductive Hormones

Puberty may begin early in tall overweight children with advanced skeletal age. Kaplowitz et al. recently demonstrated that obesity is an important contributing factor to the earlier onset of puberty in girls (266). Pubertal elevations of follicular-stimulating hormone (FSH) have been observed in the 7–9-year-old girls, without any changes in luteinizing hormone (LH) levels (266). This is usually complicated by an adiposity-related decrease in circulating concentrations of sex hormone-binding globulin (SHBG). This results in a higher fraction of free or unbound serum sex steroids that are more bioactive than the ones in lean subjects (266). In general, the SHBG abnormalities correlate with the degree of obesity, which are reversed with weight loss (266). Low serum estradiol levels and elevated progesterone levels have been observed in young prepubertal and early pubertal obese girls compared to age-matched lean girls (266).

The emergence of hyperandrogenism in pubertal girls may be associated with rapid weight gain, signs of hirsutism or virilism, and irregular menstrual periods (47). This is usually accompanied by hyperinsulinemia and insulin resistance with or without glucose intolerance. There is strong evidence that insulin exerts a regulatory effect on ovarian androgen synthesis (48). In fact, a positive correlation between the degrees of hyperinsulinemia and hyperandrogenism can be found in obese women (49).

Since insulin is believed to effect its regulatory action through LH on ovarian function, some obese patients may also present with polycystic ovaries and abnormally elevated serum LH, low follicle-stimulating hormone (FSH), and high free testosterone levels.

Obese adolescent boys appear to have an attenuated testicular response to human chorionic gonadotropin (HCG). This is probably an artifact of decreased/ro SHBG. Indeed, Glass et al. (235) demonstrated that despite a decrease in SHBG levels and increased percentage free testosterone, the free testosterone levels were normal. Serum dihydrotestosterone levels remain normal in obese subjects. Aromatization of androgens to estrogens by adipose tissue, in males, appears to be enhanced without any evidence of clinical feminization (235). However, free and total testosterone levels may be diminished in morbidly obese males. This is commonly associated with decreased gonadotropin levels, suggesting some degree of hypogonadotropic hypogonadism (158). These alterations in pituitary and gonadal hormones return to normal range with weight loss (159).

Precocious puberty may lead to obesity. Children with precocious puberty prior to treatment show no differences in regard to lean or fat mass. However, during treatment with gonadotropin-releasing hormone (GnRH) over for several years, these children end up with a reduction of lean mass and increased fat mass. This may be due to a shortening of the prepubertal growing period and by the so-called menopausal effect of the treatment. After treatment these children end up with a greater amount of fat mass, which may lead to obesity (267, 268). In another study both boys and girls with precocious puberty had BMI scores above the 85th percentile prior to and during treatment with GnRH. After treatment the scores still remained above the 85th percentile, indicating obesity. These results suggest that children with precocious puberty are prone to obesity. Furthermore, treatment of precocious puberty with GnRH does not itself contribute to obesity.

XI. HYPOTHALAMUS

Lesions of the ventromedial area of the hypothalamus (VMH) may result form inflammatory processes such as encephalitis, arachnoiditis, tuberculosis, or trauma, or malignancy (Fröhlich syndrome) (269, 270). Children with hypothalamic obesity may present with a history of foraging and stealing foods. They have a voracious appetite and may display frequent tantrums if food is denied. In children, craniopharyngioma is the most common CNS tumor that leads to hypothalamic and pituitary dysfunction (271). Hypothalamic obesity is often coupled with other hypothalamic–pituitary disturbances, which may exacerbate the obesity (e.g., growth hormone deficiency or hypothyroidism), but the obesity resists treatment with hormonal replacement (272, 273). It is believed that hypothalamic injury leads to alterations in the appetite center, which can cause hyperphagia and obesity (274). However, there is increasing evidence that the hyperinsulinemia seen in this disorder plays a role in the development of obesity. An animal model of VMH damage results in hyperphagia, obesity, hyperinsulinemia, and insulin resistance (275, 276). It is believed that VMH damage causes a disinhibition of vagal tone (277) at the pancreatic beta cell, which leads to insulin hypersecretion and resultant obesity (278). Lustig et al. (279) recently dem-

onstrated that children with hypothalamic obesity have excessive insulin secretion during a standard oral glucose tolerance test (279). They also observed that treatment of these children with octreotide, a long-acting somatostatin receptor agonist (280), attenuated hyperinsulinemia in these children and promoted weight loss. These investigators concluded that normalization of insulin secretion may be an effective therapeutic strategy in children with this syndrome.

Alterations in dopamine systems and/or abnormalities of monamines can cause various types of hyperphagia (281). On the other hand, serotonin is believed to act as a satiety factor and an inhibitor of feeding reward in the hypothalamus (282). The role of other humoral signals in regulation of appetite and body adiposity has been extensively studied (283, 284). For instance, it has been thought that a number of gut hormones (i.e., cholecystokinin) feed back to appetite-controlling areas of the CNS in the regulation of meal size and frequency (284, 285). A study by Stromayer et al. (285) demonstrated that administration of a cholecystokinin (CCK) antagonist L364,718 resulted in increased daily food intake in lean but not obese Zucker rats. This is consistent with other observations that CCK decreases appetite, and that satiety deficit in obese rats contributes to overeating in these animals.

The composition of food has been proposed to affect brain neurotransmitter metabolism in some individuals. For instance, individuals referred to as "carbohydrate cravers" have been described to binge on high-carbohydrate foods during the early evening and night (286). However, most individuals seem to prefer high-fat low-sugar foods because of their high palatability. Unfortunately, high-fat meals result in less intense satiety than high-carbohydrate meals of equal caloric value (287).

Finally, mild obesity may occur in adolescent patients with Klinefelter (288) and Turner syndromes (289) with primary hypogondism. It is believed that hypogonadism results in excessive deposition of fat due to the deficiency of anabolic hormones, which are responsible for the growth of muscle. In Klinefelter syndrome, this effect is enhanced by the unopposed influence of estrogen, leading to further fat accumulation in the hips and buttocks to produce the charactcristic eunuchoid appearance.

XII. TREATMENT MODALITIES

The main goal of therapy should be to achieve the objective of lifelong weight control. Therefore, it is important to know the child's pattern of growth and weight gain. In general, any therapeutic approach for childhood obesity should be designed to induce decreased energy intake and increase energy expenditure while maintaining normal growth. Intervention to induce weight loss must consider all of the factors believed to cause obesity and the treatment modalities that have been effective. Since most of our present experience in the treatment of obesity centers

on environmental and behavioral factors, these represent
the primary areas of intervention. Genetic factors also play
a very significant role in obesity and can help to identify
the child at risk. This allows for early intervention in a
child predisposed to obesity and is indicated before obesity reaches extreme proportions. Furthermore, any form
of treatment for obesity should take into account potential
underlying medical conditions (i.e., hypotonia) that may
frustrate or render it ineffective. Therefore, the therapeutic
plan should be individualized to reach its desired goal.

There are some indications that successful treatment
of pediatric obesity is possible. It has been reported by
two studies that one-third of the children initially treated
maintained their reduced weight after 5 and 10 years. Furthermore, preadolescent children showed better responses
to initial treatment and maintenance of long-term weight
loss (290). These studies are encouraging, but more research needs to be conducted to determine compliance
with treatment and maintenance of weight loss into adulthood (290).

A number of treatment modalities for childhood obesity exist. However, prior to initiation of any form of therapy, a comprehensive medical evaluation is indicated.
This should comprise information on the rate of growth,
developmental milestones, and family history. The latter
is essential to identify those with parental obesity, hypertension, diabetes mellitus, hyperlipidemia, and thyroid
dysfunction. Furthermore, the assessment should include
nutritional, psychological, and physical fitness evaluations
as well. Obese children are not overnourished in all aspects. Indeed, the reverse may be true as excess calorie
intake increases other nutrient requirements that are not
necessarily provided by the diet. For example, obesity is
often associated with mineral and vitamin deficits (343).
It has been reported that a subgroup of obese adolescents
and adults (5–43%) engages in binge eating (291). Those
who do are described as rigid dieters and under tremendous psychological stress. These individuals have a higher
drop out rate from weight reduction programs than those
who do not binge.

XIII. DIETS

A. Dietary Intake

The role of dietary intake in obesity remains controversial,
although new data have shed more light on this problem.
Obese patients often claim that they do not ingest excess
food (292). These patients often seek medical evaluation
for failure to lose weight despite a history of severe caloric restriction. There are no differences in resting energy
expenditure nor in metabolic rates between diet-sensitive
and diet-resistant obese individuals. However, differences
in lean body mass account for the variations in weight
reduction induced by dietary intake restrictions in obese
individuals. They are frequently thought to be hyperme-

tabolic and are often treated with thyroid or other hormones to facilitate weight loss. This is neither safe nor
necessary; moreover, the observed minus the total predicted energy expenditure vary in relation of weight progression (293). Patients who gain weight increase their
metabolic rate whereas those who are on diets and are
losing weight may reduce their energy expenditure by
10–20%. Thus the results of dietary efforts can only be
successful if the reduced intakes are accompanied by increased energy expenditures to overcome the metabolic
adaptations that occur with dieting.

Obese individuals may reduce nutrient intake without
weight loss. The possible explanations for this failure include an energy intake significantly higher than reported
and a low total energy expenditure. A number of studies
have demonstrated that obese individuals tend to under-
report food intake compared to normal-weight subjects
(294–296). Indeed, careful metabolic balance studies in
some obese adults have shown a failure to lose weight
despite self-reported low caloric intakes. This may be due
to substantial misreporting of food intake and physical
activity and not to an abnormality in thermogenesis (296).
However, the problem is often confounded in the clinical
setting by the difficulties in assessing food intake and food
efficiency.

A high susceptibility to obesity may also be the result
of unlimited availability of palatable and high-calorie-den-
sity foods. Laboratory adult rats fed a "supermarket diet"
consisting of high-carbohydrate/high-fat foods (i.e., chocolate chip cookies, marshmallows, peanut butter etc.),
gained 2.5 times more weight than normal controls (297).
In some animals, the weight gain was not reversed after
the rat was switched back to chow. It is believed that
supermarket diets increase the number and size of fat
cells.

Dietary composition and different rates of nutrient
utilization of ingested diets can influence body weight
maintenance. Using indirect calorimetric technique in
nonobese males, Flatt et al. (298) demonstrated that under
sedentary conditions, ingested carbohydrates are quickly
metabolized while the rate of fat oxidation remains unchanged. Moreover, it has been suggested that the body
tightly regulates carbohydrate balance for up to 36 h after
ingestion and is not affected by alteration in the body's
fat balance (299). On the other hand, fat balance is believed to be regulated over a varying long term and it may
take several days before the fat balance adjusts to new
levels of fat ingestion. Thus, it is believed that excessive
fat consumption over a long period of time will result in
a positive fat balance and weight gain (300, 301). Therefore, a number of medical organizations including the
American Heart Association (302) and the American Diabetes Association (303) currently recommend consumption of low-fat diets in the prevention and treatment of
obesity. However, the relationship between the dietary fat
and obesity has recently been questioned (304–306) since

both cross-sectional and longitudinal analyses have failed to show a consistent association between dietary fat and body fat (307, 308). Furthermore, recent studies indicate that weight loss on low-fat diets is usually modest and transient (304, 309). It is also noteworthy that the rate of obesity has continued to rise in the United States despite reported reduction in mean fat intake over the past 30 years, from 42% to about 34% of dietary calories (306, 307, 310, 311).

Glycemic index (GI) is another dietary factor that may influence body weight. Glycemic index is a property of carbohydrate-containing food that describes the rise of blood glucose after a meal (312). The GI of a meal is determined mainly by the amount of carbohydrate content and by other dietary factors affecting food digestibility, gastrointestinal motility, or insulin secretion (including carbohydrate type, food structure, fiber, protein, and fat) (313–316). The average American diet contains starchy foods that are primarily refined grain products, cereals, and potatoes and have a high GI. In contrast, vegetables, legumes, and fruits have generally a low GI (317). It has been suggested that a potential adverse consequence of the decrease observed in mean fat intake in recent years is a concomitant increase in dietary GI. A reduction of dietary fat tends to cause a compensatory increase in sugar and starch intake (318–320). In fact, a rise in total carbohydrate consumption and GI of American diets, over the past 2 decades, has been reported (307, 318, 320). Since fat slows gastric emptying (315), carbohydrate absorption from low-fat meals may be accelerated.

High-carbohydrate diets have been demonstrated to increase basal plasma insulin levels in animals and humans (321, 322). It has also been shown that marked obesity is associated with elevated basal plasma insulin secretory response to glucose and protein (323, 324). The hyperinsulinemia of obesity has been regarded as a compensatory adaptation to the peripheral insulin resistance characteristics of the obese state (325). Since the diets of moderately obese individuals are excessive in both total calories and in the quantity of carbohydrate ingested, the hyperinsulinemia of obesity may also be a consequence of these dietary factors rather than merely a secondary response to insulin resistance. Indeed, it has recently been shown that voluntary intake after a high-GI meal was 53% greater that after a medium-GI meal, and 81% greater than after a low-GI meal. In addition, compared with the low-GI meal, the high-GI meal resulted in higher serum insulin levels, plasma glucagon levels, postabsorptive plasma glucose, and serum fatty acids levels, along with an elevation in plasma epinephrine (326). It is, therefore, likely that the slower absorption of glucose after ingestion of high-GI meals induces a sequence of hormonal and metabolic changes that promote excessive food intake in obese adolescents. Recently, Spieth et al. suggested that a low-glycemic-index diet in the treatment of childhood obesity resulted in greater weight loss than a standard reduced-fat diet (327). Long-term effects and safety of this diet needs to be evaluated in children.

The traffic-light diet is another approach that may be suitable for preschool and preadolescent children. This consists of a 900–1300 kcal/day diet of "tagged" foods designed to meet the age recommendations for appropriate nutrient intake using the basic four food groups outlined in the food guide pyramid. These diet groups fit food into three categories: green foods (go) can be consumed in unlimited amounts; yellow foods (caution) have average nutritional values within their group, and red foods (stop) provide less nutrient density per calorie because of high fat or simple carbohydrate content (328, 329). Combined with a comprehensive treatment protocol, this diet has been found to reduce obesity and change eating habits in preadolescent children (329–332). Furthermore, weight loss up to 10 years has been maintained when the traffic light diet was combined with behavioral, exercise, and familial components of a comprehensive treatment program (333, 334).

B. Very-Low-Calorie Diets

The national task force on the prevention and treatment of obesity published a report on the efficacy of very-low-calorie diets on weight reduction (335). Although rapid weight loss could be achieved, the long-term evolution of obese patients on these diets was disappointing. Slowly but surely they regained their weight and by 1–5 years they were of the same weight as before the treatment, regardless of the diet given.

There are few studies documenting the success of structured programs for treating childhood obesity that encompass just the use of very-low-calorie diets. Low-carbohydrate diets are usually high in protein and fat. They involve intake of large amounts of meat and restrict carbohydrate-containing foods such as fruits, vegetables, and grain products. The high intake of fat in such diets can increase the risk of coronary heart disease and other problems such as gallstones and high cholesterol. The body depends heavily on its fat stores for energy while on a low-carbohydrate diet. This can lead to ketosis. The rapid weight loss on these diets is composed of 60–70% water and the dieters often regain weight rapidly once normal eating is resumed (336, 337). Very-low-calorie restriction using a protein-sparing, modified fast (PSMF) diets (400–800 kcal/day) is designed to produce rapid weight loss of up to 5 lb (2.3 kg per week), while preserving vital lean body mass. The protein is provided as lean meat or fish, or in a milk or egg-based liquid formula. It has been suggested that these diets spare body protein by decreasing insulin levels and enhancing fat breakdown (338), while inhibiting the release of amino acids from muscle (339). However, in the past several deaths have been associated with the use of these formulas (298). Moreover, these quick-fix weight-loss schemes may be unsafe for use in children and do not promote healthy eating behavior for long-lasting weight control.

Nutritionally balanced very-low-calorie diets, combined with exercise, may improve the outcomes in structured obesity treatment programs for children (340, 341). In one study obese adolescents entered a structured 10 week program that included exercise and behavior modification, along with a very-low-calorie diet. After 10 weeks BMI decreased from 33.8 to 29.6. Fat mass was reduced without decrements in both lean body mass or energy expenditure (342). In another study by the same investigators, 87 obese children from 7 to 17 years old participated in a year-long program similar to that described above. The results were the same and weight and body fat loss were maintained for 1 year. These results suggest that a multidisciplinary structured program to treating obese children that is maintained for long periods of time may yield positive results. However, it is important to reiterate that energy intake, not energy consumption or distribution of calories, determines weight loss (343). Therefore a balanced diet that provides a reduced intake is preferable because it achieves long-term weight control with healthier eating behaviors as described below.

C. Food Management

Many special diets and dietary regimens have been used in the management of obesity. Diets are most likely to succeed if they are individualized according to current eating patterns, degree of motivation, intellect, amount of family support, and financial considerations. Therefore, a management approach to food intake is preferable to a diet prescription. A well-balanced calorie restrictive intake that provides all the necessary nutrients is the most effective and safest treatment for obesity. The reduction in caloric intake should be based on the weight history of the child in conjunction with usual calorie intake, body size, rate of growth, degree of adiposity, desired weight, and estimated daily activity level. As a general rule moderately obese children should be placed on an energy intake and exercise level that will slow weight gain in accordance with age and growth. In specific instances, to allow for parental or patient desires, it may be appropriate to design a nutrient intake to induce a slight weight loss. To accomplish this goal, it can be assumed that 1 lb of fat represents 3500 kcal.

Initially a 10% calorie reduction in the usual nutrient intake is recommended. The food choices must be individualized to the taste and preferences of the family and the patient with the aim of meeting all the dietary goals and guidelines. This should be achieved gradually to ensure compliance while appropriate eating patterns are established. It is important to correct all potential nutritional deficits at the beginning of the treatment and to monitor any alteration that may develop throughout the follow-up period. Obese children are not overnourished in all aspects, just in energy. They often ingest inappropriate in-

takes, which may lead to essential nutritional deficits (343) or other alterations (i.e., hypertriglyceridemia).

The following is an example of an initial approach to the treatment of an obese adolescent.

A 14-year-old boy with a weight of 72 kg and a BMI 28 was examined because of obesity. The initial nutritional evaluation documented that he was ingesting the diet shown in Table 1. This diet is not unusual for an adolescent boy and is typical of this age group (344). Analysis of the diet reveals that he was ingesting 3200 kcal (44.5 kcal/kg/day), which is 128% of that recommended for his age. He was also ingesting 44% of the total calories from fat; 14.6% of the total calories from saturated fat and 723 mg cholesterol, all being very high. He also had a high sodium intake of 4739 mg, almost double than that recommended for his age.

Although his intake was very inappropriate, treatment was started with a slight modification to improve compliance. By eliminating one doughnut and switching from regular soda to diet soda, his energy intake was reduced to the level necessary to avoid weight gain and maintain his current weight (38.5 kcal/kg/day). By simply eliminating those two items from the diet, there was a drop in calorie intake of 433 kcal/day. Of course, other inappropriate dietary habits were not corrected, although cholesterol intake dropped by 19 mg/day. Once the patient adjusts to these simple changes, further work will be necessary to improve upon the excess fat intake and reduce the amount of saturated fat from the diet. Patients who do not comply with simple measures might not necessarily learn to improve their nutritional habits for life.

Table 1 Typical Intake of an Adolescent Evaluated for Obesity

	Energy (kcal)
Breakfast	
Two sausages and 2 eggs	300
Coffee (1 cup)	0
Whole milk (1 cup)	150
Fruit juice (1 cup)	110
Lunch	
McDonald's Quarter Pounder	525
French fries (10 stripes)	160
Soda (1 can)	148
Dinner	
Half chicken breast	220
Baked potato (1)	220
Salad with dressing (8 oz)	85
Daily snack	
Donuts (2)	570
Chocolate chip cookies (3)	185
Ice cream (1 cup)	270
Potato chips (10 pieces)	105
Total	3207

Another example is a 50 kg 5-year-old patient with a BMI of 37. The patient and the family were highly motivated to cease excess body weight gain and to improve upon the biochemical abnormalities detected in the work up (i.e., hyperinsulinemia). It has recently been demonstrated that hyperinsulinemia in obesity is more resistant to weight loss than normoinsulinernic obesity in children (41). Her caloric intake was reported to be 1400–1500 kcal/day. This level of caloric uptake was not excessive for maintenance of body weight (30 kcal/kg/day). However, it contained a high proportion of dietary fats. A realistic goal for her was set at 10% of body weight loss and then weight maintenance until her weight would catch up with her height and normalize the height-to-weight ratio. This was a long-term plan that would require a successful attempt at 3 years of body maintenance.

Food management was initiated without reducing the total calories, since her total daily caloric intake did not appear to be excessive for weight. Instead, her food choices were modified to reduce the fat intake. She was placed on a 1500 kcal meal plan with decreased fat content (30%) while increasing complex carbohydrates. This included increasing vegetables in her diet and substituting low-calorie snacks for high-fat foods. She was given three meals and three snacks daily. It is well recognized that frequent meals are more effective for weight control than one large meal (345). Therefore, diets that consist of one or two large meals per day were discouraged.

Day-to-day variations in caloric consumption are characteristic of normal eating patterns and thus they should be allowed as long as they are within an acceptable range. For example, it would be appropriate for Julie, on a 1500 kcal meal plan, to have a range of intakes from approximately 1200 to 1800 kcal/day. While assessment of the rate of weight loss and growth is important, periodic assessment of nutrient composition of the diet is essential. This is particularly important for such micronutrients as calcium, iron, magnesium, copper, zinc, folacin, and vitamins, since these are very likely to be deficient on a restricted dietary intake (345).

XIV. EXERCISE

Dietary management of childhood obesity should always be combined with an exercise program. However, exercise should be prescribed on an individual basis. An exercise program based upon the initial fitness level (346) with a slow progression of the intensity, frequency, and duration is required to achieve the goal of weight control. For instance, morbidly obese children may achieve maximal energy expenditure during a brisk walk, since prescriptions for more demanding physical activities like jogging are likely to be impossible at the start. Resistance training may also be a suitable component of a structured obesity treatment program. One study found that weight loss was maintained for up to 1 year in obese preadolescents after completing a 10-week program that included resistance training combined with a low-calorie diet, behavior modification, aerobic and flexibility exercises. Furthermore, compliance with the exercise regimen was 100% (347). Physical activity has a significant influence on energy expenditure and the energy cost for most activities is generally greater for heavier people. There is also some evidence that increased activity in the obese individual may decrease appetite while increasing metabolic rate. Both obese and lean individuals experience a 19–30% decrease in resting metabolic rate within 24–48 h following caloric restriction (336). Thus caloric restriction without an increase in physical activity may not result in continued weight loss. Regular aeroboic exercise combined with energy restriction will result in greater reductions in body weight than dieting alone (301).

Intermittent exercise and use of home exercise equipment are effective in inducing and maintaining weight loss (348). Individuals who used the equipment longer were those who lost more weight and sustained their weight loss for longer periods of time. The type of exercise is also important: long bouts of exercise of greater intensity were more beneficial. The benefits transcend those of body weight. The relationship between cardiorespiratory fitness and mortality in normal-weight, overweight, and obese men was clear (212). Fitness is an independent predictor of health, comparable to diabetes mellitus, cholesterol levels, hypertension, and smoking.

However, by simply engaging in leisure-time physical activity major benefits may be attained. This is often not achieved, since most persons trying to lose weight are not using a recommended combination of reducing calorie intake and engaging in leisure-time physical activity (150 minutes per week) (349). In the patients mentioned above on dietary treatment, if they added to their treatment regimen a habit of walking 20 min/day they would enhance their energy expenditure by 5.8 kcal/min. In other words, they would spend 116 kcal/day above the dietary restriction, therefore increasing weight loss and enhancing their health. The amount of energy necessary for various physical activities is shown in Table 2.

XV. FAMILY INVOLVEMENT

Supportive counseling and reinforcement can help set the goals for health professionals, patient, and parent, allowing for long-lasting results and avoidance of failure and frustration. Refusal to adhere to a weight-reduction plan may be due to lack of family support, insufficient motivation, or other psychological stresses. For instance, it has been demonstrated that children of married parents lose weight at higher rates than those of divorced parents (328). When a weight-reduction plan has been recommended, conflicts frequently arise between the patient and nondieting family members regarding the degree of dietary restriction and who is permitted to eat different foods.

Table 2 Energy Expenditure in Occupational, Recreational, and Sports Activities (kcal/min) for a 50 kg Individual

Activity	Calories expended (50 kg/110 lb)
Basketball	6.9
Cycling	
Leisure	5.9
Racing	8.5
Computer typing	1.4
Dancing	
Ballroom	2.6
Vigorous	8.4
Eating (sitting)	1.2
Football	6.6
Gymnastics	3.3
Swimming	
Backstroke	8.5
Breast stroke	8.1
Crawl, fast	7.8
Crawl, slow	6.4
Tennis	5.5
Volleyball	2.5
Fishing	3.1
Gardening: Mowing	5.6
Marching	7.1
Running: 8 min/mile	10.8
Sitting quietly	1.1
Skiing (hard snow): Moderate speed	6.0
Walking (comfortable pace)	
Fields and hillsides	4.1
Grass track	4.1
Writing (sitting)	1.5

Energy expenditure is related to the size of the individual and should therefore be related to body weight. The usual dietary energy allowance for children 4–18 years varies between 34 and 82 kcal/kg/day. For competitive and long endurance exercises in children, energy expenditure should be increased by 17.6–52.8 kcal/kg/day above usual.

Dietary restriction should never be introduced in a punitive fashion. In some cases, the obese child and the entire family may adhere to a diet similar in composition if not quantity. Participation of the entire family should help minimize the feelings of isolation of the obese child. It has been shown that family involvement is essential for the success of any obesity treatment plan. Children whose families are involved in their treatment protocol lose more weight and maintain it for more prolonged periods that those whose families are not participatory (333). Eating patterns, food choices, and other behavioral factors of importance in obesity are family characteristics.

Dietary management and physical exercise are essential components for the development of effective treatment. The area of greatest concern for psychologists is how to get children to alter food intake and activity behaviors. Because the primary focus is on changing the child's behavior, parenting skills represent an integral component of the intervention. Stimulus-control procedures in the behavioral control of overeating have led to the development of several behavioral techniques for the treatment of obesity which include self-monitoring of body weight and/or food intake, goal setting, reward and punishment, aversion therapy, social reinforcement, and stimulus control. Several of these modifications have been found to be effective with children (328–334). These interventions are based on the assumptions that the obese child is an overeater who is hypersensitive to food stimuli and can be trained to behave like a nonobese person and subsequently lose weight. Moreover, positive family support has been shown to improve the degree of immediate and long-term weight loss in children and adolescents (330–332).

Any program designed specifically for treating obese children must include a group format with individualized counseling, parent participation, frequent sessions over a long period of time, appropriate exercise, and changes in the home environment to reinforce changes in the child's lifestyle. The behavior modification sessions should include self-monitoring, goal setting and contracting, parenting skills training, skills for managing the high-risk situation, and skills for maintenance and relapse prevention (340).

XVI. OTHER THERAPIES

A. Drugs

Long-term use of medications to suppress appetite or antiobesity pills are not usually indicated in the treatment of pediatric obesity. Studies involving the use of anorectic drugs alone or in combination with behavior therapy have demonstrated that weight loss is no greater than when behavior therapy was used alone. When the drugs were stopped, the weight was regained more rapidly (338). Furthermore, the effectiveness of appetite-suppressant drugs (i.e., amphetamines) appears to decrease with time and there may be side effects. The addictive potential of amphetamines and the risk of depression associated with fenfluramine have resulted in the minimal use of these agents in children and adolescents. The use of serotonin agonists such as fluoxetine and fenfluramine in the short term has proven useful as an adjunct in weight-loss programs for children and adolescents (342, 350). These drugs seem to decrease appetite and carbohydrate craving. Although they are by no means the solution to weight loss, they may help individuals at the beginning of a weight loss program by suppressing appetite. They must be used with caution and for a very limited time (351). In fact, serious side effects such as pulmonary hypertension and valvular heart lesions have been associated with the use of fenfluramine and its derivative, dexfenfluramine, in combination with another appetite suppressant (i.e., phentermine) (352). Recently, a new selective serotonin reuptake inhibitor, sibutramine (Meridia), has been shown to be effective in weight reduction trials in obese adults without significant adverse effects. However, the safety and efficacy of this agent have yet to be evaluated in obese children and adolescents.

Another potential antiobesity medication is metformin, an antihyperglycemic drug, that has been reported to enhance insulin sensitivity leading to reduced appetite and body weight in obese children and adults (353). Fremark et al. recently demonstrated that a 6 month trial of metformin treatment (500 mg twice daily) in a group of obese adolescents caused significant reductions in BMI, fasting glucose, and insulin compared to a placebo group (353). In a 2 month study, Metformin (850 mg twice daily) in a group of adolescents on a hypocaloric diet caused significant reductions in weight, fasting insulin, leptin, and lipids compared to a placebo group (354). The use of diazoxide, an inhibitor of glucose-mediated insulin secretion, in a group of hyperinsulinemic obese adults was recently shown to be effective in short-term weight reduction with few adverse effects (355). Daily subcutaneous administration of octreotide (somatostatin analogue), an inhibitor of pancreatic insulin secretion, to a group of children and adolescents with hypothalamic obesity secondary to cancer therapy likewise resulted in significant reduction in body weight over a 6 month period (279). The results of these studies imply that attenuation of hyperinsulinemia of obesity may be of therapeutic benefit in the management of this disorder. However, long-term efficacy and safety of these agents have yet to be evaluated in children.

B. Fat and Sugar Substitutes

Bulking agents and nonprescription diet aids, such as methylcellulose and other noncaloric bulk materials, have also been used in experimental and clinical attempts to inhibit food intake. The rationale for the use of such agents is that they swell in the stomach and supposedly give a feeling of satiety. Indeed, several lines of evidence suggest that dietary fiber may play a key role in the regulation of circulating insulin levels. Dietary fiber reduces insulin secretion by slowing the rate of nutrient absorption following a meal (312, 313). In the experimental setting, insulin sensitivity increases (314) and body weight decreases (315) in animals fed high-fiber diets. In addition, a recent study revealed that fiber consumption predicted insulin levels, weight gain, and other cardiovascular heart disease (CVD) risk factors more strongly than total or saturated fat consumption. Therefore, high-fiber diets (10–15 g/day) may protect against obesity and CVD by lowering insulin levels (316).

The use of inhibitors of digestive enzymes, such as intestinal lipase and disaccharidase, in obese and diabetic adult patients has been shown to be beneficial for weight reduction and improved glycemic control (356, 357). For instance, a gastrointestinal lipase inhibitor (Orlistat) has been reported to be of potential benefit by reducing fat absorption from the intestinal tract in obese adults undergoing significant weight reduction (356). However, undesirable side effects such as diarrhea and flatulence were frequently observed in these patients. This was accompanied by reduction in the levels of fat-soluble vitamins A, D, and E, which can be prevented by multivitamin supplementation. The safety and efficacy of the latter have yet to be evaluated in pediatric patients.

There are many misconceptions about the benefit of foods containing nonnutritive sweeteners. Currently, three nonnutritive sweeteners are approved for use in the United States: saccharin, aspartame, and acesulfame K. Other sweeteners include sorbitol, mannitol, and xylitol. Many obese individuals consume foods containing these sweeteners, thinking they are reducing their caloric intake. However, many of these foods either contain the same amount of or more calories than their regular sweetened counterparts. For example, dietetic chocolate contains 168 calories per 2 oz serving. Regular sweetened chocolate only contains 150 calories for a similar-sized serving (358). Therefore, without proper advice from a dietician, many obese individuals may be overconsuming calories by including dietetic foods in their diets. These foods also tend to be more expensive.

C. Surgery

There are very few applications of surgical procedures in the management of pediatric obesity. Four types of surgical procedures have been used to change eating behavior: jejunoileal and gastric bypass, gastric plication, and jaw wiring. The jejunoileal bypass procedures are usually followed by a large weight loss. However, significant complications including diarrhea, vitamin D deficiency with osteomalacia, vitamin B_{12} and folate deficiencies, renal (oxalate) calculi, hyperuricemia, and liver disease follow these procedures (359). A second procedure is the gastric bypass, which appears to be effective in producing weight loss without serious late complications seen with the jejunoileal procedure (360). Gastric plication (gastroplasty), involving a stapling procedure, is also widely used. Following the gastric bypass or gastroplasty procedure, patients food intake is decreased by the sensation of fullness. They also show less anxiety, depression, irritability, and preoccupation with food during weight loss compared with their weight-reduction attempts before the surgical procedure (361). In controlled studies gastric bypass appears slightly more effective than gastroplasty. Although successful initially in almost all patients, the failure rate for both procedures is high (up to 50%) (362). These procedures should be considered carefully in a select group of adolescents with significant medical complications who have been frequently unsuccessful in losing weight with other conventional therapies.

D. New Therapies

The administration of exogenous leptin has been shown to result in loss of body fat in animals with elevated leptin levels (364), as well as in humans with leptin deficiency, by reducing food intake (365). Recently, Heymsfield et al. demonstrated that a 6 month administration of subcutaneous recombinant leptin in high dosages induced weight loss in some obese adults with elevated endogenous leptin concentrations who were maintained on a eucaloric diet (365). However, they suggested that additional research into the potential role for leptin and related hormones in the treatment of human obesity was needed; the medication is not the magic bullet for most obese patients.

E. Kids Weight Down Program

A program specifically designed for treating childhood obesity must be the best approach to dealing with obesity in children. A Kids Weight Down Program may include staff consisting of a registered dietician, child psychologist, physician, and exercise physiologist. The program should require that parents participate in their child's treatment. Treatment is begun after a preliminary physical exam and laboratory testing that includes a lipid profile. Treatment may consist of one or two sessions per week, for 10 weeks, for both children and parents. All medical assessments are repeated at the end of the treatment period to determine compliance and progress.

The treatment regimen consists of a moderate weight-reducing diet along with an exercise program. The recommended energy intake consists of a 10% reduction diet as the main dietary prescription, as described above. This dietary prescription should not depend on any fad diets or eliminate any ethnic or cultural foods normally consumed by the families. As part of the weekly sessions, the children must exercise twice a week under the supervision of an exercise physiologist. The child's sessions must also include lessons and games to teach the importance of an appropriate nutritionally balanced diet for weight loss. The goal should be to make the sessions enjoyable for children as well as convey knowledge about the importance of losing excess body weight. The parents' sessions consist of education about the importance of family participation in the child's treatment. Each week parents may discuss problems/solutions associated with the progress of the child's treatment. This should include some of the problems encountered in changing the family dynamics in order to foster a positive influence on the child's treatment. Having parents' sessions, separate from the children, enabled them to support one another and allow open discussion about the problems of treating an obese child. The program is usually successful for a short duration.

However, the importance of long-term follow-up and management can never be stressed enough.

The unique program suggested above is costly because of the high demand for specialized personnel. Insurance companies usually do not provide any reimbursement for participation in such a program.

XVII. YO-YO WEIGHT CYCLING

Weight cycling has a profound effect on body composition and its metabolic efficiency (366). Weight loss followed by regain results in loss from muscle, regained as fat; increased risk of heart disease; and frustration (201, 202). Chronic dieters learn to cope with dieting. They develop a very efficient metabolism and maintain their weight with fewer and fewer calories with each attempt to lose weight. There is loss of muscle mass as a result of body composition changes during weight cycling. The increased fat mass leads to elevation of basal insulin and lipoprotein lipase levels (367), resulting in more fat deposition. In addition to changes in the body composition, the patient becomes psychologically frustrated as he or she fails to achieve the desired weight loss. The outcome is a patient who ingests very few calories and yet cannot lose weight.

Chronic dieters may also be increasing their risk for heart disease more than if excess weight remained at a stable level. Dieting leads to fat mobilization and during the regaining phase, fat deposition in the arteries. The regained weight is more likely to be distributed in the upper body where it is potentially more harmful (96) and associated with a higher incidence of heart disease and glucose intolerance (104). Appropriate strategies to avoid weight cycling should be considered at the beginning of a child's weight-reduction program. When a child is ready to participate in a weight reduction program, it should represent a serious commitment of all involved.

XVIII. PREVENTION

The successful treatment of childhood and adolescent obesity is an effective approach to the prevention of severe adult disease. Long-term follow-up of children treated with diet, exercise, and behavior modification has shown significantly lower weights 5–10 years later than for children treated in other ways (332, 333, 368). However, not all obese children who were treated successfully initially were able to maintain their reduced relative body weight. Nevertheless, none of these studies has had similar design and/or control populations, making a critical comparison very difficult. In addition, the increasing prevalence of childhood and adolescent obesity suggests that even the most successful treatment may be of limited benefit if it relies on the traditional doctor/patient interaction model. Furthermore, the metabolic phenotype (i.e., hyperinsulinemia) and family history of type 2 diabetes (369), hypertension and/or hyperlipidemia, may play a major role in a patient's response to conventional weight management strategies. Therefore, development of effective methods for weight reduction should be continued and multidisciplinary research to identify factors that prevent relapses should be encouraged.

Children should be encouraged to develop healthy eating habits and exercise patterns that prevent excessive weight gain. This is especially important for children in high-risk groups, for instance, with obese parents and those who are overweight by the time they enter school (370). Health professionals should inform parents of the potential risks and provide instructions on preventive measures at an early age. The introduction of a variety of nutritious foods to children's diets will lead to the development of healthy eating practices in children and adolescents. These foods should include an assortment of fresh or frozen vegetables and legumes; dairy products; fresh fruits; breads (preferably whole grain); and pastas, rice, cereals, and other grain products. Sweets and other nutrient-poor foods should be allowed in limited amounts that do not interfere with the child's consumption of basic foods. With relatively free access to these highly palatable choices (i.e., caloric-dense snacks), the chances of overeating are increased and may encourage the development of obesity in predisposed children. However, these changes have not been very successful in preventing the increase in obesity in children. Other lifestyle changes may be important in resolving this problem. A more appropriate approach should include reduction of sedentary activities such as television viewing and video game use. In a comprehensive study, 198 third and fourth grade students were organized into two groups. One group served as the control while the intervention group participated in a 6 month course geared toward reduction in television viewing, video tape, and game use. After completion of the course, the BMI of the intervention group was reduced from 18.8 to 18.1 kg/m². Furthermore, triceps skinfold thickness, waist circumference, and waist-to-hip ratio showed similar positive changes. Moreover, children in the intervention group self-reported fewer hours watching television while consuming meals in front of the television. However, no changes were found between the two groups in regard to high-fat food intake, physical activity, and cardiorespiratory fitness. These results suggest that just reducing television viewing and video game use contribute to positive changes in obesity indices in children (371).

Primary public health measures are critical to formulate a sound approach to the prevention of obesity in children. It is the responsibility of schools and government agencies, as well as food industries, to support measures that can improve the food habits and exercise patterns of children and adults. The schools should play an active role in providing healthy food choices in the cafeteria and provide appropriate exercise programs for normal-weight and obese children separate from competitive athletics. Government and local authorities can insist that schools implement and promote physical fitness programs and provide easy access to exercise facilities in the community. The media should assume a responsible position with regard to idealized concepts of beauty by appropriate programming and feeding of messages to children and to society at large.

XIX. FINAL CONSIDERATIONS

Obesity and significant comorbidities are reaching epidemic proportions among children. A variety of genetic, environmental, and other factors account for the development of obesity. Understanding leptin's role in regulating food intake and energy expenditure is an important discovery. It has been identified as a component of the pathophysiological alterations in this entity, including hyperinsulinemia and its complications. Inborn alterations of leptin have also been identified in individuals with severe morbid obesity. However, most obese populations exhibit various degrees of leptin desensitization. Early recognition of excessive weight gain in relation to linear growth is important and should be closely monitored by pediatricians and health care providers. The use of BMI percentiles may also help to identify children at risk and quantify the severity of obesity. Prevention is critical, since effective treatment of this disease is limited. Food management and increased physical activity must be encouraged, promoted, and prioritized to protect children. Dietary practices must foster moderation and variety, with a goal of setting the appropriate eating habits for life. Advocacy is needed to elicit insurance coverage of the disease.

ACKNOWLEDGMENT

This work was supported in part by NIH grant (#1R41HD/DK38180-01A2) and by Pediatric Sunshine Academics.

REFERENCES

1. Popkin BM. The nutrition transition in low-income countries: an emerging crisis. Nutr Rev 1994; 52:285–298.
2. Hodge AM, Dowse GK, Zimmet PZ, Collins VR. Prevalence and secular trends in obesity in Pacific and Indian Ocean island populations. Obes Res 1995; 2:77S–87S.
3. Troiano RP, Flegal KM. Overweight children and adolescents: description, epidemiology, and demographics. Pediatrics 1998; 101:497–504.
4. Kuczmarski RJ, Flegal KM, Campbell SM, Johnson CL. Increasing prevalence of overweight among US adults: The National Health and Nutrition Examination Surveys, 1960 to 1991. JAMA 1994; 272:205–211.
5. Merritt RJ. Obesity. Curr Probl Pediatr 1982; 12:1–58.
6. Stunkard A, Burt V. Obesity and the body image. II. Age at onset of disturbances in body image. Am J Psychiatry 1967; 123:1443–1447.

7. Stark O, Atkins E, Wolff OH, Douglas JW. Longitudinal study of obesity in the National Survey of Health and Development. Br Med J (Clin Res Ed) 1981; 283:13–17.

8. Kopelman. Obesity as a medical problem. Review. Nature 2000; 404:635–642.

9. Daher M. World Health Report. J Med Liban 1998; 46:212–217.

10. Seidell JC. Obesity: a growing problem. Acta Paediatr 1999; 88:S46–S50.

11. Gray GA. Contemporary Diagnosis and Management of Obesity. Newtown, PA: Handbooks in Health Care, 1998:120.

12. Williams DP, Going SB, Lohman TG, Harsha DW, Srinivasan SR, Webber LS, Berenson GS. Body fatness and risk for elevated blood pressure, total cholesterol, and serum lipoprotein ratios in children and adolescents. Am J Public Health 1992; 82:358–363.

13. Vanhalla MJ, Vanhalla PT, Keinanen-Kiukaanniemi SM, Kumpusalo EA, Takala JK. Relative weight gain and obesity as a child predict metabolic syndrome as an adult. Int J Obes 1999; 23:656–659.

14. Tracey VV, De NC, Harper JR. Obesity in respiratory infection in infants and young children. Br Med J 1971; 1:16–18.

15. Rosenbloom AL, Joe JR, Young RS, Winter WE. Emerging epidemic of type 2 diabetes in youth. Diabetes Care 1999; 22:345–354.

16. Kelsey JL, Acheson RM, Keggi KJ. The body build of patients with slipped capital femoral epiphysis. Am J Dis Child 1972; 124:276–281.

17. Kling TF Jr. Angular deformities of the lower limbs in children. Orthop Clin North Am 1987; 18:513–527.

18. Wadden TA, Stunkard AJ. Psychopathology and obesity. Ann NY Acad Sci 1987; 499:55–65.

19. Gortmaker SL, Must A, Perrin JM, Sobol AM, Dietz WH. Social and economic consequences of overweight in adolescence and young adulthood. N Engl J Med 1993; 329:1008–1012.

20. Reaven GM. Role of insulin resistance in human disease. Diabetes 1988; 37:1595–1607.

21. Webber LS, Srinivasan SR, Wattigney WA, Berenson GS. Tracking of serum lipids and lipoproteins from childhood to adulthood: the Bogalusa heart study. Am J Epidemiol 1991; 133:884–899.

22. Webber LS, Cresanta JL, Voors AW, Berenson GS. Tracking of cardiovascular disease risk factor variables in school-age children. J Chron Dis 1983; 36:647–660.

23. Stary HC. Evolution and progression of atherosclerotic lesions in coronary arteries of children and young adults. Arteriosclerosis 1989(suppl 1)9:I19–I32.

24. Berenson GS, Wattigney WA, Tracy RE, Newman WP 3rd, Srinivasan Dalferes ER Jr, Strong JP. Atherosclerosis of the aorta and coronary arteries and cardiovascular risk factors in persons aged 6 to 30 years and studied at necropsy (The Bogalusa Heart Study). Am J Cardiol 1992; 70:851–858.

25. Must A, Jacques PF, Dallal GE, Bajema CJ, Dietz WH. Long-term morbidity and mortality of overweight adolescents. A follow-up of the Harvard Growth Study of 1922 to 1935. N Engl J Med 1992; 327:1350–1355.

26. Moran JR, Ghishan FK, Halter SA, Greene HL. Steatohepatitis in obese children: a cause of chronic liver dysfunction. Am J Gastroenterol 1983; 78:374–377.

27. Bennion LJ, Knowler WC, Mott DM, Spagnola AM, Bennett PH. Development of lithogenic bile during puberty in Pima Indians. N Engl J Med 1979; 300:873–876.

28. Liddle RA, Goldstein RB, Saxton J. Gallstone formation during weight-reduction dieting. Arch Intern Med 1989; 149:1750–1753.

29. Dietz WH Jr. Obesity in infants, children and adolescents in the United States. I. Identification, natural history and aftereffects. Nutr Res 1981; 1:117–137.

30. Williams B. Insulin resistance and syndrome X. Lancet 1994; 344:521–524.

31. Arsalanian S, Suprasongsin C. Insulin sensitivity, lipids, and body composition in childhood: is "syndrome X" present? J Clin Endocrinol Metab 1996; 81:1058–1062.

32. Steinberger J, Moorehead C, Katch V, Rochini AP. Relationship between insulin resistance and abnormal lipid profile in obese adolescents. J Pediatr 1995; 126:690–695.

33. Chen W, Srinivasan SR, Elkasababny A, Berenson GS. Cardiovascular risk factor clustering features of insulin resistance syndrome (syndrome X) in a biracial (black-white) population of children, adolescents, and young adults. Am J Epidemiol 1999; 150:666–674.

34. Glaser NS. Non-insulin-dependent diabetes mellitus in childhood and adolescence. Pediatr Clin North Am 1997; 44:307–337.

35. Dean HE, Mundy RLL, Moffatt M. Non-insulin-dependent diabetes mellitus in Indian children in Mannitoba. Can Med Assoc J 1992; 147:52–57.

36. Dean H. NIDDM-Y in First Nation children in Canada. Clin Pediatr (Phila) 1998; 37:89–96.

37. Pinhas-Hamiel O, Dolan LM, Daniels SR, Standiford D, Khoury PR, Zeitler P. Increased incidence of non-insulin-dependent diabetes mellitus among adolescents. J Pediatr 1996; 128:608–615.

38. Kitagawa T, Owada M, Urakami T, Tajima N. Epidemiology of type 1 (insulin-dependent) and type 2 (non-insulin-dependent) diabetes mellitus in Japanese children. Diabetes Res Clin Pract 1994; 24(suppl)S7–S13.

39. Kitagawa T, Owada M, Urakami T, Yamauchi K. Increased incidence of non-insulin-dependent diabetes mellitus among Japanese school children correlates with an increased intake of animal protein and fat. Clin Pediatr 1998; 37:111–115.

40. Martin MM, Martin AL. Obesity; hyperinsulinism, and diabetes mellitus in childhood. J Pediatr 1973; 82:192–201.

41. Rosenbloom AL. Age-related plasma insulin response to glucose ingestion in children and adolescents. IRCS Metab Nutr: Pediatr 1974; 2:1210–1214.

42. Mallory GB Jr, Fiser DH, Jackson R. Sleep-associated breathing disorders in morbidity obese children and adolescents. J Pediatr 1989; 115:892–897.

43. Teran-Santos J, Jimenez-Gomez A, Cordero-Guevara J. The association between sleep apnea and the risk of traffic accidents. Cooperative Group Burgos-Santander. N Engl J Med 1999; 340:847–851.

44. Shelton KE, Gay SB, Hollowell DE, Woodson H, Suratt PM. Mandible enclosure of upper airway and weight in obstructive sleep apnea. Am Rev Respir Dis 1993; 148:195–200.

45. Horner RL, Mohiaddin RH, Lowell DG, Shea SA, Burman ED, Longmore DB, Guz A. Sites and sizes of fat deposits around the pharynx in obese patients with obstructive sleep apnea and weight matched controls. Eur Respir J 1989; 2:613–622.

46. Shepard JW Jr. Cardiopulmonary consequences of obstructive sleep apnea. Mayo Clin Proc 1990; 65:1250–1259.

47. Ciampelii M, Fulghesu AM, Cucinelli F, Pavone V, Ronsisvalle E, Guido M, Caruso A, Lanzone A. Impact of insulin and body mass index on metabolic and endocrine variables in polycystic ovary syndrome. Metabolism 1999; 48:167–172.

48. Pasquali R, Casimirri F. The impact of obesity on hyperandrogenism and polycystic ovary syndrome in premenopausal women. Clin Endocrinol (Oxf) 1993; 39:1–16.

49. Singh KB, Mahajan DK, Wortsman J. Effects of obesity on the clinical and hormonal characteristics of the polycyctic ovary syndrome. J Reprod Med 1994; 39:805–808.

50. Staffieri JR. A study of social stereotype of body image in children. J Pers Soc Psychol 1967; 7:101–104.

51. Davison KK, Birch LL. Weight status, parent reaction, and self-concept in five-year-old girls. Pediatrics 2001; 107:46–53.

52. Birch LL, Fisher JO. Mothers' child-feeding practices influence daughters' eating and weight. Am J Clin Nutr 2000; 71:1054–1061.

53. Vander Wall JS, Thelen MH. Eating and body image concerns among obese and average weight children. Addit Behav 2000; 25:775–778.

54. Stunkard A, Mendelson M. Obesity and the body image. 1. Characteristics of disturbances in the body image of some obese persons. Am J Psychiatry 1967; 123:1296–1300.

55. Monello LF, Mayer F. Obese adolescent girls: an unrecognized "minority" group? Am J Clin Nutr 1963; 13:35–39.

56. Canning H, Mayer J. Obesity: its possible effect on college acceptance. N Engl J Med 1996; 275:1172–1174.

57. Thompson D, Edelsberg J, Kinsey KL, Oster G. Estimated economic costs of obestity to U.S. business. Am J Health Promot 1998; 13:120–127.

58. Birmingham CL, Muller JL, Palepu A, Spinelli JJ, Anis AH. The cost of obesity in Canada. Can Med Assoc J 1999; 160:483–488.

59. Pronk NP, Goodman MJ, O'Connor PJ, Martinson BC. Relationship between modifiable health risks and short-term health care charges. JAMA 1999; 282:2235–2239.

60. Pronk NP, Boucher J. Systems approach to childhood and adolescent obesity prevention and treatment in a managed care organization. Int J Obes Rel Metab Disord 1999; 2:S38–S42.

61. Pugliese MT, Lifshitz F, Grad G, Fort P, Marks-Katz M. Fear of obesity: a cause of short stature and delayed puberty. N Engl J Med 1983; 309:513–518.

62. Moses N, Banilvy M, Lifshitz F. Fear of obesity among adolescent girls. Pediatrics 1989; 83:33–398.

63. Richardson SA, Goodman N, Hastorf H, et al. Cultural uniformity in reaction to physical disabilities. Am Sociol Rev 1961; 26:241–247.

64. Neumark-Sztainer D, Hannan P. Weight-related behaviors among adolescent girls and boys: Results from a national survey. Arch Pediatr Adolesc Med 2000; 154:569–577.

65. Abramovitz B, Birch L. Five-year-old girls' ideas about dieting are predicted by their mothers' dieting. J Am Diet Assoc 2000; 100:1157–1163.

66. Schur E, Sanders M, Steiner H. Body dissatisfaction and dieting in young children. Int J Eat Disord 2000; 27:74–82.

67. Stice E, Agras W, Hammer L. Risk factors for the emergence of childhood eating disturbances: a five-year prospective study. Int J Eat Disord 1999; 25:375–387.

68. Johnson S, Birch L. Parents' and children's adiposity and eating style. Pediatrics 1994; 94:653–661.

69. Hood MY, Moore LL, Sundarajan-Ramamurti A, Singer M, Cupples LA, Ellison RC. Parental eating attitudes and the development of obesity in children. The Framingham Children's Study. Int J Obes 2000; 24:1319–1325.

70. Lifshitz F. Fear of obesity in childhood. Ann NY Acad Sci 1993; 699:230–236.

71. Flier JS. Metabolic importance of acanthosis nigracans. Arch Dermatol 1985; 121:193–194.

72. Lifshitz F, Tarim O, Smith MM. Nutrition in adolescence. Review. Endocrinol Metab Clin North Am 1993; 22:673–683.

73. Hamill PV, Drizd TA, Johnson CL, Reed RB, Roche AF, Moore WM. Physical growth: National Center for Health Statistics percentiles. Am J Clin Nutr 1979; 32:607–629.

74. Pugliese M, Lifshitz F, Fort P, Recker B, Ginsberg L. Pituitary–hypothalamic response in adolescents with growth failure due to fear of obesity. J Am Coll Nutr 1987; 6:113–120.

75. Lifshitz F, Moses N, Cervantes C, Ginsberg L. Nutritional dwarfing in adolescents. Semin Adolesc Med 1987; 3:255–266.

76. Neumark-Sztainer D, Rock CL, Thornquist MD, Cheskin LJ, Neuhouser ML, Barnett MJ. Weight-control behaviors among adults and adolescents: associations with dietary intake. Prev Med 2000; 5:381–391.

77. Kreipe RE. Eating disorders in adolescents and older children. Pediatr Rev 1999; 12:410–421.

78. Hammer LD, Kraemer HC, Wilson DM, Ritter PL, Dornbusch SM. Standardized percentile curves of body-mass index for children and adolescents. Am J Dis Child 1991; 145:259–263.

79. Pi-Sunyer FX. Obesity. In: Shils ME, Young VR, eds. Modern Nutrition in Health and Disease. Philadelphia: Lea & Febiger, 1988:795–816.

80. National Center for Health Statistics, U.S. Department of Health, Education and Welfare: NCHS growth curves for children: birth to 18 years. Series H, No. 165, DHEW Publication No. (PHS) 78-1650, 1977.

81. Franklin MF. Comparison of weight and height relations in boys from 4 countries. Am J Clin Nutr 1999; 70:157S–162S.

82. Bellizzi MC, Dietz WH. Workshop on childhood obesity: summary of the discussion. Am J Clin Nutr 1999; 70:173S–175S.

83. Malina RM, Katzmarzyk PT. Validity of the body mass index as indicator of the risk and presence of overweight in adolescents. Am J Clin Nutr 1999; 70:131S–136S.

84. Dietz WH, Bellizzi MC. Introduction: the use of body mass index to assess obesity in children. Am J Clin Nutr 1999; 70:123S–125S.

85. Durnin JV, Womersley J. Body fat assessed from total body density and its estimation from skinfold thickness: measurements on 481 men and women aged from 16 to 72 years. Br J Nutr 1974; 32:77–97.

86. Must A, Dallal GE, Dietz WH. Reference data for obesity: 85th and 95th percentiles of body mass index (wt/ht2) and triceps skinfold thickness. Am J Clin Nutr 1991; 53:839–846.

87. Guo SM, Roche AF, Houtkooper L. Fat-free mass in children and young adults predicted from bioelectric impedance and anthropometric variables. Am J Clin Nutr 1989; 50:435–443.

88. Houtkooper LB, Going BS, Lohman TG, Roche AF, Van Loan M. Bioelectrical impedance estimation of fat-free mass in children and youth: a cross-validation study. J Appl Physiol 1992; 72:366–373.

89. Wells JC, Fuller NJ, Dewit O, Fewtrell MS, Elia M, Cole TJ. Four-component model of body composition in children: density and hydration of fat-free mass and comparison with simpler models. Am J Clin Nutr 1999; 69:904–912.

90. Czinner A, Varady M. Quantitative determination of fatty tissue on body surface in obese children by ultrasound method. Padiatr Padol 1992; 27:7–10.

91. Armellini F, Zamboni M, Rigo L, Bergamo-Andreis IA, Robbi R, De Marchi M, Bosello O. Sonography detection of small intra-abdominal fat variations. Int J Obes 1991; 15:847–852.

92. Ellis KJ. Measuring body fatness in children and young adults: comparison of bioelectric impedance analysis, total body electrical conductivity, and dual-energy X-ray absorptiometry. Int J Obes Rel Metab Disord 1996; 20:866–873.

93. Kohrt WM. Preliminary evidence that DEXA provides an accurate assessment of body composition. J Appl Physiol 1998; 84:372–377.

94. Paradisi G, Smith L, Burtner C, Leaming R, Garvey WT, Hook G, Johnson A, Cronin J, Steinberg HO, Baron AD. Dual energy X-ray absorptiometry assessment of fat mass distribution and its association with the insulin resistance syndrome. Diabetes Care 1999; 22:1310–1317.

95. Kvist H, Chowdhury B, Grangard U, Tylen U, Sjostrom L. Total and visceral adipose-tissue volumes derived from measurements with computed tomography in adult men and women: predictive equations. Am J Clin Nutr 1988; 48:1351–1361.

96. Ross R, Shaw KD, Martel Y, de Guise J, Avruch L. Adipose tissue distribution measured by magnetic resonance imaging in obese women. Am J Clin Nutr 1993; 57:470–475.

97. Fiorotto ML, Cochran WJ, Klish WJ. Fat-free mass and total body water of infants estimated from total body electrical conductivity measurements. Pediatr Res 1987; 22:417–421.

98. Megan AM, Gomez TG, Bernauer EM, Mole PM. Evaluation of a new air displacement plethysomgraph for measuring human body composition. Med Sci Sport Exerc 1995; 27:1686–1691.

99. de Ridder CM, de Boer RW, Seidell JC, Nieuwenhoff CM, Jeneson JA, Bakker CJ, Zonderland ML, Erich WB. Body fat distribution in pubertal girls quantified by magnetic resonance imaging. Int J Obes Relat Metab Disord 1992; 16:443–449.

100. Lockner DW, Heyward VH, Baumgartner RN, Jenkins KA. Comparison of air-displacement plethysmography, hydrodensitometry, and dual X-ray absorptiometry for assessing body composition of children 10 to 18 years of age. Ann NY Acad Sci 2000; 904:72–78.

101. Kissebah AH, Vydelingum N, Murray R, Evans DJ, Hartz AJ, Kalkhoff RK, Adams PW. Relation of body fat distribution to metabolic complications of obesity. J Clin Endocrinol Metab 1982; 54:254–260.

102. Evans DJ, Hoffmann RG, Kalkhoff RK, Kissebah AH. Relationship of body fat topography to insulin sensitivity and metabolic profiles in premenopausal women. Metabolism 1984; 33:48–75.

103. Kalkhoff RK, Hartz AH, Rupley D, Kissebah AH, Kelber S. Relationship of body fat distribution to blood pressure, carbohydrate tolerance, and plasma lipids in healthy obese women. J Lab Clin Med 1983; 102:621–627.

104. Peiris AN, Hennes MI, Evans DJ, Wilson CR, Lee MB, Kissebah AH. Relationship of anthropometric measurements of body fat distribution to metabolic profile in premenopausal women. Acta Med Scand Suppl 1988; 723:179–188.

105. Peiris AN, Struve MF, Mueller RA, Lee MB, Kissebah AH. Glucose metabolism in obesity: influence of body fat distribution. J Clin Endocrinol Metab 1988; 67:760–767.

106. Zamboni M, Armellini F, Milani MP, Todesco T, De Marchi M, Robbi R, Montresor G, Bergamo AI, Bosello O. Evaluation of regional body fat distribution: comparison between W/H ration and computed tomography in obese women. J Intern Med 1992; 232:341–347.

107. Garn SM, Sullivan TV, Hawthorne VM. Fatness and obesity of the parents of obese individuals. Am J Clin Nutr 1989; 50:1308–1313.

108. Roberts SB, Savage J, Coward WA, Chew B, Lucas A. Energy expenditure and intake in infants born to lean and overweight mothers. N Engl J Med 1988; 318:461–466.

109. Ravussin E, Burnand B, Schutz Y, Jequier E. Twenty-four-hour energy expenditure and resting metabolic rate in obese, moderately obese, and control subjects. Am J Clin Nutr 1982; 35:566–573.

110. Dewey KG, Heinig MJ, Nommsen LA, Peerson JM, Lonnerdal B. Breast-fed infants are leaner than formula-fed infants at 1 y of age: the DARLING study. Am J Clin Nutr 1993; 57:140–145.

111. Wells JC, Stanley M, Laidlaw AS, Day JM, Davies PS. Energy intake in early infancy and childhood fatness. Int J Obes Relat Metab Disord 1998; 22:387–392.

112. Davis PS, Wells JC, Fieldhouse CA, Day JM, Lucas A. Parental body composition and infant energy expenditure. Am J Clin Nutr 1995; 61:1026–1029.

113. Cole CR, Rising R, Hakim A, Danon M, Mehta R, Choudhury S, Sundaresh M, Lifshitz F. Comprehensive assessment of the components of energy expenditure in infants using a new infant respiratory chamber. J Am Coll Nutr 1999; 18:233–241.

114. Zurlo F, Lillioja S, Puente AED, Nyomba BL, Raz I, Saad FM, Swinburn BA, Knowler WC, Bogardus C, Ravussin E. Low ratio of fat to carbohydrate oxidation as a predictor of weight gain: study of 24-h RQ. Am J Physiol 1990; 259:E650–E657.

115. Rising R, Keys A, Ravussin E, Bogardus C. Concomitant interindividual variation in the body temperature and metabolic rate. Am J Physiol 1992; 263:E730–E734.

116. Rising R, Fontvieille AM, Larson DE, Spraul M, Bogardus C, Ravussin E. Racial difference in body core temperature between Pima Indian and Caucasian men. Int J Obes Rel Metab Disord 1995; 19:1–5.

117. Spraul M, Ravussin E, Fontvieille AM, Rising R, Larson DE, Anderson EA. Reduced sympathetic nervous activity. A potential mechanism predisposing to body weight gain. J Clin Invest 1993; 92:1730–1735.

118. Kramer MS, Barr RG, Leduc DG, Boisjoly C, McVey-White L, Pless IB. Determinants of weight and adiposity in the first year of life. J Pediatr 1985; 106:10–14.

119. Cutting TM, Fisher JO, Grimm-Thomas K, Birch LL. Like mother, like daughter: familial patterns of overweight are mediated by mothers' dietary disinhibition. Am J Clin Nutr 1999; 69:608–613.

120. Drabmam RS, Cordua GD, Hammer D, Jarvie GJ, Horton W. Developmental trends in eating rates of normal and overweight preschool children. Child Dev 1979; 50:211–216.

121. Agras WS, Kraemer HC, Berkowitz RI, Korner AF, Hammer LD. Does a vigorous feeding style influence early development of adiposity? J Pediatr 1987; 110:799–804.

122. Hill JO, Peters JC. Environmental contributions to the obesity epidemic. Science 1998; 280:1371–1374.

123. Udal JN, Harrison GG, Vaucher Y, Walson PD, Morrow G III. Interaction of maternal and neonatal obesity. Pediatrics 1978; 62:17–21.

124. Vohr BR, McGarvey ST. Growth patterns of large-for-gestational-age and appropriate-for-gestational-age infants of gestational diabetic mothers and control mothers at age 1 year. Diabetes Care 1997; 20:1066–1072.

125. Vohr BR, McGarvey ST, Tucker R. Effects of maternal gestational diabetes on offspring adiposity at 4–7 years of age. Diabetes Care 1999; 22:1284–1291.

126. Ravussin E, Lillioja S, Anderson TE, Christin L, Bogardus C. Determinants of 24-hour energy expenditure in man. Methods and results using a respiratory chamber. J Clin Invest 1986; 78:1568–1578.

127. Griffiths M, Payne PR. Energy expenditure in small children of obese and nonobese parents. Nature 1976; 260: 698–700.

128. Gauthier BM, Hickner JM, Ornstein S. High prevalence of overweight children and adolescents in the practice partner research network. Arch Pediatr Adolesc Med 2000; 154:625–628.

129. Stunkard AJ, Srensen TI, Hanis C, Teasdale TW, Chakraborty R, Schull WJ, Schulsinger F. An adoption study of human obesity. N Engl J Med 1986; 314:193–198.

130. Stunkard AJ, Harris JR, Pedersen NL, McClearn GE. The body-mass index of twins who have been reared apart. N Engl J Med 1990; 322:1483–1487.

131. Bray GA. The inheritance of corpulence. In: Cioffi LA, James WPT, Van Itallie TB, eds. The Body Weight Regulatory System: Normal and Disturbed Mechanisms. New York: Raven Press, 1981:61–64.

132. Heitmann BL, Harris JR, Lissner L, Pedersen NL. Genetic effects on weight change and food intake in Swedish adult twins. Am J Clin Nutr 1999; 69:597–602.

133. Flier JS. Leptin expression and action: new experimental paradigms. Proc Natl Acad Sci USA 1997; 94:4242–4245.

134. Flier JS. Clinical review 94: what's in a name? In search of leptin's physiologic role. J Clin Endocrinol Metab 1998; 83:1407–1413.

135. Frederich RC, Hamann A, Anderson S, Lollmann B, Lowell BB, Flier JS. Leptin levels reflect body lipid content in mice: evidence for diet-induced resistance to leptin action. Nat Med 1995; 1:1311–1314.

136. Smith SR. The endocrinology of obesity. Endocrinol Metab Clin North Am 1996; 25:921–942.

137. Bjorbaek C, Elmquist JK, Frantz JD, Shoelson SE, Flier JS. Identification of SOCS-3 as a potential mediator of central leptin resistance. Mol Cell 1998; 1:619–625.

138. Emilsson U, Liu YL, Cawthorne MA, Morton NM, Davenport M. Expression of the functional leptin receptor mRNA in pancreatic islets and direct inhibitory action of leptin on insulin secretion. Diabetes 1997; 46:313–316.

139. Fehmann HC, Bode HP, Ebert T, Karl A, Göke B. Interaction of GLP-1 and leptin at rat pancreatic β-cells: effects on insulin secretion and signal transduction. Hormo Metab Res 1997; 29:572–576.

140. Zhao AZ, Bornfeldt KE, Beavo JA. Leptin inhibits insulin secretion by activation of phosphodiesterase 3B. J Clin Invest 1998; 102:869–873.

141. Kieffer TJ, Heller RS, Leech CA, Holz GG, Habener JF. Leptin suppression of insulin secretion by the activation of ATP-sensitive K+ channels in pancreatic beta cells. Diabetes 1997; 46:1087–1093.

142. Seufert J, Kieffer TJ, Leech CA, Holz GG, Moritz W, Ricordi C, Habener JF. Leptin suppression of insulin secretion and gene expression in human pancreatic islets: implication for the development of adipogenic diabetes mellitus. J Clin Endocrinol Metab 1999; 84:670–676.

143. Zhang Y, Proenca R, Maffei M, Barone M, Leopold L, Friedman JM. Positional cloning of the mouse obese gene and its human homologue. Nature 1994; 372:425–432.

144. Masuzaki H, Ogawa Y, Isse N, Satoh N, Okazaki T, Shigemoto M, Mori K, Tamura N, Hosoda K, Yoshimasa Y, et al. Human obese gene expression—adipocyte-specific expression and regional differences in the adipose tissue. Diabetes 1995; 44:855–858.

145. Halaas JL, Boozer C, Blair-West J, Fidahusein N, Denton DA, Friedman JM. Physiological response to long-term peripheral and central leptin infusion in lean and obese mice. Proc Natl Acad Sci USA 1997; 94:8878–8883.

146. Ahima RS, Prabakaran D, Mantzoros C, Qu D, Lowell B, Maratos-Flier E, Flier JS. Role of leptin in the neuroendocrine response to fasting. Nature 1996; 382:250–252.

147. Ioffe E, Moon B, Connolly E, Friedman JM. Abnormal regulation of leptin gene in the pathogenesis of obesity. Proc Natl Acad Sci USA 1998; 95:11852–11857.

148. Fei H, Okano HJ, Li C, Lee GH, Zhao C, Darnell R, Friedman JM. Anatomic localization of alternatively spliced leptin receptors (Ob-R) in mouse brain and other tissues. Proc Natl Acad Sci USA 1997; 94:7001–7005.

149. Friedman JM. The alphabet of weight control. Nature 1997; 385:119–120.

150. Stephens TW, Basinski M, Bristow PK, Bue-Valleskey JM, Burgett SG, Craft L, Hale J, Hoffmann J, Hsiung HM, Kriauciunas A, et al. The role of neuropeptide Y in the antiobesity action of the obese gene product. Nature 1995; 377:530–532.

151. Schwartz MW, Seeley RJ, Campfield LA, Burn P, Baskin DG. Identification of targets of leptin action in rat hypothalamus. J Clin Invest 1996; 98:1101–1106.

152. Rothwell NJ. Central effects of CRF on metabolism and energy balance. Neurosci Biobehav Rev 1990; 14:263–271.

153. Saladin R, De Vos P, Guerre-Millo M, Leturque A, Girard J, Staels B, Auwerx J. Transient increase in obese gene expression after food intake or insulin administration. Nature 1995; 377:527–529.

154. Zheng D, Jones JP, Usala SJ, Dohm GL. Differential expression of OB messenger RNA in rat adipose tissues in response to insulin. Biochem Biophys Res Commun 1996; 218:434–437.

155. Boden G, Chen X, Mozzoli M, Ryan I. Effect of fasting on serum leptin in normal human subjects. J Clin Endocrinol Metab 1996; 81:3419–3423.

156. Considine RV, Sinha MK, Heiman ML, Kriauciunas A, Stephens TW, Nyce MR, Ohannesian JP, Marco CC, McKee LJ, Bauer TL, et al. Serum immunoreactive-leptin concentrations in normal-weight and obese humans. N Engl J Med 1996; 334:292–295.

157. Ravussin E, Pratley RE, Maffei M, Wang H, Friedman JM, Bennett PH, Bogardus C. Relatively low plasma leptin concentrations precede weight gain in Pima Indians. Nat Med 1997; 3:238–240.

158. Strobel A, Issad T, Camoin L, Ozata M, Strosberg AD. A leptin missense mutation associated with hypogonadism and morbid obesity. Nat Genet 1998; 18:213–215.

159. Clement K, Vaisse C, Lahlou N, Cabrol S, Pelloux V, Cassuto D, Gourmelen M, Dina C, Chambaz J, Lacorte

JM, Basdevant A, Bougneres P, Lebouc Y, Froguel P, Guy-Grand B. A mutation in the human leptin receptor gene causes obesity and pituitary dysfunction. Nature 1998; 392:398–401.

160. Maffei M, Stoffel M, Barone M, Moon B, Dammerman M, Ravussin E, Bogardus C, Ludwig DS, Flier JS, Talley M, et al. Absence of mutations in the human ob gene in obese/diabetic subjects. Diabetes 1996; 45:679–682.

161. Clement K, Garner C, Hager J, Philippi A, LeDuc C, Carey A, Harris TJ, Jury C, Cardon LR, Basdevant A, Demenais F, Guy-Grand B, North M, Froguel P. Indication for linkage of the human OB gene region with extreme obesity. Diebetes 1996; 45:687–690.

162. Reed DR, Ding Y, Xu W, Cather C, Green ED, Price RA. Extreme obesity may be linked to markers flanking the human OB gene. Diabetes 1996; 45:691–694.

163. Comuzzie AG, Hixson JE, Almasy L, Mitchell BD, Mahaney MC, Dyer TD, Stern MP, MacCluer JW, Blangero J. A major quantitative trait locus determining serum leptin levels and fat mass is located on human chromosome 2. Nat Genet 1997; 15:273–276.

164. Fan W, Boston BA, Kesterson RA, Hruby VJ, Cone RD. Role of melanocortinergic neurons in feeding and the agouti obesity syndrome. Nature 1997; 385:165–168.

165. Hakansson ML, Brown H, Ghilardi N, Skoda RC, Meister B. Leptin receptor immunoreactivity in chemically defined target neurons of the hypothalamus. J Neurosci 1998; 18:559–572.

166. Krude H, Biebermann H, Luck W, Horn R, Brabant G, Gruters A. Severe early-onset obesity, adrenal insufficiency and red hair pigmentation caused by POMC mutations in humans. Nat Genet 1998; 19:155–157.

167. Satoh N, Ogawa Y, Katsuura G, Numata Y, Masuzaki H, Yoshimasa Y, Nakao K. Satiety effect and sympathetic activation of leptin are mediated by hypothalamic melanocortin system. Neurosci Lett 1998; 249:107–110.

168. Friedman JM, Halaas JL. Leptin and the regulation of body weight in mammals. Nature 1998; 395:763–770.

169. Havel PJ, Kasim-Karakas S, Mueller W, Johnson PR, Gingerich RL, Stern JS. Relationship of plasma leptin to plasma insulin and adiposity in normal weight and overweight women: effects of dietary fat content and sustained weight loss. J Clin Endocrinol Metab 1996; 81: 4406–4413.

170. Leroy P, Dessolin S, Villageois P, Moon BC, Friedman JM, Ailhaud G, Dani C. Expression of ob gene in adipose cells. Regulation by insulin. J Biol Chem 1996; 271: 2365–2368.

171. Caro JF, Sinha MK, Kolaczynski JW, Zhang PL, Considine RV. Leptin: the tale of an obesity gene. Diabetes 1996; 45:1455–1462.

172. Saad MF, Khan A, Sharma A, Michael R, Riad-Gabriel MG, Boyadjian R, Jinagouda SD, Steil GM, Kamdar V. Physiological insulinemia acutely modulates plasma leptin. Diabetes 1998; 47:544–549.

173. Lahlou N, Landais P, De Boissieu D, Bougneres PF. Circulating leptin in normal children and during the dynamic phase of juvenile obesity: relation to body fatness, energy metabolism, caloric intake and sexual dimorphism. Diabetes 1997; 46:989–993.

174. Chehab FF, Lim ME, Lu R. Correction of the sterility defect in homozygous obese female mice by treatment with the human recombinant leptin. Nat Genet 1996; 318: 318–320.

175. Cioffi JA, Shafer AW, Zupancic TJ, Smith-Gbur J, Mikhail A, Platika D, Snodgrass HR. Novel B219/OB receptor isoforms: possible role of leptin in hematopoiesis and reproduction. Nat Med 1996; 2:585–589.

176. Haynes WG, Morgan DA, Walsh SA, Mark AL, Sivitz WI. Receptor-mediated regional sympathetic nerve activation by leptin. J Clin Invest 1997; 100:270–278.

177. Schwartz MW, Baskin DG, Bukowski TR, Kuijper JL, Foster D, Lasser G, Prunkard DE, Porte D Jr, Woods SC, Seeley RJ, Weigle DS. Specificity of leptin action on elevated blood glucose levels and hypothalamic neuropeptide Y gene expression in ob/ob mice. Diabetes 1996; 45: 531–535.

178. Chen G, Koyama K, Yuan X, Lee Y, Zhou YT, O'Doherty R, Newgard CB, Unger RH. Disappearance of body fat in normal rats induced by adenovirus-mediated leptin gene therapy. Proc Natl Acad Sci USA 1996; 93:14795–14799.

179. Zhou YT, Shimabukuro M, Koyama K, Lee Y, Wang MY, Trieu F, Newgard CB, Unger RH. Induction by leptin of uncoupling protein-2 and enzymes of fatty acid oxidation. Proc Natl Acad Sci USA 1997; 94:6386–6390.

180. Kojima M, Hosoda H, Date Y, Nakazato M, Matsuo H, Kangawa K. Ghrelin is a growth-hormone-releasing acylated peptide from stomach. Nature 1999; 402(6762): 656–660.

181. Nakazato M, Murakami N, Date Y, Kojima M, Matsuo H, Kangawa K, Matsukura S. A role for ghrelin in the central regulation of feeding. Nature 2001; 409:194–198.

182. Tschop M, Smiley DL, Heiman ML. Ghrelin induces adiposity in rodents. Nature 2000; 407:908–913.

183. Tschop M, Weyer C, Tataranni PA, Devanarayan V, Ravussin E, Heiman ML. Circulating ghrelin levels are decreased in human obesity. Diabetes 2001; 50:707–709.

184. Siiteri PK. Adipose tissue as a source of hormones. Am J Clin Nutr 1987; 45:277S–282S.

185. Bjorntorp P. The regulation of adipose tissue distribution in humans. Int J Obes Rel Metab Disord 1996; 20:291–302.

186. Sethi J, Hotamisligil GS. The role of TNFa in adipocyte metabolism. Semin Cell Dev Biol 1999; 10:19–29.

187. Hotamisligil GS, Arner P, Caro JF, Atkinson RL, Spiegelman BM. Increased adipose tissue expression of tumor necrosis factor-alpha in human obesity and insulin resistance. J Clin Invest 1995; 95:2409–2415.

188. Yudkin JS, Stehouwer CD, Emeis JJ, Coppack SW. C reactive protein in healthy subjects: associations with obesity, insulin resistance, and endothelial dysfunction: a potential role for cystokines originating from adipose tissue? 1999; 19:972–978.

189. Shimomura I, Funahashi T, Takahashi M, Maeda K, Kotani K, Nakamura T, Yamashita S, Miura M, Fukuda Y, Takemura K, Tokunaga K, Matsuzawa Y. Enhanced expression of PAI-1 in visceral fat: possible contributor to vascular disease in obesity. 1996; 2:800–803.

190. Weyer C, Funahashi T, Tanaka S, Hotta K, Matsuzawa Y, Pratley RE, Tataranni PA. Hypoadiponectinemia in obesity and type 2 diabetes: Close association with insulin resistance and hyperinsulinemia. J Clin Endocrinol Metab 2001; 86:1930–1935.

191. Bray GA, Dahms WT, Swerdloff RS, Fiser RH, Atkinson RL, Carrel RE. The Prader-Willi syndrome: a study of 40 patients and a review of the literature. Medicine (Baltimore) 1983; 62:59–80.

192. Widhalm K, Veitt V, Isigler K. Evidence for decreased energy expenditure in the Prader-Labhart-Willi syndrome: assessment by means of the Vienna calorimeter. Proc Int Cong Nutr 1981;

193. Schoeller DA, Levitksy LL, Bandini LG, Dietz WW, Walczak A. Energy expenditure and body composition in Prader-Willi syndrome. Metabolism 1988; 37:115–120.

194. Ledbetter DH, Riccardi VM, Airhart SD, Strobel RJ, Keenan BS, Crawford JD. Deletions of chromosome 15 as a cause of the Prader-Willi syndrome. N Engl J Med 1981; 304:325–329.

195. Bauman ML, Hogan GR. Laurence-Moon-Biedl syndrome. Report of two unrelated children less than 3 years of age. Am J Dis Child 1973; 126:119–126.

196. Spiegel AM. Pseudohypoparathyroidism. In: Scriver CR, Beadet AL, et al., eds. The Metabolic Basis of Inherited Disease. New York: McGraw-Hill, 1989:2013–2027.

197. Maxfield E, Konishi F. Patterns of food intake and physical activity in obesity. J Am Diet Assoc 1966; 49:406–408.

198. Roberts SB, Savage J, Coward WA, Chew B, Lucas A. Energy expenditure and intake in infants born to lean and overweight mothers. N Engl J Med 1988; 318:461–466.

199. Ravussin E, Lillioja S, Knowler WC, Christin L, Freymond D, Abbott WG, Boyce V, Howard BV, Bogardus C. Reduced rate of energy expenditure as a risk factor for body-weight gain. N Engl J Med 1988; 318:467–472.

200. Dwyer JT, Feldman JJ, Mayer JK. Adolescent dieters: who are they? Physical characteristics, attitudes and dieting practices of adolescent girls. Am J Clin Nutr 1967; 20:1045–1056.

201. Rossner S. Weight cycling a "new" risk factor? J Intern Med 1989; 226:209–211.

202. Steen SN, Oppliger RA, Brownell KD. Metabolic effects of repeated weight loss and regain in adolescent wrestlers. JAMA 1988; 260:47–50.

203. Bray GA. Lipogenesis in human adipose tissue: some effects of nibbling and gorging. J Clin Invest 1972; 51:537–548.

204. Fabry P, Tepperman J. Meal frequency a possible factor in human pathology. Am J Clin Nutr 1970; 23:1059–1068.

205. Dietschy JM, Brown MS. Effect of alterations of the specific activity of the intracellular acetyl CoA pool on apparent rates of hepatic cholesterogenesis. J Lipid Res 1974; 15:508–516.

206. Lakshmanan MR, Nepokroeff CM, Ness GC, Dugan RE, Porter JW. Stimulation by insulin of rat liver b-hydroxy-b-methylglutaryl coenzyme A reductase and cholesterol-synthesizing activities. Biochem Biophys Res Commun 1973; 50:704–710.

207. Jenkins DJ, Wolever TM, Vuksan V, Brighenti F, Cunnane SC, Rao AV, Jenkins AL, Buckley G, Patten R, Singer W, et al. Nibbling verses gorging: metabolic advantages of increased meal frequency. N Engl J Med 1989; 321:929–934.

208. Acheson K, Jequier E, Wahren J. Influence of B-adrenergic blockade on glucose-induced thermogenesis in man. J Clin Invest 1983; 72:981–986.

209. Odeleye OE, de Courten M, Pettitt DJ, Ravussin E. Fasting hyperinsulinemia is a predictor of increased body weight gain and obesity in Pima Indian children. Diabetes 1997; 46:1341–1345.

210. Bogardus C, Lillioja S, Mott D, Reaven GR, Kashiwagi A, Foley FE. Relationship between obesity and maximal insulin-stimulated glucose uptake in vivo and in vitro in Pima Indians. J Clin Invest 1984; 73:800–805.

211. Bandini LG, Schoeller DA, Dietz WH. Energy expenditure in obese and nonobese adolescents. Pediatr Res 1990; 27:198–203.

212. Wei M, Kampert JB, Barlow CE, Nichaman MZ, Gibbons LW, Paffenbarger RS Jr, Blair SN. Relationship between low cardiorespiratory fitness and mortality in normal-weight, overweight, and obese men. JAMA 1999; 282:1547–1553.

213. Rowland TW. Exercise and Children's Health. Champaign, IL: Human Kinetics Books, 1990:356.

214. Goran MI, Gower BA, Nagy TR, Johnson RK. Developmental changes in energy expenditure and physical activity in children: evidence for a decline in physical activity in girls before puberty. Pediatrics 1998; 101:887–891.

215. Garcia AW, Broda MA, Frenn M, Coviak C, Pender NJ, Ronis DL. Gender and developmental differences in exercise beliefs among youth and prediction of their exercise behavior. J School Health 1995; 65:213–219.

216. Bullen BA, Reed RB, Mayer J. Physical activity of obese and nonobese adolescent girls appraised by motion picture sampling. Am J Clin Nutr 1964; 14:211–223.

217. Waxman M, Stunkard AJ. Caloric intake and expenditure of obese boys. J Pediatr 1980; 96:187–193.

218. Maffeis C, Schutz Y, Schena F, Zaffanello M, Pinelli L. Energy expenditure during walking and running in obese and nonobese prepubertal children. J Pediatr 1993; 123:193–1999.

219. Prentice AM, Lucas A, Vasquez-Velaquez L, Davies PS, Whitehead RG. Are current dietary guidelines for young children a prescription for overfeeding? Lancet 1988; 2:1066–1069.

220. Energy and protein requirements. Report of a joint FAO/WHO ad hoc expert committee. Rome, March 22 to April 2, 1971. FAO Nutr Meet Rep Ser 1973; (52):1–118.

221. Goran MI, Carpenter WH, Poehlman ET. Total energy expenditure in 4-to-6-yr-old children. Am J Physiol 1993; 264:E706–E711.

222. Fontvielle AM, Harper IT, Ferraro RT, Spraul M, Ravussin E. Daily energy expenditure by five-year-old children measured by doubly labeled water. J Pediatr 1993; 123:200–207.

223. Gorn GJ, Goldberg ME. Behavioral evidence for the effects of televised food messages on children. J Consumer Res 1982; 9:200–205.

224. Klesges RC, Shelton ML, Klesges LM. Effects of television on metabolic rate: potential implications for childhood obesity. Pediatrics 1993; 91:281–286.

225. Jeffrey DB, McLellarn RW, Fox DT. The development of children's eating habits: the role of television commercials. Health Ed Q 1982; 9:174–189.

226. Williams TM, Handford AG. Television and other leisure activities. In: Williams TM, ed. The Impact of Television: A Natural Experiment in Three Communities. Orlando, FL: Academic Press, 1986:143–213.

227. Dietz WH Jr, Gortmaker SL. Do we fatten our children at the television set? Obesity and television viewing in children and adolescents. Pediatrics 1985; 75:807–812.

228. Andersen RE, Crespo CJ, Bartlett SJ, Cheskin LJ, Pratt M. Relationship of physical activity and television watching with body weight and level of fatness among children: results from the Third National Health and Nutrition Examination Survey. JAMA 1998; 279:938–942.

229. Polonsky KS, Given BD, Van Cauter E. Twenty-four-hour profiles and pulsatile patterns of insulin secretion in normal and obese subjects. J Clin Invest 1988; 81:442–448.

230. Kashiwagi A, Verso MA, Andrews J, Vasquez B, Reaven G, Foley FE. In vitro insulin resistance of human adipo-

cytes isolated from subjects with noninsulin-dependent diabetes mellitus. J Clin Invest 1983; 72:1246–1254.

231. Caro JF, Dohm LG, Pories WJ, Sinha MK. Cellular alterations in liver, skeletal muscle, and adipose tissue responsible for insulin resistance in obesity and type II diabetes. Diabetes Metab Rev 1989; 5:665–689.

232. Schade DS, Eaton RP. Dose response to insulin in man: differential effects on glucose and ketone body regulation. J Clin Endocrinol Metab 1977; 44:1038–1053.

233. Le Stunff C, Bougneres PF. Time course of increased lipid and decreased glucose oxidation during early phase of childhood obesity. Diabetes 1993; 42:1010–1016.

234. Randle PJ, Garland PB, Hales CN, Newsholme EA. The glucose fatty-acid cycle: its role in insulin sensitivity and the metabolic disturbance of diabetes mellitus. Lancet 1963; 1:758–789.

235. Glass AR. Endocrine aspects of obesity. Med Clin North Am 1989; 73:139–160.

236. Rosenbaum M, Leibel RL. Pathophysiology of childhood obesity. Adv Pediatr 1988; 35:73–137.

237. Olefsky JM. Decreased insulin binding to adipocytes and circulating monocytes from obese subjects. J Clin Invest 1976; 57:1165–1172.

238. Odeleye OE, de Courten M, Pettitt DJ, Ravussin E. Fasting hyperinsulinemia is a predictor of increased body weight gain and obesity in Pima Indian children. Diabetes 1997; 46:1341–1345.

239. DeFronzo RA, Ferrannini E, Simonson DC. Fasting hyperglycemia in non-insulin-dependent diabetes mellitus: contributions of excessive hepatic glucose production and impaired tissue glucose uptake. Metabolism 1989; 38: 387–395.

240. Kida K, Wantabe N, Fujisawa Y, Goto Y, Matsuda H. The relation between glucose tolerance and insulin binding to circulating monocytes in obese children. Pediatrics 1982; 70:633–637.

241. Rossell R, Gomis R, Casmitjana R, Segura R, Vilardell E, Rivera F. Reduced hepatic insulin extraction in obesity relationship with plasma insulin levels. J Clin Endocrinol Metab 1983; 56:608–611.

242. Peiris AN, Mueller RA, Smith GA, Struve MF, Kissebah AH. Splanchnic insulin metabolism in obesity. Influence of body fat distribution. J Clin Invest 1986; 78:1648–1657.

243. Svedberg J, Bjorntorp, Smith U, Lonnroth P. Free-fatty acid inhibition of insulin binding, degradation, and action in isolated rat hepatocytes. Diabetes 1990; 39:570–574.

244. Svedberg J, Bjorntorp P, Smith U, Lonnroth P. Effect of free fatty acids on insulin receptor binding and tyrosine kinase activity in hepatocytes isolated from lean and obese rats. Diabetes 1992; 41:294–298.

245. Felber JP, Ferrannini E, Golay A, Meyer HU, Theibaud D, Curchod B, Maeder E, Jequier E, DeFronzo RA. Role of lipid oxidation in pathogenesis of insulin resistance of obesity and type II diabetes. Diabetes 1987; 36:1341–1350.

246. Lillioja S, Bogardus C, Mott DM, Kennedy AL, Knowler WC, Howard BV. Relationship between insulin-mediated glucose disposal and lipid metabolism in man. J Clin Invest 1985; 75:1106–1115.

247. Daneman D, Drash AL, Lobes LA, Becker DJ, Baker LM, Travis LB. Progressive retinopathy with improved control in diabetic dwarfism (Mauriac's syndrome). Diabetes Care 1981; 4:360–365.

248. Jabbar M, Pugliese M, Fort P, Recker B, Lifshitz F. Excess weight and precocious pubarche in children: altera-

249. Freedman DS, Srinivasan SR, Burke GL, Shear CL, Smoak CG, Harsha DW, Webber LS, Berenson GS. Relation of body fat distribution to hyperinsulinemia in children and adolescents: the Bogalusa Heart Study. Am J Clin Nutr 1987; 46:403–410.

250. Forbes GB. Influence of nutrition. In: Forbes GB, ed. Human Body Composition: Growth, Aging, Nutrition and Activity. New York: Springer-Verlag, 1987:209–247.

251. Loche S, Cappa M, Borrelli P, Faedda A, Crino A, Cella SG, Corda R, Muller EE, Pintor C. Reduced growth hormone response to growth hormone-releasing hormone in children with simple obesity: evidence for somatomedin-C mediated inhibition. Clin Endocrinol 1987; 27:145–153.

252. Leroith D. Insulin-like growth factors. N Engl J Med 1997; 336:633–637.

253. Attia N, Tamborlane WV, Heptulla R, Maggs D, Grozman A, Sherwin RS, Caprio S. The metabolic syndrome and insulin-like growth factor I regulation in adolescent obesity. J Clin Endocrinol Metab 1998; 83:1467–1471.

254. Minuto F, Barreca A, Del Monte P, Fortini P, Resentini M, Morabito F, Giordano G. Spontaneous growth hormone and somatomedin-C-insulin-like growth factor-I secretion in obese subjects during puberty. J Endocrinol Invest 1988; 11:489–494.

255. Suikkari AM, Koivisto VA, Rutanen EM, Yki-Jarvinen H, Karonen SL, Seppala M. Insulin regulates the serum level of low molecular weight plasma insulin-like growth factor binding proteins. J Clin Endocrinol Metab 1988; 66: 266–271.

256. Suikkari AM, Koivisto VA, Koistinen R, Seppala M, Yki-Jarvinen H. Dose-response characteristics for suppression of low molecular weight plasma insulin-like growth factor-binding protein by insulin. J Clin Endocrinol Metab 1989; 68:135–140.

257. Holly JM, Smith CP, Dunger DB, Edge JA, Biddlecombe RA, Williams AJ, Howell R, Chard T, Savage MO, Rees LH, et al. Levels of the small insulin-like growth factor-binding protein are strongly related to those of insulin in prepubertal and pubertal children but only weakly so after puberty. J Endocrinol 1989; 121:383–387.

258. Holly JMP. The physiological role of IGFBP-1. Acta Endocrinol (Copenh) 1991; 124:55–60.

259. Rosskamp R, Becker M, Soetadji S. Circulating somatomedin-C levels and the effect of growth hormone and somatostation-like plasma levels of growth hormone and somatostation-like immunoreactivity in obese children. Eur J Pediatr 1987; 146:48–50.

260. Kopeleman PG, Weaver JV, Noonan K. Abnormal hypothalamic function and altered insulin secretion and IGFBP-1 binding in obesity. Int J Obes 1990; 14:S75–S79.

261. Novak LP, Hayles AB, Cloutier MD. Effect of HGH on body composition of hypopituitary dwarfs. Four-compartment analysis and composite body density. Mayo Clin Proc 1972; 47:241–246.

262. Amador M, Ramos LT, Morono M, Hermelo MP. Growth rate reduction during energy restriction in obese adolescents. Exp Clin Endocrinol 1990; 96:73–82.

263. Epstein LH, Valoski A, McCurley J. Effect of weight loss by obese children on long-term growth. Am J Dis Child 1993; 147:1076–1080.

264. AvRuskin TW, Pillai S, Kasi K, Juan C, Kleinberg DL.

tions of adrenocortical hormones. J Am Coll Nutr 1991; 4:289–296.

Decreased prolactin secretion in childhood obesity. J Pediatr 1985; 106:373–378.

265. Kyle LH, Ball MF, Doolan PD. Effect of thyroid hormone on body composition in myxedema and obesity. N Engl J Med 1966; 275:12–17.

266. Kaplowitz PB, Slora EJ, Wasserman RC, Podlow SE, Herman-Giddens ME. Earlier onset of puberty in girls: Relation to increased body mass index and race. Pediatrics 2001; 108:347–353.

267. Chiumello G, Brambilla P, Guarneri MP, Russo G, Manzoni P, Sgaramella P. Precocious puberty and body composition: effects of GnRH analog treatment. J Pediatr Endocrinol Metab 2000; 13:S791–S794.

268. Palmert MR, Mansfield MJ, Crowley WF Jr, Crigler JF Jr, Crawford JD, Boepple PA. Is obesity an outcome of gonadotropin-releasing hormone agonist administration? Analysis of growth and body composition in 110 patients with central precocious puberty. J Clin Endocrinol Metab 1999; 12:4480–4488.

269. Bray G, Gallagher TF Jr. Manifestations of hypothalamic obesity in man: a comprehensive investigation of eight patients and a review of the literature. Medicine (Baltimore) 1975; 54:301–330.

270. Didi M, Didock E, Davies HA, Oligvy-Stuart AL, Wales JKH, Shalet SM. High incidence of obesity in young adults after treatment of acute lymphoblastic leukemia of childhood. J Pediatr 1995; 127:63–67.

271. Stahnke N, Grubel G, Langestein I, Willig RP. Long-term follow-up of children with craniopharyngioma. Eur J Pediatr 1984; 142:179–185.

272. Thomsett MJ, Conte FA, Kaplan SL, Grumbach MM. Endocrine and neurologic outcome in childhood craniopharyngioma: review of effect of treatment in 42 patients. J Pediatr 1980; 97:728–735.

273. Sorva R. Children with craniopharyngioma: early growth failure and rapid postoperative weight gain. Acta Paediatr Scand 1988; 77:587–592.

274. Sklar CA. Craniopharyngioma: endocrine sequalae of treatment. Pediatr Neurosurg 1994; 21:120–123.

275. Jeanrenaud B. An hypothesis on the aetiology of obesity: dysfunction of the central nervous system as a primary cause. Diabetologia 1985; 28:502–513.

276. Powley TL, Laughton W. Neural pathways involved in the hypothalamic integration of autonomic responses. Diabetologia 1981; 20:378–387.

277. Ionescu E, Rohner-Jeanrenaud F, Berthoud HR, Jeanrenaud B. Increases in plasma insulin levels in response to electrical stimulation of the dorsal motor nucleus of the vagus nerve. Endocrinology 1983; 112.904–910.

278. Rohner-Jeanrenaud F, Jeanrenaud B. Involvement of the cholinergic system in insulin and glucagon oversecretion of genetic preobesity. Endocrinology 1985; 116:830–834.

279. Lustig RH, Rose SR, Burghen GA, Velasquez-Mieyer P, Broome DC, Smith K, Li H, Hudson M, Heideman RL, Kun LE. Hypothalamic obesity caused by cranial insult in children: altered glucose and insulin dynamics and reversal by somatostatin agonist. J Pediatr 1999; 135:162–168.

280. Koontz AJ, MacDonald LM, Schade DS. Octreotide: a long-acting inhibitor of endogenous hormone secretion for human metabolic investigations. Metabolism 1994; 43:24–31.

281. Blundell JE. Impact of nutrition on the pharmacology of appetite. Some conceptual issues. Ann NY Acad Sci 1989; 575:163–170.

282. Samanin R, Garattini S. Serotonin and the pharmacology of eating disorders. Ann NY Acad Sci 1989; 575:194–208.

283. Bray GA. Peptides affect the intake of specific nutrients and the sympathetic nervous system. Am J Clin Nutr 1992; 55:265S–271S.

284. Woods SC, West DB, Stein LJ, McKay LD, Lotter EC, Porte SG, Kenney NJ, Porte D Jr. Peptides and the control of meal size. Diabetologia 1981; 20:S305–S313.

285. Stromayer AJ, Greenberg D, Von Heynr, Dornstein L, Balkman C. Blockade of cholecystokinin (CCK) satiety in genetically obese Zucker rats (abstract). Soc Neurosci 1988; 14:1196.

286. Wurtman JJ. Disorders of food intake. Excessive carbohydrate snack intake among a class of obese people. Ann NY Acad Sci 1987; 499:197–202.

287. Drewnoswki A, Greenwood MR. Cream and sugar: human preferences for high-fat goods. Physiol Behav 1983; 30:629–633.

288. Ratcliffe SG, Bancroft J, Axworthy D, McLaren W. Klinefelter's syndrome in adolescence. Arch Dis Child 1982; 57:6–12.

289. Polychronakos C, Letarte J, Collu R, Ducharme JR. Carbohydrate intolerance in children and adolescents with Turner syndrome. J Pediatr 1980; 96:1009–1014.

290. Epstein LH, Valoski AM, Kalarchian MA, McCurley J. Do children lose and maintain weight easier than adults: a comparison of child and parent weight changes from six months to ten years. Obes Res 1995; 3:411–417.

291. Lowe MR, Caputo GC. Binge eating in obesity. Toward the specification of predictors. Int J Eating Disord 1991; 10:49–55.

292. Schoeller DA. How accurate is self-reported dietary energy intake? Nutr Rev 1990; 48:373–379.

293. Leibel RL, Rosenbaum M, Hirsch J. Changes in energy expenditure resulting from altered body weight. N Engl J Med 1995; 332:621–628.

294. Mertz W, Tsui JC, Judd JT, Reiser S, Hallfrisch J, Morris ER, Steele PD, Lashley E. What are people really eating? The relation between energy intake derived from estimated diet records and intake determined to maintain body weight. Am J Clin Nutr 1991; 54:291–295.

295. Bandini LG, Schoeller DA, Cyr HN, Dietz WH. Validity of reported energy intake in obese and nonobese adolescents. Am J Clin Nutr 1990; 52:421–425.

296. Lichtman SW, Pisarska K, Berman ER, Pestone M, Dowling H, Offenbacher E, Weisel H, Heshka S, Matthews DE, Heymsfield SB. Discrepancy between self-reported and actual caloric intake and exercise in obese subjects. N Engl J Med 1992; 327:1893–1898.

297. Sclafani A, Springer D. Dietary obesity in adult rats: similarities in hypothalamic and human obesity syndromes. Physiol Behav 1976; 17:461–471.

298. Flatt JP, Ravussin E, Acheson KJ, Jequier E. Effects of dietary fat on postprandial substrate oxidation and on carbohydrate and fat balances. J Clin Invest 1985; 76:1019–1024.

299. Schutz Y, Flatt JP, Jequier E. Failure of dietary fat intake to promote fat oxidation: a factor favoring the development of obesity. Am J Clin Nutr 1989; 50:307–314.

300. Golay A, Bobbioni E. The role of dietary fat in obesity. Int J Obes Rel Metab Disord 1997; 21:S2–S11.

301. Rolls BJ, Shide DJ. The influence of dietary fat on food intake and body weight. Nutr Rev 1992; 50:283–290.

302. America Heart Association. Dietary guidelines for healthy American adults: a statement for health professionals

from the nutrition committee, American Heart Association. Circulation 1996; 94:1795–1800.

303. American Diabetes Association. Nutrition recommendations and principles for people with diabetes mellitus. Diabetes Care 2000; 23:S43–S46.

304. Katan MB, Grundy SM, Willett WC. Should a low-fat, high-carbohydrate diet be recommended for everyone? Beyond low-fat diets. N Engl J Med 1997; 337:563–566.

305. Larson DE, Hunter GR, Williams MJ, Kekes-Szabo T, Nyikos I, Goran MI. Dietary fat in relation to body fat and intraabdominal adipose tissue: a cross-sectional analysis. Am J Clin Nutr 1996; 64:787–788.

306. Allred JB. Too much of a good thing? An overemphasis on eating low-fat foods may be contributing to the alarming increase in overweight among US adults. J Am Diet Assoc 1995; 95:417–418.

307. Nicklas TA. Dietary studies of children: The Bogalusa Heart Study experience. J Am Diet Assoc 1995; 95:1127–1133.

308. Kant AK, Graubard BI, Schatzkin A, Ballard-Barbash R. Proportions of energy intake from fat and subsequent weight change in the NHANES 1 epidemiologic follow-up study. Am J Clin Nutr 1995; 61:11–17.

309. Lissner L, Heitman BL. Dietary fat and obesity: evidence from epidemiology. Eur J Clin Nutr 1995; 49:79–90.

310. Lenfant C, Ernst N. Daily dietary fat and total energy intakes—Third National Health and Nutrition Examination Survey, phase 1, 1988–1991. MMWR 1994; 43:116–117.

311. Stephen AM, Wald NJ. Trends in individual consumption of dietary fat in the United States, 1920–1984. Am J Clin Nutr 1990; 52:457–469.

312. Wolever TM, Jenkins DJ, Jenkins AL, Josse RG. The glycemic index: methodology and clinical implications. Am J Clin Nutr 1991; 54:846–854.

313. Bjork I, Granfeldt Y, Liljeberg H, Tovar J, Asp N-G. Food properties affecting the digestion and absorption of carbohydrates. Am J Clin Nutr 1994; 59:699S–705S.

314. Granfeldt Y, Hagander B, Bjork I. Metabolic responses to starch in oat and wheat products. On the importance of food structure, incomplete gelatinization or presence of viscous dietary fiber. Eur J Clin Nutr 1995; 49:189–199.

315. Welch IM, Bruce C, Hill SE, Read NW. Duodenal and ileal lipid suppresses postprandial blood glucose and insulin responses in man: possible implications for dietary management of diabetes mellitus. Clin Sci 1987; 72:209–216.

316. Trout DL, Behall KM, Osilesi O. Prediction of glycemic index for starchy foods. 1993; 58:873–878.

317. Foster-Powell K, Miller JB. International tables of glycemic index. Am J Clin Nutr 1995; 62:871S–890S.

318. Stephen AM, Sieber GM, Gerster YA, Morgan DR. Intake of carbohydrate and its components—international comparisons, trends overtime, and effects of changing to low-fat diets. Am J Clin Nutr 1995; 62:851S–867S.

319. Nicklas TA, Webber LS, Koschak ML, Berenson GS. Nutrient adequacy of low fat intakes for children: the Bogalusa Heart Study. Pediatrics 1992; 89:221–228.

320. Popkin BM, Haines PS, Patterson RE. Dietary changes in older Americans 1977–1987. Am J Clin Nutr 1992; 55:823–830.

321. Grey NJ, Goldring S, Kipnis DM. The effect of fasting, diet, and actinomycin D on insulin secretion in the rat. J Clin Invest 1970; 49:881–889.

322. Grey NJ, Kipnis DM. Effect of diet composition on the hyperinsulinemia of obesity. N Engl J Med 1971; 285:827–831.

323. Bagdade JD, Bierman EL, Porte D Jr. The significance of basal insulin levels in the evaluation of the insulin response to glucose in diabetic and nondiabetic subjects. J Clin Invest 1967; 46:1549–1557.

324. Floyd JC Jr, Fajans SS, Conn JW, Khoph RF, Rull J. Stimulation of insulin secretion by amino acids. J Clin Invest 1966; 1487–1502.

325. Rabinowitz D, Zierler KL. Forearm metabolism in obesity and its response to intra-arterial insulin. Characterization of insulin resistance and evidence for adaptive hyperinsulinism. J Clin Invest 1962; 41:2173–2181.

326. Ludwig DS, Majzoub JA, Al-Zahrani A, Dallal GE, Blanco I, Roberts SB. High glycemic index foods, overeating, and obesity. Pediatrics 1999; 103:E26.

327. Spieth LE, Harnish JD, Lenders CM, Raezer LB, Pereira MA, Hangen SJ, Ludwig DS. A low-glycemic index diet in the treatment of pediatric obesity. Arch Pediatr Adolesc Med 2000; 154:947–951.

328. Epstein LH, Valoski A, Koeske R, Wing RR. Family-based behavioral weight control in obese young children. J Am Diet Assoc 1986; 86:481–484.

329. Valoski A, Epstein LH. Nutrient intake of obese children in a family-based behavioral weight control program. Int J Obes 1990; 14:667–677.

330. Epstein LH, Wings RR, Steranchak L, Dickson B, Michelson J. Comparison of family based behavior modification and nutrition education for childhood obesity. J Pediatr Psychol 1980; 5:25–36.

331. Epstein LH, Valoski AM, Vara LS, McCurley J, Wisniewski L, Kalarchian MA, Klein KR, Shrager LR. Effects of decreasing sedentary behavior and increasing activity on weight change in obese children. Health Psychol 1995; 14:109–115.

332. Epstein LH, Valoski A, Wing RR, McCurley J. Ten-year follow-up of behavioral family-based treatment for obese children. JAMA 1990; 264:2519–2523.

333. Epstein LH, Valoski AM, Wing RR, McCurley J. Ten year outcomes of behavioral family-based treatment for childhood obesity. Health Psychol 1994; 13:373–383.

334. Sothern MS, von Almen TK, Schumacher HD, Suskind RM, Blecker U. A multidisciplinary approach to the treatment of childhood obesity. Del Med J 1999; 71:255–261.

335. National Task Force on the Prevention and Treatment of Obesity, National Institutes of Health. Very low-calorie diets. JAMA Review 1993; 270:967–974.

336. Andersen T, Backer OG, Stokholm KH, Quaade F. Randomized trial of diet and gastroplasty compared with diet alone in morbid obesity. N Engl J Med 1984; 310:352–356.

337. Wadden TA, Stunkard AJ. Controlled trial of very low calorie diet, behavior therapy, and their combination in the treatment of obesity. J Consult Clin Psychol 1986; 54:482–488.

338. Flatt JP, Blackburn GL. The metabolic fuel regulatory system: implications for protein-sparing therapies during caloric deprivation and disease. Am J Clin Nutr 1974; 27:175–187.

339. Sherwin RS, Hendler RG, Felig P. Effect of ketone infusion on amino acid and nitrogen metabolism in man. J Clin Invest 1975; 55:132–1390.

340. Robinson TN. Behavioural treatment of childhood and adolescent obesity. Int J Obes Rel Metab Disord 1999; 2:S52–S57.

341. Sothern MS, Loftin M, Suskind RM, Udall JN Jr, Blecker

U. The impact of significant weight loss on resting energy expenditure in obese youth. J Invest Med 1999; 47:222–226.

342. Boeck MA. Safety and efficiency of fluoxetine in morbidly obese adolescent females. Int J Obes 1991; 15(suppl 3):60.

343. Golay A, Allaz AF, Ybarra J, Bianchi P, Saraiva S, Mensi N, Gomis R, de Tonnac N. Similar weight loss with low-energy food combining or balanced diets. Int J Obes Rel Metab Disord 2000; 24:492–496.

344. Mahan K, Escott-Stump S. Krauses's Food Nutrition and Diet Therapy. Philadelphia: WB Saunders, 1996:463–469.

345. Apfelbaum M, Bostarron J, Lacatis D. Effect of caloric restriction and excessive caloric intake on energy expenditure. Am J Clin Nutr 1971; 24:1405–1409.

346. Hagan RD, Upton SJ, Wong L, Whittam J. The effects of aerobic conditioning and/or caloric restriction in overweight men and women. Med Sci Sports Exerc 1986; 18:87–94.

347. Sothern MS, Hunter S, Suskind RM, Brown R, Udall JN Jr, Blecker U. Motivating the obese child to move: the role of structured exercise in pediatric weight management. South Med J 1999; 92:577–584.

348. Jakicic JM, Winters C, Lang W, Wing RR. Effects of intermittent exercise and use of home exercise equipment on adherence, weight loss, and fitness in overweight women: a randomized trial. JAMA 1999; 282:1554–1560.

349. Serdula MK, Mokdad AH, Williamson DF, Galuska DA, Mendlein JM, Heath GW. Prevalence of attempting weight loss and strategies for controlling weight. JAMA 1999; 282:1353–138.

350. Selikowitz M, Sunman, Pendegast A, Wright S. Fenfluramine in Prader-Willi syndrome: a double blind, placebo controlled trail. Arch Dis Child 1990; 65:112–114.

351. Oleandri SE, Maccario M, Rossetto R, Procopio M, Grottoli S, Avogadri E, Gauna C, Ganzaroli C, Ghigo E. Three-month treatment with metformin or dexfenfluramine does not modify the effects of diet on anthropometric and endocrine-metabolic parameters in abdominal obesity. J Endocrinol Invest 1999; 22:134–140.

352. Abenhaim L, Moride Y, Brenot F, Rich S, Benichou J, Kurz X, Higenbottam T, Oakley C, Wouters E, Aubier M, Simonneau G, Begaud B. Appetite-suppressant drugs and the risk of primary pulmonary hypertension. N Engl J Med 1996; 335:609–616.

353. Freemark M, Bursey D. The effect of metformin on body mass index and glucose tolerance in obese adolescents and fasting hyperinsulinemia and a family history of type 2 diabetes. Pediatrics 2001; 107:E55.

354. Kay JP, Alemzadeh R, Langley G, D'Angelo L, Smith P, Holshouser S. Beneficial effects of Metformin in normoglycemic morbidly obese adolescents. Metabolism 2001; 50:1457–1461.

355. Alemzadeh R, Langley G, Upchurch L, Smith P, Slonim AE. Beneficial effect of diazoxide in obese hyperinsulinemic adults. J Endocrinol Metab 1998; 83:1911–1915.

356. Matsuo T, Odaka H, Ikeda HE. Effect of an intestinal disccharidase inhibitor (AO-128) on obesity and diabetes. Am J Clin Nutr 1992; 55:314S–317S.

357. James WP, Avenell A, Broom J, Whitehead J. A one-year trial to assess the value of orlistat in the management of obesity. Int J Obes Rel Metab Disord 1997; 21:S24–S30.

358. Wunschel IM, Sheikholislam BM. Is there a role for dietetic foods in the management of diabetes and/or obesity? Diabetes Care 1978; 1:247–249.

359. O'Leary JP. Gastrointestinal malabsorptive procedures. Am J Clin Nutr 1992; 55:567S–570S.

360. Alden JF. Gastric and jejunoileal bypass: a comparison in the treatment of morbid obesity. Arch Surg 1997; 112:799–806.

361. Saltzstein EC, Gutmann MC. Gastric bypass for morbid obesity; preoperative and postoperative psychological evaluation of patients. Arch Surg 1980; 115:21–23.

362. Freeman JB, Burchett H. Failure rate with gastric partitioning for morbid obesity. Am J Surg 1977; 112:799–806.

363. Bray GA, Gray DS. Treatment of obesity: an overview. Diabetes Metab Rev 1988; 4:653–679.

364. Pelleymounter MA, Cullen MJ, Baker MB, Hecht R, Winters D, Boone T, Collins F. Effects of the obese gene product on body weight regulation in ob/ob mice. Science 1995; 269:540–543.

365. Heymsfield SB, Greenberg AS, Fujioka K, Dixon RM, Kushner R, Hunt T, Lubina JA, Patane J, Self B, Hunt P, McCamish M. Recombinant leptin for weight loss in obese and lean adults. JAMA 1999; 282:1568–1575.

366. Ravussin E, Burnand B, Schutz Y, Jequier E. Energy expenditure before and during energy restriction in obese patients. Am J Clin Nutr 1985; 41:753–759.

367. Brownell KD, Greenwood MR, Stellar E, Sharager EE. The effects of repeated cycles of weight loss and regain in rats. Physiol Behav 1986; 38:459–464.

368. Nuutienen O, Knip M. Long-term weight control in obese children: persistence of treatment outcome and metabolic changes. Int J Obes 1992; 16:279–287.

369. Sigal RJ, El-Hashimy M, Martin BC, Soeldner JS, Krolowski AS, Wanam JH. Acute postchallenge hyperinsulinemia predicts weight gain. Diabetes 1997; 46:1025–1029.

370. Black O, James WPT, Besser CM. A report of the Royal College of Physicians. J R Coll Physicians Long 1983; 17:5–65.

371. Robinson TN. Reducing children's television viewing to prevent obesity: a randomized controlled trial. JAMA 1999; 282:1561–1567.

35

Hyperlipoproteinemias in Children and Adolescents

Kurt Widhalm
University of Vienna, Vienna, Austria

I. INTRODUCTION

A body of evidence now shows that elevated levels of plasma cholesterol, especially low-density lipoprotein (LDL) cholesterol, are associated with an increased probability of premature cardiovascular disease in the adult. This is particularly true for subjects with the most common familial hypercholesterolemia (a dominant disorder of the lipoprotein metabolism) who usually have a manifest atherosclerosis in the fourth to fifth decade. There is also no doubt that atherosclerosis starts in childhood and therefore preventive measures should be initiated as early as possible to prevent progression of the disease.

Hyperlipoproteinemias are biochemical abnormalities in which one or more lipids/lipoproteins is either elevated or has an abnormal composition. It should be the goal of any pediatrician or general physician to detect these abnormalities during childhood in order to start as early as possible with preventive therapeutic measures.

It is not well established that early reduction of atherogenic lipoproteins is associated with delayed development of atherosclerosis; however, many facts from adult studies support this theory very strongly. Nevertheless, the power of knowledge from intervention studies in adult population would not allow for randomized studies in the pediatric age group because of ethical concerns.

In this chapter the main focus will be on the clinical aspects of diagnostic and therapeutic procedures for lipoprotein disorders in children.

II. LIPOPROTEIN BACKGROUND AND BASICS

There is a strong relationship between the intake of fats, in particular saturated fats, and the development of premature cardiovascular diseases. One of the main mechanisms involved in that process is most probably the concentration and composition of plasma lipoproteins. These particles are responsible for the transport of lipids after absorption from the gut to the liver and to the organs (Fig. 1).

Figure 1 shows clearly that cholesterol and triglycerides are ingested into the gastrointestinal tract and are converted to chylomicrons. These triglyceride-rich particles are taken up by the liver by means of a specific apo E receptor and are secreted as very-low-density lipoproteins (VLDL) into the circulation. These particles are converted to the short-lived intermediate-density lipoproteins (IDL), which are formed into low-density lipoproteins (LDL), which are smaller, denser, and contain more cholesterol. These most atherogenic vehicles are taken up by the liver by means of LDL receptors and, to a smaller extent, by a nonreceptor pathway by the so-called scavenger cells.

The smallest lipoproteins, high-density lipoproteins (HDL), are partly responsible for the transport of LDL back to the liver.

The classification and composition of the various lipoproteins are shown in Table 1.

In regard to the atherogeneity of the various plasma lipoproteins, there is enough evidence, both on a pathophysiological and on a epidemiological level, that the most pathogenic particles are LDL, and, to a lesser extent, VLDL. In contrast, HDL particles have a protective function against atherogenesis: subjects with high HDL levels are rarely affected with cardiovascular diseases. However, subjects with low levels are considered to be at higher risk, even if they have normal cholesterol concentrations.

If total and LDL cholesterol levels are elevated, fatty streaks and fibrous plaques develop in nonhuman primates, mainly due to diets high in saturated fatty acids and cholesterol. In adults, but also in adolescents, the amount of saturated fat in the diet influences the concentration of serum cholesterol strongly. However, it seems very likely that genetic factors also are involved in the regulation of cholesterol metabolism, because there are

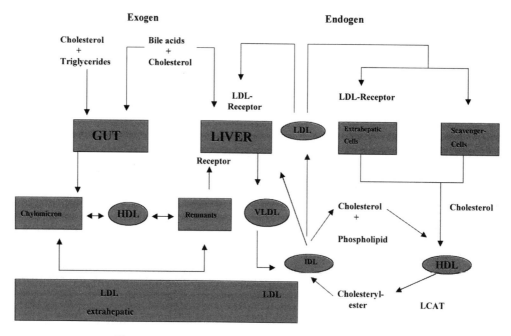

Figure 1 Schematic pathway of lipids and lipoprotein.

considerable differences in the effect of diet on the levels of plasma lipoproteins.

Intervention studies in adults have clearly shown that lowering blood cholesterol levels is associated with a reduction of coronary heart disease. This association has not yet been found in children; most probably it will be very difficult to carry out a study to establish a direct scientific evidence for this relation.

Thus, several indirect data are available to support the hypothesis, which means that lowering of elevated plasma lipoproteins, mainly LDL cholesterol, is indicated even in the pediatric age group.

First, there is clear evidence that early coronary atherosclerosis often begins in childhood and adolescence and is directly related to high serum total cholesterol, LDL cholesterol, VDL cholesterol, and low HDL levels.

Second, children and adolescents from families with a higher incidence of premature coronary heart diseases often have elevated total cholesterol and LDL cholesterol levels.

Third, there is a strong familial aggregation of total, LDL, and HDL cholesterol levels in children and their parents.

Finally, among the genetically based disorders of lipoprotein metabolism, the most common are familial hypercholesterolemia and familial combined hyperlipidemia. In affected families premature cardiovascular diseases are much more frequently diagnosed than in families with desirable cholesterol concentrations.

Lipoprotein disorders are therefore, from a preventive point of view, very important and can be diagnosed in children. This should encourage the enforcement of therapeutic and preventive strategies for the whole family.

III. DEFINITION OF HYPERLIPOPROTEINEMIA/ DYSLIPOPROTEINEMIA

The concentration mainly of total cholesterol and triglycerides in plasma or within the various lipoprotein particles is the basis of laboratory diagnosis of hyperlipidemia or hyperlipoproteinemia. Usually levels exceeding the 95th percentile or below the 5th percentile are considered abnormal. In most studies the Lipid Research Clinics Program (LRCP)-levels were used as reference guidelines for children and adults (Table 2).

According to the Expert Panel on Blood Cholesterol Level in Children and Adolescents of the National Cholesterol Education Program and the American Academy of Pediatrics, children with a parental history of elevated total cholesterol levels (>240 mg/dl) should be tested for their cholesterol levels. Children with other risk factors or with incomplete family history should be screened by the pediatrician.

Children with total cholesterol levels less than 170 mg/dl have optimal levels and do not require intervention. Children with cholesterol levels between 170 and 200 mg/dl should undergo another cholesterol measurement and the two values should be averaged. If this level is greater than 170 mg/dl, a lipid profile is recommended. On the other hand, this expert panel has recommended

Table 1 Lipoprotein Classification

Chylomicrons	
Density (g/ml)	0, 95
Diameter (nm)	75–1200
Origin	Intestine
Chol	5
TG	90
Phospholipids and proteins	5
Very-low-density lipoprotein	
Density (g/ml)	0, 95–1006
Diameter (nm)	30–80
Origin	Liver
Chol	13
TG	65
Phospholipids and proteins	22
Intermediate-density lipoprotein	
Density (g/ml)	1006–1019
Diameter (nm)	25–35
Origin	Liver, VLDL
Chol	35
TG	40
Phospholipids and proteins	25
Low-density lipoprotein	
Density (g/ml)	1019–1063
Diameter (nm)	18–25
Origin	Liver, VLDL, IDL
Chol	43
TG	10
Phospholipids and proteins	47
High-density lipoprotein	
Density (g/ml)	1063–121
Diameter (nm)	5–12
Origin	Liver, intestine, other
Chol	18
TG	2
Phospholipids and proteins	80

that all children with a family history of premature coronary heart disease (before the age of 55 years in a parent or grandparent) should undergo a complete lipoprotein profile.

Thus, the discriminating parameter is the LDL cholesterol concentration: if this is >130 mg/dl, it is considered to be elevated. Levels <110 mg/dl are considered to be acceptable. Levels between 110 and 130 mg/dl are described as borderline.

IV. FAMILIAL HYPERCHOLESTEROLEMIA

This disorder was described as early as 1938 by the Norwegian physician Carl Müller as an inborn error of metabolism, which is characterized by increased blood cholesterol levels and by premature myocardial infarction.

From the genetic and pathophysiological point of view, two major forms can be identified; the heterozygous and the severe homozygous type.

A. Heterozygous

Heterozygous patients are carriers of one mutant of the LDL receptor gene and are found in the general population with a frequency of about 1 in 500. Therefore this disorder is among the most frequent known inborn errors of metabolism. Affected subjects often have approximately doubled LDL cholesterol levels even after birth and experience their first heart attack between the 30th and the 40th year of life. For the clinical diagnosis it is essential to know about related problems (cardiovascular diseases, sudden cardiac death, peripheral vascular disease, hypercholesterolemia).

Children and adolescents with FH commonly do not present any symptoms or signs, thus it is not easy to make an appropriate diagnosis. It is also not easy to involve those subjects in therapeutic programs because they feel completely healthy.

B. Homozygous

Homozygous subjects with FH (prevalence 1:1,000,000) carry two gene mutants from their parents, who both must have hypercholesterolemia. They exhibit a 6–10-fold elevated LDL cholesterol concentration from birth, develop cutaneous and tendinous xanthomas, and suffer fatal heart attacks due to progressive atherosclerosis.

The breakthrough work of Brown and Goldstein showed that subjects heterozygous for FH carry approximately 50% of the LDL receptors in the liver that are responsible for the catabolism of LDL particles. Homozygotes do not have any LDL receptors, or they are not functional.

During the last few years researchers have found many different mutations that are partly responsible for different steps in the uptake of LDL particles. With the use of various techniques it is possible to differentiate between defects on the LDL receptor promotor, the 18 LDL R genexons, the corresponding intron-splice sequences, or the Codon 3500 region where Apo B is located.

So far, no clinical consequences can be drawn from results based on molecular diagnosis. However, preliminary findings indicate that there could be some relation between genotype and phenotype. It could be shown by recent studies that children with total cholesterol and LDL cholesterol levels in the so-called normal range with borderline levels can be diagnosed as being affected with FH on the basis of molecular diagnostic procedures.

V. TREATMENT

The goal of treatment of young subjects with heterozygous FH is to lower elevated LDL cholesterol levels to-

Table 2 Lipid Research Clinics Program Percentile Levels Defining Hyperlipoproteinemia (mg/dl)

	Total triglyceride					Total cholesterol				
	5th	Mean	75th	90th	95th	5th	Mean	75th	90th	95th
Cord	14	34	—	—	84	42	68	—	—	103
1–4 yr										
Male	29	56	68	85	99	114	155	170	190	203
Female	34	64	74	95	112	112	156	173	188	200
5–9 yr										
Male	28	52	58	70	85	125	155	168	183	189
Female	32	64	74	103	126	131	164	176	190	197
10–14 yr										
Male	33	63	74	94	111	124	160	173	188	202
Female	39	72	85	104	120	125	160	171	191	205
15–19 yr										
Male	38	78	88	125	143	118	153	168	183	191
Female	36	73	85	112	126	118	159	176	198	207

	Low-density lipoprotein cholesterol					High-density lipoprotein cholesterol[a]				
	5th	Mean	75th	90th	95th	50th	10th	25th	Mean	95th
Cord	17	29	—	—	50	13	—	—	35	60
1–4 yr										
Male	—	—	—	—	—	—	—	—	—	—
Female	—	—	—	—	—	—	—	—	—	—
5–9 yr										
Male	63	93	103	117	129	38	42	49	56	74
Female	68	100	115	125	140	36	38	47	53	73
10–14 yr										
Male	64	97	109	122	132	37	40	46	55	74
Female	68	97	110	126	136	37	40	45	52	70
15–19 yr										
Male	62	94	109	123	130	30	34	39	46	63
Female	59	96	111	29	137	35	38	43	52	74

[a]Note that different percentiles are listed for HDL cholesterol.

wards a normal range. The cornerstone of therapy is diet, which should be characterized by a low content of saturated fats and an increased content of mainly monounsaturated fats. In general, these diets contain less animal products and more fruits, vegetables, and cereals. They are also recommended for the general population in order to avoid diet-dependent health problems such as obesity, hypertension, and elevated plasma cholesterol levels, among others.

Using such a diet, many of the affected children and adolescents can achieve a lowering of total cholesterol and LDL cholesterol in the range of 10–15%.

In few studies a substitution of soy protein for animal protein has further decreased LDL cholesterol; however, up to now no food-products are available in many coun-

tries in order to enable families to introduce such diets. If the LDL cholesterol level cannot be lowered adequately by dietetic changes (into the range of 130–160 mg/dl), the use of drugs should be carefully considered. In children older than 10 years with high LDL cholesterol levels (>190 mg/dl or >160 mg/dl) and a family history of cardiovascular diseases after a 3–6 month diet period, the administration of bile-acid resins seems to be indicated. These drugs, which are not absorbed from the gastrointestinal tract, are not very palatable and therefore only a few children and adolescents adhere to this type of drug treatment. Reported results range between 15 and 25% LDL cholesterol reduction. Even in children who were placed on these drugs from years, no impairment of growth or development has been observed. However, it would seem advantagous to add mainly fat-soluble vitamin supplements in order to ensure adequate vitamin nutrition.

The use of the widely used statins (inhibitors of the 3-hydroxy-methylglutaryl-COA-reductase), which are the standard drugs for treatment of adults, is restricted to few trials.

These drugs are not generally licensed for subjects under the age of 18 years. However, it has been shown very clearly that even their use over years is not associated with any adverse effects on growth, development, or other variables. Furthermore, no serious side effects have been reported, whereas the LDL cholesterol-lowering effects range between 20 and 35%. These drugs might be also the agents of choice in adolescents with markedly elevated LDL cholesterol levels, because there are no other regimens currently available or on the horizon for the near future. For patients with extremely high LDL cholesterol levels and those with homozygous forms of FH, repeated LDL apheresis can be effective treatment.

In some patients liver transplantation and concomitant liver–heart transplantations have been performed to remove the organ responsible for the metabolic disorder. Gene therapy has been performed in some affected subjects; however, this type of treatment seems to be far from introduction into routine use. It has also not been possible so far to achieve longterm LDL cholesterol reductions.

VI. FAMILIAL COMBINED HYPERLIPIDEMIA

This type of lipoprotein disorder is relatively common (3–5:1,000) and is inherited as an autosomal dominant trait. In affected families different types of hyperlipidemias can be observed. One-third of the subjects present with hypercholesterolemia, one third with isolated hypertriglyceridemia, and one third have both elevated cholesterol and triglyceride levels.

Patients with this disorder usually have LDL particles that are enriched with Apo B, thus estimation of Apo B might differentiate between FCH and the familial hypertriglyceridemia. Subjects with FCH have an increased risk for cardiovascular diseases; however, the risk seems to be lower than in patients with FH.

Treatment consists of institution of a classic low-fat (saturated fats ↓, monounsaturated fats ↑, low cholesterol) diet; in some patients drugs are necessary, in which cases statins and fibrates are commonly used. There are very few reports detailing pediatric patients. Even the diagnosis is not very easy in this age group, because the lipid and lipoprotein pattern is not fully developed, as in adults.

VII. HYPERTRIGLYCERIDEMIA/ CHYLOMICRONEMIA SYNDROME

Familial hypertriglyceridemia, which is characterized by an increased concentration of VLDL particles, presents very rarely in children. If it does, the association with overnutrition and obesity is not uncommon. In such cases reduction in energy intake is important, and the intake of saturated fats should be lowered as well.

Excessive forms of hypertriglyceridemia (former type I or type V hyperlipidemia) are rare and characterized by markedly increased concentrations of triglycerides through the presence of chylomicrons. The lack of lipoprotein-lipase or the activating enzyme (Apo C-II) is responsible for this disorder.

Patients with this disorder often have triglyceride levels of 1000 mg/dl and even higher, which causes a milky plasma. The risk for atherosclerosis is relatively low; however, in some cases pancreatitis can occur as a complication. In some patients a strongly fat-restricted diet can achieve marked reduction of triglycerides, but in many of the affected subjects a sustained lowering of triglycerides cannot be attained. Diets containing MCT are not really established, whereas some attempts with fish oil (w-3-fatty acids) have been made. Drugs are not indicated for treatment of patients.

REFERENCES

1. PDAY Research Group: Natural history of aortic and coronary atherosclerotic lesions in Youth. Findings from the PDAY Study. Atheroscler Thromb 1993; 13:1291–1298.
2. Strong JP, Malcolm GT, McMahan CA, et al. Prevalence and extent of atherosclerosis in adolescents and young adults. Implications for Prevention from the Pathobiological Determinants of atherosclerosis in Youth Study. JAMA 199; 281:727–735.
3. American Academy of Pediatrics. Committee on Nutrition. Cholesterol in childhood. Pediatrics 1998; 101:141–147.
4. Hooper L, Summerbell CD, Higgins JPT, et al. Dietary fat intake and prevention of cardiovascular disease: systematic review. Br Med J 2001; 322:757–763.
5. Kwiterovich PO Jr. Identification and treatment of heterozygous familial hypercholesterolemia in children and adolescents. Am J Cardiol 1993; 72:30B–37B.
6. Williams RR, Hunt SC, Schumacher C, et al. Diagnosing heterozygous familial hypercholesterolemia using new practical criteria validated by molecular genetics. Am J Cardiol 1993; 72:171–176.
7. Assouline L, Levy E, Feoli-Fonseca JC, et al: Familial hypercholesterolemia: molecular, biochemical, and clinical characterization of a French-Canadian Pediatric Population. Pediatrics 1995; 96:239–246.
8. Griffin TC, Christoffer KK, Brians HJ, et al. Family history evaluation as a predictive screen for childhood hypercholesterolemia. Pediatrics 1989; 884:365–373.
9. Nissen HK, Guldberg P, Hansen AB, et al. Clinically applicable mutation screening in familial hypercholesterolemia. Human Mutat 1996; 8:168–177.
10. Tonstad S. A rational approach to treating hypercholesterolemia in children. Drug Safety 1997; 16:330–341.
11. Widhalm K, Brazda G, Schneider B, et al. Effect of soy protein diet versus standard low fat, low cholesterol diet on lipid and lipoprotein levels in children with familial or polygenic hypercholesterolemia. J Pediatr 1993; 123:30–34.

12. Stein EA,, Illingworth DR, Kwiterovich PO Jr, et al. Efficacy and safety of lovastatin in adolescent males with heterozygous familial hypercholesterolemia. A randomized controlled trial. JAMA 1999; 281:137–144.

13. The Writing Group for the DISC collaborative Research Group. Efficacy and safety of lowering dietary intake of fat cholesterol in children with elevated low-density lipoprotein cholesterol. JAMA 1995; 273:1429–1435.

14. Widhalm K, Koch S, Pakosta R, et al. Serum lipids, lipoproteins and apolipoproteins in children with and without family history of premature coronary heart disease. J Am Coll Nutr 1992; 11:32s–35s.

15. Cortner JA, Coates PM, Liacomas CA, et al. Familial combined hyperlipidemia in children: clinical expression, metabolic defects, and management. J Pediatr 1993; 123:177–184.

36

Endocrine Disorders After Cancer Therapy

Raphaël Rappaport and Elisabeth Thibaud
Hôpital Necker–Enfants Malades, Paris, France

I. INTRODUCTION

Advances in the treatment of malignant diseases have resulted in a dramatic fall in mortality rates for most of them, which means that an increasing number of survivors may have to cope with the late effects of cancer treatment. The protocols used include surgery, tumor-targeted radiotherapy, chemotherapy, and total-body irradiation and/or intensive chemotherapy followed by bone marrow transplantation. There has now been a sufficient follow-up interval for most conditions and for the current therapeutic regimens, so that most children can be followed with a prospective view of most potential complications. Appropriate therapeutic decisions can therefore be taken to avoid or minimize severe complications such as dwarfism or abnormal pubertal development. Although the primary goal is still to cure the malignant disease, knowledge of the side effects of treatment should contribute to the choice of any new therapeutic protocol.

According to the British National Registry of Childhood Tumors, acute leukemias, mostly lymphoblastic leukemias occurring in early childhood, account for one-third of all registrations. Lymphomas, most frequently non-Hodgkin's type, account for a further 10% with a higher incidence in late childhood. Brain and spinal tumors make up 25% of all tumors, and retinoblastoma, which is often bilateral and familial, is a major condition requiring cranial irradiation in infants. Most of these tumors require high dosages of radiation, which severely damage the hypothalamus and pituitary gland. The remaining childhood cancers include gonadal, bone and soft tissue sarcomas, and embryonal tumors, such as Wilms' tumors and neuroblastoma (1).

Because most children with malignant diseases are treated according to nationally or internationally driven protocols in pediatric oncology centers, it has now become clear that the most constructive evaluation and follow-up of survivors might be undertaken by a combined endocrinology and oncology clinic. Most treatment protocols combine chemotherapy and irradiation, but chemotherapy is becoming an important and sometimes exclusive form of treatment for many conditions. It is therefore important to consider the detailed structure of a given treatment for each child, focusing on the location of the radiation fields causing direct damage to endocrine glands or to the skeleton, and on the use of cytotoxic chemotherapy that could be responsible for direct damage to the gonads (Table 1). In general, the time at which the late endocrine effects may occur is variable.

II. GROWTH

Growth depends on growth hormone secretion and the timing of puberty but also on a number of factors unrelated to pituitary deficiency, such as chemotherapy, associated acute and chronic disease effects, and exposure of cartilage plates to irradiation, as seen in children with spinal or total-body irradiation. Spontaneous growth after cranial irradiation is shown in Figure 1.

A. After High-Dosage Cranial Irradiation

Radiation doses in excess of 3000 cGy reduce final height in most children. The height loss is progressive, reaching about 1 standard deviation (SD) before puberty and 2 SD at final height. Growth retardation develops more rapidly, within 2 years, in patients given 4500 cGy or more. Bone age is delayed, and typical features of GH deficiency may appear in prepubertal patients (2).

B. After Low-Dosage Cranial Irradiation

Variable patterns of growth have been reported. Typically, there is a moderate height reduction during the acute phase of the disease and the associated induction chemotherapy. This is followed by a subnormal or normal

Table 1 Targets Critical to Growth According to Irradiation Protocols

	Cranial	Craniospinal	Total body
Growth hormone[a]	++	++	+
Sex steroids[b]	+	+	+
Thyroid hormone[b]	+	++	++
Skeleton		++	+

[a]Hypothalamic and pituitary defect.
[b]Primary and/or secondary defects according to radiation protocols.

growth rate until puberty. An additional height loss of 1 SD may occur during puberty (2). A few patients have shown normal growth after irradiation, despite a GH deficiency (3). The overall mean loss in adult height in patients treated with cranial doses of 1800–2400 cGy varies from 0.9 to 1.4 SD (4–6). Final short stature is more likely to occur after intensive induction chemotherapy in children irradiated at a younger age, if puberty began earlier, and in patients with familial short stature. Because GH deficiency remains the prime candidate as a cause of growth retardation, all children should be tested for GH secretion before and at onset of puberty if they demonstrate a significant decrease in linear growth. This issue is even more critical in patients, most frequently girls, presenting with sexual precocity. These irradiated patients are prone to obesity in the long-term with increased circulating leptin levels independent of GH status (7).

C. After Spinal or Total-Body Irradiation

Some protocols include extensive skeletal irradiation, and these patients are exposed to more severe and early

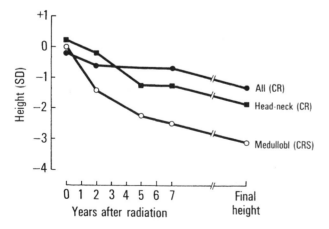

Figure 1 Mean prepubertal height changes after cranial and craniospinal irradiation and final heights in patients treated for leukemia, head and neck tumors, or medulloblastoma. (From Ref. 61.)

growth retardation. One group of patients includes those given spinal irradiation (generally 2400 cGy) in addition to cranial irradiation for medulloblastoma. They may lose up to 2 SD of height within 2 years following irradiation and have a mean final height loss of 2–3 SD, with a short upper segment largely attributed to the lack of spinal growth (8, 9). Children irradiated before age 6 years are more severely affected. Some degree of reduced spinal growth and disproportion also occurs after whole-abdomen or, more rarely, after flank irradiation, as performed for abdominal malignancies, such as Wilms' tumors (10). Total-body irradiation as conditioning for bone marrow transplantation is another therapy that leads to growth retardation unrelated to GH deficiency. It is increasingly used as the ultimate therapy in leukemia and in some nonmalignant diseases (11, 12). The outcome of growth in these patients depends on the radiation dosage and its fractionation (13). An immediate growth retardation is observed in patients given a single 1000 cGy dose. The more recent protocols with fractionated doses of 800–1000 cGy have little impact on short-term growth. Final height has been reported to decrease by 1 SD with diminished sitting height. GH deficiency was found in 30% of these patients, with some improvement in GH production over the years (14).

Difference in treatment protocols may explain some discrepancy among reported data. Other factors such as prolonged corticosteroid therapy, renal failure, and chronic graft-vs.-host disease may also contribute to growth retardation. The frequency and severity of GH deficiency depend on the radiation protocols, and GH may not play a major role in the growth disturbance of these patients (13, 15–17). Growth retardation may be caused by several factors, the most important being direct skeletal irradiation, so that the contribution of GH deficiency to a decreased growth rate remains difficult to assess. In adult long-term survivors serum insulin-like growth factor 1 (IGF-1) values were only partly correlated with GH secretion. Normal IGF-1 levels were found in contrast with evidence of GH deficiency (18, 19) and could be explained by increased adiposity. Primary thyroid insufficiency occurs in most patients given total-body irradiation. Elevated plasma TSH appears within 2 years, but fewer than 10% of patients have overt hypothyroidism. Most boys and girls irradiated before puberty develop primary gonadal failure with elevated luteinizing hormone (LH) and follicle-stimulating hormone (FSH) levels. Delayed or absence of sex steroid secretion then contributes to growth retardation at the age of puberty and requires replacement therapy.

D. After Chemotherapy

The effect of chemotherapy on growth is difficult to assess because many factors, such as differences among protocols, infection, poor nutrition, and the disease itself, may play a role. These patients do not develop GH deficiency after treatment by chemotherapy alone, but the moderate, early growth retardation, as reported in children also irradiated for leukemia (20) or cranial tumors (9), may be related to the induction chemotherapy and caused by a transient insensitivity to growth hormone (21). However, a recent study showed that the final height of patients treated for leukemia with chemotherapy alone was normal (6). There may even be catch-up growth in immunodeficient growth-retarded children after preparative chemotherapy for bone marrow transplantation (13). Because some data still suggest that chemotherapy has a moderately detrimental effect on growth (5), follow-up of all patients remains necessary. However, growth is unlikely to be a critical issue in nonirradiated patients.

III. PUBERTY

A surprising finding is that children who have received cranial irradiation may present with early or true precocious puberty (22, 23). This is in contrast with the delayed puberty usually accompanying idiopathic GH deficiency. Early puberty occurred in girls after cranial irradiation for leukemia, and the children who had been irradiated when very young tended to have the earliest puberty (24, 25). This is an important consideration because of the risk of excessive bone maturation and early epiphyseal closure. It also tends to narrow the window of opportunity to treat with human growth hormone (hGH) before secretion of sex steroids. Puberty not only occurs earlier but it is shortened with early menarche (26). The final height loss may even be more severe if full-blown precocious puberty is associated with untreated GH deficiency. In patients with optic glioma presenting with precocious puberty at the time of irradiation, the persistence of a normal growth rate within 1 or 2 years after cranial radiation may be misinterpreted, and excessive progression of bone age will lead to early cessation of growth. Growth hormone testing is then necessary 1 year after irradiation to unmask any associated GH deficiency and allow GH therapy to begin (27).

In contrast, gonadotropin deficiency may develop within a few years after high-dosage cranial radiation for tumors, as indicated by arrested puberty, primary amenorrhea in girls, and absence of LH and FSH response to an LH-releasing hormone (LHRH) stimulation test (28). Some girls suffer only from menstrual irregularities, and their impact on fertility has not been documented. Gonadotropin deficiency is usually associated with GH deficiency and moderate hyperprolactinemia, a combination indicating multiple hypothalamic pituitary deficiencies.

IV. GROWTH HORMONE SECRETION

The first case of induced hypopituitarism after cranial radiation for a tumor distant from the hypothalamic–pituitary region was reported in 1966 (29). Growth hormone deficiency is at present the most common pituitary defect occurring after radiation (Table 2). The hypothalamus is more radiosensitive than the pituitary gland, so that GH deficiency is probably caused by a dysfunction of GH-releasing hormone (LHRH) somatostatin control. This may explain the differences observed between spontaneous and pharmacologically stimulated GH secretion, as well as the persistence of normal GH responses to the GHRH stimulation test (31, 33). Experimental studies in monkeys (32) and the changes observed in the other anterior pituitary functions in adult patients (33) support such a hypothesis. The severity and frequency of pituitary defects vary according to the initial disease and its specific therapeutic regimens, but the radiation dosage effectively delivered to the hypothalamic–pituitary region defines the risk factor. It depends on the total dosage, the number of fractions, and the duration of treatment: a given dose delivered in a shorter time period is more likely to cause GH deficiency than one delivered over a long period (2, 34). Assessment of GH secretion requires a pharmacological GH stimulation test (35). If growth is retarded despite normal GH peak responses, it has been suggested that one

Table 2 Endocrine Abnormalities After External Cranial Irradiation in Patients Evaluated at Least 4 Years After Irradiation[a]

Cause	Cases (n)	Frequency of cases with endocrine abnormality (%)				
		GH deficiency		Thyroid[b]	ACTH	LHRH[c]
		Complete	Partial			
Leukemia, 24 Gy	86	30	22	2	0	3
Face and neck tumors, 25–45 Gy	56	46	22	35	7	16
Medulloblastoma, 25–45 Gy	59	52	24	47	8	20
Optic glioma, 45–55 Gy	39	77	23	46	3	40

[a]Expressed as percentage of affected cases in each patient group. GH deficiency; complete, after stimulation, GH peak <5 ng/ml; partial, 5–8 ng/ml. ACTH, adrenocorticotropic hormone.
[b]Includes elevated plasma TSH after direct thyroid irradiation.
[c]LH/FSH deficiency or precocious puberty. Evaluated in patients reaching pubertal age. Does not include primary gonadal failure.
Source: From Ref. 2.

should measure the spontaneous GH secretion during the night. If the later is subnormal, one may consider a partial GH deficiency. This condition has been described as GH neurosecretory dysfunction, and may essentially occur after low-dosage irradiation (36). Plasma IGF-1 measurement is a convenient screening method: in patients irradiated with doses higher than 3000 cGy, IGF-1 values correlated with spontaneous GH secretion (18). However, normal IGF-1 concentrations may be observed in patients with partial GH deficiency after low-dosage cranial irradiation (19). The level of IGF-1 is therefore difficult to interpret since many of these patients are moderately obese (37). Repeated GH testing may be necessary is some cases before GH deficiency is diagnosed, in patients treated with low-dosage radiation. In any case, GH responses and IGF-1 values must be interpreted according to the pubertal status of the patient (2).

GH deficiency occurs in about 75% of children treated with cranial doses between 3000 and 4500 cGy. All children irradiated with higher dosages are affected and eventually develop panhypopituitarism. The greater the radiation dosage, the earlier the GH deficiency develops, with intervals ranging from 1 year in patients irradiated with 4000 cGy for cranial tumors to more than 4 years in leukemic patients (2). The age at time of cranial irradiation is another important risk factor: younger children are more vulnerable (38). It is therefore recommended that cranial irradiation be delayed whenever possible until the child is over 3 years old. Children treated for acute leukemia with radiation doses of 2400 cGy or less do not always develop GH deficiency, and the deficiency may be restricted to the pubertal period (39). Whereas complete GH deficiency is not reversible, the long-term outcome of partial GH deficiency, as observed in patients treated with low-dosage cranial irradiation, is not firmly established. This may be partly because of difficulties in quantitatively assessing GH secretion (30). The anterior pituitary function should nevertheless be re-evaluated in these patients after adolescence to provide a reference for further follow-up during adulthood.

After total-body irradiation preparing for bone marrow transplantation, the risk of GH deficiency depends on the radiation protocol (13, 15, 17, 40). A single dose of 1000 cGy, less commonly used, generally impairs GH secretion. Doses over 700 cGy, even fractionated, induce a 50% risk of GH deficiency. Generally there seems to be no correlation between GH secretion and growth, at least during the first few years following irradiation (13). This is not surprising, because many other causative factors may play a role.

V. THYROID

The reported incidence of central hypothyroidism after cranial irradiation depends on the diagnostic criteria since most patients do not develop overt clinical hypothyroid-ism. Even low free T4 (FT4) with normal or low thyroid-stimulating hormone (TSH) is observed in only a small percentage of patients, in the high-risk group (2). In a recent study, because of the lack of overt clinical presentation, the incidence of TSH dysregulation was assessed by combining three criteria: basal FT4, TSH response to thyrotropin-releasing hormone (TRH), and nocturnal TSH surge. Using such sensitive biological criteria it was shown that 92% of the patients with central hypothyroidism would have remained undiagnosed by evaluation of baseline thyroid function tests alone. In patients treated with 3000 cGy or more or total-body irradiation its frequency reached 39%; after lower-dosage radiation the percentage was decreased to 8%, by 10 years after tumor diagnosis (41). Mixed central and primary hypothyroidism is expected to occur if the thyroid was also irradiated. The TSH deficiency may occur even before GH deficiency, although undiagnoscd by thc conventional insensitive tests (41) (Table 2).

The incidence of central hypothyroidism is related to the total radiation dose. Chemotherapy with busulfan and cyclophosphamide may exacerbate the effects of irradiation. Transient hypothyroidism has also been reported during induction chemotherapy with L-asparaginase (42). The issue of latent central hypothyroidism is complex. One may consider that it should be treated with L-thyroxine to optimize spontaneous or hGH-treated growth as well as intellectual and school performance of affected children. More studies are needed to evaluate replacement therapy in these cases. Primary hypothyroidism due to direct thyroid irradiation is diagnosed by TSH elevation. It is found in patients irradiated for Hodgkin's disease or after craniospinal irradiation. Hyperfractionation of radiation therapy lowers its incidence in the long term (43).

The risk of benign nodules or thyroid cancer in later adult life is increased after radiation of the neck. Because low-dosage thyroid radiation exposure (up to 500 cGy) is a known cause of neoplasm, both head and neck therapeutic irradiation must be considered as a risk factor. Although most data are derived from patients treated for Hodgkin's disease (44), children given spinal or total-body irradiation should also be evaluated through adulthood. Ultrasonography of the thyroid is more sensitive than physical palpation. However, it is so sensitive and nodules are so prevalent in the normal population that great caution is needed in interpreting the results. Serum thyroglobulin levels correlate with the number of nodules (45). Surgery is a difficult decision. Therefore, it is important to inform all patients of the need for prolonged follow-up. It has been suggested that thyroxine therapy, at dosages that suppress TSH secretion, would help avoid recurrence after surgery of nodules (33).

VI. GONADAL AND REPRODUCTIVE FUNCTION

Risk factors for gonadal toxicity include local irradiation, type and dosage of chemotherapy, age, pubertal status, and gender of the patient (Table 3). There are important differences between male and female gametogenesis and its relationship to gonadal endocrine function.

A. Girls

The ovocyte during postnatal life is resistant to chemotherapy. However, if ovocytes are damaged or destroyed by anticancer therapy, reduction in their number results in absence of puberty or, at a later age, in temporary or permanent cessation of ovulation with shortening of the reproductive period.

Chemotherapy-related damage to the ovary depends on the drug, its dosage, and age of the patient: gonadotoxic effects increase with age. They are minimal in prepubertal girls who have a greater reserve of germ cells and primary follicles. Alkylating agents, such as cyclophosphamide at a total dosage greater than 20 g or 500 mg/kg (46) and high-dosage busulfan permanently suppress ovarian function. Combination chemotherapy regimens have generally less effect on ovarian function in adolescent girls than in adult women. However, little is known about ovarian damage in prepubertal girls: if treated for leukemia a favorable outcome was reported (26, 47, 48). In Hodgkin's disease mechlorethamine, oncovin (vincristine), procarbazine, prednisone (MOPP) and mechlorethamine, vinblastine, procarbazine, prednisone

Table 3 Current Chemotherapy Agents Cytotoxic for the Testis and Ovary

Chemotherapy	Disease
Alkylating agents	
Cyclophosphamide	Lymphoblastic leukemia
	Non-Hodgkin's lymphoma
	Various tumors
Ifosfamide	Soft tissue tumors
	Ewing sarcoma
	Nephroblastoma
Melphalan	Bone marrow transplantation
Busulfan	Bone marrow transplantation
	Chronic myeloid leukemia
Dacarbazine (DTIC)	Soft tissue tumors
Carmustine (BCNU)	Hodgkin's disease
	Brain tumors
Lomustine (CCNU)	Hodgkin's disease
Semustine (methyl-CCNU)	Brain tumors
Other agents	
Cytarabine (cytosine arabinoside)	Lymphoblastic leukemia
Vincristine	Various tumors
Vinblastine (VLB)	Hodgkin's disease
Procarbazine	Hodgkin's disease
Cisplatin (cis-DDP)	Various tumors

(MVPP) regimens, which induce a high incidence of transient or permanent amenorrhea in adults, have little effect on ovarian function in girls providing they did not undergo additional pelvic irradiation (49, 50). In contrast, a favorable outcome was reported after Adriamycin (doxorubicin), bleomycin, vinblastine, dacarbazine (ABVD) regimen (51).

Ovarian function may be severely impaired by irradiation with fractionated doses over 700 cGy, with complete destruction of the ovocytes at 2000 cGy (52) as used in patients treated for abdominal, pelvic, or genital tumors, and Hodgkin's disease. Primary ovarian dysfunction may also occur in patients who received spinal irradiation with scattered irradiation to the ovaries (53). Ovarian transposition before abdominal irradiation has been shown to protect patients from ovarian failure if performed before puberty (54).

Total body irradiation (TBI) as conditioning for bone marrow transplantation induces a high risk of ovarian failure. Permanent and total damage to the ovary occurs in girls given high dosages of busulfan, often associated with cyclophosphamide (55, 56). In contrast, chemotherapy regimens excluding busulfan have a favorable outcome. Young age at TBI and fractionated irradiation are associated with increased ovarian recovery. However, the time required for recovery may vary up to 7 (57) or 10 years (58). Transient increase in plasma gonadotropins, and ultimate recovery, were observed in 35% of the girls treated with TBI for leukemia (59). When estrogen replacement therapy is given, it should therefore be stopped periodically to detect any ovarian recovery.

Future fertility is the main issue in these patients. The prospects for normal fertility are favorable in girls treated with nonintensive chemotherapy for leukemia (60, 61) or with nitrosureas for brain and spinal tumors. There is a poor correlation between plasma gonadotropin levels and fertility: amenorrheic girls with persistently elevated plasma gonadotropins may become pregnant. Presently there is no evidence, in spite of favorable animal studies, that suppression of gonadal activity during anticancer therapy decreases the risk of gonadal toxicity.

In a recent study, a global fertility deficit of 23% was observed in women treated during childhood with alkylating agents and abdominal–pelvic irradiation with large variations according to treatment regimens (62). Radiation is the most deleterious factor. It also damages the uterus and its vascularization, which may result in a high frequency of miscarriages or premature births with a higher frequency in girls receiving TBI before puberty (56, 60, 63). These lesions are more severe when girls were treated in early childhood (64, 65). There is no increased frequency of congenital malformations. Because of uterine atrophy, as shown by reduced uterine length and endometrial thickness at ultrasound examination, some women are also unlikely to benefit from in vitro fertilization with donor ovocytes (66). Estrogen replacement therapy may be inadequate to generate normal uterine growth (67).

Strategies to preserve fertility are available: ovarian tissue cryopreservation is being adopted by expert centers. However, there is no evidence of its ultimate efficacy in humans (68) despite favorable reports in experimental studies (69).

Clinical evaluation of ovarian activity is easy in cases with complete gonadal failure. It is less precise in patients with secondary amenorrhea with elevated FSH and LH plasma concentrations. The latter may be the only sign of ovarian dysfunction observed during posttreatment follow-up. Estrogen and progesterone replacement therapy is necessary to feminize these patients fully and allow normal pubertal growth. However, breast atrophy may result from scattered irradiation after whole abdominal or flank irradiation performed before puberty. It may require cosmetic surgery for correction (64).

B. Boys

The germinal epithelium is more sensitive to irradiation than Leydig cells. In prepubertal boys local doses between 300 and 1000 cGy, as delivered during abdominal or low spinal irradiation (craniospinal irradiation may result in a scattered dose to the gonad), induce a transient or permanent rise in serum FSH at time of puberty with later oligospermia or azoospermia and reduced testicular volume (70). Germ cell dysfunction occurs after total body irradiation, single or fractionated, with a high risk of azoospermia (59). Recovery of germ cell function is rare, even more so after fractionated irradiation (71). When irradiated during puberty, similar data were reported; recovery of gametogenesis is not assured and may occur years later.

Chemotherapy is essentially aggressive to germ cells. It includes alkylating agents, procarbazine, vinblastine, cytarabin, and cisplastin (Table 3). Except for the very aggressive intensive cytotoxic chemotherapy with high dosages of cyclophosphamide or busulfan, there are remarkable individual variations that may not be predictable and long-term follow-up is necessary. The elevation of serum FSH is consistent with germinal damage (72). Each regimen used in the management of a given cancer should be evaluated for its potential harm to the gonads. For instance, the effects of cyclophosphamide on sperm density are proportional to the dosage given before adulthood (73). A total dosage of 200 mg/kg or more is followed by evidence of germ cell damage, probably more extensive if treated after the onset of puberty; the prognosis of fertility is poor in most patients (74). Combination chemotherapy (such as MOPP or MVPP to treat Hodgkin's disease), regimens are generally more gonadotoxic than individual agents. Therefore, new regimens with low gonadal toxicity are being developed (75).

The Leydig cell function, in general, is preserved. Testosterone secretion and pubertal development are normal following local irradiation with doses inferior to 2000 cGy or total body irradiation although elevated serum LH with normal testosterone values may be observed in some cases. Only males who received high-dosage testicular irradiation after one leukemia relapse experience testicular failure and require androgen replacement therapy (76).

VII. OTHER ENDOCRINE COMPLICATIONS

Deficiency in adrenocorticotrophic hormone (ACTH) and secondary adrenal insufficiency with clinical symptoms are rare complications that occur after high doses of cranial radiation for the treatment of brain tumors. In children this may cause hypoglycemia if combined with severe GH deficiency. It may occur as early as the first 2 years after radiotherapy (33). If early morning plasma cortisol levels are low and do not respond to insulin-induced hypoglycemia, hydrocortisone replacement therapy is required.

Hyperprolactinemia (usually below 100 ng/ml) after high-dosage cranial irradiation occurs during adolescence or adulthood without any clinical expression. It is an additional indicator of hypothalamic damage (33).

Cranial irradiation is never accompanied by posterior pituitary dysfunction. Calcium homeostasis remains normal although primary hyperparathyroidism had been reported to rarely occur after low-dosage neck irradiation. There is no reported evidence of primary endocrine pancreas or adrenal dysfunction after abdominal irradiation.

VIII. FOLLOW-UP AND MANAGEMENT

Long-term assessment of oncology patients is required for growth, puberty, fertility, and other late endocrine complications. Adult endocrinologists should now focus on GH-deficiency-related symptoms, obesity, bone mineral density decrease, intellectual cognitive functions, and sexual life of the survivors. Regular checkups are necessary to decide upon replacement treatment.

A. Growth Hormone Replacement Therapy

It is easy to decide after cranial irradiation for brain and facial tumors because GH therapy is generally severe. Recombinant growth hormone given at the usual dosage of 0.1 iv/kg/day (about 0.025 mg/kg/day) produces a significant improvement in growth rate. According to earlier reports, the long-term results and final heights achieved have been disappointing (77–79). One factor may have had negative effects when compared with patients with idiopathic GH deficiency: some patients had early or precocious puberty, which accelerated the skeletal maturation more quickly than the increase in growth rate. Failure to catch up with normal height may also have been related to low hGH dosage in some studies. It is therefore essential to commence hGH therapy as soon as GH deficiency and growth retardation are documented, but preferably not less than 2 years after the primary treatment, except for severe cases.

This issue is more complex in patients treated for

leukemia with low dosages of cranial irradiation. In this group GH therapy should be started before puberty only if the height loss exceeds 1 SD, because some patients maintain normal growth rates for several years until puberty despite a GH deficiency, and at time of onset of puberty if short stature and severe GH deficiency predict significant adult height loss. Again, early or precocious puberty is an additional risk factor of short stature. LHRH analog therapy should then be considered in association with the hGH treatment. In this group of patients most authors restrict the use of hGH and/or LHRH analog therapy to GH-deficient patients most at risk of final short stature because of familial short stature, cranial irradiation at a younger age, and/or early puberty. Whatever the cranial radiation dosage, those who have received additional spinal irradiation have a poor response to hGH treatment (79, 80). The same suboptimal growth response occurs after high-dosage total-body irradiation.

In patients with cranial irradiation, there is now sufficient evidence that growth can be improved by hGH therapy. Combination with LHRH analog allows these patients to reach height in the normal range, although frequently lower than calculated target height (81, 82). Reduced final height remains a critical problem in patients with craniospinal or total body irradiation.

One major concern is the potential oncogenic effect of hGH treatment. However, there is at present no evidence that hGH promotes leukemia or tumor relapse (83). A high rate of secondary malignancies has been reported in children treated before age of 3 years with alkylating agents and etoposide with or without irradiation (84). Continuation of GH therapy after final height is reached is being evaluated. These adults are often obese, with poor physical performance. However, the need for prolonged hGH therapy in adulthood may be questionable in patients who do not show profound GH deficiency. Reduced trabecular and cortical bone mineral density after cranial irradiation was observed during chemotherapy and does not seem to be correlated with the GH status. It requires follow-up in later life and appropriate intervention (85).

B. Other Issues

At present, GH replacement therapy with conventional doses is well defined and other issues should be given priority in the long term and according to the oncology therapy. Thyroid nodules occur after many years. Gonadal failure requires replacement therapy. Risk of damage to fertility can be anticipated but long-term evaluations are still necessary in patients of both genders. Skeletal dysplasia may be secondary to irradiation and appropriate replacement sex steroid therapy is necessary to minimize loss of bone mineral density. On all issues parents and patients should be warned and helped in order to face potential problems after cure of the cancer.

C. Intellectual and Neuropsychological Risks

The risk of intellectual dysfunction has been recognized for a long time and a comprehensive analysis was provided by Duffner (86) in the early 1990s. With the protocols followed at that time, precise conclusions were presented. The most important variable was age at time of diagnosis and treatment: children younger than 3 years had significantly lower IQs than patients treated at older ages. This led practitioners to postpone cranial irradiation and to treat with postoperative chemotherapy in an attempt to delay radiation until the children could better tolerate its effects. A second risk factor is large-volume irradiation, with significant changes in IQ scores documented after whole-brain irradiation. The dosage of radiation that produces neuropsychological sequelae is not precisely known.

More recent studies have shown that only-chemotherapy protocols among leukemic children had modest late effects on nonverbal cognitive skills, particularly among girls (87). However, sequelae including language and education disabilities were reported when leukemic children received cranial irradiation (24 cGy or 18 cGy) (88). Impaired academic achievement was reported as well after central nervous system (CNS) chemotherapy prophylaxis in these patients. More recent studies have shown that only-chemotherapy protocols among leukemic children had modest late effects on nonverbal cognitive skills, particularly among girls.

Children with medulloblastoma treated with irradiation at high dosages most frequently show severe neuropsychological deficit, requiring specific support (89). Over time, deficits in nonverbal and information processing skills may increase (90).

Survivors of pediatric bone marrow transplantation are being more precisely evaluated and a recent study concluded that with or without TBI, bone marrow transplantation entails minimal neurocognitive sequelae in patients who are 6 years of age or older at therapy (91). Because there is a significant incidence of learning disabilities after cranial irradiation, early and appropriate monitoring of cognitive skills may improve the neurocognitive future of these patients.

REFERENCES

1. Stiller CA. Aetiology and epidemiology. In: Plowman PN, Pinkerton CR, eds. Paediatric Oncology. Clinical Practice and Controversies. London: Chapman and Hall Medical, 1992: 1–24.
2. Rappaport R, Brauner R. Growth and endocrine disorders secondary to cranial irradiation. Pediatr Res 1989; 25:561–567.
3. Shalet SM, Price DA, Beardwell CG, Morris Jones PH, Pearson D. Normal growth despite abnormalities of growth hormone secretion in children treated for acute leukemia. J Pediatr 1979; 94:719–722.

4. Schriock EA, Schell MJ, Carter M, Hustu O, Ochs JJ. Abnormal growth patterns and adult short stature in 115 long-term survivors of childhood leukemia. J Clin Oncol 1991; 9:400–405.

5. Sklar C, Mertens A, Walter A, et al. Final height after treatment for childhood acute lymphoblastic leukemia: comparison of no cranial irradiation with 1800 and 2400 centigrays of cranial irradiation. J Pediatr 1993; 123:59–64.

6. Katz JA, Pollock BH, Jacaruso D, Morad A. Final attained height in patients successfully treated for childhood acute lymphoblastic leukemia. J Pediatr 1993; 123:546–552.

7. Birkebaek NH, Fisker S, Clauseu N, Tuovinen V, Sindet-Pedersen S, Christiansen JS. Growth and endocrinological disorders up to 21 years after treatment for acute lymphoblastic leukemia in childhood. Med Pediatr Oncol 1998; 30(6):351–356.

8. Shalet SM, Gibson B, Swindell R, et al. Effect of spinal irradiation on growth. Arch Dis Child 1987; 62:461–464.

9. Brauner R, Rappaport R, Prevot C, et al. A prospective study of the development of GH in children given cranial irradiation, and its relation to statural growth. J Clin Endocrinol Metab 1989; 68:346–351.

10. Wallace WHB, Shalet SM, Morris Jones PH, et al. Effect of abdominal irradiation on growth in boys treated for a Wilms' tumour. Med Pediatr Oncol 1990; 18:441–446.

11. Borton MM, Rimm AA. Increasing utilization of bone marrow transplantation. Transplantation 1986; 42:229–234.

12. Sanders JE, Pritchard S, Mahoney P, et al. Growth and development following marrow transplantation for leukemia. Blood 1986; 68:1129–1135.

13. Brauner R, Fontoura M, Zucker JM, et al. Growth and growth hormone secretion after bone marrow transplantation. Arch Dis Child 1993; 68:458–463.

14. Holm K, Nysom K, Rasmussen MH, Hertz H, Jacobsen N, Skakkebaek NE, Krabbe S, Müller J. Growth, growth hormone and final height after BMT. Possible recovery of irradiation induced growth hormone insufficiency. Bone Marrow Transplant 1996; 18:163–170.

15. Borgström B, Bolme P. Growth and growth hormone in children after bone marrow transplantation. Horm Res 1988; 30:98–100.

16. Hovi L, Rajantie J, Perkkio M, Sainio K, Sipilä I, Siimes MA. Growth failure and growth hormone deficiency in children after bone marrow transplantation for leukemia. Bone Marrow Transplant 1990; 5:183–186.

17. Ogilvy-Stuart AL, Clark DJ, Wallace WHB, et al. Endocrine deficit after fractionated total body irradiation. Arch Dis Child 1992; 67:1107–1110.

18. Acherman JC, Hindmarsh PC, Brook CG. The relationship between the growth hormone and insulin-like growth factor axis in long-term survivors of childhood brain tumours. Clin Endocrinol (Oxf) 1998; 49:639–645.

19. Tillman V, Shalet SM, Price DA, Wales JKH, Pennells L, Soden J, Gill MS, Whatmore AJ, Clayton PE. Serum insulin-like growth factor-I, IGF binding protein-3 and IGFBP-3 protease activity after cranial irradiation. Horm Res 1998; 50:71–77.

20. Kirk JA, Raghupathy P, Stevens MM, et al. Growth failure and growth hormone deficiency after treatment for acute lymphoblastic leukemia. Lancet 1987; 1:190–193.

21. Nivot S, Benelli C, Clot JP, et al. Non parallel changes of GH and IGF-1, IGFBP-3, GHBP, after craniospinal irradiation and chemotherapy. J Clin Endocrinol Metab 1994; 78:597–601.

22. Brauner R, Czernichow P, Rappaport R. Precocious puberty after hypothalamic and pituitary irradiation in young children. N Engl J Med 1984; 311:920.

23. Pasqualini T, Escobar ME, Domene H, Sackmann-Muriel F, Pavlovsky S, Rivarola MA. Evaluation of gonadal function following long-term treatment for acute leukemia in girls. Am J Pediatr Hematol Oncol 1987; 9:15–22.

24. Leiper AD, Stanhope R, Kitching P, Chessels JM. Precocious and premature puberty associated with the treatment of acute lymphoblastic leukaemia. Arch Dis Child 1987; 62:1107–1112.

25. Uruena M, Stanhope R, Chessels JM, Leiper AD. Impaired pubertal growth in acute lymphoblastic leukaemia. Arch Dis Child 1990; 66:1403–1407.

26. Quigley C, Cowell C, Jimenez M, et al. Normal or early development of puberty despite gonadal damage in children treated for acute lymphoblastic leukaemia. N Engl J Med 1989; 321:143–151.

27. Brauner R, Malandry F, Rappaport R, et al. Growth and endocrine disorders in optic glioma. Eur J Pediatr 1990; 149:825–828.

28. Rappaport R, Brauner R, Czernichow P, et al. Effect of hypothalamic and pituitary irradiation on pubertal development in children with cranial tumors. J Clin Endocrinol Metab 1982; 54:1164–1168.

29. Tan BC, Kunaratnam N. Hypopituitarism dwarfism following radiotherapy for nasopharyngeal carcinoma. Clin Radiol 1996; 17:302–304.

30. Blatt J, Bercu BB, Gillin JC, Mendelson WB, Poplack DG. Reduced pulstatile growth hormone secretion in children after therapy for acute lymphoblastic leukemia. J Pediatr 1984; 104:182–186.

31. Crosnier H, Brauner R, Rappaport R. Growth hormone response to growth hormone releasing hormone (hp GHRH 1-44) as an index of growth hormone secretory dysfunction after prophylactic cranial irradiation for acute lymphoblastic leukemia (24 grays). Acta Paediatr Scand 1988; 77:681–687.

32. Chrousos GP, Poplack D, Brown T, O'Neill D, Schwade J, Bercu BB. Effects of cranial radiation on hypothalamic-adenohypophyseal function: abnormal growth hormone secretory dynamics. J Clin Endocrinol Metab 1982; 54:1135–1139.

33. Constine LS, Woolf PD, Cann D, et al. Hypothalamic–pituitary dysfunction after radiation for brain tumors. N Engl J Med 1993; 328:87–94.

34. Shalet SM, Beardwell CG, Pearson D, Morris-Jones PH. The effect of varying doses of cerebral irradiation on growth hormone production in childhood. Clin Endocrinol (Oxf) 1976; 5:287–290.

35. Rose SR, Ross JL, Uriarte M, Barnes KM, Cassorla FG, Cuttler GB. The advantage of measuring stimulated as compared with spontaneous growth hormone levels in the diagnosis of growth hormone deficiency. N Engl J Med 1988; 319:201–207.

36. Bercu BB, Shulman D, Root AW, Spiliotis BE. Growth hormone (GH) provocative testing frequently does not reflect endogenous GH secretion. J Clin Endocrinol Metab 1986; 63:709–716.

37. Davies HA, Didcock E, Didi M, Ogilvy-Stuart A, Wales JKH, Shalet SM. Growth, puberty and obesity after treatment for leukaemia. Acta Paediatr Suppl 1995; 411:45–50.

38. Brauner R, Czernichow P, Rappaport R. Greater susceptibility to hypothalamopituitary irradiation in younger children with acute lymphoblastic leukemia. J Pediatr 1986; 108:332.

39. Moell C, Garwicz S, Westgren U, Wiebe T, Albertsoon-Wikland K. Suppressed spontaneous secretion of growth hormone in girls after treatment for acute lymphoblastic leukemia. Arch Dis Child 1989; 64:252–258.

40. Sanders JE, Buckner CD, Sullivan KM, et al. Growth and development in children after bone marrow transplantation. Horm Res 1988; 30:92–97.

41. Rose SR, Lustig RH, Pitukcheewanont P, Broome DC, Burghen GA, Li H, Hudson MM, Kun LE, Heideman RL. Diagnosis of hidden central hypothyroidism in survivors of childhood cancer. J Clin Endocrinol Metab 1999; 84:4472–4479.

42. Ferster A, Glinoër D, Van Vliet G, Otten J. Thyroid function during L-asparaginase therapy in children with acute lymphoblastic leukemia: difference between induction and late intensification. Am J Pediatr Hematol Oncol 1992; 14:192–196.

43. Oberfield SE, Chin D, Uli N, David R, Sklar C. Endocrine late effects of childhood cancers. J Pediatr 1997; 131:37–41.

44. Schimpff SG, Diggs CH, Wiswell JG, et al. Radiation-related thyroid dysfunction: implications for the treatment of Hodgkin's disease. Ann Intern Med 1980; 92:91–98.

45. Schneider AB, Bekerman C, Leland J, Rosengarten J, Hyun H, Collins B, Shore-Freedman E, Gierlowski TC. Thyroid nodules in the follow-up of irradiated individuals: comparison of thyroid ultrasound with scanning and palpation. J Clin Endocrinol Metab 1997; 82:4020–4027.

46. Sanders JE and the Seattle Marrow Transplant Team. The impact of marrow transplant preparative regimens on subsequent growth and development. Semin Hematol 1991; 28:244–249.

47. Wallace WHB, Shalet SM, Tetlow LJ, Morris Jones PH. Ovarian function following the treatment of childhood acute lymphoblastic leukaemia. Med Pediatr Oncol 1993; 21:333–339.

48. Mills JL, Fears TR, Robison LL, Nicholson HS, Sklar CA, Byrne J. Menarche in a cohort of 188 long-term survivors of acute lymphoblastic leukemia. J Pediatr 1997; 131:598–602.

49. Clark ST, Radford JA, Crowther D, Swindell R, Shalet SM. Gonadal function following chemotherapy for Hodgkin's disease: a comparative study of MVPP and a seven-drug hybrid regimen. J Clin Oncol 1995; 13:134–139.

50. Ortin TT, Shostak CA, Donaldson SS. Gonadal status and reproductive function following treatment for Hodgkin's disease in childhood: the Stanford experience. Int J Radiat Oncol Biol Phys 1990; 19:873–880.

51. Viviani S, Santoro A, Ragni G, Bonfante V, Bestetti O, Bondonna G. Gonadal toxicity after combination chemotherapy for Hodgkin's disease. Comparative results of MOPP vs ABV. Eur J Cancer Clin Oncol 1985; 21:601–605.

52. Wallace WHB, Shalet SM, Hendry JH, et al. Ovarian failure following abdominal irradiation in childhood: the radiosensitivity of the human ovocyte. Br J Radiol 1989; 62:995–998.

53. Livesey EA, Brook CGD. Gonadal dysfunction after treatment of intracranial tumours. Arch Dis Child 1988; 63:495–500.

54. Thibaud E, Ramirez M, Brauner R, et al. Preservation of ovarian function by ovarian transposition performed before pelvic irradiation during childhood. J Pediatr 1992; 121:880–884.

55. Sanders JE, Hawley J, Levy W, et al. Pregnancies following high dose cyclophosphamide with or without high-dose busulfan or total-body irradiation and bone marrow transplantation. Blood 1996; 87:3045–3052.

56. Thibaud E, Rodriguez-Macias K, Trivin C, Esperou H, Michon J, Brauner R. Ovarian function after bone marrow transplantation during childhood. Bone Marrow Transplant 1988; 21:287–290.

57. Sanders JE, Buckner CD, Amos D, et al. Ovarian function following marrow transplantation for aplastic anemia or leukemia. J Clin Oncol 1988; 6:813–818.

58. Spinelli S, Chiodi S, Bacigalupo A, et al. Ovarian recovery after total body irradiation and allogeneic bone marrow transplantation: long-term follow up of 79 females. Bone Marrow Transplant 1994; 14:373–380.

59. Saragoglou K, Boulad F, Gillio A, Sklar C. Gonadal function after bone marrow transplantation for acute leukemia during childhood. J Pediatr 1997; 130:210–216.

60. Byrne J, Mulvihill JJ, Myers MH, et al. Effects of treatment on fertility in long-term survivors of childhood or adolescent cancer. N Engl J Med 1987; 317:1315–1321.

61. Green DM, Hall B, Zevon A. Pregnancy outcome after treatment for acute lymphoblastic leukaemia during childhood or adolescence. Cancer 1989; 64:2335–2339.

62. Chiarelli AM, Marrett LD, Darlington G. Early menopause and infertility in females after treatment for childhood cancer diagnosed in 1964–1988 in Ontario, Canada. Am J Epidemiol 1999; 150:245–254.

63. Li FP, Cambrere K, Gelber RD, et al. Outcome of pregnancy in survivors of Wilms' tumor. JAMA 1987; 257:216.

64. Bath LE, Critchley HOD, Chambers SE, Anderson RA, Kelnar CJH, Wallace WHB. Ovarian and uterine characteristics after total body irradiation in childhood and adolescence: response to sex steroid replacement. Br J Obstet Gynaecol 1999; 106:1265–1272.

65. Critchley HOD. Factors of importance for implantation and problems after treatment for childhood cancer. Med Pediatr Oncol 1999; 33:9–14.

66. Critchely HOD, Wallace WHB, Mamtora H, Higginson J, Shalet SM, Anderson DC. Ovarian failure after whole abdominal radiotherapy: the potential for pregnancy. Br J Obstet Gynaecol 1992; 99:392–394.

67. Holm K, Nysom K, Brocks V, Hertz H, Jacobsen N, Müller J. Ultrasound B-mode changes in the uterus and ovaries and Doppler changes in the uterus after total body irradiation and allogeneic bone marrow transplantation in childhood. Bone Marrow Transplant 1999; 23:259–263.

68. Rutherford AJ, Gosden RG. Ovarian tissue cryopreservation: a practical option? Acta Paediatr Suppl 1999; 88:13–19.

69. Salle B, Lornage J, Demirci B, et al. Restoration of ovarian steroid secretion and histologic assessment after freezing, thawing, and autograft of a hemi-ovary in sheep. Fertil Steril 1999; 72:366–370.

70. Shalet SM, Beardwell CG, Jacobs HS, Pearson D. Testicular function following irradiation of the human prepubertal testis. Clin Endocrinol (Oxf) 1978; 9:483–490.

71. Sklar C. Growth and endocrine disturbances after bone marrow transplantation in childhood. Acta Paediatr Suppl 1995; 411:57–61.

72. Shalet SM. Disorders of gonadal function due to radiation and cytotoxic chemotherapy in children. Adv Intern Med Pediatr 1989; 58:1–21.

73. Lentz AD, Bergstein J, Steffes MW, et al. Postpubertal evaluation of gonadal function following cyclophosphamide therapy before and during puberty. J Pediatr 1977; 91:385–394.

74. Wallace WHB, Shalet SM, Lendon M, Morris Jones PH. Male fertility in long-term survivors of acute lymphoblastic leukaemia in childhood. Int J Androl 1991; 14:312–319.

75. Yeung SCJ, Chiu AC, Vassilopoulou-Sellin R, Gagel RF. The endocrine effects of nonhormonal antineoplastic therapy. Endocr Rev 1998; 19:144–172.

76. Brauner R, Czernichow P, Cramer P, Schaison G, Rappaport R. Leydig-cell function in children after direct testicular irradiation for acute lymphoblastic leukemia. N Engl J Med 1983; 309:25–28.

77. Clayton PE, Shalet SM, Price DA. Growth response to growth hormone therapy following cranial irradiation. Eur J Pediatr 1988; 147:593–596.

78. Lannering B, Albertsson-Wikland K. Improved growth response to GH treatment in irradiated children. Acta Paediatr Scand 1989; 78:562–567.

79. Sulmont V, Brauner R, Fontoura M, et al. Response to growth hormone treatment and final height after cranial or craniospinal irradiation. Acta Paediatr Scand 1990; 79:542–549.

80. Clayton PE, Shalet SM, Price DA. Growth response to growth hormone therapy following craniospinal irradiation. Eur J Pediatr 1988; 147:597–601.

81. Adan L, Souberbielle JC, Zucker JM, Pierre-Kahn A, Kalifa C, Brauner R. Adult height in 24 patients treated for growth hormone deficiency and early puberty. J Clin Endocrinol Metab 1997; 82:229–233.

82. Adan L, Sainte-Rose C, Souberbielle JC, Zucker JM, Kalifa C, Brauner R. Adult height after growth hormone (GH) treatment for GH deficiency due to cranial irradiation. Med Pediatr Oncol 2000; 34:14–19.

83. Ogilvy-Stuart AL, Ryder WDJ, Gattamaneni HR, Clayton PE, Shalet SM. Growth hormone and tumour recurrence. Br Med J 1992; 304:1601–1605.

84. Duffner PK, Krischer JP, Horowitz ME, Cohen ME, Burger PC, Friedman HS, Kun LE. Second malignancies in young children with primary brain tumors following treatment with prolonged postoperative chemotherapy and delayed irradiation: a Pediatric Oncology Group study. Ann Neurol 1998; 44:313–316.

85. Brennan BM, Rahim A, Adams JA, Eden OB, Shalet SM. Reduced bone mineral density in young adults following cure of acute lymphoblastic leukaemia in childhood. Br J Cancer 1999; 79:1859–1863.

86. Duffner PK, Cohen ME. Long-term consequences of CNS treatment for childhood cancer, Part II: Clinical consequences. Pediatr Neurol 1991; 7:237–242.

87. Brown RT, Sawyer MG, Antoniou G, Toogood I, Rige M. Longitudinal follow-up of the intellectual and academic functioning of children receiving central nervous system —prophylactic chemotherapy for leukemia: a four-year final report. J Dev Behav Pediatr 1999; 20:373–377.

88. Smibert E, Anderson V, Godber T, Ekert H. Risk factors for intellectual and educational sequelae of cranial irradiation in childhood acute lymphoblastic leukaemia. Br J Cancer 1996; 73:825–830.

89. Copeland DR, deMoor C, Moore BD, Ater JL. Neurocognitive development of children after a cerebellar tumor in infancy: a longitudinal study. J Clin Oncol 1999; 17:3476–3786.

90. Anderson VA, Godber T, Smibert E, Weiskop S, Ekert H. Cognitive and academic outcome following cranial irradiation and chemotherapy in children: a longitudinal study. Br J Cancer 2000; 82:255–262.

91. Phipps S, Dunavant N, Srivastava DK, Bowman L, Mulhern RK. Cognitive and academic functioning in survivors of pediatric bone marrow transplantation. J Clin Oncol 2000; 18:1004–1011.

37

Endocrine Alterations in Human Immunodeficiency Virus Infections

Robert Rapaport and Daphne Sack-Rivers
Mount Sinai School of Medicine, New York, New York, U.S.A.

I. INTRODUCTION

On June 5, 2001, acquired immunodeficiency syndrome (AIDS) turned 20. AIDS has claimed more than 21 million lives, including more Americans than died in World War I and World War II combined (1).

The first cases of AIDS in children were reported in 1983 (2,3). Since the beginning of the epidemic, 4.3 million children have died and 1.4 million children less than 15 years of age are infected with human immunodeficiency virus (HIV) (4). Approximately 70% of all cases of AIDS occur in sub-Saharan Africa, where it is estimated that 1:4 adults is HIV-seropositive. Other regions struggling with substantial rates of new infections are the Caribbean, Southeast Asia, and Eastern Europe (1). AIDS has evolved into two distinct epidemics: a horizontal epidemic in adults, spread by sexual contact or shared needles; and a vertical epidemic in which infected mothers give birth to infected children. Since the number of HIV-infected women will continue to increase because of both intravenous drug use and heterosexual transmission, many more cases of AIDS in children are expected to occur (5).

Most cases of pediatric HIV infection worldwide are a result of perinatal transmission. During the year 2000 alone 600,000 children became infected with HIV-1 through mother-to-child transmission (4). Of pediatric HIV cases reported in children less than 13 years of age in the United States, 88% were acquired perinatally; 2% were caused by infection via blood and blood products in individuals with clotting disorders, such as hemophilia; and 10% were classified as other or not reported (6). In the United States there has been a dramatic reduction in mother-to-child HIV transmission rates, from a high of 2500 in 1992 to fewer than 400 perinatal infections in 1998. This decline reflects the Public Health Service's recommendations made in 1994 and 1995 for routine HIV counseling and voluntarily testing for all pregnant women, and for offering zidovudine to infected women during pregnancy and delivery, and for the infant after birth (6–8). A longitudinal follow-up study of the Pediatric AIDS Clinical Trials Group Protocol 076 (PACTG 076), revealed that there were no adverse outcomes with respect to growth, cognitive/developmental function, immune function, cancers, or mortality for uninfected PACTG 076 children treated with zidovudine in utero compared to a placebo group (7,8).

The situation is less fortunate in the developing world. Mother-to-child transmission is the major mode of HIV-1 infection in children. Approximately 1600 children are infected daily with HIV (9,10). Viral burden, immunocompetence in the mother, obstetric factors, as well as other unknown inherited factors influence the risk of transmission.

In the United States, improvements in the means of detecting and treating HIV infections have lead to improvements in the quality of life and survival of infected children. As these children survive longer, the effects of HIV infections on various organ systems become more apparent. It is therefore imperative to detect and treat HIV-related complications as early and effectively as possible.

The endocrine alterations observed in HIV-infected children may be caused by the direct effects of HIV infections, the severe often-debilitating chronic disease that results from infection with the HIV and/or accompanying opportunistic infections or neoplasms, or the therapeutic agents used to treat HIV-infected children.

Evidence for alterations in the endocrine system by HIV disease derives from pathological studies of autopsy material as well as from in vitro and in vivo studies and clinical trials. In this section we review existing evidence of endocrine system alterations in patients infected with HIV, with special emphasis on studies relating to HIV-infected children.

II. GROWTH

The effect of HIV infection on growth in children is expressed differently during the different stages of development.

Markson et al. (11) examined factors associated with low birth weight (LBW) in HIV-infected patients and compared them to a control group. The study population consisted of 772 HIV-infected women; 2377 women served as controls. Women who were HIV-positive had a 29% chance of delivering a LBW infant compared to a 9.3% chance for the control group. Delivery of a LBW infant was also strongly associated with illicit drug use, maternal smoking, and African-American vs. non-Hispanic white ethnicity. When they compared the odds of delivering a LBW infant among full-term deliveries, they found that HIV-infected women were three times as likely to deliver a LBW infant. After adjusting for the effects of smoking, illicit drug use, maternal risk factors, and health care delivery, HIV-infected women are at an increased risk of delivering a LBW infant.

Weng et al. (12) evaluated the effect of perinatal HIV-1 transmission and birth outcomes, such as birth weight, gestational age, head circumference, and weight/head ratio. Some 627 women and their infants were analyzed; 318 women were HIV-seropositive and 309 women were seronegative. Unadjusted mean birth weight of HIV-uninfected infants was 235 g more than HIV-infected infants. When the infants were evaluated at the end of the neonatal period, HIV-infected infants' weight was lower than the weight of HIV-negative infants born to HIV-positive mothers. The adjusted birth weight was found to be 96 g less in the infected than in the uninfected group. Maas et al. (13) studied prospectively the effects of maternal HIV infection on fetal development and neonatal morbidity in 17 neonates and 37 controls, of whom 21 were exposed to opiates. They concluded that prenatal exposure to opiates and nicotine but not HIV infection resulted in fetal growth retardation and neonatal morbidity.

Results from prospective cohort studies of pregnancy outcomes of HIV-infected mothers in the United States indicate that HIV-infected newborns weigh 0.28 kg less and are 1.64 cm shorter than HIV-exposed but uninfected controls (14). A total of 282 patients were enrolled in this study, of whom 59 were infected with HIV and 223 were not. When re-evaluated at age 18 months, the HIV-infected infants were 0.7 kg lighter and 2.2 cm shorter than the HIV-exposed uninfected children. Therefore, mother-to-child transmission of HIV is associated with a decrease in birth weight of the infant. The effect of HIV infection is on par with other determinants of birth weight, such as primiparity and gender, and somewhat lower than the effect of maternal smoking during pregnancy.

In conclusion, infants with perinatal acquired HIV tend to be shorter and have a lower birth weight. Most of these studies were done prior to the use of Zidovudine, which has been shown to cause an increase in weight (15).

Johnson et al. (16) evaluated prospectively 20 children born to HIV-infected mothers for 18 months. All infants had normal birth weights, suggesting no effect of HIV exposure on intrauterine growth. By the end of the first year of life 12 children had no evidence of infection. None of them was considered to have failure to thrive. Of the eight infected children, four (50%) exhibited growth failure, two developing a syndrome of growth failure, dermatitis, and early death. The authors' conclusion was that the growth failure accompanying HIV infection appears to be postnatal in origin.

In a group of children age 4–24 months with perinatally acquired infection, 10 who had antigen-induced lymphocyte proliferation were found to grow normally, in contrast to 8 children with absent antigen-induced lymphoproliferation, 7 of whom had failure to thrive (17).

McKinney et al. (18) compared 62 HIV-infected with 108 uninfected children $<25\frac{1}{2}$ months of age. The weight for length scores through the first 2 years of life were comparable in the two populations, suggesting that the HIV-infected children were not abnormally lean or wasted. However, the uninfected population was significantly longer (higher length for age scores) at 4–24 months of age than the infected children. However, the study did not take into account that 73% of the infected children had received antiretroviral treatment (Zidovudine), which has been shown to result in increased weight (Table 1).

de Martino et al. (19) studied 32 congenitally acquired HIV-infected prepubertal children, classified as Centers for Disease Control (CDC) clinical category C, who were taking two nucleoside reverse transcriptase inhibitors. The control group consisted of 248 HIV-negative children. All children were evaluated for 12 months. The height, height velocity, bone age, insulin growth factor 1, (IGF-1), and IGF-binding protein-3 (IGFBP-3) of the HIV-positive group were lower than those of controls. They also had higher spontaneous and phytohemagglutinin-stimulated interleukin-6 (IL-6) release. This was inversely correlated with height velocity, bone age, IGF-1, and IGFBP-3, suggesting that IL-6 overproduction may be a mechanism of IGF-1 and IGFBP-3 downregulation, which causes the impaired linear growth in children with perinatal HIV-infection.

In children with HIV infections, poor growth has been a consistent finding. Of the first 15 children with AIDS reported in 1983, 13 (87%) were described as having failure to thrive (FTT) (2,3). A subsequent report described FTT in 14 of 14 infants less than 7 months of age with AIDS (20). The poorly defined term FTT has been a frequently reported characteristic of infants and children with AIDS. A dysmorphic syndrome noted in HIV-infected children and named HIV embryopathy by some had, as its most commonly found feature, FTT or poor growth (21). Reviews of large numbers of HIV-infected children have consistently commented on the occurrence of poor growth in the affected children (22–25).

Table 1   Birth Weight (Wt) and Length (L) in Perinatally Acquired HIV Infection vs. HIV-Negative Infants

Reference	N	%	Diagnosis	L (cm)	Wt (kg)	Remarks
11	NA	29	HIV+	NA	LBW	9.3% born to HIV-negative mothers had LBW.
12	48	100	HIV+	NA	−0.154	206 uninfected infants born to HIV-positive mothers were 0.154 kg more at birth.
14	59	100	HIV+	−1.64	−0.28	At birth, compared to HIV-negative infants.
	59	100	HIV+	−2.2	−0.7	At age of 18 months compared to HIV-negative infants.
16	20	100	a	normal	normal	At birth.
	8	75	HIV+	NA	NA	At 12 months, 2/8 died.

[a] At birth could not establish diagnosis.
NA, not available.

The cause of growth failure of most HIV-infected children is not known. Johann-Liang et al. (26) evaluated 23 prepubertal congenitally HIV-infected children aged 1.3–13.2 years. They observed that HIV-infected children had significantly lower IGF-1 levels compared with age- and gender-matched controls. When compared with HIV-infected children with normal growth, the group with growth impairment had lower IGF-1 levels, severe immune suppression, increased viral burden, increased IL-6 activity, and decreased total serum protein.

We evaluated 31 children with symptomatic HIV infections. We found that as a group they were not smaller than average. When individual patients were evaluated, however, we found that about 1:6 of the HIV-infected children were underweight (weight < 3%), and one-third had height and weight velocities <3%. Those children who had more opportunistic infections and lower CD4 lymphocyte counts tended to grow most poorly. A substantial number of patients had abnormal thyroid function test results, IGF-1, and cortisol levels. Urinary growth hormone excretion was increased in the patients as a group (27).

In a retrospective analysis of 198 children enrolled in the Children's Hospital of New Jersey AIDS program, sufficient data for growth analysis were found in 122 subjects. Poor growth, defined as weight or height <5% based on National Center for Health Statistics (NCHS) data, was noted in 10 of 22 infants less than 2 years of age, 5 of whom were girls. Of these, eight had heights and weights <5%. Among boys older than 2 years, 15 of 49 had poor growth, 6 having low weights and heights, 7 only low heights, and 2 low weights. These data confirm our earlier finding that height was more affected than weight in HIV-infected children, suggesting that nutritional factors alone could not explain the growth failure. CD4 cell counts were lower and the incidences of opportunistic infections were higher in poorly growing children. The incidence of progressive encephalopathy was not related to the children's growth patterns (28).

Jospe and Powell reported an 8-year-old girl with growth hormone deficiency (29). Laue et al. (30) studied nine children with severe growth failure, with heights between 2 and 5 standard deviations (SD) below the mean. All children had normal levels of IGF-1, and eight of nine had normal growth hormone responses to stimulation tests with arginine and levodopa. Thyroid and adrenal function tests were by and large normal in these children and could therefore not provide an explanation for their growth failure. Schwartz et al. (31), also found normal growth hormone response to glucagon stimulation in 12 short children with average heights of 2.23 SD below the mean. Serum IGF-1 levels were low. Lepage et al. (32) compared 16 HIV-seropositive children 5–12 years of age with perinatally acquired disease in Kigali, Rwanda, with age- and gender-matched seronegative children. Of 16 patients, 12 had short stature, and 7 had low weight for age. Mean IGF-1 concentrations were lower in patients (n = 11) than controls, but basal (unstimulated) growth hormone levels were not different between the two groups.

Rondanelli et al. (33), looked at the circadian secretion of growth hormone (GH), IGF-1, cortisol, adrenocorticotropin (ACTH), and thyroid-stimulating hormone (TSH) in HIV-infected children. Twenty-seven prepubertal children participated in the study, of whom 14 were well-nourished HIV-seropositive and 13 were clinically healthy children chosen as controls. They demonstrated that throughout the 24 h period plasma GH, cortisol, and ACTH levels were similar and fell within normal limits in HIV-seropositive and healthy controls. Serum TSH levels were similar, except at 2400 h, when the TSH levels were significantly lower in the HIV-seropositive children than in the healthy children. Bone age and chronological age ratio were below 1.0 in 10 of the 14 children (71%), 4 of the 14 children had height <3rd percentile, 2 of 14 children had weight <3rd percentile, and mean basal IGF-1 levels were below normal range for 12 of 14 children. At all time points the IGF-1 circadian profile was significantly lower in HIV-seropositive children than in the control group.

Carey et al. (34) studied 1338 HIV-infected children aged 3 months to 15 years, who participated in a multicenter pediatric AIDS clinical trials to assess their somatic growth and to construct age-specific growth velocity norms. They found that there were consistent deficits in

Table 2 Growth Disturbances Observed in HIV-Infected Children

Reference	N	Height < 5%	Weight < 5%	Height velocity < 3%	Weight velocity < 3%
27	31		19% < 3%	10%	10%
28	22 < 2 yr	45%	45%	NA	NA
28	49 > 2 yr	26%	16%	NA	NA
33	14	29%	14%	NA	NA
34	1338 (3 m–15 yr)	33% < 3%	20 < 3%	NA	NA

NA, not available.

growth velocities among HIV-infected children. Approximately 33% of height and 20% of weight age- and gender-corrected velocity measurements were below the 3% percentile. These normalized growth velocities are useful means of following the growth of pediatric AIDS patients (Table 2,3).

Children with hemophilia provide a unique population for the study of the effects of HIV infection on growth. In one study, 3 of 22 boys had growth failure: 2 had low IGF-1 levels and possible neurosecretory dysregulation of growth hormone secretion (35). In another study, Jason et al. (36) noted a decline in weight percentiles in 41 children with hemophilia following the diagnosis of HIV infection. They suggested that the effect of HIV infection on weight might precede both the clinical and laboratory alterations of the immune deficiency.

Brettler et al. (37) found that growth failure, defined as decrease of more than 15 percentile points in height or weight for age for 2 consecutive years, was predictive of the development of symptoms in HIV-positive children with hemophilia. The growth failure in many cases predated the lowering in CD4 levels, generally thought to be a prognostic indicator of disease progression. In a multicenter Hemophilia Growth and Development Study, entry data revealed that, adjusted for age, HIV-positive subjects were three times as likely as HIV-negative subjects to have height for age decrement (38). Gertner et al. (39) studied a cohort of 300 boys with hemophilia. Those who were infected (62% of the total) had lower age-adjusted heights and weights than the uninfected boys. Despite decrements in growth parameters, the HIV-infected group had no evidence of wasting or malnutrition. The growth

failure was postulated to be caused by delays in pubertal maturation, reflected by delays in bone age and by differences in testosterone or sex-hormone-binding globulin secretion.

The Hemophilia Growth and Development Study (40) evaluated growth and hormone correlates in 207 HIV-positive and 126 HIV-negative males for a period of 3.5 years. Eighty-nine of 207 HIV-positive males and 31 of the 126 HIV-negative males were further evaluated according to the study protocol; subjects who demonstrated declines in height for age (measurement <5th percentile with two previous heights >10th percentile), who had not achieved Tanner stage IV level by age 15 years or who had abnormal growth velocity. IGF-1 levels were normal for age in both subgroups. In participants with abnormal growth, 47% of HIV-positive and 17% of HIV-negative had an abnormal response to growth hormone (GH) stimulation test (a value <10 ng/ml). For the entire HIV-positive population, no correlation was found between growth hormone response to stimulation test and state of immunodeficiency (CD4 count <200 vs. >200). There were no abnormalities in IGF-1 and/or thyroid function tests, and there was no correlation with CD4 count.

Another longitudinal study of the Hemophilia Growth and Development Study evaluated the association between plasma HIV RNA and CD4 T lymphocytes and height, weight, skeletal maturation, testosterone levels, and height velocity in children and adolescents with hemophilia. Two hundred and seven boys participated for a period of 7 years. They found that any increments in viral load led to decrease in both height and weight. Furthermore, participants with a baseline viral load >3125 copies/ml, had sig-

Table 3 Growth Disturbances and Hypothalamic–Pituitary Axis in HIV-Infected Children

Reference	N	Height SD below mean	IGF-I	Response to stimulation test
26	23	NA	Low	NA
30	9	2–5	100% normal	89% normal response
31	12	2.23	100% low	100% normal response
32	16	NA	69% low	NA

NA, not available.

nificant delays in achieving maximum height velocity and lower maximum velocity when compared with participants with lower viral load. A decrement of 100 cell/ml of CD4 was associated with a 2.51 cm decrement in height, 3.83 kg decrease in weight, and decreases in bone age and testosterone level. Baseline immune function was more important in predicting the outcome than were the changes from baseline (41) (Table 4).

The growth abnormalities in HIV-infected children were thought by many researchers to be due to inadequate caloric intake. Malnutrition and evidence of carbohydrate malabsorption as detected by lactose hydrogen breath tests and D-xylose absorption studies are common in HIV-infected children; these abnormalities do not seem to be predictive of or correlated with growth failure (42,43). Henderson et al. (44) studied the effect of tube feeding in 18 HIV-infected children who presented with growth failure. The study ranged from 2 to 24 months (median of 8.5 m). They observed increased weight, weight for height, and arm fat area. Tube feeding did not result in significant increase in height for age, or arm muscle area. This suggested that other variables are involved in growth. It is apparent that there are decrements both in weight and height in HIV-infected children, but malnutrition could not be directly tied to the growth abnormalities. One of the reasons is that abnormalities of growth have been observed in nourished HIV-infected children.

The results of the study by Johann-Liang et al. (26) demonstrated that total energy expenditure by HIV-infected children does not differ from energy expenditure of noninfected children. They found that a hypermetabolic state is not the basis for the growth impairment observed in HIV-infected children. Arpadi et al. (45) assessed whether elevated resting energy expenditure (REE) might contribute to the poor growth observed in HIV-infected children. In contrast to studies performed on HIV-infected adults, in which increased REE was observed, children with HIV-associated growth failure tended to have reduced levels of energy expenditure compared with children with normal growth rates.

We have measured serum and cerebrospinal fluid (CSF) levels of tumor necrosis factor (TNF) in children with HIV infections and without progressive encephalopathy (PE). We found that neither serum nor CSF levels of TNF were correlated with the degree of cachexia (wasting) in these children. Serum but not CSF TNF levels were increased in the children who had PE (46).

Miller et al. (47) studied the effect of protease inhibitors (PI) on growth and body composition in HIV-infected children. Sixty-seven HIV-infected children were evaluated for a period of 2.4 years. At baseline, the children were 1.2 SD below in weight and 1.4 SD below in height. The study results reconfirm the finding that in children treated with PIs there is a significant improvement in weight, moderate improvement in weight-for-height, and a borderline improvement in height. Furthermore, there was a significant decrease of virus load and improvement of CD4 T lymphocyte count.

The increased use of PIs and highly active antiretroviral therapy (HAART) has reduced both short-term morbidity and mortality in HIV-infected pediatric patients. The virus is not eradicated from the body and therapy is required for life. During the late 1990s there was a surge of reports (48–51) describing the toxicities that have emerged in adult patients who were treated with antiretroviral therapies, of which the most common is lipodystrophy syndrome (LDS). Lipodystrophy syndrome is characterized by body composition changes, including the development of an enlarged posterior cervical fat pad, increased truncal adiposity, breast enlargement, peripheral fat loss, and facial fat atrophy. This syndrome is also characterized by insulin resistance, hyperglycemia, and hypertriglyceridemia (52).

The cause of LDS remains controversial. Most studies, in adults, indicate that this syndrome is associated with the use of PIs (48,51). On the other hand, there have been some publications in which LDS has been described in patients not taking PIs and not treated with HAART protocols (53). Publications documenting prevalence of the syndrome have been conflicting as well. Some authors

Table 4   Growth Impairment in HIV-Infected Boys with Hemophilia

Reference	HIV-positive	HIV-negative
35	3/22: growth failure 2/22: low IGF-1 levels	NA
36	Observed decline in weight percentiles	NA
38	Three times more likely to have height for age decrements	NA
39	186/300: lower age-adjusted height and weight	114/300: normal age-adjusted height and weight
40	89/207: response to GH stimulation test <10 ng/ml Normal IGF-1 values in entire cohort	31/126: response to GH stimulation test <10 ng/ml Normal IGF-1 values in entire cohort

41	Decrements of 100 cell/ml of CD4
	    2.51 cm decrement in height
	    3.83 kg decrease in weight
		NA

NA, not available.

report a prevalence of 83% in patients taking PIs (54), yet others report a prevalence of only 12% (55). Lipid abnormalities are common and they constitute part of the syndrome. Papadopoulos et al. (56) demonstrated that hypertriglyceridemia is more common than hypercholesterolemia.

Hypertriglyceridemia has been described commonly in patients with AIDS, but it was found not to be related to degree of wasting as measured by total body potassium as an index of body cell mass (57). The role of cytokines as potential mediators of the wasting syndrome was also investigated. In AIDS, TNF and haptoglobin levels were not increased, but interferon-alpha (IFN-alpha) and C-reactive protein were. Levels of these cytokines, however, were not related to plasma cholesterol, high-density lipoprotein cholesterol, or free fatty acids. Plasma triglycerides were correlated with IFN-alpha levels only. The decrease in cholesterol and cholesterol-containing lipoprotein in AIDS precedes the appearance of hypertriglyceridemia and is unrelated to IFN-alpha or triglyceride levels (58).

Arpadi et al. (59) studied LDS in children. They evaluated 28 prepubertal children and found that 8 of 28 had extremity lipoatrophy with trunk fat accumulation. Lipodystrophy was associated with the use of Stavudine (a nucleoside reverse transcriptase inhibitor) or PIs. However, no information was available about whether these children had insulin resistance or increased risk of cardiovascular disease due to hypertriglyceridemia, similar to the presentation in adults. Wedekind and Pugatch (60) have observed this syndrome in three HIV-infected children. The patient they describe is an 8-year-old girl who was observed to have thinning of the extremities and an increase in abdominal girth.

Rietschel et al. (61) studied growth hormone dynamics in 21 HIV-infected subjects with lipodystrophy, 20 HIV-infected subjects without lipodystrophy, and 20 healthy controls. Subjects underwent an extensive metabolic and endocrine work-up that included lipid profiles, measurement of hemoglobin A1C (HgbA1C), free testosterone, viral load and CD4 cell counts, and urine free cortisol levels. Participants also underwent OGTT, GH sampling every 20 min from 2000 h to 0800 h to determine the IGF-1 axis. The body mass index (BMI) and age were similar between the subgroups; viral load and CD4 cell count were not significantly different between groups. No significant differences were observed in HgbA1C, fasting glucose, and urine free cortisol; free testosterone was normal in the lipodystrophy group and was found not to differ significantly from the control group. However, high-density lipoproteins (HDL) were decreased and triglycerides and cholesterol were increased in patients with lipodystrophy compared to the other two groups. Insulin area under curve was increased as well in the lipodystrophy group compared to the other two groups. Findings regarding GH parameters were as follows: mean overnight

GH concentrations, basal GH concentrations, and pulse amplitude were reduced in the lipodystrophy group, whereas GH pulse frequency did not differ among the three groups. Using a cutoff response of normal GH response to stimulation of 3 ng/ml, 33% of lipodystrophy group demonstrated GH response below cutoff, 10% of control had such a value, and the group of HIV-infected without lipodystrophy had 0 subjects. This study links reduced GH dynamics with increased visceral adiposity in lipodystrophic men infected with HIV.

Publications supporting the use of GH in adults have raised the question of whether HIV-infected adults with lipodystrophy would benefit from GH therapy. Lo et al. (62) evaluated eight men with HIV-associated visceral adiposity. The men were on a daily dosage of 3 mg GH for 6 months. At 6 months there was a significant decrease in posterior cervical fat pad, visceral adipose tissue, and an increase in lean body mass (63–65).

Helle et al. (66) evaluated the relation of immune parameters, virus load, clinical stage, and wasting to several parameters of the IGF system in 76 patients with HIV, of whom 37 had developed AIDS. IGF-binding protein-2 and IGF-binding-protein-3 protease activity were increased in subjects with AIDS compared with other HIV-infected individuals and controls. These parameters correlated positively with virus load and TNF-alpha and negatively to CD4 and CD8 cell counts. IGF-2 was decreased in AIDS patients compared to HIV-infected individuals and controls. Furthermore, AIDS patients with wasting had lower IGF-2 levels and higher IGF-binding-protein-2 levels than other AIDS patients.

In conclusion, HIV infection does affect growth either prenatally (low birth weight, length) or postnatally. Sometimes the effect of HIV infection can become apparent only later in childhood. Results of studies are sometimes conflicting because of differences in study protocols, medications, and treatment strategies, and due to variability among the manifestations of HIV infection in individuals. Pediatricians need to be aware that a child who is failing to grow normally might have a chronic condition such as HIV infection. Furthermore, with the advances in treatment, HIV is becoming a chronic disease with major endocrine effects on growth. Pinto et al. (67) report two HIV-infected prepubertal children who were treated with growth hormone for 3 years. In one child height increased from −3.6 SD to −2.0 SD below the mean and in the second child height increased from −4.7 SD to −1.9 SD.

Studies in adults are not always applicable to the special considerations that need to be addressed in the pediatric population. Future research and advances in the field may unmask the whole spectrum of HIV infection and its effect on growth and development.

III. ADRENAL FUNCTION

In patients with HIV infections, the adrenal gland has been a frequently studied endocrine organ. Earlier studies concentrated on pathological evaluations of adrenal gland involvement in autopsy specimens. More recently, in vivo studies of adrenal function have been undertaken, but mostly in adults.

Pathological studies have demonstrated frequent involvement of the adrenal glands, most commonly by opportunistic infection, such as *Cytomegalovirus* (CMV), *Mycobacterium*, cryptococci, *Toxoplasma*, and *Pneumocystis*. Neoplasms, such as lymphoma and Kaposi's sarcoma, have also been shown to affect the adrenal glands. The frequency of adrenal gland involvement on autopsy material varies from 36 to 90% (68–76). A pattern of adrenal gland involvement with the medulla being the site of primary involvement and with areas of focal and generalized hemorrhage affecting both medulla and cortex initially described by Reichert et al. (68), has been repeatedly reported ever since. The adrenal gland is the most common extrapulmonary site of CMV infection (70).

Glasgow et al. (73) found CMV adrenalitis in 21 of 41 cases examined and widespread lipid depletion in most cases (a nonspecific finding on autopsies of critically ill patients). The adrenal cortical involvement was limited to 10% of the cortex in most, and fewer than 70% of all, cases. In an attempt to establish clinicopathological correlation, 32 cases were also analyzed for signs and symptoms of adrenal insufficiency. Common findings were hyponatremia (75%), hypotension (34%), hypokalemia (19%), hyperkalemia (16%), vomiting, diarrhea, and fever (percentage not specified). No patient had hyperpigmentation. Morning levels of serum cortisol were normal or elevated in five of five patients. One of two patients tested had a subnormal increase in cortisol after ACTH infusion. Despite significant pathological adrenal abnormalities, no clinical adrenal insufficiency was documented. The degree of adrenal cortical damage seen was considered less than that usually associated with adrenal insufficiency.

Pulakhandman and Dincsoy (77) found CMV infections in half of 74 autopsied cases of AIDS. Of those 37 cases, the adrenal gland was most commonly affected of all organs (84%) compared with the lungs being affected in 55% of cases. CMV inclusions were found in endothelial, cortical, and medullar cells. The CMV adrenalitis was diffuse in 10 cases and focal in 20. Analysis of the clinical data in 30 subjects revealed no findings related to the adrenal pathology, with the possible exception of serum sodium–potassium ratio of less than 30 in those with more severe adrenal pathology.

Adrenal function has been among the most commonly studied clinical endocrine parameters. Many of the signs and symptoms characteristic of adrenal insufficiency are seen in severely ill patients with HIV infections. However, definite adrenal insufficiency is rare in subjects with AIDS. The results of many studies of adrenal function in subjects with AIDS vary depending on the nature of the subjects studied, the severity of the disease, the concomitant intercurrent illnesses and medications to which they are exposed, and the means of adrenal testing: baseline or stimulated levels of glucocorticoids and/or ACTH.

Most studies of adrenal function were performed in adults with HIV infections. Early reports documented both normal and diminished cortisol responses to ACTH in patients with AIDS (78–82). Membreno et al. (83) studied 74 randomly selected hospitalized patients with AIDS and 19 patients with AIDS-related complex (ARC). Based on subnormal cortisol responses to ACTH stimulation, four patients with AIDS were diagnosed as having adrenal insufficiency. Mean basal cortisol levels were higher in patients with AIDS than in healthy individuals, but ACTH-stimulated cortisol responses were not different from normal. However, stimulated levels of 17-deoxysteroid levels (corticosterone and 18-OH-deoxycorticosterone [18-OHDOC]) were lower than normal. Patients with ARC responded in similar manner to those with AIDS. Based on these findings the authors suggested that impaired 17-deoxysteroid levels, especially 18-OHDOC, might be a "harbinger of progressive adrenal disorder." Plasma ACTH levels were normal in patients with adrenal insufficiency, suggesting a possible pituitary defect in these patients. Administration of the hypothalamic factor corticotropin-releasing hormone (CRH) resulted in subnormal 18-OHDOC responses in two patients. The authors advanced the hypothesis that HIV pituitary infection could lead to selective hypopituitarism and hypoadrenalism, with subsequent HIV adrenal infection leading to complete adrenal insufficiency.

Dobs et al. (84) reported normal cortisol responses to ACTH in 36 of 39 ambulatory patients with AIDS. Merenich et al. (85), although finding no clinical evidence of endocrine disorder, reported lower baseline cortisol and aldosterone and ACTH-stimulated cortisol levels in 40 symptomatic HIV-infected men compared with 27 HIV-infected age-matched control subjects; 1 patient had low cortisol and also low ACTH-stimulated aldosterone levels.

HIV-infected subjects have been reported to have lower responses in cortisol and/or ACTH to cold stress (86) or tetanus toxoid administration (87). Several investigators, however, have reported elevated baseline levels (88–90) or 24 h secretion (91) of cortisol and/or ACTH.

Catania et al. (92) compared propiomelanocortin-derived peptides and cytokines in 80 patients with AIDS and in 80 normal subjects. Average plasma alpha-melanocyte-stimulating hormone levels were higher in the AIDS patients, but mean levels of cortisol, ACTH, beta-endordorphins, interleukin-1 (IL-1), IL-6, and tumor necrosis factor were not different between the two groups.

In a prospective study of 98 HIV-infected patients Raffi et al. (93) found only 4 patients with low baseline and 7 with low ACTH-stimulated cortisol levels. Only two were believed to have adrenal insufficiency.

Eledrisi and Verghese (94) described three patients with AIDS who had clinical features suggestive of adrenal insufficiency, with a normal ACTH stimulation test. Fol-

lowing repeat testing, the diagnosis of adrenal insufficiency was made in one of the patients. The other two
cases required the overnight metyrapone test to confirm
the diagnosis. All three patients showed an improvement
in their clinical condition following glucocorticoid therapy. Adrenal insufficiency can be a complication of HIV
infection, and health care professionals should have a high
index of suspicion of subtle adrenal dysfunction.

To explain further the effect of HIV infection on the
hypothalamic–pituitary–adrenal (HPA) axis, Azar and
Melby (95) administered ovine CRH (oCRH) to 25 ambulatory HIV-infected patients without AIDS and 10 normal volunteers. Six patients had diminished cortisol and
ACTH responses to CRH, 6 had low cortisol and normal
ACTH responses, and 13 had normal cortisol and ACTH
responses. They suggested enhanced hypothalamic CRH
production in HIV infections as a possible explanation for
their results. Complex interaction between the immune
and HPA axis, mediated by cytokines and perhaps lym-
phocyte-produced ACTH, has been postulated by some to
explain the mechanisms by which HIV infections may affect adrenal function (96,97).

Hyponatremia has been reported in 30% to more than
50% of hospitalized patients with AIDS (98). In most patients, however, the hyponatremia has been thought to be
caused by renal and/or gastrointestinal losses and the syndrome of inappropriate secretion of antidiuretic hormone
(99–101). Hyporeninemic hypoaldosteronism (102) and
also mineralocorticoid deficiency have been reported in
patients with AIDS (103). However, the adrenal mineralocorticoid pathway is normal in both the baseline and
ACTH-stimulated states in most HIV-infected patients
(88,93).

Serum levels of dehydroepiandrosterone have been
reported to be decreased in HIV-infected patients, to correlate with CD4 levels, and to be a reliable predictor of
the progression of HIV infection to AIDS (104–107).

Norbiato et al. (108) reported nine patients with AIDS
and characteristic clinical features of adrenal insufficiency
with elevated cortisol levels, suggesting resistance to glucocorticoids by abnormal glucocorticoid receptors on lymphocytes.

In children with symptomatic HIV infections ($n =
28$), we measured morning serum cortisol levels and
found that the lowest levels occurred in those with the
lowest CD4 levels. ACTH tests performed on two children
with the lowest cortisol levels were normal, suggesting
normal adrenal glucocorticoid function. In several ill children with AIDS suspected of having adrenal insufficiency,
we found normal baseline cortisol levels in all. In four
subjects ACTH-stimulated cortisol responses were normal, excluding the diagnosis of adrenal insufficiency
(27,109).

Oberfield et al. (110) found normal or slightly elevated baseline and ACTH-stimulated cortisol levels, with
mildly diminished stimulated serum deoxycorticosterone
and corticosterone levels in 12 HIV-infected children, 2

of whom were receiving ketoconazole, a drug known to
inhibit adrenal function. Laue et al. (30) reported normal
cortisol response to ACTH in eight of nine children with
AIDS; the 1 patient with a subnormal response was receiving treatment with ketoconazole. Schwartz et al. (31)
found normal cortisol responses to glucagon stimulation
in 12 of 12 HIV infected children.

IV. THYROID

During the course of HIV infections, the thyroid gland
has been reported to be affected either directly or indirectly. The mechanisms that can contribute to thyroid
gland involvement include infections (111,112), neoplastic
processes (113), changes in thyroid hormone secretion and
binding (114–116), and drugs used to treat HIV-infected
patients (117–119).

In autopsy specimens, thyroid pathology has been described in 10–14% of cases analyzed. Cytomegalovirus
inclusions, Kaposi's sarcoma, and cryptococcal infections
in the thyroid have been reported (70–72,111,119). Fine-
needle aspiration of an area of decreased thyroid uptake
in an individual with biochemical but not clinical evidence
of hypothyroidism revealed *Pneumocystis carinii* infection (112). Following antibiotic therapy, the goiter decreased in size and thyroid function tests became normal.

Clinically significant evidence of hypothyroidism in
individuals with HIV disease has been rare. However,
many reports have attested to altered biochemical parameters of thyroid function in subjects with HIV infections,
especially AIDS. The incidence of clinical or subclinical
hypothyroidism in studies of large series of patients was
as low as 1% (114,115). The most consistent abnormalities described have been low levels of triiodothyronine
(T3), especially in the more severely ill patients, and elevated levels of thyroxine-binding globulin (TBG)
(85,114–116,120–124). The lowering of serum T3 levels
suggested biochemical thyroid picture noted in ill patients
with nonthyroid disease. Some authors have correlated
low T3 levels with severity of the critical illness and mortality among hospitalized patients with AIDS (120,122).
In a minority of patients with symptomatic HIV infections, exaggerated TSH responses to thyrotropin-releasing
hormone (TRH) administration have been reported, suggesting a so-called hypothyroid-like regulation of the hypothalamic–pituitary–thyroid axis in subjects with stable
HIV infections (85,123).

Blethen et al. (125) studied the effect of perinatally
acquired HIV infection on thyroid function (Table 5).
They evaluated 53 children born to HIV-infected mothers
and 17 healthy controls. T4, T3, TSH, and TBG levels
were obtained from prepubertal healthy controls and the
HIV-infected children. The group of HIV-infected was organized into subgroups according to the CDC criteria. Of
the 53 children, 16 had maternally-derived antibodies to
HIV and no evidence of HIV infection (13 of them seroreverted), 6 were HIV antibody positive, 8 were HIV

Table 5 Thyroid Abnormalities Observed in HIV-Infected Children

Reference	N	Diagnosis	T4 (FT4)	T3 (TT3)	TSH	TBG
132	53	23/53: AIDS	Increased in 9%	Low in 9%	Increased in 22%	Increased in 44%
33	9	HIV-positive	NA	NA	NA	Increased in 100%
134	56	Perinatal HIV	FT4: decreased	TT3: decreased	Increased	Increased

NA, not available.

antibody positive with nonspecific symptoms such as fever or "failure to thrive," and 23 were classified with AIDS. In the subgroup of children with AIDS, 15 of 23 had at least one measure of thyroid function outside of the normal range for healthy children. The abnormalities observed were elevated TBG in 10, elevated TSH in 5 (none of these children had goiter or antithyroid antibodies), low T3 in 2, and elevated T4 in 2. In the subgroup of P1 and P2, only two patients had abnormal thyroid levels, and each was acutely ill at the time. The findings of this study differ from what is known in HIV-infected adults in two aspects. First, in stage P1 and P2 TBG levels remain normal, whereas in adults TBG are higher even at stage P1 (120). Second, in adults the increase in TBG is followed by an increase of T4. In children with AIDS, T4 levels were not increased compared to healthy children or to other HIV-infected children.

The presence of antithyroid autoantibodies in perinatally HIV-infected children was evaluated by Fundaro et al. (126) in 80 children: 58 born to HIV-infected mothers and 22 healthy children. Eighteen of 58 children born to HIV-infected mothers seroreverted and 40 children remained seropositive and were classified according to the CDC clinical criteria: 7 asymptomatic (stage N), and 33 symptomatic (stage A, B, C). In this study they evaluated T3, T4, TSH, free T3 (FT3), FT4, TSH, antithyroglobulin autoantibodies (TGAb), and antithyroid peroxidase autoantibodies (TPOAb). None of the children had either clinical symptoms of thyroid disease or enlargement of the gland at the time of the study. Of the symptomatic children 34% were TgAb-positive and all were TPOAb-negative. Antibodies were not found in any of the asymptomatic children, seroreverted subjects, or healthy controls. The finding of autoantibodies was not correlated with worsening immune stages and was not associated with clinical signs or symptoms of thyroiditis. Increased TSH values were observed more frequently in the symptomatic HIV-infected children. When this group was subclassified according to immune status, a positive correlation was found between immune status and TSH values. High TSH values were found more frequently in the stages with moderate or severe immunosuppression. In the healthy control group there was no increase of TBG, but an increase of TBG was observed in 68% of HIV-infected children.

Chiarelli et al. (127) studied retrospectively 109 prepubertal children (56 children with perinatal HIV infection and 53 healthy age-matched children) for the following: total T4 (TT4), FT4, total T3 (TT3), FT3, reverse triiodothyronine (rT3), TSH, thyroglobulin (TG), TBG, CD4+ cell counts, and viral load, as well as antibodies: antithyroglobulin, antimicrosomal, thyroid peroxidase, and thyrotropin receptor. They found that TT3, TT4, FT4, and TG were significantly reduced in children with HIV infection when compared with controls, and that rT3, TBG, and TSH were increased. In all determinations autoantibodies were negative in the HIV-infected children. Their findings suggest that thyroid dysfunction precedes the worsening of the clinical course of the disease in HIV-infected children. Thyroid dysfunction correlates with disease severity and it can be observed early in the course of perinatal HIV infection.

We observed one child with AIDS and evidence of primary hypothyroidism in whom treatment with replacement doses of thyroid hormone resulted in improvement in growth velocity (128). In children with symptomatic HIV infections we noted transiently abnormal thyroid function test results in 3 of 20 patients. Serum levels of T3 and free thyroxine did correlate with an index of weight retardation: chronological age minus weight age (27). Hypothyroidism in one of nine short children with AIDS, along with elevated TBG levels in all nine, and evidence of possible central hypothyroidism (based on timed hourly TSH measurements), were reported by Laue et al. (30). Among 12 clinically and biochemical euthyroid children with AIDS, Schwartz et al. (31) reported elevated TSH responses to TRH in 5.

The results of the Hemophilia Growth and Development Study (40) revealed that in 99% of 321 subjects, including HIV-negative and HIV-positive subgroups, thyroid function tests (T4, T3, TSH) were normal for age. Subtle abnormalities of thyroid function were not investigated in this study, but even in HIV-positive boys with growth abnormalities thyroid function was normal for age. In conclusion, thyroid function can be altered in the course of HIV infection. The results from the different studies are somewhat inconsistent. The most common findings were decreased T3 and elevated TBG values.

V. GONADS

The vast majority of information regarding gonadal function in HIV-infected individuals is from studies performed in adult men and women and from autopsy material derived from adult men. Reports have included normal (68) to atrophic testicular volume (70–72), as well as evidence of infiltration by CMV (68,70,129), Kaposi's sarcoma (68), toxoplasmosis (129,130), tuberculosis (130), retrovirus-like particles (131), and neoplasm (132). On histological examination, the testes exhibit evidence of peritubular fibrosis, arrest of spermatogenesis, germ cell degeneration and loss of seminiferous tubules and basement membranes, epididymal obstruction, prostatic inclusion, and Leydig cell atrophy (68,70–72,133–137). The presence of focal HIV-associated proteins, such as HIV P17, was documented by anti-HIV P17 monoclonal antibodies in testes and prostate (136). The possibility of immune-mediated gonadal destruction was not substantiated in one study in which immune complex deposits were found not to be increased in the testes of homosexual AIDS patients compared with those of a control group of heterosexual men without AIDS (135).

Studies of the effects of HIV infection on hypothalamic–pituitary–gonadal function have been performed mostly in adult men. Most have shown some degree of hypogonadism, especially in the most severely affected individuals. Conflicting data exist regarding the causes of the hypogonadism as primary, gonadal, or hypothalamic–pituitary in origin. Clinical evidence of hypogonadism as reflected by a history of decreased libido and impotence was reported in 28 of 42 and 14 of 42 ambulatory patients with AIDS, respectively (84). Of the HIV-infected men, 38% had low serum testosterone levels, the majority having low baseline serum gonadotropin levels. Human chorionic gonadotropin stimulation in two men resulted in normal testosterone responses, attesting to a normal testicular ability to produce testosterone. In seven of eight men, gonadotropin-releasing hormone (GnRH) stimulation resulted in normal gonadotropin responses, suggesting that the gonadal dysfunction was hypothalamic in origin. In contrast, Croxson et al. (138) described low testosterone levels accompanied by high levels of LH and follicle-stimulating hormone (FSH) in patients with AIDS, suggestive of the diagnosis of primary hypogonadism.

Rietschel at al. (139) investigated the prevalence of hypogonadism in HIV-infected men receiving HAART, or PI, nucleoside reverse transcriptase inhibitor, or nonnucleoside reverse transcriptase inhibitor compared to healthy controls. The prevalence of hypogonadism was ∼20% in all medication groups. Testosterone levels and free testosterone levels were not different between the groups.

Decreased basal and also mean 24 h plasma testosterone levels have been reported by some (93,110). One study has documented elevated free testosterone levels and exaggerated LH responses to GnRH (85). Martin et al. (140) reported that HIV-positive patients had 39–51% higher levels of sex-steroid-binding proteins than HIV-negative control subjects. Isolated LH deficiency (141) and transient gynecomastia (142) have been described.

Grinspoon and others (144,146) have studied hormonal changes in patients with HIV infection and lipodystrophy. In men with lipodystrophy, with hypogonadism, it has been shown that the administration of testosterone led to improvements in lean body mass, indexes of insulin sensitivity, and the sense wellbeing. HIV-infected women with lipodystrophy have increased androgen levels (147). Thirty-nine women were evaluated: 9 HIV-positive with lipodystrophy, 14 HIV-positive without lipodystrophy, and 16 healthy age- and BMI-matched women served as controls. Total testosterone and free testosterone levels were increased in the HIV-positive group. Sex-hormone-binding globulin levels were not significantly different between the HIV-positive group and control, but were significantly lower in the lipodystrophic group than in the HIV-positive patients without lipodystrophy.

Gonadal function has not been systematically investigated in children with HIV infections. Gertner et al. (39) documents pubertal delay accompanied by bone age delay in HIV-positive poorly growing boys with hemophilia. de Martino et al. (148) studied the onset of puberty and its progression in 212 (107 girls; 105 boys) children with perinatal HIV infection. The age of onset of puberty in girls was delayed by about 2 years and 12–15 months in boys. The progression of puberty was also prolonged in both girls and boys. More studies are needed to identify and examine gonadal function in children of all ages with HIV infections.

VI. PANCREAS

Anatomical evidence for pancreatic involvement by HIV or associated organisms has been more common than clinical evidence of either exocrine or endocrine pancreatic deficiencies (149).

Pancreatic lesions as a result of HIV, CMV, toxoplasmosis, Kaposi's sarcoma, lymphoma, and pancreatitis have been reported in autopsy material in approximately half of the patients with AIDS. The most frequent damage to the pancreas in AIDS patients is drug-induced, especially by the nucleoside analog Diadanosine (DDI) and pentamidine used for prophylaxis of *Pneumocystis carinii* (71,72,150). Clinical correlation in one of these studies (150) revealed no evidence of hyperglycemia. One report described the development of insulin-dependent diabetes mellitus in two HIV-infected, drug-addicted subjects in whom neither anti-insulin nor anti-islet-cell antibodies were detected (151). In most HIV-infected patients normal glucose levels were found (84). Hommes et al. (152) used the euglycemic clamp technique to measure insulin sensitivity and clearance in 10 HIV-infected stable patients and 10 healthy control subjects. They found increased rates of insulin clearance and increased peripheral tissue sensitivity in the HIV-infected men.

Chehter et al. (153) conducted a prospective study of 109 postmortem AIDS patients and 38 controls. Pancreatic involvement was observed in 91% of the cases, but none was symptomatic. The changes, based on morphological characteristics, had no correlation with clinical or laboratory features.

Sentongo et al. (154) studied the association among steatorrhea, growth, and immunological status in children with perinatally acquired HIV infection. They postulated that the steatorrhea observed in HIV-infected children was due to exocrine pancreatic insufficiency (EPI). In their sample of 44 children with perinatally acquired HIV infection, there was a high prevalence of steatorrhea (39%) that was neither secondary to EPI nor associated with impaired growth, HIV RNA virus load, CD4 status, or the type of antiviral regimen used. The clinical significance of steatorrhea remained unclear.

Clinical presentation of acute pancreatitis in HIV-infected patients is similar to that of immunocompetent patients. Evidence of pancreatitis has not generally been reported, although Zazzo et al. (155), in a prospective study of 35 consecutive patients with AIDS admitted to an intensive care unit, found evidence of acute pancreatitis with elevated levels of amylase and lipase in 16. Of these patients, eight died and had documentation on autopsy of pancreatic infection by CMV, *Candida*, and cryptococci. Because of the lack of sufficient clinical warning signs of pancreatitis, the authors suggest laboratory measurements of amylase and lipase in critically ill HIV-infected patients. Pancreatitis has also been reported in one 3-year-old HIV-positive child (156,157).

Miller et al. (158) reported that 9 of 53 children with AIDS developed acute pancreatitis during a 6 year period. The risk of pancreatitis was greatest in patients who received pentamidine and had CD4 counts <100 cell/mm.

In conclusion, the most consistent finding in acute pancreatitis in HIV-infected patients is serum amylase and lipase values greater than three times the upper limit of normal (157).

VII. PARATHYROID

Lesions of the parathyroid glands have been reported in autopsy studies (70,72), but parathyroid dysfunction has been reported extremely infrequently. Hypercalcemia with low serum levels of parathyroid hormone and calcitriol has been described in two patients with AIDS and disseminated CMV infection (159). The hypercalcemia improved with calcitriol treatment in one patient. It was postulated by the authors that the hypercalcemia might have been caused by increased osteoclast-mediated bone resorption resulting from disseminated CMV infection with accompanying renal insufficiency. Six patients with AIDS-associated lymphoma were found to have hypercalcemia (n = 4) or hypercalcuria (n = 2), presumably because of the

deregulated synthesis of a compound such as 1,25-dihydroxyvitamin D (160).

Aukurst et al. (161) report that HIV patients with advanced clinical disease have a decreased or normal serum calcium, decreased PTH, and decreased serum 1,25-(OH)2D. They also found a decrease of osteocalcin and elevated C-telopepetide level. These findings suggest that during advanced HIV-related disease there is a disturbance of bone metabolism. This disturbance was correlated with increased activity of the TNF system. Patients with advanced HIV-related disease receiving HAART therapy had a marked rise in serum osteocalcin. This finding suggests a synchronization of the bone remodeling process during the HAART therapy. It is unclear whether the benefit is due to the HAART, the decrease of TNF, or decreased viral load.

VIII. PROLACTIN

Because of the potential immune-regulatory property of prolactin (162,163), serum prolactin levels were studied in HIV-infected individuals. Compared with HIV-negative homosexual, bisexual, or heterosexual controls, serum prolactin levels were normal in HIV-infected men, including those with AIDS (164,165).

Hutchinson et al. (166) reported four women with galactorrhea and hyperprolactinemia as an isolated endocrine abnormality following use of PIs. The mechanism underlying these findings is unclear, yet it is known that the use of PI has been linked to other endocrine abnormalities such as hyperlipidemia, diabetes mellitus, and insulin resistance.

IX. HYPOTHALAMUS AND PITUITARY

The effects of HIV infections on the central nervous system have been the subjects of numerous reports (167). Nevertheless, specific pathological documentation of lesions in the hypothalamus or pituitary of affected individuals has been rare. So-called panhypopituitarism secondary to toxoplasmosis (168) and posterior pituitary lesions in HIV-infected children with disseminated CMV (76) have been reported.

Yanovski et al. (169) postulated that the increase of abdominal adipose tissue found in HIV-infected subjects treated with PIs could be due to abnormalities in adrenal function. They designed a study to evaluate the HPA, in HIV-infected men and women receiving the PI regimen, patients with Cushing syndrome, and healthy controls. Patients on the PI regimen had normal diurnal cortisol secretion, cortisol secretory dynamics after oCRH, cortisol-binding globulin levels, and glucocorticoid number and affinity. The abnormalities noted were increased basal and CRH-stimulated plasma ACTH and 24 h urinary 17-

OHCS excretion, and decreased urinary free cortisol. The study design did not include any HIV-infected patients who were not receiving PI treatment; therefore the changes observed, although coinciding with PI treatment, could not be solely ascribed to the use of PI. They suggested that the increased intra-abdominal adiposity, dyslipidemia, and insulin resistance without total body weight gain was a distinct yet undefined form of hypercortisolism unrelated to HPA axis.

Evidence of specific hypothalamic–pituitary dysfunction in endocrine organs was reviewed in previous sections.

X. ENDOCRINE ALTERATIONS SECONDARY TO TREATMENT

In HIV-infected children and adults, the effects of the various treatment regimens employed may also cause endocrine dysfunction. These effects must be separated from endocrine defects caused by HIV and related opportunistic infections.

Hypothyroidism has been reported as a result of drugs that affect cytochrome P450 enzyme systems, such as ketoconazole (117,170) and rifampin (118), as well as interferon treatment (171,172).

Hypoadrenalism may result from ketoconazole (173–175) or rifampin (176,177) treatment. Hypogonadism and gynecomastia in men have also been noted during ketoconazole treatment (178,179). Hypoglycemia has been reported in patients with AIDS treated with pentamidine (180–183) and trimethoprim–sulfamethoxazole (184). Hyponatremia has been associated with pentamidine (185) and vidarabine (186) therapy. Hypocalcemic tetany secondary to magnesium loss has been noted during amphotericin B and aminoglycoside treatment (187). Hyperkalemia was reported in a patient with AIDS to be a result of the sodium channel inhibitory effects of trimethoprim (188).

With the increased use of PI in the treatment of HIV-infected adults, a number of studies have reported LDS and hyperinsulinemia (49,50,54,55). It is unclear whether or how PI treatment causes LDS and hyperglycemia. Hadigan et al. (189) reported hyperinsulinemia and increased truncal adiposity in HIV-infected men receiving a nucleoside reverse transcriptase protocol who were not receiving PI therapy. They found that testosterone replacement in hypogonadal men improved insulin sensitivity.

There are some reports in the literature on the development of diabetes mellitus in HIV-infected individuals (190–192). Abdel-Khalek et al. (191) reported new-onset diabetes mellitus in an 18-year-old girl with HIV. She presented with polydipsia and polyuria with nonketotic hyperglycemia. Pancreatic islet cell antibodies were negative and she had normal basal C-peptide levels, normal serum lipase and amylase, and normal BMI. She was treated initially with 1.15–1.38 U/kg/day; her HbA1c at diagnosis was 7.6%. Later, she had hyperglycemia with serum glucose concentrations above 400 mg/dl and her HBA1c value rose to 13.6%; she required an insulin dosage of 2.22 U/kg/d.

In another publication, Lee et al. (192) reported an HIV-positive patient who presented with a random blood glucose level of 493.2 mg/dl and a 3 week history of polyuria, polydipsia, and polyphagia, with weight loss, fatigue, weakness, and blurry vision. The patient had no symptoms of infection at presentation. The patient was treated with oral hypoglycemic agents and insulin. These medications were discontinued gradually as his blood glucose level declined. Significant decrease in blood glucose values was observed when the patient discontinued all antiretroviral medications. Overall, the incidence of diabetes has not increased substantially. Some reports associate the development of diabetes with the use of PI (190–192). The likely explanation seems to be increase in insulin resistance during PI treatment only (192).

XI. FUTURE HORMONAL THERAPY IN HIV INFECTIONS

Considerable attention has focused on reversal of the weight loss and wasting accompanying AIDS. Therapeutic strategies have involved the use of appetite stimulants, such as megesterol acetate; anticytokine-directed supplements, such as dietary N-3 fatty acids; anabolic agents, such as steroids and growth hormone; and metabolic inhibitors, such as hydrazine sulfate (193,194).

The most extensive experience with megestrol acetate in adults has been summarized elsewhere (195–197). Clarick et al. (198) evaluated 19 HIV-infected children (11 boys and 8 girls) with a median age of 89 months (range, 28–192) who were treated with megestrol acetate for a median duration of 7 months (range, 3–11 months). Megestrol acetate treatment led to significant weight gain without linear growth acceleration.

Growth hormone and IGF-1 have been utilized in HIV-infected patients. In a prospective double-blind clinical trial, five patients each were assigned randomly to treatment with GH at either 5.0 or 2.5 mg every other day (199). Of the 10, 3 withdrew because of opportunistic infections. In the remaining patients, all of whom also received zidovudine, the higher dosages of GH reversed the pretreatment weight loss by increasing lean body mass and total body water, and decreasing total body fat and urinary nitrogen excretion. Muscle power and endurance also improved. Fasting plasma glucose, insulin, and C peptide levels increased in all. CD4 cell counts did not change. During treatment one patient became p24 antigen-positive. The short-term beneficial effects were noted only with use of the higher GH dosages.

In a short-term, carefully conducted clinical trial, Mulligan et al. (200) administered GH, 0.1 mg/kg/day for

7 days, to six HIV-positive men with an average weight loss of 19% and six healthy HIV-negative subjects. Treatment resulted in an increase in body weight, nitrogen retention, increased energy expenditure, lipid oxidation, and glucose flux, and decreased protein oxidation in both groups. These short-term effects of increases in protein anabolism and protein-sparing lipid oxidation, should they be sustained during long-term treatment, were postulated to result in increased total body cell mass.

Lieberman et al. (201) found that a single injection of GH administered to 21 patients with AIDS resulted in a smaller increase in IGF-1 than in 23 age-matched controls, suggesting partial resistance to GH in AIDS. In 10 subjects low-dosage but not high-dosage IGF-1 administration for 10 days resulted in only a transient anabolic effect, as demonstrated by a transient increase in nitrogen retention.

Waters et al. (63) studied 60 patients with AIDS wasting receiving 1.4 mg GH once a day, 5 mg IGF-1 twice a day, 5 mg IGF-1 twice a day and 1.4 mg GH once a day, and a placebo group. At 6 weeks, lean body mass increased and fat mass decreased in the groups receiving GH, IGF-1, or both. The improvements observed persisted at 12 weeks only in the group receiving GH and IGF-1 therapy. Ellis et al. (64) conducted a double-blind, placebo-controlled study in which 44 HIV-infected men received GH/IGF-1 treatment and 22 HIV-infected men received placebo treatment. The treatment group received 0.34 mg GH twice a day and 5.0 mg IGF-1 twice a day. The study duration was 12 weeks. At 6 weeks, GH/IGF-1 group had a significant increase in fat free-mass and a substantial decrease in fat. At 12 weeks, the loss of fat remained significant, whereas the increase in fat-free mass was lost in many of the subjects. The loss of body fat was not observed in the placebo group.

Lo et al. (62) studied the effect of 3 mg GH daily in eight men with HIV-associated fat accumulation. In six subjects who completed 6 months of study, GH treatment decreased total body fat and increased lean body mass. At 1 month of treatment insulin sensitivity and glucose tolerance worsened, but these improved towards baseline by 6 months.

Several studies of GH treatment are underway. Pinto et al. (67) reported two HIV-infected prepubertal children who were treated with GH for 3 years. In one child height increased from −3.6 SD to −2.0 SD below the mean and in the second child height increased from −4.7 SD to −1.9 SD.

Gonadal steroid hormone replacement has been used with increasing success in HIV-positive patients. Decreases in gonadal function have been widely reported in adults. Men with AIDS had a significant reduction in testosterone secretion despite normal gonadotropin response to testing.

Grinspoon et al. (144,146,202) report the beneficial effect of exogenous testosterone administration for hy-

pogonadal men with lipodystrophy. Patients receiving therapy had an increase in lean body mass, weight gain, and a decrease in the incidence of depression. Overall, their wellbeing, as measured by the Beck Depression Inventory, improved with testosterone replacement therapy. In women, administration of a lower dosage of testosterone (150 and 300 μg/day) led to normalization of serum testosterone levels, weight gain, and improvement in their quality of life (203).

Studies are underway to evaluate the long-term complications associated with PI therapy. As reported in other sections, the LDS might be associated with progression of atherosclerosis, cardiovascular disease, and complications that can be attributed to hyperinsulinemia. As the management of HIV-infected individuals continues to improve, we can look forward to newer, more innovative, and specifically targeted interventions to address even the hormonal dysfunction of these patients.

XII. CONCLUSION

From the initial description in the literature on June 5th, 1981, there have been many advances in the field of HIV/AIDS. There have been numerous advances in the areas of epidemiology, management, prevention, and prophylaxis of HIV disease globally. Much effort is currently being focused on prevention strategies, with vaccines playing a potentially pivotal role. Some phase III trials of vaccines have already started. Yet HIV/AIDS continues to spread. Reports indicate that rate of HIV infection from heterosexual sex is soaring among US teenaged girls. Clinicians need to promote intensive, focused, appropriate HIV prevention efforts among adolescent women.

Endocrine effects of HIV infection are not often easily recognized by clinical signs and/or symptoms, or baseline hormonal evaluation, or even stimulation tests. Therefore, health care providers need to have a high index of suspicion for possible endocrine abnormalities secondary to HIV infection and/or its treatment. Persistent and careful investigations may eventually disclose the endocrine abnormalities, the treatment of which should improve patients' quality of life.

The evaluation and treatment of endocrine alterations in subjects with HIV infections will continue to become an increasingly important clinical and investigational area of pediatric endocrinology.

REFERENCES

1. Sepkowitz KA. AIDS—The first 20 years. N Engl J Med 2001; 344(23):1764–1772.
2. Oleske J, Minnefor A, Cooper R Jr, et al. Immune deficiency syndrome in children. JAMA 1983; 249:2345–2349.
3. Rubinstein A, Sicklick M, Gupta A, et al. Acquired immunodeficiency with reversed T4/T8 ratios in infants born

to promiscuous and drug addicted mothers. JAMA 1983; 249:2350–2356.

4. UNAIDS, WHO. AIDS epidemic update: December 2000. Geneva: Joint United Nations Programme on HIV/ AIDS, 2000.

5. Grubman S, Conviser R, Oleske J. HIV infections in infants, children and adolescents. In: Wormser GP, ed. AIDS and other Manifestations of HIV Infections. 2nd ed. New York: Raven Press, 1992:201–216.

6. CDC update: a glance at the HIV epidemic. Medline December 2000.

7. Sperling RS, Shapiro DE, Delifraissy JF, et al. Safety of the maternal-infant zidovudine regimen utilized in the Pediatric AIDS Clinical Trial Group 076 Study. AIDS 1998; 12:1805–1813.

8. Oleske J, et al. Lack of long-term effects of in utero exposure to zidovudine among uninfected children born to HIV-infected women. JAMA 1999; 281:151–157.

9. Mofenson LM, McIntyre JA. Advances and research directions in the prevention of mother-to-child HIV-1 transmission. Lancet 2000; 355:2237–2244.

10. Dabis F, Leroy V, Salamon R, et al. Preventing mother-to-child transmission of HIV-1 in Africa in the year 2000. AIDS 2000; 14:1017–1026.

11. Markson LE, Turner BJ, Houchens R, Silverman NS, Cosler L, Taki BK. Association of maternal HIV infection with low birth weight. J Acquir Immune Defic Syndr Hum Retrovirol 1996; 1;13(3):227–234.

12. Weng S, Bulterys M, Chao A, Stidely A, Dushimimana A, Mbatutso E, Saah A. Perinatal HIV-1 transmission and intrauterine growth: A cohort study in Butare, Rwanda. Pediatrics 1998; 102(2).

13. Maas U, Kattner E, Koch S, Schafer A, Obladen M. Fetal development and neonatal morbidity in infants of HIV-positive mothers. Monatsschr Kinderheilkd 1990; 138: 799–802.

14. Moye J Jr, Rich KC, Kalish LA, Sheon AR, Diaz C, Cooper ER, Pitt J, Handelsman E. Natural history of somatic growth in infants born to women infected by human immunodeficiency virus. J Pediatr 1996; 128:58–66.

15. McKinney RE, Maha MA, Connor EM, et al. A multi-center trial of oral zidovudine in children with advanced human immunodeficiency virus disease. N Engl J Med 1991; 324:1018–1025.

16. Johnson JP, Nair P, Hines SE, et al. Natural history and serologic diagnosis of infants born to human immuno-deficiency virus-infected women. Am J Dis Child 1989; 143:1147–1153.

17. Blanche S, Le Keist F, Fischer A, et al. Longitudinal study of 18 children with perinatal LAV/HTLV II infection: attempts at prognostic evaluation. J Pediatr 1986; 109:965–970.

18. McKinney RE, Wesley J, Robertson R. Effect on human immunodeficiency virus infection on the growth of young children. J Pediatr 1993; 123:579–582.

19. de Martino M, Galli L, Chiarelli F, Verrotti A, Rossi ME, Bindi G, Galluzzi F, Salti R, Vierucci A. Interleukin-6 release by cultured peripheral blood mononuclear cells inversely correlates with height velocity, bone age, insulin-like growth factor-I, and insulin-like growth factor binding protein-3 serum levels in children with perinatal HIV-1 infectio. Clin Immunol 2000; 94(3):212–218.

20. Scott GB, Buck BE, Leterman JG, Bloom FL, Parks WO. Acquired immunodeficiency syndrome in infants. N Engl J Med 1984; 12(310):76–81.

21. Marion RW, Wiznia AA, Hutcheon RG, Rubinstein A. Human T-cell lympho-tropic virus type III (HTLV-III) embryopathy. Am J Dis Child 1986; 140:638–640.

22. Rubinstein A. Pediatric AIDS. Curr Probl Pediatr 1986; 16(7):379–380.

23. Shannon KM, Ammann AJ. Acquired immune deficiency syndrome in children. J Pediatr 1985; 106(332):42.

24. Falloon J, Eddy J, Wiener L, Pizzo PA. Human immunodeficiency virus infection in children. J Pediatr 1989; 114:1–30.

25. Kamani N, Lightman H, Leiderman MS, Kirlov LR. Pediatric acquired immunodeficiency syndrome-related complex: clinical and immunologic features. J Pediatr Infect Dis 1998; 7:383–388.

26. Johann-Liang R, O'Neill L, Cervia J, Haller I, Giunta Y, Licholai T, Noel GJ. Energy balance, viral burden, insulin-like growth factor-1, interleukin-6, and growth impairment in children infected with human immunodeficiency virus. AIDS 2000; 14:683–690.

27. Rapaport R, McSherry G, Connor E, et al. Growth and hormonal parameters in symptomatic human immunodeficiency virus (HIV) infected children (abstract). Pediatr Res 1989; 25:187A.

28. Rapaport R, Sills I, Figueroa W, Hoyt I, Mintz M. Growth failure (GF) in HIV infected children (HIV-IC) (abstract). Pediatr Res 1993: 33:82A.

29. Jospe N, Powell KR. Growth hormone deficiency in an 8-year-old girl with human immunodeficiency virus infection. Pediatrics 1990; 86:309–312.

30. Laue L, Pizzo PA, Butler K, Cutler GB Jr. Growth and neuroendocrine dysfunction in children with acquired immunodeficiency syndrome. J Pediatr 1990; 117:541–545.

31. Schwartz LJ, Louis Y, Wu R, Wiznia A, Rubinstein A, Saenger P. Endocrine function in children with human immunodeficiency virus infection. Am J Dis Child 1991; 145:330–333.

32. Lepage P, Van de Perre P, Van Vliet G, et al. Clinical and endocrinologic manifestations in perinatally human immunodeficiency virus type-1 infected children aged 5 years or older. Am J Dis Child 1991; 145:1248–1251.

33. Rondanelli M, Caselli D, Maccabruni A, et al. Involvement of hormonal circadian secretion in the growth of HIV-infected children. AIDS 1998; 12:1845–1850.

34. Carey VJ, Yong FH, Frenkel LM, McKinney RE Jr. Pediatric AIDS prognosis using somatic growth velocity. AIDS 1998; 12:1361–1369.

35. Kaufman FR, Gomperts ED. Growth failure in boys with hemophilia and HIV infection. Am J Pediatr Hematol Oncol 1989; 11:292–294.

36. Jason J, Gomperts E, Lawrence DN, et al. HIV and hemophilic children's growth. J Acquir Immune Defic Syndr 1989; 2:277–282.

37. Brettler DB, Forsberg A, Bolivar E, Brewster F, Sullivan J. Growth failure as a prognostic indicator for progression to acquired immunodeficiency syndrome in children with hemophilia. J Pediatr 1990; 117:584–588.

38. Hilgartner MW, Donfield SM, Willoughby A, et al. Hemophilia growth and development study. Am J Pediatr Hematol Oncol 1993; 15:208–217.

39. Gertner JM, Kaufman FR, Donfield SM, et al. Delayed somatic growth and pubertal development in human immunodeficiency virus-infected hemophiliac boys: hemophilia growth and development study. J Pediatr 1994; 124(6):896–902.

40. Kaufman FR, Gertner JM, Sleeper LA, Donfield SM, and the Hemophilia Growth and Development Study. Growth

hormone secretion in HIV-positive versus HIV-negative hemophilic males with abnormal growth and pubertal development. J Acquir Immune Defic Syndr 1997; 15(2): 137–144.

41. Hilgartner MW, Donfield MS, Lynn HS, Hoots WK, Gomperts ED, et al. The effect of plasma human immunodeficiency virus RNA and CD4+ T lymphocytes on growth measurements of hemophilic boys and adolescents. Pediatrics 2001; 107(4)e56.

42. Miller TL, Ovav EJ, Martin SR, Cooper ER, McIntosh K, Winter HS. Malnutrition and carbohydrate malabsorption in children with vertically transmitted human immunodeficiency virus 1 infection. Gastroenterology 1991; 100:1296–1302.

43. Brief critical reviews. Is malabsorption an important cause of growth failure in HIV-infected children? Nutr Rev 1991; 49:341–343.

44. Henderson RA, Saavedra JM, Perman JA, Hutton N, Livingston RA, Yolken RH. Effect of enteral tube feeding on growth of children with symptomatic human immunodeficiency virus infection. J Pediatr Gastroenterol Nutr 1994; 18(4):429–434.

45. Arpadi SM, Cuff PA, Kotler DP, Wang J, Bamji M, Lange M, Pierson RN, Matthews DE. Growth velocity, fat-free mass and energy intake are inversely related to viral load in HIV-infected children. J Nutr 2000; 130:2498–2502.

46. Mintz M, Rapaport R, Oleske JM, et al. Elevated serum levels of tumor necrosis factor are associated with progressive encephalopathy in children with acquired immunodeficiency syndrome. Am J Dis Child 1989; 143: 171–174.

47. Miller TL, Mawn BE, Orav J, Wilk D, Geoffrey A, et al. The effect of protease inhibitor therapy on growth and body composition in human immunodeficiency virus type 1-infected children. Pediatrics 2001; 107(5):e77.

48. Ho TTY, Chan KCW, Wong KH. Abnormal fat distribution and use of protease inhibitors. Lancet 1998; 351: 1736–1737.

49. Dube M, Johnson D, et al. Protease inhibitor-associated hyperglycemia. Lancet 1997; 350:713–714.

50. Carr A, Samaras K, et al. Pathogenesis of HIV-protease inhibitor-associated peripherl lipodystrophy, hyperlipidemia and insulin resistance. Lancet 1998; 351:1881–1883.

51. Sullivan AK, Nelson MR. Marked hyperlipidemia on ritonavir therapy. AIDS 1997; 11:938–939.

52. Grinspoon S. Endocrine disorders and therapeutic strategies in AIDS. Post Graduate Course in Clinical Endocrinology 2001. Boston, MA: Mass. General Hospital/Harvard Medical School April 2–6, 2001.

53. Lo J, Mulligan K, et al. "Buffalo hump" in men with HIV-1 infection. Lancet 1998; 351:867–870.

54. Carr A, Samaras K, Thorisdottir A, Kauffman GR, Chisolm DJ, Cooper DA. Diagnosis, prediction, and natural course of HIV-1 protease-inhibitor associated lipodystrophy, hyperlipidemia and diabetes mellitus: a cohort study. Lancet 1999; 353:2093–2099.

55. Bonnet E, Cuzin L, et al. Associated lipodystropy metabolic disorders due to protease inhibitors containing regimens. Abstract 12299, 12th World AIDS Conference, Geneva, June 28–July 3, 1998.

56. Papadopoulos A, Vangelopoulou E, et al. Serum lipid changes in HIV-infected patients under combination therapy containing a protease inhibitor. Abstract 60118, 12th World AIDS Conference, Geneva, June 28–July 3, 1998.

57. Grunfeld C, Kotler DP, Hamadeh R, Tierney A, Wang J, Pierson RN. Hypertriglyceridemia in the acquired immunodeficiency syndrome. Am J Med 1989; 86:27–31.

58. Grunfeld C, Pang M, Doerrler W, Shigenaga JK, Jensen P, Feingold KR. Lipids, lipoproteins, triglycerides clearance, and cytokines in human immunodeficiency virus infection and the acquired immuno-deficiency syndrome. J Clin Endocrinol Metab 1992; 74:1045–1052.

59. Arpadi SM, Cuff PA, Horlick M, Wang J, Kotler DP. Lipodystrophy in HIV-infected children is associated with high viral load and low CD4+-lymphocyte count and CD4+-lymphocyte percentage at baseline and use of protease inhibitors and stavudine. J Acquir Immune Defic Syndr 2001;27(1):30–34.

60. Wedekind CA, Pugtach D. Lipodystrophy syndrome in children infected with human immunodeficiency virus. Pharmacotherapy 2001; 21(7):861–866.

61. Rietschel P, Hadigan C, Corcoran C, Stanley T, Neubauer G, Gertner J, Grinspoon S. Assessment of growth hormone dynamics in human immunodeficiency virus-related lipodystrophy. J Clin Endocrinol Metab 2001; 86(2):504–510.

62. Lo JC, Mulligan K, Noor MA, Schwartz JM, Halvorsen RA, Grunfeld C, Schambelan M. The effects of recombinant human growth hormone on body composition and glucose metabolism in HIV-infected patients with fat accumulation. J Clin Endocrinol Metab 2001; 86(8):3480–3487.

63. Waters D, Danska J, Hardy K, Koster F, Qualls C, Nickell D, et al. Recombinant human growth hormone, insulin-like growth factor 1, and combination therapy in AIDS associated wasting. Ann Intern Med 1996; 125:865–872.

64. Ellis KJ, Lee PDK, Pivarnik JM, Bukar JG, Gesundheit N. Changes in body composition of human immunodeficiency virus-infected males receiving insulin-like growth factor 1 and growth hormone. J Clin Endocrinol Metab 1996; 81(8):3033–3038.

65. Mynarcik DC, Frost RA, Lang CH, DeCristofaro K, McNurlan MA, et al. Insulin-like growth factor system in patients with HIV infection: effects of exogenous growth hormone administration. J Acquir Immune Defic Syndr 1999; 22:49–55.

66. Helle SI, Ueland T, Ekse D, Froland SS, Holly JMP, Lonning PE, Aukrust P. The insulin-like growth factor system in HIV infection: Relations to immunological parameters, disease progression, and antiretroviral therapy. J Clin Endocrinol Metab 2001; 86(1):227–233.

67. Pinto G, Blanche S, Thiriet I, Souberielle JC, Goulet O, Brauner R. Growth hormone treatment of children with human immunodeficiency virus-associated growth failure. Eur J Pediatr 2000; 159(12):937–938 (Letter).

68. Reichert CM, O'Leary TJ, Levens DL, Simrell CR, Macher AM. Autopsy pathology in the acquired immune deficiency syndrome. Am J Pathol 1983; 112:357–382.

69. Tapper ML, Rotterdam HZ, Lerner CW, Al'Khafaji K, Seitzman PM. Adrenal necrosis in the acquired immunodeficiency syndrome. Ann Intern Med 1984; 100:239–241.

70. Welch K, Finkbeiner W, Alpers CE, et al. Autopsy findings in the acquired immune deficiency syndrome. Ann Intern Med 1984; 100:239–240.

71. Mobley K, Rotterdam HZ, Lerner CW, Tapper ML. Autopsy findings in the acquired immunodeficiency syndrome. Pathol Annu 1985; 20:45–65.

72. Niedt GW, Schinella RA. Acquired immunodeficiency syndrome. Arch Pathol Lab Med 1985; 109:727–734.

73. Glasgow BJ, Steinsapir KP, Anders K, Layfield LJ. Adrenal pathology in the acquired immune deficiency syndrome. Am J Clin Pathol 1985; 84:594–597.

74. Weiss CD. The human immunodeficiency virus and the adrenal medulla. Ann Intern Med 1986; 105:300.

75. Laulund S, Visfeldt J, Klinken L. Patho-anatomical studies in patients dying of AIDS. Acta Pathol Microbiol Immunol Scand [A] 1986; 94:201–221.

76. Joshi VV, Oleske JM, Saad S, Connor EM, Rapkin RH, Minnerfor AB. Pathology of opportunistic infections in children with acquired immune deficiency syndrome. Pediatr Pathol 1986; 6:145–150.

77. Pulakhandam U, Dincsoy HP. Cytomegaloviral adrenalitis and adrenal insufficiency in AIDS. Am J Clin Pathol 1990; 93:651–656.

78. Klein RS, Mann DN, Freidland GH, Surks MI. Adrenocortical function in the acquired immunodeficiency syndrome. Ann Intern Med 1983; 99:566.

79. Greene LW, Cole W, Greene JB, et al. Adrenal insufficiency as a complication of the acquired immunodeficiency syndrome. Ann Intern Med 1984; 101:497–498.

80. Guenthner EE, Rabinowe SL, Van Niel A, Naftilan A, Dluhy RG. Primary Addison's disease in a patient with the acquired immuno-deficiency syndrome. Ann Intern Med 1984; 100:847–848.

81. Salik JM, Kurtin P. Severe hyponatremia after colonoscopy preparation in a patient with the acquired immune deficiency syndrome. Am J Gastroenterol 1985; 80:177–179.

82. Bleiweiss IJ, Pervez NK, Hammer GS, Dikman SH. Cytomegalovirus-induced adrenal insufficiency and associated renal cell carcinoma in AIDS. Mt Sinai J Med 1986; 53:676–679.

83. Membreno L, Irony I, Dere W, Klein R, Biglieri EG, Cobb E. Adrenocortical function in acquired immunodeficiency syndrome. J Clin Endocrinol Metab 1987; 65:482–487.

84. Dobs AS, Dempsey MA, Ladenson PW, Polk BP. Endocrine disorders in men infected with human immunodeficiency virus. Am J Med 1988; 84:611–616.

85. Merenich JA, McDermott MT, Asp AA, Harrison SM, Kidd GS. Evidence of endocrine involvement early in the course of human immuno-deficiency virus infection. J Clin Endocrinol Metab 1990; 70:566–571.

86. Kumar M, Kumar AM, Morgan R, Szapocznik J, Eisdorfer C. Abnormal pituitary–adrenocortical response in early HIV-1 infection. J Acquir Immune Defic Syndr 1993; 6:61–65.

87. Catania A, Manfredi MG, Airaghi L, et al. Delayed cortisol response to antigenic challenge in patients with acquired immunodeficiency syndrome. Ann NY Acad Sci 1992; 650:202–204.

88. Verges B, Chavanet P, Desgres J, et al. Adrenal function in HIV infected patients. Acta Endocrinol (Copenh) 1989; 121:633–637.

89. Christeff N, Gharakhanian S, Thobie N, Rozenbaum W, Nuenez EA. Evidence for changes in adrenal and testicular steroids during HIV infection. J Acquir Immune Defic Syndr 1992; 5:841–846.

90. Malone JL, Oldfield EC, Wagner KF, et al. Abnormalities of morning serum cortisol levels and circadian rhythms of CD4 lymphocyte counts in human immunodeficiency virus type 1-infected adult patients. J Infect Dis 1992; 156:185.

91. Villette JM, Dourin P, Doinel C, et al. Circadain variations in plasma levels of hypophyseal adrenocortical and testicular hormones in men infected with human immunodeficiency virus. J Clin Endocrinol Metab 1990; 70:572–577.

92. Catania A, Airaghi L, Manfredi MG et al. Proopiomelanocortin-derived peptides and cytokines: relations in patients with acquired immunodeficiency syndrome. Clin Immunol Immunopathol 1993; 66:73–79.

93. Raffi F, Brisseau JM, Planchon B, Remi JP, Barrier JH, Grolleau JY. Endocrine function in 98 HIV-infected patients: a prospective study. AIDS 1991; 5:729–733.

94. Eledrisi MS, Verghese AC. Adrenal insufficiency in HIV infection: a review and recommendations. Am J Med Sci 2001; 321(2):137–144.

95. Azar ST, Melby JC. Hypothalamic-pituitary-adrenal function in non-AIDS patients with advanced HIV infection. Am J Med Sci 1993; 305:321–325.

96. Gonovan DS, Dluhy RG. AIDS and its effect on the adrenal gland. Endocrinologist 1991; 1:227–232.

97. Grinspoon S, Bilezikian JP. HIV disease and the endocrine system. N Engl J Med 1992; 32:1360–1365.

98. Vitting KE, Gardenswartz MH, Zabetakis PM, et al. Frequency of hyponatremia and nonosmolar vasopressin release in the acquired immunodeficiency syndrome. JAMA 1990; 263:973–978.

99. Agarwal A, Soni A, Ciechanowsky M, Chander P. Treser G. Hyponatremia in patients with the acquired immunodeficiency syndrome. Nephron 1989; 53:317–321.

100. Cusano AJ, Thies HL, Siegal FP, Dreisbach AW, Maesaka JK. Hyponatremia in patients with acquired immune deficiency syndrome. J Acquir Immune Defic Syndr 1990; 3:949–953.

101. Tang WW, Kaptein EM, Feinstein EI, Massry SG. Hyponatremia in hospitalized patients with acquired immune deficiency syndrome. Am J Med 1993; 94(2):169–174.

102. Kalin MF, Poretsky L, Seres DS, Zumoff B. Hyporeninemic hypoaldo-steronism associated with acquired immune deficiency syndrome. Am J Med 1987; 82:1035–1038.

103. Guy RJC, Turberg Y, Davidson RN, Finnerty G, MacGregor GA, Wise PH. Mineralocorticoid deficiency in HIV infection. Br Med J 1989; 298:496–497.

104. Merril CR, Harrington MG, Sunderland T. Plasma dehydroepiandrosterone levels in HIV infection. JAMA 1989; 261:1149.

105. Jacobson MA, Fusaro RE, Galamarini M, Lang W. Decreased serum dehydroepiandrosterone is associated with an increased progression of human immunodeficiency virus infection in men with CD4 cell counts of 200–499. J Infect Dis 1991; 164:864–868.

106. Mulder JW, Jos Frissen PH, Krijen P, et al. Dehydroepiandrosterone as predictor for progression to AIDS in asymptomatic human immunodeficiency virus-infected men. J Infect Dis 1992; 165:413–418.

107. Wisniewski TL, Hilton CW, Morse EV, Svec F. The relationship of serum DHEA-S and cortisol levels to measures of immune function in human immunodeficiency virus-related illness. Am J Med Sci 1993; 305:79–83.

108. Norbiato G, Bevilacqua M, Vago T, et al. Cortisol resistance in acquired immunodeficiency syndrome. J Clin Endocrinol Metab 1992; 74:608–613.

109. Rapaport R, McSherry G, Connor E, Oleske J. Neuroendocrine function in acquired immunodeficiency syndrome (letter). J Pediatr 1991; 118:828.

110. Oberfield SE, Kairman R, Bakshi S, et al. Steroid response to adrenocorticotropin stimulation in children with

human immunodeficiency virus infection. J Clin Endocrinol Metab 1990; 70:578–581.

111. Frank TS, LiVolsi VA, Connor M. Cytomegalovirus infection of the thyroid in immunocompromised adults. Yale J Biol Med 1987; 60:1–8.

112. Battan R, Mariuz P, Raviglione MC, Sabatini MT, Muller MP, Poretsky L. *Pneumocystis carinii* infection of the thyroid in a hypothyroid patient with AIDS: diagnosis by fine needle aspiration biopsy. J Clin Endocrinol Metab 1991; 72:724–726.

113. Krauth PH, Katz JF. Kaposi's sarcoma involving the thyroid in patients with AIDS. Clin Nucl Med 1987; 12:848–849.

114. Bourdoux PP, deWit SA, Servais GM, Clumeck N, Bonnyns MA. Biochemical thyroid profile in patients infected with the human immunodeficiency virus. Thyroid 1991; 1:147–149.

115. Tang WW, Kaptein EM. Thyroid hormone levels in the acquired immunodeficiency syndrome (AIDS) or AIDS-related complex. West J Med 1989; 151:627–631.

116. Lambert M, Zech F, DeNayer P, Jamez J, Vandercam B. Elevation of serum thyroxine-binding globulin associated with the progression of human immunodeficiency virus infection. Am J Med 1990; 89:748–751.

117. Kitching NH. Hypothyroidism after treatment with ketoconazole. Br Med J 1986; 293:993–994.

118. Isley WL. Effect of rifampin therapy on thyroid function tests in a hypothyrois patient on replacement L-thyroxine. Ann Intern Med 1987; 107:517–518.

119. Machac J, Nejatheim M, Goldsmith SJ. Gallium citrate uptake in cryptococcal thyroiditis in a homosexual male. J Nucl Med Allied Sci 1985; 29:283–285.

120. LoPresti JS, Fried JC, Spencer CA, Nicoloff JT. Unique alterations of thyroid hormone indices in the acquired immunodeficiency syndrome (AIDS). Ann Intern Med 1989; 110:970–975.

121. Feld-Rasmussen U, Sestoft L, Berg H. Thyroid function tests in patients with acquired immune deficiency syndrome and healthy HIV 1-positive out-patients. Eur J Clin Invest 1991; 21:59–63.

122. Fried JC, LoPresti JS, Micon M, Bauer M, Tuchschmidt JA, Nicoloff JT. Serum triiodothyronine values: prognostic indicators of acute mortality due to Pneumocystis carinii pneumonia associated with the acquired immunodeficiency syndrome. Arch Intern Med 1990; 150:406–409.

123. Hommes MJT, Romijn JA, Endert E, et al. Hypothyroid-like regulation of the pituitary–thyroid axis in stable human immunodeficiency virus infection. Metabolism 1993; 42: 556–561.

124. Sato K, Ozawa M, Demura H. Thyroid function in the acquired immunodeficiency syndrome (AIDS). Ann Intern Med 1989; 111:857–858.

125. Blethen SL, Nachman S, Chasalow FI. Thyroid function in children with perinatally acquired antibodies to human immunodeficiency virus. J Pediatr Endocrinol 1994; 7(3): 201–204.

126. Fundaro C, Oliveri A, Rendeli C, Genovese O, Martino AM, et al. Occurrence of anti-thyroid autoantibodies in children vertically infected with HIV-1. J Pediatr Endocrinol Metab 1998; 11:745–750.

127. Chiarelli F, Galli L, Verrotti A, et al. Thyroid function in children with perinatal human immunodeficiency virus type 1 infection. Thyroid 2000; 10(6):499–505.

128. Rapaport R, McSherry G. Unpublished data. 1993.

129. Chabon AB, Stenger RJ, Grabstald H. Histopathology of

testes inacuired immunodeficiency syndrome (AIDS). Urology 1987; 29:658–663.

130. Nistal M, Santana A, Paniagna R, Palacios J. Testicular toxoplasmosis in two men with the acquired immunodeficiency syndrome (AIDS). Arch Pathol Lab Med 1986; 110:744–746.

131. Lectsas G, Houff S, Macher A, et al. Retrovirus-like particles in salivary glands, prostate and testes of AIDS patients. Proc Soc Exp Biol Med 1985; 178:653–655.

132. Tessler AN, Cantanese A. AIDS and serous cell tumors of the testes. Urology 1987; 30:203–204.

133. Yoshikawa T, Truong LD, Fraire AE, Kim HS. The spectrum of histopathology of the testis in acquired immunodeficiency syndrome. Mod Pathol 1989; 2:233–238.

134. De Paepe ME, Waxman M. Testicular atrophy in AIDS: a study of 57 autopsy cases. Hum Pathol 1989; 20:210–214.

135. De Paepe ME, Vuletin JC, Lee MH, Rojas-Corona RR, Waxman T. Testicular atrophy in homosexual AIDS patients. Hum Pathol 1989; 20:572–578.

136. Da Silva M, Shevchuk MM, Cronin WJ, et al. Detection of HIV-related protein in testes and prostates of patients with AIDS. Am J Clin Pathol 1990; 93(2):196–201.

137. Dalton ADA, Harcout-Webster JN. The histopathology of the testis and epididymis in AIDS—A post-mortem study. J Pathol 1991; 163(1):47–52.

138. Croxon TS, Chapman WE, Miller LK, Levit CD, Senie R, Zumoff B. Changes in the hypothalamic-pituitary-gonadal axis in human immuno-deficiency virus-infected homosexual men. J Clin Endocrinol Metab 1989; 68: 317–321.

139. Rietschel P, Corcoran C, Stanley T, et al. Prevalence of hypogonadism among men with weight loss related to human immunodeficiency virus infection who were receiving highly active antiretroviral therapy. Clin Infect Dis 2000; 31:1240–1244.

140. Martin ME, Benassayag C, Amiel C, Canton P, Nunez EA. Alterations in the concentrations and binding properties of sex steroid binding protein and corticosteroid-binding globulin in HIV+ patients. J Endocrinol Invest 1992; 15:597–603.

141. Garavelli PL, Azzini M, Boccalatte G, Rosti G. Isolated LH deficiency in an AIDS patient (letter). J Acquir Immune Defic Synd 1990; 3:547.

142. Couderc LJ, Clauvel JP. HIV-infection-induced gynecomastia. Ann Intern Med 1987; 107:257.

143. Macallan DC. Wasting in HIV infection and AIDS. J Nutr 1999; 129(1):238S–242S.

144. Grinspoon S, Corcoran C, Stanley T, et al. Effects of androgen administration on the growth hormone-insulin-like growth factor I axis in men with acquired immunodeficiency syndrome wasting. J Clin Endocrinol Metab 1998; 83(12):4251–4256.

145. Hadigan C, Corcoran C, Stanley T, et al. Fasting hyperinsulinemia in human immunodeficiency virus-infected men: relationship to body composition, gonadal function, and protease inhibitor use. J Clin Endocrinol Metab 2000; 85(1):35–41.

146. Grinspoon S, Corcoran C, Stanley T, et al. Effects of hypogonadism and testosterone administration on depression indices in HIV-infected men. J Clin Endocrinol Metab 2000; 85(1):60–65.

147. Hadigan C, Corcoran C, Piecuch S, Rodriguez, Grinspoon S. Hyperandrogenemia in human immunodeficiency virus-infected women with the lipodystrophy syndrome. J Clin Endocrinol Metab 2000; 85(10):3544–3550.

148. De Martino M, Tovo PA, Galli L, Gabiano C, Chiarelli F, Zappa M, Gattinara GC, Bassetti D, Giacomet V, Chiappini E, Duse M, Garetto S, Caselli D. Puberty in perinatal HIV-1 infection: a multicentre longitudinal study of 212 children. AIDS 2001; 15:1527–1534.

149. Schwartz MS, Brandt LJ. The spectrum of pancreatic disorders in patients with the acquired immune deficiency syndrome. Am J Gastroenterol 1989; 84:459–462.

150. Brivet F, Coffin B, Bedossa P, et al. Pancreatic lesions in AIDS (letter). Lancet 1987; 2:1212.

151. Vendrell J, Nubiola A, Goday A, et al. HIV and the pancreas (letter). Lancet 1987; 2:1212.

152. Hommes MJ, Romijn JA, Endert E, Eeftinck Schattenkerk JKM, Sauerwein HP. Insulin Sensitivity and insulin clearance in human immunodeficiency virus-infected men. Metabolism 1991; 40:651–656.

153. Chehter EZ, Longo MA, Laudanna AA, Duarte MIS. Involvement of the pancreas in AIDS: a prospective study of 109 post-mortems. AIDS 2000; 14:1879–1886.

154. Sentongo TA, Rutstein RM, Stettler N, et al. Association between steatorrhea, growth, and immunologic status in children with perinatally acquired HIV infection. Arch Pediatr Adolesc Med 2001; 155:149–153.

155. Zazzo JF, Pichon F, Regnier B. HIV and the pancreas (letter). Lancet 1987; 2:1212.

156. Torre D, Montanari M, Fiore GP. HIV and the pancreas (letter). Lancet 1987; 2:1212.

157. Dassopoulos T, Ehrenpreis ED. Acute pancreatitis in human immunodeficiency virus-infected patients: a review. Am J Med 1999; 107:78–84.

158. Miller TL, Winter HS, Luginbuhil LM, et al. Pancreatitis in pediatric human immunodeficiency virus infection. J Pediatr 1992: 120:223–227.

159. Zaloga GP, Chernow B, Eil C. Hypercalcemia and disseminated cyto-megalovirus infection in the acquired immunodeficiency syndrome. Ann Intern Med 1985; 102:331–333.

160. Adams JS, Fernandez M, Gacad MA, et al. Vitamin D metabolite-mediated hypercalcemia and hypercalciuria patients with AIDS- and non-AIDS-associated lymphoma. Blood 1989; 73:235–239.

161. Aukrust P, Haug CJ, Ueland T, et al. Decreased bone formative and enhanced resorptive markers in human immunodeficiency virus infection: indication of normalization of the bone-remodeling process during highly active antiretroviral therapy. J Clin Endocrinol Metab 1999; 84(1):145–150.

162. Berczi I. Pituitary hormones and immune function. Acta Paediatr Suppl 1997; 423:70–75.

163. Berczi I, Chalmers IM, Nagy E, Warrington RJ. The immune effects of neuropeptides. Baillieres Clin Rheumatol 1996; 10(2):227–257 Abstract.

164. Chernow B, Schooley RT, Dracup K, Napolitano LM, Stanford GG, Klibanski A. serum prolactin concentrations in patients with the acquired immunodeficiency syndrome. Crit Care Med 1990; 18:440–441.

165. Gorman JM, Warne PA, Begg MD, et al. Serum prolactin levels in homosexual and bisexual men with HIV infection. Am J Psychiatry 1992; 149:367–370.

166. Hutchinson J, Murphy M, Harries R, Skinner CJ. Galactorrhoea and hyperprolactinaemia associated with protease-inhibitors. Lancet 2000; 356:9234–9237.

167. Mintz M. Neurologic abnormalities. In: Yogev IR, Connor E, eds. Management of HIV infection in infants and children. Chicago: Mosby Year Book 1992; 247–287.

168. Milligan SA, Katz MS, Craven PC, Strandberg DA, Russell IJ, Becker RA. Toxoplasmosis presenting as panhypopituitarism in a patient with acquired immunodeficiency syndrome. Am J Med 1984; 77:760–764.

169. Yanovski JA, Miller KD, Kino T, Friedman TC, Chrousos GP, Tsigos C, Falloon J. Endocrine and metabolic evaluation of human immunodeficiency virus-innfected patients with evidence of protease inhibitor-associated lipodystrophy. J Clin Endocrinol Metab 1997; 84(6):1925–1931.

170. Tanner AR. Hypothyroidism after treatment with ketoconazole. Br Med J 1987; 294:125.

171. Fentiman IS, Thomas BS, Balkwill FR, Rubens RD, Hayward JL. Primary hypothyroidism associated with interferon therapy of breast cancer. Lancet 1985; 1:1166.

172. Burman P, Trotterman TH, Oberg K, Karlsson FA. Thyroid autoimmunity in patients on long-term therapy with leukocyte-derived interferon. J Clin Endocrinol Metab 1986; 63:1086–1090.

173. Sonino N. The use of ketoconazole as an inhibitor of steroid production. N Engl J Med 1987; 317:812–818.

174. Tucker WS Jr, Snell BB, Island DP, Gregg CR. Reversible adrenal insufficiency induced by ketoconazole. JAMA 1985; 253:2413–2414.

175. Best TR, Jenkins JK, Murphy FY, Nicks SA, Bussell MD, Vesely DL. Persistent adrenal insufficiency secondary to low-dose ketoconazole therapy. Am J Med 1987; 82:676–680.

176. Elansary EH, Earis JE. Rifampicin and renal crisis. Br Med J 1983; 286:1861–1862.

177. Kryiazopoulou V, Parparadi O, Vagenaskis AG. Rifampicin induced renal crisis in Addison patients receiving corticosteroid replacement therapy. J Clin Endocrinol Metab 1984; 59:1204–1206.

178. Pont A, Graybill JR, Crayen PC, et al. High dose ketoconazole therapy and renal and testicular function in humans. Arch Intern Med 1984; 144:2150–2153.

179. Pont A, Goldman ES, Sugar AM, Siiteri PK, Stevens DA. Ketoconazole-induced increase in estriol-testosterone ratio. Arch Intern Med 1985; 145:1429–1431.

180. Ganada OP. Pentamidine and hypoglycemia. Ann Intern Med 1984; 100:464.

181. Stahl-Bayliss CM. Pentamidine-induced hypoglycemia in patients with the acquired immune deficiency syndrome. Clin Pharmacol Ther 1986; 39:271–275.

182. Perronne C, Bricaire F, Leport C, Assan D, Vilde JL, Assan R. Hypoglycemia and diabetes mellitus following parenteral pentamidine mesylate treatment in AIDS patients. Diabetic Med 1990; 7:585–589.

183. Hauser L, Sheehan P, Simpkins H. Pancreatic pathology in pentamidine-induced diabetes in acquired immunodeficiency syndrome patients. Hum Pathol 1991; 22:926–929.

184. Gordin FM, Simon GL, Wofsy CB, Mills J. Adverse reactions to trimethoprim-sulfamethoxazole in patients with the acquired immunodeficiency syndrome. Ann Intern Med 1984; 100:495–499.

185. Andersen R, Boedicker M, Ma M, Goldstein EJ. Adverse reactions associated with pentamidine isothionate in AIDS patients: recommendations for monitoring therapy. Drug Intell Clin Pharm 1986; 20:862–868.

186. Semel JD, McNerney JJ Jr. AIADH during disseminated herpes varicella-zoster infections: relationship to vidarabine therapy. Am J Med Sci 1986; 291:115–118.

187. Davies SV, Murray JA. Amphotericin B, aminoglycoside,

and hypomagnesemic tetany. Br Med J 1986; 292:1395–1396.

188. Choi MJ, Fernandez PC, Coupaye-Gerard B, D'Andrea D, Szerlip H, Kleyman TR. Brief report: Trimethoprim-induced hyperkalemia in a patient with AIDS. N Engl J Med 1993; 328:703–706.

189. Hadigan C, Miller K, Corcoran C, Anderson E, Basgoz N, Grinspoon S. Fasting hyperinsulinemia and changes inregional body composition in human immunodeficiency virus-infected women. J Clin Endocrinol Metab 1999; 84(6):1932–1937.

190. Yarasheski KE, Tebas P, Sigmund CM, Dagogo-Jack S, Cryer PE, Powderly WG. Insulin resistance in HIV-protease inhibitor-associated diabetes. Interscience Conference on Antimicrobial Agents and Chemotherapy September 1998; 38:390(abstract I-90).

191. Abdel-Khalek I, Moallem HJ, Fikrig S, Castells S. New onset diabetes mellitus in HIV-positive adolescent. AIDS Patient Care STDS 1998; 12(3):167–169

192. Lee ECC, Walmsley S, Fantus IG. New-onset diabetes mellitus associated with protease inhibitor therapy in an HIV-positive patient: case report and review. Can Med Assoc J 1999; 161:1614 Medline.

193. Hellerstein MK, Kahn J, Mudie H, Viteri F. Current approach to the treatment of human immunodeficiency virus-associated weight loss: pathophysiologic considerations and emerging management strategies. Semin Oncol 1990; 17:17–30.

194. Loprinzi CL, Ellison NM, Goldberg RM, Michalak JC, Burch PA. Alleviation of cancer anorexia and cachexia: studies of the Mayo Clinic and the North Central Cancer Treatment Group. Semin Oncol 1990; 17:8–12.

195. Aisner J, Parnes H, Tait N, et al. Appetite stimulation and weight gain with megestrol acetate. Semin Oncol 1990; 17:2–7.

196. Von Roenn JH, Murphy RL, Wegener N. Megestrol acetate for treatment of anorexia and cachexia associated with human immunodeficiency virus infection. Semin Oncol 1990; 17:13–16.

197. Coltman CA, Abrams JS, Aisner J, et al. (panel participants). Therapy to promote weight gain in cancer and acquired immunodeficiency syndrome patients: a panel discussion (Part I). Semin Oncol 1990; 17:34–37.

198. Clarick RH, Hanekom WA, Yogev R, Chadwick EG. Megestrol acetate treatment of growth failure in children infected with human immunodeficiency virus. Pediatrics 1997; 99(3):354–357.

199. Krentz AJ, Koster FT, Crist DM, et al. Anthropometric, metabolic, and immunological effects of recombinant human growth hormone in AIDS and AIDS-related complex. J Acquir Immune Defic Syndr 1993; 6:245–251.

200. Mulligan K, Grunfeld C, Hellerstein MK, Nesse RA, Schambelan M. Anabolic effects of recombinant human growth hormone in patients with wasting associated with human immunodeficiency virus infection. J Clin Endocrinol Metab 1993; 77:956–962.

201. Lieberman SA, Butterfield GE, Harrison D, Hoffman AR. Anabolic effects of recombinant insulin-like growth factor-I in cachectic patients with the acquired immunodeficiency syndrome. J Clin Endocrinol Metab 1994; 78:404–410.

202. Grinspoon S, Corcoran C, Anderson E, Hubard J, Stanley T, et al. Sustained anabolic effects of long-term androgen administration in men with AIDS wasting. Clin Infect Dis 1999; 28:634–636.

203. Miller K, Corcoran C, Armstrong C, Caramelli K, et al. Transdermal testosterone administration in women with acquired immunodeficiency syndrome wasting: a pilot study. J Clin Endocrinol Metab 1998; 83(8):2717–2725.

38

Hypertension in Children: Endocrine Considerations

Julie R. Ingelfinger

Harvard Medical School, Massachusetts General Hospital for Children, Massachusetts General Hospital, and New England Journal of Medicine, Boston, Massachusetts, U.S.A.

I. INTRODUCTION

This chapter reviews pediatric hypertension caused either by endocrine abnormalities or by mutations in genes modulated by endocrine systems. Endocrine-related hypertension has been thought to account for a minority of those cases of childhood hypertension due to definable causes. However, considering an endocrine cause whenever a child presents with hypertension is mandatory, since certain identifiable conditions will otherwise be overlooked. Delineating the pathogenesis and pathophysiology of hypertension is particularly important in managing a child or adolescent with elevated blood pressure; the more specific the diagnosis, the less the likelihood of prescribing empirical and often futile regimens. The more focused treatment can be, the less the risk of assigning a child to nonspecific pharmacotherapy, with unknown long-term effects, including those on growth and development.

II. NORMAL BLOOD PRESSURE AND ITS DEFINITION

Hypertension is defined by levels above the 95th centile for age, taking into consideration height and weight centiles as well. To facilitate categorizing blood pressure as normal or elevated, the National Heart, Lung, and Blood Institute (NHLBI) Task Force in Blood Pressure Control in Childhood issued an update in 1996 that provides tables according to height centiles (Table 1) (1–3). The Task Force data, pooled from measurements in over 12,000 pediatric subjects, is helpful as a guideline. But the aware clinician must understand that these norms are based on in-office seated blood pressure determinations and do not take into account changes with posture, activity, time of day, or various stresses that occur in daily life (4–6).

If one suspects secondary hypertension, a problem in interpreting an in-office blood pressure by norms is that epidemiologically based normal blood pressure data do not reflect what may occur in an abnormal state (5). For example, if one looks at blood pressure measurements among children and adolescents with renovascular hypertension, as was done by Hiner and Falkner (6), one sees that virtually all subjects have markedly elevated blood pressure. Furthermore, the diurnal pattern of blood pressure elevation in some forms of hypertension may be importantly distinct from a normal blood pressure pattern.

In recent years, much has been learned both about normal blood pressure in disparate ethnic groups and the circadian rhythm of blood pressure response. The reader is referred to reviews on the subject (7–12).

III. CAUSES OF HYPERTENSION

As noted in the Second Task Force report (2), most pediatric hypertension is not endocrine in nature, yet considering definable causes that are related to adrenal, thyroid, pituitary and other endocrine organs may identify a cause for hypertension. Children with specific endocrine disorders and syndromes may have a known increased risk of hypertension and will be able to benefit from specific therapy. Table 2a lists the most common causes of hypertension in each childhood age group; Table 2b lists those endocrine causes of hypertension most commonly seen in children.

IV. COMPLICATIONS OF HYPERTENSION: PATTERNS AND DIAGNOSIS

By the time a child is referred to a pediatric endocrinologist for evaluation of hypertension, it is likely that she or he has already been assessed by a primary care physician, and, possibly, by other specialists such as a pediatric cardiologist or nephrologist. Thus, some referrals

Table 1a Blood Pressure Levels for the 95th Percentile of Blood Pressure for Girls Aged 1–17 Years by Percentile of Height

Age	Blood pressure percentile[a]	Systolic blood pressure by percentile of height (mmHg)[b]							Diastolic blood pressure by percentile of height (mmHg)[b]						
		5%	10%	25%	50%	75%	90%	95%	5%	10%	25%	50%	75%	90%	95%
1	95th	101	102	103	104	105	107	107	57	57	57	58	59	60	60
2	95th	102	103	104	105	107	108	109	61	61	62	62	63	64	65
3	95th	104	104	105	107	108	109	110	65	65	65	66	67	67	68
4	95th	105	106	107	108	109	111	111	67	67	68	69	69	70	71
5	95th	107	107	108	110	111	112	113	69	70	70	71	72	72	73
6	95th	108	109	110	111	112	114	114	71	71	72	73	73	74	75
7	95th	110	110	112	113	114	115	116	73	73	73	74	75	76	76
8	95th	112	112	113	115	116	117	118	74	74	75	75	76	77	78
9	95th	114	114	115	117	118	119	120	75	76	76	77	78	78	79
10	95th	116	116	117	119	120	121	122	77	77	77	78	79	80	80
11	95th	118	118	119	121	122	123	124	78	78	79	79	80	81	81
12	95th	120	120	121	123	124	125	126	79	79	80	80	81	82	82
13	95th	121	122	123	125	126	127	128	80	80	81	82	82	83	84
14	95th	123	124	125	126	128	129	130	81	81	82	83	83	84	85
15	95th	124	125	126	128	129	130	131	82	82	83	83	84	85	86
16	95th	125	126	127	128	130	131	132	83	83	83	84	85	86	86
17	95th	126	126	127	129	130	131	132	83	83	83	84	85	86	86

[a]Blood pressure percentile was determined by a single measurement.
[b]Height percentile was determined by standard growth curves.
Source: Adapted from Ref. 3.

Table 1b Blood Pressure Levels for the 95th Percentile of Blood Pressure for Boys Aged 1–17 Years by Percentile of Height

Age	Blood pressure percentile[a]	Systolic blood pressure by percentile of height (mmHg)[b]							Diastolic blood pressure by percentile of height (mmHg)[b]						
		5%	10%	25%	50%	75%	90%	95%	5%	10%	25%	50%	75%	90%	95%
1	95th	98	99	101	102	104	106	106	55	55	56	57	58	59	59
2	95th	101	102	104	106	108	109	110	59	59	60	61	62	63	63
3	95th	104	105	107	109	111	112	113	63	63	64	65	66	67	67
4	95th	106	107	109	111	113	114	115	66	67	67	68	69	70	71
5	95th	108	109	110	112	114	115	116	69	70	70	71	72	73	74
6	95th	109	110	112	114	115	117	117	72	72	73	74	75	76	76
7	95th	110	111	113	115	116	118	119	74	74	75	76	77	78	78
8	95th	111	112	114	116	118	119	120	75	76	76	77	78	79	80
9	95th	113	114	116	117	119	121	121	76	77	78	79	80	80	81
10	95th	114	115	117	119	121	122	123	77	78	79	80	80	81	82
11	95th	116	117	119	121	123	124	125	78	79	79	80	81	82	83
12	95th	119	120	121	123	125	126	127	79	79	80	81	82	83	83
13	95th	121	122	124	126	128	129	130	79	80	81	82	83	83	84
14	95th	124	125	127	128	130	132	132	80	81	81	82	83	84	85
15	95th	127	128	129	131	133	134	135	81	82	83	83	84	85	86
16	95th	129	130	132	134	136	137	138	83	83	84	85	86	87	87
17	95th	132	133	135	136	138	140	140	85	85	86	87	88	89	89

[a]Blood pressure percentile was determined by a single measurement.
[b]Height percentile was determined by standard growth curves.
Source: Adapted from Ref. 3.

Table 1c Blood Pressure Levels for the 90th Percentile of Blood Pressure for Girls Aged 1–17 Years by Percentile of Height

Age	Blood pressure percentile[a]	Systolic blood pressure by percentile of height (mmHg)[b]							Diastolic blood pressure by percentile of height (mmHg)[b]						
		5%	10%	25%	50%	75%	90%	95%	5%	10%	25%	50%	75%	90%	95%
1	90th	97	98	99	100	102	103	104	53	53	53	54	55	56	56
2	90th	99	99	100	102	103	104	105	57	57	58	58	59	60	61
3	90th	100	100	102	103	104	105	106	61	61	61	62	63	63	64
4	90th	101	102	103	104	106	107	108	63	63	64	65	65	66	67
5	90th	103	103	104	106	107	108	109	65	66	66	67	68	68	69
6	90th	104	105	106	107	109	110	111	67	67	68	69	69	70	71
7	90th	106	107	108	109	110	112	112	69	69	69	70	71	72	72
8	90th	108	109	110	111	112	113	114	70	70	71	71	72	73	74
9	90th	110	110	112	113	114	115	116	71	72	72	73	74	74	75
10	90th	112	112	114	115	116	117	118	73	73	73	74	75	76	76
11	90th	114	114	116	117	118	119	120	74	74	75	75	76	77	77
12	90th	116	116	118	119	120	121	122	75	75	76	76	77	78	78
13	90th	118	118	119	121	122	123	124	76	76	77	78	78	79	80
14	90th	119	120	121	122	124	125	126	77	77	78	79	79	80	80
15	90th	121	121	122	124	125	126	127	78	78	79	79	80	81	82
16	90th	122	122	123	125	126	127	128	79	79	79	80	81	82	82
17	90th	122	123	124	125	126	128	128	79	79	79	80	81	82	82

[a]Blood pressure percentile was determined by a single measurement.
[b]Height percentile was determined by standard growth curves.
Source: Adapted from Ref. 3.

Table 1d Blood Pressure Levels for the 90th Percentile of Blood Pressure for Boys Aged 1–17 Years by Percentile of Height

Age	Blood pressure percentile[a]	Systolic blood pressure by percentile of height (mmHg)[b]							Diastolic blood pressure by percentile of height (mmHg)[b]						
		5%	10%	25%	50%	75%	90%	95%	5%	10%	25%	50%	75%	90%	95%
1	90th	94	95	97	98	100	101	102	50	51	52	53	54	54	55
2	90th	98	99	100	102	104	105	106	55	55	56	57	58	59	59
3	90th	100	101	103	105	107	108	109	59	59	60	61	62	63	63
4	90th	102	103	105	107	109	110	111	62	62	63	64	65	66	66
5	90th	104	105	106	108	110	112	112	65	65	66	67	68	69	69
6	90th	105	106	108	110	111	113	114	67	68	69	70	70	71	72
7	90th	106	107	109	111	112	114	115	69	70	71	72	72	73	74
8	90th	107	108	110	112	*114*	*115*	116	71	71	72	73	74	75	75
9	90th	109	110	112	113	115	117	117	72	73	73	74	75	76	77
10	90th	110	112	113	115	117	118	119	73	74	74	75	76	77	78
11	90th	112	113	115	117	119	120	121	74	74	75	76	77	78	78
12	90th	115	116	117	119	121	123	123	75	75	76	77	78	78	79
13	90th	117	118	120	122	124	125	126	75	76	76	77	78	79	80
14	90th	120	121	123	125	126	128	128	76	76	77	78	79	80	80
15	90th	123	124	125	127	129	131	131	77	77	78	79	80	81	81
16	90th	125	126	128	130	132	133	134	79	79	80	81	82	82	83
17	90th	128	129	131	133	134	136	136	81	81	82	83	84	85	85

[a]Blood pressure percentile was determined by a single measurement.
[b]Height percentile was determined by standard growth curves.
Source: Adapted from Ref. 3.

Table 2a Most Common Causes of Hypertension in Each Age Group

Age group	Causes
Neonate	Coarctation of the aorta
	Renal artery thromboembolism
	Renal artery stenosis
	Congenital renal abnormalities
Infancy to 6 years	Renal parenchymal disease (including structural, inflammatory disease and tumors)
	Coarctation of the aorta
	Renal artery stenosis
6–10 years	Renal parenchymal disease (including structural, inflammatory disease and tumors)
	Renal artery stenosis
	Primary hypertension
Adolescence	Primary hypertension
	Renal parenchymal disease

Source: Ref. 2.

will be made for children who have findings in their history, physical examination, or laboratory data that specifically suggest an endocrine cause of hypertension. Other referrals, however, will be de novo, or will be children who have been found to have hypertension in the course of treatment or evaluation for a known endocrinopathy. Prompt and focused evaluation of elevated blood pressure is critical, given the potential complications of pediatric hypertension.

Certain findings in a hypertensive child imply a role for an endocrinologist. An endocrinologist's first approach should be to seek historical facts that suggest a familial endocrinopathy associated with hypertension, the taking of medications that would be associated with endocrine-mediated hypertension (e.g., steroids or sympathomimetic agents), or an endocrine diagnosis known to be associated with hypertension (e.g., Turner syndrome). Physical examination will, of course, focus the evaluation further, in that findings may clearly suggest a particular endocrine diagnosis (clinical hyper- or hypothyroidism, Cushing syndrome). The blood pressure should be determined in both arms and one leg, and postural changes should be noted. Blood pressure after exercise, as well as at several points in the day, may also be helpful. Ambulatory blood pressure monitoring (ABPM) may be helpful in assessing circadian rhythm and particular patterns that could be associated with endocrine hypertension.

Laboratory data help to hone in on specific forms of hypertension. Thus, the initial endocrine assessment should focus on seeking signs of catecholamine-mediated hypertension, glucocorticoid-related hypertension, or thyroid-mediated hypertension (which are discussed at length in other chapters). Next, a plasma renin level, examined

Table 2b Endocrine Causes of Hypertension Seen in Children

Congenital adrenal hyperplasia
  11-β-hydroxylase deficiency
  3-β hydroxysteroid dehydrogenase
  17-α-hydroxylase deficiency
Hyperaldosteronism and hyperaldosterone-like conditions
  Aldosterone-producing adenoma
  Hyperplasia
  Glucocorticoid-responsive aldosteronism
  Apparent mineralocorticoid excess
Salt Handling
  Liddle syndrome
  Pseudohypoaldosteronism II (Gordon Syndrome)
Catecholamine-mediated
  Pheochromocytoma
  Neuroblastoma
Cushing syndrome
  Exogenous (due to medication)
  Central
  Adrenal
Thyroid
  Hyperthyroidism
  Hypothyroidism
Parathyroid
  Hyperparathyroidism
  Hypoparathyroidism (related to therapy)
Turner syndrome
PCOS/Metabolic Syndrome
Diabetes mellitus
Iatrogenic
  Glucocorticoid
  Calcium-phosphorus mediated
  Catecholamine-mediated
  Thyroid hormone mediated
  Hormone replacement therapy

together with a measure of sodium excretion and a plasma potassium level, should provide a basis for a focused endocrine assessment (13–16). A high plasma renin level is unlikely to be associated with endocrine hypertension, although secondary aldosteronism will accompany renovascular hypertension. If plasma renin activity or concentration is low, one should then consider an underlying hormonal basis. As can be seen in Table 3, those forms of low-renin hypertension that have been fully defined are due to mutations on autosomal chromosomes and thus occur equally in males and females (16). Each will be considered in turn. It has been proposed that, in fact, many more cases of so-called primary hypertension may be associated with partial defects in steroidogenesis or factors that control steroid effects.

The diagnostic considerations include a variety of inherited disorders that have a very low plasma renin activity as a cardinal feature. These include steroid enzyme

Table 3 Low-Renin Hypertension

Signs and symptoms	Hormonal findings	Source	Genetics	Comment
Steroidogenic enzyme defects				
Steroid 11β-hydroxylase deficiency	$\Downarrow$ PRA and aldo; high serum androgens/urine 17 ketosteroids; elevated DOC and 11-deoxycortisol	Adrenal: zona fasciculata	CYP11B1 mutation (encodes cytochrome P$_{450}$11β/18 of ZF); impairs synthesis of cortisol and ZF 17-deoxysteroids	Hypertensive virilizing CAH; most patients identified by time they are hypertensive. Increased BP may also occur from medication side effects.
Steroid 11α-hydroxylase/17,20-lyase deficiency	$\Downarrow$ PRA and aldo; low serum/urinary 17-hydroxysteroids; decreased cortisol; $\Uparrow$ corticosterone (B), and DOC in plasma; serum androgens and estrogens very low; serum gonadotrophins very high	Adrenal: zona fasciculata; Gonadal: interstitial cells (Leydig's in testis; theca in ovary)	CYP17 mutation (encodes cytochrome P$_{450}$C17) impairs cortisol and sex steroid production	CAH with male pseudohermaphroditism; female external genital phenotype in males; primary amenorrhea in females
Hyperaldosteronism				
Primary aldosteronism	$\Downarrow$ PRA; $\Uparrow$ plasma aldosterone, 18-OH- and 18 oxoF; normal 18-OH/aldo ratio	Adrenal adenoma: clear cell tumor with suppression of ipsilateral ZG	Unknown; very rare in children; female:male ratio is 2.5–3/1	Conn syndrome with aldo producing adenoma; muscle weakness and low K+ in sodium-replete state
Adrenocortical hyperplasia	As above; source of hormone established by radiology or scans	Adrenal: focal or diffuse adrenal cortical hyperplasia	Unknown	As above
Idiopathic primary aldosteronism	High plasma aldo; elevated 18-OHF/aldo ratio	Adrenal: hyperactivity of ZG of adrenal cortex	Unknown	As above
Deoxycorticosterone-producing tumor	High plasma DOC	Adrenal: adenoma/carcinoma	Unknown	As above
Dexamethasone-suppressible hypertension				
Glucocorticoid-remediable aldosteronism (GRA)	Plasma and urinary aldo responsive to ACTH; dexamethasone suppressible within 48 h; $\Uparrow$ urine and plasma 18OHS, 18-OHF, and 18 oxoF	Adrenal: abnormal presence of enzymatic activity in adrenal ZF, allowing completion of aldo synthesis from 17-deoxy steroids	Chimeric gene that is expressed at high level in ZF (regulated like CYP11B1) and has 18-oxidase activity (CYP11B2 functionality)	Hypokalemia in sodium-replete state
Apparent mineralocorticoid excess (AME)				
	$\Uparrow$ plasma ACTH and secretory rates of all corticosteroids; nl serum F (delayed plasma clearance)	$\Uparrow$ plasma F bioactive in periphery (F$\rightarrow$B) of bi-dir. 11βOHSD or slow clearance by 5 α/β reduction to allo dihydro-F	Type 2 11βOHSD mutations	Cardiac conduction changes; LVH, vessel remodeling; some calcium abnormalities; nephrocalcinosis; rickets
Nonsteroidal defects				
Liddle syndrome	Low plasma renin, low or normal K+; negligible urinary aldosterone	Not a disorder of steroidogenesis but of transport	Autosomal dominant abnormality in epithelial sodium transporter, EnaC, in which channel is constitutively active	Responds to triamterene
Pseudohypoaldosteronism II-Gordon syndrome	Low plasma renin, normal or elevated K+	Not a disorder of steroidogenesis but of transport	Autosomal dominant abnormality in WNK1 or WNK4	Responds to thiazides

Source: Adapted from Ref. 142.

abnormalities, as well as abnormalities in transporters or in modulating genes. Yiu et al. (13) developed an algorithm for thinking about these entities, which are accompanied by low plasma renin activity (Fig. 1). The algorithm is based on the fact that a number of hypertensive syndromes share a low plasma renin as a common feature. Most are inherited either as an autosomal dominant, in which case family history is positive, or as an autosomal recessive, in which case family history is lacking.

V. STEROIDOGENIC ENZYME DEFECTS

As noted in Chapters 6 and 7, steroids are produced in the adrenal cortex, which is divided into zones: the zona glomerulosa (ZG, outer zone), zona fasciculata (ZF, middle zone), and zona reticularis (ZR, inner zone). Normally, the ZG and ZF are functionally separate. Cortisol is synthesized under the control of adrenocorticotropin (ACTH) in the ZF, while aldosterone is synthesized primarily under the influence of angiotensin II and potassium in the ZG. ACTH normally has only a secondary effect on the synthesis of aldosterone. However, when any of the enzymes that control cortisol biosynthesis is defective or acts abnormally, the feedback relationships between the hypophysis and the adrenal are interrupted, with a resultant increase in plasma ACTH. Figure 2 depicts steroidogenesis, indicating enzyme defects that can be associated with hypertension, and Figure 3 indicates regulation of aldosterone biosynthesis.

Congenital adrenal hyperplasia (CAH) is the general term used to describe enzyme defects that can occur in steroid biosynthesis, each causing a characteristic profile of plasma and urinary steroids together with a specific clinical manifestation (15,16). These defects all are autosomal recessive, have varying frequency, and have a spectrum of clinical manifestations. Any of the enzymes that are part of the pathways of steroidogenesis may have a mutation, most commonly 21-hydroxylase, not generally associated with hypertension. Enzymes with mutations that are associated with hypertension include (in order of frequency) 11-β hydroxylase >> 3β-hydroxysteroid dehydrogenase>>>17α-hydroxylase and cholesterol desmolase. A net salt-retaining propensity and hypertension occur in patients with the 11-β hydroxylase and 3β-hydroxysteroid dehydrogenase defects. It is also important to remember that individuals with CAH may develop hypertension owing to overzealous replacement therapy.

A. Steroid 11-β-Hydroxylase Deficiency

Hypertension is one of the cardinal features of 11-β hydroxylase deficiency (16–21), as the abnormal adrenal steroid pattern leads to mineralocorticoid excess, the physiology of which includes decreased renal sodium excretion with consequent volume expansion and hypertension.

The virilization seen in 11-β-hydroxylase deficiency and its management are discussed at length in Chapters 6 and 7; virilization is universal in this condition. Unless the mother is treated during pregnancy, an affected female fetus will have ambiguous or masculinized external genitalia, owing to excess of adrenal androgens, while the baby's internal organs will be normal. After birth affected males and females develop progressive penile or clitoral enlargement, respectively, along with rapid somatic growth. If appropriate treatment is not initiated, early closure of epiphyses will lead to short final stature.

Hypertension is common but not universal in 11β-hydroxylase deficiency, usually noted in later childhood or adolescence, and this hypertension often has an inconsistent relation to the biochemical profile (15,16). Hypokalemia is only variably present, although it should be remembered that potassium depletion and sodium retention may not be reflected by serum or plasma potassium values, owing to shifts from intracellular potassium to the extracellular space. Thus, total body potassium may be markedly depleted, yet serum or plasma potassium may be in the normal range. The production and release of renin are suppressed by the volume expansion. Furthermore, aldosterone production is decreased with relative decrease in circulating potassium. However, in some circumstances, the characteristic findings of low renin and elevated aldosterone have been absent (20,22–24).

Therapy of 11-β-hydroxylase deficiency should be focused on normalizing steroids. Thus, glucocorticoid administration will not only normalize cortisol function but should also reduce ACTH secretion and levels to normal, which should remove the drive for oversecretion of deoxycorticosterone (DOC). Such therapy usually cures the hypertension (17). However, if hypertension is marked, antihypertensive therapy should be used in this disorder until good control of hypertension is obtained.

Variants of 11-β-hydroxylase deficiency have been reported and likely relate to the several mutations that can cause the syndrome. For example, Zachman et al. (21) found an individual in whom 11β-hydroxylation was inhibited for 17-α-hydroxylated steroids but in whom there was intact 17-deoxysteroid hydroxylation. Multiple mutations affecting the expression of the CYP11B1 gene have been described; these include frameshifts, point mutations, extra triplet repeats, and stop mutations (22–26). A distinct hypotensive disorder, called corticosterone methyloxidase type II, occurs when a mutation affects CYP11B2 (aldosterone synthase). This abnormality leads to a clinical problem of terminal aldosterone synthesis and thus is accompanied by salt wasting and hypotension.

B. Steroid 17α-Hydroxylase Deficiency

The adrenals and gonads are both affected when the enzyme 17α-hydroxylase is abnormal, because a dysfunctional 17α hydroxylase enzyme results in decreased production of both cortisol and sex steroids (the production of which requires the 17,20 lyase function of the same enzyme) (16,17,28–30). An affected individual, irrespective of genetic sex, appears phenotypically female, and puberty does not occur. In fact, diagnosis too often occurs late: at puberty, when primary amenorrhea and lack of secondary sexual characteristics are noted (16,17,28–30). Another mode of presentation for affected children is with the presence of an inguinal hernia. Patients are usually both hypertensive and hypokalemic, owing to huge overproduction of corticosterone (compound B). The biochemical aspects of these defects are described more completely in the chapters on CAH.

This rare type of hypertension was first described in a female patient by Biglieri et al. (28), and then in a feminized male by New (29), although it has since been described in well over 100 patients (31–34). Treatment is effective if glucocorticoid replacement is initiated before puberty, but this may not always correct the hypertension. If replacement therapy fails to correct the elevated blood pressure, appropriate pharmacotherapy should be used to lower the blood pressure to maintain it within the normal ranges for age and size.

VI. PRIMARY ALDOSTERONISM: ALDOSTERONE-PRODUCING ADENOMA AND BILATERAL ADRENAL HYPERPLASIA

Aldosterone-producing adenomas (APAs) are rare in children, but they do occasionally occur, most often as solitary masses (16,35–42). Although rare (10% of total), bilateral masses may also occur. Occasionally such adenomas produce DOC rather than aldosterone. The hallmarks include hypokalemia and hypertension, and the optimal method for diagnosis can be complex and controversial, even among adults. Rather than primary aldosteronism secondary to adenomas, it is far more likely that a child will have bilateral renal hyperplasia (42).

Diagnosis should be possible when the studies for an APA fail to find a definite lesion. The number and type of tests (some invasive) are similar for APA and hyperplasia. ACTH sensitivity is assessed by suppression of the adrenal glands. Assessment of aldosterone levels, not only peripherally but also using bilateral adrenal vein sampling, may be helpful. Imaging studies including ultrasonography (41), computed tomography (CT) (43), scintigraphy

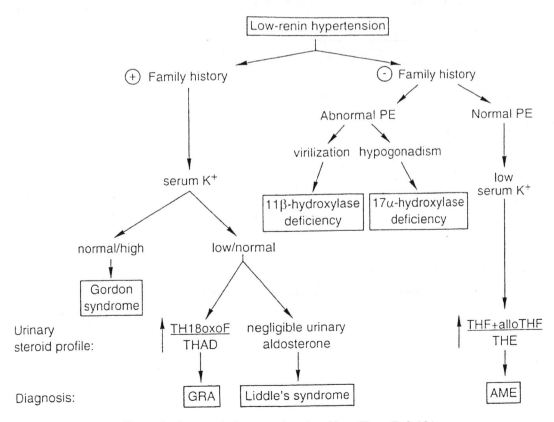

Figure 1 Low-renin hypertension algorithm. (From Ref. 13.)

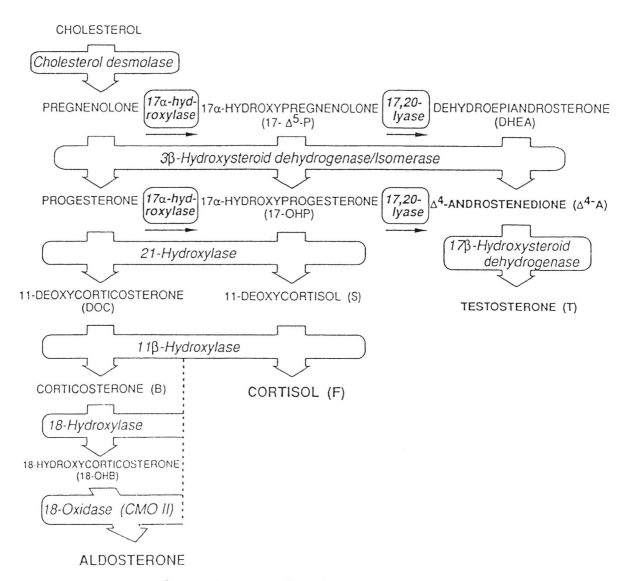

Figure 2   Steroid biosynthesis. (Reproduced from Ref. 142.)

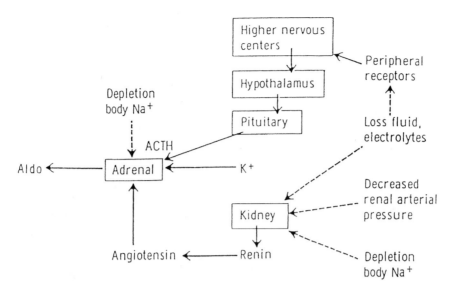

Figure 3 Aldosterone regulation. (Reproduced from Ref. 142.)

using radioiodocholesterol (44), and nuclear magnetic resonance (NMR) imaging (45) have all been used.

When APA is present, surgery is indicated (16). Surgical therapy with total or subtotal adrenalectomy for bilateral adrenal hyperplasia has been advocated, but hypertension may either continue or return. Instead, management using the nonspecific mineralocorticoid antagonist spironolactone may be more effective (16,37). Eplerenone is the first of the more specific aldosterone receptor antagonists and may prove to have a useful role (46).

VII. GLUCOCORTICOID-RESPONSIVE ALDOSTERONISM: DEXAMETHASONE-SUPPRESSIBLE HYPERALDOSTERONISM (OMIM #103900)

Glucocorticoid-responsive aldosteronism (GRA) was first reported by Sutherland et al. (47) and New et al. (48) in 1966–1967, as a novel form of increased aldosterone secretion accompanied by suppressed renin and treatable by dexamethasone. It is listed in the Online Mendelian Inheritance in Man (OMIM) as #103900. (OMIM can be accessed at http://www.ncbi.nlm.nih.gov/Omim.) This condition, which is inherited as autosomal dominant (49), has been reported in numerous pedigrees (50–54), and has now been identified as due to a chimeric gene duplication (the fusion of 11β-hydroxylase and aldosterone synthase genes from an unequal crossing-over event) (55,56), leading to the regulation of aldosterone synthesis and secretion solely by corticotropin instead of by angiotensin II and potassium (54,57–59). The chimeric gene product converts cortisol to 18-hydroxy and 18-oxo metabolites (60–63).

In patients with GRA both serum and urine aldosterone levels are generally elevated, but not invariably so.

However, pathognomonic findings are generally that the urinary cortisol metabolites TH18oxoF and 18-hydroxycortisol are very high in GRA, and the ratio of TH18oxoF/tetrahydroaldosterone (THAD) is elevated. A commercially available urinary steroid profile can differentiate GRA patients from those with apparent mineralocorticoid excess (AME) or Liddle syndrome (Nichols Institute, San Juan Capistrano, CA) (63). Specific genetic testing is both sensitive and specific.

Patients have excessive aldosterone secretion, which leads to salt and water retention, plasma volume expansion, and then hypertension. When hypertension occurs, as it often does in GRA, glucocorticoid suppression can control the hypertension. GRA appears to be rare, yet it still is not often considered in the course of an evaluation of pediatric hypertension. Affected individuals often have a family history of severe so-called essential hypertension that has resisted therapy, or of family members who had early cardiovascular events including stroke and myocardial infarction.

Dluhy et al. recently reviewed the medical records of 20 children from 10 unrelated pedigrees of GRA to assess their course (64). Sixteen of the 20 developed hypertension, as early as 1 month of age. An interesting finding was that four were not hypertensive. Half of those with hypertension had conditions controllable with monotherapy [glucocorticoid suppression or aldosterone receptor/amiloride-sensitive epithelial sodium channel (ENaC) antagonists]. The rest required combination therapy, and three of those were unable to achieve blood pressure control.

Neither hypokalemia nor suppressed plasma renin activity is necessarily present at diagnosis, and thus this diagnosis might be entertained more frequently than it has been. Dexamethasone and other glucocorticoids usually control the hypertension quite easily in young individuals with GRA, although adults with this chimeric gene may not experience resolution of their hypertension when diagnosis has been delayed.

VIII. APPARENT MINERALOCORTICOID EXCESS (OMIM #218030)

Apparent mineralocorticoid excess (AME) is marked by low-renin hypertension accompanied by hypokalemia and metabolic alkalosis (22). The syndrome was first delineated in 1977 by New et al. during their evaluation of a young Native American girl from the Zuni tribe who presented with this clinical picture (65,66). The hypertension in AME is severe, often accompanied by early end-organ damage (67). Although initial therapy with spironolactone frequently is effective, patients may well become refractory, and there is an absence of 11-β-hydroxysteroid dehydrogenase. The presence of 11-β-hydroxysteroid dehydrogenase is necessary for the prevention of mineralocorticoid activity of cortisol. When this enzyme is low or absent, cortisol-mediated hypertension can occur. In AME, cortisol acts as if it were a potent mineralocorticoid.

The microsomal enzyme 11β-hydroxysteroid dehydrogenase (11β-HSD) interconverts the active 11-hydroxyglucocorticoids to their inactive keto-metabolites. Both aldosterone and cortisol have an affinity for the mineralocorticoid receptor and, under usual circumstances, 11β-HSD is protective, preventing binding of cortisol to the mineralocorticoid receptor. In AME, the slow metabolism of cortisol to the biologically inactive cortisone, with a prolonged cortisol half-life (68,69), causes cortisol to act as a potent mineralocorticoid. The metabolism of cortisone to cortisol, however, is normal.

There are two kinetically distinct forms of the 11-β-HSD enzyme. 11-β-HSD1 is widely distributed and, while its Km for cortisol is an order of magnitude higher than 11-β-HSD2, it is NADP-preferring, and mainly acts as a reductase. In contrast, 11-β-HSD2 is present mainly in epithelia that transport sodium. It has a high affinity for cortisol and requires nicotinamide adenine dinucleotide (NAD). It is involved in sodium transport, predominantly in the kidney distal tubule. The clinical findings suggest that the 11β-hydroxysteroid dehydrogenase enzyme is abnormal in AME (70,71). It was postulated that patients with AME had a loss of mineralocorticoid receptor specificity such that cortisol could bind to the mineralocorticoid receptor (MR) and act as a mineralocorticoid. Although defective 11β-HSD seemed a likely explanation, the first form of this enzyme found was normal. However, it is now known that an abnormality in the type 2 isoform of 11β-HSD is mutated in patients with AME (72–76). To date, many distinct mutations have been reported. These have been shown to impair the conversion of cortisol to cortisone.

Classic AME generally presents in early life and is associated with failure to thrive, severe hypertension, and persistent polydipsia. The patients are volume expanded and respond to dietary sodium restriction. Plasma renin activity is impressively decreased. The diagnosis can be made biochemically by obtaining the ratio of cortisol to cortisone in the urine. There is an abnormal urinary ratio of tetrahydrocortisol/tetrahydrocortisone (THF/THE), with a predominance of THF. The generation of cortisone from cortisol after 11-tritiated cortisol is injected is only 0–6%, compared to normal: 90–95% (77).

Complications of hypertension in these children often include cardiovascular ravages of hypertension. In addition, some patients develop nephrocalcinosis and renal failure (78). Early diagnosis can do much to ameliorate the situation, if the hypertension can be controlled.

A mild form of AME has been reported in a Mennonite kindred, in whom there is a P227L mutation in the HSD11B2 gene (79,80). In 2001 New et al. reported two sisters from the Iroquois Nation who appear to have resistance to multiple steroids (81). The proband was referred with mild hypertension as a possible patient with AME, yet she had resistance to glucocorticoids, mineralocorticoids, and androgens (81). Despite significantly elevated glucocorticoid levels, she had no cushingoid features and no evidence of masculinization, although her androgen levels were elevated (81). It was proposed that these two young women may have a coactivator defect (81).

Hypertension without the characteristic findings of AME has recently been described in a heterozygous father and homozygous daughter who have mutations in 11β-HSD2 (82). Studies in patients with hypertension suggest a deficiency in 11β-HSD2 activity, along with abnormalities that may be genetically determined (83) The 11β-HSD2 gene appears to confer specificity for the aldosterone receptor.

Licorice-induced hypertension has a pathogenesis similar to that seen in AME (79,80,84). Glycerrhetinic acid, which is the active component of licorice, inhibits 11β-hydroxysteroid dehydrogenase, leading to increased stimulation of the mineralocorticoid receptor (84).

IX. MUTATIONS IN RENAL TRANSPORTERS CAUSING LOW-RENIN HYPERTENSION

A. Pseudohypoaldosteronism Type II: Gordon Syndrome (OMIM #145260)

Pseudohypoaldosteronism type II (PHAII) is an autosomal dominant condition associated with hyperkalemia, acidemia, and hypertension along with increased salt reabsorption by the kidney (13,85–87). The condition is also known as Gordon syndrome or familial hyperkalemia and is listed as OMIM #145260. A hallmark of this disease is low renin hypertension and improvement with the use of thiazide diuretics or with triamterene. Aldosterone receptor antagonists do not correct the abnormalities. The pathogenesis remained elusive for a long time, although the physiological studies and response to diuretics strongly indicated a defect in renal ion transport in the presence of normal glomerular filtration rate.

Genes for PHAII were mapped to chromosomes 17, 1 or 12 (88–90). A PHAII kindred in which linkage analysis suggested that the involved area was the most telomeric 2-centimorgan segment of chromosome 12p [lod score 5.07] was recently found to have abnormalities in the WNK1 gene. The WNK genes, a family of serine-threonine kinases, are named WNK because they have no lysine, the symbol for which is "K." The mutations are large intronic deletions that increase WNK1 gene expression. Another family has been found with mutations in WNK4, which is on chromosome 17. These mutations are missense. WNK1 is widely expressed in the body, while WNK4 is mainly expressed in kidney, localized to tight junctions. It is thought that abnormalities in WNKs change the way potassium and and hydrogen are handled in the collecting duct, thus increasing salt resorption and intravascular voloume. How this occurs is not clear. It is unlikely that these kinases simply increase the activity of ENaC. More likely they either increase transcellular chloride conductance in the collecting duct, or increase paracellular chloride conductance. This may increase salt resoprtion and intravascular volume, and dissipate the electrical gradient and decrease K+ and H+ secretion. They might also lead to constitutive increase in activity of the Na−Cl cotransporter in the collecting duct or increase its activity in the distal convoluted tubule.

The lesson inherent in the association of WNK kinases with PHAII is that many individuals with low-renin primary hypertension respond to treatment with thiazide diuretics. Might these people have variants in WNK1 or WNK4 that predispose to hypertension? There are some data from linkage studies that suggest such an association might be important (90). Furthermore, the WNK kinases and their signaling pathways may be a fruitful target for future development of antihypertensive drugs.

B. Liddle Syndrome (OMIM #177200)

In 1963 Liddle (91) described early onset of hypertension with hypokalemia in a family who had low renin and aldosterone concentrations. Inheritance was autosomal dominant. Inhibitors of renal epithelial sodium transport, such as triamterene, worked well in controlling hypertension, but inhibitors of the mineralocorticoid receptor did not. A general abnormality in sodium transport seemed apparent, as the red blood cell transport systems were not normal (92). The concept that a major abnormality was present in renal salt handling was fostered by the fact that a patient with Liddle syndrome who needed a renal transplant experienced normalization of the blood pressure and serum potassium after the procedure (93).

The abnormality in Liddle syndrome thus looked like aldosterone excess yet had very low aldosterone levels as well as renin (94–96). Many patients have low potassium

levels, but not all do. Mineralocorticoid-dependent sodium transport within the renal epithelia needs activation of the epithelial sodium channel. The α, β, and γ subunits have been cloned and characterized. The β and γ subunits are found close to each other on chromosome 16. Mutations in these subunits have been identified in Liddle syndrome. More information can be found in OMIM, in which Liddle syndrome is listed as OMIM 177200.

X. CUSHING SYNDROME AND HYPERTENSION

Glucocorticoid excess leads to the well-described syndrome of weight gain, linear height growth attenuation, myopathy, centripetal obesity, striae, moon facies, and buffalo hump (97–100). Hypertension is part of this constellation, whether the syndrome is due to exogenous glucocorticoid therapy or to endogenous hypercortisolism from a variety of causes. The hypertension improves upon control of the underlying cause (and therapy is discussed in Chapter 6, 30). The hypertension should be controlled while the cause is being evaluated and treated.

XI. HYPERTENSION IN PHEOCHROMOCYTOMA AND NEURAL CREST TUMORS

Hypertension is nearly universal in pediatric pheochromocytoma, and management is discussed in Chapter 8, Disorders of the Adrenal Medulla: Catecholamine-Producing Tumors in Childhood. Several points concerning the hypertension in children with pheochromocytoma are worth emphasizing in this chapter as well (101–117). The hypertension seen in children and adolescents with pheochromocytoma is often constant rather than episodic; thus the diagnosis should always be ruled out in a child with marked hypertension.

Management of hypertension in a child with pheochromocytoma should be classified into the preoperative phase, intraoperative phase, and postoperative phase. Preoperatively, it is worthwhile to be certain the child's blood pressure is controlled and the child stable before surgery is attempted. The dosages of medications used are listed in Table 4. As was pointed out in Chapter 8, although alpha blockade is thought to be important, beta-adrenoceptor blockade should not be used as sole therapy, because it fails to prevent the effects of catecholamine at alpha-adrenoceptors and may cause severe hypertension.

Some sources suggest inducing volume expansion along with blood pressure control in the preoperative period, to prevent intraoperative volume instability (103,107).

Preoperatively it is wise to premedicate to avoid anxiety, which itself may precipitate catecholamine release and crisis. Perioperatively, it is important to consider the use of nonexcitatory neuromuscular medications. Fentanyl and droperidol should be avoided because they may lead

Table 4 Treatment of Catecholamine Excess: Oral Medications to Use Preoperatively

Drug	Indications/pharmacokinetics	Dose	Preparation
α-Adrenergic blockers			
Phenoxybenzamine	Long half-life	Start at 10 mg bid $\rightarrow$ 20–40 mg bid or tid	10 mg capsules
Prazosin	Selective α_1-antagonist; short half-life	1 mg q 8 h, up to 20 mg/day	1, 2, 5 mg capsules
β-Adrenergic blockers: Don't use before full α-blockade			
Propranolol	Nonselective β-antagonist; may induce wheezing; biologic half-life ~4 h	1 mg/kg/dose bid to qid	10, 20, 40, 60, 80 mg tabs
Propranolol-long acting	Same as propranolol	1 mg/kg/day	60, 80 mg capsules
Atenolol	Selective β_1-antagonist; 50% absorbed orally; peaks at 2–4 h, half-life 6–7 h; oral duration 24 h	1–2 mg/kg qd	25, 50, 100 mg tablets
α/β-Adrenergic blockade			
Labetalol	Combined blocker; limited pediatric information	3–4 mg/kg/day in two divided doses; increase to 40 mg/kg/day orally	100, 200, 300 mg tablets
Competitive inhibitor of tyrosine hydroxylase			
Metyrosine (Demser)	Competitive inhibitor of tyrosine hydroxylase	250 mg bid to qid	250 mg capsules

to catecholamine release. Atropine is also contraindicated, since this agent may lead to tachycardia in the presence of elevated blood catecholamines.

Monitoring arterial pressure and the cardiogram is essential during surgery, and providing muscle relaxants prior to intubation is important. Anesthesia with isofluorance or enflurane is usual and well tolerated. If a hypertensive crisis occurs during surgery, prompt therapy with intravenous phentolamine or nitroprusside is essential, as well as control of any arrhythmias that may develop. In addition to phentolamine and nitroprusside, the calcium channel blocker nicardipine has been used with success, as have labetalol, esmolol, nitroglycerine, and the dopamine 1 agonist fenoldopam.

In a recently published series from the Mayo Clinic, the majority of patients were given isoflurane for their primary volatile anesthetic, and 61% were given succinylcholine as a muscle relaxant. Most required intraoperative antihypertensive use (82%), and 45% required the use of vasopressors.

Postoperatively blood pressure normalizes in most children with resectable tumors. However, about 25% of adults do not, likely because most have concomitant primary hypertension. Those children who require continued antihypertensive therapy after resection generally have tumors that are not fully resectable, or have malignant pheo-

chromocytoma. In such situations a combination of alpha and beta blockade can control blood pressure. Metyrosine (Demser) is also useful for inhibiting catecholamine synthesis. The calcium channel blocker nifedipine is successful in decreasing clinical symptoms.

XII. HYPERTENSION IN THYROID DISEASE

Hypertension is widely stated to occur in conditions of both hyperthyroidism (118–120) and hypothyroidism (121), not surprisingly via distinctly different mechanisms. A considerable body of experimental data demonstrates that models of hyperthyroidism are accompanied by hypertension. For example, a model of hyperthyroidism in which rats are rendered thyrotoxic by injection of 0.1 mg/kg/24 h of L-thyroxine is accompanied by both hypertension and left ventricular hypertrophy. Activation of the renin–angiotensin system appears important in this form of hypertension, which is ameliorated by the angiotensin II antagonist (e.g., valsartan). Conversely, an older literature showed that spontaneously hypertensive rats had a propensity to thyroid functional abnormalities.

Clinical hypertension as part of hyperthyroidism is widely known (118–120). Treatment of the hypertension with antihypertensive agents generally proves successful.

This form of hypertension has been reported in neonates with hyperthyroidism as well as in older children. The circadian rhythm in hyperthyroidism appears to vary compared to normal, with a failure to exhibit nocturnal decrease (dipping) in blood pressure. Systolic hypertension as an isolated finding is more common than elevation of both systolic and diastolic hypertension, particularly in young patients. Increased cardiac output with decreased total peripheral resistance are observed.

Hypothyroidism has long been reported as associated with hypertension (121). However, few data truly support this claim. Rather, studies note left ventricular hypertrophy post hoc, in autopsy studies, or make this claim without providing control subjects. Therapy of the thyroid deficiency generally decreases the blood pressure for most individuals. The clinical findings include increased sympathetic nervous system tone, with an augmented alpha-adrenergic responsiveness. Cardiac output tends to be decreased, while peripheral resistance is increased. If hypertension is present, it is most often diastolic in nature. Once the hypothyroidism is corrected, patients can generally be weaned from hypotensive therapy.

XIII. HYPERPARATHYROIDISM AND HYPERTENSION

Hypertension is a frequent occurrence with hyperparathyroidism (122,123). Studies that have considered mechanisms suggest that intracellular ionized calcium is elevated and regulated abnormally in this condition. Iatrogenic hypertension may occur, since therapy may have side effects leading to hypertension. Patients with hypoparathyroidism, if treated to excess with vitamin D analogs and calcium, may likewise become hypertensive.

XIV. PREVENTION OF HYPERTENSION AND ENDOCRINE SYSTEMS

A. Expectable Hypertension in the Course of Prescribed Therapy

No discussion of hypertension in children is complete without some mention of iatrogenic forms of hypertension. A number of medications commonly used in endocrine practice may lead to hypertension: including glucocorticoids and mineralocorticoids, thyroid replacement, and estrogen–progestin combinations (124). Thus, the alert clinician prescribing such medication will monitor any individual for whom such medications are prescribed. The self-prescription or inadvertent exposure of patients to such compounds can also result in elevated blood pressure.

Glucocorticoid-related hypertension is extremely common among those taking such preparations for prolonged time periods. A recent publication noted that 88% of children receiving glucocorticoids were hypertensive

(125). The hypertension related to glucocorticoid use appears irrespective of indication and has been reported among children with neurological, renal, pulmonary, and GI disease. Given a necessary course of steroids, it is imperative that blood pressure be monitored and treated as needed until the glucocorticoid treatment can be discontinued.

B. Expectable Hypertension in the Course of a Known Diagnosis

Certain endocrine diagnoses are associated with hypertension. A child with Turner syndrome has a definitive chance of renovascular hypertension, owing to renal artery abnormalities or to renal malrotation and anatomical anomalies (126). Children with disorders of calcium regulatory hormones may develop hypercalcemia and hypercalciuria, and nephrocalcinosis with attendant renal calcification and hypertension (127). Children from families with a familial endocrinopathy should be evaluated carefully, given the frequency of neural crest tumors.

Diabetes may be associated with microalbuminuria early, and endocrinologists should, from all that is now known, monitor children with diabetes for microalbuminuria, renal function, and blood pressure. Renoprotective treatment may well be indicated (128–130).

The endocrine diagnoses for which monitoring blood pressure levels should be part of routine care are listed in Table 3.

XV. PRIMARY HYPERTENSION: HOW OFTEN ENDOCRINE?

About 25% of the adult population has hypertension, and many hypertensive individuals have salt sensitivity: blood pressure increases with a high-salt intake and decreases with a lowered salt intake. The delineation of several monogenic forms of low-renin hypertension have raised questions of whether some individuals with so-called primary hypertension might have abnormalities in genes that lead to mendelian forms of low-renin hypertension. Such mutations might not lead inevitably to hypertension but might cause a predisposition to hypertension. Recent studies of individuals with primary hypertension have detected certain polymorphisms that appear to be associated with differences in function of 11-β hydroxysteroid dehydrogenase-2. Some publications suggest that individuals with either a polymorphism in 11-β-HSD2 or who have an increased cortisol half-life seem to respond differently from others with respect to salt sensitivity. Such findings suggest that some forms of primary hypertension may be differentiated from others by their 11-β-HSD-2 activity (83,131,132,134). Since not all studies (133) support such findings, this remains an area of continuing consideration.

Table 5a Oral and Topical Hypertensives

Medication type	Drug	Route	Dosage	Adverse effects	Contraindication	Comment
Vasodilator	Minoxidil	PO	0.2 mg/kg to start	Fluid retention, reflex tachycardia	Need to get BP controlled immediately; catecholamine-mediated hypertension	May help in urgencies
	Hydralazine	PO	0.75–3.0 mg/kg/day	Vasodilation	Tachycardia; sensitivity to hydralazine	Unstable in suspension; consider periodic ANA testing
Beta blockers	Propranolol	PO	0.5–1.90 mg/kg/day divided q 6 h	Bradycardia, CHF, intensification of AV block; mental depression, visual disturbances, nightmares, hallucinations; bronchospasms; GI symptoms	Asthma, CHF, sinus bradycardia, liver disease, cardiogenic shock, diabetes (?), pheochromocytoma	May mask signs of hypoglycemia or hyperthyroidism; available in long-acting form
	Atenolol	PO	Once daily, 50 mg qd (adult)	Fewer side effects than nonselective beta blockers	Can consider using in patients with reactive airway disease	Relatively cardioselective
	Metoprolol	PO	1 mg/kg every 12 h	Fewer side effects than other beta blockers	Beta blocker of choice in asthma	Relatively cardioselective
	Nadolol	PO	1 mg/kg/24 h	Same as other beta blockers, but less severe	Beta blocker of choice in asthma	Longer duration of action permits once/day dosing
Angiotensin-converting enzyme inhibitors	Captopril	PO	0.05–0.15 mg/kg/dose (low end in infants)	Hyperkalemia, proteinuria, cough, rash, marrow suppression	Use with caution in renal artery disease (bilateral), do not use in pregnancy, or in anyone who has had angioeurotic edema	More rapid onset than other ACE inhibitors
	Enalapril	PO	0.05–0.15 mg/kg/day	Similar to captopril	Similar to captopril, but longer acting. Not sulfur-containing, so perhaps fewer side effects	
Calcium channel blockers	Nifedipine	PO	0.25 mg/kg/dose, every 4–6 h	Vasodilation, tachycardia, nausea, vomiting, sweating, cardiac problems	Use with caution in heart failure	Absorption not affected by food
	Verapamil	PO	4–10 mg/kg/day, given 3x/day	Similar to nifedipine		Absorption delayed by food
	Isradipine	PO	0.05–0.83 mg/kg/day	Similar to nifedipine		Can be put into suspension
Alpha blockers	Prazosin	PO	1 mg to a max of 20 mg q 24 h	Orthostatic hypotension, lethargy, sedation and fatigue		First-dose hypotension may occur
	Phenoxybenzamine	PO	0.2 mg/kg/24 h	Orthostatic hypotension, nasal congestion		Specific for catecholamine excess
Central adrenergic stimulators	Clonidine	PO or patch	0.05 mg/kg/ bid to max 2.4 mg/24 h	Lethargy, sedation, dry mouth, (?) retinal degeneration		

Source: Adapted from Ref. 141.

Table 5b Parenteral and Sublingual Drugs for Use in Hypertensive Emergencies

Medication	Route	Dosage	Onset of action	Peak/duration	Adverse effects	Contraindication	Comments
Sodium nitroprusside (Nipride)	IV infusion	0.3–10 µg/kg/min	Immediate	1–2 min/2–3 min	Thiocyanate toxicity	Hepatic insufficiency	Photosensitive preparation; shield from light
Labetalol	IV bolus	0.5 mg/kg over 2 min; if no response, double dosage and repeat q 10 min to max dosage of 5 mg/kg	1–5 min	5 min/variable (generally 2–6 h)	Postural hypotension; neurological symptoms; nausea and vomiting	Bronchial asthma; CHF	
Nifedipine	Sublingual	0.25 mg/kg q 4–6 h	10–15 min	60–90 min/variable, usually 2–4 h	Vasodilatation, headache, cardiac events if preceding heart failure	Cardiomyopathy; concomitant use of beta blockers; cimetidine (relative)	Cardiac concerns less relevant in children than in adults
Esmolol	IV	500 µg/kg over 30 s, and then infusion of 25 µg/kg/min increasing dosage (e.g., 4 min to max 300 µg/kg/min)	1 min	mins/mins	Hypotension, CNS effects, nausea		Good drug for hypertension intraoperatively
Enalaprilat	IV, over 5 min	0.04–0.8 mg/kg/dose (child); 0.01 mg/kg starting (neonate)	15 min	1–4 h/variable	Hypotension, oliguria, hypokalemia	Renal failure, dehydration	Rx hypotension with volume
Diazoxide	IV bolus	1–3 mg/kg repeated every 5–15 min until control BP	1–5 min	1–5 min/variable (usually <12 h)	Arrhythmias, hyperglycemia, sodium and water retention	Thiazide sensitivity, diabetes, coarctation	May need diuretics to prevent fluid retention; unpredictable blood pressure drop may occur
Phentolamine	IV bolus	0.05–0.1 mg/kg	Within 30 s	2 min/5–30 min	Tachycardia, arrhythmia, marked hypotension		Specific for pheo.

Source: Adapted from Ref. 141.

Table 5c Diuretic Agents

Medication	Dosage	Onset	Peak/duration	Adverse effects	Relative contraindication
Furosemide (Lasix)	1–2 mg/kg (max, 6 mg/kg/24h)	Oral: 1–2 h IV: 5 min (child); 1 h (neonate)	1–2 h/4–6 h 30 min/2 h (child); 1–2 h/5–6 h (neonate)	Hyperuricemia, hyperglycemia, hypokalemia, hyponatremia, fluid depletion, ototoxicity	Sulfonamide sensitivity, anuria, metabolic alkalosis
Ethacrynic acid (Edecrin)	1 mg/kg (max, 25 mg total/day)	Oral: ~30 min IV: 15–30 min	2 h/6–8 h 45 min/3h	Same as for furosemide; ototoxicity more	Anuria, metabolic alkalosis
Bumetanide (Bumex)	Newborn: 0.01–0.05 mg/kg q 24 h Child: 0.015–0.1 mg/kg/dose q 6–24 h	Oral: 30–60 min IV: minutes	Oral: 4–6 h duration; IV: 30–60 min dur'n	Similar to furosemide; GI discomfort	As for furosemide
Hydrochlorothiazide (HydroDiuril)	2 mg/kg bid	Oral: 2 h	4 h/6–12 h	Electrolyte depletion; hyperuricemia; hypoglycemia	Anuria, sulfonamide sensitivity
Spironolactone (Aldactone)	1–3.3 mg/kg q 6, 8, or 12 h	Oral: gradual	3 d/2–3 d	Hyperkalemia, gynecomastia	Anuria, hyperkalemia, decreasing renal function
Metolazone (Zaroxolyn, Diulo, Mykrox)	1 mg/kg	Oral: gradual	Gradual	Similar to thiazide; also bloating, chest pain, chills	Anuria

Source: Adapted from Ref. 141.

XVI. TREATMENT

Current evidence supports the concept that blood pressure should be well within normal ranges among adults. For example, the risk of cardiovascular events among adults is higher among individuals with high normal blood pressure than in those with midrange or low–normal blood pressure (135). While no such data yet exist for children, it is more likely than not that stringent blood pressure control is important, particularly for children with health problems that can be associated with hypertension. Thus, it is reasonable to control blood pressure into the normal range in any infant, child, or adolescent with hypertension.

A primary endocrinopathy should be treated. If blood pressure is elevated, either because full therapy is not yet being administered or because therapy includes medications that can raise blood pressure, additional therapy in the form of antihypertensive treatment is indicated. Table 5 lists current oral and intravenous medications for hypertension and dosages (136–141). One should note that specific pediatric indications are presently evolving, as a result of the Food and Drug Administration's Modernization Act of 1997, which has mandated antihypertensive trials in children (137–139).

REFERENCES

1. Report of the Task Force on Blood Pressure Control in Children. Pediatr 1977; 59(Suppl 5):797–820.
2. Task Force on Blood Pressure Control in Children. Report of the second task force on blood pressure control of children. Pediatrics 1987; 79:1–25.
3. National High Blood Pressure Education Program Working Group on Hypertension Control in Children and Adolescents. Update on the 1987 task force report on high blood pressure in children and adolescents: a working group report from the National High Blood Pressure Education Program. Pediatrics 1996; 98:649–658.
4. Goonasekera CDA, Dillon MJ. Measurement and interpretation of blood pressure. Arch Dis Child 2000; 82: 261–265.
5. Kay JD, Sinaiko AR, Daniels SR. Pediatric hypertension. Am Heart J 2001; 142:422–432.
6. Hiner LB, Falkner B. Renovascular hypertension in children. Pediatr Clin North Am 1993; 40(1):123–140.
7. Soergel M, Kirschstein M, Busch C, Danne T, Gellermann J, Holl R, et al. Oscillometric twenty-four-hour ambulatory blood pressure values in healthy children and adolescents: a multicenter trial incuding 1141 subjects. J Pediatr 1997, 130:178–184.
8. Sorof JM, Portman RJ. Ambulatory blood pressure measurements. Curr Opin Pediatr 2001; 13(2):133–137.
9. Flynn JT. Impact of ambulatory blood pressure monitor-

ing on the management of hypertension in children. Blood Press Monit. 2000; 5(4):211–216.

10. Lurbe E, Redon J. Diagnosis of high blood pressure in children by means of ambulatory blood pressure monitoring. Curr Hypertens Rep 2001; 3:89–90.

11. Koch VH, Colli A, Saito MI, Furusawa EA, Ignes E, Okay Y, Mion D Jr. Comparison between casual blood pressure and ambulatory blood pressure monitoring parameters in healthy and hypertensive adolescents. Blood Press Monit 2000; 5(5-6):281–289.

12. Khan IA, Gajaria M, Stephens D, Balfe JW. Ambulatory blood pressure monitoring in children: a large center's experience. Pediatr Nephrol 2000; 14:802–805.

13. Yiu VW, Dluhy RG, Lifton RP, Guay-Woodford LM. Low peripheral plasma renin activity as a critical marker in pediatric hypertension. Pediatr Nephrol 1997; 11:343–346.

14. Pratt JH. Low-renin hypertension: more common than we think? Cardiol Rev 2000; 8:202–206.

15. Warnock DG. Genetic forms of human hypertension. Curr Opin Nephrol Hypertens 2001; 138:715–720.

16. New MI, Wilson RC. Steroid disorders in children: congenital adrenal hyperplasia and apparent mineralocorticoid excess. Proc Natl Acad Sci USA 1999; 96:12790–12797.

17. New MI, Seaman MP. Secretion rates of cortisol and aldosterone precursors in various forms of congenital adrenal hyperplasia. J Clin Endocrinol Metab 1970; 30:361.

18. New MI, Levine LS. Hypertension of childhood with suppressed renin. Endocrinol Rev 1980; 1:421–430.

19. New MI, Levine LS. Congenital adrenal hyperplasia. Adv Hum Genet 1973; 4:251–326.

20. Mimouni M, Kaufman H, Roitman A, Morag C, Sadan N. Hypertension in a neonate with 11 beta-hydroxylase deficiency. Eur J Pediatr 1985; 143:231–233.

21. Zachmann M, Vollmin JA, New MI, Curtius C-C, Prader A. Congenital adrenal hyperplasia due to deficiency of 11-hydroxylation of 17α-hydroxylated steroids. J Clin Endocrinol Metab 1971; 33:501.

22. Cerame BI, New MI. Hormonal hypertension in children: 11β-hydroxylase deficiency and apparent mineralocorticoid excess. J Pediatr Endocrinol 2000; 13:1537–1547.

23. White PC, Dupont J, New MI, Lieberman E, Hochberg Z, Rosler A. A mutation in CYP11B1 [Arg448His] associated with steroid 22β-hydroxylase deficiency in Jews of Moroccan origin. J Clin Invest 1991; 87:1664–1667.

24. Curnow KM, Slutker L, Vitek J, et al. Mutations in the CYP11B1 gene causing congenital adrenal hyperplasia and hypertension cluster in exons 6,7 and 8. Proc Natl Acad Sci USA 1993; 90:4552–4556.

25. Skinner CA, Rumsby G. Steroid 11β-hydroxylase deficiency caused by a 5-base pair duplication in the CYP11B1 gene. Hum Mol Genet 1994; 3:377–378.

26. Helmberg A, Ausserer B, Kofler R. Frameshift by insertion of 2 basepairs in codon 394 of CYP11B1 causes congenital adrenal hyperplasia due to steroid 11β-hydroxylase deficiency. J Clin Endocrinol Metab 1992; 75:1278–1281.

27. Pascoe L, Curnow KM, Slutsker L, et al. Mutations in the human CYP11B2 [aldosterone synthase] gene causing corticosterone methyloxidase II deficiency. Proc Natl Acad Sci USA 1992; 89:4996–5000.

28. Biglieri EG, Herron MA, Brust N. 17-hydroxylation deficiency. J Clin Invest 1966; 45:1946.

29. New MI. Male pseudohermaphroditism due to 17-α-hydroxylase deficiency. J Clin Invest 1970; 49:1930.

30. Mantero F, Scaroni C. Enzymatic defects of steroidogenesis: 17α-hydroxylase deficiency. Pediatr Adolesc Endocrinol 1984; 13:83–94.

31. Wit JM, van Roermund HPC, Oostdik W, et al. Heterozygotes for 17α-hydroxylase deficiency can be detected with a short ACTH test. Clin Endocrinol 1988; 28:657–664.

32. Matteson KJ, Picado-Leonard J, Chung BC, Mohandas TK, Miller W. Assignment of the gene for adrenal P450c17 to human chromosome 10. J Clin Endocrinol Metab 1986; 63:789.

33. Fan Y-S, Sasi R, Lee C, Winter JSD, Waterman MR, Lin CC. Localization of the human CYP17 gene (cytochrome P45017a) to 10q24.3 by fluorescence in situ hybridization and simultaneous chromosome banding. Genomics 1992; 14:1110–1111.

34. Wilson RC, Nimkarn S, New MI. Apparent mineralocorticoid excess. Trends Endocrinol Metab 2001; 12(3):104–111.

35. Labhart A. Adrenal cortex. In: Labhart A, ed. Clinical Endocrinology: Theory and Practice. New York: Springer-Verlag, 1974:332–339.

36. Stewart PM. Mineralocorticoid hypertension. Lancet 353: 1341–1347.

37. Conn JW. Primary aldosteronism, a new clinical entity. J Lab Clin Med 1955; 45:3–17.

38. Young WF. Primary aldosteronism: update on diagnosis and treatment. Endocrinologist 1997; 7:213–221.

39. Kelch RP, Connors MH, Kaplan SL, Biglieri EG, Grumbach MM. A calcified aldosterone-producing tumor in a hypertensive, normokalemic prepubertal girl. J Pediatr 1973; 83:432.

40. Bryer-Ash M, Wilson D, Tune BM, Rosenfeld RG, Shochat SJ, Luetscher JA. Hypertension caused by an aldosterone-secreting adenoma. Am J Dis Child 1984; 138: 673–676.

41. Decsi J Soltesz G, Harangi F, Nemes J, Szabo M, Pinter A. Severe hypertension in a ten-year-old boy secondary to an aldosterone-producing tumor identified by adrenal sonography. Acta Pediatr Hung 1986; 27:233–238.

42. Oberfield SE, Levine LS, Firpo A, et al. Primary hyperaldosteronism in childhood due to unilateral macronodular hyperplasia. Hypertension 1984; 6:75–84.

43. Prosser PR Sutherland CM, Scullin DR. Localization of adrenal aldosterone adenoma by computerized tomography. N Engl J Med 1979; 300:1278–1279.

44. Weinberger MH, Grim CE, Hollifield JW, et al. Primary aldosteronism: diagnosis, localization and treatment. Ann Intern Med 1979; 90:386–395.

45. Hietakorpi S, Korhonen T, Aro A, et al. The value of scintigraphy and computed tomography for the differential diagnosis of primary hyperaldosteronism. Acta Endocrinol 1986; 113:118–122.

46. Delyani JA, Rocha R, Cook CS, Tobert DS, Levin S, Roniker B, Workman DL, Sing YL, Whelihan B. Eplerenone: a selective aldosterone receptor antagonist (SARA). Cardiovasc Drug Rev 2001; 19(3):185–200.

47. Sutherland DJ, Ruse JL, Laidlaw JC. Hypertension, increased aldosterone secretion and low plasma renin activity relieved by dexamethasone. Can Med Assoc J 1966; 95:1109–1119.

48. New MI, Peterson RE. A new form of congenital adrenal hyperplasia. J Clin Endocrinol Metab 1967; 27:300–305.

49. New MI, Oberfield SE, Levine LS, Dupont B, Pollack M, Gill JR, Bartter FC. Demonstration of autosomal

dominant transmission and absence of HLA linkage in dexamethasone-suppressible hyperaldosteronism. Lancet 1980; 1:550–551.

50. Miura K, Yoshinaga K, Goto K, Katsushima I, Maebashi M, Demura H, Iino M, Demura R, Torikai T. A case of glucocorticoid-responsive hyperaldosteronism. J Clin Endocrinol Metab 1968; 28(12):1807–1815.

51. New MI, Siegal EJ, Peterson RE. Dexamethasone-suppressive hyperaldosteronism. J Clin Endocrinol Metab 1973; 37:93–100.

52. Giebink GS, Gotlin RW, Biglieri EG, Katz FH. A kindred with familial glucocorticoid-suppressible aldosteronism. J Clin Endocrinol Metab 1973; 36:715–723.

53. Grim CE, Weinberger MH. Familial dexamethasone-suppressible hyperaldosteronism. Pediatrics 1980; 65:597–604.

54. Oberfield SE, Levine LS, Stoner E, Chow D, Rauh W, Greig F, Lee SM, Leightner E, Witte E, New MI. Adrenal glomerulosa function in patients with dexamethasone-suppressible normokalemic hyperaldosteronism. J Clin Endocrinol Metab 1981; 53:158–164.

55. Lifton RP, Dluhy RG, Powers M, Rich GM, Cook S, Ulick S, Lalouel MA. Chimeric 11b-hydroxylase/aldosterone synthase gene causes GRA and human hypertension. Nature 1992; 355:262–265.

56. Lifton RP, Dluhy RG, Powers M, Rich GM, Gutkin M, Fallo F, Gill JR, Feld L, Ganguly A, Laidlaw JC, Murnaghan DJ, Kaufman C, Stockigt JR, Ulick S, Lalouel MA. Hereditary hypertension caused by chimeric gene duplications and ectopic expression of aldosterone synthetase. Nature Genet 1992; 2:66–74.

57. Gill JR Jr, Bartter FC. Overproduction of sodium-retaining steroids by the zona glomerulosa is adrenocorticotropin-dependent and mediates hypertension in dexamethasone-suppressible aldosteronism. J Clin Endocrinol Metab 1981; 53:331–337.

58. Gomez-Sanches CE, Gill JR Jr, Ganguly A, Gordon RD. Glucocorticoid-suppressible aldosteronism: a disorder of the adrenal transitional zone. J Clin Endocrinol Metab 1988; 67:444–448.

59. Ulick S, Chan CK, Gill JR Jr, et al. Defective fasciculate zone function as the mechanism of glucocorticoid-remediable aldosteronism. J Clin Endocrinol Metab 1990; 71:1151–1157.

60. Ulick S, Chu MD. Hypersecretion of a new cortico-steroid, 18-hydroxycortisol in two types of adrenocortical hypertension. Clin Exp Hypertens 1982; Suppl 9/10:1771–1777.

61. Ulick S, Chu MD, Land M. Biosynthesis of 18-oxocortisol by aldosterone-producing adrenal tissue. J Biol Chem 1983; 258:5498–5502.

62. Gomez-Sanchez CE, Montgomery M, Ganguly A, et al. Elevated urinary excretion of 18-oxocortisol in glucocorticoid-suppressible aldosteronism. J Clin Endocrinol Metab 1984; 59:1022–1024.

63. Shackleton CH. Mass spectrometry in the diagnosis of steroid-related disorders and in hypertension research. J Steroid Biochem Mol Biol 1993; 45:127–140.

64. Dluhy RG, Anderson B, Harlin B, Ingelfinger J, Lifton R. Glucocorticoid-remediable aldosteronism is associated with severe hypertension in early childhood. J Pediatr 2001; 138(5):715–720.

65. New MI, Levine LS, Biglieri EG, Pareira J, Ulick S. Evidence for an unidentified ACTH-induced steroid hormone causing hypertension. J Clin Endocrinol Metab 1977; 44:924–933.

66. New MI, Oberfield SE, Carey RM, Greig F, Ulick S, Levine LS. A genetic defect in cortisol metabolism as the basis for the syndrome of apparent mineralocorticoid excess. In: Mnatero F, Biglieri EG, Edwards CRW, eds. Endocrinology of Hypertension. Serono Symposia No. 50. New York: Academic Press, 1982:85–101.

67. Downey MK, Riddick L, New MI. Apparent mineralocorticoid excess: a genetic form of fatal low-renin hypertension. Program and Abstracts, American Society of Hypertension, Second World Congress on Biologically Active Atrial Peptides, New York, May 1987.

68. Ulick S, Ramirez LC, New MI. An abnormality in steroid reductive metabolism in a hypertensive syndrome J Clin Endocrinol Metab 1977; 44:799–802.

69. Ulick S, Levine LS, Gunczler P, et al. A syndrome of apparent mineralocorticoid excess associated with defects in the peripheral metabolism of cortisol. J Clin Endocrinol Metab 1979; 44:757–764.

70. Lakshmi V, Monder C. Evidence for independent 11-oxidase and 11-reductase activities of 11b-hydroxysteroid dehydrogenase: enzyme latency, phase transitions, and lipid requirements. Endocrinology 1985; 116:552–560.

71. Werder EA, Zachmann M, Vollmin JA, Veyrat R, Prader A. Unusual steroid excretion in a child with low renin hypertension. Res Steroids 1974; 6:385–389.

72. White PC, Munte T, Agarwal AK. 11β-Hydroxysteroid dehydrogenase and the syndrome of apparent mineralocorticoid excess. Endocr Rev 1997; 18:135–156.

73. Ferrari P, Lovati E, Frey FJ. The role of the 11β-hydroxysteroid dehydrogenase type 2 in human hypertension. J Hypertens 2000; 18:241–248.

74. Obeyesekere VR, Ferrari P, Andrews RK, Wilson RC, New MI, Funder J, Krozowski ZS. The R337C mutation generates a high Km 11 beta-hydroxysteroid dehydrogenase type II enzyme in a family with apparent mineralocorticoid excess. J Clin Endocrinol Metab 1995; 80:3381–3383.

75. Ferrari P, Obeyesekere VR, Li K, Wilson RC, New MI, Funder JW, Krozowski ZS. Point mutations abolish 11 beta-hydroxysteroid dehydrogenase type II activity in three families with the congenital syndrome of apparent mineralocorticoid excess. Mol Cell Endocrinol 1996; 119:21–24.

76. Mune T, Rogerson FM, Nikkila H, Agarwal AK, White PC. Human hypertension caused by mutations in the kidney isozyme of 11 beta-hydroxysteroid dehydrogenase. Nat Genet 1995; 10:394–399.

77. Azar M, Krozowski Z, Funder JW, Shackelton CHL, Bradlow HL, Wei J, Hertecant J, Moran A, Neiberger RE, Balfe JW, Fattah H, Daneman D, Akkurt HI, DeSantis C, New MI. Examination of genotype and phenotype relationships in 14 patients with apparent mineralocorticoid excess. J Clin Endocrinol Metab 1998; 83:2244–2254.

78. Moudgil A, Rodich G, Jordan SC, Kamil ES. Nephrocalcinosis and renal cysts associated with apparent mineralocorticoid excess syndrome. Pediatr Nephrol 2000; 15(1-2):60–62.

79. Mercado AB, Wilson RC, Chung KC, Wei J-Q, New MI. Prenatal treatment and diagnosis of congenital adrenal hyperplasia owing to steroid 21-hydroxylase deficiency. J Clin Endocrinol Metab 1995; 80:2014–2020.

80. Ugrasbul F, Wiens T, Rubinstein P, New MI, Wilson RC. Prevalence of mild apparent mineralocorticoid excess in Mennonites. J Clin Endocrinol Metab 1999; 84:4735–4738.

81. New MI, Nimkarn S, Brandon DD, Cunningham-Rundles

S, Wilson RC, Newfield RS, Vandermeulen J, Barron N, Russo C, Loriaux DL, O'Malley B. Resistance to multiple steroids in two sisters. J Steroid Biochem Mol Biol 2001; 76:161–166.

82. Li A, Li KXZ, Marui S, Krozowski ZS, Batista MC, Whorwood C, Arnhold IJP, Shackleton CHL, Mendonca BB, Stewart PM. Apparent mineralocorticoid excess in a Brazilian kindred: hypertension in the heterozygote state. J Hypertens 19997; 15:397–1402.

83. Ferrari P, Krozowski Z. Role of the 11b-hydroxysteroid dehydrogenase in blood pressure regulation. Kidney Int 2000; 57:1374–1381.

84. Stewart PM, Wallace AM, Valentino R, Burt D, Shakleton CHL, Edwards CRW. Mineralocorticoid activity of liquorice: 11β-hydroxysteroid dehydrogenase deficiency comes of age. Lancet 1987; 2:821–823.

85. Gordon RD, Klemm SA, Tunny TJ, Stowasser M. Genetics of primary aldosteronism. Clin Exp Pharmacol Physiol 1994; 21(11):915–918.

86. Schambelan M, Sebastian A, Rector FC Jr. Mineralocorticoid-resistant renal hyperkalemia without salt wasting (type II pseudohypoaldosteronism): role of increased renal chloride reabsorption. Kidney Int 1981; 19:716.

87. Take C, Ikeda K, Kurasawa T, Kurokawa K. Increased chloride reabsorption as an inherited renal tubular defect in familial type II pseudohypoaldosteronism. N Engl J Med 1991; 324:472–476.

88. Mansfield TA, Simon DB, Farfel Z, Bia M, Tucci JR, Lebel M, Gutkin M, Vialettes B, Christofilis MA, Kauppinen-Makelin R, Mayan H, Risch N, Lifton RP. Multilocus linkage of familial hyperkalaemia and hypertension, pseudohypoaldosteronism type II, to chromosomes 1q31-42 and 17p11-q21. Nat Genet 1997; 16:202–205.

89. Erdogan G, Corapciolgu D, Erdogan MF, Hallioglu J, Uysal AR. Furosemide and dDAVP for the treatment of pseudohypoaldosteronism type II. J Endocrinol Invest 1997; 20:681–684.

90. Wilson FH, Disse-Nicodeme S, Choate KA, Ishikawa K, Nelson-Williams C, Desitter I, Gunel M, Milford DV, Lipkin GW, Achard J-M, Feely MP, Dussol B, Berland Y, Unwin RJ, Mayan H, Simon DB, Farfel Z, Jeunemaitre X, Lifton RP. Human hypertension caused by mutations in WNK kinases. Science 2001; 293:1107–1112.

91. Liddle GW, Bledsoe T, Coppage WS. A familial renal disorder simulating primary aldosteronism ut with negligible aldosterone secretion. Trans Assoc Am Physicians 1963; 76:199–213.

92. Wang C, Chan TK, Yeung RT, Coghlan JP, Scoggins BA, Stockigt JR. The effect of triamterene and sodium intake on renin, aldosterone, and erythrocyte sodium transport in Liddle's syndrome. J Clin Endocrinol Metab 1981; 52:1027–1032.

93. Botero-Velez M, Curtis JJ, Warnock DG. Brief report: Liddle's syndrome revisited—a disorder of sodium reabsorption in the distal tubule. N Engl J Med 1994; 330:178–181.

94. Shimkets RA, Warnock DG, Bositis CM, et al. Liddle's syndrome: heritable human hypertension caused by mutations in the β subunit of the epithelial sodium channel. Cell 1994; 79:407–414.

95. Hansson JH, Nelson-Williams C, Suzuki H, et al. Hypertension caused by a truncated epithelial sodium channel gamma subunit: genetic heterogeneity of Liddle syndrome. Nat Genet 1995; 11:76–82.

96. Rossier BC. 1996 Homer Smith Award Lecture: cum grano salis: the epithelial sodium channel and the control of blood pressure. J Am Soc Nephrol 1997; 8:980–992.

97. Treadwell BLJ, Sever ED, Savage O, Copeman WSC. Side effects of long term treatment with corticosteroids and corticotrophin. Lancet 1964; 1:1121–1123.

98. Gomez-Sanchez CE. Cushing's syndrome and hypertension. Hypertension 1986; 8:258–264.

99. Ritchie CM, Sheridan B, Fraser R, Hadden DR, Kennedy AL, Riddell J, Atkinson A. Studies on the pathogenesis of hypertension in Cushing's disease and acromegaly. Q J Med 1990; 280:855–867.

100. Saruta T, Suzuki H, Handa M, Igarashi Y, Kondo K, Senba S. Multiple factors contribute to the pathogenesis of hypertension in Cushing's syndrome. J Clin Endocrinol Metab 1986; 62:275–279.

101. Mircescu H, Wilkin F, Paquette J, Oligny LL, Decaluwe H, Gaboury L, Nolet S, Van Vliet G, Deal C. Molecular characterization of a pediatric pheochromocytoma with suspected bilateral disease. J Pediatr 2001; 138(2):269–73.

102. Kinney MA, Warner ME, vanHeerden JA, Horlocker TT, Young WF Jr, Schroeder DR, Maxson PM, Warner MA. Perianesthetic risks and outcomes of pheochromocytoma and paraganglioma resection. Anesth Analg 2000; 91(5):1118–1123.

103. Reddy VS, O'Neill JA Jr, Holcomb GW III, Neblett WW III, Pietsch JB, Morgan WM III, Goldstein RE. Twenty-five-year surgical experience with pheochromocytoma in children. Am Surg 2000; 66(12):1085–1091.

104. Chen TY, Liang CD, Shieh CS, Ko SF, Kao ML. Reversible hypertensive retinopathy in a child with bilateral pheochromocytoma after tumor resection. J Formos Med Assoc 2000; 99(12):945–947.

105. Lertakyamanee N, Lertakyamanee J, Somprakit P, Nimmanwudipong T, Buranakitjaroen P, Bhavakula K, Sindhavananda K. Surgery and anesthesia for pheochromocytoma—a series of 40 operations. J Med Assoc Thai 2000; 83(8):921–927.

106. Radmayr C, Neumann H, Bartsch G, Elsner R, Janetschek G. Laparoscopic partial adrenalectomy for bilateral pheochromocytomas in a boy with von Hippel-Lindau disease. Eur Urol 2000; 38(3):344–348.

107. Hack HA. The perioperative management of children with phaeochromocytoma. Paediatr Anaesth 2000; 10(5):463–476.

108. Ross JH. Pheochromocytoma. Special considerations in children. Urol Clin North Am 2000; 27(3):393–402.

109. Laporte R, Godart F, Breviere GM, Vaksmann G, Francart C, Rey C. [Severe arterial hypertension and pheochromocytoma in childhood. Case report and review of the literature]. [French] Arch Mal Coeur Vaiss 2000; 93(5):627–630.

110. Ferragut J, Caimari M, Rituerto B, Gomez-Rivas B, Herrera M, Alonso F. Pheochromocytoma and clear-cell renal carcinoma in a child with von Hippel-Lindau disease: a patient report. J Pediatr Endocrinol 1999; 12(4):579–582.

111. Hack HA, Brown TC. Preoperative management of phaeochromocytoma—a paediatric perspective. [letter; comment]. Anaesth Intensive Care 1999; 27(1):112–113.

112. Clements RH, Goldstein RE, Holcomb GW III. Laparoscopic left adrenalectomy for pheochromocytoma in a child. J Pediatr Surg 1999; 34(9):1408–1409.

113. Pretorius M, Rasmussen GE, Holcomb GW. Hemodynamic and catecholamine responses to a laparoscopic adrenalectomy for pheochromocytoma in a pediatric patient. Anesth Analg 1998; 87(6):1268–1270.

114. Eder U, Fischer-Colbrie R, Kogner P, Leitner B, Bjellerup P, Winkler H. Levels and molecular forms of chromogranins in human childhood neuroblastomas and ganglioneuromas. Neurosci Lett 1998; 253(1):17–20.

115. Favia G, Lumachi F, Polistina F, D'Amico DF. Pheochromocytoma, a rare cause of hypertension: long-term follow-up of 55 surgically treated patients. World J Surg 1998; 22(7):689–694.

116. Russell WJ, Metcalfe IR, Tonkin AL, Frewin DB. The preoperative management of phaeochromocytoma. Anaesth Intensive Care 1998; 26(2):196–200.

117. Maher ER, Kaelin WG Jr, Basset A, Blanc J, Messas E, Hagege A, Elghazi, JL. Renin–angiotensin system contribution to cardiac hypertrophy in experimental hyperthyroidism: an echocardiographic study. J Cardiovasc Pharmacol 2001; 37:163–172.

118. Schonwetter BS, Libber SM, Jones MD Jr, Park KJ, Pictnick LP. Hypertension in neonatal hyperthyroidism Am J Dis Child 1983; 137:954–955.

119. Minami N, Imai Y, Abe K, Munakata M, Sakurada T, Yamamoto M, Yoshida K, Sekino H, Yoshinaga K. The circadian variation of blood pressure and heart rate in patients with hyperthyroidism. Tohoku J Exp Med 1989; 159:185–193.

120. Saito I, Saruta T. Hypertension in thyroid disorders. Endocrinol Metab Clin North Am 1994; 23:379–386.

121. Streeten DH Anderson GH Jr, Howland T, Chiang R, Smulyan H. Effects of thyroid function on blood pressure. Recognition of hypothyroid hypertension. Hypertension 1988; 11:78–83.

122. Lind L, Ridefelt P, Rastad J, Akerstrom G, Ljunghall S. Relationship between abnormal regulation of cytoplasmic calcium and elevated blood pressure in patients with primary hyperparathyroidism. J Hum Hypertens 1994; 8: 113–118.

123. Lind L, Ljunghall S. Blood pressure reaction during the intraoperative and early postoperative periods in patients with primary hyperparathyroidism. Exp Clin Endocrinol 1994; 102:409–413.

124. Scuteri A, Bos AJ, Brant LJ, Talbot L, Lakatta EG, Fleg JL. Hormone replacement therapy and longitudinal changes in blood pressure in postmenopausal women. Ann Intern Med 2001; 135(4):229–238.

125. Covar RA, Leung DY, McCormick D, Steelman J, Zeitler JP, Spahn JD. Risk factors associated with glucocorticoid-induced adverse effects in children with severe asthma. J Allergy Clin Immunol 2000; 106:651–659.

126. Nathwani NC, Unwin R, Brook CG, Hindmarsh PC. The influence of renal and cardiovascular abnormalities on blood pressure in Turner syndrome. Clin Endocrinol 2000; 52(3):371–377.

127. Jorde R, Sundsfjord J, Haug E, Bonaa KH. Relation between low calcium intake, parathyroid hormone, and blood pressure. Hypertension 2000; 35(5):1154–1159.

128. Balkau B, Tichet J, Caces E, Vol S, Eschwege E, Cahane M. Insulin dose and cardiovascular risk factors in type 1 diabetic children and adolescents.Diabete Metab 1998; 24(2):143–150.

129. Sochett EB, Poon I, Balfe W, Daneman D. Ambulatory blood pressure monitoring in insulin-dependent diabetes mellitus adolescents with and without microalbuminuria. J Diabetes Complications 1998; 12(1):18–23.

130. Madacsy L, Yasar A, Tulassay T, Korner A, Kelemen J, Hobor M, Miltenyi M. Relative nocturnal hypertension in children with insulin-dependent diabetes mellitus. Acta Paediatr 1994; 83(4):414–417.

131. Ferrari P, Lovati E, Frey FJ. The role of the 11beta-hydroxysteroid dehydrogenase type 2 in human hypertension. J Hypertens 2000; 18(3):241–248.

132. Donovan SJ. 11 beta-Hydroxysteroid dehydrogenase: a link between the dysregulation of cortisol metabolism and hypertension. Br J Biomed Sci 1999; 56(3):215–225.

133. Brand E, Kato N, Chatelain N, Krozowski ZS, Jeunemaitre X, Corvol P, Plouin PF, Cambien F, Pascoe L, Soubrier F. Structural analysis and evaluation of the 11beta-hydroxysteroid dehydrogenase type 2 (11beta-HSD2) gene in human essential hypertension. J Hypertens 1998; 16(11):1627–1633.

134. Bjorntorp P, Holm G, Rosmond R, Folkow B. Hypertension and the metabolic syndrome: closely related central origin? Blood Pressure 2000; 9(2-3):71–82.

135. Vasan RS, Larson MG, Leip E, Evans JC, O'Donnell CJ, Kannel WB, Levy D. Impact of high normal blood pressure on the risk of cardiovascular disease. N Engl J Med 2001; 345:1291–1297.

136. Wells TG. Trials of antihypertensive therapies in children. Blood Pressure Monit 1999; 4(3-4):189–192.

137. Chesney RW, Adamson P, Wells T, Wilson JT, Walson PD. The testing of antihypertensive medications in children: report of the Antihypertensive Agent Guidelines Subcommittee of the Pediatric Pharmacology Research Units. Pediatrics 2001; 107(3):558–561.

138. Sinaiko AR, Lauer RM, Sanders SP. End points for cardiovascular drug trials in pediatric patients. Am Heart J 2001; 142(2):229–232.

139. Temple ME, Nahata MC. Treatment of pediatric hypertension. Pharmacotherapy 2000; 20(2):140–150.

140. Adelman RD, Coppo R, Dillon MJ. The emergency management of severe hypertension. Pediatr Nephrol 2000; 14(5):422–427.

141. Ingelfinger JR. Hypertensive Emergencies in Infants and Children. In: Grenvik A, Ayres SM, Holbrook PR, Shoemaker WC, eds. Textbook of Critical Care. 4th ed. Philadelphia: WB Saunders, 2000:1087–1098.

142. New MI, Crawford C, Virdis R. Low resin hypertension in childhood. In: Lifshitz F, ed. Pediatric Endocrinology, 3d ed. New York: Marcel Dekker, 1996:776.

39

Dietary Supplements to Enhance Athletic Performance

Alan D. Rogol
University of Virginia, Charlottesville, and Medical College of Virginia, Richmond, Virginia, U.S.A.

I. INTRODUCTION

Ergogenic aids (from the Greek, *ergon*, meaning work) are ingested to enhance energy utilization by producing more, better controlling its expenditure, or increasing efficiency of use. It is apparent that true athletic success stems primarily from a combination of genetic endowment, training, technique, equipment, and proper nutrition. The ingestion of nutritional supplements may play only a small, mainly insignificant, role in the outcome of athletic endeavors. What do athletes want? They want enhanced athletic performance and many believe that one way, perhaps a shortcut, is to take nutritional supplements. Extracting and extrapolating from a wide variety of sources, it appears that the athlete truly desires increased strength, power, and endurance; as well as salutary alterations in body composition: increased lean body (muscle) mass and decreased fat mass as quickly as possible, and faster and more complete recovery from exercise (training) and competition to achieve the goal of improved performance at subsequent competitions.

These are issues for athletes of both genders and almost all ages; however, there are additional issues when the adolescent athlete is considered. Normal physiological growth should occur during the time of adolescence. This topic is covered extensively in other portions of this text. In general the linear growth rate is relatively constant at 5.5 cm/year during childhood. It continues at this rate until just before the pubertal growth spurt. This physiological event has significant variability in both *timing* and *tempo* and may be of special importance to athletes in certain sports that may select for the smaller and more delayed body type, for example, gymnastics and the lightweight wrestler. It is against the norm that one must explain variations in adolescent development in those who train for athletics and competition and in addition may take dietary supplements.

Nutritional supplements come in many varieties and forms: foods, vitamins, antioxidants, and anabolics, to mention only a few. A critical historical fact is a change in the level of scrutiny by the U.S. Food and Drug Administration (FDA). The Dietary Supplement Health and Education Act of 1994 defined a food supplement as ... "any product that contains a vitamin, a mineral, an amino acid, an herb or other botanical; or a concentrate, metabolite, constituent, extract or combination of any of these ingredients." Virtually overnight an exponentially growing multibillion dollar industry was spawned. In the following sections I shall review information on two herbals (ephedra and ginseng), creatine, and some anabolics including dehydroepiandrosterone (DHEA), androstenedione, and growth hormone. Growth hormone and the more potent anabolic steroids are administered parenterally and are not so readily available as the three agents noted above; however, I shall very briefly review some of the agents that act in the growth hormone–insulin-like growth factor-1 (IGF-1) system.

II. DIETARY SUPPLEMENTS: HERBAL PRODUCTS

Because of the Dietary Supplement Health Education Act in 1994 herbs and other botanicals are not subject to the stringent premarketing safety (and efficacy) evaluations that apply to other foods (and drugs). They are not subject to FDA regulation, but fall under the jurisdiction of the Federal Trade Commission. Claims are made that such products will favorably alter body composition: increase lean body mass, decrease fat mass, and perhaps alter the regional distribution of body fat. In addition, supplements are taken to decrease fatigue, permit more intensive workouts, and aid in the recovery from these intensive bursts of muscle use to allow energy expenditure for the next training session. The message of the utility (even necessity) of these ergogenic aids is heard by the adolescent athlete who seeks athletic success, often as an avenue for social acceptance. Proper training technique includes strength training and proper nutrition; the purveyors of dietary supplements know that the message that their products can be part of the overall route to athletic success will be understood.

Although there are many herbal products for which claims are made for ergogenic properties, I shall review only two, ephedra and ginseng, for which there is some significant scientific information as ergogenic aids for humans who exercise.

III. EPHEDRA

Chinese ephedra (*Ephedra sinica*) (1) or ma huang has a long tradition (more than 5000 years) of use as treatment for respiratory ailments. Although many ingredients are found in ephedra extracts, the active pharmacological agents are ephedrine and its related alkaloids pseudoephedrine, norephedrine, and norpseudoephedrine. These and the synthetic ephedrine alkaloids are ingredients of many prescription and over-the-counter pharmaceutical products. Many of the dietary supplements today actually contain *added* synthetic ephedrine alkaloids or are combined with other stimulants, (e.g., caffeine) and thus are not really comparable to the original Chinese herbal extracts, especially with reference to the dosages of the active ephedrine alkaloid ingredients. These latter are more likely to mimic the effects of ephedrine and cause adverse events (See below), especially when combined with caffeine.

There have been several studies of the acute effects of the ephedra alkaloids on exercise performance, but the dosages often are in excess of those "recommended" for daily use. These have evaluated time to exhaustion or muscle strength. Most have shown no significant effects, except for a rise in peak systolic blood pressure (2,3). However, when combined with a high dosage of caffeine, Bell and colleagues (4) were able to determine a statistically significant increase in time to exhaustion in a cycle ergometer trial.

The ephedra alkaloids found in many dietary supplements are banned substances for some amateur and professional sporting events. After these supplements are taken, their metabolites are excreted into the urine in amounts sufficient to be detected by the usual testing procedures.

A disadvantage of the use of supplements containing ephedra, ephedra extract, or ma huang is their propensity to untoward reactions. Reports to the FDA and Poison Control Centers include many cardiovascular toxic effects including cardiac arrhythmias, myocardial infarctions, and stroke, with a number of these events being fatal. Haller performed a review of the cardiovascular and central nervous system (CNS) events associated with dietary supplements containing ephedra alkaloids. Benowitz (5) found hypertension as the single most frequent adverse event followed by tachycardia and palpitations. Although these cardiovascular events and those related to the CNS did not occur with great frequency, the authors suggested that they could be devastating in *vulnerable* individuals. Central nervous system adverse events include agitation, mania, psychoses, and dependence. Although many may have followed so-called improper dosage of the supplement, the amounts taken were well within the range of those who use these dietary supplements. It is important to note that the content of ephedra alkaloids in herbal dietary supplements varied over a very wide range. In one review Gurley and co-workers (6) found lot-to-lot variations in the contents of (−)-ephedrine, (+)-pseudoephedrine, and (−)-methylephedrine of greater that 180%, 250%, and 1000%, respectively. (+)-Norpseudoephedrine, a schedule IV substance, was an ingredient of a number of the supplements tested. A majority of the products had major discrepancies (>20%) in the amounts of ephedra alkaloids actually contained and those claimed on the label. Such products *can* be very dangerous even if "used as directed," given the wide variations in ingredient content.

IV. GINSENG

Ginseng (1) usually refers to the Chinese or Korean preparation of *Panax ginseng*. It is used as a dietary and medicinal product in most of Asia, in the form of root, root extract, or root powder. The root contains multiple glycosylated steroidal saponins as *likely* active agents. Although used to improve general health (*Qi*, life energy) some more recent studies have focused on its effect on exercise performance. Some properly controlled studies have shown statistically significant improvements in physical performance (e.g., increased aerobic capacity and muscle strength) after 6 weeks of ingesting ginseng root powder (7). A number of other studies have shown small or nonsignificant changes in the cardiovascular and respiratory systems, especially in untrained, older subjects and in larger trials. It is difficult to find evidence for a salutary effect on athletic performance in the younger, training competitive athlete.

The untoward effects from the usual dosages are not prominent and it is often difficult to separate those effects (e.g., CNS stimulation) from those of the added "contaminants," such as caffeine or ephedra alkaloids (see above). No metabolites that appear on the banned list for athletes are excreted in the urine of those who take ginseng preparations.

V. CREATINE

Creatine (8–12) is a nutrient found naturally in various foods, for example, meat and fish. It is also available as a nutritional concentrated supplement that is not on the banned list, that is, it is "legal." Its main source in the diet is fish and red meat and is found almost exclusively in skeletal muscle, where it is one of the main energy sources available to fuel the energy bursts for explosive contractions, such as those in jumping and weight training. The idea is to match ATP supply to ATP demand. Creatine exists mainly in two forms: creatine and creatine phosphate for the storage of energy in muscle. Within the muscle, 60–70% exists as creatine phosphate, which is unable to pass through biological membranes, and thus is osmotically active.

$$PCr^{2-} + ADP^{3-} + H^+ \leftrightarrow ATP^{4-} + Cr$$

Creatine kinase

Why would an athlete supplement his or her diet with creatine? For those whose athletic endeavors include the generation of explosive power, the more phosphocreatine (PCr) stored, the more power one might generate. From the ergogenic viewpoint, the resynthesis of PCr could be the critical factor during sustained, very-high-intensity exercise. Thus the rationale for its use is based on supplementation to increase resting levels of creatine phosphate and free creatine to increase the regeneration of ATP to *delay* fatigue, and thus improve athletic performance. Depletion of phosphocreatine, especially in fast type II muscle fibers, and subsequent declines in force production are thus delayed. Investigation has focused on activities that require short or repeated bouts of energy expenditure. In fact, several laboratory studies have shown small but statistically significant increases in cycle ergometer performance (13–16); however, no studies have shown the effectiveness of creatine supplementation in subjects less than 18 years old. Others have not been able to replicate such results.

Orally ingested creatine is completely absorbed intact from the gastrointestinal tract. It is delivered to the skeletal muscle for storage, where it can quickly rephosphorylate ADP to ATP (See above) to fuel muscular contraction and stimulate myosin heavy-chain (protein) synthesis. The daily requirement is approximately 2 g/day for a 70 kg person. Approximately half comes from in vivo production and the other half from dietary sources. The most popular supplements are administered as a loading dose of 20–25 g for 2–5 days, followed by 2–5 g/day as maintenance. The more that is ingested, the less is synthesized.

Which teenaged athletes take creatine supplements and why do they take them? Metzl and colleagues surveyed a group of high school athletes and found that slightly fewer than 6% (but many more among 11th and 12th grade students) admitted taking creatine supplements (16). Boys were almost five times more likely than girls to supplement with creatine and the older athletes more likely than the younger athletes. Use was significantly more likely among strength-dependent athletes, for example, football players, wrestlers, ice hockey players, and lacrosse players. The surveys indicated that those who took the supplement expected enhanced athletic performance (~75%), improved appearance (~60%: a not inconsequential reason for adolescents to take many types of supplements even among nonathletes), improved endurance (~45%), and improved speed (~40%). Ray and colleagues have also recently reported similar results (17).

Because these supplements are not necessarily made under "Good Manufacturing Practices" as our prescription drugs are, one is not assured of the potency of the product nor what other chemicals might be contained in the product. The FDA does not necessarily test these products. Most of the creatine is excreted in the urine; however, as an osmotically active substance it draws in water leading to several of its side effects: weight gain, edema, and muscle cramps. Gastrointestinal (GI) cramps are also common. In fact it is the cramping in muscle and in the GI tract that has limited its use.

VI. ANABOLIC STEROIDS

Anabolic steroids are used to increase lean tissue mass and to reduce body fat. In addition to enhanced athletic performance, athletes claim that supplementation with these compounds increases strength and weight as well as aggressiveness to permit longer and more intense workouts. Anabolic effects of androgens occur in the nonreproductive tissues and include an increase in muscle mass; acceleration of bone growth before epiphyseal closure in the adolescent; increase in bone density; stimulation of red blood cell production, as noted by increases in the circulating hemoglobin level and hematocrit; laryngeal enlargement and vocal cord thickening; and decrease in body fat (18). Androgenic effects are those that reflect the development of the primary sexual characteristics: changes in genital size and function, spermatogenesis, and sexual hair. Of some interest as well are the anticatabolic effects (19), perhaps acting by blocking the glucocorticoid receptor that might permit more rapid recovery from previous training or more intensive training sessions. There are at least two well-controlled clinical trials that show unequivocal efficacy of moderately increased levels of testosterone (20,21).

The rationale for using anabolic, androgenic steroids includes the following (22):

The clear differential in athletic performance between men and women depends in the main on differences in body composition; on average, the lean body mass is 30% greater in men.

The obvious anabolic effects resulting from the physiological increases in testosterone during male pubertal development.

The production of undoubted anabolic and ergogenic effects by physiological dosages of testosterone in hypogonadal men.

The assumption that use of supraphysiological dosages of testosterone or more potent synthetic analogs would increase muscle bulk and improve athletic performance in *eugonadal* adult men.

The assumption that anabolic effects can be separated from the virilizing effect by use of *pure anabolic* agents.

The rationale may be correct, but the assumptions have in the main yet to be realized, because only one androgen receptor has been identified. I shall not consider the injectable anabolic steroids since these are really not dietary supplements. I shall consider both dehydroepiandrosterone and androstenedione below, because they are both widely available and used, as is creatine, by adolescent athletes.

VII. DEHYDROEPIANDROSTERONE

Dehydroepiandrosterone (DHEA) and its sulfate (DHEAS) are the most abundant circulating steroid hormones, with daily secretory rates of almost 30 mg/day in the adult. In addition they are precursors to both androgens and estrogens. The circulating levels change remarkably over the normal life span: in the fetus these steroids are precursors for placental estrogens. The levels then decline until midchildhood when they begin to slowly rise during a process called *adrenarche*, which may be heralded by the appearance of pubic hair, hence an often-used synonym: *pubarche*. This small rise is followed by a continued rise to a peak in the young adult. After that, the levels decline steadily to 20–25% of the maximum. This natural decline has become a target of nutritional supplementation: that is, to the suggestion that DHEA might attenuate or reverse some of the effects of aging. The aim of this supplementation is to again raise the levels of circulating DHEA to those of the young adult.

For adolescents the goal must be quite different, since it is during this period that DHEA and DHEAS levels are close to their highest. The aim must be to increase the levels of the more anabolic steroids, since the potency of DHEA is weak as an androgen (23). Despite being banned as a pharmaceutical by the FDA in 1996, DHEA has been resurrected as a nutritional supplement (so-called nutriceutical). In young men neither single doses of DHEA (50 mg) nor 150 mg/day during an 8 week resistance training protocol raised testosterone or free testosterone levels (24). Levels of DHEA and androstenedione were raised as a positive control for drug absorption. The levels of gonadotropins did not decrease as they would were a sufficiently potent anabolic steroid administered (for example, testosterone). The levels of testosterone and its free fraction also did not change. Thus, there were no discernable effects on the hypothalamic–pituitary–gonadal axis from these amounts of DHEA.

Common side effects of potent anabolic steroid administration include liver enzyme elevations and a dysli-

pidemia characterized by an increase in low-density lipoprotein (LDL)-cholesterol and a decrease, often marked, in high-density lipoprotein (HDL)-cholesterol. No alterations in the lipid profile or hepatic enzyme profile of the subjects were found. All subjects increased the amount of weight lifted, but there was no difference between those who ingested DHEA and those receiving placebo. The muscle fiber cross-sectional area of the type II fibers increased with resistance training, but there were no differences between the groups of subjects receiving DHEA and placebo. These data in young males (although not adolescents) make it unlikely that the usual amounts of DHEA supplementation will have an anabolic effect that will lead to increases in athletic performance above those gained by diligent training and a proper diet.

DHEA may have a role in patients with adrenal insufficiency, because the usual replacement therapy with glucocorticoids and mineralocorticoids does not address the issue of decreased adrenal androgens. Arlt and colleagues made a strong case for DHEA replacement therapy in women with adrenal insufficiency (25).

VIII. ANDROSTENEDIONE

Androstenedione is an anabolic steroid that is a precursor to both testosterone and estradiol. It is itself a weak androgen and poorly converted to more potent androgens; however, because of the hype engendered following its use by Mark McGwire during his spectacular season of hitting home runs for the St. Louis Cardinals, it received much undeserved press from which the manufacturers reaped an extraordinary financial benefit. Several well-done studies (See below) have been unable to find credible evidence for an anabolic effect.

Oral androstenedione administered at 100 or 300 mg/day to 20–40-year-old or 30–56-year-old men raised androstenedione concentrations in all. A total of 97 subjects were enrolled in two separate studies (26,27). The intersubject variability was remarkably high. Although there was no increase in total testosterone concentration in the older men, there were increases in free testosterone and estradiol levels. There was a 30% increase in total testosterone level in the younger men; however, this rise was accompanied by a 150% rise in circulating estradiol levels. When conjugated steroid hormone levels were assessed, the increases in excretion rates of these steroid hormone metabolites increased markedly (far out of proportion to the circulating levels of testosterone) as did circulating levels of testosterone *glucuronide* (28). Despite these changes in circulating steroid hormone levels, there were no changes in gonadotropin levels, indicating a minimal, if any, effect on the hypothalamic–pituitary–gonadal axis. Thus the ingested steroid is largely metabolized to its glucuronide conjugate and other metabolites before it is released into the general circulation. In an additional well-controlled study, the ingestion of androstenedione did not stimulate muscle protein anabolism across the thigh muscles in young healthy men (29). In contrast to studies with DHEA, the levels of HDL cholesterol declined slightly in the older men.

There have been no credible studies in adolescent athletes nor do I think that one could ethically be done. The overwhelming preponderance of the evidence in younger and older adults does not indicate a salutary effect on strength or athletic performance. On the other hand, many athletes are taking androstenedione at unknown dosages and a product of unknown purity and with many other "chemical" preparations. However, some of the impurities may be on the banned list, as was found for a nandrolone metabolite contaminating an over-the-counter preparation of androstenedione (30). I suspect that no major harm is being done to the adolescent except for the cost of the product (and the resulting expensive urine), while the producers are making large profits.

IX. GROWTH HORMONE AND INSULIN-LIKE GROWTH FACTOR 1

Growth-hormone-deficient subjects are weaker and their body composition has a higher percentage of fat than normals of the same body mass index. Therapy with growth hormone (GH) increases strength and lean body mass. All of these are desired effects in athletes. Growth hormone is also likely to promote the anabolic state. Whether GH will have these effects in highly trained athletes who already have a larger lean body mass, increased strength, and little adipose tissue remains an open question. There are no comprehensive studies of highly trained athletes receiving GH supplementation. Growth hormone certainly has been used in otherwise normal individuals, including some with constitutional delay of growth and adolescence, with obvious additional benefit over and above that of puberty itself. Growth hormone is expensive (perhaps $2,000–$5,000 per month, depending on the dose) and many counterfeit products exist.

Another approach to increasing circulatory GH levels is to use GH secretagogues: compounds that *transiently* raise GH levels by a direct action on the pituitary or indirectly via stimulating GH-releasing hormone or inhibiting somatostatin. These include the drugs levodopa, clonidine, and perhaps glucagons and vasopressin. More to the point of supplementation would be the use of the amino acids arginine, ornithine, lysine, and tryptophan. Under controlled conditions (often very high dosages given intravenously), these amino acids have the capacity to release a large pulse of GH acutely. However, because of an absolute and then a relative refractory period for the next (spontaneous) GH pulse, it is unlikely that the overall GH secretory rate is increased for the full 24 h. The feedback loops conspire to downregulate endogenous GH release to compensate for the large additional, pharmacologically induced, GH spike.

Although insulin-like growth factor 1 (IGF-1) theoretically might deliver what the athlete desires, that is, an anabolic but nonandrogenic activity, there are two major impediments to its widespread use: hypoglycemia from large bolus injections and availability (and cost). There simply is not a large enough supply of the peptide available and what is touted to be rhIGF-1 may be counterfeit. There are no studies of IGF-1 to show an effect on athletic performance or on strength, aerobic capacity, body composition, or bone mass in athletes. Theoretically, IGF-1 ought to be anabolic in adolescents, but does it cause more than the natural changes surrounding peak height velocity?

X. CONCLUSIONS

Supplementation (doping) in an attempt to increase athletic performance has been used for centuries: potions, caffeine, adrenergics, strychnine, amphetamines, anabolic steroids, and peptides related to the growth hormone–IGF axis have been used. Irrespective of the choice of the class of the compound or specific agent, the science usually greatly trails the hype and agents' subsequent use. Some, in fact are proven effective, for example, testosterone (20,21), but the majority of supplements have not been shown to increase anything, let alone athletic performance.

The use of drugs to enhance athletic performance is on the rise as more products become available not only to aid performance but also to avoid detection in those venues where drug testing is performed. One will note that the issues of fairness, ethics, addiction, and the roles of the enablers—coaches, trainers, and the medical community—have not been considered in this chapter. These issues as a group are critical challenges to sport in general, but are of even greater import as they apply to the adolescent athlete whose growth, body composition, and sexual development is not only incomplete but also at a critical stage. Psychosocial development is also at a vulnerable state as the adolescent is trying to become an adult with a set of moral and ethical values. What lifetime messages do we transmit by condoning these behaviors?

REFERENCES

1. Bucci LR. Selected herbals and human exercise performance. Am J Clin Nutr 2000; 72(suppl):624S–636S.
2. Sidney KH, Lefcoe NM. The effects of ephedrine on the physiological and psychological responses to submaximal and maximal exercise in man. Med Sci Sports Exerc 1977; 9:95–99.
3. Gillies H, Derman WE, Noakes TD, et al. Pseudoephedrine is without ergogenic effects during prolonged exercise. J Appl Physiol 1996; 81:2611–2617.
4. Bell DG, Jacobs I, Zamecnik J. Effects of caffeine, ephedrine and their combination on time to exhaustion during high-intensity exercise. Eur J Appl Physiol 1998; 77:427–433.

5. Haller CA, Benowitz NL. Adverse cardiovascular and central nervous system events associated with dietary supplements containing ephedra alkaloids. N Engl J Med 2000; 343:1833–1838.

6. Gurley BJ, Gardner SF, Hubbard MA. Content versus label claims in ephedra-containing dietary supplements. Am J Health Syst Pharm 2000; 15:963–969.

7. McNaughton L, Egan G, Caelli G. A comparison of Chinese and Russian ginseng as ergogenic aids to improve various facets of physical fitness. Int Clin Nutr Rev 1989; 90:32–35.

8. Benzi G, Ceci A. Creatine as nutritional supplementation and medicinal product. J Sport Med Phys Fitness 2001; 41:1–10.

9. Feldman EB. Creatine: a dietary supplement and ergogenic aid. Nutr Rev 1999; 57:45–50.

10. Juhn MS, Tarnopolsky M. Oral creatine supplementation and athletic performance: a critical review. Clin J Sports Med 1998; 8:286–297.

11. Williams MH, Kreider RB, Branch JD. Creatine: The Power Supplement. Champaign, IL: Human Kinetics, 1999.

12. Kraemer WJ, Volek JS. Creatine supplementation: its role in human performance. Clin Sports Med 1999; 18:651–666.

13. Jacobs I, Bleue S, Goodman J. Creatine ingestion increases anaerobic capacity and maximal accumulate oxygen deficit. Can J Appl Physiol 1997; 22:231–243.

14. Prevost MC, Nelson AG, Morris GS. Creatine supplementation enhances intermittent work performance. Res Q Exerc Sport 1997; 68:233–240.

15. Smith JC, Stephens DP, Hall EL, et al. Effect of oral creatine ingestion of parameters of the work rat-time relationship and time to exhaustion in high-intensity cycling. Eur J Appl Physiol 1998; 77:360–365.

16. Metzl JD, Small E, Levine SR, Gershel JC. Creatine use among young athletes. Pediatrics 2001; 108:421–425.

17. Ray TR, Eck JC, Covington LA, et al. Use of oral creatine as an ergogenic aid for increased sports performance: perceptions of adolescent athletes. South Med J 2001; 94:608–612.

18. Rogol AD, Yesalis CE: Anabolic-androgenic steroids and athletes: What are the issues: J Clin Endocrinol Metab 1997; 74:465–469.

19. Haupt H. Anabolic steroids and growth hormone. Am J Sports Med 1999; 21:468–473.

20. Bhasin S, Storer TW, Berman N, et al. The effects of supraphysiological doses of testosterone on muscle size and strength in normal men. N Engl J Med 1996; 335:1–7.

21. Bhasin S, Woodhouse L, Casaburi R, et al. Testosterone dose–response relationships in healthy young men. Am J Physiol 2001; 281:E1172–E1181.

22. Wu FCW. Endocrine aspects of anabolic steroids. Clin Chem 1997; 43:1289–1292.

23. Baulieu EE. Dehydroepiandrosterone (DHEA): a fountain of youth? J Clin Endocrinol Metab 1996; 81:3147–3151.

24. Brown GA, Vukovich MD, Sharp RL, et al. Effect of oral DHEA on serum testosterone and adaptations to resistance training in young men. J Appl Physiol 1999; 87:2274–2283.

25. Arlt W, Callies F, van Vlijmen JC, et al. Dehydroepiandrosterone replacement in women with adrenal insufficiency. N Engl J Med 1999; 341:1013–1020.

26. Brown GA, Vukovich MD, Martini ER, et al. Endocrine responses to chronic androstenedione intake in 30- to 56-year old men. J Clin Endocrinol Metab 2000; 85:4074–4080.

27. Leder BZ, Longcope C, Catlin DH, et al. Oral androstenedione administration and serum testosterone concentrations in young men. JAMA 2000; 283:779–782.

28. Leder BZ, Catlin DH, Longcope C, et al. Metabolism of orally administered androstenedione in young men. J Clin Endocrinol Metab 2001; 86:3654–3658.

29. Rasmussen BB, Volpi E, Gore DC, Wolfe RR. Androstenedione does not stimulate muscle protein anabolism in young healthy men. J Clin Endocrinol Metab 2000; 85:55–59.

30. Catlin DH, Leder BZ, Ahrens B, et al. Trace contamination of over-the-counter androstenedione and positive urine test results for a nandrolone metabolite. JAMA 2000; 284:2618–2621.

40

Using the Web to Obtain Information on Genetic and Hormone Disorders

John A. Phillips III

Vanderbilt University School of Medicine and Meharry Medical College, Nashville, Tennessee, U.S.A.

I. INTRODUCTION

New findings on the genetic basis of endocrine disorders are reported at an ever-increasing rate in a growing variety of books, journals, and other periodicals. Unfortunately, access to this and other current information on clinical and laboratory findings of familial endocrine disorders, and who performs genetic tests, cannot be found in a single journal or text. Electronic databases are now providing medical professionals rapid access to the bulk of current information and data. These electronic databases can also be searched in an interactive way for conditions that cause symptoms and signs, to permit generation of differential diagnoses that will often include rare or recently discovered disorders that many endocrinologists probably have never encountered. Access to and use of these databases can enable all endocrinologists to more frequently diagnose cases and be aware of subtleties that differentiate alternative diagnoses. These are important reasons to use electronic databases. This chapter provides information on how to use the World Wide Web for information about genetic and hormone disorders.

A. Online Mendelian Inheritance in Man

Online Mendelian Inheritance in Man (1) (OMIM) is maintained by the National Center for Biotechnology Information (NCBI). It is available without charge at http://www.ncbi.nlm.nih.gov/Omim. It is updated daily. In March 2001, 12,379 entries were included. A wealth of information is contained about the history, signs, symptoms, diagnosis, management, and research findings in these 12,379 genes and genetic disorders, as are detailed gene and disease focused maps. Access through hyperlinks to a variety of Web sites is another important strength. These hyperlinks include MEDLINE, GenBank retrieval system, Human Gene Nomenclature Home Page,

Online Mendelian Inheritance in Animals, The Alliance of Genetic Support Groups, The Cardiff Human Gene Mutation Database, MitoMap (the Emory University mitochondrial genome database), and databases on genes that cause retinal diseases, and a variety of other locus-specific databases. The utility of these databases and their hyperlinks in clinical applications will be illustrated in this chapter.

B. Frequently Used Terms Related to the Web

Knowing the definitions of terms that will be helpful in using the World Wide Web (WWW) is a good first step in learning how to use Web.

E-mail: Abbreviation for electronic mail. The use of a network to send and receive messages.

HTML: Abbreviation for hypertext markup language, which enables authors to insert hyperlinks. Clicking on a hyperlink displays another HTML document. Therefore, in a hypertext system one can navigate by clicking hyperlinks, which produces a display of another document that also contains selected hyperlinks.

Http: The Internet standard supporting exchange of information on the WWW. Http enables the embedding of hyperlinks in Web documents. Http also defines the process by which a Web client uses a Web browser program to generate a request for information and send it to a Web server, which is a program designed to respond to Http requests and provide the desired information.

Hypertext: A computer text form that allows readers, by clicking on the hyperlink, to display another HTML document that may also contain hyperlinks to other related documents.

Internet: The worldwide system of linked computer networks that facilitates data communication services such as remote log on, file transfer, e-mail, the WWW, and news groups. The Internet assigns every connected computer a unique Internet address so that any two connected computers can locate each other on a network and exchange data.

Log on/log off: The processes of establishing/terminating a connection with a network or computer.

Netscape Communicator: A package including a popular Web browser called Netscape Navigator that is available for Microsoft Windows, Macintosh computers, and a variety of Unix workstations.

Online information service: America Online (AOL) is an example of a for-profit firm that makes current news, stock quotes, and other information available to subscribers over standard telephone lines.

Surfing the net: Exploring the WWW by following a series of hyperlinks of interest to the surfer.

URL: Abbreviation for uniform resource locator. On the WWW, URLs are a string of characters that precisely identifies an Internet's resource types and locations. The following fictitious URL identifies a WWW document (http://www.genetic.edu). http:// indicates the domain name of the computer on which it is stored; (www.genetic.edu), fully describes the document's location. In addresses, small letters (www and http) are used. In abbreviations not pertaining to addresses, capital letters may be used (WWW, Http, and HTTP).

Web (World Wide Web, WWW): A global hypertext system that uses the Internet-linked computer network to facilitate data communication.

Web browser: A program that runs on an Internet-connected computer and provides access to the WWW.

Web server: A program that accepts Http-formatted requests for information. The server processes these requests and sends the requested document to the connected computer requesting the information.

Web site: A set of related documents making up a hypertext presentation on the WWW. A Web site usually has a welcome or home page that serves as the initial document. By following instructions on the home page, one can select and gain access to the information and data included in the web site.

II. USING THE WEB TO OBTAIN INFORMATION FOR DYSMORPHIC PATIENTS

A newborn baby is suspected of having some form of dwarfism. Ventriculomegaly and short limbs, as detected by fetal ultrasound, were noted at 20 weeks gestation. Chromosome studies from amniocentesis revealed a 46, XY pattern without any abnormalities noted. The fetal head size at 30 weeks' gestation as noted on ultrasound was stated to be 35 weeks. The ventriculomegaly had resolved, and the limb lengths were those expected at 29 weeks. Physical examination detected macrocephaly, macroglossia, downward slanting palpebral fissures, cataracts, and syndactyly of the second and third fingers. Blood glucose was 28 mg/% (low).

The attending neonatologist believes that the baby "looks funny" and wants to know if you, the consulting physician, think the baby has a syndrome. He wants to know if the infant has this syndrome, how to confirm it, and what is the expected prognosis?

You, as the consulting physician, are unaware of this constellation of clinical findings and/or what syndrome might be present but must solve the problem. You decide to carry out a systematic search to obtain a list of possible syndromes that share the infant's signs and symptoms. To do this, the first step is to carry out a keyword search. Since the WWW might contain helpful information, you initiate a search beginning with the OMIM database. Using the computer in the nursery, you open Netscape Communicator, America Online, or any Web browser available on the computer, and type in the OMIM URL or address: http://www.ncbi.nlm.nih.gov/Omim. The OMIM homepage appears on the computer screen and you click on "Search the OMIM Database," and then enter "macrocephaly" as a search term and press the "enter" key. Ninety-nine disorders in OMIM have macrocephaly listed. This is too many items to consider, so you repeat the search using "cataract" as a finding, and 206 matching entries appear. This number of disorders is also too long, so you search using "syndactyly." Your third search produces 184 matching entries—again too many. You then decide to find out how many disorders have both macrocephaly and cataract by typing both macrocephaly and cataract, leaving a space between the two words (macrocephaly cataract) as a search string.

Only 11 entries are listed as having both of these findings (see Fig. 1). These are #109400 basal cell nevus syndrome (BCNS); *120140 collagen, type II, ALPHA-1; COL2A1, #30700 hydrocephalus due to congenital stenosis of aqueduct of Sylvius, HSAS1, HSAS, HYCX; #156550 Kniest dysplasia; #194050 Williams-Beuren syndrome, WBS; *#231675 glutaricaciduria IIC; *231680 glutaricaciduria IIA; *300005 methyl-CpG-binding protein 2, MECP2; #300279 mental retardation, X-linked, with progressive spasticity; #301050 Alport syndrome, X-linked, ATS; #312870 Simpson-Golabi-Behmel syndrome, type 1, SGBS1. Note that the entry numbers are in hypertext (color) on the screen. By clicking on any of these hypertext *numbers*, each corresponding entry is automatically opened. To narrow further the number of matches and focus your search, you add "syndactyly" and enter

OMIM Home	Search

Select Entries from OMIM --
Online Mendelian Inheritance in Man

11 entries found, searching for "macrocephaly cataract"

#109400 BASAL CELL NEVUS SYNDROME; BCNS
*120140 COLLAGEN, TYPE II, ALPHA-1; COL2A1
#307000 HYDROCEPHALUS DUE TO CONGENITAL STENOSIS OF AQUEDUCT
HSAS1; HSAS; HYCX
#156550 KNIEST DYSPLASIA
#194050 WILLIAMS-BEUREN SYNDROME; WBS
*231675 GLUTARICACIDURIA IIC
*231680 GLUTARICACIDURIA IIA
*300005 METHYL-CpG-BINDING PROTEIN 2; MECP2
#300279 MENTAL RETARDATION, X-LINKED, WITH PROGRESSIVE SPASTICITY
#301050 ALPORT SYNDROME, X-LINKED; ATS
#312870 SIMPSON-GOLABI-BEHMEL SYNDROME, TYPE 1; SGBS1

Figure 1 OMIM page shows results of search initiated using "macrocephaly cataract" as a search string.

"macrocephaly cataracts syndactyly" as a search string. Only one OMIM entry is listed for all three of these findings: #312870 Simpson-Golabi-Behmel syndrome, type 1; SGBS1.

You have done something remarkable. In less than 2 min, you have logged onto and searched a large electronic database of genetic and endocrine disorders to generate a successive series of progressively refined differential diagnoses. You open the single file (#312870 SGBS1) that matches your search criteria (macrocephaly cataracts syndactyly) by clicking your mouse on it, and the first of seven pages of information on SGBS1 appears on the screen for review (see Fig. 2). The clinical synopsis under Table of Contents or the complete text of this entry can then be reviewed. Note in Figure 2 that the Database Links below the Table of Contents provide immediate access to other databases, including MEDLINE. If you click on the MEDLINE database link, you will automatically see 28 publications on SGBS1. To see the abstract of any of these, you can click on the author's name in hypertext. To see all articles that, in turn, are related to each publication, you can click on "See Related Articles," which is also in hypertext. Using these hypertext links, you can obtain, select, and print the abstracts of any of the numerous articles that constitute the published knowledge about this disorder.

Since SGBS1 is a rare disorder that you may have not seen previously, you want to know if there are laboratories that can provide confirmatory tests. The GeneTests database available at http://www.genetests. org/servlet/access is a directory of laboratories that provide testing for genetic disorders (see list of selected Web sites below). After you register with GeneTests, you are given a password for professional users. Using this password, you can access and search the GeneTests database for Simpson-Golabi-Behmel syndrome to find labs that provide either clinical or research testing for this disorder. In a matter of a very few minutes, you have generated a working diagnosis (SGBS1); obtained information about the pathogenesis, mode of inheritance, and findings associated with SGBS1; and gained access to a lab that can help confirm the working diagnosis. Using this information that you obtained from the Web in just a few minutes, you feel much better prepared to talk with the neonatologist and the baby's parents who are waiting for your opinions.

III. HOW TO GENERATE A DIFFERENTIAL DIAGNOSIS FOR A FAMILY HAVING UNUSUAL ENDOCRINE PROBLEMS

A 15-month-old boy is referred to you by his pediatrician who suspects he has growth hormone deficiency. The child weighed 3.2 kg at full term following an uncomplicated pregnancy, labor, and vaginal delivery. His height SDS is now −3.2, and his length since 5 months has become progressively retarded. Your examination shows the child is proportionate and his height and weight are commensurate with each other. You note that his extremities appear normal in length, and you do not detect any kyphosis, limitation of joint motion, or dysmorphic features. His bone age is delayed greater than −2 SD. You see no skeletal abnormalities. The serum thyroxin level is abnormally low, but the levels of electrolytes, glucose, urea nitrogen, bicarbonate and anion gap, calcium, phos-

| OMIM Home | Search | Comments |

#312870 SIMPSON-GOLABI-BEHMEL SYNDROME, TYPE 1; SGBS1

Alternative titles; symbols

SGBS
BULLDOG SYNDROME
DYSPLASIA GIGANTISM SYNDROME, X-LINKED; DGSX
GOLABI-ROSEN SYNDROME
SIMPSON DYSMORPHIA SYNDROME; SDYS

TABLE OF CONTENTS

- TEXT
- REFERENCES
- CONTRIBUTORS
- CREATION DATE
- EDIT HISTORY
- CLINICAL SYNOPSIS

Database Links

| MEDLINE | Protein | DNA | Genome | LocusLink | Gene Map | Coriell | Nomenclature |

Gene Map Locus: Xq26

Note: pressing the 🔦 symbol will find the citations in MEDLINE whose text most closely matches the text of the preceding OMIM paragraph, using the Entrez MEDLINE neighboring function.

TEXT

A number sign (#) is used with this entry because of evidence that some cases of the Simpson-Golabi-Behmel overgrowth syndrome are caused by mutation in the gene for glypican-3 (300037), which maps to Xq26. A second SGBS locus (SGBS2; 300209), located on Xp22, was identified by gene mapping (Brzustowicz et al., 1999). 🔦

In 2 males, sons of sisters, Simpson et al. (1975) observed a 'new' dysmorphism with the following features: broad stocky appearance, distinctive facies (large protruding jaw, widened nasal bridge, upturned nasal tip), enlarged tongue, and broad, short hands and fingers. Intelligence was normal. The family referred to the appearance as 'bulldog'-like. In infancy hypothyroidism was suggested, but this was excluded by laboratory tests. Close linkage with the Xg blood group locus was excluded. Kaariainen (1981) told me of a tall (192 cm) 40-year-old man with operated pectus excavatum, ventricular septal defect, central cleft of the lower lip, peculiar cup-shaped ears with knobbiness and nodularity, short clubbed terminal phalanges, low-pitched voice, and cataracts developing at age 35. The parents, who came from different parts of Finland, were 170 and 160 cm tall. A brother, height 180 cm, died at age 18 years of ventricular septal defect and pulmonary hypertension. He looked like the surviving brother and quite different from other members of the family. Kaariainen (1982) concluded that the disorder is the

Figure 2 OMIM page shows first of seven pages of information on Simpson dysmorphia syndrome. Note Database Links below Table of Contents that provide immediate access to other databases, including MEDLINE.

phorus, and urine pH are all within normal limits. A 16-year-old full sister reportedly had "panhypopituitarism" and she "didn't go through puberty." She was treated with "growth hormone, thyroid hormone and other shots to make her grow and go through puberty." The results of previous endocrine blood tests on the 15-month-old show low serum levels of gonadotropins and thyroxin. Combined pituitary hormone deficiency is a logical diagnosis for the 15 month old, since there is failure of response to growth-hormone-releasing hormone (GHRH), thyroid-releasing hormone (TRH), and leuteinizing-hormone-releasing hormone (LHRH), and the magnetic resonance imaging (MRI) study reveals a hypocellular pituitary. This working diagnosis also fits with the information known about his 16-year-old sister.

You decide to perform a keyword search to produce a differential diagnosis. To utilize the WWW to obtain information on familial hormone deficiencies, you carry out this search of the OMIM database. To do this, you log onto the OMIM Home Page by entering the URL: http://www.ncbi.nlm.nih.gov/Omim. You then click on "Search the OMIM Database" with the mouse and enter "gh" as a search term. Using gh as the search term gives 49 hits (see Fig. 3). If you search using both gh and thyroid (gh thyroid), only 11 disorders appear on the screen (see Fig. 4). Finally, if you add gonadotropin to your keyword search (gh thyroid gonadotropin) only three OMIM entries match: *173110 POU domain, class 1, transcription factor 1; POU1F1; #262600 pituitary dwarfism III; *601538 PROPHET OF PIT1, paired-like homeodomain transcription factor; PROP1 (see Fig. 5).

The first entry (*173110 POU domain, class 1, transcription factor 1; POU1F1) contains information about the PIT1 transcription factor and includes the following interesting paragraph under Clinical Features

"Mutations of the POU1F1 gene in the human and Pit1 in the mouse are responsible for pleiotropic deficiencies of growth hormone, prolactin, and thyroid-stimulating hormone, while the production of adrenocorticotrophic hormone, luteinizing hormone (LH; 152780), and follicle-stimulating hormone (FSH; 136530) are preserved. On the other hand, patients with combined pituitary hormone deficiency due to homozygosity or compound heterozygosity for inactivating mutations of PROP1 (601538) cannot produce LH and FSH at a sufficient level and do not enter puberty spontaneously (Wu et al., 1998)."

This latter entry sounds like a very good match to the signs and symptoms of your patient.

The second entry (#262600 pituitary dwarfism III) also contains interesting information in its first paragraph

Many patients classified as exhibiting panhypopituitarism probably have combined pituitary hormone deficiency with sparing of adrenocorticotro-

pin. Mutations causing combined pituitary hormone deficiency have been described in the PIT1 (173110), PROP1 (601538), HESX1 (601802), and LHX3 (600577) genes. In addition to manifestations of the deficiency of pituitary hormones, the LHX3 mutations are associated with rigid cervical spine, and the HESX1 is associated with septooptic dysplasia (182230).

The third entry (*601538 PROPHET OF PIT1, paired-like homeodomain transcription factor; PROP1) includes, as its first paragraph,

PROP1 has both DNA-binding and transcriptional activation ability. Its expression leads to ontogenesis of pituitary gonadotropes, as well as somatotropes, lactotropes, and caudomedial thyrotropes. Inactivating mutations of PROP1 which have an autosomal recessive mode of inheritance, cause deficiencies of luteinizing hormone (LH; 152780), follicle-stimulating hormone (FSH; 136530), growth hormone (GH; 139250), prolactin (PRL; 176760), and thyroid-stimulating hormone (TSH; 188540).

This entry sounds like the best match for the signs and symptoms of your patient.

Since this case fits the findings reported for PROP1 mutations, you decide to review the 1998 article by Wu et al. On the Web, you can obtain a copy of the abstract of this paper by clicking the mouse on either of the following: Wu et al., 1998 hypertext at the end of the paragraph cited above; or Wu et al., 1998 hypertext in either the PIT1 (173110) or PROP1 (601538) entries. Then click on the PubMed ID (9462743) that follows the reference that appears. You will then see the abstract of the reference on your screen and you can print it. Since this is a PubMed document, you can also save it as a file on your computer as shown at the bottom of the page, or you can order a complete copy through Lonesome Doc as shown at the top. You can also obtain copies of articles by clicking on MEDLINE under "Database Links" that are just below the Table of Contents of each entry (see Fig. 2). If you do a PubMed search for "gh thyroid gonadotropin familial" you will immediately find 16 related articles, of which two of the first three contain information that you may find helpful in your further evaluation and treatment of your new patient (see Fig. 6). As in the first case, you can carry out a GeneTests search to find a lab that can carry out molecular analysis of the PROP1 gene (see GeneTests in the list of selected Web sites below).

Now you have a working diagnosis (PROP1 defects), information on the pathogenesis, mode of inheritance, the findings associated with the disorder, and a way to find a lab that could be used to help confirm your working diagnosis. Obviously, with this information in hand you feel better prepared to talk with your patient's parents and answer their questions.

| OMIM Home | Search |

Select Entries from OMIM --
Online Mendelian Inheritance in Man

49 entries found, searching for "gh"

*139250 GROWTH HORMONE 1; GH1
*600946 GROWTH HORMONE RECEPTOR; GHR
#262500 PITUITARY DWARFISM II
*150200 CHORIONIC SOMATOMAMMOTROPIN HORMONE 1; CSH1
245590 LARON SYNDROME, TYPE II
*139191 GROWTH HORMONE-RELEASING HORMONE RECEPTOR; GHRHR
*102200 ACROMEGALY
*139190 GROWTH HORMONE-RELEASING HORMONE; GHRH
*601538 PROPHET OF PIT1, PAIRED-LIKE HOMEODOMAIN TRANSCRIPTION FACTOR; PROP1
#262400 PITUITARY DWARFISM I
*173110 POU DOMAIN, CLASS 1, TRANSCRIPTION FACTOR 1; POU1F1
*603515 CHORIONIC SOMATOMAMMOTROPIN HORMONE-LIKE 1; CSHL1
#173100 PITUITARY DWARFISM DUE TO ISOLATED GROWTH HORMONE DEFICIENCY, AUTOSOMAL DOMINANT
#262600 PITUITARY DWARFISM III
*307800 HYPOPHOSPHATEMIA, X-LINKED
*139320 GUANINE NUCLEOTIDE-BINDING PROTEIN, ALPHA-STIMULATING ACTIVITY POLYPEPTIDE 1; GNAS1
*176761 PROLACTIN RECEPTOR; PRLR
*605353 GHRELIN
*147440 INSULIN-LIKE GROWTH FACTOR I; IGF1
*118820 CHORIONIC SOMATOMAMMOTROPIN HORMONE 2; CSH2
#170500 HYPERKALEMIC PERIODIC PARALYSIS; HYPP
#246200 LEPRECHAUNISM
#262650 PITUITARY DWARFISM IV
*603967 SODIUM CHANNEL, VOLTAGE-GATED, TYPE IV, ALPHA SUBUNIT; SCN4A
*601898 GROWTH HORMONE SECRETAGOGUE RECEPTOR; GHSR
*601663 ESTROGEN RECEPTOR 2; ESR2
*312000 PANHYPOPITUITARISM; PHP
*188545 THYROTROPIN-RELEASING HORMONE RECEPTOR; TRHR
*176640 PRION PROTEIN; PRNP
*147620 INTERLEUKIN 6; IL6
*146732 INSULIN-LIKE GROWTH FACTOR-BINDING PROTEIN 3; IGFBP3
*141900 HEMOGLOBIN--BETA LOCUS; HBB
*133430 ESTROGEN RECEPTOR 1; ESR1
*192340 ARGININE VASOPRESSIN; AVP
#100800 ACHONDROPLASIA; ACH
#602579 CONGENITAL DISORDER OF GLYCOSYLATION, TYPE Ib
*600577 LIM HOMEO BOX GENE 3; LHX3
*600239 G PROTEIN-COUPLED RECEPTOR 1; GPR1

Figure 3 OMIM page shows results of search initiated using "gh" as a keyword.

```
┌─────────────┐┌──────────┐
│ OMIM Home   ││  Search  │
└─────────────┘└──────────┘
```

Select Entries from OMIM --
Online Mendelian Inheritance in Man

11 entries found, searching for "gh thyroid"

---

*139250 GROWTH HORMONE 1; GH1
*173110 POU DOMAIN, CLASS 1, TRANSCRIPTION FACTOR 1; POU1F1
#262500 PITUITARY DWARFISM II
*601538 PROPHET OF PIT1, PAIRED-LIKE HOMEODOMAIN TRANSCRIPTION FACTOR;
PROP1
*139320 GUANINE NUCLEOTIDE-BINDING PROTEIN, ALPHA-STIMULATING ACTIVITY
POLYPEPTIDE 1; GNAS1
#118450 ALAGILLE SYNDROME; AGS
#262600 PITUITARY DWARFISM III
*133430 ESTROGEN RECEPTOR 1; ESR1
*188545 THYROTROPIN-RELEASING HORMONE RECEPTOR; TRHR
*600239 G PROTEIN-COUPLED RECEPTOR 1; GPR1
*602663 PREPROPROLACTIN-RELEASING PEPTIDE

Figure 4 OMIM page shows results of search done using "gh thyroid" as a search string.

IV. HOW TO OBTAIN INFORMATION ON A CASE OF ENDOCRINE NEOPLASIA

You are asked to see a 42-year-old woman who has a widely metastatic pheochromocytoma. Her history shows that her father was diagnosed with medullary carcinoma of the thyroid at 20 years of age. His thyroidectomy was complicated by severe hypertension, which led to the discovery of his also having had a pheochromocytoma. You perform a keyword search to produce a differential diagnosis. You carry out this search of the OMIM database using the terms "medullary carcinoma thyroid pheochromocytoma" and obtain nine matching entries (see Fig. 7).

The first matching entry (#171400 multiple endocrine neoplsia, type II; MEN2) contains the following information in its introduction:

> A number sign (#) is used with this entry because of evidence indicating that MEN2A results from mutation in the RET oncogene (164761). Multiple endocrine neoplasia, type IIA, is an autosomal dominant syndrome of multiple endocrine neoplasms, including medullary thyroid carcinoma, pheochromocytoma, and parathyroid adenomas.

This suggests that you should consider MEN2, which is caused by mutations in the RET gene.

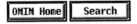

```
┌─────────────┐┌──────────┐
│ OMIM Home   ││  Search  │
└─────────────┘└──────────┘
```

Select Entries from OMIM --
Online Mendelian Inheritance in Man

3 entries found, searching for "gh thyroid gonadotropin"

---

*173110 POU DOMAIN, CLASS 1, TRANSCRIPTION FACTOR 1; POU1F1
#262600 PITUITARY DWARFISM III
*601538 PROPHET OF PIT1, PAIRED-LIKE HOMEODOMAIN TRANSCRIPTION FACTOR;
PROP1

Figure 5 OMIM page shows results of search initiated using "gh thyroid gonadotropin" as a search string.

| NCBI *PubMed* | **PubMed QUERY** | PubMed ? |

| Details | gh thyroid gonadotropin familial | Search | Clear |

Click here to enter the new PubMed System

Docs Per Page: 20 ▼ Entrez Date limit: No Limit ▼

16 citations found

| Display | Abstract report ▼ | for the articles selected (default all).

| Order | documents on this page through Loansome Doc

☐ Rosenbloom AL, et al.   [See Related Articles]
Clinical and biochemical phenotype of familial anterior hypopituitarism from mutation of the PROP1 gene.
J Clin Endocrinol Metab. 1999 Jan;84(1):50-7.
PMID: 9920061; UI: 99116789.

☐ Fofanova OV, et al.   [See Related Articles]
Rarity of PIT1 involvement in children from Russia with combined pituitary hormone deficiency.
Am J Med Genet. 1998 Jun 5;77(5):360-5. Review.
PMID: 9632165; UI: 98293954.

☐ Wu W, et al.   [See Related Articles]
Mutations in PROP1 cause familial combined pituitary hormone deficiency.
Nat Genet. 1998 Feb;18(2):147-9.
PMID: 9462743; UI: 98122575.

☐ Irie Y, et al.   [See Related Articles]
Screening for PIT1 abnormality by PCR direct sequencing method.
Thyroid. 1995 Jun;5(3):207-11.
PMID: 7580269; UI: 96082752.

☐ Terao S, et al.   [See Related Articles]
[Disturbance of hypothalamic-pituitary hormone secretion in familial chorea-acanthocytosis].
No To Shinkei. 1995 Jan;47(1):57-61. Japanese.
PMID: 7669403; UI: 95399007.

☐ Yagi H, et al.   [See Related Articles]
Familial congenital hypopituitarism with central diabetes insipidus.
J Clin Endocrinol Metab. 1994 Apr;78(4):884-9.
PMID: 8157716; UI: 94209376.

☐ Links TP, et al.   [See Related Articles]
Growth hormone-, alpha-subunit and thyrotrophin-cosecreting pituitary adenoma in familial setting of pituitary tumour.
Acta Endocrinol (Copenh). 1993 Dec;129(6):516-8.
PMID: 8109184; UI: 94152205.

Figure 6 PubMed page shows results of search done using "gh thyroid gonadotropin familial" as a search string.

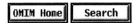

Select Entries from OMIM --
Online Mendelian Inheritance in Man

9 entries found, searching for "medullary carcinoma thyroid pheochromocytoma"

[#171400](#) MULTIPLE ENDOCRINE NEOPLASIA, TYPE II; MEN2
[*164761](#) RET PROTOONCOGENE; RET
[#155240](#) MEDULLARY THYROID CARCINOMA, FAMILIAL; MTC
[#171300](#) PHEOCHROMOCYTOMA
[#162300](#) MULTIPLE ENDOCRINE NEOPLASIA, TYPE IIB; MEN2B
[*256700](#) NEUROBLASTOMA
[*118910](#) CHROMOGRANIN A; CHGA
[219080](#) CUSHING DISEASE, ADRENAL
[#142623](#) HIRSCHSPRUNG DISEASE

Figure 7 OMIM page shows results of search initiated using "medullary carcinoma thyroid pheochromocytoma" as a search string.

The second matching entry (*164761 RET protoon-cogene; RET) begins with the following information:

Mutations in the RET gene are associated with the disorders multiple endocrine neoplasia, type IIA (MEN2A; 171400), multiple endocrine neoplasia, type IIB (MEN2B; 162300), Hirschsprung disease (HSCR; aganglionic megacolon; 142623), and medullary thyroid carcinoma (MTC; 155240).

Since a RET gene mutation seems likely, before you see your patient you want to know if there are laboratories that can provide confirmatory tests. To get this information you access and search the GeneTests database for MEN2 and find the addresses, phone, and fax numbers of several labs that provide testing for this disorder. This testing involves sequencing of exons 10, 11, 13, 14, and 16 of the RET proto-oncogene, which include the sites of common mutations that cause MEN2. In a matter of a very few minutes, you have generated a working diagnosis (MEN2); obtained information concerning the pathogenesis, mode of inheritance, and the findings associated with MEN2; and gained access to a lab that can help confirm your working diagnosis. Having this information you feel much better prepared to talk with your new patient to address her questions about the risk of her children having a genetic predisposition to medullary thyroid carcinoma or pheochromocytoma. If she is found to have an identifiable RET mutation, testing of her children would be possible. If they test positive, prophylactic resection of their thyroids could be offered as well as frequent screening for pheochromocytomas.

V. SELECTED WEB SITES ON GROWTH AND HORMONE DISORDERS

American Diabetes Association (http://www.diabetes.org). For professionals as well as lay individuals. http://www.childrenwithdiabetes.com/index_cwd.htm is the online community for kids, families, and adults.

Chromosomal Variation in Man (http://www.wiley.com/products/subject/life/borgaonkar/access.html). A catalog of chromosomal variants and anomalies that includes citations on all common and rare chromosomal alterations, phenotypes, and abnormalities in humans. The database is organized by variations and anomalies, numerical anomalies, and chromosomal breakage syndromes.

Cytogenetic resources (http://www.kumc.edu/gec/geneinfo.html). Database of normal and abnormal karyotypes, empirical risks for chromosome abnormalities, and maps of genes on chromosomes.

Dysmorphic Human-Mouse Homology database (DHMHD) (http://www.hgmp.mrc.ac.uk/DHMHD/dysmorph.html). Searchable database of phenotypic features that generates differential diagnoses of syndromes, and genetic and cytogenetic disorders.

Endocrine Society (http://www.endo-society.org/). Information on the Endocrine Society, fellow societies, organizations, and patient education groups as well as resources for scientists and physicians.

GeneMap'99 (http://www.ncbi.nlm.nih.gov/genemap/). Includes the locations of more than 30,000 genes and provides an early glimpse of some of the most important pieces of the genome.

GeneTests (http://www.genetests.org/servlet/access). Contains a medical genetics laboratory directory, genetics clinic directory, and disease information through companion site (GeneClinics).

Genetic Alliance (http://www.geneticalliance.org). Disease information as well as genetic support groups to voice the common concerns of children, adults, and families living with, and at risk for, genetic conditions.

Genetic Conditions/Rare Conditions Support Groups and Information Page (http://www.kumc.edu/gec/support). For professionals, educators, and individuals seeking information on genetic disorders, birth defects, and chromosomal disorders

Genetics Education Center (http://www.kumc.edu/gec/geneinfo.html). Contains information on genetic conditions; clinical genetics resources; clinical genetic centers, departments, and clinics; genetics education center; genetic courses, lectures, and educational materials; ethical, legal, and social implications of the human genome project; genetic computer resources.

Glossary of Genetic Terms (http://www.kumc.edu/gec/glossary.html). Contains a variety of sites that define and illustrate genetic terms useful to clinicians, educators, and the lay public.

Human Genome Project Information (http://www.ornl.gov/hgmis/). Contains information and educational materials on the Human Genome Project, including pertinence to clinical medicine and ethical, legal, and social issues.

Human Growth Foundation (http://www.hgfound.org/). A lay organization established for parents and friends of children with various growth disturbances including overgrowth, growth hormone deficiency, Turner syndrome, and others.

Information for Genetic Professionals (http://www.kumc.edu/gec/geneinfo.html). Contains information on cancer, cytogenetics, genetics, hyperlipidemia, neurogenetics, single-gene disorders, support groups, and genetic tests.

International Society for Pediatric and Adolescent Diabetes (http://www.ispad.org). News, membership roster, meeting dates.

Lawson Wilkins Pediatric Endocrine Society (http://lwpes.org). News, job listings.

Magic Foundation (http://www.magicfoundation.org). A lay organization established for parents and friends of children with various growth disturbances including overgrowth, growth hormone deficiency, Turner syndrome, and others.

March of Dimes (http://modimes.org). Information on birth defects for professionals and families.

MEDLINE PubMed (http://www.ncbi.nlm.nih.gov). Provides access to a cornucopia of scientific and medical publications in a searchable format. It is available on the Web site of National Center for Biotechnology Information.

National Association for Rare Disorders (NORD) (http://www.NORD-rdb.com/~orphan). Database of rare disorders includes symptoms, causes, diagnostic tests, and treatment for families and professionals.

National Human Genome Research Institute (NHGRI) (http://www.nhgri.nih.gov/). Contains information on the Human Genome Project and ethical, legal, and social implications.

NCBI Education (http://www.ncbi.nlm.nih.gov/Education/index.html). Contains PubMed and other tutorials.

NCBI Site Map (http://www.ncbi.nlm.nih.gov/Sitemap/index.html). Contains over 60 links to databases including genes and diseases, gene maps, mutation databases, OMIM PubMed, and educational sites.

Neurofibromatosis Homepage (http://nf.org). Contains information about neurofibromatosis and contacts for related resources.

OMIM (http://www.ncbi.nlm.nih.gov/Omim). Online Mendelian Inheritance in Man contains textual information, pictures, and reference information on genes and genetic disorders containing clinical findings, references, and gene maps. OMIM has many links to NCBI's Entrez database of MEDLINE articles and sequence information, and many links to other databases.

Policy Statements from the American Academy of Pediatrics (http://www.aap.org/policy/pprgtoc.html). Contains policy statements and guidelines on diagnosis and treatment of genetic disorders as well as newborn screening.

Policy Statements from the American College of Human Genetics (http://www.faseb.org/genetics/acmg/pol-menu.htm). Contains a variety of policy statements about genetic diseases, genetic testing, and treatment of genetic disorders.

Primer on Molecular Genetics (http://www.ornl.gov/hgmis/publicat/primer/intro.html). A Department of Energy site that contains information on molecular genetics, genetic testing, and the Human Genome Project.

Quackwatch (http://www.quackwatch.com/). Information on health fraud and quackery as well as alternative treatment, such as nutritional supplements for Down syndrome.

Rare Genetic Diseases in Children (http://mcrcr2.med.nyu.edu/murphp01/lysosome/lysosome.htm). Intends to publicize, educate, and refer those interested in or concerned about the various lysosomal storage diseases.

Simulated Genetic Counseling Session (http://www. kumc.edu/gec/gcsim.html). Online simulated session that illustrates the process of genetic counseling.

VI. CONCLUSIONS

The World Wide Web is here to stay. It offers access to a wealth of information on and differential diagnoses for complex genetic and endocrine problems. In addition, to information for the physician, the WWW can also provide access to specialized lab tests and educational materials for patients and their families. It behooves every physician to capitalize on the resources that computer technology can provide. As is true for most things in life, some effort must be expended to develop the expertise to accomplish these goals. We hope that the material in this chapter will help readers to succeed in using the WWW to obtain information on genetic and hormone disorders.

REFERENCES

1. Online Mendelian Inheritance in Man (OMIM). Baltimore, MD: McKusick-Nathans Institute for Genetic Medicine, Johns Hopkins University; and Bethesda, MD: National Center for Biotechnology Information, National Library of Medicine, 2001; http://www.ncbi.nlm.nih.gov/omim/
2. Webster's New World Pocket Internet Directory and Dictionary. New York: Simon & Schuster, 1997.
3. MIM Number: 312870: 12/8/1999. Online Mendelian Inheritance in Man, OMIM. Baltimore, MD: Johns Hopkins University.
4. MIM Number: 173110: 11/20/2000. Online Mendelian Inheritance in Man, OMIM. Baltimore, MD: Johns Hopkins University.
5. Wu W, Cogan JD, Pfaffle RW, Dasen JS, Frisch H, O'Connell SM, Flynn SE, Brown MR, Mullis PE, Parks JS, Phillips JA III, Rosenfeld MG. Mutations in PROP1 cause familial combined pituitary hormone deficiency. Nat Genet 1998; 18:147–149.

41

Hormone Measurements and Dynamic Tests in Pediatric Endocrinology

Adriana A. Carrillo
University of Miami School of Medicine, Miami, Florida, U.S.A.

Fred Chasalow
Maimonides Medical Center, Brooklyn, New York, U.S.A.

I. INTRODUCTION

Measurement of hormones has had a tremendous impact on the diagnosis of endocrine disorders. Quantification of basal hormone levels in a serial manner at different diurnal or night-sleep hours provides understanding in physiological and pathological endocrine events. However, differentiation between normal and abnormal endocrine function may require dynamic tests to determine if feedback mechanisms are intact. By providing a stimulatory agent such as medication, stimulation tests are used to document hormonal deficiency as in presence of growth hormone deficiency, adrenal insufficiency, or gonadal failure. Suppression tests are performed to determine the presence of hormonal excess by evaluating functionality of feedback mechanism, as in Cushing's syndrome and in acromegaly. The individual performing a test is referred to the pertinent chapter in this book for an extensive review of indications, precautions, and interpretations of results.

II. ROLE OF THE LABORATORY

A. General Considerations in Interpreting Test Results

Several steps are needed to interpret test results, as well as consideration of the units and reference values given by the laboratory. First, the units reported can be classified into two types: (1) mass-based units, usually used for small molecules, such as steroids and thyroid hormones; and (2) standard preparation-based units, usually used for

proteins. Both of these have specific problems. Most small molecules are generally reported in mass units (e.g., ng/dl). The pure materials are readily available and inexpensive; test solutions of known concentration can be compared from laboratory to laboratory. Some laboratories report results as ng/dl, and others use ng/ml. The *S*ystem *I*nternational (SI) *is* an effort to standardize scientific nomenclature. Small molecules are now being reported in SI units (moles per liter). When peptide hormones assays were first established, pure materials were not readily available and each laboratory generated its own standard. To solve this problem, groups with international support (National Institutes of Health and/or the World Health Organization) made large standard preparations and defined the amount of active hormone present as an International Unit (IU). As needed, a vial of the standard, with a defined concentration in IU/l would be reconstituted. Over time, the original international standards were depleted and new standards were collected, but the new standards did not have exactly the same amount of hormone as the old. Thus, depending upon when a particular laboratory established its assay, the normal values in IU will be different, but each is properly called an International Unit. Hence, knowing that a hormone is reported as IU/l does not specify the normal or expected values.

Another source of differences in laboratory results is microheterogenicity. Many peptide hormones are glycoproteins with variable amounts of carbohydrate groups, perhaps a partial cause of inactive or hyperactive molecules. Because the epitopes frequently overlap with the glycosyl groups, specific antibodies may be more (or less) immunoreactive with the active hormone or with metabolites or fragments, and the different standards may also be more or less contaminated with metabolites or fragments. As a consequence, the microvariation, immunoreactivity, and bioactivity correlate to a variable extent. In summary, it is not sufficient to report results as IU/l because different IUs are in use. This problem becomes more important if an endocrinologist is using several different laboratories, perhaps because of third-party payment or requirements.

The reference values are provided by the laboratory and are used for comparison with a test result rather than to identify normal from abnormal values. To have statistical validity, reference values should be established from a sample of 100–200 individuals without disease. The reference range is calculated considering 95% of all values ±2 standard deviations (SD). It is assumed that the sample population has a normal gaussian distribution. If a test result is not between the reference parameters, different possibilities such as disease, individual variation, different populations, or use of medications may be considered to determine if further action is needed. Reference values including conventional, SI values and conversion factors are available in Addendum 1.

B. Assay Format and Design

The most commonly used format (1) for antibody-based assays is displacement analysis. With this format, a limited amount of antibody is allowed to bind to a limited amount of specific tracer for the hormone, the antibody-bound tracer is separated from the free tracer, and the antibody-bound tracer is quantitated. If the tracer is a radioactive hormone, then the assay is classified as a radioimmunoassay (RIA); if the tracer is a hormone coupled to an enzyme, then the assay is classified as an enzyme immunoassay. If the tracer is a fluorescent compound, then the assay might be classified as fluorescent immunoassay. In each format, a standard curve is generated by adding known amounts of unlabeled hormone and determining the decrease (displacement) in tracer bound to the antibody. To determine the serum concentration of a hormone, the observed displacement is compared to the standard curve. The important points to consider are that additional amounts of antibody (or binding proteins) are present in the serum or that there are closely related forms of the hormone in the serum, then the assay result is unreliable. The forms can be closely related steroids for a steroid assay; glycoproteins with differences in glycosyl groups; closely related hormones, such as the activin-inhibin or luteinizing hormone–human chorionic gonadotropin (LH-hCG) pairs; or isoforms, such as the 20 K and 22 K isoforms of growth hormone. In each of these formats, the least analytic precision occurs at the lowest concentration of analyte. Thus, alternative methodology must be used if the clinically important analyte concentration is at the lowest range of ligand concentration. In the enzyme-linked immunosorbent assay (ELISA) format, a

small amount of hormone is prebound to each well of a 96-well plate (or to a plastic or glass tube as an alternative). Then the standards and unknowns are added. The hormone-specific antibody is added and allowed to react with both the prebound and free hormone. More is bound if there is less free hormone present. The amount of antibody bound is then quantitated by a suitable technique, typically by eliminating all unbound proteins and adding a second antibody that is specific for the first antibody and to which an active enzyme is bound. Finally, the amount of active enzyme is specifically determined in each well and compared to the known amount of hormone added and to a standard curve generated for comparison with the unknowns. This format is best used for assays to detect the presence of important compounds.

In the immunoradiometric assay (IRMA) format, one hormone-specific antibody is attached to the solid support. The standards and unknowns are added, and a second hormone-specific antibody is added. Note that the second antibody used in IRMA is ligand specific rather than specific for the first antibody, as would be the case in RIA or ELISA. The second antibody is labeled with radioactive tracer, fluorescent or other nonradioactive tracer, or an enzyme. After a suitable incubation period, all unbound materials are washed away. Only when the desired analyte forms a bridge between the (first) antibody bound to the solid support and the soluble (second) antibody is the tracer or enzyme bound to the solid support and available for detection. If a pair of epitopes is very closely spaced on a ligand of interest, then the combination of antibodies cannot be used in an IRMA. As a consequence of the format, the amount of tracer bound to the bridge is approximately proportional to the amount of ligand present. At high ligand concentrations, the amount of ligand can exceed the amount of either one of the antibodies. This leads to a so-called high-dose hook effect and results in low estimations of ligand concentration. IRMA reagents are generally more expensive than reagents suitable for displacement analysis because of the requirement for two matched specific antibodies. As a compensating advantage, however, in contrast to displacement analysis, the IRMA format has its greatest analytic precision at the lowest analyte concentrations. The improved sensitivity at low concentrations and the improved specificity inherent in the method has led to widespread replacement of kits for displacement analysis (including RIA) for all analytes large enough for the generation of suitable antibodies.

C. Assay Specificity

The specificity of an assay (2,3), defined as the precision of a method to measure correctly the indicated substance, is limited by two factors: the amount and nature of sample preparation, and the specificity of the antibody. Thus, most laboratories minimize the first factor and rely on the second as much as possible. The difference between an alcohol and a ketone (such as between androstenedione and testosterone) generally permits a 10–50-fold difference in sensitivity based on a suitable antibody (a type 2 factor). Thus, for steroids present in similar concentrations, an antibody can usually provide sufficient specificity. In patients with biosynthetic defects, however, specific intermediates may be present to 10,000-fold excess. For example, an assay kit for testosterone would not be specifically tested or approved for use in children with congenital adrenal hyperplasia. At the time of diagnosis of the non-salt-losing form (typically a boy 4–6 years of age), 17-hydroxyprogesterone levels might exceed 50,000 ng/dl. Even if the testosterone antibody had only 1% cross-reactivity with 17-hydroxyprogesterone, the contribution of 17-hydroxyprogesterone to the apparent testosterone concentration would be 500 ng/dl, a level much greater than the normal range for a 4–6-year-old boy. The large amount of 17-hydroxyprogesterone would also serve as a substrate for synthesis of testosterone. Thus, both large amounts of testosterone and a cross-reacting steroid may be contributing to the apparent hormone levels. Lack of specificity can also be compounded because of age-specific differences in secretion.

There are two different mechanisms by which binding proteins can also contribute to the lack of clinical utility of a particular assay. First, if the affinity constant of the binding protein is comparable to the affinity constant of the antibody, then it may interfere with the assay by providing additional binding sites. This would probably lead to inappropriately low hormone levels. Second, because the definition of a hormone includes passage through the blood and control of the function of a second organ, serum binding proteins (BPs) can interfere with or supplement the activity of the parent hormone. For example, some binding proteins increase the half-life of a short-lived hormone (insulin-like growth factor, IGFBP-3); others increase the amount present in the serum by increasing the solubility of a lipophilic compound (testosterone–estradiol-binding globulin); others seem to have hormonal functions of their own (corticosteroid-binding globulin). Changes in binding protein concentrations can lead to large changes in total hormone levels without corresponding changes in free levels, which are presumably the active form.

Although there is no mystery in immunoassay there are many places for error, and no single laboratory value should be considered diagnostic without confirmation.

III. PRACTICAL CONSIDERATIONS

Meticulous attention to detail, both in the selection of laboratory tests and in the test room, are the keys to a successful procedure. In particular, the most important details to evaluate are the sample size requirements, the type of tubes (e.g., serum, ethylenediamine tetraacetic acid [EDTA], or heparin) used to collect the blood, and the specific sample-processing requirements, including whether serum samples should be separated and if they could, should, or must be frozen. In consultation with the laboratory, one should determine the amount of serum required for each analyte and prepare a table listing the exact time of sampling, the analytes for that time point, and the amount of blood required by the laboratory. The proper number and type of blood collection tubes should be collected. Recall that if a mistake is made and inappropriate or inadequate blood samples are obtained, the protocol will probably have to be repeated. Finally, arrangements must be made to transport samples to the laboratory in a manner that does not lead to degradation.

A. Mechanics

Successful testing is accomplished primarily through organization before the test. A tray should be prepared to hold completed laboratory slips, the correct number and types of tubes, labels, syringes, alcohol, arm board, and tape. This allows methodical sampling throughout the test. Normal saline lock is most often used and permits an indwelling line for both withdrawal of blood samples and delivery of medication with minimal discomfort to the patient. When using heparin lock flush (10 units/ml), a maximum of 1 ml is recommended. Withdraw and discard 1.0–1.5 ml from the line before sampling; after sampling, the line may be cleared by injection of an equal volume of the normal saline or heparin solution flush. An intravenous setup is a suitable alternative but leaves the patient somewhat less comfortable during the protocol. In a child younger than 4 years of age, it is appropriate to maintain a separate intravenous line with normal saline, in addition to the heparin lock, for emergencies during potentially hazardous testing such as insulin tolerance protocols. Although this may cause some added discomfort to the patient, loss of a line is common in young children and a patent line is essential to address any untoward events.

The size of the heparin lock needle must be selected on the basis of its intended use. A 24 gauge angiocatheter needle in a scalp vein may be adequate for infusion for an infant or young child; however, it is futile to attempt to obtain multiple blood samples from such a small needle or vein. Generally, a 22 or 23 gauge angiocatheter is adequate for both infusion and sampling.

Many of the protocols for tolerance tests include an overnight fast. Because the nothing by mouth order starts after midnight, a snack should be given just before midnight, if the child is awake at that time. Otherwise, the snack should be given at bedtime. For infants and very young children, however, an overnight fast may be too long. Therefore, the fast should conform to the child's eating patterns (i.e., an infant may be on a 3–4 h feeding schedule). In general, to avoid unnecessary fasting by young children, most tolerance tests should be started as early in the morning as possible. If the test must be postponed, the child should be fed and refasted. However, if a protocol is delayed, diurnal variation must be considered in the interpretation of the results. In most cases, medications that might interfere with the test should be discontinued for at least 1 week. If this is not possible, the effects of the medication on the tolerance test must be considered when interpreting the results. Other factors, such as extreme agitation or exercise, can also affect the results and should be noted.

A critical factor when conducting a tolerance test is the total amount of blood that must be obtained if, as is usually the case, multiple samples are required. Within a 2 week period, the usual guideline is a maximum of 5% of the total blood volume, which is calculated by multiplying the body weight (kg) by 80 ml. Remember to include any other testing planned for the same time or within 2 weeks of the tolerance test. If the amount required is more than 5% of the patient's total blood volume, the protocol must be modified.

B. Person-to-Person Considerations

One of the greatest challenges is informing the parents and the child about the purposes and mechanics of the test. This must be done in terms understandable both to the parents and to the child. Allow sufficient time for questions and answers. While you are describing the test, judge whether the parents should stay in the room with the child during the test. In deciding whether to allow the parents to stay, exercise discretion on an individual basis.

C. Time-of-Day Considerations

Most protocols are usually performed in the morning. Almost all of these tests should be performed while the patient is fasting, although there might not be any physiological rationale for food restriction. As a consequence, normal and expected values are all based on testing in the morning. There are circadian rhythms in many hormonal secretion patterns that can be superimposed on other patterns. For example, LH and FSH are both secreted episodically with 90 min cycles, but the amplitude of the cycle is increased in the morning. As a consequence, pituitary responses to gonadotropin-releasing hormone (GnRH) may be different and basal testosterone levels are

higher in the morning and one cannot measure an acute response to hCG. Adrenocorticotropic hormone (ACTH) is also secreted episodically with a 90 min cycle, but episodes of secretion occur more frequently in the morning and the ratio of cortisol to adrenal androgen secretion also changes with time of day. Hence, if testing is or must be performed at times other than morning, care must be used in comparing observed values to expected values. The exception to this requirement is in young infants, in whom circadian patterns have not yet been established.

IV. PRACTICAL PROTOCOLS FOR DYNAMIC TESTING IN CHILDREN

A. Dynamic Tests for Growth Hormone Deficiency

1. Screening Tests for GH Deficiency

   a. Background. The most widely used screening tests (4–8) to evaluate GH deficiency are serum insulin-like growth factor-I (IGF-I) and serum IGF-binding protein-3 (IGFBP-3) levels. IGF-I (somatomedin C or sulfation factor) is secreted in the liver and cartilage in response to GH and mediates many of the anabolic and mitogenic actions of GH. The IGFs are mostly bound to specific binding proteins designated BP-3. Serum levels of IGF-I are age-, gender-, and nutrition-dependent in normal children with a sharp increase at the time of puberty. IGF-I levels are not highly specific for GH deficiency. Low serum IGF-I levels also occur in children with GH receptor and/or postreceptor defects, thyroid disorders, delayed puberty, diabetes, and malnutrition. Serum IGFBP-3 has less age, gender, and nutrition dependence than IGF-I levels.

   b. Indications. The diagnosis of GH deficiency in childhood must be based on auxiological criteria. Candidates for evaluation of the GH–IGF–IGFBP axis include children in the lowest fifth height–growth or bone age percentiles, when proper consideration is made for family history; children with syndromes associated with short stature; children who have acute changes in their growth charts; and children who have sustained possible insults to the pituitary, such as chemotherapy, radiotherapy, or physical injury to the head.

   c. Preparation and Medication. None is needed.

   d. Sampling. A single sample is obtained at the time of a routine patient visit. There is no time of day or dietary restrictions. Some laboratories require plasma, rather than serum, for IGF-I assays. Check with the laboratory before collecting a sample. IGFBP-3 levels are determined on serum. Thus, both serum and plasma may be needed.

   e. Normal and Expected Values (IGF-I Levels). Normal levels (see Table 1) were determined by collecting samples from children of normal height. However, the de-

Table 1 Insulin-Like Growth Factor 1 (IGF-I)

Age	Males (ng/ml)	Females (ng/ml)
2 mo–6 yr	17–248	17–248
6–9 yr	88–474	88–474
9–12 yr	110–565	117–771
12–16 yr	202–957	261–1096
16–26 yr	182–780	182–780
<26 yr	123–463	123–463

From Ref. 6.

sired ideal test comparison is between children with short stature without GH deficiency and children with short stature with GH deficiency.

f. Normal and Expected Values (BP-3 Levels). The normal range is from 2.5 to 10 mg/dl, with a small dependence, compared with the normal variation in RIA or IRMA assays, on differences in age and gender. Serum levels less than 2.4 mg/dl are associated with GH deficiency. Slightly higher values occur at the time of puberty.

g. General Considerations. Although a major screening tool for diagnosing GH deficiency, IGF-I has limited sensitivity due to significant overlap with normal values. Low levels of IGF-I may be found in normal children, mainly under 5 years of age. About 50% of low levels of IGF-I are not associated with GH deficiency but with receptor and postreceptor defects. Furthermore low serum IGF-I levels with normal GH secretory dynamics may be indicative of other disorders associated with growth failure, such as nutritional inadequacies, inadequate spontaneous GH secretion, and psychosocial growth failure. Low serum IGFBP-3 levels are suggestive of GH deficiency; however, up to 43% of normal short children were reported to have low IGFBP-3 levels. In summary, IGF-I and IGFBP-3 are helpful tests in the diagnosis of severe GH deficiency, but their sensitivity and specificity are still suboptimal.

h. Basic Physiology of Growth Hormone Secretion. GH is secreted episodically with most episodes occurring during rapid eye movement sleep (Chap. 3). Serum concentrations are typically below the sensitivity of most conventional assays (<1–2 ng/ml) (9–13). Random serum samples (at least 90%) cannot be used to evaluate GH deficiency. A variety of pharmacological agents have been identified to induce GH secretion, and suitable dynamic test procedures have been developed. There are two factors necessary for the evaluation of the response to pharmacological stimuli for GH secretion: knowledge of normal and inadequate responses to the particular protocol, and laboratory selection of methods and reagents for the evaluation of serum GH levels. The pharmacodynamics of GH secretion and metabolism determine the design of the serum-sampling protocol. Episodes of active GH secretion by the pituitary last about 5–10 min, and the half-life of GH is 20–30 min. Thus, the specific protocol for a tolerance test must collect serum every 20–30 min to detect an episode of secretion.

i. Normal Values. Serum GH concentration over 10 ng/ml usually indicates adequate GH response to pharmacological stimulation. A single value over 10 ng/ml is sufficient to evaluate the response; there is not usually a second serum sample with a concentration over 10 ng/ml because GH concentration will decrease by half before the next sample is obtained. At the present time, the generally recognized criteria for GH deficiency are responses of less than 10 ng/ml (or 10 μg/l) to two different pharmacolog-

ical stimuli for GH secretion. However the interpretation of these values must be made in accordance with the child's data (see Chaps. 1–3). The stimuli can have their effects at the level of the hypothalamus, pituitary, or both. High serum glucose levels inhibit GH secretion. Thus, each protocol must also include a significant period of fasting before the test.

j. Expected Frequency of Inadequate GH Secretion in Response to a Tolerance Test. Children with Prader-Willi syndrome, Russell-Silver syndrome, Down syndrome, other syndromes associated with short stature, Turner syndrome, or a history of cranial irradiation or of treatments for leukemia have a very high frequency (perhaps up to 100%) of inadequate GH secretion. Thus, there should be a high index of suspicion for a diagnosis of GH deficiency if a child also has one of these syndromes. Children with GH deficiency frequently continue to cross growth lines on growth charts and show significant bone age delay.

k. General Considerations. The following sections describe protocols for dynamic tests to evaluate the GH secretory capacity of the pituitary gland. These tests are expensive, not free of side effects, and require special conditions. There are two major groups of GH tests: screening tests that include exercise, levodopa, and clonidine; and definite tests that comprise arginine, insulin, and glucagon tests. Two different dynamic tests, sequentially or simultaneous, are required to confirm the diagnosis of GH deficiency.

During the immediate period of prepuberty, differentiating between growth hormone deficiency and constitutional growth delay is difficult. Sex steroid priming with testosterone or estrogen administered for Tanner stage I or II is recommended before growth hormone testing. One protocol for androgen priming is the administration of 100 mg depot testosterone 7–10 days before the actual GH tolerance test. For girls and boys, some endocrinologists prime with ethynil–estradiol. The protocol we use is 0.02 mg for children less than 50 pounds (23 kg) and 0.05 mg for those over 50 pounds (23 kg) given 18 h, 12 h, and 1 h prior to start the test.

Pharmacological tests involving the use of potent medications may mask the diagnosis of partial GH deficiency. Caution must be taken in interpreting results in obese children who undergo provocative testing for GH secretion, due to a negative impact of adipose tissue on GH secretion. Table 2 shows the protocols most commonly used in the assessment of GH secretion.

2. Arginine and Combined Arginine-L-Dopa Test for GH Secretion

a. Indications. The arginine stimulant apparently works by inducing insulin secretion and dopamine acts by blocking somatostatin secretion. The combined test (14–16) thus stimulates GH secretion by two separate mech-

Table 2 Growth Hormone Stimulation Tests

Test	Dosage	Timing peak of GH	Side effect
Arginine L-dopa	Arginine hydrochloride 0.5 g/kg/IV to a maximum of 30 g over 30 min	30–60 min	Late hypoglycemia
	L-dopa 125 mg if body weight <13.5 kg 250 mg >13.5 <31.5 kg 500 mg >31.5 kg		Nauseas, emesis, headache
GHRH	1 or 2 μg/kg, IV bolus	15 or 30 min	Flushes
Glucagon	0.03 mg/kg to a maximum of 0.1 mg IM/SQ	2–3 h	Late hypoglycemia
Insulin-induced hypoglycemia	0.05–0.1 IU/kg IV bolus	30–60 min	Severe hypoglycemia requires IV glucose. Not recommended in newborn or small children
Clonidine	5 μg/kg to a maximum of 250 μg	60 min	Drowsiness, hypotension
Exercise	20 min exercise	20–40 min postexercise	Exhaustion-induced asthma

anisms. Perhaps as a consequence, the combined protocol has fewer false-positive results than when either agent is administered alone. The test is used primarily when a second pharmacological test for GH secretion is required.

b. Preparation. Nothing should be given by mouth after midnight or following bedtime snack. Have arginine prepared for administration. Plan ahead: not all pharmacies have stocks of arginine, and it may have to be specially ordered in advance.

c. Medications. After the baseline serum sample is obtained, arginine HCL (0.5 g/kg to a maximum of 30 g) is administered intravenously over a 30 min period. If the combined arginine-L-dopa protocol is used, L-dopa is administered orally (PO) immediately after the baseline blood sample is obtained. Then arginine is administered. The dose of L-dopa should be as follows: 125 mg for children less than 13.5 kg; 250 mg for children between 13.5 and 31.5 kg; and 500 mg for children over 31.5 kg.

d. Sampling. Blood for GH assay should be sampled at 0, 30, 60, 90, and 120 min.

e. Special Considerations. As with the L-dopa protocol, nausea and vomiting frequently occur in toddlers. Be prepared. Do not stop taking blood samples. Children should be recumbent and may be given water throughout the test.

3. Clonidine Stimulation Test for GH Secretion

a. Specific Indications. Clonidine is an alpha 2-adrenergic agonist (17–20) that increases the growth-hormone-releasing hormone secretion, and inhibits somatostatin-releasing inhibiting factor (SRIF). This agent is probably the best choice for avoiding false-positive results. Children who fail to secrete GH in response to phar-

macological dosages of clonidine seldom secrete GH in response to any other test.

b. Preparation. The patient should receive nothing by mouth for at least 4–6 h before the test and is generally not receiving other medications.

c. Medications. Administer clonidine, 5 μg/kg, after baseline sample is drawn, to a maximum of 250 μg.

d. Sampling. Blood for GH assay should be drawn at 0, 60, and 90 min and blood for cortisol assay at 0 and 90 min. Usually the 60 min sample has the highest amount of GH, the 90 min sample being about 30% lower.

e. Special Considerations. Clonidine is an agent that lowers blood pressure. Blood pressure should be monitored at 0, 30, 60, and 90 min. In young children, clonidine frequently causes drowsiness, which lasts for several hours. Parents should be aware of this possible, transient side effect. Patients should have a place to lie down and may sleep or lie quietly throughout the procedure. Drowsiness may prolong the fasting period and may cause hypoglycemia. The patient must be encouraged to eat or drink after the test is finished. Water may be given freely throughout the test period.

4. Dexamethasone Response Test

a. Indications. Dexamethasone (21–23) can be used to induce growth hormone secretion with the same time course as glucagon. When used in this way, dexamethasone administration has no reported side effects. This test is not widely used for clinical purposes.

b. Preparation. Patients should fast after midnight.

c. Medications. After collection of the baseline serum sample, dexamethasone (2 mg/m^2) is administered intravenously as a bolus.

d. Sampling. After bolus administration of dexamethasone, serum samples should be obtained every 30 min for 2 h, every 15 min for 2 h, and then every 30 min for the fifth hour. The serum samples may be withdrawn from a heparin lock.

e. Normal Values. A peak of GH secretion should occur between 2 and 4 h after dexamethasone administration. The peak GH concentration should exceed 5 ng/ml in normal individuals. In patients with GH deficiency, the peak response does not exceed 5 ng/ml. Patients with obesity may also respond poorly.

f. General Considerations. Patients can drink water as desired throughout the test. At the conclusion of the protocol, patients should be fed. Like the galanin test, this protocol has not been widely utilized. Additional study is necessary to improve the response pattern.

5. Exercise-Induced GH Secretion

a. Indications. This test is frequently used as a screening test (24,25) to evaluate the need for more formal testing for GH secretion. This is a suggested protocol to take advantage of an active (hyperactive) child. Use caution with exercise-challenged children.

b. Preparation. The patient should have fasted for 3–4 h before the test.

c. Medications. None are needed.

d. Sampling. The stimulus is 20 min mild exercise: going up and down stairs, running up and down the corridor, and 20 min on an exercise cycle or bicycle. Final heart beat should exceed 120 beats/min. Obtain blood samples at the end of the exercise and at 20 and 40 min after completion of exercise or severe crying episode.

e. General Considerations. Water should be provided freely, as requested. As soon as the first serum sample is obtained at the conclusion of the exercise period, the child may eat and drink as desired. Most offices do not have the equipment for an exercise test. The usual occasion to use this protocol is a chance recognition of exercise, inadvertently performed by an active young child. Although the test is simple, safe, and inexpensive, up to one-third of normal children have an absent GH response.

6. Galanin Response Test

a. Indications. Galanin is a neuropeptide (26,27) that participates in the regulation of GH secretion, apparently in the hypothalamus. Thus, the response to galanin tests the hypothalamus–pituitary secretary pathway. This test is not widely used for clinical purposes.

b. Preparation. As with most of the pharmacological tests to evaluate GH secretion, the test should be performed in the morning after an overnight fast.

c. Medication. Galanin (p-galanin 1-29; Clinalfa AG, Switzerland) is administered over 1 h as an intravenous infusion at a total dosage of 15 μg/kg body weight.

d. Sampling. After a baseline sample is obtained, the galanin infusion is started and additional serum samples are obtained every 15 min for 2 h.

e. Normal Values. The peak response occurs between 1 and 2 h after the start of the infusion. The expected peak response is a peak level greater than 5 ng/nl. Note that the expected response is lower than with many other pharmacological tests for GH secretion. Obese children respond poorly or do not respond at all.

f. General Considerations. Patients may drink water, if desired, during the test. At the conclusion of the serum-sampling protocol, patients should be allowed to eat. The only reported side effect is a temporary bad taste when the galanin infusion is started. Galanin has fewer side effects than either clonidine or insulin administration. This may be due to the fact that galanin is a natural part of the GH secretion mechanism. However, galanin is not currently approved by the Food and Drug Administration (FDA) as a pharmaceutical agent in the United States and must be obtained as part of a research protocol at this time. The protocol described here has not been standardized for using galanin as an inducer for GH secretion. Additional studies are needed to establish the validity of this test.

7. GH-Releasing Hormone Test for Pituitary Reserve for GH Secretion

a. Indications. Administration of GH-releasing hormone (GHRH) evaluates the ability of the pituitary to secrete GH directly (28–33). Due to fluctuations in somatostatin secretion, there is great variability in the GH response. Thus, inhibitors of endogenous somatostatin such us piridostigmin and arginine have been used to enhance the GH response and to reduce the intra- and interindividuality variability. If a patient secretes GH in response to GHRH but not to pharmacological stimuli that function in the hypothalamus, then a defect in the hypothalamus is indicated.

b. Preparation. The test should be performed in the morning after an overnight fast.

c. Medication. Intravenously inject human pituitary GHRH at a dosage of 1 μg/kg over a period of 1 min. The patient may experience some flushing immediately after the infusion.

d. Sampling. Serum samples for evaluation of GH should be obtained at 0, 15, 30, 45, and 60 min. Earlier protocols also collected a late sample at 90 min, but this does not seem to be needed because the peak generally occurs within the first hour after administration of GHRH.

e. Normal Values. Children with pituitary defects fail to secrete GH to a peak of 10 ng/ml. The peak serum level usually occurs in the 15 or 30 min sample.

f. General Considerations. Most individuals with idiopathic GH secretion have a defect in hypothalamic regulation of pituitary secretion of GH. Hence, most patients secrete GH in response to GHRH but do not secrete GH in response to normal physiological processes. High endogenous (or exogenous) levels of somatostatin block the effect of GHRH.

8. Glucagon Test for GH Secretion

a. Indications. This test is the best choice in young children and infants (34,35). Glucagon induces GH secretion by stimulating endogenous insulin secretion to compensate for elevated serum glucose levels. It is a good substitute for the insulin tolerance test that could be risky in newborn and small children.

b. Preparation. Give nothing by mouth after midnight. Patients must have normal glucose reserves at the start of the test.

c. Medications. After baseline sample is drawn, glucagon is administered intramuscularly (IM) or subcutaneous (SQ) at a dosage of 0.03 mg/kg to a maximum of 1 mg.

d. Sampling. For evaluation of GH secretion, serum samples should be obtained at 0, 1, 2, 2-1/2, and 3 h after administration of glucagon. For other indications for the glucagon tolerance test, different sampling protocols are required. Be sure to collect the last samples.

e. Normal Values. At least one sample with a GH concentration over 10 ng/ml of GH secretion usually occurs between 2 and 3 h after glucagon administration.

f. Specific Considerations. The administration of glucagon causes a temporary increase in serum glucose levels. As part of the rebound process, insulin is oversecreted and serum glucose levels decrease. Hence, a glucagon tolerance test cannot be used as a stimulus for GH secretion in individuals with a limited ability to secrete insulin. Young children frequently experience nausea and vomit during the course of this test. Be prepared.

9. IGF-I Generation Test

a. Indications. This procedure examines GH receptor function by evaluating its ability to increase serum IGF-I levels (36–39). This test is useful for identifying patients with GH resistance. There are major variabilities in administration of GH, timing of samples, and cutoff levels of the normal IGF-I response.

b. Preparation. No specific preparation is necessary, but an adequate diet must be maintained.

c. Medications. Daily doses (4 or 7 day protocol) of GH (0.025–0.05 mg/kg/day × 7 days or 0.1 mg/kg/day × 4 days) are given SQ. Parents or guardians may administer the additional GH injections.

d. Sampling. A baseline sample should be obtained on days 1, 5, and 8 when using dosages of 0.025 or 0.05 mg/kg/day. If the 0.1 mg/kg/day GH dosage is used, blood should be obtained before the first GH injection and 8–16 h after the fourth injection. Samples taken on intermediate days are often helpful, but are not required.

e. Normal Values. In response to GH administration, serum levels of IGF-I should triple or increase to a high normal level for age and gender. IGFBP-3 and the acid-labile subunit are measured as well.

f. General Considerations. The GH should be administered at the same time each day, either in the morning or in the evening. The dose administered is equivalent to the normal daily secretion. There are no reported side effects. Children who do not respond to GH administration with an increase in IGF-I levels are not good candidates for GH therapy.

10. Insulin Stimulation Test for GH Secretion

a. Specific Indications. This test is generally considered the gold standard (40–42), but is risky and must be done under appropriate surveillance. The mechanism of stimulation is the counterregulatory response to insulin-induced hypoglycemia. Although there are few children with responses classified as false-negative, many children have responses classified as false-positive. A false-positive response is defined as occurring in a patient who fails to secrete GH in response to insulin but secretes GH in response to other pharmacological stimuli. In contrast, a false-negative response occurs if a patient secretes GH in response to insulin but does not secrete GH in response to other pharmacological or physiological stimuli. False-positive responses may be caused by insulin insensitivity, which leads to an inadequate induced hypoglycemia. The reserve of the adrenal cortex for cortisol secretion can also be confirmed during this protocol. If cortisol reserve is adequate, then at least one sample will have a cortisol level over 20 μg/dl. This test is not recommended for newborn or small children as they are more sensitive to insulin, nor for those with suspected hypopituitarism with risk of adrenal insufficiency.

b. Preparation. Give nothing by mouth after midnight. Calibrate and prepare for use a bedside device for rapid serum glucose measurement. Prepare a 50% glucose solution, and fill a 25 ml syringe. (Fill two syringes if the patient is larger than 25 kg.) An intravenous line with saline solution should be established in small children.

c. Medications. To start the protocol in children over 4 years of age, 0.1 unit/kg regular insulin should be administered. For younger children, a dosage of 0.05 unit/

kg is usually sufficient. However, if used for infants, the dosage must be one tenth (0.01unit/kg) and must be administered under careful observation. It is preferable to use glucagon or a different provocative test.

d. Sampling. Serum samples should be obtained before insulin administration and then at 15, 30, 45, and 60 min. Serum glucose levels must be evaluated at the bedside at each time point during the protocol. Glucose levels must decrease by 50% of the initial value or to less than 40 mg/dl. However, more severe hypoglycemia must be avoided because it can lead to seizures, coma, or death.

e. Monitoring and Dangers of Hypoglycemia. At the bedside, each blood sample must be immediately evaluated for serum glucose levels. It is not sufficient to send the sample to the hospital laboratory. If a child shows symptoms of hypoglycemia (blood glucose level less than 40 mg/dl, rapid pulse, diaphoresis, hot, and lethargic) and the signs do not improve by the next scheduled blood sampling, the 50% glucose solution should be administered (1 g/kg) from the previously prepared syringes. If this occurs, do not stop collecting serum samples according to the protocol. After the test protocol is complete, either administer the glucose solution (0.5–1.0 g/kg) or require the patient to eat and ensure that a good meal is ingested and not vomited. The patient must be monitored until serum glucose levels return to normal. Water should be provided as requested.

f. Normal and Expected Values. About 20 min after the glucose nadir there should be an episode of GH secretion. The peak level should be above 10 ng/ml. In some patients the response is delayed. Children with GH deficiency have a response of less than 10 ng/ml. About 20% of children with short stature and severe bone age delay can have a false-positive response.

g. Special Considerations. For the test to be valid, serum glucose levels must decrease more than 50% from the baseline or to less than 40 mg/dl. If signs of severe hypoglycemia occur, administer glucose but continue to collect serum for GH assay. Children with GH deficiency frequently have enhanced response to insulin, thus making them more likely to have an episode of severe hypoglycemia. Hence, this test requires the presence of either an experienced nurse or a physician.

Shah et al. (37) recently reported three cases of iatrogenic illness as a result of tolerance tests for GH deficiency (two with insulin and one with glucagon). Two of the three children died as a result of hyperglycemic hyperosmolar coma, perhaps as a result of inappropriate management after the test. Both children who died were shown to have GH deficiency when the serum obtained during the test was analyzed. Examination of the case reports suggests that the coma may have been avoided had immediate, appropriate action (not overreaction) been taken by an attending physician. In each case, analysis of serum samples showed severe hyperglycemia as a con-

sequence of excessive administration of glucose to treat hypoglycemia or rebound hypoglycemia induced by the tolerance test.

11. L-dopa Stimulation Test for GH Secretion

a. Indications. This test is frequently used (43) as the second test necessary to confirm the diagnosis of GH deficiency.

b. Preparation. Give nothing by mouth after midnight on the night before the test.

c. Medications. L-dopa is given orally immediately after the baseline blood sample is obtained. The dosage is as follows: 125 mg for children less than 13.5 kg; 250 mg for children between 13.5 and 31.5 kg; and 500 mg for children over 31.5 kg.

d. Sampling. Draw blood for GH assay at 0, 30, 60, 90, and 120 min.

e. Normal Values. At least one serum value should be above 10 ng/ml. Usually, the samples with high levels of GH are the last samples collected during the protocol.

f. Expected Values. If there is no sample with a concentration of GH greater than 10 ng/ml, then the test is diagnostic for GH deficiency.

g. Special Concerns. Nausea and vomiting frequently occur in toddlers. Be prepared. Do not stop taking blood samples. Children should be recumbent and may be given water throughout the test.

12. Overnight Test for Spontaneous GH Secretion

a. Indications. This procedure is used to evaluate spontaneous GH secretion rather than secretion in response to pharmacological stimulation (44,45). This is the diagnostic test necessary to document inadequate spontaneous GH secretion or a neurosecretory defect in GH secretion. This test is not used as often as it was used in the past due to the cost, including admitting the patient to the hospital overnight.

b. Preparation. Patients can be tested in the hospital or at home with the aid of an experienced home care service. In either case, patients should go to bed at the usual time but not later than 11 p.m. A heparin lock can be used to cause the least disturbance in sleep pattern.

c. Medication. No medication is needed as part of the tolerance test.

d. Sampling. Serum samples should be obtained every 20 min from 8 p.m. to 8 a.m., a total of 37 samples over 12 h.

e. Normal Values. There are two criteria for evaluating the adequacy of overnight GH secretion: mean levels, and number and height of episodes of secretion. The mean level is the simple average of the 37 samples collected. This is a representation of the total amount of GH secreted during the 12 h period. The evaluation of normal values is confounded by practical and ethical considerations: Institutional Review Boards (IRBs) do not permit testing truly normal individuals. With this caveat, most reports suggest a normal lower limit of the mean about 3 ng/ml. Means below this limit probably indicate inadequate physiological secretion.

The second method of evaluating results is after deconvolution analysis using the Veldhuis and Johnson cluster analysis program. The program permits the evaluation of the number of episodes of secretion and the half-life of serum GH. There should be 6–10 episodes of secretion, with at least four peaks over 10 ng/ml. Fewer peaks of lower peak height are consistent with the diagnosis of inadequate spontaneous secretion or neurosecretory defect.

f. Special Concerns. In view of the large number of samples collected and the general limitation of using no more than 5% of total blood volume for laboratory testing in any 2 week period, it is frequently necessary to limit the amount of serum obtained in each sample. Hence, it is necessary to discuss with the laboratory the absolute minimum amounts of blood necessary for each sample. For example, if the laboratory requests 1 ml serum for a GH assay, then each sample collected must have 2 ml whole blood and the total volume collected is about 75 ml. If the patient weighs 10 kg, then total blood volume is only approximately 800 ml and the amount necessary would represent almost 10% of the total, which is an unacceptable proportion. This test is difficult to perform, expensive, and unspecific. No normative data for comparison purposes are available yet.

13. Combined Hormonal Stimulation Test

a. Indication. The combined hormonal stimulation test (CHST) is used for evaluation of the pituitary function by combined sequential hormonal administration in children with pathological short stature (46). As many as 30% of patients with growth hormone deficiency may have associated pituitary deficiencies. The CHST includes simultaneous assessment of the following axes: growth, thyroid, gonadal, and adrenal. In prepubertal children, the assessment of the gonadal axis can be eliminated unless LH and FSH deficiencies are suspected.

b. Preparation. Indicate nothing by mouth after midnight on the night before the test.

c. Medications. Sequential administration of insulin, thyrotropin-releasing hormone, gonadotropin-releasing hormone, and levodopa is required. First 0.1 unit/kg body weight of regular insulin is infused intravenously (IV) over 90 s. This is followed by 100 μg of gonadorelin IV (10 μg/kg, max 100 μg), and protirelin (7 μg/kg to a maximun of 400 μg IV) over 90 s. Afterward L-dopa is given orally at the dosage of 125 mg for children < 13.5

kg, 250 mg for children between 13.5 and 31.5 kg, and 500 mg for children > 31.5 kg.

d. Sampling. The following table illustrates timing for measurements of glucose, growth hormone, TSH, LH, FSH and prolactin.

Time (min)	Glucose	GH	Cortisol	FSH	LH	TSH	Prolactin
0	X	X	X	X	X	X	X
20	X	X					
45	X	X		X	X		
60	X	X	X				
90	X			X	X		
120	X					X	

e. Special Concerns. For detailed information about specific monitoring of each test, see the pertinent section in this chapter. Special attention must be given to hypoglycemia induced by insulin. There should also be an assessment of the amount of blood required for all these tests and the cost of performing them.

f. Normal Results. Normal values for each test are described in each specific section elsewhere in this chapter.

g. Special Considerations. There are potential modifications to this test. The first is to perform the full CHST as described but store the samples for measurement of TSH, LH, FSH, and prolactin until GH deficiency is confirmed, thereby reducing the expenses if the diagnosis is not growth hormone deficiency. The second modification is to select who will undergo the thyrotropin-releasing hormone and/or gonadotropin releasing hormone test. These tests provide an effective means of evaluating multiple pituitary functions in 2 h.

B. Tests for Thyroid Function

1. Calcium-Pentagastrin Test

a. Indications. This test is generally used for the detection of thyroid medullary carcinoma (47,48) as part of the work-up for multiple endocrine neoplasia (MEN) syndrome. In patients with MEN who are at high risk for the disorder, this test should be repeated on a yearly basis to confirm that thyroid medullary carcinoma has not recurred.

b. Preparation. Patients should fast after midnight or bedtime snack; water is permitted as desired. The test should be performed with the patient in a supine position.

c. Medications. Elemental calcium (2 mg/kg) is infused intravenously over 1 min; pentagastrin (0.5 μg/kg) is administered as a bolus immediately thereafter.

The elemental calcium content of some common calcium salts is calcium gluconate, 10%; calcium lactate, 13%; and calcium chloride, 27%.

d. Sampling. Serum samples for calcitonin are obtained at 0, 1, 2, 3, 5, and 10 min after administration of both stimulants.

e. Normal Values. Normal values should be established in conjunction with the laboratory.

f. Expected Values. An increase of five times over the baseline level during the test is diagnostic of medullary thyroid carcinoma.

g. General Considerations. The test protocol leads to some minor discomfort. Infusion of calcium may be accompanied by a mild generalized flush or feeling of warmth, the urge to urinate, and a sensation of gastric fullness. These symptoms are self-limited and usually do not last longer than 5 min. Pentagastrin may cause some discomfort in the pharynx and substernal and retrosternal areas, a sense of gastric fullness, abdominal cramping and nausea, and dyspepsia. These symptoms also last less than 2 min. It is extremely important to maintain patent intravenous access during the calcium infusion; infiltration of calcium into subcutaneous tissue can cause tissue necrosis.

Screening for DNA mutations of the RET proto-oncogene is more sensitive in detecting medullar carcinoma (Chapter 8). Measurement of plasma calcitonin after calcium and pentagastrin provocative testing is still used for detecting persistent or recurrent medullary thyroid carcinoma (MTC) postoperatively.

2. Thyroid Suppression Test

a. Indications. This test is used in the diagnosis of thyrotoxicosis (49,50). Radioiodine uptake by the thyroid gland should be decreased by exogenous thyroid hormone administration in a properly functioning gland. If uptake continues after treatment with thyroid hormone, then the gland is autonomous and the patient is at risk for thyrotoxicosis.

b. Preparation. Medications that affect thyroid function should be discontinued at least 1 week before the test.

c. Medications. Triiodothyronine (75 μg; Cytomel) is given orally daily (25 μg PO three times per day) for 7–10 days.

d. Sample. Radioactive iodine uptake studies should be performed before and after treatment.

e. Normal Values. Radioactive iodine uptake in the thyroid should decrease by 50% of the initial value. Failure to suppress is indicative of an autonomous gland.

f. General Considerations. No side effects of this test have been reported. However, the test is contraindicated during pregnancy.

3. TRH Test

a. Indications. The first generation of assays could only quantitate TSH levels greater than 1 mIU/l. In many cases, however, a TSH test does not differentiate between hyperthyroidism and euthyroidism. In response to thyrotropin-releasing hormone (TRH) TSH is secreted, reaching a maximal level 5–10 times the basal TSH level. Thus, during a TRH tolerance test in euthyroid individuals (51,52), serum TSH increases into the range that could be detected by the assay methodology even though the basal level could not be detected. In contrast, the TSH levels in individuals with hyperthyroidism remained undetectable or very nearly so. With the new third- and fourth-generation TSH tests, it is possible to evaluate very low levels of TSH, and TRH is not longer used to evaluate hyperthyroidism. At the present time, TRH tolerance tests are used primarily for evaluation of prolactin secretion or secondary hypothyroidism.

b. Preparation. The patient should discontinue all thyroid medication and chronic aspirin therapy for at least 1 week before the test.

c. Medication. TRH (7 μg/kg up to a maximum of 400 μg) should be administered intravenously over 90 s.

d. Sampling. Samples should be collected before the administration of TRH and at 15 min intervals for 1 h after treatment. Baseline samples should be assayed for triiodothyronine and thyroxine. All the samples should be assayed for TSH and prolactin.

e. Normal Results. TSH should increase to 5–10 times higher than the basal level. Prolactin levels should increase to three to five times over basal levels, with the peak secretion 15–30 min after TRH administration.

f. Expected Values. Individuals with hyperthyroidism or secondary hypothyroidism do not raise their TSH levels into the normal range. High basal prolactin levels without increase during the tolerance test are suggestive, but not diagnostic, of prolactinoma.

g. General Considerations. TRH may cause an increase in blood pressure and is contraindicated in patients with hypertension or cardiovascular disease. During the infusion of TRH subjects may feel a strong urge to urinate. Thus it is useful to suggest that patients urinate before the start of the protocol. Other side effects of TRH infusion are nausea, vomiting, and facial flushing. These effects only last for 30–90 s. Because of the nausea, an overnight fast or omission of the last meal should be considered, although this is not specifically required for the test.

C. Tests for Parathyroid Function

The following protocols were used to evaluate parathyroid function before the availability of RIA tests for parathyroid hormone (PTH). At present, these protocols are occasionally used to detect and evaluate minimal degrees of dysfunction, perhaps associated with partial resistance to PTH or partial protein S deficiency.

1. Ethylenediaminetetraacetic Acid Infusion Test (53,54)

a. Indications. This test is a direct method for detecting disorders of the parathyroid gland, including both hypoparathyroidism and pseudohypoparathyroidism in its different forms. Ethylenediamine tetraacetic acid (EDTA) is a calcium-specific chelating agent. It is metabolized by excretion in urine with its chelated cations, mostly calcium. Thus, the infusion of EDTA leads to a decrease in serum calcium levels; the response to this stimulus forms the test. Under the regulation of hormones secreted by the parathyroid gland, normal individuals respond to its stimulus by mobilization of calcium stores and restoration of serum calcium levels within 12 h.

b. Preparation. Patients should fast overnight before the test and should be recumbent for the duration of the test.

c. Medication. Intravenous infusion of 50 mg/kg trisodium EDTA in 300 ml 5% dextrose over 1 h period is used. To reduce discomfort at the site of infusion, procaine hydrochloride (1 or 2%) or lidocaine should be added to the infusion. Care should be taken to ensure that the tubing is primed with the anesthetic before the administration of EDTA.

d. Sampling. Draw blood for calcium immediately before EDTA infusion, immediately after infusion, and at 4, 8, and 12 h after the start of the infusion. Serum samples may also be assayed directly for parathyroid hormone and calcitonin to differentiate the basis for the disorder.

e. Normal Values. Preinfusion calcium values should be within the normal range for the laboratory. Post-infusion levels should fall immediately by 2–3 mg/dl. The failure of calcium levels to return to preinfusion levels within 12 h after EDTA infusion is indicative of the lack of proper function of the parathyroid hormone. Further tests may be necessary to identify the exact nature of the disorder.

f. General Considerations. Patients in whom calcium stores may be challenged should be monitored carefully until normal serum calcium levels are restored. Paresthesias of the face and extremities may occur, and patients should be forewarned. Positive Chvostek's and/or Trousseau's signs may be seen at any time in the 24 h period. Patients should be observed carefully for signs of tetany; appropriate measures must be taken should tetany or seizures ensue.

2. Ellsworth-Howard Test

a. Indications. The test is used to differentiate between hypoparathyroidism and pseudohypoparathyroidism (55,57).

b. Preparation. All supplemental medications used to treat hypoparathyroidism and pseudohypoparathyroidism, such as calcium or vitamin D, should be withheld for 8–12 h before the testing period. Patients should be fasted over the same period.

c. Medications. Over a 15 min period, PTH 200–300 IU is administered intravenously in 50 ml normal saline with 0.5% human serum albumin.

d. Sampling. Collect urine 1 h before PTH infusion and for 5 h afterward. Assay for cyclic AMP.

e. Expected Values. Expected values are listed in Table 3.

D. Tests for Prolactin Secretion

1. Dopamine Inhibition of Prolactin Secretion

a. Indications. Dopamine normally inhibits prolactin secretion (58). Thus, this test is used when hypersecretion of prolactin is suspected.

b. Preparation. Give nothing by mouth from midnight or after the bedtime snack.

c. Medication. L-dopa is given PO immediately after the baseline blood sample is obtained. The dosage is as follows: 125 mg for children less than 13.5 kg; 250 mg for children between 13.5 and 31.5 kg; and 500 mg for children over 31.5 kg.

d. Sampling. Draw blood for prolactin assay at 0, 40, 60, 90, 120, and 180 min after administration of L-dopa. In view of the method of evaluation of the result, two baseline samples should be obtained: one 15 min before and the second just before the administration of L-dopa.

e. Normal Values. Prolactin levels should decrease to less than 50% of the baseline value within 1–3 h. Lack of suppression suggests autonomous or hypersecretion of prolactin.

f. General Considerations. Nausea and vomiting frequently occur in toddlers. Be prepared. Do not stop taking blood samples. Children should be recumbent and may be given water throughout the test.

Table 3 Expected cAMP Values After PTH

Diagnosis	Cyclic AMP after PTH infusion (μmol)
Normal adults	3.90 ± 0.35
Pseudohypoparathyroidism	0.63 ± 0.12
Idopathic hypoparathyroidism	4.43 ± 0.54
Pseudopseudohypoparathyroidism	2.98 ± 0.49

2. TRH-Induced Prolactin Secretion

a. Indications. This test is often used to confirm abnormalities of prolactin secretion (59). Although the mechanism is unknown, TRH stimulates prolactin secretion.

b. Preparation. The patient should be off all thyroid medication and chronic aspirin therapy for at least 1 week before the test. For their own comfort, patients should be requested to urinate before the start of the test.

c. Medication. After collection of a baseline sample, TRH (7 μg/kg up to a maximum of 400 μg) should be administered intravenously over 90 s.

d. Sampling. Serum should be collected every 15 min for 1 h after administration of TRH. The samples should be assayed for prolactin.

e. Normal Values. In children, prolactin levels should increase three- to fivefold during the test. The peak usually occurs at 15 or 30 min. Men have a similar response. In women, the increase can be somewhat larger.

f. General Considerations. TRH may cause an increase in blood pressure and is contraindicated in patients with hypertension or cardiovascular disease. Because during the infusion of TRH subjects may feel a strong urge to urinate, it is useful to suggest urination before the start of the protocol. Other side effects of TRH infusion are nausea, vomiting, and facial flushing. These effects only last for 30–90 s. Because of the nausea, an overnight fast or omission of the last meal should be considered, although it is not directly required for the test.

E. Tolerance Tests for Adrenal Cortex Function

1. Basic Physiology of Adrenal Cortex Function

ACTH has two major effects on the adrenal cortex: it serves as a growth factor, and it stimulates the secretion of steroids. Within 15 min of an endogenous or exogenous episode of ACTH secretion, the adrenal cortex secretes cortisol in large amounts and smaller amounts of androgens and intermediates. At the time of biochemical adrenarche, the reticularis increases the production of DHEA, but the serum level of DHEA-S is not increased during an ACTH-stimulatory episode. Tolerance testing for the adrenal cortex primarily involves testing for the adequacy of cortisol production and for excessive production of either intermediates of cortisol production or adrenal androgens other than DHEA-S. Evaluating the adequacy of cortisol production is one of the main purposes of ACTH tolerance testing. Following are specific protocols to evaluate different aspects of adrenal function.

2. Dexamethasone Suppression Test (Overnight)

a. Indications. This test is a screening test for Cushing's syndrome or excessive cortisol and/or androgen production (60,61). In women or girls with hirsutism, it can also be used to differentiate between the ovary and the adrenal as the source of excess androgen production. If the source of excess androgen production is the ovary or autonomous adrenal function, then androgen levels are not suppressed by overnight dexamethasone suppression. (Chap. 6).

b. Preparation. No specific preparation is needed. The test need not be performed in the hospital. Dexamethasone can be provided to the parent, administered at the proper time at home, and the child brought for serum collection the following morning.

c. Medication. For children over 25 kg, prescribe 1 mg dexamethasone at bedtime. For children smaller than 25 kg, administer 0.5 mg dexamethasone at bedtime.

d. Samples. A single serum sample is obtained between 8 and 9 a.m.

e. Normal Values. The morning serum cortisol level should be less than 2 μg/dl.

f. Expected Values. In the absence of extenuating circumstances, serum cortisol levels in excess of 2 μg/dl are abnormal and a physiological basis should be explored. Children with Cushing's syndrome may have cortisol levels after dexamethasone suppression as low as 4 μg/dl in the early course. This level should slowly increase under the continuing ACTH-induced hyperplasia.

g. General Considerations. Most texts and review articles suggest cutoff values of 5–10 μg/dl. However, these values were obtained with chemical tests for cortisol that were less specific than the RIAs now used. The use of 2 μg/dl (more than 2.5 standard deviations above the mean) might result in a few more false-positive results, but it leads to fewer false-negative ones, which is the real purpose of a screening test.

Dexamethasone suppresses ACTH secretion and therefore prevents its function as a growth factor for the adrenal cortex. Repeated administration leads to inadequate adrenal reserves.

3. Dexamethasone Suppression Test (High-Dosage)

a. Indications. This test is used to define further the control of cortisol secretion for individuals who do not have adequate suppression with the overnight dexamethasone test (62,63).

b. Preparation for Part 1. No specific preparation is needed.

c. Medication for Part 1. Dexamethasone, 20 μg/kg per day, to a maximum of 0.5 mg/dose, is given PO every 6 h for 2 days beginning on day 3 of the test. Older children and adults may be given 0.5 mg every 6 h for eight doses.

d. Sampling for Part 1. The 24 h urine collections are started on day 1. Each urine sample should be assayed for 17-ketogenic steroids, urinary free cortisol, and creatinine. Serum should be collected each morning and assayed for DHEA-S and cortisol.

e. Normal Values for Part 1. The 17-ketogenic steroids should fall to ≤7 mg/day (≤3 ≤mg/g creatinine) by the day of the test. Urinary free cortisol should be suppressed by more than 50% in normal subjects.

f. General Considerations for Part 1. Food and water should be available as desired throughout the test period. The test can be done on an outpatient basis. Patients who do not suppress the urinary free cortisol levels should be tested with high dosages of dexamethasone (part 2 of the protocol). In general, if the results are not available or are ambiguous, part 2 of the protocol should be performed immediately.

g. Preparation for Part 2. Part 2 should be performed immediately after completion of part 1 as days 5 and 6 of the combined protocol.

h. Medication for Part 2. Dexamethasone, 2 mg/dose, is given PO every 6 h for 2 days beginning on day 5 of test.

i. Sampling for Part 2. The 24 h urine samples are collected on days 5 and 6. Each urine sample should be assayed for 17-ketogenic steroids, urinary free cortisol, and creatinine. Serum should be collected each morning and assayed for DHEA-S and cortisol.

j. Normal Values for Part 2. The 17-ketogenic steroids and urinary free cortisol should be suppressed by more than 50% even in subjects with adrenal hyperplasia or Cushing's syndrome. In patients in whom they are not suppressed during part 2 of the protocol, the presence of an independent, steroid-producing tumor must be explored.

4. Low-Dosage ACTH Stimulation Test

a. Indications. This test is used to evaluate the integrity of the hypothalamic–pituitary–adrenal axis adrenal reserve (64,65). Evidence supporting the use of a low-dose (1 μg) ACTH test rather than the standard ACTH test (250 μg) has increased over the past years. A low-dose ACTH test has more sensitivity in detecting subtle states of adrenal insufficiency and provides more physiological concentration of ACTH.

b. Preparation. The patient should be off medications that interfere with ACTH secretion (glucocorticosteroids) for at least 1 week before the test. If the patient has been receiving chronic steroid treatment, the withdrawal process may take a few months.

c. Medications. In the morning, after collecting baseline serum samples, a single intravenous bolus of 1 μg Cortrosyn is administered. Although a 1 μg ampule would be desirable, this presentation is not available. We advise dilution by the pharmacist following an established protocol. Dilute the 250 μg vial with 10 ml NaCl (25

μg/ml) and take an aliquot of 0.2 ml. Diluted to 1 ml, this will yield a final concentration of 1 μg/ml. Glass or plastic tubes can be used.

d. Sampling. Baseline sample and additional sample at 30 min will be sent for cortisol measurement. Some authors recommend a single sample at 30 min.

e. Normal Values. Various cutoff set points of serum cortisol levels have been proposed to indicate normal adrenal function. However, a cutoff of 600 nmol/l (22 μg/dl) is an optimal level with 100% sensitivity and 83% specificity. High sensitivity of a test is preferred in life-threatening conditions such as adrenal insufficiency.

5. Standard-Dose ACTH Stimulation Test

a. Indications. This protocol is used to evaluate the adequacy of cortisol secretion and adrenal reserve, primarily to eliminate a diagnosis of Addison's disease or congenital ACTH unresponsiveness (66–69).

b. Preparation. The patient should be off medications that interfere with ACTH secretion, especially high-dose glucocorticoids or other steroids. High-dose steroids must be discontinued for at least 1 week to permit restoration of the normal biosynthetic reserve.

c. Medications. In the morning, after collection of baseline serum samples, a single intravenous bolus of 0.25 mg Cortrosyn is administered.

d. Sampling. Before the administration of Cortrosyn, a baseline sample is obtained. An additional sample is collected 30 min after administration of Cortrosyn. Each sample is assayed for cortisol, 17-hydroxyprogesterone, progesterone, and 17-hydroxypregnenolone. The exact interval between the administration of ACTH and the second sample must be noted.

e. Normal and Expected Values. Cortisol levels should exceed 16 μg/dl in either the baseline or post-ACTH sample. Cortisol levels may not be decreased in individuals with 21-hydroxylase deficiency. For evaluation of 21-hydroxylase deficiency, the sum of the increase in progesterone and 17-hydroxyprogesterone concentrations is divided by the time between the samples. Individuals who are heterozygous for the congenital adrenal hyperplasia (CAH) trait have responses between 9 to 30 ng/dl/min. Increases below 7 ng/ml/h are typical of normal homozygous individuals. For evaluation of 3,β-hydroxysteroid dehydrogenase deficiency, the ratio of 17-hydroxypregnenolone to 17-hydroxyprogesterone levels is considered. Normal individuals have a ratio of less than 10, and higher ratios are considered diagnostic.

f. General Considerations. However, because of the variable timing of the morning endogenous ACTH secretary episodes and the secretion of ACTH when a child is frightened, the baseline values are often already stimulated. Therefore a dexamethasone suppression test should be continued as described below.

6. Dexamethasone-Suppressed ACTH Stimulation Test

a. Indications. This protocol differs from the simple ACTH stimulation test by the administration of a single dose of dexamethasone at bedtime before the test (70,71). This step serves to block the normal morning episodes of ACTH secretion and eliminates the continuing secretion of cortisol and its intermediates. As a consequence, before the administration of ACTH, the adrenal cortex synthesizes and secretes only small amounts of steroids. Without the dexamethasone treatment, the so-called white coat syndrome (fear of doctors) experienced by many children leads to immediate ACTH secretion and thus to high levels of steroids in the baseline samples. In fact, on many occasions, the baseline samples have higher levels of steroids than the samples obtained after ACTH administration. In contrast, after dexamethasone pretreatment, the presence of steroids in the baseline samples can be attributed either to gonadal secretion or to ACTH-independent pathways. The protocol is used to confirm a suspected diagnosis of complete or partial steroid biosynthetic defects. The phenotype characteristic of heterozygote carriers for 21-hydroxylase deficiency can also be identified. The dexamethasone pretreated protocol was specifically developed to overcome the variation in baseline steroid intermediate levels caused by uncontrolled endogenous episodes of ACTH secretion.

b. Preparation. A single dose of dexamethasone ($0.5\ \mu g/m^2$) is administered just before the subject goes to bed, usually between 10 and 11 p.m. Patients should fast from the time of dexamethasone treatment until the completion of the test. Water may be consumed as desired. Menstruating women should be tested in the follicular phase of the cycle.

c. Medications. In the morning, after collection of baseline serum samples, a single intravenous bolus of 0.25 mg Cortrosyn is administered.

d. Sampling. Two baseline samples are obtained 15 min and right before the administration of Cortrosyn. Additional samples are collected 30, 45, and 60 min after the administration of Cortrosyn.

e. Normal and Expected Values. The test is evaluated by considering the difference between the baseline and stimulated samples of steroid levels. The baseline level is obtained by averaging the two baseline samples; the stimulated level is the average of the two highest samples obtained after Cortrosyn administration. As a consequence of the continued function of the long-acting synthetic glucocorticoid, the morning episodes of ACTH secretion do not occur. Thus, baseline levels of steroid intermediates are not elevated. Expected values are listed in Table 4.

f. General Considerations. Girls (but not boys) with idiopathic, premature adrenarche frequently have re-

sponse phenotypes similar to those of carriers for 21-hydroxylase deficiency. It is not clear whether the genotype is also similar to that of carriers for 21-hydroxylase deficiencies. About 15% of girls with features of hyperandrogenism have steroid secretary patterns typical of nonclassic 21-hydroxylase or 3,β-hydroxysteroid dehydrogenase deficiency. When older populations are tested, the frequency of deficiency syndromes decreases, perhaps because of prior identification of severely affected individuals.

After dexamethasone suppression, there are four common causes of elevated baseline levels of cortisol, androgens, or steroid intermediates: the subject did not take the dexamethasone; breakthrough ACTH secretion; gonadal secretion of steroids; and lack of regulatory control, perhaps caused by Cushing's syndrome. If the subject does not take the dexamethasone, the baseline samples are frequently similar to stimulated values. Ovarian secretion of 17-hydroxyprogesterone, DHEA, and androstenedione is most common in patients with polycystic ovarian disorder or during the luteal phase of the menstrual cycle. The source of excess steroids in the baseline samples can be attributed to the ovary if the cortisol level is less than 2 $\mu g/dl$ or less than 5 $\mu g/dl$ in a woman taking birth control pills. Finally, with the exceptions noted, baseline cortisol levels in excess of 2 $\mu g/dl$ are suggestive of Cushing's syndrome. Thus, the addition of dexamethasone pretreat-

Table 4 Expected Steroid Values

Steroid	Baseline levels	Stimulated levels
Normal individuals		
Cortisol ($\mu g/dl$)	≤ 2	12–24
17-Hydroxyprogesterone (ng/dl)	≤ 50	50–150
Androstenedione (ng/dl)	≤ 50	50–200
Dehydroepiandrosterone (ng/dl)	≤ 200	400–800
Heterozygote for 21-hydroxylase deficiency		
Cortisol ($\mu g/dl$)	≤ 2	12–24
17-Hydroxyprogesterone (ng/dl)	≤ 50	150–500
Androstenedione (ng/dl)	≤ 50	50–200
Dehydroepiandrosterone (ng/dl)	≤ 200	900–1300
Individuals with 21-hydroxylase deficiency		
Cortisol ($\mu g/dl$)	≤ 2	12–24
17-Hydroxyprogesterone (ng/dl)		≥ 2000
Androstenedione (ng/dl)	≤ 50	50–200
Dehydroepiandrosterone (ng/dl)	≤ 200	900–1300
Individuals with 3 β-hydroxysteroid dehydrogenase deficiency		
Cortisol ($\mu g/dl$)	≤ 2	12–24
17-Hydroxyprogesterone (ng/dl)	≤ 50	150–500
Androstenedione (ng/dl)	≤ 50	50–200
Dehydroepiandrosterone (ng/dl)	≤ 400	1600–8000

ment the night before the administration of ACTH increases the validity of the entire Cortrosyn tolerance test procedure.

7. Metyrapone Test

a. Indications. Metyrapone blocks the conversion of 11-deoxycortisol (compound S or cortexolone) to cortisol (72–74). The test is used to assess pituitary ACTH reserve, adrenal insufficiency, and the extent of adrenal suppression for patients receiving prolonged glucocorticoid therapy for any reason.

b. Warning. For patients in whom adrenal insufficiency (Addison's disease) is suspected, an appropriate steroid medication should be kept at bedside in case of an adverse reaction.

c. Preparation. The patient should be off all medications that interfere with ACTH production, including glucocorticoids, drugs that accelerate the action of metyrapone (such as diphenylhydantoin), and drugs that alter the concentration of 17-ketogenic steroids, such as penicillin and its variants.

d. Medication and Sampling: 24 h Test. Metyrapone, 300 mg/m^2 in children or 750 mg in adults, is orally administered every 4 h for six doses. Basal 24 h urine should be collected before the administration of metyrapone and for the next 3 days. The urine is assayed for creatinine and for 17-hydroxycorticosteroids. Serum should be obtained 4 h after the last dose of metyrapone and assayed for ACTH, cortisol, and 11-deoxycortisol.

e. Normal Values: 24 h Test. In normal individuals, 17-hydroxycorticosteroids levels should be greater than 9 mg/m^2/24 h during the metyrapone treatment. Plasma cortisol levels should be less than 8 μg/dl, and 11-deoxycortisol levels should exceed 10 μg/dl.

f. Medication and Sampling. Single-dose test. Metyrapone, 30 mg/kg to a maximum of 1 g, is administered as a single oral dose at midnight. Serum should be obtained at 8 a.m. and assayed for ACTH, cortisol, and 11-deoxycortisol.

g. Normal Values: Single-Dose Test. The results of the test should be considered in the following order: First, ACTH levels should be elevated. Inadequate ACTH secretion suggests inadequate pituitary reserve for secretion of ACTH. Second, cortisol levels should be less than 8 μg/dl; higher levels suggest inadequate therapy (rapid metabolism) or excessive production of cortisol, perhaps caused by Cushing's syndrome. Third, 11-deoxycortisol levels should exceed 10 μg/dl; lower levels suggest adrenal insufficiency, caused by either lack of recovery from high-dosage therapy or Addison's disease.

h. General Considerations. Hypotension and vomiting may occur during the administration of metyrapone. Transient vertigo may be avoided by administering the drug with milk or a meal. Patient's activity should be mild throughout the day of drug treatment.

F. Tests for Pheochromocytoma

This diagnosis is frequently suspected but is actually very rare in children. In this disorder, catecholamine secretion from the adrenal medulla no longer responds to proper hormonal regulation (Chap. 8).

1. Clonidine Suppression Test

a. Indications. Clonidine suppresses catecholamines arising from the sympathetic neuroendocrine system but not from a pheochromocytoma (75,76).

b. Preparation. Nothing should be given by mouth after midnight or for 10–12 h before the test. B-adrenergic-blocking drugs should be discontinued 48 h before the test; concomitant administration of these drugs can lead to severe bradycardia and decreased cardiac output. Adequate hydration must be maintained (or restored) before the test because of the possibility of potentiating hypovolemia.

c. Medication. Clonidine, 0.005 mg/kg to a maximum of 0.25 mg, is administered as a single oral dose.

d. Sampling. Draw blood for measurement of free catecholamines (epinephrine and norepinephrine) at 0, 1, 2, and 3 h after clonidine administration.

e. Normal Values. By 3 h after clonidine treatment, circulating catecholamine levels should decrease to less than 500 pg/ml. Failure to suppress the circulating levels is usually diagnostic of pheochromocytoma.

f. General Considerations. Because of the hypotensive effects of clonidine, blood pressure should be monitored during the protocol and the patient should be in a supine position. Patients may become very drowsy 30–45 min after clonidine administration. Various clinical laboratories have different instructions for the handling of blood plasma for catecholamine assay. Refer to the specific laboratory you intend to use and their protocol.

2. Glucagon Test

a. Preparation. The patient should rest quietly in a supine position without environmental stress or distraction (77). A heparin lock should be established at least 30 min before the start of the test.

b. Medication. After collection of baseline blood pressure data and serum, the test is started by the intravenous administration of 0.5 mg glucagon.

c. Sampling. Blood pressure should be determined 10 and 5 min before glucagon administration and after 5, 10, 20, 25, and 30 min of glucagon. Plasma should be collected for catecholamine levels at 0, 5, and 10 min after glucagon administration.

d. Normal Values. In normal patients, there should not be a rise in blood pressure. If a 0.5 mg dose of glucagon does not produce a rise in blood pressure, the test can be repeated with 1 mg glucagon administered as an intravenous bolus. A significant elevation in blood pressure and catecholamines for 5–15 min after glucagon administration is indicative of pheochromocytoma.

e. General Considerations. Patients must be supine throughout the test period. Performing the test in a darkened room without disturbance is often helpful. Various clinical laboratories have different instructions for the handling of blood plasma for catecholamine assay. Refer to the specific laboratory you intend to use and their protocol.

G. Test for Acromegaly: Glucose Test for Suppression of GH Secretion

a. Indications. Individuals with autonomous GH secretion do not blunt GH response to hyperglycemia as occurs physiologically (78). This response is indicative of GH excess, including acromegaly. It should be noted that young infants and diabetics in poor control often have paradoxical GH secretion. Elevated levels of IGF-I (>2 SD) are considered a good initial screening test suggestive of GH excess. It is important to use age-referenced comparative values, especially when evaluating adolescents who have highest levels among all age groups (Chap. 5).

b. Preparation. Overnight fast is prescribed before the test.

c. Medication. After collection of a baseline serum sample, glucose, 1.75 g/kg body weight to a maximum of 75 g, is given by mouth (Glucola, Trutol, or Dextol Cola is commonly used).

d. Sampling. Serum should be obtained for glucose and GH at the time of glucose administration and every 30 min for 2 h.

e. Normal Values. GH levels should decrease to less than 5 ng/ml. GH levels above 10 ng/ml confirm a diagnosis of GH excess. Values between 5 and 10 ng/ml are inconclusive.

f. General Considerations. As desired, patients can drink water and walk during the protocol.

H. Tests for Regulation of Serum Glucose Levels

1. Glucose Tolerance Tests

a. Indications. This test is useful for the evaluation of impaired glucose tolerance and insulin resistance or hypersensitivity (79,80). The test must include insulin levels to make an accurate diagnosis. A new cutoff point of less than 109 mg/dl is considered the upper limit of normal fasting plasma glucose level (FPG). Impaired fasting glucose (IFG) corresponds to a range of 110–126 mg/dl. FPG greater than 126 mg/dl indicates a provisional diagnosis of diabetes mellitus, and must be confirmed on a separate day. If the FPG is <126 mg/dl and there is a high suspicion for diabetes, an oral glucose tolerance test (OGTT) is indicated. The intravenous protocol should be reserved for patients with gastrointestinal disturbances or intolerance to oral glucose load. The intravenous protocol may also be preferred when assessing insulin secretion reserve or residual function of β-pancreatic cell in patients at high risk of developing diabetes or in patients with diabetes if indicated.

b. Preparation. For 3 days before the test, patients should be on a high-carbohydrate diet (at least 60% of calories from carbohydrates). Patients should fast after midnight or after a bedtime snack the night before the test. Medications that may act as hyper- or hypoglycemic agents should be discontinued.

c. Medication: Oral Protocol. After the baseline serum sample is obtained, glucose solution, 1.75 g/kg body weight to a maximum of 75 g, is administered as an oral solution. Trutol, Glucola, and Dextol Cola are commonly used commercial solutions.

d. Sampling: Oral Protocol. Draw blood for glucose and insulin at 0, 30, 60, 90 min, and at 2, 3, and 4 h after glucose administration. Urine is measured for sugar and acetone at each void throughout the protocol.

e. Expected Values: Oral Protocol. The criteria established by the National Diabetes Data Group in 1979 have been revised by an International Expert Committee sponsored by the American Diabetes Association.

- 2 h postload plasma glucose levels less than 140 mg/dl are normal.
- 2 h postload plasma glucose levels greater than 140 but less than 200 mg/dl indicate an impaired glucose tolerance test.
- 2 h postload glucose levels higher than 200 mg/dl indicate a provisional diagnosis of diabetes mellitus.

Impaired fasting glucose and impaired glucose tolerance tests are associated with insulin resistance, obesity, dyslipidemia of the high-triglyceride and/or low-HDL type, and hypertension.

f. Medication: Intravenous Protocol. After the baseline serum sample is obtained, glucose, 0.5 g/kg body weight, is given as an intravenous bolus over a 3–4 min period. It is preferable to have two separate intravenous lines, one for infusion of glucose and one for obtaining blood samples. The first line may be discontinued after the infusion is complete.

g. Sampling: Intravenous Protocol. Draw blood for glucose and insulin at 0, 1, 3, 5, 10, 20, 30, 45, and 60 min after the start of the glucose infusion.

h. Normal Values: Intravenous Protocol. For quantitative evaluation of the first-phase insulin response

(FPIR), the parameter used is the sum of plasma insulin values for 1 and 3 minutes (designated insulin [1′ + 3′]). Normal values for individuals over 8 years of age are insulin (1′ + 3′) > 100 μU/mL. Normal values for individuals between 3 and 8 years of age are insulin Σ (1′ + 3′) > 60 μU/ml. Individuals at high risk for developing diabetes mellitus have a low FPIR (<48 μU/ml).

The disappearance curve of glucose is plotted as a function of time on semilogarithmic paper and the K value (glucose disappearance rate) determined. K = 0.693 $\times$ 100/T$_{1/2}$ where T$_{1/2}$ is time in minutes for the glucose to fall to half of its initial value. A K value less than 1.4 indicates impaired glucose tolerance in persons less than 50 years of age. Insulin levels should reach their peak within 10 min of the start of the infusion.

i. General Considerations. Patients may drink water and move about freely during the test. The test should be postponed until 2 weeks after any acute illness. There is a risk of hyperosmolality in patients with elevated baseline blood glucose levels.

2. Hypoglycemia Workup

a. Indications. The following plan is valuable when evaluating hypoglycemia in children (81–83). Hyperinsulinemia, glycogen storage disease, factitious hypoglycemia, carnitine deficiency, fatty acid oxidation disturbance, and inborn errors of metabolism are indications for the use of this workup. The protocol evaluates metabolic changes that occur during a fast.

b. Preparation. The test should be conducted under close supervision. For younger children, maintain a separate intravenous line with 0.25 normal saline, in addition to the heparin lock, both for hydration and to ensure a patent venous line other than the heparin lock. The patient should be on a high-carbohydrate diet (60% of calories from carbohydrates) for 3 days. The diet should include frequent feedings. No high-fat foods should be allowed on the evening before the start of the test, and the patient should fast after midnight or bedtime snack. Test and prepare a bedside device to measure glucose (Dextrostix, Chemstrip bG, or equivalent). In anticipation of hypoglycemia, have at hand syringes prepared with glucagon, 30 μg/kg, and 50% glucose, 1 ml/kg body weight.

c. Medications. Glucagon, 30 μg/kg to a maximum of 1 mg, is administered by slow intravenous push.

d. Sampling.

Part 1. Approximately 4 h after fast is begun collect baseline blood sample and administer the first glucagon challenge. The baseline serum should be assayed for glucose at bedside and the hypoglycemia panel (insulin, GH, cortisol, venous blood gases, phosphorus, uric acid, lactate, alanine, ketones, β-hydroxybutyrate, free fatty acids, carnitine, and glucagon) at 5, 15, 30, and 60 min after

glucagon administration, draw and test blood for glucose and insulin.

Part 2. All urine is collected and evaluated for ketones and specific gravity. Every 2 h blood should be collected and assayed for glucose at bedside. Every 4 h blood should be collected and assayed for glucose and hypoglycemia panel at bedside.

Part 3. If at any time blood glucose is less than 40 mg/dl in whole blood (or less than 45 mg/dl in serum or plasma) with or without symptoms, then confirm with laboratory glucose measurement and assay for the hypoglycemia panel. Terminate the test with a 50% glucose solution, 1 ml/kg as an intravenous push over a couple of minutes. If severe symptomatic hypoglycemia and/or convulsions occur at any point, collect the serum sample and terminate the fast at once by administering the 50% glucose solution, 1 ml/kg intravenously. The serum should be assayed for the hypoglycemia panel and electrolytes.

If no hypoglycemia occurs within 24 h of the first glucagon test, perform a second glucagon tolerance test and terminate the protocol. If no hypoglycemia occurs but the patient develops metabolic acidosis (HCO$_3$ less than 15 mEq/l, with or without normal pH), repeat the glucagon tolerance test and terminate the test.

Part 4. After the fast, you may consider the following additional tolerance tests needed for further evaluation of defective gluconeogenesis: 0.5 g/kg alanine, 1.0 g/kg glycerol, and 1.0 g/kg fructose. In each case blood should be collected at 0, 15, 30, 45, 60, and 120 min after administration and assayed for glucose, serum ketones, lactic acid, and β-hydroxybutyrate.

e. Normal Values. Glucose levels should remain above 40 mg/dl throughout the 24 h fast. Episodes of hypoglycemia are considered abnormal at any time throughout the test, whether or not there are symptoms. Episodes of GH secretion greater than 10 ng/ml should follow about 20 min after any hypoglycemic episodes. Cortisol levels of 8–20 μg/dl are normal under nonstressful conditions. Under the conditions of this fast, levels should increase by 10 μg/dl or exceed 20 μg/dl. In samples obtained during hypoglycemic episodes, low glucose-insulin ratios (ratio of 3 vs. ratio of 6 as observed in normal individuals) are indicative of hyperinsulinism. The concentration of metabolites must be considered to evaluate the pathophysiology of hypoglycemia in other patients.

f. General Consideration. Only children over 4 years of age should be submitted to the full 24 h fast protocol. Patients must remain quiet but can sit in a chair or lie down, as they desire. They can drink water and use the bathroom freely. The intravenous infusion rate should be adjusted according to water intake. Parents should be encouraged to remain with the child, if this will lower the child's stress. If the patient fails to develop ketonuria during the test, the possibility of surreptitious food intake should be considered. Glucagon may cause some mild abdominal discomfort and/or nausea. Hence, it should be administered by slow intravenous push. The patient should be checked frequently for vital signs and symptoms of hypoglycemia, including convulsions, stupor, tremors, coma, or decreased blood pressure. A flow sheet should be maintained and all data recorded as rapidly as possible.

I. Tests for Gonadal Function

1. Acute Response to hCG Administration

a. Indications. This protocol is useful to confirm the diagnosis of nonclassic 17-ketosteroid reductase deficiency, typically in a teenage boy with severe gynecomastia (84,85).

b. Preparation. The test should be performed in the morning. Patients should eat a normal breakfast and can continue to eat and drink as desired and as appropriate.

c. Medications. At bedtime at home, the patient should take 1 mg dexamethasone. In the morning (about 9 a.m.), the patient should receive 4000 IU hCG as an intramuscular injection.

d. Samples. Serum samples should be obtained before the administration of hCG and 2, 4, 6, 24, and 48 h later.

e. Normal Values. In normal males, the testosterone–androstenedione ratio increases in response to hCG. The final testosterone levels should exceed 300 ng/dl, which are adult normal levels. In patients with partial 17-ketosteroid reductase deficiency, the sum of testosterone and androstenedione concentrations equals the adult normal levels, but the ratio is about equal rather than in excess of 4:1.

f. General Considerations. The two major sources of androstenedione are the adrenal gland and the testis. Administration of dexamethasone serves to eliminate secretion from the adrenal and thus permits monitoring of testicular synthesis.

Compared with testosterone, androstenedione is the preferred substrate for aromatization. Thus, the excess production of androstenedione leads to excess production of estrogens and the development of gynecomastia. Many boys at puberty develop mild gynecomastia that disappears as testosterone production increases. In normal individuals, the 17-ketosteroid dehydrogenase is substrate- (androstenedione) and product- (testosterone) activated, thus leading to complete conversion of androstenedione to testosterone. However, the enzyme of some individuals does not have the proper kinetic properties and does not fully convert all androstenedione to testosterone. The incomplete deficiency disorder is inherited as an autosomal recessive trait. This test helps to identify these patients.

2. Tonic Response to hCG Administration

a. Indications. This test is used to aid in the diagnosis of vanishing testis syndrome, disorders of steroidogenesis, micropenis, ambiguous genitalia, or other circumstances in which there is a question about normal testicular function (86,87).

b. Preparation. No specific preparation is needed.

c. Medication. Four daily doses of hCG (5000 IU/m^2 per dose) are administered as intramuscular injections. Alternative protocols use only 3000 IU/m^2 every day or every other day

d. Samples. A baseline serum sample and a stimulated sample obtained 24 h after the last dose of hCG should be assayed for testosterone and androstenedione.

e. Normal Values. Testosterone should increase to normal adult levels or greater than 300 ng/dl. Androstenedione should not exceed one-quarter of the observed testosterone level.

f. General Considerations. Prolonged administration of hCG can lead to bone age advancement. Progesterone or other intermediates can be assayed if the testosterone response is inadequate.

3. Gonadotropin Sleep Study

a. Indications. This test is useful in patients with suspected polycystic ovarian disease and in suspected cases of precocious puberty (88,89).

b. Preparation and Medication. None is needed.

c. Sampling. Sample serum for LH and FSH from the heparin lock every 20 min, overnight for up to 12 h. In small children for whom the amount of blood drawn may be a critical factor, the test may be modified by limiting the period of sample collection and increasing the interval to 30 min.

d. Normal Values. Normal, prepubertal children have no nocturnal episodes of gonadotropin secretion.

e. General Considerations. There are no side effects of this protocol.

4. GNRH (Factrel) Response Test

a. Indications. The response to the administration of gonadotropin-releasing hormone is useful for evaluating the role of pituitary dysfunction in children with premature or delayed puberty (90–93). Tolerance test responses can be used to differentiate central nervous system dysfunction from peripheral dysfunction in patients with both premature and delayed puberty. In children with premature puberty, peripheral dysfunction (testotoxicosis, McCune-Albright syndrome, and ovarian follicular cysts) is frequently associated with hypogonadotropism, whereas hypergonadotropism can be caused by central nervous system dysfunction (hamartoma or craniopharyngioma). In contrast, in children with delayed puberty, peripheral dysfunction is associated with hypergonadotropinism (Turner syndrome) and hypogonadotropism suggests dysfunction in the central nervous system (Kallman syndrome, Prader-Willi syndrome, and constitutional delay). The test is also useful in evaluating the extent of damage caused by radiation or chemotherapy in children with leukemia or brain tumors. In this group, the results can indicate the need for endocrine replacement therapy.

b. Preparation. Although not required, many physicians request that the patient fast overnight before the test and the test be performed in the morning. Certainly, there is time-of-day variation in the secretory pattern for LH and FSH, and most of the normal data have been collected in this manner. Thus, using a consistent protocol makes easier the comparison of results to previous studies.

c. Medications. Administer an intravenous bolus dose of 10 μg/kg to a maximun of 100 μg GNRH (Factrel, Ayerst Laboratories, New York, NY).

d. Sampling. Baseline samples ($n = 2$) should be obtained 15 min apart before the administration of the GNRH. Stimulated samples should be obtained 15, 30, 45, 60, and 90 min after treatment. For comparison with published values, the baseline samples and the three highest stimulated samples should be averaged. This protocol minimizes slight variations in secretary pattern and in laboratory values.

e. Normal Values. The response pattern changes with age, gender, and development. After 6 months of age and before puberty, basal levels for both LH and FSH are frequently less than 2 IU/l. Stimulated levels less than 5 IU/l are indicative of hypogonadotropism, and levels in excess of 50 IU/l are indicative of hypergonadotropinism. With a few exceptions, the increase in both gonadotropins should be similar in magnitude. Girls within a year of menarche often have FSH levels about twice those of LH. Individuals with mild or partial steroid biosynthetic defects often have higher LH than FSH levels.

f. General Considerations. Patients need not remain seated but can walk about during the test. There are many units for LH and FSH. Be sure to check that the units reported by the laboratory are the same units used for reporting normal values.

J. Test for Diabetes Insipidus: Water Deprivation Test

a. Indications. This protocol is most useful in the diagnosis of diabetes insipidus and in differentiating among neurogenic (hypothalamic central) diabetes insipidus, nephrogenic (renal) diabetes insipidus, and primary polydipsia (inappropriate thirst mechanism or psychogenic diabetes insipidus).

b. Preparation. No special preparation is necessary. Treatment for diabetes insipidus with vasopressin, desmopressin (DDAVP), or analogs should be discontinued 48–72 h before the protocol. Careful attention to the possibility of dehydration should be given after the medications are stopped.

c. Medication. After obtaining the first pair of urine and plasma samples, water and food are restricted for 3 h. At the end of the period of restriction, a second pair of urine and plasma samples is obtained. No food or drink may be consumed during the protocol.

d. Sampling. Paired samples are evaluated for urine osmolality (Uosm) and plasma osmolality (Posm).

e. Normal Values. At any time during the protocol, baseline Uosm in excess of 400 mOsm/kg with normal Posm (between 275 and 300 mOsm/kg) eliminates a diagnosis of diabetes insipidus. Baseline Uosm less than 300 mOsm/kg with normal Posm is consistent either with overhydration or with diabetes insipidus. After the 3 h water-deprivation period, individuals with overhydration or with diabetes insipidus may still have Uosm less than 30 mOsm/kg. However, individuals with overhydration have Posm between 275 and 290 mOsm/kg while Posm remains above 290 mOsm/kg in individuals with diabetes insipidus.

f. General Considerations. Some physicians have extended the period of water deprivation to 7 h or even longer. However, care must be taken to ensure that the patient does not ingest water surreptitiously and/or does not become dehydrated.

Addendum 1 Reference Table for the Conversion of Current Units to SI Units

Substance	Conventional unit (CU)	Conversion factor (CF)	SI unit (Cu × CF)
Aldosterone	ng/dl	0.027	nmol/l
Androstenedione	ng/dl	0.0349	nmol/l
Andosterone	ng/dl	0.0349	nmol/l
Corticosterone	ng/ml	2.89	nmol/l
Cortisol	μg/dl	27.59	nmol/l
18-0H-corticosterone	ng/dl	27.9	pmol/l
DHEA	ng/dl	0.0347	nmol/l
DHEAS	μg/dl	0.026	μmol/l
11-deoxicorticosterone	ng/dl	0.0303	nmol/l
11-Deoxicortisol	ng/dl	0.02886	nmol/l
Dehydrotestosterone	ng/dl	0.0344	nmol/l
17-β-Estradiol (E2)	ng/dl	36.71	pmol/l
Estriol (E3)	μg/l	3.47	nmol/l
Estrone (E1)	pg/ml	3.70	nmol/l
FSH	mIU/ml	1	IU/ml
Glucose	mg/dl	0.0555	mmol/l
Growth hormone	ng/ml	1	mg/l
17-hydroxyprogesterone	ng/dl	0.03029	nmol/l
Insulin-like growth factor-I	ng/ml	0.1307	nmol/l
LH	mIU/ml	1	IU/ml
Parathyroid hormone intact	pg/ml	0.1053	pmol/l
Progesterone	ng/dl	0.0318	nmol/l
Renin (plasma rennin activity)	ng/ml/h	1	mg/l/h
Testosterone	ng/dl	0.03467	nmol/l
Testosterone, free	pg/ml	3.4673	pmol/l
Thyroglobulin	pg/ml	1	mg/l
TSH	mIU/ml	1	mIU/l
Thyroid of radioactive iodine	%	0.01	
Thyrotropin releasing hormone	pg/ml	2.759	pmol/l
Thyroxine total	μg/dl	12.9	nmol/l
Thyroxine free	ng/dl	12.9	pmol/l
Transcortin	mg/dl	10	mg/l
Triiodothyronine total	ng/dl	0.0154	nmol/l
Triiodothyronine free	pg/dl	× 0.01536	pmol/l
Urine			
Cathecolamine fractionated:			
Norepinephrine	mg/24 h	5.911	nmol/24 h
Epinephrine	μg/24 h	5.458	nmol/24 h
Dopamine	μg/24 h	6.528	nmol/24 h
17-hydroxycorticosteroids	mg/day	2.759	mmol/day
17-ketosteroids (urine)	mg/24 h	2.76	μmol/24 h

REFERENCES

1. Chasalow FI, Ginsberg LJ. Laboratory aids and tolerance in pediatric endocrinology: a practical approach. In: Lifshitz F. Textbook of Pediatric Endocrinology. 3rd ed. New York: Marcel Dekker, 1996:861.
2. Blum WF, Hom N, Kratzsch J, et al. Clinical studies of IGF-BP-3 by radioimmunoassay. Growth Regul 1993; 3: 100–104.
3. Martin JL, Baxter RC. Insulin-like growth factor binding protein-3: biochemistry and physiology. Growth Regul 1992; 2:88–99.
4. Leung KC, Ho KK. Measurement of growth hormone, insulin-like growth factor I and their binding proteins:

the clinical aspects. Clin Chim Acta 2001; 313:119–123.

5. Shalet SM, Toogood A, Rahim A, and Brennan B. The diagnosis of growth hormone deficiency in children and adults. Endocrinol Rev 1998; 19(2):202–223.

6. Keefer JF. Endocrinology. In: The Harriet Lane Handbook. 15th ed. St. Louis: Mosby, 2000:216.

7. Lofqvist C, Andersson E, Gelander L, Rosberg S, Blum WF, Wikland KA. Reference values for IGF-I throughout childhood and adolescence: a model that accounts simultaneously for the effect of gender, age and puberty. J Clin Endocrinol Metab 2001; 86:5870–5876.

8. Chrysis DC, Alexandrides TK, Koromantzou E, Georgopoulos N, Vassilakos P, Kiess W, Kratsch J, Beratis NG, Spiliotis BE. Novel application of IGF-I and IGFBP-3 generation tests in the diagnosis of growth hormone axis disturbances in children with beta-thalassaemia. Clin Endocrinol (Oxf) 2001; 54(2):253–259.

9. Reiter EO, Morris AH, MacGillivray MH, Weber D. Variable estimates of serum growth hormone concentrations by different radioassay systems. J Clin Endocrinol Metab 1988; 66:68–71.

10. Ceiniker AC, Chen AB, Wert RM, Sherman BM. Variability in the quantitation of circulating growth hormone using commercial immunoassays. J Clin Endocrinol Metab 1989; 68:469–476.

11. Gonc EN, Yordam N, Kandemir N, Alikasifoglu A. Comparison of stimulated growth hormone levels in primed versus unprimed provocative tests. The effect of various testosterone doses on growth hormone levels. Horm Res 2001; 56:32–37.

12. Rosenfield RL, Furlanetto RW. Physiologic testosterone or estradiol induction of puberty increases plasma somatomedin C. J Pediatr 1985; 107:415–417.

13. Martinez AS, Domene HM, Ropelato MG, Jasper HG, Pennisi PA, Escobar ME, Heinrich JJ. Estrogen priming effect on growth hormone (GH) provocative test: a useful tool for the diagnosis of GH deficiency. J Clin Endocrinol Metab 2000; 85(11):4168–4172.

14. Weldon VV, Gupta SK, Klingensmith G, et al. Evaluation of growth hormone release in children using arginine and L-dopa in combination. J Pediatr 1975; 87:540–544.

15. Alba-Roth J, Muller OA, Schopohl J, Von Werder K. Arginine stimulates growth hormone secretion by suppressing endogenous somatostatin secretion. J Clin Endocrinol Metab 1988; 67:1186–1189.

16. Mauras N, Walton P, Nicar M, Welch S, Rogol AD. Growth hormone stimulation testing in both short and normal statured children: use of an immunofunctional assay. Pediatr Res 2000; 48:614–618.

17. Lanes R, Recker B, Fort P, Lifshitz F. Low dose oral clonidine a simple and reliable growth hormone screening test. Am J Dis Child 1985; 139:87–88.

18. Fraser NC, Seth J, Brown S. Clonidine is a better test for growth hormone deficiency than insulin hypoglycemia. Arch Dis Child 1983; 58:355–358.

19. Philippi H, Pohlenz J, Grimm W, Koffler T, Schonberger W. Simultaneous stimulation of growth hormone, adrenocorticotropin and cortisol with L-dopa/L-carbidopa and propranolol in children of short stature. Acta Paediatr 2000; 89:442–446.

20. Huang C. Hypoglycemia associated with clonidine testing for growth hormone deficiency. J Pediatr 2001; 139:323–324.

21. Pineda J, Dieguez C, Casanueva FF, Martul P. Decreased growth hormone response to dexamethasone stimulation test in obese children. Acta Paediatr 1994; 83:103–105.

22. Martul P, Pineda J, Pombo M, Penalva A, Bokser L, Dieguez C. New diagnostic tests of GH reserve. J Pediatr Endocrinol 1993; 6:317–323.

23. Casanueva FF, Burguera B, Alvarez CV, Zugaza JL, Pombo M, Dieguez. Corticoids as a new stimulus of growth hormone secretion in man. J Pediatr Endocrinol 1992; 5:85–90.

24. Eisenstein E, Plotnick L, Lanes R, Lee P, Migeon C, Kowarski AA. Evaluation of the growth hormone exercise test in normal and growth hormone deficient children. Pediatrics 1978; 62:526.

25. Buckler JMH. Plasma growth hormone response to exercise as a diagnostic aid. Arch Dis Child 1973; 48:565–567.

26. Loche S, Cella SG, Puggione R, Stabilini L, Pintor C, Muller EE. The effects of galanin secretion on growth hormone secretion in children of normal and short stature. Pediatr Res 1989; 26:316–319.

27. Bauer FE, Rokaeus A, Jomvall H, McDonald TJ, Mutt V. Growth hormone release in man induced by galanin, a new hypothalamic peptide. Lancet 1986; 2:192–195.

28. Takano K, Hizuka N, Shizume L, et al. Plasma growth hormone (GH) response to GH-releasing factor in normal children with short stature and patients with primary dwarfism. J Clin Endocrinol Metab 1984; 58:236–241.

29. Butenandt 0. Diagnostic value of growth hormone-releasing hormone tests in short children. Acta Paediatr Scand (Suppl) 1989; 349:93–99.

30. Martha PM, Blizzard RM, McDonald JA, Thomer MO, Rogol AD. A persistent pattern of varying pituitary responsiveness to exogenous growth hormone (GH) releasing hormone in GH deficient children: evidence supporting periodic somatostatin secretion. J Clin Endocrinol Metab 1988; 67:449–454.

31. Gelato MC, Malozowski S, Caruso-Nicoletti M, et al. Growth hormone (GH) responses to GH-releasing hormone during pubertal development in normal boys and girls: comparison to idiopathic short stature and GH deficiency. J Clin Endocrinol Metab 1986; 63:174–179.

32. Maghnie M, Salati B, Bianchi S, Rallo M, Tinelli C, Autelli M, Aimaretti G, Ghigo E. Relationship between the morphological evaluation of the pituitary and the growth hormone (GH) response to GH-releasing hormone plus arginine in children and adults with congenital hypopituitarism. J Clin Endocrinol Metab 2001; 86:1574–1579.

33. Schmiegelow M, Lassen S, Poulsen HS, Feldt-Rasmussen U, Schmiegelow K, Hertz H, Muller J. Growth hormone response to a growth hormone-releasing hormone stimulation test in a population-based study following cranial irradiation of childhood brain tumors. Horm Res 2000; 54:53–59.

34. Leong KS, Walker AB, Martin I, Wile D, Wilding J, MacFarlane IA. An audit of 500 subcutaneous glucagon stimulation tests to assess growth hormone and ACTH secretion in patients with hypothalamic-pituitary disease. Clin Endocrinol 2001; 54:463–468.

35. Mitchell ML, Savin CT. Growth hormone responses to glucagon in diabetic and non-diabetic persons. Isr J Med Sci 1972; 8:867.

36. Furlanetto RW, Underwood LE, VanWyk JJ, D'Ercole AJ. Estimation of somatomedin C levels in normals and patients with pituitary disease by radioimmunoassay. J Clin Invest 1977; 50:648–657.

37. Plotnick LP, Van Meter QL, Kowarski AA. Human growth hormone treatment of children with growth failure and normal growth hormone level by radioimmunoassay: lack of correlation with somatomedin generation. Pediatrics 1983; 71:324–327.

38. Jorgensen JOL, Blum WF, Moller N, Ranke MB, Christiansen JS. Short-term changes in serum insulin-like growth factors (IGF) and IGF binding protein 3 after different modes of intravenous growth hormone (GH) exposure in GH-deficient patients. J Clin Endocrinol Metab 1991; 72:582–587.

39. Buckway CK, Guevara-Aguirre J, Pratt KL, Burren CP, Rosenfeld RG. The IGF-I generation test revisited: a marker of growth hormone insensitivity. J Clin Endocrinol Metabol 2001; 86:5176–5183.

40. Shah A, Stanhope R, Mathew D. Hazards of pharmacological tests of growth hormone secretion in childhood. Br Med J 1992; 304:173–174.

41. Greenwood FC, Landon J, Stamp TCB. The plasma sugar, free fatty acid cortisol and growth hormone response to insulin in control subjects. J Clin Invest 1966; 45:429–436.

42. Brauman H, Gregoire F. The growth hormone response to insulin induced hypoglycemia in anorexia nervosa and control underweight or normal subjects. Eur J Clin Invest 1975; 5:289–295.

43. Weldon VV, Gupta SK, Haymond MW, et al. The use of L-dopa in the diagnosis of hyposomatropinism in children. J Clin Endocrinol Metab 1973; 36:42–46.

44. Veldhuis JD, Johnson ML. A novel general biophysical model for simulating episodic endocrine gland signaling. Am J Physiol 1988; 255:E740–E759.

45. Tapanainen P, Rantala H, Leppaluoto J, Lautala P, Kaar M-L, Knip M. Nocturnal release of immunoreactive growth-hormone releasing hormone and growth hormone in normal children. Pediatr Res 1989; 26:404–409.

46. Pugliese M, Lifshitz F, Fort P, Cervantes C, Recker B, Ginsberg L. Pituitary function assessment in short stature by a combined hormonal-stimulation test. Am J Dis Child 1987; 141:556–561.

47. Verges B, Boureille F, Goudet P, Murat A, Beckers A, Sassolas G, Cougard P, Chambe B, Montvernay C, Calender A. Pituitary disease in MEN type 1 (MEN1): data from the France-Belgium MEN1 multicenter study. J Clin Endocrinol Metab 2002; 87(2):457–465.

48. Brandi ML, Gagel RF, Angeli A, Bilezikian JP, Beck-Peccoz P, Bordi C, Conte-Devolx B, Falchetti A, Gheri RG, Libroia A, Lips CJ, Lombardi G, Mannelli M, Pacini F, Ponder BA, Raue F, Skogseid B, Tamburrano G, Thakker RV, Thompson NW, Tomassetti P, Tonelli F, Wells SA Jr, Marx SJ. Guidelines for diagnosis and therapy of MEN type 1 and type 2. J Clin Endocrinol Metab 2001; 86: 5658–5671.

49. Burke G. The triiodothyronine suppression test. Am J Med 1967; 42:600–608.

50. Ramos CD, Zantut-Wittmann DE, Tambascia MA, Assumpcao L, Etchebehere EC, Camargo EE. Thyroid suppression test with L-thyroxine and [99mTc] pertechnetate. Clin Endocrinol 2000; 52(4):471.

51. Whitley RJ. Thyrotropin-releasing hormone (TRH) stimulation test. Am Assoc Clin Chem Endocr In-Service Training Contin Educ 1993; 11:207–209.

52. Spencer CA, Schwarzbein D, Guttler RB, et al. Thyrotropin (TSH)-releasing hormone stimulation test responses employing third and fourth generation TSH assays. J Clin Endocrinol Metab 1993; 76:494–498.

53. Marx SJ. Hyperparathyroid and hypoparathyroid disorders. N Engl J Med 2000; 343:1863–1875.

54. Jones KH, Fourman P. Edetic acid test of parathyroid insufficiency. Lancet 1963; 2:119–121.

55. Ellsworth R, Howard JE. Studies on the physiology of the parathyroid glands. VII. Some responses of normal human kidneys and blood to intravenous parathyroid extracts. Bull Johns Hopkins Hosp 1934; 55:296.

56. Chase LR, Melson GL, Aurbach GD. Pseudohypoparathyroidism: defective excretion of 3′,5′-AMP in response to parathyroid hormone. J Clin Invest 1969; 48:1832–1844.

57. Mikati MA, Melham RE, Najjar SS. The syndrome of hyperostosis and hyperphosphatemia. J Pediatr 1981; 99: 900–904.

58. Buckman M, Kaminsky N, Conway M, et al. Utility of L-dopa and water loading in evaluating hyperprolactinemia. J Clin Endocrinol Metab 1973; 36:911–919.

59. Foley TP, Jacobs LS, Hoffman W, et al. Human prolactin and thyrotropin concentrations in normal and hypopituitary children before and after administration of synthetic TRH. J Clin Invest 1972; 51:2143–2150.

60. Blethen SL, Chasalow FI. Overnight dexamethasone suppression test: normal responses and the diagnosis of Cushing's syndrome. Steroids 1989; 54:185–193.

61. Savage MO, Lienhardt A, Lebrethon MC, Johnston LB, Huebner A, Grossman AB, Afshar F, Plowman PN, Besser GM. Cushing's disease in childhood: presentation, investigation, treatment and long-term outcome. Horm Res 2001; 55 Suppl 1:24–30.

62. Liddle GW. Test of pituitary-adrenal suppressibility in the diagnosis of Cushing's syndrome. J Clin Endocrinol 1960; 20:1539.

63. Newell-Price J, Grossman AB. The differential diagnosis of Cushing's syndrome. Ann Endocrinol (Paris) 2001; 62(2):173–179.

64. Abdu TA, Clayton RN. Comparison of the low dose short Synacthen test (1 μg), the conventional short synacthen tests (250 μg), and the insulin tolerance test for assessment of the hypothalamo-pituitary-adrenal axis in patients with pituitary disorders. J Clin Endocrinol Metab 1999; 84: 838–843.

65. Thaler LM, Blevins L. The low dose (1 μg) adrenocorticotropin stimulation test in the evaluation of patients with suspected central adrenal insufficiency. J Clin Endocrinol Metab 1998; 83:2726–2729.

66. Temeck W, Pang S, Nelson C, New MI. Genetic defects of steroidogenesis in premature adrenarche. J Clin Endocrinol Metab 1987; 64:609–617.

67. Childs DF, Bu'lock DE, Anderson DC. Adrenal steroidogenesis in heterozygotes for 21-hydroxylase deficiency. Clin Endocrinol (Oxf) 1979; 11:391–398.

68. Gutai P, Kowarski AA, Migeon CJ. The detection of heterozygote carrier for congenital virilizing adrenal hyperplasia. J Pediatr 1977; 90:924–929.

69. Granoff AB, Chasalow FI, Blethen SL. 17-Hydroxyprogesterone responses to adrenocorticotrophin in children with premature adrenarche. J Clin Endocrinol Metab 1985; 60:409–415.

70. Yanovski JA, Cutler GB Jr, Chrousos GP, Nieman LK. The dexamethasone-suppressed corticotropin-releasing hormone stimulation test differentiates mild Cushing's disease from normal physiology. J Clin Endocrinol Metab 1998; 83:348–352.

71. Hawkins LA, Chasalow FI, Blethen SL. The role of adrenocorticotrophin testing in evaluating girls with prema-

ture adrenarche and hirsutism/oligomenorrhea. J Clin Endocrinol Metab 1992; 74:248–253.

72. Liddle GW, Estep HL, Kendall KW, et al. Clinical application of a new test of pituitary reserve. J Clin Endocrinol 1959; 19:875.

73. Gold EM, Kent JR, Forsharn PH. Clinical use of a new diagnostic agent methoapyrapone (SU-4885), in pituitary and adrenocortical disorders. Ann Intern Med 1961; 54: 175.

74. Sparks LL, Smile RP, Pilots FC, Forsham PH. Experience with a rapid oral methadone test and the plasma ACTH content in determining the cause of Cushing's syndrome. Metabolism 1969; 18:175–192.

75. Schulman D, Zamanillo J, Lowitt S, et al. Effect of clonidine upon anterior pituitary function and plasma catecholamine concentrations in short children and adolescents. J Pediatr Endocrinol 1985; 1:211–216.

76. Mannelli M, Ianni L, Cilotti A, Conti A. Pheochromocytoma in Italy: a multicentric retorspective study. Euro J of Endocrinol 1999; 141:619–624.

77. LeFebvre PJ, Cession-Fossion A, Luyckx AS. Glucagon test for phaeochromocytoma. Lancet 1966; 2:1366.

78. Murray RD, Peacey SR, Rahim A, Toogood AA, Thorner MO, Shalet SM. The diagnosis of growth hormone deficiency (GHD) in successfully treated acromegalic patients. Clin Endocrinol (Oxf) 2001; 54:37–44.

79. Rosenbloom AL, Wheller L, Bianchi R, Chin FT, Tiwary CM, Grgic A. Age-adjusted analysis of insulin responses during normal and glucose tolerance tests in children and adults. Diabetes 1975; 24:820–828.

80. American Diabetes Association. Screening for Diabetes (Position Statement) Diabetes Care 2002; 25:S21–S24.

81. Cornblath M, Schwartz R. Disorders of Carbohydrate Metabolism in Infancy. Philadelphia: WB Saunders, 1976: 355–361.

82. Comblath M, Poth M. Hypoglycemia. In: Kaplan S, ed. Clinical Pediatric and Adolescent Endocrinology. Philadelphia: WB Saunders, 1982:157–170.

83. Stanley CA, Baker L. Hyperinsulinism in infants and children: diagnosis and therapy. Adv Pediatr 1976; 23:324–325.

84. Rogers DG, Chasalow FI, Blethen SL. Partial deficiency in 17-ketosteroid reductase deficiency presenting as gynecomastia. Steroids 1985; 45:195–200.

85. Saez JM, Bertand J. Studies on testicular function in children: plasma concentrations of testosterone, dehydroepian-

drosterone and its sulfate before and after stimulation with human chorionic-gonadotropin. Steroids 1968; 12:749–761.

86. Chasalow FI, Blethen SL, Marr HB, French FS. An improved method for evaluating testosterone biosynthetic defects. Pediatr Res 1984; 18:759–763.

87. Zachmann M. Evaluation of gonadal function in childhood and adolescence. Helv Pediatr Acta (Suppl) 1974; 34:53–62.

88. Matthews MJ, Parker DC, Rebar RW, et al. Sleep associated gonadotropin and oestradiol patterns in girls with precocious sexual development. Clin Endocrinol (Oxf) 1982; 17:601–607.

89. Zung A, Raisin A, Zadik Z, Chen M. Nocturnal integrated gonadotropin concentrations in evaluating pubertal transition in girls. J Pediatr Endocrinol Metab 2000; 13:417–423.

90. Roth JC, Kelch SL, Kaplan SI, Grumbach MM. FSH and LH responses to luteinizing hormone releasing factor in prepubertal and pubertal children, adult males, and patients with hypogonadotropic and hypergonadotropic hypogonadism. J Clin Endocrinol Metab 1972; 35:926–930.

91. Partsch CJ, Hummetink R, Lorenzen F, Sippell WG. Significance of the LHRH test in diagnosis of premature sexual development in girls: the stimulated LH/FSH ratio differentiates between central precocious puberty and premature thelarche. Monatsschr Kinderheilkd 1989; 137:284–288.

92. Job JC, Gamier PE, Chaussain JL, Milhaud G. Elevation of serum gonadotropins (LF and FSH) after releasing hormone (LH-RH) in normal children and patients with disorders of puberty. J Clin Endocrinol Metab 1972; 35:473–476.

93. Chasalow FI, Granoff AB, Tse TF, Blethen SL. Adrenal steroid secretion in girls with pseudoprecocious puberty due to autonomous ovarian cysts. J Clin Endocrinol Metab 1986; 63:82.

94. Richman RA, Post EM, Notman DD, Hochberg Z, Moses AM. Simplifying the diagnosis of diabetes insipidus in children. Am J Dis Child 1981; 135:839–841.

95. Frasier SD, Kutnik LA, Schmidt RT, Smith FG. A water deprivation test for the diagnosis of diabetes insipidus in children. Am J Dis Child 1967; 114:157–160.

96. Robertson GL. Diagnosis of diabetes insipidus. Horm Res 1985; 13:176–189.

42

Reimbursement Issues in Endocrinology: A Coding Supplement

Bridget F. Recker
Staten Island University Hospital, Staten Island, New York, U.S.A.

I. REIMBURSEMENT

There are many so many issues related to reimbursement that simply thinking about reimbursement could fill you with dread. The complexities of practicing medicine, coding your services, and being reimbursed for your services has led to the creation of many separate businesses. How then can any practitioner not become overwhelmed with the task?

There are over 7000 current procedural terminology (CPT) codes and the International Classification of Diseases 10 (ICD-10) is already in use. As soon as you learn to assimilate all you need to know about documentation, billing, and reimbursement, new, improved coding is implemented. The basis for all coding and reimbursement is reflected in the patients' medical record documentation. If it is not written down as being assessed, discussed, or performed, it was not done. With audits being done routinely by third-party payers, the failure to recognize this important factor and respond to it can be costly.

A sure sign that this problem is greater than us is the number of companies that have sprung up to address your practice nightmares. Companies that teach, assess, implement, and provide the actual services included in medical practice management increase annually. Medicine has led to the creation of an entire industry. I think the industries supporting medical practices are doing better than the medical practices, for they will not provide the service without definite reimbursement dollars from the practice. Unfortunately, medical practices are having greater fiscal management problems than ever. When did you lose control over your fate?

II. CPT CODING

The CPT codes for medical and healthcare services change annually. Many books define these codes and give some examples. Since the codes are updated annually, you need a new guidebook annually. If there is a new book with updated codes and new rules, you have to learn how to use them to your benefit. As you can see, without a lot of work and learning, you can never know all about coding.

CPT Codes are standardized five-digit codes describing the services provided during health care/medical encounters. Each encounter needs to be clearly documented in the patient's medical record. Documentation that reflects the stated billed codes must be written. The fact that a code is published does not ensure that all insurers you deal with will accept that code. Also, some patients' policies may specifically exclude certain codes.

Making matters more mystifying is that some insurance companies have created their own internal codes that relate to published CPT codes. However, you are not given the road map with which to decipher their system. When a submitted code is queried or denied, it becomes more difficult to understand what has been denied and what has been approved for payment. With the CPT codes being updated annually, little lag time is given for correct coding. These updates attempt to stay current with trends in clinical practice by adding, updating, and revising codes to reflect changing technology and practice. Once a code has been changed, you have a specific period of time in which to update your billing system. When staff or billing services do not make the appropriate changes, financial difficulties ensue. For instance, Medicare gives you a definite date after which a code that has been changed will no longer be recognized for reimbursement. After that time, you are not able to appeal or recoup your loses. Why would Medicare standards be important to you? Because most third-party payers follow Medicare rules within a short period of time.

The reimbursement schedule for services (CPT codes) is driven by the Resource-Based Relative Value System (RBRVS). These values are also updated annually and published in the *Federal Register*. The Health Care Financing Administration (HCFA) introduced RBRVS in 1992 to quantify health care and equalize reimbursement. Under this system a national standardized fee schedule for payments to physicians was enacted. In 2001 HCFA's name changed and is now known as the Centers for Medicare and Medicaid Services (CMS).

The RBRVS incorporates the cost of resources required including time, mental effort, practice overhead, stress, technical skill, and malpractice costs. All of Medicare fees as well as the greater portion of private insurer fees are now based on this system. Many third-party payers including Medicaid programs and managed care organizations are using variations of the Medicare RBRVS to determine physician reimbursement and capitation rates. Since the RBRVS fee schedule was developed for Medicare originally, particular pediatric CPT codes and practice expense issues were not addressed. Work on this issue continues by the American Academy of Pediatrics. CPT codes are the property of the American Medical Association.

There are also modifiers involved in CPT coding and these are added like a suffix to a word. Success with CPT modifier reporting requires a thorough review of CPT guidelines and some detective work to identify heath plan requirements for specific modifier codes. The modifier that should be used most frequently is −25. It identifies an evaluation and management service separately provided on the same day as a procedure. You should be using this modifier more than you think. You should use a separate ICD9 code for the office visit and the procedure. There are also HCPCS codes, which represent nonphysician services such as medications, intravenous (IV) solutions of varying volumes, sterile trays, supplies, and durable medical equipment.

Handheld personal digital assistants (PDAs) can be used with CPT software to customize practice coding, improve record keeping (particularly in-patient data), and improve billing. You can have at your fingertips the fields necessary to capture important patient data and the coding necessary to define your encounter. The downloading capabilities will forever free you from those little note pads you try to keep track of and submit to the practice billing office in a timely manner.

III. ICD-9 (ICD-10 COMING)

The International Classification of Diseases (ICD-9) (1) documents specific diagnoses, signs, and symptoms. Codes for special screening states, accidents, injuries, or adverse events are included. ICD was developed by the World Health Organization to accumulate and analyze international morbidity and mortality data. In 1989, the government mandated the use of ICD-9 coding. It describes the clinical situation the patient is in, thus giving third-party payers a clinical picture of the individual. The ICD code establishes the link with the CPT code. For instance, a CPT code for a thyroid biopsy would never be reimbursed for an individual seen with an ICD code for a foot infection. The link between these two entities does not exist and the medical necessity of the procedure is not established. ICD-9 is also updated annually with changes, and now the new version of this the ICD-10 is on our doorstep. ICD-9 and HCPCS codes are maintained and regulated by CMS.

As an example, you see a patient every few months or so for evaluation and management of hypothyroidism. The simple ICD-9 code for this encounter and the one most frequently used by most practitioners is 245.2 or Hashimoto's disease. But did the patient raise any other issues you considered or evaluated such as brittle nails (703.8), dry skin (701.1), puffy eyes (374.82), hair loss (704.00), tiredness (780.79), abnormal weight gain (783.1), or throat pain (784.1)? Perhaps one of the later issues required the greatest amount of thought and discussion but you did not address the issue in the medical documentation for the patient. Maybe one of the later issues should have been the diagnostic code for the encounter, followed by the hypothyroid code. Such inclusions could support the need for a higher use of evaluation and management codes, requested follow-up appointments, and laboratory evaluations.

The ICD for mortality has been modified approximately every 10 years. The ICD-10 is the first revision since 1979. Revisions are necessary for the same reason that CPT codes are revised: to reflect changing medical science and technology. ICD-10 varies from the previous version (2) in detail: double the number of categories listed, a change to alphanumeric coding, rearrangement of chapters, addition of chapters, titles for cause of death have been changed, and conditions reordered. Some of the coding rules have also changed. Further information on the states' implementation of ICD-10 can be found at the NCHS website.

IV. LINKING CPT AND ICD CODING

Creating the link between CPT codes and ICD codes is essential for practice survival. If you provide prolonged attendance to a patient, it must be linked to a specific event. For instance, if a patient experiences hypotension during an arginine test, the ICD code for this occurrence would be related to E944.5: an adverse effect of arginine in therapeutic use. If a child experienced nausea or vomiting following levodopa administration, it would be a toxic effect of levodopa: E936.4.

Evaluations of medical practices are challenging, time-consuming, and costly. Clinicians do not always attend to economic evaluations and this may lead to overlooked clinical benefits and needless costs. Practitioners need to be well informed and remain current in their knowledge of CPT and ICD coding. The individual who signs the bill is ultimately responsible for any bill submitted in their name. This responsibility lasts beyond the signature and encompasses the entire billing process. Practitioners need to audit their billing processes and react to discovered inconsistencies. This in itself will improve reimbursement.

V. COLLECTIONS

The collection process begins at the front desk. The importance of this step in providing care and expecting to be reimbursed for your skill is frequently undervalued. Practices such as mailing a new patient packet prior to an individual's first office contact or requesting that an individual arrive early to complete necessary paperwork can save time and prevent errors. Patients need to be clearly informed in a professional manner as to exactly what the office policy is regarding payment and reimbursement. The patient information sheet should be reviewed and any areas that have been omitted or are unclear should be clarified. The front desk staff sets the tone for your office. A calm, professional, relaxed manner will aid in collecting needed payments from patients. The practice expectations should be clearly stated, with all options for payment given at the time of service.

Patient intake is the most important time frame for timely reimbursement. Having correct information at the start of every encounter will hasten reimbursement. Forms, which maximize patient responsibility, must be completed annually. Employees must be trained in the correct policies and procedures of the office billing system. They must be held responsible for knowing them and for adhering to them. Control of patients at the front desk is of paramount importance. Communication skills are essential for discussing billing issues with patients and gaining an understanding of and cooperation with even the most unreasonable and difficult individuals encountered in the process. Linking the salaries of individuals specifically involved with the billing process to reimbursement (accounts receivable) seems a win–win arrangement.

Talking money is extremely difficult and uncomfortable for most practitioners. Yet this is an extremely essential skill. Presenting programs that may not be covered by insurers should not determine their fate. Learning how to talk to customers about these programs and get them

to commit to them can be as easy as selling vitamins. When you know that an insurer does not cover a particular service, let the patient know this up front and resolve the payment problem prior to delivering the service rather than after the service is given. There is a high price to pay for insurance snags and the duplicate work effort required of your staff handling these issues.

Requesting payment in the right manner with the right approach is essential and should be the only behavior you accept from the front desk staff. It is difficult to understate the importance of this step. If reimbursement for provided services is denied due to improper patient information, the only one to blame for the delay in payment is you. A copy of your practice's general billing policies should be given to patients both new and established. Policies should include the law regarding waiving copayments and deductibles and any other insurer-specific payments. Exemptions to these policies due to financial hardship would need to be clearly written and documentation provided to analyze the situation fully.

VI. DENIAL AND APPEAL

Claims are denied at an almost predictable rate. Claims are denied with the knowledge that most denials are accepted by practices without queries or action. It is assumed that medical providers do not have the time, knowledge, or experience to investigate the reason for or purpose of the claims denial. Delayed insurance payments weaken your practice financially. A thoughtful, established plan to avoid this occurrence should be in place.

Explanations of benefits (EOBs) often state only "claim denied" and you have to guess at the reason for the denial. Not accepting the statement that a claim is denied is worth the time and effort to reply aggressively. EOBs must be reviewed on a regular basis in order to keep current with your practice reimbursement expectations. A thorough review of EOBs will help to identify the particular insurer or code that is leading to decreased revenues. Tackling the major problem and resolving it can only spur you on to taking greater control of your practice's future.

Numerous denials are overturned following the first appeal letter. However, if not overturned you must continue to file appeals until you receive an acceptable answer. It is important to keep the appeal active until it is resolved. Once a practitioner or practice is noted to be persistent regarding appeals, the carrier begins to recognize them as someone who will follow through on the appeal process. In this case, if cloudy issues arise on your claims, they will most likely be paid so that the insurer does not hear from you.

If your appeal was reviewed and remains denied, you should request other individuals to review it, such as the company president or legal counsel. Your letters to them should be concise and state your case clearly. The person reviewing your claim may not have enough knowledge of your specialty to have made an informed decision. You may have other cases in which the same insurer approved such treatment. You should try to speak on equal terms to those in control of the appeal. Once an appeal moves up to the next level, you must be diligent in addressing issues on a like plane: physician to physician, or physician to president or legal counsel, not physician to administrative assistant or clerk. Recognizing that you are extremely busy and time pressured, the importance of this task cannot fall to anyone other than you. If it is not important enough for you to get on the telephone, it will probably not be important enough for them to reverse their decision on the denial. You can also petition for a face-to-face meeting, with support personnel invited, to further address the issue under consideration. It is always prudent to request a written response to all issues and to keep all communication filed.

As an example, arginine 10% intravenous solution used in growth hormone evocative testing is an unlisted drug in the CPT codes. If filed electronically, this charge will automatically be denied as all unlisted codes are. This claim must go to paper to be considered. Along with the drug, the package label's administration instructions clearly state that the patient must be placed at bed rest for at least 30 min prior to the infusion. This additional 30 min of professional time should therefore be included in the fees for the test.

Another line of financial fallout is underpayment of claims. Medical reimbursement rates are readily accessible to the public. Many companies can provide average reimbursement rates (fee analyzers) broken down by CPT code, medical specialty, and geographic location. Software programs are also available to assist in this effort. This is a robust tool to evaluate underpayment on claims. This information can be used to appeal poorly paid claims by attaching a letter with the usual and customary rate and the reimbursed fee received. Knowledge of this method of practice fee-setting is a concise way to negotiate with third-party payers. It allows for an actual cost of your services for each CPT code; this is then used in contract negotiation. As your malpractice or overhead increases, these increases can be factored into the CPT codes equally. The recovered amounts can be amazing. Looking for denied claims is not enough; you must look for paid but lowered rates.

Timely filing is of the utmost importance. Filing deadlines are becoming shorter and shorter.

VII. CONTRACTING

Conduct a managed care contract review. Providers should understand the contract requirements and not participate in those plans that result in additional costs. Review, and get clarification if needed on, questionable terminology and the dispute resolution procedures. When you sign

your name on the annual contract with third-party payers, have you reviewed those fees for the services you provide most along with evaluation and management codes? Often when you are in larger practice groups, the decision-makers for the group are only interested in the higher reimbursed codes (such as surgical ones). Yet when your specialty is reviewed, your receivables vs. cost are questioned. Maybe your evocative/suppressive testing codes have been repeatedly denied or rates decreased without you being aware of it. The fees for the codes you use most are the ones you must review before signing any annual contract. The information you receive may eventually lead your practice toward participating in plans that will support your practice's future as well as your patients' care.

VIII. CHART REVIEWS

Third-party payers and managed care organizations are conducting chart reviews and grading physicians on their findings. They are only interested in what was actually written down—documented—in the medical chart. They rate their reviews on the quality of the care you provide. They look for continuity of care including follow up and review of all received reports and records. Audits can lead to fines equal to or greater than the overpayment the reviewers believe you received. The process takes time and creates an enormous amount of stress for you and your staff. Preprinted flow sheets and checklists, which correspond to evaluation and management code components, will help avoid undercoding and overcoding errors. Remember: if it is not documented, it was not done.

IX. STIMULATION TESTING

Receiving reimbursement for stimulation/evocative testing is a function of staffing, setting, time, and the payer. It is a constant struggle in most offices to test patients in a safe environment and receive reimbursement for your time, knowledge, blocking of the test room, and monitoring. Although the American Association of Clinical Endocrinologists (AACE) has the creation of an evocative/suppressive testing code (CPT) on their agenda of tasks to accomplish, it is not at the forefront of current discussions.

A standardized protocol for the evocative/suppressive testing should be in place. Space and time for performing the test should be available. There are many facets to an evocative/suppressive test, including:

Intravenous access
Administration of agents of stimulation/suppression and flush solutions for multiple draws (intravenous, subcutaneous, oral)
Repeated line access
Timed specimen collection
Patient monitoring

Example: Evocative/Suppressive Test Coding

Arginine/Growth Hormone Evocative Test

CPT code	Description
99211–99215	Office/outpatient evaluation and management; established patient
−25 modifier	Separate E&M same day as procedure
90780	IV infusion; up to 1 h
±90781	IV infusion; each additional hour to 8 h (i.e., normal saline drip infusion during test)
J3490	Unlisted drug—Arginine
90784	IV injection—× how many times
J1642	Heparin lock drug—× how many times/units
99000	Handling/transport of specimens

When a physician, nurse practitioner or physician's assistant performs the testing, the prolonged services codes can also be used based on the amount of total face-to-face time delivered.

Know the rules for coding evocative/suppressive testing. Supplies and drugs should be coded, physician attendance if required should be documented and coded, prolonged physician attendance codes are not reported separately if prolong infusion codes are used, and J codes are used to report injectables. It is better to give the patient a prescription for the medications to be used to cut down on practice expenses and the reimbursement follow up.

If reimbursement for testing in your practice area is insufficient, you may need to consider other options. One option is to meet with and negotiate with the insurer to evaluate the issue further. Provide information concerning the medical necessity of the procedure, the testing protocols, and any supporting information relating to specific patient cases. You may need to write a letter to the medical director of the health care plan clearly stating the need and the amount of financial remuneration requested. If the reimbursement dilemma cannot be resolved, a practice policy will have to be decided upon defining under which circumstances testing for membes of those insurers are performed.

X. DIABETIC EDUCATION

Many health plans have limited or no coverage for diabetes training and supplies. Some providers have agreements with insurers to provide for these services. Companies are reviewing outcome measures of diabetes programs such as hemoglobin A1C, eye evaluations, lipid management, and timely monitoring of diabetes complications. They are making reimbursement based on chart audits of these elements. The problems are great and the possible solutions worrisome.

As Medicare sets guidelines for reimbursement linked with American Diabetes Association recognition programs, there are other movements afoot. Pharmacists, in many instances, are being given the pivotal role in diabetes education. Mississippi pharmacists are receiving payments from Medicaid for providing diabetes care to patients. A major insurer in New Jersey that covers near 1 million lives has contracted with a network of pharmacists for diabetes self-management education. The Department of Veterans Affairs is already using its pharmacists to manage diabetes as well as other chronic diseases. The move is on to improve patient outcomes while providing services, especially in the chronic disease management arena. Codes and reimbursement rates are being established for pharmacists. They will not need years of study or extensive knowledge of diabetes to reach a level of skill necessary to provide and be recognized for reimbursement dollars. Pharmacists' time will be valued and compensated. This recognition for pharmacy reimbursement has become known as medication therapy management services (MTMS). The American Society of Consultant Pharamcists has developed a new payment formula for Medicare/Medicaid pharmacy services (3). The fee would be derived by recognizing the product cost, administrative overhead, dispensing fee, and professional services. Does this sound familiar? HCFA appears willing to accept pharmacists as providers of disease management services. The American Medical Association administers the CPT codes and will therefore work with the pharmacy organizations to develop billing codes.

An article in *Drug Topics* (4) reported some interesting findings. Pharmacists responding to a questionnaire (17% response rate) reported that 52% had stopped doing business with a third-party payer. The reason cited by 89% of these pharmacists was low reimbursement rates. Additional issues noted included slow or no payment along with restrictive formularies. Does any of this sound familiar? Eight out of 10 pharmacists reported that their business did not suffer due to this decision. It would probably not be a surprise to find out the payers pharmacists had the most problems with.

What the pharmacies are experiencing with reimbursement issues mimics the experiences of medical practitioners. They are hiring more technicians and less experienced pharmacists as they face a greater volume of work. In many instances, they cannot even afford to hire more technicians. The pharmacists are looking into other areas, including providing immunizations and vaccinations to customers. As physicians struggle with time and effort involved in providing diabetes education, you must wonder if they are aware of the silently evolving change in the future of diabetes education. Do we want to turn this important responsibility as well as others over to local pharmacists?

XI. CLINICAL TRIALS

Whether or not to participate in clinical trials becomes a resource vs. cost and balanced budget decision. Although

Table 1

Code	Diagnosis	4th digit code	5th digit
240	Goiter, simple—4th digit required	240.0	
	Goiter, unspecified—4th digit required	240.9	
241	Nontoxic nodular goiter—4th digit required		
	Nontoxic uninodular goiter	241.0	
	Nontoxic multinodular goiter	241.1	
	Unspecified nontoxic nodular goiter	241.9	
242	Thyrotoxicosis with or without goiter—4th and 5th digit required		
	Without mention of thyrotoxic crisis or storm		0
	With mention of thyrotoxic crisis or storm		1
	Neonatal thyrotoxicosis	775.3	
	Toxic diffuse goiter	242.0	0 or 1
	Toxic uninodular goiter	242.1	0 or 1
	Toxic multinodular goiter	242.2	0 or 1
243	Congenital hypothyroidism		
	Congenital dyshormonogenic goiter	246.1	
244	Acquired hypothyroidism—4th digit required		
245	Thyroiditis—4th digit required		
	Acute thyroiditis	245.0	
	Subacute thyroiditis	245.1	
	Chronic lymphocytic thyroiditis	245.2	
250	Diabetes mellitus—4th and 5th digit required		
	Hypoglycemia in infant of diabetic mother	775.0	
	Neonatal diabetes mellitus	775.1	
	Nonclinical diabetes	790.2	
	Type II—not stated as uncontrolled		0
	Type I—not stated as uncontrolled		1
	Type II—uncontrolled		2
	Type I—uncontrolled		3
	Diabetes mellitus without mention of complication	250.0	
	Diabetes with ketoacidosis; without mention of coma	250.1	
	Diabetes with hyperosmolarity	250.2	
	Diabetes with other coma	250.3	
	Diabetes with renal manifestations; use additional codes to specify manifestation	250.4	
	Diabetes with ophthalmic manifestations; use additional codes to specify manifestation	250.5	
	Diabetes with neurological manifestations; use additional codes to specify manifestation	250.6	
	Diabetes with peripheral circulatory disorders; use additional codes to specify manifestation	250.7	
	Diabetes with other specified manifestations; such as diabetic hypoglycemia, hypoglycemic shock—use additional codes to specify manifestation	250.8	
	Diabetes with unspecified complications	250.9	
251	Other disorders of pancreatic internal secretion—4th digit required		
252	Disorders of parathyroid gland—4th digit required		
	Hyperparathyroidism	252.0	
	Hypoparathyroidism	252.1	
	Other specified disorders of parathyroid gland	252.8	
	Unspecified disorder of parathyroid gland	252.9	
253	Disorders of the pituitary gland and its hypothalamic control—4th digit required		
	Acromegaly and gigantism	253.0	
	Other and unspecified anterior pituitary hyper function	253.1	
	Panhypopituitarism/hypopituitarism	253.2	
	Pituitary dwarfism; isolated deficiency of GH, Lorain-Levi dwarfism	253.3	
	Other anterior pituitary disorders; isolated or partial deficiency of an anterior pituitary hormone other than growth hormone	253.4	
	Diabetes insipidus	253.5	

Table 1   Continued

Code	Diagnosis	4th digit code	5th digit
	Nephrogenic diabetes insipidus	588.1	
	Other disorders of neurohypophysis	253.6	
	Iatrogenic pituitary disorders	253.7	
	Other disorders of the pituitary and other syndromes of diencephalohypophyseal origin	253.8	
	Unspecified; dyspituitarism	253.9	
255	Disorders of adrenal glands—4th digit required		
	Cushing's syndrome; adrenal hyperplasia due to excess ACTH, ectopic ACTH syndrome, iatrogenic syndrome of excess cortisol, overproduction of cortisol	255.0	
	Hyperaldosteronism	255.1	
	Adrenogenital disorders; Adrenogenital syndromes, CAH	255.2	
	Other corticoadrenal over activity	255.3	
	Corticoadrenal insufficiency; Addisonian crisis, Addison's disease NOS	255.4	
256	Ovarian dysfunction—4th digit required		
	Hyperestrogenism	256.0	
	Other ovarian hyperfunction	256.1	
	Postablative ovarian failure	256.2	
	Other ovarian failure; delayed menarche, ovarian hypofunction, primary ovarian failure NOS	256.39	
	Polycystic ovaries	256.4	
	Hirsutism	704.1	
257	Testicular dysfunction—4th digit required		
	Testicular hyperfunction	257.0	
	Postablative testicular hypofunction	257.1	
	Other testicular hypofunction; defective biosynthesis of testicular androgen, eunuchoidism, failure, testicular hypogonadism	257.2	
	Other testicular dysfunction; Goldberg-Maxwell syndrome, male pseudohermaphroditism with testicular feminization, testicular feminization	257.8	
	Unspecified testicular dysfunction	257.9	
	Undescended testis—5th digit required	752.5	1
	Retractile testis—5th digit required	752.5	2
	Other specified anomaly of genital organs/anarchism—4th digit required	752.8	
	Hypospadias—5th digit required	752.6	1
	Epispadias—5th digit required	752.6	2
	Micropenis—5th digit required	752.6	4
	Hidden penis—5th digit required	752.6	5
	Hypospadias—4th digit required	752.7	
258	Polyglandular dysfunction and related disorders—4th digit required		
259	Other endocrine disorders—4th digit required		
	Delay in sexual development and puberty; not elsewhere classified; delayed puberty	259.0	
	Precocious sexual development and puberty, not elsewhere classified; sexual precocity NOS or constitutional, idiopathic, cryptogenic	259.1	
	Carcinoid syndrome	259.2	
	Ectopic hormone secretion, not elsewhere classified; ectopic ADH, ectopic hyperparathyroidism	259.3	
	Dwarfism, not elsewhere classified	259.4	
	Gynecomastia/hypertrophy of the breast	611.1	
	Nutritional deficiencies		
260	Kwashiorkor		
261	Nutritional marasmus		
262	Other severe, protein–calorie malnutrition		
263	Other and unspecified protein–calorie malnutrition—4th digit required		
	Malnutrition of moderate degree; with biochemical changes in electrolytes, lipids, blood plasma	263.0	
	Malnutrition of mild degree	263.1	

Table 1 Continued

Code	Diagnosis	4th digit code	5th digit
	Arrested development following protein–calorie malnutrition; nutritional dwarfism, physical retardation due to malnutrition	263.2	
268	Vitamin D deficiency—4th digit required		
	Vitamin D-resistant: osteomalacia, rickets	275.3	
	Rickets, active	268.0	
	Rickets, late effect	268.1	
	Osteomalacia, unspecified	268.2	
270	Disorders of amino acid transport and metabolism—4th digit required		
271	Disorders of carbohydrate transport and metabolism—4th digit required		
272	Disorders of lipoid metabolism—4th digit required		
783	Symptoms—4th and 5th digit required for some		
	Anorexia; loss of appetite	783.0	
	Anorexia nervosa	307.1	
	Abnormal weight gain	783.1	
	Obesity—5th digit required	278.0	0
	Morbid obesity	278.0	1
	Localized adiposity/fat pad	278.1	
	Acanthosis nigricans	701.2	
	Striae	701.3	
	Fatigue/lethargy	780.7	9
	Pallor	782.6	1
	Flushing	782.6	2
	Abnormal loss of weight	783.2	1
	Underweight	783.2	2
	Feeding problem, infant	783.3	
783	Lack of normal physiological development in childhood		
	Abnormal posture	781.9	2
	Unspecified, inadequate development, lack of development	783.4	0
	Failure to thrive; failure to gain weight	783.4	1
	Delayed milestones; late walker, late talker	783.4	2
	Short stature; growth failure, growth retardation, lack of growth, physical retardation—includes constitutional short stature, stature inconsistent with chronological age	783.4	3

many practitioners would like to participate, the task becomes too great for the time involved. Bennett et al. (5) reported findings suggesting that phase II and III clinical trials resulted in a modest increase in cost over standard treatment. Policy makers have also decided to support clinical trial reimbursement initiatives. You have to think and decide which resources you can assign to a clinical trial protocol. There is a lot of responsibility and work involved in these protocols; entering into an agreement should be thoughtfully considered before starting protocols in your practice. The principal investigator's history of participation in clinical trials is extremely important. Your first attempts should be carefully done with few queries or problems in completing the study. It is also essential that you meet your agreed-upon quota of study subjects. Sponsors are very interested in this factor when reviewing your application to be an investigator in their trial. Sponsors are looking for investigators with good

clinical practice and a certificate in Human Subjects Protection. A good history of successful completion of clinical trials greatly increases your chances by reputation in being awarded further clinical trials from sponsors. You have to start slowly with careful planning and this part of your practice will grow over time into a rewarding part of your practice.

XII. WHAT IS NEEDED?

A sign stating "Wanted: trained coders only" is needed. You and your billing staff need to attend courses, including the Medicare courses, to keep updated on coding and reimbursement issues. The practice should have a code fee profile based on its RBRVS incorporating the cost of resources for your practice in your geographic area. Any investment that increases receivables for your practice is a sound investment. There are many links on the Internet where you can find easily accessible information and companies that address this issue.

XIII. FREQUENTLY USED DIAGNOSED CODES FOR THE PEDIATRIC ENDOCRINE PRACTICE

This list is a quick list of common codes used in a pediatric endocrine practice (see Table 1). It does not adequately represent the many different presentations a child or young adult might bring to your attention nor are all possible diagnoses mentioned. Please refer to official sources for further definitions and instructions on use of these codes.

REFERENCES

1. ICD.9.CM Expert for Physicians, Vols 1,2. 2002; Ingenix, 2001.
2. A guide to state implementation of ICD-10 for mortality part II: applying comparability ratios. National Center for Health Statistics, Centers for Disease Control and Prevention. 2000; December 4.
3. Gebhart F. Time short for setting up R.Ph. reimbursement system, say experts. Drug Topics 2001; May 7.
4. Levy S. The good, the bad, and ugly. Drug Topics 2001; September 3.
5. Bennett CL, Adams JR, Knox KS, Kelahan AM, Silver SM, Bailes JS. Clinical trials: are they a good buy? J Clin Oncol 2001; 19(23):4330–4339.

43

Reference Charts Used Frequently by Endocrinologists in Assessing the Growth and Development of Youth

Adriana A. Carrillo
University of Miami School of Medicine, Miami, Florida, U.S.A.

Bridget F. Recker
Staten Island University Hospital, Staten Island, New York, U.S.A.

I. STANDARDS OF GROWTH AND DEVELOPMENT

A. Neonates

Figure 1 Curve of birth weight against gestational age.
Figure 2 Curve of length and head circumference against gestational age.
Figure 3 Growth curves of infants with low birth weight.
Figure 4 Growth curves of infants with low birth weight (not corrected for gestational age).
Figure 5 Phallic lengths of premature and full-term infants.
Figure 6 Phallic diameters of premature and full-term infants.
Figure 7 Ratio of clitoral diameter to infant's weight plotted against menstrual age.

B. Infants

Figure 8 Weight of infants breastfed at least 12 months: boys and girls.
Figure 9 Length of infants breastfed at least 12 months: boys and girls.
Figure 10 Head circumference of infants breastfed at least 12 months: boys and girls.

C. Females

Figure 11 Length and weight for age: birth to 36 months.
Figure 12 Head circumference for age and weight for length: birth to 36 months.
Figure 13 Height and weight for age: 2–20 years.
Figure 14 Height/weight percentiles.
Figure 15 Height velocity.
Figure 16 Height and pubertal development.

Figure 17 Body mass index for age.
Figure 18 Progression of puberty: staging of breast and pubic hair.
Figure 19 Mean height and standard deviation, 2–18 years.
Figure 20 Prediction of adult height from the height and the age at menarche.

D. Males

Figure 21 Length and weight for age: birth to 36 months.
Figure 22 Head circumference for age and weight for length: birth to 36 months.
Figure 23 Height and weight for age: 2–20 years.
Figure 24 Height/weight percentiles.
Figure 25 Height velocity.
Figure 26 Height and pubertal development.
Figure 27 Body mass index for age.
Figure 28 Progression of puberty: staging of genitalia and pubic hair.
Figure 29 Mean height and standard deviation: 2–18 years.
Figure 30 Penile growth: birth to adolescence.
Figure 31 Testicular growth: 4–18 years.
Figure 32 Testicular volume: birth to 16 years.

II. MISCELLANEOUS STANDARDS

Figure 33 Arm span in relation to age and standing height: birth to 20 years.
Figure 34 Upper to lower segment ratio, both sexes: birth to 16 years.
Figure 35 Sitting height in relation to age and standing height: birth to 20 years.
Figure 36 Average anthropometric measurements.

969

III. STANDARD GROWTH CHARTS FOR CHILDREN WITH GENETIC OR PATHOLOGICAL CONDITIONS

I. STANDARDS OF GROWTH AND DEVELOPMENT

A. Neonates: Figures 1–7

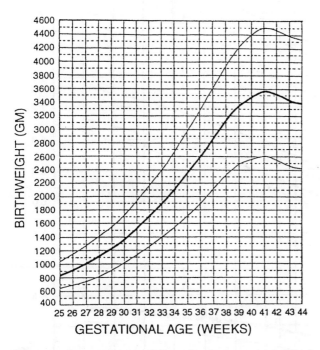

Figure 1 Smoothed curve values for the mean ± 2 SD of birth weight against gestational age. (From Usher R, McLean F. Intrauterine growth of live-born Caucasian infants at sea level: standards obtained from measurements in 7 dimensions of infants born between 25 and 44 weeks of gestation. J Pediatr 1969; 74(6):901–910.)

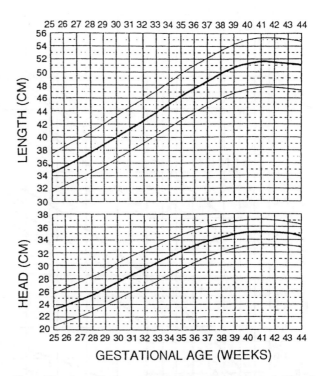

Figure 2 Smoothed curve values for the mean ± 2 SD of crown–heel length and head circumference against gestational age. (From Usher R, McLean F. Intrauterine growth of live-born Caucasian infants at sea level: standards obtained from measurements in 7 dimensions of infants born between 25 and 44 weeks of gestation. J. Pediatr 1969; 74(6):901–910.)

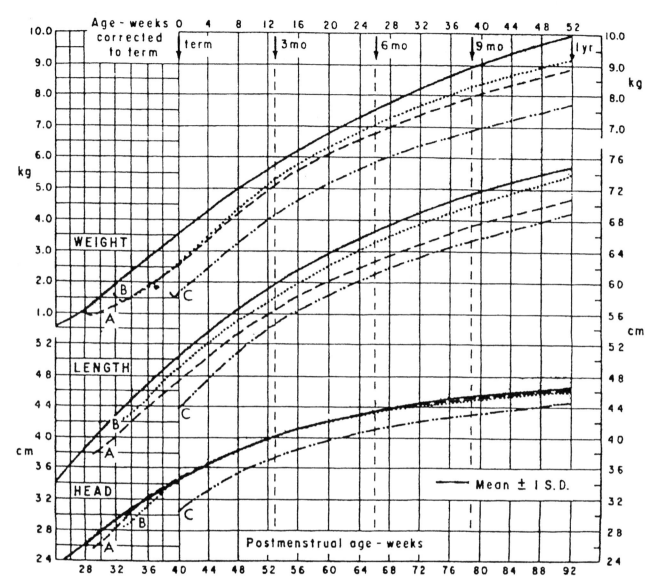

Figure 3 Mean growth curves of three groups of low-birth-weight infants. (A) Very premature and appropriate in size. (B) Moderately premature and appropriate in size. (C) Full-term but severely undergrown. These curves are plotted against the gestation age for that group. (From Babson SG. Growth of low birth weight infants. J Pediatr 1970; 77(1):11–18.)

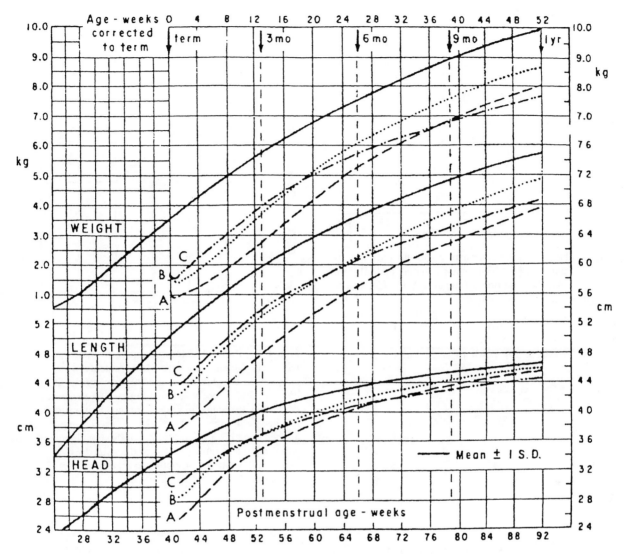

Figure 4 Growth curves of three groups of low-birth-weight infants plotted without correction for gestational age. (From Babson SG. Growth of low-birth-weight infants. J Pediatr 1970; 77(1):11–18.).

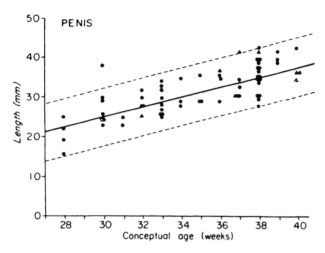

Figure 5   Phallic length of premature and full-term infants. Stretched phallic length of 63 normal premature and full-term male infants (●), showing lines of mean ± 2 SD. Correlation coefficient is 0.80. Superimposed are data for two small-for-gestational-age infants (△), seven large-for-gestational-age infants (▲), and four twins (■), all of which are in the normal range. (From Feldman KW, Smith DW. Fetal phallic growth and penile standards for newborn male infants. J Pediatr 1975; 86(3):395–398.)

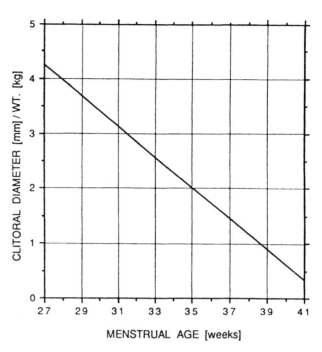

Figure 7   Ratio of clitoral diameter to infant's weight plotted against menstrual age. Measurements were made with calipers on 69 premature and 90 term infants in the first 3 days of life. There was no difference in measurements between black infants and white infants. Clitoral diameter had reached term size by 27 weeks' menstrual age. Clitoral diameter varied from 2 to 6 mm, but did not change with menstrual age. The ratio of clitoral diameter to body showed a significant negative correlation to menstrual age. (From Riley WS, et al. J Pediatr 1980; 96:918.)

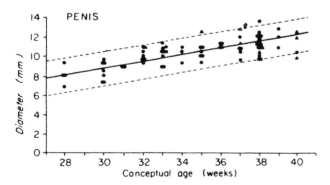

Figure 6   Phallic diameter of premature and full-term infants. Phallic diameter of 63 normal premature and full-term male infants (●), showing lines of mean ± 2 SD. Correlation coefficient is 0.82. Superimposed are data for two small-for-gestational-age infants (△), seven large-for-gestational-age infants (▲), and four twins (■), all of which are in the normal range. (From Feldman KW, Smith DW. Fetal phallic growth and penile standards for newborn male infants. J Pediatr 1975; 86(3):395–398.)

B. Infants: Figures 8–10

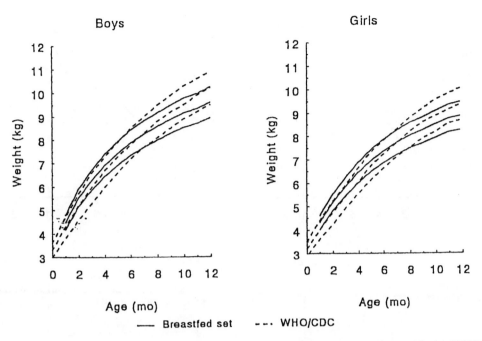

Figure 8 Weight quartiles of infants breastfed at least 12 months (n = 226) in comparison with the WHO/CDC reference (1986). (From Dewey KG, Peerson LA, Brown KH, et al. Pediatrics 1995; 96:495.)

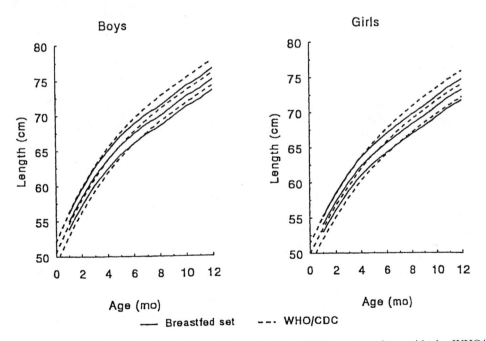

Figure 9 Length quartiles of infants breastfed at least 12 months (n = 226) in comparison with the WHO/CDC reference (1986). (From Dewey KG, Peerson LA, Brown KH, et al. Pediatrics 1995; 96:495.)

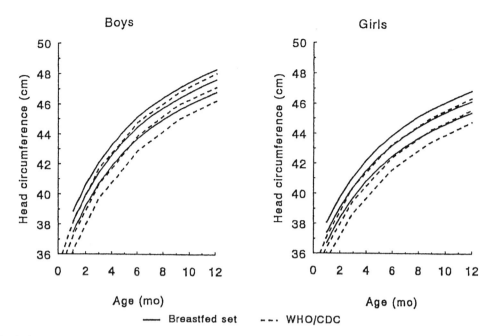

Figure 10 Head circumference quartiles of infants breastfed at least 12 months (n = 226) in comparison with the WHO/CDC reference (1986). (From Dewey KG, Peerson LA, Brown KH, et al. Pediatrics 1995; 96:495.)

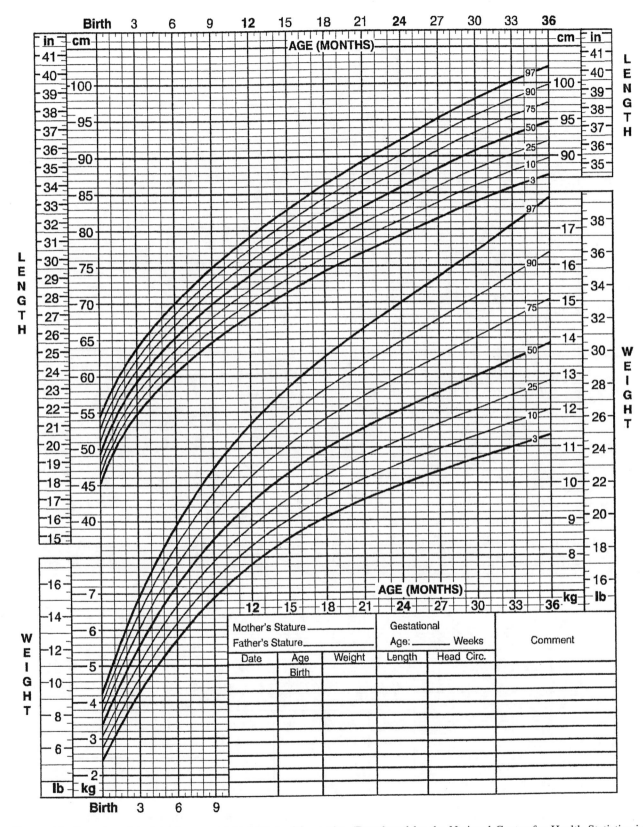

Figure 11 Length and weight for age, girls: birth to 36 months. (Developed by the National Center for Health Statistics in collaboration with the National Center for Chronic Disease Prevention and Health Promotion (2000); http://www.cdc.gov/growthcharts.)

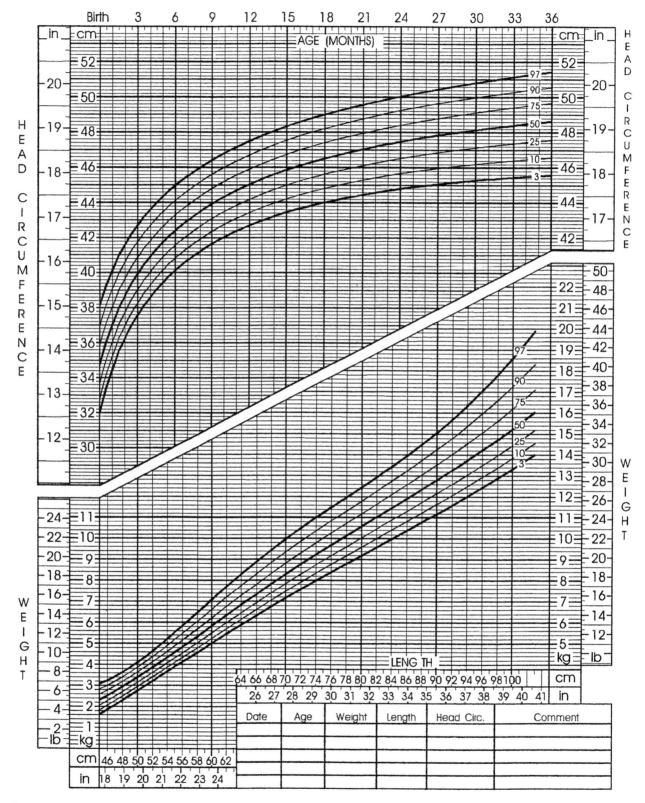

Figure 12   Head circumference for age and weight for length, girls: birth to 36 months. (Developed by the National Center for Health Statistics in collaboration with the National Center for Chronic Disease Prevention and Health Promotion (2000); http://www.cdc.gov/growthcharts.)

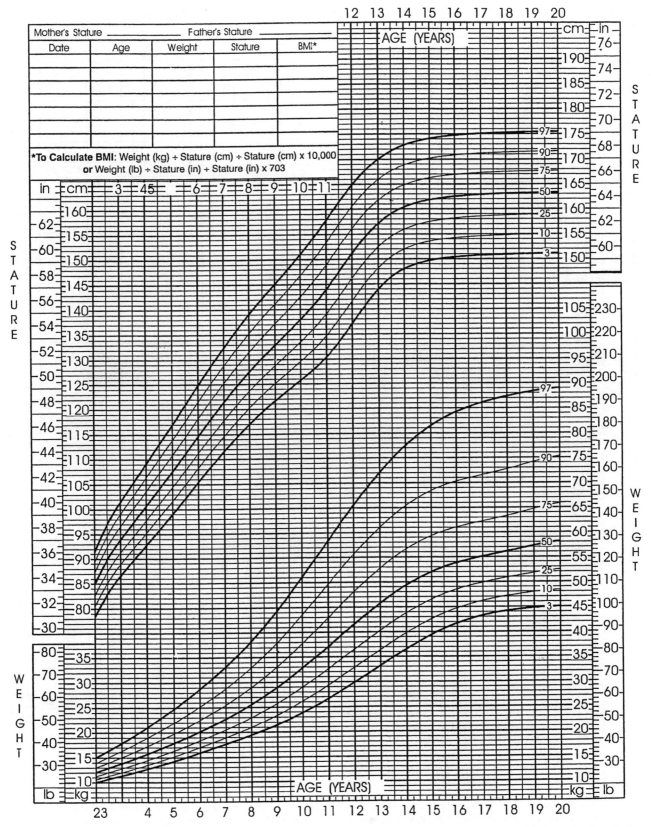

Figure 13 Stature for age and weight, girls: 2–20 years. (Developed by the National Center for Health Statistics in collaboration with the National Center for Chronic Disease Prevention and Health Promotion (2000); http://www.cdc.gov/growthcharts.)

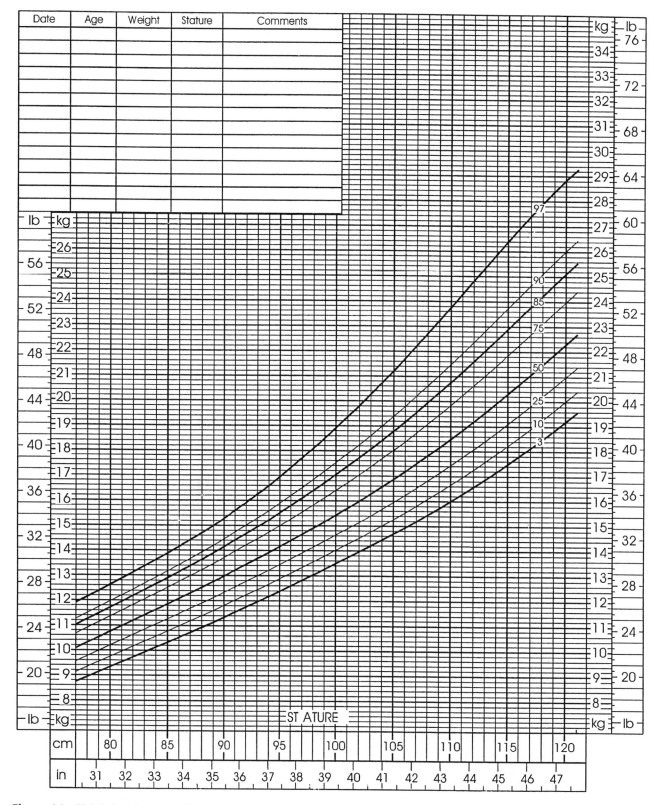

Figure 14 Height/weight percentiles, girls. (Developed by the National Center for Health Statistics in collaboration with the National Center for Chronic Disease Prevention and Health Promotion (2000); http://www.cdc.gov/growthcharts.)

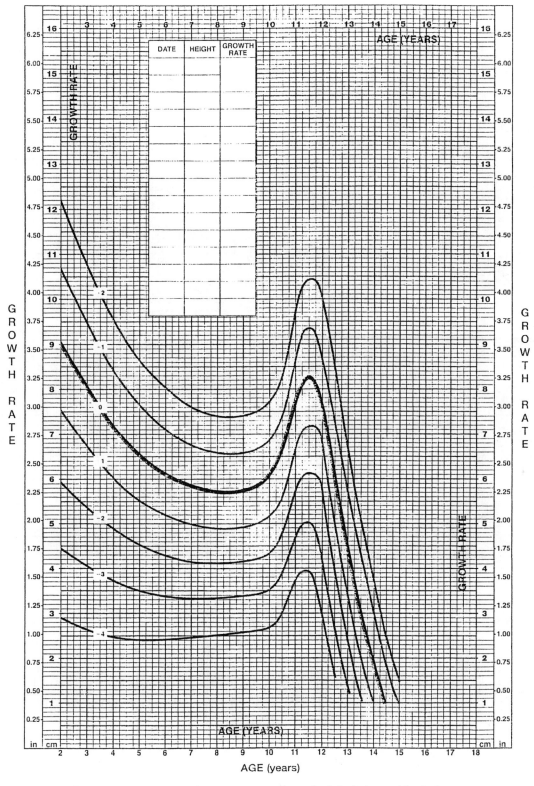

Figure 15 Yearly growth rate, means and standard deviations, girls: 2–5 years.

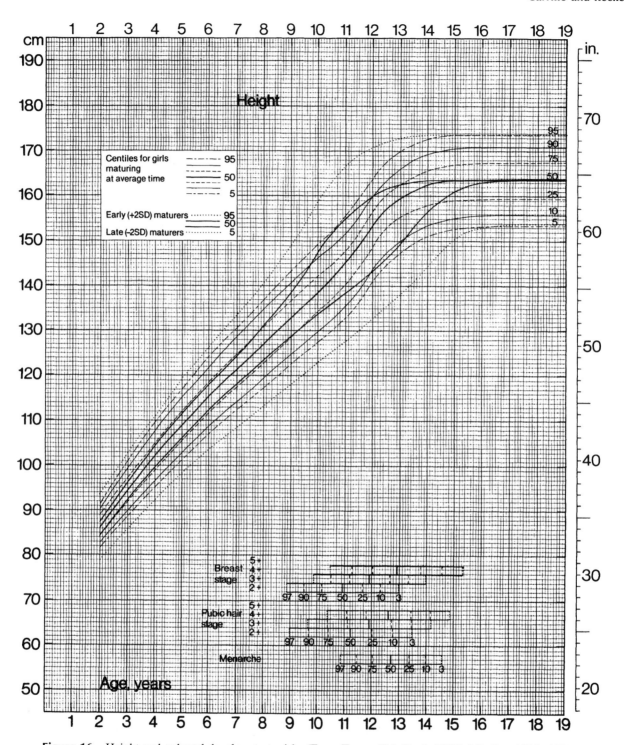

Figure 16 Height and pubertal development, girls. (From Tanner JM, Davis PSW. J Pediatr 1985; 107.)

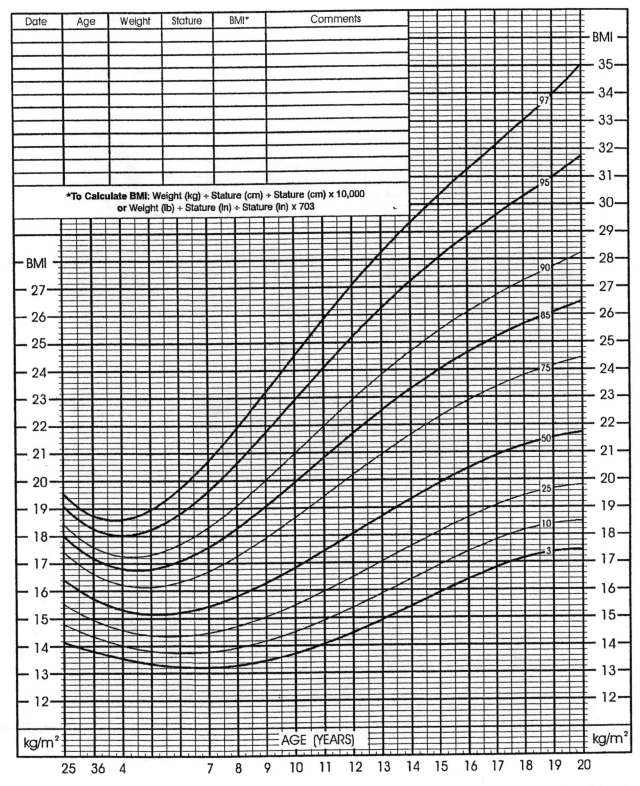

Figure 17   Body mass index for age, girls: 2–20 years. (Developed by the National Center for Health Statistics in collaboration with the National Center for Chronic Disease Prevention and Health Promotion (2000); http://www.cdc.gov/growthcharts.)

Typical Progression of Female Pubertal Development

Pubertal development in size of female breasts.

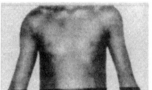 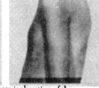

Stage 1. The breasts are preadolescent. There is elevation of the papilla only.

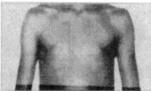 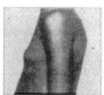

Stage 2. Breast bud stage. A small mound is formed by the elevation of the breast and papilla. The areolar diameter enlarges.

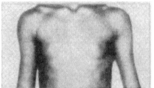 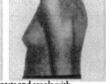

Stage 3. There is further enlargement of breasts and areola with no separation of their contours.

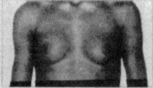 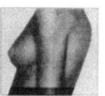

Stage 4. There is a projection of the areola and papilla to form a secondary mound above the level of the breast.

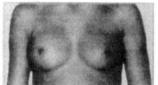 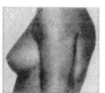

Stage 5. The breasts resemble those of a mature female as the areola has recessed to the general contour of the breast.

Pubertal development of female pubic hair.

Stage 1. There is no pubic hair.

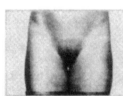 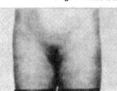 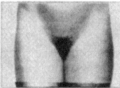 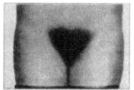

Stage 2. There is sparse growth of long, slightly pigmented, downy hair, straight or only slightly curled, primarily along the labia.

Stage 3. The hair is considerably darker, coarser, and more curled. The hair spreads sparsely over the junction of the pubes.

Stage 4. The hair, now adult in type, covers a smaller area than in the adult and does not extend onto the thighs.

Stage 5. The hair is adult in quantity and type, with extension onto the thighs.

Figure 18 Typical progression of pubertal development, girls. (Reproduced with permission from Ross Laboratories, Columbus, Ohio 43216. © Ross Laboratories.)

Age	Height	s.d.	Age	Height	s.d.	Age	Height	s.d.	Age	Height	s.d.
2.0	86.80	3.16	7.0	120.60	5.35	12.0	151.50	7.11	17.0	163.10	6.32
2.1	87.39	3.18	7.1	121.19	5.39	12.1	152.15	7.13	17.1	163.17	6.30
2.2	87.99	3.20	7.2	121.77	5.42	12.2	152.79	7.16	17.2	163.23	6.28
2.3	88.62	3.22	7.3	122.35	5.45	12.3	153.41	7.18	17.3	163.29	6.25
2.4	89.28	3.25	7.4	122.92	5.49	12.4	154.02	7.21	17.4	163.34	6.22
2.5	90.00	3.28	7.5	123.50	5.53	12.5	154.60	7.23	17.5	163.40	6.20
2.6	90.77	3.32	7.6	124.08	5.58	12.6	155.15	7.24	17.6	163.46	6.18
2.7	91.59	3.37	7.7	124.66	5.63	12.7	155.68	7.25	17.7	163.52	6.17
2.8	92.43	3.42	7.8	125.24	5.68	12.8	156.18	7.25	17.8	163.58	6.16
2.9	93.27	3.48	7.9	125.82	5.73	12.9	156.65	7.24	17.9	163.64	6.15
3.0	94.10	3.53	8.0	126.40	5.78	13.0	157.10	7.23	18.0	163.70	6.14
3.1	94.90	3.58	8.1	126.98	5.82	13.1	157.52	7.22			
3.2	95.67	3.63	8.2	127.56	5.86	13.2	157.92	7.21			
3.3	96.42	3.68	8.3	128.14	5.89	13.3	158.30	7.19			
3.4	97.16	3.72	8.4	128.72	5.93	13.4	158.66	7.18			
3.5	97.90	3.77	8.5	129.30	5.96	13.5	159.00	7.17			
3.6	98.65	3.82	8.6	129.88	6.00	13.6	159.32	7.16			
3.7	99.40	3.87	8.7	130.45	6.03	13.7	159.63	7.15			
3.8	100.14	3.92	8.8	131.03	6.07	13.8	159.91	7.14			
3.9	100.88	3.97	8.9	131.61	6.10	13.9	160.17	7.13			
4.0	101.60	4.01	9.0	132.20	6.14	14.0	160.40	7.11			
4.1	102.30	4.05	9.1	132.79	6.17	14.1	160.60	7.09			
4.2	102.98	4.08	9.2	133.39	6.21	14.2	160.77	7.07			
4.3	103.66	4.12	9.3	133.99	6.24	14.3	160.92	7.04			
4.4	104.33	4.15	9.4	134.59	6.28	14.4	161.06	7.01			
4.5	105.00	4.19	9.5	135.20	6.32	14.5	161.20	6.99			
4.6	105.68	4.23	9.6	135.81	6.37	14.6	161.33	6.97			
4.7	106.36	4.28	9.7	136.43	6.42	14.7	161.47	6.95			
4.8	107.05	4.33	9.8	137.05	6.47	14.8	161.59	6.92			
4.9	107.73	4.39	9.9	137.67	6.52	14.9	161.70	6.90			
5.0	108.40	4.44	10.0	138.30	6.57	15.0	161.80	6.87			
5.1	109.06	4.49	10.1	138.93	6.61	15.1	161.88	6.84			
5.2	109.71	4.54	10.2	139.57	6.66	15.2	161.94	6.80			
5.3	110.35	4.59	10.3	140.21	6.69	15.3	162.00	6.76			
5.4	110.98	4.64	10.4	140.85	6.72	15.4	162.05	6.72			
5.5	111.60	4.68	10.5	141.50	6.75	15.5	162.10	6.69			
5.6	112.21	4.72	10.6	142.15	6.77	15.6	162.16	6.66			
5.7	112.81	4.75	10.7	142.81	6.79	15.7	162.22	6.64			
5.8	113.41	4.79	10.8	143.46	6.82	15.8	162.28	6.62			
5.9	114.01	4.82	10.9	144.34	6.84	15.9	162.34	6.60			
6.0	114.60	4.86	11.0	144.80	6.87	16.0	162.40	6.57			
6.1	115.20	4.90	11.1	145.48	6.91	16.1	162.46	6.53			
6.2	115.80	4.95	11.2	146.16	6.95	16.2	162.51	6.49			
6.3	116.40	5.00	11.3	146.84	6.99	16.3	162.57	6.45			
6.4	117.00	5.06	11.4	147.52	7.02	16.4	162.63	6.41			
6.5	117.60	5.11	11.5	148.20	7.05	16.5	162.70	6.38			
6.6	118.20	5.16	11.6	148.87	7.07	16.6	162.78	6.36			
6.7	118.81	5.21	11.7	149.54	7.08	16.7	162.86	6.35			
6.8	119.41	5.26	11.8	150.19	7.09	16.8	162.94	6.34			
6.9	120.01	5.31	11.9	150.85	7.10	16.9	163.02	6.33			

Figure 19 Mean height and SD, girls: 2–18 years. (From Hamill PVV, Dzird TA, Johnson CL, Reed RR, Roche AF. NCHS growth curves for children from birth to 18 years: United States. DHEW publication (PHS) 78-1650. Washington DC: US Government Printing Office; Vital Health Stat 1977; (11) 165:1–74.)

Prediction of height

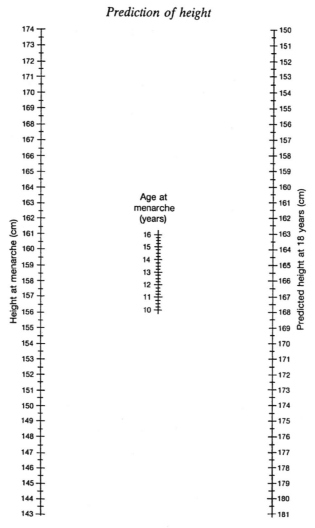

Figure 20   Nomogram for the prediction of adult height from the height and age at menarche. (From Harriet Lane Handbook, 1975, by permission.)

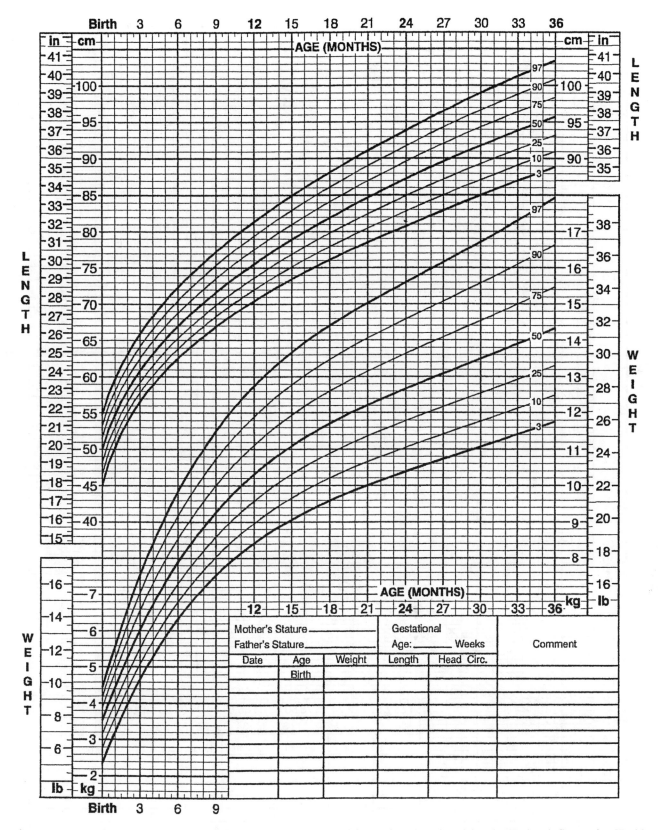

Figure 21 Length for age and weight for age, boys: birth to 36 months. (Developed by the National Center for Health Statistics in collaboration with the National Center for Chronic Disease Prevention and Health Promotion (2000); http://www.cdc.gov/growthcharts.)

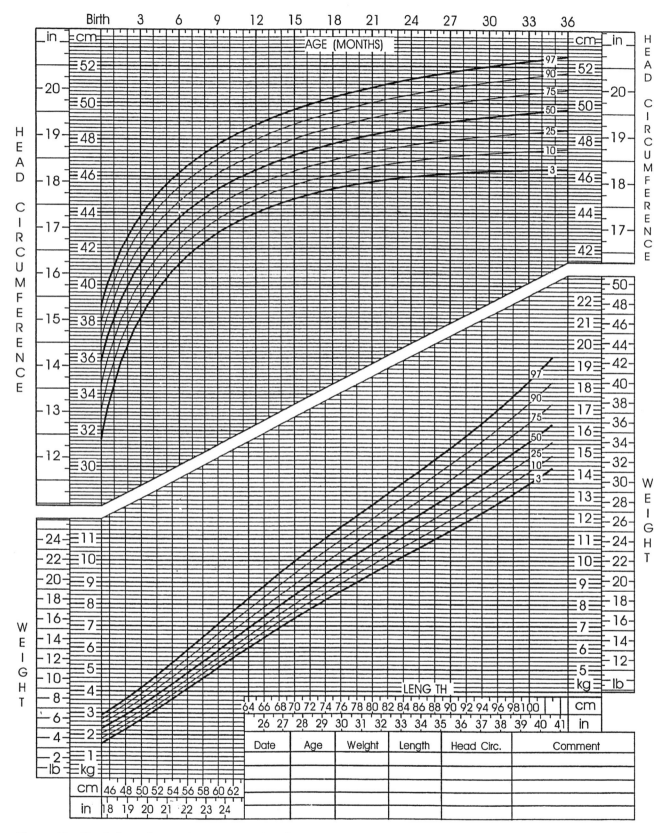

Figure 22 Head circumference for age and weight for length, boys: birth to 36 months. (Developed by the National Center for Health Statistics in collaboration with the National Center for Chronic Disease Prevention and Health Promotion (2000); http://www.cdc.gov/growthcharts.)

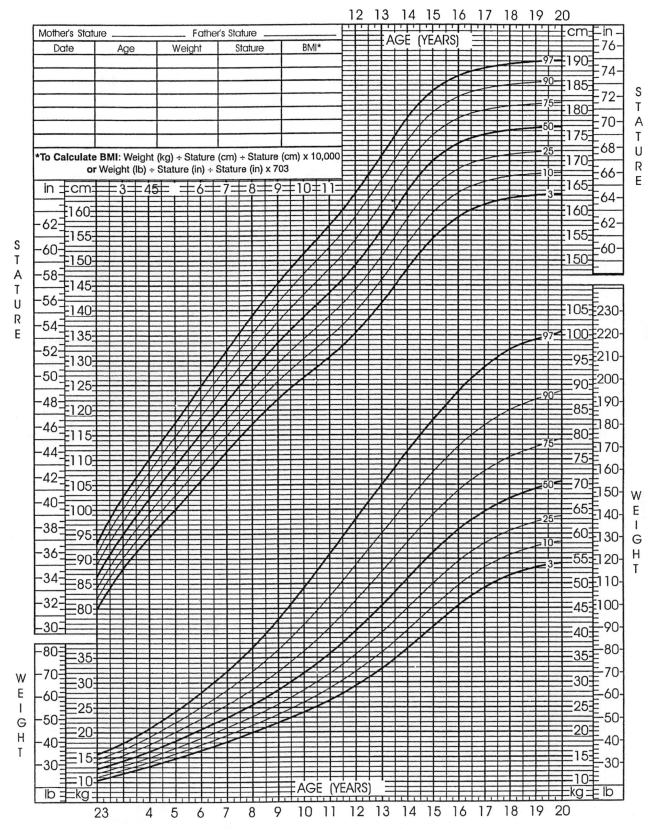

Figure 23 Stature for age and weight for age, boys: 2–20 years. (Developed by the National Center for Health Statistics in collaboration with the National Center for Chronic Disease Prevention and Health Promotion (2000); http://www.cdc.gov/growthcharts.)

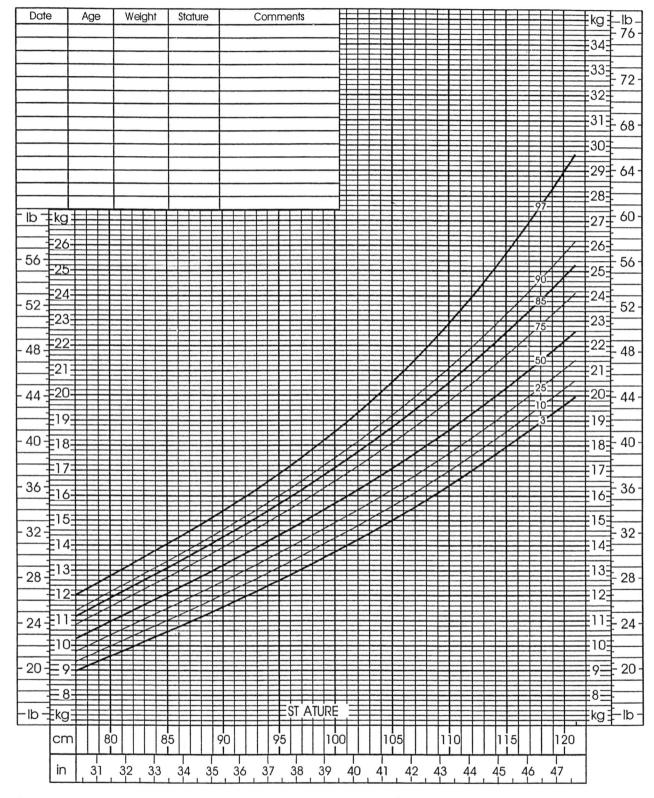

Figure 24 Height/weight percentiles, boys. (Developed by the National Center for Health Statistics in collaboration with the National Center for Chronic Disease Prevention and Health Promotion (2000); http://www.cdc.gov/growthcharts.)

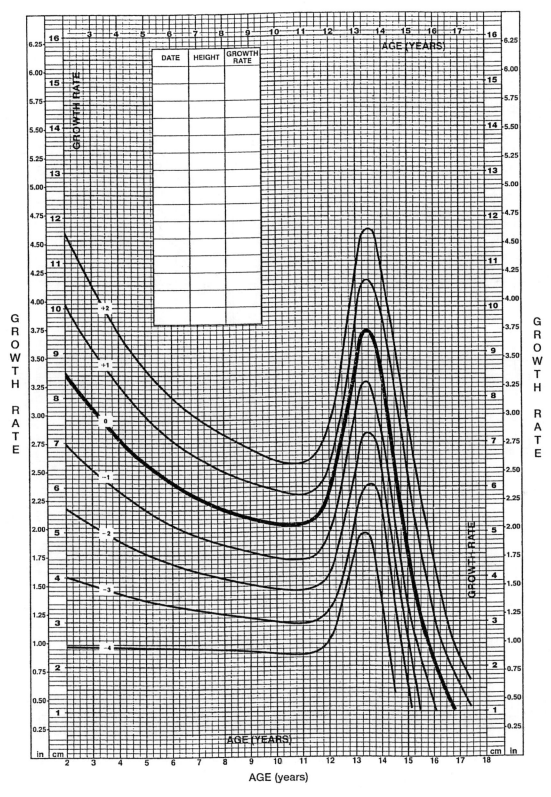

Figure 25 Yearly growth rate, means and standard deviations, boys: 2–18 years.

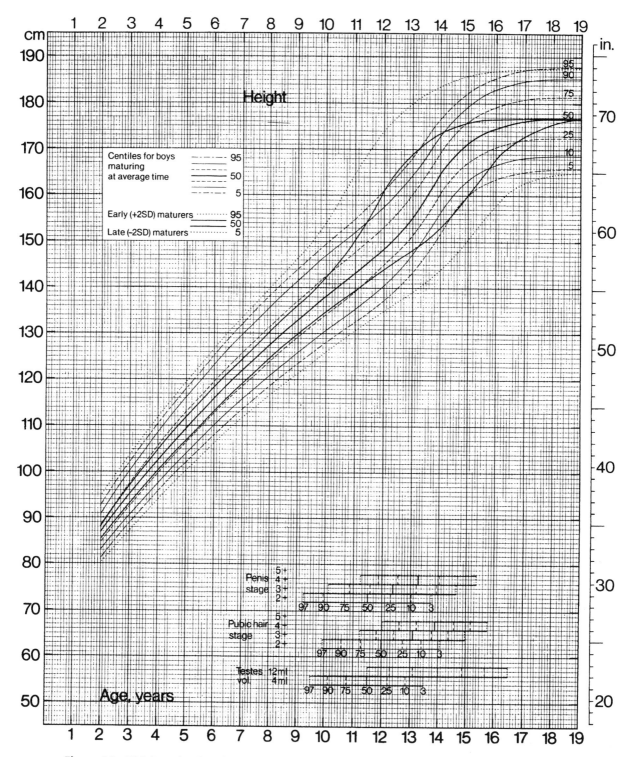

Figure 26 Height and pubertal development, boys. (Tanner JM, Davis PSW. J Pediatr 1985; 107.)

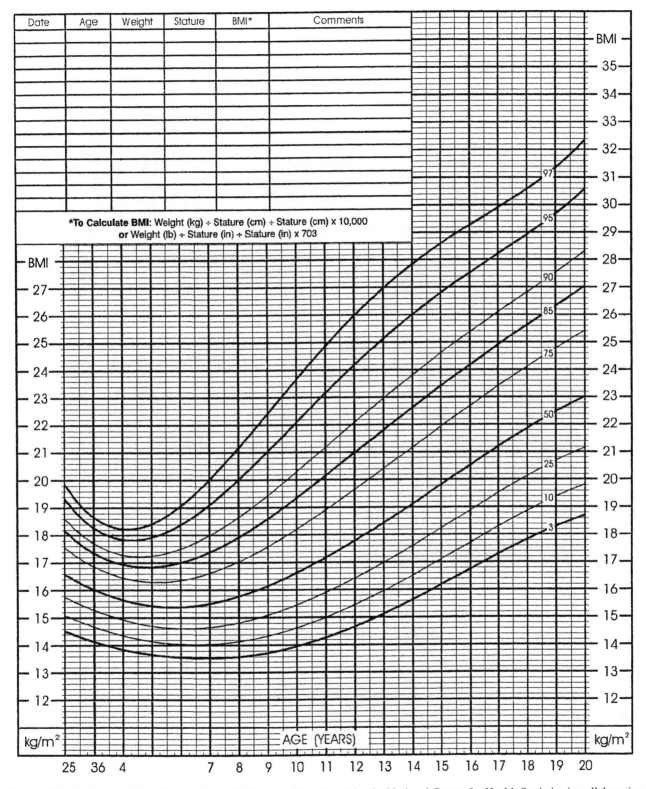

Figure 27 Body mass index for age, boys: 2–20 years. (Developed by the National Center for Health Statistics in collaboration with the National Center for Chronic Disease Prevention and Health Promotion (2000); http://www.cdc.gov/growthcharts.)

Typical Progression of Male Pubertal Development

Pubertal development in size of male genitalia.

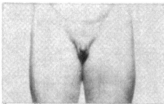

Stage 1. The penis, testes, and scrotum are of childhood size.

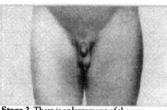

Stage 2. There is enlargement of the scrotum and testes, but the penis usually does not enlarge. The scrotal skin reddens.

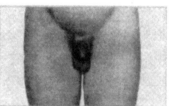

Stage 3. There is further growth of the testes and scotum and enlargement of the penis, mainly in length.

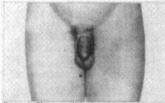

Stage 4. There is still further growth of the testes and scrotum and increased size of the penis, especially in breadth.

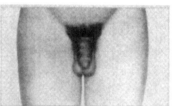

Stage 5. The genitalia are adult in size and shape.

Pubertal development of male pubic hair.

Stage 1. There is no pubic hair.

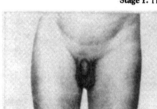

Stage 2. There is sparse growth of long, slightly pigmented, downy hair, straight or only slightly curled, primarily at the base of the penis.

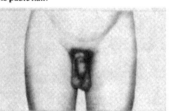

Stage 3. The hair is considerably darker, coarser, and more curled. The hair spreads sparsely over the junction of the pubes.

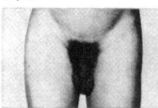

Stage 4. The hair, now adult in type, covers a smaller area than in the adult and does not extend onto the thighs.

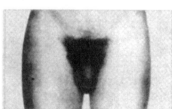

Stage 5. The hair is adult in quantity and type, with extension onto the thighs.

Figure 28 Typical progression of pubertal development, boys. (Reproduced with permission from Ross Laboratories, Columbus, Ohio 43216. © Ross Laboratories.)

Age	Height	s.d.	Age	Height	s.d.	Age	Height	s.d.	Age	Height	s.d.
2.0	86.80	2.61	7.0	121.70	5.29	12.0	149.70	7.36	17.0	176.20	6.87
2.1	87.47	2.50	7.1	122.24	5.30	12.1	150.34	7.44	17.1	176.33	6.83
2.2	88.15	2.40	7.2	122.78	5.31	12.2	150.97	7.52	17.2	176.45	6.80
2.3	88.86	2.34	7.3	123.33	5.33	12.3	151.61	7.60	17.3	176.55	6.78
2.4	89.61	2.35	7.4	123.87	5.34	12.4	152.28	7.69	17.4	176.64	6.76
2.5	90.40	2.43	7.5	124.40	5.35	12.5	153.00	7.78	17.5	176.70	6.75
2.6	91.25	2.60	7.6	124.93	5.36	12.6	153.77	7.88	17.6	176.74	6.74
2.7	92.14	2.84	7.7	125.45	5.37	12.7	154.57	7.97	17.7	176.77	6.74
2.8	93.06	3.10	7.8	125.97	5.38	12.8	155.38	8.07	17.8	176.79	6.74
2.9	93.99	3.37	7.9	126.48	5.39	12.9	156.16	8.17	17.9	176.80	6.75
3.0	94.90	3.59	8.0	127.00	5.41	13.0	156.90	8.27	18.0	176.80	6.75
3.1	95.79	3.75	8.1	127.52	5.43	13.1	157.57	8.36			
3.2	96.65	3.86	8.2	128.04	5.45	13.2	158.18	8.45			
3.3	97.49	3.93	8.4	128.56	5.48	13.3	158.75	8.52			
3.4	98.30	3.97	8.4	129.08	5.50	13.4	159.32	8.58			
3.5	99.10	4.01	8.5	129.60	5.53	13.5	159.90	8.63			
3.6	99.88	4.06	8.6	130.12	5.56	13.6	160.51	8.66			
3.7	100.64	4.11	8.7	130.64	5.58	13.7	161.14	8.68			
3.8	101.40	4.17	8.8	131.16	5.60	13.8	161.79	8.69			
3.9	102.15	4.24	8.9	131.68	5.63	13.9	162.45	8.69			
4.0	102.90	4.32	9.0	132.20	5.65	14.0	163.10	8.69			
4.1	103.65	4.40	9.1	132.72	5.67	14.1	163.74	8.69			
4.2	104.41	4.48	9.2	133.23	5.70	14.2	164.38	8.68			
4.3	105.15	4.56	9.3	133.75	5.72	14.3	165.00	8.67			
4.4	105.89	4.63	9.4	134.27	5.75	14.4	165.60	8.65			
4.5	106.60	4.68	9.5	134.80	5.78	14.5	166.20	8.63			
4.6	107.29	4.72	9.6	135.33	5.81	14.6	166.78	8.60			
4.7	107.96	4.74	9.7	135.87	5.84	14.7	167.35	8.55			
4.8	108.61	4.76	9.8	136.41	5.88	14.8	167.91	8.51			
4.9	109.26	4.78	9.9	136.95	5.92	14.9	168.46	8.45			
5.0	109.90	4.80	10.0	137.50	5.96	15.0	169.00	9.39			
5.1	110.55	4.83	10.1	138.05	6.00	15.1	169.53	8.33			
5.2	111.19	4.86	10.2	138.60	6.05	15.2	170.05	8.26			
5.3	111.84	4.90	10.3	139.16	6.10	15.3	170.56	8.19			
5.4	112.47	4.94	10.4	139.72	6.15	15.4	171.04	8.11			
5.5	113.10	4.98	10.5	140.30	6.20	15.5	171.50	8.02			
5.6	113.72	5.01	10.6	140.89	6.25	15.6	171.93	7.93			
5.7	114.32	5.04	10.7	141.48	6.31	15.7	172.35	7.83			
5.8	114.92	5.06	10.8	142.09	6.37	15.8	172.74	7.73			
5.9	115.51	5.09	10.9	142.69	6.43	15.9	173.12	7.63			
6.0	116.10	5.11	11.0	143.30	6.50	16.0	173.50	7.54			
6.1	116.69	5.14	11.1	143.91	6.58	16.1	173.87	7.46			
6.2	117.28	5.16	11.2	144.52	6.66	16.2	174.24	7.38			
6.3	117.86	5.19	11.3	145.13	6.75	16.3	174.58	7.31			
6.4	118.44	5.21	11.4	145.76	6.84	16.4	174.91	7.24			
6.5	119.00	5.23	11.5	146.40	6.93	16.5	175.20	7.17			
6.6	119.55	5.25	11.6	147.05	7.02	16.6	175.46	7.10			
6.7	120.09	5.26	11.7	147.72	7.11	16.7	175.68	7.04			
6.8	120.63	5.27	11.8	148.39	7.19	16.8	175.88	6.98			
6.9	121.16	5.28	11.9	149.05	7.28	16.9	176.05	6.92			

Figure 29 Mean height and SD, boys: 2–18 years. (From Hamill PVV, Dzird TA, Johnson CL, Reed RR, Roche AF. NCHS growth curves for children from birth to 18 years: United States. DHEW publication (PHS) 78-1650. Washington DC: US Government Printing Office; Vital Health Stat 1977; (11) 165:1–74.)

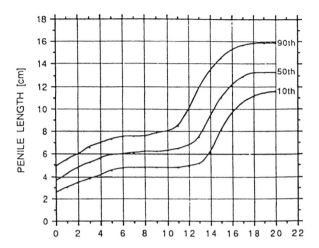

Figure 30 Penile growth in stretched length from the pubic ramus to the tip of the glans; from infancy into adolescence. (From Schonfield WA. Am J Dis Child 1943; 65:535.)

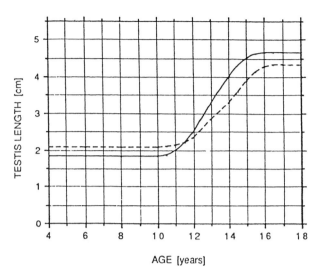

Figure 31 Testicular growth in length, adapted from normal standards of testicular volume: 4–18 years. (Solid line from data in Zurich; broken line from data of Laron A, Zilka E. J Clin Endocrinol Metab 1969; 29:1409; adapted from data of Praeder A. Recognizable Patterns of Human Malformation, 3rd ed. Philadelphia: WB Saunders, 1982.)

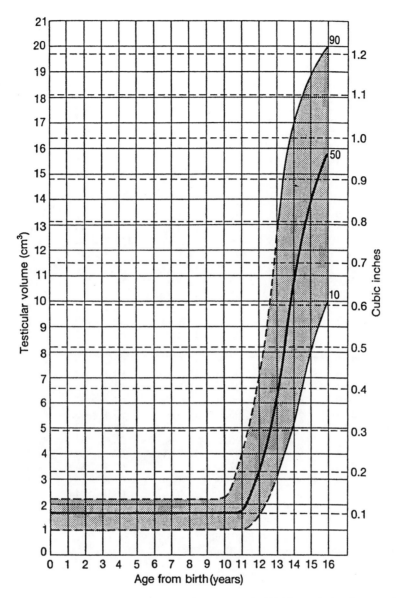

Figure 32 Testicular volume, birth to 16 years. (From Zachmann et al. (1974), and Goodman and Gorlin (1983), by permission.)

II. MISCELLANEOUS STANDARDS: FIGURES 33–49

Age	Height (In.) M	Height (In.) F	Span Absolute M	Span Absolute F	Span Relative M	Span Relative F	Age	Height (In.) M	Height (In.) F	Span Absolute M	Span Absolute F	Span Relative M	Span Relative F
Birth	20.2	19.9	19.3	18.9	95.7	95.2	7½ Yrs.	48.2	47.9	47.6	47.0	98.7	98.1
1 Mo.	21.9	21.5	21.0	20.5	95.7	95.2	8 Yrs.	49.2	48.9	48.8	48.1	99.1	98.3
2 Mos.	23.1	22.7	22.1	21.6	95.7	85.2	8½ Yrs.	50.2	49.9	50.0	49.2	99.6	98.6
3 Mos.	24.1	23.7	23.1	22.6	95.8	95.3	9 Yrs.	51.2	50.9	51.2	50.3	100.0	98.8
4 Mos.	25.0	24.6	24.0	3.4	95.8	95.3	9½ Yrs.	52.2	51.9	52.4	51.4	100.4	99.0
5 Mos.	25.7	25.3	24.6	24.1	95.8	95.3	10 Yrs.	53.2	53.0	53.6	52.6	100.7	99.2
6 Mos.	26.4	26.0	25.3	24.8	95.8	95.3	10½ Yrs.	54.2	54.1	54.7	53.8	100.9	99.4
7 Mos.	27.1	26.6	26.0	25.4	95.9	95.4	11 Yrs.	55.2	55.3	55.8	55.1	101.2	99.6
8 Mos.	27.6	27.1	26.5	25.9	95.9	95.4	11½ Yrs.	56.2	56.5	56.9	56.3	101.4	99.8
9 Mos.	28.1	27.6	26.9	26.3	95.9	95.4	12 Yrs.	57.1	57.6	58.0	57.6	101.6	100.0
10 Mos.	28.6	28.1	27.4	26.8	95.9	95.9	12½ Yrs.	58.0	58.7	59.1	58.7	101.8	100.1
11 Mos.	29.1	28.6	27.9	27.3	96.0	95.5	13 Yrs.	58.9	59.7	60.1	59.9	102.0	100.3
12 Mos.	29.5	29.0	28.3	27.7	96.0	95.5	13½ Yrs.	59.8	60.6	61.1	60.9	102.2	100.4
15 Mos.	30.7	30.2	29.5	28.9	96.1	95.6	14 Yrs.	60.7	61.4	62.1	61.7	102.3	100.6
18 Mos.	31.9	31.4	30.7	30.0	96.2	95.7	14½ Yrs.	61.6	62.0	63.1	62.4	102.5	100.7
21 Mos.	32.9	32.4	31.7	31.0	96.3	95.7	15 Yrs.	62.4	62.5	64.0	63.0	102.6	100.8
24 Mos.	33.9	33.4	32.6	32.0	96.3	96.8	15½ Yrs.	63.2	62.9	64.9	63.5	102.7	100.9
30 Mos.	35.7	32.1	34.4	33.7	96.4	96.0	16 Yrs.	64.0	63.2	65.8	63.0	102.8	101.0
36 Mos.	37.3	30.7	30.0	35.0	96.6	96.2	16½ Yrs.	64.7	63.5	66.6	64.2	102.9	101.0
42 Mos.	38.8	38.2	37.5	36.5	96.8	96.4	17 Yrs.	65.4	63.7	67.4	64.4	103.0	101.2
48 Mos.	40.2	39.6	39.0	38.2	97.0	96.6	17½ Yrs.	66.0	63.9	68.1	64.6	103.1	101.2
54 Mos.	41.5	40.9	40.3	39.6	97.2	96.8	18 Yrs.	66.6	64.0	68.7	64.8	103.2	101.3
60 Mos.	42.7	42.2	41.6	40.9	97.4	97.0	18½ Yrs.	67.1	64.0	69.3	64.8	103.3	101.3
5½ Yrs.	43.9	43.4	42.8	42.2	97.6	97.2	19 Yrs.	67.5	64.0	69.8	64.8	103.4	101.3
6 Yrs.	45.0	44.6	44.0	43.4	97.8	97.4	19½ Yrs.	67.8	64.0	70.1	64.8	103.4	101.3
6½ Yrs.	46.1	45.7	45.2	44.6	98.1	97.6	20 Yrs.	68.0	64.0	70.4	64.8	103.5	101.3
7 Yrs.	47.2	46.8	46.4	48.9	98.4	97.8							

Figure 33 Arm span in relation to age and standing height: birth to 20 years. (From Engelbach W. Endocrine Medicine. Courtesy of Charles C Thomas, Publisher, Springfield, Illinois, 1932.)

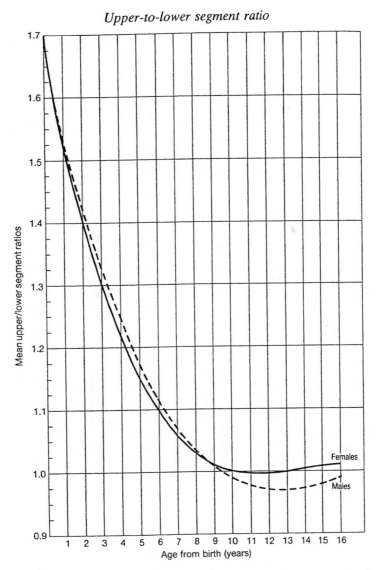

Figure 34 Upper to lower segment ratio, both sexes: birth to 16 years. (From Harriet Lane Handbook, 1975, by permission.)

Age	Standing height (In.)		Sitting height, absolute		Sitting height, relative	
	M	F	M	F	M	F
Birth	20.2	19.9	13.6	13.4	67.3	67.3
1 Month	21.9	21.5	14.6	14.4	66.7	66.8
2 Months	23.1	22.7	15.3	15.1	66.2	66.3
3 Months	24.1	23.7	15.8	15.6	65.6	65.7
4 Months	25.0	24.6	16.3	16.1	65.1	65.2
5 Months	25.7	25.3	16.6	16.4	64.6	64.7
6 Months	26.4	26.0	16.9	16.7	64.1	64.2
7 Months	27.1	26.6	17.3	17.0	63.8	63.9
8 Months	27.6	27.1	17.5	17.2	63.4	63.5
9 Months	28.1	27.6	17.7	17.4	63.1	63.2
10 Months	28.6	28.1	18.0	17.7	62.8	62.9
11 Months	29.1	28.6	18.2	17.9	62.6	62.7
12 Months (1 yr)	29.5	29.0	18.4	18.1	62.3	62.4
15 Months	30.7	30.2	18.9	18.6	61.6	61.7
18 Months	31.9	31.4	19.4	19.1	60.9	61.0
21 Months	32.9	32.4	19.8	19.5	60.3	60.4
24 Months (2 yrs)	33.9	33.4	20.3	20.0	59.8	59.9
30 Months	35.7	35.1	21.0	20.7	58.9	59.0
36 Months (3 yrs)	37.3	36.7	21.7	21.4	58.2	58.3
42 Months	38.8	38.2	22.3	22.0	57.6	57.6
48 Months (4 yrs)	40.2	39.6	22.9	22.5	57.0	56.9
54 Months	41.5	40.9	23.4	23.1	56.5	56.4
60 Months (5 yrs)	42.7	42.2	23.9	23.6	56.0	55.9
5½ Years	43.9	43.4	24.4	24.1	55.6	55.5
6 Years	45.0	44.6	24.9	24.6	55.2	55.2
6½ Years	46.1	45.7	25.3	25.1	54.9	54.9
7 Years	47.2	46.8	25.8	25.5	54.6	54.5
7½ Years	48.2	47.9	26.2	26.0	54.3	54.2
8 Years	49.2	48.9	26.6	26.4	54.1	54.0
8½ Years	50.2	49.9	27.1	26.9	53.9	53.8
9 Years	51.2	50.9	27.5	27.3	53.7	53.6
9½ Years	52.2	51.9	27.9	27.7	53.4	53.3
10 Years	53.2	53.0	28.3	28.1	53.2	53.0
10½ Years	54.2	54.1	28.8	28.6	53.0	52.8
11 Years	55.2	55.3	29.2	29.1	52.9	52.6
11½ Years	56.2	56.5	29.6	29.7	52.7	52.6
12 Years	57.1	57.6	30.0	30.3	52.6	52.6
12½ Years	58.0	58.7	30.4	30.9	52.5	52.7
13 Years	58.9	59.7	30.9	31.5	52.4	52.8
13½ Years	59.8	60.6	31.3	32.0	52.3	52.8
14 Years	60.7	61.4	31.7	32.5	52.3	52.9
14½ Years	61.6	62.0	32.2	32.8	52.4	52.9
15 Years	62.4	62.5	32.8	33.0	52.5	52.9
15½ Years	63.2	62.9	33.3	33.2	52.6	52.9
16 Years	64.0	63.2	33.7	33.4	52.7	52.9
16½ Years	64.7	63.5	34.1	33.5	52.8	52.9
17 Years	65.4	63.7	34.5	33.6	52.8	52.8
17½ Years	66.0	63.9	34.8	33.7	52.8	52.8
18 Years	66.6	64.0	35.1	33.8	52.7	52.8
18½ Years	67.1	64.0	35.3	33.8	52.6	52.8
19 Years	67.5	64.0	35.5	33.8	52.6	52.8
19½ Years	67.8	64.0	35.6	33.8	52.5	52.8
20 Years	68.0	64.0	35.7	33.8	52.5	52.8

Figure 35 Sitting height in relation to age and standing height: birth to 20 years. (From Engelbach W. Endocrine Medicine. Courtesy of Charles C Thomas, Publisher, Springfield, Illinois, 1932.)

| | Boys | | | | | Girls | | | | | Both sexes | | Span Difference span minus height | |
| Age yrs. | Height | | Weight | Lower segment | Ratio | Height | | Weight | Lower segment | Ratio | Head | Chest | Male | Female |
	cm	Annual incr.	kg	cm	U/L	cm	Annual incr.	kg	cm	U/L	cm	cm	cm	cm
Birth	50.8		8.4	18.8	1.70	50.8		3.2	18.8	1.70	35	35	−2.5	−2.5
½	67.8		8.5	25.7	1.62	65.8		7.7	25.3	1.60	43.4	44	−2.5	−3.0
1	76.1	25.3	10.8	30.0	1.54	74.2	23.4	9.9	20.4	1.52	46.5	47	−2.5	−3.3
1½	81.9		12.2	32.8	1.50	80.0		11.3	32.5	1.46	48.0	48	−2.7	−3.3
2	87.4	11.4	13.2	36.1	1.42	86.1	11.9	12.5	36.7	1.41	49.0	50	−3.0	−3.5
2½	92.2		14.8	38.9	1.37	91.1		13.6	38.9	1.34			−3.0	−3.8
3	96.4	9.0	15.8	41.0	1.35	95.4	9.3	14.7	41.5	1.30	50.0	52	−2.7	−4.0
3½	100.2		16.3	43.6	1.30	99.5		15.9	43.8	1.27			−2.7	−4.0
4	104.0	7.6	17.3	46.4	1.24	103.3	7.9	16.9	46.5	1.22	50.5	53	−3.0	−3.8
4½	107.6		18.4	48.5	1.22	107.2		18.1	49.0	1.19			−3.0	−3.5
5	110.7	6.7	19.4	50.6	1.19	110.6	7.3	10.2	51.4	1.15	50.8	55	−3.3	−3.5
6	117.7	7.0	21.9	55.5	1.12	117.6	7.0	21.9	56.0	1.10	51.2	56	−2.5	−3.3
7	123.8	6.1	21.6	60.0	1.07	123.8	6.2	21.7	60.1	1.06	51.6	57	−2.5	−2.0
8	120.9	6.1	27.6	61.0	1.03	120.8	6.0	28.1	64.2	1.02	52.0	50	−1.8	−1.8
9	135.4	5.5	31.0	67.0	1.02	135.4	5.6	31.6	67.3	1.01		60	0	−1.2
10	141.0	5.0	34.8	70.8	0.99	141.0	5.6	35.4	70.5	1.00	58.0	61	0	−1.0
11	145.9	4.9	38.8	73.7	0.95	147.7	6.7	40.1	74.2	0.90			0	0
12	151.4	5.5	43.2	76.4	0.98	154.2	0.5	45.5	77.5	0.99	53.2	66	+8.0	0
13	157.5	6.1	47.9	80.0	0.97	150.5	5.3	50.1	79.7	1.00			+3.3	0
14	161.8	7.3	54.0	83.6	0.97	102.9	3.4	54.5	80.6	1.01	54.0	72[a]	+3.3	0
15	171.1	6.3	60.0	86.3	0.95	104.8	1.9	57.4	81.5	1.01			+4.3	+1.2
16	175.2	4.1	64.4	88.0	0.99	165.5	0.7	59.2	81.9	1.01	55.0	77[a]	+4.6	+1.2
17	176.6	1.4	66.9	88.8	0.99	165.5	0	60.5	81.9	1.01	55.4	82[a]	+5.8	+1.2

[a]Males only.

Figure 36 Average anthropometric measurements. (From Wilkins, Lawson. The Diagnosis and Treatment of Endocrine Disorders in Childhood and Adolescence. Courtesy of Charles C. Thomas, Publisher, Springfield, Illinois, 1966.)

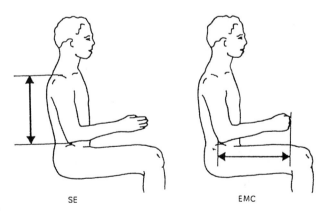

SE   EMC

Figure 37 Measurement of shoulder-to-elbow length (SE) and elbow-to-end-of-third metacarpal length (EMC) is shown using an anthropometer. SE is the distance between the shoulder and the tip of the elbow; EMC is the distance between the tip of the elbow and the distal end of the third metacarpal on a closed fist. (From Tanner JM, Davies PSW. J Pediatr 1985; 107:317–327.)

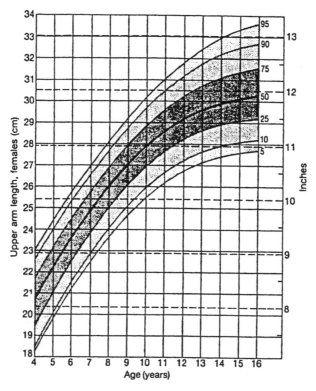

Figure 38   Upper arm length, girls: 4–16 years. (From Manila RM, Hamill PVV, and Lemeshow S. Manual of physical status and performance in childhood. 1973; 1B:1048; New York: Plenum Press.)

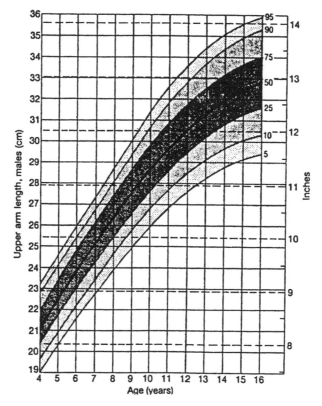

Figure 39   Upper arm length, girls: 4–16 years. (From Manila RM, Hamill PVV, and Lemeshow S. Manual of physical status and performance in childhood. 1973; 1B:1048; New York: Plenum Press.)

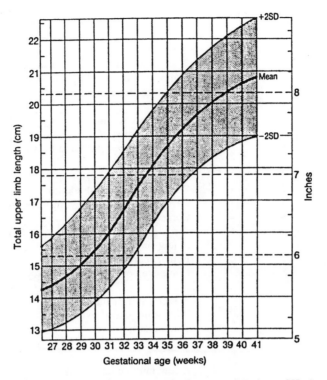

Figure 40 Total upper limb length at birth. (From Sivan Y, Merlob P, and Reisner SH. Am J Dis Child 1983; 137:829.)

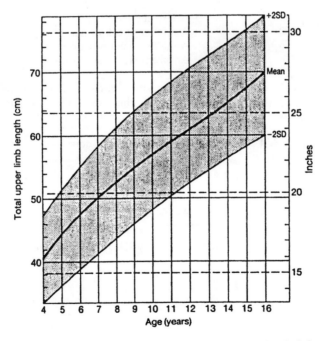

Figure 41 Total upper limb length, both sexes, 4–16 years. (From Martin and Saller. Lehrburch der Anthropologie, Stuttgart: Gustave Fische.)

Site	Grade	Definition
1. Upper lip	1	A few hairs at outer margin.
	2	A small moustache at outer margin.
	3	A moustache extending halfway from outer margin.
	4	A moustache extending to midline.
2. Chin	1	A few scattered hairs.
	2	Scattered hairs with small concentrations.
	3 & 4	Complete cover, light and heavy.
3. Chest	1	Circumareolar hairs.
	2	With midline hair in addition.
	3	Fusion of these areas, with three-quarter cover.
	4	Complete cover.
4. Upper back	1	A few scattered hairs.
	2	Rather more, still scattered.
	3 & 4	Complete cover, light and heavy.
5. Lower back	1	A sacral tuft of hair.
	2	With some lateral extension.
	3	Three-quarter cover.
	4	Complete cover.
6. Upper abdomen	1	A few midline hairs.
	2	Rather more, still midline.
	3 & 4	Half and full cover.
7. Lower abdomen	1	A few midline hairs.
	2	A midline streak of hair.
	3	A midline band of hair.
	4	An inverted V-shaped growth.
8. Arm	1	Sparse growth affecting not more than a quarter of the limb surface.
	2	More than this: cover still incomplete.
	3 & 4	Complete cover, light and heavy.
9. Forearm	1, 2, 3, 4	Complete cover of dorsal surface; 2 grades of light and 2 of heavy growth.
10. Thigh	1, 2, 3, 4	As for arm.
11. Leg	1, 2, 3, 4	As for arm.

Figure 42 Hair-grading system. (From Rerriman D, Gallwey JD. J Clin Endocrinol Metab 1961; 21:1440–1447.)

PRIMARY (DECIDUOUS) TEETH

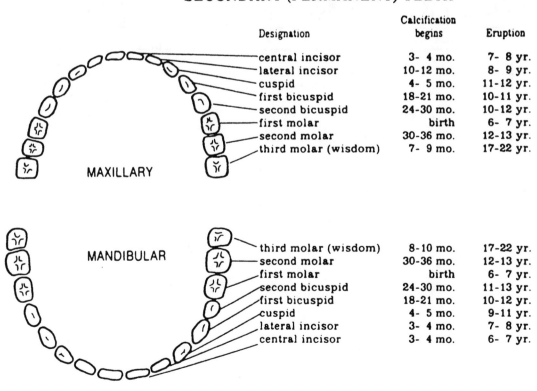

Designation	Calcification (fetal month)	Eruption (months)	Shedding (years)
central incisor	5	6- 8	7- 8
lateral incisor	5	8-11	8- 9
cuspid	6	16-20	11-12
first primary molar	5	10-16	10-11
second primary molar	6	20-30	10-12

MAXILLARY

Designation	Calcification (fetal month)	Eruption (months)	Shedding (years)
second primary molar	6	20-30	11-13
first primary molar	5	10-16	10-12
cuspid	6	16-20	9-11
lateral incisor	5	7-10	7- 8
central incisor	5	5- 7	6- 7

MANDIBULAR

DESIGNATION OF TEETH

$$\frac{211111 | 101112}{211110 | 11111}$$

Deciduous teeth designated by 1; permanent teeth by 2, missing teeth by 0. Upper row indicates maxillary teeth, lower row of numbers indicates mandibular teeth. Vertical line locates the midline.

SECONDARY (PERMANENT) TEETH

Designation	Calcification begins	Eruption
central incisor	3- 4 mo.	7- 8 yr.
lateral incisor	10-12 mo.	8- 9 yr.
cuspid	4- 5 mo.	11-12 yr.
first bicuspid	18-21 mo.	10-11 yr.
second bicuspid	24-30 mo.	10-12 yr.
first molar	birth	6- 7 yr.
second molar	30-36 mo.	12-13 yr.
third molar (wisdom)	7- 9 mo.	17-22 yr.

MAXILLARY

Designation	Calcification begins	Eruption
third molar (wisdom)	8-10 mo.	17-22 yr.
second molar	30-36 mo.	12-13 yr.
first molar	birth	6- 7 yr.
second bicuspid	24-30 mo.	11-13 yr.
first bicuspid	18-21 mo.	10-12 yr.
cuspid	4- 5 mo.	9-11 yr.
lateral incisor	3- 4 mo.	7- 8 yr.
central incisor	3- 4 mo.	6- 7 yr.

MANDIBULAR

Figure 43 Development of dentition. (From Simon FA, Stevenson RE. Pediatric Patient Care. University of Texas Press, 1975.)

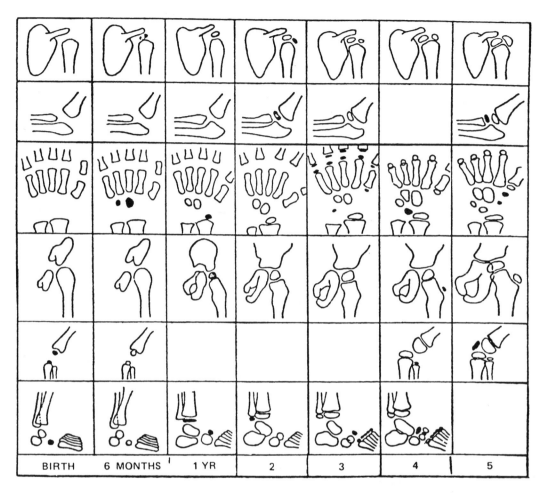

Figure 44 Chronological order of appearance of osseous centers, birth to 5 years. (From Wilkins, Lawson. Diagnosis and Treatment of Endocrine Disorders in Childhood and Adolescence. Courtesy of Charles C Thomas, Publisher, Springfield, Illinois, 1966.)

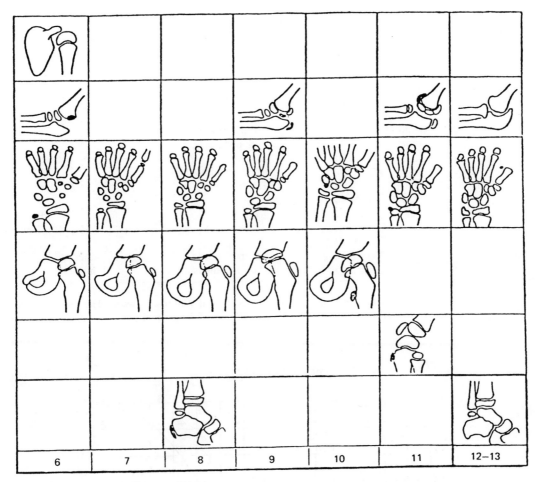

Figure 45 Chronological order of appearance of osseous centers, 6–13 years. (From Wilkins, Lawson. The Diagnosis and Treatment of Endocrine Disorders in Childhood and Adolescence. Courtesy of Charles C Thomas, Publisher, Springfield, Illinois, 1966.)

	12 Yrs.	13 Yrs.	14 Yrs.	15 Yrs.	16 Yrs.	17 Yrs.	18 Yrs.
Shoulder							Head of humerus Great tuberosity
Elbow	Trochlen & capitelium	Olecranon	Ext. epicondyle Head of radius				
Hand		Styloid of ulna		Ep. metacarpals & phalanges			Ep. radius & ulna
Hip				Head of femur Trochanters			
Knee							Ep. femur, tibia & fibula
Foot	Ep. os raleis			Ep. metatarsals & phalanges		Ep. tibia & fibula	

Figure 46 Chronological order of union of epiphysis with diaphysis. (From Wilkins, Lawson. The Diagnosis and Treatment of Endocrine Disorders in Childhood and Adolescence. Courtesy of Charles C Thomas, Publisher, Springfield, Illinois, 1966.)

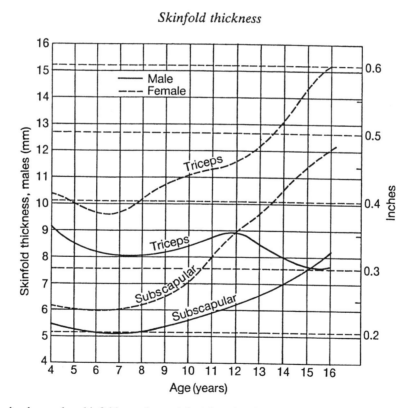

Figure 47 Triceps and subcapsular skinfolds, males and females: 4–16 years. (From Schulueter K, Funfack W, Pachalay J, and Weber B. Eur J Pediatr 1976; 123:255.)

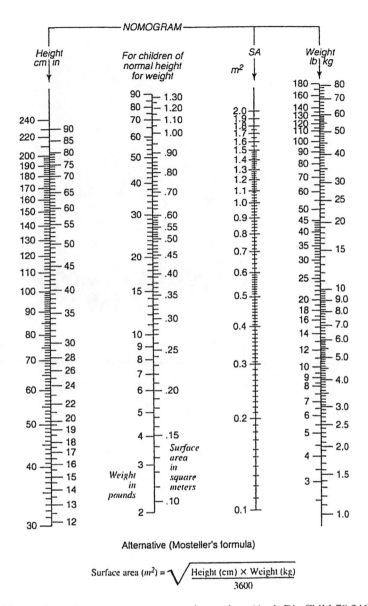

Figure 48   Body surface area nomogram and equation. (Arch Dis Child 70:246, 1994.)

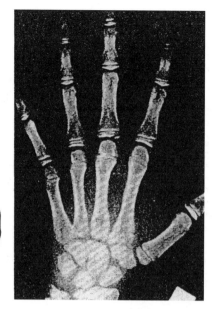

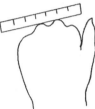

Figure 49 A straight ruler is applied against the distal ends of the third, fourth, and fifth metacarpals of a tightly closed fist. The clinical observation of brachymetacarpia V was confirmed radiologically when the fifth metacarpal bone failed to intercept a straight line connecting the distal ends of the third and fourth metacarpal bones by more than 2 mm. (Tanner JM, Davies PSW. J Pediatr 1985; 107:317–327.)

III. STANDARD GROWTH CHARTS FOR CHILDREN WITH GENETIC OR PATHOLOGICAL CONDITIONS: FIGURES 50–90

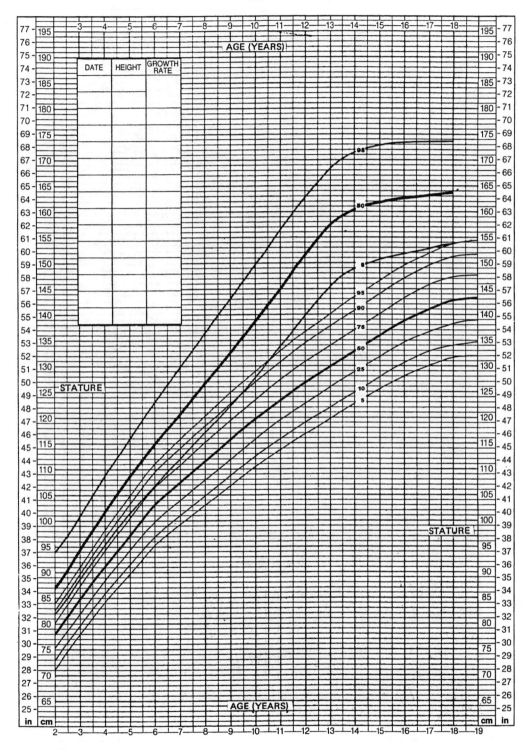

Figure 50 Growth chart for Turner syndrome compared to normal female growth. The solid line shows growth in normal girls; percentiles derived from the National Center for Health Statistics. The broken line shows growth in untreated Turner syndrome girls; percentiles derived from Lyon AJ, Preece MA, Grant DB. Arch Dis Child 1985; 60:932–935. (© Genetech, Inc., 1987. All rights reserved.)

1011

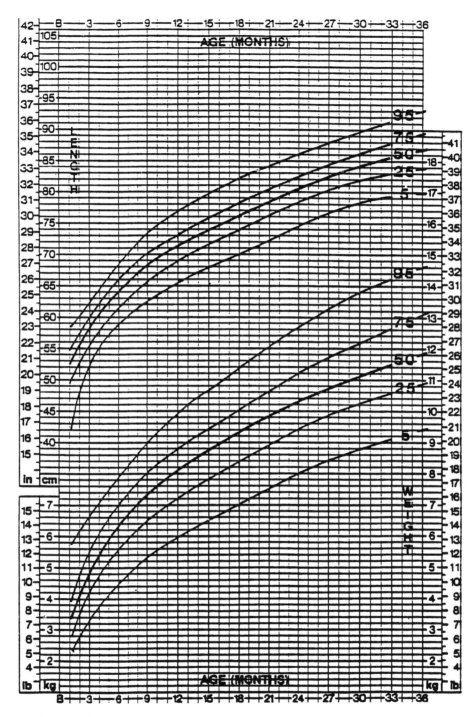

Figure 51 Height and weight for Down syndrome, boys: birth–36 months. (Reproduced by permission of Pediatrics 1988; 81:102.)

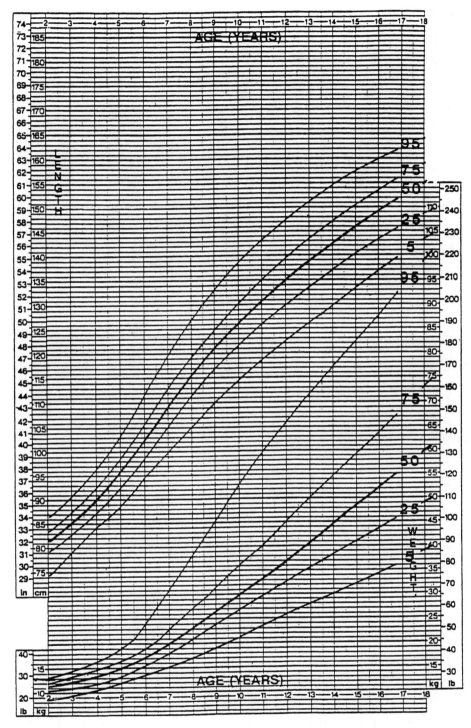

Figure 52 Height and weight for Down syndrome, boys: 2–18 years. (Reproduced by permission of Pediatrics 1988; 81:102.)

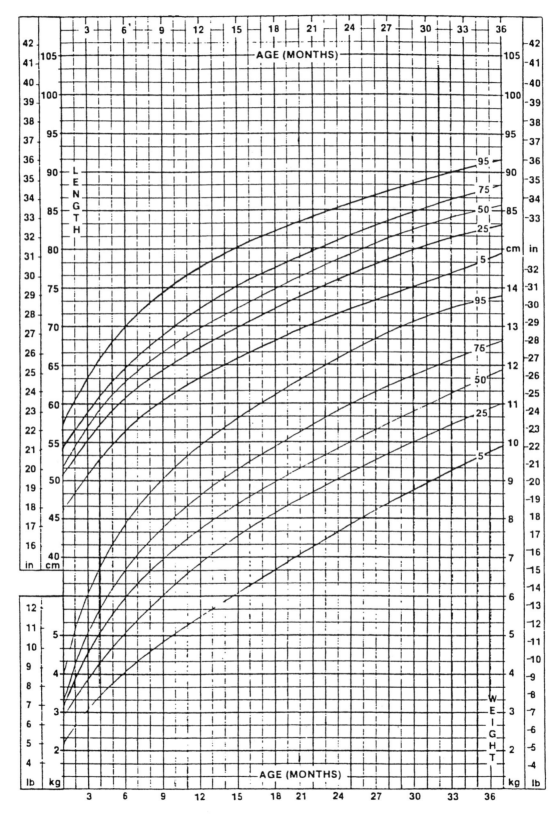

Figure 53 Height and weight for Down syndrome, girls: birth–36 months. (Reproduced by permission from Pediatrics 1988; 81:102.)

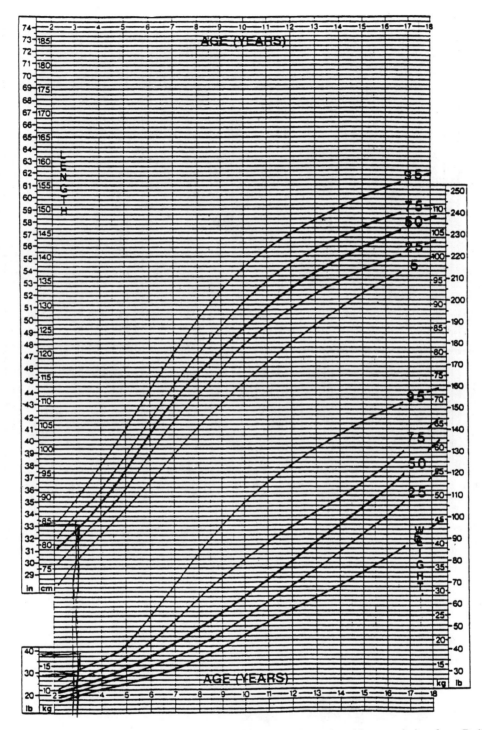

Figure 54   Height and weight for Down syndrome, girls: 2–18 years. (Reproduced by permission from Pediatrics 1988; 81: 102.)

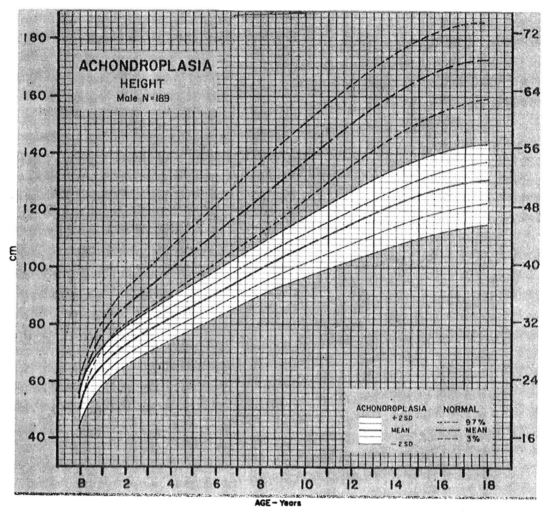

Figure 55 Height curve for achondroplasia compared to normal height curve, boys. (From J Pediatr 1978; 93(3):435–438.)

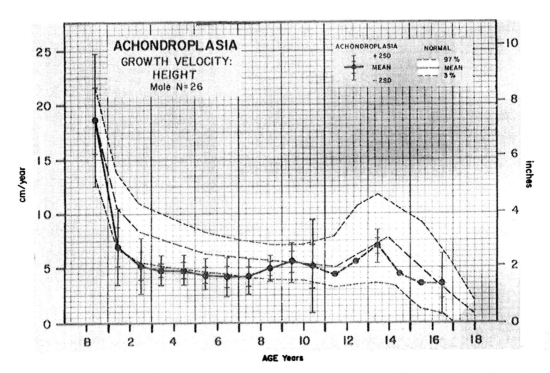

Figure 56 Height velocity for achondroplasia compared to normal height velocity standard, boys. (From J Pediatr 1978; 93(3): 435–438.)

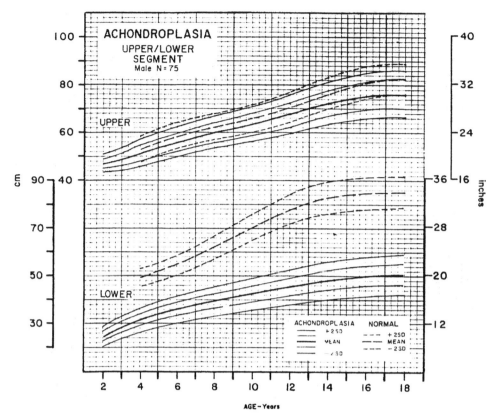

Figure 57 Upper and lower segment lengths for achondroplasia compared to normal segment lengths, boys. (From J Pediatr 1978; 93(3):435–438.)

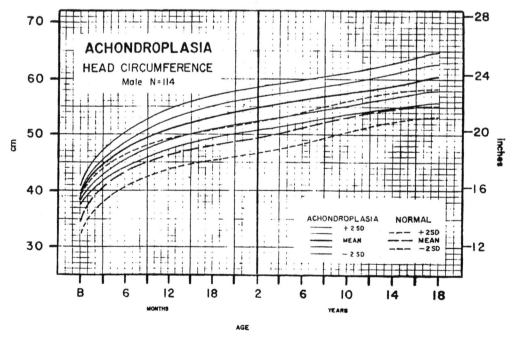

Figure 58 Head circumference for achondroplasia compared to normal head circumference, boys. (From J Pediatr 1978; 93(3): 435–438.)

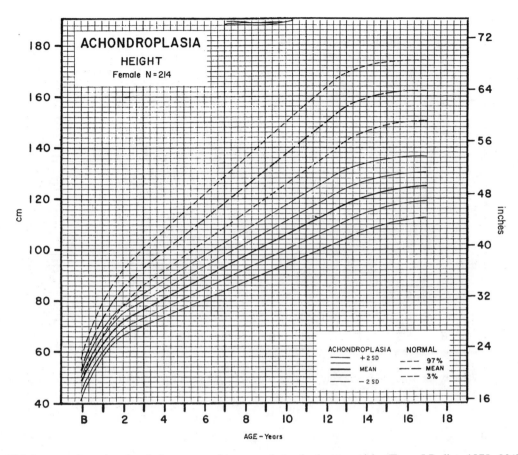

Figure 59 Height curve for achondroplasia compared to normal standard curve, girls. (From J Pediatr 1978; 93(3):435–438.)

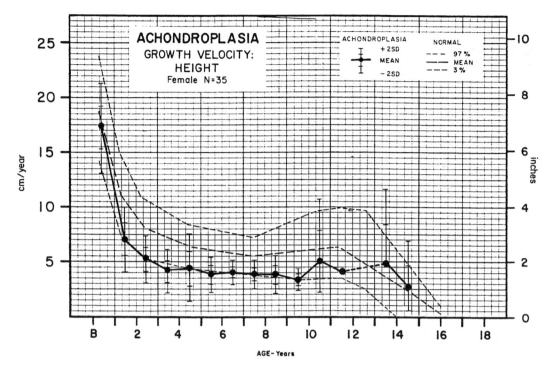

Figure 60 Height velocity for achondroplasia compared to normal height velocity standard, girls. (From J Pediatr 1978; 93(3): 435–438.)

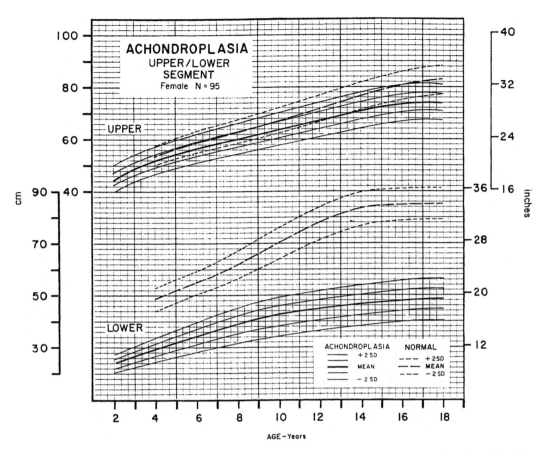

Figure 61 Upper and lower segment lengths for achondroplasia compared to normal segment lengths, girls. (From J Pediatr 1978; 93(3):435–438.)

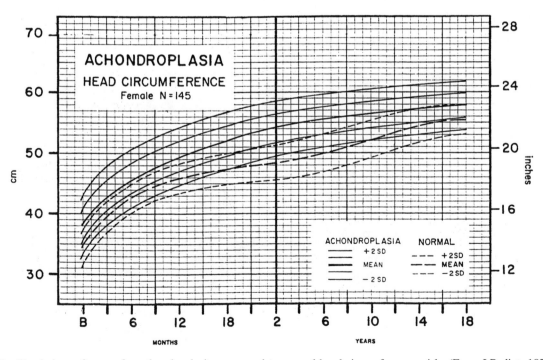

Figure 62 Head circumference for achondroplasia compared to normal head circumference, girls. (From J Pediatr 1978; 93(3): 435–438.)

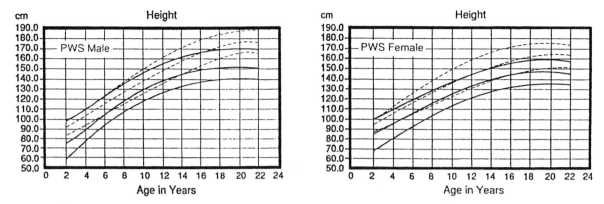

Figure 63 Curves for height of males and females with Prader-Willi syndrome (solid lines) and healthy individuals (broken lines). (From Pediatrics 1991; 88:853.)

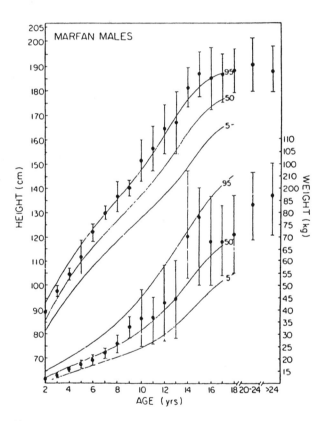

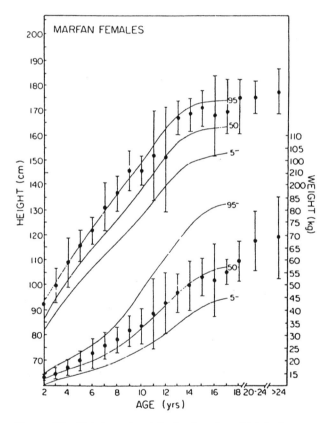

Figure 64 Height and weight for males with Marfan syndrome, superimposed on normal growth curves (5th, 50th, and 95th percentiles). Cross-sectional and longitudinal data from 200 White patients with Marfan syndrome were used. Patients were not treated with hormones. Bars shown ± 1 standard deviation. (From Pyeritz RE. Marfan syndrome. In: Principles and Practice of Medical Genetics. New York: Churchill Livingstone, 1983.)

Figure 65 Height and weight for females with Marfan syndrome, superimposed on normal growth curves (5th, 50th, and 95th percentiles). Cross-sectional and longitudinal data from 200 White patients with Marfan syndrome were used. Patients were not treated with hormones. Bars shown ± 1 standard deviation. (From Pyeritz RE. Marfan syndrome. In: Principles and Practice of Medical Genetics. New York; Churchill Livingstone, 1983.)

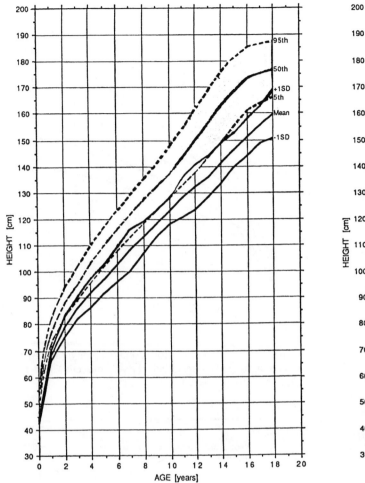

Figure 66 Growth curve for height in males with Noonan syndrome (solid lines) compared to normal values (dashed lines). Data obtained in 64 Noonan syndrome males from a collaborative retrospective review. (From Witt DR, et al. Clin Genet 1986; 30:150.)

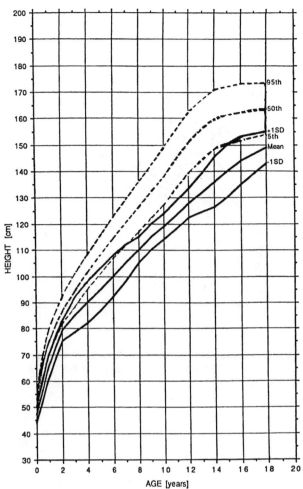

Figure 67 Growth curve for height in females with Noonan syndrome (solid lines) compared to normal values (dashed lines). Data obtained in 48 Noonan syndrome females from a collaborative retrospective review. (From Witt DR, et al. Clin Genet 1986; 30:150.)

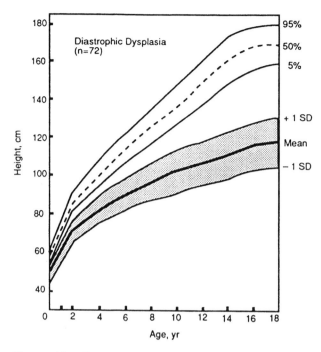

Figure 68 Growth curve for diastrophic dysplasia, no gender specified. (From Am J Dis Child 1983; 136:316–319. © AMA.)

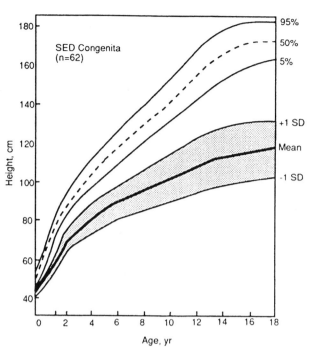

Figure 69 Growth curve for spondyloepiphyseal dysplasia congenita, no gender specified. (From Am J Dis Child 1983; 136:316–319. © AMA.)

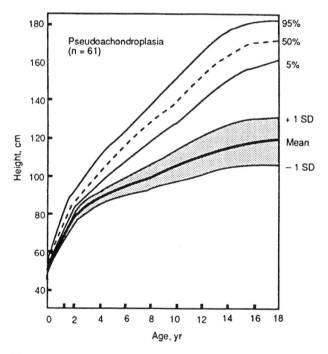

Figure 70 Growth curve for pseudoachondroplasia, no gender specified. (From Am J Dis Child 1983; 136:316–319. © AMA.)

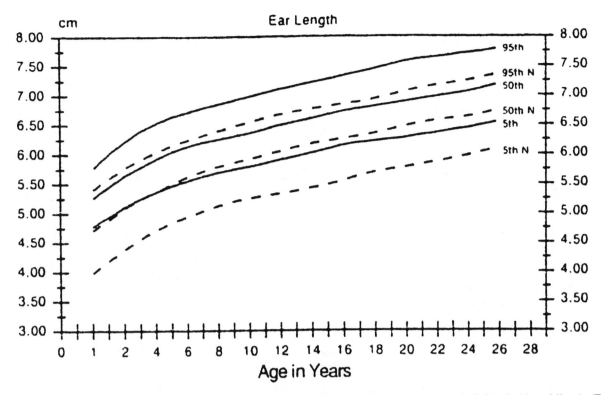

Figure 71   Curves for ear length of males with fragile X syndrome (solid lines) and normal individuals (dotted lines). (From Butler MG, Brunschwig A, Miller LK, et al. Pediatrics 1992; 89:1059–1062.)

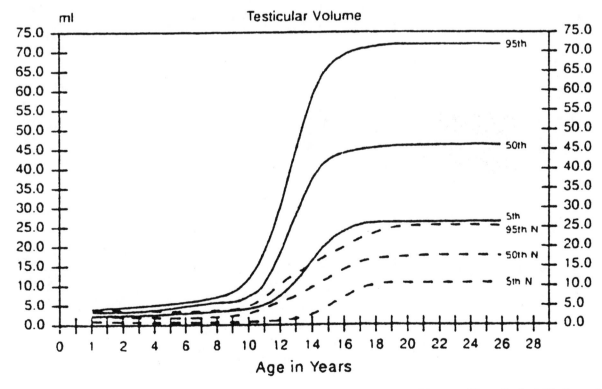

Figure 72   Curves for testicular volume of males with fragile X syndrome: birth to 28 years. (From Butler MG, Brunschwig A, Miller LK, et al. Pediatrics 1992; 89:1059–1062.)

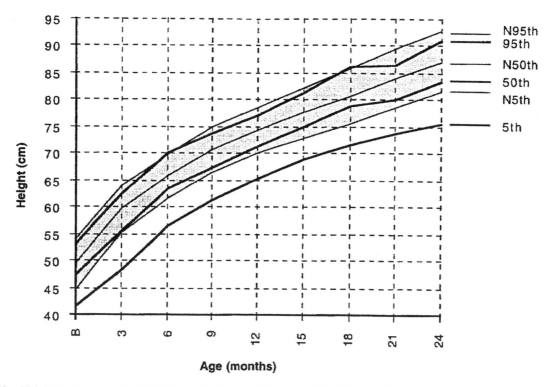

Figure 73   Height in females with CDCS from birth to age 24 months (thick lines). The normal growth curve is shaded. (From Marinescu RC, Mainardi PC, Collins MR, et al. Am J Med Genet 2000; 94:153.)

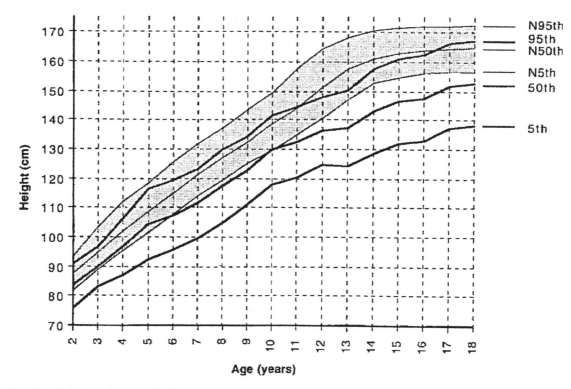

Figure 74   Height in females with CDCS from 2 to 18 years (thick lines). The normal growth curve is shaded. (From Marinescu RC, Mainardi PC, Collins MR, et al. Am J Med Genet 2000; 94:153.)

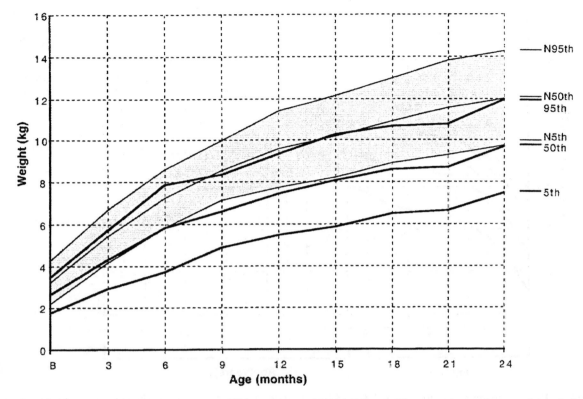

Figure 75 Weight in females with CDCS from birth to 24 months (thick lines). The normal growth curve is shaded. (From Marinescu RC, Mainardi PC, Collins MR, et al. Am J Med Genet 2000; 94:153.)

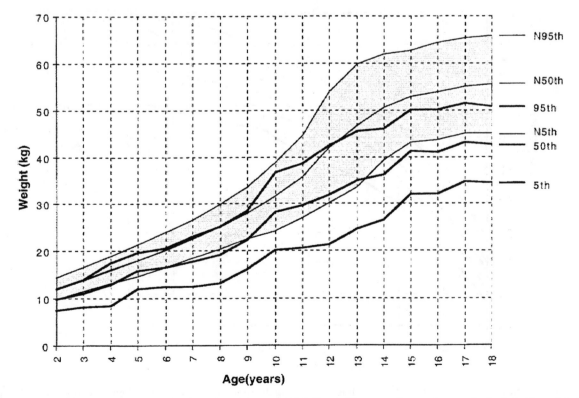

Figure 76 Weight in females with CDCS from 2 to 18 years (thick lines). The normal growth curve is shaded. (From Marinescu RC, Mainardi PC, Collins MR, et al. Am J Med Genet 2000; 94:153.)

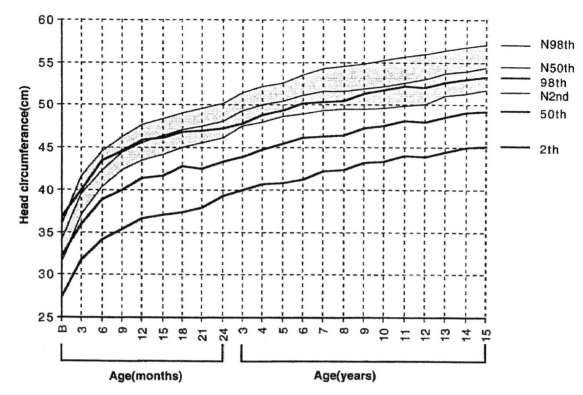

Figure 77 Head circumference in females with CDCS from birth to 15 years (thick lines). The normal growth curve is shaded. (From Marinescu RC, Mainardi PC, Collins MR, et al. Am J Med Genet 2000; 94:153.)

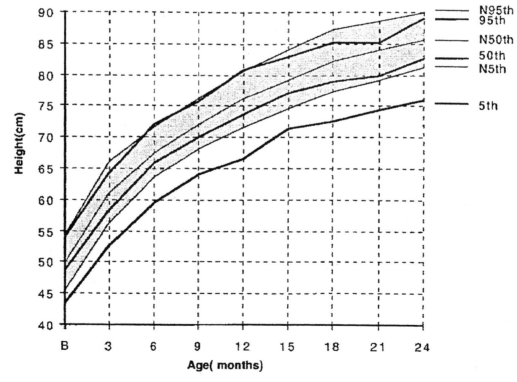

Figure 78 Height in males with CDCS from birth to age 24 months (thick lines). The normal growth curve is shaded. (From Marinescu RC, Mainardi PC, Collins MR, et al. Am J Med Genet 2000; 94:153.)

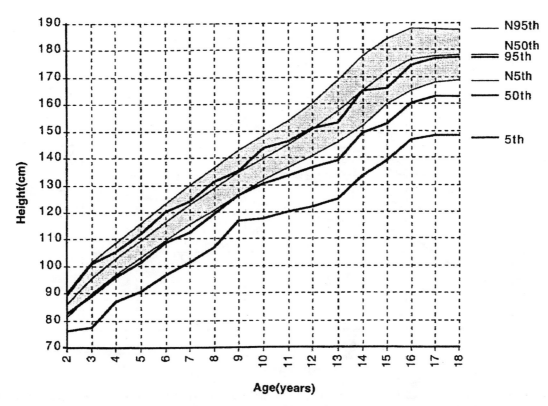

Figure 79 Height in males with CDCS from 2 to 18 years (thick lines). The normal growth curve is shaded. (From Marinescu RC, Mainardi PC, Collins MR, et al. Am J Med Genet 2000; 94:153.)

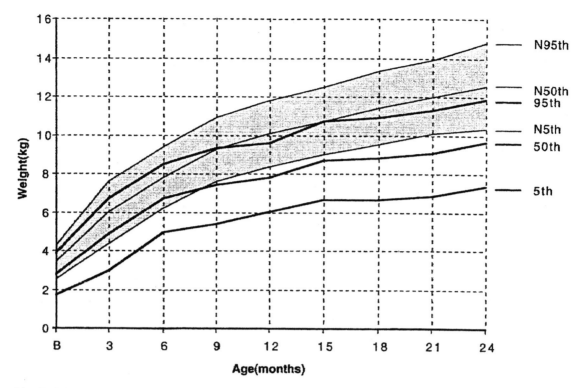

Figure 80 Weight in males with CDCS from birth to 24 months (thick lines). The normal growth curve is shaded. (From Marinescu RC, Mainardi PC, Collins MR, et al. Am J Med Genet 2000; 94:153.)

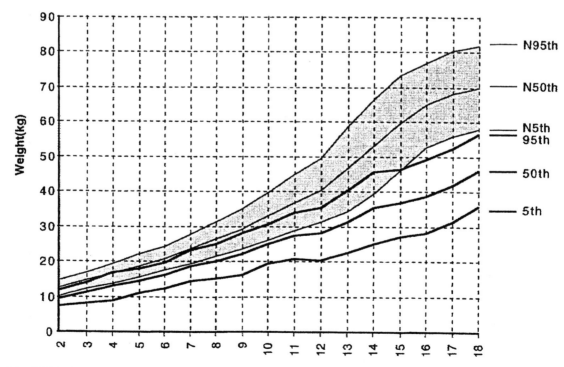

Figure 81 Weight in males with CDCS from 2 to 18 years (thick lines). The normal growth curve is shaded. (From Marinescu RC, Mainardi PC, Collins MR, et al. Am J Med Genet 2000; 94:153.)

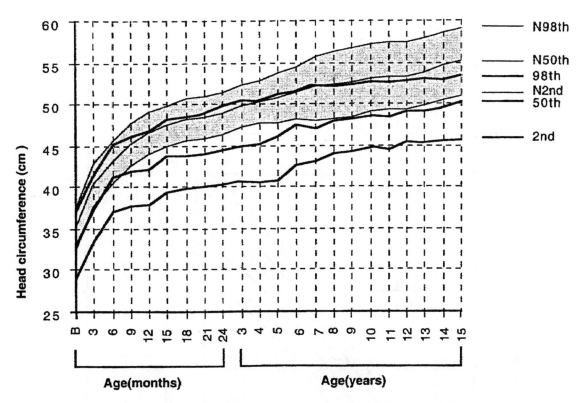

Figure 82 Head circumference in males with CDCS from birth to 15 years (thick lines). The normal growth curve is shaded. (From Marinescu RC, Mainardi PC, Collins MR, et al. Am J Med Genet 2000; 94:153.)

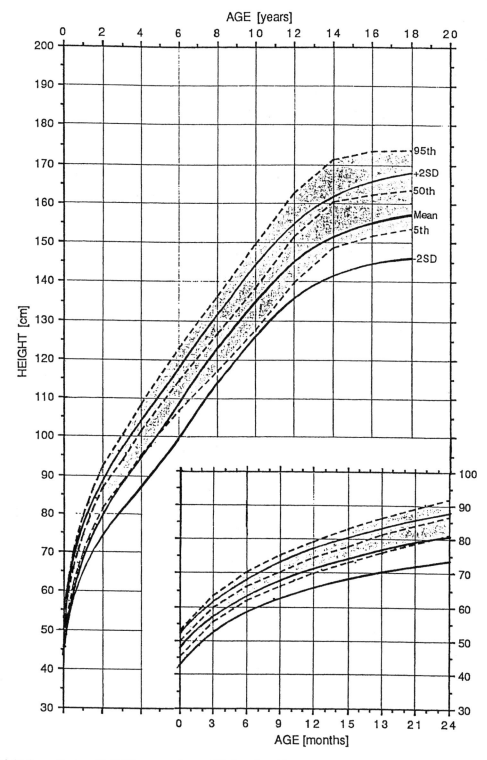

Figure 83 Height for patients with Williams syndrome (61 females, 47 males). Normal curves, dashed lines; affected patients, solid lines. (Reprinted with permission from Saul RA, Geer JS, Seaver LH, Phelan MC, Sweet KM, Mills MS. *Growth References: Third Trimester to Adulthood.* Greenwood, SC: Greenwood Genetic Center; 1998.)

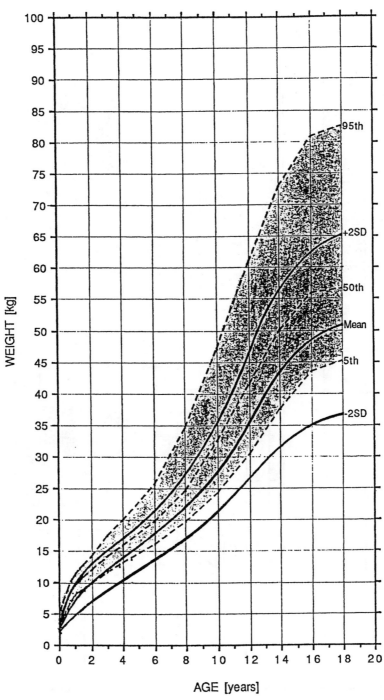

Figure 84 Weight for females with Williams syndrome. Normal curves, dashed lines; affected patients, solid lines. (Reprinted with permission from Saul RA, Geer JS, Seaver LH, Phelan MC, Sweet KM, Mills MS. *Growth References: Third Trimester to Adulthood.* Greenwood, SC: Greenwood Genetic Center; 1998.)

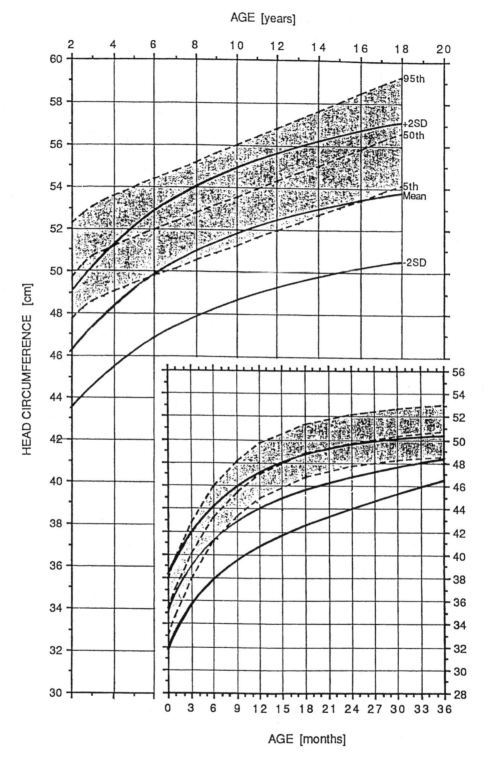

Figure 85 Head circumference for females with Williams syndrome. Normal curves, dashed lines; affected patients, solid lines. (Reprinted with permission from Saul RA, Geer JS, Seaver LH, Phelan MC, Sweet KM, Mills MS. *Growth References: Third Trimester to Adulthood.* Greenwood, SC: Greenwood Genetic Center; 1998.)

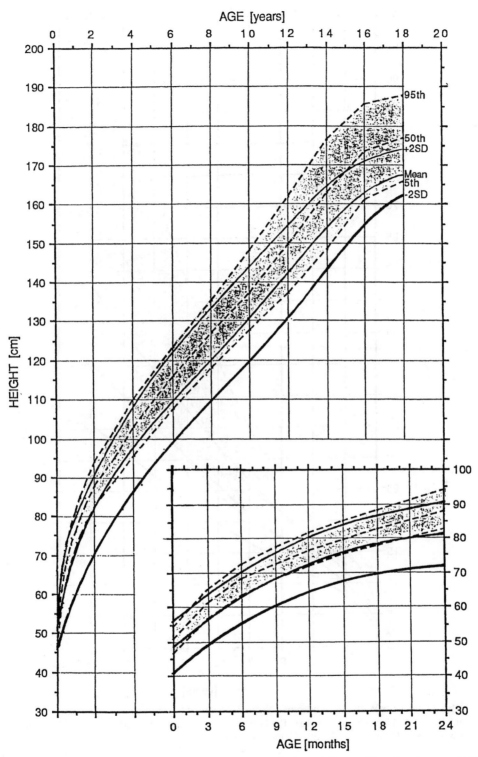

AGE [years]

HEIGHT [cm]

AGE [months]

Figure 86 Height for males with Williams syndrome. Normal curves, dashed lines; affected patients, solid lines. (Reprinted with permission from Saul RA, Geer JS, Seaver LH, Phelan MC, Sweet KM, Mills MS. *Growth References: Third Trimester to Adulthood.* Greenwood, SC: Greenwood Genetic Center; 1998.)

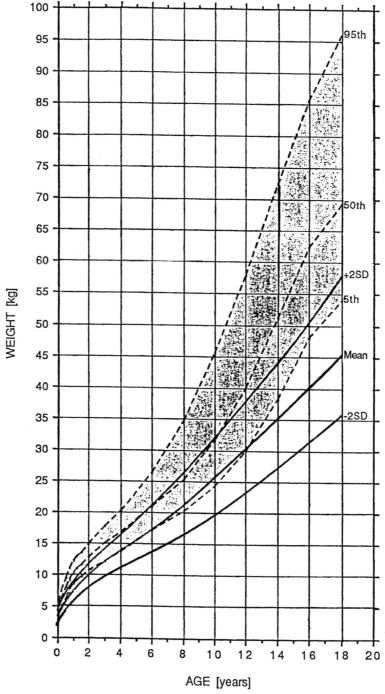

Figure 87 Weight for males with Williams syndrome. Normal curves, dashed lines; affected patients, solid lines. (Reprinted with permission from Saul RA, Geer JS, Seaver LH, Phelan MC, Sweet KM, Mills MS. *Growth References: Third Trimester to Adulthood.* Greenwood, SC: Greenwood Genetic Center; 1998.)

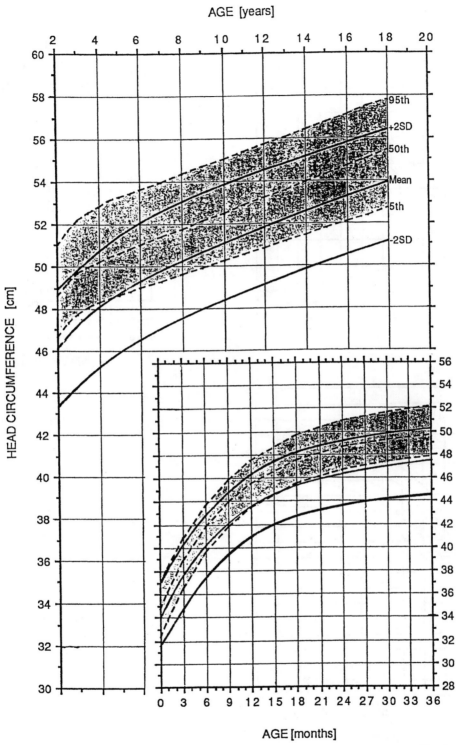

AGE [years]

HEAD CIRCUMFERENCE [cm]

AGE [months]

Figure 88 Head circumference for males with Williams syndrome. Normal curves, dashed lines; affected patients, solid lines. (Reprinted with permission from Saul RA, Geer JS, Seaver LH, Phelan MC, Sweet KM, Mills MS. *Growth References: Third Trimester to Adulthood.* Greenwood, SC: Greenwood Genetic Center: 1998.)

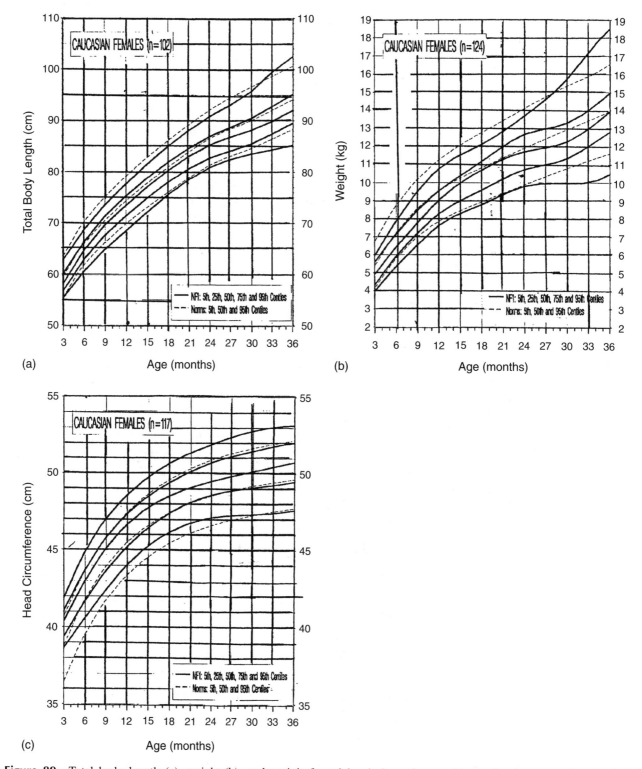

Figure 89 Total body length (a), weight (b), and occipitofrontal head circumference (c) centiles by age in females 3–36 months. NF1 patient measurements are from the National Foundation International Database. Unaffected norms are from the National Center for Health Statistics and the Fels Institute.

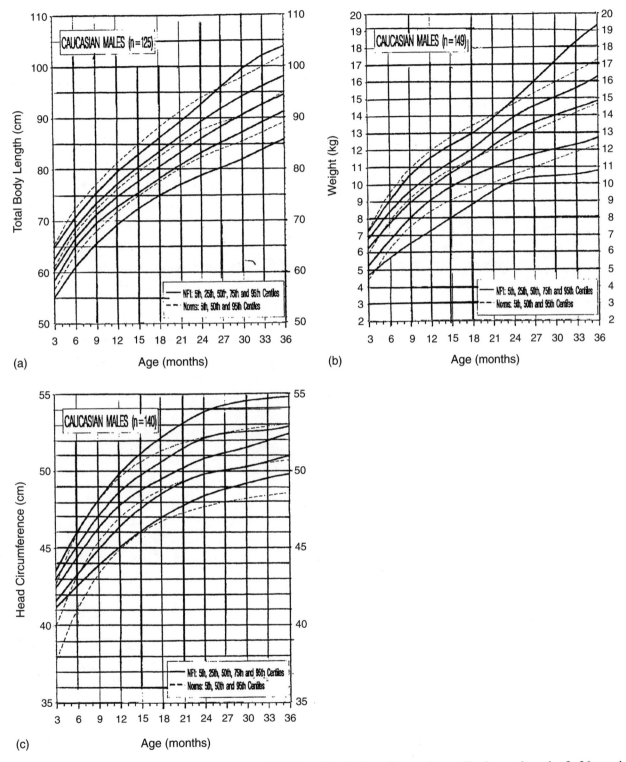

Figure 90 Total body length (a), weight (b), and occipitofrontal head circumference (c) centiles by age in males 3–36 months. NF1 patient measurements are from the National Foundation International Database. Unaffected norms are from the National Center for Health Statistics and the Fels Institute.

Index